HUMAN PHYSIOLOGY
for Medical Students

HUMAN PHYSIOLOGY
for Medical Students

As per the Competency-based Medical Education Curriculum (NMC)

SECOND EDITION

N Geetha MBBS MD (Physiology)
Professor and Head
Department of Physiology
and Vice Principal
Government Medical College
Kollam, Kerala, India

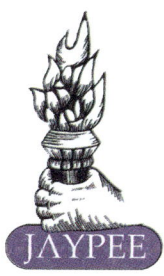

JAYPEE BROTHERS MEDICAL PUBLISHERS
The Health Sciences Publisher
New Delhi | London

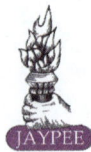 **Jaypee Brothers Medical Publishers (P) Ltd**

Headquarters
Jaypee Brothers Medical Publishers (P) Ltd
EMCA House, 23/23-B
Ansari Road, Daryaganj
New Delhi 110 002, India
Landline: +91-11-23272143, +91-11-23272703
+91-11-23282021, +91-11-23245672
Email: jaypee@jaypeebrothers.com

Corporate Office
Jaypee Brothers Medical Publishers (P) Ltd
4838/24, Ansari Road, Daryaganj
New Delhi 110 002, India
Phone: +91-11-43574357
Fax: +91-11-43574314
Email: jaypee@jaypeebrothers.com

Overseas Office
J.P. Medical Ltd
83 Victoria Street, London
SW1H 0HW (UK)
Phone: +44 20 3170 8910
Fax: +44 (0)20 3008 6180
Email: info@jpmedpub.com

Website: www.jaypeebrothers.com
Website: www.jaypeedigital.com

© 2023, Jaypee Brothers Medical Publishers

The views and opinions expressed in this book are solely those of the original contributor(s)/author(s) and do not necessarily represent those of editor(s) and publisher of the book.

All rights reserved. No part of this publication may be reproduced, stored or transmitted in any form or by any means, electronic, mechanical, photocopying, recording or otherwise, without the prior permission in writing of the publishers.

All brand names and product names used in this book are trade names, service marks, trademarks or registered trademarks of their respective owners. The publisher is not associated with any product or vendor mentioned in this book.

Medical knowledge and practice change constantly. This book is designed to provide accurate, authoritative information about the subject matter in question. However, readers are advised to check the most current information available on procedures included and check information from the manufacturer of each product to be administered, to verify the recommended dose, formula, method and duration of administration, adverse effects and contraindications. It is the responsibility of the practitioner to take all appropriate safety precautions. Neither the publisher nor the author(s)/editor(s) assume any liability for any injury and/or damage to persons or property arising from or related to use of material in this book.

This book is sold on the understanding that the publisher is not engaged in providing professional medical services. If such advice or services are required, the services of a competent medical professional should be sought.

Every effort has been made where necessary to contact holders of copyright to obtain permission to reproduce copyright material. If any have been inadvertently overlooked, the publisher will be pleased to make the necessary arrangements at the first opportunity.

Inquiries for bulk sales may be solicited at: jaypee@jaypeebrothers.com

Human Physiology for Medical Students
First Edition: 2021
Second Edition: **2023**
ISBN: 978-93-5465-892-1
Printed at: Samrat Offset Pvt. Ltd.

Dedicated to

Karthika Sanker, the youngest doctor in the family.

Preface to the Second Edition

Editing and expanding a book that has been well received by the target audience is a challenging task. On one hand you need to make additions and modifications that keep the book updated and current and on the other hand, you must preserve what worked with the original so that the readers are not disappointed so, you must balance both while ensuring that the book doesn't turn voluminous.

This book would serve as a reference to more mature doctors, and practitioners without a glitch. However, my focus, as ever has been on first year students who need an uncluttered book which focuses on the basics. They are my target audience, and at every juncture, when faced with a choice between making the book a holistic reference and making it a go to study material for the young doctors in their first year, I have favoured the latter option.

I have received many constructive criticisms for my first book and this has helped me understand what was needed to be changed. Errors were flagged and pointers were given by my colleagues and readers which helped me perfect the book further.

I wish to hear from you about what you found lacking, and what could have been better. Kindly write to me at geethaphysiology@gmail.com.

I extend my gratitude to Shri Jitendar P Vij (Group Chairman), Mr Ankit Vij (Managing Director), Mr MS Mani (Group President) of Jaypee Brothers Medical Publishers (P) Ltd, and all the staff especially, Dr Madhu Choudhary (Director–Educational Publishing), Ms Pooja Bhandari (Production Head), Ms Sunita Katla (Executive Assistant to Group Chairman and Publishing Manager), Ms Samina Khan (Executive Assistant to Director–Educational Publishing), Mr Rajesh Sharma (Production Coordinator), Ms Seema Dogra (Cover Visualizer), Mr Binay Kumar (Proofreader), Mr Om Prakash Mishra (Typesetter), Mr Rakesh Verma (Graphic Designer), who tried their best to bring out the book at short notice. Above all, I thank Dr Aditya Tayal (Team Leader-UG Publishing), who was instrumental in ensuring timely completion of the work.

N Geetha

Preface to the First Edition

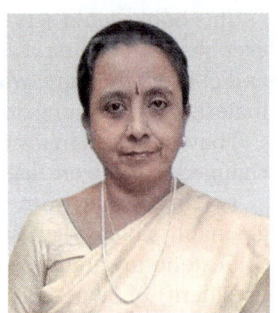

When I set about writing my first book in 2006, I never thought that I would still be writing in 2021. I owe this plethora of literature to the immense encouragement and creative criticism, I received till date from colleagues and students alike. Fourteen years down the lane, my fundamental goal remains the same. Make something that is simple enough for the young doctor to comprehend yet elegant enough for learner to use as a tool for the future.

This book is the result of over thirty years of teaching experience. However, it would not be a stretch to claim that I, as an author have matured over the past fourteen years. I believe that the readers of my first book would find a familiar style in this book, but will also notice the more mature distillation of the information within. While my first book was intended as a textbook which would be easy to learn and reproduce, this book serves as a tool for the exam but also aspires to double as a reference for the mature doctors. The focus, however, is still firmly on the first year medical students who wishes to understand the basics of the topic without being subject having too much information. Therefore, the diagrams, as with all my works, are hand-drawn and easy to reproduce, and the text is simple and exam-oriented.

While no pains have been spared by me to ensure that the material is free from error, it is invariable that some mistakes may have been crept. Since this book is a completely a new work; the end-product of a complete overhaul of the materials in my possession, I earnestly encourage criticism and comments which would help me and the editors in fine-tuning it. The greatest joy for me as an author is to hear what my colleagues, young and old alike, have to say about the book. Anyone welcome to contact me at geethaphysiology@gmail.com.

First of all, I thank almighty God. It would be amiss if I do not thank my postgraduate fellows for providing me immense support. Their aid and efforts were invaluable and helped me finalize this book at a pace I could not have imagined ten years back. It is truly an honor to have you on my side. I hope you enjoyed reading the work at least half as much as I enjoyed writing it. I am indebted to all my colleagues who provided me with the clinical photographs used in the book.

I extend my gratitude to Shri Jitendar P Vij (Group Chairman), Mr Ankit Vij (Managing Director), and Mr MS Mani (Group President) of Jaypee Brothers Medical Publishers (P) Ltd, and all the staff especially Dr Madhu Choudhary (Publishing Head–Education), Ms Pooja Bhandari (Production Head), Ms Sunita Katla (Executive Assistant to Group Chairman and Publishing Manager), Ms Samina Khan (Executive Assistant to Publishing Head–Education), Mr Rajesh Sharma (Production Coordinator), Ms Seema Dogra (Cover Visualizer), Mr Binay Kumar (Proofreader), Mr Rohit Sharma (Typesetter), Mr Rajesh Gurkundi (Graphic Designer), who tried their best to bring out the book at short notice. Above all, I thank Dr Astha Sawhney (Development Editor), who was instrumental in ensuring timely completion of the work. Her enthusiasm and passion is quite infectious.

Before closing, a word to my young reader who has stepped into the world of medicine, fresh out of school. Every amazing, intimidating, successful doctor you see in your med-school once stood where you are standing now, as student. At the end, what we did with our life is a sum total of what we do with our days. This is my legacy. What will be yours?

N Geetha

Contents

Section 1: General Physiology

1. **Introduction to Physiology and General Principles in Physiology** — 1
   - PH, Acid/Base and Buffer *1*
   - Acid-base Disorders (Acidosis and Alkalosis) *2*
   - Osmosis *3*
   - Osmotic Pressure *3*
   - Osmolality and Osmolarity *3*
   - Tonicity *3*
   - Diffusion *4*
   - Forces Acting on Ions *5*

2. **The Body Fluid Compartments** — 7
   - Total Body Water *7*
   - Distribution of Body Fluids *7*
   - Measurement of Body Fluid Volumes *8*
   - Body Electrolytes *8*
   - Intravenous Fluid Therapy *8*

3. **Homeostasis** — 11
   - Control Systems of the Body *11*
   - Feedback Systems *12*
   - Role of Different Systems in the Body in Homeostasis *13*
   - Homeostatic Imbalance *13*

4. **Cell Physiology** — 15
   - Parts of a Cell *15*
   - Plasma Membrane *15*
   - Cytoplasm *15*
   - Nucleus *15*
   - Plasma Membrane *15*

   Cytoplasm *17*
   - Cytosol *17*
   - Cell Organelles *19*

   Nucleus *22*
   Genetics *22*
   - Genes *22*
   - Genetics and Disease *23*
   - Cloning *25*

   Cell Division *26*
   - Somatic Cell Division *26*
   - Reproductive Cell Division or Meiosis *27*

   Apoptosis *29*
   - Mechanism of Apoptosis *29*
   - Significance of Apoptosis *29*

   Intercellular Connections *30*
   - Cell Adhesion Molecules *30*
   - Intercellular Connections *30*

5. **Transport Processes across Cell Membrane** — 34
   - Types of Transport across Cell Membrane *34*

6. **Nerve Physiology and Bioelectrical Potentials** — 44

   Neuron *44*
   - Classification of Neurons *44*
   - Morphology of a Typical Neuron *45*
   - Processes of the Neuron *46*
   - Properties of Nerve Fibers *48*

   Bioelectrical Potentials *48*
   - Resting Membrane Potential *48*
   - Graded Potentials *50*
   - Action Potential *50*
   - Excitability *54*
   - Conduction of Nerve Impulse or Propagation of Action Potential *56*
   - Classification of Nerve Fibers *57*
   - Nerve Injury *58*
   - Response of Neurons to Injury *58*
   - Injury to the Axon *59*

7. **Skeletal Muscle Physiology** — 65
   - Skeletal Muscle *65*
   - Motor Point and Motor Unit *72*
   - Electromyography *73*
   - Muscle Metabolism and Energy Source *73*
   - Applied Physiology *75*

8. **Neuromuscular Junction or Myoneural Junction** — 79
   - Structure of Neuromuscular Junction *79*
   - Effects of Denervation of Muscle *82*

9. **Cardiac Muscle** — 85
   - Structure of Cardiac Muscle *85*
   - Electrical Activity of Cardiac Muscle *85*
   - Properties of Cardiac Muscle *88*

10. **Smooth Muscle** — 90
    - Functional Anatomy *90*
    - Neuromuscular Junction in Smooth Muscle *91*
    - Electrical Responses in Smooth Muscle *91*
    - Ionus *92*
    - Mechanism of Smooth Muscle Contraction and Relaxation *92*
    - Length–Tension Relationship in Smooth Muscle *93*
    - Similarities between Cardiac and Visceral Smooth Muscle *93*

Contents

Section 2: Hematology

11. Blood — 99
- Circulating Body Fluids 99
- Blood 99

12. Plasma — 102
- Composition 102
- Plasma Proteins 102
- Plasmapheresis 103
- Albumin-globulin Ratio 104

13. Red Blood Corpuscles or Erythrocytes and Hemoglobin — 106
- Morphology of Mature RBC 106
- Packed Cell Volume or Hematocrit 107
- Special Properties of Erythrocytes 108
- Metabolism in RBC 110
- RBC Count 111
- Hemoglobin 111
- Blood Indices 113
- Life Span of RBC 114
- Destruction of RBC 114
- Hematopoiesis 116
- Erythropoiesis 116
- Erythropoietin 119
- Factors Regulating Erythropoiesis 120
- Anemia 122

14. White Blood Corpuscles or Leukocytes — 131
- Granulocytes 132
- Agranulocytes 133
- Properties of Leukocytes 134
- Functions of Leukocytes 134
- Disorders of Phagocytic Function 135
- Variations in WBC Count 136
- Leukopoiesis 138

15. Spleen and Reticuloendothelial System — 141
- Spleen 141
- Reticuloendothelial System or Tissue Macrophage System 142

16. Immune System — 144
- Cytokines, Chemokines and the Complement System 144
- Immune Response 146
- Immunity 146
- Innate Immunity 147
- Development of Immune System 148
- Acquired Immunity or Specific Immunity 150
- Humoral Immunity 153
- Immunological Memory 155
- Immunological Tolerance or Recognition of Self 156
- Immunological Disorders 157

17. Platelets — 159
- Structure of Platelet 159
- Variations in the Platelet Count 160
- Properties of Platelets 160
- Functions of Platelet 162
- Von Willebrand Factor 162
- Thrombopoiesis 162

18. Hemostasis — 164
- Primary Hemostasis 164
- Secondary Hemostasis 165
- Factors that Prevent Intravascular Coagulation or Intravascular Anticoagulants 169
- Fibrinolytic System 170
- Fibrinolysis Inhibitors 171
- Anticoagulants 171
- Bleeding Disorders 172
- Purpura 174
- Thromboembolic Conditions in Human 174

19. Tissue Fluid and Lymph — 177
- Tissue Fluid 177
- Lymph 179

20. Blood Volume — 183
- Measurement of Blood Volume 183
- Variations in Blood Volume 183
- Regulation of Blood Volume 184

21. Blood Groups and Blood Transfusion — 186
- ABO Blood Group System 186
- RH System 190
- Blood Transfusion 193

Section 3: Cardiovascular System

22. Functional Anatomy of the Heart — 201
- Heart 202
- Specialized Excitatory and Conducting System of Heart 205
- Properties of Cardiac Muscle 208

23. Recording of Electrical Activity of Heart — 210
- Electrocardiography 210
- Electrocardiogram 212
- Normal Pattern of ECG 213
- Intervals in ECG 214
- Pattern of ECG in Other Leads 215
- Mean Electrical Axis 215
- Clinical Application of ECG 217

24. Cardiac Cycle — 224
- Phases of Cardiac Cycle 224
- Pressure Changes during Cardiac Cycle 227
- Volume Changes during Cardiac Cycle 229
- Heart Sounds 230

25. Hemodynamics — 234
- Relation between Pressure, Flow and Resistance 235
- Methods for Measuring Blood Flow 235
- Laminar Flow 235
- Flow Continuity Equation 235
- Critical Velocity 236
- Circulation Time 237
- Resistance to Flow of Blood 237
- Tests to Assess Cardiac Function 240

26. Heart Rate — 243
- Factors Affecting Heart Rate 243
- Afferents to the Cardiac Centers 246

- Chemical Factors Affecting Heart Rate *249*
- Physical Factors *250*
- Age and Sex *250*
- Regulation of Heart Rate *250*
- Regulation of Transplanted Heart *250*
- Sympathovagal Balance *250*
- Heart Rate Variability *251*

27. Cardiac Output 253
- Measurement of Cardiac Output *253*
- Variations in Cardiac Output *255*
- Cardiac Reserve *255*
- Factors Affecting Cardiac Output *255*
- Regulation of Cardiac Output *255*
- Regulation of Stroke Volume *255*
- Regulation of Heart Rate *257*
- Neural Factors *257*
- Physical Factors Regulating Heart Rate *257*

28. Vascular System and Arterial Blood Pressure 261
- Vascular System *261*
- Arterial Blood Pressure *263*
- Measurement of Arterial Blood Pressure *264*
- Variations in Blood Pressure *264*
- Determinants of Arterial Blood Pressure *266*
- Regulation of Peripheral Resistance *267*
- Regulation of Blood Pressure *270*
- Factors Affecting Blood Pressure *271*
- Factors Affecting Cardiac Output *271*
- Factors Affecting Peripheral Resistance *271*
- Circulatory Shock *272*
- Cardiac Failure or Heart Failure *275*

29. Arterial and Venous Pulse 281
- Arterial Pulse *281*
- Jugular Venous Pulse *283*

30. Cardiovascular Adjustments in Exercise 285
- Increase in Sympathetic Discharge *285*
- Increase in Arterial Pressure *285*
- Increase in Cardiac Output *286*
- Local Mechanisms *286*
- Effect of Training *286*

31. Effect of Acceleratory Forces on Circulatory System 288
- Effects of Positive "G" On Circulatory System *288*
- Effects of Negative "G" *288*
- Effect of Gravity on Circulatory System *288*
- Compensatory Cardiovascular Adjustments in Prolonged Standing *289*
- Effects of Zero Gravity in the Body (Weightlessness) *289*

32. Circulation through Special Regions 290
- Capillary Circulation *290*
- Structural Organization of Capillaries *290*
- Cutaneous Circulation *292*
- Coronary Circulation *293*
- Measurement of Coronary Blood Flow *294*
- Cerebral Circulation *299*
- Splanchnic Circulation *303*
- Intestinal Microcirculation *303*
- Hepatic Portal Circulation *304*
- Fetal Circulation *305*

Section 4: Respiratory System

33. Structure and Functions of Respiratory System 313
- Functions of the Respiratory Tract *313*
- Functional Anatomy of the Respiratory System *315*
- Innervation of Lungs *318*
- Bronchoscopy *318*
- Bronchography *318*
- Pleura *318*
- Blood Supply to Lungs *319*

34. Mechanics of Ventilation 321
- Patterns of Breathing *321*
- Boundaries of the Thoracic Cage *321*
- Muscles of Respiration *321*
- Mechanism of Ventilation of Lungs *322*
- Movements of the Thoracic Cage *322*
- Breath Sounds *322*
- Pressure Changes during Respiratory Cycle *324*
- Elastic behavior of Lungs or Reasons for Recoil of Lung *325*
- Surfactant *325*
- Application of Law of Laplace in Lung *327*
- Alveolar Stability *327*
- Effects of Cigarette Smoking *327*

35. Methods of Study of Respiratory Movements 331
- Direct Technique to Study Respiratory Movements *331*
- Indirect Techniques *331*
- Lung Volumes and Capacities *332*
- Pulmonary Ventilation and Alveolar Ventilation *335*
- Respiratory Dead Space *336*
- Compliance (Pressure–Volume Relationship) *337*
- Work of Breathing *339*

36. Pulmonary Circulation 343
- Pulmonary Blood Pressure *344*
- Measurement of Pulmonary Blood Flow *345*
- Regional Variation in Distribution of Ventilation and Perfusion *345*
- Effect of Gravity in Pulmonary Circulation *346*
- Relationship between Pulmonary Artery Pressure and Pulmonary Venous Pressure in Pulmonary Capillary Blood Flow *347*
- Ventilation-perfusion Ratio *348*

37. Pulmonary Gas Exchange 351
- Partial Pressure of Gases *351*
- Techniques of Collection of Alveolar Air or Sampling of Alveolar Air *351*
- Methods of Analysis of the Collected Alveolar Gas *352*
- Reasons for the Difference in the Composition of Atmospheric Air and Alveolar Air *352*
- Mechanism of Gas Exchange at Lung Level (External Respiration) *352*
- Internal Respiration *354*

- Respiratory Quotient or Respiratory Exchange Ratio *355*

38. Transport of Gases — 357
- Transport of Oxygen *357*
- Carbon Dioxide Transport *361*

39. Regulation of Respiration — 366
Neural Control of Respiration *366*
- Voluntary Control *366*
- Automatic Control *366*
- Reflex Control of Respiration *368*

Chemical Regulation of Respiration *370*
- Chemoreceptors *370*
- Interaction of Chemical Factors in Regulation of Respiration *374*
- Abnormalities in Regulation of Respiration *375*
- Hypoxia *378*
- Cyanosis *381*

40. Environmental Physiology — 386
- High Altitude Physiology *386*

Effects of Barometric Pressure on Respiratory System *386*
- Effects of Decreased Barometric Pressure *386*
- Factors other than Barometric Pressure at High Altitude *388*
- Effects of Increased Barometric Pressure *388*
- Barotrauma *390*

Space Physiology *390*
- Weightlessness in Space *390*
- Diseases due to Ionizing Radiation *392*

41. Respiratory Adjustments in Exercise — 395
- Fatigue *397*

42. Artificial Respiration and Cardiopulmonary Resuscitation — 398
- Cardiopulmonary Resuscitation *399*

43. Pulmonary Function Tests — 401

Section 5: Gastrointestinal System

44. Introduction to Digestive System — 405
- Functions of Gastrointestinal System *405*
- Digestion *406*
- Innervation of Gut *407*
- Gut-brain Axis *409*

45. Salivary Glands and Esophagus — 413
- Functional Anatomy *413*
- Histology of Salivary Gland *413*
- Blood Supply *414*
- Innervation of Salivary Glands *415*
- Composition of Saliva *416*
- Functions of Saliva *416*
- Mechanism of Secretion of Saliva *417*
- Regulation of Salivary Secretion *418*
- Nature of Saliva *418*
- Salivary Reflexes *418*
- Disturbances of Salivary Secretion *419*
- Esophagus *420*

46. Stomach — 422
- Functions of Stomach *422*
- Functional Anatomy of Stomach *422*
- Histology *423*
- Gastric Mucosal Barrier *424*
- Innervation of Stomach *425*
- Gastric Juice *425*
- Phases of Gastric Juice Secretion *429*
- Gastrin *430*
- Abnormalities of Gastric Secretory Function *432*

47. Exocrine Pancreas — 438
- Innervation *438*
- Composition of Pancreatic Juice *438*
- Mechanism of Secretion of Pancreatic Juice *440*
- Regulation of Secretion of Pancreatic Juice *440*
- Phases of Pancreatic Juice Secretion *441*

48. Liver and Biliary System — 443
- Functions of Liver *443*
- Biliary System *444*
- Jaundice or Icterus *446*
- Regulation of Biliary Secretion *447*
- Gallbladder *447*
- Investigations of Liver and Gallbladder *448*

49. Small Intestine — 451
- Functional Anatomy *451*
- Parts of Small Intestine *451*
- Small Intestinal Juice or Succus Entericus *452*
- Functions of Small Intestine *452*
- Regulation of Small Intestinal Secretion *453*

50. Large Intestine — 455
- Dietary Fiber *456*

51. Movements of Gastrointestinal Tract — 459
- Types of Movements *459*
- Gastric Movements *462*
- Movements of Small Intestine *464*
- Movements of Large Intestine *466*
- Defecation *466*

52. Digestion and Absorption of Food — 469
- Digestion and Absorption of Carbohydrates *469*
- Digestion and Absorption of Proteins and Nucleic Acids *471*
- Vitamins *474*

53. Gastrointestinal Hormones — 477
- Amine Precursor Uptake and Decarboxylation (APUD) Cells *477*
- Incretins *477*
- Glucagon-like Peptide-I *478*
- Glucose-dependent Insulinotropic Polypeptide *478*

Section 6: Renal Physiology

54. Functional Anatomy of Kidney — 483
- Kidney *483*

55. Mechanism of Formation of Urine — 494
- Glomerular Filtration *494*
- Glomerular Filtration Rate *495*

56. Lower Urinary Tract — 519
- Innervation of the Bladder 519
- Micturition 520
- Abnormalities of Bladder Function 521
- Cystometry 521
- Diuresis and Diuretics 522

57. Renal Function Tests — 524
- Urine Analysis 524
- Blood Examination 525
- Miscellaneous Tests 525

Section 7: Skin and Temperature Regulation

58. Skin — 529
- Structure of Skin 529
- Appendages of Skin 529
- Blood Supply of the Skin 531
- Skin Color 531
- Functions of Skin 531

59. Temperature Regulation — 533
- Measurement of Body Temperature 533
- Mechanisms of Heat Gain and Heat Loss from the Body 534
- Variations in Body Temperature 540
- Effects of Exposure of the Body to Extremes of Temperature 542

Section 8: Endocrine System

60. Organization of the Endocrine System — 547
- Relation between Endocrine System and Nervous System 548
- Endocrine Glands 548
- Radioimmunoassay 550
- Clinical Syndromes Related to Endocrine Functions 550

61. Mechanism of Cellular Action of Hormones — 552
- Hormone Receptors 552

Intercellular Communication 554

- G-Proteins 554
- Mechanism by which Combination of Hormone with Receptor Triggers Cellular Function 555
- Genomic and Nongenomic Effects of Hormones 561
- Regulation of Hormone Secretion 561

62. Anterior Pituitary Gland and Hypothalamus — 565
- Pituitary Gland 565
- Hormones of the Pituitary Gland 566
- Anterior Pituitary 567
- Physiology of Growth and Development 573
- Hypothalamus 579

63. Posterior Pituitary — 582
- Hormones of Posterior Pituitary 582
- Oxytocin 584

64. Pineal Gland — 587
- Functional Anatomy 587
- Circadian Rhythm 589

65. Thyroid Gland — 591

66. Calcium and Phosphate Homeostasis — 608
- Physiology of Bone 608
- Body Calcium 609
- Phosphorus Metabolism 610
- Parathyroid Glands 610
- Parathormone 610
- Calcitriol or 1,25- Hydroxycholecalciferol 615

67. Adrenal Gland — 620
- Functional Anatomy of Adrenal Gland 620
- Glucocorticoids 622
- Mineralocorticoids 628
- Adrenal Medulla 632

68. Endocrine Pancreas — 640
- Functional Anatomy 640
- Insulin 641
- Obesity and Metabolic Syndrome or Syndrome-X 648
- Houssay Animal 649
- Glucagon 649
- Somatostatin 649
- Pancreatic Polypeptide 650
- Control of Blood Glucose 650

69. Other Endocrine Organs and Local Hormones — 654
- Thymus 654
- Kidney 655
- Heart 656
- Local Hormones 656
- Endothelium 658
- Endothelins 659

Section 9: Reproductive System

70. Introduction to Reproductive Physiology — 663
- Characteristics which Differentiate an Adult Human Male from an Adult Female 663

71. Sexual Development in the Embryo — 665
- Sex Determination 665
- Sex Differentiation 666
- Abnormalities in Sexual Differentiation 668
- Puberty 670

72. Male Reproductive System — 673
- Functional Anatomy of Male Reproductive System 673
- Spermatogenesis 674
- Erection and Ejaculation 677
- Endocrine Function of Testis 678

73. Female Reproductive System — 684
- Functional Anatomy 684
- Secondary Sexual Organs in Female 685
- Oogenesis 685
- Female Reproductive Cycle or Menstrual Cycle 686
- Changes in the Breast 690
- Endocrine Function of Ovary 690
- Control of Ovarian Function 693
- Abnormalities of Menstruation 694
- Tests of Ovulation 696

- Menopause 696
- Physiology of Human Sexual Responses 696

74. Fertilization and Pregnancy 701
- Changes in the Sperm before Fertilization 701
- Fertilization 702
- Functions of Placenta 703
- Pregnancy Tests 705
- Amniocentesis 706
- Parturition or Labor 706
- Puerperium 707

75. Cardiorespiratory Adjustments of the Baby after Birth 710
- Respiratory Adjustments after Birth 710
- Cardiovascular Adjustments 710

76. Lactation 711
- Milk Secretion 712
- Milk Ejection 712
- Lactation and Menstruation 712

77. Contraception and Infertility 714
- Contraception 714
- Infertility 717

Section 10: Nervous System

78. Organization of Nervous System 721
- Functions of Nervous System 721
- Organization of Nervous System 722
- Basis of Neural Activity 722
- Centers of Nervous System 723
- Processing of Sensory Information 723
- Functional Anatomy of the Brain 724
- Cranial Nerves 724
- Structure of Central Nervous System 724
- Structure of Spinal Cord 726

79. Physiology of Nervous System 731
- Synapse 731
- Mechanism of Transmission at the Excitatory Chemical Synapse 734
- Electrical Events at Synapses 735
- Properties of Synapse 736
- Effect of Environmental Factors on Synaptic Transmission 742
- Neurotransmitters and Neuromodulators 742

80. Reflex Action 747
- Reflex ARC 747
- Classification of Reflexes 748
- General Properties of Reflexes 757

81. Sensory Division of Nervous System 761
- Sensation 761
- Sensory Receptors 762
- Pacinian Corpuscle 763
- Generator Potential or Receptor Potential 763
- Properties of Receptors 764
- Sensory Unit 764
- Intensity Discrimination by Cerebral Cortex 765
- Weber-Fechner Law 765
- Coding of Sensory Information (Sensory Coding) 765
- Muller's Doctrine of Specific Nerve Energies 766
- Law of Projection 766
- Cortical Plasticity 766
- Superficial Senses 766
- Cortical Sensations 767
- Lateral Inhibition or Surround Inhibition 767
- Synthetic Cutaneous Senses 768

82. Ascending Sensory Pathways 770
- Dorsal Column Pathway or Medial Lemniscal System 771
- Spinothalamic Pathway or Anterolateral System 771
- Ascending Tracts of Spinal Cord 772
- Sensory Tracts 773
- Nonsensory Tracts 773
- Sensory Cortical Area 774
- Sensory Association Area 775
- Sense of Touch 775
- Pathway for Temperature Sensation 778
- Kinesthetic Sensation (Kinesthesia) or Proprioception 779
- Itching and Tickling 780
- Visceral Sensations 781
- Pain Sensation 781

83. Thalamus 794
- Functional Anatomy of Thalamus 794
- Anatomical Classification of Thalamic Nuclei 794
- Functional Classification of Thalamic Nuclei 795
- Connections of Thalamus 795
- Functions of Thalamus 795
- Lesions of Thalamus 796

84. Motor Division of Nervous System 798
- Somatic Nervous System 798
- Muscle Tone 798
- Upper Motor Neuron Pathways 799
- Voluntary Motor Activity 800
- Motor Areas of Cerebral Cortex 801
- Mirror Neurons 801
- Pyramidal Tract 801
- Extrapyramidal Tracts 804
- Cortically Originating Extrapyramidal Fibers 804
- Applied Physiology 805

85. Lesions of Spinal Cord 810
- Types of Lesions of Spinal Cord 810
- Complications of Spinal Cord Transection 812
- Section of Posterior Nerve Root in Spinal Cord 813
- Section of Anterior Nerve Root 813
- Section of Peripheral Nerve 813
- Diseases Affecting Spinal Cord 813

86. Basal Ganglia or Basal Nuclei 815
- Functional Anatomy 815
- Connections of Basal Ganglia 816
- Putamen Circuit and the Caudate Circuit 819
- Functions of Basal Ganglia 820
- Effects of Lesions of Basal Ganglia 820
- Parkinson's Disease or Paralysis Agitans 820
- Huntington's Disease 822
- Hemiballism or Hemiballismus 823

- Wilson's Disease or Progressive Hepatolenticular Degeneration 823
- Kernicterus 823

87. Cerebellum — 825
- Functional Anatomy 825
- Parts of Cerebellum 825
- Phylogenetic Classification 826
- Functional Classification 826
- Cerebellar Cortex 826
- Connections of Cerebellum 828
- Peduncles of Cerebellum 829
- Functions of Cerebellum 830
- Lesions of Cerebellum 831

88. Reticular Formation — 835
- Connections of Reticular Formation 835
- Functions of Reticular Formation 836

89. Vestibular Apparatus — 838
- Functional Anatomy of Vestibular Apparatus 838
- Vestibular Pathway 841
- Mechanism of Control of Equilibrium 841
- Functions of Vestibular Apparatus 842
- Vestibular Function Tests 843
- Vestibular Dysfunction 844
- Effects of Removal of Vestibular Apparatus 844

90. Posture and Equilibrium — 845
- Postural Reflexes 845

91. Cerebral Cortex — 849
- Functional Anatomy of Cerebral Cortex 849
- Methods of Study of Cerebrocortical Function 851
- Functionally Important Areas of Cerebral Cortex 852

92. Hypothalamus — 855
- Functional Anatomy 855

93. Limbic System — 860
- Parts of Limbic System 860
- Functions of Limbic System 861

94. Autonomic Nervous System — 863
- General Organization of ANS 863
- Functional Anatomy of Sympathetic Nervous System 864
- Functional Anatomy of Parasympathetic Nervous System 865
- Types of Transmission in the Autonomic Nervous System 866
- Functions of Autonomic Nervous System 869
- Disorders of Autonomic Nervous System 870
- General Adaptation Syndrome 870

95. Electroencephalography, Sleep, Yoga and Meditation — 873
- Electroencephalography 873
- Sleep 874
- Physiology of Sleep-Wake Cycles 877
- Yoga and Meditation 878

96. Higher Functions of Brain — 882
- Unconditioned Reflex 882
- Conditioned Reflex 882
- Learning and Memory 884
- Thought 886
- Neuroplasticity or Cortical Plasticity 886
- Speech and Language 887
- Intercortical Transfer of Learning 889

97. Cerebrospinal Fluid — 891
- Anatomy of the Ventricles of Brain and their Connections 891
- Cerebrospinal Fluid 892

Section 11: Special Senses

98. Vision — 901
- Functional Anatomy of Eyeball 901
- Ophthalmoscopy 904
- Contents of the Eyeball 904
- Intraocular Pressure 905
- Glaucoma 905
- Lens 906
- Vitreous Body 906
- Extraocular Muscles 906
- Lacrimal Apparatus 907
- Physical Optics 907
- Refractive Index 908
- Refractive Power 908
- Refraction in the Eye 909
- Accommodation 909
- Near Response or Near Reflex 910
- Optical Defects in the Eye 912
- Optical Aberrations 913
- Cataract 914
- Visual Acuity (Resolving Power of Eye) 914
- Field of Vision or Visual Field 915
- Retina 917
- Visual Receptor Mechanism 920
- Electrophysiological Changes in Retinal Receptors 922
- Experimental Evidence to Show that Rods are Responsible for Dim Light Vision 923
- Adaptation in the Visual System 924
- Lateral Inhibition in the Visual Pathway 926
- Visual Pathway 927
- Lesions of Visual Pathway 930
- Pupillary Reflexes 930
- Color Vision 932
- Mechanism of Color Vision 933
- Theories of Color Vision 933
- Tests for Color Vision 935
- Color Blindness 935
- Electroretinogram 937
- Visual Evoked Potential 937

99. Audition — 943
- Functional Anatomy of the Ear 943
- Physiology of Hearing or Audition 949
- Mechanism of Hearing 951
- Mechanism of Appreciation of Frequency, Intensity and Localization of Sound 952
- Auditory Pathway 954
- Cochlear Microphonics 956
- Applied Aspects 957
- Hearing Aids 958
- Audiometry 959

100. **Gustation or Taste Sensation** 965
- Taste Buds 965
- Taste Pathway 966
- Basic Taste Modalities or Primary Taste Sensations 967
- Abnormalities of Taste Sensation 968

101. **Olfaction** 969
- The Olfactory Apparatus 969
- Olfactory Pathway 971
- Vomeronasal Organ 973
- Variations in the Sense of Smell 973

Section 12: Integrated Physiology

102. **Integrated Physiology** 977
- Physiology of Infancy 977
- Applied Physiology 978
- Physiology of Aging 979
- Free Radicals and Antioxidants 980
- Brain Death 982
- Cardiorespiratory and Metabolic Adjustments during Exercise 982
- Cardiorespiratory Changes in Isotonic and Isometric Exercises 984
- Effect of Exercise Under Different Environmental Conditions (Heat and Cold) 985
- Consequences of Sedentary Life Style 985

Important Questions 987

Index 1015

Abbreviations

2,3-DPG (2,3-BPG)	2,3-Diphosphoglycerate (2,3-Biphosphoglycerate)	BV	Blood volume
Aa	Amino acid	CABG	Coronary artery bypass grafting
Ab	Antibody	CAD	Coronary artery disease
ABP	Androgen binding protein	CAMP	Cyclic adenosine-3',5'-monophosphate
ACC	Anodal closing contraction	CAT	Computed axial tomography
ACD	Acid-citrate-dextrose	CAT scan	Computed axial tomography scan
ACE	Angiotensin converting enzyme	CCC	Cathodal closing contraction
ACh	Acetylcholine	CCF	Congestive cardiac failure
ACTH	Adrenocorticotropic hormone	CCK-PZ	Cholecystokinin-pancreozymin
ADH	Antidiuretic hormone	CCP	Critical closing pressure
ADP	Adenosine diphosphate	CFF	Critical fusion frequency
ADS	Anatomical dead space	CFTR	Cystic fibrosis transmembrane conductance regulator
Ag	Antigen	CFU	Colony-forming units
AHG	Antihuman globulin	CGRP	Calcitonin-gene-related peptide
AIDS	Acquired immunodeficiency syndrome	CHP	Capsular hydrostatic pressure
AIF	Apoptosis inducing factor	CIC	Cardioinhibitory center
ANP	Atrial natriuretic peptide	CLIP	Corticotropin like intermediate lobe peptide
ANS	Autonomic nervous system	CLP	Common lymphoid progenitor cell
AP	Action potential	CMP	Common myeloid progenitor cell
APC	Antigen presenting cell	CNS	Central nervous system
APD	Acid peptic disease	CoA	Coenzyme A
APO-1	Apoptosis antigen 1	CO	Carbon monoxide; cardiac output
APTT	Activated partial thromboplastin time	COHb	Carbonmonoxyhemoglobin
APUD cell	Amine precursor uptake and decarboxylation cell	COMT	Catecholamlne-O-methyl transferase
ARAS	Ascending reticular activating system	COPD	Chronic obstructive pulmonary disease
ARDS	Adult respiratory distress syndrome	CPD-A	Citrate phosphate dextrose-adenine
ARP	Absolute refractory period	CPK	Creatine phosphokinase
ASD	Atrial septal defect	CRH	Corticotropin releasing hormone
ATP	Adenosine triphosphate	CRO	Cathode ray oscilloscope
AV node	Atrioventricular node	CRP	C-reactive protein
AV valve	Atrioventricular valve	CSF	Cerebrospinal fluid; colony stimulating factor
BBB	Blood-brain barrier	CT	Collecting tubule
BCOP	Blood colloidal osmotic pressure	CV	Closing volume
BDG	Bilirubin diglucuronide	CVLM	Caudal ventrolateral medulla
BER	Basic electrical rhythm	DB	Decibel
BFU-E	Burst forming unit-erythroid	DCT	Distal convoluted tubule
BFU	Burst forming units	DHEA	Dehydroepiandrosterone
BMD	Becker muscular dystrophy	DHPRs	Dihydropyridine receptors
BMR	Basal metabolic rate	DIC	Disseminated intravascular coagulation
BPA	Burst promoting activity	DIFP	Di-isopropyl fluorophosphate
BP	Blood pressure	DMN	Dorsal motor nucleus
		DMT-1	Divalent metal transporter-1

DNA	Deoxyribonucleic acid		GnRH	Gonadotropin releasing hormone
DNS	Dextrose-normal saline		GPI	Glycosyl phosphatidylinositol
DOPA	Dihydroxyphenylalanine		HAg	H antigen
DPP-4	Dipeptidyl peptidase-4		HbA1c	Glycated hemoglobin
DRG	Dorsal respiratory group		Hb	Hemoglobin
ECF	Extracellular fluid		HBE	His bundle electrogram
ECG	Electrocardiogram		HbO_2	Oxyhemoglobin
ECL cells	Enterochromaffin-like cells		hCG	Human chorionic gonadotropin
EDRF	Endothelium derived-relaxing factor		hCS	Human chorionic somatomammotropin
EDTA	Ethylenediaminetetraaceticacid		HDL	High-density lipoprotein
EDV	End-diastolic volume		HDN	Hemolytic disease of newborn
EEG	Electroencephalogram		HGP	Human Genome Project
EF	Ejection fraction		HHb	Reduced hemoglobin
EJP	Excitatory junctional potentials		HIV	Human immunodeficiency virus
EMG	Electromyogram		HLA	Human leukocyte associated antigen
ENaC	Epithelial Na^+ channel		HMP	Hexose monophosphate
E neurons	Expiratory neurons		HMW-K	High molecular weight kininogen
ENS	Enteric nervous system		HPNS	High pressure nervous syndrome
EPO	Erythropoietin		HRV	Heart rate variability
EPP	Endplate potential		HSC	Hematopoietic stem cell
EPSP	Excitatory postsynaptic potential		I-neurons	Inspiratory neurons
Eq	Equivalent		ICF	Intracellular fluid
ERCP	Endoscopic retrograde cholangiopancreatography		IC	Inspiratory capacity
ERG	Electroretinogram		ICP	Isovolumetric contraction phase
ERPF	Effective renal plasma flow		ICSH	Interstitial cell stimulating hormone
ERV	Expiratory reserve volume		IF	Intrinsic factor
ESR	Erythrocyte sedimentation rate		IFN-α	Interferon-α
ESV	End-systolic Volume		IGF	Insulin-like growth factor
FDP	Fibrinogen degradation product		Ig	Immunoglobulin
FEV-1	Forced expiratory volume in one second		IHD	Ischemic heart disease
FEV	Forced expiratory volume		IJP	Inhibitory junctional potentials
FFP	Fresh frozen plasma		IL	Interleukin
FRC	Functional residual capacity		IMN	Infectious mononucleosis
FSH	Follicle stimulating hormone		INR	International normalized ratio
FVC	Forced vital capacity		IPSP	Inhibitory postsynaptic potential
G-CSF	Granulocyte colony stimulating factor		IRS	Inspiratory ramp signal
GABA	Gamma-aminobutyric acid		IRV	Inspiratory reserve volume
GBHP	Glomerular blood hydrostatic pressure		IUCD	Intrauterine contraceptive device
GERD	Gastroesophageal reflux disease		IVC	Inferior vena cava
GFR	Glomerular filtration rate		IVF	Intravenous fluid
g	Gram		IVP	Intravenous pyelogram
GH	Growth hormone		JAMs	Junctional adhesion molecules
GHIH	Growth hormone inhibiting hormone		JGA	Juxtaglomerular apparatus
GHRH	Growth hormone releasing hormone		JVP	Jugular venous pulse
GIFT	Gamete intrafallopian transfer		Kf	Ultrafiltration coefficient
GIP	Gastric inhibitory peptide		LDH	Lactate dehydrogenase
GIP	Glucose-dependent insulinotropic polypeptide		LDL	Low-density lipoprotein
GIT	Gastrointestinal tract		LEMS	Lambert-Eaton myasthenic syndrome
GLP-I	Glucagon-like peptide-I		LES	Lower esophageal sphincter
GLUT	Glucose transporter		LFT	Liver function test
GM-CSF	Granulocyte-macrophage colony stimulating factor		LH	Luteinizing hormone

LHRH	Luteinizing hormone releasing hormone	PAM	Pulmonary alveolar macrophage
LISS	Low-ionic strength saline	PAMs	Pulmonary alveolar macrophages
LP	Lumbar puncture	PAT	Paroxysmal atrial tachycardia
LQTS	Long QT syndrome	PBI	Protein-bound iodine
M-CSF	Macrophage colony stimulating factor	PCR	Polymerase chain reaction
MAO	Monoamine oxidase	PCV	Packed cell volume
MBC	Maximum breathing capacity	PDA	Patent ductus arteriosus
MBP	Major basic protein	PDGF	Platelet-derived growth factor
MCHC	Mean corpuscular hemoglobin concentration	PET	Positron emission tomography
MCH	Mean corpuscular hemoglobin	P factor	Pain producing substance
MCV	Mean corpuscular volume	PFTs	Pulmonary function tests
MEPP	Miniature endplate potential	PGO	Ponto-geniculo-occipital spikes
mEq/L	Milliequivalents per litre	PG	Prostaglandin
MHC	Major histocompatibility complex	pH	Hydrogen ion concentration
MI	Myocardial infarction	PHSC	Pluripotent hematopoietic stem cells
min	Minutes	Pi	Inorganic phosphate
MIS	Mullerian inhibiting substance	PL	Platelet phospholipid
MIT	Monoiodotyrosine	PNS	Peripheral nervous system
MMC	Migrating motor complex or migrating myoelectrical complex	POMC	Pro-opiomelanocortin
		PPH	Postpartum hemorrhage
m	Meter	PPS	Plasma protein solution
mm Hg	Millimeters of mercury	PRC	Packed red cells
MPF	Maturation promoting factor	PRCV	Packed red cell volume
MRI	Magnetic resonance imaging	PRH	Prolactin releasing hormone
mRNA	Messenger RNA	PRL	Prolactin
MSH	Melanocyte-stimulating hormone	PRP	Platelet-rich plasma
ms	Milliseconds	PS	Precursor substance
mV	Millivolt	PST	Proximal straight tubule
MW	Maximum voluntary ventilation	PTA	Plasma thromboplastin antecedent (clotting factor XI)
MW	Molecular weight	PTCA	Percutaneous transluminal coronary angioplasty
NADPH	Nicotinamide adenine dinucleotide phosphate	PTH	Parathyroid hormone
NE	Norepinephrine	PT	Prothrombin time
NK cells	Natural killer	PTT	Partial thromboplastin time
NMJ	Neuromuscular junction	PVN	Posteroventral nucleus
NO	Nitric oxide	RBC	Red blood cell
NPY	Neuropeptide Y	RDS	Respiratory dead space
NRDS/IRDS	Neonatal or infant respiratory distress syndrome	RDS	Respiratory distress syndrome
NREM	Nonrapid eye movement sleep	REM sleep	Rapid eye movement sleep
NSAID	Nonsteroidal anti-inflammatory drug	RER	Rough endoplasmic reticulum
NS	Normal saline	RFLP	Restriction fragment length polymorphism
NSR	Normal sinus rhythm	Rh factor	Rhesus factor
NT	Neurotransmitter	RIA	Radioimmunoassay
NTS	Nucleus of tractus solitarius	RISA	Radioiodinated serum albumin
ORS	Oral rehydration solution	RL	Ringer lactate
Osm	Osmoles	RMP	Resting membrane potential
PIH	Prolactin inhibiting hormone	RMV	Respiratory minute volume
P_{50}	Partial pressure of O_2 at which hemoglobin is half saturated with O_2	RNA	Ribonucleic acid
		RPF	Renal plasma flow
PAF	Platelet activating factor	rpm	Revolutions per minute
PAH	Para-aminohippuric acid	RQ	Respiratory quotient
PAI	Plasminogen activator inhibitor	rRNA	Ribosomal RNA

RR	Respiratory rate	TGF-β	Transforming growth factor-β
RVLM	Rostral ventrolateral medulla	TLC	Total lung capacity
RV	Residual volume	TmG	Transport maximum for glucose
RYR	Ryanodine receptors	Tm	Renal tubular maximum
s/sec	Seconds	TNF	Tumor necrosis factor
SA node	Sinoatrial node	TPL	Thromboplastin
SCUBA	Self-contained underwater breathing apparatus	TPO	Thrombopoietin
SDA	Specific dynamic action	TRH	Thyrotropin-releasing hormone
SEC	Series elastic component	TRIM	Transfusion-related immune modulation
SERCA	Sarcoplasmic or endoplasmic reticulum Ca^{2+} ATPase	TSH	Thyroid-stimulating hormone
SER	Smooth endoplasmic reticulum	TTX	Tetrodotoxin
SGLT	Sodium-dependent glucose transporter	TV	Tidal volume
SGOT	Serum glutamate-O-methyl transferase	u-PA	Urokinase-type plasminogen activator
SGOT	Serum glutamic-oxaloacetic transaminase	UDPGA	Uridine diphosphoglucuronic acid
SGPT	Serum glutamate pyruvate transaminase	USS	Ultrasound scan
SIDS	Sudden infant death syndrome	UV	Ultraviolet
SLE	Systemic lupus erythematosus	VAT	Ventricular Activation Time
SLV	Semilunar valves	VC	Vital capacity
SNO-Hb	S-nitrosohemoglobin	VIP	Vasoactive intestinal polypeptide
SPECT	Single photon emission CT scan	VLDL	Very low density lipoprotein
STAT	Signal transducer and activation of transcription	VMA	Vanillylmandelic acid
STEMI	ST-elevation myocardial infarction	VMC	Vasomotor center
SVC	Superior vena cava	VPLN	Ventral posterolateral nucleus of thalamus
SV	Stroke volume	VPMN	Ventral posteromedial nucleus of thalamus
t-PA	Tissue plasminogen activator	VPN	Ventral posterior nucleus (also called posteroventral nucleus PVN)
T4	Thyroxine		
TBG	Thyroxine binding globulin	VRG	Ventral respiratory group
TBW	Total body water	VSD	Ventricular septal defect
TCOP	Tubular colloid osmotic pressure	V	Volts
TCR	T cell receptor	vWF	von Willebrand's factor
TFPI	Tissue factor pathway inhibitor	WBC	White blood cell

Competency Table

Number	Competency: The student should be able to	Core(Y/N)	Chapter Number	Page Number
PY1.1	Describe the structure and functions of a mammalian cell	Y	4	15
PY1.2	Describe and discuss the principles of homeostasis	Y	3	11
PY1.3	Describe intercellular communication	Y	61	554
PY1.4	Describe apoptosis – programmed cell death	Y	4	29
PY1.5	Describe and discuss transport mechanisms across cell membranes	Y	5	34
PY1.6	Describe the fluid compartments of the body, its ionic composition and measurements	Y	2 20	7 183
PY1.7	Describe the concept of pH and Buffer systems in the body	Y	1	1
PY1.8	Describe and discuss the molecular basis of resting membrane potential and action potential in excitable tissue	Y	6	48
PY2.1	Describe the composition and functions of blood components	Y	11	99
PY2.2	Discuss the origin, forms, variations, and functions of plasma proteins	Y	12	102
PY2.3	Describe and discuss the synthesis and functions of hemoglobin and explain its breakdown. Describe variants of hemoglobin	Y	13	111
PY2.4	Describe RBC formation (erythropoiesis and its regulation) and its functions	Y	13	116
PY2.5	Describe different types of anemias and jaundice	Y	13 48	122 446
PY2.6	Describe WBC formation (granulopoiesis) and its regulation	Y	14	138
PY2.7	Describe the formation of platelets, functions, and variations	Y	17	159
PY2.8	Describe the physiological basis of hemostasis, and anticoagulants. Describe bleeding and clotting disorders (Hemophilia, purpura)	Y	18	164
PY2.9	Describe different blood groups and discuss the clinical importance of blood grouping, blood banking and transfusion	Y	21	186
PY2.10	Define and classify different types of immunity. Describe the development of immunity and its regulation	Y	16	146
PY2.12	Describe test for ESR, osmotic fragility, hematocrit. Note the findings and interpret the test results, etc.	Y	13	107 108 110
PY3.1	Describe the structure and functions of a neuron and neuroglia; Discuss nerve growth factor and other growth factors/cytokines	Y	6	44
PY3.2	Describe the types, functions and properties of nerve fibers	Y	6	44
PY3.3	Describe the degeneration and regeneration in peripheral nerves	Y	6	58
PY3.4	Describe the structure of neuro-muscular junction and transmission of impulses	Y	8	79
PY3.5	Discuss the action of neuro-muscular blocking agents	Y	8	81
PY3.6	Describe the pathophysiology of myasthenia gravis	Y	8	82
PY3.7	Describe the different types of muscle fibers and their structure	Y	7	65
PY3.8	Describe action potential and its properties in different muscle types (skeletal and smooth)	Y	7 10	68 91
PY3.9	Describe the molecular basis of muscle contraction in skeletal and in smooth muscles	Y	7 10	69 92
PY3.10	Describe the mode of muscle contraction (isometric and isotonic)	Y	7	71
PY3.11	Explain energy source and muscle metabolism	Y	7	73
PY3.12	Explain the gradation of muscular activity	Y	7	75

Competency Table

Number	Competency: The student should be able to	Core(Y/N)	Chapter Number	Page Number
PY3.13	Describe muscular dystrophy: myopathies	Y	7	75
PY3.17	Describe strength-duration curve	Y	6	55
PY4.1	Describe the structure and functions of digestive system	Y	44	405
PY4.2	Describe the composition, mechanism of secretion, functions, and regulation of saliva, gastric, pancreatic, intestinal juices and bile secretion	Y	45 46 47 48 49 50	416 425 438 444 452 455
PY4.3	Describe GIT movements, regulation and functions. Describe defecation reflex. Explain role of dietary fiber	Y	50 51	456 459
PY4.4	Describe the physiology of digestion and absorption of nutrients	Y	52	469
PY4.5	Describe the source of GIT hormones, their regulation and functions	Y	53	477
PY4.6	Describe the Gut-Brain axis	Y	44	409
PY4.7	Describe and discuss the structure and functions of liver and gallbladder	Y	48	443, 447
PY4.8	Describe and discuss gastric function tests, pancreatic exocrine function tests and liver function tests	Y	47 48	441 448
PY4.9	Discuss the physiology aspects of: peptic ulcer, gastroesophageal reflux disease, vomiting, diarrhea, constipation, adynamic ileus, Hirschsprung's disease	Y	46 51	432 463, 466
PY5.1	Describe the functional anatomy of heart including chambers, sounds; and pacemaker tissue and conducting system	Y	22	202
PY5.2	Describe the properties of cardiac muscle including its morphology, electrical, mechanical and metabolic functions	Y	9 22	85 208
PY5.3	Discuss the events occurring during the cardiac cycle	Y	24	224
PY5.4	Describe generation, conduction of cardiac impulse	Y	22	205
PY5.6	Describe abnormal ECG, arrhythmias, heart block and myocardial infarction	Y	23	212 217
PY5.7	Describe and discuss hemodynamics of circulatory system	Y	25	234
PY5.8	Describe and discuss local and systemic cardiovascular regulatory mechanisms	Y	26 28	243 261
PY5.9	Describe the factors affecting heart rate, regulation of cardiac output and blood pressure	Y	26 27 28	243 253 263
PY5.10	Describe and discuss regional circulation including microcirculation, lymphatic circulation, coronary, cerebral, capillary, skin, fetal, pulmonary and splanchnic circulation	Y	19 32 36	179 290 343
PY5.11	Describe the patho-physiology of shock, syncope and heart failure	Y	28	272
PY5.12	Record blood pressure and pulse at rest and in different grades of exercise and postures in a volunteer or simulated environment	Y	29	281
PY5.16	Record arterial pulse tracing using finger plethysmography in a volunteer or simulated environment	N	29	281
PY6.1	Describe the functional anatomy of respiratory tract	Y	33	315
PY6.2	Describe the mechanics of normal respiration, pressure changes during ventilation, lung volume and capacities, alveolar surface tension, compliance, airway resistance, ventilation, V/P ratio, diffusion capacity of lungs	Y	34 35 36 37	322 331 348 351
PY6.3	Describe and discuss the transport of respiratory gases: Oxygen and Carbon dioxide	Y	38	357
PY6.4	Describe and discuss the physiology of high altitude and deep sea diving	Y	40	386
PY6.5	Describe and discuss the principles of artificial respiration, oxygen therapy, acclimatization and decompression sickness	Y	39 40 42	380 389 398
PY6.6	Describe and discuss the pathophysiology of dyspnea, hypoxia, cyanosis asphyxia; drowning, periodic breathing	Y	39	378
PY6.7	Describe and discuss lung function tests and their clinical significance	Y	43	401
PY7.1	Describe structure and function of kidney	Y	54	483

Competency Table

Number	Competency: The student should be able to	Core(Y/N)	Chapter Number	Page Number
PY7.2	Describe the structure and functions of juxtaglomerular apparatus and role of renin-angiotensin system	Y	54	487
PY7.3	Describe the mechanism of urine formation involving processes of filtration, tubular reabsorption and secretion; concentration and diluting mechanism	Y	55	494
PY7.4	Describe and discuss the significance and implication of renal clearance	Y	55	496, 509
PY7.5	Describe the renal regulation of fluid and electrolytes and acid-base balance	Y	55	498
PY7.6	Describe the innervations of urinary bladder, physiology of micturition and its abnormalities	Y	55, 56	509, 519
PY7.7	Describe artificial kidney, dialysis and renal transplantation	Y	55	514
PY7.8	Describe and discuss renal function tests	Y	57	524
PY7.9	Describe cystometry and discuss the normal cystometrogram	Y	56	521
PY8.1	Describe the physiology of bone and calcium metabolism	Y	66	608
PY8.2	Describe the synthesis, secretion, transport, physiological actions, regulation and effect of altered (hypo and hyper) secretion of pituitary gland, thyroid gland, parathyroid gland, adrenal gland, pancreas and hypothalamus	Y	62, 63, 65, 66, 67, 68	565, 579, 582, 591, 610, 620, 640
PY8.3	Describe the physiology of thymus and pineal gland	Y	64, 69	587, 654
PY8.4	Describe function tests: Thyroid gland; adrenal cortex, adrenal medulla and pancreas	Y	65, 67, 68	599, 620, 640
PY8.5	Describe the metabolic and endocrine consequences of obesity and metabolic syndrome, stress response. Outline the psychiatry component pertaining to metabolic syndrome	Y	68	648
PY8.6	Describe and differentiate the mechanism of action of steroid, protein and amine hormones	Y	61	552, 555
PY9.1	Describe and discuss sex determination; sex differentiation and their abnormiities and outline psychiatry and practical implication of sex determination	Y	71	665
PY9.2	Describe and discuss puberty: onset, progression, stages; early and delayed puberty and outline adolescent clinical and psychological association	Y	71	670
PY9.3	Describe male reproductive system: functions of testis and control of spermatogenesis and factors modifying it and outline its association with psychiatric illness	Y	72	673
PY9.4	Describe female reproductive system: (a) functions of ovary and its control; (b) menstrual cycle—hormonal, uterine and ovarian changes	Y	73	684
PY9.5	Describe and discuss the physiological effects of sex hormones	Y	72, 73	678, 690
PY9.6	Enumerate the contraceptive methods for male and female. Discuss their advantages and disadvantages	Y	77	714
PY9.7	Describe and discuss the effects of removal of gonads on physiological functions	Y	72	680
PY9.8	Describe and discuss the physiology of pregnancy, parturition and lactation and outline the psychology and psychiatry—disorders associated with it	Y	74, 76	701, 706, 711
PY9.9	Interpret a normal semen analysis report including (a) sperm count, (b) sperm morphology, and (c) sperm motility, as per WHO guidelines and discuss the results	Y	72	678
PY9.10	Discuss the physiological basis of various pregnancy tests	Y	74	705
PY9.11	Discuss the hormonal changes and their effects during perimenopause and menopause	Y	73	696
PY9.12	Discuss the common causes of infertility in a couple and role of IVF in managing a case of infertility	Y	77	717
PY10.1	Describe and discuss the organization of nervous system	Y	78	721
PY10.2	Describe and discuss the functions and properties of synapse, reflex, receptors	Y	79, 80, 81	731, 747, 761

Competency Table

Number	Competency: The student should be able to	Core(Y/N)	Chapter Number	Page Number
PY10.3	Describe and discuss somatic sensations and sensory tracts	Y	80 81 82	747 761 770
PY10.4	Describe and discuss motor tracts, mechanism of maintenance of tone, control of body movements, posture and equilibrium and vestibular apparatus	Y	84 89 90	798 838 845
PY10.5	Describe and discuss structure and functions of reticular activating system, autonomic nervous system (ANS)	Y	88 94	835 863
PY10.6	Describe and discuss spinal cord, its functions, lesion and sensory disturbances	Y	85	810
PY10.7	Describe and discuss functions of cerebral cortex, basal ganglia, thalamus, hypothalamus, cerebellum and limbic system and their abnormalities	Y	83 86 87 91 92 93	794 815 825 849 855 860
PY10.8	Describe and discuss behavioral and EEG characteristics during sleep and mechanism responsible for its production	Y	95	873
PY10.9	Describe and discuss the physiological basis of memory, learning and speech	Y	96	882
PY10.13	Describe and discuss perception of smell and taste sensation	Y	100 101	965 969
PY10.14	Describe and discuss patho-physiology of altered smell and taste sensation	Y	100 101	965, 968 973
PY10.15	Describe and discuss functional anatomy of ear and auditory pathways and physiology of hearing	Y	99	943
PY10.16	Describe and discuss pathophysiology of deafness. Describe hearing tests	Y	99	957
PY10.17	Describe and discuss functional anatomy of eye, physiology of image formation, physiology of vision including color vision, refractive errors, color blindness, physiology of pupil and light reflex	Y	98	901
PY10.18	Describe and discuss the physiological basis of lesion in visual pathway	Y	98	930
PY10.19	Describe and discuss auditory and visual evoke potentials	Y	99	960
PY11.1	Describe and discuss mechanism of temperature regulation	Y	59	534
PY11.2	Describe and discuss adaptation to altered temperature (heat and cold)	Y	59	540
PY11.3	Describe and discuss mechanism of fever, cold injuries and heat stroke	Y	59	540
PY11.4	Describe and discuss cardio-respiratory and metabolic adjustments during exercise; physical training effects	Y	30 41 102	285 395 977
PY11.5	Describe and discuss physiological consequences of sedentary lifestyle	Y	102	977
PY11.6	Describe physiology of infancy	N	102	977
PY11.7	Describe and discuss physiology of aging; free radicals and antioxidants	N	102	977
PY11.8	Discuss and compare cardio-respiratory changes in exercise (isometric and isotonic) with that in the resting state and under different environmental conditions (heat and cold)	Y	102	977
PY11.11	Discuss the concept, criteria for diagnosis of brain death and its implications	Y	102	977
PY11.12	Discuss the physiological effects of meditation	N	95	878
PY11.14	Demonstrate basic life support in a simulated environment	Y	42	399

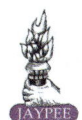

TOP DOC BANE WOHI
JISKA GUIDE HO SAHI

diginerve
A Jaypee Initiative

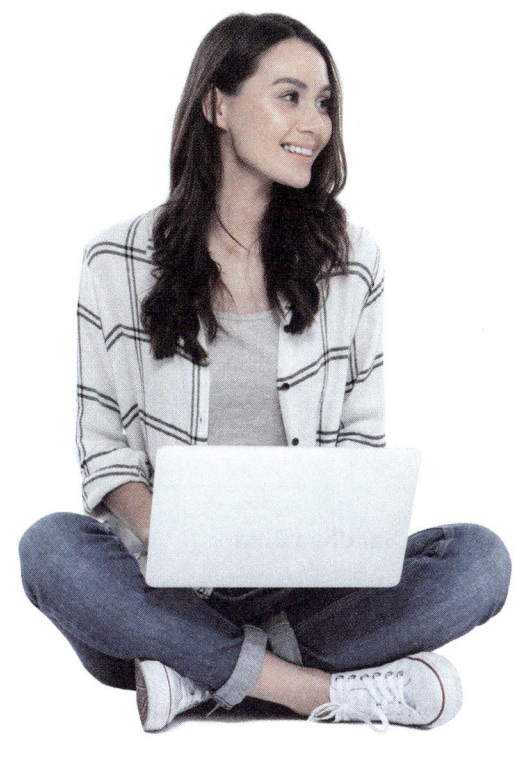

YOUR GUIDE AT EVERY STEP

Expert Knowledge Anytime, Anywhere

SCAN QR CODE
FOR MORE DETAILS

WHY CHOOSE US

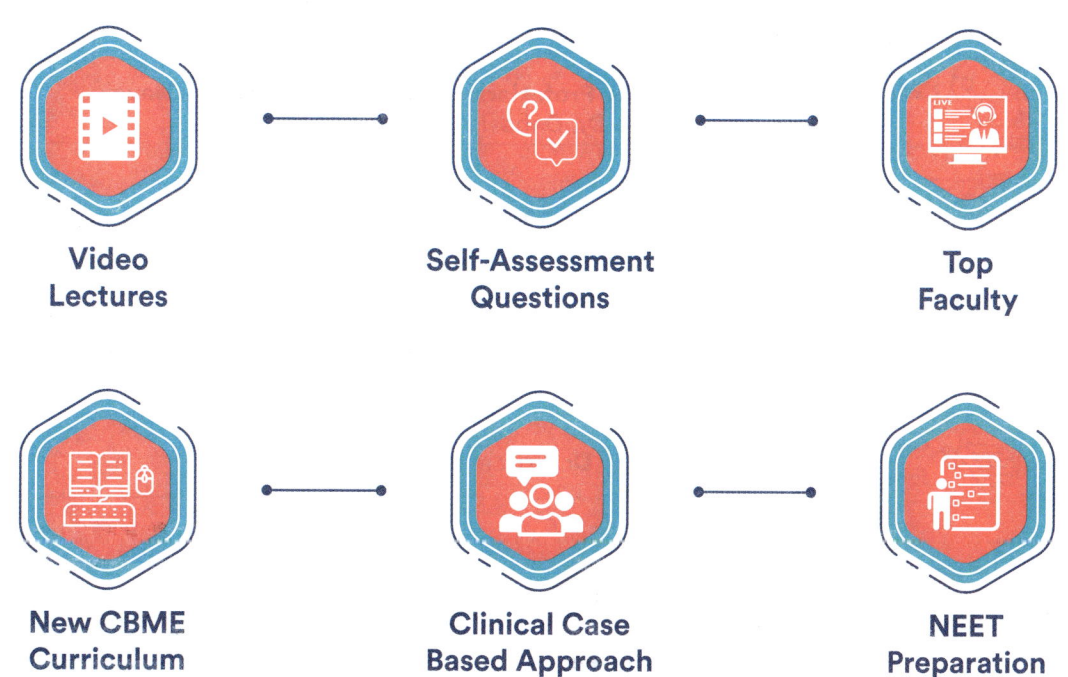

- Video Lectures
- Self-Assessment Questions
- Top Faculty
- New CBME Curriculum
- Clinical Case Based Approach
- NEET Preparation

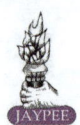

TOP DOC BANE WOHI JISKA GUIDE HO SAHI | **diginerve** — A Jaypee Initiative

Video Lectures | Notes | Self-Assessment
UnderGrad Courses Available

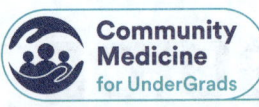 **Community Medicine** for UnderGrads — by Dr. Bratati Banerjee

Forensic Medicine & Toxicology for UnderGrads — by Dr. Gautam Biswas

 Medicine for UnderGrads — by Dr. Archith Boloor

 Microbiology for UnderGrads — by Dr. Apurba S Sastry, Dr. Sandhya Bhat & Dr. Deepashree R

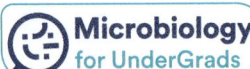 **OBGYN** for UnderGrads — by Dr. K. Srinivas

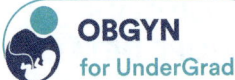 **Ophthalmology** for UnderGrads — by Dr. Parul Ichhpujani & Dr. Talvir Sidhu

 Orthopaedics for UnderGrads — by Dr. Vivek Pandey

 Pathology for UnderGrads — by Prof. Harsh Mohan, Prof. Ramadas Nayak & Dr. Debasis Gochhait

 Pediatrics for UnderGrads — by Dr. Santosh Soans & Dr. Soundarya M

 Pharmacology for UnderGrads — by Dr. Sandeep Kaushal & Dr. Nirmal George

 Surgery for UnderGrads — by Dr. Sriram Bhat M (SRB)

 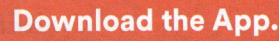 Download the App.

*T&C Apply

Contact: +91 8800 418 418
marketing@diginerve.com

SECTION 1: GENERAL PHYSIOLOGY

CHAPTER 1

Introduction to Physiology and General Principles in Physiology

LEARNING OBJECTIVES

Must know
- Define pH and explain the mechanisms operating in the body to maintain normal pH

Desirable to know
- Define diffusion, osmosis, osmotic pressure and tonicity
- Define the units for measuring the concentration of solutes
- Explain Donnan membrane equilibrium, Nernst equation and Goldman-Hodgkin-Katz equation

INTRODUCTION

Medical physiology or **human physiology** deals with the study of the structure and functions of the molecules, cells, tissues, organs and organ systems in the human body. It also deals with the biophysical and the biochemical processes that support body's function. All these functions are controlled by the genome. A **tissue** is a collection of cells that have similar structure and function. **Organs** are made up of one or more types of tissues. In the human body there are multiple organ systems like the musculoskeletal system for support and movement; the respiratory system to take up O_2 and eliminate CO_2; gastrointestinal system to digest and absorb food; excretory system to remove wastes; cardiovascular system to distribute nutrients, O_2 and the products of metabolism; reproductive system to perpetuate the species; and nervous and endocrine systems to coordinate and integrate the functions of the other systems.

Almost all branches of medicine are related to physiology. Pathogenesis, clinical manifestation, diagnosis and management of all diseases have a physiological basis. Action of all drugs also has a physiological basis. Knowledge of physiology also helps to promote community health. So a basic knowledge in physiology is essential for all successful physicians. The basis of yoga practices is also physiology; hence a physiologist has a holistic knowledge of the working of the body. The Nobel Prize in the field of medical sciences has been designated as '**Nobel Prize in Physiology and Medicine**'. This shows the importance of physiology in medicine and it beings the core subject of medical research.

pH, ACID/BASE AND BUFFER

PY1.7: Describe the concept of pH and buffer systems in the body.

pH of a Solution

The pH of a solution is defined as the negative logarithm of the [H^+] (hydrogen ion concentration) in the solution. The pH of pure water at 25°C is 7. At this pH, H^+ and OH^- ions are present in equal numbers. A solution with a pH below 7 is acidic and with pH above 7 is alkaline or basic. Acidic solution contains more H^+ than OH^-. For each pH unit less than 7, the [H^+] is increased tenfold and for each pH unit above 7, the [H^+] is decreased tenfold. For example, at pH 7, the [H^+] is 10^{-7} mol/L and when the pH is decreased to 6, the [H^+] becomes 10^{-6} mol/L, i.e., the [H^+] is increased tenfold.

The pH of a solution is said to be neutral, i.e., 7 when the concentration of H^+ and OH^- are equal, e.g., pure water. The maintenance of a stable hydrogen ion concentration in the body fluids is essential to life. *The normal pH of blood ranges between 7.35 and 7.45.* Enzymatic activity and protein structure are very sensitive to pH changes. Body pH is maintained normal by the buffering capacity of the body fluids.

Acids, Bases and Buffers

Molecules that act as H^+ donors in solution are considered acids, while those that tend to remove H^+ from solution are bases. Acids turn blue litmus paper red, while bases turn red litmus paper blue. Strong acids like HCl or strong bases like NaOH dissociate completely in water. For example,

HCl dissociates to form H^+ and Cl^-. Whereas, weak acids like carbonic acid (H_2CO_3) and weak bases dissociate incompletely in water. So they contribute relatively few H^+ or take away few H^+ from solution. For example, H_2CO_3 dissociates to form H^+ and HCO_3^-.

A **buffer** is a substance which when present in a solution reduces any change in the pH of the solution when acid or alkali is added to it. pH is the negative logarithm of the hydrogen ion concentration [H^+]. Buffer has the ability to bind or release H^+ in solution keeping the pH of the solution relatively constant despite addition of acid or base. The pH of blood and body fluids is maintained constant at 7.4 ± 0.05 although acid metabolites like lactic acid, CO_2, etc., are continually being formed in the tissues. The pH of the extracellular fluid (ECF) that is compatible with life ranges from 7 to 7.7.

Buffers in Blood

Buffers in blood include hemoglobin, plasma proteins and H_2CO_3/HCO_3^- system.

- **Plasma proteins** are effective buffers because, both their free carboxyl (COOH) and their free amino (NH^+) groups dissociate:
  $RCOOH \leftrightarrow RCOO^- + H^+$
  $RNH_3^+ \leftrightarrow RNH_2 + H^+$
- Since **hemoglobin** molecule contains 38 histidine residues and is present in large amounts in blood, hemoglobin has 6 times the buffering capacity of plasma proteins. The buffer system is provided by the dissociation of the imidazole groups of the histidine residues in hemoglobin. Reduced hemoglobin is a good proton acceptor and oxyhemoglobin is a good proton donor.
  $HHb \leftrightarrow H^+ + Hb^-$
  $HHb + O \rightarrow HbO + H^+$
- Third major buffer system in blood is the **carbonic acid-bicarbonate** system. This is one of the most effective buffer systems in the body. If H^+ is increased, the equilibrium shifts to left and most of the added H^+ is removed from blood.
  $H_2CO_3 \leftrightarrow H^+ + HCO_3^-$

Interstitial Fluid Buffer System

The main interstitial fluid buffer system is H_2CO_3/HCO_3^- system.

Intracellular Fluid Buffer Systems

- Protein buffer system
  $H_{Protein} \leftrightarrow H^+ + Protein^-$
- Phosphate system
  The components of this system are dihydrogen phosphate ($H_2PO_4^-$) which acts as weak acid and monohydrogen phosphate (HPO_4^{2-}) which acts as weak base.
  HPO_4^{2-} can act as weak base and can buffer H^+ released by strong acids such as HCl
  $H^+ + HPO_4^{2-} \leftrightarrow H_2PO_4^-$
  $H_2PO_4^-$ can act as weak acid and can buffer strong bases like OH^-
  $OH^- + H_2PO_4^- \rightarrow H_2O + HPO_4^{2-}$

Buffers in Cerebrospinal Fluid and Urine

The principal buffers in **cerebrospinal fluid (CSF) and urine** are bicarbonate and phosphate buffer systems. Buffer system in urine also includes NH_3/NH_4^+ buffer system (*refer* renal physiology).

ACID-BASE DISORDERS (ACIDOSIS AND ALKALOSIS)

There will be a relative excess of acid (acidosis) or base (alkalosis) in the body when the blood is outside the normal pH range (7.35–7.45). This will impair the delivery of O_2 to and removal of CO_2 from the tissues. There are a number of disease conditions in the body that can interfere with the pH control of the body. Acid-base disorders that result from respiration to alter CO_2 concentration are called **respiratory acidosis and respiratory alkalosis (Table 1.1)**. Respiratory acidosis can be relieved by restoring ventilation. Treatment of the underlying cause is very important.

Non-respiratory disorders that affect H^+ and HCO_3^- concentration in blood are referred to as **metabolic acidosis and metabolic alkalosis**. This can be caused by electrolyte disturbances, severe vomiting or diarrhea, ingestion of certain drugs and toxins, kidney disease and metabolic disorders like diabetes mellitus. Bicarbonate is used in the treatment of acute metabolic acidosis.

Table 1.1: Acidosis and alkalosis.				
	Respiratory acidosis	*Respiratory alkalosis*	*Metabolic acidosis*	*Metabolic alkalosis*
pH	Decreased	Increased	Decreased	Increased
Plasma HCO_3^-	Moderately increased	Decreased	Decreased	Increased
Arterial PCO_2	Increased (48 mm Hg)	Decreased (27 mm Hg)	Normal (40 mm Hg)	Normal
Causes	Decreased alveolar ventilation Decreased diffusing capacity Ventilation-perfusion mismatch	Increased alveolar ventilation	Accumulation of acids as in renal failure and diabetes mellitus Loss of HCO_3^- as in severe diarrhea	Loss of acid (vomiting) or increased HCO_3^- intake

Compensatory Responses of the Body in Acid-Base Disturbances

❖ Intracellular and extracellular buffering
❖ Changes in ventilation
❖ Renal adjustments.

Intracellular and Extracellular Buffering

The HCO_3^- buffer system is the principal ECF buffer.

$$CO_2 + H_2O \leftrightarrow H_2CO_3 \leftrightarrow H^+ + HCO_3^-$$

Plasma proteins also have a role in buffering excess H^+ in the ECF.

In intracellular buffering H^+ moves into the cell and it combines with HCO_3^-, PO_4^{3-} and histidine group of proteins.

Reduced hemoglobin is a very good proton acceptor.

Changes in Ventilation

Changes in PCO_2 alter blood pH. When PCO_2 increases it leads to respiratory acidosis.

Chemoreceptors in the medulla sense changes in PCO_2 and H^+ concentration and alter the rate of respiration. In metabolic acidosis there is increase in H^+ concentration which increases ventilation and washes out CO_2 leading to decrease in PCO_2. In diabetic ketosis where there is metabolic acidosis the patient develops deep and rapid breathing known as **Kussmaul breathing.**

Renal Mechanism

When there is acidosis the kidneys excrete more acid mainly by the increased synthesis and excretion of NH_4^+. The secretion of H^+ by the nephron is stimulated and more of new HCO_3^- is generated because of increased excretion of H^+. This new HCO_3^- increases the plasma HCO_3^- level, thereby increasing the buffering capacity of blood.

Opposite of the above mechanisms occur in alkalosis.

■ OSMOSIS

Osmosis is defined as the movement of water molecules (solvent) across a semipermeable membrane from a region of its higher concentration to an area of its lower concentration. When a solution is separated from pure water by a membrane that is permeable to water but not to the solute (semipermeable membrane), water molecules diffuse down their concentration gradient into the solution. This is an important factor in physiologic processes.

■ OSMOTIC PRESSURE

The movement of solvent molecules to a region of greater solute concentration can be prevented by applying pressure to the more concentrated solution. This pressure, necessary to prevent the movement of solvent molecules into the solution, is called **osmotic pressure**. Normally, the osmotic pressure of intracellular fluid is same as the osmotic pressure of interstitial fluid or extracellular fluid (ECF). As the osmotic pressure on both sides of the cell membrane is the same, the cell volume remains relatively constant. Osmotic pressure depends on the number of particles present in the solution, i.e., the number of molecules or ions rather than the type of particles. The colloid osmotic pressure due to the plasma colloids like albumin, globulin, etc., in blood is called the **oncotic pressure**.

■ OSMOLALITY AND OSMOLARITY

A **mole** is a gram molecular weight of a substance, i.e., the molecular weight of the substance in grams. For example, the gram molecular weight of a substance divided by the number of particles the molecule liberates in solution. For example, when one molecule of NaCl dissolves in water, it dissociates into Na^+ and Cl^- ions, so that each molecule of NaCl supplies two freely moving particles. 1 milli Osm (mOsm) is 1/1000 of 1 Osm.

Osmolarity is the number of osmoles per liter of solution, whereas osmolality is the number of osmoles per kilogram of solvent. Osmotically active substances are dissolved in water in the body and the density of water is 1. So, 1 L of water is equal to 1 kg of water and hence osmolality is expressed in mOsm per liter of water. Normal osmolality of plasma is 290 mOsm/L. Out of this, 270 mOsm in each liter is contributed by Na^+, Cl^- and HCO_3^-. Other cations and anions in plasma make a relatively small contribution. Plasma proteins contribute to less than 2 mOsm/L because of their very high molecular weights. Nonelectrolytes of plasma like glucose and urea contribute to osmolality of about 5 mOsm/L. But their contribution to osmolality can become quite large in hyperglycemia or uremia. Total plasma osmolality is important in assessing dehydration, overhydration, and other fluid and electrolyte abnormalities. Since the volume of the solution is altered by temperature and different kinds of solutes, osmolarity is also affected. Whereas, osmolality is little affected by these factors and so it is considered as the physiologically preferred unit. One equivalent (Eq) is one mol of an ionized substance divided by its valence. One mol of NaCl dissociate into 1 Eq of Na^+ and 1 Eq of Cl^-. One equivalent of Na^+ = 23 g. Milliequivalent (mEq) is 1/1000 of 1 Eq. Normal plasma sodium level is expressed as 145 mEq/L.

■ TONICITY

The term **tonicity** is used to describe the osmolality of a solution relative to plasma. Na^+ is the major contributor to the tonicity of ECF. Tonicity is a measure of the ability of the solution to change the volume of cells by altering their water content. Solutions that have the same osmolality as that of plasma are said to be **isotonic** to that of plasma, e.g., 0.9% sodium chloride and 5% dextrose in water are isotonic. Isotonic solution maintains the normal shape and volume of cells. Solutions with greater osmolality are **hypertonic**; and those with lesser osmolality are **hypotonic**. Pure water is very hypotonic. When cells are suspended in hypotonic solution, the cells swell due to endosmosis, and when cells are suspended in hypertonic solution, the cells shrink due to exosmosis.

APPLIED PHYSIOLOGY

Hypertonic solution like mannitol is given intravenously in cerebral edema, where there is excess interstitial fluid in brain.
When the blood becomes hypertonic, the excess interstitial fluid enters the blood and relieves the edema of brain. Kidneys will excrete the excess water present in blood.
Hypotonic solution can be used to treat patients with dehydration. When blood becomes hypotonic, water moves from blood across the capillary wall into the concentrated interstitial fluid and from there into the dehydrated cells to rehydrate them.

DIFFUSION

Passage of gases, ions or molecules from a region of higher concentration to a region of lower concentration without the expenditure of energy is called **diffusion**. It is directly proportional to the concentration gradient inside and outside the membrane (Ci–Co), cross-sectional area across which diffusion is taking place (A) and solubility (s), and inversely proportional to the thickness of membrane (t) and square root of molecular weight (MW) of the substance. This is **Fick's law of diffusion**.

$$D \alpha = \frac{(Ci - Co) \times A \times s}{t \times \sqrt{MW}}$$

Nonionic Diffusion

Some weak acids and bases are readily soluble in cell membranes in the undissociated form, whereas they cannot cross membranes in the charged (dissociated) form. If such undissociated substances diffuse from one side of the membrane to the other and then dissociate, it cannot further cross the membrane. In such conditions, there will be appreciable net movement of the undissociated substance from one side of the membrane to the other. This phenomenon is called **non-ionic diffusion**. For example, NH_3 is produced in the kidneys by the metabolism of amino acid glutamine. Since NH_3 is lipid soluble, it freely passes through the tubular membrane. In the tubular fluid it reacts with H^+ to form NH_4^+. NH_4^+ does not enter the cell since it is polarized. The process by which NH_3 is secreted into the tubular fluid and then changed to NH_4^+ for maintaining the concentration gradient for the diffusion of more NH_3 into the tubular fluid is called nonionic diffusion.

Donnan Membrane Equilibrium

When two solutions are separated by a membrane and if an ion on one side of the membrane cannot diffuse through the membrane, the distribution of other ions to which the membrane is permeable occurs according to the calculations of Donnan. For example, the negative charge of a non-diffusible anion hinders diffusion of the diffusible cations and favors diffusion of the diffusible anions.

In **Figure 1.1A**, compartment 'X' contains K^+ and protein anion (A^-) and compartment 'Y' contains K^+ and Cl^-. Protein anion (A^-) having high molecular weight cannot diffuse across the membrane but K^+ and Cl^- are freely permeable. From compartment 'X', K^+ can diffuse freely but A^- cannot.

From compartment 'Y' both K^+ and Cl^- can diffuse freely. Assume that the concentrations of the anions and cations on the two sides are initially equal **(Fig. 1.1A)**. Cl^- diffuses down its concentration gradient from compartment Y to X, and some K^+ moves with the negatively charged Cl^- because of its opposite charge.

$$[K^+_x] + [Cl^-_x] + [A^-_x] > [K^+_y] + [Cl^-_y]$$

We can see that when equilibrium is reached, more osmotically active particles are on side X than on side Y. Donnan and Gibbs showed that in the presence of a non-diffusible ion, the diffusible ions distribute themselves so that at equilibrium their concentration ratios are equal. That is, the products of the diffusible electrolytes in both the compartments will be equal. In **Figure 1.1B**, 9×4 in X = 6×6 in Y).

$$\frac{[K^+_x]}{[K^+_y]} = \frac{[Cl^-_y]}{[Cl^-_x]}$$

Cross multiplying,

$$[K^+_x][Cl^-_x] = [K^+_y][Cl^-_y]$$

This is **Gibbs-Donnan equation**. It holds for any pair of cations and anions of the same valence.

Donnan equation also states that the electrical neutrality in each compartment should be maintained. The number of cations should be equal to the number of anions. In **Figure 1.1B**, number of cations is 9 and the number of anions is also 9 (5 + 4) in compartment X. In compartment Y, the number of cations is 6 and anions is also 6.

To summarize:
- The products of diffusible ions in both compartments are equal.
- The electrical neutrality of each compartment is maintained.
- The total number of an ion before and after equilibrium is the same.
- When there is non-diffusible anion on one side of the membrane, the diffusible cations are more and diffusible anions are less on that side.

Application of Donnan Effect in the Body

- Because of charged protein anions (A^-) in the cells, there are more osmotically active particles in the cells than in the interstitial fluid. As a result, osmosis occurs across the plasma membrane making the cells swell. This normally does not occur in the body because of the activity of Na^+-K^+

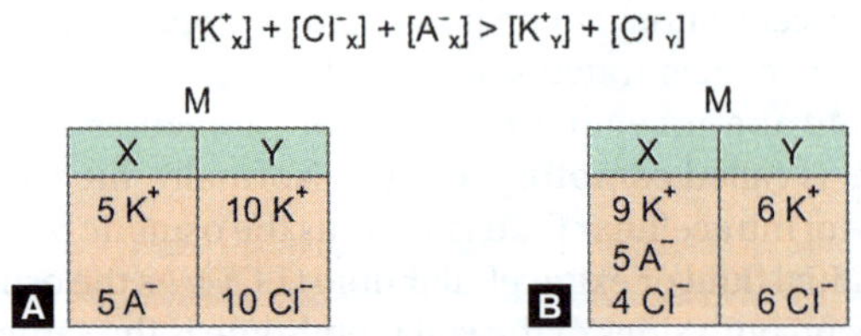

$$[K^+_x] + [Cl^-_x] + [A^-_x] > [K^+_y] + [Cl^-_y]$$

	M			M	
	X	Y		X	Y
	5 K^+	10 K^+		9 K^+	6 K^+
				5 A^-	
A	5 A^-	10 Cl^-	B	4 Cl^-	6 Cl^-

Figs. 1.1A and B: Donnan membrane equilibrium: (A) Before equilibrium is reached; (B) After equilibrium is reached.
(M: membrane; X and Y: compartments; A^-: protein anion)

ATPase which pumps Na⁺ back out of the cells. Thus normal cell volume depends on Na⁺-K⁺ ATPase.

- ❖ At equilibrium the distribution of permeable ions across the cell membrane is asymmetric. As a result an electrical difference exists across the cell membrane at rest (resting membrane potential) whose magnitude can be determined by the Nernst equation.
- ❖ Because there are more proteins in plasma than in interstitial fluid, there is a Donnan effect on ion movement across the capillary wall.
- ❖ The pH is lower in the cells in tissues than in the surrounding fluids due to the higher concentration of protein anions within the cells.
- ❖ The pH of red blood cells is lower than that of plasma due to the very high concentration of negative non-diffusible hemoglobin ions. The concentration of H⁺ will be higher within the cell.
- ❖ The chloride shift in erythrocytes as well as the higher concentration of chloride in CSF is also due to Donnan effect.

FORCES ACTING ON IONS

The forces acting across the cell membrane on each ion can be analyzed mathematically. K⁺ ions are present in higher concentration in the intracellular fluid (ICF) than in the extracellular fluid (ECF), and they tend to diffuse along this concentration gradient out of the cell. The interior of the cell becomes negative and the exterior positive. So the efflux of K⁺ slows down because its electrical gradient is in the opposite (inward) direction and consequently equilibrium is reached in which the tendency of K⁺ to move out of the cell is balanced by its tendency to move into the cell. The membrane potential at which this equilibrium exists is the equilibrium potential for K⁺. Its magnitude can be calculated from the Nernst equation. Similarly the equilibrium potential for Na⁺ and Cl⁻ can be calculated.

Nernst Equation

Nernst potential refers to the relation of the diffusion potential to the concentration difference of a particular ion. The diffusion potential across a membrane that exactly opposes the net diffusion of a particular ion through the membrane is called Nernst potential for that ion. The magnitude of the Nernst potential is determined by the ratio of the concentrations of that specific ion on the two sides of the membrane. The greater this ratio, the greater will be the tendency for the ion to diffuse in one direction. **Nernst equation** given below can be used to calculate the Nernst potential for any univalent ion at normal body temperature. While using this formula, it is usually assumed that the potential in the extracellular fluid outside the membrane remains at zero potential so that the Nernst potential is the potential inside the membrane.

Nernst potential in millivolts

$$= \pm 61 \times \log \frac{\text{Concentration of the ion inside}}{\text{Concentration outside}}$$

The sign of the potential is positive (+) if the ion diffusing from inside to outside is a negative ion and it is negative (-) if the ion is positive. In the case of resting membrane potential of nerve fiber membrane, the ion diffusing to the outside is K⁺ and so the Nernst potential for K⁺ will be a negative value. The concentration of K⁺ is very high inside the membrane and very low outside. If we assume that the membrane is permeable only to K⁺, but not to any other ion, there is a strong tendency for K⁺ to diffuse to the outside through the membrane. As they do so they carry positive charges to the outside, creating electropositivity outside the membrane and electronegativity inside the membrane. The potential difference generated between the inside and outside of the membrane is called **diffusion potential**. This potential becomes great enough to block further net K⁺ diffusion to the exterior even though the net potassium ion concentration gradient across the membrane is high. If the concentration of potassium ions on the inside of the membrane is 10 times that on the outside, the log of 10 is 1 and so, the Nernst potential for K⁺ is calculated to be –61 millivolts inside the membrane.

Diffusion potential for K⁺ in millivolts =
$$-61 \times \log 10 = -61 \times 1 = -61 \, mV$$

Thus, Nernst equation is applicable only if the membrane is permeable to one monovalent ion but not to any other ions. **Table 1.2** shows the calculated equilibrium potential for ions taking into consideration their concentrations inside and outside the cell. For example,

$$E_K = -61.5 \log \frac{[K_o^+]}{[K_i^+]} = -90 \, mV \text{ at } 37°C$$

Goldman-Hodgkin-Katz Equation

When a membrane is permeable to several different ions, the diffusion potential that develops can be calculated by the Goldman-Hodgkin-Katz equation. It depends on three factors:
1. The electrical charge of each ion (+ or -)
2. The permeability of the membrane to each ion (P)
3. The concentration of each ion (C) on the inside (i) and outside (o) of the membrane

In the case of neurons and muscle cells, the most important diffusible ions involved in the development of membrane potentials are Na⁺, K⁺ and Cl⁻, i.e., two univalent positive ions and one univalent negative ion are involved. The concentration gradient of each of these ions across the membrane helps in determining the voltage of the membrane potential (**Table 1.2**).

The voltage is also determined by the permeability of the membrane to that particular ion. For example, in excitable cells, K⁺ is more permeable than Na⁺ since it has leak

Table 1.2: Equilibrium potential of different ions calculated by Nernst equation in spinal motor neurons.

Ion	Concentration (mmol/L of water)		Equilibrium potential (mV)
	Inside cell	Outside cell	
Na⁺	15	150	+60
K⁺	150	5.5	–90
Cl⁻	9	125	–70

channels and has high permeability since the hydrated ion diameter is less when compared to sodium. Protein anion is impermeable because of its large size.

A positive ion concentration gradient from inside the membrane to the outside causes electronegativity inside the membrane. This is because the excess positive ions diffuse to the outside when their concentration is higher inside than outside. This carries positive charges to the outside but leaves non-diffusible negative ions on the inside, creating electronegativity on the inside. The opposite effect occurs if the gradient is for a negative ion. That is, a chloride ion gradient from outside the membrane to inside causes negativity inside the cell because excess negatively charged chloride ions diffuse to the inside, while leaving the non-diffusible positive ions on the outside.

Goldman-Hodgkin-Katz equation is (in the equation, 'o' denotes concentration of the ion in the outside of the cell and 'i' denotes concentration of the ion in the inside of the cell):

Diffusion potential (EMF) in millivolts

$$= -61.5 \times \log \frac{C_{Nai}{}^+P_{Na}{}^+ + C_{Ki}{}^+P_K{}^+ + C_{Clo}{}^-P_{Cl^-}}{C_{Nao}{}^+P_{Na}{}^+ + C_{Ko}{}^+P_K{}^+ + C_{Cli}{}^-P_{Cl^-}}$$

■ MULTIPLE CHOICE QUESTIONS

1. Normal blood pH is:
   a. 7.2
   b. 7.3
   c. 7.4
   d. 7.7

2. Nernst equation deals with:
   a. Oxygen uptake
   b. Chloride shift
   c. Cellular ATP levels
   d. Plasma bicarbonate level

3. Potassium is maximally present in:
   a. Cell
   b. Plasma
   c. Interstitium
   d. Bone

4. The equilibrium potential calculated by Nernst equation for chloride ions in the mammalian spinal neuron is:
   a. −70 mV
   b. −90 mV
   c. +60 mV
   d. +90 mV

5. The most effective buffer system in the body is:
   a. Hemoglobin
   b. Ammonia mechanism
   c. Bicarbonate-carbonic acid system
   d. Plasma proteins

6. Metabolic acidosis leads to:
   a. Increased Na⁺ reabsorption
   b. Decreased K⁺ excretion
   c. Increased K⁺ excretion
   d. Increase in arterial PCO_2

7. Causes of respiratory alkalosis include the following, *except:*
   a. Increased alveolar ventilation
   b. Decreased alveolar ventilation
   c. Respiratory center depression
   d. Increase in plasma HCO_3^-

8. The FALSE statement regarding diffusion is:
   a. Diffusion is directly proportional to the solubility of the substance
   b. It is inversely proportional to the thickness of the membrane
   c. It is directly proportional to the square root of the molecular weight of the substance
   d. It is directly proportional to the concentration gradient across the membrane

9. The diffusion potential of K⁺ calculated by Nernst equation is:
   a. +60 mV
   b. −90 mV
   c. −70 mV
   d. +90 mV

10. Secretion of NH_3 into the renal tubular fluid and converting it into NH_4^+ is an example of:
    a. Facilitated diffusion
    b. Secondary active transport
    c. Active transport
    d. Nonionic diffusion

11. During buffering H⁺ combines with which group of proteins?
    a. Histidine
    b. Valine
    c. Leucine
    d. Serine

ANSWERS

1. c   2. b   3. a   4. a   5. c
6. b   7. a   8. c   9. b   10. d
11. a

The Body Fluid Compartments

CHAPTER 2

LEARNING OBJECTIVES
- Name the different fluid compartments of the body and describe their measurements
- Mention the role of electrolytes in the body

INTRODUCTION

PY1.6: Describe the fluid compartments of the body, its ionic composition and measurements.

The two major body fluid compartments are extracellular fluid and intracellular fluid. All the cells in the body are surrounded by a fluid called **extracellular fluid (ECF)** from which cells take up O_2 and nutrients needed for their functioning and discharge metabolic waste products produced within the cell. The extracellular fluid contains the ions and nutrients needed by the cells and is known as **internal environment** of the body or **milieu interieur**. The composition of ECF closely resembles that of sea water in which, presumably all life originated. The ECF is divided into the interstitial fluid, the circulating blood plasma and the lymph. Body fluid inside the cells is called **intracellular fluid (ICF)**.

For homeostasis, the volume and composition of the body fluids should be maintained constant. There should be a balance between fluid intake and fluid loss from the body. Otherwise the body fluid volumes may increase or decrease. Water is added to the body by ingestion and it is also synthesized in the body by oxidation of carbohydrates. Water is lost from the body by insensible water loss (through lungs and skin) of which we are not consciously aware of, by sweating, and water lost through feces and urine.

Body is formed of solids and fluids. In a young adult, 18% of the body weight is constituted by protein and related substances, 7% by minerals and 15% by fat. The remaining 60% is water; two-third of this fluid is intracellular and one-third is extracellular fluid. Approximately 25% of the ECF is in the vascular system (plasma is 5% of body weight) and 75% outside the blood vessels (interstitial fluid which is 15% of body weight). The total blood volume (plasma + formed elements of blood) is about 8% of body weight. Inappropriate compartmentalization of the body fluids can result in edema.

TOTAL BODY WATER

For an adult, total body water (TBW) is 70 mL/100 g of tissue. In a man weighing 70 kg, it is about 42 L. 55% of TBW is present intracellularly and 45% in the **extracellular fluid (ECF)** compartment. TBW is less in women than in men due to relatively greater amount of adipose tissue in females. The value decreases with age in both sexes. TBW is distributed into two main compartments of body fluids, ECF and ICF, separated by a semipermeable membrane. The water molecule (H_2O) has the following properties relevant to physiology:
- Water is an ideal solvent for physiological reactions
- It has a high surface tension
- It has a high heat of vaporization and heat capacity
- It has a high dielectric current. It serves as a solvent; it provides optimal heat transfer and conduction of current.

DISTRIBUTION OF BODY FLUIDS

Body fluids are mainly divided into ECF and **intracellular fluid (ICF)**. ECF is divided into two components: the interstitial fluid and blood plasma (**Flowchart 2.1**). The interstitial fluid is that part of the ECF that is outside the vascular system and forms the internal environment. It bathes the cells. **Transcellular fluid** is also part of body fluid, but its volume when compared to ECF and ICF, is very small.

Body fluids are:
- Interstitial fluid including lymph (8 L)
- Plasma (3 L)
- Intracellular fluid (24 L)
- Transcellular fluids (2 L)
  - Cerebrospinal fluid (CSF)
  - Intraocular fluid
  - Gastrointestinal secretions
  - Pleural, pericardial and peritoneal fluid

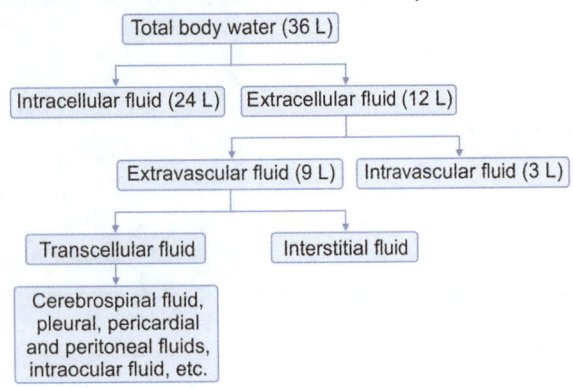

Flowchart 2.1: Distribution of body fluids.

- Synovial fluid
- Fluid in urinary tract.

MEASUREMENT OF BODY FLUID VOLUMES

Measurement of Total Body Water

Total body water is measured using dilution principle. A marker is injected that will be evenly distributed in all the compartments of body fluids. To measure TBW, the marker should diffuse freely not only in the water outside the cells, but also should cross the cell membrane and reach intracellular fluid.

The concentration of the marker in the plasma is measured and from this value the TBW can be calculated. The markers used are:

- Deuterium oxide (D_2O or ^2H_2O) or heavy water
- Radioactive water or tritium oxide (^3H_2O)
- Antipyrine, a lipid soluble substance, which can rapidly penetrate cell membranes and distribute itself uniformly throughout the intracellular and extracellular compartments.

Technique

A known quantity of labeled water (D_2O) is injected intravenously as an isotonic solution of NaCl. It mixes freely with the water in the body in a few hours. After 2 hours, blood sample is taken and the concentration of labeled water is measured. As some marker is lost through urine, urine is also collected and concentration of D_2O in urine is determined. For example, if 100 mL of D_2O was infused intravenously into a 70 kg man and if the concentration of D_2O was found to be 0.0025 mL/mL of plasma and urine concentration 0.5 mL after 2 hours, then TBW can be calculated as follows:

$$TBW = \frac{100 \text{ mL} - 0.5 \text{ mL}}{0.0025 \text{ mL/mL}} = 39.8 \text{ L or}$$

$$= \frac{39.8 \times 100}{70} = 57\% \text{ of body weight}$$

Measurement of ECF Volume

Extracellular fluid (ECF) volume is measured using inulin, which is a polysaccharide. Other substances used are mannitol, thiosulfate and sucrose. These substances cannot enter the cells, but can freely cross the capillary membrane and thus distribute evenly in the ECF compartments. Normal ECF volume in a 70 kg man is about 15 L.

Absolute ECF volume is less in children and so, *dehydration develops more rapidly and is more severe in children.*

Measurement of Plasma Volume

Plasma volume is measured using dyes like Evans blue (T-1824) that bind specifically to plasma proteins. It will not diffuse into the interstitium. Plasma volume can also be measured by injecting serum albumin labeled with radioactive iodine (^{131}I-albumin). (For details of measurement of blood volume, *refer* Chapter 20).

Measurement of Interstitial Fluid Volume

Interstitial fluid volume is calculated by subtracting the plasma volume from the ECF volume.

Interstitial fluid volume = ECF volume – Plasma volume

Measurement of ICF Volume

Intracellular fluid volume is calculated by subtracting the ECF volume from total body water.

ICF volume = TBW – ECF volume

BODY ELECTROLYTES

Electrolytes are molecules that dissociate in water to their cation and anion equivalents, for e.g., NaCl splits to form Na^+ and Cl^-. Because of their net charge on water molecules, these electrolytes do not re-associate in water. Electrolytes constitute 7% of total body weight. The important electrolytes are Na^+, K^+, Ca^{2+}, Mg^{2+}, Cl^-, and HCO_3^-. The electrolytes and other charged compounds like proteins are unevenly distributed in the body fluids and this plays an important role in physiology. The distribution of electrolytes in the ECF and ICF is given in Chapter 6, **Table 6.1**.

Functions of Electrolytes in the Body

- Maintenance of acid-base balance.
- Maintenance of normal osmolality and volume of body fluids.
- Ions like Na^+, Ca^{2+}, K^+, Cl^-, etc., affect excitability of cells.
- Helps in muscle contraction
- Buffering of body fluids
- Formation of bones and teeth.

INTRAVENOUS FLUID THERAPY

Intravenous fluid (IVF) therapy is usually done in hospitals. Appropriate intravenous fluid is administered for different disease conditions. If inappropriate fluid is administered, it can result in electrolyte imbalance mainly sodium imbalance. Severe electrolyte imbalance can lead to serious neurological conditions and can even lead to death. So an understanding of the different types of intravenous fluids and how to choose the appropriate fluid is necessary.

CHAPTER 2 ⮕ The Body Fluid Compartments

Indications
* To replace lost fluid as in burns, vomiting, diarrhea, etc.
* To supply daily needs as a maintenance measure, e.g., when the patient is advised nil orally before or after certain surgeries or in unconscious patients
* To replace fluid in times of dehydration as in fever
* For the treatment of hypovolemic shock
* In acid-base and electrolyte abnormalities.

The different types of intravenous fluids used are:
* Normal saline (NS)
* Dextrose-normal saline (DNS)
* Ringer lactate (RL)
* 5% dextrose.

Precautions in Fluid Therapy
* IVF is prescribed only after assessing the status of the patient like hydration, electrolyte, acid-base status, etc., and other diseases like diabetes mellitus, congestive cardiac failure, renal failure, etc.
* Before administration, the amount of fluid required should be calculated. Based on the deficit, appropriate intravascular fluid should be selected.
* Rate of fluid administration is important. For acute fluid losses and in severe dehydration quick replacement is necessary. In chronic losses, fluid therapy should be done with caution.

Selection of IVF in Common Clinical Problems
* Hypovolemic shock—normal saline or ringer lactate
* Diarrhea—Ringer lactate
* Vomiting—normal saline
* Diarrhea + vomiting—Ringer lactate or normal saline with potassium supplementation.

Hyponatremia—treatment depends on hydration status:
* Hyponatremia with dehydration—normal saline or Ringer lactate
* With hypervolemia—fluid restriction along with loop diuretic
* With normal blood volume—3% saline is used.

Complications of IVF Therapy
* Hypersensitivity reaction
* Infection
* Fluid overload.

MULTIPLE CHOICE QUESTIONS

1. Total blood volume is about:
   a. 5% of body weight
   b. 8% of body weight
   c. 10% of body weight
   d. 6% of body weight

2. The percentage of ECF constituted by blood is:
   a. 20%   b. 40%
   c. 55%   d. 45%

3. Total body water of newborn is what percent of body weight?
   a. 60%   b. 70%
   c. 80%   d. 90%

4. The percentage of body weight constituted by water in an adult is:
   a. 60%   b. 70%
   c. 80%   d. 90%

5. Compared with intracellular fluid, extracellular fluid has:
   a. A greater osmolarity
   b. A lower sodium ion concentration
   c. A lower K^+ concentration
   d. A lower Cl^- concentration

6. The percentage of body weight constituted by ECF is:
   a. 10%   b. 20%
   c. 33%   d. 60%

7. Most accurate measurement of ECF volume can be done by using:
   a. Sucrose   b. Mannitol
   c. Inulin   d. Aminopyrine

8. All the following are used to measure total body water, *except*:
   a. Heavy water (D_2O)   b. Tritium oxide
   c. Aminopyrine   d. Evan's blue (T-1824)

9. The substance that can most accurately measure ECF volume is:
   a. Heavy water   b. Evan's blue
   c. Inulin   d. Sucrose

10. The primary force that moves water molecules from plasma to the interstitial fluid is:
    a. Filtration
    b. Facilitated diffusion
    c. Co-transport with sodium
    d. Active transport

11. Ringer lactate contains all, *except*:
    a. Chloride
    b. Sodium
    c. Bicarbonate
    d. Potassium

12. Content of Na^+ in Ringer lactate solution is:
    a. 154 mEq/L   b. 121 mEq/L
    c. 130 mEq/L   d. 144 mEq/L

13. D_2O (deuterium oxide) is used to measure volume of:
    a. Blood   b. Total body water
    c. Extracellular fluid d. Intracellular fluid

14. Normal plasma sodium concentration is:
    a. 120 mEq/L   b. 3.5 mEq/L
    c. 140 mEq/L   d. 110 mEq/L

15. Most accurate measurement of ECF volume can be done by using:
    a. Sucrose   b. Mannitol
    c. Inulin   d. Aminopyrine

SECTION 1 — General Physiology

16. The properties of water includes all the following, *except:*
    a. It has a low surface tension
    b. It has high latent heat of vaporization
    c. It has high dielectric current
    d. It is an ideal solvent

ANSWERS

1. b	2. a	3. c	4. a	5. c
6. b	7. c	8. d	9. c	10. a
11. c	12. c	13. b	14. c	15. c
16. a				

CHAPTER 3

Homeostasis

LEARNING OBJECTIVES

Must know
- Define homeostasis
- Discuss the different feedback systems operating in the body to maintain homeostasis with examples
- What is the role of various body systems in homeostasis?

■ INTRODUCTION

PY1.2: Describe and discuss the principles of homeostasis.

Animals have two environments: the milieu exterior that physically surrounds the whole organism; and the internal environment in which the tissues and cells of the organism live. The internal environment is the extracellular fluid. The extracellular fluid (ECF) contains ions and nutrients needed by the cells to maintain cell life and is called the **internal environment** of the body. The cells in a multicellular organism live in a relatively constant internal environment despite changes in the external environment of the organism. The internal environment in which the body cells survive is called **milieu interieur** coined by the French physiologist, **Claude Bernard**. The actual environment of the cells of the body is the interstitial fluid component of ECF. Maintenance of the constancy of this fluid is necessary for the normal functioning of the cells. Maintaining nearly constant conditions in the internal environment by various physiologic adjustments is referred to as **homeostasis**, coined by American physiologist, **Walter B Cannon** in 1929. It is the condition of equilibrium in the body's internal environment. This state is achieved by the interplay of various regulatory processes in the body. Functions performed by all organs and tissues of the body together with nervous, hormonal and local control systems help to maintain the relatively constant conditions. Buffering properties of body fluids, renal and respiratory adjustments are examples of homeostatic mechanisms.

Most important aspect of homeostasis is maintaining the volume and composition of body fluids (intracellular fluid and extracellular fluid) within a narrow range. This is achieved by varying the permeability of biological membranes to fluids, electrolytes, nutrients, and metabolites. Thus, even distribution of these substances across the various body fluid compartments is achieved.

Whenever there is disturbance of homeostasis, the regulating systems bring the internal environment back into balance. This is mainly achieved by nervous system and endocrine system by *negative feedback mechanisms*. There are also positive feedback mechanisms operating in the body. The nervous system regulates homeostasis by sending information in the form of nerve impulses to the organs that correct the disturbance in homeostasis. Endocrine system secretes hormones into the bloodstream, which lead to restoration of homeostasis. The nervous system regulates many muscular and secretory activities of the body, whereas the endocrine system regulates many metabolic functions.

The body is protected by the **immune system and the integumentary system**. The immune system consists of white blood cells, reticuloendothelial cells, thymus and the lymphatic system that protect the body from pathogens. It destroys the invaders by phagocytosis or by producing antibodies which destroy the invader. Immune system also helps to distinguish its own cells from foreign cells and substances. The integumentary system includes skin and its various appendages. Skin protects the deeper tissues and organs of the body and forms a boundary between the outside world and the body's internal environment. Skin has an important role in temperature regulation and excretion of wastes and it also act as a sense organ.

■ CONTROL SYSTEMS OF THE BODY

There are thousands of control systems operating in the body to maintain health. In the absence of any one of these control systems, serious disruption of body function or death can result. The genetic control systems operate in all cells to help control intracellular and extracellular functions. Other control systems operate to control the functions of different organs and systems of the body. The vital parameters are regulated by more systems of the body. If one system fails,

Table 3.1: Normal values and normal ranges of the important variables in the body.

Variable	Normal value	Normal range	Unit
Venous O_2	40	35–45	mm Hg
Venous CO_2	45	35–45	mm Hg
Na^+	142	138–146	mmol/L
K^+	4.2	3.8–5	mmol/L
Ca^{2+}	1.2	1–1.4	mmol/L
Cl^-	106	103–112	mmol/L
HCO_3^-	24	24–32	mmol/L
Plasma glucose	90	75–95	mg/dL
Body temperature	98.4	98–98.8	°F
pH	7.4	7.3–7.5	

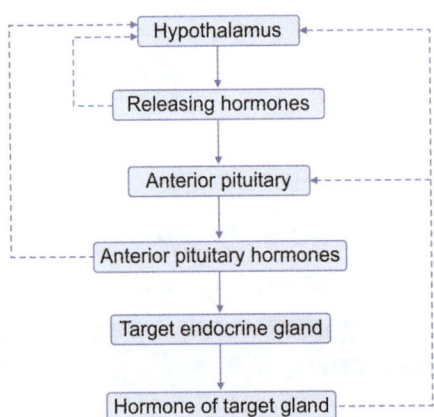

Flowchart 3.1: Negative feedback mechanism in regulation of hormone secretion. Dashed line denotes inhibition at various levels in the feedback loop.

others help to maintain homeostasis. Tightly controlled parameters of the body include regulation of arterial pressure, blood volume, plasma levels of O_2, glucose, K^+, Ca^{2+}, H^+ and HCO_3^-.

The important constituents and the physical characteristics of the extracellular fluid have very narrow normal ranges (Table 3.1). Values outside these ranges may even lead to death. For example, an increase in body temperature of 7°C from normal can increase cellular metabolism to an extent to destroy the cells. A decrease in potassium ion concentration to less than one-third of normal can lead to paralysis as a result of the inability of nerves to carry impulses. On the other hand, an increase in potassium level to two times the normal can depress the myocardium. Most of the control systems operate by feedback mechanisms.

FEEDBACK SYSTEMS

A **feedback system** is a cycle of events, which continuously monitors and evaluates any change in the internal environment and brings it back to normal. The basic components of a feedback system include receptor, control center, and effector. The **receptor** monitor changes in the internal environment. The monitored variables include body temperature, blood pressure, blood glucose, etc. The **control center** receives inputs from receptors in the form of nerve impulses or hormones. **Effector** receives input from the center and produces a response that corrects the disturbance in homeostasis. Every organs or tissues in the body act as the receptor. **Feedback systems** can produce either negative feedback or positive feedback (Flowchart 3.1).

Negative Feedback System

If the response reverses the original disturbance to normal, then the system is **negative feedback** system. Deviations from a given normal set point are detected by the sensor, and the signals from the sensor trigger compensatory changes that continue until the set point is again reached. *The action of the negative feedback system stops as soon as the internal environment is brought back to normal.* Here the response will be negative to the initiating stimulus. Most control systems of the body operate on the principle of negative feedback.

Examples of negative feedback systems are:
* Decrease in the body temperature is sensed by the brain, which sends nerve impulses to the skeletal muscles. The resulting shivering increases the body temperature bringing it back to normal. Shivering stops when the body temperature comes to normal value.
* A high blood pressure leads to a series of mechanisms to lower the blood pressure to normal or a low blood pressure leads to a series of reactions that increases the pressure to normal. In both instances, the effects are negative with respect to the initiating stimulus.
* When there is increase in blood sugar, there is increased secretion of insulin from the pancreas. Insulin helps in the transport of glucose into the cell and thus decreases blood sugar level back to normal. On the contrary, when there is decrease in blood glucose, there is decreased secretion of insulin and increased secretion of glucagon. This will increase blood glucose to normal level.
* Whenever there is increase in the concentration of a particular hormone of the pituitary, by negative feedback mechanisms there will be inhibition of secretion of the concerned releasing hormone from the hypothalamus and the hormone level comes back to normal. For example if there increase in the blood level of ACTH, there will be feedback inhibition of CRH release from the hypothalamus which is exerted by ACTH itself.

Positive Feedback System

If the response reinforces or intensifies the initial change or disturbance, then the system is operating by **positive feedback mechanism**. It cannot be controlled unless interrupted by some mechanisms outside the system. For example, in the progressive stage of circulatory shock, the positive feedback mechanism operating worsens the condition finally leading to death.

Severe fall in BP → decreased cardiac output → decreased coronary blood flow ↓
Decreased cardiac output ← Myocardial depression
↑ (from Severe fall in BP)

Other examples of positive feedback mechanisms are:
- **Blood coagulation:** Coagulation of blood progresses in a positive feedback manner unless it is interrupted by the anticlotting mechanisms like fibrinolytic system. Once there is damage to blood vessel, platelets adhere to the site which releases chemicals that attract more and more platelets to the site of damage. One clotting factor when activated will cause activation of other clotting factor and so on till a large quantity of clotting factors get activated in a positive feedback manner. The activated clotting factors act as enzymes for the activation of others. Excessive spread of clot is usually prevented by the fibrinolytic system.
- **Parturition reflex** (*refer* Chapter 61 Fig. 61.7)
- **Excitation of excitable cells:** Opening of sodium channels during depolarization of a nerve or muscle cell further activates opening of more and more sodium channels so that there is explosive entry of sodium ions into the cell leading to the depolarization phase of the action potential in the cell. This is referred to as **Hodgkin's cycle**. Entry of sodium ions into the cell stops because of the closure of the sodium channel.

(For details of feedback systems *refer* Chapter 61).
- **LH surge** during menstrual cycle: Low levels of estrogen exerts a negative feedback effect on LH secretion from the anterior pituitary. But very high levels of estrogen maintained for a certain period of time will increase LH secretion leading to LH surge, which is followed by ovulation.
- **Activation of digestive enzymes:** Activation of digestive enzymes like trypsin leads to further activation of inactive enzymes to active forms.

ROLE OF DIFFERENT SYSTEMS IN THE BODY IN HOMEOSTASIS

Each and every tissues of the body contribute to homeostasis. For example:
- Circulatory system plays the most important role in transporting the extracellular fluid (ECF) to all parts of the body thus helping in the exchange of substances between ECF and ICF. This help to maintain the volume of different fluid compartments within normal range.
- Acid-base balance is maintained by respiratory system, kidney, blood, and other buffer systems in the body. The pH of the ECF has to be maintained at 7.4 for the proper functioning of the tissues. Acidosis or alkalosis affects tissues markedly.
- Nervous system and endocrine system have a very important role in homeostasis by feedback mechanisms. The nervous system regulates muscular and secretory activities of the body, whereas the endocrine system regulates many metabolic functions. Neuroendocrinology means the study of the interactions of the endocrine and nervous system in the maintenance of homeostasis. ANS operating at a subconscious level regulates the vegetative functions of the body essential for homeostasis like movements of GIT, secretion by many of the body's glands, pumping activity of heart, etc. Whenever there is rise or fall in blood pressure, many neural and hormonal mechanisms come into play to restore blood pressure within the normal range.
- Water and electrolyte balance is maintained by kidneys, skin, lungs and digestive system.
- Bone tissue contributes to homeostasis of the body by providing support, protection and production of blood cells and storage of minerals. Skeletal muscles and bone help the organism to move around for protection against adverse surroundings and to obtain food.
- Muscular tissue and liver produce heat and maintain body temperature. Skin has an important role in maintaining normal body temperature at 37°C. When there is an increase in body temperature, there is cutaneous vasodilatation and increased sweating. In times of hypothermia, the body tries to decrease heat loss by cutaneous vasoconstriction and tries to increase heat production by shivering.
- The digestive system contributes to homeostasis by digesting food, absorbing nutrients, water, vitamins, minerals, etc., for growth and functioning of body tissues and by eliminating waste products. The liver changes the chemical composition of many nutrients absorbed from the GIT to more usable forms. It also eliminates certain waste products produced in the body and toxic substances that are ingested.
- Adequate amount of O_2 should be made available to the cells for the metabolism of nutrients. Simultaneously CO_2 and waste products must be removed from the body. Respiratory system is concerned with the supply of O_2 and removal of CO_2. Kidneys and other excretory organs remove metabolic and other waste products from the body.
- The immune system protects the body from pathogens, such as bacteria, virus, parasites and fungi. It also helps to distinguish its own cells from foreign cells and substances.

HOMEOSTATIC IMBALANCE

Homeostatic imbalance occurs when the body functions are disrupted. Disease is a state of disrupted homeostasis. From psychological point of view also body's balance can be disrupted. Diseases such as diabetes mellitus, dehydration, hyperthermia, or hypothermia, heart failure and hypertension are examples of the consequence of homeostatic imbalance and inability of the negative feedback mechanism to bring back physiological parameters to normal levels.

Even in the presence of disease, homeostatic mechanisms continue to operate and maintain vital functions through various compensatory mechanisms. Sometimes, homeostasis when disturbed cannot be brought back to normal by the regulatory systems. For example, chronic illnesses like cancer, or AIDS disrupt the body's ability to function properly and it is difficult to return to a homeostatic state. Aging is a cause of homeostatic imbalance as the control mechanisms of the feedback loops lose their efficiency. If homeostatic imbalance is moderate, a disease may be the result but if it is severe, death may result. Heart failure is a cause of death in old age where a positive feedback loop sets in. Diabetes occurs when the control mechanisms for insulin secretion fails. An imbalance in energy homeostasis leads to obesity and cachexia.

Disease is characterized by recognizable set of signs and symptoms. **Signs** include fever, swelling, increase or decrease in blood pressure, paralysis, etc. **Symptoms** include loss of appetite, vomiting, headache, anxiety, breathlessness, etc. As age advances, the body's responses to restore homeostasis progressively decline. This is the reason for the changes occurring in old age. Dysfunction of the homeostasis of cell number is a major factor in aging. For example, there is a reduction in the cell number in some skeletal muscles.

■ MULTIPLE CHOICE QUESTIONS

1. The term homeostasis was coined by:
   a. Claude Bernard
   b. WB Cannon
   c. Hans Berger
   d. Emil Theodor Kocher

2. Which of the following is NOT an example of positive feedback?
   a. Hodgkin's cycle
   b. Blood coagulation
   c. Parturition
   d. Regulation of ACTH secretion

3. The following is an example of negative feedback:
   a. Increase in insulin secretion in hyperglycemia
   b. Activation of clotting factors
   c. LH surge before ovulation
   d. Na^+ influx during action potential

4. The following are symptoms of disease, *except:*
   a. Vomiting
   b. Pain
   c. Pitting edema
   d. Loss of appetite

5. The internal environment of the body is constituted by:
   a. Interstitial fluid
   b. Blood
   c. Plasma
   d. Intracellular fluid

6. The term milieu interieur was coined by:
   a. Claude Bernard
   b. WB Cannon
   c. Charles Darwin
   d. William Harvey

ANSWERS

1. b   2. d   3. a   4. c   5. a
6. a

Cell Physiology

CHAPTER 4

LEARNING OBJECTIVES

Must know
- Describe the structure and functions of a mammalian cell
- Discuss the functions of the cell organelles and its clinical importance
- Draw the electron microscopic structure of a typical mammalian cell
- Describe the structure of the cell membrane and enumerate the functions of cell membrane proteins
- Explain the functions of proteasomes and its clinical importance
- Explain the steps in apoptosis and its clinical significance
- Briefly mention the different intercellular junctions and their functions

Desirable to know
- Describe mitosis and meiosis with the help of diagrams
- Explain human genome project
- Describe the types of mutations
- Discuss cloning and DNA fingerprinting

■ INTRODUCTION

PY1.1: Describe the structure and functions of a mammalian cell.

Cell theory, proposed by German physiologists **Matthias Schleiden** and **Theodor Schwann**, states that all living things are made up of cells and it is the basic structural, functional and smallest living unit of the body. In 1665, **Robert Hook** coined the word 'cell.' About 200 different types of specialized cells are present in the body. Each type of cell performs a particular function. Size of the different cells varies depending on the function. The cell with the largest diameter is an oocyte with a diameter of about 140 mm. Longest cells are neurons in the pyramidal tract reaching the sacral segments of spinal cord. There are about 100 trillion cells in the human body, the most abundant being red blood corpuscles (25 trillion). Almost all cells of the body have the ability to reproduce, except most of the neurons (bipolar neurons of olfactory mucosa and hippocampal neurons can regenerate).

Cell biology is the study of cellular structure and function.

■ PARTS OF A CELL

The parts of a cell include:
- Plasma membrane or cell membrane
- Cytoplasm
- Nucleus.

■ PLASMA MEMBRANE

Each cell is enclosed by a membrane called plasma membrane, which separates intracellular fluid from extracellular fluid. It is a **selectively permeable** membrane, which regulates transport of substances into and out of the cell. It allows some substances to pass through it and excludes others. The permeability can be varied due to the presence of ion channels and other transport proteins. The nucleus and other organelles are also surrounded by a membrane.

■ CYTOPLASM

Cytoplasm consists of all the contents of cell between the plasma membrane and nucleus. It is divided into **cytosol** and **organelles**. Cytosol is the fluid portion of cytoplasm containing water, solutes, suspended particles, etc. Organelles, also known as **little organs**, have characteristic shape and perform specific functions, e.g., ribosome, endoplasmic reticulum, Golgi complex, lysosome, peroxisomes, mitochondria, etc. **(Fig. 4.1)**.

■ NUCLEUS

Nucleus contains most of the DNA in the cell. It contains chromosomes and each chromosome contains thousands of hereditary units called genes that control all the functions of the cell.

■ PLASMA MEMBRANE

Structure of Cell Membrane

Under electron microscopy, cell membrane is a three-layered structure showing an outer electron dense layer, middle electron loosened layer and inner electron dense layer. **Osmium tetroxide** is the fixative used in electron microscopy.

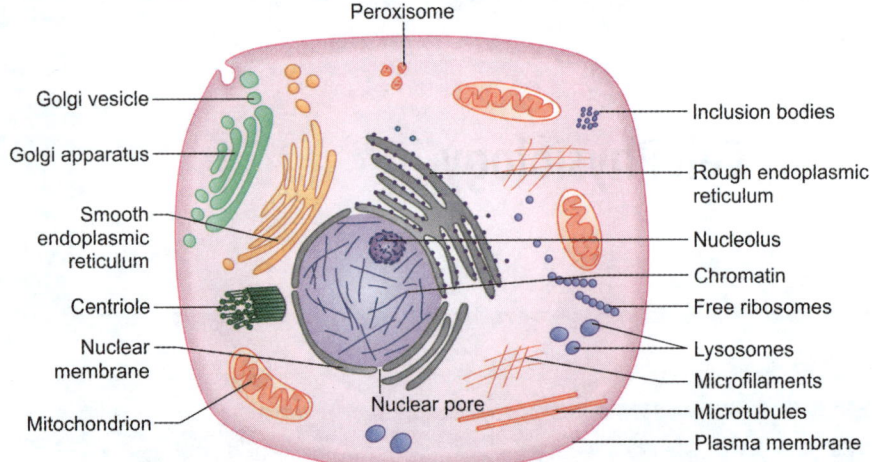

Fig. 4.1: Electron microscopic structure of cell.

Thickness of the cell membrane is about 7.5 nm or 75 angstroms [A⁰]. Membrane is primarily **lipoprotein** in nature and sometimes it may be **glycoprotein**. The approximate composition is 55% proteins, 25% phospholipids, 13% cholesterol, 4% other lipids and 3% carbohydrate.

The lipids are **phospholipids, cholesterol** and **sphingomyelin**. Phospholipids are **phosphatidylcholine, phosphatidylserine** and **phosphatidylethanolamine**. The shape of the phospholipid molecule is roughly that of a clothes-pin. The head end of the molecule contains a phosphate portion and is relatively soluble in water and is called **polar or hydrophilic end**. The tail portion is relatively insoluble and is called **nonpolar or hydrophobic end**. The uncharged hydrophobic end resides within the depth of the cell membrane and the charged hydrophilic end is exposed to the ECF and cytoplasm (**Fig. 4.2**).

There are different proteins embedded in the cell membrane. Proteins may be **integral proteins or peripheral proteins**. Integral proteins exist as separate globular units and pass through the membrane. Peripheral proteins stud the inside and outside of the membrane. The proteins are held to the cell surface by *glycosyl phosphatidylinositol* (GPI) anchors. When the protein extends throughout the thickness of the membrane, it is called **transmembrane protein channel**. The amount of protein varies significantly with the function of the cell but makes up an average 50% of the mass of the membrane.

Plasma membranes are dynamic structures because most of the membrane lipids and membrane proteins rotate easily and move sideways in their own half of the lipid bilayer. They seldom move from one half of the bilayer to the other. Therefore, the halves of the membrane bilayer remain asymmetric. Cholesterol molecules are dissolved in the lipid bilayer and it controls much of the fluidity of the membrane. The structure of cell membrane is referred to as **fluid mosaic model**. This fluidity helps the cell to undergo significant changes in shape (during cell movement, cell division, endocytosis, exocytosis, etc.) without affecting their structural integrity.

> In vitro fertilization (IVF) is possible because of the **plasma membrane fluidity**. A sperm cell can be injected into an oocyte through a tiny syringe in IVF. The puncture site seals spontaneously because of the fluid nature of the cell membrane. This property of lipid bilayer also helps in cloning experiments, where the nucleus is removed from a cell and replaced by another.

Functions of Cell Membrane

❖ Protection of the cell contents: Cell membrane forms a physical barrier between the intracellular and extracellular compartments.
❖ Maintains the structural integrity of the cell and provide shape to the cell.

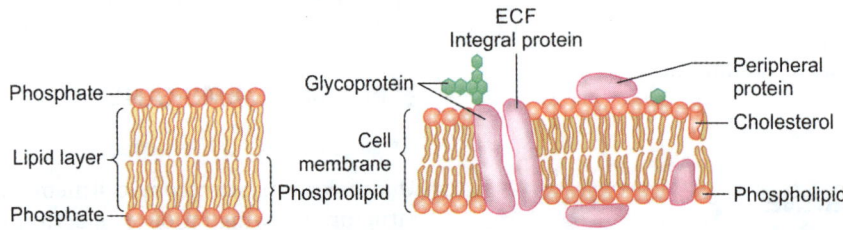

Fig. 4.2: Structure of cell membrane.

- Cell membrane being a selectively permeable membrane helps in the transport of substances across it and helps to maintain the composition of intracellular fluid and extracellular fluid constant.
- Gases like oxygen, carbon dioxide, nitrogen; lipids, steroid hormones, etc., can move freely across the cell membrane.
- It helps in endocytosis and exocytosis.
- It contributes to intercellular connections.
- The cell membrane proteins serve several functions (details are given below).

Functions of Cell Membrane Proteins

- *Structural proteins or integral proteins* contribute to the structure of cell membrane.
- Some cell membrane proteins are *cell adhesion molecules* that anchor cells to their neighbors or to the basal lamina, e.g., integrin, cadherin, selectin, etc.
- Some proteins function as *pumps* for active transport of substances in the direction opposite to their electrochemical gradients for diffusion, e.g., Na^+-K^+ pump.
- *Some integral proteins act as carrier proteins* for the transport of substances which could not penetrate the lipid bilayer, down their electrochemical gradient, e.g., glucose transporters (GLUT).
- *Proteins act as ion channels* which permit the passage of ions into or out of the cell when activated, e.g., Na^+ channel, Ca^{2+} channel, etc.
- Aquaporins are membrane proteins present in most cells, which act as *water channels* permitting high rate of water flow through the membrane.
- Peripheral proteins act as *enzymes*, catalyzing chemical reactions on the membrane surface. For example, the enzymes located on the side of the intestinal cells that faces the lumen of the intestine, break down small polysaccharides into simple sugars or break down polypeptides to amino acids so that they can be transported into the cells.
- Some membrane proteins act as *receptor sites* for hormones and neurotransmitters, e.g., acetyl choline (ACh) receptor, insulin receptor, etc. Integral proteins act as receptors for water-soluble hormones like peptide hormones which cannot penetrate the cell membrane. They help to relay the signal from the extracellular part of the receptor to the interior of the cell. Thus they provide a means of conveying information about the environment to the interior of the cell.
- Membrane proteins like glycoproteins and glycolipids act as *cell identity markers*. ABO blood group antigens on the RBC membrane, major histocompatibility complex (MHC) protein, etc., are the examples.
- Glycoproteins function as antigens in antibody processing and also help in distinguishing self from non-self.

CYTOPLASM

Cytoplasm consists of **cytosol and cell organelles**.

CYTOSOL

Fluid portion of cytoplasm, which constitutes 55% of total cell volume, is called **cytosol**; 75–90% of cytosol is composed of water and the rest by solids. The solids include ions, glucose, amino acids, fatty acids, proteins, lipids, enzymes, ATP, waste products, etc. It also contains stored foods like glycogen granules, lipid droplets, etc., which are called **cell inclusions**. Most of the chemical reactions in the cell occur in the cytosol.

Cell inclusions are chemical substances produced by the cell and are not bound by membrane, e.g., **melanin** in skin, hair, eye, etc., protect body from harmful ultraviolet rays of sun. **Glycogen** is a polysaccharide stored in liver, skeletal muscle, uterus, vagina, etc., which is broken down to glucose in times of need. **Triglycerides** are stored in adipocytes (fat cells) and are broken down to release energy. It constitutes 95% of the cell mass of adipocyte.

Proteins constitute 10–20% of the cell mass. They are divided into structural and functional proteins. Structural proteins are present in the cell in the form of long filaments which form the cytoskeleton in the cell. Functional proteins are mainly the enzymes of the cell which catalyze intracellular chemical reactions.

Cytoskeleton

Cytoskeleton is a network of different kinds of protein filaments present in the cytosol. It provides a structural framework for the cell. It also helps in the movement of organelles in the cell, movement of chromosomes during cell division and also helps in the phagocytic activity. Three types of filaments contribute to cytoskeleton:
1. Microfilaments
2. Intermediate filaments
3. Microtubules

Microfilaments

Microfilaments are the thinnest elements which are long solid fibers about 5–9 nm in diameter. They are composed of two F-actin strands that are coiled helically. It provides mechanical support and helps in the movement of the cell. Microfilaments are anchored to the plasma membrane by anchoring proteins. They are abundant at the zonula adherens.

The molecular motor of microfilament is myosin. Microfilaments help in muscle contraction, cell division, movement of phagocytes to the sites of inflammation, etc. Microfilaments also support microvilli of epithelial cells of the intestinal mucosa.

Intermediate Filaments

Intermediate filaments are thicker than microfilaments with a diameter of 8–14 nm. They are made up of **cytokeratin** in epithelial cells and **vimentin** is a major intermediate filament in fibroblasts. They serve as the flexible scaffolding for the cell, giving structural strength to it. They help to stabilize the position of organelles like nucleus where they connect the nuclear membrane to the cell membrane. Intermediate filaments are also present in desmosomes. In the absence of intermediate filaments, cells rupture more easily, and when they are abnormal, blistering of the skin is seen.

Microtubule

Microtubule is the **largest** cytoskeletal component. They are long, unbranched hollow tubes about 15–20 nm in diameter composed of the protein, **tubulin** (α-tubulin and β-tubulin subunits). Centrosome is the site of formation of microtubules. A third subunit, γ-tubulin, is associated with the production of microtubules in centrosomes. Functions of microtubules are:

- They help to maintain cell shape and also help in the movement of secretory vesicles and mitochondria from one part of the cell to another. Movement is associated with molecular motors called **kinesins** and **dyneins**. These proteins help to propel substances and organelles along a microtubule. Cargo can be transported in either direction on microtubules.
- They form mitotic spindle and participate in the movement of chromosomes during cell division.
- They also help in the movement of cilia and flagella.

> **APPLIED ASPECT**
>
> Anti-cancerous drugs like **vincristine** destroy microtubules in the highly mitotic tumor cells and thus prevent cell division and further growth of the tumor. Colchicine and vinblastine prevent microtubule assembly. Paclitaxel (Taxol), the anticancer drug, binds to microtubules and make them so stable that organelles cannot move. Mitotic spindle cannot be formed and the cells die.

Molecular Motors

Molecular motors are 100–500-kDa ATPases that move proteins, organelles and other cell parts (collectively referred to as cargo) to all parts of the cell. Each consists of two domains. First domain attach to the cargo at one end and at the other end, the second domain, i.e., the head binds to microtubules or actin polymers. Head part has ATPase activity. Hydrolysis of ATP in their heads causes the molecules to move. There are three super families of molecular motors; kinesins (associated with mitosis and meiosis), dyneins (in cilia and flagella) and myosin (in muscle contraction).

Diseases associated with molecular motor dysfunction include Charcot Marie tooth type 2A, polycystic kidney disease, retinitis pigmentosa, lissencephaly, primary ciliary dyskinesia or Kartagener's syndrome and myosin storage myopathy.

Functions of Molecular Motors

- Transport of vesicles in the cytoplasm
- Ciliary movement and movement of mucus on epithelium
- Movement of chromosomes during cell division
- Movement of myofilament during muscle contraction.

Molecular motors are also classified as:
- **Microtubule-based molecular motors** produce motion along microtubules, e.g., conventional kinesin and dyneins.
- **Actin-based molecular motors** produce motion along, actin, e.g., myosin I to V involved in muscle contraction and cell migration.

Kinesin

Conventional form of kinesin is double headed and tends to move its cargo towards the positive ends of microtubules (orthograde). In neurons, kinesin bound vesicles move from microtubular (negative) ends originating at the centromere in the cell body towards the positive end in axons. This is known as anterograde fast axonal transport. Some kinesins are associated with mitosis and meiosis.

Dynein

Dyneins are the fastest molecular motors which move at a speed of 14 μm/sec as compared to kinesin which move cargo at a rate of 2 μm/sec. Dyneins are of two types: **Cytoplasmic form and axonemal form.** Cytoplasmic dynein move particles and membranes to the negative end of the microtubules, i.e., retrograde motion from periphery to center of cell. It helps in positioning Golgi complexes and other organelles in the cell. It is also involved in movement of chromosomes and positioning mitotic spindle for cell division. Axonemal dynein oscillates and is responsible for the beating of flagella and cilia. They have microtubular "9+2" arrangement.

Myosin

The multiple forms of myosin are divided into 18 classes. It is an actin-based molecular motor. Myosin I to V are the main actin-based molecular motors. Myosin molecules are tadpole shaped with head and tail and a total length of 150 nm. Head is 15–25 nm long and 4 nm thick. Tail is 1.5–2 nm thick. Both muscle myosin and non-muscle myosin show binding to actin to form actomyosin. It contains Ca^{2+} activated ATPase. Myosin constitutes 54% of myofibril with molecular weight 450,000. The heads of myosin molecule binds to actin and produce motion by bending their neck regions around pivot point called hinge region. Thus they perform functions like

- Muscle contraction
- Contraction of intestinal villi
- Cell migration.

Cilia and Flagella

Cilia and flagella are motile processes of cells. Both have the same diameter, but flagella are about 10 times longer. Cilia usually occur in large numbers on cell surface, while flagella are usually limited to one or two per cell. Mucociliary transport seen in the respiratory tract is a function of cilia. Movement of sperm is due to flagellar action.

Dynein is the molecular motor responsible for the beating of cilia and flagella.

> Primary ciliary dyskinesia refers to a group of inherited disorders that limit ciliary structure and function. In Kartagener's syndrome, the molecular motor protein dynein responsible for ciliary beating and flagellar movement is absent congenitally. These patients suffer from airway obstruction and infection (bronchiectasis), infertility due to lack of sperm motility, etc.

CELL ORGANELLES

An **organelle** is a membrane-bound structure present in the cytoplasm, which can be isolated by ultracentrifugation. It includes the mitochondria, endoplasmic reticulum, Golgi apparatus, peroxisome, and lysosome. *The nucleolus, ribosomes, and cytoskeleton proteins are not considered as organelles because they are not membrane bound.* Different types of reactions occur in different organelles. Each organelle has its own enzymes, which carry on specific cell reactions. The number and type of organelles depend on the functional state of the cell. Some consider nucleus as a large organelle **(Fig. 4.1)**.

Centrosome

Centrosome consists of a pair of **centrioles** and **pericentriolar material**. The centrioles are cylindrical structures, and each is composed of nine clusters of 3 microtubules arranged in a circular pattern. Pericentriolar material contains hundreds of ring-shaped complexes composed of protein **tubulin**. These proteins play a critical role in cell division. The centrosome is also called microtubule-organizing center. When a cell divides, the centrosomes duplicate themselves and the pairs move apart to form the poles of the mitotic spindles, which are made of microtubules. *Neurons lack centrosome and hence, cannot divide.*

Ribosomes

Ribosomes are small granules, which contain ribosomal RNA (rRNA) and many proteins. The rRNA is synthesized by DNA in the nucleolus. Ribosomes are the site of protein synthesis in the cell. Ribosomes are of two types: **free ribosomes** present in the cytoplasm and **bound ribosomes** located in the rough endoplasmic reticulum. Free ribosomes synthesize cytoskeletal proteins and other cytoplasmic proteins such as hemoglobin. Bound ribosomes synthesize all membrane proteins and most of the proteins that are secreted by the cell.

> The ribosomes of eukaryotes and prokaryotes are different. Hence, in bacterial infections, antibiotics are able to selectively inhibit the prokaryotic ribosomes of the bacteria but not of the human cells. Thus, only the bacteria are destroyed following antibiotic therapy.

Endoplasmic Reticulum

Endoplasmic reticulum is a system of membrane-enclosed channels of varying shapes, called *cisterns*. Endoplasmic reticulum is continuous with the nuclear membrane. Two types of endoplasmic reticulum are **rough endoplasmic reticulum (RER)** studded with ribosomes and **smooth endoplasmic reticulum (SER)**, which has no ribosomes attached to it. RER synthesizes proteins and helps in the storage of proteins as glycoproteins.

SER is the site of synthesis of fatty acids, phospholipids, steroids, etc. Steroid secreting cells are rich in SER. In skeletal and cardiac muscle cells, SER is called sarcoplasmic reticulum, from which Ca^{2+} is released during muscle contraction. SER is also the site of detoxification of drugs and poisons, especially in liver cells. *Glucose 6-phosphatase is the marker enzyme for SER.*

Golgi Apparatus

Golgi apparatus is an organelle with **secretory activity**. In secretory cells, Golgi complex is extensive. It consists of flattened sacs called **cisterns**, which are arranged in the form of a pile of plates. Associated with cisterns are **Golgi vesicles**. The Golgi complex processes and delivers proteins and lipids to plasma membrane and also forms lysosome and secretory vesicles. The secretory vesicles bud off from the cistern into the cytoplasm and are finally exocytosed to the cell exterior.

Most of the substances synthesized in the smooth endoplasmic reticulum enter the Golgi apparatus. The substances are modified and encased in vesicles for secretion. Raw proteins are modified and carbohydrates are added to them. The substances include hormones, enzymes, etc. In addition to processing the substances already formed in the endoplasmic reticulum, Golgi apparatus also synthesize substances that cannot be formed in the endoplasmic reticulum like hyaluronic acid and chondroitin sulphate.

Lysosomes

Lysosomes discovered by Belgian biologist, Christian de Duve (Nobel prize in physiology in 1974) are membrane-enclosed vesicles, which are budded off from the Golgi complex. It is present in nearly all animal cells and forms the **digestive apparatus** of the cell. Lysosomal enzymes are synthesized in the RER and then processed by the Golgi apparatus. There are about 40 different types of hydrolytic enzymes inside the lysosomes contained in small granules 5–8 μm in diameter. Lysosomal enzymes are utilized for digesting large molecules of proteins, polysaccharides, fats and nucleic acids. *The marker enzyme for lysosome is acid phosphatase.*

The interior of lysosome is acidic due to the presence of active H^+ pumps in the membrane, which pump H^+ into the lysosomes from the cytosol. The lysosomal pH is 5, which is the optimum pH for the activity of lysosomal enzymes.

Functions of Lysosomes

- Lysosomes remove old and worn out organelles by **autophagy**. Sometimes, lysosomal enzymes destroy the host cell by a process called **autolysis** when damaged cells cannot be repaired. Lysosomal enzymes released at the site of inflammation help to digest cellular debris, bacteria, etc., and prepare the area for repair.
- The granules of neutrophils, eosinophils and basophils are actually lysosomes. Bacteria, worn out cells, viruses, etc., engulfed by phagocytosis by neutrophils, macrophages, etc., form phagosome and it fuses with the lysosomal membrane. The lysosomal enzymes digest the ingested material and the residue is excreted out by exocytosis. Sometimes in some cells the residual body remains as **lipofuscin granules** and it contributes to cell aging. By determining the amount of lipofuscin in a cell, the age of the cell can be determined.

- Apoptosis by lysosomal enzymes is often important in the process of development. For example, in the embryonic stage, the hands are webbed till lysosomes digest the tissues between the fingers. Lysosomes also help in the regression of tissues like uterus after delivery, muscles after long period of inactivity, etc.

Lysosomal storage disorders: There are many diseases due to faulty lysosomes. When a lysosomal enzyme is congenitally absent, it results in one of a group of disorders called **lysosomal storage disorders**. In this condition, lysosomes become engorged with indigestible substrates. There are over 50 such diseases. For example, **Tay-Sachs disease** is due to congenital absence of a lysosomal enzyme, hexosaminidase-A, which breaks down a membrane glycolipid, ganglioside (GM2) present in nerve cells. GM2 accumulates in Tay-Sachs disease, which leads to impaired nerve function like mental retardation and blindness due to the engorgement of brain cells with the lipid. Others include **Fabry disease** caused by deficiency of α-galactosidase and **Gaucher's disease** caused deficiency of β-galactocerebrosidase. In **Niemann-Pick disease**, there is deficiency of acid sphingomyelinase and sphingomyelin accumulates in lysosomes. The symptoms are related to the organ in which sphingomyelin accumulates. Main features are hepatosplenomegaly, thrombocytopenia, ataxia, dysarthria, dementia and seizures.

Peroxisomes

Peroxisomes or microbodies are single membrane bound organelles present in all eukaryotic cells except RBCs. They are named peroxisomes because they perform hydrogen peroxide based respiration. Due to their small size, they are called microbodies. They are similar to lysosomes, but smaller in size (0.5 μm in diameter). They are rich in enzymes like peroxidase, catalase, D-amino acid oxidase and to a lesser extent urate oxidase **(Table 4.1)**. They contain nearly 50 metabolic enzymes that oxidize various organic substances producing H_2O_2. *Marker enzymes for peroxisomes are catalase and urate oxidase.*

Peroxisomes are formed from endoplasmic reticulum and after 4–5 days they are destroyed by autophagy. The enzymes of peroxisomes are synthesized from ribosomes of endoplasmic reticulum. Proteins are also directed into peroxisomes by the help of protein chaperons called peroxins which are coded by PEX genes. There are about 32 **peroxins** which carry about peroxisomal function inside the organelle.

Peroxisomes are present in plenty in the liver and tubular epithelial cells of kidney. In the liver peroxisomes detoxify alcohol and other harmful compounds. For example, catalase is an enzyme, which uses H_2O_2 to oxidize toxic substances present in blood like phenol, formic acid, formaldehyde, etc., especially in the liver and kidney. Drugs used for lowering blood lipids like clofibrate, causes an increase in the number of peroxisomes and these drugs are referred to as peroxisome proliferators.

Functions of Peroxisomes

It include both catabolic and anabolic functions:
- Oxidation of very long chain fatty acids (more than 22 carbon atoms) like phytanic acid which cannot be directly performed in the mitochondria occurs in the peroxisomes. They are converted to medium and short chain fatty acids.
- Oxidation of ceruloplasmin and release of copper
- Oxidation of purine and release of uric acid
- D-amino acids like D-aspartate are oxidized in peroxisomes by D-amino oxidase (most of the human amino acids are L amino acids)
- Polyamine oxidation
- Reduction of H_2O_2 by catalase present in peroxisomes to reduce oxidative stress. 40% of protein in peroxisome is catalase which converts excess H_2O_2 to water and oxygen.
- It plays a key role in the production and scavenging of reactive oxygen species.
- About half of the alcohol ingested is detoxified by the peroxisomes of liver cells.
- Peroxisomes also have **anabolic functions** like synthesis of plasmalogens (a class of glycerophospholipids required for the proper function of integral membrane proteins and for the generation of lipid second messengers), bile acids, etc. Myelin sheath contains higher concentration of plasmalogens (80–90%) and hence peroxisomal disorders present with neurological abnormalities.

APPLIED ASPECT

Mutations in the gene coding peroxisomal enzymes result in peroxisome biogenesis disorders (PBD) collectively called **Zellweger spectrum disorders.** It includes Zellweger syndrome (most severe form), neonatal adrenoleukodystrophy (intermediate form) and infantile Refsum disease (the mildest form). Zellweger spectrum disorders are caused by defects in any one of the 13 genes, termed PEX genes, required for the normal formation and functions of peroxisomes. The disease can affect most organs of the body.

Zellweger syndrome or cerebrohepatorenal syndrome: Average lifespan is 5–7 months. It is characterized by craniofacialdysmorphia and neurological abnormalities. Biochemical abnormalities include increased conjugated bilirubin, increased serum iron, hypoprothrombinemia and increased serum transaminase.

Neonatal adrenoleukodystrophy (NALD) is characterized by demyelination of white matter, atrophy of adrenal cortex, etc. There will be hypotonia, convulsions, absent grasp reflex, bronzing of skin, etc.

Infantile Refsum disease (IRD) is the mildest variant of the peroxisome biogenesis disorder characterized by hypotonia, retinitis pigmentosa, developmental delay, sensorineural hearing loss and liver dysfunction. It is due to accumulation of phytanic acid. Recent studies show that altered function of peroxisomes also plays a role in the development of **Alzheimer's disease, Parkinson's disease and multiple sclerosis.**

Table 4.1: Differences between lysosomes and peroxisomes.

Lysosomes	Peroxisomes
Larger	Smaller
Formed from Golgi apparatus	Formed by self-replication or budding from smooth ER
Digestive organ of cell	Detoxifying organ of the cell
Contain hydrolases	Contain oxidases and catalase and form H_2O_2
Help in intracellular digestion of food, bacteria, damaged cell structures, etc.	Along with catalase, help in the detoxification of injurious substances

Mitochondria

Mitochondria are filamentous or sausage-shaped organelle present in the cytoplasm of cells. The size, shape and the number of mitochondria in a cell depend on the type of the tissue and the activity of the cell. They are ovoid bodies having a diameter of 0.5 to 1 μm and a length between 2 to 7 μm. The number of mitochondria per cell varies from one to 10,000 depending on the cell functions; average per cell is around 200. It is a double-layered organelle; the outer layer is smooth and the inner membrane is arranged in a series of folds called **cristae**. The cavity of mitochondrion is filled with matrix.

The smooth outer membrane contains 50% lipids, cholesterol and phosphatidyl inositol. It has an integral protein called **porin** through which molecules with molecular weight less than 10,000 can diffuse freely. Outer membrane also contains enzymes involved in oxidation of epinephrine, degradation of tryptophan, elongation of fatty acids, etc. The inner membrane is not smooth, but folded inwards to form cristae. It contains more than 100 different polypeptides and a high protein/lipid ratio. It is devoid of cholesterol, but contains an unusual phospholipid **cardiolipin**. Inner membrane is impermeable and molecules and ions require special membrane transporters to gain entrance to the matrix. Inner membrane cristae are covered by particles of 8.5 nm size called elementary or F1 particles which are regularly spaced on the inner surface of the membrane. There are about 10^4 to 10^5 elementary particles per mitochondrion. These represent a special ATPase involved in coupling of oxidation and phosphorylation. The enzymes on the inner mitochondrial membrane are present in a highly organized, repetitive pattern of subunits, which facilitate sequential catalytic reactions.

Matrix has gel-like consistency owing to the presence of high concentration of water-soluble proteins. The enzymes in the matrix are involved in citric acid cycle and protein and lipid synthesis.

The matrix also contains ribosomes, RNA and DNA. Mitochondrial DNA is of maternal origin and this DNA can undergo self-replication and when required can form a second or third mitochondria. The enzymes needed for oxidative phosphorylation are coded by the mitochondrial DNA which is a double-stranded circular molecule containing approximately 16,500 base pairs. Other mitochondrial enzymes are synthesized in ribosomes in the cytoplasm and transported into the mitochondria. The mitochondria have machinery to synthesize protein necessary for proliferation of mitochondria and RNA. Human mitochondrial DNA encodes 2 ribosomal RNAs and 22 t-RNA that are used in protein synthesis. 5–10% of protein synthesis in the organelle is carried out by its own machinery.

Functions of Mitochondria

- Mitochondria are called the **powerhouses** of the cell since 95% of ATP is formed in them by **oxidative phosphorylation.** Main function of mitochondria is energy production by phosphorylation of ADP and generation of ATP (via TCA cycle), which forms the energy currency of the cell. Thus it helps in regulating cellular metabolism.
- Metabolic functions other than TCA cycle include beta oxidation of fatty acids, ketone body formation, urea synthesis, pyrimidine synthesis and gluconeogenesis.
- The inner membrane of mitochondria contains certain proteins involved in uptake and release of calcium ions and thus they play an important role in regulating the concentration of calcium in the cytosol. It acts as a reservoir of Ca^{2+} particularly in osteoblasts and calcifying tissue (the endoplasmic reticulum is the main site of cellular storage of calcium).
- Has a role in apoptosis. Cytochrome C released from mitochondria activates caspases and trigger apoptosis when cells are deprived of growth factors and other surviving signals.
- It helps in the production of heat (non-shivering thermogenesis which occurs in brown fat). The process is controlled by a protein called **thermogenin (UCP1)** present in brown fat.
- Recent studies show that it has a role in systemic inflammatory response. At the site of tissue damage, release of mitochondrial particles activates the immune system.

> **APPLIED ASPECT**
>
> Mitochondria contain mitochondrial DNA and so **can replicate** and increase their number. *Mitochondrial genes are inherited from the mother in contrast to nuclear genes, which are inherited from both parents*. The head of the sperm that penetrates the ovum lacks mitochondria. Mitochondria have an ineffective DNA repair system, and the mutation rate for mitochondrial DNA is over 10 times the rate for nuclear DNA. It leads to many diseases affecting organs with high metabolic requirement like heart and muscle. Here there will be abnormality in the production of ATP. Depending on the tissue affected, symptoms include altered motor control, gastrointestinal dysfunction, altered growth, visual or hearing problems, susceptibility to infections, cardiac, liver and respiratory diseases. Mitochondrial DNA abnormalities lead to diseases like Leber's hereditary optic neuropathy, cardiomyopathy; mitochondrial encephalopathy, lactic acidosis and stroke (MELAS); Pearson's syndrome characterized by pancreatic insufficiency, lactic acidosis and pancytopenia; metabolic syndrome (type II diabetes mellitus), etc.
>
> **Mitochondrial theory of aging:** Since mitochondrial DNA is not protected by histones unlike nuclear DNA, they are most likely to get damaged by aging. Also since they are the major sources of reactive oxygen species, they are likely to be a major site of oxidative damage. This also contributes to aging.

Proteasomes

Lysosomes degrade proteins delivered to them in vesicles, which are phagocytosed from outside. Sometimes, the proteins formed in the cytoplasm also need to be removed from the cell. **Proteasomes** are tiny structures in the cell that cause continuous destruction of abnormal proteins and those proteins that are not needed, produced inside the cell. Up to 30% of newly produced proteins in the body are abnormal. Mutant or viral proteins formed in the cells are recognized by T lymphocytes and digested in the proteasomes.

If the proteins that are necessary for a particular metabolic pathway are not degraded after they have accomplished their function, the reactions continue and do not stop. So, such proteins should be destroyed. Each cell contains thousands of proteasomes in the cytosol and in the nucleus. They split unwanted proteins into small peptides and finally the peptides are broken down to amino acids and recycled for the synthesis of new proteins.

Ubiquitin

Ubiquitin is a 74-amino acid polypeptide that helps in the degradation of abnormal proteins in 26S proteasomes. Up to 30% of newly produced proteins are abnormal. Old normal proteins should also be removed from the cell. The process of conjugation of the unwanted protein to ubiquitin is called **ubiquitination**. This binding marks the particular protein for degradation which occurs in proteolytic particles called proteasomes. There is a balance between the rate of production of a protein and its destruction by a carefully regulated process. Ubiquitin conjugation plays a major role in this process. It also has a major role in the regulation of cell cycle.

> **APPLIED PHYSIOLOGY**
>
> In **Parkinson's disease and Alzheimer's disease**, the proteasomes fail to degrade unwanted, abnormal proteins and clumps of these proteins accumulate in the brain cells leading to the symptoms. In **cystic fibrosis**, proteasomes fail to degrade an abnormal membrane transporter protein, which pumps Cl⁻ out of certain cells. This results in defective transport of ions and fluid across plasma membrane, leading to accumulation of thick mucus outside certain cells. This mucus clogs airways leading to dyspnea, blocks pancreatic ducts leading to indigestion, etc. In familial Parkinson's disease, some of the genes coding for ubiquitin are found to be mutated.

NUCLEUS

Nucleus is present in almost all cells of the body, except some cells like mature red blood cells. The functions of nucleus are control of cellular activity and production of ribosomes in the nucleolus. Usually, one nucleus is present in each cell but there are exceptions. Skeletal muscle cells have more than one nucleus. Nucleus consists mainly of the chromosomes. Except in germ cells, the chromosomes occur in pairs, one from each parent. Each chromosome consists of a long strand of DNA.

A double-layered membrane called **nuclear envelope** separates nucleus from cytoplasm. The outer membrane is continuous with rough endoplasmic reticulum (RER). **Nuclear pores** are openings present in the nuclear envelope, which control the movement of substances across nuclear membrane **(Fig. 4.1)**. Messenger RNA (mRNA) molecules move from nucleus into cytoplasm through these pores by active transport. Certain proteins in the cytoplasm can enter into the nucleus through these pores. Transport through the nuclear pores requires proteins called **importins and exportins**.

The nucleus contains one or more nucleoli whose function is to produce ribosomes. It contains the genes for ribosome synthesis. **Nucleolus** is not enclosed by a membrane and contains protein, DNA and RNA. It is the site of synthesis of r-RNA. It is prominent in muscle and liver cells, which are active in protein synthesis. Nucleoli disappear during cell division.

GENETICS

Human somatic cells contain **46 chromosomes**, 23 from each parent. Each chromosome is made up of long **DNA** molecule coiled together in the form of a **double helix** to which several proteins are incorporated. This complex of DNA, proteins, especially **histones**, and RNA forms **chromatin**.

Chromatin is made up of bead-like structures called **nucleosome**, which consists of double-stranded DNA wrapped around a core of 8 proteins called **histones**, which help in the coiling and folding of DNA. Just before cell division, the DNA replicates and the loops condense to form a pair of **chromatids**, which constitute a chromosome.

■ GENES

Nucleus contains the hereditary units called **genes**, which control cellular activities. They are arranged in chromosomes. Protein-coding portions of gene are called **exons**. Only 3% of human genome is exon. The remaining 97% is made up of **introns**. This 97% is sometimes called **junk DNA**. The number of nucleotides in each gene varies. The average gene consists of 3000 nucleotides. The largest known human gene codes for the protein, **dystrophin** and has 2.4 million nucleotides.

The total genetic information present in a cell or an organism is its **genome**. Total number of genes in the human genome is about 35,000–45,000 in a single set of 23 chromosomes. The study of the relationships between the genome and the biological functions of an organism is called **genomics**. Genomic medicine aims to detect and treat genetic diseases like hypertension, obesity, diabetes and cancer at an early stage.

Genotype and Phenotype

Genetic makeup of an individual is **genotype**, e.g., 44,XY, 44,XX, 44,XXY, 44,XO, etc. Actual characteristic manifested by the individual is **phenotype**, e.g., male or female. Normally, genotype and phenotype will be the same, i.e., for male phenotype, genotype will be 44,XY and in normal females, genetic pattern will be 44,XX. But genotype and phenotype will be different in pseudohermaphroditism. In female pseudohermaphroditism, phenotype will be that of female and genetic pattern will be that of male, i.e., XY pattern.

Modes of Inheritance

Autosomal inheritance: A trait may be transmitted by a gene or genes located on one or more of the 22 pairs of autosomes. Autosomal transmission may be autosomal dominant or autosomal recessive.

Sex-linked inheritance: Some traits are transmitted by sex chromosomes and such traits are called sex-linked characters. It may be sex-linked dominant or recessive inheritance. Example for X-linked dominant inheritance is vitamin D-resistant rickets. X-linked recessive inheritance includes red–green color blindness and hemophilia.

GENETICS AND DISEASE

Technological advances, such as **polymerase chain reaction (PCR)** and **automated DNA sequencing** and rapid progress in the **Human Genome Project (HGP)** have contributed a lot to our understanding of the disease etiology and pathogenesis. About 10% of hospital admissions involve genetic diseases. It is estimated that 3% of pregnancies result in a child with a genetic disease.

Many chromosomal and metabolic disorders can be diagnosed using genetics. For example, Down's syndrome, Turner syndrome, etc., can be diagnosed using **cytogenetics**. Several genetic causes of obesity have been identified.

Identification of defective genes can pinpoint cellular pathway involved in the physiologic process. Disorders such as hypertension, asthma, diabetes, cardiovascular diseases and mental illness are affected by genetic background.

Most genetic diseases are caused by an alteration in the DNA sequence that alters the synthesis of a single gene product.

Some genetic diseases are caused by:
- Chromosome rearrangements that result in deletion or duplication of a group of closely linked genes.
- Mistakes during mitosis or meiosis that result in an abnormal number of chromosomes per cell.

Human Genome Project (HGP), 1990–2003

The goal of HGP was to identify the entire 3 billion nucleotide sequence of the human genome by 2003. It also aimed at classifying common diseases based on the underlying genetic differences and to use this information to guide treatment. Genetic differences are likely to be a major determinant of susceptibility to conditions such as diabetes, hypertension, schizophrenia, etc.

The project was conceived in 1984 and officially started in October 1990. It was an international venture involving research group of six countries—USA, UK, France, Germany, Japan and China. Several laboratories, large number of scientists and technicians from various disciplines were also involved. This collaborative venture was named International Human Genome Sequencing Consortium and was headed by Francis Collins.

A second human genome project was set up by a private company, Celera Genomics of USA in 1990 headed by Crag Venter. On 26th June 2000, Francis Collins and Crag Venter in the presence of the US President jointly announced working drafts of human genome sequence. This date will be remembered as one of the most important dates in the history of science. The detailed results were published in February 2001.

Mapping of Human Genome

The most important objective of human genome project was to construct a series of maps for each chromosome.
- Cytogenetic map—this is the map of the chromosome in which active genes respond to a chemical dye and display themselves as bands on chromosome.
- Gene linkage map—a chromosome map in which active genes are identified by locating closely associated marker genes. Most commonly used DNA markers are RFLP, VNTRS and STRS.
- Restriction fragment map—here random DNA fragments are sequenced.
- Physical map—this is the ultimate map of chromosome with highest resolution base sequence. Physical map depicts location of active genes and number of bases between active genes.

About 90% of human genome has been sequenced. It composed of 3.2 billion base pairs of which only a small fraction represents actual genes, while the rest is due to gene-related sequences like introns, pseudogenes and intergeneric DNA. Only 1.1–1.5% of human genome codes for proteins. This represents exons of genome.

The number of proteins in human cells is about 80,000–100,000. The results of HGP announced that there are about 30,000–40,000 genes. The fact that the number of genes is much lower than protein suggests RNA editing (RNA processing), so that single mRNA may code for more than one protein.

Major Highlights of the Draft

- The draft represents about 90% of entire human genome
- The remaining 10% of the genome sequences are at the very ends of the chromosomes, telomeres and around centromeres
- Human genome is composed of 3.2 billion base pairs
- Approximately 1.1–1.5% genome codes for proteins
- Approximately 24% of total genome is composed of introns, which split coding regions (exons) and appear as repeating sequences with no specific functions.
- The number of protein coding genes is about 30,000–40,000.
- An average gene consists of 3,000 bases, the sizes however vary greatly. Dystrophin gene is the largest known human gene with 2.4 million bases.
- Chromosome 1, the largest human chromosome contains highest number of genes (2,968) while Y chromosome has the lowest number.
- Genes and DNA sequences associated with many diseases, such as breast cancer, muscle diseases, deafness and blindness have been identified.
- Repeated sequences constitute about 50% of human genome.
- 97% of genome has no known function.
- Between different individuals DNA differs only by 0.2% or 1 in 500 bases.
- More than 3 million single nucleotide polymorphism have been identified.
- Human DNA is about 98% identical to that of chimpanzees.
- About 200 genes are similar to that found in bacteria.

Benefits of Human Genome Project

- Identification of human genes and their functions
- Understanding polygenic disorders like cancer
- Gene therapy
- Improved the diagnosis of diseases
- Helps in the development of pharmacogenomics
- Genetic basis of psychiatric diseases
- Better understanding of developmental biology
- Comparative genomics
- Development of biotechnology.

Ethics and Human Genome

There is possibility that individuals with substandard genome sequences may be discriminated. Human genome identification may also promote racial discrimination by categorizing persons with good and bad genome sequences.

Genetic Mutation

Mutation is defined as a biochemical event in which there is change in the primary nucleotide sequence of DNA regardless of its functional consequences. After replication of DNA, daughter DNA molecules carrying mutation segregate and appear in the next generation.

Mutagens are agents which increase DNA damage or cell proliferation and cause increase rate of mutations. X-ray, gamma rays, ultraviolet rays, etc., are well-known mutagens. Lethal mutations are incompatible with the life of the cell or the organism.

Some mutations may be lethal, others less harmful and some may confer an evolutionary advantage. Thus, mutation represents an important cause of **genetic diversity** as well as **disease**. Only some mutations result in a clinically abnormal phenotype.

Mutation can occur in the sperm or ovum and these mutations can be transmitted to the progeny. Mutations can also occur during embryogenesis or in somatic tissue. Mutations that occur during the development lead to **mosaicism**, a situation in which tissues are composed of mutant and non-mutant cells with different genetic constitutions.

Mutation can involve the entire genome or it can be structural alterations in chromosomes or individual genes. Single gene disorders include *Duchenne's muscular dystrophy, cystic fibrosis and hemophilia.* Mutations in collagen genes lead to osteogenesis imperfecta.

Types of Mutations

Substitution, addition (insertion) or deletion of a codon produces mutations.
- Base substitution mutation
- Deletion
- Insertion.

Base Substitution Mutation

It may be single base mutation or point mutation. A point mutation is defined as a change in a single nucleotide. It can be **transition** (a given pyrimidine changed to another pyrimidine or purine changed to another purine) or **transversion** (pyrimidine changed to purine or purine to pyrimidine). The point mutation in the DNA is transcribed and translated, so that the defective gene produces an abnormal protein.

Deletion

- **Large gene deletion:** It can be entire gene deletion, e.g., alpha thalassemia or it can be partial, e.g., hemophilia.
- **Deletion of a codon:** This leads to missing of one amino acid in the protein, e.g., cystic fibrosis.
- **Deletion of a single base:** This leads to frame shift effect (*refer* frame shift mutation).

Insertion or Addition

- **Single base addition** leads to frame shift effect
- **Trinucleotide expansion:** There will be repetition of trinucleotides. The severity of the condition will be increased as the number of repeats is more. For example, in Huntington's chorea, CAG trinucleotides are repeated 30 to 300 times.
- **Duplications:** Gene duplications occur during unequal crossing over of chromosomes during meiosis. This plays an important role in evolution.

Effects of Mutation

Silent Mutation

If the changed nucleotide base is in the third position of the codon, there may be no detectable functional consequences. For example, if CUA is mutated to CUC, both code for leucine and there will be no change.

Missense Mutation

In missenced mutation, a different amino acid is incorporated at corresponding site of protein molecule. It can be:
- Acceptable mutation
- Partially acceptable mutation
- Unacceptable or non-acceptable mutation
  - In **acceptable type**, one amino acid is replaced by another which has similar functional group as the original one. There will be no functional consequences. It can be detected by electrophoresis. For example, in hemoglobin Hikari, the beta chain of the hemoglobin, position 61 is replaced by asparagine (AAU) instead of glycine (AAA). This variant is functionally normal. This type of mutation is also called **conserved substitution**.
  - In **partially acceptable type**, the hemoglobin is partially functional even though it is abnormal. For example in hemoglobin S, the sixth position of the beta chain is replaced by valine instead of glutamic acid. Here the normal codon GAG is changed to GUG (transversion). HbS has subnormal function and leads to sickle cell anemia.
  - In the **non-acceptable type** or unacceptable type the protein formed is non-functional and the condition is incompatible with normal life. For example, in HbM, in the alpha chain of hemoglobin, 58th position histidine

is replaced by tyrosine (CAU to UAU, substitution). The ferrous ion gets oxidized to ferric form and this leads to methemoglobinemia. Methemoglobin cannot transport oxygen and this leads to severe cyanosis.

Nonsense Mutation

Nonsense mutation is also known as **terminator codon mutation**. A nonsense codon will appear resulting in premature termination of amino acid sequence producing a fragment of protein which is functionless. When a coding codon is mutated to form a terminal codon, it leads to premature termination of the protein (UAC which codes for tyrosine to UAA which is a terminal codon). As a result, the functional activity of the protein will be destroyed, e.g., beta thalassemia. In another case, a terminator codon may be mutated into a coding codon. This results in the elongation of the protein to produce **run on polypeptide,** e.g., UAA to CAA.

Frame Shift Mutation

Frame shift mutation result from deletion or insertion of nucleotide bases in gene. From that point onwards, the reading frame shifts leading to altered nucleotide sequence of mRNA. Deletion of single nucleotide from coding strand of gene results in altered reading frame of mRNA. This change is not recognized since there is no punctuation in the reading of codons. A completely irrelevant protein with altered amino acid sequence is produced. For example:

UUU**U**UCUAGUGAU if in this sequence the fourth **U** is deleted it becomes UUU UCU AGU GAU, etc., instead of UUU UUC UAG, etc. Thus a major alteration in the amino acid sequence of protein is found.

Similarly, insertion of one or two nucleotides will lead to distortion of the reading frame of mRNA. Useless proteins are produced. For example:

In UUU U**A**GC AUU UGA, if **A** is inserted as shown, it becomes UUU U**A**G CAU UUG and so on.

Suppressor t-RNA

Due to mutation, abnormally functioning t-RNA molecules are formed and some are capable of suppressing the effects of mutations in distant structural genes. These suppressor t-RNAs are a result of alterations in their anticodon regions and suppress missense mutation, nonsense mutation and frame shift mutation.

Conditional Mutation

Conditional mutations are manifested only when circumstances are appropriate. Most of the spontaneous mutations are conditional. The resistance acquired by bacteria when treated with antibiotics for a long time is due to spontaneous conditional mutations. In a patient with tuberculosis some of the bacteria in the lung may be resistant to one antituberculous drug. So if only this drug is given to the patient, there will be overgrowth of the resistant bacteria. To avoid this, two antituberculous drugs are given in combination. Thus one drug will destroy the other drug resistant mutant bacilli and vice versa.

Beneficial Mutations

Beneficial spontaneous mutations are the basis of evolution. Beneficial mutants are artificially selected in agriculture.

Carcinogenic Effect

Some of the mutations may alter the regulatory mechanisms. Such a mutation in a somatic cell may result in uncontrolled cell division leading to cancer.

■ CLONING

Cloning means development of many identical copies of a molecule, cell or organism. Types of cloning include:
❖ Gene cloning or DNA cloning or recombinant DNA technology
❖ Reproductive cloning
❖ Therapeutic cloning
❖ Tissue culture

Recombinant DNA Technology or Genetic Engineering

Genetic engineering includes the artificial synthesis, modification, removal, addition and repair of DNA to get a desired and useful phenotype. Genes from other organisms can be inserted into a variety of host cells like bacteria and thus the host organism can produce proteins, which it normally does not synthesize. Such organisms are called **recombinants** and their DNA is called **recombinant DNA** (a combination of DNA from different sources) or hybrid DNA. DNA is isolated and manipulated by end-to-end joining of DNA sequence from different sources. This DNA has both human and bacterial sequence. Now, this host cell will synthesize the proteins specified by the new gene that was introduced. The field of recombinant DNA technology is called **genetic engineering**. It involves the transfer of specific genes from one organism to another by the use of appropriate enzymes called endonucleases like restriction endonucleases (act on DNA at specific sites), DNA ligase, DNA polymerase and reverse transcriptase.

Uses of Genetic Engineering

❖ Recombinant bacteria can produce large quantities of therapeutic substances like insulin, calcitonin, human growth hormone, interferon, interleukins, antiviral substances, anticancerous substances, erythropoietin, clotting factor VIII, vaccines, etc.
❖ It helps to understand the molecular basis of a number of diseases like sickle cell anemia, thalassemia, etc.
❖ Recombinant DNA technology helps in the diagnosis of several infectious diseases, in predicting genetic disorder carrier parents, etc.
❖ **Gene therapy** is used to replace a faulty gene by a normal healthy functional gene (therapeutic gene). Gene therapy is defined as the delivery of nucleic acids to alter or prevent a pathologic process. It is used in the treatment of a wide range of disorders, such as inherited monogenic disorders, cancer, sickle cell anemia, neurodegenerative diseases and infections. Gene therapy in cancer has great potentiality.

A **vector or vehicle** is required to transfer a gene into an appropriate cell. Two major classes of vectors are used for transferring nucleic acid into cells. They are **viral and non-viral vectors**. Viral vectors have been genetically engineered and the viruses like retrovirus, lentivirus and adenovirus transfer the therapeutic nucleic acids into the cells through a process called transduction. Non-viral vectors consist of nucleic acids that are complexed with other chemicals to facilitate gene transfer.

Reproductive Cloning

Reproductive cloning is a technology used to produce an organism that has the same nuclear DNA as another existing organism. In this technique, the genetic material is transferred from the nucleus of a donor adult cell to an ovum whose nucleus alone is removed. This reconstructed ovum is stimulated by appropriate means to divide. When the cloned embryo reaches a particular stage of division, it is transferred to the uterus of another animal where it continues to develop till birth. The first clone developed was a sheep named **Dolly**, who was created from a cell taken from the parent's udder, in 1997.

Therapeutic Cloning

Therapeutic cloning refers to the production of human embryos for research purposes and **not to create a cloned human being**. Stem cells are isolated from the embryo (produced by the above method) in the blastocyst stage of development. These stem cells can be used to generate virtually any type of specialized cell in the human body. Stem cells can be used as replacement cells to treat heart disease, Alzheimer's disease, cancer, etc.

Tissue Culture

Certain cells when grown in a suitable medium can produce similar cells indefinitely. This technique is a useful substitute for laboratory animals and thus obeys the rules and regulations put forward by SPCA. The effect of hormones, drugs like antibiotics, etc., on different tissues can be studied by this technique.

DNA Fingerprinting

DNA fingerprinting is a technique to ascertain whether a person's DNA matches the DNA obtained from samples like blood stain, hair, semen, etc. In each person, certain DNA segments contain base sequences that are repeated several times. These short sequences (10–60 base pairs long) of repetitive DNA that show greater variation from one person to another than other parts of the genome are called **minisatellites**. Both the number of repeat copies in one region and the number of regions subject to repeat are different from one person to another. DNA fingerprinting simultaneously detects lots of minisatellites in the genome to produce a pattern unique to an individual. This is a DNA fingerprint. The probability of two people with the same DNA fingerprint is very small. Identical twins may have the same DNA fingerprint. DNA fingerprinting was invented in 1984 by Sir Alec Jeffreys. DNA fingerprinting is done by **restriction fragment length polymorphism (RFLP) analysis** using restriction enzymes.

Uses

- To identify crime victims as RFLP analysis can be carried out on small specimens of semen, blood, hair, or other tissues.
- To determine paternity in cases of disputed paternity. Possibility of RFLP match due to chance is only 1 in 10 lakhs.
- Used in the study of animal and human evolution. It also helps to determine whether two people have a common ancestor.
- Help in identifying the chromosomal location of genes responsible for hereditary diseases.

CELL DIVISION

Cell division is the process of formation of new cells from pre-existing cells. Damaged, diseased and worn out cells must be replaced by cell division. An adult loses billions of cells from different parts of the body per day. Cell division is also essential for tissue growth and for the formation of new germ cells. Types of cell division are:
- Somatic cell division
- Reproductive cell division.

SOMATIC CELL DIVISION

In somatic cell division, a parent cell divides to produce two identical daughter cells with the genetic constitution same as that of the parent cell, i.e., the daughter cells contain same number of chromosomes as that of the parent cell. Each human cell, except gametes, contains 23 pairs of chromosomes. In a pair, one chromosome is contributed by the mother and the other by the father and they are called **homologous chromosomes**. The daughter cells will be morphologically and physiologically similar.

Cell Cycle (Fig. 4.3)

Cell cycle is the growth and division of a single cell into two daughter cells. A cell normally divides after a certain period of its growth. The cell division takes place when the cell has grown to its maximum size. Each cell has two phases in its life cycle:
a. Interphase
b. Cell division or mitotic phase

Interphase

The stage of a cell in between divisions is called interphase. During this stage, replication of DNA, centrosome and centrioles occur and the cell grows and prepares for cell division. The RNA and proteins necessary for the doubling of all cellular components are manufactured in this phase. Microscopically, the cell has a well-defined nuclear envelope, nucleoli and chromatin. The chromosomes are not visible in this phase. Interphase is divided into three phases:

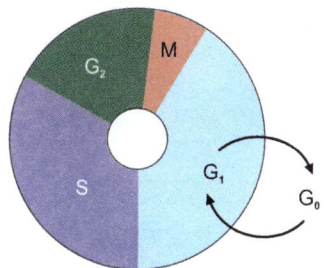

Fig. 4.3: Cell cycle.
(S: DNA synthesis; M: mitosis [cell division]; G_0: quiescent phase; G_1: growth; G_2: growth and preparation for mitosis)

1. G_1 phase (gap or growth phase) and G_0 phase
2. S phase (synthesis phase)
3. G_2 phase

G_1 and G_0 Phase

This phase occurs immediately after cell division. Growth of the cell, metabolism and production of substances necessary for cell division occur in this phase. The duration of this phase varies in different situations. It is very short in embryonic cells and cancerous cells. It is also less in rapidly dividing cells like cells of bone marrow, germinal layers of skin, epithelium of gut, etc.

Cells that do not divide are permanently arrested in the G_1 phase and is termed **G_0 phase**. Neurons, heart muscle cells and skeletal muscle cells are in the G_0 phase, i.e., they do not divide because they are permanently arrested in the G_0 phase after birth.

S Phase or Synthesis Phase

Chromosomes and centrosome replicate in this phase, which is the longest phase. The original DNA molecule becomes 2 DNA molecules. Once a cell enters S phase, it is committed to undergo cell division.

G_2 Phase

G_2 phase is another period of growth of the cell. Centriole divides to form a new pair.

Mitotic Phase or M Phase

The cell division occurring in the somatic cell is called mitosis. The daughter cells produced are quantitatively similar. This phase consists of two stages **(Fig. 4.4)**:
1. Nuclear division or karyokinesis
2. Cytoplasmic division or cytokinesis.

Nuclear Division or Karyokinesis: Stages

1. Prophase
2. Metaphase
3. Anaphase
4. Telophase

Prophase: This is the **longest** phase in karyokinesis. The chromatin fibers condense and shorten to form chromosome, which consists of two **chromatids**. The constriction that holds the chromatids together is the **centromere**. In late prophase, tubulin (microtubules) in the pericentriolar material of centrosome form mitotic spindle that gets attached to centromere. As the microtubules increase in length, the centrosomes are pushed to the poles of the cell. The nucleolus disappears and nuclear membrane breaks down. The chromosomes now lie in the cytoplasm without any definite arrangement.

Metaphase: The chromosomes move towards the center of the cell. The centromeres get arranged at the exact center of the mitotic spindle and this part forms the equatorial plane. The chromosomes become visible in this stage.

Anaphase: This is the **shortest** phase in karyokinesis. The centromeres split longitudinally and the two members of the chromatid pair move towards the opposite poles of the cell. The separated chromatids are called **daughter chromosomes**. The daughter chromosomes are pulled to the opposite poles of the cell by the contraction of the fibers of the spindle attached to centromere.

Telophase: The identical sets of chromosomes at each pole of the cell uncoil and form chromatin threads. The nuclear envelope forms around each chromatin mass, nucleoli reappear and mitotic spindle disappears.

Cytoplasmic Division or Cytokinesis

Cytokinesis begins in late anaphase or early telophase of mitosis. A slight indentation of the plasma membrane called cleavage furrow appears midway between the centrosomes (equatorial plane) and extends around the periphery of the cell. The plasma membrane is pulled progressively inward due to contraction of the actin and myosin filaments in the contractile ring. The contraction ring constricts the center of the cell and ultimately pinches the cell into two **(Fig. 4.4)**. When cytokinesis is completed, the cell enters the interphase stage of next cell cycle.

■ REPRODUCTIVE CELL DIVISION OR MEIOSIS

The division of germ cells is called meiosis. It involves reduction in the number of chromosomes to half the original number. Male and female reproductive cells divide meiotically to form gametes, which fuse to form a diploid organism. Meiosis is divided into two stages **(Fig. 4.5)**:
1. Meiosis I
2. Meiosis II.

Meiosis I

Karyokinesis of meiosis I is divided into:
❖ Prophase I
❖ Metaphase I
❖ Anaphase I
❖ Telophase I

Prophase I

This is the longest phase. There is increase in the volume of nucleus. The homologous chromosomes, one derived from each parent, pair along their entire length. By this pairing,

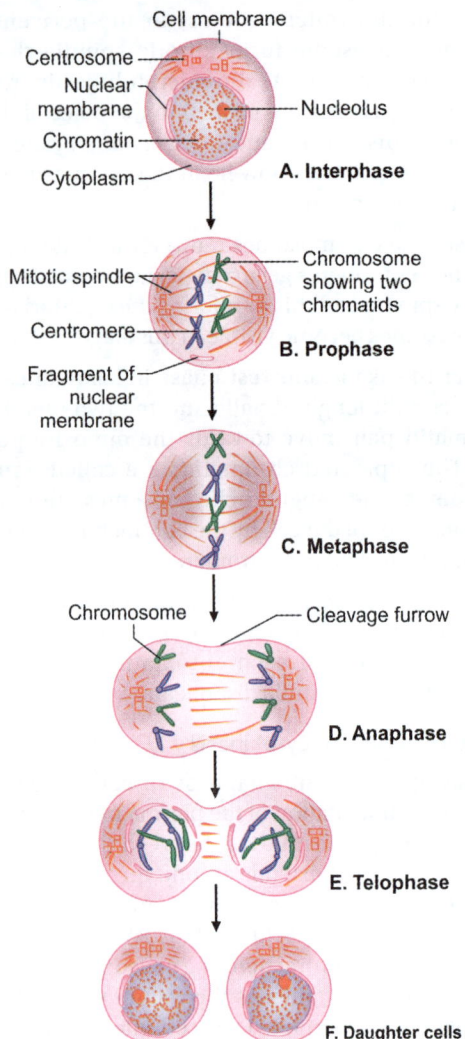

Fig. 4.4: Somatic cell division (two diploid identical daughter cells are formed).

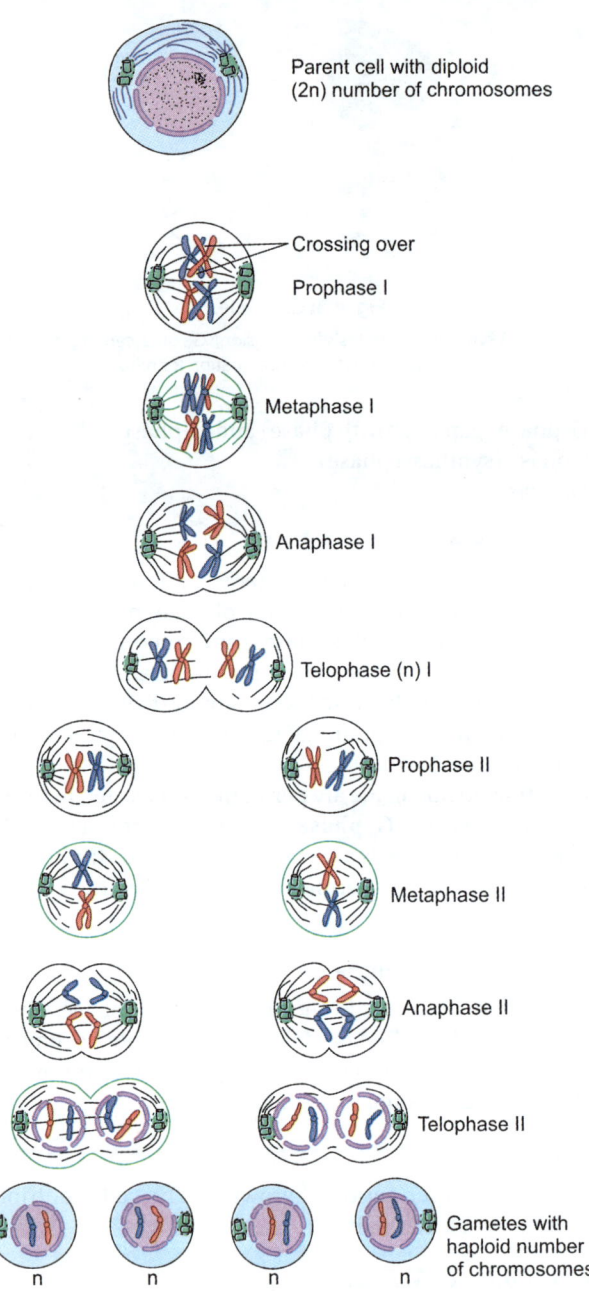

Fig. 4.5: Meiosis or reproductive cell division (meiosis occurs in two stages—meiosis I and meiosis II designated as I and II respectively).

each gene is brought into close contact with its allele located on the homologous chromosome.

Individual chromosome of each pair splits longitudinally into two similar chromatids. Thus, each group, which initially consisted of two homologous chromosomes, becomes 4 chromatids (tetrad). Enzymes called endonucleases break chromatids into segments and the segments rejoin. During this re-joining, exchange of genetic material between chromatids occurs. This process is called **crossing over**. This is followed by separation of the paired chromosomes, which is called **disjunction**. The homologous chromosomes in a bivalent separate. The nuclear envelope and nucleolus disappear. Spindle fibers originate from the poles.

Metaphase I

Spindle formation is completed and chromosomes get arranged at the equator of the spindle.

Anaphase I

The two chromosomes of each bivalent move along the spindle to the opposite poles. The diploid number of chromosomes is reduced to haploid number.

Telophase I

The chromosomes at each pole form chromatin fiber. Nucleolus and nuclear membrane reappear and two haploid daughter nuclei are formed (**Fig. 4.5**).

Cytokinesis or cytoplasmic division is similar to that occurring in somatic cell division.

Meiosis II

This is similar to somatic cell division, but the two daughter cells are quantitatively and qualitatively different from the parent cell before meiosis I. This is due to reduction division and **crossing over (Fig. 4.5)**.

Significance of Meiosis

- Four haploid daughter cells are formed from a single diploid cell.
- Each cell forms a gamete. The diploid number is restored when the gametes fuse during fertilization, so that continuity of species is maintained. Thus, a constant chromosome number is maintained in successive generations.
- Due to crossing over, genetic variation is possible.

Control of Cell Growth and Division

Homeostasis is maintained only when there is a balance between cell proliferation and cell death. Certain cells can reproduce rapidly, but its proliferation should be checked. For example, liver cells can reproduce rapidly even if a large part of liver tissue is removed surgically. The multiplication normally stops when the normal liver mass is attained. Growth factors like **maturation promoting factor (MPF)** are the regulatory factors for cell division. MPF induces cell division. **Tumor-suppressor genes** produce proteins that normally inhibit cell division.

The size of the cell is determined by the amount of DNA in the nucleus. When the desired size is attained by the cell, DNA stops replication. The cell size can be increased experimentally by arresting mitosis using a drug, **colchicine**. Colchicine acts by destroying the mitotic spindle. So, replication of DNA continues and more of RNA and cell proteins accumulate in the cell leading to an increased size of the cell.

APOPTOSIS

PY1.4: Describe apoptosis—programmed cell death.

Cell death is also regulated. **Apoptosis** (dropping off) is an orderly, genetically programmed normal type of cell death in which the cell's own genes are responsible for cell death. Apoptosis is also referred to as **programmed cell death**. Apoptosis removes the cells that are not required and regulates the number of cells in a tissue, and is also responsible for eliminating cancer cells. It is a normal process occurring in the body during life. Growth and differentiation needs reshaping of different organs and tissues. Apoptosis-mediating genes (suicidal genes or oncosuppressor genes) are c-fos, p53, Rb (retinoblastoma oncosuppressor protein). Rb protein is the product of an oncosuppressor gene. It is so named, because it was isolated from patients suffering from retinoblastoma, a cancer arising from the retina. Certain tumor antigens derived from viruses may combine with Rb. Then, Rb protein cannot inhibit cell cycle, leading to continuous cell division and cancer.

MECHANISM OF APOPTOSIS

Certain genes are responsible for producing enzymes that damage the cell. **Caspases** are a group of cysteine proteases which exist in cells as inactive proenzyme. When activated, caspases cause DNA fragmentation, cytoplasmic and chromatin condensation and membrane bleb formation. Finally, phagocytes ingest the dying cells and cell debris. Caspase activation is facilitated by **cytochrome C** and a protein called **smac/DIABLO.**

Inflammatory responses are not seen in apoptosis. No leakage of cell contents occurs and neighboring cells remain healthy. Whereas in necrosis, which is a pathological type of cell death, the healthy cells are destroyed in an unregulated manner, surrounding tissue is affected, and inflammatory responses are present. *Necrosis is referred to as cell murder, whereas apoptosis is cell suicide*. Apoptosis is stimulated by the following:

- **Fas**, a transmembrane protein, which is present in natural killer cells and T lymphocytes.
- Tumor necrosis factor (TNF).
- **p53 protein** produced by the *p53* gene.
- Free radicals.

Apoptosis is completed in four phases.
1. Induction
2. Initiation
3. Execution
4. Disposal

Induction phase is the stage of gene activation through signal transduction. Two important activating factors are Fas-antigen and TNF. *p53* gene (tumor suppressor gene) produces p53 antigen, which exerts an anticancer activity by activating apoptosis. Apoptosis inducing factor (AIF) is produced by damaged mitochondrial membranes. Proapoptotic factors like ultraviolet light, oxidants, cytokines, neurotoxins, etc., damage the mitochondrial membrane.

In the **initiation phase**, the activated gene initiates a proteolytic cascade involving at least 10 proteases called *caspases* (cysteine aspartase). They cleave their target proteins at aspartic acids.

The **execution phase** completes the death program. The dying cell shrinks and loses its contact with neighboring cells. The cell DNA gets fragmented. Nucleus and cytoplasm eventually break up into small cell remnants called *apoptotic bodies*.

In the **disposal phase**, the apoptotic bodies are either phagocytosed or are shed from the epithelial surface.

SIGNIFICANCE OF APOPTOSIS

- In the immune system, apoptosis helps to eliminate inappropriate clones of lymphocytes that are likely to react with 'self'.

- In fetal life, apoptosis is responsible for the removal of webs between the fingers, and regression of Wolffian or Mullerian duct system in the course of sexual differentiation.
- In adults, apoptosis is responsible for the cyclic breakdown of endometrium leading to menstruation and regression of incompletely developed Graafian follicles in the ovary after ovulation.
- Rapid turnover of enterocytes of intestine is due to apoptosis of mucosal cells as they reach the tip of the villus.
- Death of a large number of neurons in the central nervous system that do not make appropriate synaptic contact with their target organs occur by apoptosis.
- Drugs used for the treatment of cancer induce apoptosis in cancer cells.
- Apoptosis also has a role in degeneration and regeneration of neurons.

APPLIED PHYSIOLOGY

Abnormalities in genes that regulate apoptosis are associated with many diseases like autoimmune diseases, cancer and neurodegenerative diseases like Alzheimer's disease. **Tumor suppressor genes** produce proteins that inhibit cell division. Cancers are produced when tumor suppressor genes are damaged. Tumor suppressor gene called *p53* on chromosome 17 is an **oncosuppressor protein** which is very important in preventing cancer. It is so named because it is a protein with 53kD size, having 393 amino acids. Loss of function of this gene leads mainly to tumor of breast and colon. It is seen that *p53* gene is mutated in up to 50% of cancer patients. Function of *p53* is to arrest cell division in G_1 phase. This allows enough time for any damage to DNA that has occurred to be repaired. It increases the production of a 21-kDa protein that blocks two cell cycle enzymes. This slows the cycle and permits repair of mutations and other defects in the DNA. It also induces apoptosis in cells where DNA is abnormal and repair is not possible. So, *p53* **is called guardian angel of the genome**. In most cancer cells, the *p53* gene is mutated or non-functional.

INTERCELLULAR CONNECTIONS

Cell junctions are contact points between the cell membrane of adjacent cells of a tissue **(Fig. 4.6)**. In the tissues and organs of the body, the cells should be held together and so, they must be connected. A group of proteins called **cell adhesion molecules** (CAMs) help to hold cells in their place in the tissue. Some CAMs span the cell membrane and connect the fibers of the cytoskeleton inside the cell to the extracellular fibers of the matrix. This anchors the cells in place. Some cell junctions provide channels for ions and molecules to pass from cell to cell.

CELL ADHESION MOLECULES

Cell adhesion molecules are important parts of intercellular connections. They attach cells to the basal lamina and to each other. The important CAMs are **integrins, immunoglobulins of IgG superfamily, cadherins** and **selectins**. They are important in the embryonic development and formation of nervous system and other tissues. In adults, they hold tissues together. They play an important role in inflammation and wound healing. They may pass through the cell membrane and get connected to the cytoskeleton inside the cell. Some bind to similar CAMs on the adjacent cell. Many of the CAMs bind to **laminins** in the extracellular matrix. During apoptosis, the cells lose their contact with the extracellular matrix *via* the CAMs. Interactions between integrins and the cytoskeleton are involved in cell movement.

INTERCELLULAR CONNECTIONS

There are two types of intercellular connections:
1. Connections that fasten the cells to one another and to the surrounding tissues, which include tight junctions, desmosomes, zonula adherens, hemidesmosomes and focal adhesions.
2. Connections that permit transfer of ions and molecules from one cell to another, like gap junctions.

Tight Junctions or Zonula Occludens

Tight junctions connect apical margins of adjacent cells to one another strongly. They are seen in the epithelium of gastric and intestinal mucosa, urinary bladder, renal tubules and choroid plexus. The composition of membrane transport proteins in the brush border that faces the lumen of the intestine and the renal tubule is different from the transport protein composition of the basolateral plasma membrane of the cell. The tight junctions that join the epithelial cells prevent mixing of the transport protein of the luminal and basolateral plasma membrane.

Due to the presence of tight junctions, transepithelial transport (movement of substances from one side of epithelium to the other) of substances occurs through ion channels and transport proteins present in different parts of the cell membrane, in a regulated manner. It also provides strength and stability to the tissues. Tight junctions are made up of **ridges**, half from one cell and half from the other. The ridges adhere so strongly that there will be no space between the cells at the tight junctions **(Fig. 4.6)**. **Occludin, junctional adhesion molecules (JAMs) and claudins** are the three main families of transmembrane proteins that contribute to the tight junction.

Tight junction prevents the passage of substances between cells and also prevents leaking of the secretions of these cells into the surrounding area. For example, the tight junctions seen in the gastric epithelium normally prevent back diffusion of H^+ into the gastric mucosa from the gastric lumen. But in gastric ulcer, the tight junctions are disrupted and there will be back diffusion of H^+ from the gastric lumen leading to hypochlorhydria.

Zonula Adherens

Zonula adherens is a continuous structure on the basal side of the zonula occludens. It contains the cell adhesion molecule, **cadherins**. Zonula adherens is a major site of attachment of intracellular microfilaments.

Desmosomes

Desmosomes are apposed thickenings of membranes of two adjacent cells. At the thickened part, the intercellular space contains **cadherins (Fig. 4.6)**. They attach cells to one another and are mainly seen between cells of epidermis and cardiac muscle cells. Desmosomes prevent cells from pulling apart during contraction, especially in cardiac muscle cells.

Hemidesmosomes

Hemidesmosomes appear like half desmosomes and they anchor cells to the basement membrane and not to each other. The cell adhesion molecules involved are **integrins** and not cadherins **(Fig. 4.6)**. On one side, the integrins are connected to the intermediate filament made up of the protein, **keratin**. On the other side, integrins are attached to the protein **laminins** present in the basal lamina.

Focal Adhesions

Focal adhesions attach cells to the basal lamina. They are associated with actin filaments inside the cell and they play an important role in cell movement.

Gap Junctions

Gap junctions form tunnels that join the cytoplasm of two cells. They also fuse the plasma membranes into a single structure. Normally, the width of the intercellular space is 25 nm. But at gap junctions, the intercellular space narrows to 3 nm.

Units called **connexons** line up in the cell membrane of each cell that contributes to the gap junction. Each connexon is made up of 6 protein subunits called **connexins (Fig. 4.6)**. The subunits surround a channel of diameter 2 nm and the channel of the connexon of one cell is continuous with the channel in the connexon of the adjacent cell at the gap junction. This permits substances to pass from one cell into the adjacent one without entering the ECF. For example, ions, sugars, amino acids, other solutes with molecular weight up to 1000 Da and certain chemical messengers pass from one cell to another through the gap junctions. As it allows ions to pass from one cell to the next cell, it helps in rapid propagation of electrical activity from cell to cell in certain tissues like cardiac muscle.

> Mutation in the genes coding for the connexins leads to almost 20 different diseases. For example, X-linked **Charcot-Marie-Tooth disease** is a peripheral neuropathy associated with mutation of one particular connexin gene. Other diseases include erythrokeratoderma (a skin disorder), inherited deafness, cataract, idiopathic atrial fibrillation, etc.

MULTIPLE CHOICE QUESTIONS

1. **The structure in the cell that is concerned with synthesis of ribosomes is:**
   a. Nucleolus
   b. Endoplasmic reticulum
   c. Golgi apparatus
   d. Centriole

2. **The correct sequence of cell cycle is:**
   a. G_0-G_1-S-G_2-M
   b. G_0-G_1-G_2-S-M
   c. G_0-M-G_2-S-G_1
   d. G_0-G_1-S-M-G_2

3. **Hemoglobin is synthesized by:**
   a. Rough endoplasmic reticulum
   b. Free ribosomes
   c. Mitochondria
   d. Golgi apparatus

4. **Storage site of Ca^{2+} inside the cell:**
   a. Rough endoplasmic reticulum
   b. Smooth endoplasmic reticulum
   c. Golgi apparatus
   d. Secretory vesicles

5. **The organelle in the cell that contains DNA is:**
   a. Peroxisome
   b. Proteasome
   c. Mitochondrion
   d. Ribosome

6. **The organelle that removes toxic hydrogen peroxide formed in the cell:**
   a. Peroxisome
   b. Lysosome
   c. Proteasome
   d. Golgi apparatus

7. **The cell organelle which contains enzymes concerned with citric acid cycle and respiratory chain oxidation is:**
   a. Rough endoplasmic reticulum
   b. Smooth endoplasmic reticulum
   c. Golgi apparatus
   d. Mitochondrion

8. **The cell organelle that is referred to as the digestive system of the cell is:**
   a. Peroxisome
   b. Lysosome
   c. Proteasome
   d. Golgi apparatus

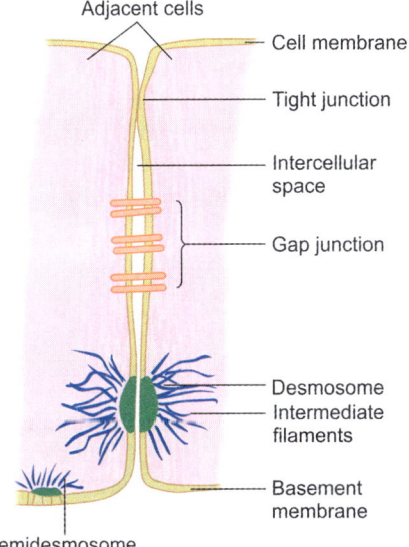

Fig. 4.6: Intercellular connections.

SECTION 1 ⊃ General Physiology

9. The portion of DNA required to synthesize a single protein or polypeptide is called:
   a. Genome
   b. Gene
   c. Nucleosome
   d. Chromatin

10. Reperfusion injury is caused by:
    a. Vitamin E
    b. Superoxide ion
    c. Calcium ion
    d. Magnesium ion

11. True about glutathione reductase:
    a. Sulphur containing enzyme
    b. Important in methemoglobinemia
    c. Free radical scavenger
    d. All of the above

12. All the following statements regarding mitochondrial DNA are correct, *except*:
    a. It is the only non-chromosomal DNA in human cells
    b. Mitochondrial DNA is always maternally inherited
    c. It is a small closed-circular double helix molecule
    d. All children from affected mother will not inherit the disease

13. The long and short arm of chromosomes are designated respectively as:
    a. p and q arms
    b. m and q arms
    c. q and p arms
    d. l and s arms

14. Which of the following was the first bacterium to have complete mapping of chromosomes?
    a. *E. coli*
    b. *H. pylori*
    c. *Vibrio*
    d. *H. influenzae*

15. All the following cell types contain the enzyme telomerase which protect the length of telomeres at the end of chromosomes, *except*:
    a. Germinal cells
    b. Somatic cells
    c. Hemopoietic cells
    d. Tumor cells

16. Protein synthesis occurs in:
    a. Smooth endoplasmic reticulum
    b. Golgi bodies
    c. Rough endoplasmic reticulum
    d. Lysosomes

17. True about mitochondria:
    a. Site of ATP synthesis
    b. Isolation is done by hydrolysis in alkaline pH
    c. Protein synthesis
    d. Fatty acid synthesis

18. Specific role of endoplasmic reticulum is:
    a. Lipid biosynthesis
    b. Lipid catabolism
    c. Maintenance of calcium store
    d. Pentose phosphate pathway

19. Catabolism of H_2O_2 is carried out by:
    a. Peroxisomes
    b. Mitochondria
    c. Endoplasmic reticulum
    d. Lysosomes

20. In dividing cells, spindle is formed by:
    a. Ubiquitin
    b. Tubulin
    c. Laminins
    d. Keratin

21. Cell shape and motility are provided by:
    a. Microfilaments
    b. Microtubules
    c. Golgi apparatus
    d. Mitochondria

22. The following phases of cell cycle are fixed in duration, *except*:
    a. G_1
    b. G_2
    c. S
    d. M

23. Plasma membrane is mainly composed of:
    a. Cholesterol
    b. Carbohydrate
    c. Phospholipid
    d. Protein

24. The percentage of carbohydrate present in cell membrane is:
    a. 3%
    b. 13%
    c. 55%
    d. 25%

25. Function of phospholipid in cell membrane are all, *except*:
    a. Cell to cell variation
    b. Signal transduction
    c. Maintain fluidity of membranes
    d. Enzyme activation at membrane surface

26. True about lipid bilayer of cell membrane:
    a. Asymmetrical arrangement of cell membrane component
    b. Lateral diffusion of ions
    c. Symmetrical arrangement of cell membrane components
    d. Not made up of amphipathic lipids

27. In cell membrane, following are true, *except*:
    a. Lipids are regularly arranged
    b. Lipids are symmetrical
    c. Proteins displaced laterally
    d. Membrane lipids are amphipathic

28. Which of the following membrane has the highest protein content per gram tissue?
    a. Inner mitochondrial membrane
    b. Outer mitochondrial membrane
    c. Plasma membrane
    d. Myelin sheath

29. Peripheral proteins in RBC are all, *except*:
    a. Anion exchange protein
    b. Spectrin
    c. Ankyrin
    d. Actin

30. Integrity of RBC membrane is maintained by:
    a. Spectrin
    b. Laminins
    c. Collagen
    d. Elastin

31. The lipid bilayer of cell membrane exists as:
    a. Solid
    b. Semisolid
    c. Gel
    d. Fibers

32. Correct statement about biological membrane is:
    a. They have a symmetric bi-leaflet structure
    b. The constituent lipid and protein moieties are held together by covalent interaction
    c. They are rigid assemblies of protein, lipid and carbohydrate
    d. Their lipid moieties are amphipathic in nature

33. On weight basis, the cell membrane contains protein and lipid in the ratio of:
    a. 1 : 2   b. 1 : 1
    c. 2 : 1   d. 4 : 1

34. Gap junctions are present in:
    a. Choroid plexus
    b. Skeletal muscle
    c. Renal tubular epithelium
    d. Smooth muscle

35. The molecular motor involved in the movement of cilia and flagella is:
    a. Dynein   b. Kinesin
    c. Myosin   d. Actin

36. Site of protein synthesis is:
    a. Nucleus
    b. Ribosomes
    c. Proteasomes
    d. Golgi complex

37. All the following are functions of mitochondria, *except*:
    a. Protein synthesis
    b. Urea synthesis
    c. Ketone body formation
    d. Glycogen synthesis

38. DNA replication occurs in:
    a. Nucleus
    b. Rough endoplasmic reticulum
    c. Smooth endoplasmic reticulum
    d. Golgi apparatus

39. Asymmetry of cell membrane in the inner and outer surfaces is attributed to all the following, *except*:
    a. Irregular distribution of proteins within the cell membrane
    b. External location of carbohydrate attached to membrane protein
    c. Location of specific enzymes exclusively on the inside or outside of the membrane
    d. Presence of transmembrane protein channels

40. Which of the following does not have antioxidant properties?
    a. Vitamin C   b. Zinc
    c. Selenium   d. Magnesium

41. The most reactive oxygen free radical is:
    a. Hydroxyl free radical
    b. Superoxide free radical
    c. Hydrogen peroxide free radical
    d. Nitric oxide radical

42. The antioxidant enzyme is:
    a. Cytochrome oxidase
    b. Xanthine oxidase
    c. Superoxide dismutase
    d. Cyclooxygenase

43. Zinc is present in all, *except*:
    a. Cytochrome oxidase
    b. Carbonic anhydrase
    c. LDH
    d. Alcohol dehydrogenase

44. Cytochrome oxidase contains:
    a. Zn   b. Cu
    c. Iron d. Manganese

45. Iron is present in all, *except*:
    a. Cytochrome oxidase
    b. Catalase
    c. Peroxidase
    d. Carbonic anhydrase

46. Degradation of substances takes place in which part of the cell:
    a. Mitochondria
    b. Nucleus
    c. Endoplasmic reticulum
    d. Lysosomes

47. Transfer of genetic material by means of bacteriophage is known as:
    a. Transformation
    b. Conjugation
    c. Transduction
    d. Translation

48. Finger printing method was first used in:
    a. India   b. Japan
    c. China   d. USSR

ANSWERS

1. a	2. a	3. b	4. b	5. c
6. a	7. d	8. b	9. b	10. b
11. c	12. d	13. c	14. d	15. b
16. c	17. a	18. b	19. a	20. b
21. b	22. a	23. d	24. a	25. a
26. a	27. b	28. a	29. a	30. a
31. c	32. d	33. b	34. d	35. a
36. b	37. d	38. a	39. d	40. d
41. a	42. c	43. a	44. b	45. d
46. d	47. c	48. a		

Transport Processes Across Cell Membrane

CHAPTER 5

LEARNING OBJECTIVES

Must know
- Describe the different transport mechanisms across cell membrane
- Explain the mechanism of endocytosis and its applied aspects
- Know the different ion channels and explain channelopathies
- Differentiate between primary and secondary active transport
- Explain the mechanism of exocytosis

Desirable to know
- Describe patch clamp technique and voltage clamp technique

INTRODUCTION

PY1.5: Describe and discuss transport mechanisms across cell membranes.

Substances move across the cell membrane mainly by passive transport and active transport. In passive transport substances move across the cell membrane without the expenditure of energy. It includes osmosis and diffusion. Active transport requires energy in the form of ATP. Substances can also be transported across the cell membrane by exocytosis and endocytosis.

TYPES OF TRANSPORT ACROSS CELL MEMBRANE

- Osmosis
- Diffusion
- Active transport
- Endocytosis
- Exocytosis

Osmosis

Osmosis is defined as the movement of water molecules (solvent) in a solution across a selectively permeable membrane from a region of its higher concentration to an area of its lower concentration or osmosis is the movement of solvent from a solution with a lower concentration of solutes to a solution with higher concentration of solutes when both the solutions are separated by a selectively permeable membrane. For example, if pure water is separated from sodium chloride solution by a *selectively permeable membrane*, water molecules move from pure water to sodium chloride solution across the membrane. In other words osmosis occurs from the pure water into the sodium chloride solution. The membrane is said to be selectively permeable because it is readily permeable to water but much less so to sodium and chloride ions. The amount of pressure required to stop osmosis is called the *osmotic pressure* of the sodium chloride solution (for details *refer* Chapter 1). The most abundant substance that moves across the cell membrane is water.

During osmosis, water molecules pass through the plasma membrane in two ways:
1. By moving through the lipid bilayer because of their small size and high kinetic energy.
2. By moving through **aquaporins**, which are membrane proteins functioning as water channels.

Diffusion

Passage of ions or molecules from a region of higher concentration to a region of lower concentration without the expenditure of energy is called **diffusion**. It is directly proportional to the concentration difference, area and solubility, and inversely proportional to the thickness of membrane and square root of molecular weight of the substance. This is **Fick's law of diffusion**. Diffusion occurs either through the lipid matrix or through transmembrane protein channels.

1. *Diffusion through lipid matrix*: The lipid bilayer is freely permeable to water because the molecules are small and have high kinetic energy. It is also permeable to urea. Its permeability to other substances depends on their size, lipid solubility and charge. Non-polar, uncharged, hydrophobic substances like oxygen, carbon dioxide, nitrogen, fatty acids, alcohol, steroid hormones, etc., pass easily through the lipid matrix. These substances

do not contribute to the tonicity of body fluids as plasma membrane is permeable to these substances. The lipid bilayer is impermeable to ions and charged or polar molecules like glucose (exceptions are water and urea).

2. *Diffusion through ion channels or transmembrane protein channels*: Ions like Na^+, K^+, Ca^{2+}, Cl^-, etc., can cross the cell membrane only through some channels in the cell membrane. Different types of protein channels are present, open type or those that can be closed. Open channels are also called **leak channels**, e.g., K^+ channel.

Ion Channels

Ion channels are integral proteins that span the entire width of the membrane, through which ions pass without crossing the lipid bilayer. Many of the protein channels are highly selective and permits only specific ions to pass through. The part of the protein, which closes the channel is called **gate**. It can be opened or closed in response to a specific stimulus and it occurs in three ways:
1. Voltage gating
2. Ligand gating
3. Mechanical gating

Voltage Gating

Variation in the voltage across the cell membrane can open or close the gate. This is called **voltage gating** and the channels are **voltage gated channels**. These channels are involved in the production and propagation of action potential in excitable tissues. In the nerve membrane, there is only voltage gating. A collection of charged amino acids within voltage-dependent channels detects changes in voltage and induces a conformational change in the channel to alter ion permeability.

Ligand Gating

Attachment of a ligand/chemical to the gate can open it and is called **ligand gating**. The ligand may be a hormone or neurotransmitter. Binding sites for neurotransmitters such as glutamate, gamma amino butyric acid (GABA), glycine, acetyl choline, etc., exist on ligand-gated channels. When these sites are occupied by the ligand, it induces a conformational or chemical bonding change in the protein molecule that opens the gate. Ligand gating is seen mainly at the synapses. The ligands can be intracellular or extracellular ligands and the channels are called intracellular or extracellular ligand gated channels. **Extracellular ligands** can be neurotransmitters or hormones. For example nicotinic acetyl choline receptor on the motor end-plate opens the acetylcholine channel with a pore diameter of 0.65 nm when acetyl choline binds with it. The inside of the pore is negatively charged and it becomes permeable to positive ions smaller than this diameter, e.g., Na^+. **Intracellular ligands** are intracellular signaling molecules such as cAMP, IP_3, etc. For example, in the SA node of heart, gates on the sodium channels open when there is increase in the intracellular cAMP level.

Mechanical Gating

Some cation channels are opened by mechanical stimuli like stretch, touch, sound waves, etc. These are **mechanically gated channels**. Examples are ion channels on the hair cells in the cochlea, stretch sensitive channels in ventricular muscle and smooth muscles of intestine.

Study of Ion Channels

Patch Clamp Technique

The ion channels were studied in detail by *patch clamp technique* devised by **Erwin Neher and Bert Sakmann**. They were awarded Nobel Prize in 1991. Patch clamp technique is used to measure and study the ionic currents through membrane ion channels and electrogenic membrane transporters in isolated living cells or tissues. With patch clamp technique, it is possible to record the conductance of a single ion channel.

A small fine polished glass micropipette with a tip diameter of about 1 µm is pressed against the cell membrane of an excitable cell. When a little suction is applied through the pipette, a high resistance seal is formed around the tip of the pipette. Thus, a patch of the membrane under the tip of the pipette is sealed or clamped **(Fig. 5.1)**. The result is a seal with extremely high resistance (gigaohm seal) between the inside and outside of the pipette. The clamped patch of the cell membrane contains only about 1–5 ion channels which allow their detailed biophysical study. The micropipette is filled with a fluid whose composition is similar to extracellular fluid. The pipette also contains a metal microelectrode connected to a recording device, which can record the potential across the sealed patch. The number and type of channels on the clamped patch can be studied by varying the voltage, neurotransmitter concentration, and by using specific blocking drugs.

Types of Patch Clamping

- ❖ **Cell-attached patch clamp:** The patch of the cell membrane remain attached to the cell and the cell is kept intact.
- ❖ **Whole-cell patch**: The patch still attached to the rest of the cell membrane can be sucked out with the micropipette. The electrode can then be introduced into the cell for whole cell recording.

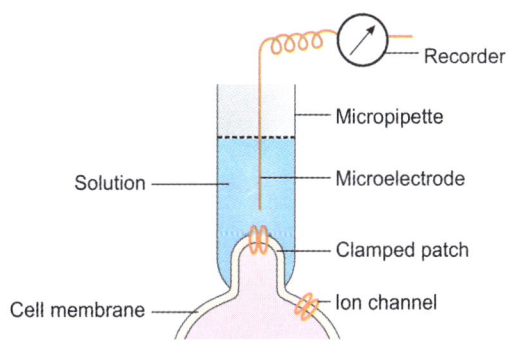

Fig. 5.1: Patch clamp.

❖ **Inside-out patch**: The patch of the membrane at the end of the pipette is torn away from the cell. The pipette with its sealed patch is then inserted into a solution whose concentrations of ions can be altered as desired. Also the voltage between the two sides of the membrane (one side facing the micropipette and the other side facing the outside solution) can be set or 'clamped' to a given voltage.

Types of Ion Channels

Sodium Channel

Na$^+$ channel is a tetramer and the subunits surround an aqueous pore of about 0.5 nm in diameter. The channel is a protein with molecular weight 200,000. The hydrated ion diameter of Na$^+$ is 0.36 nm. Na$^+$ channel has an *activation gate* in the outer side of the cell membrane and an *inactivation gate* in the interior of the cell membrane. Na$^+$ channel is closed from the outside by the activation gate and the inactivation gate remains open in the resting state of the cell. Recent view is that, there are also leak channels for Na$^+$ **(Fig. 5.2A)**.

The number of sodium channels varies in different areas:
❖ In unmyelinated nerve—110/square mm of membrane
❖ At the node of Ranvier—2000–12,000/square mm of membrane

The number and distribution of sodium channels in tissues can be determined using toxins that specifically block sodium channels. These toxins are tagged to a suitable label and the distribution of the label is analyzed to study the channel. *Na$^+$ channel blockers are tetrodotoxin (TTX) and saxitoxin (STX)*.

> **APPLIED PHYSIOLOGY**
> TTX is a lethal neurotoxin present in the viscera of Japanese puffer fish. It combines with sodium channel and renders it unable to open. Saxitoxin is produced by red colored dinoflagellates that are responsible for producing **red tides** in the sea.

Potassium Channel

Potassium channels also have a tetrameric structure consisting of four identical protein subunits surrounding a central pore. At the top of the channel pore are pore loops that form a narrow selectivity filter. This filter is lined by carbonyl oxygen which interacts with the hydrated potassium ions. This interaction leads to the shedding of the water molecules bound to the potassium ions permitting the dehydrated potassium ions to pass through the channel.
❖ Hydrated ion diameter of K$^+$ —0.24 nm
❖ Channel diameter—0.3 nm.

Structurally there are two types of K$^+$ channels in the cell membrane. One type is always open called leak channel and the other type is closed from inside **(Figs. 5.2B and C)**. Functionally there are three types of potassium channels **(Table 5.1)**.

K$^+$ channel blockers are *Tetraethyl ammonium (TEA) and 4-Amino pyridine (4AP)*.

Calcium Channel

Calcium channel is closed from outside in the resting state **(Fig. 5.2D)**. The different types of calcium channels are given in **Table 5.2**.

Ca^{2+} channel blockers are *verapamil and nifedipine*.

> K$^+$ is 50–100 times more permeable than Na$^+$. Na$^+$ is 100 times more permeable than Ca^{2+}. Ca^{2+} is the least permeable ion of the three.

Table 5.1: Types of potassium channels depending on the function.

Type of K$^+$ channel	Function
Delayed outward rectifier K$^+$ channel	Involved in the repolarization phase of action potential
Ca^{2+} dependent K$^+$ channel	Activated when there is increased intracellular Ca^{2+} due to repeated firing, involved in hyperpolarization
Inward rectifier (anomalous rectifier) K$^+$ channel	Prevent excessive loss of K$^+$ during repetitive activity and helps to maintain equilibrium potential of K$^+$ close to the resting membrane potential

Table 5.2: Types of Ca^{2+} channels.

Type of Ca^{2+} channel	Location	Function
L-type (long duration)	Cardiac muscle	Excitation-contraction coupling
T-type (transient)	SA node, neurons	Repetitive firing of impulses
N-type	Presynaptic terminal	Release of neurotransmitter (NT)
P/Q type	Purkinje cell and granule cell of cerebellum	NT release
R-type	Granule cell of cerebellum	NT release

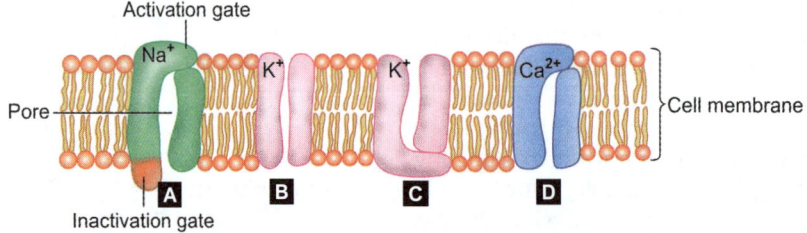

Figs. 5.2A to D: Transmembrane protein channels: (A) Sodium channel; (B) Potassium leak channel; (C) Gated K$^+$ channel; (D) Calcium channel.

Other Ion Channels

- **Epithelial Na⁺ channel (ENaC)** is seen mainly in the principal cells in the collecting duct of kidney.
- **Ryanodine receptors** (RYR) are Ca^{2+} channels in the sarcoplasmic reticulum.
- **Chloride channels** (voltage gated) may be dimers or pentamers.
- **Ligand gated Cl⁻ channels** are present in $GABA_A$ and glycine receptors.

> **Epithelial sodium channels** (ENaCs) are made up of three subunits; α, β and γ subunits. The α-subunit transports Na⁺. Addition of β and γ-subunits increases Na⁺ transport through the α-subunit. ENaCs are inhibited by the diuretic amiloride which binds to the α-subunit. So these channels are also called amiloride-inhibitable Na⁺ channels. ENaCs are found in the apical membrane of the epithelial cells in kidney, colon, lung and brain.

Channelopathies

Channelopathies include a wide range of disease that affects ion channels of both excitable and non-excitable tissues. In excitable tissues it can cause periodic paralysis, myasthenia gravis (ligand gated cation channels are affected), myotonia (K⁺ channel), malignant hyperthermia (Ca^{2+} channel), long QT syndrome, convulsions, etc. In non-excitable cells channelopathies can produce cystic fibrosis (Cl⁻ channel), Bartter syndrome (K⁺ channel), etc.

- **Cystic fibrosis**: This is a chloride channel disease and is the most common inherited ion channel disease. It is an autosomal recessive disorder where, cystic fibrosis transmembrane conductance regulator (CFTR) gene on chromosome 7 is affected. It is a multisystem disease. There will be raised transepithelial electrical potential difference. Upper respiratory tract disease is common causing chronic sinusitis, nasal obstruction, rhinorrhea, nasal polyps, etc. There are abnormalities in both active sodium absorption and active chloride secretion in the epithelia. This leads to dehydration of the airway surfaces causing thickening of the mucus and its adhesion to the airway surface.

  In the exocrine pancreas, the absence of CFTR Cl⁻ channel in the apical membrane of the epithelium of pancreatic duct limits the function of apical Cl⁻-HCO^- exchanger to secrete HCO_3^- and Na⁺ into the duct. It leads to retention of the enzymes and ultimately destruction of the pancreatic tissue.

  More than 95% of male cystic fibrosis patients are azoospermic and more than 20% female patients are infertile. The thick cervical mucus blocks sperm migration and there will be fallopian tube abnormalities.

- **Bartter's syndrome:** This results from mutations affecting any of the ion transport proteins in the thick ascending limb of loop of Henle like Na⁺-K⁺-Cl⁻ cotransporter, apical K⁺ channel, basolateral Cl⁻ channel, etc. It results in NaCl wasting, hypercalciuria, hypokalemia and mild hypomagnesemia.

- **Long QT syndrome** where Na channel is affected is characterized by ventricular fibrillation and sudden death.

- Other channelopathies include **hyperkalemic periodic paralysis** (myotonia and paralysis), **Liddle syndrome** (hypertension, hypokalemia, low renin, low aldosterone), **episodic ataxia** type I (choreoathetotic movements) and type II (nystagmus, vertigo, vomiting, progressive cerebellar signs), **Lambert-Eaton syndrome** characterized by muscle weakness (presynaptic Ca^{2+} channels at the neuromuscular junction are affected).

> The smaller an ion, the stronger is its electric field. Smaller ions like Na⁺ have stronger effective electric fields and attract water more strongly. This strong electrostatic attraction for water causes sodium to have a larger water shell. So hydrated Na⁺ is larger than the hydrated K⁺ and so Na⁺ channel has a larger diameter than K⁺ channel.

Factors which influence the passage of charged ions through transmembrane protein channels are listed below.

- Charge of the ion and diameter of the channel pore
- Charges lining the interior of the protein channel. If the interior of the channel is lined by negative charge, cation can pass through with ease, and if lined by positive charge, anion can pass through easily. For example, the inner surface of the Na⁺ channel is lined by amino acids that are strongly negatively charged. This strong negative charge can pull small dehydrated sodium ions into these channels. Actually because of this charge difference, the sodium ions are pulled away from their hydrating water molecules and only the dehydrated ion will pass through the channel into the cell.
- Concentration difference of the ion between the inside and outside of the membrane
- Channel specificity which depends on the different selectivity filters formed by pore loops at the entrance of the protein channel. These filters determine the specificity of various channels for particular ions such as Na⁺, K⁺, Ca^{2+}, etc. that gain access into the channels.

Facilitated Diffusion or Facilitated Transport

Solutes that are too polar or highly charged or too big cannot diffuse through the lipid bilayer or transmembrane protein channels. These solutes cross the membrane by facilitated diffusion. This requires a **carrier protein**, which binds to the solute and this is followed by some conformational changes in the carrier protein and the carrier carries the substance into or out of the cell. Facilitated diffusion allows passage of substances into and out of the cell depending on their concentration gradient and *it does not require energy*. The graphs showing simple diffusion and facilitated diffusion is shown in **Figure 5.3**.

Maximum rate at which facilitated diffusion can occur through the membrane is called **transport maximum (T_m or V_{max})**. The rate of diffusion cannot rise greater than the V_{max} level even though the concentration gradient of the diffusing substance is high across the membrane **(Fig. 5.3)**.

V_{max} depends on the number of transporters present on the plasma membrane. Once all the transporters are occupied by

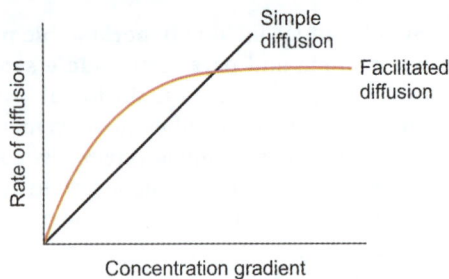

Fig. 5.3: Simple diffusion and facilitated diffusion.

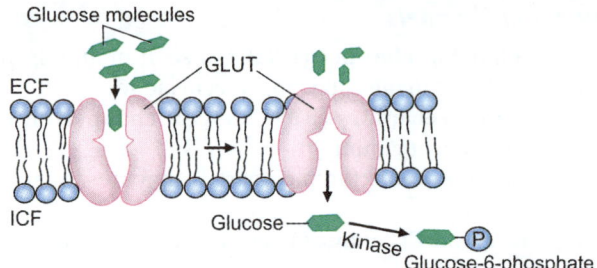

Fig. 5.4: Facilitated diffusion of glucose with the help of glucose transporter (GluT).

Table 5.3: Comparison of simple diffusion and facilitated diffusion.	
Simple diffusion	**Facilitated diffusion**
Movement occurs along the concentration gradient	Movement occurs along concentration gradient
Energy not required	Energy not required
Carrier protein not required	Requires carrier protein
No saturation kinetics. Rate of diffusion increases proportionately with the concentration of the diffusing substance **(Fig. 5.3)**	Obey saturation kinetics. Has a transport maximum (V_{max}) and there will be no increase in diffusion once saturation is reached
Small, lipid-soluble substances are transported, e.g., CO_2, O_2, alcohol	Transports large, lipid insoluble molecules, e.g., glucose, amino acids
No competitive inhibition since there are no carrier proteins	Competitive inhibition may be present. If the competing substance has a similar structure to the substance to be normally transported by the carrier protein, then there will be competitive inhibition

the solute, the transport maximum is reached. Comparison between simple diffusion and facilitated diffusion is given in **Table 5.3**.

Substances transported by facilitated diffusion include glucose, fructose, galactose, vitamins, etc. Glucose is transported into the cell from the interstitial fluid by glucose transporters called GLUT. Insulin increases the transport maximum of glucose in many tissues by increasing the number of glucose transporters in the plasma membrane of these cells. Once glucose is inside the cell, hexokinase converts glucose to glucose 6-phosphate. This reaction keeps the intracellular concentration of glucose low so that, glucose does not diffuse out of the cell. It also favors facilitated diffusion of more glucose into the cells by producing a concentration gradient (**Fig. 5.4**).

Factors Affecting Facilitated Diffusion

* Concentration gradient across the membrane.
* Greater the temperature more will be the diffusion.
* Rate at which the complex breaks down depends on the enzyme activity.
* Number of carriers present and the rapidity with which the carrier can move.
* Presence of inhibitors to the carrier protein.

Active Transport

The passage of substances against their electrical and chemical gradients at the expenditure of energy is **active transport**. The energy is provided by the hydrolysis of ATP in primary active transport. The energy stored in an ionic concentration gradient produced by primary active transport is the source of energy in secondary active transport. Both processes require a **carrier protein**. The cellular activities in the body that require energy include muscle contraction, movement of chromosomes during cell division, movement of structures within cells, transport of substances across cell membrane, synthesis of substances within the cell, etc. Actively transported substances include Na^+, K^+, H^+, Ca^{2+}, I^-, Cl^-, etc.

> **APPLIED PHYSIOLOGY**
>
> Poisons like cyanide are lethal because they inhibit ATP production in the cells and thus shut down all active transport processes in cells throughout the body.

Primary Active Transport

In primary active transport, the carrier protein involved is called **pump** and it involves *energy expenditure*. The energy comes mostly from the hydrolysis of ATP. *40% of ATP produced in a cell is utilized for primary active transport*. The enzymes, which catalyze the hydrolysis of ATP, are called ATPases. In primary active transport, ATP is hydrolyzed by the pumps (carrier proteins) itself and hence the pumps are also called ATPases.

Different types of ATPases are:

a. Na^+-K^+ ATPase
b. H^+-K^+ ATPase in the gastric mucosa and renal tubules
c. Ca^{2+} ATPase pumps Ca^{2+} out of cells
d. Na^+-H^+ ATPase
e. Proton ATPases acidify intracellular organelles like lysosome and Golgi complex

Na^+-K^+ Pump or Na^+-K^+ ATPase

The sodium-potassium pump was discovered in 1957 by the Danish scientist **Jens Christian Skou** and was awarded Nobel Prize in 1997. **Sodium-potassium adenosine triphosphatase (Na^+-K^+ ATPase)** has two subunits, α- and β-**subunits**. α-subunit has the ATPase activity and β-subunit is a glycoprotein. Both subunits extend through the cell membrane. Separation of subunits eliminates activity of the pump. α-subunit has intracellular Na$^+$ and ATP binding sites and a phosphorylation site. It also has extracellular binding sites for K$^+$ and ouabain **(Fig. 5.5)**. **Ouabain** and digitalis glycosides are drugs, which can inhibit the activity of Na$^+$-K$^+$ ATPase. The endogenous ligand of the ouabain-binding site is unsettled. *One-third of our energy expenditure is for the activity of Na$^+$-K$^+$ pump and in neurons, it accounts for 70% of the energy utilized.* This pump accounts for a large part of the basal metabolism.

The function of Na$^+$-K$^+$ pump is to pump out excess Na$^+$ from the intracellular fluid and to draw in K$^+$ into the intracellular fluid from the ECF. For every 3 ions of Na$^+$ extruded, 2 ions of potassium are drawn in. The pump is activated when the concentration of sodium inside the cell increases. When activated, 3 sodium ions bind to the Na$^+$ binding site and ATP binds to the ATP binding site of the α-subunit. This ATP is hydrolyzed to ADP and inorganic phosphate, liberating large quantities of energy, which is utilized for pumping out sodium. The phosphate group is transferred to aspartic acid residue in the phosphorylation site of the alpha subunit. This causes a change in the configuration of the protein, extruding 3 Na$^+$ to the ECF. 2 K$^+$ then bind extracellularly to the protein, dephosphorylating the α-subunit (aspartic acid-phosphate bond is hydrolyzed) and the ATPase shifts back to the first conformational state, releasing 2 K$^+$ ions into the cytoplasm. It is therefore said to have a **coupling ratio** of 3:2.

Na$^+$-K$^+$ pump is called an **electrogenic pump** because it is capable of producing an electrical gradient across the cell membrane. When it moves three positive charges out of the cell, only two positive charges move in.

Depolarization of the cell membrane activates the Na$^+$ pump, whereas hyperpolarization leads to reduced activity of the pump. Thus, the sodium pump is regulated by *negative feedback* mechanism. The amount of Na$^+$ extruded by the cell is regulated in a feedback manner by the amount of Na$^+$ present in the cell. Whenever there is increase in intracellular Na$^+$ concentration, the pump is activated. It also maintains normal tonicity across the plasma membrane, so that the cell size is not altered. If the Na$^+$ concentration inside the cell increases, it leads to osmosis of water into the cell and swelling of the cells. Other factors increasing the activity of the pump are thyroid hormones, aldosterone and insulin. Ouabain and related digitalis glycosides which inhibits the pump are used in the treatment of heart failure. Dopamine also inhibits the activity of the pump.

> **APPLIED ASPECT**
>
> The Na$^+$-K$^+$ pump stops functioning when the cell is cooled. The storage of blood in the blood bank at 4°C makes the pump inactive so that plasma contains excess K$^+$ and the interior of RBC contains excess Na$^+$. This is a dangerous situation; this fact should be remembered during blood transfusion, as it leads to hyperkalemia. **Digitalis**, a drug used in the management of congestive cardiac failure (CCF), causes inhibition of Na$^+$-K$^+$ pump so that Na$^+$ exit is decreased. This causes an increase in the intracellular Na$^+$ concentration, decreasing the Na$^+$ gradient across the cell membrane. This decreases Na$^+$ influx and thus decreases Ca^{2+} efflux through Na$^+$-Ca^{2+} exchange antiport in the cell membrane of myocardial cell. This causes an increase in the intracellular Ca^{2+} leading to increased contractility of the myocardium **(Fig. 5.6)**.

Secondary Active Transport

In some tissues, the active transport of Na$^+$ into the ECF by Na$^+$-K$^+$ pump is coupled to the transport of other substances across the cell membrane against their concentration gradient. When Na$^+$ is pumped out into the ECF, the intracellular Na$^+$ concentration falls and a Na$^+$ gradient is produced across the cell membrane. Here, the free energy stored in the Na$^+$ gradient thus produced, is used to transport substances like amino acids, monosaccharides, ions, etc., against their concentration gradient into the cell. The energy for the transport is not directly obtained from ATP hydrolysis. This is **secondary active transport (Figs. 5.7A and B)**.

Secondary active carrier-mediated transport represents a combination of primary active transport and facilitated diffusion, for example, Na$^+$-glucose symport across intestinal mucosal cells. The primary active transport of Na$^+$ into the lateral interstitial space by Na$^+$-K$^+$ ATPase lowers the intracellular Na$^+$ concentration. This will draw in more Na$^+$ into the cell from the lumen along its concentration gradient by facilitated co-transport with glucose. The carrier protein (Na$^+$-glucose co-transporter) will function only if both Na$^+$ and glucose get attached to the carrier. Glucose can move into the cell against its concentration gradient so long as Na$^+$ diffuses into the cell along its concentration gradient. Na$^+$-K$^+$ pump maintains a low concentration of Na$^+$ in the intracellular fluid. Secondary active transport is possible only if intracellular Na$^+$ is kept at low levels. As glucose enters the

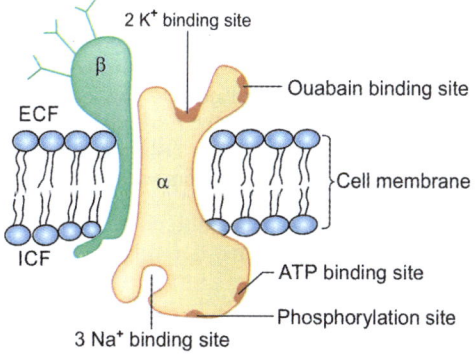

Fig. 5.5: Sodium-potassium pump.

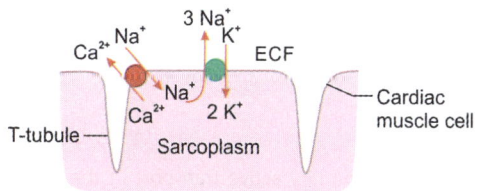

Fig. 5.6: Na$^+$-Ca^{2+} countertransport in cardiac muscle (secondary active transport of Ca^{2+}).

cell against its concentration gradient, indirectly powered by Na$^+$-K$^+$ ATPase, it is called secondary active transport of glucose. Secondary active transport may be symport, e.g., Na$^+$-glucose symport and Na$^+$-amino acid symport in the renal tubular cells and intestinal mucosal cells. Other substances carried by Na$^+$ co-transport (symport) are Cl$^-$, iodide, iron and urate ions.

Secondary active transport can also occur by antiport mechanism, e.g., **Na$^+$-Ca^{2+} antiport** in myocardial cells (**Fig. 5.6**) and **Na$^+$-H$^+$ antiport** (**Fig. 5.7B**) in the renal tubular cells. In the above examples, Ca^{2+} and H$^+$ are transported out of the cell by secondary active transport. Antiport in the membrane of cardiac muscle cells exchanges intracellular Ca^{2+} for extracellular Na$^+$. For one Ca^{2+} extruded out of the cell, 3 Na$^+$ will enter the cardiac cell.

Types of Transport Depending on the Direction of Transport

- **Uniport:** Here, the carrier protein transports one substance in one direction, e.g., glucose transport through glucose transporters (GLUT) in the basal membrane of intestinal epithelial cell into the interstitial space.
- **Symport:** Here, the carrier protein transports two substances in one direction and the transport occurs only if the two substances are attached to the carrier, e.g., Na$^+$ co-transport of glucose or amino acid across the intestinal mucosa.
- **Antiport:** The carrier protein transports one substance in one direction and another substance in the opposite direction, e.g., Na$^+$-H$^+$ counter-transport in the proximal tubules of kidney move Na$^+$ from the lumen to the interior of tubular cells and H$^+$ is counter transported into the lumen. Another example is Na$^+$-Ca^{2+} counter-transport in the cardiac muscle, where Na$^+$ moves into the cell and Ca^{2+} is counter transported to the outside (**Fig. 5.6**).

Active transport, passive transport, facilitated diffusion and secondary active transport are together shown in **Figure 5.8**.

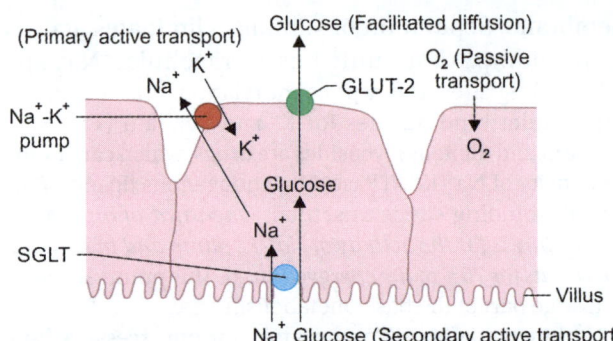

Fig. 5.8: Passive transport, facilitated diffusion, primary active transport, secondary active transport in the intestinal epithelial cell.
(SGLT: sodium dependent glucose transporter; GLUT-2: glucose transporter-2)

Endocytosis

Endocytosis is the process by which cells take up macromolecules and large particles that cannot enter the cell by diffusion or active transport. The process requires ATPase, Ca^{2+} and microfilaments. There are three types of endocytosis:
1. Receptor-mediated endocytosis
2. Phagocytosis
3. Pinocytosis

Receptor-mediated Endocytosis

Receptor-mediated endocytosis is a highly specific type of endocytosis by which cells take up **specific ligands** for which the cell membrane bears specific receptors. *A specific molecule that binds to a receptor is called the ligand of that receptor.* The receptors for these ligands are concentrated in specific areas of the cell membrane called **clathrin-coated pits**. The pits also contain actin and myosin filaments. These are invaginations in the cell membrane that are coated on the cytoplasmic side with a filamentous material called clathrin, a peripheral membrane protein. The cell membrane fuses around the receptor-ligand complex in the pit forming a vesicle, which gets pinched off into the cytoplasm called **clathrin-coated vesicle**. This process requires Ca^{2+} and energy supplied by ATP. The clathrin coat gets separated and the vesicle fuses with an endosome or lysosome, which contains enzymes that breakdown the substance endocytosed (**Fig. 5.9**).

For example, cells take up cholesterol contained in low-density lipoprotein (LDL), transferrin, certain vitamins, antibodies, and hormones by this mechanism.

> Human immunodeficiency virus (HIV) enters the helper T-cell *via* receptor-mediated endocytosis after binding to a receptor in the helper T-cell membrane called CD4. This leads to acquired immunodeficiency syndrome (AIDS). Viruses causing hepatitis and poliomyelitis also gain access into the cell by receptor-mediated endocytosis. Iron toxicity also occurs with excessive uptake through endocytosis.

Phagocytosis

Phagocytosis is the process by which aged and worn-out cells, bacteria, viruses, dead tissue, etc., are engulfed by **phagocytes** of the body, such as neutrophils and

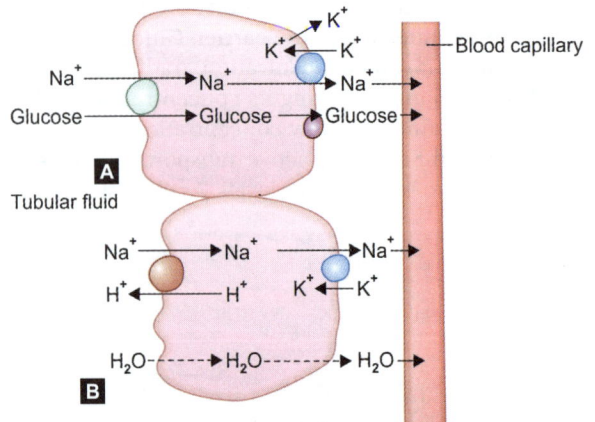

Figs. 5.7A and B: Secondary active transport in the renal tubular cells: (A) Glucose-sodium symport; (B) Na$^+$-H$^+$ antiport (glucose and H$^+$ are transported by secondary active transport).

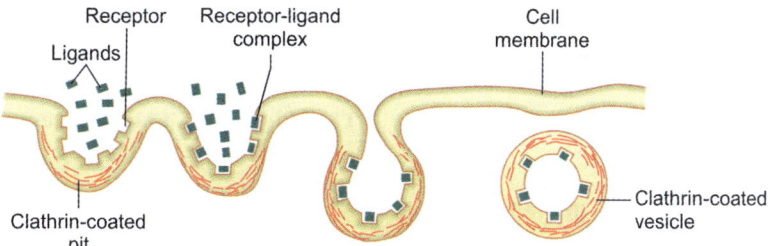

Fig. 5.9: Receptor-mediated endocytosis.

macrophages. Phagocytosis begins when the particle makes contact with the cell membrane receptor protein. This part of the plasma membrane then invaginates and the invagination is pinched off into the cell forming **phagosome**, leaving the cell membrane intact. Phagosome fuses with lysosome and the enzymes break down the ingested material.

Pinocytosis

In pinocytosis, the only difference from phagocytosis is that the substance ingested is in solution and hence *pinocytic vesicle is not visible under the microscope.* Solutes in ECF like amino acids, fatty acids, etc., enter the cell by pinocytosis. *No receptor proteins are involved in pinocytosis.*

Exocytosis

Exocytosis is the process for release of macromolecules from cells to the exterior. Exocytosis requires *calcium and energy.* Substances produced in the endoplasmic reticulum move to the Golgi apparatus and from there secretory vesicles are budded off. These vesicles move to the cell membrane and fuse with it. The area of fusion breaks down leaving the contents to the outside. The membrane of the vesicle becomes part of the cell membrane **(Fig. 5.10)**. Thus, exocytosis increases the surface area of the cell membrane and this may lead to increase in the size of the cell. But part of the cell membrane is being removed by endocytosis and this *exocytosis–endocytosis coupling maintains the surface area of the cell membrane constant.*

Exocytosis is also known as reverse pinocytosis or emeiocytosis. This is the mechanism by which substances synthesized within the secretory cells like digestive enzymes, hormones, mucus, etc., and neurotransmitters from nerve cells are secreted out of the cell. These are exocytosed only when the cell is stimulated. Some of the exocytosed molecules attach to the cell surface and become peripheral proteins, e.g., antigens. Some become part of extracellular matrix, e.g., collagen and glycosaminoglycan.

Transcytosis

In transcytosis, vesicles undergo endocytosis on one side of a cell, and then undergo exocytosis on the opposite side of the cell. Hence, transcytosis is also called **vesicular transport** or **cytopempsis**. For example, transport of substances like nutrients across the endothelial cells of blood vessels to the interstitial fluid, transfer of antibodies across placenta from maternal circulation to fetal circulation, etc. occur by transcytosis. In transcytosis, the transport mechanism makes use of coated vesicles that appear to be coated with **caveolin**. Caveolin is a protein that resembles **clathrin**, which is involved in endocytosis.

MULTIPLE CHOICE QUESTIONS

1. **Which of the following is true about Na^+-K^+ pump?**
   a. K^+ is pumped against the gradient
   b. 2 K^+ are exchanged with 5 Na^+
   c. Hypercalcemia causes arrest in Na^+-K^+ pump
   d. Decrease in intracellular Na^+ increases activity of the pump

2. **True regarding transport across a cell membrane is:**
   a. Cl^- with glucose transport
   b. Na^+ with glucose antiport
   c. Na^+ with glucose symport
   d. K^+ with glucose symport

3. **The sodium-potassium pump is an example of:**
   a. Active transport
   b. Passive transport
   c. Facilitated diffusion
   d. Osmosis

4. **True statement about Ca^{2+} transport across cell membrane:**
   a. Calcium-calmodulin mediated
   b. Maintain intracellular Ca^{2+} 1,000 times higher than extracellular Ca^{2+}
   c. Requires hydrolysis of ATP
   d. It is a symport

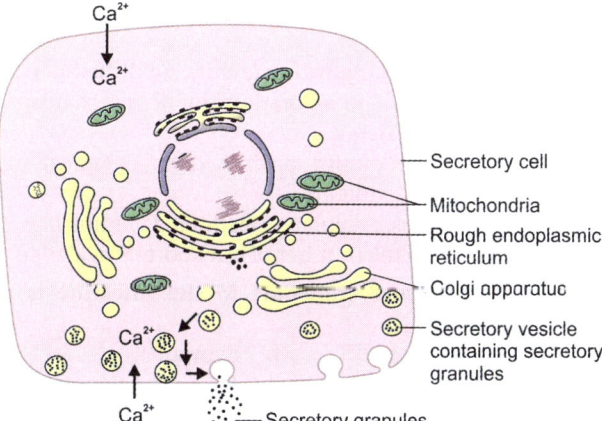

Fig. 5.10: Mechanism of secretion by emeiocytosis in a secretory cell.

5. Which of the following substances act to increase the release of Ca²⁺ from endoplasmic reticulum?
   a. Inositol triphosphate
   b. Parathyroid hormone
   c. 1,25-dihydroxycholecalciferol
   d. Diacylglycerol

6. All the following are true about facilitated diffusion, *except*:
   a. Occur in the direction of concentration gradient
   b. Does not require energy
   c. Occur in direction opposite to electrical gradient
   d. Facilitated by charge of molecule

7. All the following transport processes follow saturation kinetics, *except*:
   a. Facilitated diffusion
   b. Na⁺-Ca²⁺ exchanger
   c. Simple diffusion
   d. Na⁺ coupled active transport

8. Active transport across cell membrane is mediated by:
   a. G-proteins
   b. Na⁺-K⁺ ATPase
   c. Carrier protein
   d. Channel protein

9. Exocytosis is:
   a. Extrusion of cell bound vesicles
   b. Intrusion of liquid particles
   c. Intrusion of solid particles
   d. Intrusion of both solid and liquid particles

10. Clathrin is used in:
    a. Exocytosis
    b. Receptor mediated endocytosis
    c. Cell to cell adhesion
    d. Ion transport

11. Fusion of part of a cell membrane occur in all the following, *except*:
    a. Cell division
    b. Endocytosis
    c. Exocytosis
    d. Emeiocytosis

12. Sodium channels are specifically blocked by:
    a. Nifedipine
    b. Tetrodotoxin
    c. Choline
    d. Verapamil

13. Emeiocytosis or reverse pinocytosis requires which ion?
    a. Na⁺
    b. K⁺
    c. Ca²⁺
    d. Mg²⁺

14. Plasma K⁺ constitutes what percentage of total body potassium?
    a. 0.4%
    b. 7.6%
    c. 10.4%
    d. 89.6%

15. For Na⁺-K⁺ pump the coupling ratio is:
    a. 1:1
    b. 2:3
    c. 3:2
    d. 1:4

16. Most important intracellular anion is:
    a. Proteins
    b. HCO_3^-
    c. Cl^-
    d. PO_4^{3-}

17. Chemical gradient across cell membrane is maintained chiefly by:
    a. Na⁺
    b. Ca²⁺
    c. K⁺
    d. Cl⁻

18. The ion channels in excitable cells are lined by:
    a. Cephalins
    b. Proteins
    c. Lipids
    d. Carbohydrates

19. When water is moving in one direction, it tends to drag along some molecules of solute. This is called:
    a. Filtration
    b. Osmosis
    c. Donnan effect
    d. Solvent drag

20. The lipid bilayer of cell membrane is most permeable to:
    a. Potassium
    b. Sodium
    c. Glucose
    d. Urea

21. The major driving force for the formation of membrane lipid bilayer is:
    a. Hydrogen bonding
    b. Hydrophobic interactions
    c. Van der Waal forces
    d. Starling's forces

22. Tetrodotoxin blocks:
    a. Na⁺ channel during action potential
    b. K⁺ channel during action potential
    c. Na⁺ channel during resting state
    d. K⁺ during resting state

23. Diffusion through a membrane is affected by all, *except*:
    a. Temperature
    b. Membrane pore size
    c. Size of the particle
    d. Concentration gradient across the membrane

24. Which of the following require energy?
    a. Simple diffusion
    b. Facilitated diffusion
    c. Passive transport
    d. Active transport

25. True statement regarding facilitated diffusion is:
    a. Does not follow saturation kinetics mechanism
    b. Requires energy
    c. Substances move against their chemical and electrical gradient
    d. Hormones regulate facilitated diffusion by changing the number of transporters available

26. Sodium-glucose transport in the intestine is an example of:
    a. Uniport
    b. Symport
    c. Antiport
    d. Primary active transport

27. The following statements regarding endocytosis are true, *except*:
    a. Pinocytosis means cellular uptake of fluid and fluid contents
    b. Phagocytosis is a property of all cells
    c. Most endocytic vesicles fuse with primary lysosomes to form secondary lysosomes
    d. Clathrin is involved in receptor mediated endocytosis

28. The activity of Na^+-K^+ pump is an example of:
    a. Uniport
    b. Antiport
    c. Symport
    d. Secondary active transport

29. The primary force that moves water molecules from plasma to the interstitial fluid is:
    a. Filtration
    b. Facilitated diffusion
    c. Co-transport with sodium
    d. Active transport

30. The single most important factor determining diffusion across a membrane is:
    a. Molecular weight
    b. Thickness of the membrane
    c. Concentration gradient
    d. Lipid solubility

31. Diffusion through a biological membrane is affected by all, *except*:
    a. Temperature
    b. Membrane pore size
    c. Size of the particle
    d. Concentration gradient across the membrane

32. The most important process for transcapillary exchange is:
    a. Diffusion
    b. Endocytosis
    c. Active transport
    d. Exocytosis

33. All are involved in phagocytosis, *except*:
    a. Recognition and attachment
    b. Engulfment
    c. Pavementing of cells
    d. Killing and degradation

34. Movement of water molecules across a semipermeable membrane from a less concentrated solution to a more concentrated solution is called:
    a. Facilitated diffusion
    b. Active transport
    c. Secondary active transport
    d. Osmosis

ANSWERS

1. a	2. c	3. a	4. c	5. a
6. c	7. c	8. c	9. a	10. b
11. a	12. b	13. c	14. a	15. c
16. a	17. c	18. b	19. d	20. d
21. b	22. a	23. c	24. d	25. d
26. b	27. b	28. b	29. a	30. c
31. c	32. a	33. c	34. d	

Nerve Physiology and Bioelectrical Potentials

CHAPTER 6

LEARNING OBJECTIVES
Must know
- Describe the structure of a neuron with the help of a diagram
- Know the classification of neurons
- Describe the types, functions and properties of nerve fibers
- Describe the ionic basis of resting membrane potential
- Explain the ionic basis of action potential in a nerve fiber
- Understand the differences between graded potential and action potential
- Know the difference between myelination in peripheral and central nervous system
- Mechanism of conduction of impulse in myelinated and unmyelinated nerve fibers
- Describe the mechanism of degeneration and regeneration in peripheral nerve

Desirable to know
- Discuss the measurement of resting membrane potential
- Describe the recording of action potential
- Discuss the role of different ions in the excitability of excitable tissues
- Describe compound action potential recorded from a peripheral nerve
- Functions of nerve growth factor

INTRODUCTION

The nervous system is composed of neurons and neuroglial cells. Neurons are excitable cells which can respond to a stimulus by producing action potentials. These action potentials can be transmitted along the nerve fiber. Neuroglial cells are not excitable and so cannot produce action potentials. In this chapter, the structure and functions of neurons is dealt with.

Nervous system has three basic functions. They are:
1. **Sensory function:** Nervous system can sense stimuli from within the body and outside the body.
2. **Integrative function:** It analyzes and stores sensory information and makes appropriate decisions.
3. **Motor function:** It responds to stimuli.

NEURON

PY3.1: Describe the structure and functions of neuron. Discuss nerve growth factor.
PY3.2: Describe the types, functions and properties of nerve fibers.

Neuron is the **structural and functional unit** of nervous system. The specialized function of neuron is integration and transmission of nerve impulses.

Human central nervous system (CNS) consists of about 10^{11} neurons and 10–50 times more number of **glial cells** or supporting cells. A neuron contains a cell body and its processes; axon and dendrites. Some neurons are less than 1 mm in length, whereas some are the longest cells in the body, measuring about 1 meter in length.

Peripheral nerve is the collective term used for the 12 pairs of cranial nerves and 31 pairs of spinal nerves. Each peripheral nerve consists of parallel bundles of nerve fibers, which may be afferent or efferent axons; may be myelinated or unmyelinated. They are supported by connective tissue sheaths which also supports associated blood vessels and lymph vessels. The outer most sheath, which surrounds the peripheral nerve, is called **epineurium.** Within this sheath are bundles of nerve fibers, each of which is surrounded by connective tissue sheath called **perineurium.** Each individual nerve fiber is surrounded by **endoneurium.**

CLASSIFICATION OF NEURONS

Structural Classification

Based on the Number of Processes Extending from the Cell Body

According to this, neurons are classified into unipolar, bipolar, multipolar and anaxonic neuron (**Fig. 6.1**).

All neurons contain only one axon, but dendrites may be one or many.

Unipolar Neuron

True unipolar neurons are seen only in the embryonic life of human beings. In adults, it is present only in the

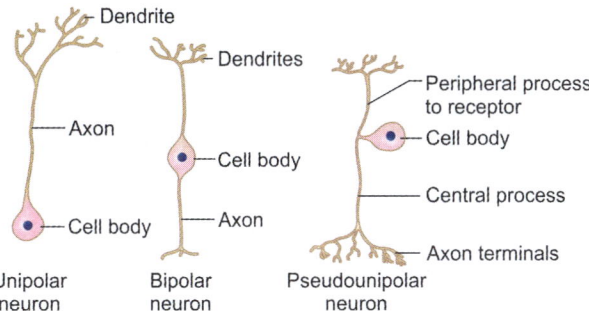

Fig. 6.1: Types of neurons based on structure.

mesencephalic nucleus of the 5th cranial nerve. Structurally, dorsal root ganglion cell is unipolar, but functionally, it is referred to as **pseudounipolar** as one process arises from the cell body, which divides to form two processes; one going to the periphery (receptor) bringing sensory information from the receptors (functioning as dendrite) and the other entering the spinal cord (functioning as axon). Pseudounipolar neuron is also classified as a subclass of bipolar neuron.

Bipolar Neurons

In bipolar neurons, dendrite arises from one pole and axon arises from the opposite pole. Bipolar neurons are present in the retina, vestibular ganglion, spiral ganglion of cochlea and olfactory neuroepithelium.

Multipolar Neurons

In multipolar neurons, axon and dendrites arise from different points of the cell body. Examples are anterior horn cell of spinal cord, Purkinje cell of cerebellar cortex, pyramidal cell of motor cortex, neurons in the spinal nucleus of trigeminal nerve, etc.

Anaxonic Neuron

Sometimes, axon may be absent in the neuron or it cannot be differentiated from the dendrites. These axons communicate through their dendrites through dendro-dendritic connections. Some anaxonic neurons are found in the brain and retina. For example, amacrine cells of retina, granule cells of brain and periglomerular cells in the olfactory bulb belong to this group. They usually act as interneurons which connect two neurons. They are not motor or sensory neurons.

Based on the Length of the Neuron

Depending on the length of the axon, neurons are classified into:
- **Golgi type I neurons or projection neurons** are large cells with long axons. They constitute the peripheral nerves and the long tracts of the brain and spinal cord.
- **Golgi type II neurons or local circuit neurons** are small neurons, which are stellate shaped with short axons or without axons. The axon does not leave that part of the gray matter in which the cell body lies. These neurons are found in the retina, cerebellar cortex and cerebral cortex. They may be of different shapes and all have numerous radiating processes, which give them a stellate or star-shaped appearance.

Functional Classification

Sensory or Afferent Neuron

The sensory neurons transmit sensory impulses from receptors to the CNS.

Motor or Efferent Neurons

Motor neurons convey motor nerve impulses from CNS to the effector organs.

Association Neurons or Interneurons

Association neurons include all other neurons that are not specifically sensory or motor. 90% of neurons are association neurons or interneurons.

MORPHOLOGY OF A TYPICAL NEURON

Anterior horn cell of spinal cord is considered as a typical neuron (**Fig. 6.2**).

Neuron is composed of:
- A **cell body or soma** which is the metabolic center of the neuron
- **Dendrites** that branch extensively which receive inputs to the neuron
- The **initial segment** of the axon where the action potential is initiated
- A long **axon** that conducts the action potentials to the nerve terminal.

Nerve Cell Body or Soma

Cell body is referred to as the metabolic center of the neuron. It contains the following structures: nucleus, Nissl granules and all cell organelles, except centrosome. Centrosome necessary for mitosis is absent in the mature neuron. *As there is no centrosome in the neuron, regeneration of the cell body is not possible and formation of new neurons stops in the intrauterine life.*

The cell body is present only in the following areas of the nervous system:
- Gray matter of brain and spinal cord
- Nuclei of brain
- Ganglia of the peripheral nervous system

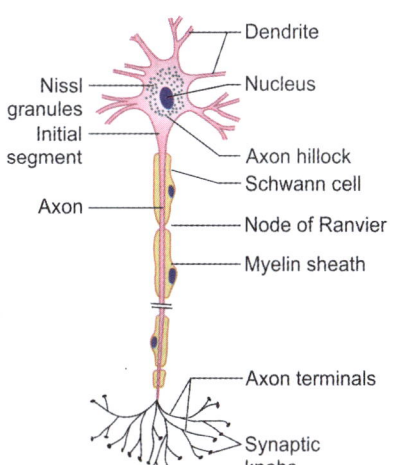

Fig. 6.2: Structure of a motor neuron (multipolar neuron).

Nucleus

Nucleus occupies the central part of soma and usually contains one nucleolus.

Nissl Granules or Nissl Bodies

Nissl granules are present all over the cell body, except axon hillock. They are organelles containing **ribosome** or they are stacks of rough endoplasmic reticulum. The number and size of Nissl granules depend on the functional state of the cell. When the cell is highly active or injured or fatigued, disintegration of Nissl granules occur called **chromatolysis**. The function of Nissl granules is to synthesize the proteins necessary for the neuron.

Mitochondria

Mitochondria are present in the cell body as well as in the axon in plenty. They supply energy for the cell.

Neurofibrils

Neurofibrils are thread-like structures seen in the soma, axon and dendrite. They provide support and shape to the cell.

Lipofuscin

Lipofuscin is a harmless pigment, which is a by-product of neuronal lysosomal activity and its concentration increases as age advances.

PROCESSES OF THE NEURON

The nerve cell processes are **dendrites** and **axon**. Dendrites bring information towards the cell body and hence sensory in function. Unlike the axon hillock, the proximal part of the dendrite contains Nissl granules, endoplasmic reticulum and Golgi apparatus. Axon takes away information from the cell body and hence motor in function. Nerve fiber is a general term for any neuronal process, i.e., dendrite or axon. A **nerve** is a bundle of many nerve fibers in the peripheral nervous system, e.g., ulnar nerve, radial nerve, etc. Most of the nerves have both sensory and motor fibers. A **tract** is a bundle of nerve fibers in the central nervous system, e.g., pyramidal tract.

Nerve fibers, which carry impulses to the central nervous system (CNS), are called **afferent fibers**. Those which carry impulses from the CNS to the periphery are called **efferent fibers**. A pure sensory nerve contains only afferent fibers and a motor nerve contain only efferent fibers. A mixed nerve contains fibers of both types.

Axon

The portion of the cell body from which axon arises is slightly thickened and is called **axon hillock**. Nissl granules, endoplasmic reticulum and Golgi apparatus are absent in the axon hillock. The part of the axon between the axon hillock and the beginning of myelin sheath is called **initial segment**. **Trigger zone** is the junction of the axon hillock and the initial segment. *Impulse or action potential arises in the neuron from the trigger zone or the initial segment in the axon as this part has the lowest threshold of excitation*. In myelinated nerve fibers, the axon is covered by a **myelin sheath** distal to the initial segment. The axon possesses branches known as **collaterals**. The axon and collaterals divide into terminal branches, each ending in a number of **synaptic knobs** or terminal buttons or axon telodendria. These knobs contain vesicles in which the **synaptic transmitters** secreted by nerves are stored. Many neurons contain two or even three neurotransmitters, which may be excitatory or inhibitory to the postsynaptic cell.

The axon cylinder contains axoplasm in the interior. Axoplasm contains mitochondria, neurofibrils, microtubules, vesicles, etc. *Nissl granules are absent in the axon*. Substances synthesized in the cell body are transported by **orthograde transport** or axonal flow to the axon terminals by two systems:

1. **Slow axonal transport system**, which transports materials at a slow speed (1–10 mm/day) and substances are transported in one direction only, i.e., from cell body to axon terminals.
2. **Fast axonal transport system**, which transports substances at a faster speed (200–400 mm/day) with the help of 2 **molecular motors** called **dynein and kinesin**, which are transport proteins.

In **retrograde transport**, where substances are transported in the opposite direction, i.e. from the nerve ending to the cell body, the transport is fast and it occurs through microtubules at a speed of about 200 mm/day. Some materials taken up at the nerve ending like nerve growth factor; used synaptic vesicles, etc. are transported to the cell body by this route. This is also the route by which certain viruses and toxins reach the nerve cell body (rabies, tetanus, etc.).

Distal to the initial segment in most neurons, axon is covered by **myelin sheath**, a protein–lipid complex made up of many layers of cell membrane of **Schwann cells**. Schwann cells are glial cells found along peripheral nerves. Axons covered by myelin sheath are called **myelinated fibers** and others are called **unmyelinated fibers**.

The myelin sheath is absent at the **nodes of Ranvier**. These are gaps in between Schwann cells that are about 1 mm apart. At the node of Ranvier, the axon is covered by a thin sleeve of **basal lamina**. Outer to the basal lamina is the **endoneurium**, the connective tissue layer surrounding the axon. In the CNS, myelination is carried out by **oligodendrocytes**.

Myelination of Neurons

Myelination in the Peripheral Nervous System

The peripheral nerves are the cranial and the spinal nerves. **Myelination or myelinogenesis** means formation of myelin sheath around axon. The **Schwann cells** are responsible for myelination in the peripheral nervous system. The Schwann cell rotates round the axis cylinder about 100 or even more times so that concentric layers of cell membrane are wrapped round the axis cylinder. There is no cytoplasm in between the layers and later these concentric layers fuse to form a lipid-rich membrane called **myelin sheath**. The outermost layer of the Schwann cell forms the **neurilemma**. The nucleus and

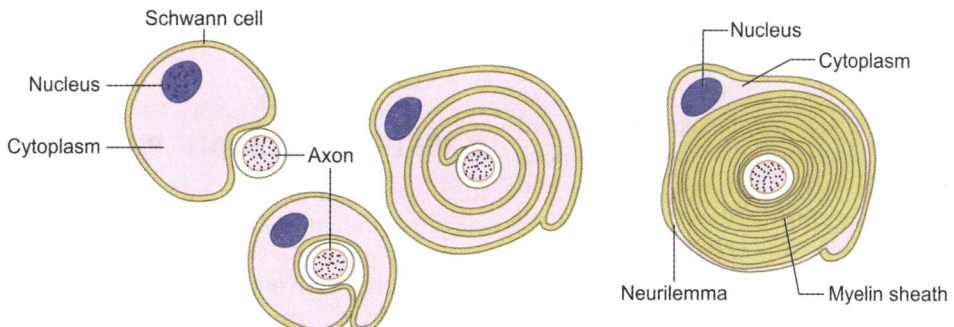

Fig. 6.3: Myelination in a peripheral nerve fiber.

the cytoplasm of the Schwann cell are present between the neurilemma and the myelin sheath **(Fig. 6.3)**. Externally, the Schwann cell is covered by a **basal lamina** and the endoneurium.

Persistence of the basal lamina and endoneurium after nerve injury serves to guide the regenerating axons along the right path.

Sensory fibers start myelination from 4th to 5th month of the intrauterine life. Motor fibers start myelination by 2 months of infancy and continue up to the 2nd year of life. *It is only after the completion of myelination that a neuron becomes fully functional.* As myelination is still in progress during infancy, an infant's responses to stimuli are not as rapid and coordinated as those of an older child.

Myelination in the CNS

Schwann cells are found only in the peripheral nerves. The myelin sheath in the CNS is formed by **oligodendrocytes** (neuroglial cells). Myelination in the spinal cord starts at about the 4th month of intrauterine life and the sensory fibers are myelinated first. The last to be myelinated are the descending motor fibers.

Myelination of brain begins in the basal ganglia by about the 6th month of intrauterine life. At birth, the brain is largely unmyelinated. After birth, corticobulbar, corticospinal, tectospinal and cortico-ponto-cerebellar fibers begin to myelinate. The corticospinal fibers start to myelinate at about 6 months after birth and the process is completed only by the end of the 2nd year.

As oligodendrocytes have several processes, unlike Schwann cells, they can form myelin on different axons. A single oligodendrocyte can form myelin on as many as 60 nerve fibers. Unlike Schwann cells in the peripheral nervous system, oligodendrocytes and their associated axons are not surrounded by a basement membrane. Thus, regeneration after injury is not possible in the axons of CNS. Myelination of axons increases their speed of conduction, but greatly increases their diameter. Motor neurons to muscles and sensory proprioceptive fibers from muscles are heavily myelinated because speed of conduction of impulse is very important in these fibers. Inside the brain, neurons are thinly myelinated or unmyelinated because neurons travel short distances and hence speed is less important. 50% of fibers in the pyramidal tract are unmyelinated.

All mammalian neurons are not myelinated. *Nerve fibers less than 1 mm in diameter are unmyelinated.* In unmyelinated fibers, many axons are buried within a Schwann cell. The unmyelinated fibers in the nervous system are:
1. Postganglionic autonomic fibers
2. Somatic nerves less than 1 mm in diameter

Functions of Myelin

- Myelin sheath forms insulation for the axon. It confines the nerve impulse to individual fibers and thus prevents cross stimulation of adjacent axons.
- Helps in the conduction of impulses at a faster rate
- Helps in regeneration of nerve fiber after injury

Diseases Affecting Myelin Sheath

Normal conduction of action potentials depends on the insulating properties of myelin. So any defect in the myelin sheath can lead to major neurological conditions.

- In an autoimmune disorder called **multiple sclerosis**, there is patchy destruction of myelin in the CNS; herein conduction of impulses is greatly affected in the demyelinated axons. This leads to neurological symptoms like paralysis and altered (paresthesia) or lost sensations. Optic neuritis leads to blurred vision, central scotoma and change in color perception. There will be painful eye movements, dysarthria and dysphagia. Multiple sclerosis can be due to genetic causes or environmental causes. Environmental causes include exposure to viruses such as Epstein-Barr virus and those viruses causing measles, herpes, chickenpox or influenza. Antibodies and white blood cells attack myelin, causing inflammation and injury to the myelin sheath and eventually destroy the nerve that it surrounds. Loss of myelin leads to leakage of K^+ through voltage gated channels leading to hyperpolarization and failure to conduct impulses. The condition is diagnosed by magnetic resonance imaging which reveals multiple scarred areas or plaques in the brain. Corticosteroids and β-interferons suppress inflammation and immune response and thus reduce the severity and slow the progression of the disease.
- A membrane protein called **myelin protein zero (P_0)** is necessary for the compaction of the layers of the myelin sheath. P_0 and a hydrophobic protein PMP22 are components of myelin sheath in the peripheral nervous system. Autoimmune reactions to these proteins cause **Guillain-Barre syndrome**, a peripheral demyelinating neuropathy. Various mutations in the myelin protein genes cause **peripheral neuropathies** that disrupt myelin and cause axonal degeneration, e.g., **Charcot-Marie-Tooth disease.**

Dendrite

Other than axon, neuron has 5–7 processes called dendrites that extend outward from the cell body and arborize extensively. The difference between the axon hillock and the proximal part of the dendrite is that the axon hillock does not contain Nissl granules, endoplasmic reticulum and Golgi apparatus, whereas, the proximal dendrite contains all these structures. In the cerebral and cerebellar cortex, the dendrites have small knobby projections called **dendritic spines**.

Neurons generally have four important zones **(Fig. 6.2)**:
1. A receptive or dendritic zone where potential changes generated in the synapse are integrated. The potential changes may be excitatory postsynaptic potential (EPSP) or inhibitory postsynaptic potential (IPSP).
2. The initial segment in spinal motor neurons or the initial node of Ranvier in cutaneous sensory neurons where propagated impulses or action potentials are generated.
3. An axonal process that transmits propagated impulses to the nerve ending.
4. The nerve endings, where action potentials cause the release of synaptic transmitters.

PROPERTIES OF NERVE FIBERS

- **Excitability** denotes the ease with which an action potential can be produced in the nerve.
- **Conductivity** is the self-propagating process in a nerve, by which an action potential is actively conducted at a constant amplitude and velocity along the axon to the nerve terminal.
- **All or none law**: An adequate stimulus gives a maximum response in a single nerve fiber under a given set of experimental conditions.
- **Refractory period**: During the rising and much of the falling phases of the spike potential, the neuron is refractory to stimulation.
- **Adaptation**: The nerve fiber quickly adapts itself. Due to this property, there is no excitation during the passage of a constant current. Only when the strength is altered or the current is made or broken does excitation takes place.
- **Accommodation**: If a stimulus of stronger strength is applied very slowly to a nerve fiber, there will be no response. Only an abruptly rising strength of current can produce a response.
- **Indefatigability**: Nerve is not fatigued even if it is stimulated repeatedly.

BIOELECTRICAL POTENTIALS

PY1.8: Describe and discuss the molecular basis of resting membrane potential and action potential in excitable tissue.

Most animal cells maintain an electrical potential difference (voltage) across their cell membrane. There are three types of membrane potentials:

1. Resting membrane potential (RMP)
2. Graded potential
3. Action potential (AP)

RESTING MEMBRANE POTENTIAL

Resting membrane potential (RMP) is defined as the electrical potential difference existing *just across* the cell membrane in the resting state of the cell with the interior of the cell negative and the outside positive. It is always denoted by a **minus sign**, signifying that the cytoplasm is electrically negative relative to the extracellular fluid. A cell that exhibits a membrane potential is a **polarized** cell **(Fig. 6.4)**.

The magnitude of RMP varies from tissue to tissue ranging from –9 to –100 mV. RMP of nerve fiber is –70 mV. That is, the potential inside the fiber is 70 millivolts more negative than the potential in the extracellular fluid outside the fiber. It can be measured with an electrode inside and another electrode outside the cell membrane. This type of recording is called **monophasic recording**. Studies were done in the long axons of squid, Loligo (squid giant axon), whose axons are about 1 mm in diameter. Electrophysiological studies in the skeletal muscle fiber were studied in **frog's sartorius muscle**.

Recording of RMP

Monophasic method alone can measure RMP. It is recorded with one electrode inside and another outside the cell membrane connected to a **cathode ray oscilloscope**.

Ionic Basis of RMP or Genesis of RMP or Production of RMP

Two factors are responsible for the production of RMP:
1. Diffusion of ions across the cell membrane
2. Electrogenic pump

Diffusion of Ions Across the Cell Membrane

Diffusion of ions across the cell membrane depends on two factors:
1. Differential concentration of ions across the cell membrane
2. Differential permeability of ions

The composition of the major ions in the intracellular and the extracellular fluid are entirely different **(Table 6.1)**. Initially, there is no potential difference across the cell membrane. K^+ has a **leak channel** and has high permeability and mobility through the membrane. The permeability of the plasma membrane to K^+ is 50–100 times more than that

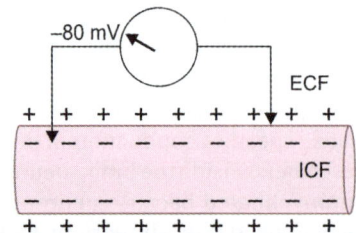

Fig. 6.4: Membrane potential in a polarized cell.

Table 6.1: Distribution of ions across the cell membrane at rest.		
Ion	ICF (mmol/L of H_2O)	ECF (mmol/L of H_2O)
Na^+	15	150
K^+	150	5.5
Cl^-	9	125
Ca^{2+}	0.0001	1.2
Protein anion	65	<5
Mg^{2+}	58	3
HCO_3^-	10	28
PO_4^{3-}	75	4

of sodium. So, K^+ moves from inside to outside according to the concentration gradient. This process is called **efflux** of potassium. This efflux of K^+ upsets the electrical equilibrium both inside and outside the membrane. There are two ways in which this can be prevented:
1. An anion should come along with K^+ to the outside.
2. A cation should come from outside to inside of the membrane.

Na^+ cannot come to the inside because the channel is closed in the resting state of the cell. Ca^{2+} channel is also closed from outside in the resting state. Na ions are subjected to two forces:
1. Concentration gradient
2. Electrical gradient

Therefore, Na^+ come and lines the outside of the membrane. Inside the cell, the anions are Cl^- and protein anion (A^-). Cl^- has to move against a concentration gradient. Protein anions cannot go out because they are very large. So the protein anions come and stay close to the inside of the cell membrane with the cation just outside the membrane, thus creating a charge difference across the membrane called resting membrane potential. It is also called **diffusion potential or potassium potential or equilibrium potential**. Since, the RMP is close to the equilibrium potential for potassium it is also called potassium potential. The equilibrium potential of sodium is calculated to be +60 mV. This is far away from the RMP calculated for an excitable cell (*Refer* Nernst potential Chapter 1).

Further efflux of K^+ stops when the positive charges outside gain sufficient strength to repel the positive ions. The resting membrane potential represents a state of equilibrium at which the driving force for the membrane permeable ions to move down their concentration gradients across the membrane is equal and opposite to the driving force for these ions to move down their electrical gradients.

Role of Electrogenic Pump or Na^+-K^+ ATPase

Na^+ pump is said to be **electrogenic** because it contributes to the negativity of RMP by pumping out 3 Na^+ in exchange for only 2 K^+, thus contributing to the charge difference. Of the total –70 mV RMP in a neuron, only –3 mV is due to the activity of Na^+-K^+ pump. But, the role of sodium pump is very significant because *RMP is maintained constant by sodium pump* although RMP is produced by the exit of potassium ions. Some amount of Na^+ leaks into the cell in the resting state. This excess Na^+ is pumped out against its electrochemical gradient by Na^+-K^+ ATPase so that the RMP of a particular cell is maintained constant. It is proved that there are leak channels for Na^+, through which some amount of Na^+ leaks into the cell in the resting state. This excess Na^+ is pumped out by Na^+-K^+ pump and thus it plays an important role in maintaining the RMP that has already been established by the exit of K^+.

Experimental Evidence to Show that K^+ is Responsible for the Production of RMP

When Na^+ concentration outside the cell was varied, RMP did not change. This shows that sodium has no role in the production of RMP. When K^+ concentration was varied in the extracellular fluid, RMP changed. The change in RMP was proportional to the change in the logarithmic concentration of K^+ outside the cell. If the extracellular level of K^+ is increased (hyperkalemia), the resting potential move closer to the threshold for eliciting an action potential and the neuron become more excitable (the RMP will be less negative). If the extracellular level of K^+ is decreased (hypokalemia), the membrane potential is reduced and the neuron becomes hyperpolarized and less excitable.

Measurement of Resting Membrane Potential

Very small quantities of electrical potential have to be measured. Most of the fibers have very small size. So the electrode should be very small. One electrode has to be introduced into the cell. Another electrode called the indifferent electrode is placed in the extracellular fluid, and the potential difference between the inside and outside of the fiber is measured using an appropriate voltmeter. This *monophasic method alone can measure RMP.*

There are three components for measuring RMP:
1. Electrode
2. Amplifier
3. Recording device

Electrodes

Two electrodes are necessary. The electrode introduced into the interior of the cell is called **ultra- microelectrode or recording electrode**. It has a tip diameter of 0.25 micrometer and a resistance of more than a million Ohms. The other electrode called **indifferent electrode** is placed outside the cell membrane.

Amplifier

The two electrodes are connected to a **biological amplifier** or differential amplifier, which amplifies biological signals alone and unwanted signals will be rejected. The RMP will be amplified. The biological amplifier amplifies potential changes 1000 times or more.

Recording Device

The recording device used is **cathode ray oscilloscope (CRO)**. This device can convert electrical signals into visible record.

CRO consists of a special type of tube with a narrow and a broad end, and vacuum inside the tube. At the narrow end is a cathode. In front of the cathode are two anodes. Cathode and anode are connected to a power supply. When high voltage is applied, cathode is heated and emits electrons.

The principle is **thermionic emission**. Electrons emitted are collimated, focused and brought to a narrow beam by anode. This beam is accelerated towards the fluorescent screen at the broad end of the tube by **accelerating anode** placed behind the screen. When electrons strike the screen, it is seen as a visible spot of light on the screen (**Fig. 6.5**).

Any changes in the potential occurring in the nerve are recorded as vertical deflections of the beam, as it moves across the tube. The screen is graduated in the X- and Y-axes. X-axis represents time, and Y-axis represents the amplitude of the signal. When the two electrodes are outside the cell membrane, there is no deflection and the beam moves only in the horizontal direction. When one electrode is introduced into the cell, there is a downward deflection and so far as the electrode is inside the cell the deflection remains the same (**Fig. 6.6A**).

Stimulus

Stimulus is a sudden change in the environment, which produces a response in the cell depending on the strength of the stimulus. There are different types of stimuli like mechanical, electrical, chemical, thermal, osmotic, etc. Depending on the strength of the stimulus, two types of responses are produced.

1. Local, non-propagated potentials called graded potentials.
2. Propagated potentials called action potentials.

GRADED POTENTIALS

Graded potential or local response is a small deviation from RMP, which is caused by an appropriate stimulus. As the potential is proportional to the strength of the stimulus, it is called graded potential. When the strength of the stimulus is increased, the magnitude of graded potential also increases. Depending on the location and type of stimulus, graded potentials are of different types:

1. Postsynaptic potential (EPSP or IPSP) is seen at the synapse and endplate potential at the neuromuscular junction (*refer* page 80).
2. Receptor potential or generator potential generated during the transduction of sensory stimuli in sensory receptors (*refer* page 763).
3. Electrotonic potential depending on whether the cathode or anode is the stimulating electrode (*refer* page 56).

A graded potential may make the membrane either more polarized, i.e., more negative than the resting potential or less polarized, i.e., less negative than the resting level. Polarization more negative than the resting level is called **hyperpolarization** and polarization less negative than the resting level is referred to as **depolarization**. Graded potentials vary in amplitude depending on the strength of the stimulus. The current formed here is localized, i.e., it spreads along the membrane of the excitable cell only for a few μm with **decrement**, i.e., it is not propagated. Its magnitude decreases with time as well as with distance from the point and time of origin (**Table 6.2**). The distance over which the potential change decreases to 37% of its maximal value is called **length constant or space constant**. For a mammalian nerve or muscle fiber, the length constant is 1–3 mm. Local responses can be added together to get a greater response (refer electrotonic potentials).

ACTION POTENTIAL

Action potential is a sequence of rapidly occurring changes in the membrane potential, i.e., depolarization and repolarization, in an excitable cell, when a stimulus of sufficient strength is applied. The nerve transmits information in the form of nerve impulse called action potential. *Action potential is the universal language of the nervous system.* The size and shape of action potential differ from one excitable tissue to another. For example, in nerve and skeletal muscle fibers, it is a *spike potential*, whereas in ventricular muscle fiber and visceral smooth muscle, it is a *plateau potential*.

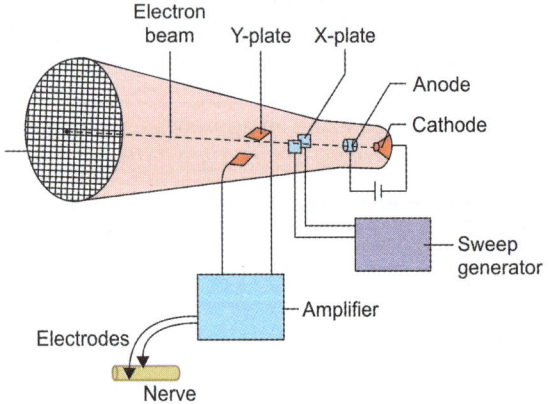

Fig. 6.5: Cathode ray oscilloscope.

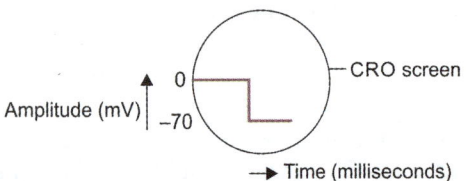

Fig. 6.6A: Resting membrane potential recorded from a nerve fiber on a CRO screen. RMP –70 mV.

Table 6.2: Differences between action potential and graded potential (local response).

S. No.	Action potential	Graded potential (local response)
1.	Always a depolarizing potential	Can be depolarizing or hyperpolarizing potential
2.	Large response with reversal of polarity of membrane potential	Small response with no reversal of polarity
3.	Propagated along the entire length of the excitable cell without decrement	Localized or nonpropagated. It is conducted with decrement (reduction in magnitude) for a very short distance
4.	The size and shape of the action potential remains the same as it travels along the fiber, i.e., AP has a constant amplitude for a given cell	It has variable amplitude, the size of the potential decreases with distance
5.	Obey all or none law, i.e., the size of the AP does not increase with increase in stimulus strength	Does not obey all or none law, the amplitude of graded potential is proportional to strength of stimulus
6.	Exhibit refractory period so cannot be summated	Do not exhibit refractory period so they can be summated
7.	Duration is less, about ½ to 2 milliseconds in a nerve	Duration is much longer, about milliseconds to minutes

Recording of Action Potential

- **Monophasic recording:** One electrode is placed inside and another outside the cell membrane.
- **Biphasic recording:** Both electrodes are placed outside the cell membrane.

Monophasic Action Potential from a Single Nerve Fiber

Excitation occurs at the cathode when a stimulus is applied and it is propagated. **Excitation** denotes the process of producing an action potential in an excitable cell. The impulse or action potential is normally conducted along the axon to the nerve terminals. The electrical events in neurons are rapid and so it is measured in **milliseconds (ms)** and the potential changes being small are measured in **millivolts (mV)**.

Conduction is an active, self-propagating process and the impulse moves along the nerve at a constant amplitude and velocity.

When a stimulus is applied, a brief irregular deflection of the baseline is recorded on the CRO, known as **stimulus artifact (Fig. 6.6B)**. This is due to current leakage from the stimulating electrodes to the recording electrodes. It marks the point of application of the stimulus on the cathode ray screen. This is followed by an isoelectric-potential interval called **latent period**. Latent period ends with the start of action potential. Latent period denotes the time taken by the impulse to travel from the point of stimulation to the recording electrodes. It is directly proportional to the distance between the stimulating and recording electrodes and inversely proportional to the conduction velocity.

Velocity of conduction of impulse in the axon can be calculated if the duration of latent period and distance between the stimulating and recording electrodes are known.

$$\text{Velocity} = \frac{\text{Distance between stimulating and recording electrodes}}{\text{Latent period}}$$

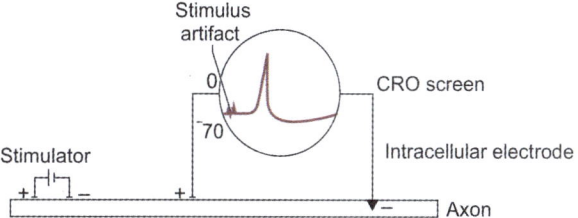

Fig. 6.6B: Monophasic recording from an axon. Note that the baseline starts at –70 mV.

For example, if distance between the electrodes is 5 cm and latent period 0.5 millisecond, then velocity of conduction in the fiber is:

$$\frac{5 \text{ cm}}{0.5 \text{ millisecond}} = 100 \text{ m/sec}$$

Voltage Clamp Technique

Hodgkin and Huxley gave explanation of the ionic basis of action potential in 1950 by using **voltage clamp technique**. Voltage clamp measures currents across cell membrane and is used to understand the functioning of excitable cells. In this technique, the membrane potential can be maintained at a predetermined level of depolarization by passing current across the cell membrane by specialized electronic methods. This clamps the cell membrane at a desired constant voltage called **clamping voltage.** The current-voltage relationships of membrane channels can then be studied. While holding the membrane voltage at a set level, the transmembrane ion currents which are required to maintain that voltage can be measured.

Advantages of voltage clamp technique:
- The duration of action potential is very brief. So, it is impossible to make reliable observation about current flow. In voltage clamp technique, any membrane potential can be maintained for any desired length of time.
- Action potential is an all-or-none phenomenon. So all the events cannot be dissected and studied. In this technique, the membrane potential in millivolts can be clamped at –60 mV, –40 mV, –20 mV, 0 mV, +20 mV, +40 mV and +60 mV.

Ionic Basis of Action Potential

Depolarization

When a stimulus of sufficient strength is applied to a nerve, the nerve becomes active and there is slight opening of sodium channel. This is called **sodium channel activation**. Na⁺ will pass from outside to inside according to electrical and concentration gradient. The potential changes from –70 to a less negative value. As more and more Na⁺ enters the cell, the gates open more and more widely and the potential goes more and more to the positive side setting up a **positive feedback loop**. At a critical voltage of –55 mV, there is sudden wide opening of Na⁺ channel. This critical voltage is called **firing level or threshold potential**. At the firing level, the membrane permeability of Na⁺ is increased to about 5000 times. Gradual change of potential from resting stage to firing level is called **partial or slow depolarization (Fig. 6.7)**.

At the firing level, there is explosive entry of Na⁺ into the cell. The potential goes to the positive side for a brief period. This phase is called **depolarization phase** (the resting cell is said to be in a polarized state). The membrane potential moves towards the equilibrium potential for Na⁺ (+60 mV) but does not reach it during action potential. This is because the increase in Na⁺ conductance is short lived.

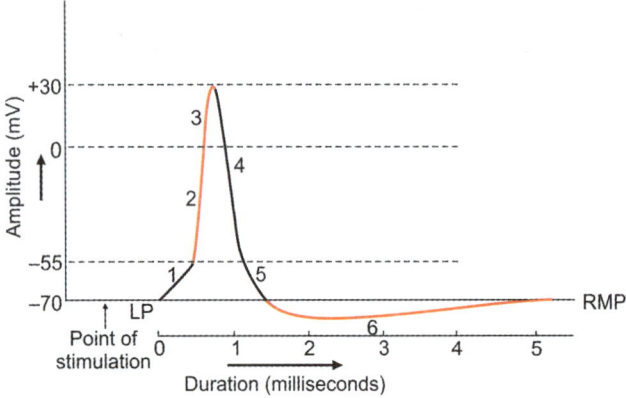

Fig. 6.7: Monophasic recording of nerve action potential latent period (LP). Numbers denote: (1) Slow depolarization; (2) Rapid depolarization; (3) Reversal of polarity; (4) Rapid repolarization; (5) After-depolarization; (6) After-hyperpolarization.

Going of the potential to the positive side is called **reversal of polarity**. The inside becomes positive and outside negative at the point of stimulation. When a sodium channel is completely open, about 20,000 Na⁺ flow across the membrane.

Next change is the closure of inactivation gate of Na⁺ from inside, which is a slow process. Increase in Na⁺ permeability is short lived. The reasons are:

❖ As soon as the activation gate of Na⁺ starts opening, the inactivation gate starts to close. The opening of the activation gate of Na⁺ is quick, while the closure of the inactivation gate is a delayed process. So, for a brief period, the channel is fully opened.

❖ Another reason is that as Na+ enters the cell, the interior becomes positively charged and this resists further entry of Na⁺ **(Fig. 6.8A)**.

Along with Na⁺ channels, Ca²⁺ channels also open during cellular excitation, allowing calcium ions to enter the cell from outside according to concentration gradient. Opening of calcium channels is a very slow process and the role of calcium channel is more important in cardiac and smooth muscle cells.

Repolarization

Repolarization is initiated by the closure of Na⁺ channel from inside by the inactivation gate. The opening of K⁺ channels from inside of the membrane coincides with the closure of the inactivation gate of Na⁺. Both these processes contribute to repolarization of the membrane. According to the concentration gradient, K⁺ goes from inside to outside and causes rapid repolarization. Towards the end of the repolarization phase, the process is slowed down and this phase is called **after-depolarization or negative after-potential**. This is due to the accumulation of K⁺ just outside the cell membrane, thereby slowing down the efflux of K⁺ **(Fig. 6.8B)**. The voltage gated K⁺ channels bring the action potential to an end and cause closure of their gates through a **negative feedback process.** The repolarization phase overshoots to the negative side to some extent and this is called **after-hyperpolarization or positive after-potential**. This is because it takes a longer time for the K⁺ gates to close.

At the end of action potential, the Na⁺-K⁺ pump will function to re-establish the concentration gradient because

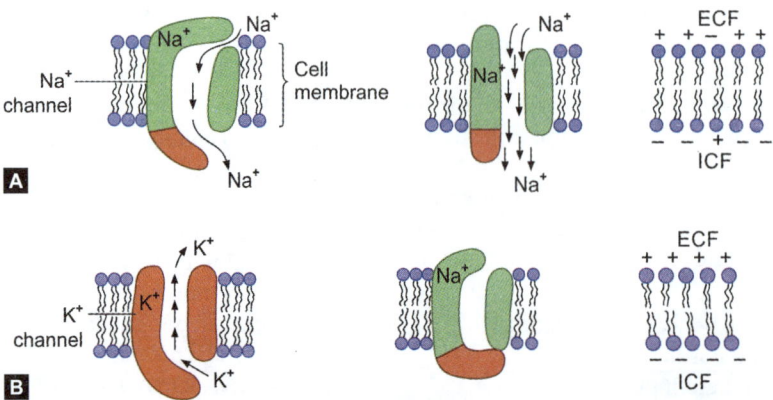

Figs. 6.8A and B: Ionic basis of action potential: (A) Depolarization; (B) Repolarization.

there is some excess Na⁺ inside the cell and excess K⁺ outside the cell membrane. Action potential in nerve fiber is also called **spike potential** because it resembles a spike.

As long as the inactivation gate of Na⁺ remains closed, the membrane cannot be activated further. After the repolarization of the membrane, the inactivation gate opens and comes to the resting state. Then the membrane becomes excitable and another action potential can be produced. That is the reason why *one action potential must be completed before a second one can be induced*. Action potential cannot be fused or superimposed on each other. This is the reason for the lack of responsiveness of an excitable cell during an action potential referred to as the *refractory period*.

> *Although Na⁺ enters the nerve cell and K⁺ leaves it during an action potential, very few ions actually move across the membrane. It has been estimated that only 1 in 100,000 K⁺ cross the membrane during repolarization to change the membrane potential from +30 millivolt (peak of action potential) to –70 mV (resting potential).*

Experimental Evidence to Show that Na⁺ is Responsible for the Production of Action Potential

Decreasing the extracellular sodium concentration decreases the size of action potential, but has little effect on the RMP.

Changes in Na⁺ and K⁺ Conductance during the Action Potential (Fig. 6.9)

Inference from the **Figure 6.9** is listed below.
- Sodium conductance increases with the start of depolarization phase.
- It also starts decreasing before depolarization is complete.
- Sodium conductance comes back to the resting level when repolarization is almost complete.
- Potassium conductance starts increasing when sodium conductance starts falling.
- Potassium conductance comes back to the resting level only towards the end of after-hyperpolarization.

Intensity Discrimination by the Sensory System

Although action potentials are of the same size, the intensity of the stimulus can be appreciated by the sensory system due to variation: (a) in the frequency of impulses, and (b) in the number of sensory neurons activated by the stimulus.

Biphasic Recording of Action Potential

If both the recording electrodes are placed on the surface of the axon, there is no potential difference between them at rest. So the graph in the cathode ray screen starts from zero baseline. In monophasic recording, graph starts from –70 mV.

When the nerve is stimulated and an impulse is conducted past the two electrodes, a characteristic sequence of potential changes occur called biphasic action potential (**Fig. 6.10**):
1. Activity has not reached the recording electrode.
2. Impulse has reached the first recording electrode, which becomes negative with respect to the other causing a positive deflection.
3. Action potential spreads between the two recording electrodes. Both the electrodes become positive, and graph reaches the baseline followed by an isoelectric interval. The duration of the isoelectric interval is proportionate to the speed of conduction of the nerve and the distance between the recording electrodes. When conduction velocity is very high and the distance between the two electrodes is very small, there will be no isoelectric segment.
4. Action potential has reached the second recording electrode, which becomes negative with respect to the first and a downward deflection is produced.
5. Action potential has passed the region where recording electrodes are placed, and the graph comes to the baseline.

Recording of Action Potential in a Mixed Nerve

Peripheral nerves are made up of many axons bound together in a fibrous envelope called epineurium. Potential changes recorded extracellularly from such nerves represent the algebraic sum of the action potentials of many axons. The pattern of action potential obtained from a mixed nerve is called **compound action potential or multipeaked action potential**. This pattern is obtained when recording electrodes are kept at a greater distance from the stimulating electrodes (**Fig. 6.11**). The stimulus that produces excitation of all the axons in a mixed nerve is called the maximal stimulus.

The different peaks in the compound action potential represent action potentials obtained from different nerve fibers in the mixed nerve, which have different conduction velocity and different threshold of excitation. The fastest conducting fibers produce the first peak and the rest by those,

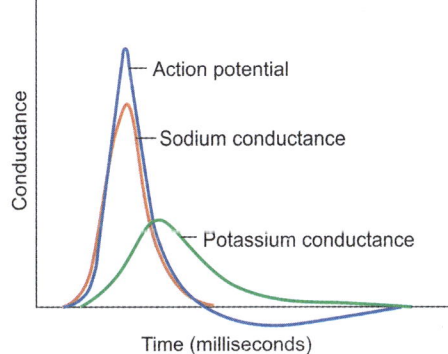

Fig. 6.9: Changes in sodium and potassium conductance during an action potential in nerve.

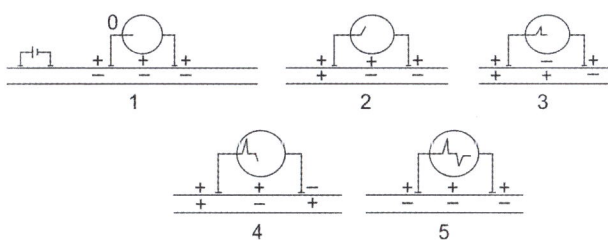

Fig. 6.10: Biphasic recording of action potential from an axon. Note that the baseline starts at zero potential since there is no potential difference between the electrodes at rest.

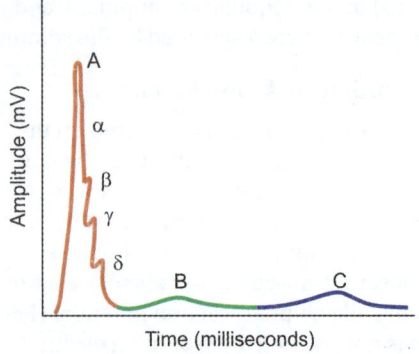

Fig. 6.11: Compound action potential.

which are having conduction velocities lesser and lesser, respectively. There are three main waves in compound action potential recording. They are A, B and C waves. **A wave** has four subunits—α, β, γ and δ waves **(Fig. 6.11)**.

'A' wave represents activity in myelinated axons and 'C' wave in unmyelinated axons. The 'B' wave represents activity in both types of nerve fibers.

Clinical Importance of Action Potential

ECG, EMG, ERG, EEG, etc., are basically action potentials.

■ EXCITABILITY

Cells which have the ability to be electrically excited by electrical, chemical or mechanical stimuli resulting in the generation of action potentials are referred to as **excitable cells**. Examples are neurons, skeletal, smooth and cardiac muscle cells. *Excitability of a tissue is the ease with which excitation or action potentials can be produced.* In order to produce an action potential, the membrane potential should reach the firing level from resting level. Nearer the resting membrane potential to firing level, greater will be the excitability.

Role of Different Ions on the Excitability of Excitable Tissues

- When the concentration of Na^+ in the extracellular fluid (ECF) increases, there is increase in excitability and the amplitude of action potential increases.
- An increase in Ca^{2+} concentration in the ECF decreases the excitability. This is because Ca^{2+} is a **membrane stabilizer** and when its concentration is increased in the ECF, Ca^{2+} binds with the gate of Na^+ channel making it more difficult to open. The ease with which RMP changes to firing level is excitability. So, when Ca^{2+} is increased, the Na^+ channel opens slowly, thus decreasing the excitability.
- When Ca^{2+} concentration in the ECF is decreased; the excitability of the neuron and muscle cells is increased. This is by decreasing the amount of depolarization necessary to initiate the changes in the Na^+ and K^+ conductance that produce the action potential. This is the cause for tetany in hyperventilation, during which,

the ionic calcium level falls due to alkalosis, which leads to increase in excitability.
- When K^+ concentration is decreased in ECF, there is a decrease in excitability. The reason is that when K^+ concentration outside decreases, the concentration gradient of K^+ across the membrane is more and so more of K^+ goes out causing more negativity inside or hyperpolarization.
- When K^+ concentration is increased in ECF, there is increase in excitability due to less negativity inside the cell and the RMP moves closer to the threshold of excitation.

Characteristics of the Electrical Stimulus Used for Excitation

Commonly used stimulus in experimental studies is electrical. A special type of stimulus is used called **square wave pulse** from an electronic stimulator. The number of pulses in 1 sec is frequency. Strength and duration of the pulse can be varied. The stimulus should be of sufficient strength and duration to produce an action potential.

According to strength, stimuli are divided into:
- Threshold stimulus
- Sub-threshold stimulus
- Supra-threshold stimulus
- Maximal stimulus
- Supra-maximal stimulus
- **Threshold stimulus:** The strength of stimulus is just sufficient to bring the RMP to firing level and produce an action potential.
- **Sub-threshold stimulus:** The strength is less than the threshold stimulus. Although it does not produce an action potential, it brings the membrane potential nearer to the firing level. This state of the cell is called local excitatory state or local response (refer local response).
- **Supra-threshold stimulus:** The strength of stimulus is more than the threshold value. It will not produce a further increase in the amplitude of action potential. Inference is that the function of stimulus is just to bring the membrane potential to the firing level. Once firing level is reached, the rest occur automatically. This phenomenon is called **all-or-none phenomenon**.

All-or-none law states that a stimulus capable of producing an action potential will produce the maximum possible amplitude of action potential. All-or-none law is applicable only to a **single nerve fiber or cell**. When a mixed nerve is stimulated, it will not obey all-or-none law. Similarly, a single skeletal muscle fiber and not the whole muscle will obey all-or-none law.
- **Maximal stimulus:** It is that strength of the stimulus, which will excite all the axons in a mixed nerve. A number of nerve fibers, which differ in the threshold of excitation, are present in a mixed nerve. A low threshold of excitation means greater excitability. As the strength of the stimulus applied to a mixed nerve is increased gradually, the fibers with least threshold of excitation will get excited first and slowly more fibers with greater threshold of excitation will

be stimulated and finally, at a particular strength, all the fibers of the nerve will be stimulated and this strength is called maximal stimulus.
- **Supra-maximal stimulus:** The strength is more than maximal stimulus and it has no additional effect.

Duration of the Stimulus

Threshold strength should be of sufficient duration to produce an action potential. Strength is inversely proportional to duration of application of stimulus, i.e., **strength ∝ 1/duration.**

As the strength is increased, it needs to be applied for a less duration. If the strength is low, it should be applied for a longer period of time to produce an action potential.

Strength-Duration Curve or Excitability Curve

PY3.17: Describe strength-duration curve.

Threshold intensity is the minimal intensity of the stimulating current which when applied for a given duration will just produce an action potential. The threshold intensity varies with the duration of application of stimulus. The relation between the strength and the duration of a threshold stimulus is called **strength-duration curve.** Strength-duration curve is plotted to study the response of a nerve when the strength and duration of the stimulus are changed **(Fig. 6.12).**

There is a minimum strength of the stimulus below which it will not be effective although applied for infinite duration of time. There is also a minimum duration below which the strongest stimulus will not be effective.
- **Rheobase:** The minimum threshold strength, which can produce an action potential, is called rheobase.
- **Utilization time:** Duration for which rheobase strength should be applied to produce an action potential is called utilization time.
- **Chronaxie:** Duration for which twice the rheobase strength has to be applied to produce an action potential is called chronaxie. Chronaxie is a measure of the excitability of the tissue. Greater the chronaxie, lesser will be the excitability.

Values of Chronaxie for Different Tissues
- Nerve fiber—0.1 millisecond
- Skeletal muscle fiber—0.25-1 milliseconds
- Cardiac muscle—1-3 milliseconds.

Rate of rise of strength of the stimulus is important in producing an action potential. Slowly rising currents fail to produce action potential in nerve because the nerve adapts to the applied stimulus. This is called **adaptation**. *Only an abruptly rising strength of current can produce an action potential.*

Reasons
- When strength is gradually increased, the inside gate of sodium closes, while the outside gate opens. This is voltage inactivation. So, the membrane potential does not reach the firing level and an action potential does not occur. The nerve adapts to the applied stimulus. This is **accommodation**.
- When depolarization is produced slowly, the opening of potassium channels balances the gradual opening of Na⁺ channels. Thus, the potential does not reach the firing level.

Refractory Period

Refractory period is the period during which the excitability of excitable tissue is decreased. During the rising and much of the falling phases of the spike potential, the neuron is refractory to stimulation **(Fig. 6.13)**.

Refractory period is divided into:
1. Absolute refractory period (ARP)
2. Relative refractory period

Absolute Refractory Period

Absolute refractory period (ARP) is the period during which, the strongest stimulus cannot produce an action potential. It extends from firing level to 1/3rd of repolarization. ARP is due to voltage inactivation of Na⁺ channels. The inactivation gates of Na⁺ channels close soon after the activation gates open. Once the sodium channels are inactivated, the membrane must be repolarized towards the normal RMP before the

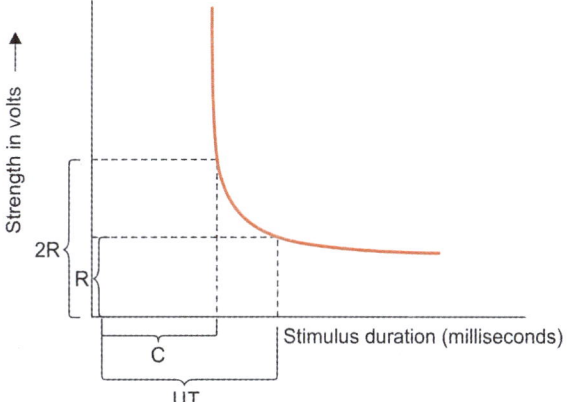

Fig. 6.12: Strength-duration curve.
(R: rheobase strength; UT: utilization time)

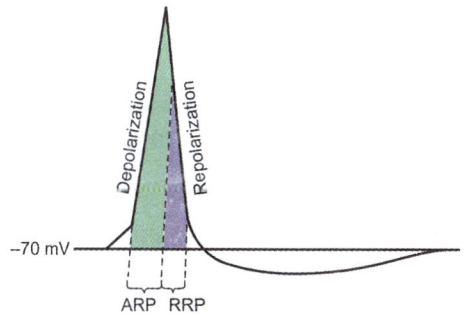

Fig. 6.13: Nerve action potential showing refractory period.
(ARP: absolute refractory period; RRP: relative refractory period)

channels can be reopened. After the repolarization of the membrane, the inactivation gate open and comes to the resting state. Refractory period makes a continuous excitatory state of a nerve impossible and limits the frequency of the impulses.

In large diameter axon, ARP is about 0.4 millisecond (ms), i.e., the nerve can transmit 2500 impulses/sec. In small diameter fibers, ARP is 4 ms and so they can transmit only 250 impulses/sec. Thus, depending on the duration of absolute refractory period, the frequency of action potentials can vary. *We are able to differentiate between different types of stimuli of varying intensity due to the difference in the frequencies of action potentials.*

Relative Refractory Period

Relative refractory period is the period during which, a stronger than normal stimulus can produce excitation. It extends from 1/3rd of repolarization to the start of after-depolarization. Throughout the relative refractory period, the conductance of potassium is elevated and this opposes the depolarization of the membrane. Furthermore, during this period, some Na$^+$ channels are still voltage inactivated. So, a stronger than normal stimulus is required to open the critical number of sodium channels needed to produce an action potential.

In the after-depolarization phase, excitability of the tissue is increased or threshold is decreased.

During after-hyperpolarization, excitability is decreased because membrane potential is more negative inside, i.e., it is farther away from the firing level.

Electrotonic Potentials

Although sub-threshold stimulus does not produce an action potential, it has an effect on the membrane potential. Recording electrodes are used to measure the potential difference near the anode and the cathode and thus can study the potentials produced. It is seen that a depolarizing potential is produced at the cathode called **catelectrotonic potential**, and a hyperpolarizing potential called **anelectrotonic potential** is recorded at the anode. Cathode is the stimulating electrode. Both catelectrotonic and anelectrotonic potentials are localized or non-propagated.

When the cathodal stimulation is great enough to produce about 15 mV of depolarization, i.e., when the membrane potential reaches –55 mV, a propagated action potential occur (Fig. 6.14).

CONDUCTION OF NERVE IMPULSE OR PROPAGATION OF ACTION POTENTIAL

Conduction through an Unmyelinated Axon

The principal function of neuron is to transmit nerve impulse in the form of action potential. Conduction of impulse is an active and self-propagating phenomenon.

Once an action potential is produced, it spreads automatically. *Group C fibers are unmyelinated fibers.*

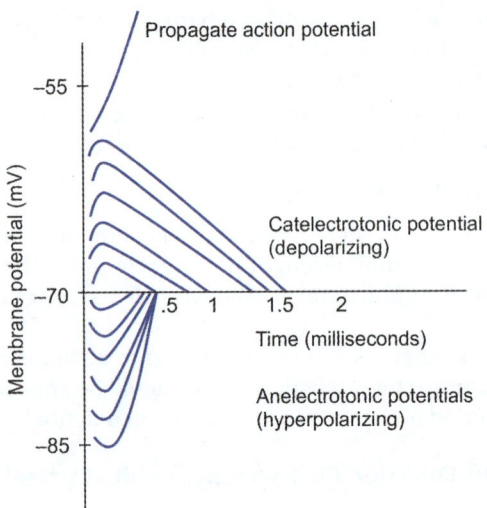

Fig. 6.14: Electrotonic potentials.

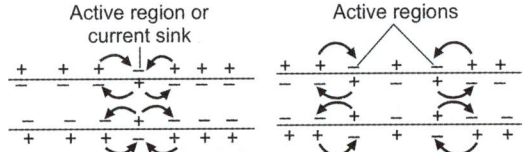

Fig. 6.15: Conduction of nerve impulse through an unmyelinated axon showing local circuit current flow.

The region where excitation is produced in the axon is called **active region**. Outside the membrane, current flows from the neighboring inactive region into the active region, whereas inside the membrane, current flows from active to inactive region. Active region is also called **current sink** (Fig. 6.15). This type of circular current flow is called **local circuit current flow or electrotonic conduction**. The current flow from inside to outside at the two neighboring areas will open up the sodium channels at these points and action potentials are produced. Neighboring regions become active regions and the process is repeated by setting a series of local circuit current flow and action potential spread throughout the membrane.

At the same time, repolarization also starts at the point of stimulation and spreads in both directions. If the axon is stimulated at the center, impulses travel in both directions. Conduction towards the effector organ is called **orthodromic conduction**, and conduction towards the cell body is called **antidromic conduction**. Once initiated, a moving impulse does not depolarize the area behind it to the firing level because this area is in the refractory period. In the intact body, action potentials generated at the **initial segment** will move only in one direction, i.e., towards its termination. An antidromic impulse will fail to pass the first synapse because synapses unlike axons permit conduction in one direction only.

Conduction in a Myelinated Nerve Fiber

Myelin is an effective insulator and current flow through it is negligible. When the nerve is stimulated in the center,

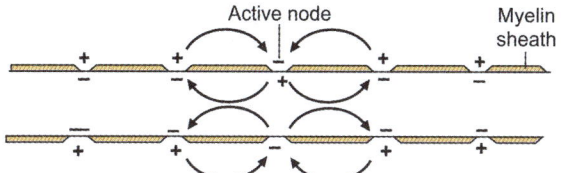

Fig. 6.16: Conduction of nerve impulse in a myelinated axon showing saltatory conduction.

action potential is generated only at the node of Ranvier. Here, instead of active region it is called as **active node**. From neighboring inactive nodes, current will flow into the active nodes outside the membrane and from active node to inactive node inside the membrane, thus setting up a local circuit current flow **(Fig. 6.16)**.

At the two inactive nodes, current flow from inside to outside will open up sodium channels and action potentials are produced at the two neighboring nodes. The process is repeated and impulse is conducted by jumping from one node to another, and this type of conduction in a myelinated fiber is called **saltatory conduction** (saltare means to leap). Saltatory conduction occurs in both the peripheral and central nervous system.

Merits of Saltatory Conduction

- In myelinated nerve fiber, only the nodes are depolarized. In unmyelinated fiber, it is point-to-point conduction. So, conduction through myelinated fiber is 50–100 times faster than in unmyelinated fiber.
- Saltatory conduction is also more energy efficient. As only small regions of the membrane depolarize, there is minimal inflow of sodium and less ATP is used by sodium pump to maintain the RMP.
- Also the large increase in membrane resistance due to myelin sheath minimizes loss of current across the leaky axonal membrane and forces the current to flow longitudinally along the inside of the fiber. *In an autoimmune demyelinating disease like multiple sclerosis, the myelin is lost progressively and there will be loss of membrane resistance. As a result, K+ leaks through voltage-gated channels leading to hyperpolarization. There will be failure of conduction of action potentials leading to weakness.*

CLASSIFICATION OF NERVE FIBERS

Depending on Conduction Velocity and Fiber Diameter by Erlanger and Gasser (Table 6.3)

Erlanger and Gasser divided mammalian nerve fibers into A, B and C groups, further subdividing A group into α, β, γ and δ fibers. In **Table 6.3**, the various fiber types are listed with their diameters, conduction velocity and functions.

Numerical Classification of Sensory Nerve Fibers

Numerical classification of sensory nerve fibers is shown in **Table 6.4**.

Table 6.3: Erlanger and Gasser classification of nerve fibers.

Fiber type	Function	Diameter (µm)	Conduction velocity (m/sec)
Aα	Proprioception, somatic motor	12–20	70–120
Aβ	Touch, pressure	5–12	30–70
Aγ	Motor to muscle spindle	3–6	15–30
Aδ	Pricking pain, cold crude touch	2–5	12–30
B	Preganglionic autonomic fibers	<3	3–15
C-dorsal root	Burning pain, temperature, reflex responses	0.4–1.2	0.5–2
C-sympathetic	Postganglionic sympathetic fibers	0.3–1.3	0.7–2.3

Table 6.4: Numerical classification of sensory nerve fibers.

Number	Origin	Fiber type
Ia	Muscle spindle (annulospiral ending)	Aα
Ib	Golgi tendon organ	Aβ
II	Muscle spindle (flower spray ending), touch, pressure	Aγ
III	Pricking pain, cold receptors	Aδ
IV	Burning pain, temperature	C-dorsal root

Classification Depending on Myelination

- Myelinated (medullated)
- Unmyelinated (non-medullated)

Functional Classification (Fig. 6.17)

- Sensory
- Motor

Factors Influencing the Velocity of Conduction in a Nerve Fiber

- **Myelination**: Myelinated fibers conduct impulses 50–100 times faster than unmyelinated fibers. The high conduction velocity produces reflexes that are fast enough to avoid dangerous stimuli.
- **Fiber diameter**: Greater the diameter of the fiber, greater will be the velocity of conduction of action potentials. This is because the internal resistance of the axoplasm is inversely related to the internal cross sectional area of the axon. As the radius increases, the axoplasm along the length of the nerve fiber becomes less resistant to conduction.
- **pH**: Increase in pH within physiological limits increases the velocity of conduction.
- **Temperature**: Increase in the temperature within physiological limits increases the velocity of conduction. Cold decreases the conduction velocity. Application of ice over the injured area reduces pain by decreasing the velocity of conduction through the pain fibers.
- **Anesthetics**: Decrease the velocity of conduction.

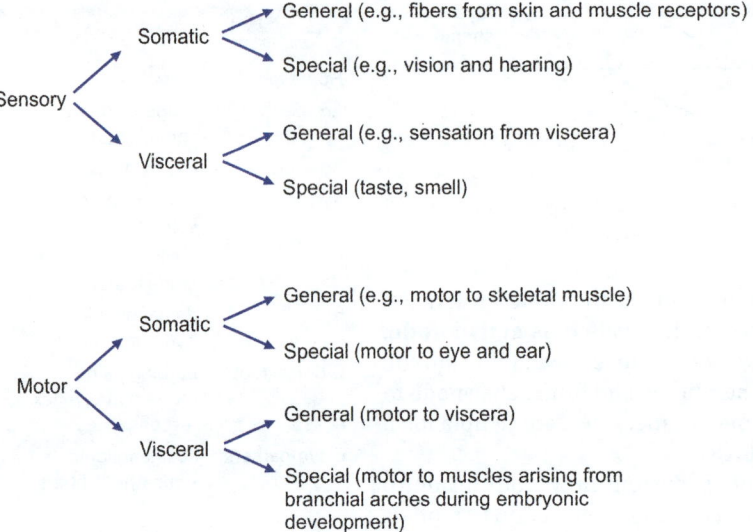

Fig. 6.17: Functional classification of nerve fibers.

Effect of Hypoxia, Pressure and Anesthetics on Various Classes of Fibers in Peripheral Nerves

B-fibers are most susceptible to **hypoxia** and C-fibers least. **Pressure** on a nerve can cause loss of conduction in large diameter motor, touch and pressure fibers while pain sensation remains relatively intact. There will be numbness of the hand in individuals who sleep with their arms under their head because A-fibers are affected. **Local anesthetics** depress transmission in unmyelinated group C nociceptive fibers first. This is followed by sequential loss of sensitivity to temperature, touch and deep pressure. Motor fibers are the most resistant to the actions of local anesthetics. Local anesthetics like procaine, lidocaine, etc., can act by blocking the opening of voltage-gated sodium channels so that pain impulses do not reach the central nervous system.

NERVE INJURY

> **PY3.3:** Describe the degeneration and regeneration in peripheral nerves.

Types of Nerve Injury

Peripheral nerves include 12 pairs of cranial nerves and 31 pairs of spinal nerves. A nerve can get damaged by various means:
- Transection
- Crush injury
- Injected toxins or neurotoxic drugs like quinine and tetracycline
- Medical conditions like leprosy, diabetes mellitus
- Radiation

Classification of Nerve Injury

Nerve injury is classified into three types according to Seddon (1944). They are:
- **Neuropraxia**—occurs due to minor nerve stretch or pressure causing ischemic injury to the nerve. It results in conduction block without causing any structural damage to the nerve. Recovery occurs spontaneously within a few weeks and is complete.
- **Axonotmesis**—occurs due to excessive stretch, crush injury, etc. to a nerve. The basal lamina of Schwann cells and other sheaths are all intact even though axons are damaged. It results in Wallerian degeneration. Nerve regeneration is easier because of the intact nerve sheaths but may take many months. Complete recovery may not occur.
- **Neurotmesis**—occurs as a result of penetrating injury to the nerve. Here, both the nerve and the nerve sheaths are disrupted due to complete section of the nerve trunk. Wallerian degeneration occurs. Spontaneous recovery is not possible and nerve repair is required.

Depending on the extent of injury, nerve injury is classified into two types:
1. **Mild injury**, e.g., a nerve subjected to pressure for a long time, temporary cessation of blood supply to a nerve.
2. **Severe injury**, e.g., crush injury, cut injury.

RESPONSE OF NEURONS TO INJURY

Injury to the Nerve Cell Body

Severe damage of the nerve cell body leads to degeneration of the entire neuron. The tissue macrophages remove the debris and the local fibroblasts replace the neuron with scar tissue.

Effect of Cutting a Peripheral Nerve

When a nerve is cut, it will have two parts; a **proximal part** attached to the cell body and a **distal part** not attached to the cell body. Changes mainly occur in the cell body and in the distal stem. Changes may or may not occur in the proximal stem. Degeneration in the distal part is called **anterograde degeneration** and that in the proximal part is called **retrograde degeneration**.

Axon is a part of the neuron and it is the cell body that maintains the structural and functional integrity of the axon. All necessary proteins responsible for maintaining the integrity of the axon are synthesized in the cell body and are transported along the axon by means of **axoplasmic flow.** This is the reason for the changes in the distal stem (Wallerian degeneration) when a nerve degenerates.

■ INJURY TO THE AXON

When an axon is bisected completely, certain physical and chemical changes occur in the nerve. Changes occur in two stages **(Figs. 6.18A to C):**
1. Stage of degeneration
2. Stage of regeneration

Stage of Degeneration

If the axon is injured, degenerative changes will occur in the distal segment, proximal segment and in the cell body.

Changes in the Cell Body (Figs. 6.18A to C)

❖ 24–48 hours after injury there will be disintegration of Nissl granules into fine dust referred to as **chromatolysis.** Degree of chromatolysis is more in motor neurons.
❖ Golgi apparatus fragments and decreases in number.
❖ The cell body swells up and becomes rounded due to increased fluid content.
❖ The neurofibrils disappear and nucleus becomes displaced towards the cell margin.
❖ Withdrawal of the synaptic terminals from the cell body and dendrites of the injured neuron or its separation from the cell by the interposition of a glial cell (synaptic stripping).
❖ Sometimes, the nucleus may be completely extruded out of the cell, resulting in death of the nerve cell.

Changes in the Distal Segment or Wallerian Degeneration (Anterograde Degenerative Changes)

Degenerative changes occurring in the distal end of the injured neuron are referred to as **Wallerian degeneration.** This was described by **Sir Augustus Waller** and hence the name. The changes spread distally from the site of lesion and include its termination.

1. Within 24 hours of injury, the axon become swollen and fragments into short lengths. The entire axon gets destroyed within a week.
2. Within 10 days, the myelin sheath disintegrates and oily droplets appear within the Schwann cell cytoplasm. Later the droplets get extruded from the Schwann cell and are subsequently phagocytosed by tissue macrophages. Enlargements appear along the myelin sheath, giving it a beaded appearance. Within 30 days, the myelin is denatured chemically.
3. At the site of injury, the nucleus of Schwann cells divides rapidly and form parallel cords of cells within the persisting basement membrane. These cells secrete enzymes, which accelerate myelin degeneration.
4. Within 3 months, macrophages from the endoneurium invade the injured area and phagocytose the degenerating myelin sheath and axon fragments. Only the endoneural tube or the neurilemmal sheath and the contained cords of Schwann cells are left behind **(Figs. 6.18A to C).** This is referred to as **band fiber.**
5. Up to 3 days after injury, the distal segment can conduct impulses, but changes in the action potential occur within 2 days. After 5 days, there is complete loss of conduction of action potential.

Chemical destruction of myelin lasts for 8–32 days after injury. It includes hydrolysis of myelin sheath and the products are cerebroside, sphingomyelin, cholesterol esters and fatty acids. Free cholesterol completely disappears.

If regeneration does not occur, the axon and the Schwann cells will be replaced by fibrous tissue produced by local fibroblasts.

Wallerian degeneration can be demonstrated by **Marchi technique.** The degenerated nerve fiber takes up a black color after staining.

Changes in the Proximal Segment

Change in the proximal stem is similar to the change in the distal cut end and is called **retrograde degeneration.** The changes in the proximal segment extend only up to the first node of Ranvier or up to the nearest collateral. Retrograde

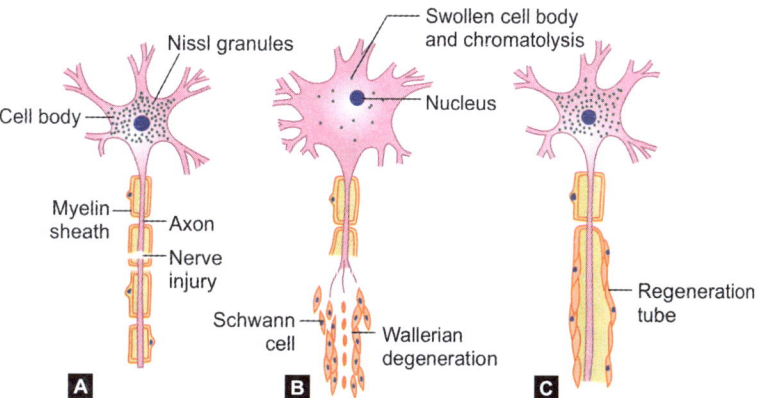

Figs. 6.18A to C: Degeneration and regeneration in an injured nerve fiber in peripheral nervous system: (A) Injured neuron; (B) Changes in the cell body and distal segment; (C) Regeneration.

degeneration occurring in a neuron after its axon is cut is due to deficiency of the trophic factors that are derived from the target organs at the distal end of the axon.

Stage of Regeneration

Mammalian neurons have very limited powers of regeneration. By 6 months of age, all neurons lose their ability to divide.

Conditions for Regeneration in an Injured Nerve

- Regeneration of a nerve fiber occurs only if the neurilemma and endoneurium are intact.
- Regeneration is not possible if the gap between the cut ends is too large, i.e., more than 3 mm.
- It is not possible for neurons in the central nervous system to regenerate (reasons are given below).
- Regeneration is also not possible if nucleus is extruded from the cell.
- Regeneration is not possible, if the cut ends of the nerve are displaced, i.e., if they are not in the same line.
- Sensory fibers regenerate faster than the motor fibers.
- If a mixed nerve is completely cut, chances of recovery are less because of the incorrect destination of the regenerating fibers.
- Regeneration is difficult if there is infection at the site of wound.

It is not possible for neurons in the central nervous system to regenerate because of the following reasons:

- CNS myelin is a potent inhibitor of axonal growth.
- The CNS axons have no neurilemmal sheath or endoneural tubules to guide the regenerating axons. Oligodendrocytes have no basement membrane, whereas Schwann cells have a basement membrane.
- Failure of oligodendrocyte to form cell cords to bridge the gap at the site of injury through which the axon can regenerate. At the site of injury, Schwann cells in the peripheral nerves differentiate into thin elongated cells that can bridge up the gap up to 3 cm.
- Formation of scar tissue at the site of injury by astrocyte proliferation, activation of microglia, scar formation, inflammation and invasion of immune cells create an inappropriate environment for regeneration in the CNS.
- Deficiency of nerve growth factors like **laminins and neurotrophins** that are needed for regeneration.
- Production of nerve growth-inhibiting factors by neuroglial cells inhibits regeneration in CNS.

If the conditions are favorable for regeneration, it begins about 20 days after the injury and is almost complete by 80 days.

Regenerative Changes in the Cell Body

First change is reappearance of Nissl granules and Golgi apparatus. Cell regains its normal size and nucleus returns to the central position. Repair of the cell body occurs even if the axon does not regenerate **(Figs. 6.18A to C)**.

Changes in the Distal Segment

- The Schwann cells on either side of the injured site multiply by mitosis and grow towards each other and form a **regeneration tube** or ghost tube across the cut end. They can bridge up the gap up to 3 cm.
- Hundreds of neurofibrils start growing from the tip of the axis cylinder (central axon) of the proximal stem called **regenerative sprouting or axonal spouting**. This results from growth-promoting factors secreted by Schwann cells that attract axons toward the distal stump. The neurofibrils grow at a rate of 3–4 mm/day towards the distal stem. There are inhibitory factors present in the perineurium that inhibit the neurofibrils from leaving the nerve.
- 2–3 weeks after the injury, the regeneration tube contains a number of developing neurofibrils. Eventually, one single fibril grows towards the distally located receptors or effectors (muscle or gland).
- This neurofibril will increase in diameter and myelin sheath starts appearing in approximately 15 days. Myelination is completed by 1 year. Final diameter attained is 80–85% of normal.
- Once the regenerated axon reaches its target, a new functional connection (e.g., neuromuscular junction) is formed.
- Sensory or motor connections are re-established within 80 days of injury. Although anatomical regeneration is complete, functional recovery occurs only after a long period. Full recovery is not possible for example; fine motor control may be permanently impaired.

Administering **neurotrophins** like nerve growth factor can accelerate regeneration. Neurotrophins are proteins synthesized in neurons, muscles, glands, Schwann cells and astrocytes, which help in the neuronal development, growth, survival and repair of neurons. Commercial preparation of nerve growth factor is extracted from snake venom. Regeneration can also be accelerated if the cut ends are approximated surgically. Use of non-steroidal anti-inflammatory drugs (NSAIDs) like ibuprofen can overcome the factors that inhibit axonal growth following injury.

There is a better chance of regeneration in crush injury than in cut injury as the neurilemmal sheath and endoneurium are intact.

Signs of Regeneration

- **Tinel's sign:** On gently tapping over the course of the nerve from distal to proximal part, a sensation of current or hyperesthesia is felt in the area of the skin supplied by the injured nerve. A distal progression of the level at which this sign is elicited suggests regeneration.
- **Motor examination:** When a peripheral nerve undergoes regeneration, muscles supplied nearest to the site of injury are the first to recover. This is noticed by the ability of the muscles to contract. The muscles in the more distal area begin to contract as they become innervated one after another (**motor march**).

❖ **Electrodiagnostic test:** This test helps in predicting nerve recovery even before it is apparent clinically. It includes electromyography (EMG), recording of strength duration curve (S-D curve) and nerve conduction studies.
  ■ **EMG** is the graphic recording of the electrical activity of a muscle during rest and during activity. In a normal muscle, there will be no activity at rest and the electrical activity increases progressively as the intensity of the muscular activity increases. But in a denervated muscle, spontaneous electrical activity is recorded even at rest.
  ■ **S-D curve** is the graphic representation of the excitability of muscles and nervous tissue at rest. A small strength of current can excite a normal muscle. In a denervated muscle, the excitation is possible only on direct stimulation of muscle fibers which needs a higher strength of current.
  ■ **Nerve conduction studies** measure the velocity of conduction of impulse in a nerve. A stimulating electrode is applied over a point on the nerve trunk and the response is picked up by an electrode kept at a distance or directly over the muscle. Normal conduction velocity of a motor nerve is 70 m/sec.

> If no connection is established between the proximal and distal cut ends, the sprouting neurofibrils coalesce or get tangled to form a tumor-like mass or a ball-shaped mass called **neuroma**. This is a very painful mass, especially when the neuroma is formed in a sensory nerve, which is commonly seen in amputation stumps. Sometimes neuroma causes a tingling sensation if tapped or if pressure is applied.

Nerve Growth Factor

Nerve growth factor is a neuropeptide (neurotrophin) involved in the regulation of growth, proliferation, maintenance and survival of certain neurons in central nervous system and peripheral nervous system. *It is the first neurotrophic factor discovered in 1950.* It also helps in the repair of myelin sheath during nerve regeneration. Studies have shown that peripherally innervated tissues produce and release NGF which is retrogradely transported by specific receptors to the neuron to provide a protective action and functional neuronal integrity. Reduced transport of NGF by this way can lead to damage of neurons as seen in peripheral neuropathies. Administration of NGF can promote peripheral nerve growth and reestablish the functional activity of peripheral nerve fibers and damaged neurons. But it has side effects. Topical application of NGF as a healing-promoting agent on cutaneous, corneal and pressure ulcers is found to be successful and have no systemic or local adverse side effects. Low level of NGF is seen in diseases like atherosclerosis, depression, Alzheimer's disease, type 2 diabetes mellitus and metabolic syndrome. Exercise increases NGF level. In autoimmune diseases, after brain injury and in patients with chronic pain, the NGF level is found to be increased.

Trans-neuronal Degeneration

If an afferent nerve fiber is cut, the degenerative changes are also seen in the neuron with which the afferent nerve fiber synapses (which suffers no direct damage). This is called trans-neuronal degeneration. For example, chromatolysis occurs in the cells of lateral geniculate body when optic nerve is cut. Retrograde trans-neuronal degeneration is also seen.

Changes Occurring in the Skeletal Muscles Supplied by the Cut Motor Nerve

❖ Impulse transmission is decreased in the muscle.
❖ Muscle tone decreases and the muscle become flaccid.
❖ Paralysis occurs if there is no regeneration of the nerve.
❖ Fibrillation potentials can be recorded by electromyography.
❖ If there is no regeneration, muscle atrophies.
❖ Reaction of degeneration will be present (*Refer* Chapter 8).

MULTIPLE CHOICE QUESTIONS

1. **What is true regarding resting membrane potential of nerve?**
   a. Can be measured by applying electrode over the nerve fiber
   b. Potassium ion mainly contributes to RMP
   c. Equal to RMP of muscle
   d. Reduction in RMP inhibits a voltage dependent increase in Na$^+$ permeability

2. **Action potential is:**
   a. Decremental phenomenon
   b. Does not obey all or none phenomenon
   c. K$^+$ goes from ECF to ICF
   d. Threshold stimulus is required

3. **Orthodromic conduction means:**
   a. Conduction of impulse towards the axon terminal
   b. An axon can conduct impulse in both directions
   c. The jumping of depolarization from node to node
   d. Conduction of impulse towards the cell body

4. **Chronaxie is:**
   a. Magnitude of current
   b. Time taken to respond to a current strength equal to rheobase
   c. Time taken to respond to current strength double the rheobase
   d. Velocity of nerve conduction

5. **Rapid repolarization phase in action potential of cardiac muscle is due to:**
   a. Decreased permeability of K$^+$
   b. Closure of Na$^+$ channels
   c. Decreased intracellular Ca^{2+}
   d. Na$^+$-K$^+$ pump inactivation

SECTION 1 → General Physiology

6. **True about C type of nerve fiber is:**
   a. Most susceptible to hypoxia
   b. Unmyelinated
   c. Preganglionic autonomic
   d. Not for temperature and pain senses

7. **All the following are associated with nerve transmission, *except*:**
   a. Na⁺
   b. K⁺
   c. Cl⁻
   d. Mg²⁺

8. **Resting membrane potential in nerve fiber:**
   a. Is equal to the potential of ventricular muscle fiber
   b. Can be measured by surface electrodes
   c. Increases as extracellular K⁺ increases
   d. Depends upon K⁺ equilibrium

9. **False about saltatory conduction:**
   a. Occurs in non-myelinated nerves
   b. Depends on nodes of Ranvier
   c. It is a fast process
   d. Less energy is consumed

10. **The true statement regarding action potential in a nerve is:**
    a. Depolarization is a result of outward movement of potassium ions
    b. Action potential occurs due to rapid opening of Na⁺ channels
    c. Resting membrane potential is –90 mV
    d. Action potential occurs when the potential reaches a threshold at –65 mV

11. **The first change to occur in the distal segment of cut nerve is:**
    a. Axonal degeneration
    b. Myelin cell degeneration
    c. Multiplication of Schwann cell
    d. Loss of conduction of impulse

12. **After nerve injury, complete functional recovery occurs approximately by:**
    a. Two months
    b. Four months
    c. Six months
    d. One year

13. **Maximum velocity of conduction occurs in which fibers:**
    a. B-fibers
    b. Aα-fibers
    c. Sympathetic fibers
    d. C-fibers

14. **Resting membrane potential is established by all the following, *except*:**
    a. Selective permeability of cell membrane
    b. Differential concentration of ions inside and outside the membrane
    c. Sodium-potassium pump
    d. Fluidity of cell membrane

15. **Major intracellular cation is:**
    a. Na⁺
    b. K⁺
    c. Ca²⁺
    d. Mg²⁺

16. **When RMP changes from –80 to –60:**
    a. Threshold of action potential increases
    b. Threshold of action potential decreases
    c. Threshold remains constant
    d. None of these

17. **The most susceptible fiber to hypoxia is:**
    a. Type A fiber
    b. Type B fiber
    c. Type C fiber
    d. All are equally sensitive

18. **Nissl granules are composed of:**
    a. Rough endoplasmic reticulum
    b. Nerve cell vesicles
    c. Aggregated mitochondria
    d. Deposits of pigmented granules

19. **ATP needs:**
    a. Calcium
    b. Magnesium
    c. Manganese
    d. Zinc

20. **Spike duration is maximal in which nerve fiber:**
    a. A-alpha
    b. A-beta
    c. A-delta
    d. C-fiber

21. **Non-myelinated fibers differ from myelinated axons in that they:**
    a. Are more excitable
    b. Lack node of Ranvier
    c. Are not associated with Schwann cells
    d. Are not capable of regeneration

22. **Group B nerve fibers are situated in:**
    a. Muscle spindles
    b. Fibers carrying pain sensation
    c. Preganglionic autonomic fibers
    d. Postganglionic autonomic fibers

23. **Group B nerve fibers are:**
    a. Sympathetic preganglionic
    b. Sympathetic postganglionic
    c. Parasympathetic preganglionic
    d. Parasympathetic postganglionic

24. **Group A fibers are most susceptible to:**
    a. Pressure
    b. Hypoxia
    c. Local anesthetics
    d. Temperature

25. **The intrafusal fibers of skeletal muscles are innervated by which type of motor neuron?**
    a. Alpha fibers
    b. Beta fibers
    c. Gamma fibers
    d. Delta fibers

26. **Nerve fibers involved in proprioception is:**
    a. Type A fiber
    b. Type B fiber
    c. Type C fiber
    d. Type IV fiber

27. **If a subject complains of paresthesia following nerve compression, the type of nerve fiber affected is:**
    a. A-alpha
    b. A-alpha and delta
    c. Type C
    d. Type B

28. Neuronal degeneration is seen in all the following, *except*:
    a. Crush nerve injury   b. Fetal development
    c. Senescence   d. Neuropraxia
29. First change observed in the distal part of a cut nerve is:
    a. Axonal degeneration
    b. Sprouting
    c. Myelin degeneration
    d. Schwann cell proliferation
30. The first change occurring in the proximal part of a sharp cut nerve is:
    a. Schwann cell proliferation
    b. Degeneration of myelin sheath
    c. Chromatolysis
    d. Degeneration of neurolemma
31. Lowest threshold potential in a motor nerve fiber is at:
    a. Dendrite   b. Body
    c. Axon hillock   d. Axon
32. Initiation of nerve impulse occurs at the initial segment because:
    a. It has a lower threshold than the rest of the axon
    b. It is unmyelinated
    c. Neurotransmitter release occur here
    d. It has long refractory period
33. Which is true regarding nerve conduction?
    a. All or none phenomenon
    b. Conduction independent of amplitude
    c. Propagated action potential is generated in dendrites
    d. Faster in unmyelinated fibers
34. Which of the following is true about propagated nerve action potential?
    a. Decremental
    b. Not affected by hypoxia
    c. Fastest in C fibers
    d. Affected by membrane capacitance
35. A travelling nerve impulse does not depolarize the area immediately behind it, because:
    a. It is hyperpolarized
    b. It is refractory
    c. It is not self-propagating
    d. The conduction is always orthodromic
36. True about nerve impulse is:
    a. Travels in one direction along axon
    b. If current is increased slowly nerve responds faster
    c. Travels in one direction at the synapse
    d. Travels with the speed of electric current
37. Most diffusible ion in an excitable tissue is:
    a. Sodium   b. Potassium
    c. Phosphate   d. Chloride
38. Excitable tissue at rest is least permeable to:
    a. Na^+ b. K^+
    c. Ca^{2+} d. Cl^-
39. The nerve fiber which is the thickest in human is that which carries the sense of:
    a. Touch   b. Pain
    c. Proprioception d. Temperature
40. Which type of nerve fiber is blocked maximally by pressure:
    a. C-fibers   b. A-alpha fibers
    c. A-beta fibers d. A-gamma fibers
41. In a neuron the impulse is generated at the:
    a. Dendritic tree b. Cell body
    c. Axon hillock   d. Initial segment
42. First change to occur in the distal segment of cut nerve is:
    a. Myelin degeneration
    b. Axonal degeneration
    c. Mitosis of Schwann cell
    d. Sprouting
43. The afferent nerve fibers which are most sensitive to local anesthetics belong to group:
    a. Aα   b. B
    c. C   d. Aβ
44. The rapid repolarization phase of nerve action potential is due to increased permeability of:
    a. Calcium ion   b. Sodium ion
    c. Potassium ion d. Chloride ion
45. Chronaxie is increased in the following condition:
    a. When the excitability of the tissue is low
    b. When the threshold of excitation is decreased
    c. When local excitatory state is present
    d. When the membrane potential is nearer to the firing level
46. Non-myelinated nerve axons differ from myelinated nerve fiber in that they:
    a. Are more excitable
    b. Lack nodes of Ranvier
    c. Conduct relatively faster
    d. Are not associated with Schwann cells
47. Resting membrane potential of skeletal muscle is about:
    a. –90 mV   b. –60 mV
    c. –70 mV   d. –55 mV
48. Action potentials are produced by:
    a. Na^+ influx   b. Na^+ and K^+ influx
    c. K^+ influx   d. K^+ efflux
49. In excitable cells, repolarization is closely associated with:
    a. Na^+ influx   b. K^+ efflux
    c. Na^+ efflux   d. K^+ influx
50. Sodium channels are specifically blocked by:
    a. Nifedipine   b. Tetrodotoxin
    c. Choline   d. Tetraethyl ammonium
51. The slowest conduction velocity is found in the following type of nerve fibers:
    a. Aα   b. Aγ
    c. B   d. C

52. **Resting membrane potential of a neuron is:**
    a. −90 mV
    b. −60 mV
    c. −70 mV
    d. −55 mV

53. **RMP is close to the isoelectric potential of:**
    a. K⁺
    b. Cl⁻
    c. Na⁺
    d. Ca²⁺

54. **During depolarization, there is a sharp increase in the permeability of the cell membrane to:**
    a. K⁺
    b. Cl⁻
    c. Na⁺
    d. HCO_3^-

55. **Synaptic conduction is mostly orthodromic because:**
    a. Dendrites cannot be depolarized
    b. Once repolarized, the area cannot be depolarized
    c. The strength of antidromic impulse is less
    d. Chemical mediator is localized only in the presynaptic terminal

56. **Which of the following statement is true for excitatory post-synaptic potential?**
    a. Is self-propagating
    b. Show all or none response
    c. Is proportional to the amount of transmitter released by the presynaptic neuron
    d. Is inhibitory to presynaptic terminal

57. **Synaptic potentials can be recorded by:**
    a. Patch clamp technique
    b. Voltage clamp technique
    c. Microelectrode
    d. EEG

58. **Compared with intracellular fluid, extracellular fluid has:**
    a. A greater osmolarity
    b. A lower sodium ion concentration
    c. A lower K⁺ concentration
    d. A lower Cl⁻ concentration

59. **Chronaxie of a tissue is the measurement of:**
    a. Strength of current
    b. Velocity of conduction
    c. Duration of application of stimulus
    d. Excitability

60. **The number of sodium channels per µm² of membrane in myelinated nerve fiber is maximum at the:**
    a. Axon hillock
    b. Axon terminal
    c. Node of Ranvier
    d. Cell body

61. **The type of nerve fiber most susceptible to local anesthetics is:**
    a. B group
    b. Aα group
    c. Aβ group
    d. C group

62. **The velocity of conduction is fastest in nerve carrying:**
    a. Motor information
    b. Pain sensation
    c. Temperature sensation
    d. Autonomic information

63. **Action potential recorded from a mixed nerve fiber is of:**
    a. Spike type
    b. Plateau type
    c. Compound type
    d. Rhythmic type

64. **Rheobase indicates:**
    a. Magnitude of the current
    b. Rate of discharge
    c. Velocity of nerve conduction
    d. Specificity of impulse transmission

65. **The ion that is responsible for the production of resting membrane potential is:**
    a. Na⁺
    b. K⁺
    c. Ca²⁺
    d. Cl⁻

66. **Regarding action potential all the statements are true, *except*, that it:**
    a. Is a self-propagating process
    b. Can be elicited by a threshold stimulus
    c. Is a graded potential
    d. Has a refractory period

67. **Gradual change of potential from resting state to firing level in a nerve fiber is called:**
    a. Reversal of polarity
    b. After depolarization
    c. After hyper polarization
    d. Partial depolarization

68. **Velocity of conduction of impulse is maximal in:**
    a. Aα nerve fiber
    b. Aβ fiber
    c. B fiber
    d. C fiber

69. **The relation between nerve thickness and conduction velocity is:**
    a. Parabolic
    b. Hyperbolic
    c. Linear
    d. No relation

ANSWERS

1. b	2. d	3. a	4. c	5. b
6. b	7. d	8. d	9. a	10. b
11. a	12. d	13. b	14. d	15. b
16. b	17. b	18. a	19. a	20. d
21. b	22. c	23. a	24. a	25. c
26. a	27. a	28. d	29. a	30. c
31. c	32. a	33. a	34. d	35. b
36. c	37. b	38. a	39. c	40. c
41. d	42. b	43. c	44. c	45. a
46. b	47. a	48. a	49. b	50. b
51. d	52. c	53. b	54. c	55. d
56. c	57. c	58. c	59. d	60. c
61. d	62. a	63. c	64. a	65. b
66. c	67. d	68. a	69. a	

Skeletal Muscle Physiology

CHAPTER 7

LEARNING OBJECTIVES

Must know
- Describe the structure of a skeletal muscle fiber
- Describe the properties of skeletal muscle
- Describe excitation-contraction coupling and the molecular basis of skeletal muscle contraction and relaxation
- Distinguish between isotonic and isometric contraction
- Define refractory period and its significance
- Define oxygen debt and its significance

Desirable to know
- Explain heat production in muscles
- Causes of fatigue
- Describe muscular dystrophy

INTRODUCTION

PY3.7: Describe the different types of muscle fibers and their structure.

Muscles constitute 50% of our body weight. Like neurons, muscle cells can be excited to produce an action potential. Unlike neurons, they have a contractile mechanism that is activated by the action potential. Muscles are classified into:
- Skeletal muscle—40% of body weight
- Cardiac and smooth muscle—10%.

SKELETAL MUSCLE

Skeletal muscles are voluntary striated muscles attached to bones by means of tendons on both ends. In a cross section, a muscle shows large number of muscle fibers (**Fig. 7.1A**). The muscle fibers are arranged in parallel between the tendons. Each muscle fiber is composed of numerous myofibrils (**Fig. 7.1B**). Under electron microscopy, each myofibril is made up of thick and thin filaments (**Fig. 7.1C**).

Each muscle fiber is a single muscle cell, multinucleated, long, cylindrical, striated and surrounded by a cell membrane called **sarcolemma** (**Fig. 7.2**). During intrauterine life, a skeletal muscle fiber is formed by the fusion of a large number of small mesodermal cells called **myoblasts**. Therefore, a single mature skeletal muscle fiber contains numerous nuclei. After birth, the muscle loses its ability to divide and so the number of muscle fibers remains almost constant throughout life. Hyperplasia (increase in the number of cells) occurs rarely in skeletal muscle and this is due to the persistence of a few myoblasts referred to as **satellite cells**. Cytoplasm of a muscle fiber is called **sarcoplasm**. The endoplasmic reticulum is highly developed and is called **sarcoplasmic reticulum**.

Innervation of Skeletal Muscle

The nerve supplying a muscle contains motor and sensory fibers.

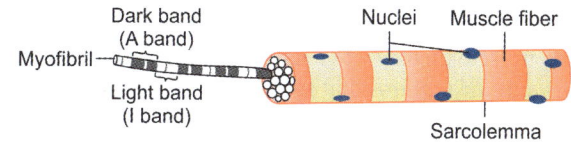

Fig. 7.2: Structure of a skeletal muscle fiber and a myofibril. Note the striation and multiple nuclei in the muscle fiber.

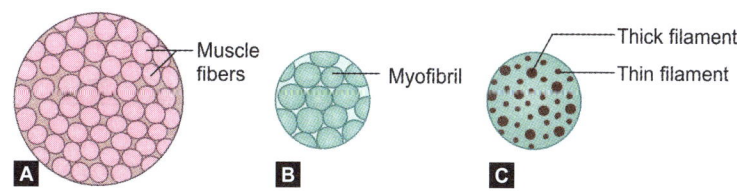

Figs. 7.1A to C: Cross section of: (A) Skeletal muscle; (B) Skeletal muscle fiber; (C) Myofibril.

Motor Fibers to Skeletal Muscle

❖ Large α-myelinated fibers
❖ Small γ-myelinated fibers
❖ Fine unmyelinated fibers, which are postganglionic autonomic efferents that supply smooth muscles in the walls of the blood vessels of muscles.

Sensory Fibers

❖ Myelinated fibers originating in the annulospiral and flower spray endings of muscle spindle.
❖ Myelinated fibers from Golgi tendon organ.
❖ Myelinated and non-myelinated fibers from sensory endings in the connective tissue of muscle.

Muscle Proteins

Muscle proteins are of three groups:
1. Contractile proteins
2. Regulatory or relaxing proteins
3. Structural proteins

Contractile proteins in the skeletal muscle are **myosin** and **actin**.

Relaxing proteins are **tropomyosin** and **troponin**. Troponin is made up of three subunits: troponin I, troponin T and troponin C.

Structural Proteins: Structural proteins are of many types, the important being **titin, myomesin, desmin, dystrophin** and α-**actinin**. The structural proteins contribute to the stability, elasticity and extensibility of the myofibril.

Titin is the largest known protein that is found abundantly in the skeletal muscle. Each titin molecule extends from the Z disc to the M line and thus helps to stabilize the position of the thick filament in the sarcomere **(Fig. 7.3)**. Titin is highly elastic towards its attachment to the Z line and it can stretch to 4 times its resting length and then can spring back to its original length. Thus, it accounts for the elasticity and extensibility of the myofibrils. The sarcomere returns to its resting length after contraction because of this elastic component of muscle. Titin contains two folded domains which unfold when the muscle is stretched initially and so there will be relatively little resistance. With further stretch, there is rapid increase in resistance. Other elastic components of the muscle include connective tissue around the muscle fibers and the tendons that attach muscle to bone.

Myomesin is a structural protein present in the M line, which binds M line to titin and also connects the adjacent thick filaments to one another.

Desmin binds Z-lines to the plasma membrane.

Dystrophin is the anchor protein, which provides structural support and strength to the myofibril. Dystrophin is connected to laminins present in the basal lamina matrix through proteins present in the sarcolemma.

Dystrophin forms a rod that connects the actin filament to the transmembrane protein, β-**dystroglycan** in the sarcolemma by means of smaller proteins in the sarcoplasm called **syntrophins.** Dystroglycan-β is connected to dystroglycan-α outside the cell membrane which in turn is connected to laminins in the extracellular matrix. The dystroglycans are also associated with transmembrane glycoproteins called **sarcoglycans**. This dystrophin-glycoprotein complex adds strength to the muscle by connecting the actin filament to the extracellular matrix. Abnormalities in the gene coding for dystrophin are associated with different forms of *muscular dystrophy.*

α-actinin crosslinks the actin filaments in the area of **Z line** (*refer* Fig. 7.6).

Electron Microscopic Structure of a Myofibril

When a myofibril is examined under electron microscope, alternating dark and light bands are seen. Dark band is called **A band** (anisotropic band) and light band is called **I band** (isotropic band). Junction between A and I band is called AI junction **(Fig. 7.4)**.

At the center of the A band, there is a comparatively lighter area called **H band**. At the center of the H band is a dark line called **M line**; it is so called because it is seen at the middle of the sarcomere. At the center of the I band, there is a dark line called **Z line**. The area between two adjacent Z lines is called a **sarcomere**. *Sarcomere is the functional unit of a muscle fiber* **(Figs. 7.5 and 7.6)**.

Sarcolemma

Sarcolemma is the cell membrane, which covers the muscle fiber and also dips deep into the muscle fiber at the **AI junctions**. These invaginations are called **transverse tubules or T tubules** and it contains extracellular fluid. They have a large number of branches. Branches of the T tubules cover or encircle the myofibril at different points, i.e., the T system forms a grid perforated by individual myofibrils. It is through the T tubules that the action potential reaches the interior of the muscle fiber.

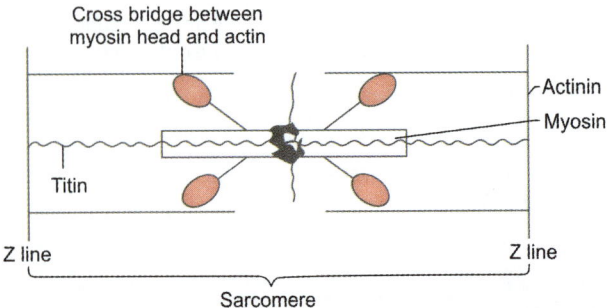

Fig. 7.3: Actin and myosin forming cross bridges.

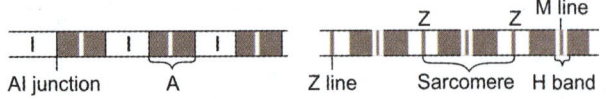

Fig. 7.4: Electron microscopic structure of myofibril (longitudinal section).

(A: A-band; I: I-band; Z: Z-line)

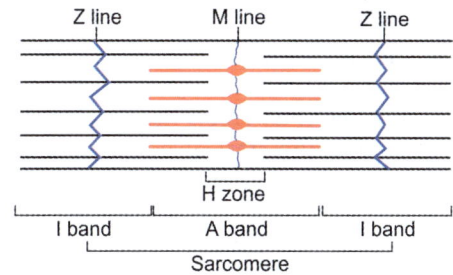

Fig. 7.5: Structure of a sarcomere.

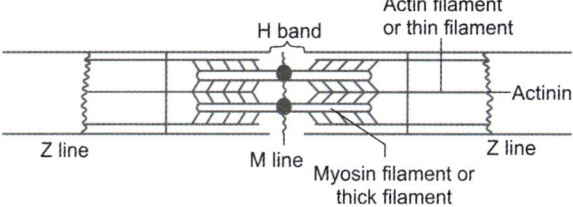

Fig. 7.6: Detailed structure of sarcomere (part of myofibril between two Z-lines) showing cross bridges.

Sarcoplasmic Reticulum

Sarcoplasmic reticulum forms **longitudinal tubules or L tubules**. This also has a large number of branches. They extend the whole length of the sarcomere and when they reach the T tubule they fuse and form enlargements called **terminal cisterns**. The junction of the T tubule and cisterns is known as a **triad (Fig. 7.7)**. This area has a very important role in the transmission of action potential. Sarcoplasmic reticulum contains large quantity of calcium ions and calcium binding protein called **calsequestrin**. As Ca^{2+} is sequestered by calsequestrin, the concentration of Ca^{2+} inside the sarcoplasmic reticulum is 10,000 times higher than in the sarcoplasm when the muscle fiber is relaxed. When an action potential reaches the triad, large amounts of Ca^{2+} will be released from the cistern. This has a very important role in muscle contraction. Both T and L tubules together form the **sarcotubular system**.

Thick and Thin Filaments

The peculiar arrangement of thick and thin filaments is responsible for the striations seen in muscle fiber. The thick filaments, which are about twice the diameter of the thin filaments, are made up of myosin molecules. The thin filaments are made up of actin, tropomyosin and troponin.

The thick filaments are lined up to form 'A' band. The thin filament overlaps the thick filament for a short distance. H band is formed by the absence of overlapping when the muscle is relaxed. The width of the H zone depends on the contractile state of the muscle. When the muscle contracts the H zone disappears. I band is formed of thin filaments only. When a transverse section through the A band is taken, it is seen that under electron microscope each thick filament is surrounded by 6 thin filaments and 1 thin filament by 3 thick filaments (*refer* **Fig. 7.1C**).

Structure of Myosin

The form of myosin in the muscle is myosin-II with two globular heads and a long tail. It is made up of 2 heavy chains and 4 light chains. The heads contain an actin binding site and a catalytic site that hydrolyses ATP **(Fig. 7.8)**.

In skeletal muscles, about 300 myosin molecules form a single thick filament. The myosin molecules are arranged symmetrically on either side of the center of the sarcomere. M line is due to a central bulge in each of the thick filaments **(Fig. 7.9)**.

Structure of Thin Filament

The actin filaments or thin filaments are polymers made up of 2 actin chains. The actin molecules are globular units called **G actins** arranged in the form of 2 strands, wound around one another to form a **double helical structure**. Each G

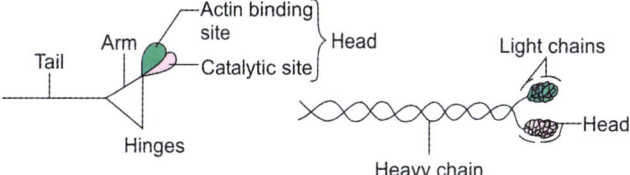

Fig. 7.8: Structure of myosin molecule.

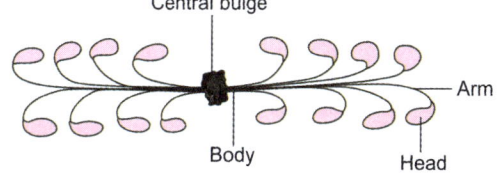

Fig. 7.9: Structure thick filament of myobril.

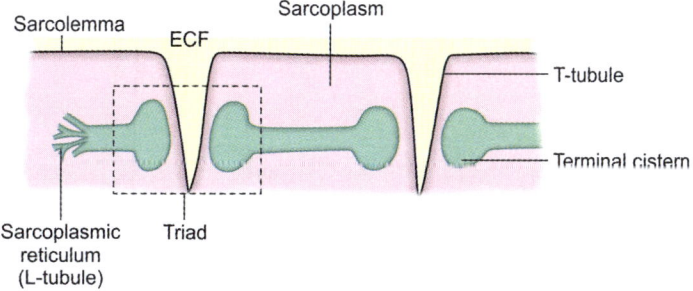

Fig. 7.7: Sarcotubular system in skeletal muscle.

actin contains a site where ADP is present called **active site**, because it is the site where myosin head gets attached during muscle contraction.

Tropomyosin molecules are long filaments located in the groove between the two chains of actin. It is arranged in such a way that during resting stages all the active sites of actin filaments is covered. Each thin filament contains about 300–400 actin molecules and 40–60 tropomyosin molecules. The tropomyosin strands are held in position by troponin molecules.

Troponin molecules are small globular units located at intervals along the tropomyosin molecules. Troponin is composed of 3 subunits troponin T, troponin I and troponin

C. **Troponin T** binds the other troponin components to tropomyosin. **Troponin I** inhibits the interaction of myosin with actin. **Troponin C** contains binding sites for Ca^{2+} that initiates muscle contraction **(Fig. 7.10)**.

Electrical Activity in Skeletal Muscle

> **PY3.8:** Describe action potential and its properties in different muscle types.

An artificial stimulus is applied to a single skeletal muscle fiber and a monophasic recording is taken.
- RMP: –90 mV
- Firing level: –50 mV
- Duration of action potential: 2–4 millisec
- Absolute refractory period: 1–3 millisec
- Conduction velocity: 3–5 m/sec
- Chronaxie: 0.25–1 millisec

Ionic basis of RMP and action potential is the same as that of nerve fiber *(refer: nerve action potential)*.

Properties of Skeletal Muscles

- Excitability and contractility
- Refractory period
- Tone
- Conductivity
- Extensibility and elasticity

Excitability and Contractility

Muscles are excitable tissues, i.e., they can respond to an adequate stimulus by contraction. When a muscle is given a single induction shock, it immediately contracts which is immediately followed by relaxation. This is called simple muscle twitch.

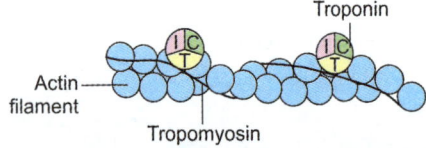

Fig. 7.10: Structure of thin filament of myofibril showing the arrangement of actin, tropomyosin and the three subunits of troponin (I, C and T).

Simple Muscle Twitch

A single action potential causes a brief contraction followed by relaxation of the muscle. This response is called a **simple muscle twitch (Fig. 7.11)**. The twitch starts about 2 milliseconds after the start of depolarization of the membrane and before repolarization is complete **(Fig. 7.12)**. Correlation between electrical and mechanical events in the skeletal muscle is shown in **Figure 7.12**. The twitch duration varies with the type of the muscle.
- Fast muscles involved in fine, rapid, precise movement—7.5 milliseconds
- Slow muscles involved in strong, gross, sustained movement—100 milliseconds

Refractory Period

Refractory period is the period during which the muscle does not respond to a second stimulus after stimulation (details in page no 56).

Muscle Tone

Reflex sustained and partial contraction of the muscle at rest is referred to as muscle tone (details in page no 812).

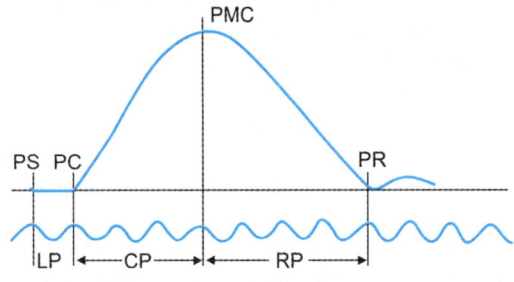

Fig. 7.11: Simple muscle twitch. One wave in the time tracing corresponds to 0.1 second.

(PS: point of stimulation; PC: point of contraction; PMC: point of maximum contraction; PR: point of relaxation; LP: latent period; CP: contraction period; RP: relaxation period)

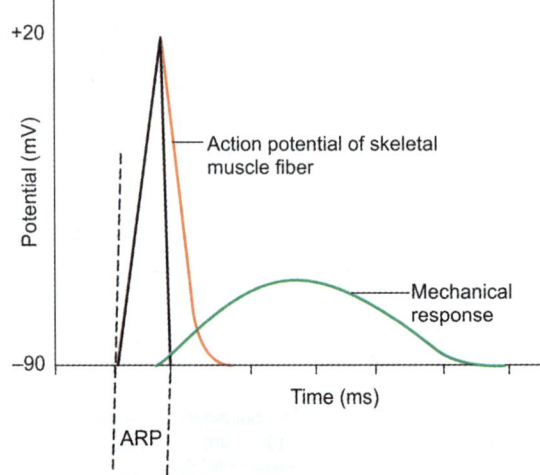

Fig. 7.12: Correlation between electrical and mechanical events in skeletal muscle.

Conductivity

Once stimulated the muscle fiber can conduct impulses throughout the sarcolemma.

Extensibility and Elasticity

A muscle can be stretched within physiological limits. When the tension is released it moves back to its original position.

Molecular Basis of Skeletal Muscle Contraction or Excitation-Contraction Coupling

> **PY3.9:** Describe the molecular basis of muscle contraction in skeletal muscle.

Excitation-contraction coupling refers to the events between the generation of sarcolemmal action potential (excitation) and the release of Ca^{2+} from the terminal cisterns into the sarcoplasm, which, in turn, leads to muscle contraction.

In the resting muscle, troponin I is tightly bound to actin, and tropomyosin covers the active site of actin. *Thus, the troponin–tropomyosin complex constitutes a relaxing protein that inhibits the interaction between actin and myosin.* During activity, action potential passes through the T tubules and reaches the triad. Depolarization of the T tubule membrane activates the sarcoplasmic reticulum *via* **dihydropyridine receptors (DHPRs)**, which are voltagegated Ca^{2+} channels in the T tubules. It causes release of large amounts of Ca^{2+} from the cisterns into the sarcoplasm. The Ca^{2+} channel in the sarcoplasmic reticulum that releases Ca^{2+} into the sarcoplasm is called **ryanodine receptor (RyR)** which is ligand gated Ca^{2+} channel where Ca^{2+} is the ligand. DHP receptors in the T tubule and ryanodine receptors in the terminal cisternal membrane are located very close to each other and the protein chains of DHPR and RYR are mechanically interlocked in skeletal muscle **(Fig. 7.13)**. So stimulation of DHPRs directly activates the RyRs and cause release of Ca^{2+}. (But in cardiac muscle, activation of DHPRs leads to influx of Ca^{2+} from the extracellular fluid in the T tubules and this Ca^{2+} stimulates the RyRs which leads to release of Ca^{2+} from the sarcoplasmic reticulum. This is also referred to as **Ca^{2+}-induced Ca^{2+} release**).

The released Ca^{2+} diffuses to the thick and thin filaments and this Ca^{2+} initiates contraction. Ca^{2+} combines with the C part of troponin. This weakens the binding of troponin-I to actin and the tropomyosin moves laterally due to some conformational change occurring in it. This movement uncovers the active sites of actin filament. *When one troponin binds with Ca^{2+}, 7 myosin-binding sites are uncovered in the actin filament.* ATP is then split and contraction occurs. The process by which depolarization of muscle fiber initiates contraction is called **excitation-contraction coupling**. *Calcium ions are the linking or coupling material between excitation and contraction.*

Mechanism of Skeletal Muscle Contraction

Shortening of the contractile elements in the muscle occurs by the sliding of the thin filaments over the thick filaments. This is called **sliding filament theory or walk along mechanism or Ratchet mechanism**.

The length of the A band remains constant during contraction. When the muscle contracts, the Z lines move closer together and the thin filaments from the opposite ends of the sarcomere approach each other towards the M line and may even overlap if shortening is marked.

Summary of the events during muscle contraction are:
- At rest, the myosin head contain tightly bound ADP and inorganic phosphate (Pi). The myosin head is said to be in the cocked position at rest.
- Following an action potential in the muscle membrane, sarcoplasmic Ca^{2+} is increased and Ca^{2+} binds to troponin C
- Combination of Ca^{2+} with troponin C exposes the active sites of actin filament.
- Myosin head gets attached to the active site or myosin-binding site of actin to form cross bridges.
- When this attachment occurs, the ADP attached to the myosin head is released. This causes a conformational change in the myosin head and the myosin head bends on the rest of the myosin molecule towards the center of the sarcomere. This movement is possible because of the hinge present between the head and arm of the myosin molecule.
- This causes the actin filaments to be pulled towards the center of the sarcomere from both sides. It seems that the myosin heads attach to and walk along the thin filaments at both ends of the sarcomere and hence called **walk along mechanism**. The Z lines come closer. The bending of the myosin head is known as **power stroke (Figs. 7.14A to C)**, and this process requires energy. This energy is provided by the **stored energy** during the hydrolysis of ATP in the previous cycle. Each power stroke shortens the muscle by 10 nm (1%).
- Bending of the head exposes the other part of the head having ATPase activity. This site combines with ATP molecule and **hydrolysis of ATP occurs**. But the ADP and the phosphate group are still attached to the myosin head till the next power stroke when this energy is utilized for the power stroke. The combination of ATP with the myosin head helps in the detachment of head of myosin from the actin filament. ATP is hydrolyzed releasing Pi and the head comes back to the original state and the process is called **re-cocking of the myosin head (Figs. 7.14A to C)** and one

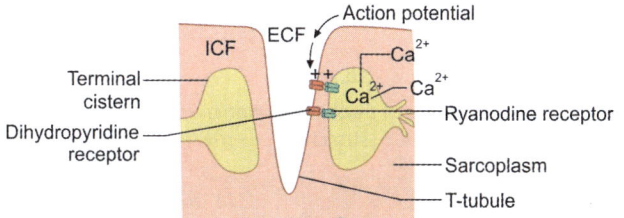

Fig. 7.13: Excitation-contraction coupling in skeletal muscle. When an action potential reaches T-tubule the dihydropyridine receptor get stimulated which in turn directly stimulates ryanodine receptors in the terminal cisterns of the sarcoplasmic reticulum. This causes release of Ca^{2+} into the sacroplasm and this Ca^{2+} initiates muscle contraction.

(ECF: extracellular fluid; ICF: intracellular fluid)

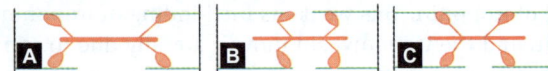

Figs. 7.14A to C: Mechanism of muscle contraction: (A) Myosin head attached to active site of actin; (B) Power stroke; (C) Re-cocking of head (note that the sarcomere length decreases with each cycle and the Z lines come closer).

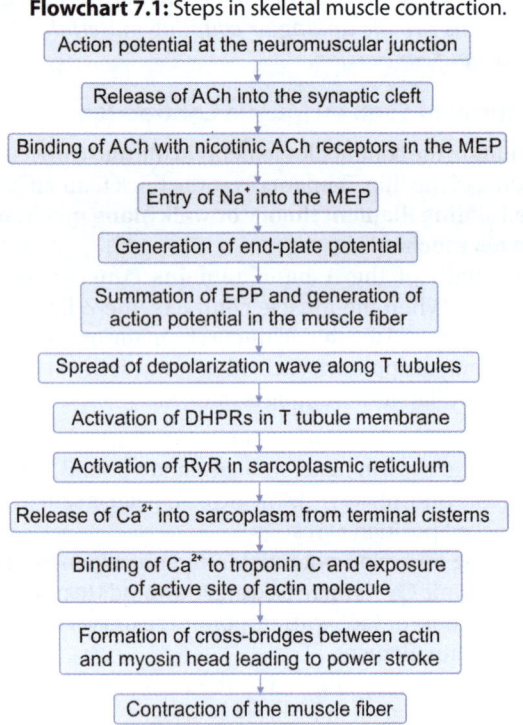

(MEP: motor endplate; EPP: end-plate potential; DHPR: dihydropyridine receptor; RyR: ryanodine receptor)

cycle is completed. Summary of muscle contraction as in **Flowchart 7.1.**

❖ When the head goes back, it again gets attached to another myosin binding site of actin and the process continues as long as the sarcoplasmic Ca²⁺ level is high and sufficient ATP is available. This leads to gross muscle contraction. This whole process cycles about **5 times/sec** during a rapid contraction. Each contraction cycle utilizes one molecule of ATP.

When the muscle fiber starts to shorten, it first causes a stretch of the elastic components of muscle like titin, connective tissue around the muscle fibers and tendons, which attach the muscle to bone. The tension produced in the muscle during contraction initially causes these elastic components to stretch a little, but after a limit these elastic components become taut and produce a pull on the bones *and cause movement. Movement occurs only in isotonic contraction.* In **isometric contraction**, the tension generated by the actin–myosin interaction is not adequate to move the load on the muscle.

Changes in the Sarcomere During Moderate and Severe Contraction

In moderate contraction, H zone disappears and the sarcomere length decreases to 2 µm from 2.5 µm, which is the resting length of the sarcomere. In severe contraction, actin filaments overlap and instead of H zone, a darker area is seen **(Figs. 7.15A to C)**.

When the muscle is maximally stretched, the sarcomere length comes to about 3.5 µm **(Fig. 7.16)**.

Mechanism of Muscle Relaxation

Relaxation requires energy, and so, like contraction this is also an active process. ATP provides energy for both contraction and relaxation. When action potential in the muscle membrane stops, Ca²⁺ is actively transported back into the sarcoplasmic reticulum and is stored in the terminal cisterns until released by the next action potential. The pump involved is **sarcoplasmic or endoplasmic reticulum Ca²⁺ ATPase (SERCA)** present in the membrane of sarcoplasmic reticulum. Inside the sarcoplasmic reticulum, a calcium binding protein called **calsequestrin** is present, which binds Ca²⁺ and favors further entry of Ca²⁺ into the sarcoplasmic reticulum. As a result, the concentration of Ca²⁺ in the sarcoplasmic reticulum is 10,000 times more than in the sarcoplasm in a relaxed muscle fiber. When the Ca²⁺ level falls sufficiently in the sarcoplasm, the troponin–tropomyosin complex slides back and it covers the myosin binding sites of actin filament and the muscle relaxes completely **(Flowchart 7.2)**.

If the transport of Ca²⁺ into the sarcoplasmic reticulum is inhibited, relaxation does not occur, although there are no action potentials. It leads to sustained contraction of the muscle fiber called **contracture**.

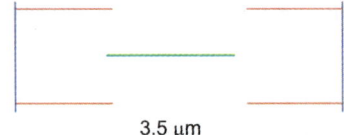

Fig. 7.16: Appearance of sarcomere when muscle is maximally stretched.

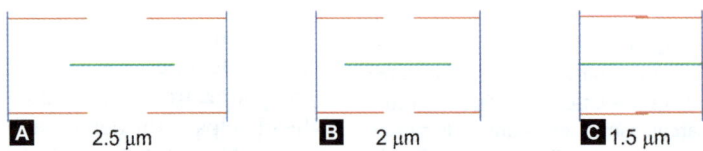

Figs. 7.15A to C: Changes in the sarcomere length during contraction in skeletal muscle: (A) At rest; (B) In moderate contraction; (C) In severe contraction.

Flowchart 7.2: Mechanism of skeletal muscle relaxation.

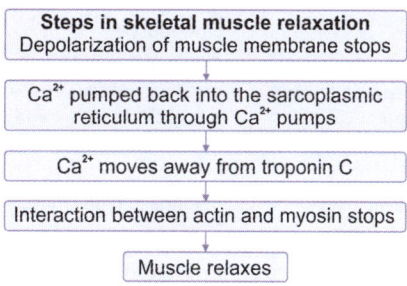

Rigor and Rigor Mortis

The sources of energy in muscle are ATP and creatine phosphate. When muscle fibers are completely depleted of ATP and creatine phosphate, they develop a state of extreme rigidity called **rigor**. In rigor, almost all the myosin heads attach to actin in an abnormal, fixed and resistant way. When this occurs after death, the condition is called **rigor mortis**.

3–4 hours after death, all the muscles of the body go into a state of contracture even without action potential. This is rigor mortis. This is because after death, the membrane of sarcoplasmic reticulum becomes leaky and Ca^{2+} leaks out of sarcoplasmic reticulum into the sarcoplasm and causes contraction. As ATP synthesis does not occur, the cross bridges cannot detach from actin and so relaxation is not possible. This leads to the state of rigidity. The muscles remain in rigor until the muscle proteins are destroyed by the lysosomal enzymes (**auto-digestion**). This occurs 15–24 hours after death.

Types of Muscle Contraction (Table 7.1)

PY3.10: Describe the mode of muscle contraction (isotonic and isometric).

- Isotonic contraction
- Isometric contraction

In isotonic contraction, change in the length of the muscle occurs, but tension remains constant. External work is done only in isotonic muscle contraction, e.g., while lifting a small weight by bending the elbow; the contraction of the biceps muscle can be seen.

In isometric contraction, length remains constant, but the tension rises due to the formation of cross bridges between actin and myosin and due to stretching of the elastic components, such as tendons. This is possible due to the presence of elastic and viscous elements in series with the contractile elements. The stretching of the series elastic component compensates the shortening produced by the contractile component. Thus, the length does not change. No external work is done by the muscle, but the muscle becomes hard, hot and expends energy, e.g., while trying to lift a very heavy weight from the ground, the muscle will not contract sufficiently and the weight does not move, but the tension rises considerably.

Length–Tension Relationship in Skeletal Muscle

The tension that a muscle develops varies with the length of the muscle fiber. This relationship can be studied in a whole skeletal muscle preparation. The muscle is fixed between two points. Changing the distance between its two attachments can vary the length of the muscle. Change in tension is recorded using a force transducer.

As soon as the muscle is stretched, the tension rises. This is **passive tension**. Fix the muscle at that length and stimulate it. The muscle contracts isometrically and the increase in tension is recorded and the value obtained is **total tension**. The difference between total tension and passive tension is the amount of tension actually generated by the contractile process at that length. This is called **active tension**. The passive and active tensions are measured for varying lengths of the muscle (**Fig. 7.17**). Rupture of the muscle occurs when it is stretched beyond a limit.

Passive tension rises slowly at first and then rapidly as the muscle is stretched. The total tension curve rises to a maximum and then falls until it reaches the passive tension curve. At a particular length of the muscle, the active tension developed is maximal and above or below this level the active tension falls. The length at which active tension is maximum is called **resting length (Fig. 7.17)**. In the body, at rest, the skeletal muscles are in the resting length, when the tension developed can be maximal.

Similar curves are obtained when single muscle fibers are studied. A single muscle fiber is isolated and stimulated and changes in tension and length are studied. When a muscle fiber contracts isometrically, the tension developed is proportionate to the number of cross linkages between actin and myosin molecules (**Fig. 7.18**). In the figure, at point D, tension is zero because no cross bridges are formed between myosin head and active site of actin filament. As the length is decreased, tension rises and when the length of the

Table 7.1: Differences between isometric and isotonic muscle contraction.	
Isometric contraction	**Isotonic contraction**
No shortening of the muscle occurs and hence no movement occurs at the joint	Shortening of the muscle occurs and hence movement occurs
Shortening of the contractile component is compensated by stretching of the series elastic component (SEC), so length remains the same	Shortening of contractile component is not associated with significant stretching of SEC
No external work is done as there is no muscle shortening	External work is done due to shortening of the muscle
Tension in the muscle rises due to stretching of SEC	No rise in tension in muscle as SEC is not stretched significantly
Heat released is less and is therefore more energy efficient	Heat released is more due to the release of the heat of shortening, so less energy efficient
Function is mostly to stabilize the joints	Functional role in movement at different joints

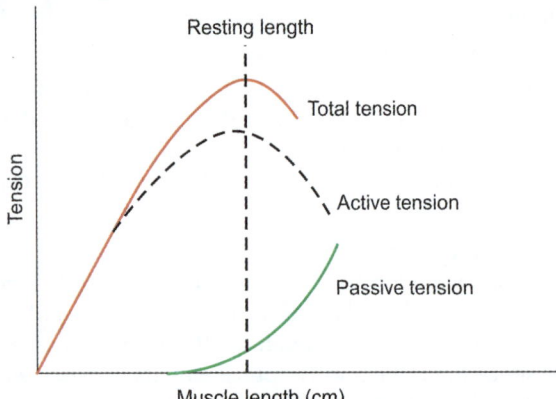

Fig. 7.17: Length-tension relationship in skeletal muscle.

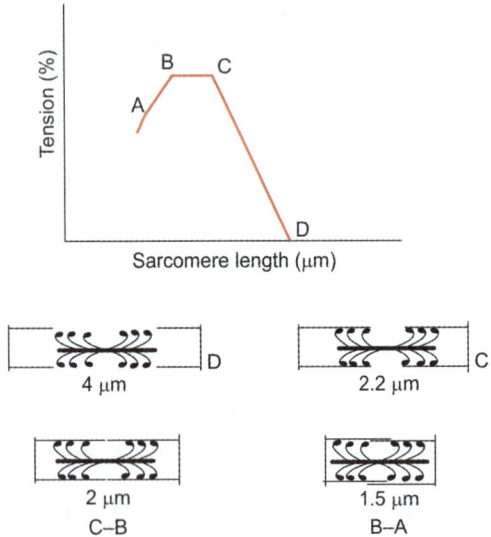

Fig. 7.18: Length-tension relationship in muscle fiber.

Table 7.2: Differences between fast muscle and slow muscle.	
Fast muscle	**Slow muscle**
Called **white muscle** as it is pale in color because of low myoglobin content. Contains extensive sarcoplasmic reticulum	Called **red muscle** as they have greater capillary density, more myoglobin content and very large number of mitochondria
Belongs to type IIB fibers	Belongs to type I muscle fibers
Twitch duration: 7.5 ms	Twitch duration: 100–200 ms
Involved in fine, rapid, precise movement, which is of short duration	Involved in strong, gross, slow, sustained contraction of long duration
Only 3–6 fibers/motor unit	Contain 120–160 fibers/motor unit
Easily fatigued due to lactic acidosis resulting from anaerobic metabolism	Resistant to fatigue
Creatine kinase level very high	Creatine kinase level low
Glycogen content is high and can derive energy both by aerobic and anaerobic glycolysis, e.g., muscles of eye, hand, etc.	Glycogen content is low and energy is derived mainly by aerobic cellular respiration, e.g., muscles concerned with maintenance of posture like the long muscles of the back
Resting blood flow is 2–4 mL/100 g/min	Resting blood flow is 30 mL/100 g/min
Constitutes ¾th of the total muscle mass	Constitutes 1/4th of the muscle mass
Shows rapid phasic contractions	Shows steady prolonged contractions as they are concerned with the maintenance of posture

sarcomere is 2.2 µm maximum numbers of cross-linkages is formed between actin and myosin as seen in point C. When the length is decreased to 2 µm, there is no additional increase in tension. The tension remains steady between points C and B at a maximum value. When the sarcomere length is decreased to less than 2 µm, there is overlapping of actin filaments and the number of cross-bridges formed will be less. So, tension starts falling from B to A.

Starling's Law

*Starling's law states that the force of contraction of a skeletal muscle is proportional to the initial length of the muscle fiber **within physiological limits***. When the initial length is increased, force of contraction also increases.

Types of Skeletal Muscles and Muscle Fibers

The two main types of muscles are **fast muscles and slow muscles (Table 7.2)**. Muscles contain three main types of fibers: Type I, Type IIA and IIB fibers. In humans, type IIA fibers are infrequent. Although the number of muscle fibers per motor unit is high in slow muscles, all the units do not contract simultaneously. This is referred to as **asynchronous contraction** and because of this, they are not easily fatigued. This is very important in posture controlling muscles.

■ MOTOR POINT AND MOTOR UNIT

Motor point is that point on the skin, which when stimulated by an active electrode gives the maximum contraction of the underlying muscle. It usually corresponds to the area of entry of the nerve into the muscle. The nerve supply and blood supply to a muscle enter it at a more or less constant position called **neurovascular hilus**.

A motor nerve contains a large number of nerve fibers and each nerve fiber divides into a number of terminal branches.

Each terminal branch will make contact with a single muscle fiber at its center so that the action potential can spread equally in both directions along the muscle membrane. A single motor neuron with all the muscle fibers supplied by its terminal branches is called a **motor unit (Fig. 7.19)**. The number of muscle fibers in a motor unit varies. In muscles concerned with fine, precise, graded movements, there are only 3–6 fibers per motor unit. For example, fast muscles, such as muscles of larynx that control voice production has only 2–3 muscle fibers per motor unit. In slow muscles, such as biceps and gastrocnemius, there are as many as 2000–3000 muscle fibers in some motor units.

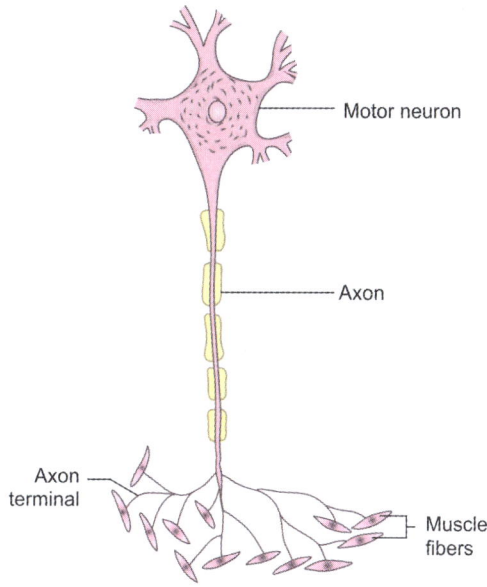

Fig. 7.19: Motor unit.

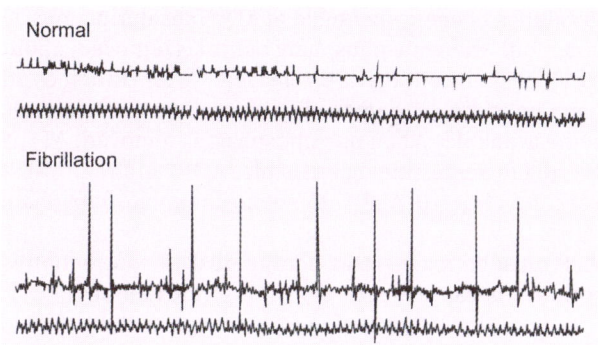

Fig. 7.20: EMG at rest showing normal pattern (above) and fibrillation potentials (below).

Each spinal motor neuron innervates only one kind of muscle fiber, i.e., all the muscle fibers in a motor unit are of the same type. All the muscle fibers of a motor unit contract and relax together, but all of them are not found together. Instead, they are dispersed throughout the muscle.

Muscle **tone** is a small amount of tension maintained in the muscles at rest due to weak involuntary contraction of motor units. There is alternate contraction and relaxation of small groups of motor units at rest and their activity is maintained by neurons in the brain and spinal cord. Muscle tone is also exhibited by smooth muscles. The tone of the smooth muscle of blood vessels is very important in maintaining normal blood pressure.

ELECTROMYOGRAPHY

Recording of electrical activity of muscle on a CRO is electromyography. The instrument is called **electromyograph** and the record obtained **electromyogram**.

Electromyograph consists of electrodes, amplifier, CRO, electronic stimulator, photographic device, loudspeaker, tape recorder, etc.

Principle

When the muscle is in the relaxed state, no potentials are recorded, as it is electrically silent. When an action potential moves through the muscle fibers, some amount of energy is transmitted to the skin. When large number of muscle fibers contract, a summated effect can be recorded from the skin and potential with greater amplitude is obtained. In EMG, both visual and audio display of electrical activity is obtained.

Electrodes

Electrodes are used to pick up the electrical activity from the muscle. Two types of electrodes are used:

1. Surface disk electrodes
2. Needle electrodes

Surface disk electrode is placed on the skin and summated potentials from groups of muscle fibers can be recorded. Needle electrodes are very fine needles, which can be introduced into a single fiber or between 2 or 3 fibers. The record obtained depends on the number of muscle fibers involved. Thus, the recording can be monophasic, biphasic and polyphasic.

Loudspeaker makes the sounds associated with muscular contractions audible. Tape recorder helps to store the signals. Photographic device takes photographs from the oscilloscope and stores it.

Uses of EMG

- Helps in the diagnosis of neuromuscular disorders.
- Neuropathy can be distinguished from myopathy.
- Helps to distinguish between diseases of central nervous system and peripheral nervous system.
- Help to assess the prognosis of neuromuscular diseases, i.e., to check whether the patient is responding to treatment.
- Helps in nerve conduction studies. Conduction velocity is decreased in peripheral neuropathy.
- Normally at rest no spontaneous electrical activity is recorded from the muscle. Following denervation of muscle due to spinal cord lesions, abnormal spontaneous activities, such as fibrillation potentials and fasciculation potentials can be recorded during the resting phase (Fig. 7.20).

MUSCLE METABOLISM AND ENERGY SOURCE

PY3.11: Explain energy source and muscle metabolism.

Adenosine Triphosphate

Muscle contraction requires energy and the immediate source of this energy is the energy-rich organic phosphate derivative in the muscle, adenosine triphosphate (ATP). ATP is the only energy source that can be used directly for muscle contraction. The bonds attaching the last two phosphate radicals to the adenosine molecule are high energy phosphate bonds. Each of these bonds stores about

7300 calories of energy per mole of ATP. Thus during muscle contraction, when one phosphate radical is removed, about 7300 calories of energy are released. When the second phosphate radical is removed, still another 7300 calories become available. When one phosphate is removed, ATP is converted to adenosine diphosphate (ADP) and removal of the second converts ADP into adenosine monophosphate (AMP).

ATP must be regenerated continuously if contraction is to continue because muscle stores very little amount of ATP. The amount of ATP present in muscles can sustain muscle contraction only for a few seconds.

Muscle fibers can produce ATP in three ways:
1. By direct phosphorylation of ADP by creatine phosphate (**phosphocreatine-creatine system**)
2. By anaerobic cellular respiration (**glycogen-lactic acid system**)
3. By aerobic cellular respiration (**aerobic system**)

Creatine Phosphate-Creatine System

Much of the energy for ATP synthesis in the muscle comes from **creatine phosphate or phosphocreatine**. *Creatine phosphate is a high energy molecule found only in muscle fibers and using creatine phosphate for ATP production is unique to muscle fibers.* Creatine phosphate is 3–6 times more plentiful than ATP in the sarcoplasm of a relaxed muscle fiber. At rest, the muscle fibers contain more ATP than needed for resting metabolism. The excess ATP is used to synthesize creatine phosphate.

$$\text{Creatine} + \text{ATP} \xrightarrow{\text{Creatine kinase}} \text{Creatine phosphate} + \text{ADP}$$

When muscle contraction occurs, the above reaction is reversed and new ATP molecules are formed and are used for contraction. When creatine phosphate decomposes to creatine and phosphate ion, about 10,300 calories of energy is released. This energy is used to reconstitute the high-energy bond of ATP. The energy transfer from creatine phosphate to ATP occurs within a small fraction of a second.

Resynthesis of ATP and creatine phosphate occur by the breakdown of glucose to carbon dioxide and water. Glucose in the blood stream enters the muscle cells during exercise and is degraded to pyruvate. Another source of intracellular glucose is the stored glycogen in the muscle. If adequate oxygen is present, pyruvate enters the citric acid cycle and is metabolized to carbon dioxide and water. This process is called **aerobic glycolysis**. This process liberates sufficient energy to form large quantities of ATP from ADP. At rest and in mild-to-moderate exercise 95% of ATP used up comes from aerobic metabolism. It occurs in the mitochondria and the pathway is called **oxidative phosphorylation**. Glucose is broken down completely to CO_2 and water. It provides 36 ATP per glucose molecule. The sources of oxygen for the muscle are oxygen diffusing from blood and oxygen released from myoglobin.

$$\text{Glucose} + 2\,\text{ATP} \xrightarrow{O_2} 6\,CO_2 + 6\,H_2O + 40\,\text{ATP} + \text{Heat}$$

Glycogen Lactic Acid System

The stored glycogen in the muscle can be split into glucose and the glucose can be used for energy. The initial stage of this process (glycolysis) occurs without the use of oxygen and so it is called **anaerobic metabolism.** During glycolysis, each glucose molecule is split into two pyruvic acid molecules and four ATP molecules are formed. If oxygen supply is insufficient, pyruvate does not enter citric acid cycle, but is reduced to lactic acid. This is **anaerobic glycolysis**. Lactic acid diffuses into the interstitial fluid and into the blood stream. The accumulation of lactic acid leads to muscle fatigue.

Thus when muscle glycogen is transformed to lactic acid, considerable amounts of ATP are formed without consumption of oxygen. When large amount of ATP is required for short periods of muscle contraction, anaerobic glycolysis can be used as a rapid source of energy.

$$\text{Glucose} + 2\,\text{ATP} \xrightarrow{\text{Anaerobic}} 2\,\text{Lactic acid} + 4\,\text{ATP}$$

Skeletal muscle also takes up free fatty acids from the blood and oxidizes them to CO_2 and water via aerobic cellular respiration.

$$\text{Free fatty acid} \xrightarrow{O_2} CO_2 + H_2O + 100\,\text{ATP}$$

Heat Production in the Muscle

- **Resting heat** is the heat given off at rest from the muscle, and is produced by the basal metabolic processes occurring in the muscle, especially for the activity of Na^+-K^+ pump to maintain resting membrane potential.
- **Activation heat** is the heat produced in the stimulated muscle before shortening. This heat is the byproduct of energy used in the release of calcium from the terminal cisterns and binding of calcium with troponin.
- **Shortening heat** is the heat released during muscle shortening. It depends on the degree and velocity of shortening. As there is no shortening in isometric contraction, there is no shortening heat associated with it.
- **Initial heat** is the heat produced in excess of the resting heat during contraction. It includes activation heat and shortening heat.
- **Recovery heat**: During recovery, i.e., following muscle contraction, heat production in excess of the resting heat continues for as long as 30 minutes. This is the **recovery heat** or delayed heat and is the heat liberated by the metabolic processes that restore the muscle to the pre-contraction state. Recovery heat is equal to the initial heat.
- **Maintenance heat** occurs in tetanic contractions.

Oxygen Debt

During muscular exercise, energy needs are met from ATP and creatine phosphate stores and by aerobic breakdown of glucose. Some amount of energy is also released by the anaerobic breakdown of glucose to lactic acid. After exercise, lactic acid is converted back into pyruvic acid by heart, liver, kidney, and skeletal muscle. Pyruvic acid is used for ATP production *via* aerobic cellular respiration. **Oxygen debt** (coined by AV Hill) is the extra amount of oxygen consumed during the recovery period of exercise above the resting oxygen consumption. Oxygen debt is also referred to as **recovery oxygen uptake**. After exercise, during the recovery period, extra oxygen is consumed for the following reasons:

- To oxidize excess lactic acid formed during exercise. It is first converted to pyruvic acid, which is then oxidized to CO_2 and H_2O.
- To replenish ATP and creatine phosphate stores.
- To replace oxygen that was removed from myoglobin.
- Rise in temperature during exercise increases metabolic rate and so O_2 consumption is increased till temperature comes back to normal.
- Catecholamines released during exercise also stimulate metabolic rate and so O_2 consumption is increased.
- Heart rate and respiratory rate remain high for some time after exercise and the cardiac muscle and respiratory muscles continue to consume more O_2 after exercise.

Muscle Fatigue

Muscle fatigue is defined as a subjective sensation of the feeling of tiredness after prolonged activity, where the muscles are unable to contract forcefully. Fatigue is due to changes occurring in the muscle fibers and in severe cases there will be muscle damage. Certain types of muscle fibers fatigue more quickly than others, e.g., fast muscles fatigue more easily but posture-controlling muscles get fatigued very slowly. This is because all the motor units in the muscle are not stimulated at the same time. If this occurs, the movements will be jerky instead of being smooth. Normally, while some motor units are contracting, others will be relaxed and this alternately contracting motor units delays muscle fatigue. This is referred to as **asynchronous muscle contraction** and this helps in the sustained contraction of postural muscles. When the force of contraction is to be increased, more number of motor units is activated and is called **motor unit recruitment**.

Causes of Muscle Fatigue

- Depletion of ATP and creatine phosphate within muscle fibers
- Inadequate release of calcium from the sarcoplasmic reticulum
- Hypoxia
- Depletion of nutrients, such as glycogen
- Acidosis due to increase in the lactic acid content
- Increase in the temperature
- Inadequate release of acetylcholine at the neuromuscular junction (NMJ)
- Continuous stimulation of brain by impulses from the muscles, causing neuronal fatigue
- There is reduction in critical fusion frequency (CFF) in fatigue. When a skeletal muscle is stimulated repetitively, so that, the successive stimuli fall during the contraction period of previous contraction complete fusion of mechanical events occurs. The resulting state of continuous contraction of the muscle is called **tetanus**. The minimum frequency at which tetanus develops is called **critical fusion frequency**. For mammalian skeletal muscle, CFF is 50–100 stimuli/sec. In fatigue, it is less.

Gradation of Muscular Activity

PY3.12: Explain the gradation of muscular activity.

The contraction in the whole muscle is graded by variation in the number of muscle fibers involved. By a weak stimulus, only few fibers become excited when compared with maximal or submaximal stimuli. On minimal voluntary contraction, when EMG is recorded, only a single or two motor units are stimulated. With progressive increase in voluntary contraction, the firing rates of small units increases until it reaches a certain frequency, when larger units are recruited. During maximal contraction, many motor units are recruited.

■ APPLIED PHYSIOLOGY

PY3.13: Describe muscular dystrophy; myopathies.

Muscular Dystrophy; Myopathies

Myopathies or skeletal muscle disorders include structural changes or functional impairment of muscles. Features of myopathies include proximal limb weakness with normal reflexes and sensations. Examples of myopathies include myasthenia gravis, hypokalemic or hyperkalemic periodic paralysis, poliomyelitis, mitochondrial myopathy, etc. Myopathies can be hereditary as in Duchenne muscular dystrophy.

Muscular dystrophy refers to diseases that cause progressive weakness of skeletal muscles. The prominent cause for muscular dystrophy is mutations in the genes coding for the various components of the dystrophin-glycoprotein complex.

Dystrophin is a structural protein of the muscle fiber localized on the inner surface of the sarcolemma. This protein keeps the muscle cell membrane from breaking or tearing when the muscles contract or relax. The gene coding for this protein is located in the short arm of X-chromosome. Dystrophin binds to **F-actin** and to β-**dystroglycan**. The β-dystroglycan complexes to α-**dystroglycan** which in turn binds to laminin in the extracellular matrix. The transmembrane **sarcoglycan** protein also binds to dystrophin. These five proteins complex tightly with each other. This complex confer stability to the sarcolemma. Deficiency of one member of the complex may cause abnormalities in other components affecting the structural integrity of the muscle.

Myopathies may be structural myopathies where the genes coding for the structural proteins get mutated or metabolic myopathies.

Structural Myopathies

Duchenne Muscular Dystrophy

The dystrophin gene is one of the largest genes in the body and mutations can occur at different sites in it. Duchenne

muscular dystrophy or **pseudohypertrophic muscular dystrophy** is a serious condition where there is mutation of the gene that encodes the dystrophin protein. Dystrophin protein is absent in the muscle in this condition.
- This is an **X-linked recessive** disorder.
- The child falls frequently once it starts walking.
- Loss of muscle strength is progressive.
- There will be hypertrophy of the affected muscles like calf muscles
- Walking becomes difficult as age advances.
- Death occurs by the age of 30 years

Becker Muscular Dystrophy

Becker Muscular Dystrophy (BMD) named after German doctor **Peter Emil Becker** is a genetic, degenerative disease primarily affecting voluntary muscles. This is a condition where dystrophin is present but altered or reduced in amount. It is a less severe disease and the course of the disease is slower. The muscles become weaker and smaller. Boys are affected mainly but some females can be affected. Many females act as carriers. It has an **X-linked recessive** inheritance. The patients live up to mid-forties. The principal cause of death is heart failure from dilated cardiomyopathy.

Limb-Girdle Muscular Dystrophies

This condition is associated with mutation of the genes coding for the sarcoglycans or other components of the dystrophin-glycoprotein complex. It includes a group of diseases that cause weakness and wasting of the muscles in the arms and legs. The proximal muscles are mostly affected like muscles of shoulders, upper arms, pelvic area and thighs.

Metabolic Myopathies

Metabolic myopathies are rare genetic diseases that affect metabolism. Mutation in genes that code for various enzymes involved in the metabolism of carbohydrates, fats and proteins to CO_2 and H_2O in the muscle and production of ATP can cause metabolic myopathies like **McArdle syndrome** where there is lack of enzyme that assists carbohydrate metabolism. In **Pompe disease**, there is deficiency of acid maltase. The affected muscles cannot convert fuel into energy and thus cannot function. **Mitochondrial metabolic myopathy** results from a lack of a particular enzyme normally present in the mitochondria, the energy producing parts of the cells.

Manifestations are exercise intolerance, fatigue, muscle cramps, breathing difficulty and muscle breakdown due to accumulation of toxic metabolites. Muscle breakdown releases muscle proteins into the bloodstream, which may cause severe kidney damage. Metabolic myopathy can cause a serious reaction to general anesthesia called **malignant hyperthermia**.

■ MULTIPLE CHOICE QUESTIONS

1. **Force generating proteins are:**
    a. Myosin and myoglobin
    b. Dynein and kinesin
    c. Calmodulin and G-protein
    d. Troponin

2. **When tetanizing stimuli are given to a muscle, increased response is due to:**
    a. Recruitment phenomenon
    b. Increased Ca^{2+} influx into muscle fiber
    c. Contraction of different muscle fibers at different places
    d. All of the above

3. **All the following are true about striated muscle, *except*:**
    a. ATP and creatine phosphate are responsible for structural alterations in muscle
    b. Calcium combines with troponin and causes change in tropomyosin
    c. The T-tubules are modified endoplasmic reticulum
    d. The endoplasmic reticulum in muscle is called as sarcoplasmic reticulum

4. **All the following are associated with actin filament, *except*:**
    a. G-actin
    b. Tropomyosin
    c. Troponin
    d. Tapaicin

5. **Best method to increase muscle strength is:**
    a. Isometric exercise
    b. Isotonic exercise
    c. Electrical stimulation
    d. Aerobic exercise

6. **Among the muscles, skeletal muscle is the most excitable tissue because:**
    a. There are two T tubules per sarcomere and has well developed sarcoplasmic reticulum
    b. Is supplied by large myelinated nerve fibers
    c. Is regulated by nerves
    d. Chronaxie is longer

7. **Regarding skeletal muscle contraction true is:**
    a. H band increases
    b. I band increases
    c. Both H and I decrease
    d. Both remain constant

8. **False about excitatory postsynaptic potential is:**
    a. It is localized
    b. Can be summated
    c. Weans in exponential rate
    d. Hyperpolarization occurs

9. **All are true regarding muscle contraction, *except*:**
    a. A band remain unchanged
    b. H zone disappears
    c. I band become wider
    d. Two Z lines come closer

10. **Which protein prevents muscle contraction by covering the active sites of actin filament?**
    a. Troponin
    b. Calmodulin
    c. Myosin
    d. Tropomyosin

11. The action of tropomyosin is:
    a. Help in the interaction of actin and myosin
    b. Cover myosin binding sites in actin filament at rest
    c. Slides over myosin during contraction
    d. Causes calcium release

12. The force of muscle contraction can be increased by all the following, *except*:
    a. Increasing the frequency of activation of motor units
    b. Increasing the number of motor units activated
    c. Increasing the amplitude of action potentials in the motor neurons
    d. Recruiting larger motor units

13. Twitch of a single motor unit is called:
    a. Myoclonic jerk   b. Fasciculation
    c. Tremor   d. Chorea

14. During skeletal muscle contraction there is no change in the length of:
    a. A band   b. I band
    c. H zone   d. Sarcomere

15. During muscle contraction:
    a. Width of I band increases
    b. Width of A band increases
    c. Z lines come closer
    d. Actin filaments move apart

16. The correct statement regarding action potential in skeletal muscle is:
    a. Has a prolonged plateau phase
    b. Is not essential for contraction
    c. Spreads to all parts of the muscle through T-tubules
    d. Ca^{2+} has a very important role in the depolarization phase

17. The cross-bridges of the sarcomere in the skeletal muscle are made up of:
    a. Troponin   b. Tropomyosin
    c. Actin   d. Myosin

18. Depolarization of the T tubule membrane of skeletal muscle activate the sarcoplasmic reticulum via:
    a. Ryanodine receptor
    b. Dihydropyridine receptor
    c. Muscarinic receptor
    d. Nicotinic receptor

19. At the resting length of the skeletal muscle, which of the following is maximum?
    a. Total tension   b. Active tension
    c. Passive tension   d. Resting tension

20. The relaxing protein in mammalian skeletal muscle include:
    a. Actin   b. Troponin
    c. Tropomyosin   d. Calmodulin

21. The following are true of isometric contraction, *except*:
    a. The muscle does not shorten
    b. The tension in the muscle increases
    c. Work is done
    d. Heat is liberated

22. The function of tropomyosin in skeletal muscle include:
    a. Produce shortening by sliding on actin
    b. Bind with myosin during contraction
    c. Acts as a relaxing protein at rest
    d. Generates ATP during contraction

23. All the following statements regarding skeletal muscles are correct, *except*:
    a. It is a true syncytium
    b. It is under voluntary control
    c. It depends on electrical stimuli from neurons to elicit contraction
    d. Relaxation of skeletal muscle is a passive process

24. All are true regarding skeletal muscle contraction, *except*:
    a. H band decreases
    b. Z lines come closer
    c. A band decreases
    d. Length of the sarcomere decreases

25. The cross bridges of the sarcomere in skeletal muscle is formed of:
    a. Actin   b. Myosin
    c. Troponin   d. Tropomyosin

26. The function of tropomyosin in skeletal muscle is:
    a. Releases calcium after initiation of contraction
    b. Bind to myosin during contraction
    c. Act as a relaxing protein at rest covering the active sites of actin filament
    d. Binds to calcium and initiates contraction

27. High twitch muscle fibers in comparison to low twitch muscle fibers are having more:
    a. Mitochondria   b. cAMP
    c. Cytoplasm   d. Enzymes

28. In severe exercise muscle spasm occurs due to:
    a. Accumulation of K^+
    b. Accumulation of acetylcholine
    c. Accumulation of Ca^{2+}
    d. Depletion of ATP

29. When a muscle is stimulated, the Ca^{2+} stored in the sarcoplasmic reticulum is released by activating:
    a. Ryanodine receptors
    b. Dihydropyridine receptors
    c. Myosin light chain kinase
    d. Phosphodiesterase

30. The band in the muscle fiber that disappears on muscle contraction:
    a. A band   b. I band
    c. H band   d. M band

31. All the following statements regarding skeletal muscle contraction are true, *except*:
    a. Depends on action potential
    b. Recruitment of more number of fibers produces more contraction

c. Increase in the strength of action potential increases contraction
d. Increased availability of Ca^{2+} increases contraction

32. **Best method to increase the muscle strength is:**
    a. Isometric exercise
    b. Isotonic exercise
    c. Aerobic isotonic exercise
    d. Electrical stimulation

33. **Isotonic contraction differs from isometric contraction in that in the former:**
    a. Heat of activation is greater
    b. Muscle uses more high energy phosphate bonds
    c. Muscle is less efficient
    d. Recovery heat is less

34. **The source of ATP for skeletal muscle at rest is:**
    a. Phosphoryl creatine
    b. Free fatty acid
    c. Glucose
    d. Proteins

35. **When a skeletal muscle shortens in response to a stimulus, there is:**
    a. Decrease in the length of I and H band
    b. Decrease in the length of A band
    c. Decrease in the length of A and I bands
    d. Increase in the width of H zone

ANSWERS

1. b	2. b	3. c	4. d	5. a
6. a	7. c	8. d	9. c	10. d
11. b	12. c	13. b	14. a	15. c
16. c	17. d	18. b	19. b	20. a
21. c	22. c	23. d	24. c	25. b
26. c	27. a	28. d	29. a	30. c
31. c	32. b	33. b	34. c	35. a

Neuromuscular Junction or Myoneural Junction

CHAPTER 8

LEARNING OBJECTIVE
Must know
- Describe the structure of neuromuscular junction (NMJ)
- Mechanism of transmission of impulse across neuromuscular junction
- Classify neuromuscular blockers and mention their mechanism of action
- Describe the pathophysiology of myasthenia gravis
- Physiological basis of denervation hypersensitivity

STRUCTURE OF NEUROMUSCULAR JUNCTION

PY3.4: Describe the structure of neuromuscular junction and transmission of impulses.

As the axon supplying a skeletal muscle approaches the muscle, it loses its myelin sheath and divides into a number of terminal branches and each branch supplies a single muscle fiber. The junction between the branch of axon and the skeletal muscle fiber is called **neuromuscular junction (NMJ)** or **myoneural junction (Fig. 8.1)**.

When the nerve enters the muscle fiber, its tip enlarges to form a knob called **end foot** or **terminal button**. The synaptic knob dips into the muscle membrane and the membrane of the synaptic knob is called **presynaptic membrane** or prejunctional membrane. Membrane thickening seen in the presynaptic membrane is called **active zone**. The active zone contains many proteins and rows of Ca^{2+} channels. The neurotransmitters are released at the **release sites** in the active zone. In most of the muscles, one single muscle fiber contains only one NMJ.

The thickened portion of the muscle membrane of the NMJ is called **motor endplate** or **sole plate** or **post-junctional membrane**. Between the pre-junctional and post-junctional membranes is a small gap called **synaptic cleft** or neuromuscular cleft, which is about 50–100 nm wide. This cleft contains ECF and spongy reticular fibers to which acetylcholine esterase is attached. The motor endplate is thrown into folds or palisades called **subneuronal clefts** or **palisades** or **junctional folds**, which increase the surface area of motor endplate. The synaptic knob contains many small, **clear vesicles** 40 nm in diameter, which contain the neurotransmitter **acetylcholine (Fig. 8.1)**. Each nerve terminal contains about 300,000 vesicles and each vesicle contains about 10,000 acetylcholine molecules. Acetylcholine is synthesized in the nerve ending itself

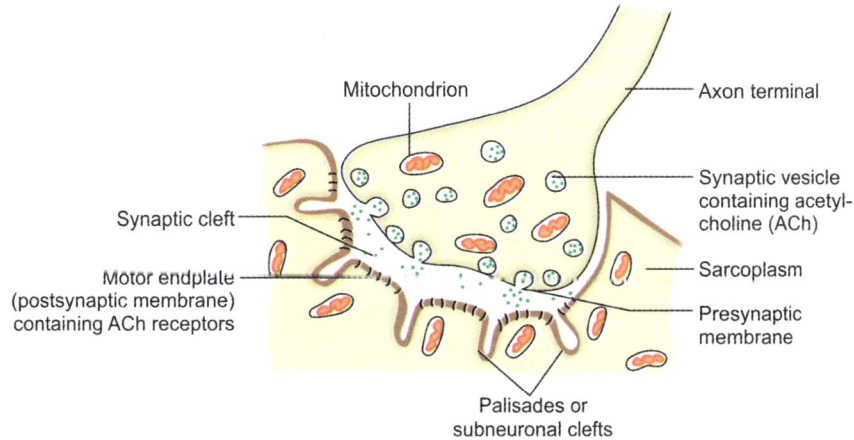

Fig. 8.1: Structure of neuromuscular junction.

and a small quantity is transmitted from the axon. *Neurons are the only cells in the body that can synthesize ACh*. Choline is not synthesized in the nerve ending, but enters the nerve ending by reuptake from the synaptic cleft.

$$\text{Choline + Acetyl-CoA} \xrightarrow{\text{Choline acetyltransferase}} \text{Acetylcholine}$$

Acetylcholine Receptors

Acetylcholine receptors are of two kinds, **nicotinic receptors** and **muscarinic receptors**. The motor endplate contains nicotinic acetylcholine receptors.

Acetylcholine receptors are studied in detail using snake venom neurotoxins that tightly bind to ACh receptors. For example, α-**toxin** in cobra venom binds to acetylcholine binding sites on ACh receptor and prevents ACh from binding to the receptor. This leads to paralysis.

Transmission of Action Potential at the NMJ

There is no anatomical continuity between nerve ending and the muscle fiber. *Action potential can never cross the NMJ.* Here, the transmission is **chemical** in nature. The presynaptic membrane communicates with the postsynaptic membrane by releasing a chemical called **neurotransmitter**. So NMJ is a chemical synapse. The nerve endings act as transducers converting electrical energy into chemical energy at the NMJ.

When an action potential reaches the nerve terminal, the presynaptic membrane becomes highly permeable to Ca^{2+}. Large amounts of Ca^{2+} enter into the synaptic knob from the synaptic cleft. This Ca^{2+} causes release of acetylcholine into the cleft by **emeiocytosis or exocytosis**. Each nerve impulse releases about 300–600 acetylcholine vesicles. The amount of ACh released at the NMJ is about 10 times more than that required to produce an action potential in the postsynaptic membrane. This is known as **safety factor** at NMJ. Excess ACh will be easily hydrolyzed by **acetylcholine esterase** and this prevents repetitive stimulation of the muscle fiber.

Receptors, which can combine with acetylcholine molecules present on the motor endplate of the postsynaptic membrane, are called **nicotinic acetylcholine receptors**. Acetylcholine receptors are also ligand-gated ion channels. When two molecules of acetylcholine combine with this receptor, some conformational changes occur in the receptor and the ion channel which is a part of the receptor opens (**ligand gating**). There is influx of cations, especially Na^+ into the motor endplate producing a depolarizing potential called **endplate potential**, which is a graded potential or local response. EPP is called a non-propagated change although it spreads along the membrane for some distance and for some time. *A change is called propagated only if it spreads from point to point without alteration.* EPP is a decremental potential. Action potential spreads without decrement and hence it is said to be propagated.

The magnitude of the EPP depends on the number of sodium ions entering the muscle fiber. This depends on the amount of acetylcholine released, which in turn depends on the frequency with which action potentials reach the axon terminal. When the summated endplate potential reaches firing level an action potential is produced in the muscle. Action potentials spread in both directions along the entire muscle fiber, which in turn initiates muscle contraction. The sequence of events takes about 5–10 milliseconds.

Endplate potential alone can be studied by giving blocking agents like **D-tubocurarine**. Action potential can be blocked in this way and EPP alone can be studied. Differences between action potential and endplate potential are given in **Table 8.1**.

After activation, cholinergic receptors are rapidly inactivated, reducing sodium entry. They remain inactive until acetylcholine dissociates from the receptor. Acetylcholine will be destroyed by an enzyme called **acetylcholine esterase**, which is found abundantly in the synaptic cleft and choline will be reabsorbed into the nerve terminal. Thus, the action of acetylcholine is short lived, i.e., ½ life is 1 ms. Destruction of acetylcholine is important because it prevents undue prolongation of the action of acetylcholine.

$$\text{Acetylcholine} \xrightarrow{\text{Acetylcholine esterase}} \text{Acetate + choline}$$

An average human motor endplate contains about 10^7–10^8 acetylcholine receptors. So the quantity of acetylcholine required for combination with receptor is about 100 million.

Miniature Endplate Potential (MEPP)

At rest, small quanta or packets of acetylcholine are released from the presynaptic membrane into the synaptic cleft producing a minute depolarizing potential called miniature EPP, which is only about 0.5 mV in amplitude. The size of the quanta of acetylcholine released varies directly with the Ca^{2+} concentration and inversely with the Mg^{2+} concentration at the motor endplate. The miniature EPP is very minimum and not sufficient to produce EPP. A large number of MEPP can be summated to produce an action potential when it reaches –50 mV which is the firing level.

Drugs and Toxins Acting on the NMJ

I. *Facilitatory drugs*
   - Acetylcholine-like action
     - Carbachol
     - Nicotine
     - Succinylcholine in low-to-moderate doses
   - Anticholine esterases
     - Physostigmine
     - Neostigmine

Table 8.1: Differences between action potential and endplate potential.

Endplate potential (EPP)	Action potential (AP)
It is a local event, hence not propagated	Once developed will be propagated
Does not show all-or-none phenomenon; stronger the stimulus, greater will be the response	Obeys all-or-none phenomenon
Precedes action potential	Follows endplate potential

- Di-isopropyl fluorophosphate (DIFP)
- Organophosphorus compounds (Tic 20)
- Organochloride compounds (Folidol)

II. *Neuromuscular blocking drugs*
- Curare and Gallamine
- Botulinum toxin

Drugs blocking acetylcholine receptors in the NMJ are classified into two:
1. **Non-depolarizing neuromuscular blockers**: d-tubocurarine, α-bungarotoxin.
2. **Depolarizing neuromuscular blockers**: Succinylcholine and anticholinesterases in high dosage.

> Succinylcholine in low-to-moderate doses causes muscle spasm as it has acetylcholine-like action when it binds to acetylcholine receptors in the motor endplate. But in high dosage, it induces desensitization of ACh-gated channels with consequent paralysis. So succinylcholine is used commonly as a muscle relaxant during abdominal surgery and during electro-convulsion treatment (to reduce violent movements during the procedure).

Facilitatory Drugs

Drugs Having Acetylcholine-like Action

These drugs behave like acetylcholine. They combine with acetylcholine receptors and cause contraction of muscle fiber, but they are resistant to the action of acetylcholine esterase. Therefore, their action is much more prolonged than that of ACh. In small doses, these drugs produce muscle spasm by binding to ACh receptors in the motor endplate. But in large doses, they produce flaccid paralysis because the muscle remains in a state of depolarization for a longer time and is refractory to any stimulus. This is due to desensitization of ACh-gated channels in the motor endplate. This is called **depolarizing block**. So succinylcholine is used in anesthesia as a muscle relaxant. *Thus, succinylcholine in low doses is a neuromuscular facilitatory drug, whereas in high doses, it is a depolarizing neuromuscular blocker.*

Anticholinesterases

Anticholinesterases are drugs that bind to acetylcholine esterase and inactivate it thereby preventing it from hydrolyzing acetylcholine in the synaptic cleft. Thus, it prolongs the half-life of acetylcholine. This leads to accumulation of large amounts of ACh in the myoneural cleft. In small doses, they produce spasm due to an increased availability of acetylcholine, which leads to prolonged depolarization. In large doses, they produce **depolarizing block**. The motor endplate becomes inexcitable due to Na^+ channel desensitization. Desensitization occurs in a ligand-gated channel when the ligand remains attached to the channel receptor for several milliseconds. Anticholine esterase drugs are of two types:
1. Reversible agents
2. Irreversible agents

Reversible Anticholine Esterases

The action of physostigmine and neostigmine is reversible and they are competitive inhibitors of acetylcholine esterase. These drugs get hydrolyzed by acetylcholine esterase within a few hours. Thus acetylcholine esterase becomes available for hydrolyzing acetylcholine. Reversible inhibitors are used in the treatment of myasthenia gravis and curare poisoning.

Irreversible Anticholine Esterases

Insecticides like organophosphates, and **nerve gas** (DIFP) bind to cholinesterase so tightly that the block is irreversible. They are poorly hydrolyzed by acetylcholine esterase and so they remain attached to acetylcholine esterase molecule for several weeks. Ach esterase will not be available to bind and hydrolyze Ach. This causes channel desensitization of the motor endplate due to continuous action of Ach. So, irreversible anticholinesterases produce deadly paralysis and death is due to paralysis especially of respiratory muscles.

Neuromuscular Blocking Drugs

> **PY3.5:** Discuss the action of neuromuscular blocking agents.

1. *Non-depolarizing neuromuscular blocker*
2. *Depolarizing neuromuscular blocker*

Non-depolarizing neuromuscular blocker

D-tubocurarine or curare

Curare is extracted from a plant and is used by Red Indians as an arrow poison. Curare produces **non-depolarizing block** unlike succinylcholine, which produces depolarizing block. Structurally, **d-tubocurarine**, the active principle of curare, is similar to acetylcholine. So there is competitive inhibition of acetylcholine. Curare binds to ACh receptors on the motor endplate, but do not depolarize the motor endplate, as it has no intrinsic activity. But, it keeps the ACh receptors blocked. The affinity of curare for acetylcholine receptor is very high, but as the curare-receptor complex has no action, the muscle goes into flaccid paralysis.

(α-**Bungarotoxin** found in the venom of krait produces non-depolarizing block similar to that of curare.)

Treatment for Curare Poisoning

Neostigmine is used as an antidote for curare poisoning. In competitive inhibition, when the substrate concentration is increased, the activity of inhibitor decreases. Neostigmine increases the concentration of acetylcholine at the motor endplate by inhibiting acetylcholine esterase. D-tubocurarine leaves the receptor and acetylcholine combines with the receptor as the substrate concentration is high. So the block produced by tubocurarine is a reversible block.

Depolarizing Neuromuscular Blocker

Drugs like succinylcholine has acetylcholine like action. But it is poorly inactivated by acetylcholine esterase and therefore has a very prolonged action as compared to acetylcholine. In high doses it causes channel desensitization of the ACh-gated channels leading to paralysis. The channel remains desensitized long after the succinylcholine molecules detach from ACh receptors.

Botulinum Toxin

Botulinum toxin is a bacterial toxin produced by *Clostridium botulinum*. It inhibits the release of acetylcholine by exocytosis at the nerve terminals of the NMJ and parasympathetic cholinergic synapses. It is best known for producing food poisoning. This toxin leads to **flaccid paralysis**. Death results from paralysis of the respiratory muscles.

Applied Physiology

- **Botulinum toxin (Botox)** is the first bacterial toxin to be used as medicine. It acts as a long-acting muscle relaxant whose effect lasts for 3–4 months. It is used therapeutically in conditions of muscle hyperactivity as in squint due to spasm of extra-ocular muscle. Injection of small doses of botulinum toxin into the lower esophageal sphincter relieves spasm in achalasia cardia. It is also used for cosmetic purposes to relax muscles that cause facial wrinkles and in skeletal deformities that occur due to muscle spasm.
- **α-Latrotoxin** is the toxin of black widow spider *Lactrodectus mactans*. It binds to receptors in the presynaptic membrane and results in massive Ca^{2+} influx and secretion of large amount of ACh into the myoneural cleft. This leads to muscle spasm and death results due to severe spasm of the respiratory muscles.

Diseases Affecting the NMJ

> **PY3.6:** Describe the pathophysiology of myasthenia gravis.

- **Myasthenia gravis**: It is a rare, serious and sometimes fatal disease in which skeletal muscles are weak and easily fatigued. The disease is caused by the formation of circulating antibodies, which destroy the **nicotinic acetylcholine receptors** on the motor endplate of NMJ. Therefore, it is considered as an **autoimmune disease**. ACh receptor antibodies are demonstrated by radioimmunoassay in the serum of 90% of patients with myasthenia gravis. Histologically, the number of sub-neuronal clefts is decreased and there is widening of the synaptic cleft. In adults, with myasthenia gravis, about 70% of patients show hyperplasia of the thymus gland. Excessive synthesis of thymic hormone, thymopoietin may contribute to the autoimmune response. Thymopoietin binds to the ACh receptors to inactivate them. It is seen that surgical removal of thymus is of benefit in these patients.
  Treatment: **Neostigmine**, which increases the availability of ACh in the synaptic cleft, is the drug of choice. High dose of **cortisol** is also given to suppress antibody production (immunosuppressant). Plasmapheresis also helps to remove the autoantibodies. Thymectomy is done in patients with thymoma.
- **Lambert-Eaton myasthenic syndrome (LEMS)**: LEMS resembles myasthenia gravis. Here, muscle weakness is caused by autoantibodies against one of the voltage-gated Ca^{2+} channels in the nerve ending at the NMJ. This decreases the normal Ca^{2+} influx at the synaptic knob that causes acetylcholine release. The deficiency of ACh results in muscle weakness. Aminopyridines, which block the voltage-gated K^+ channels on the nerve terminals, is of limited use in LEMS. These drugs prolong action potential in the nerve terminal, which results in greater Ca^{2+} influx and release of more ACh into the cleft.

EFFECTS OF DENERVATION OF MUSCLE

- Fibrillation
- Denervation hypersensitivity or supersensitivity
- Fasciculation
- Muscle atrophy

Fibrillation

In the intact body, skeletal muscle contracts only if its motor nerve supply is stimulated. Destruction of this nerve supply leads to abnormal excitability of the muscle and fine, irregular **contractions of the individual fibers** called fibrillation. Fibrillation is seen for several weeks after injury and then ceases as the muscle cells atrophy. Such contractions are not visible grossly, but fibrillation potentials can be recorded by electromyography using needle electrodes (*refer* **Fig. 7.20**). If the motor nerve regenerates, these potentials disappear. Fibrillation is due to denervation hypersensitivity.

Denervation Hypersensitivity or Supersensitivity

When degeneration of a motor nerve supplying a skeletal muscle occurs, the muscle gradually becomes **hypersensitive to acetylcholine**. This is called *denervation hypersensitivity*. Here, a minimum quantity of acetylcholine can produce stimulation of the muscle. The synthesis of acetylcholine receptors at the motor endplate increases and the already existing ones become activated. Denervation hypersensitivity disappears if the skeletal muscle atrophies. Denervation hypersensitivity is also seen in denervated smooth muscles and exocrine glands (except sweat glands). Denervated smooth muscle does not atrophy, but becomes hypersensitive to the chemical mediators.

Causes of Hypersensitivity

- *Upregulation of receptors*: When there is deficiency of a chemical messenger, there will be an increase in the number of receptors. Normally, only the motor endplate contains acetylcholine receptors; but in denervated muscle, the area of the muscle membrane sensitive to acetylcholine increases because of **upregulation of receptors**.
- If the neurotransmitter is norepinephrine, in addition to upregulation of receptors there is reduction in the reuptake of norepinephrine into the presynaptic membrane as the ending of the cut nerve degenerates. Norepinephrine, reaching the synaptic cleft from other sources, stimulates the noradrenergic receptors on the postsynaptic membrane and the effect will be greater.

Fasciculations

Intact motor nerve supply is required for the organization of the muscle endplate and for the clustering of cholinergic receptors to that region. Receptors belonging to denervated fibers fail to cluster and become spread across the muscle membrane. Muscle fibers within a denervated motor unit may then discharge spontaneously; giving rise to visible twitches called fasciculations. These are jerky, visible contractions (twitching) of **groups of muscle fibers.** It can also be as a result of pathologic discharge of spinal motor neurons. It is seen in diseases affecting the anterior horn cells; e.g., in poliomyelitis, the anterior horn cell is destroyed and there will be spontaneous discharge of impulses causing fasciculation.

Muscle Atrophy and Reaction of Degeneration

When there is permanent loss of motor nerve supply to a muscle, the muscle shows flaccid paralysis and atrophies. Atrophy of muscle is called **muscle wasting**. Motor nerves exert trophic influences on the muscles they innervate. Denervated muscles undergo marked atrophy, losing more than half of their original bulk in 2–3 months. The size of the muscle decreases. This is not due to decrease in the number of muscle fibers but due to decrease in the diameter of the fibers. Individual fibers separate and dissolution of the contents occurs and the fiber becomes a tube-like structure. The reflexes are lost. The paralyzed muscle ceases to respond to faradic stimuli after 4–7 days of nerve injury. After 10 days, the muscle responds only sluggishly to galvanic stimulation and the strength of the current must be greater than that required for a normally innervated muscle. This altered response of muscle to electrical stimulation is known as **reaction of degeneration**.

In reaction of degeneration, anodal closing contraction (ACC) will be greater than cathodal closing contraction (CCC). But in a normal muscle, CCC will be greater than ACC. The muscle is stimulated with two electrodes, one electrode acts as active electrode and this is kept at the motor point. It is the point at which the nerve enters the muscle. The other electrode, which is called the indifferent electrode is kept over the muscle on a flat surface of the body. Electrode at the motor point can be made anode or cathode. First, apply galvanic current and give a make shock after closing the circuit with motor point as anode and record the effect. Make shock is given because break shock is more powerful than make shock and may injure the nerve. Similarly, stimulate with motor point as cathode and record the contraction. In normal muscles, it is seen that CCC>ACC, but in reaction of degeneration, ACC>CCC.

Muscle Hypertrophy

Hypertrophy is the increase in the muscle size due to forceful muscular activity, especially isometric exercises. There is slight increase in the number of muscle fibers due to the presence of satellite cells referred to as **hyperplasia**, but the main change is increase in the diameter of the fibers already present. There is increase in the amount of sarcoplasmic reticulum, mitochondria, glycogen, lipids, ATP content, and phosphocreatine. Myofibrils, i.e., thick and thin filaments also increase in size and number. As hypertrophied muscle contains more myofibrils, they are capable of more forceful contraction. The strength and size of the skeletal muscles can be increased by isometric exercises but the muscle should contract to at least 75% of its maximum tension to hypertrophy. Weak muscular activity although prolonged does not produce hypertrophy.

Cardiac muscle hypertrophy is seen when the load on the heart is chronically increased as in hypertension. It is also seen in muscular dystrophy, which is due to alteration in the various proteins in the contractile apparatus like dystrophin.

MULTIPLE CHOICE QUESTIONS

1. **Miniature endplate potential:**
   a. Is inhibited by anticholineesterase
   b. Occurs in resting muscle
   c. Causes depolarization of muscle
   d. Occurs in working muscle

2. **The motor endplate contains how many nicotinic acetylcholine receptors approximately?**
   a. 1 million   b. 10 million
   c. 20 million   d. 50 million

3. **Entry of which ion into the presynaptic membrane causes release of neurotransmitter into the synaptic cleft at the neuromuscular junction:**
   a. Sodium ions   b. Potassium ions
   c. Calcium ions   d. Chloride ions

4. **Myasthenia gravis may be associated with:**
   a. Drug intake
   b. Viral infection
   c. B-lymphocyte dysfunction
   d. Thymoma

5. **Synaptic transmission in autonomic ganglia is due to:**
   a. Adrenergic receptors
   b. Nicotinic receptors
   c. Muscarinic receptors
   d. Dopaminergic receptors

6. **The neurotransmitter present at the neuromuscular junction in skeletal muscle:**
   a. Dopamine   b. Epinephrine
   c. Acetylcholine   d. Norepinephrine

7. **Which of the following is a presynaptic blocking agent of neuromuscular junction?**
   a. D-tubocurarine b. Succinylcholine
   c. Botulinum toxin d. Physostigmine

8. **A patient complains of muscle weakness. On administration of neostigmine it disappears. The mechanism of action of the drug is:**
   a. It blocks action of acetylcholine
   b. It interferes with the action of amine oxidase

c. It interferes with the action of carbonic anhydrase
d. It interferes with the action of acetylcholine esterase

9. Enzyme involved in acetylcholine synthesis is:
   a. Choline esterase
   b. Pseudocholine esterase
   c. Choline acetyltransferase
   d. Transaminase

10. Neostigmine decreases muscular weakness by:
    a. Blocking the action of acetylcholine
    b. Stimulating the action of norepinephrine
    c. Interfering with the action of choline esterase
    d. Increasing the synthesis of acetylcholine

11. The endplate potential at the neuromuscular junction:
    a. Obeys all or none law
    b. Can be easily recorded
    c. Is a localized potential
    d. Is a hyperpolarizing potential

12. Neostigmine act by:
    a. Increasing the number of acetylcholine receptors
    b. Inhibiting acetylcholine metabolism
    c. Accelerating acetylcholine metabolism
    d. Decreasing the number of acetylcholine receptors

13. Shortest acting skeletal muscle relaxant is:
    a. Succinylcholine   b. D-tubocurarine
    c. Metacholine   d. Botulinum toxin

14. Curare in therapeutic doses:
    a. Decreases the amplitude of skeletal muscle contraction
    b. Prevents propagation of action potential in skeletal muscle
    c. Enhances the action of choline esterase
    d. Enhances the action of catecholamines

15. Endplate potential is characterized by:
    a. Propagation
    b. All or none law
    c. Depolarization
    d. Hyperpolarization

16. Which action is caused by acetylcholine through nicotinic receptors?
    a. Contraction of skeletal muscles
    b. Decrease in heart rate
    c. Secretion of saliva
    d. Contraction of pupils

17. Spontaneous release of acetylcholine at the neuromuscular junction produces:
    a. Miniature endplate potential
    b. Action potential
    c. Post-tetanic potential
    d. Resting membrane potential

18. Myasthenia gravis is a disorder of:
    a. Motor neuron
    b. Neuromuscular junction
    c. Peripheral nerve
    d. Spinal cord

ANSWERS

1. b	2. d	3. c	4. d	5. b
6. c	7. c	8. d	9. c	10. c
11. c	12. b	13. a	14. a	15. c
16. a	17. a	18. b		

Cahpter 9: Cardiac Muscle

LEARNING OBJECTIVES

Must know
- Describe the structure of cardiac muscle
- Describe the ionic basis of ventricular action potential with the help of a diagram
- Ionic basis of nodal action potential and causes of prepotential
- Enumerate the properties of cardiac muscle
- Explain length-tension relationship in cardiac muscle

STRUCTURE OF CARDIAC MUSCLE

PY5.2: Describe the properties of cardiac muscle including its morphology, electrical, mechanical and metabolic functions.

Cardiac muscle is striated, involuntary muscle composed of a branching network of muscle fibers. Each muscle fiber is about 80 μm in length and 15 μm broad. Cardiac muscle fiber has a single centrally placed nucleus and the fibers are interconnected. Sarcomere is the functional unit of the muscle fiber. Cardiac muscle does not have the capacity to regenerate because of the lack of stem cells and absence of mitosis in the mature cardiac muscle fibers. So, after myocardial infarction, the infarcted tissue can only be replaced by fibrous scar tissue. The myocardial cells are divided into two groups:

1. **Working myocardial cells**, which include atrial and ventricular musculature. Their function is to contract.
2. **Pacemaker cells and conducting cells**: They do not contract, but can generate impulse and conduct it to different parts of heart.

The myocardial cells are connected to one another end to end by special junctions called **intercalated discs**, which are irregular transverse thickenings of the muscle membrane held together by desmosomes. They are present at the Z lines. The pull of one contractile unit can be transmitted along its axis to the next. There are **gap junctions** between adjacent cells, which allow action potentials to spread immediately from one cardiac muscle fiber to another. Thus, the cells act as a single unit or **functional syncytium (Fig. 9.1A)**.

ELECTRICAL ACTIVITY OF CARDIAC MUSCLE

Working Myocardial Cell

Monophasic recording from a single ventricular muscle fiber is taken.

Different Values for Cardiac Muscle

- RMP: minus 90 mV (– 90 mV)
- Duration of action potential: 250 ms
- Amplitude: 105–110 mV
- Absolute refractory period: 200 ms

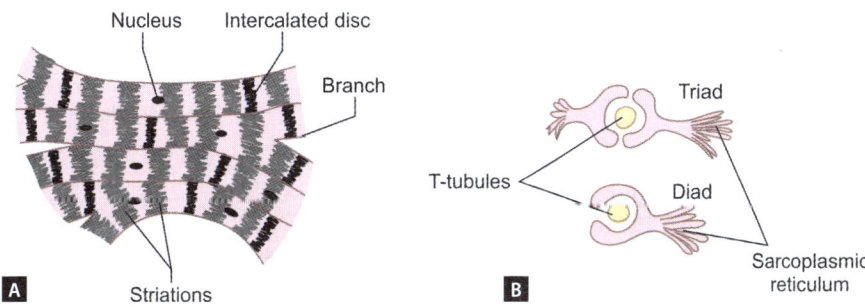

Figs. 9.1A and B: (A) Structure of cardiac muscle; (B) Sarcoplasmic reticulum in cardiac muscle fiber forming triad and diad around T-tubule.

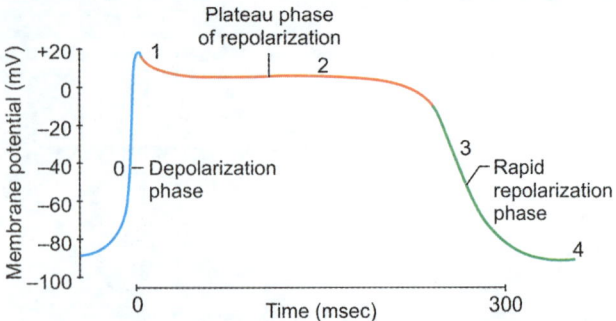

Fig. 9.2: Action potential recorded from a ventricular muscle fiber.

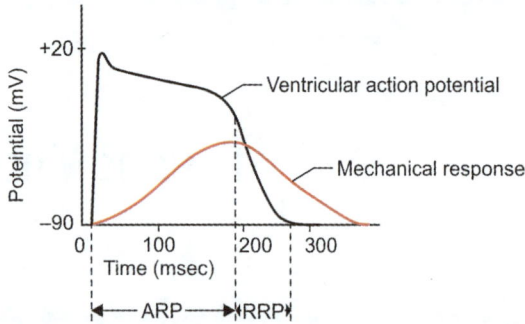

Fig. 9.3: Refractory period in cardiac muscle action potential.
[ARP: absolute refractory period (200 msec); RRP: relative refractory period]

- Chronaxie : 1–3 ms
- Conduction velocity : 1 m/sec

Ionic Basis of Action Potential

Action potential is divided into different phases (**Fig. 9.2**):
- **Phase 0:** Depolarization
- **Phase 1:** Initial rapid repolarization
- **Phase 2:** Plateau phase
- **Phase 3:** Late rapid repolarization
- **Phase 4:** Resting level or baseline

Phase 0: This phase is due to opening of voltage-gated sodium channel and explosive entry of Na^+ into the cell. Slow Ca^{2+} channels also open when the membrane potential reaches –30 to –40 mV. Duration is 2 ms.

Phase 1: This phase is due to closure of Na^+ channel and Cl^- influx. There is also slow increase in K^+ permeability.

Phase 2: This is due to slower but prolonged opening of voltage-gated Ca^{2+} channels through which Ca^{2+} and Na^+ ions enter. So these channels are also called Na^+-Ca^{2+} channels. At the same time, there is also increase in K^+ permeability and K^+ goes out of the cell. The efflux of equal number of cations balances the influx of cation and hence a plateau phase is obtained.

Phase 3: This is due to closure of Ca^{2+} channels and sudden rapid efflux of K^+ through K^+ channels.

Phase 4: The membrane pump starts functioning and re-establishes the resting potential. Most of the excess Ca^{2+} that has entered the cell mainly during phase 2 are eliminated principally by a $3Na^+$-$1Ca^{2+}$ antiporter, which exchanges 3 Na^+ for 1 Ca^{2+} by secondary active transport. The energy is obtained by the primary active transport of Na^+ by Na^+-K^+ pump. Some of the Ca^{2+} are eliminated by an ATP-driven sarcolemmal Ca^{2+} pump. *There is no after-hyperpolarization in cardiac muscle.*

The repolarization time decreases as the heart rate increases. At a heart rate of 75/min, the duration of action potential is 250 ms. When it becomes 200 beats/min, the duration become 150 ms.

Contractile Response and Refractory Period in Ventricular Muscle

Absolute refractory period is much longer in the cardiac muscle. It lasts for about 200 ms, i.e., it extends from firing level to ½ of phase 3. Towards the end of action potential, a stronger stimulus can produce an action potential. This is **relative refractory period**, whose duration is about 50 ms. In the intact heart, whole of action potential is refractory and hence it is referred to as **functional refractory period** (**Fig. 9.3**). Because of long refractory period, summation and tetanus of the type seen in skeletal muscle does not occur in cardiac muscle. *This is a safety measure because tetanization of cardiac muscle leads to death.*

Electrical Activity in the Nodal Tissue or Pacemaker Potential of Sinoatrial Node

Pacemaker tissue has an unsteady membrane potential. RMP is –55 mV. It does not remain steady at this potential but slowly depolarizes. When the potential reaches –40 mV, an action potential is generated (**Fig. 9.4**). So, SA node is called **pacemaker tissue**. The property of self-generation of action potential by spontaneous depolarization is called **automaticity**. Cardiac muscle is not dependent on its nerve supply for contraction. Velocity of conduction in SA node is 0.05 m/s.

Ionic Basis of Nodal Action Potential

The action potential in the nodal tissue is largely due to Ca^{2+} with little contribution by Na^+ influx. The membrane of pacemaker tissue is leaky to Na^+, and so Na^+ enters the cell even in the resting state. Potential becomes less negative and when it reaches –40 mV Ca^{2+} channels open and Ca^{2+} and Na^+ enter the cell. As the Ca^{2+} channels are slow channels, there is

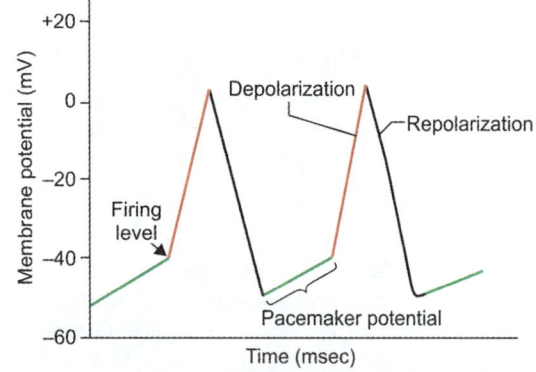

Fig. 9.4: Action potential recorded from SA node.

no sharp, rapid depolarizing spike. Repolarization starts when Ca^{2+} channels close and K^+ channel open. Towards the end of action potential, Na^+ channels open, depolarization starts and the process is repeated. SA node functions throughout life. The potential change from resting level to firing level is called **prepotential or pacemaker potential**.

Causes of Prepotential
- Hyperpolarization induced influx of Na^+
- Decrease in K^+ permeability
- Increase in Ca^{2+} permeability (Ca^{2+} channel blockers abolish prepotential)

There are two types of Ca^{2+} channels in heart: **Transient channel (T channel)** and **Long lasting channel (L channel)**. T channels open during prepotential and opening of the L channels produce the impulse (*refer* pacemaker potential—**Chapter 22**).

The slope of the prepotential determines heart rate and the slope is affected by sympathetic and parasympathetic stimulation.

- If the **vagus** nerve is stimulated, the membrane becomes hyperpolarized and the prepotential becomes less steep and the heart rate decreases. The slope of the prepotential is decreased because the acetylcholine released at the nerve ending increases K^+ conductance and slows the opening of Ca^{2+} channels. This action is mediated by **M2 muscarinic receptors**, which open a special set of K^+ channels *via* G protein. In addition, activation of M2 receptors decreases cAMP in the cells and this slows opening of L-Ca^{2+} channels. Stimulation of right vagus slows the heart rate by inhibiting SA node, and left vagus slows AV nodal conduction. Strong vagal stimulation may even stop the heart.
- If **sympathetic** cardiac nerves are stimulated, the prepotential becomes steeper and heart rate increases. Norepinephrine secreted by the sympathetic endings facilitates the opening of Ca^{2+} channels. Norepinephrine binds to $β_1$-**receptors** and the resulting increase in intracellular cAMP facilitates the opening of L-channels increasing intracellular Ca^{2+} and the rapidity of the depolarization phase of the impulse. The rise in the level of cAMP activates cAMP-dependent protein kinase, which in turn promotes phosphorylation of the L-type Ca^{2+} channels in the cell membrane and thus increases the influx of Ca^{2+} into the cells.
- The rate of discharge of the nodal tissue is influenced by temperature and drugs. Increase in temperature within physiological limits increases heart rate by increasing the metabolism in the nodal tissue.
- $Ca2+$ channel blockers and digitalis depress the nodal tissue and decrease heart rate. Effect is similar to vagal stimulation particularly on the AV node.

Sarcotubular System
The T tubules are very large in cardiac muscle and they are present at the Z lines. Sarcoplasmic reticulum is highly developed and the ends encircle the T tubules forming a **diad or triad (Fig. 9.1B)**.

Excitation-Contraction Coupling in Cardiac Muscle
Excitation-contraction coupling is similar to that of skeletal muscle. T tubules are present at the Z lines in cardiac muscle. When an action potential reaches the T tubules, there is activation of **dihydropyridine channels** in the T tubule. This causes influx of extracellular Ca^{2+} into the sarcoplasm. It is this Ca^{2+} that triggers the release of stored Ca^{2+} from the sarcoplasmic reticulum. T tubules of cardiac muscle also contain mucopolysaccharides that bind an abundant store of Ca^{2+} ions. This Ca^{2+} also diffuses into the sarcoplasm when an action potential reaches the T-tubules. Ca^{2+} influx is a slow process and this is responsible for the plateau phase of action potential in the cardiac muscle. The period for which Ca^{2+} remains in the sarcoplasm in the cardiac muscle is 200–300 ms; whereas in the skeletal muscle, it is 1/30 sec.

The muscle proteins are myosin, actin, tropomyosin, and troponin. Another protein called **dystrophin** is present, which is also present in the skeletal muscle. It is a large protein and it helps in coordinated contraction of muscle.

Mechanism of muscle contraction is same as that of skeletal muscle (*refer* skeletal muscle).

Mechanism of Relaxation of Cardiac Muscle
Relaxation of cardiac muscle occurs in diastole when the Ca^{2+} ions are extruded out of the cardiac muscle fiber by a Na^+-Ca^{2+} **antiport** mechanism operating in the sarcolemma. Relaxation is also aided by **phospholamban** present in the sarcoplasmic reticulum especially on beta adrenergic stimulation (Refer the box).

By the Na^+-Ca^{2+} antiport mechanism, when one Ca^{2+} is extruded out of the myocardial cell, two Na^+ ions enter the cell. The gradient for the entry of Na^+ into the cell is created by Na^+-K^+ ATPase present in the cell membrane. Thus, the extrusion of Ca^{2+} out of the myocardial cell is an example of *secondary active transport mechanism* (*refer* **Fig. 5.6**). Cardiac glycosides like **digitalis**, which increase myocardial contractility act by inhibiting this secondary active transport of Ca^{2+} out of the cell. As the intracellular Ca^{2+} concentration is increased by digitalis, there is increase in the myocardial contractility and is of great benefit in treating congestive cardiac failure.

> **Phospholamban** is an integral membrane protein present in the sarcoplasmic reticulum that regulates the Ca^{2+} pump in cardiac muscle. It is a key regulator of cardiac contractility. In its dephosphorylated state, it decreases sarcoplasmic reticulum Ca^{2+} sequestration by inhibiting **sarcoplasmic reticulum Ca^{2+}-ATPase (SERCA)**. Upon phosphorylation in response to increase in cAMP, mediated through β-adrenergic stimulation, the inhibitory effect of phospholamban on the function of SERCA is relieved. The increased activity of cardiac sarcoplasmic reticulum Ca^{2+} transport system lowers the cytoplasmic Ca^{2+} levels and leads to cardiac muscle relaxation. Beta adrenergic stimulation increases the force of contraction of the cardiac muscle and at the same time it also increases the rate of relaxation of cardiac muscle. The accelerated rate of cardiac contraction is due to increased Ca^{2+} influx through the sarcolemmal channel protein from the extracellular fluid. Whereas the accelerated rate of relaxation following β-adrenergic stimulation is as a result of increased rate of Ca^{2+} uptake into the sarcoplasmic reticulum in response to phosphorylation of phospholamban present in the cardiac sarcoplasmic reticulum.

Cardiac muscle is not fatigued due to the following reasons:
- ❖ Cardiac muscle has abundant blood supply and very high oxygen extraction. The local metabolites that produce fatigue are immediately washed off due to high blood flow.
- ❖ There are numerous large mitochondria and very high myoglobin content.
- ❖ Lactic acid production is very less because, less than 1% of the total energy liberated is provided by anaerobic metabolism. In other words, cardiac muscle depends greatly on aerobic cellular respiration to generate ATP.
- ❖ Under resting conditions, 70% of the caloric need of the human heart is provided by oxidative metabolism of fat instead of carbohydrate. One molecule of fatty acid when metabolized aerobically releases 100 ATP molecules. Circulating free fatty acids account for 50% of the lipid utilized.
- ❖ Lactic acid released from the skeletal muscles into the blood during exercise is used by cardiac muscle to synthesize ATP. Cardiac muscle is capable of converting lactic acid to pyruvic acid, which, in turn, enters the citric acid cycle to produce ATP.
- ❖ The absolute refractory period of cardiac muscle is very long. Thus, it does not respond to tetanizing stimuli and so tetanus and fatigue do not occur in cardiac muscle.

Length–Tension Relationship in the Cardiac Muscle

The initial length of cardiac muscle fiber is determined by the degree of diastolic filling of the heart. **Frank Starling's law** of the heart states that greater the end-diastolic volume greater will be the force of contraction **within physiological limits**. Whenever force of contraction has to be increased, there is increase in venous return to the heart. This increases the end-diastolic volume so that the initial length of the fiber is increased. When the length of the muscle fiber exceeds the physiological limit, force of contraction decreases **(Fig. 9.5)**.

Another way of increasing the force of contraction is by increasing the contractility of the myocardium. This property of increasing the contractility is called **inotropic effect**. This increase in the force of contraction occurs without a change in the muscle length. Contractility is increased in mental excitation and following administration of catecholamine.

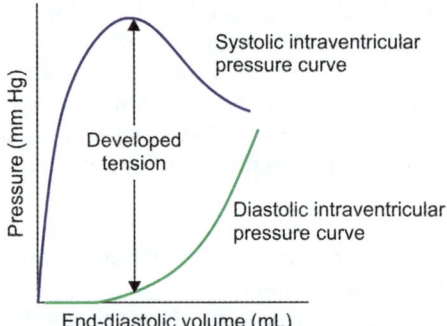

Fig. 9.5: Length-tension relationship in cardiac muscle.

Force of myocardial contraction is decreased when Ca^{2+} channel blockers like verapamil are given.

Differences between skeletal muscle and cardiac muscle are shown in **Table 9.1**.

Comparison of action potentials in nerve fiber, skeletal muscle fiber and cardiac muscle fiber is shown in **Figure 9.6**.

PROPERTIES OF CARDIAC MUSCLE (REFER CHAPTER 22)

- ❖ Excitability or irritability (Bathmotropism)
- ❖ Automaticity and rhythmicity (Chronotropism)
- ❖ Conductivity (Dromotropism)
- ❖ Contractility (Inotropism)
- ❖ Distensibility

MULTIPLE CHOICE QUESTIONS

1. Slow repolarization phase of cardiac muscle is due to:
    a. Slow Ca^{2+} channel
    b. Slow Na^+ channel
    c. Na^+-K^+ pump inactivation
    d. Decreased permeability of K^+
2. Rapid depolarization in cardiac muscle is due to:
    a. Ca^{2+} b. Na^+
    c. K^+ d. Mg^{2+}

Table 9.1: Differences between skeletal muscle and cardiac muscle.		
S. No.	Skeletal muscle	Cardiac muscle
1.	Voluntary in action	Involuntary in action
2.	It helps in movement, maintenance of posture and thermogenesis	Help in pumping of blood to all parts of the body
3.	A single cell is multinucleated, cylindrical, unbranched and long and the fibers are arranged parallel to each other. Mitochondria are small and less numerous than cardiac muscle. Length of the fibers varies from few mm to 30 cm and diameter varies from 10–100 μm	A single cell is branched, short, interconnected end to end by intercalated disks, contains a single nucleus and mitochondria are larger and more numerous. The fibers are about 50–100 μm long and 15 μm in diameter
4.	Mainly attached to bones by tendons	Confined to heart walls and not attached to bones
5.	Do not function as a syncytium because there is no anatomic or functional connection between the cells	Function as a syncytium since the cells are interconnected by low resistance bridges
6.	Innervation from the somatic nervous system	Innervation is through autonomic nervous system
7.	T tubules are more abundant, narrow and are present at the AI junction	T tubules are less in number but wider and are present at the Z lines
8.	Sarcotubular system forms a triad. There will be two triads per sarcomere	Sarcotubular system form triad or diad. There is only one triad or diad per sarcomere

Contd...

Contd...

S. No.	Skeletal muscle	Cardiac muscle
9.	T tubules contain voltage gated dihydropyridine receptors	T tubules contain Ca^{2+} gated dihydropyridine receptors
10.	Action potential is of spike type	Action potential is of plateau type
11.	Ca^{2+} for contraction is released only from the sarcoplasmic reticulum and the intracellular Ca^{2+} reserve is more	Ca^{2+} for contraction enters the sarcoplasm both from sarcoplasmic reticulum and extracellular fluid because the intracellular Ca^{2+} reserve is less as the sarcoplasmic reticulum is small
12.	Duration of action potential is 2–4 ms	Duration of action potential is 250–300 ms
13.	Absolute refractory period is very short and so summation and tetanization is possible	Duration of absolute refractory period is 200 ms and so summation and tetanus is not possible
14.	Do not exhibit autorhythmicity. Contract only on nervous stimulation	Exhibit autorhythmicity due to the presence of pacemaker cells
15.	The descending limb of Starling curve is due to decrease in the number of cross bridges between actin and myosin	The descending limb is due to disruption of myocardial fibers and not due to decrease in the number of cross bridges
16.	Easily fatigued	Not fatigued
17.	Twitch duration is less	Twitch duration is more because Ca^{2+} channels in the sarcolemma remains open for a longer time and Ca^{2+} remains in the sarcoplasm for a longer time
18.	Aerobic and anaerobic glycolysis can generate ATP	Depends mainly on aerobic cellular respiration for ATP. So cardiac muscle cannot withstand hypoxia
19.	All or none law is applicable only to a single muscle fiber	All or none law is applicable to the entire atria or entire ventricular syncytium
20.	Mechanical response begins after the end of repolarization phase of action potential	Mechanical response overlaps the electrical response for the whole period

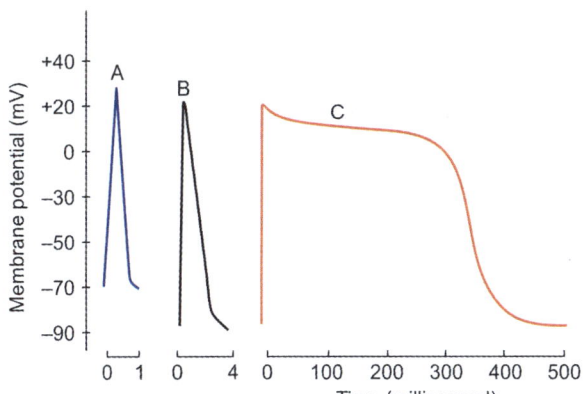

Fig. 9.6: Comparison of action potentials A: Nerve fiber; B: Skeletalmuscle fiber; C: Ventricular muscle fiber.

3. **Plateau phase of cardiac muscle action potential is due to:**
   a. Na^+ influx
   b. K^+ influx
   c. Na^+-Ca^{2+} slow channel
   d. Na^+ efflux

4. **Gap junctions:**
   a. Are absent in cardiac muscle
   b. Are absent in smooth muscle
   c. Provide a pathway for the rapid spread of action potential from one cardiac muscle fiber to another
   d. Has little functional importance in visceral smooth muscle

5. **Sarcotubular system in cardiac muscle is present at:**
   a. Z-line
   b. A-I junction
   c. M line
   d. Actin-myosin junction

6. **It is not possible to tetanize:**
   a. Skeletal muscle
   b. Cardiac muscle
   c. Visceral smooth muscle
   d. Multiunit smooth muscle

7. **The property by which force of contraction of the myocardium is increased is called:**
   a. Dromotropism
   b. Inotropism
   c. Chronotropism
   d. Bathmotropism

8. **The ions that are responsible for the plateau phase of ventricular action potential are:**
   a. Ca^{2+} and K^+
   b. Ca^{2+} and Cl^-
   c. Na^+ and K^+
   d. Na^+ and Cl^-

9. **The following are features of cardiac muscle, *except*:**
   a. Tetanization
   b. All or none phenomenon
   c. Functional syncytium
   d. Prepotential

10. **The function of phosphorylated phospholamban in cardiac muscle is:**
    a. Inhibition of Na^+-K^+ pump
    b. Sequestrate Ca^{2+} into sarcoplasmic reticulum
    c. Increase cytoplasmic Ca^{2+}
    d. Increase Ca^{2+} influx from extracellular fluid

ANSWERS

1. a 2. b 3. c 4. c 5. a
6. b 7. b 8. a 9. a 10. b

Smooth Muscle

CHAPTER 10

LEARNING OBJECTIVES
- Compare and contrast the types of smooth muscles
- Describe the types of action potentials recorded in smooth muscles
- Explain the molecular basis of smooth muscle contraction and relaxation
- Define plasticity with example

FUNCTIONAL ANATOMY

Like cardiac muscle, smooth muscles are **involuntary muscles**. They are also known as **plain muscles** because they have no cross striations. The muscle proteins are **actin, myosin** and **tropomyosin**. *Troponins are not demonstrated in smooth muscle.* The actin and myosin molecules are arranged in a **random manner**, i.e., not in a regular pattern. This is the reason for the absence of cross striations. Each smooth muscle cell is spindle shaped and contains only one nucleus. Here, instead of Z lines, the actin filament is attached to structures called **dense bodies** present in the cytoplasm by means of α-actinin. The dense bodies are, in turn, attached to the cell membrane (**Fig. 10.1C**).

Unlike skeletal and cardiac muscles, smooth muscle tissue in some areas can regenerate. Smooth muscle fibers, such as those in the uterus have the capacity for division and thus can grow by hyperplasia. Also, the smooth muscle stem cells called **pericytes** present in capillaries and small veins can divide and produce new smooth muscle cells.

Types of Smooth Muscles

- Visceral smooth muscle or single-unit smooth muscle
- Multiunit smooth muscle

Visceral Smooth Muscle

Visceral smooth muscle resembles the cardiac muscle. They are found as **sheets** of muscle fibers and large number of muscle fibers contract as a single unit. Hence, the name **single-unit smooth muscle**. Adjacent muscle fibers are connected by **gap junctions** so that action potential from one cell can quickly pass into the neighboring cells. Thus, it acts as a **functional syncytium** (**Fig. 10.1A**). The visceral smooth muscle does not depend on its nerve supply for contraction. Even when completely denervated, these smooth muscles continue to contract because they can generate their own rhythm. The nerves can only modify the activity of visceral smooth muscle. Stretch is the stimulus for the contraction of these muscles and they exhibit **spontaneous contraction.** Visceral smooth muscles are present in the walls of hollow organs, such as stomach, intestine, uterus, gallbladder, urinary bladder, ureter, etc. Since they are present in many visceral organs, they are called **visceral smooth muscles**.

Multiunit Smooth Muscle

Multiunit smooth muscle resembles skeletal muscle, but is not under voluntary control. They are composed of discrete small groups of muscle fibers without interconnecting bridges or gap junctions (**Fig. 10.1B**).

Each fiber can contract independently. They mainly depend on their nerve supply for contraction. They cannot generate their own impulses and do not function as a syncytium. They do not contract when stretched and rarely exhibit spontaneous contraction, e.g., ciliary muscle of eye, muscle of iris, piloerector muscle of skin, large airways to the lungs, large arteries, etc.

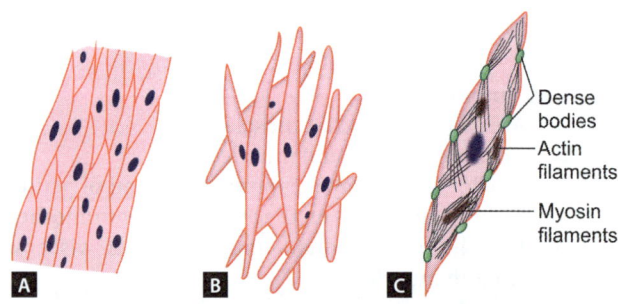

Figs. 10.1A to C: (A) Visceral smooth muscle; (B) Multiunit smooth muscle; (C) Structure of a single smooth muscle cell.

NEUROMUSCULAR JUNCTION IN SMOOTH MUSCLE

Neuromuscular junction is not well developed in smooth muscle and there are no recognizable endplates. The nerve fibers run along the membranes of the muscle cells. Branches of neurons supplying smooth muscle have a beaded appearance due to the presence of swellings along their course called **varicosities**. These varicosities contain vesicles, which contain neurotransmitters (**Fig. 10.2A**). There are about 20,000 varicosities per neuron. In sympathetic fibers, varicosities contain dense core vesicles, which contain the neurotransmitter norepinephrine. Parasympathetic fibers contain varicosities, which contain clear vesicles containing acetylcholine. When an action potential is generated in the nerve, neurotransmitter is released at each varicosity. Thus, one nerve terminal innervates many effector cells. This is called **synapse en passant**; where one nerve ending comes into contact with one cell and then passes on to make contact with other cells. In the case of skeletal muscle, one nerve ending innervates a single muscle fiber. The junction between the autonomic nerve and the smooth muscle cell is called **neuroeffector junction**.

In multiunit smooth muscle innervation by nerve fibers is almost similar to that of skeletal muscle. It is not under voluntary control. Each multiunit smooth muscle cell has en passant endings of nerve fibers (**Fig. 10.2B**). But in visceral smooth muscle, there are en passant endings on fewer cells, with excitation spreading to other cells by gap junctions.

ELECTRICAL RESPONSES IN SMOOTH MUSCLE

PY3.8: Describe action potentials in smooth muscle.

Electrical stimulation of smooth muscle produces various types of action potentials, such as spike potential, plateau potential, etc. Resting membrane potential is –60 to –50 mV. Some smooth muscles are self-excitatory. Spontaneous electrical activity in the form of **slow waves** is present in some smooth muscles without any stimulus. This is due to waxing and waning of the activity of sodium pump. Slow wave is not an action potential, but it can initiate action potentials if it reaches the firing level.

Table 10.1: Differences between visceral smooth muscle and multiunit smooth muscle.

Visceral smooth muscle	Multiunit smooth muscle
Resembles cardiac muscle	Resembles skeletal muscle
Found as sheets of muscle fibers and function as a syncytium	Discrete small groups of muscle fibers, which do not function as a syncytium
Can generate its own rhythm and does not depend on nerve supply for contraction	Depend on their nerve supply for contraction
Stretch is a stimulus for contraction	Do not contract when stretched
Exhibit spontaneous contraction	Do not show spontaneous contraction
Synapse en-passant present	Synapse en-passant absent
Plateau potential recorded from a single fiber	Spike-shaped potential recorded from a single fiber

Arteriolar smooth muscle is a combination of visceral and multiunit smooth muscle.

The differences between visceral smooth muscle and multiunit smooth muscle are shown in **Table 10.1**.

Sarcotubular System in Smooth Muscle

T tubules are absent. The sarcoplasmic reticulum is poorly developed. Therefore, the smooth muscles mainly depend on extracellular Ca^{2+} for contraction.

Nerve Supply of Smooth Muscle

Smooth muscles are supplied by postganglionic autonomic nerve fibers, which are **unmyelinated**. Sympathetic fibers release norepinephrine at their nerve endings and parasympathetic fibers release acetylcholine. One division is stimulatory in action and the other inhibitory in action. In visceral smooth muscle, parasympathetic fibers have a stimulatory action and sympathetic stimulation have inhibitory action. In multiunit smooth muscle, the actions vary depending on the site. In visceral smooth muscles, norepinephrine produces inhibitory potentials. Norepinephrine has both α and β actions. β-action is mediated *via* cAMP and cause increased intracellular binding of Ca^{2+}, thereby decreasing the Ca^{2+} content. α-action is associated with increased Ca^{2+} efflux from muscle cells. So, there is a decrease in the frequency of spikes and thus it is inhibitory in action.

Acetylcholine produces excitatory potentials. Effect is mediated *via* phospholipase-C and inositol triphosphate (IP_3), which increases intracellular Ca^{2+}. Spikes become more frequent, which increases tonic tension and the number of rhythmic contractions.

Depolarizing **excitatory junctional potentials (EJP)** occur when excitatory nerves are stimulated and hyperpolarizing **inhibitory junctional potentials (IJP)** occur when inhibitory neurons to smooth muscle are stimulated.

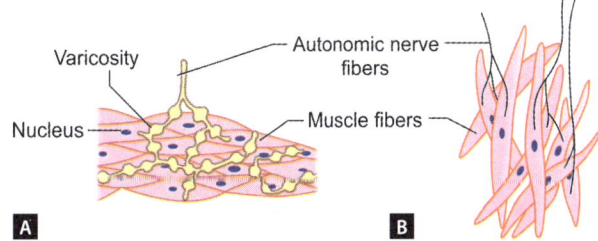

Figs. 10.2A and B: Structure and innervation of smooth muscle: (A) Visceral smooth muscle showing synapse en-passant; (B) Multiunit smooth muscle.

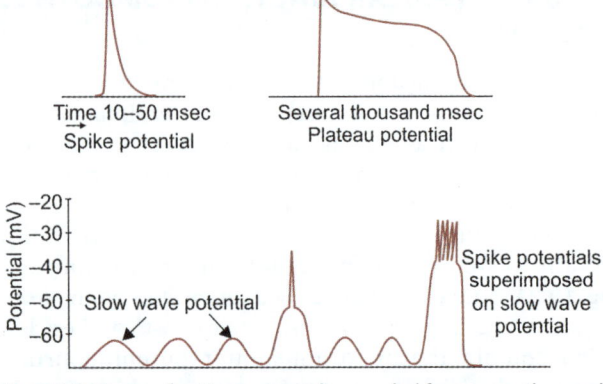

Fig. 10.3: Types of action potentials recorded from smooth muscles. Slow waves are not action potentials.

Stretch is a stimulus for visceral smooth muscle. When stretched, the mechanically gated Na+ channels open and when the potential reaches –35 mV, a spike potential is superimposed on a slow wave. When the potential reaches –20 mV, more number of spike potentials will be superimposed on a slow wave. So, slow waves are called pacemaker waves (**Fig. 10.3**).

Tonic and Phasic Smooth Muscles

Smooth muscles that remain contracted most of the time and relax only in response to inhibitory stimuli are called **tonic smooth muscles**. Smooth muscles of gastrointestinal (cardiac sphincter, pyloric sphincter, etc.) and urogenital sphincters (internal urethral sphincter) are examples of tonic smooth muscles.

Smooth muscles that remain mostly relaxed and contract only in response to excitatory stimuli are called **phasic smooth muscles**. Muscles forming the walls of gastrointestinal tract (stomach, intestine, etc.) and urogenital tracts (ureter, urinary bladder, etc.) are examples of phasic smooth muscles.

■ TONUS

The visceral smooth muscles show continuous, irregular contractions that are independent of their nerve supply. This maintained state of partial contraction is called **tonus or tone**. Stretch is followed by a depolarizing membrane potential leading to an increase in the frequency of spikes and an increase in the tone. The action of acetylcholine in visceral smooth muscle is similar.

Epinephrine and norepinephrine produce hyperpolarization and the spikes decrease in frequency and the muscle relaxes or tonus decreases.

■ MECHANISM OF SMOOTH MUSCLE CONTRACTION AND RELAXATION

PY3.9: Describe the molecular basis of muscle contraction in smooth muscle.

Types of Excitation Contraction Coupling in Smooth Muscle

There are three different ways in which the smooth muscle excitation can be coupled to its contraction.
1. In **electromechanical coupling**, smooth muscle is excited through sarcolemmal depolarization. The voltage-gated Ca^{2+} channels in the sarcolemma open up and Ca^{2+} moves into the sarcoplasm from ECF and bring about contraction.
2. In **pharmacomechanical coupling**, the muscle is excited by chemical agents in the absence of membrane depolarization. Neurotransmitters and hormones bind to ligand-gated Ca^{2+} channels on the sarcolemma and open them up, allowing ECF Ca^{2+} to enter the smooth muscle cell leading to muscle contraction.
3. In **mechanomechanical coupling**, smooth muscles are excited by stretch, which opens up stretch sensitive Ca^{2+} channels on the sarcolemma.

Smooth Muscle Contraction

The smooth muscle membrane contains a large number of voltage-gated Ca^{2+} channels and very few voltage- gated Na^+ channels. Excitation–contraction coupling is different in smooth muscle. When an action potential reaches the muscle, along with Na^+ channel voltage- gated Ca^{2+} channels also open. There is influx of Ca^{2+} and Na^+ into the cell from ECF. As the smooth muscle cell is small, Ca^{2+} entering the cell can easily diffuse within the myofibril. Troponin is absent in smooth muscle. One of the light chains of myosin head called **regulatory chain of myosin** in the smooth muscle must be phosphorylated for activation of myosin ATPase. Ca^{2+} combines with a Ca^{2+} binding protein called **calmodulin**, which is similar to troponin C. When calmodulin-Ca^{2+} complex is formed, it activates the enzyme calmodulin-dependent **myosin light chain kinase**, which is present on the regulatory chain of myosin. This enzyme catalyzes phosphorylation of myosin regulatory chain. Phosphorylation of the regulatory chain of myosin head initiates ATPase activity and permits actin–myosin interaction. Actin slides on myosin producing smooth muscle contraction (**Flowchart 10.1**). The Ca^{2+} remains in the sarcoplasm of smooth muscle from 200 ms to several seconds.

Smooth Muscle Relaxation and Latch Mechanism

For smooth muscle relaxation to occur, the phosphorylated myosin head should be dephosphorylated. **Dephosphorylation** requires another enzyme called **myosin light chain phosphatase**, which splits phosphate from the myosin head during relaxation. Ca^{2+}–calmodulin complex dissociates releasing Ca^{2+}. During relaxation of smooth muscle, Ca^{2+} is pumped out of the smooth muscle by Ca^{2+} pump present on the smooth muscle membrane. This pump functions very slowly and so relaxation is also a slow process in smooth muscle (**Flowchart 10.1**).

Sometimes, the dephosphorylated myosin cross bridges remain attached to actin for some time even after decrease

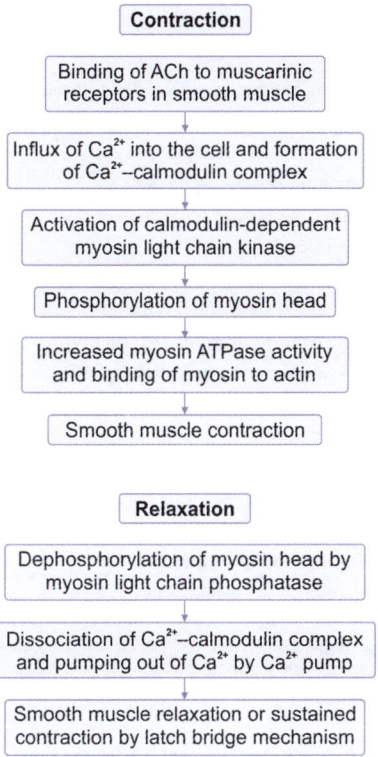

Flowchart 10.1: Sequence of events in contraction and relaxation of smooth muscle.

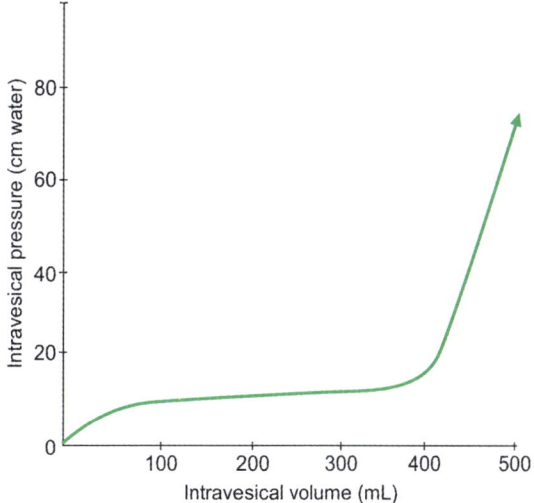

Fig. 10.4: Cystometrogram; length-tension relationship in urinary bladder (plasticity).

in intracellular Ca^{2+}. This causes sustained contraction with little expenditure of energy. This is due to a **latch bridge** mechanism in smooth muscle. Such a muscle cannot generate active tension and move a load, but can effectively resist passive stretching because of the actin–myosin bonds. Smooth muscles are mostly found in the walls of hollow viscera that must resist excessive stretching rather than actively move a load. This is especially important in vascular smooth muscle that must resist excessive stretching.

LENGTH–TENSION RELATIONSHIP IN SMOOTH MUSCLE

Plasticity

There is no orderly arrangement of actin and myosin filaments in smooth muscle. When the visceral smooth muscle is stretched, it develops the passive tension, which rises immediately. But if the muscle is held at the greater length after stretching, the tension gradually comes back to the resting prestretch level. Again when the length is increased (within physiological limits), tension rises and then falls. This phenomenon is called **stress relaxation or plasticity**. Rearrangement of bonds between actin and myosin molecules is the cause for return of tension after stretch.

Thus, smooth muscle behaves more like a viscous mass than a rigidly structured tissue because of this property. After a particular length, the tension rises steadily.

When the length is decreased, tension falls but soon comes back to normal. This is called **reverse stress relaxation**. Unlike striated muscle, smooth muscle can contract up to 70% of their initial length without much change in the tension developed. In other words, whether actively contracted or passively stretched, the smooth muscle fiber tends to behave as if it is always at its resting length.

These properties of smooth muscle are of great importance in urinary bladder. Study of the relationship between length and tension in urinary bladder is called **cystometrogram** (**Fig. 10.4**). The bladder can accommodate large volumes of urine because of the plasticity of the bladder wall (*refer* Chapter 49). Stomach also accommodates food because of this property of smooth muscle. However, a point is eventually reached at which the tension in the organ rises and it contracts.

SIMILARITIES BETWEEN CARDIAC AND VISCERAL SMOOTH MUSCLE

❖ Involuntary in action
❖ Unstable membrane potentials present
❖ Act as functional syncytium
❖ Exhibits plateau potential
❖ Independent of their nerve supplies; nerves only modify their action
❖ Regulated by autonomic nervous system and hormones
❖ Exhibit auto rhythmicity

Differences between skeletal muscle and visceral smooth muscle is given in **Table 10.2**.

Differences between cardiac muscle and visceral smooth muscle is given in **Table 10.3**.

Table 10.2: Differences between skeletal muscle and visceral smooth muscle.	
Skeletal muscle	**Visceral smooth muscle**
Voluntary muscle	Involuntary muscle
Attached to bones by tendons	Not attached to bones
Single fiber is large, cylindrical and multinucleate (10–30 cm in length)	Small, spindle shaped and uninucleate (0.02–0.5 mm in length)
Well-developed T tubules	No T tubules
Has Z discs	Has only dense bodies which are analogous to Z disks
Actin filaments are arranged in a parallel manner	Actin filaments radiate from the dense bodies
Ratio of actin to myosin filaments is approximately 2:1	Ratio of actin to myosin is 12:1
Calcium binding protein is troponin	Calmodulin serves the role of troponin
Has well-developed neuromuscular junction	No definite motor end plate and synapses are called synapse en-passant
Following excitation, quick onset of contraction and relaxation	Have delayed onset of contraction and relaxation
RMP is –90 mV	Has unsteady RMP which ranges from –20 to –65 mV
Na^+-K^+ pump contributes very little to RMP	Na^+-K^+ pump makes a significant contribution to RMP
Slow wave potential absent	Exhibit slow wave potentials
Action potential is spike potential with duration 2–4 ms	Spike (10–50 ms) or plateau potential (several thousand ms)
More energy required for contraction	Have lower energy requirements for contraction
Phosphorylation of myosin head is not necessary for contraction	Phosphorylation of myosin head should occur for contraction
Latch mechanism absent	Latch mechanism present
Can contract only up to 30% of its initial length	Contract up to 70% of their initial length
Does not exhibit plasticity and reverse stress relaxation	Exhibit plasticity and reverse stress relaxation

Table 10.3: Differences between cardiac and visceral smooth muscle.	
Cardiac muscle	**Visceral smooth muscle**
• Striated, orderly arrangement of actin and myosin filaments • Responses are phasic, i.e., contraction alternating with relaxation • Increase in intracellular cyclic AMP increases the force of contraction • Do not exhibit plasticity • Sarcotubular system well developed • No synapse en-passant • Troponin is present • Phosphorylation of myosin head is not necessary for contraction • Relaxation is a fast process and the duration depends on the heart rate • Single cell is branched and cylindrical in shape	• Nonstriated • Contraction is often tonic because of latch bridge mechanism • Cyclic AMP relaxes visceral smooth muscle because it inhibits the phosphorylation of myosin light chain kinase • Exhibits plasticity • Sarcotubular system poorly developed with no T tubules • Synapse en-passant present • Troponin absent instead calmodulin is present • Phosphorylation of myosin head is necessary for contraction • Relaxation is a very slow process • Single cell is small, un branched and spindle shaped

MULTIPLE CHOICE QUESTIONS

1. **The resting membrane potential of smooth muscle is:**
   a. –20 to –30 mV
   b. –50 to –70 mV
   c. –70 to –90 mV
   d. –90 to –110 mV

2. **Calmodulin activates:**
   a. Muscle phosphorylase
   b. Protein kinase
   c. 2,3 BPG
   d. Glucokinase

3. **Plasticity is shown by:**
   a. Visceral smooth muscle
   b. Multiunit smooth muscle
   c. Skeletal muscle
   d. Cardiac muscle

4. **A unique characteristic of smooth muscle is that:**
   a. Calcium is not required for contraction
   b. It can sustain a contraction for prolonged periods
   c. Repetitive contractions are not possible
   d. Myosin filaments are not required

5. **In smooth muscle, excitation contraction coupling is triggered by binding of Ca^{2+} with:**
   a. Troponin
   b. Calmodulin
   c. Tropomyosin
   d. Actin

6. **All the following about visceral smooth muscle are true, *except* that it:**
   a. Has a stable membrane potential
   b. Shows continuous irregular contractions
   c. Contracts on stretching
   d. Shows basic electrical rhythm

7. **All the following are calcium binding proteins in the body, *except*:**
   a. Troponin
   b. Tropomyosin
   c. Calmodulin
   d. Calbindin

8. Smooth muscle proteins include all the following, *except*:
   a. Actin
   b. Myosin
   c. Tropomyosin
   d. Troponin

9. All the following statements are true regarding muscle contraction, *except*:
   a. Myosin in smooth muscle must be phosphorylated for activation of myosin ATPase
   b. Phosphorylation and de-phosphorylation of myosin occur in skeletal muscle
   c. Excitation-contraction coupling in visceral (unitary) smooth muscle occur at a delay of 500 ms
   d. En-passant ending of nerve fibers are present in all cells of visceral smooth muscle

10. The time from initial depolarization to initiation of contraction (excitation–contraction coupling) in visceral smooth muscle is:
    a. 10 ms
    b. 50 ms
    c. 100 ms
    d. 500 ms

11. Troponin is absent in which type of muscle fiber:
    a. Skeletal
    b. Smooth
    c. Atrial
    d. Ventricular

12. The following statements regarding smooth muscles are true, *except*:
    a. They can divide
    b. Have well-developed sarcotubular system
    c. Cross striations are absent
    d. Calcium combines with calmodulin

13. Action of calmodulin is:
    a. Through calcium dependent kinase
    b. Through calmodulin dependent kinase
    c. Through cAMP dependent kinase
    d. Through cGMP dependent kinase

14. True regarding excitation contraction coupling in smooth muscle is:
    a. Presence of troponin is essential
    b. Sustained contraction occurs with high calcium concentration
    c. Phosphorylation of actin is required for contraction
    d. Presence of intracellular calcium is essential to cause muscle contraction

15. Multiunit smooth muscles are present in the wall of:
    a. Stomach
    b. Large blood vessels
    c. Intestine
    d. Gallbladder

16. Largest smooth muscle is present in:
    a. Pregnant uterus
    b. Aorta
    c. Urethra
    d. Small intestine

17. All are features of smooth muscle fibers, *except*:
    a. Spindle shaped
    b. Unbranched
    c. Multinucleated
    d. Non-striated

ANSWERS

1. b   2. a   3. a   4. b   5. b
6. a   7. b   8. d   9. d   10. d
11. b   12. b   13. b   14. d   15. b
16. a   17. c

FILL IN THE BLANKS/GIVE THE NORMAL VALUES/NAME THE FOLLOWING

1. Ion channels are **transmembrane** proteins that allow selective entry of various ions.
2. Proteins that form water channels in the cell membrane: **Aquaporins**.
3. The major protein of RBC membrane: **Spectrin**.
4. Part of cell membrane that mediate cellular attachment to the extracellular matrix: **Integrins**.
5. Molecular motors are **ATPases** that moves proteins, organelles and other cell parts to all parts of the cell.
6. Molecular motors that produce motion along microtubules: **Dyneins and kinesins**.
7. Molecular motors that produce motion along actin: **Myosin molecules**.
8. Molecular motor involved in the movement of cilia and flagella: **Dynein**.
9. During cell division, mitotic spindle is formed by **microtubules**.
10. Organelle where protein synthesis occur: **Rough endoplasmic reticulum**.
11. Organelle concerned with steroid synthesis, synthesis of fatty acids and detoxification of substances: **Smooth endoplasmic reticulum**.
12. The power houses of cells: **Mitochondria**.
13. Enzymes involved in citric acid cycle and oxidative phosphorylation are present in **mitochondria**.
14. DNA synthesis occurs in which phase of cell cycle?: **S phase**.
15. Percentage of body weight constituted by water of body weight: **60%**.
16. Percentage of ECF constituted by plasma: **25%**.
17. Percentage of body weight constituted by intracellular fluid: **40%**.
18. The percentage of body weight constituted by proteins in an average young adult: **18%**.
19. ECF volume is measured using **inulin**.
20. Plasma volume is measured using **Evan's blue (T-1824)**.
21. Most abundant anion in the ICF: **protein**.
22. Most abundant anion in ECF: **Cl^-**.
23. The potential difference across the inside and outside of cell membrane under resting condition is called **resting membrane potential (RMP)**.
24. Ions responsible for the development of RMP: **K^+**.
25. RMP of a nerve fiber: **70 mV**.
26. Activity of Na^+-K^+ pump is stimulated by increased intracellular **Na^+** concentration and inhibited by **ouabain** and digoxin.

27. Na⁺-K⁺ pump or Na⁺-K⁺ ATPase extrudes 3 Na⁺ from the cell and take **2 K⁺** into the cell.
28. Most diffusible ion in an excitable tissue: **Potassium ion**.
29. Inside the cell, calcium is stored in the **endoplasmic reticulum** and **mitochondria**.
30. **Diffusion** is the process by which solute particles move from a more concentrated area to a less concentrated area to bring a uniform concentration throughout.
31. The single most important factor determining diffusion across a biological membrane: **Concentration gradient**.
32. Facilitated diffusion is one in which a carrier protein move substances in the direction of electrochemical gradient without the expenditure of energy.
33. Hormones regulate facilitated diffusion by changing the number of **transporters** available.
34. The time taken by an excitable tissue to respond to current strength double the rheobase: **Chronaxie**.
35. Chronaxie of a tissue is a measure of **excitability** of the tissue.
36. Conduction is blocked maximally by pressure in which type of nerve fibers: **Aβ**.
37. Local anesthetics block conduction maximally in **C type** nerve fibers.
38. The most susceptible nerve fiber to hypoxia: **B type fiber**.
39. Greater the diameter of the nerve fiber **greater** is the speed of conduction of impulse.
40. The part of the neuron that has the highest concentration of Na⁺ channel: **initial segment**.
41. Tetrodotoxin specifically blocks **Na⁺ channels** during excitation.
42. The thickest nerve fiber in humans is concerned with **proprioception**.
43. Miniature end-plate potential occurs in resting muscle and is due to release of small quantity of **acetylcholine** into the synaptic cleft.
44. Maximum velocity of conduction of impulse is seen in Aα nerve fibers.
45. **T-tubules** are formed by invaginations of the sarcolemma.
46. T-tubule of sarcotubular system in cardiac muscle is present at **Z-line**.
47. In skeletal muscle, the T-tubule is present at the **A-I junction**.
48. The L-tubules in muscle fiber are modified **endoplasmic reticulum**.
49. Depolarization of the T tubule membrane activates the sarcoplasmic reticulum via **dihydropyridine** receptors.
50. Calcium ions stored in the sarcoplasmic reticulum are released (calcium induced calcium release) by activating **ryanodine** receptors.
51. The structural and functional unit of nervous system: **Neuron**.
52. A threshold stimulus produces action potential where as a sub-threshold stimulus produces a **local response**.
53. In a myelinated nerve fiber, the number of Na⁺ channels per unit area of membrane is maximal at the **node of Ranvier**.
54. Depolarization in a nerve fiber is due to opening of **sodium** channels.
55. Gradual change of potential from the resting state to firing level in a nerve fiber is called **partial depolarization**.
56. Repolarization in a nerve fiber is due to **K⁺** efflux.
57. Hyperpolarization in an excitable tissue decreases its **excitability**.
58. Saltatory conduction is seen in **myelinated** nerve fibers.
59. Type of nerve fibers that are unmyelinated: **C type**.
60. Myelination is the function of **Schwann** cell in peripheral nervous system and **oligodendrocytes** in CNS.
61. **Vitamin B₁** is necessary for complete oxidation of pyruvic acid and lactic acid in a nerve.
62. Neurotransmitter at the neuromuscular junction: **Acetyl choline**.
63. Enzyme involved in acetyl choline synthesis: **Choline acetyltransferase**.
64. Acetylcholine is destroyed by **acetylcholinesterase** in the synaptic cleft.
65. Myasthenia gravis is due to destruction of **nicotinic acetylcholine** receptors in the motor end plate by autoantibodies.
66. Myasthenia gravis is treated by using **acetylcholinesterase** inhibitors like neostigmine.
67. Spontaneous release of acetylcholine at the NMJ produces **miniature end-plate potential**.
68. Transmission of impulse away from the cell body is called **orthodromic conduction**.
69. Transmission of impulse towards the cell body is called **antidromic conduction**.
70. Type of degeneration occurring in the distal stump of the cut nerve fiber: **Wallerian degeneration**.
71. Disintegration of Nissl granules in the nerve cell body due to injury or fatigue is called **chromatolysis**.
72. For regeneration to occur, the distance between the cut ends of the nerve fiber should be less than **3 mm**.
73. **Denervation hypersensitivity** in smooth muscle is due to increased sensitivity of the postsynaptic membrane to the neurotransmitter.
74. Denervated exocrine glands except **sweat glands** shows hypersensitivity.
75. Compound action potential is recorded in a mixed nerve that contain a group of nerve fibers with different **conduction velocities**.
76. Cardiac muscle and visceral smooth muscles act as functional syncytium due to the presence of **gap** junctions.
77. Structural and functional unit of muscle fiber: **Sarcomere**.

78. The area between two Z-lines in a myofibril: **Sarcomere**.
79. During muscle contraction there is no change in the length of **A** band.
80. In the resting state of the muscle, one tropomyosin molecule covers **seven** myosin binding sites on actin filament.
81. RMP of skeletal muscle and working cardiac muscle fiber is **–80 to –90 mV**.
82. RMP of pace maker cell in heart is **–50 mV**.
83. **Starling's law** states that force of contraction is directly proportional to the initial length of the muscle within physiological limits.
84. In **isotonic** muscle contraction tone remains the same but the length decreases.
85. A muscle fails to respond to a second stimulus of any strength if it is in the **absolute refractory** period.
86. During the **relative refractory** period, a second stimulus of greater intensity will produce a response in the excitable tissue.
87. A **motor unit** is a single motor neuron and all the muscle fibers it supplies.
88. Contractile proteins in muscle: **Actin and myosin**.
89. Relaxing proteins in skeletal muscle: **Troponin and tropomyosin**.
90. In the smooth muscle, **troponin** is absent instead calcium binding protein, calmodulin is present.
91. Thick filament of skeletal muscle fiber is made up of **myosin** molecules.
92. Thin filament of skeletal muscle is made up of **actin, troponin and tropomyosin** molecules.
93. The length of the muscle at which it develops maximum active tension: **Optimum length**.
94. Maximum shortening that can occur is **30%** of total length of the muscle.
95. The site of fatigue in an intact animal: **Synapse**.
96. **Rigor mortis** is due to depletion of high energy phosphate compounds in the skeletal muscle after death.
97. In Duchene's muscular dystrophy, **dystrophin** is absent in muscles.
98. When the motor nerve to a skeletal muscle is cut, it leads to **flaccid** paralysis of the muscle.
99. Recording of the electrical activity of skeletal muscle: **Electromyography**.
100. **Phosphorylation** of myosin head is necessary for smooth muscle contraction.
101. **Dephosphorylation** of myosin head is necessary for smooth muscle relaxation.
102. Smooth muscle does not restore original length immediately after relaxation due to **latch bridge** mechanism.
103. Plasticity is a property exhibited by **visceral smooth** muscles.

CLINICAL CASE SCENARIO

1. A 35-year-old lady complains of muscle fatigue on exertion, generalized skeletal muscle weakness especially of the extremities and drooping of eyelids. There is improvement of symptoms after a period of rest. The symptoms worsen towards evening. She gives a history of autoimmune disorder in the family. To confirm the diagnosis, the physician treats her with an anticholinesterase inhibitor. She reports that there is considerable relief in her symptoms.
    a. What is your probable diagnosis?
    b. Explain the pathophysiology of the condition.
    c. Name the drugs used for the treatment of the above condition stating their mechanism of action.
    d. With the help of a diagram, explain the mechanism of transmission of impulse at the neuromuscular junction.

SECTION 2 HEMATOLOGY

Blood

CHAPTER 11

LEARNING OBJECTIVES

Must know
- Describe the composition and functions of blood
- Mention the conditions where viscosity of blood is altered
- Enumerate the factors affecting the viscosity of blood

CIRCULATING BODY FLUIDS

The circulatory system is the transport system that supplies O_2 and nutrients to the tissues and returns CO_2 and other waste products of metabolism to the excretory organs. Circulating body fluids include **blood and lymph** that flows through a closed system of vessels. **Hematology** is the study of body fluids like blood and lymph.

BLOOD

PY2.1: Describe the composition and functions of blood components.

Blood is a **unique connective tissue** because it is a fluid. It is a suspension of cells in plasma with dissolved proteins. Some consider blood as an organ kept in the liquid state. It is a **fluid connective tissue**, which is red colored, opaque and alkaline in reaction. Arterial blood is bright red due to the presence of oxyhemoglobin and venous blood is dark red due to the presence of reduced hemoglobin. Volume of blood in an average adult man is about 5–6 L, which comes to about 8% of the body weight.

Functions of Blood

- Transport of respiratory gases
- Nutritive function
- Excretory function
- Protective function
- Acid–base balance
- Water balance
- Transport of substances like hormones, enzymes, etc.
- Maintenance of blood pressure and osmotic pressure
- Prevention of blood loss
- Storage function
- Regulation of body temperature.

- **Transport of respiratory gases:** Blood carries O_2 from alveoli to the tissues where metabolism occurs. Final products of metabolism like CO_2 are taken from tissues to lungs by blood where it is eliminated.
- **Nutritive function:** The final products of digestion, such as glucose, amino acids, fatty acids; minerals, vitamins, etc., from the alimentary tract enter blood and reach the tissues. Blood also carries nutritive materials from storage depots like liver to various tissues.
- **Excretory function:** Waste products of metabolism, such as urea, uric acid, creatinine, etc., are carried by blood to the excretory organs, such as kidney, skin, etc.
- **Protective function:** Leukocytes protect body from invading organisms. Lymphocytes play an important role in cellular and humoral immunity. Blood also contains antibodies, antitoxins, etc., involved in defense mechanism.
- **Acid–base balance:** Buffers of blood, such as hemoglobin, plasma proteins, HCO_3^- etc., maintain the pH of the body constant at 7.4.
- **Water balance:** There is constant exchange of fluid between the intravascular and extravascular compartments across the blood vessel wall. This helps in maintaining the water and electrolyte balance of the body.
- **Transport function:** Blood acts as a vehicle, which transports hormones, antibodies, enzymes, metals, etc., to the target tissues.
- **Maintenance of blood pressure and osmotic pressure:** Blood maintains the blood pressure at 120/80 mm Hg by various mechanisms. The plasma proteins are responsible for maintaining the osmotic pressure constant.
- **Prevention of blood loss:** Since blood has the property of **coagulation**, blood loss from the body can be prevented during injury.
- **Storage function:** Blood serves as the immediate source of substances, such as water, glucose, proteins, Na^+, K^+, etc., required by the tissues especially in emergency conditions, such as starvation.

- **Regulation of body temperature**: Body temperature is maintained constant at 37°C mainly by blood due to constant circulation of blood throughout the body.

The main constituent of blood is water and water has certain physical properties, such as:
1. High-specific heat
2. High thermal conductivity
3. High latent heat of evaporation.

A man of average weight generates about 3000 k calories of heat per day. The body temperature may rise to 100–150°C if the tissues had low specific heat. Water due to its high specific heat can absorb a large amount of heat and thus prevent sudden increase in body temperature. **Specific heat** of a substance is the number of calories of heat required to raise the temperature of one gram of the substance by one degree centigrade.

Water has the capacity to conduct heat from deeper tissues to superficial tissues, such as skin and thus increases the rate of evaporation.

As water has high latent heat of evaporation, a large amount of heat is lost from the skin and lungs by evaporation, decreasing the body temperature.

Composition of Blood

Blood is composed of plasma and blood cells (**Flowchart 11.1**). Gases present in blood are O_2, CO_2 and N_2.

Physical Properties of Blood

- Color and appearance—red and opaque
- Taste—salty
- pH—7.4
- Specific gravity—1.050–1.060
- Viscosity—3.5–5.4 times more viscous than water.

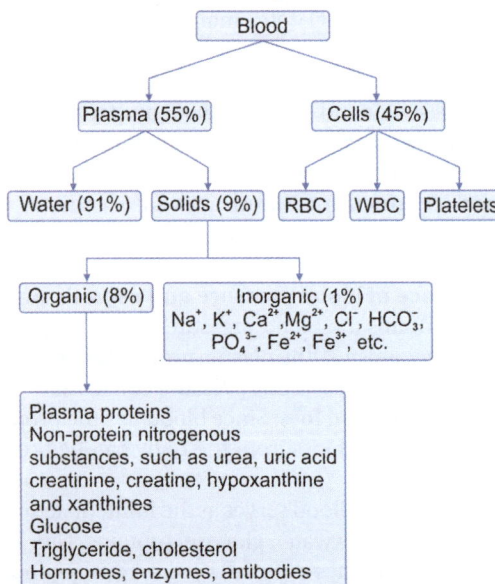

Flowchart 11.1: Composition of blood.

Specific Gravity

Specific gravity of blood is defined as the ratio of weight of blood to the weight of an equal volume of water at 4°C (the density of water is maximum at 4°C). Specific gravity of blood is determined mainly by the hemoglobin and plasma protein concentration.

Factors Affecting Specific Gravity

- RBC count
- Hemoglobin concentration
- Plasma protein concentration
- Water content of blood.

Normal Values of Specific Gravity

- Specific gravity of whole blood: 1.050–1.060
- Specific gravity of plasma: 1.025–1.030
- Specific gravity of blood cells: 1.085–1.090.

Variations in Specific Gravity

Physiological Increase

- Newborn
- High altitude
- Males
- After exercise.

Physiological Decrease

- Females
- During pregnancy
- In excess water intake, etc.

Pathological Increase

- Polycythemia
- Hemoconcentration as in dehydration (diarrhea, vomiting, burns)
- Hyperproteinemia.

Pathological Decrease

- Anemia
- Hypoproteinemia
- Renal diseases with albuminuria
- Increase in glucocorticoid hormone level.

Viscosity

Viscosity is the internal frictional resistance offered by the different particles of blood, as it flows through blood vessels. Relative viscosity of blood is 3.5–5.4, i.e., blood is 3.5–5.4 times more viscous than water. Viscosity of plasma is about 1.5 times that of water.

Factors Affecting Viscosity

- Hematocrit value (ratio of red blood cells to plasma volume)—increase in hematocrit value increases viscosity, e.g., polycythemia.
- Increase in the concentration of plasma proteins increases viscosity

- Increase in the temperature decreases viscosity
- Hypercapnia increases viscosity
- Increase in the velocity of blood flow decreases viscosity
- Shape of blood cells—if there is an alteration from normal shape as in microcytes and spherocytes, there will be an increase in viscosity
- Viscosity of venous blood is more than that of arterial blood because red blood cells are larger in venous blood because of water and chloride shift (*refer* page 361).

Physiologic Significance of Viscosity

Viscosity is one of the most important factors that determine the peripheral resistance of blood, which in turn affects the blood pressure. For example, in polycythemia, blood viscosity may increase to about 10. This means that ten times as much pressure is required to force blood as to force water through the same vessel.

Variations in Viscosity

Increase in Viscosity

- Polycythemia, leukemia
- Hyperproteinemia, hemoconcentration
- Decrease in temperature
- Hypercapnia (increase in PCO_2 of blood)
- Hereditary spherocytosis
- Venous blood, due to increased size of red blood cells in venous blood
- Males, due to increase in RBC count.

Decrease in Viscosity

- Anemia
- Hypoproteinemia, hemodilution
- Increase in temperature
- Hypocapnia (decrease in PCO_2)
- Arterial blood when compared to venous blood in the same individual
- About 25% less in capillary blood than in blood in large arteries due to plasma skimming (*refer* page 238)
- Females.

MULTIPLE CHOICE QUESTIONS

1. **Viscosity of blood is:**
   a. Same as that of ECF
   b. 10 times that of urine
   c. 5-6 times more than that of water
   d. 5-6 times less than that of water

2. **Which of the following situations will lead to increased viscosity of blood?**
   a. Fasting state   b. Hypoglycemia
   c. Multiple myeloma   d. Amyloidogenesis

3. **When osmotic fragility is normal, RBCs begin to hemolyse when suspended in:**
   a. 0.33% saline   b. 0.48% saline
   c. 0.9% saline   d. 1.2% saline

4. **Decrease in viscosity is seen in:**
   a. Increase in body temperature
   b. Decrease in body temperature
   c. Males when compared to females
   d. Hypercapnia

5. **Increase in specific gravity occurs in:**
   a. Pregnancy   b. Dehydration
   c. Hypoproteinemia   d. Albuminuria

ANSWERS

1. c   2. c   3. b   4. a   5. b

Plasma

CHAPTER 12

LEARNING OBJECTIVES

Must know
- Name the plasma proteins and explain their functions
- Explain the importance of plasmapheresis
- Significance of albumin-globulin ratio
- Enumerate the causes of hyperproteinemia and hypoproteinemia

INTRODUCTION

The fluid portion of blood is plasma. It is a clear straw-colored fluid, which constitutes 55% of the blood volume. The normal plasma volume is about 5% of body weight, i.e., about 3500 mL in a 70 kg man. Serum is the fluid part of blood after coagulation of blood.

COMPOSITION

About 91–92% of plasma is water and the rest is constituted by ions, inorganic and organic molecules. Inorganic materials are Na^+, K^+, Ca^{2+}, Mg^{2+}, I, F, Cu, P, etc.

Organic substances include proteins, urea, uric acid, bilirubin, creatinine, glucose, lipids, hormones, antibodies, enzymes, etc.

Normal Plasma Values

- Sodium : 135–145 mEq/L
- Potassium : 3.5–5 mEq/L
- Calcium : 8.5–10.5 mg/dL
- Phosphorus : 3–4.5 mg/dL
- Magnesium : 1.5–2 mEq/L
- Fasting glucose : 70–110 mg/dL
- Cholesterol : 160–200 mg/dL
- Urea : 8–25 mg/dL
- Uric acid : 2–8 mg/dL
- Creatinine : 0.6–1.5 mg/dL
- Creatine : 1–2 mg/dL
- Bilirubin: 0.2–0.8 mg/dL.

PLASMA PROTEINS

PY2.2: Describe the origin, forms, variations and functions of plasma proteins.

Total plasma protein concentration is 6–8 g/100 mL of blood. It is classified into two:

I. Major fraction
  - Albumin: 3.5–5 g/dL
  - Globulin: 1.5–3 g/dL
  - Fibrinogen: 0.3 g/dL
II. Minor fraction
  - Prothrombin: 0.04 g/dL
  - Nucleoproteins
  - Enzymes

Albumin

- Molecular weight: 69,000
- Site of synthesis: Liver
- Rate of synthesis: 200–400 mg/kg body weight/day
- About 80% of osmotic pressure of blood is exerted by albumin, as it has the highest concentration.

Globulin

Molecular weight: 90,000–150,000
Globulin fraction is subdivided into:
1. α-globulin
    - $α_1$
    - $α_2$
2. β-globulin
    - $β_1$
    - $β_2$
3. γ-globulin

Site of synthesis: α and β fractions synthesized in the liver, spleen and bone marrow; and γ globulin is synthesized in plasma cells derived from B lymphocytes and lymphoid tissue.

Fibrinogen

- Molecular weight: 3,40,000
- Site of synthesis: Liver
- Fibrinogen helps in the coagulation of blood.

Protein Complexes

In blood, there are certain complexes of proteins, such as:
- Glycoproteins, e.g., haptoglobin, which combines with hemoglobin.
- Lipoproteins, such as LDL, HDL, VLDL, etc.
- Metalloproteins, such as transferrin, which transport iron and ceruloplasmin, which combines with copper.

Methods of Separation of Plasma Proteins

- Precipitation method in which the salt used is ammonium sulfate or sodium sulfate.
- Ultracentrifugation
- Fractional precipitation
- Electrophoresis: Different types of electrophoresis are:
  - Tiselius method
  - Paper electrophoresis
  - Agar or cellulose acetate electrophoresis
  - Immunoelectrophoresis

In electrophoresis, the rate of migration of different proteins depends on their surface charges, molecular weight and shape. Depending on the rate of mobility, different fractions of proteins form different bands. From this, the relative amount of plasma proteins can be found out **(Fig. 12.1)**.

Functions of Plasma Proteins

- Maintenance of osmotic pressure of blood
- Immunity
- Coagulation of blood
- Transport function
- Maintenance of blood viscosity
- Acid-base balance
- Rouleaux formation
- Reserve protein in times of starvation
- Nourishment of tissue cells by trephones.
- **Maintenance of colloidal osmotic pressure of blood:** The plasma proteins are responsible for maintaining the normal osmotic pressure of blood because the capillaries are relatively impermeable to them. The osmotic pressure exerted by plasma proteins is called **oncotic pressure or colloidal osmotic pressure**. The normal osmotic pressure of blood is **25–30 mm Hg** across the capillary wall. This pressure pulls water from the interstitial tissue to blood and thus maintains blood volume and fluid balance between blood and tissue fluid. *About 80% of the total osmotic pressure exerted by plasma protein is contributed by albumin because of its least molecular weight and maximum concentration.* Since they are freely permeable across capillary wall, crystalloids, such as urea, glucose, etc., does not contribute to the capillary osmotic pressure.
- **Immune function:** Antibodies or immunoglobulins are γ globulins, which react with antigens present in microorganisms, thus destroying them.
- **Coagulation of blood and fibrinolysis:** During coagulation, soluble fibrinogen is converted to insoluble fibrin, which forms the clot. This prevents bleeding. Fibrinolytic factors, such as fibrinolysin are also plasma proteins.
- **Transport or carrier function:** Albumin, α-globulin, and β-globulin transport hormones, enzymes, CO_2, vitamins, drugs, bile pigments, calcium, copper, free hemoglobin, etc., by combining loosely with these agents. Transcobalamin transports vitamin B_{12}, ceruloplasmin transports copper, haptoglobin transports free hemoglobin, albumin transports various drugs and bilirubin and transferrin transports iron. Hormone-binding proteins are thyroxine-binding globulin, transcortin (cortisol), etc. The carrier function of plasma proteins helps in prolonging the half-life of hormones in blood. It also prevents the rapid filtration of hormones through the glomeruli.
- **Maintenance of normal viscosity of blood:** Viscosity is one important factor that maintains normal blood pressure. *Fibrinogen and globulin provide maximum viscosity to blood because of their large size and asymmetrical shape.* Thus, they provide resistance to the flow of blood through blood vessels.
- **Acid-base balance:** The plasma proteins are responsible for 15% of the buffering capacity of blood because of their *amphoteric nature, i.e.,* they behave as acids or bases depending on the conditions. Plasma proteins are soluble in water and their polar residues comprise both positive (NH_3^+) and negative (COO^-) groups. In acidic pH, the plasma proteins acts as base and accept protons and in alkaline pH, it acts as acid and can donate proton. Thus they maintain the pH of blood at 7.4.
- **Prevention of rouleaux formation:** Fibrinogen and globulin favor rouleaux formation in vivo. Albumin inhibits rouleaux formation. ESR depends on the concentration of fibrinogen in plasma. More the rouleaux formation more will be the ESR. In conditions where the fibrinogen concentration is more as in acute inflammation, malignancy, etc. ESR will be more.
- **Reserve proteins:** Plasma proteins serve as reserve proteins in times of starvation, protein energy malnutrition, etc.
- **Nourishment of tissue cells by trephones:** Trephones are substances produced by leukocytes from plasma proteins. It promotes cell growth.

PLASMAPHERESIS

Plasmapheresis is the procedure for collecting plasma from donors without depleting their blood cells. Whole blood is withdrawn and the plasma is separated from the cells by centrifugation. The cells are then returned to the circulatory system of the donor. Plasmapheresis is done in

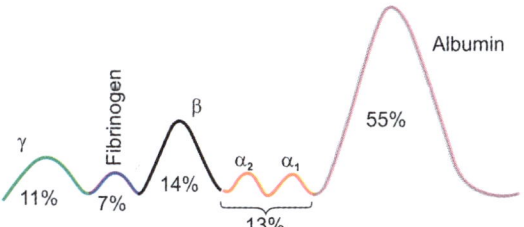

Fig. 12.1: Relative amount of plasma proteins in paper electrophoresis.

severe cases of autoimmune disorders, such as **myasthenia gravis** to get rid of the excess antibodies from blood. After removing the plasma, blood cells are reconstituted in saline, plasma expander, such as albumin or donor plasma before being returned to the patient. In this way, IgG is removed and the ACh receptor antibody level falls in patients with myasthenia gravis. A course of plasmapheresis consisting of approximately 40–50 mL/ kg plasma exchange daily for 4–5 days is usually used for treating **Guillain-Barre syndrome**, a demyelinating disease.

Plasmapheresis was previously done as an experimental procedure in animals by Whipple to demonstrate the *importance of plasma proteins in the body*. Some amount of blood is withdrawn and is centrifuged. The cells are then washed in saline so that all plasma proteins are removed.

The cells are then suspended in Ringer-Locke fluid, which is a nutrient fluid for mammalian cells. The protein- free cells in the nutrient fluid devoid of protein are re- injected into the animal. The procedure is repeated so that the plasma protein level is decreased very much. If the protein depletion is very severe, the animal was unable to survive and it died. But if the animal is provided with protein-rich diet containing all the 10 essential amino acids, recovery occurs within 7–14 days. This occurs only if the protein depletion was not that severe.

ALBUMIN-GLOBULIN RATIO

Normal value: 1.7–2.

Reversal of albumin-globulin ratio is seen in chronic liver diseases (due to decreased synthesis of albumin), chronic renal diseases with albuminuria and in autoimmune diseases where there is increase in the γ globulin fraction. Reversal of albumin-globulin ratio may be normal in old age due to decreased synthesis of albumin.

Variations in Plasma Protein Level

Hypoproteinemia (Decrease in the Levels of Plasma Proteins)

Hypoproteinemia is seen when there is increased loss or decreased synthesis of plasma proteins. It is seen in the following conditions:
- Hemorrhage and burns
- Pregnancy (due to hemodilution)
- Malnutrition, starvation and malabsorption of proteins
- Chronic liver diseases where there is decreased synthesis of plasma proteins.
- Renal diseases, such as nephrotic syndrome where there is increased loss of proteins through urine.

Hyperproteinemia

Hyperproteinemia is a rare condition and is seen in:
- Dehydration (due to hemoconcentration)
- Acute inflammatory conditions and malignancies where there is increased synthesis of acute phase proteins, such as C-reactive proteins, haptoglobin, fibrinogen, globulins, etc.
- *Multiple myeloma* is a condition where the plasma cells secrete large amounts of immunoglobulins resulting in *hypergammaglobulinemia*. It is associated with increased levels of Bence-Jones proteins.

Hypoalbuminemia

Hypoalbuminemia is seen in:
- Hemodilution
- Burns
- Liver and renal diseases
- Malnutrition.

Agammaglobulinemia

Agammaglobulinemia is congenital, total absence of γ globulin. Immunity is decreased leading to recurrent infections.

Hypergammaglobulinemia

- Multiple myeloma
- Systemic lupus erythematosus (SLE), an autoimmune disorder
- Acute and chronic infections
- Lymphatic leukemia.

Hyperfibrinogenemia

- Pregnancy
- Menstruation
- Malaria
- Malignancy.

MULTIPLE CHOICE QUESTIONS

1. Normal albumin-globulin ratio is:
    a. 2:1
    b. 1.7:1
    c. 1:1.7
    d. 1:2
2. The oncotic pressure of plasma is contributed mainly by:
    a. Albumin
    b. Fibrinogen
    c. Prothrombin
    d. Immunoglobulin
3. Oncotic pressure of plasma is important because:
    a. It retains fluid inside the vascular system
    b. It favors filtration across capillary wall
    c. It maintains acid-base balance
    d. It prevents proteinuria
4. Albumin which is an important factor in maintaining osmotic pressure, has:
    a. Low molecular weight and high blood concentration
    b. Low molecular weight and low blood concentration
    c. High molecular weight and low blood concentration
    d. High molecular weight and high blood concentration
5. In pregnancy:
    a. Plasma fibrinogen levels are increased
    b. Fibrinogen levels are decreased

c. Thyroglobulin level is decreased
d. IgD is markedly increased

6. **Which is true about serum albumin?**
   a. Contributes maximally to plasma oncotic pressure
   b. Freely permeable in kidney
   c. Not synthesized in liver
   d. Increases ESR

7. **Which of the following is not primarily a function of blood plasma?**
   a. Transport of hormones
   b. Transport of antibodies
   c. Transport of chylomicrons
   d. Maintenance of RBC size

8. **All the statements regarding albumin are correct, *except*:**
   a. It is the smallest of the plasma proteins
   b. It contributes to 80% of oncotic pressure
   c. Behaves as an anion at the pH of blood
   d. It is involved in the transport of O_2

9. **All the following statements regarding globulin are correct, *except*:**
   a. It decreases viscosity of blood
   b. It is bigger than albumin
   c. It helps in the transport of iron
   d. Gamma globulin act as antibodies

10. **The function of plasma protein includes:**
    a. Helps to prevent edema
    b. Helps to decrease blood pressure
    c. Decrease viscosity of blood
    d. Increases lymph flow

11. **The following plasma proteins are synthesized in the liver, *except*:**
    a. Fibrinogen   b. Gamma globulin
    c. Prothrombin   d. Albumin

12. **Plasmapheresis is done for treating:**
    a. Malaria   b. Renal failure
    c. Chronic infections d. Myasthenia gravis

13. **Maximum viscosity of blood is contributed by:**
    a. Albumin   b. Electrolytes
    c. Prothrombin   d. Fibrinogen

14. **The percentage of plasma constituted by water normally is:**
    a. 70%   b. 91%
    c. 80%   d. 96%

15. **The normal level of plasma fibrinogen is:**
    a. 3 mg/dL   b. 0.3 mg/dL
    c. 0.3 g/dL   d. 3 g/dL

16. **Albumin contributes to oncotic pressure of plasma by:**
    a. 80%   b. 20%
    c. 50%   d. 90%

ANSWERS

1. b	2. a	3. a	4. a	5. a
6. a	7. c	8. d	9. a	10. a
11. b	12. d	13. d	14. b	15. c
16. a				

Red Blood Corpuscles or Erythrocytes and Hemoglobin

CHAPTER 13

LEARNING OBJECTIVES

Must know
- Describe the stages of erythropoiesis
- Enumerate the functions of erythrocytes
- Explain the factors affecting erythropoiesis
- List the variations in red blood cell count
- Describe the synthesis and functions of hemoglobin
- Explain the steps in the breakdown of hemoglobin
- Explain the etiological classification of anemia
- Describe the different types of anemia
- Classify jaundice and mention their differences
- Define polycythemia and discuss its pathophysiology

Desirable to know
- Factors affecting ESR
- Describe hemoglobinopathies
- Sources and actions of erythropoietin
- Differentiate between reticulocyte response and reticulocyte crisis

MORPHOLOGY OF MATURE RBC

Red blood corpuscles or *erythrocytes* are disc-shaped **non-nucleated** elements of blood. They are also devoid of organelles like mitochondria and ribosomes. 90% of the energy requirement of RBC is through anaerobic metabolism and 10% energy is supplied by aerobic or pentose-phosphate cycle. Mature red cell is not capable of protein synthesis since they have no ribosomes. Red color is due to the presence of red pigment, hemoglobin, in the cytoplasm. Presence of nucleated erythrocytes in the peripheral smear suggests an underlying disease. *Hemoglobin forms 95% of the dry weight of an erythrocyte.* Blood group antigens are present on the RBC membrane. Carbonic anhydrase constitutes about 4% of the red cell protein.

- **Normal shape:** Biconcave or disc shaped or dumb-bell shaped **(Fig. 13.1A)**.
- **Size:** 7.2–7.5 μm in diameter, 2 μm thick at the periphery and 1 μm thick at the center **(Fig. 13.1B)**.
- **Surface area:** 120 μm^2
- **Volume:** 90 μm^3

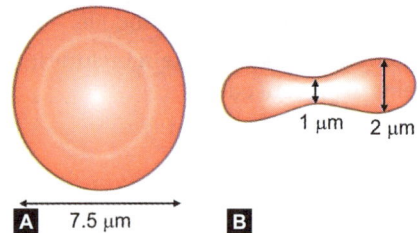

Figs. 13.1A and B: Morphology of red blood corpuscle: (A) Surface view; (B) Side view.

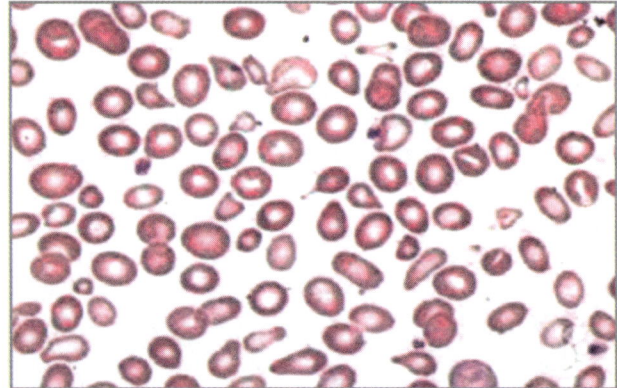

Fig. 13.2: Peripheral smear showing anisopoikilocytosis (note the difference in the size and shape of RBCs).

Variations in the Size and Shape of Erythrocytes (Fig. 13.2)

Variation in the size of RBC is called **anisocytosis**; e.g., in pernicious anemia, the cell size is increased and the cells are called **macrocytes**, whereas in iron deficiency anemia, the cells are small and are called **microcytes**.

Variation in the shape of RBC is called **poikilocytosis**, e.g., in sickle cell anemia, erythrocytes are sickle shaped or comma shaped. It may be spherical in spherocytosis and oval shaped in ovalocytosis or elliptocytosis. RBC become crenated when suspended in hypertonic solution.

Advantages of Biconcave Shape

- Biconcave shape provides larger surface-to-volume ratio when compared to the spherical shape. This is necessary for rapid exchange of gases and diffusion of other substances across the RBC membrane.
- Because of the **flexible** shape, erythrocytes can squeeze through very small capillaries, which are as narrow as 3 μm in diameter.
- Due to lack of mitochondria, erythrocytes do not consume any of the O_2 that they transport.
- Considerable alteration in the cell volume is possible because of the biconcave shape. This prevents the erythrocytes from rupturing when increase in the volume of the cell occurs or in other words, RBC can withstand considerable changes in the osmotic pressure.

Red Cell Membrane

The red cell membrane consists of lipid bilayer and interval proteins attached to an underlying protein skeleton. The protein skeleton helps to maintain the shape of the red cell. The protein skeleton consists of a two-dimensional mesh of **spectrin** tetramers and oligomers, cross linked by **protein 4.1 (Beatty's protein)** and **ankyrin**. Spectrin is a cytoskeletal protein that forms a scaffolding and plays an important role in maintaining cell membrane integrity and cytoskeletal structure. Ankyrin, a peripheral protein located on the inside of the cell membrane mediate the attachment of integral membrane protein to the spectrin-actin cytoskeleton. Ankyrin has binding sites for the beta-subunit of spectrin. The protein skeleton is attached to the membrane by the binding of spectrin to ankyrin, and of ankyrin to another integral protein of erythrocyte called **band-3** which is an anion exchanger. Abnormalities of the membrane proteins lead to early destruction of erythrocytes as occurs in spherocytosis. There will be loss of biconcave shape and defective deformation of the RBCs while passing through blood vessels of smaller diameter. Because of the flexible biconcave shape, erythrocytes can squeeze through very small capillaries normally.

Factors Maintaining Biconcave Shape of RBC

- **Spectrin, ankyrin, actin** and other cytoskeletal proteins of RBC plays important role in maintaining the integrity of RBC membrane. Ankyrin plays a very important role in the maintenance of the biconcave shape of the erythrocyte.
- Albumin adsorbed to the RBC membrane helps to maintain the shape.
- Decrease in the cell volume by removing intracellular structures, especially nucleus gives it the biconcave shape.

■ PACKED CELL VOLUME OR HEMATOCRIT

PY2.12: Describe the test for ESR, osmotic fragility, hematocrit.

Hematocrit or packed cell volume (**PCV**) expresses the proportion of the blood sample occupied by the formed elements of blood. It refers to the percentage of RBC, WBC and platelets in the whole blood. As the volume of WBC and platelets is very less (only about 1% of the volume of blood), for practical purposes, PCV is considered to be the volume of **packed red cell volume (PRCV)** i.e., the fraction of the total column of blood occupied by RBCs. But in conditions like leukemia where WBC count is significantly increased, PCV will differ from that of PRCV.

- Normal value of PCV is approximately 45%
- In adult males: 47%
- In adult females: 42%
- In newborn: 55%.

Determination of PCV

Principle

A known volume of anticoagulated blood is taken in a specialized graduated tube and centrifuged for a sufficient length of time. Due to centrifugal force, the blood cells get packed at the bottom of the tube leaving clear plasma at the top **(Fig. 13.3)**. RBCs have the highest density and are seen as the bottom layer.

Apparatus

- Wintrobe's hematocrit tube
- Van Allen's hematocrit tube
- Micro-hematocrit tube.

After centrifugation, blood gets separated into three layers:
1. Upper layer of straw colored plasma about 55 mm thick.
2. A grayish white, thin layer of platelets and leukocytes just below the plasma layer called buffy coat layer, which is normally 1 mm thick.
3. A bottom layer of red blood cells packed together, about 45 mm in length. A dark line separates the buffy coat layer from red cell layer **(Fig. 13.3)**. This is due to the presence of reduced hemoglobin in the red cells that are lying next

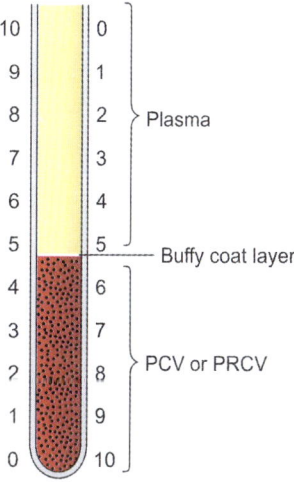

Fig. 13.3: Wintrobe's hematocrit tube showing packed cell volume (PCV) or packed red cell volume (PRCV) buffy coat layer and plasma layer.

to leukocytes. O_2 is being utilized by the leukocytes for their metabolism.

PCV is determined as follows:

$$PCV = \frac{45 \times 100}{100} = 45\%$$

Packed Red Cell Volume

The length of the lower layer in the hematocrit tube up to the dark line is taken as PRCV and it is expressed in percentage. PRCV is determined only in cases of thrombocytosis and leukemia. In leukemia, PCV may be normal, but PRCV will be very low because of severe anemia.

Significance of Hematocrit

- **Plasma layer** is straw colored normally, but there will be a red tinge in hemolysis, deep yellow or brown-green in jaundice, milky and opaque in lipemia.
- **Buffy coat layer** is normally 1 mm thick, which means that the blood contains 10,000 leukocytes per cubic mm of blood. *0.1 mm of the buffy coat layer corresponds to 1000 WBC.* It is increased in leukocytosis and leukemia.
- **Red cell volume (PCV)** can be found out.

Variations in PCV (Figs. 13.4A and B)

Increase in PCV is seen in:
- Polycythemia
- Chronic heart disease and chronic lung disease
- Hemoconcentration as in diarrhea, dehydration, etc.
- Venous blood when compared to arterial blood in the same individual.
- In newborn PCV is approximately 55% and this value falls to about 35% at 2 months of age. Adult values are reached at puberty

Decrease in PCV is seen in:
- Anemia
- Hemodilution as in pregnancy
- Leukemia

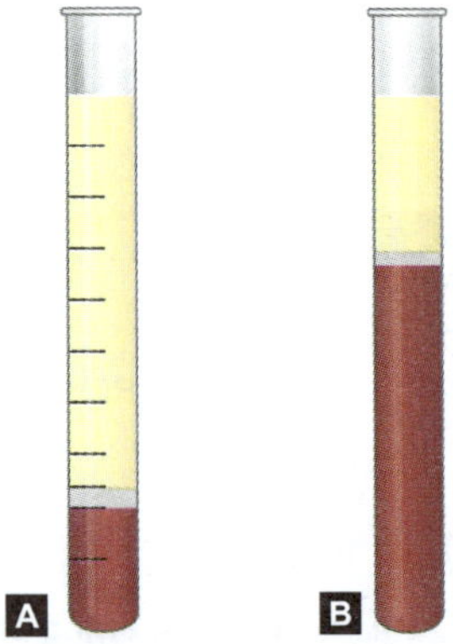

Disadvantages
- Reading error is more
- Hematocrit value gives only the concentration of red cells, i.e., the red cells present in a particular volume of blood. It does not give an idea of the total red cell mass. For example, in hypovolemic shock due to hemorrhage, the PCV will be normal but the total red cell mass is drastically reduced.
- About 2% of plasma remains trapped in between the red cells after centrifugation. This will be more if the red cells are of abnormal shape as in spherocytosis. The true hematocrit value can be found out by using a correction factor.

True hematocrit = Obtained hematocrit × 0.98
(Correction factor)

■ SPECIAL PROPERTIES OF ERYTHROCYTES

- Rouleaux formation
- Erythrocyte sedimentation rate (ESR)
- Red cell fragility.

Rouleaux Formation

When fresh blood is examined under the microscope, erythrocytes are seen grouped together attached at their broad surfaces like a pile of coins. This phenomenon is called rouleaux formation **(Fig. 13.5)**. This is a reversible phenomenon and is different from agglutination in which there is irreversible clumping of RBC.

Rouleaux formation does not occur in the body during life under physiological conditions because:
- Blood is in constant motion.
- Surface of RBC membrane is negatively charged due to the presence of **sialic acid** in the cell membrane. So, there is repulsion of erythrocytes.

Erythrocyte Sedimentation Rate

PY2.12: Describe the test for ESR, osmotic fragility, hematocrit.

Blood is a suspension of cells in plasma. ESR is a measure of the suspension stability of blood.

Figs. 13.4A and B: (A) PCV in anemia; (B) PCV in polycythemia.

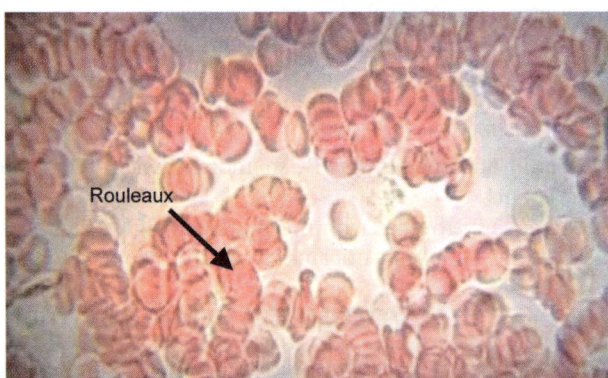

Fig. 13.5: Fresh blood under the microscope (note the biconcave shape of erythrocytes and rouleaux formation).

Definition

Depth in millimeters of clear plasma formed at the top of a vertical column of anticoagulated blood kept undisturbed for 1 hour in a tube of standard dimensions (2.5 mm inner diameter, 200 mm height) is called erythrocyte sedimentation rate (ESR) **(Figs. 13.6A and B)**. It is expressed in mm at the end of the first hour.

Normal Values

- *Male*: 2–4 mm in the 1st hour
- *Female*: 4–8 mm in the 1st hour
- *Infants*: 0.5 mm in the 1st hour
- *Old age*: 20 mm in the 1st hour.

Methods of Determination of ESR

- Westergren's method
- Wintrobe's method
- Esrite method.

Factors Affecting ESR

- *Rouleaux formation*: The red blood cells align themselves side by side forming stacks called Rouleaux (*See* **Fig. 13.5**). The protein coating of red cells plays a major role in rouleaux formation. More the rouleaux formation more will be the ESR because it gravitates to the bottom at a much higher speed due to increased mass than individual cells.
- *Plasma proteins*: Fibrinogen and globulin neutralize the surface charges of RBCs and this accelerates rouleaux formation and thus increases ESR. But, increase in albumin decreases ESR.
- *Plasma lipids*: Increase in lecithin decreases ESR and increase in cholesterol increases ESR.
- *Body temperature*: Increase in temperature increases ESR.
- *Viscosity of blood*: Increase in viscosity decreases ESR. ESR is low in polycythemia where viscosity is high and ESR is high in anemia where viscosity is low.
- *Specific gravity*: Increase in specific gravity decreases ESR.
- *RBC count*: Increase in RBC count decreases ESR; e.g., in polycythemia there is decrease in ESR, whereas in anemia there is increase in ESR (except spherocytic anemia where ESR is decreased due to defective Rouleaux formation).
- *Size and shape of RBC*: Variation in the normal shape (sickle cell anemia, spherocytosis, etc.,) and increase in cell size decreases ESR.
- *Position of the tube*: If the apparatus is kept inclined, ESR will be increased.

Variations in ESR

- **Physiological increase** is seen in females in the reproductive age group, during pregnancy, menstruation, etc.
- **Physiological decrease** is seen in males, newborn, etc.
- Pathological increase:
  - Acute and chronic infections (globulin, fibrinogen and products of tissue destruction increase rouleaux formation). ESR is very high in septicemia and tuberculosis.
  - Collagen disorders like systemic lupus erythematosus (SLE) due to increase in globulin.
  - Malignancy (due to products of tissue destruction and increased fibrinogen).
  - Renal diseases decrease erythropoiesis due to decreased erythropoietin secretion.
  - Anemia, especially iron deficiency anemia (in sickle cell anemia and spherocytic anemia, ESR is decreased because of defective rouleaux formation).
- Pathological decrease:
  - Allergy
  - Polycythemia
  - Sickle cell anemia and spherocytic anemia

Clinical Significance of ESR

ESR is a measure of the presence of disease processes within the body.

- ESR helps in the **diagnosis** of diseases to some extent along with other parameters. As ESR is elevated in many diverse pathological conditions, it has little diagnostic value of its own.
- Serial estimations of ESR in a patient help to assess the **prognosis** of a disease, i.e., prediction of the probable course of a disease in an individual and the chances of recovery. For example, if the initial value of ESR in a patient suffering from tuberculosis was 90 mm in the 1st hour and after antituberculous treatment for 1 month, if the ESR has decreased to 40 mm in the 1st hour, it shows that the patient is responding very well to the treatment. Otherwise, the drug regimen should be changed. Another situation is, if a patient is suffering from a chronic disease and if the ESR is increasing rapidly, it denotes that the disease is progressing rapidly.
- It helps to diagnose hidden diseases like cancer.
- Helps in the **differential diagnosis** of benign and malignant tumors. In malignancy, ESR is very much increased.

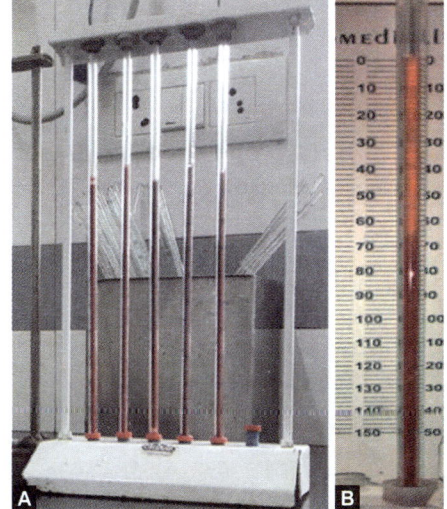

Figs. 13.6A and B: (A) Westergren's pipettes mounted on the Westergren's stand; (B) ESR in Esrite tube (note the ESR is 70 mm in the first hour and the plasma is tinted red due to hemolysis).

- Helps to assess the **severity** of a disease. If the extent of inflammatory process is very high, ESR will also be very high. Any acute stress to the body like trauma, infection, malignancy, etc. induces a reaction called **acute-phase response**. This response enhances release of inflammatory cytokines which stimulate the liver to secrete proteins called **acute phase proteins** like fibrinogen. This leads to increase in ESR.
- ESR is routinely done in all hematological disorders.
- ESR also helps in distinguishing functional disorders (psychological disorders) from organic diseases affecting body structures.

Red Cell Fragility

PY2.12: Describe the test for ESR, osmotic fragility, hematocrit.

Definition

Fragility is the ease with which red cell membrane is broken leading to the release of hemoglobin. Rupture of RBC and release of hemoglobin into the plasma is called **hemolysis**. Fragility is of two types:
1. Osmotic fragility
2. Mechanical fragility.

Osmotic Fragility

0.9% sodium chloride solution (normal saline) is isotonic with plasma. Red blood cells shrink in solutions with osmotic pressure greater than this and swell in solutions with osmotic pressure less than normal saline. When suspended in hypotonic solution, red cells swell and finally rupture (hemolyse) releasing hemoglobin, which colors the supernatant solution red.

The ease with which erythrocytes rupture or hemolyse when suspended in hypotonic solution is called **osmotic fragility**.

Normal value: Hemolysis starts in 0.45% and is completed in 0.35% sodium chloride solution.

Mechanical Fragility

The ease with which RBCs rupture when subjected to mechanical stress is called **mechanical fragility**. The RBCs become more brittle due to pathological changes in the red cell membrane and due to other red cell disorders. The red cells are subjected to mechanical stress, as they pass through capillaries and trabeculae of spleen and the abnormal cell becomes more fragile than the normal cell. For example, in sickle cell anemia, the cells are sickle shaped at low PO_2 and have a high mechanical fragility. However, the osmotic fragility of the sickle cells is normal or even low.

Variation in Fragility of RBC

Increase in fragility is seen in spherocytosis, purpura, mismatched blood transfusion, glucose-6-phosphate dehydrogenase (G-6-PD) deficiency, and in venous blood when compared to arterial blood (due to Hamberger phenomenon).

Decrease in fragility is seen in iron deficiency anemia, thalassemia and pernicious anemia. The osmotic fragility of sickle cell is normal or even low but they have high mechanical fragility. Because of the abnormal shape, the sickle cells are subjected to deforming mechanical stresses as they pass through capillaries and may rupture.

Hemolysins

Hemolysins are substances that produce hemolysis. Hemolysins may be chemical or biological agents.
- *Chemicals*: Ether, chloroform, bile salts, acids, alkali, drugs like aspirin, etc., produce hemolysis.
- *Biological hemolysins*: Toxins of bacteria, snake venom, etc., produce hemolysis. Venom of cobra and certain insects contains lecithinase, which dissolves lecithin present in the red cell membrane, so that they are easily ruptured.

■ METABOLISM IN RBC

Metabolic activity in RBC is low and it consumes very little oxygen. RBC can utilize only glucose for energy. 90% of glucose in the RBC is utilized for ATP production through anaerobic glycolysis. This is because mitochondria are absent in the mature RBC. A major portion of this energy is utilized to pump out Na^+ by sodium-potassium pump. Otherwise, it may result in hemolysis as water enters the RBC by osmosis if Na^+ content is high (Na^+ and Ca^{2+} are present in very small amount or are absent inside the RBC). Rest of the energy is utilized to maintain the integrity of the RBC membrane and to maintain iron in hemoglobin in the reduced form.

90% of glycolysis occurs through **anaerobic** glycolytic pathway known as **Embden-Meyerhof pathway**, but the glycolytic step catalyzed by phosphoglycerate kinase is bypassed **(Flowchart 13.1)**. Two molecules of ATP are generated from each molecule of glucose. The

Flowchart 13.1: Steps in the formation of 2,3 DPG in red blood cells (note that the glycolytic step is bypassed).

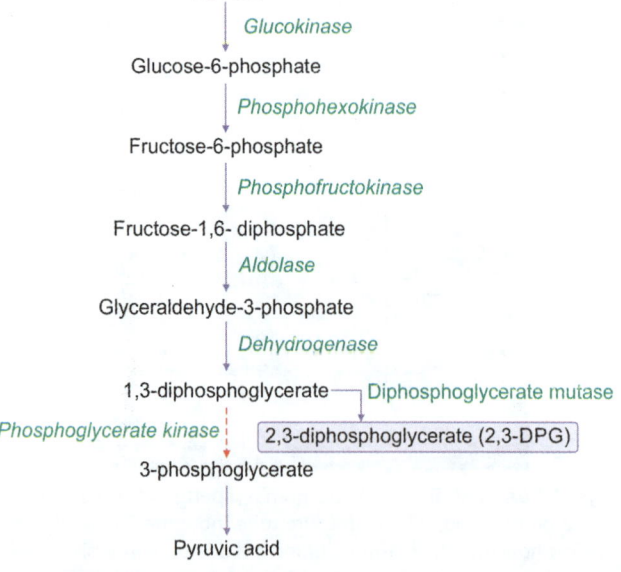

significance of this modified pathway is the production of **2,3-diphosphoglycerate (2,3-DPG)**, which influences the oxygen affinity of hemoglobin. Acidity decreases 2,3-DPG production in the red cell by inhibiting glycolysis, and hypoxia increases 2,3-DPG by inhibiting Krebs cycle. Hormones that increase 2,3-DPG are thyroid hormones, growth hormone and androgens. 2,3-DPG is also known as 2,3-bisphosphoglycerate (2,3-BPG).

10% of glycolysis in RBC occurs through the **pentose phosphate pathway or hexose monophosphate (HMP) shunt**. It generates NADPH, which is needed for the reduction of glutathione and reduced glutathione protects hemoglobin against oxidation.

RBC COUNT

Apparatus used to determine RBC count is called **hemocytometer**.

Normal Count

- *Male*: 5–6.5 million cells/mm^3 or μL of blood
- *Female*: 4.5–5.5 million cells/mm^3 of blood
- *Infants*: 6–8 million/mm^3 of blood.

Variations in the RBC Count

Increase in the RBC count is called **polycythemia** and decrease in the count is called **anemia**.

Physiological Increase in the RBC Count

- **Age**: Count is high in infants and decreases as age advances. At birth, count is 8–10 million/mm^3 of blood. Within 10 days after birth, the count decreases due to rapid destruction of erythrocytes which in turn causes a slight increase in the serum bilirubin level. This is the reason for the **physiological jaundice** seen in newborn.
- **Sex**: Count is more in adult males than in females due to the effect of androgen.
- **Altitude**: At high altitude, RBC count is more due to hypoxic stimulation of erythropoiesis.
- In muscular exercise and emotional states, count is high due to sympathetic stimulation, which causes release of stored RBC, especially from the spleen.
- After meals, there is a slight increase in the RBC count.

Physiological Decrease in the RBC Count

- High barometric pressure as at depths causes decrease in count due to increase in the PO$_2$ of blood.
- During sleep.
- In pregnancy, there is a relative reduction in RBC count due to hemodilution.

Pathological Increase in the RBC Count

Increase in RBC count is called **polycythemia,** which may be:
- Primary polycythemia or polycythemia vera
- Secondary polycythemia.

Polycythemia Vera

Polycythemia vera is a *malignant condition of red bone marrow*. It is always associated with increase in leukocyte count. RBC count will be >14 million/mm^3 of blood.

Secondary Polycythemia

It is secondary to other pathological conditions, which produce a state of chronic hypoxia like:
- Chronic lung diseases
- Congenital heart disease
- Carbon monoxide poisoning
- Repeated small hemorrhages, which stimulates erythropoiesis
- Phosphorus and arsenic poisoning
- **Relative polycythemia** is seen in conditions, which produce hemoconcentration.

Pathological Decrease in the RBC Count

Abnormal decrease in RBC count is called anemia, e.g., iron deficiency anemia, pernicious anemia, thalassemia, hemolytic anemia, etc.

HEMOGLOBIN

> **PY2.3:** Describe and discuss the synthesis and functions of hemoglobin and explain its breakdown. Describe variants of hemoglobin.

Hemoglobin is the red coloring pigment and the O$_2$ binding protein of RBC. It forms 95% of the dry weight of RBC. The function of hemoglobin is to carry O$_2$ and CO$_2$. It is a conjugated protein with molecular weight 65,000. In lower animals, hemoglobin is seen dissolved in plasma, but in higher animals, it is confined to the RBC. If hemoglobin is found in plasma as free hemoglobin, it leads to the following problems:
- It increases the viscosity of blood leading to an increase in the blood pressure.
- Increase in the osmotic pressure of blood.
- Hemoglobin from plasma will be filtered across the capillary walls to the interstitial fluid.
- Free hemoglobin will be filtered and excreted by the kidneys leading to hemoglobinuria and precipitation of hemoglobin in the renal tubules leading to renal failure and anuria.
- Free hemoglobin will be rapidly destroyed by the reticuloendothelial cells leading to increase in the bilirubin content of blood and **acholuric jaundice** (jaundice with excessive amount of unconjugated bilirubin in plasma and without bilirubin in the urine).

Normal Hemoglobin Content

- At birth: 23–25 g% (high due to high RBC count)
- Adult male: 14–16 g%
- Adult female: 12–15 g%.

The amount of hemoglobin in a 70 kg man comes to about 900 g.

Functions of Hemoglobin

- It helps in the transport of O_2 from lungs to tissues by forming oxyhemoglobin
- Helps in the transport of CO_2 from tissues to lungs by forming carbaminohemoglobin
- It acts as a buffer to maintain the normal pH of blood. Hemoglobin being a protein is responsible for 70% of the buffering capacity of whole blood.
- The β-chain of hemoglobin has an additional nitric oxide (NO) binding site. The affinity of hemoglobin for NO is increased by O_2. So hemoglobin binds with NO in the lungs and releases it in the tissues where it promotes vasodilatation.

Structure of Hemoglobin

Hemoglobin is a globular molecule made up of 4 subunits. Each subunit contains a heme part conjugated to a polypeptide. Heme is an iron-containing **porphyrin derivative**. The polypeptides form the globin portion of the hemoglobin molecule. There are two pairs of polypeptides in each hemoglobin molecule. Adult hemoglobin is referred to as **HbA**, which contains 2α and 2β chains. Thus, HbA is designated as $\alpha_2\beta_2$. About 2.5% of hemoglobin in circulation is **HbA$_2$**, which contains 2α and 2δ chains designated as $\alpha_2\delta_2$. **HbF** is the hemoglobin present in the fetus, which contains 2α and 2γ chains designated as $\alpha_2\gamma_2$. Synthesis of β-chains normally begins about 6 weeks before birth, and HbA usually replaces almost all the HbF by the time an infant is 6 months old.

Blood also contain very small amounts of HbA derivatives like HbA$_{1c}$, which has a glucose attached to the β chain. Significance of this is that its level in the blood gives an indication of the severity of diabetes mellitus and is a measure of glucose control in diabetes.

Heme belongs to a compound called **porphyrin**. The characteristic feature of porphyrin is that it combines with metals like iron, copper, magnesium, etc. Protoporphyrin is a cyclic compound formed of 4 pyrrole rings connected by methene bridges. Iron is present in the center of the porphyrin ring in the **ferrous (Fe^{2+})** form. It has 2 primary and 4 secondary valencies. One valency is bound to polypeptide chain of globin and the other to O_2, which is a loose and reversible combination **(Fig. 13.7)**. The other valencies are attached to the nitrogen atom of each pyrrole ring.

In one molecule of hemoglobin there are 4 heme subunits. So, one molecule of hemoglobin can combine with 4 molecules of O_2 **(Fig. 13.7)**. Each RBC contains about 280 million hemoglobin molecules.

Embryonic hemoglobins are **Gower I, Gower II and Portland**. They are found only during the first 3 months of fetal development. Heme is also part of the structure of **myoglobin, neuroglobin, cytochrome C, etc.**

Reactions of Hemoglobin or Derivatives of Hemoglobin

- **Oxyhemoglobin** (HbO$_2$): Oxygenation of hemoglobin leads to the formation of oxyhemoglobin.

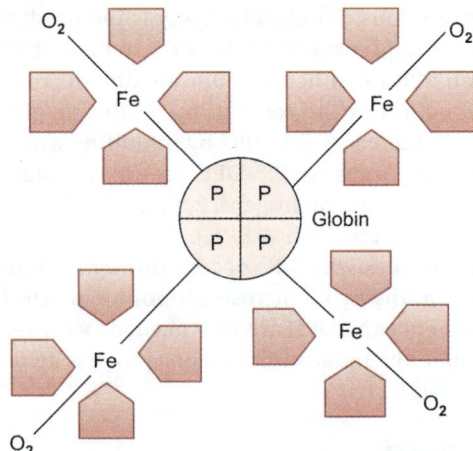

Fig. 13.7: Structure of oxyhemoglobin.

- **Carbaminohemoglobin** (HbNHCOOH): When hemoglobin combines with CO_2, carbaminohemoglobin is produced. CO_2 binds to the terminal NH_2 groups of valine in the polypeptide chain.
- **Carboxyhemoglobin** or **carbonmonoxyhemoglobin (COHb)**: The affinity of hemoglobin for CO is 200 times more than that of its affinity for O_2 and combination of hemoglobin with CO produces carboxyhemoglobin.
- **Sulfhemoglobin**: Combination of hemoglobin with H_2S produces sulfhemoglobin.
- **Methemoglobin** (HbOH): When blood is exposed to oxidizing agents like potassium ferricyanide, ferrous ion (Fe^{2+}) gets oxidized to ferric ion (Fe^{3+}) forming methemoglobin. When it is present in large amounts, it causes discoloration of skin resembling cyanosis. Normally, some amount of methemoglobin is produced in the body. Only about 1.5% of total hemoglobin is in the methemoglobin state and it is incapable of binding O_2. **NADH-methemoglobin reductase** (a heme containing enzyme) present in the RBC converts methemoglobin back to hemoglobin. Congenital absence of this enzyme leads to **hereditary methemoglobinemia**. In this condition, methemoglobin represents 25% or more of the total hemoglobin. This leads to decrease in the oxygen carrying capacity leading to tissue hypoxia.
- **Reduced hemoglobin**: When O_2 is released from oxyhemoglobin, it forms reduced hemoglobin. Increased amount of reduced hemoglobin in the blood leads to **cyanosis**.
- **Buffering of hydrogen ions**: H^+ binds to the NH group of the intermediate histidine residues of hemoglobin to form NH_2. Binding of O_2 to hemoglobin releases H^+.
- **Glycated hemoglobin (HbA1c)**: When glucose gets attached to the terminal valine in the β-chain of hemoglobin A, it forms glycated hemoglobin. The amount of glycated hemoglobin is proportionate to the blood glucose concentration and is normally about 5%. It serves as an index of long-term control of diabetes mellitus. Since, the glucose remains attached to hemoglobin till the red blood cell is destroyed (life span of RBC is 120 days), the level of glycated hemoglobin reflects the average blood glucose

level over the past 3 months. If the level is more than 7% it is abnormal.
- ❖ **Reaction with 2,3-DPG**: Only a single molecule of 2,3-DPG binds to a molecule of hemoglobin. Binding of hemoglobin with 2,3-DPG makes it difficult for O_2 to bind to hemoglobin and shifts the O_2 dissociation curve to the right.
- ❖ **Reaction with nitric oxide (NO)**: Oxyhemoglobin acts as a carrier of NO in the form of S-nitrosothiol, on the cysteine residues on the β-chain. This is called **S-nitrosohemoglobin (SNO-Hb)**. When hemoglobin releases O_2, NO is also released. Thus in regions where PO_2 is low, this NO produces vasodilatation and increase blood flow.

Synthesis of Hemoglobin

Hemoglobin synthesis occurs in the cytoplasm of the **intermediate normoblast** during erythropoiesis. Globin synthesis begins in the proerythroblast stage. Heme is synthesized in the mitochondria from succinyl CoA and glycine. First protoporphyrin-IX is formed into which ferrous ion gets incorporated to form heme catalyzed by the enzyme heme synthetase. Globin part of hemoglobin is synthesized in the ribosome from amino acids. By the end of orthochromatic erythroblast stage, hemoglobin synthesis is complete. 0.3 g of hemoglobin is destroyed and 0.3 g is synthesized every hour. Chromosome 16 controls synthesis of alpha-globin chain and chromosome 11 controls synthesis of beta-globin chains.

Abnormalities of Hemoglobin Production

- ❖ Hemoglobinopathies
- ❖ Thalassemias

In hemoglobinopathies, abnormal polypeptide chains are produced but in thalassemia, polypeptide chains are normal in structure, but produced in decreased amounts or sometimes absent.

Hemoglobinopathies

Hemoglobinopathies refer to abnormalities in the amino acid sequence of the polypeptide chains of hemoglobin. About 1000 abnormal hemoglobins have been detected in man. Many of the abnormal hemoglobins are harmless.

Letters designates abnormal hemoglobin. For example, HbC, D, E, G, I, J, S, etc., are abnormal hemoglobins. Abnormal hemoglobins differ from normal hemoglobin in the structure of polypeptide chain.

In **sickle cell anemia**, the abnormal hemoglobin is **HbS**. In HbS, α chains are normal but the β chains are abnormal. In the β chain, glutamic acid residue in the 6th position is replaced by valine. HbS polymerizes at low O_2 tension causing the cells to become sickle shaped and increase hemolysis. This leads to sickle cell anemia. Sickling occurs only in cells with deoxygenated hemoglobin. A sickle cell is more fragile than a normal erythrocyte. The cells have a tendency to stick to one another, which increases blood viscosity favoring thrombosis or blockage of blood vessels. The sickle cell gene confers resistance to one type of malaria and is common in the black population of Africa.

Thalassemia

Thalassemia refers to the reduced synthesis or absence of a pair of polypeptide chains of hemoglobin due to defects in the regulatory portion of the globin genes. The affected polypeptide has a normal sequence of amino acids. Two types of thalassemias are:
- ❖ α-thalassemia: The number of α chain is decreased or absent.
- ❖ β-thalassemia: β chain is decreased or absent and this is the common type.

■ BLOOD INDICES

The features of RBC such as volume, number and color indicate the quality of blood and these features are referred to as blood indices. The blood indices are calculated from packed cell volume, hemoglobin concentration and the red cell count. The various blood indices are:
- ❖ Mean corpuscular volume (MCV)
- ❖ Mean corpuscular hemoglobin (MCH)
- ❖ Mean corpuscular hemoglobin concentration (MCHC)

Mean Corpuscular Volume

MCV is the average volume of the red cells. It is calculated by dividing PCV in 100 mL of blood by RBC count in 100 mL of blood. It is expressed in femtoliters (fL) or μm^3. Normal value is 87–90 μm^3 (fL) and the RBCs are referred to as normocytes. Cells with MCV more than 95 fL are called macrocytes and RBCs with MCV less than 80 fL are called microcytes. MCV is increased in megaloblastic anemia due to folic acid deficiency and in pernicious anemia due to vitamin B_{12} deficiency. MCV is decreased in iron deficiency anemia, sideroblastic anemia, anemia due to chronic blood loss (bleeding piles, hookworm infestation, etc.,) and in thalassemia.

$$MCV = \frac{PCV \text{ in } 100 \text{ mL of blood}}{RBC \text{ count in } 100 \text{ mL of blood}} \text{ or}$$

$$\frac{PCV \text{ in } 100 \text{ mL} \times 10}{RBC \text{ count in millions/mm}^3} = \frac{45 \times 10}{5} = 90 \text{ fL}$$

Mean Corpuscular Hemoglobin

MCH is the average mass of hemoglobin in picograms contained in each red cell. It is calculated by dividing hemoglobin content in 100 mL of blood by RBC count in 100 mL of blood. Normal value is 30 pg (picogram) and the RBCs are referred to as normochromic. It ranges from 27 to 32 pg. Cells with MCH less than 25 pg are referred to as hypochromic. MCH is increased in megaloblastic anemia and it is decreased in microcytic hypochromic anemia (iron deficiency anemia, copper deficiency).

$$MCH = \frac{\text{Hemoglobin in g}/100 \text{ mL}}{RBC \text{ count in } 100 \text{ mL of blood}}$$

Mean Corpuscular Hemoglobin Concentration

MCHC is expressed in percentage. It is the amount of hemoglobin per 100 mL of RBC.

Normal value is 34 g/dL (32–38 g/dL) or 34%. For example, if hemoglobin content is 15 g% and PCV 45%.

$$MCHC = \frac{\text{Hemoglobin in g/100 mL}}{\text{PCV in 100 mL}} \times 100$$

$$= \frac{15 \times 100}{45}$$

$$= 33.3\% \text{ (g of Hb/100 mL of RBC)}$$

MCHC is decreased in iron deficiency anemia but it is normal in megaloblastic anemia (vitamin B_{12} and folic acid deficiency).

If MCHC is within normal range, RBCs are said to be normochromic. Decrease in MCHC is referred to as hypochromia. Iron deficiency anemia is referred to as microcytic hypochromic anemia. Pernicious anemia is macrocytic normochromic anemia. In pernicious anemia, MCV and MCH are increased; MCHC is normal. Macrocytic hypochromic anemia is seen when there is combined deficiency of iron and folic acid or vitamin B_{12}.

Anemia can never be hyperchromic because MCHC can never be more than 38% with the exception of hereditary spherocytosis and some cases of homozygous sickle cell disease.

LIFE SPAN OF RBC

Average life span of RBC in adult is **120 days** after they are released from the bone marrow into the circulatory system. Life span of RBC in newborn is 100 days. It is determined by **radioisotope method**. In this method, about 15 mL of blood is withdrawn from an individual. RBCs are tagged with radioactive substances like radioactive iron or radioactive chromium. The tagged RBCs are injected back into the same individual. Blood samples are collected from the individual every day and the radioactivity is determined. The rate of loss of radioactivity is measured. It is seen that the radioactivity falls to zero at about 120 days. Another method to determine the life span of RBC is **differential agglutination** method. The life span of erythrocytes is found to be reduced in conditions, such as hereditary spherocytosis, sickle cell anemia, thalassemia, glucose-6-phosphate dehydrogenase deficiency, pyruvate kinase deficiency, etc.

DESTRUCTION OF RBC

Old erythrocytes are destroyed in the **reticuloendothelial system**, especially in the spleen. So, *spleen is referred to as the graveyard of RBCs*. Old RBCs become fragile due to decreased NADPH activity. The fragile membrane of old RBC ruptures when they pass through very small capillaries and release hemoglobin. The hemoglobin is taken up by the reticuloendothelial cells (tissue macrophages) where the globin portion of hemoglobin molecule is split off to form heme. The tetrapyrrole ring structure of heme is broken by oxidation of one of its methene (=CH) bridges by **heme oxygenase** and the four pyrrole groups become arranged as a straight chain. This is the green iron-containing compound biliverdin. Fe^{3+} and **CO** are formed as by product in the process. Biliverdin is acted upon by **NADPH-dependent biliverdin reductase** to form **bilirubin (Fig. 13.8)**. When 1 g of hemoglobin is destroyed, 35 mg of bilirubin is formed.

Globin is degraded into amino acids, which enters the amino acid pool of plasma. Iron is released into circulation and carried to the bone marrow or to other tissues, where it combines with apoferritin to form ferritin, which is the storage form of iron. CO is an intercellular messenger, like NO.

Normal bilirubin level is 0.2–0.8 mg/100 mL of blood. When it becomes more than 2 mg/100 mL of blood, the condition is called **jaundice**.

Bilirubin enters the circulation and in combination with albumin reaches the liver. Binding of bilirubin with albumin prevents its excretion by the kidneys through urine. In the liver, bilirubin splits off from albumin and enters the hepatic cells. In the hepatocytes, bilirubin is conjugated with 2 molecules of uridine diphosphoglucuronic acid (UDPGA) to form **bilirubin diglucuronide** by the enzyme UDP-glucuronosyl transferase. This enzyme is located in the smooth endoplasmic reticulum. Bilirubin diglucuronide (BDG) is the water-soluble **conjugated bilirubin**, which is excreted through bile. Some of the conjugated bilirubin escapes into general circulation and is excreted by kidneys as urine bilirubin. Some of the unconjugated free bilirubin enters the blood stream and form free bilirubin. When the total bilirubin content of blood is estimated, both conjugated and free bilirubin levels are taken into consideration. The **van den Bergh test** helps to determine the type of bilirubin present in the serum.

In the intestine, BDG is acted upon by bacterial enzymes in the terminal ileum and large intestine to form **urobilinogen**. Some of the urobilinogen enters portal circulation and reaches the liver. This is known as **enterohepatic circulation** of bile pigments. Some urobilinogen escapes into general circulation and is excreted through urine as urinary urobilinogen. When exposed to the outside, urobilinogen gets oxidized to urobilin. Rest of the urobilinogen present

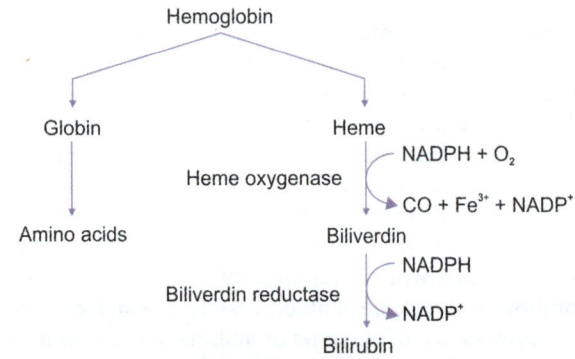

Fig. 13.8: Conversion of hemoglobin to bilirubin in the reticuloendothelial cells.

in the large intestine is converted to **stercobilinogen** and is excreted through feces (20–250 mg/day). It is oxidized to stercobilin and this gives golden yellow color to feces (**Fig. 13.9**).

Conjugated bilirubin is water-soluble and is excreted through urine. But, unconjugated bilirubin is insoluble and hence not excreted through urine. The reason is unconjugated bilirubin is bound to albumin and so it is not filtered by the kidneys. In conditions like **Gilbert's syndrome and Crigler-Najjar syndrome**, there is unconjugated hyperbilirubinemia. Urine does not contain bile pigments and hence called **acholuric jaundice**.

Enterohepatic Circulation

The circular route of substances from the intestine to the liver through the portal circulation and then through bile back to the intestine is called **enterohepatic circulation** of substances (**Fig. 13.9** shows enterohepatic circulation of urobilinogen). Substances that undergo enterohepatic circulation are bile salts, bile pigments (urobilinogen), iodide excreted through bile, adrenocortical and other steroid hormones and a number of drugs. Enterohepatic circulation of bile salt is very important in fat digestion and absorption.

Physiological Jaundice

Yellowish discoloration of skin and mucous membrane seen in newborn within 2–3 days of birth is called physiological jaundice. It usually disappears in 2 weeks. Causes are:
1. The RBC count in the newborn is high and there will be increased destruction of red cells after birth leading to increase in the serum bilirubin and appearance of jaundice.
2. During intrauterine life, bilirubin in fetal circulation is removed by the placenta. After birth, it takes time for the liver to take up the function of conjugation of bilirubin and its excretion through bile completely. This is particularly seen in premature babies having hepatic immaturity.

Physiological jaundice is treated by *phototherapy* with white light. Exposure of the body to white light leads to photo isomerization of bilirubin to water-soluble **lumirubin**. Lumirubin can be easily excreted through bile without conjugation. Exposure to light also causes oxidation of bilirubin to a colorless compound.

Importance of Iron in the Body

65–70% of the total body iron is present in hemoglobin. Iron is also necessary for the formation of **myoglobin, cytochrome oxidase, peroxidase, catalase,** etc. Total body iron comes to about 3–5 g depending on the sex and body weight. It is more in males, which comes to an average of 3.8 g (**Table 13.1**).

Iron is absorbed from duodenum and proximal jejunum in the ferrous form. Dietary iron is mainly in the ferric form and it is converted to ferrous form by acidic pH.

Phosphates and phytic acid inhibit iron absorption from the intestine. Phosphate forms insoluble ferric phosphate. Phytic acid present in cereals converts both ferrous and ferric ion into phytates and thus inhibits iron absorption. Vitamin C increases iron absorption. In the blood, Fe^{2+} is converted to Fe^{3+} which combines with the iron transport protein **transferrin**. Iron is stored in the reticuloendothelial cells and hepatocytes. Iron is stored mainly as **ferritin** and small

Table 13.1: Distribution of iron in the body.	
Sites of iron	**Amount**
Hemoglobin	2.3 g
Ferritin and hemosiderin	1 g
Myoglobin	0.5 g
Plasma iron	3–4 mg

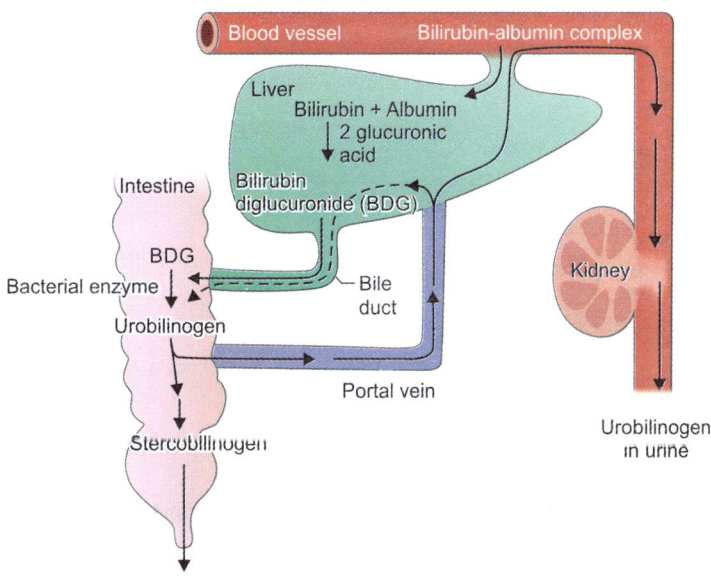

Fig. 13.9: Fate of bilirubin in the liver and enterohepatic circulation of urobilinogen formed in the intestine.

amounts as **hemosiderin**. The amount of iron in the body is controlled by a feedback mechanism. **Apoferritin** is the limiting factor of iron absorption.

Deficiency of iron in the body leads to **iron deficiency anemia**. *Gastrectomy also leads to iron deficiency anemia.*

This is because HCl present in gastric juice converts ferric ion into ferrous form. Iron can be absorbed by the intestinal mucosal cells only in the ferrous form.

Increased deposition of iron, especially in the liver, pancreas and skin leads to **hemochromatosis**. As pancreas is affected, it leads to diabetes and the diabetes seen in hemochromatosis is called **Bronze diabetes**.

HEMATOPOIESIS

Formation of all the cells present in blood in general is termed **hematopoiesis**. The process of differentiation from stem cell to mature erythrocyte is called **erythropoiesis**, to mature leukocyte is called **leukopoiesis** and development of platelets is called **thrombopoiesis**. The rates at which the blood cells are produced are regulated in healthy individuals to match the rates at which they leave the circulation. The balance between production and elimination is disturbed in pathological conditions. More than 100 billion cells are produced in the bone marrow every day.

Pluripotent long-term hematopoietic stem cells (LT-HSCs) are a population of multipotent adult stem cells found in the bone marrow which are capable of self-renewal. After differentiation, it becomes **pluripotent short-term hematopoietic stem cells (ST-HSCs)** which give rise to committed stem cells or **progenitors**, which after proliferation differentiate into lineages that in turn give rise to burst-forming units (BFU) or colony-forming units (CFU). Each CFU ultimately produce one or a limited number of mature blood cells. Cytokines like colony stimulating factors (CSF) guide the development of each lineage from progenitor cells. They are granulocyte-macrophage colony stimulating factor (GM-CSF), granulocyte colony stimulating factor (G-CSF), macrophage colony stimulating factor (M-CSF), interleukin-3 (IL-3), IL-5, thrombopoietin (TPO) and erythropoietin (EPO) **(Fig. 13.10)**.

Hematopoietic Niche

All blood cells originate from the **hematopoietic stem cell (HSC)**. For proper self-renewal of its population and differentiation of HSC progenitor cells to different blood cells, the HSC requires a specialized microenvironment. This special microenvironment in the bone marrow is termed the **hematopoietic stem cell niche**. HSC niche provides cytokines and cell signaling molecules necessary for the differentiation of HSCs throughout life. Except fishes, HSCs are maintained in the niche of the bone marrow of all vertebrates including mammals. Disturbances in this niche environment leads to pathological conditions.

HSC niche is divided into two types:
1. **Endosteal niche**, which includes the outer edge of the bone marrow that contains osteocytes, bone matrix, quiescent HSCs and high concentration of calcium ions.
2. **Perivascular niche**, which includes the inner core of the bone marrow that contains actively dividing HSCs, reticular cells and mesenchymal stem cells.

Osteoblasts in the bone marrow interact with the HSCs and provide proliferative signals and thus maintain their differentiation potential. It is seen that increase in the number of osteoblasts increases the number of HSCs.

Mutations in the osteoblastic lineage cells can result in malignant hematopoiesis leading to conditions like leukemia.

ERYTHROPOIESIS

PY2.4: Describe RBC formation (erythropoiesis and its regulation) and its functions.

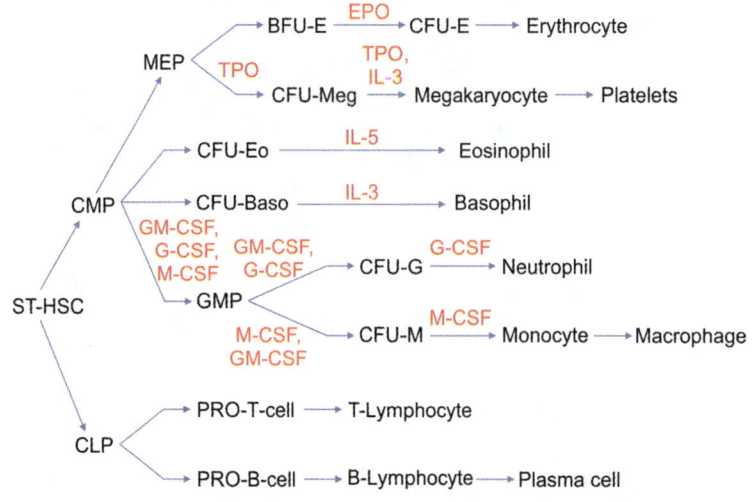

Fig. 13.10: Steps in hematopoiesis.

(ST-HSC: pluripotent short-term hematopoietic stem cell; CMP: common myeloid progenitor cell; CLP: common lymphoid progenitor cell; PRO: progenitor; MEP: megakaryocyte-erythroid progenitor; CFU: colony forming unit; GM: granulocyte-macrophage; G: granulocyte; M: macrophage; IL: interleukin; TPO: thrombopoietin; EPO: erythropoietin)

The entire process by which red cells are formed in the body is termed **erythropoiesis**. It includes origin, development and maturation of erythrocytes. Various control mechanisms regulate erythropoiesis so that the red cell mass in the body remains constant.

Sites of Erythropoiesis

Intrauterine Life
- Mesoblastic phase
- Hepatic phase
- Myeloid phase.

Mesoblastic Phase
Mesoblastic phase starts in the 3rd week of intrauterine life in the mesoderm of yolk sac and continues up to the 3rd month. This is the stage where intravascular erythropoiesis occurs.

Hepatic Phase
From the 2nd month up to delivery, liver produces RBCs and peak is seen during the 5th and 6th month. Spleen is also involved in erythropoiesis between 3rd and 7th month.

Myeloid Phase
From the 5th month onwards, bone marrow is the chief site of erythropoiesis **(Fig. 13.11)**.

After Birth
After birth, red bone marrow alone is concerned with erythropoiesis. Bone marrow consists of red marrow and yellow marrow. Red marrow is active and yellow marrow is inactive due to fat deposition.

Up to 5 years after birth, the marrow in all the bones of the body is red. By the age of 5 years, fat cells begin to appear and the red marrow in the bones gradually is replaced by yellow fatty marrow. The replacement occurs first in the bones of the hands and feet and then in the bones of the arms and legs from the distal to the proximal ends. By 6–20 years, red marrow is present only in long bones and in membranous bones.

After the age of 20 years, red marrow is present only at the upper ends of long bones like humerus and femur and in membranous bones like sternum, ribs, scapula, ilium, skull and vertebrae. When there is an increased demand of RBCs, the yellow marrow is capable of reverting back to active red marrow. When bone marrow is destroyed or fibrosed, **extramedullary hematopoiesis** occurs, i.e., in adults at times of need, liver and spleen also produce RBCs.

Bone Marrow
Bone marrow is one of the largest and one of the most active organs in the body. Its weight is equal to the weight of liver. An adult of average height has about 3–4 L of bone marrow. Total volume of **red marrow** in adults is about 1–2 L and hematopoiesis occurs in the red marrow. The rest of the bone marrow is **yellow marrow**. It serves as a reserve space into which hemopoietic tissue can expand in response to increased demand for blood cell production as in severe anemia. Yellow marrow consists mainly of adipose cells. Fat, especially triglycerides, stored in the adipose cells in the yellow marrow are an important chemical energy reserve. *Extramedullary (in spleen, liver, etc.) hematopoiesis* also occurs in adults in pathological situations where there is an increased demand of red cells.

75% of active marrow is involved in producing white blood cells, i.e., **myeloid series** and 25% produce red cells, i.e., **erythroid series**, thus forming a ratio 3:1, whereas in the peripheral blood, ratio of white cell to red blood cell is 1:700. This difference is because of the fact that the life span of RBC is far greater than that of WBC.

Bone marrow stem cells are the primitive cells in the bone marrow, which give rise to blood cells. The stem cells are capable of **self-replication**, i.e., they can divide and form more stem cells. They are also capable of **differentiation and commitment**, i.e., they can differentiate into specialized cells called **progenitor cells**. Different peptides called cytokines are involved in directing the dividing stem cells down a particular path of development **(Table 13.2)**.

Bone marrow stem cells also give rise to osteoclasts, Kupffer cells, mast cells, dendritic cells, Langerhans cells, etc. In cases of complete destruction of bone marrow, bone marrow transplantation can be done. The best source of the hemopoietic stem cell is umbilical cord blood.

Stages of Erythropoiesis
Erythropoiesis involves a number of cells of different stages of maturation, starting with the first stem cell progeny, i.e., CFU-E, committed to erythroid differentiation and ending with the mature circulating red blood cell **(Fig. 13.13)**. The entire mass of these erythroid cells is termed **erythron**.

All blood cells are produced in the bone marrow from precursors known as **uncommitted pluripotent hematopoietic stem cells (PHSC)**. The uncommitted stem cells are not designed to form a particular type of blood cell. These cells differentiate into progenitor cells for different blood cells. Progenitor cells possess the ability to give rise to clones or group of cells and so they are also called colony forming unit-stem cell (CFU-S). When the cells are designed to form a particular type of blood cell, the stem cells are called

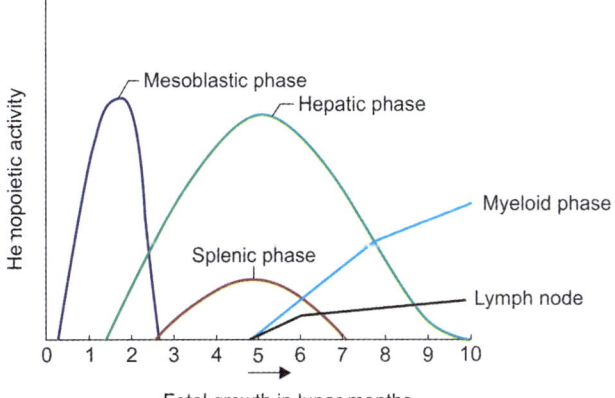

Fig. 13.11: Hemopoiesis during the fetal life.

SECTION 2 → Hematology

Table 13.2: Cytokines that regulate hematopoiesis.

Cytokine	Cell lines stimulated
IL-1	• Erythrocyte • Granulocyte • Megakaryocyte • Monocyte
IL-3	• Erythrocyte • Granulocyte • Megakaryocyte • Monocyte
IL-4	Basophil
IL-5	Eosinophil
IL-6	• Erythrocyte • Granulocyte • Megakaryocyte • Monocyte
IL-11	• Erythrocyte • Granulocyte • Megakaryocyte
Erythropoietin	Erythrocyte
GM-CSF	• Erythrocyte • Granulocyte • Megakaryocyte
G-CSF	Granulocyte
M-CSF	Monocyte
Thrombopoietin	Megakaryocyte

(IL: interleukin; CSF: colony stimulating factor; G: granulocyte; M: macrophage).

Table 13.3: Differences between CFU-E and BFU-E.

BFU-E	CFU-E
Large colonies containing about 500–5000 progenitor cells	Small colonies containing about 60–70 nucleated progenitor cells
Not differentiated	Progenitor cells differentiated
Erythropoietin is necessary only during its later stages of development	Erythropoietin is very essential for its further development. Administration of erythropoietin leads to expansion of CFU-E compartment
For cellular proliferation burst promoting activity (BPA), a substance produced by lymphocytes and macrophages is necessary	BPA not necessary for further development

committed hematopoietic stem cell. Committed stem cells are of two types:
1. Common lymphoid progenitor cell (CLP) or lymphoid stem cell, which give rise to lymphocytes.
2. Common myeloid progenitor cell (CMP) which gives rise to blood cells other than lymphocytes (*See* **Fig. 13.10**).

Burst forming unit-erythroid (BFU-E) is an erythroid progenitor that is very immature and is considered as a progenitor of CFU-E. BFU-E differentiates into CFU-E by about 6–7 days (**Table 13.3**). Presence of ferritin helps to distinguish erythrocyte precursors from other immature cells.

From CFU-E, by differentiation blast cells are produced. The first identifiable blast cell in erythropoiesis is pronormoblast. For identification, cells are stained with **Leishman's stain** (**Figs. 13.12 and 13.17B**).

Pronormoblast or Proerythroblast (Fig. 13.12)
❖ Round or oval in shape
❖ 15–20 μm in diameter
❖ Large nucleus, which occupies 80% of cell and contains 2–3 nucleoli
❖ Thin rim of cytoplasm is seen
❖ Ferritin molecules are present
❖ After repeated cell division, pronormoblast differentiates into basophilic normoblast.

Basophilic Normoblast or Early Normoblast
❖ 12–17 μm in diameter
❖ Nucleus smaller with no nucleoli

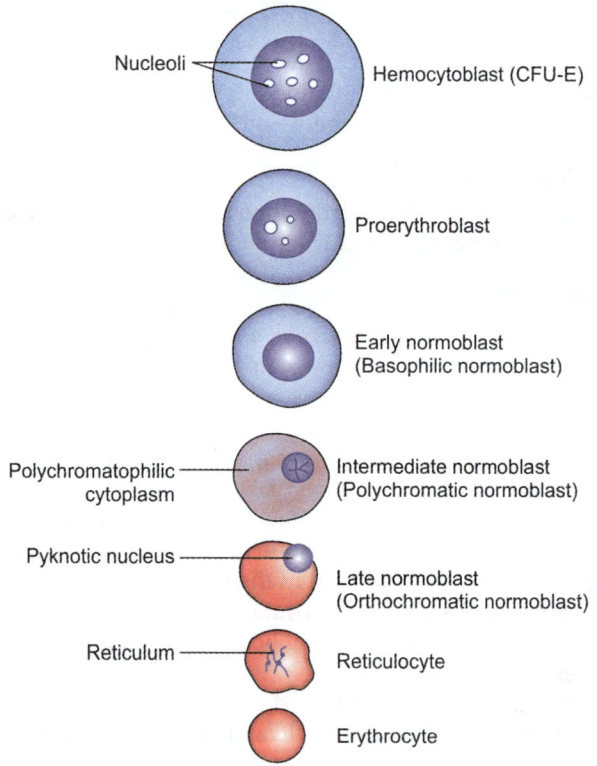

Fig. 13.12: Stages of erythropoiesis: The size of the cell decreases in each stage. Nucleus is extruded in late normoblast stage.

❖ Chromatin condensation seen
❖ Cytoplasm more and deeply basophilic due to increased number of ribosomes; hemoglobin is absent.

Polychromatophilic Normoblast or Intermediate Normoblast
❖ 12–15 μm in diameter
❖ Nucleus very small and assumes a cart wheel appearance.
❖ Chromatin condensation more
❖ Cytoplasm shows both pink and blue areas. Pink color is due to increase in the hemoglobin content

- Number of mitochondria decreases
- *Mitosis stops in this phase* due to inactivation of chromosomes.

Orthochromatic Normoblast or Late Normoblast

Late normoblast is 8–12 μm in diameter, and is the smallest of the nucleated precursors of RBC. Cytoplasm is pink and hemoglobin synthesis is almost complete. Nucleus undergoes pyknotic degeneration and it shrinks and becomes irregular. Finally, the nucleus is extruded out of the cell. Orthochromatic normoblast cannot synthesize DNA because nucleus is completely inactive and therefore cannot divide. Mechanism of inactivation of nucleus is by the following mechanism:

- Hemoglobin enters the nucleus through nuclear pores and it reacts with nucleohistones leading to chromosomal inactivation and condensation. Rate of hemoglobin synthesis determines the number of cell divisions and the ultimate size of the erythrocyte. For example, in iron deficiency anemia, cells are microcytic because it takes a longer time to reach the critical hemoglobin concentration and so, more cell divisions occur before nuclear inactivation. The resulting cell will be small or microcyte.
- When erythropoiesis is stimulated, macrocytes result because, the critical hemoglobin concentration is attained at an earlier stage, leading to earlier nuclear degeneration and decrease in the number of cell divisions.

This is the reason why *MCHC remains relatively constant even though the erythrocyte size varies greatly.*

Reticulocyte

Reticulocyte is 8 μm in diameter, irregular and polylobulated due to extrusion of nucleus. Cytoplasm contains small amount of basophilic material consisting of remnants of organelles like ribosomes, mitochondria and Golgi complex. Reticulocyte cannot be seen in a Leishman-stained blood smear. **Supravital staining** with brilliant cresyl blue causes ribosomal RNA to precipitate into a network of blue strands, hence the name reticulocyte **(Fig. 13.13)**.

As RNA is present, they are still able to synthesize hemoglobin. As the reticulocyte matures, the organelles decrease in number. Mitochondria disappear first and ribosomes are the last to disappear. The unneeded cellular components are discarded by **autophagosomes** or secondary lysosomes. Reticulocyte becomes mature RBC within 32–48 hours. Reticulocytes remain in the bone marrow till mature because of their adhesive property. They have a coating of globulin, especially transferrin.

Normal Reticulocyte Count

1. Adult: 0.5–1% of the RBC count
2. Fetus: 30–50%
3. At birth: 2–6% and 1 week after birth count comes to adult level.

Variation in the Reticulocyte Count

Increase in the reticulocyte count is called **reticulocytosis**. It is seen in conditions of increased erythropoietic activity. For

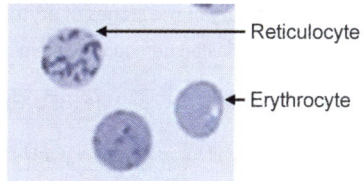

Fig. 13.13: Reticulocyte.

example, in hypoxia, hemolytic anemia, during treatment of deficiency anemia, and after splenectomy there will be an increase in reticulocyte count.

The reticulocytes are normally trapped in the trabeculae of spleen where they mature into RBC in a day or two and enter circulation once again. After splenectomy, this does not occur and hence an increase in the reticulocyte count is seen.

Decrease in the reticulocyte count is called **reticulocytopenia**. It is seen in aplastic anemia, myxedema and in hypopituitarism.

Clinical Importance of Reticulocyte Count

- Regeneration of bone marrow can be tested, i.e. reticulocyte count provides useful information about the bone marrow's capacity to synthesize and release red cells in response to a physiologic challenge, such as anemia.
- Helps to diagnose aplastic anemia.
- Helps to diagnose deficiency of vitamin B_{12} and folic acid.
- **Reticulocyte response** is a good indication of improvement during treatment for anemia.
- In hemolytic anemia, there is increase in the reticulocyte count due to their premature release from bone marrow into circulation under the effect of erythropoietin in response to increased demand. This is **reticulocyte crisis**. These reticulocytes are larger and less mature.

Mature Erythrocyte

Mature RBC is 7.2–7.5 μm in diameter with biconcave shape. As ribosomes are absent, mature red cells cannot synthesize hemoglobin. One pronormoblast gives rise to 8–32 mature RBCs.

Summary of the stages of erythropoiesis is given in **Flowchart 13.2.**

Duration of Various Phases in Erythropoiesis

- BFU-E to CFU-E: 6–8 days
- BFU-E to erythroblast: 12–15 days
- CFU-E to erythroblast: 5–7 days
- Proerythroblast to mature RBC: 7 days and this is the maturation time
- Reticulocyte to mature RBC: 32–48 hours.

ERYTHROPOIETIN

Erythropoietin (EPO) is a hormone with molecular weight 34,000, glycoprotein in nature and contains 165 amino acid residues and four oligosaccharide chains.

1. Normal value: 5–30 milliunits/mL of plasma.
2. Site of production: 85% produced by **kidney** and 15% from the **liver**.
3. Site of destruction: Liver.

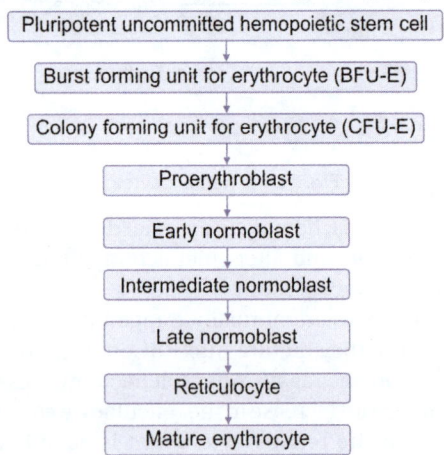

Flowchart 13.2: Summary of the stages of erythropoiesis.

Mechanism of Secretion of EPO

The interstitial cells in the peritubular capillary bed of kidney and the perivenous hepatocytes in the liver secrete EPO. This peptide regulates red cell production by a feedback system. When there is reduction in the concentration of hemoglobin (anemia) in the blood flowing through the kidney, it leads to reduction in the tissue O_2 tension in the kidney. This stimulates erythropoietin secretion, which in turn stimulates erythropoiesis in the bone marrow. *Thus, hypoxia is the most potent stimulus for EPO secretion*. This is the reason for the polycythemia observed in normal individuals residing at high altitude where PO_2 is low. Also in patients suffering from cardiopulmonary disorders, such as bronchial asthma, right- to-left shunt, etc., erythropoietin secretion is high due to chronic hypoxia. Production of EPO can be experimentally induced by renal artery constriction, which proves that erythropoietin is produced from the kidney.

When the hemoglobin level rises, the kidney produces less erythropoietin and the erythropoietic activity of the marrow decreases.

Actions of Erythropoietin (EPO)

- Erythropoietin increases the number of erythropoietin-sensitive committed stem cells in the bone marrow. Erythroid progenitor cells differentiate into pronormoblast under the influence of EPO. This increases the size of the erythron and increases red blood cell production, which leads to increase in the tissue O_2 level. Maximum EPO activity and sensitivity to EPO is seen during the conversion of CFU-E to pronormoblast. Activity is seen up to orthochromatic stage. CFU-E contains the highest density of EPO receptors on their membrane and they depend on EPO for their survival. In the absence of EPO, erythroid cells die.
- EPO increases hemoglobin synthesis and potentiates the activity of δ-amino levulinic acid synthetase.
- EPO decreases maturation time of RBC.
- It stimulates the release of mature erythrocytes from bone marrow into general circulation
- EPO receptor has tyrosine kinase activity, and it activates a cascade of serine and threonine kinases, resulting in inhibited apoptosis of red cells
- In addition to erythroid cells, EPO affects megakaryocytes and their progenitors CFU-MK. Following EPO administration an increase in platelet count is also seen.

Regulation of EPO Secretion

The stimuli that increase EPO secretion are hypoxia, androgens and cobalt salts. Catecholamines via β– adrenergic receptors facilitate erythropoietin secretion. The sensor that regulates EPO secretion is a heme protein that in the deoxy form stimulates and in the oxy form inhibits transcription of the erythropoietin gene to form erythropoietin mRNA.

Variation in Erythropoietin Secretion

EPO secretion is increased in:
- Hypoxia
- Renal artery constriction by serotonin, norepinephrine, etc.
- Hemolytic anemia
- Blood loss
- cAMP, NAD and NADP increase EPO secretion.

EPO secretion is decreased in:
- Cirrhosis liver
- Renal failure
- Increased RBC count as in blood transfusion.

FACTORS REGULATING ERYTHROPOIESIS (TABLE 13.4)

Following are the factors that regulate erythropoiesis:
- Hemopoietic growth factors like burst promoting activity (BPA)
- Erythropoietin
- Hormones
- Metals
- Lipids and proteins
- Vitamins
- Maturation factors.
- **Burst promoting activity (BPA)** is a substance produced by lymphocytes and macrophages, which is necessary for the proliferation and growth of BFU-E, e.g., interleukins

Table 13.4: Factors affecting erythropoiesis.

General factors	Maturation factors	Factors necessary for hemoglobin synthesis
Erythropoietin	Folic acid	Proteins
Hormones like androgen, estrogen, thyroxine, growth hormone, prolactin, ACTH	Vitamin B_{12}	Iron
Lipids	Intrinsic factor of Castle	Copper
Growth factors like interleukins (IL3, IL6, IL11)		Cobalt and nickel
		Vitamin B, C, D and E

(IL). The ILs involved in erythropoiesis are IL-3, IL-6 and IL-11.
- ❖ **Erythropoietin (EPO)** is secreted in response to hypoxia mainly by the kidneys. It stimulates the formation and release of new RBCs into circulation (explain the mechanism of action of EPO).
- ❖ **Hormones affecting erythropoiesis**
  - **Androgens**: Androgens increase EPO secretion and this is the reason for increased RBC count in adult males when compared to females.
  - **Estrogen**: It decreases the sensitivity of progenitor cells to EPO and decrease RBC count. Estrogen also inhibits the synthesis of globin in the liver.
  - **Thyroxine**: Thyroxine increases tissue metabolism and tissue hypoxia leading to decreased O_2 tension and increased EPO secretion. Anemia is a feature in hypothyroidism and polycythemia is a feature in hyperthyroidism.
  - **Adrenocorticotropic hormone (ACTH) and adrenocortical steroids** increase EPO secretion leading to increased RBC count. Polycythemia is a prominent feature in Cushing's syndrome.
  - **Growth hormone and prolactin** increase EPO secretion.
  - **Vasopressin, serotonin and norepinephrine** cause renal artery constriction leading to local tissue hypoxia in the kidney, thus stimulating EPO secretion.
- ❖ **Metals**: Iron, copper and cobalt are very essential for erythropoiesis. Copper is necessary for the absorption and utilization of iron. Copper is necessary for the incorporation of iron into protoporphyrin during the final stages of the synthesis of heme. Cobalt is an ingredient of vitamin B_{12}.
- ❖ **Lipids and proteins**: Amino acids are necessary for the synthesis of globin part of hemoglobin. Lipids and proteins are necessary for the normal integrity of cell membrane and stroma of erythrocytes.
- ❖ **Vitamins**: Vitamins B, C, D and E are necessary for normal erythropoiesis. Vitamin C helps in the conversion of ferric ion to ferrous form. It is necessary for facilitating iron turnover in the body. In scurvy, a disease due to vitamin C deficiency, anemia is a feature.
- ❖ Vitamin E deficiency leads to reduced resistance of erythrocytes to oxidative stress, i.e., vitamin E has antioxidant effect. Vitamin B_6 or pyridoxine is important because, pyridoxal-6-phosphate is a co-enzyme in the synthesis of δ-aminolevulinic acid. This is the first step in the biosynthesis of protoporphyrin ring, four of which combine to form the porphyrin molecule of hemoglobin.
- ❖ **Maturation factors**
  - Vitamin B_{12}
  - Folic acid

Vitamin B_{12} or Cyanocobalamin

- ❖ Source: Dietary sources are milk, meat, liver, etc. Bacterial flora of large intestine synthesizes vitamin B_{12}.
- ❖ Daily requirement in adult is 1–2 µg.
- ❖ Deficiency of vitamin B_{12} leads to **pernicious anemia**.

Absorption of Vitamin B_{12}

Vitamin B_{12} is also known as **extrinsic factor or antipernicious factor**. For the absorption of B_{12} from the intestine, **intrinsic factor of Castle** secreted by the parietal cells of stomach is necessary. Intrinsic factor combines with B_{12} to form a complex. This complex attaches to receptors in the ileal mucosa, which contain **cubulin**, a high-affinity apolipoprotein and cubulin is responsible for the uptake of the complex into the enterocyte by endocytosis. After absorption, B_{12} is transported in combination with **transcobalamin II**. Vitamin B_{12} is stored in the liver.

The extrinsic (vitamin B_{12}) and intrinsic factors are together called hematinic principle.

Actions of B_{12}

Vitamin B_{12} increases DNA synthesis and decreases the maturation time of RBC. It interacts with folic acid in the synthesis of DNA **(Fig. 13.14)**. In B_{12} deficiency, maturation time is increased and the number of cells is decreased and the cells will be large leading to megaloblastic anemia or pernicious anemia. Neurological symptoms are more in B_{12} deficiency.

Folic Acid

- ❖ Source: Leafy vegetables, yeast, pulses and liver.
- ❖ Daily requirement in adult is 100 µg.

Actions of Folic Acid

Folic acid is also essential for DNA synthesis and RBC maturation. In plasma, folic acid is present in the form of methyl tetrahydrofolate. It is changed to tetrahydrofolate in a pathway that requires vitamin B_{12}. The methyl group is transferred to homocysteine, which forms methionine and this reaction occurs only in the presence of vitamin B_{12}. Finally, uridine monophosphate is converted to d-thymidine monophosphate necessary for the synthesis of DNA **(Fig. 13.14)**. DNA synthesis is decreased leading to *megaloblastic anemia in folic acid deficiency*.

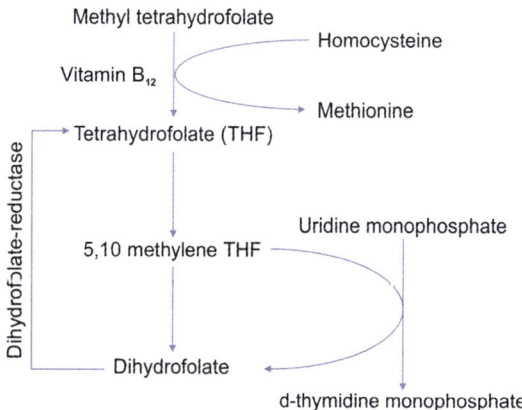

Fig. 13.14: Interaction between vitamin B_{12} and folic acid in the synthesis of DNA.

ANEMIA

PY2.5: Describe different types of anemia and jaundice.

Definition

Anemia is a condition where the hemoglobin content of the blood is below the normal level for the age and sex of the subject. Thus, *an adult male is said to be anemic when his hemoglobin falls below 13 g/dL and an adult female is said to be anemic when her hemoglobin falls below 11.5 g/dL*. The RBC count may or may not be reduced in anemia. The RBC count may be normal in certain anemia like iron deficiency anemia. But here, the hemoglobin present in the individual cells is significantly reduced. There is a drastic reduction in the RBC count in aplastic anemia, pernicious anemia, etc.

Depending on the hemoglobin content, anemia is graded as:
- **Mild anemia**, where the hemoglobin content is 10–11 g%.
- **Moderate anemia**, where the hemoglobin content is 7–8 g%.
- **Severe anemia**, when the hemoglobin content falls below 6 g%.

The commonly occurring deficiency anemia can be grouped into two categories:
1. Anemia caused by lack of maturation factors (Vitamin B_{12} and folic acid), which is usually macrocytic normochromic. Here MCHC will be normal but MCH and MCV may be increased.
2. Anemia caused by iron deficiency; the type will be microcytic hypochromic anemia.

In anemia, the O_2 carrying capacity of blood is reduced. Anemia is not a disease by itself, but it is only a sign of the presence of disease. The correct treatment requires an understanding of the pathogenesis of the condition. For example, in hemodilution as in pregnancy, the hemoglobin content will be low for that age and sex. But, there may not be any pathology. In hemoconcentration, as in dehydration, if the hemoglobin content is estimated it will be more than normal. In certain deficiencies like iron deficiency, in renal diseases where erythropoietin secretion may be inadequate, hemolysis, bleeding, etc., the hemoglobin content will be reduced. So, the treatment should be aimed at the cause.

Signs and Symptoms of Anemia

- Pallor of skin and mucous membrane is the most evident sign of anemia **(Figs. 13.15A and B)**.
- Anemia reduces oxygen carrying capacity of blood, resulting in tissue hypoxia. Hypoxia produces symptoms like easy fatigability, breathlessness, palpitation, etc.
- Decrease in viscosity of blood and increase in cardiac output produces turbulence of blood during its passage through the heart producing cardiac murmurs.
- Dry skin, brittle nails, glossitis (inflammation of tongue; **Fig. 13.16**), atrophy of papillae of tongue, restlessness, etc., are other features.

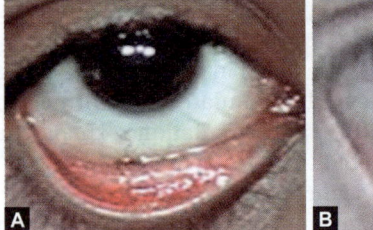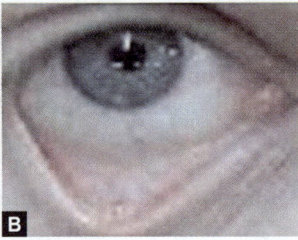

Figs. 13.15A and B: Appearance of palpebral conjunctiva: (A) Normal color; (B) Anemia.

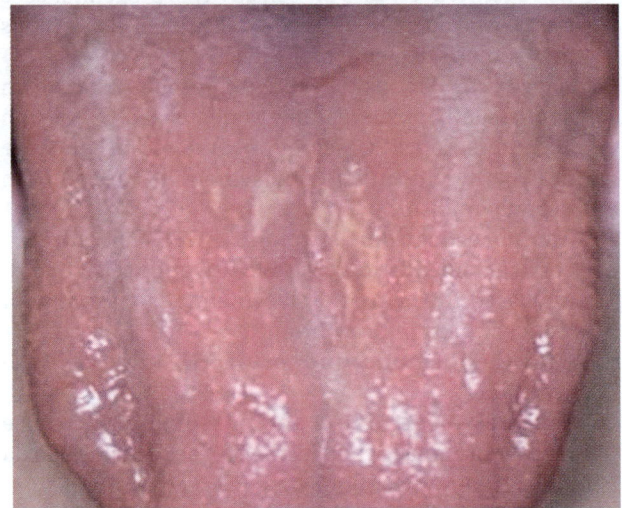

Fig. 13.16: Inflammation of tongue (glossitis) in severe anemia.

Blood Picture

Blood picture depends on the cause of anemia.
- In *megaloblastic anemia*, there is marked macrocytosis, anisocytosis, and poikilocytosis; there will also be neutropenia and thrombocytopenia as DNA synthesis is impaired.
- In *iron deficiency anemia*, RBCs are microcytic and hypochromic in the blood smear. MCH and MCHC are reduced. RBC count may or may not be normal.
- In *hemolytic anemia*, reticulocyte count is increased. Few immature RBCs may also be seen in the peripheral smear.

Etiological Classification of Anemia (Depending on the Cause) (Flowchart 13.3)

I. **Hemolytic anemia (due to increased destruction of RBC)**
   - Intracorpuscular defects:
     - Abnormality in RBC membrane as in hereditary spherocytosis
     - Disorders of glycolysis due to enzyme defect like G_6PD deficiency
     - Abnormality in globin structure of hemoglobin as in thalassemia, sickle cell anemia, etc.
   - Extracorpuscular defects:
     - Incompatible blood transfusion
     - Infections like malaria

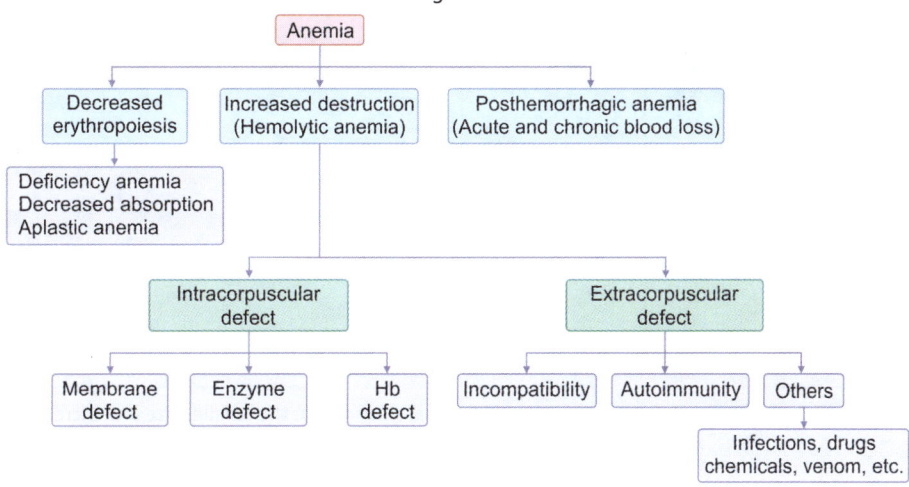

Flowchart 13.3: Etiological classification of anemia.

- Autoimmune hemolytic anemia
- Drugs
- Snake venom

II. **Anemia due to defective formation of RBC**
- Deficiency of essential substances like iron, folic acid, vitamin B_{12}, protein, Co, Cu, vitamin B6, etc.
- Defective absorption of essential substances.
  For example, intrinsic factor deficiency leads to pernicious anemia; HCl and vitamin C deficiency leads to iron deficiency anemia. These are due to defective absorption of B_{12} and iron.
- Atrophy of bone marrow leads to aplastic anemia. Causes are drugs like sulfa group, ionizing radiation in the treatment for cancer, malignancy of bone marrow as multiple myeloma, etc.

III. **Post-hemorrhagic anemia**
- Acute blood loss following accident, childbirth, etc.
- Chronic blood loss as in hookworm infestation, which is the most common cause of anemia in children, bleeding piles, bleeding peptic ulcer, etc.

Classification of Anemia Depending on Morphology

Morphological classification is based on MCV and MCHC:
1. Normocytic normochromic anemia as in acute hemorrhage, aplastic anemia, etc.
2. Macrocytic normochromic anemia as in pernicious anemia.
3. Microcytic hypochromic anemia as in iron deficiency anemia, chronic hemorrhage, thalassemia, etc.
4. Microcytic normochromic anemia is seen in copper deficiency.
5. Macrocytic hypochromic anemia (dimorphic anemia) is seen in combined iron and folic acid deficiency.

Iron Deficiency Anemia

Iron deficiency anemia is the most common nutritional deficiency disorder. It is common in women in the reproductive age group and during periods of active growth like infancy and childhood. The body of a healthy adult contains 4–5 g of iron, which is present in hemoglobin (70%), ferritin and hemosiderin (20%), myoglobin (5%), and the rest in the intracellular enzymes like catalase, cytochrome oxidase and peroxidase. Site of absorption of iron is duodenum (details of iron absorption are dealt with in the gastrointestinal system).

Causes of Iron Deficiency Anemia

- Defective absorption of iron due to HCl and vitamin C deficiency
- Dietary deficiency of iron
- Increased loss of iron as in hemorrhage following injury, menorrhagia (excessive menstrual bleeding), bleeding piles (hemorrhoids)
- Increased requirement as in children, in pregnancy, menstruating females
- Prematurity leads to anemia. The fetus stores iron in the liver during the last weeks of pregnancy and this iron is used for hemoglobin synthesis during the first 6 months of extra uterine life. Stored iron is less in premature infants and so they develop anemia. Breast milk contains very little iron and the baby depends on the stored iron for hemoglobin synthesis till weaning.

Signs and Symptoms

Pallor due to deficiency of hemoglobin, edema, glossitis, koilonychia (dry spoon-shaped nails), dyspnea (difficulty in breathing) due to anemic hypoxia, palpitation (awareness of one's own heart beat), easy fatigability due to muscle hypoxia, restlessness, confusion and drowsiness due to cerebral hypoxia.

Blood Examination

- RBC count low
- Erythrocytes small (microcytes) and pale in blood picture **(Fig. 13.17A)**
- Anisocytosis and poikilocytosis

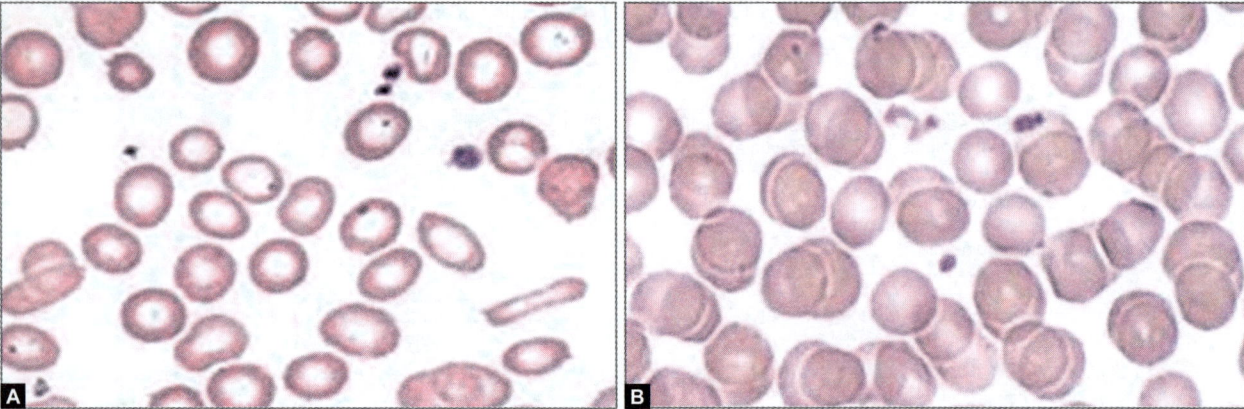

Figs. 13.17A and B: (A) Smear showing iron deficiency anemia; (B) Normal smear (note the smaller size and increase in central pallor of red cells in iron deficiency anemia).

- Hemoglobin content low
- Blood indices like MCV, MCH and MCHC are decreased.

Treatment

- Oral preparation is *ferrous sulfate*
- Parenteral preparation is *iron-dextran complex*, which is given by deep intramuscular injection in severe cases of anemia
- Treat the underlying cause like worm infestation by deworming.

Pernicious Anemia

Cause of pernicious anemia is lack of **intrinsic factor of Castle** leading to defective absorption of vitamin B_{12} in the distal ileum. Intrinsic factor is produced by the parietal cells of the stomach. The deficiency of intrinsic factor may be due to *gastrectomy, atrophy of gastric mucosa, autoimmune destruction of parietal cells (Addisonian pernicious anemia) and carcinoma stomach*. In 50% of cases, anti-intrinsic factor antibodies are present in the serum. Vitamin B_{12} deficiency due to inadequate dietary intake is rare, because the minimum daily requirement is low and it is found in most foods of animal origin. It may be seen in strict vegetarians. Deficiency of vitamin B_{12} leads to *defective DNA synthesis* and abnormally large cells of erythrocyte series called **megaloblasts**. Defective absorption of vitamin B_{12} is also seen in diseases of distal ileum.

Signs and Symptoms

- Glossitis and atrophy of lingual papilla
- Features of achlorhydria
- **Subacute combined degeneration** in the nervous system. There is destruction of myelin sheath in pernicious anemia leading to neuritis. This may extend up to dorsal column and lateral column and sensations will be affected.
- Loss of appetite (anorexia)
- Fatigue.

Blood Picture (Figs. 13.18A and B)

Macrocytes are seen in circulation. Peripheral smear shows large, immature, red cells called **megaloblasts**. The size of RBC comes to about 9–11 μm. RBC count will be less than 1 million/mm³ of blood. MCV and MCH will be increased, but the MCHC will be normal and hence pernicious anemia is referred to as **macrocytic normochromic anemia**. MCHC is normal because there is increase in both MCV and MCH. Bone marrow is stimulated due to severe anemia and red marrow extends towards the shaft of long bones referred to as **hyperplasia of bone marrow**. Reticulocyte count will be increased. Because of large cells, there is increased hemolysis

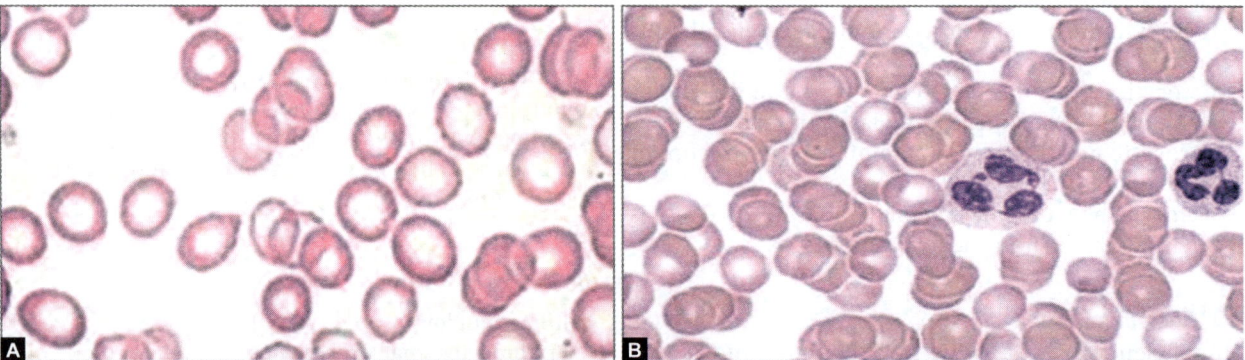

Figs. 13.18A and B: (A) Peripheral smear showing macrocytic anemia; (B) Normal red blood cells (note the large size, increase in central pallor and decrease in the number of erythrocytes in macrocytic anemia).

in spleen, liver and bone marrow leading to **jaundice**. Platelet count and WBC count is decreased because much of the bone marrow is involved in erythropoiesis.

Treatment of Pernicious Anemia

Vitamin B_{12} injection is given. Oral B_{12} is not effective because, it cannot be absorbed from the gastrointestinal tract due to deficiency of intrinsic factor or due to defective absorption. Treatment of pernicious anemia with B_{12} prevents further progression of neuronal degeneration, but cannot reverse the damage already made. Hence, this anemia is called pernicious anemia, which means *destructive or injurious anemia*. The changes in the stomach remain unaffected by B_{12} administration.

Reticulocyte Response

Following B_{12} injection in pernicious anemia, reticulocytes start to appear in circulation by 4–5 days and maximum is reached by 10 days. This is **reticulocyte response** and it is taken as the earliest sign of clinical improvement. There will be increase in the number of circulating reticulocytes up to 30–40%. Extent of reticulocyte response is inversely proportional to the RBC count before treatment.

Reticulocyte Crisis

In conditions of acute hemolysis or in periods of recovery from severe anemia, the RBC production is sharply increased and the reticulocyte count may go up to 25–30%. This is known as **reticulocyte crisis**. During the course of pernicious anemia, there will be periods of remission and relapse. The increase in the reticulocyte count seen during periods of remission is also called reticulocyte crisis.

Folic Acid Deficiency

Folic acid deficiency also leads to megaloblastic anemia where the cells are larger in size. Causes for folate deficiency include inadequate dietary intake, malabsorption, and increased demand as in pregnancy and lactation and use of drugs like methotrexate and contraceptive pills.

There is inter-relationship between the actions of vitamin B_{12} and folic acid. In the plasma, folic acid is present as **methyl tetrahydrofolate**. For the conversion of methyl tetrahydrofolate to **tetrahydrofolate**, vitamin B_{12} is essential. Methyl tetrahydrofolate is converted to active folate co-enzymes necessary for the synthesis of DNA (*refer* **Fig.13.14**). Thus, in B_{12} deficiency, folic acid is not metabolized and so a combined deficiency is seen. Thus, folate deficiency leads to megaloblastic anemia. But, in B_{12} deficiency if folic acid alone is given, the neurological symptoms worsen and it is relieved only by administration of vitamin B_{12}.

Sickle Cell Anemia

Sickle cell anemia is a **homozygous** disorder that is inherited from both parents. If it is heterozygous, the condition is called **sickle cell trait**.

Sickle cell anemia is caused by a mutation in the β-globin gene that changes the amino acid glutamic acid to valine in the 6th position of β-chain of hemoglobin. This hemoglobin is called **hemoglobin S (HbS)**.

HbS polymerizes reversibly when deoxygenated to form a gelatinous network of fibrous polymers that stiffens the erythrocyte membrane.

Other changes include leakage of K^+ out of the cell, influx of Ca^{2+} and the cells become sticky. All these changes produce a characteristic sickle shape or comma shape to the RBC (**Fig. 13.19**).

As the cells are stiff and sickle shaped, they cannot easily pass through the capillaries. Due to the sticky nature of the cells, they adhere to the endothelium of small venules. These effects lead to microvascular occlusion and hemolysis, especially in the spleen. This is because blood flow through the spleen is sluggish and so, the amount of reduced hemoglobin formed will be more and there will be accelerated sickling and increased hemolysis in the spleen.

The result is **hemolytic anemia**. The vascular occlusion due to abnormal shape and stickiness leads to tissue **ischemia, acute pain and end-organ damage**. Other important findings in sickle cell anemia are reticulocytosis and the hematocrit value will be 15–30%. *In sickle cell trait, the symptoms are rarely severe.*

Thalassemia

In thalassemia, *the polypeptide chains are normal* but are produced in decreased amounts or absent due to decreased synthesis. This is because of the defects in the regulatory portion of globin genes. In β-**thalassemia**, the amount of β-chain is decreased or absent, whereas in α-**thalassemia**, α-chain is absent or decreased. β-thalassemia is of two types, thalassemia major (Mediterranean anemia or Cooley's anemia) and thalassemia minor (more common). Thalassemia syndromes are inherited **heterozygous** disorders and the features are hypochromia (decreased MCH) and microcytosis. Nucleated RBCs will be present in circulation. Hemoglobin content will be 2.5–6 g%. The patients usually present with severe anemia, jaundice and hepatosplenomegaly. Treatment of thalassemia includes repeated blood transfusion or bone marrow transplantation.

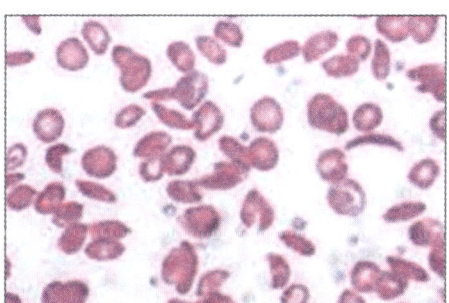

Fig. 13.19: Peripheral smear in sickle cell anemia (note the sickle shaped red cells).

SECTION 2 — Hematology

MULTIPLE CHOICE QUESTIONS

1. Sickle cell anemia is due to:
   a. Addition
   b. Deletion
   c. Point mutation
   d. None of the above

2. Maturation defect in RBC is seen in:
   a. Folic acid and vitamin B_{12} deficiency
   b. Vitamin C deficiency
   c. Vitamin D deficiency
   d. Iron deficiency

3. Earliest response to iron therapy is:
   a. Increase in hemoglobin content
   b. Reticulocytosis
   c. Increase in PCV
   d. Decrease in ESR

4. The substance that helps to distinguish erythrocyte precursors from other immature blood cells is:
   a. Ferritin
   b. Hemoglobin
   c. Hemosiderin
   d. Transferrin

5. The disorder that is referred to as Cooley's anemia is:
   a. Pernicious anemia
   b. Sickle cell anemia
   c. Thalassemia major
   d. Thalassemia minor

6. The most potent stimulus for erythropoietin secretion is:
   a. Renal failure
   b. Hypoxia
   c. Hypercapnia
   d. Liver disease

7. Erythropoietin secretion is decreased in all the following conditions, *except*:
   a. Cirrhosis liver
   b. Renal failure
   c. Polycythemia
   d. Renal artery constriction

8. In the synthesis of DNA during erythropoiesis, vitamin B_{12} is necessary for the conversion of:
   a. Methyl tetrahydrofolate to tetrahydrofolate
   b. Uridine monophosphate to d-thymidine monophosphate
   c. Dihydrofolate to tetrahydrofolate
   d. Methylene tetrahydrofolate to dihydrofolate

9. Pernicious anemia is treated by injecting:
   a. Vitamin A
   b. Iron
   c. Vitamin B_{12}
   d. Vitamin K

10. Megaloblastic anemia is characterized by all the following features, *except*:
    a. MCHC is increased
    b. RBC count is decreased
    c. Nucleated RBCs in circulation
    d. MCH is increased

11. Richest source of folate is:
    a. Liver
    b. Leafy vegetables
    c. Grains
    d. Milk

12. Pernicious anemia is due to deficiency of:
    a. Vitamin B_6
    b. folic acid
    c. Vitamin B_{12}
    d. Iron

13. Pyknotic nucleus is present in:
    a. Early normoblast
    b. Committed stem cell
    c. Reticulocyte
    d. Late normoblast

14. The only formed element of blood that divides once it leaves the red bone marrow is:
    a. Platelet
    b. Lymphocyte
    c. RBC
    d. Neutrophil

15. Normal reticulocyte count is:
    a. 0.5–1.5%
    b. 2–4%
    c. 4–8%
    d. 10–12%

16. One drop of blood is about:
    a. 1 mm^3
    b. 20 mm^3
    c. 50 mm^3
    d. 10 mm^3

17. Rate of RBC production is:
    a. 2 million/sec
    b. 2 million/min
    c. 2 million/day
    d. 2 lakhs/day

18. The percentage of weight of RBC constituted by hemoglobin is:
    a. 50%
    b. 10%
    c. 33%
    d. 45%

19. The cell that can generate ATP only anaerobically is:
    a. RBC
    b. Lymphocyte
    c. Eosinophil
    d. Platelet

20. Number of hemoglobin molecules that each RBC contain is:
    a. 28 million
    b. 280 million
    c. 28 lakhs
    d. 280 lakhs

21. Heme synthesis requires:
    a. Ferric ion
    b. Alanine
    c. Succinyl CoA
    d. Lead

22. With regard to hemoglobin, all the following statements are true, *except*:
    a. It is the major source of bile pigment
    b. Contains iron in ferrous state
    c. Is completely deoxygenated in the blood drawn from cubital vein
    d. Can be estimated by acid hematin principle

23. Life span of neonatal RBC is:
    a. 120 days
    b. 100 days
    c. 6 months
    d. 1 year

24. Biconcave shape of RBC is helpful because:
    a. Easy passage through capillaries
    b. Rouleaux formation
    c. Increased surface area for a given diameter
    d. Increased binding of oxygen

25. Increased blood viscosity and slow circulation causes:
    a. RBC rouleaux formation
    b. Increased plasma skimming
    c. Increased number of RBC in capillaries
    d. Increased hemolysis

26. Heme is converted to bilirubin mainly in:
    a. Kidney
    b. Liver
    c. Spleen
    d. Bone marrow
27. Metalloproteins is of help in jaundice by the following mechanism:
    a. Increased glucuronyl transferase activity
    b. Inhibit heme oxygenase
    c. Decrease RBC lysis
    d. Increase Y and Z receptors
28. True statement regarding iron:
    a. It is stored in ferritin
    b. It is absorbed by transferrin in the intestine
    c. Spleen is the major storage organ
    d. Ferrous ion is excreted in urine
29. The type of hemoglobin that has least affinity for 2,3-DPG is:
    a. HbA
    b. HbF
    c. HbA_2
    d. HbS
30. G-CSF and GM-CSF in hematopoiesis causes:
    a. Leukocytosis
    b. Erythrocytosis
    c. Leukopenia
    d. Thrombocytosis
31. Erythropoiesis is promoted by all the following, except:
    a. ACTH
    b. Thyroxine
    c. Estrogen
    d. Prolactin
32. Nitric oxide (NO) binding protein present in blood is:
    a. Albumin
    b. Transferrin
    c. Haptoglobin
    d. Hemoglobin
33. Thrombopoietin is produced by:
    a. Liver
    b. Spleen
    c. Lymph node
    d. Kidney
34. Normal life span of RBC is:
    a. 1–2 weeks
    b. 120 days
    c. 70 days
    d. 48 hours
35. All the following hormones maintain osmotic pressure and blood volume relatively constant, except:
    a. Aldosterone
    b. ANP
    c. ADH
    d. Adrenaline
36. MHC antigens are present in the plasma membrane of all the following cells, except:
    a. Neutrophil
    b. Lymphocyte
    c. Macrophage
    d. Erythrocyte
37. Normal ratio of RBC to WBC in the body is:
    a. 700:1
    b. 500:1
    c. 1000:1
    d. 100:1
38. All the following cells exhibit phagocytic activity, except:
    a. Monocyte
    b. Lymphocyte
    c. Eosinophil
    d. Neutrophil
39. All the following enzymes contain iron, except:
    a. Cytochrome oxidase
    b. Peroxidase
    c. Xanthine oxidase
    d. Glucuronyl transferase
40. All the following are iron binding proteins, except:
    a. Transferrin
    b. Apoferritin
    c. Hemosiderin
    d. Ceruloplasmin
41. All the following statements regarding leukocytes are true, except:
    a. Lymphocytes and monocytes possess cytoplasmic granules
    b. Neutrophils are called polymorphonuclear leukocytes
    c. Eosinophils contain histamine and heparin
    d. Increase in the number of large lymphocytes is seen in acute viral infections
42. Life span of platelet is:
    a. 5–9 days
    b. 2–4 weeks
    c. 4–6 hours
    d. 1–2 months
43. Plasma cells are transformed:
    a. Mast cells
    b. Monocytes
    c. B-lymphocytes
    d. Polymorphs
44. ESR is increased in all the following conditions, except:
    a. Pneumonia
    b. Tuberculosis
    c. SLE
    d. Polycythemia
45. Normal RBC count in an adult male is:
    a. 4.5 million/mm^3
    b. 5.5 million/mm^3
    c. 5.5 lakhs/mm^3
    d. 11,000/mm^3
46. The following statements are true of HbF, except that it:
    a. Contains 2 alpha and 2 gamma chains
    b. Is not normally present in adulthood
    c. Has high affinity for 2,3-DPG
    d. Has high affinity for oxygen
47. Iron in hemoglobin is in the ferric form in:
    a. Oxyhemoglobin
    b. Carboxyhemoglobin
    c. Carbaminohemoglobin
    d. Methemoglobin
48. During granulopoiesis, specific granules appear in:
    a. Myelocyte
    b. Promyelocyte
    c. Myeloblast
    d. Metamyelocyte
49. Deficiency of all the following can produce megaloblastic anemia, except:
    a. Vitamin B_{12}
    b. Folic acid
    c. Iron
    d. Vitamin B_{12} and folic acid
50. The type of anemia seen in nuclear maturation defect of RBC is:
    a. Microcytic hypochromic anemia
    b. Macrocytic anemia
    c. Normocytic normochromic anemia
    d. Microcytic normochromic anemia

SECTION 2 — Hematology

51. **Inheritance of hemophilia is:**
    a. X-linked recessive
    b. Autosomal recessive
    c. X-linked dominant
    d. Autosomal dominant

52. **In hemolytic jaundice all are true, *except*:**
    a. Increased stercobilin in feces
    b. Increased urobilin in urine
    c. Increased bilirubin in urine
    d. Increased conjugated bilirubin in bile

53. **Acholuric jaundice is a salient feature of:**
    a. Hemolytic jaundice
    b. Hepatocellular jaundice
    c. Obstructive jaundice
    d. Both hepatic and obstructive jaundice

54. **Absence of intrinsic factor is associated with all the following, *except*:**
    a. Hypochlorhydria
    b. Sub-acute combined degeneration of spinal cord
    c. Macrocytic anemia
    d. Microcytic anemia

55. **All the following are necessary for erythropoiesis, *except*:**
    a. Iron
    b. Cobalt
    c. Copper
    d. Chromium

56. **In blood, maximum amount of carbonic anhydrase is present in:**
    a. Red blood cells
    b. Plasma
    c. Monocytes
    d. Neutrophils

57. **Erythropoiesis is:**
    a. Stimulated by a rise in PCO_2 of arterial blood
    b. Stimulated by a fall in the PO_2 of arterial blood
    c. Stimulated by a fall in the PCO_2 of arterial blood
    d. Stimulated by a fall in pH of arterial blood

58. **Erythropoietin is secreted from all the following areas, *except*:**
    a. Kidney
    b. Liver parenchymal cells
    c. Cells of tissue macrophage system
    d. Bone marrow

59. **Erythropoietin helps in the differentiation of:**
    a. Stem cells into proerythroblast
    b. Proerythroblast to early normoblast
    c. Reticulocyte to mature erythrocyte
    d. Intermediate normoblast to late normoblast

60. **The following statements are true, *except*:**
    a. All RBCs in peripheral blood are non-nucleated normally
    b. Reticulocyte count is 1% of total RBCs in circulation
    c. RBCs obtain energy by anaerobic glycolysis
    d. RBCs obtain energy through citric acid cycle

61. **Erythropoiesis occur in the fetus in the second trimester primarily in the:**
    a. Spleen
    b. Bone marrow
    c. Liver
    d. Lymph node

62. **In adults erythropoiesis occurs in all the following areas, *except*:**
    a. Sternum
    b. Ribs
    c. Proximal ends of long bones
    d. Distal end of long bones

63. **Majority of plasma proteins are synthesized in the:**
    a. Kidney
    b. Lymph node
    c. Liver
    d. Plasma cell

64. **Vitamin B_{12} is absorbed in:**
    a. Duodenum
    b. Jejunum
    c. Proximal ileum
    d. Terminal ileum

65. **Daily requirement of vitamin B_{12} is:**
    a. 1 µg
    b. 5 µg
    c. 2 µg
    d. 1 mg

66. **Daily requirement of folic acid is:**
    a. 1 mg
    b. 100 µg
    c. 200 µg
    d. 2 mg

67. **Vitamin B_{12} deficiency is found in all the following conditions, *except*:**
    a. Gastric atrophy
    b. Malabsorption states affecting ileum
    c. Blind loop syndrome
    d. Peptic ulcer

68. **Aplastic anemia is due to deficiency of:**
    a. Intrinsic factor
    b. Vitamin B_{12}
    c. Iron
    d. Hemopoiesis in red marrow

69. **The stage of erythropoiesis at which hemoglobin appear is:**
    a. Proerythroblast
    b. Intermediate normoblast
    c. Reticulocyte
    d. Late normoblast

70. **Total blood volume in an individual is normally:**
    a. 80 mL/kg body weight
    b. 90 mL/kg body weight
    c. 50 mL/kg body weight
    d. 100 mL/kg body weight

71. **The type of bilirubin that crosses the blood-brain barrier to produce kernicterus is:**
    a. Conjugated bilirubin
    b. Unconjugated bilirubin bound to albumin
    c. Unbound unconjugated bilirubin
    d. Both conjugated and unconjugated bilirubin

72. Eosinophil differentiation factor is:
    a. IL-5   b. G-CSF
    c. IL-7   d. IL-2
73. Normal MCH is:
    a. 32–36 pg   b. 27–32 pg
    c. 80–94 pg   d. 32–36 μg
74. Fragility of red cell is increased in all the following conditions, *except*:
    a. Spherocytosis   b. Sickle cell anemia
    c. Hemolytic anemia d. Thalassemia
75. Normal half-life of platelet is:
    a. 4 days   b. 2 weeks
    c. 4 weeks   d. 12 days
76. Platelets are formed from:
    a. Megakaryocytes in bone marrow
    b. Megakaryocytes in bloodstream
    c. Megakaryoblast
    d. Macrophage
77. Smallest blood cell is:
    a. Basophil   b. Erythrocyte
    c. Small lymphocyte d. Platelet
78. Regarding RBC, all the following statements are true, *except*:
    a. Anaerobic metabolism supplies 90% of energy requirement of RBC
    b. Mature erythrocyte is incapable of protein synthesis
    c. In adults 5–10% of hemoglobin is made of HbA_2
    d. Blood group antigens are attached to the RBC membrane
79. Reticulocytes are stained with:
    a. Methyl violet b. Brilliant cresyl blue
    c. Sudan black   d. Indigo carmine
80. Shift to right in Arneth count is seen in the following condition:
    a. Neutropenia   b. Neutrophilia
    c. Leukocytosis   d. Eosinopenia
81. Of the total lymphocyte population in our body, the percentage found in blood is:
    a. 20   b. 10
    c. 5   d. 2
82. Kaposi's sarcoma is associated with:
    a. HIV infection b. Hepatitis-B
    c. COPD   d. Smoking
83. Hereditary spherocytosis is due to defect in:
    a. Spectrin   b. Inositol phosphate
    c. α-globin   d. Dystrophin
84. Normal platelet function requires:
    a. Presence of immunoglobulins
    b. Intact cell membrane
    c. Presence of sodium ions
    d. Presence of von Willebrand factor
85. Decreased MCHC is found in:
    a. Microcytic hypochromic anemia
    b. Megaloblastic anemia
    c. Sideroblastic anemia
    d. Pernicious anemia
86. Bronze diabetes is seen in:
    a. Cushing syndrome
    b. Hyperthyroidism
    c. Hemochromatosis
    d. Gigantism and acromegaly
87. The percentage of dry weight of RBC that is constituted by hemoglobin is:
    a. 95%   b. 50%
    c. 25%   d. 15%
88. The number of hemoglobin molecules that each RBC contain is:
    a. 280   b. 28,000
    c. 28 lakhs   d. 280 million
89. Heme is a part of all the following, *except*:
    a. Myoglobin   b. Neuroglobin
    c. Cytochrome C   d. Peroxidase
90. The amount of bilirubin formed when 1 g of hemoglobin is completely destroyed in the reticuloendothelial system is:
    a. 35 mg   b. 1 g
    c. 0.5 g   d. 100 mg
91. Acholuric jaundice is seen in all the following conditions, *except*:
    a. Gilbert's syndrome
    b. Crigler-Najjar syndrome
    c. Hemolytic anemia
    d. Obstructive jaundice
92. Total body iron in an adult male is about:
    a. 38 g   b. 3.8 g
    c. 38 mg   d. 380 mg
93. Absorption of iron in the GIT occurs in the:
    a. Proximal ileum
    b. Distal ileum
    c. Jejunum and ileum
    d. Duodenum and proximal jejunum
94. Limiting factor of iron absorption is:
    a. Hemosiderin
    b. Amount of iron in the intestine
    c. Apoferritin
    d. Transferrin
95. Half-life of transfused platelet is:
    a. 4 hours   b. 4 days
    c. 8 days   d. 15 days
96. Cyanosis is seen if the concentration of methemoglobin is more than:
    a. 1.5 g%   b. 2.5 g%
    c. 3 g%   d. 4 g%

SECTION 2 — Hematology

97. **Iron is stored in:**
    a. RBC
    b. Reticuloendothelial system
    c. Plasma
    d. Muscle

98. **The best method for the estimation of hemoglobin concentration in blood is:**
    a. Acid hematin method
    b. Alkali hematin method
    c. Cyanmethemoglobin method
    d. Any of the above

99. **Alkali resistant hemoglobin is:**
    a. HbA
    b. HbA1C
    c. HbS
    d. HbF

ANSWERS

1. c	2. a	3. b	4. a	5. c
6. b	7. d	8. a	9. c	10. a
11. a	12. c	13. d	14. b	15. a
16. c	17. a	18. c	19. a	20. b
21. c	22. c	23. b	24. a	25. a
26. c	27. b	28. a	29. b	30. a
31. c	32. d	33. a	34. b	35. d
36. d	37. a	38. b	39. d	40. d
41. c	42. a	43. c	44. d	45. b
46. c	47. d	48. d	49. c	50. b
51. a	52. c	53. a	54. d	55. d
56. a	57. b	58. d	59. a	60. d
61. c	62. d	63. c	64. d	65. c
66. c	67. d	68. d	69. b	70. a
71. c	72. a	73. b	74. d	75. a
76. a	77. d	78. c	79. b	80. a
81. d	82. a	83. a	84. d	85. a
86. c	87. a	88. d	89. d	90. a
91. d	92. b	93. d	94. d	95. b
96. a	97. b	98. c	99. d	

White Blood Corpuscles or Leukocytes

CHAPTER 14

LEARNING OBJECTIVES

Must know
- Describe granulopoiesis and its regulation
- Describe the properties of leukocytes
- Explain the functions of different leukocytes
- Enumerate the variations in WBC count

Desirable to know
- Describe the structure of leukocytes with the help of diagrams
- Differentiate between Arneth count and Schilling index
- Differentiate between leukemia and leukemoid reaction

■ INTRODUCTION

Leukocytes are the **nucleated, active and motile** constituents of blood and lymph. They are **colorless** because they do not contain pigments. The total **white blood corpuscles** (WBC) count ranges from 4000 to 11,000/mm³ of blood. Leukocytes are classified into:
- ❖ **Granulocytes**
  - Neutrophils
  - Eosinophils
  - Basophils
- ❖ **Agranulocytes**
  - Lymphocytes
  - Monocytes

A peripheral smear is taken and it is stained with **Leishman's stain**, which contains **eosin** and **methylene blue** in acetone-free methyl alcohol. Methylene blue is a basic stain that stains the nucleus and some cytoplasmic structures, a blue or purple color. These structures are said to be **basophilic**, e.g., DNA or RNA. Eosin is an acidic stain that stains some cytoplasmic structures an orange–red color. These structures are said to be **acidophilic**, e.g., specific granules of eosinophils. When both the basic and the acidic components of the stain, stains a cytoplasmic structure, a pink or lilac color develops. These structures are said to be **neutrophilic**, e.g., granules of neutrophils (**Fig. 14.1C**). Acetone-free methyl alcohol in the stain acts as a fixative and preservative. Fixative is a substance that preserves the

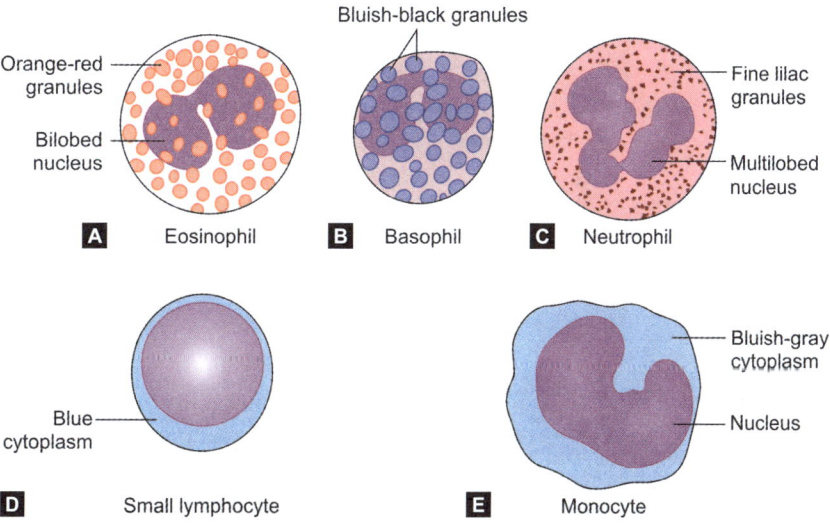

Figs. 14.1A to E: Types of white blood cells (leukocytes).

morphology of the cell or the tissue. A stained peripheral smear is shown in **Figure 14.2**.

The cytoplasm of granulocytes contains secretory granules that readily take up the stains. The granules that distinguish the different types of granulocytes are called specific granules. Monocytes and lymphocytes do not have specific granules in their cytoplasm and are therefore called agranulocytes.

■ GRANULOCYTES (FIGS. 14.1A TO E)

All granulocytes have cytoplasmic granules that contain biologically active substances involved in inflammatory and allergic reactions. The granules take up **Romanowsky stains** like Leishman stain (A Romanowsky stain is defined as any stain that contains eosin and methylene blue).

Neutrophils or Polymorphs

- **Size**: 10–14 μm
- **Shape**: No definite shape as they show amoeboid movement.
- **Nucleus** is lobulated and hence referred to as **polymorphs**. Lobes vary from 2 to 5 depending on the age of the neutrophils. The number of lobes increases as the cell becomes older. Chromatin strands connect the lobes. Nucleus is purple in color after Leishman's staining (**Fig. 14.2**).
- **Cytoplasm** is light pink in color with **lilac** colored **fine** granules, which take up both acidic and basic stain. The granules contain enzymes like *acid phosphatase, alkaline phosphatase, peroxidase, elastase, esterase, lysozyme, defensins, cathepsin, nucleosidase, etc.* Neutrophils have three granule subsets: (a) **primary** or azurophilic granules, which contain hydrolytic enzymes like elastases and myeloperoxidases, (b) **secondary** or specific granules which contain high levels of iron-binding protein called lactoferrin and (c) **tertiary** or gelatinase granules which contain matrix metalloproteinases.

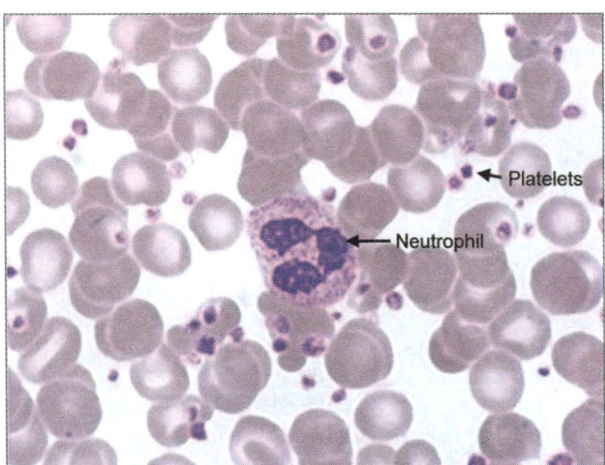

Fig. 14.2: Peripheral smear showing 1 neutrophil with multilobed nucleus; the red blood cells show central pallor due to disc shape. Rouleaux formation is also seen. The smallest purple dots are the platelets.

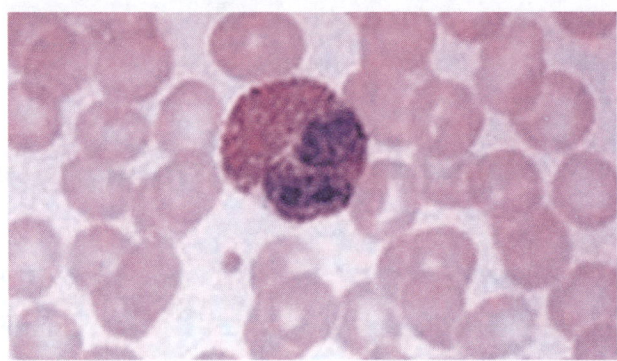

Fig. 14.3: Peripheral smear showing an eosinophil. Note the orange-red coarse granules in the cytoplasm and bilobed nucleus.

- 1–15% of neutrophils in genetic females contain a drumstick-like structure attached to the nucleus called **Barr body or sex chromatin** (*refer* **Fig. 71.2**). It represents the inactive X chromosome. This is important in medicolegal cases.
- The *average half-life of neutrophil in circulation is 6 hours*. To maintain normal neutrophil count in circulation, it is necessary to produce over 100 billion neutrophils per day.

Eosinophil

- **Diameter**: 12–15 μm.
- **Shape**: No definite shape due to amoeboid movement.
- **Nucleus**: Bilobed or spectacle-shaped, purple in color.
- **Cytoplasm** is acidophilic, which contains large, dense, **orange–red** granules with Leishman's stain (**Figs. 14.1A and 14.3**).
- The granules of eosinophil contain enzymes like *myeloperoxidase, glucuronidase, lipase, aryl sulfatase, acid phosphatase, beta-glucuronidase, cathepsins. It also contains plasminogen, histamine, eosinophil chemotactic factor of anaphylaxis, major basic protein (MBP) and eosinophil cationic protein*. Eosinophil cationic protein binds with heparin and neutralizes it. MBP in eosinophil kills organisms and it plays a key role in the eosinophil's ability to damage the helminthic larvae. Eosinophils secrete lysophospholipase, which forms **Charcot-Leyden crystals** in the pulmonary secretions of patients with asthma.
- Eosinophils are abundant in the lining of gastrointestinal tract (GIT), respiratory tract, and urinary tract. Function is defense against foreign allergic substances. For each circulating eosinophil, about 100 eosinophils are present in the tissues primarily in the skin and sub-mucosa. Like neutrophils, they have a short half-life in circulation, i.e., about 8 hours.

Basophil

Diameter: 8–10 μm.

Nucleus: Bilobed and purple in color.

Cytoplasm: It is slightly basophilic and contains numerous, large, coarse, **purplish-black** granules that obscure the nucleus (**Fig. 14.4**). Granules are water-soluble and so may get dissolved in the process of staining and washing.

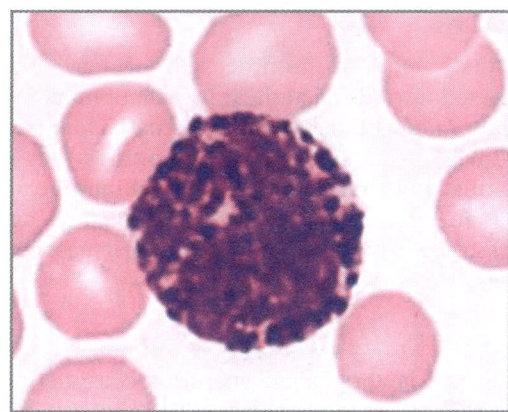

Fig. 14.4: Basophil. Note the purplish-black coarse granules obscuring the nucleus.

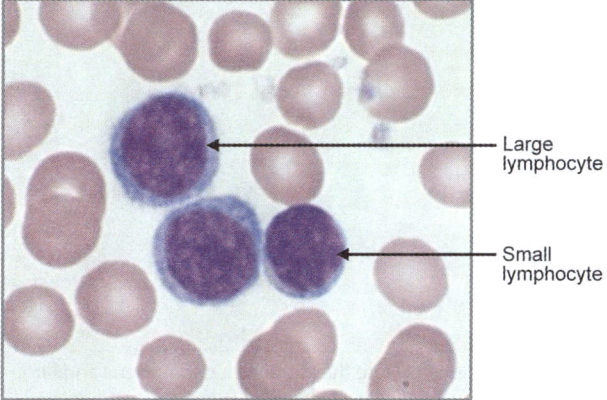

Fig. 14.5: Lymphocytes.

Granules contain *heparin, histamine, serotonin, kallikrein, platelet activating factor*, etc.

Basophils remain in the blood only for a few hours, after which they move into tissues. Their fate in the tissues is uncertain. In contrast to the earlier belief, basophils do not transform into mast cells in tissues.

Mast Cells

Mast cells are cells similar to basophils and both are derived from marrow stem cells. Mast cells are heavily granulated cells of the connective tissues, especially, beneath epithelial surfaces. They are most abundant at those places where the body comes in direct contact with the environment like lung, skin, gastrointestinal tract (GIT), etc. Mast cells participate in immune response and repair.

The mast cell granules contain heparin, histamine, leukotrienes, prostaglandins and many proteases. Like basophils, they degranulate when allergens bind to IgE molecules on their surface and fights invading parasites. Thus, it is involved in acquired immunity. Excessive mast cell degranulation produces clinical manifestation of allergy and even anaphylaxis. Leukotrienes released by the mast cell trigger the bronchospasm and the mucosal edema of bronchial asthma.

In addition to its involvement in acquired immunity, mast cells release tumor necrosis factor (TNF) in response to bacterial products by an antibody-independent mechanism. Thus, it also contributes to nonspecific innate immunity that combats infections before the development of an adaptive immune response.

■ AGRANULOCYTES

The monocytes and lymphocytes do not contain specific granules that can be stained by methylene blue and eosin. Therefore, they are called agranulocytes. They may have a few small azurophilic or primary granules.

Lymphocytes

The size of the lymphocytes varies and structurally, they are classified into small, medium and large lymphocytes (**Fig. 14.5**). Majority of lymphocytes in the peripheral blood are small lymphocytes. Lymphocyte precursors leave the bone marrow early and require extramedullary (outside the marrow) maturation to become normally functioning immune cells in the blood or lymphatic system. After birth, lymphocytes are formed in the lymph nodes, thymus and spleen from the precursor cells that came from the bone marrow and were processed in the thymus (T lymphocytes) or bone marrow (B cells). Only 2% of the lymphocytes in the body are present in the peripheral blood. The rest are in the lymphoid organs.

Diameter

- *Small lymphocyte:* 6–8 μm
- *Large lymphocyte:* 10–15 μm.

After Leishman's staining, the nucleus is deep purplish blue and is round or slightly indented. Cytoplasm forms a thin rim in small lymphocytes, but it may be abundant in large lymphocytes (**Fig. 14.1D**). Cytoplasm is basophilic and is usually devoid of visible granules. But larger cells may contain reddish–violet granules, which do not contain peroxidase, i.e., peroxidase test is negative.

Depending on the function, lymphocytes are classified into **T-lymphocytes and B-lymphocytes**. Maturation of T-lymphocytes occurs in the thymus and B-lymphocytes mature in the bone marrow and lymphoid tissue. 70–80% of circulating blood lymphocytes is T-lymphocyte and 10–15% B-lymphocytes. Remaining lymphocytes are referred to as **null cells**. These include cells like natural killer (NK) cells, which are large granular lymphocytes.

Monocytes

- **Diameter**: 15–20 μm, largest of the leukocytes.
- **Nucleus**: Kidney or horse-shoe shaped (**Figs. 14.1E and 14.6**).
- **Cytoplasm**: Muddy blue or slate grey and sometimes contain purple dust like granules called *azur granules*.

Macrophages

Macrophages are formed from monocytes which enter the tissues from blood. Monocytes enter the blood from bone marrow and circulate for 3 days. They then enter the tissues

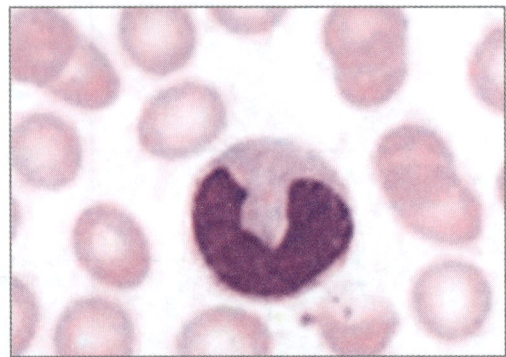

Fig. 14.6: Monocyte: Note the kidney-shaped nucleus and large size.

and develop into large **tissue macrophages** which are 20–40 µm in diameter. Their life span is about 3 months. Tissue macrophages include Kupffer cells of liver, pulmonary alveolar macrophages, microglia in the brain, etc. The tissue macrophages act as immune cells that phagocytose bacteria and other antigens and subsequently present components of these antigens to lymphocytes that further amplify and refine the immune response (*refer* Immunity, Chapter 16).

■ PROPERTIES OF LEUKOCYTES

- ❖ Margination and diapedesis
- ❖ Amoeboid movement
- ❖ Chemotaxis
- ❖ Opsonization
- ❖ Phagocytosis.

Margination and Diapedesis

Leukocytes are attracted to the endothelial surface by **selectins** (cell adhesion molecules) and they roll along it. This property is called **margination**. Endothelial selectins are markedly increased in areas of inflammation. There are pores in between endothelial cells and the leukocytes squeeze out through these pores by a process called **diapedesis**. Some products of inflammation cause vasodilatation and this increases the pore size, which promotes diapedesis (**Fig. 14.7**).

Amoeboid Movement

Leukocytes move through tissues by **amoeboid movement** by putting out pseudopodia. They move at a rate of 40 µm/minute.

Chemotaxis

Chemotaxis refers to the process by which leukocytes are attracted towards bacteria at the site of inflammation. Bacterial products interact with plasma factors and cells to produce substances called **chemokines** that attract neutrophils to the infected area. **Chemokines** include C_5a (component of complement system), leukotrienes and cytokines (polypeptides from lymphocytes, mast cells and basophils).

Opsonization

Some plasma factors called **opsonins** coat the bacteria to make them tasty to phagocytes. This property is called opsonization. The principal opsonins that coat the bacteria are IgG (a particular class of immunoglobulin), complement proteins like perforins, etc. Opsonins neutralize the negative surface charges of bacteria and they get easily bound to the surface of the phagocyte. This triggers phagocytosis, degranulation and respiratory burst.

Phagocytosis

The leukocytes can engulf bacteria and other foreign substances by **phagocytosis** to form phagocytic vacuole. The movements of the leukocytes involve microtubules and microfilaments. The granules of the leukocyte fuse with the phagocytic vacuole to form **phagosome** and the enzymes digest the bacteria.

■ FUNCTIONS OF LEUKOCYTES

Functions of Neutrophils

- ❖ The main site of action of neutrophils is in the tissues. Invasion of the body by microorganisms triggers the inflammatory response. Bone marrow is stimulated and large number of neutrophils is released into circulation. By **diapedesis** and **chemotaxis**, they reach the site of infection. The opsonin-coated bacteria bind to receptors on the neutrophil cell membrane. This increases the motor activity and the neutrophils phagocytose the bacteria to form **phagocytic vacuoles**. One neutrophil phagocytose 5–20 microbes at a time. The granules of the neutrophils discharge their contents into the phagocytic vacuoles containing the bacteria. This is known as **degranulation**. The granules also contain antimicrobial proteins called **defensins**. The proteases and the defensins in the granule digest the organism.

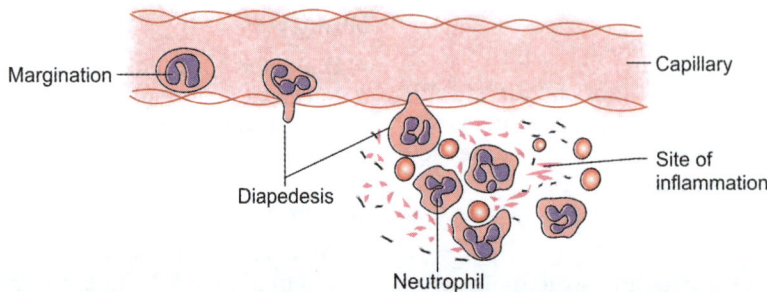

Fig. 14.7: Margination and diapedesis of neutrophil at the site of inflammation.

- **Respiratory burst**: Within seconds of stimulation of neutrophils, it also activates the cell membrane bound enzyme **nicotinamide adenine dinucleotide phosphate (NADPH) oxidase** with the production of toxic O_2 metabolites. This reaction is associated with a sharp increase in O_2 uptake and metabolism in the neutrophil called **respiratory burst**, which leads to the generation of free radical oxygen ions (O_2^-). The increased O_2 uptake is utilized for oxidation of glucose *via* the hexose monophosphate shunt, resulting in the production of NADPH.

$$NADPH + H^+ + 2O_2 \xrightarrow{NADPH\ oxidase} NADP^+ + 2H^+ + 2O_2^-$$

  O_2^- and H_2O_2 are **oxidants** and are very effective bactericidal agents. H_2O_2 is converted to H_2O and O_2 by the enzyme, **catalase**. In **amyotrophic lateral sclerosis**, this enzyme is defective and O_2^- accumulates in motor neuron and destroys them.
  Neutrophils also contain **myeloperoxidase**, which converts Cl^-, Br^-, I^-, etc., to the corresponding acids, HOCl, HOBr, etc. These are also potent oxidants.

$$H_2O_2 + 2Cl^- \xrightarrow{Myeloperoxidase} 2HOCl$$

- Neutrophil granules also contain elastases; two metalloproteinases that attack collagen and a variety of other proteases that help destroy invading organisms. All these along with O_2^-, H_2O_2 and HOCl produce a **killing zone** around the activated neutrophil, which kills the invading organisms. *Thus, neutrophils form the **first line of defence** against invading organisms.*

Functions of Monocytes

Monocytes, which form the macrophages, also act in a similar way like that of neutrophils. The diameter of the macrophage is about 80 µm and they can engulf more number of bacteria, i.e., >100 at a time. They also engulf parasites, especially malarial parasite, necrosed tissues, dead neutrophils, etc. *Monocyte thus forms the **second line of defence** against invading organism. Some organisms like Mycobacterium leprae are not destroyed by the macrophages.*

Many leukocytes are killed during inflammatory process. The dead neutrophils, macrophages, plasma leaked from capillaries, dead tissue cells, RBCs, etc., constitute **pus**. The dead leukocytes are called **pus cells**.

Functions of Eosinophils

Functions of eosinophils are same as that of neutrophils but weak. They are especially abundant in the mucosa of the gastrointestinal tract, and in the mucosa of respiratory and urinary tract. Like neutrophils, they undergo diapedesis and margination and release proteins, cytokines and chemokines that produce inflammation and kill invading organisms. Other functions of eosinophils include:

- Eosinophils play a crucial role in the host's defence against parasites. They kill parasites by releasing cationic proteins and reactive oxygen metabolites into the extracellular fluid. The granules of eosinophils contain **major basic protein (MBP)** which is toxic to parasites. They also secrete leukotrienes, prostaglandin and various other cytokines. Larval forms of parasites like filaria and schistosomes are killed by eosinophils. Eosinophils are abundant in the GIT where they defend against parasites.
- They phagocytose antigen–antibody complexes and circulating eosinophils are increased in allergic diseases like allergic asthma, hay fever, etc.
- Eosinophils suppress allergic inflammatory processes. The eosinophils are attracted to tissue sites of allergic reactions by chemotactic factors secreted by mast cells. At the site of allergic reaction, eosinophils degrade mast cell products and thereby decrease the clinical manifestations of allergic responses.
- Remove fibrin formed during inflammation.

Functions of Basophils

Basophils contain **histamine, heparin and peroxidase**. The basophils are important in healing after inflammation and are also involved in allergic reactions.

Basophils are the major source of the cytokine IL4, which stimulates B lymphocytes to produce IgE antibodies.

Basophils possess high affinity receptors for IgE and mediate **immediate-type hypersensitivity reactions** (allergic or type-I hypersensitivity response). These range from mild urticaria to severe anaphylactic shock. The specific antigen binds to IgE antibodies (IgE molecules) present on the surface of basophils. The result is the release of inflammatory mediators such as chemotactic factors, histamine, enzymes, prostaglandins, leukotrienes and platelet activating factor. *The antigens that trigger IgE formation and basophil and mast cell activation are referred to as allergens.*

Functions of Lymphocytes

- T lymphocytes mediate cellular immunity
- B lymphocytes mediate humoral immunity
- Large lymphocytes referred to as NK cells nonspecifically destroy foreign cells, tumor cells and infected cells (*Refer* Immunity, Chapter 16).

DISORDERS OF PHAGOCYTIC FUNCTION

- In **neutrophil hypomotility syndrome**, actin in neutrophil is defective and so neutrophil moves slowly.
- **Deficiency of integrins** leads to defective diapedesis of leukocytes to the site of infection. WBCs move out of blood vessels after binding to the integrins on endothelial cells. Integrins present on macrophages are necessary for their migration to the site of injury.
- In **chronic granulomatous disease**, there is failure to generate O_2^- in neutrophils and monocytes leading to inability to kill phagocytosed bacteria.
- In **glucose-6-phosphate dehydrogenase deficiency**, there will be multiple infections because NADPH production is defective leading to deficiency of O_2^-.

- In **congenital myeloperoxidase deficiency**, hypohalite ions are not formed leading to defective phagocytosis.
- **Defective chemotaxis** occurs in corticosteroid therapy, myeloid leukemia, etc., making the patient prone to recurrent infections.

VARIATIONS IN WBC COUNT

Leukocytosis

Increase in the WBC count above the upper limit of normal is called leukocytosis.

Physiological increase in the WBC count is seen:
- In newborn
- After strenuous exercise
- In pregnancy and labor
- After meals

Pathological increase in the leukocyte count is seen in:
- Acute and chronic infections
- Leukemia
- Hodgkin's disease.

Leukemia

Leukemia is a malignant condition of bone marrow where there is abnormal, uncontrolled, purposeless proliferation of the precursor cells of leukocytes. Large number of blast cells or immature cells will be seen in circulation. WBC count will be in lakhs or millions. The abnormal cells are functionless. Leukemia is classified based on the predominant cell types into myeloid (cells derived from myeloid stem cells are involved) and lymphoid leukemia (involving cells derived from lymphoid stem cells). Another classification is acute and chronic leukemia. The main types of leukemia are:
- Acute and chronic myeloid leukemia
- Acute and chronic lymphoid leukemia (**Fig. 14.8**).

Leukemoid Reaction

Leukemoid reaction is a condition where there is excessive leukocytosis resembling that of leukemia, but not having clinical features of leukemia like hepatosplenomegaly, lymphadenopathy, etc. Features of underlying disorders like severe infections, other malignant conditions, etc., will be present.

Leukopenia

Decrease in the leukocyte count below the lower limit is called **leukopenia**. Causes are:
- Bacterial infections like typhoid and paratyphoid fever; tuberculosis, brucellosis, etc.
- Viral infections like measles, influenza, hepatitis, infectious mononucleosis (IMN), AIDS, etc.
- Aplastic anemia due to bone marrow depression
- Arsenic poisoning and therapy with drugs like chloromycetin, sulfonamides, penicillin, cytotoxic drugs, antithyroid drugs, etc.
- Anaphylaxis and hypersensitivity
- Hypersplenism
- Autoimmune disorders like systemic lupus erythematosus (SLE)
- Vitamin B_{12} and folate deficiency that interferes with DNA synthesis
- Radiotherapy that causes bone marrow depression
- Autoimmune neutropenia
- Hormones like ACTH.

Variations in Counts of Different Leukocytes

Normal differential count of leukocytes in a peripheral smear is given in **Table 14.1**.

Neutrophils

Neutrophilia

Neutrophilia is increase in the neutrophil count >10,000/mm³ of blood. It is seen in the following conditions:
- Acute pyogenic bacterial infections like tonsillitis, appendicitis, septicemia, etc.
- Metabolic disturbances like diabetes mellitus, renal failure, etc.
- Necrotic lesions like myocardial infarction, burns, etc.
- Non-infective inflammatory conditions like gout, rheumatic fever, etc.
- Administration of drugs like glucocorticoids, adrenaline, etc.
- Malignancies like myeloid leukemia.

Neutropenia

Neutropenia is decrease in the neutrophil count below 2500/mm³ of blood:

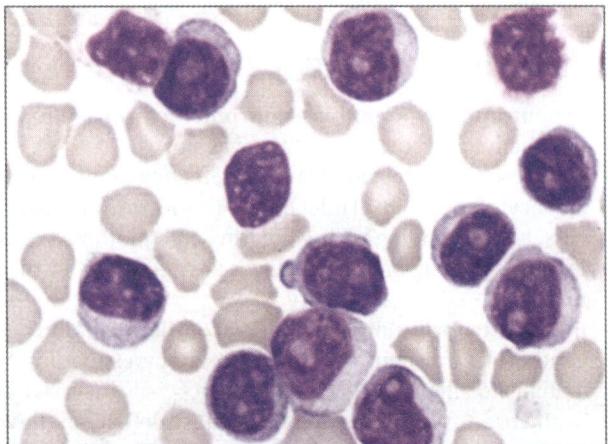

Fig. 14.8: Peripheral smear of chronic lymphoid leukemia.

Table 14.1: Differential count of leukocytes in a peripheral smear.		
Cell	**Normal range (cells/μL)**	**Total WBC (%)**
Neutrophils	3000–6000	50–70
Eosinophils	150–300	1–4
Basophils	0–100	0.4
Lymphocytes	1500–4000	20–40
Monocytes	300–600	2–8

- Bacterial infections like typhoid and paratyphoid fever, tuberculosis, etc. In typhoid and paratyphoid infections, there is depression of bone marrow and the neutrophil count falls first because its half-life in circulation is very less (only 6–7 hours). In tuberculosis, there is lymphocytosis and so a relative decrease in neutrophil count is observed.
- Viral infections like measles, influenza, hepatitis, infectious mononucleosis (IMN), AIDS, etc.
- Aplastic anemia
- Arsenic poisoning and drugs like chloromycetin, penicillin, cytotoxic drugs, etc.
- Anaphylaxis and hypersensitivity
- Hypersplenism where there is sequestration of neutrophils and also increased destruction
- Autoimmune disorders like SLE
- Vitamin B_{12} and folate deficiency
- Congenital neutropenia is found in early life and the more severely affected children die in the first 1–2 years of life from repeated infections
- In chronic granulomatous disease of childhood the neutrophil count will be normal but the neutrophils are nonfunctioning due to failure of chemotaxis or due to lack of hydrolytic enzymes which kill bacteria or due to lack of opsonization.

Eosinophils

Eosinophilia (>500/mm³)

- Allergic conditions such as bronchial asthma, hay fever, hypersensitivity reactions, drug allergy, serum sickness, urticaria
- Worm infestations, e.g., roundworm, hookworm, tapeworm, filarial worm
- Drugs like penicillin
- Skin diseases like eczema, dermatitis, scabies, etc.
- Tropical pulmonary eosinophilia and scarlet fever
- Chronic myeloid leukemia
- Infrequently in conditions like Hodgkin's disease, polyarteritis nodosa
- If the absolute eosinophil count is more than 1500/mm³ of blood, the condition is called **hypereosinophilia** e.g., eosinophilic leukemia

Eosinopenia (<50/mm³)

- Endocrine disorders like Cushing's syndrome where there is increase in glucocorticoid secretion; acromegaly, etc.
- ACTH and corticosteroid therapy; glucocorticoids cause margination and sequestration of circulating eosinophils, lowering the eosinophil count.
- Stress, as in acute infection, traumatic shock, severe exercise, burns, acute emotional stress, exposure to cold, etc.
- Aplastic anemia, systemic lupus erythematosus (**SLE**), eclampsia, etc.

Basophils

Basophilia (>100/mm³)

- Viral infections like measles, chickenpox, influenza, etc.,
- Chronic myeloid leukemia and myeloproliferative disorders
- Polycythemia vera
- Myxedema
- Ulcerative colitis
- Hypersensitivity states

Basopenia

- Cushing's disease and prolonged corticosteroid therapy
- Acute pyogenic infections associated with neutrophilia

Lymphocytes

Lymphocytosis (>4000/mm³)

- Chronic bacterial infections like tuberculosis, syphilis, etc. and acute bacterial infections like whooping cough and typhoid
- Viral infections like chickenpox, mumps, measles, influenza and viral hepatitis
- Infectious mononucleosis
- Lymphocytic leukemia
- Autoimmune conditions like myasthenia gravis and thyrotoxicosis
- Relative lymphocytosis is due to a decrease in the number of other WBCs especially neutrophils as in typhoid
- In children, lymphocyte count is high.

Lymphopenia (<1500/mm³)

- Corticosteroid and immunosuppressive therapy
- Aplastic anemia due to excessive radiation
- Acquired immunodeficiency syndrome (AIDS)
- Hypersplenism.

Monocytes

Monocytosis (>800/mm³)

Monocytosis is a rare condition, may be seen in:
- Protozoal infections like malaria; kala-azar, amoebiasis and rickettsial infections.
- Bacterial infections like tuberculosis, typhoid, syphilis, brucellosis and sub-acute bacterial endocarditis.
- Monocytic leukemia and myeloproliferative disorders.
- Collagen vascular disorders like SLE.
- Infectious mononucleosis or glandular fever and Hodgkin's disease.

Monocytopenia

It is rare and is seen in aplastic anemia.

Pancytopenia

Pancytopenia is a condition where all the formed elements of blood are reduced. It is seen in the following conditions:
- Aplastic anemia due drugs or excessive radiation
- Hypersplenism

- Disseminated tuberculosis
- In conditions of bone marrow infiltration like malignant lymphomas (Hodgkin's disease), multiple myeloma, secondary carcinoma, myelosclerosis.

Agranulocytosis or Granulocytopenia

In agranulocytosis, there is decrease in granulocyte count. So, there is relative increase in agranulocyte count and hence called **agranulocytosis**. Usually, drugs that cause bone marrow depression cause this condition.

Arneth Count

Arneth devised a technique by which neutrophils can be classified depending on the number of lobes in the nucleus. This is known as **Arneth count**. If the number of lobes is less, it comes under younger series of cells. If the number of lobes is more, the cells are older. **Shift to left**, i.e., more number of younger cells, is seen in pyogenic infections. If most of the neutrophils in peripheral blood show four or more lobes in the nucleus, it is called **shift to right**; seen in pernicious anemia, neutropenia, etc. The younger forms will be absent in conditions of neutropenia caused by diminished formation of blood cells in bone marrow (pancytopenia) as in bone marrow depression.

Younger Cells

- Single lobe—5%
- 2 lobes—30%
- 3 lobes—45%.

Older Cells

- 4 lobes—18%
- 5 lobes—2%.

Schilling Index

The bone marrow precursors of leucocytes in peripheral blood are also taken into account in finding out **Schilling index**. Schilling index is important to assess the severity of leukemia. In leukemia, the bone marrow precursors will be present in plenty in the peripheral smear. The percentages of bone marrow precursors normally present in the peripheral blood are:

- Myelocyte—0%
- Metamyelocyte—1%
- Band form—2-6%.

The rest of the granulocytes will be mature in normal states.

■ LEUKOPOIESIS

PY2.6: Describe WBC formation (granulopoiesis) and its regulation.

Formation of Granulocytes and Monocytes (Flowchart 14.1)

Colony forming unit-granulocyte monocyte (CFU- GM) is further classified into CFU-G, which forms neutrophils,

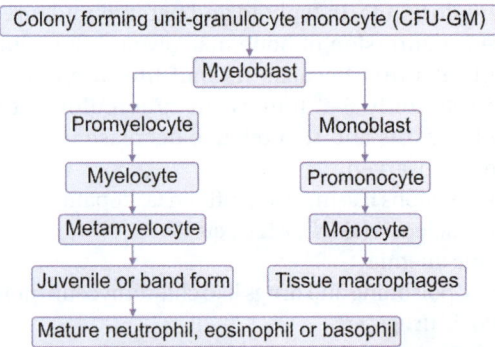

Flowchart 14.1: Stages of leukopoiesis.

CFU-E forming eosinophils, CFU-B forming basophils and CFU-M forming monocytes. Normal duration of granulopoiesis (myelopoiesis) is 12 days and the newly formed granulocytes are stored in the bone marrow. The store of granulocytes present in the marrow is 10–15 times more than those present in the circulating pool. Myeloblasts, promyelocytes and myelocytes are together known as the **proliferative or mitotic pool** and the metamyelocytes, band forms and segmented neutrophils are known as the **post-mitotic maturation pool**.

Formation of Lymphocytes

Pluripotent hemopoietic stem cells in the bone marrow differentiate into **lymphocyte stem cells**. These stem cells migrate to the **thymus** and after differentiation reach the lymphoid tissues like lymph nodes and spleen and mature to lymphocytes. Stages of lymphoid series are:

- Lymphoblast
- Prolymphocyte
- Large lymphocyte
- Small lymphocyte.

Some of the lymphocytes processed in the thymus form T-lymphocytes, which are involved in cellular immunity. Some lymphocytes processed in the liver and bone marrow gets differentiated to B-lymphocytes involved in humoral immunity. In birds, B-cell processing occurs in the **bursa of Fabricius** and hence the name B-lymphocyte. In humans, this bursa is absent.

Control of Leukopoiesis

Leukopoiesis is controlled mainly by the products of damaged leukocytes. For example, during tissue damage, infections, etc., there is increase in the production and release of leukocytes by products of injury, bacterial toxins, etc. Leukocytosis is a very important finding in infections and trauma. **Cytokines like colony stimulating factors (CSFs), interleukins and tumor necrosis factor (TNF) are responsible for the regulation of leukopoiesis.**

- **Interleukins** are cytokines expressed mainly by white blood cells. The function of interleukins are modulation of growth; differentiation and activation during inflammatory and immune responses. Fifteen different

types of interleukins are known. Those that are involved in leukopoiesis are:
a. IL-1, IL-6 and IL-3 helps in the maturation of stem cells
b. IL-5 is also called eosinophilic growth factor
c. IL-3 and IL-4 help in the development of basophils
d. IL-2 inhibits myelopoiesis (development of RBCs, platelets and granulocyte-monocyte series)

❖ Colony-stimulating factors are glycoproteins formed by monocytes and T-lymphocytes. The important colony-stimulating factors are **granulocyte-monocyte colony stimulating factor (GM-CSF), granulocyte colony stimulating factor (G-CSF) and monocyte colony stimulating factor (M-CSF)**. GM-CSF secreted by fibroblasts, vascular endothelial cells, monocytes and T-lymphocytes stimulates differentiation and proliferation of pluripotent stem cells into committed cells. They also help in the development of granulocyte and monocyte precursors into mature cells.

❖ **Tumor necrosis factor** helps in the proliferation and differentiation of stem cells.

❖ **Prostaglandins** formed from monocytes and **lactoferrin** also play a role in the regulation of leukopoiesis.

MULTIPLE CHOICE QUESTIONS

1. **Secondary granules of neutrophils contain:**
   a. Lactoferrin   b. Catalase
   c. Myeloperoxidase   d. Nucleotidase

2. **The ratio of myeloid series to erythroid series in the bone marrow is:**
   a. 3:2   b. 2:3
   c. 3:1   d. 1:3

3. **The ratio of white blood cell to red blood cell in the peripheral blood is:**
   a. 1:7   b. 1:70
   c. 1:700   d. 1:7000

4. **The process by which leukocytes are arranged along the endothelium is called?**
   a. Margination   b. Rolling
   c. Diapedesis   d. Chemotaxis

5. **Cell involved in immunity against parasitic infection is:**
   a. Neutrophil   b. Eosinophil
   c. Basophil   d. Lymphocyte

6. **Charcot-Leyden crystals are formed by:**
   a. Eosinophils   b. Neutrophils
   c. c. Lymphocytes d. Monocytes

7. **Histamine is present in all of the following cells, *except*:**
   a. Eosinophils   b. Basophils
   c. Lymphocytes   d. Mast cells

8. **The blood cell that contains heparin is:**
   a. Neutrophil   b. Eosinophil
   c. Basophil   d. Monocyte

9. **All of the following statements regarding lymphocytes are true, *except*:**
   a. Large lymphocytes may contain reddish violet granules
   b. 70–80% of circulating lymphocytes are T-lymphocytes
   c. Peroxidase test is positive
   d. Null cells include cells like natural killer cells

10. **In allergic conditions there will be:**
    a. Basophilia
    b. Eosinophilia
    c. Neutrophilia
    d. Lymphocytosis

11. **Macrophages are mature forms of:**
    a. Neutrophil   b. Monocyte
    c. Eosinophil   d. Lymphocyte

12. **Neutrophil secretes all, *except*:**
    a. Superoxide dismutase
    b. Myeloperoxidase
    c. Acid phosphatase
    d. Histamine

13. **Average half-life of neutrophil in circulation is:**
    a. 6 hours   b. 6 days
    c. 10 days   d. 15 days

14. **The function common to neutrophils, monocytes and macrophages is:**
    a. Humoral immunity
    b. Phagocytosis
    c. Liberation of histamine
    d. Destruction of old erythrocytes

15. **Correct statement regarding T-lymphocyte is:**
    a. Mature in lymph nodes
    b. Produce antibodies
    c. Responsible for humoral immunity
    d. Principal cell in lymph node cortical center

16. **Arneth count is:**
    a. Counting the lymphocytes
    b. Counting the lobes in the neutrophil
    c. Counting the granules in the eosinophil
    d. WBC counting in bone marrow

17. **All the following statements about lymphocytes are correct, *except*:**
    a. Produced by thymus, red bone marrow, spleen and lymph node
    b. Concentration falls in the blood abruptly and immune reaction is disturbed after removal of thymus in adults
    c. Probably change into plasma cells
    d. Constitute 20–40% of leukocytes

18. **Neutropenia is seen in all, *except*:**
    a. Pernicious anemia
    b. Severe bacterial infection
    c. SLE
    d. Bone marrow depression

19. Which one of the following statement regarding monocyte is incorrect?
    a. More common in blood than eosinophil and basophil
    b. Produced in the adult by bone marrow and lymph nodes
    c. Unlike neutrophil does not accumulate outside circulation in area of inflammation
    d. Not classified as a granulocyte

20. The true statement regarding lymphocyte is:
    a. All lymphocytes are released from bone marrow
    b. Interact with eosinophils to produce platelets
    c. Are unaffected by hormones
    d. Are part of body's defense against cancer

21. In parasitic infection, the following cell count is increased:
    a. Basophil
    b. Lymphocyte
    c. Eosinophil
    d. Neutrophil

22. The cell which is similar in function to mast cell is?
    a. Basophil
    b. Lymphocyte
    c. Eosinophil
    d. Monocyte

23. Delayed type of hypersensitivity reaction is mediated by:
    a. T-lymphocyte
    b. B-lymphocyte
    c. Monocyte
    d. Eosinophil

24. The property by which leukocytes can squeeze through pores in the capillary is called?
    a. Chemotaxis
    b. Opsonization
    c. Pinocytosis
    d. Diapedesis

25. Regarding monocytes, all of the following statements are correct, *except*:
    a. More common in blood than eosinophil and basophil
    b. Not classified as granulocyte
    c. Produced in the adults in the bone marrow and lymph nodes
    d. Does not accumulate outside circulation in areas of inflammation

26. Cell type which lacks HLA antigen:
    a. Monocyte
    b. Neutrophil
    c. Erythrocyte
    d. Eosinophil

27. G-CSF and GM-CSF in hematopoiesis produces:
    a. Erythrocytosis
    b. Leukocytosis
    c. Thrombocytoss
    d. Leukopenia

28. Arneth count is:
    a. Counting of lymphocytes
    b. Counting the lobes of neutrophil
    c. Counting the granules in eosinophil
    d. WBC counting in bone marrow

29. All of the following mediate anaphylaxis, *except*:
    a. Serotonin
    b. Bradykinin
    c. Prostaglandin
    d. Anaphylatoxin

30. All the following statements regarding lymphocyte are true, *except*:
    a. Produced by thymus, red bone marrow, lymph node and spleen
    b. Lymphocyte count falls abruptly and immune reaction gets disturbed after removal of thymus in adult
    c. B-lymphocyte change into plasma cell
    d. They do not perform phagocytic function

31. Slow reacting substance of anaphylaxis (SRS-A) is
    a. Prostaglandin
    b. Serotonin
    c. Histamine
    d. Leukotriene

32. Macrophages are the mature forms of:
    a. Neutrophil
    b. Basophil
    c. Monocyte
    d. Lymphocyte

ANSWERS

1. a	2. c	3. c	4. a	5. b
6. a	7. c	8. c	9. c	10. b
11. b	12. d	13. a	14. b	15. a
16. b	17. b	18. b	19. c	20. d
21. c	22. a	23. a	24. d	25. d
26. c	27. b	28. b	29. a	30. b
31. d	32. c			

Spleen and Reticuloendothelial System

CHAPTER 15

LEARNING OBJECTIVES
- Describe the functions of spleen
- Explain the functions of reticuloendothelial system

SPLEEN

Central lymphoid organs include bone marrow and thymus whereas **peripheral lymphoid organs** include spleen, lymph nodes, Peyer's patches, tonsils and adenoids. Spleen is the largest lymphoid tissue in the body, which is specialized for filtering blood. It weighs about 150 g in adult. Spleen is covered by a connective tissue capsule. The parenchymal tissue enclosed within the capsule is the **splenic pulp**. It is of two distinct types, white pulp and red pulp. **White pulp** is composed of typical lymphatic tissue, whereas **red pulp** is composed of atypical lymphatic tissue. White pulp contains lymphocytes, plasma cells and macrophages.

Red pulp consists of splenic sinuses or sinusoids and splenic cords. **Splenic sinuses** are long vascular channels 40 μm in diameter and they extend throughout the red pulp. The wall of the splenic sinuses is composed of specialized reticular cells of phagocytic type and belongs to the reticuloendothelial system. **Splenic cords** form partitions between the sinuses. These cellular cords form a spongy network of lymphatic tissue, which gradually merges into the white pulp. The blood from the splenic venous sinuses leaves the spleen through the splenic veins.

Functions of the Spleen

- Spleen plays an important role in producing blood cells in the embryo. In embryo, the red pulp contains myelocytes, erythroblasts, megakaryocytes, etc. Extramedullary hemopoiesis occurs in the spleen in adults under circumstances in which the bone marrow is unable to meet the needs.
- In humans, large number of red blood cells (RBCs) is stored in the spleen. These are released into circulation in emergency conditions like exercise, hemorrhage, etc. Spleen acts as a reservoir of blood mainly in animals like dogs. When the spleen contracts, it may release 150 mL of blood (mainly erythrocytes) into circulation in man. Sympathetic stimulation causes splenic contraction.
- Spleen also stores platelets and it contains 1/3rd of the total body platelets and a significant number of marginated neutrophils. The increase in platelet and leukocyte count seen after exercise is due to release of these sequestered cells from spleen. Splenectomy is done to increase platelet count in thrombocytopenia.
- The macrophages (reticuloendothelial cells) of splenic pulp phagocytose microorganisms like bacteria, parasites, and other foreign bodies.
- Spleen is considered as the graveyard of old or senescent blood cells and fragmented blood cells.
- Breakdown of hemoglobin and formation of bilirubin also occur in the spleen.
- Spleen is an important blood filter that removes spherocytes and other abnormal and useless red cells. It allows only normal, young, active cells to pass into the circulation.
- Spleen also plays a significant role in immune system. Spleen contains about 25% of T-lymphocytes and 15% of B-lymphocytes and forms an important site of antibody production. Numerous plasma cells are present in white pulp. It also removes antibody-coated bacteria and antibody-coated blood cells from circulation. In the absence of spleen, bacterial infections are more common and more severe. Splenectomized animals cannot be immunized against tetanus toxin.
- The deformed red cells that contain the malarial parasite are removed by the spleen.

Effects of Splenectomy (Surgical Removal of Spleen)

- Leukocytosis and thrombocytosis
- Anisocytosis and poikilocytosis
- Increased susceptibility to infections with organisms like *Streptococcus pneumoniae*
- Presence of occasional nucleated erythrocytes in peripheral blood.

RETICULOENDOTHELIAL SYSTEM OR TISSUE MACROPHAGE SYSTEM

The system is called **reticuloendothelial system** because the reticuloendothelial (RE) cells generally occupy the endothelial lining and the reticular spaces of the connective tissues. These cells develop from mesenchyme. One of the characteristic features of reticuloendothelial cells is that they can phagocytose large colloidal particles. These cells can be demonstrated by **vital staining**. The cells of the reticuloendothelial system can be stained by intravenously injecting vital dyes like **trypan blue, lithium carmine**, etc. The dye particles are engulfed only by the cells of the reticuloendothelial system. Now this system is usually referred to as the **tissue macrophage system**.

Monocytes enter the blood from the bone marrow and circulate for about 72 hours. Then they enter the tissues and become **tissue macrophages or reticuloendothelial cells**. The cells increase in size and the number of lysosomes and mitochondria increases. The tissue macrophages are of two types:
1. Mobile or wandering macrophages
2. Fixed macrophages.

Mobile or Wandering Macrophages

The **mobile or wandering macrophages** wander through the tissues and perform scavenger functions of eliminating microorganisms and other foreign particles that invade the tissues. Wandering reticuloendothelial cells include:
- Wandering histiocytes found in splenic pulp, lymph node, bone marrow, etc. Sometimes, they contain many nuclei, e.g., osteoclasts and megakaryocytes of the bone marrow.
- Monocytes are the wandering reticuloendothelial cells in blood.

Fixed Macrophages

Some of the macrophages become attached to certain tissues in the body to form **fixed macrophages**. *Fixed reticuloendothelial cells include*:
- Tissue histiocytes found in connective tissue and loose areolar tissue.
- Reticulum cells of spleen, lymph node and bone marrow.
- Reticuloendothelial cells present in the lining membrane of blood sinuses of spleen, bone marrow, adrenal cortex, pituitary and liver. In liver, they are called Kupffer cells.
- Microglia, which are small cells found in central nervous system.

The life span of tissue macrophages is about 3 months. These cells do not re-enter the circulation. Some of them form multinucleated giant cells seen in chronic inflammatory diseases, such as tuberculosis. The tissue macrophages include **Kupffer cells of liver, pulmonary alveolar macrophages (dust cells and heart failure cells), microglia in the brain, littoral cells of bone marrow, osteoclasts of bone marrow, histiocytes in connective tissue, macrophages in spleen, lymph node, etc**. All of these cells have escaped from blood. The shape of the cells varies in different sites. Histiocytes are oval shaped, macrophages in spleen are elongated, star shaped in bone marrow and lymph glands.

The tissue macrophages become activated by lymphokines liberated from T-lymphocytes. The activated macrophages migrate to the site of inflammation in response to chemotactic stimuli at the site. They phagocytose and kill the bacteria with the help of bacteriolytic substances present in the lysosomes. The process is similar to those occurring in neutrophils.

Functions of Reticuloendothelial Cells

- Defense against invading organisms such as bacteria and viruses is the most important function. They ingest and destroy the organisms by phagocytosis. During infectious states, the reticuloendothelial cells increase in number and there will be enlargement of organs like lymph node, spleen, etc., which are rich in reticuloendothelial cells. For example, there will be cervical lymphadenopathy in pulmonary tuberculosis and inguinal lymphadenopathy in infections of the lower limb.
- It processes the antigen and stimulates the production of antibody.
- Dust cells of lungs remove foreign particles entering the lungs.
- RE cells can help in repair processes and are called scavenger cells. They ingest cellular debris, fibrin, bacteria, etc., from the inflamed area and promote healing.
- It can ingest and destroy old and fragmented RBC, white blood cell (WBC) and platelets. Breakdown of hemoglobin and formation of bilirubin occurs in the reticuloendothelial cells.
- Iron released from hemoglobin is stored in the reticuloendothelial cells. They also store excess lipid and mucoproteins.
- Manufacture of plasma proteins like serum globulin to some extent.
- *Formation of tissue cells*: As the cells of the reticuloendothelial system are undifferentiated, they can be converted to ordinary connective tissue cells such as fibroblasts. This occurs during repair stage of inflammatory process.

MULTIPLE CHOICE QUESTIONS

1. All the following cells come under reticuloendothelial system, *except*:
    a. Microglia
    b. Ependymal cells
    c. Osteoclasts
    d. Pulmonary alveolar macrophages
2. Immune complexes are removed from blood by:
    a. B lymphocyte
    b. Basophil
    c. Plasma cell
    d. Kupffer cell
3. Mast cells originate from:
    a. Liver
    b. Red bone marrow
    c. Spleen
    d. Lymph node

4. **All the following statements regarding spleen in humans are correct, *except*:**
   a. Helps in the formation of RBC in intrauterine life
   b. In emergency, extramedullary hemopoiesis occurs in the spleen in adults
   c. Contains lymphoid tissue concerned with lymphocyte formation
   d. Acts as a reservoir of blood

5. **Conversion of heme to bilirubin occurs mainly in:**
   a. Kidney
   b. Liver
   c. Bone marrow
   d. Spleen

6. **Central lymphoid organ include:**
   a. Bone marrow
   b. Lymph node
   c. Spleen
   d. Tonsil

ANSWERS

1. b   2. d   3. b   4. d   5. d
6. a

Immune System

CHAPTER 16

LEARNING OBJECTIVES

Must know
- Define immunity and classify the different types of immunity
- Explain the mechanism of innate immunity
- Describe the development of immune system
- Describe humoral and cellular immunity
- Classify antibodies and give their functions
- Differentiate between primary and secondary immune responses

Desirable to know
- Understand the role of cytokines, chemokines and complement system in regulation of immunity
- Explain the role of the complement system in immunity
- Mention the mechanism of immunological tolerance

INTRODUCTION

Our body is being continuously challenged by potentially harmful invaders such as bacteria, viruses and other microorganisms. Immune system is the defense system that has evolved in vertebrates to protect them from invading pathogenic microorganisms and other foreign substances not found in human tissues. It consists of specialized cells that sense and respond to these invaders. Normally, the immune system not only protects the host from exogenous factors, such as microorganisms or toxins, but also protects the body from the attacks of endogenous factors such as cancer cells or autoimmune phenomena. The circulating immunological cells include neutrophils, eosinophils, basophils, lymphocytes and monocytes. Tissue macrophages derived from monocytes; and mast cells are also part of the immune system. Sometimes the body may face inappropriate immune attacks as in autoimmune diseases where the immune system attack body's own tissues.

CYTOKINES, CHEMOKINES AND THE COMPLEMENT SYSTEM

Cytokines, chemokines and the complement system comprise the soluble regulators of immunity.

Cytokines

Cytokines are a broad category of small proteins that are important in cell signaling and constitute one of the regulators of the immune system. They are very essential for regulation of the growth and activation of immune cells. They are included under the super family of chemokines, which are substances that attract neutrophils at the site of inflammation.

Once activated, the immune cells communicate by means of cytokines and chemokines. **Cytokines** are hormone like molecules secreted mainly by lymphocytes, mast cells and macrophages. They are also secreted by neurons, neuroglial cells and endothelial cells. Cytokines include interleukins, tumor necrosis factors-α and β, interferons, transforming growth factor-β and granulocyte-macrophage colony stimulating factor. More than 100 cytokines have been identified. The principal cytokines are listed in **Table 16.1**.

The cytokine receptor belongs to 'enzyme-linked receptor' family. When cytokine binds with its receptor, the enzyme tyrosine kinase associated with the enzyme-linked receptor is activated. It phosphorylates STAT (signal transducer and activation of transcription) which act as transcription factor (*refer* JAK-STAT pathway).

Chemokines

A superfamily of cytokines is the chemokine family. **Chemokines** are substances that attract neutrophils and other leukocytes to areas of inflammation or immune response (*refer* chemotaxis). Over 40 chemokines have now been identified. They also play a role in the regulation of cell growth and angiogenesis. The chemokine receptors are G protein-coupled receptors, which causes the migration of the leukocyte towards the source of inflammation. Cytokines and chemokines help the immune cell to kill viruses, bacteria and other foreign cells by secreting other cytokines and by activating the complement system.

Functions of Cytokines

- Interleukin-1 stimulates B lymphocytes, T lymphocytes, activates neutrophil and aids in chemotaxis and phagocytosis

CHAPTER 16 — Immune System

Table 16.1: Source and functions of different cytokines.

Cytokine	Source	Functions
IL-1	Monocytes and macrophages	Proliferation of helper T cells Act on hypothalamus and produce fever
IL-2 (T cell growth factor)	Helper T cell	Activates non-killer cells Proliferation of helper T cell and cytotoxic T cell
IL-4 (B cell stimulating factor)	Helper T cell	Stimulates B cells and causes plasma cells to secrete antibodies
IL-5	CD4 T cells and mast cells	Stimulates B cells and increases antibody production
Tumor necrosis factor (TNF)	Macrophages	Stimulates accumulation of neutrophils and macrophages at the site of inflammation
Transforming growth factor-β	T cells and macrophages	Inhibits proliferation of T cells and activation of macrophages
γ Interferon	Helper and cytotoxic T cell, non-killer cells	Stimulates phagocytosis by neutrophils and macrophages, activates NK cells, enhances both cell mediated and humoral immunity
α and β interferon	Virus infected cells	Stimulates T cell growth Activates NK cells Inhibits cell growth and suppresses formation of some tumors
Lymphotoxin	Cytotoxic T cell	Kills infected target cells by activating enzymes that cause fragmentation of DNA
Perforins	Cytotoxic T cell and NK cells	Perforates cell membrane of infected target cells and causes cytolysis
Macrophage migration inhibiting factor	Cytotoxic T cell	Prevents macrophages from leaving the site of infection
Granzymes	Cytotoxic T cell and NK cells	Stimulates apoptosis of infected target cells
Granulysin	Cytotoxic T cell	Creates holes in the microbial plasma membrane that kill the microbes

- IL-2 stimulates cytotoxic T cells and destroys tumor cells
- IL-3 is known as 'multi-colony stimulating factor'. It acts as growth factor for bone marrow stem cells.
- IL-4 helps in B lymphocyte proliferation and antibody synthesis. It is involved in allergy and nematode infection as it augments IgE synthesis.
- Tumor necrosis factor (TNF) can directly kill tumor cells and can act as endogenous pyrogen. TNF-α is implicated in the pathogenesis of rheumatoid arthritis, Crohn's disease, etc. TNF-β is implicated in the pathogenesis of multiple sclerosis, insulin-dependent diabetes mellitus, etc.
- Transforming growth factor-β act as growth factor to transform fibroblast to produce collagen and more matrix to promote wound healing. It also regulates T cell proliferation, has immunosuppressive effect and can be used as therapeutic agent in multiple sclerosis, myasthenia gravis, etc. It can inhibit thrombopoietin and prevent excess platelet production.
- Colony stimulating factor produced by T cells, B cells, macrophages, etc., can act on bone marrow to increase the production of granulocytes and monocytes.
- Interferon α and β produced by virally infected cells inhibits viral protein synthesis and induce resistance to viral infection. Interferon-γ produced by helper T cell (T_H cell) and natural killer cells (NK cells) activates macrophages and enhance killing of phagocytosed bacteria.

APPLIED ASPECT

Cytokine storm is a fatal immune reaction with highly elevated blood levels of various cytokines. Patient presents with high fever, edema, fatigue, nausea, etc. Anti-inflammatory drugs or immunosuppressants are not effective in this condition. It is seen in graft versus host disease, acute respiratory distress syndrome, septicemia, avian influenza, COVID-19, etc. In many serious COVID-19 cases, the blood contains very high levels of the immune system proteins called cytokines. Rather than just fighting the virus, these cytokines attack body's own cells and tissues leading to their damage especially the lungs. As the lung tissue breaks down, the alveoli become leaky and get filled with fluid, causing pneumonia and respiratory distress syndrome, which is fatal. The cytokine IL-6 is linked to the risk of death. Drugs that block the cytokine IL-6 receptor may be of some help.

Cytokines are used as drugs in certain conditions. Interferon-α (IFN-α) is used to treat hepatitis B, C; and AIDS, IFN-β is effective in multiple sclerosis; INF-γ is effective in chronic granulomatous disease.

Recombinant IL-11 (**Oprelvekin**) stimulates bone marrow to induce platelet production in patients undergoing chemotherapy; recombinant colony stimulating factor (**Filgrastim**) is effective in chemotherapy-induced neutropenia. It is used after hemopoietic stem cell transplantation.

Certain drugs act by blocking the action of cytokines. For example, **etanercept** (tumor necrosis factor receptor inhibitor) is used to treat rheumatoid arthritis, ankylosing spondylitis, psoriatic arthritis, etc.

IL-1 and TNF-α are shown to have a role in the development of atherosclerosis.

The Complement System

The **complement system** is a system of about 30 plasma proteins designated **C1 to C9,** many of which are enzyme precursors. C1 is further divided into C1q, C1r and C1s. Though there are more than 30 proteins (enzymes) in the complement system, only the above mentioned 11 proteins are categorized. They are named so because they complement the effects of antibodies.

Normally, the complement proteins are in the inactive state. Three different pathways or enzyme cascades activate the complement system (1) classical pathway: (2) mannose-binding lectin pathway and (3) alternative pathway. All three pathways cause the activation of the inactive complement protein C3 to active C3 (C3a). The rest of the steps are same in all pathways. C3a activates other complement proteins.

Classical Pathway

The classical pathway is triggered by antigen-antibody complexes (immune complexes). Activation of one complement protein will activate another one and so on till a large number of complement proteins get activated. This is similar to the enzyme cascade theory of the intrinsic pathway of blood coagulation. The activity of the complement system is triggered when C1 binds to the antigen–antibody complex. The activated C1, in turn, activates the other complement proteins in a series of cascade reactions. The final product of complement activation is C5b-C6-C7-C8-C9 complex and it leads to cell lysis. Many of the by-products in the pathway cause vasodilatation (C2b), chemotaxis (C5b), opsonization (C3a) and mast cell degranulation (C3b).

Mannose-binding Lectin Pathway

Mannose-binding lectin pathway is triggered when the plasma protein lectin binds with mannose groups on the surface of bacteria. This leads to activation of C3. C3a causes further activation of other complement proteins as in the classical pathway.

Alternative or Properdin Pathway

Alternative pathway is triggered by contact of a circulating protein called **factor-1** with polysaccharides present on the surface of viruses, bacteria, fungi and tumor cells. This leads to the activation of complement protein C3. **Properdin** is a circulating protein which stabilizes the activated enzyme complexes in the complement system.

Functions of the Complement System

- **Opsonization, chemotaxis and phagocytosis:** Complement proteins help in killing invading organisms by promoting opsonization, chemotaxis and phagocytosis by phagocytes (neutrophils, monocytes and macrophages). C3b activates phagocytosis by neutrophils and macrophages which engulf the bacteria to which antigen-antibody complexes are attached. This process of opsonization increases the number of bacteria destroyed by many hundred folds. C5a initiates chemotaxis of neutrophils and macrophages to migrate into the area where the antigenic agent is present.
- **Lysis of the organism:** They also lead to lysis of the microbial cells. Cell lysis is brought about by inserting proteins called **perforins** into the cell membranes of the microbes. These create holes which permit free flow of ions and thus cause disruption of the membrane polarity of the invading organism. C5bC6C7C8C9 (lytic complex) directly act on the microbial cell membrane and lead to their rupture.
- **Agglutination:** The complement products cause the invading organisms combined with the antibodies to adhere to one another leading to their agglutination and destruction.
- **Neutralization of viruses:** The complement enzymes can attack the structures of certain viruses and render them non-virulent.
- **Activation of mast cells and basophils:** Fragments of the complement system C3a, C4a and C5a activate mast cells and basophils leading to the release of histamine, heparin and other substances into the affected area. These substances can increase local blood flow and leakage of fluid and plasma proteins into the tissue leading to local tissue reaction that help to inactivate the antigenic agent.
- **Inflammatory effects:** Activation of mast cells and basophils leads to local inflammation. There will be further increase in blood flow, capillary leakage of proteins and coagulation of proteins in the tissue spaces. This prevents the movement of the invading organism to other parts.
- Complement system activates B-lymphocyte and thus facilitates humoral immunity
- They serve as a bridge from innate to acquired immunity by activating B-lymphocytes and aiding immune memory.
- Complement proteins help in the disposal of waste products (debris) after apoptosis.

IMMUNE RESPONSE

Immune response includes:
- Recognition
- Response
  - Effector response
  - Memory response

Recognition (Self/Nonself)

The immune system is able to recognize and discriminate between foreign molecules and body's own cells and proteins.

Response

Once the foreign substance is recognized by the immune system, by a variety of cells and molecules, it eliminates the foreign substance. This is known as **effector response**.

Exposure to the same foreign substance later produces a heightened immune reaction to eliminate the pathogen and prevent disease. This is called **memory response**.

IMMUNITY

PY2.10: Define and classify different types of immunity. Describe the development of immunity and its regulation.

Definition

Immunity is defined as the state of protection from infectious disease or it is the ability of the body to resist different types of foreign bodies like bacteria, virus, parasites, toxic substances, etc., which enter the body.

Immunity is of two types:
1. Innate or nonspecific immunity or natural immunity
2. Acquired or adaptive or specific immunity

Acquired immunity does not function independent of innate immunity. Both these systems work together to eliminate a foreign invader.

INNATE IMMUNITY

Innate or natural immunity is the nonspecific defense mechanisms of the body, which are present from birth. Despite the lack of specificity, innate immunity is largely responsible for protection against a large number of environmental microorganisms and foreign substances. It provides the first line of defense against infections and it also triggers the more specific acquired immune response. It comprises four types of defensive barriers:
1. Anatomic barrier
2. Physiologic barrier
3. Phagocytic barrier
4. Inflammatory barrier

Anatomic Barrier

Skin and mucous membrane form anatomic barriers. The skin and epithelial surfaces serve as the first line of defense of the innate immune system. Skin secretes sebum, which contains lactic acid and fatty acid and these are responsible for maintaining the pH of skin between 3 and 5. This protects the skin from many bacteria and fungi.

Physiologic Barrier

Temperature, HCl of stomach, saliva, tears, chemical mediators like lysozyme, interferon, basic polypeptides, complement proteins, etc., act as physiological barriers in immunity.
- **Lysozyme** is a mucolytic polysaccharide that attacks bacteria and destroy them.
- **Interferons comprise a group of proteins produced by virus-infected cells. Interferon binds to nearby cells and induces a generalized antiviral state.**
- **Basic polypeptides present in blood react with and inactivate certain types of gram positive bacteria.**
- **Complement system** is a group of about 30 normally inactive proteins present in plasma. The union of antigen with IgG or IgM antibody initiates activation of the classic complement pathway. When one complement is activated, it activates other complement proteins (complement cascades), which attack and destroy microbes.

Phagocytic Barrier

The cells that mediate innate immunity are **monocytes, neutrophils, tissue macrophages and natural killer (NK) cells**, which kill and digest the microorganisms. **NK cells** are large lymphocytes that are not T cells but are cytotoxic. Unlike T cells, they lack antigen specific T-cell receptors. They nonspecifically kill any cell that is coated with immunoglobulin (IgG). They do not require major histocompatibility complex (MHC) molecules for antigen recognition. Thus, NK cells provide innate immunity. NK cells are particularly effective against foreign cells, tumor cells and virus-infected cells. **Eosinophil** granules contain enzymes and toxic molecules that destroy larvae of helminthes.

Inflammatory Barrier

Inflammation is a form of natural immunity. Acute phase proteins like **C-reactive proteins** are released from infected tissues when there is tissue damage. These bind to the cell wall of microorganisms and this binding activates the complement system. This, in turn, causes lysis of pathogen or favors phagocytosis.

Inflammatory mediators released during immune responses include histamine, proteolytic enzymes, kinins, platelet activation factor, leukotriene, prostaglandins, thromboxane, etc. These substances cause vascular dilation and increased permeability. Vasodilation at the site of injury or infection causes entry of clotting factors from capillaries into the site of injury. This forms a clot, which walls off the injured or infected area from the rest of the body, thus preventing the spread of infection. Due to vasodilatation, there is exudation of plasma into the interstitial space and the exudate contains large number of neutrophils, which phagocytose the invading organisms.

Antigens

Substances that are recognized as foreign by the immune system and which provoke immune responses are called **antigens**. They are mostly proteins and large polypeptides. Antigens should have high molecular weight of 8000 or more. Immune responses are also formed against nucleic acids and lipids if they are in the form of conjugated proteins like lipoprotein, glycoprotein, nucleoprotein, etc. Entire microbes or parts of microbes act as antigens. Bacterial structures, such as flagella, capsule, cell wall, bacterial toxins, etc., can act as antigen. Non-microbial antigens include pollen, egg white, incompatible blood cells, transplanted tissues, etc.

Lymphocytes are responsible for mediating acquired immunity. T lymphocytes have specialized receptors for antigens. In B lymphocyte, the immunoglobulins present on the cell membrane (IgM and IgD) serve as receptors for antigens.

Hapten

Hapten is a small non-protein molecule, which by itself cannot elicit antibody production, as it has no antigenic property. But when combined with a carrier protein molecule, it forms a new antigen capable of stimulating production of specific immunoglobulins, the specificity of which depends on the hapten fraction rather than the carrier protein. The antibody can combine with the hapten directly without the help of the carrier. Some lipids and simple carbohydrates that are not antigenic are often powerful haptens. A secondary response can be elicited by a subsequent challenge by the same carrier—hapten complex, but not by the hapten combined with a different carrier. The presence of haptens in tissue proteins is one of the causes for producing autoimmunity.

Active and Passive Immunity

Depending on whether actively acquired or passively acquired, acquired immunity is classified into active immunity, which is actively acquired and passive immunity, which is passively acquired. **Active immunity** involves a direct encounter with the antigen. Here, there is development of immunological memory of the antigen so that on subsequent encounters, the response to the same antigen is more vigorous. Active immunization against a microbe can be achieved by injecting its antigens into the body.

Passive immunity is acquired without an encounter with the antigen. For example, during pregnancy, mother's antibodies cross the placenta and provide passive immunity to the fetus. Passive immunity does not confer immunological memory. Passive immunization can be achieved by injecting antibodies against specific microbial antigens.

DEVELOPMENT OF IMMUNE SYSTEM (FIG. 16.1)

In mammals, the primary lymphoid organs are the thymus and the bone marrow. The lymph nodes, spleen, and gut-associated lymphoid tissue (tonsils, Peyer's patches of the small intestine and the appendix) are the secondary lymphoid organs connected by blood and lymphatic vessels. All cells of the immune system are originally derived from the bone marrow.

During intrauterine life, lymphocyte precursors (committed lymphoid progenitor cells) come from the bone marrow and some go to the thymus and others go to the liver and spleen. Those that populate the thymus become transformed into **T lymphocytes** responsible for cellular immunity and **natural killer T cells (NKT cells)**. NKT cells are so called because they share features of both T lymphocytes and natural killer cells (NK cells). The processing in the thymus is favored by **thymosin**, a hormone produced by the thymus.

In the thymus the T lymphocytes divide rapidly and at the same time, develop extreme diversity for reacting against different specific antigens. One thymic lymphocyte develops specific reactivity against one antigen and the next lymphocyte develops specificity against another antigen. This process continues till there are thousands of different types of lymphocytes in the thymus with specific reactivity against many thousands of different antigens. These T lymphocytes leave the thymus and through the blood reach the lymphoid tissues in the body. The pre-processing of lymphocytes in the thymus occurs just before birth of the baby and continues for a few months after birth. Removal of the thymus few months before birth can prevent the development of cell-mediated immunity.

Those lymphocytes that populate the fetal liver and the bone marrow get transformed and processed into B lymphocytes and natural killer cells. After birth, processing of B lymphocytes occurs in the bone marrow. After leaving the thymus, liver and bone marrow, many of the T and B lymphocytes migrate to the lymph nodes. B lymphocytes differentiate into cells capable of producing various classes of immunoglobulins called plasma cells. Differences between T lymphocyte and B lymphocyte are given in **Table 16.2**.

Each of the preformed lymphocyte is capable of forming only one type of antibody or one type of T cell with a single type of specificity. Only one specific type of antigen can activate it. Once the specific type of lymphocyte is activated by its antigen, it reproduces enormously forming large number of lymphocytes of the same kind. If it is a B-lymphocyte, its progeny will secrete only the specific type of antibody that circulates in the body. If it is a T-lymphocyte, its progeny are specific sensitized T cells that are released into the lymph.

Table 16.2: Differences between T-lymphocytes and B-lymphocytes.

T-Lymphocyte	B-lymphocyte
Preprocessed in the thymus	Preprocessed in the liver during mid-fetal life and in the bone marrow during late fetal life and after birth
The whole cell develop reactivity against the antigen	Secrete antibodies that are the reactive agents
T-cells respond only to antigens that are bound to specific molecules called MHC proteins	B-lymphocytes can recognize intact antigens
Diversity is less when compared to B lymphocytes	They have greater diversity and form many million types of B-lymphocyte antibodies with different specific reactivity
Mediates cellular immunity	Mediates humoral immunity
They are of three types: cytotoxic, memory and helper T cells	They are of two types: plasma cells and memory B cells

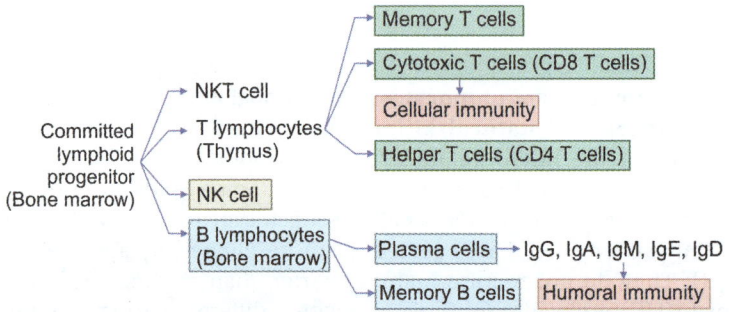

Fig. 16.1: Development of acquired immune system.
(NK: natural killer; Ig: immunoglobulin)

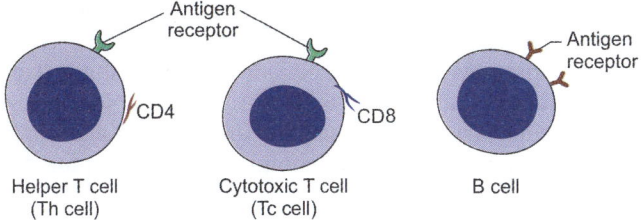

Fig. 16.2: Difference in the structure of Th cell, Tc cell and B lymphocyte.

From the lymph it reaches the general circulation. All such lymphocytes that are capable of forming one specific antibody or specific T cell are called a **clone of lymphocytes**. The lymphocytes in each clone are alike and are derived from one or a few lymphocytes of its specific type by repeated division. These mature T and B lymphocytes are highly specific and populate the lymphoid tissue.

T and B lymphocytes are morphologically similar. They can be identified only by detecting **markers** or surface antigens on their cell membrane. Markers or surface antigens on the surface of lymphocytes are assigned **clusters of differentiation (CD)** numbers. Markers on T cells include **CD8**, which is a glycoprotein closely associated with receptors of cytotoxic T cell (TC cells) and **CD4** is the marker present on helper T cell (**Fig. 16.2**).

B lymphocytes are of two types:
1. Plasma cells
2. Memory B cells

T lymphocytes are of three types:
1. Killer T cell or cytotoxic T cell (TC)
   - αβ TC
   - γδ TC
2. Helper T cell (Th)
   - T helper 1 (Th1)
   - Th2 cells
   - Th17 cells
   - T_{reg} cells (regulatory T cell)
3. Memory T cell

Cytotoxic T-cells

Cytotoxic T cells destroy transplanted cells and other foreign cells. Their development is aided and directed by helper T cells. γδ-T cells are prominent in the mucosa of gastrointestinal tract (GIT) and they form a link between the innate and acquired immune system by way of the cytokines they secrete. (NK and NKT cells are also cytotoxic lymphocytes even though they do not come under T or B types)

Helper T-cells

Helper T cells are the most numerous of the T cells. Three fourths of the T cells are T-helper cells. The lymphokines secreted by the T-helper cells are interleukin 2, 3, 4, 5, 6, granulocyte-monocyte colony-stimulating factor and interferon-γ. It is the T-helper cells that are destroyed by human immunodeficiency virus (HIV).

- **T-helper 1** (Th1) cells secrete IL-2 and γ-interferon and are concerned primarily with stimulating cellular immunity.
- **T helper 2** (Th2) cells secrete IL-4 and IL-5 and interact primarily with B cells in relation to humoral immunity.
- **Th17 cells** produce IL-6 and IL-17 in response to bacterial infections and they help to recruit neutrophils at the site of infection. They are also involved in the generation of harmful inflammatory responses that occur in autoimmune diseases.
- T_{reg} **cells** produce IL-10 to dampen T cell-driven responses. Previously they were grouped as **suppressor T cells** but now they are classified along with T-helper cells. Regulatory T cells suppress the functions of both cytotoxic and T-helper cells. This prevents the cytotoxic cells from causing excessive immune reaction that may damage body's own tissues. Regulatory T cells has an important role in limiting the ability of the immune system to attack one's own body tissues, called **immune tolerance.**

Functions of T-helper Cells

1. Stimulation of growth and proliferation of cytotoxic T cells. Interleukin 2 is responsible for this.
2. Stimulation of B-cell growth and differentiation to form plasma cells and antibodies. IL 4, 5, and 6 are responsible for this and these interleukins are called B-cell stimulating factors or B-cell growth factors.
3. Activation of macrophage system: T-helper cells activate macrophages and increase their phagocytic ability so that more bacteria are destroyed.
4. Feedback effect on T-helper cell: IL2 has positive feedback effect on stimulating activation of more helper T cells and amplify helper cell response.

Differences between helper T cell and cytotoxic T cell are given in **Table 16.3**.

> Approximately 70-80% of circulating blood lymphocytes is T cells and 10-15% is B cells; the remainder is referred to as natural killer cells (NK cells) and natural killer T cell (NKT cells). NK cells which are formed in the bone marrow are large granular lymphocytes that are not T cells, but are cytotoxic. They mediate innate immunity by releasing perforin, a pore forming protein that cause cytolysis of the invading cell. NKT cells differentiate in the thymus and shares features of both T lymphocytes and NK cells. They are also cytotoxic. Thus, there are four main types of cytotoxic lymphocytes in the body: αβ-TC, γδ-TC, NKT cell and NK cells.

Memory B Cells and T Cells

When B and T cells are activated by an antigen, some of them differentiate into memory B and T cells. These memory cells get converted to the effector cells when they come into contact with the same antigen later and an accelerated response is seen. The memory cells may live for decades. For example, immunity to measles is life-long. These cells are plentiful in the mucosa of the respiratory tract and gastrointestinal tract, which are always challenged by antigens. Chemotactic cytokines known as chemokines are involved in guiding activated lymphocytes to these locations.

Table 16.3: Difference between helper T cell and cytotoxic T cell.	
Helper T cell	**Cytotoxic T cell**
1. Contains CD4 co-receptor	1. Contains CD8 co-receptor
2. Binds to MHC-II protein	2. Binds to MHC-I protein
3. Binding promotes release of cytokines which activate lymphocytes	3. Kill target cells directly by inserting perforins and initiating apoptosis
4. Two types of helper T cells are Th1 cells which secrete IL-2 and γ-interferon concerned with cellular immunity and Th2 cells which secrete IL-4 and IL-5 concerned with humoral immunity	4. Two types are there αβ-T cells, γδ-T cells. αβ-T cells are circulating T cells which help to recognize MHC protein-antigen fragment complex. γδ-T cells are present in the mucosa of GIT and they secrete cytokines which form a link between innate and acquired immunity

ACQUIRED IMMUNITY OR SPECIFIC IMMUNITY

The ability of the body to defend itself against specific invading agents is called **specific immunity**. This capacity, which is *acquired after birth*, is also called **acquired immunity or adaptive immunity**. Acquired immunity develops only after the body is first attacked by an organism or toxin. It often takes weeks or months for the immunity to develop. It includes the ability of B-lymphocytes to produce antibodies and T-lymphocytes to produce cell surface receptors that are specific for one of the many millions of foreign substances that may invade the body. Acquired immunity is the basis of immunization which is very important in protecting human beings against several diseases and toxins.

Characteristics of Acquired Immunity

Acquired immunity is capable of specifically recognizing and selectively eliminating foreign antigens. It has the following characteristics:
1. Antigenic specificity
2. Immunologic memory
3. Self/nonself recognition.

Antigenic Specificity

Each toxin or each type of organism contains one or more specific proteins or large polysaccharides in their structure that are different from all others. These substances which are called antigens initiate the acquired immunity. Their antigenicity usually depends on regularly recurring molecular groups called **epitopes** on their surface. Antibodies are so antigen-specific that they can differentiate between two antigen molecules that differ by only a single amino acid.

When a specific antigen comes in contact with processed lymphocytes residing in the lymphoid tissue, some of the lymphocytes become activated to form activated T or B lymphocytes. The activated T cells and antibodies produced by the activated B-lymphocytes react highly specifically against the particular types of antigen that initiated their development. The mature B cell has on its cell surface membrane about 100000 antibody molecules that will react highly specifically with only one type of antigen. T-cell receptor proteins (T-cell markers) are present on the surface of the T-cell membrane and these are also highly specific for one specified activating antigen. An antigen stimulates only those lymphocytes that have complementary receptors for the antigen.

Immunologic Memory

Once an immune system has recognized and responded to an antigen, during a second encounter with the same antigen a heightened state of immune reactivity is seen.

This is termed immunologic memory (*refer* immunological memory).

Self/Nonself Recognition

The ability of the immune system to distinguish self from nonself and to respond only to nonself molecules is called self-nonself recognition. An inappropriate response to self-molecules can be a fatal autoimmune response (*refer* immunological tolerance).

Types of Acquired Immunity

Acquired immunity is of two types:
1. Cell-mediated immunity or T-cell immunity
2. Humoral immunity or B-cell immunity

In 1950, lymphocyte was identified as the cell responsible for both cellular and humoral immunity.

Cell-mediated Immunity

Cellular immunity *refers to specific acquired immunity accomplished by T lymphocytes and macrophages effective against parasites, fungi, virus, cancer cells and transplanted tissue.*

The steps in cell mediated immunity are:
a. Antigen recognition, presentation and processing
b. Activation and proliferation of T cells
c. Elimination of invader.

Antigen Recognition

An extremely large number of antigens can be recognized by the lymphocytes in the body. Stem cells differentiate into millions of T lymphocytes, each with the ability to respond to a particular antigen. T lymphocytes have specialized receptors for antigens. Cell-mediated immune response begins with activation of a small number of T lymphocytes by a particular antigen present on the surface of the antigen presenting cell (APC). Once activated, it enlarges and begins to proliferate (divide) and differentiate into cells that can recognize the same antigen. Thus, **clones** of cells (population of identical cells that can recognize the same antigen) are formed and this is referred to as **clonal selection**. Before the first exposure to a particular antigen, only a few T cells are there to recognize it. But, after an immune response has occurred, there are thousands of cells to recognize the same antigen. **Interleukin-2** is necessary for T cell proliferation. IL-2 is a hormone-like molecule secreted by helper T cell (Th cell).

Corticosteroids and cyclosporine (immunosuppressive drug used in organ transplants) suppress immune response by inhibiting the production of interleukins.

Stimulation of helper T cells (Th cells) by an antigen leads to proliferation of Th cells to form clones of Th cells that secrete IL-2 and other cytokines. It also forms clones of **memory Th cells**, which are long lived.

Lymphocyte precursors that are reactive with self- antigens are normally deleted during an immune response.

This results in **immunological tolerance**. In autoimmune diseases, antibodies are produced against cells expressing normal proteins. This leads to their destruction because immune tolerance is disrupted in autoimmune diseases.

T-cell Receptors

T-cell receptor (TCR) is a molecule found on the surface of T lymphocytes that is responsible for recognizing fragments of antigens bound to MHC molecules. T cell receptor consists of two polypeptide chains. One T cell may have as many as 100,000 receptor sites on its membrane surface. In 95% of T cells, the TCR consists of an α-chain and a β-chain complexed with CD3 molecules. CD3 is called signal transducer. The T cells expressing this receptor is called αβT cell. In 5% of T cells, the TCR consists of γ and δ chains (γδT cell). These T cells are prominent in the mucosa of the gastrointestinal tract and they form a link between the innate and acquired immune systems by way of cytokines they secrete. Association of polypeptide CD3 is required for the surface expression of TCR. Each chain of TCR is composed of 2 extracellular domains, variable region and constant region. It is the variable region that binds to MHC-peptide complex in the antigen presenting cell. Constant region is close to the cell membrane.

CD8 is present on the surface of cytotoxic T cells that bind MHC-I proteins, and CD4 is seen on the surface of helper T cells that bind MHC-II proteins. CD8 and CD4 proteins facilitate the binding of MHC proteins to the T cell receptor. The activated CD8 cytotoxic T cells kill the organism directly, whereas the activated CD4 helper T cells secrete cytokines that activate other lymphocytes.

The T cell receptors are surrounded by cell-to- cell adhesion molecules and proteins that bind to complementary proteins in the antigen presenting cell when the two cells join to form the immunological synapse. This is very essential for the activation of T cells. If this combination does not occur the T cell remains unresponsive.

Antigen Processing and Presentation

Antigens are of two types:
1. **Exogenous antigens** like bacteria, pollen, dust, toxins, etc.
2. **Endogenous antigens** like viruses that have infected cells, abnormal (mutant) proteins formed in tumor cells, etc.

For an immune response to occur, B and T cells must recognize that a foreign antigen is present. B lymphocytes can recognize and bind to antigens in extracellular fluid (ECF). T cells can only recognize fragments of antigenic proteins that have been processed and presented in association with major histocompatibility complex proteins (**MHC** proteins).

Major Histocompatibility Complex Proteins (MHC Proteins)

Major histocompatibility genes (MHC genes) are located on the short arm of chromosome 6. These genes code for specific **MHC proteins**. MHC molecules are glycoproteins, which are unique for a person except identical twins. Their function is to help T cells recognize foreign invaders. T lymphocytes fail to recognize the antigen in isolation, so the antigen has to be closely associated with MHC molecules in order to be recognized by the T-cells. The phenomenon is called **associated recognition**. The normal function of MHC-antigen complex is to help T cells recognize that an antigen is foreign i.e., non self. B-lymphocytes do not require MHC molecules for recognizing antigens.

In man, the MHC proteins are referred to as **human leukocyte associated antigen (HLA antigen)** since they were first identified on leukocytes. They are of two types:
1. Class I MHC proteins or MHC-I protein
2. Class II MHC proteins or MHC-II protein.

MHC-I protein, which is a monomer, is present in all nucleated cells in the body on their cell membranes (RBCs lack the MHC antigen). It binds with endogenous antigen (MHC antigens in transplanted tissue, mutant proteins in tumor cells, viral protein, etc.). Specific MHC molecules are responsible for graft rejection following tissue transplantation. The MHC-I molecules on the donor tissue cells themselves act as antigens called MHC antigens. When a malignant tumor develops in the body, its mutant gene codes for the synthesis of abnormal antigenic protein molecules on its cell surface. Thus, the tumor cell gets associated with MHC-I molecules and the cell will be destroyed by the cytotoxic T cell normally. When a virus invades a cell, the viral antigens get associated with class I MHC molecules and will be eliminated.

MHC-II protein, which is a heterodimer, is present in antigen presenting cells (APC), macrophages and B lymphocytes and bind with exogenous antigens like bacteria, toxins, etc. The cytotoxic T lymphocytes recognize antigen complexed to cell surface protein of MHC-I, whereas helper T cell recognize antigen complexed to cell surface protein of MHC-II. This process of dual recognition is called **MHC restriction**.

Significance of HLA Antigen or MHC Antigen

❖ HLA antigen plays an important role in immunity by recognizing foreign antigens
❖ They form important histocompatibility antigens in organ transplantation
❖ Presence of some HLA antigens is associated with susceptibility to certain diseases
❖ HLA antigen typing is used for paternity testing.

Processing of Exogenous Antigen

Antigens present outside the body cells are exogenous antigens, which are processed by antigen-presenting cells (APCs). The process of engulfing an antigen, fragmenting it and presenting the antigen fragments on the cell surface

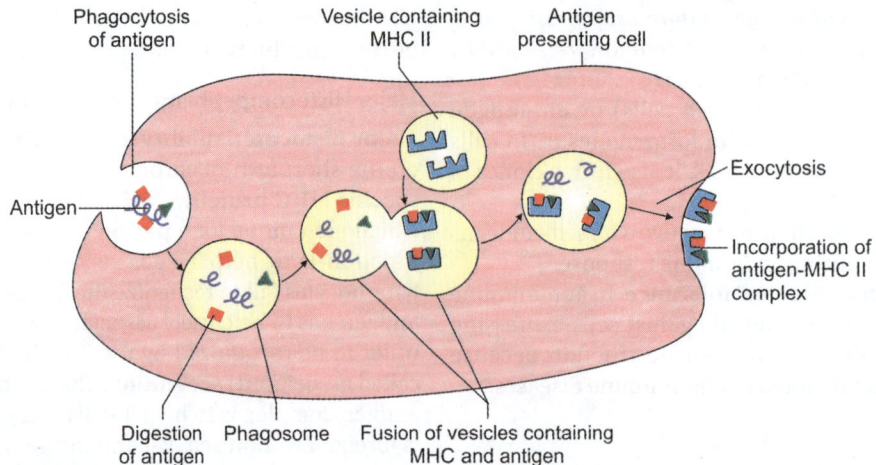

Fig. 16.3: Processing of exogenous antigen in the antigen presenting cell in cellular immunity.

in association with MHC-II molecules is called **antigen processing and presentation** and the phagocytes that process antigens are called **antigen-processing cells or antigen-presenting cells (APCs)**. APCs include specialized cells called *dendritic cells* in the lymph nodes and spleen, *Langerhans dendritic cells* in the skin, Kupffer cells of liver and microglial cells in the nervous system. Macrophages and B lymphocytes themselves can act as APCs (**Fig. 16.3**). Millions of macrophages are present in the lymphoid tissue. These line the sinusoids of the lymph nodes, spleen and other lymphoid tissues. Macrophages engulf tumor cells as well. APCs are present in plenty in areas where antigen entry into the body occurs such as skin, mucous membrane of respiratory, gastrointestinal and genitourinary tracts.

The steps in antigen processing and antigen presentation are:
1. Recognition of antigen by the APC
2. Ingestion of antigen by phagocytosis
3. Digestion of antigens into peptides by lysosomal enzymes in the APC
4. Fusion of vesicles containing peptides of the antigen and MHC-II molecules
5. Binding of peptides to MHC-II molecule
6. Insertion of antigen-MHC-II complex into the plasma membrane (**Fig. 16.3**) by exocytosis

The APC then migrates to the lymphatic tissue. This cell is recognized by a small number of helper T cells that have correctly shaped receptors called T cell receptors (TCR). That is, each TCR possess unique antigen specificity determined by the structure of the antigen binding site formed by the alpha and beta subunits of the receptor. They form immunological synapse and this interaction triggers cell-mediated response or humoral response. *The junction between the T cell and the antigen presenting cell which leads to activation of T cell and mediation of cell mediated immunity is called* **immunological synapse**. Proper immune response depends on the correct transfer of information across the synapse.

Processing of Endogenous Antigens (Fig. 16.4)

Endogenous antigen fragments combine with MHC-I molecule and the complex moves to the plasma membrane.

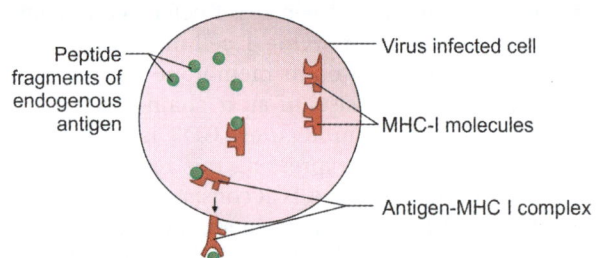

Fig. 16.4: Processing of endogenous antigen.

The peptide fragments of the antigens are generated from proteins synthesized within cells. Peptides formed inside the cell to which the host is not tolerant (e.g., mutant proteins or viral proteins) are recognized by the T lymphocytes. These proteins are digested in **proteasomes** in the cell into peptide fragments. These peptides bind to MHC-I protein to form a complex. This complex is presented on the surface of the cell by exocytosis (**Fig. 16.4**).

Activation of T Lymphocyte

Only the processed antigen can stimulate the T lymphocytes. Receptors on the T lymphocyte recognize a wide variety of MHC-antigen fragment complexes. Most of the receptors on the circulating T lymphocytes are made up of two polypeptide units designated as α and β. These cells are called $\alpha\beta$ T cells. These cells recognize the MHC protein-antigen complex.

CD4 and CD8 proteins are closely associated with the T cell receptors and may function as co-receptors for major histocompatibility complex (MHC) class I and II respectively. They occur on the surface of T cells. Based on the presence of co-receptor CD4 or CD8, there are two subsets of T cells: helper T cell (contains CD4) and cytotoxic T cell (contains CD8). Both CD4 and CD8 co-receptors facilitate the binding of MHC-antigen complex to T cell receptor (TCR). Stimulation of cytotoxic T cells (TC cells) or killer T cells requires IL-2 secreted by helper T cell (Th cell). The cytotoxic T cell recognize antigen combined with MHC-I molecules on the cells containing endogenous antigen. T cell activation is complete only if the cell-to-cell adhesion molecules and

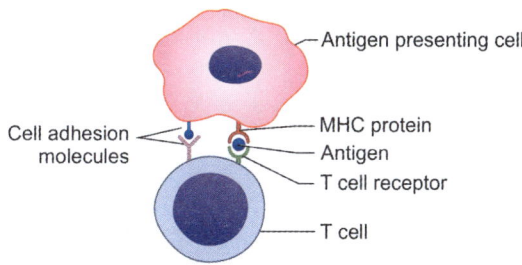

Fig. 16.5: T-cell activation and immunological synapse.

proteins that surround the TCR bind to complementary proteins present in the APC when the two cells form the **immunological synapse** (**Fig. 16.5**). Thus two signals are necessary for the activation of the T cell receptor:
1. Binding of MHC protein-antigen complex on the APC surface to the specific TCR on the T lymphocyte
2. Binding of the cell-to-cell adhesion molecules and proteins surrounding the TCR to complementary proteins in the APC (**Fig. 16.5**).

The activated CD8 cytotoxic T cell kills their targets directly, whereas the activated CD4 helper T cells secrete cytokines that activate other lymphocytes (**Fig. 16.6**). Memory T cells are programmed to recognize the original invading antigen during a second invasion.

Elimination of the Invader

Destruction of the invader by the cytotoxic T cell (TC cell) includes the following mechanisms:
1. Granules containing **perforin** undergo exocytosis from the αβTC cell (CD8 cell). Perforin forms holes in the plasma membrane of target cells. Fluid enters the cells through the holes and the cell bursts (**Fig. 16.6**).
2. TC cells secrete a toxic substance called **lymphotoxin** that destroys the target cell.
3. TC cells also secrete γ-**interferon**, which activates neutrophils and macrophages increasing their phagocytic activity (**Fig. 16.6**).

Summary of cell-mediated immunity is shown in **Figure 16.7**.

■ HUMORAL IMMUNITY

B cell becomes activated when an antigen binds to antigen receptors on B cell membrane. B cell antigen receptors are chemically similar to antibodies. These receptors will be eventually secreted as antibodies.

For proliferation and differentiation of B cell, **IL-2** secreted by helper T cell (Th cell) and **IL-1** secreted by macrophages are necessary. This activation is essential for the production of adequate quantities of antibodies by the B-lymphocyte. Activated B cells enlarge, divide and differentiate into a clone of **plasma cells** (**Fig. 16.8**). From one activated B lymphocyte, about 500 plasma cells are formed by repeated division. The plasma cells secrete **antibodies** at a rate of 2000 molecules/sec for each cell for several days or weeks. After that it dies. The antibodies or immunoglobulins are actually the secreted form of

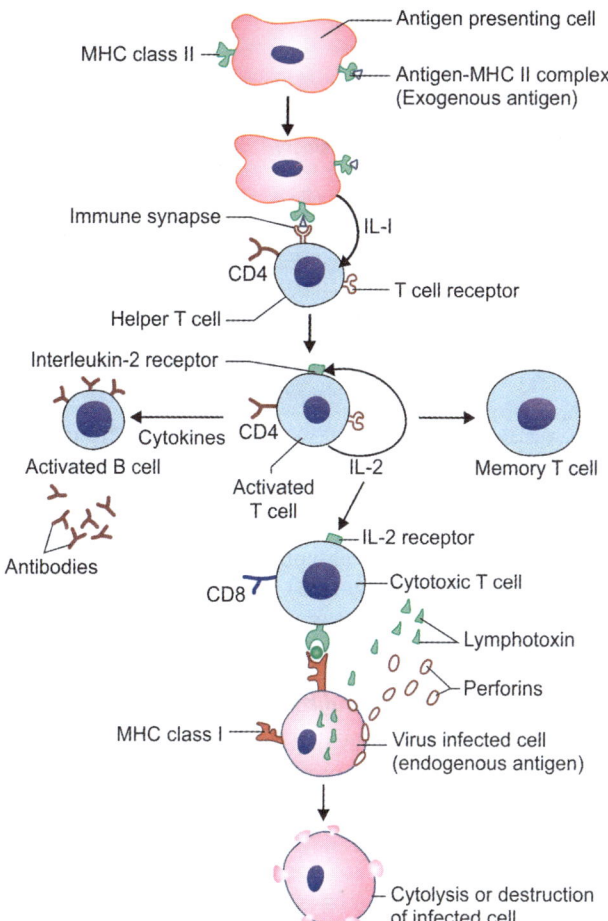

Fig. 16.6: Summary of acquired immunity IL-2 produced by activated helper T cell (CD4) acts in an autocrine manner causing the activated cell to form a clone of cells which also include memory cells. The activated CD4 cell can also cause B cell activation leading to humoral immunity or it can activate Cytotoxic CD8 cell. CD8 cell release perforins and lymphotoxins.

antigen-binding receptors on the cell membrane of B lymphocytes.

The activated B cells that do not differentiate into plasma cells remain as **memory B cells**, which respond more rapidly during a second attack by the same antigen. Numerous memory cells to a specific antigen will be present in the lymphatic tissue throughout the body. The B cells of a particular clone are capable of secreting only one kind of antibody or immunoglobulin specific to the antigen that stimulated its secretion. The antibodies enter circulation and form **antigen–antibody complexes** with the corresponding antigen. The complexes will be phagocytosed by macrophages and removed from the body.

Immunoglobulins or Antibodies

An immunoglobulin molecule is made up of 4 polypeptide chains, two heavy chains and two light chains. Disulfide bonds anchor the light chain to the heavy chain and also hold the two heavy chains together. The NH2 terminal part of the heavy chain and the light chain has a variable sequence of amino

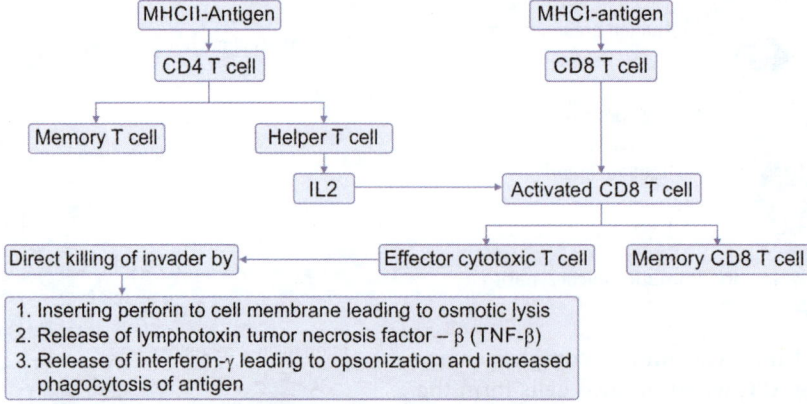

Fig. 16.7: Summary of cell mediated immunity.

acids and is therefore called the **variable region**. Variable regions are distinct for each immunoglobulin. The COOH terminal part has a relatively constant sequence and is called the **constant region** (**Fig. 16.9**). The constant regions of the different immunoglobulins are very similar. *It is the variable region that binds with specific affinity to different antigens.*

Classes of Immunoglobulins or Antibodies

Immunoglobulins are divided into 5 classes based on the differences in the constant regions of their heavy chains.

There are five types of heavy chains gamma, alpha, mu, delta and epsilon. These produce five classes of immunoglobulins namely IgG, IgA, IgM, IgD and IgE respectively.

IgG
- IgG constitutes 75% of antibodies in blood, lymph and intestine. As it is small, it readily diffuses out into the extravascular spaces where its concentration is the same as that in the plasma. Plasma concentration of IgG is 1000 mg/dL.
- It is the only antibody that crosses the placenta and confers passive immunity to the newborn in its first few weeks.
- IgG in colostrum is transferred across the gut mucosa of the neonates, which also reinforces passive immunity.
- In secondary immune response, IgG antibodies predominate.
- It provides protection against bacteria and viruses.
- It is present in milk, saliva, nasal and bronchial secretions.
- They act as opsonins for leukocyte activity

IgA
- Constitutes 15% of total antibodies
- Present in sweat, tear, saliva, mucus, colostrum, genitourinary and gastrointestinal secretions (IgA is referred to as secretory immunoglobulins, which provide secretory immunity).

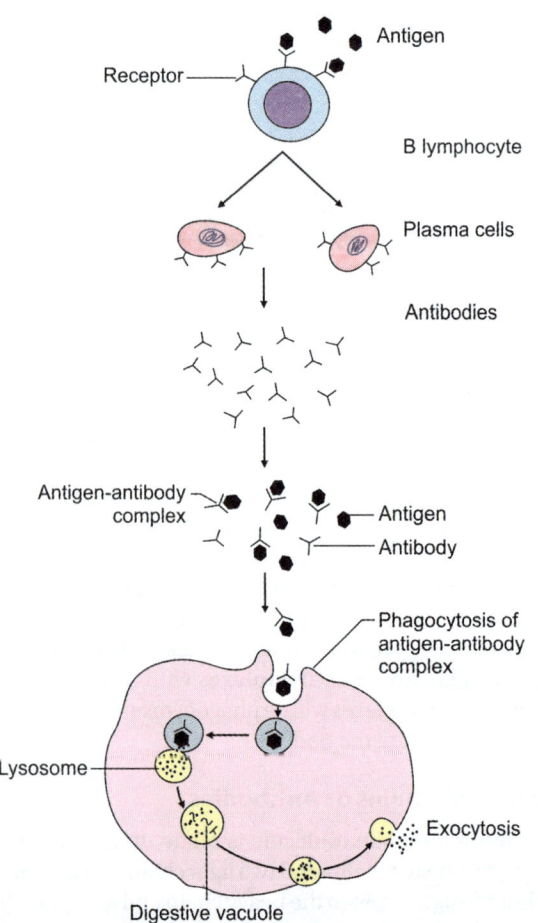

Fig. 16.8: Mechanism of humoral immunity.

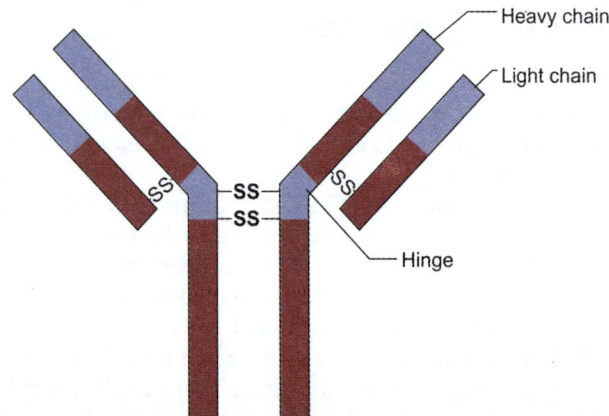

Fig. 16.9: Structure of an immunoglobulin molecule. Constant regions are colored red and variable regions are colored blue. The chains are joined by disulfide bridges.

❖ Provides localized protection on mucous membrane
❖ They cannot cross the placenta

IgM
❖ Constitute 5–10% of antibodies present in blood and lymph and is predominantly intravascular because of its large size.
❖ It is the first antibody secreted by plasma cell in the primary response.
❖ Antibodies of ABO blood group system belong to IgM class.
❖ IgM is the only immunoglobulin, which is produced before birth.

IgE
❖ Constitutes less than 0.1% in blood
❖ IgE receptors are located in mast cells and basophils.
❖ Provides protection against parasites
❖ IgE is involved in allergic reaction by releasing histamine from basophils and mast cells. They are also called reagins.

IgD
❖ Constitutes less than 1% in blood
❖ Helps in the activation of B lymphocytes by acting as antigen receptors for B cells and thus involved in antigen recognition.

Mechanism of Action of Antibodies

Direct Action
❖ Antibodies can combine with receptors in the antigen and form clumps (agglutination)
❖ When the clumps become very large it precipitates
❖ Antibodies can combine with the toxic sites of the antigen and render it nontoxic
❖ Antibodies can act as opsonins and can coat the organism and thus promote phagocytosis
❖ Certain antibodies can combine with the antigen and can lyse the cell membrane of the organism

Indirect Action
Indirect action is through activation of complement system. Activated complement produces the following effects:
❖ Opsonization and phagocytosis of the foreign substance by neutrophils and macrophages
❖ Lysis of the invading organism
❖ Agglutination of the invading organisms
❖ Complement leads to inflammatory changes in the area of invasion by the agent, which can immobilize the organisms and prevent them from invading the other parts of the body

Functions of Antibodies in General
❖ Help to neutralize antigens.
❖ Cause immobilization of bacteria.
❖ Help in the agglutination and precipitation of antigen
❖ Activation of complement system by IgG, IgA and IgM.
❖ Enhance phagocytosis by acting as opsonins.
❖ Provide fetal and newborn immunity. Maternal IgG antibodies cross placenta, and IgA and IgG antibodies present in colostrum provide passive immunity to the newborn in its first few weeks.

Table 16.4: Differences between humoral and cell-mediated immunity.

Humoral immunity	Cell-mediated immunity
Mediated by circulating antibodies produced by B lymphocytes	Mediated by T lymphocytes
B cells cannot directly kill the invader	T cells can directly the invader kill
Act by activating complement system and forming antigen–antibody complexes	Kill organisms by inserting perforins into their cell membrane and thus producing holes
Major defense against bacterial infection (extracellular bacteria) and against antigens dissolved in body fluids	Major defense against infections by viruses, fungi, bacteria (intracellular) such as tubercle bacteria and against tumor cells
No delayed reactions	Responsible for delayed allergic reactions and foreign tissue transplant rejection

Differences between humoral and cell mediated immunity is shown in (**Table 16.4**).

Warm and cold antibodies: Antigens of the ABO and Rh system can react with their corresponding antibodies at normal body temperature (optimally active at 37°C). They are called warm antibodies which belong to IgG type. But the antibodies of other blood group systems can react with their corresponding antigens only at a temperature between 5 and 20°C (optimally active at 4°C). They are called cold antibodies and they belong to IgM type.

IMMUNOLOGICAL MEMORY

Immunological memory is due to the presence of long-lived memory B and T lymphocytes. The amount of antibody in serum can be measured and is called **antibody titer**. After an initial contact with an antigen, there is a delay of one week followed by a slow rise in antibody titer. First, there is an increase in IgM titer and then IgG followed by a gradual decline. This is called **primary response** (**Fig. 16.10**) and it has a short life. Low level of antibodies can be detected in blood after about two weeks.

When the body is exposed to the same antigen again, there is rapid response i.e., within hours and the antibody titer is far greater than during primary response. It is mainly IgG antibodies that are increased in second exposure and the value declines more slowly i.e., it lasts for many months. This accelerated response is **secondary response**. Immunological memory is the basis for active immunization against infectious diseases like polio, measles, etc. The vaccine contains attenuated (weakened) or killed microorganisms and the antigen is injected in multiple doses with intervals of several months.

Prevention of Autoimmunization in the Body

Autoimmunization is prevented in the body by the following mechanisms:
❖ Lymphocytes capable of reacting to self-antigens are eliminated during differentiation of T and B cells in the thymus and bone marrow. This is called **clonal deletion**.

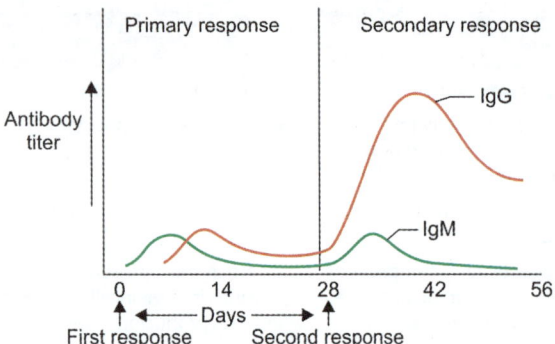

Fig. 16.10: Immunological memory.

- Suppressor T cells or Treg cells keep the autoantibodies in check and help in tolerance to self.
- Tolerance of T cells to self-antigens prevents autoantibody production by B cells. This occurs because B cells need cooperation of T cells for antibody production.
- Certain cells and substances of the body such as lens protein of the eye and sperms in the seminal vesicles, which are highly antigenic are isolated from the cells of the immune system.

> The fetus is a foreign transplant in the mother as it contains the paternal genes. It should, therefore, induce immune response in the mother leading to its rejection. This normally does not happen due to the following reasons:
> a. The placenta is resistant to immune attack because the density of MHC antigens in the trophoblast is very less leading to loss of its immunogenicity
> b. An inert coating of mucoproteins occur on the surface of the trophoblast cells
> c. The antibodies produced by the mother against the fetus are removed by the placenta, thus preventing their entry into fetal circulation
> d. Alpha-fetoprotein and progesterone produced during embryonic development are immunosuppressants
> e. Fetal T cells have suppressive effect on maternal T cells that are exposed to fetal cells.

IMMUNOLOGICAL TOLERANCE OR RECOGNITION OF SELF

Under normal circumstances, animals do not produce immunological response to their own cells or proteins. During early fetal life, i.e. during the period of immunological immaturity all potential antigens that are encountered by the cells of the body will be recognized as self. These substances will not evoke an immunological response when exposed in the post-natal life. That is, they are treated as self-antigens. After the period of immunological immaturity materials which are foreign to the body when it comes in contact with the tissues will be recognized as non-self and will evoke an immune response.

Immunological tolerance is defined as a state of unresponsiveness to an antigen which is induced by the exposure of specific lymphocytes to that particular antigen.

Self-tolerance refers to lack of responsiveness to one's own tissue antigen.

Mechanism of Self-tolerance

Self-tolerance can be:
1. Central tolerance
2. Peripheral tolerance.

Central Tolerance

Clonal deletion (negative selection)
Central tolerance is due to clonal deletion. During fetal life, the clones of T and B lymphocytes containing receptors that react against self-antigens are selectively deleted from the body in the central lymphoid organs like thymus, bone marrow or liver. So they will not be present in the post natal life to react against self-antigens. These cells undergo apoptosis by the process called negative selection or deletion.

During the period of pre-processing of the T lymphocytes in the thymus, and B lymphocytes in the bone marrow, these organs select the T and B lymphocytes which are to be released into circulation by first mixing them with all the specific self-antigens from the body's own tissues. If a lymphocyte reacts with self-antigen, it is destroyed and phagocytized. All such lymphocytes will not be released. Thus the only lymphocytes that are finally released are those that are nonreactive against body's own antigens. The thymus and the bone marrow make sure that the released T lymphocytes and the antibodies react only against foreign antigens, i.e., which are nonself.

Peripheral Tolerance

Some of the self-reactive T cells and B cells escape into the periphery where they may cause tissue injury unless destroyed by peripheral tolerance. There are several mechanisms that act in the periphery against self-reactive T and B cells. They include clonal anergy, suppression by T_{reg} cells and deletion by apoptosis.

1. *Clonal anergy*
   Clonal anergy refers to functional inactivation of lymphocytes rather than their death. When mature B and T lymphocytes come in contact with potentially antigenic substances in fetal life, they enter a prolonged hyporesponsive state without making an immune response. This is referred to as clonal anergy or immunological silence. Thus all antigenic materials both self and nonself encountered in the fetal life will not produce a response in the future. Another mechanism is by expressing inhibitory T cell receptors that limit their activation and prevent response against self-antigens.
2. *Suppression by regulatory T cells (T_{reg} cells)*
   Regulatory T cells are a population of T cells that function to prevent reaction against self-antigens. They develop in the thymus and belong to a class of helper T cell. The mechanism of action of regulatory T cells is thought to be mediated by secretion of immunosuppressive cytokines that inhibit lymphocyte activation.
3. *Deletion by apoptosis*
   Mature T cells that recognize self-antigen also receive signals to induce apoptosis by upregulation of proapoptotic factors and by mechanisms mediated by the death receptor

Fas also known as **apoptosis antigen 1 (APO-1)** which is encoded by **FAS gene**. Binding of Fas with its receptor induces apoptosis. Fas receptor belongs to the TNF-receptor superfamily. It is seen that mutation of Fas gene causes some autoimmune diseases.

Some self-antigens are hidden or sequestered from the immune system as these tissues do not communicate with blood or lymph. Such tissues are called **immune privileged** tissues, e.g., ocular lens, testes, etc. Whenever there is injury to the lens or when the blood-testis-barrier breaks down, the antigenic substances reach the blood stream and stimulate antibody production leading to destruction of the normal lens and uveitis; and destruction of germ cells of testes (orchitis) leading to sterility.

Transplantation Tolerance

Tolerance to transplanted tissues can be achieved by using monoclonal antibodies against CD4 and CD8 proteins.

IMMUNOLOGICAL DISORDERS

Acquired Immunodeficiency Syndrome

Acquired immunodeficiency syndrome (AIDS), first identified in 1981, is caused by the **human immunodeficiency virus type 1 (HIV-1),** which is a retrovirus. HIV-1 specifically infects helper T cells (**Th cells or T4 cells**), destroying them. TH cells are necessary for optimal antibody production by plasma cells and for the generation of cytotoxic T cells (TC cells). *Normal Th cell count is 1200/mm³ and in AIDS it is less than 200/mm³ of blood.*

In addition to helper T cells, monocytes also get infected with HIV-1. The virus can survive in these cells and get transported to different parts of the body like the brain and lung. Thus, monocytes serve as a major reservoir for HIV in the body. The number of circulating natural killer (NK) cells in AIDS patients is not significantly reduced but their cytotoxic ability is diminished.

The disease is characterized by severe weight loss, night sweats, swollen lymph nodes and high susceptibility to opportunistic infections. Because of reduction in immunity, these people are more prone for tuberculosis, candidiasis, fungal pneumonia and Kaposi's sarcoma (a type of skin and lymph node cancer). HIV-1 also invades brain cells causing dementia and other neuropsychiatric abnormalities in over half of the patients.

AIDS spreads by intimate homosexual or heterosexual contact, by exposure to infected blood or blood products or from mother to child during pregnancy. National AIDS Control Organization (NACO) has been set up under the Ministry of Health and Family Welfare Department.

Autoimmune Diseases

Normally during fetal life, most of the antigens in the body of the fetus are presented to the immune system of the fetus and these antigens are recognized as self-antigens. Antibodies and cytotoxic T cells are not produced after birth against self-antigens. Sometimes, the immune system fails to recognize self-antigens and produces antibodies or T cells, which attack self-antigens destroying own cells or body tissues. Thus, autoimmunity is defined as the immune response to self-antigen where *the body's immune response gets directed towards its own tissues.* According to some studies, deficiency of regulatory T cells (suppressor T cells) is probably the cause of auto-immune diseases.

Examples of autoimmune diseases are rheumatoid arthritis, systemic lupus erythematosus (SLE), autoimmune thyroiditis, Grave's disease, rheumatic fever, autoimmune hemolytic anemia and pernicious anemia, thrombocytopenic purpura, type I diabetes mellitus, myasthenia gravis, multiple sclerosis, etc.

Some antigens referred to as **hidden antigens or sequestrated antigens** are present that are never exposed to the immune system during fetal life. Immunological tolerance against such antigens does not develop in the fetus. These antigens include lens protein, sperm antigen, etc.

When these antigens get exposed to the immune system it leads to immune response, damaging the affected tissues. The lens protein may accidentally leak out during cataract surgery, which stimulates antibody production against lens protein leading to damage of the other eye as well. Another example is *orchitis* where there is infection of the testes by mumps virus leading to damage of blood-testis barrier. This leads to leakage of sperm proteins into circulation evoking an immune response against own testes destroying the germinal epithelium. This leads to sterility.

Hypersensitivity or Allergy

Allergy is defined as an acquired abnormal **hyperimmune reaction** to an agent during subsequent exposures. Any substance that produce, allergy is called an **allergen**, e.g., food substances, pollen grains, dust, drugs, certain plants, etc., act as allergens. Most common hypersensitivity reaction is type I hypersensitivity or anaphylaxis, which is mediated by IgE antibodies.

There is degranulation of mast cells resulting in release of histamine and other vasoactive substances. It is of two types, local anaphylaxis and generalized anaphylaxis. Example of local anaphylaxis is asthma and example of generalized anaphylaxis is penicillin anaphylaxis, which is a circulatory shock such as condition and requires immediate medical attention.

MULTIPLE CHOICE QUESTIONS

1. **Plasma cells are activated:**
    a. B lymphocytes
    b. T lymphocytes
    c. Macrophages
    d. Monocytes

2. **Life span of plasma cell is:**
    a. 1–2 weeks   b. 2–3 days
    c. 1 month   d. 4–5 weeks

3. Immunoglobulin that is active in type I hypersensitivity is:
   a. IgA
   b. IgE
   c. IgD
   d. IgG
4. The immunoglobulin that is present in colostrum, saliva and tear is:
   a. IgA
   b. IgE
   c. IgG
   d. IgD
5. The type of antibody that is responsible for hemolytic disease of new born due to Rh incompatibility between mother and fetus is:
   a. IgA
   b. IgE
   c. IgG
   d. IgD
6. HIV is not present in:
   a. Tears
   b. Cervical secretion
   c. Semen
   d. Blood
7. Cellular target of HIV is:
   a. CD4 helper T cell
   b. Cytotoxic T cell
   c. Memory cell
   d. CD8 cell
8. Cell mediated immunity is provided by:
   a. Macrophage
   b. T-lymphocyte
   c. B-lymphocyte
   d. Monocyte
9. T-lymphocytes differentiate into all, *except*:
   a. Helper cells
   b. Plasma cells
   c. Cytotoxic cells
   d. Suppressor cells
10. Immediate or type-I hypersensitivity responses are mediated by:
    a. Basophils
    b. Eosinophils
    c. Monocytes
    d. Neutrophils
11. Helper and cytotoxic cells belong to:
    a. T cells
    b. B cells
    c. Monocytes
    d. Macrophages
12. Immunity is not suppressed in:
    a. Liver failure
    b. Patients on ACTH therapy
    c. Anemia
    d. Renal failure
13. Antigen presenting cells are specialized cells present on all the following, *except*:
    a. Skin
    b. Lymph node
    c. Spleen
    d. Kidney
14. B-lymphocytes are associated with:
    a. CD 19
    b. CD 27
    c. CD 4
    d. CD 35
15. Macrophages are the mature forms of:
    a. Neutrophils
    b. Basophils
    c. Monocytes
    d. Lymphocytes
16. False statement regarding IgG:
    a. Pentamer with J chain
    b. No additional chain
    c. Only gamma chains as heavy chains
    d. Performs complement fixation
17. Antibodies of ABO blood group system belongs to:
    a. IgG
    b. IgM
    c. IgD
    d. IgE
18. The antibody that crosses the placenta:
    a. IgG
    b. IgM
    c. IgD
    d. IgE

ANSWERS

1. a	2. b	3. b	4. a	5. c
6. a	7. a	8. b	9. b	10. a
11. a	12. a	13. d	14. a	15. c
16. a	17. b	18. a		

Platelets

CHAPTER 17

LEARNING OBJECTIVES

Must know
- Explain the properties and functions of platelets
- Describe the formation of platelets and its variations

Desirable to know
- Functions of von Willebrand factor

INTRODUCTION

PY2.7: Describe the formation of platelets, functions and variations.

Platelets or thrombocytes are small, colorless, refractile, and **non-nucleated** fragments of large multinucleated cells in the bone marrow called megakaryocytes. Resting platelets appear as flat discs. Platelet membrane is an important source of phospholipids that are required for coagulation. These are the *smallest formed elements in circulation*. They are seen as clumps in the peripheral blood smear (*refer* **Fig. 14.2**).

- Size: 2–4 µm
- Volume: 6–8 µm³
- Count: 2–4 lakh/mm³ of blood
- Life span: 8–12 days in circulation
- Site of destruction: Spleen, liver and bone marrow.

STRUCTURE OF PLATELET (FIG. 17.1)

Cell membrane of platelet is 6 nm thick and is extensively invaginated to form a canalicular system which is in contact with plasma. It consists of outer glycocalyx layer and inner lipoprotein layer. Platelet membrane also contains **glycoproteins**, which form various receptors on platelet membrane like *receptors for collagen, ADP, fibrinogen, von Willebrand's factor (vWF)*, etc. The receptors are responsible for the adhesion of activated platelets on to the injured vessel wall especially to injured endothelial cells and exposed collagen.

Lipoprotein layer consists of phospholipid, cholesterol, glycolipid, etc. Phospholipid in platelet is also known as **platelet activating factor (PAF)** or **platelet factor-3**, a cytokine that activates intrinsic mechanism of coagulation. PAF has inflammatory activity and it also increases the

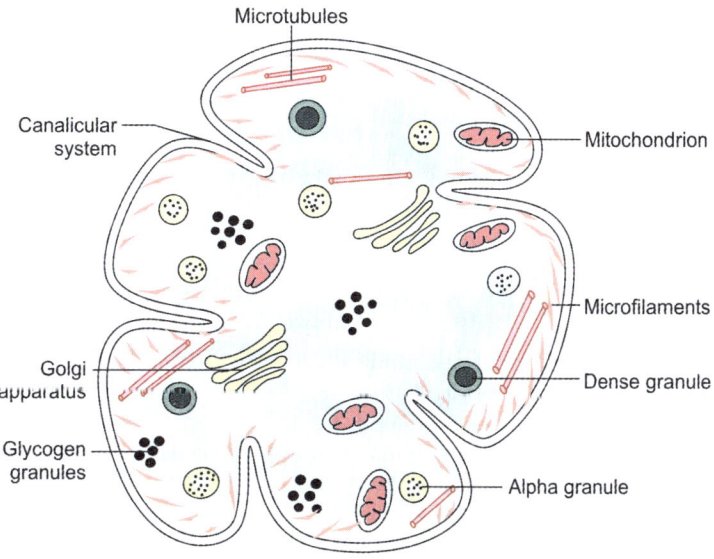

Fig. 17.1: Structure of platelet.

production of arachidonic acid derivatives like thromboxane A_2. Precursors of thromboxane A_2, prostaglandins, leukotrienes, platelet factors, etc., are also present in the platelet membrane.

Cytoplasm of platelets contains microtubules, microfilaments, endoplasmic reticulum, granules, mitochondria, lysosomes, microperoxisomes, etc. Lysosomes contain enzymes like acid hydrolases. Microperoxisomes contain catalase. Microtubules and endoplasmic reticulum store calcium. Golgi apparatus and endoplasmic reticulum synthesize various enzymes. Mitochondria and enzyme systems are capable of forming ATP and ADP. Microfilaments are made up of a protein called **actomyosin** or **thrombosthenin**, which has a structure similar to actin and myosin of skeletal muscle. Actin comprises approximately 25% of total platelet protein and tropomyosin and a-actinin comprises about 2–5% of total platelet protein. Microfilaments are seen as a ring around the periphery of platelet and are responsible for maintaining the shape of platelet. They can contract and relax, helping in the movement of platelets.

Platelets do not have deoxyribonucleic acid (DNA) and ribonucleic acid (RNA) and so, protein synthesis does not occur in the platelet. The proteins present in the platelets are synthesized in the megakaryoblast and megakaryocyte.

Granules in the platelets are of three types:
1. Dense granules
2. α-granules
3. Glycogen granules

1. **Dense granules** contain non-protein substances like ATP, ADP, pyrophosphate, serotonin, Mg^{2+}, Ca^{2+}, catecholamine, etc.
2. **Alpha-granules** are the predominant platelet granules. It contains secreted proteins other than hydrolases present in lysosomes. They include growth factors like platelet-derived growth factor (PDGF), vWF, thrombospondin, platelet factor-4 (PF-4); coagulation factors like factor V, factor XIII and fibrinogen.
   - **Platelet derived growth factor (PDGF)** helps in the proliferation of endothelial cells, vascular smooth muscle cells, glial cells and fibroblasts, and also helps in wound healing. Macrophages and endothelial cells also produce PDGF. PDGF, transforming growth factor-β and vascular endothelial growth factor in the α-granules play a role in the progression of atherosclerotic vascular lesions because of their mitotic activity.
   - **von Willebrand's factor (vWF)**, is a very large circulating glycoprotein produced by platelets as well as vascular endothelium. (details of vWF are given further)
   - **Thrombospondin** belongs to a family of secreted glycoproteins with antiangiogenic functions. They are considered as matricellular proteins that mediate cell-to-cell and cell-to-matrix interactions. This protein can bind to fibrinogen, fibronectin, laminin, collagen, etc. In platelets, it is responsible for fixation of platelet and participates in platelet plug formation. Thrombospondin synthesized in the megakaryocyte comprise 20% of the total platelet protein released in response to thrombin.
   - **Platelet factor 4** combines with heparin and inactivates it, thereby facilitating platelet aggregation.
   - About 20% of the total factor V in blood is located in the α-granules. Factor V, fibrinogen and vWF found in platelets contribute to coagulation.

VARIATIONS IN THE PLATELET COUNT

Increase in the platelet count is known as **thrombocytosis or thrombocythemia**.
❖ **Physiological increase** is seen in:
   - Violent exercise (increases platelet count due to splenic contraction)
   - Stress and administration of adrenaline causes splenic contraction which releases the stored platelets
   - High altitude
   - After meals
   - After delivery due to the trauma
❖ **Physiological decrease** is seen in the newborn
❖ **Pathological increase** (>4 lakh/mm^3 of blood).
   - Trauma and hemorrhage (increased production in response to chronic bleeding or inflammation)
   - Allergic reactions
   - Polycythemia vera
   - Myeloid leukemia (malignant proliferation of megakaryocytes)
   - After splenectomy (25–40% of platelet pool of the body is present in the spleen)
❖ **Pathological decrease** is called **thrombocytopenia** where the count will be less than 1 lakh/mm^3 of blood.
   - Purpura
   - Aplastic anemia (decreased production in the bone marrow)
   - Pernicious anemia
   - Hypersplenism (there will be increased sequestration of platelets in the spleen)
   - Drugs like aspirin
   - Increased destruction in the blood due to autoimmunity, septicemia, etc.
   - Viral infections like dengue fever, chickenpox, etc.

PROPERTIES OF PLATELETS

❖ Adhesiveness and platelet activation
❖ Aggregation

These properties help the platelets to perform their most important function of temporary **hemostasis** (prevention of bleeding), by platelet plug formation.

Adhesiveness and Activation

Endothelial cells line blood vessels internally and collagen fibers are seen sub-endothelially. Platelets do not adhere to the normal vascular lining. When blood vessel is injured, the collagen fibers are exposed to blood and the circulating vWF binds to the exposed sub-endothelial collagen fibers.

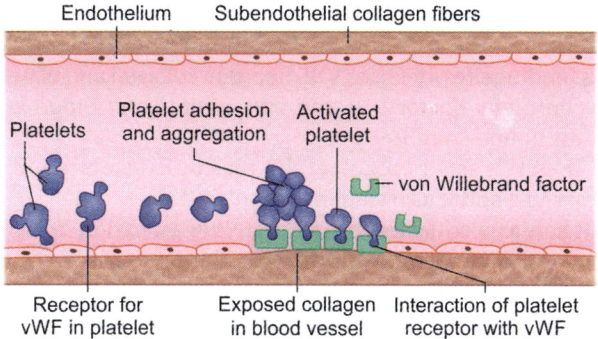

Fig. 17.2: Platelet activation when there is disruption of the endothelial lining of blood vessel. Sub-endothelial collagen get exposed to blood. von Willebrand factor (vWF) binds to the exposed collagen. Platelet receptors for vWF interact to form a complex. This leads to platelet activation, adhesion and aggregation leading to formation of platelet plug.

Activation of the platelets occurs when their receptor interact with vWF. Platelet receptors are glycoproteins in the platelet membrane belonging to integrin class of receptors. vWF binds to platelet receptor known as **glycoprotein Ib/Ia (GPIb/Ia) complex** which is a dimer of GPIb linked to GPIa.

Platelet activation refers to the rise in intracellular Ca^{2+} concentration that occurs in the platelet after it gets anchored to the sub-endothelial collagen through vWF. The rise in Ca^{2+} during platelet activation also leads to the formation of thromboxane A_2 inside the platelet. Thrombin, ADP, Ca^{2+} and thromboxane A_2 also help in platelet activation. Thus, there is a positive feedback cycle of platelet activation. When activated, the platelets collect at the site of injury, change shape, swell up, put out pseudopodia or filopodia, become sticky and release their granular contents like Ca^{2+}, ADP, serotonin, etc., by Ca^{2+} mediated exocytosis. Ca^{2+} and ADP act on nearby platelets and make them sticky. Thus, more and more platelets get attached to collagen fibers **(Fig. 17.2)**. The released ADP acts on ADP receptors on the platelet membrane to produce further accumulation of more platelets (platelet aggregation).

To summarize:
- vWF present in the blood as well as that which is released from activated platelets binds to the platelet receptor GPIb/Ia and help the platelet to adhere to the exposed collagen.
- Binding of platelet to collagen leads to a conformational change in the platelet receptor.
- This initiates an intracellular signaling cascade, which leads to **release reaction or platelet activation**.
- Transduction cascade involves activation of phospholipase C and an influx of calcium ions.
- This leads to exocytosis of dense granules, which release ADP, ATP, serotonin and Ca^{2+}.
- Exocytosis of the contents of alpha granules also occur, which contain vWF, factor V and fibrinogen.
- Platelet activation is also associated with morphological changes in the platelet and many finger-like sticky filopodia get extended from the platelet.

Flowchart 17.1: Steps in the synthesis of thromboxane A_2.

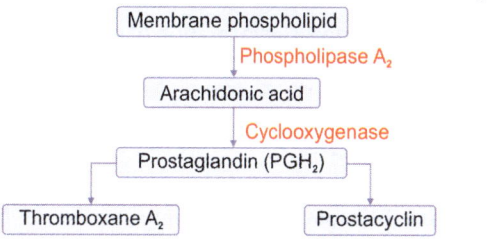

Platelet Aggregation

Aggregation involves **platelet-to-platelet adhesion**. The activated platelet activates phospholipase A_2, which acts on membrane phospholipid and releases arachidonic acid. Activated platelets also activate cyclooxygenase enzyme which break down membrane arachidonic acid to prostaglandin and then to thromboxane A_2 (TxA_2) which is also released **(Flowchart 17.1)**. ADP, serotonin, and thromboxane A_2 activate nearby platelets and they come and stick to the originally activated platelets. This process continues and the platelets aggregate to form a plug at the site of injury. An integrin on the platelet membrane binds to **thrombospondin**, an adhesive protein secreted by the platelet itself. Aggregation of platelets occurs due to the cross-linking of thrombospondin with fibrinogen. Aggregation is promoted by **platelet-activating factor (PAF)**, a cytokine secreted by neutrophils and monocytes as well as platelets. Platelet plug causes temporary arrest of bleeding **(Table. 17.1)**.

Nitric oxide (NO) generated by the endothelial cells inhibits platelet activation through cGMP as the second messenger. Endothelial NO synthase activity is increased during platelet activation. This helps in limiting platelet aggregation.

Applied Physiology

The drug aspirin inhibits the formation of thromboxane A_2, thus inhibiting platelet aggregation. Low doses of aspirin help to prevent intravascular coagulation and thrombus formation in patients who are prone to develop myocardial infarction and stroke.

Platelet membrane has receptors for ADP like $P2Y_1$, $P2Y_2$ and $P2X_1$. During vessel wall injury, the ADP released from activated platelets will cause further accumulation of more platelets leading to platelet aggregation. Several new inhibitors synthesized against the above-mentioned ADP receptors on the platelet membrane can be used in the prevention of myocardial infarction and stroke.

Table 17.1: Factors affecting platelet aggregation.

Factors favoring	Factors inhibiting
ADP, thromboxane A_2	ATP
Serotonin, platelet activating factor	PGI_2
Ca^{2+}	Aspirin, cortisol
vWF	

FUNCTIONS OF PLATELET

- Primary hemostasis by formation of platelet plug
- Promotes blood coagulation
- Clot retraction
- Phagocytosis
- Storage function
- Repair.
- **Primary hemostasis**: It means arrest of bleeding. Serotonin, released from the dense granules of platelets at the site of injury, produces vasoconstriction and thus prevents blood loss. For smaller vessels, the activated platelets are responsible for much of the vasoconstriction by releasing a vasoconstrictor substance thromboxane A_2 synthesized from membrane phospholipid. Platelet plug alone can stop bleeding if the injury is small. Thrombospondin in the platelet helps in the stabilization of platelet plug.
- **Blood coagulation**:
  - Platelet factor 3, a phospholipid released from platelet is necessary for the intrinsic mechanism of clotting.
  - Platelet factor 4 is a procoagulant and has **antiheparin** activity.
  - Platelet also releases **antiplasmin**, which inhibits early breakdown of clot.
  - Platelets entrapped in the clot release procoagulant substances like fibrin stabilizing factor (factor XIII), which produces more and more cross-linking bonds between adjacent fibrin fibers, thus helping in the stabilization of clot.
- **Clot retraction**: Platelets put forward pseudopodia, which get attached to the fibrin threads of the clot. The pseudopodia contain **thrombosthenin**, which contracts and shortens the fibrin thread. The contraction is accelerated by calcium ions released from the calcium stores in the mitochondria, endoplasmic reticulum and Golgi apparatus of the platelets. This helps to compress the fibrin meshwork into a smaller mass so that the edges of the broken vessel wall are pulled together, thus stopping bleeding. This is clot retraction. It occurs 30–60 minutes after clotting. In thrombocytopenia, the clot formed is soft and friable due to the absence of clot retraction.
- **Phagocytosis**: Platelets phagocytize carbon particles, viruses, immune complexes, etc.
- **Storage function**: Platelets are storehouses of serotonin, heparin, histamine, etc.
- **Repair**: Platelet derived growth factor (**PDGF**), being a strong mitogen, induces proliferation of fibroblasts, glial cells and endothelial cells and helps to repair the injured part of the vessel.

VON WILLEBRAND FACTOR

von Willebrand factor (vWF) is a large adhesive glycoprotein that circulates in plasma as a heterogeneous mixture of disulfide-linked multimers. Endothelial cells and megakaryocytes produce it. It is also present in the α-granules of platelets. Platelet activation results in the release of vWF from platelets. Endothelial cell vWF release is induced by histamine. vWF gene is located on chromosome 12 and vWF has binding sites for factor VIII, heparin, collagen and platelet glycoprotein. Factor VIII and vWF circulate in blood as a tightly bound complex.

The vWF acts to regulate the plasma concentration of factor VIII and it also stabilizes factor VIII in plasma. Factor VIII acts as a co-factor to accelerate the activation of factor X by activated factor IX in the coagulation cascade. Factor VIII in complex with vWF has a plasma half-life of about 12 hours whereas factor VIII alone has a half-life of only 2 hours. vWF is also an acute phase protein and the level is elevated in stress, pregnancy, surgical trauma, etc. **Von Willebrand disease** is fairly common and is seen in 1–2% of general population.

Functions of vWF

- It has a very important role in hemostasis. vWF helps in platelet adhesion to thrombogenic substances like collagen at the site of injury in the blood vessel.
- Stabilizes factor VIII and protects it from inactivation by anticoagulant protein C (APC) thus prolonging its half-life in circulation. Thus, it regulates circulating levels of factor VIII.
- vWF is a structural protein and is part of the sub-endothelial matrix.
- It acts as a bridge between platelets and promotes platelet aggregation.
- Inhibits angiogenesis.

THROMBOPOIESIS

Each day an adult human produces about 10^{11} platelets, although in times of increased demand, its production can increase tenfold or more. Formation of platelet, i.e., thrombopoiesis occurs in the red bone marrow from pluripotent hemopoietic stem cells. From pluripotent, stem cell develops committed stem cell, which differentiates into **colony forming unit (CFU) megakaryocyte (Flowchart 17.2)**.

- **Megakaryoblast** is the *first recognizable cell in the platelet series*. Cytoplasm is blue with no granules.
- **Pro-megakaryocyte** is larger and the cytoplasm shows fine granules.
- **Megakaryocytes** are large polyploid cells seen within the bone marrow. It is more than 100 μm in diameter. Polyploidy is because DNA replication occurs in the absence of nuclear or cytoplasmic division. Nucleus contains no nucleoli. Cytoplasm is blue and contains reddish granules. It puts out pseudopodia, which get pinched off, forming platelets. From a single megakaryocyte, about 1000 platelets are formed. About 30–40% of platelets, released from the bone marrow, are stored in the spleen. *This is the reason for thrombocytosis after splenectomy.*

Regulation of Thrombopoiesis

- Platelet production is regulated by the **colony stimulating factors (CSFs)** that control the production

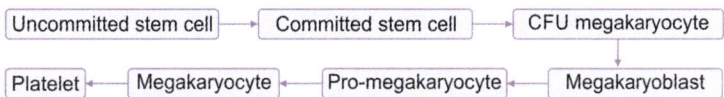

Flowchart 17.2: Steps in the formation of platelets.

of the platelet precursors in the bone marrow, known as megakaryocytes.

- ❖ **Thrombopoietin (TPO)**, a peptide secreted by liver, kidney, skeletal muscle and marrow stroma controls the maturation of megakaryocyte. In thrombocytopenia, thrombopoietin level in blood increases due to lack of negative feedback by platelets on thrombopoietin secretion. There are thrombopoietin receptors on platelets.
- ❖ **Feedback** mechanism prevents excessive thrombocytosis by depressing platelet production. This negative feedback effect on platelet production is due to the release of **transforming growth factor-β (TGF-β)** from platelets. There will be inhibition of thrombopoietin secretion. There are thrombopoietin receptors on platelets. When the number of platelets is low, less of thrombopoietin will be bound to platelets and more is available to stimulate production of platelets. Conversely, when platelet count is high, more of thrombopoietin will be in the bound form and less is available for platelet production.
- ❖ **Interleukin**-3 (IL-3), IL-6 and IL-11 are the cytokines that stimulate thrombopoiesis.

Abnormalities of Platelet Function

Decrease in Platelet Function

- ❖ *Quantitative defect*: **Thrombocytopenia**, where there is reduction in the platelet count. When platelet count is low, clot retraction is deficient and there is poor constriction of ruptured vessels. The condition is thrombocytopenic purpura characterized by easy bruisability and multiple subcutaneous hemorrhages (*refer* **Fig. 18.9**). **Purpura** is bleeding in the skin. Severe purpura is also called **purpura hemorrhagica**. In purpura, bleeding time is prolonged and clotting time is normal. Clot retraction is delayed and the clot formed is soft and friable.
- ❖ *Qualitative defect*: **Thrombasthenia**, where the platelets are abnormal, but platelet count is normal. The purpura occurring here is called *thrombasthenic purpura* (for details, *refer* Chapter 18).

Thrombocytopenia and thrombasthenia lead to purpura, bleeding in the mucosa, bleeding from nose, mouth and gastrointestinal and urinary tract. Platelet count less than 30,000/mm³ of blood leads to spontaneous bleeding. In severe cases, fundal and intracranial bleeding occur. Treatment is by fresh whole blood transfusion, splenectomy, etc.

Thrombocytosis

Thrombocytosis is increase in the platelet count. These individuals are predisposed to thrombotic events like myocardial infarction.

■ MULTIPLE CHOICE QUESTIONS

1. Which of the following promotes platelet aggregation?
   a. Prostacyclin   b. Interleukin
   c. Thromboxane A_2 d. Thrombin
2. Which of the following secretes thromboxane A2?
   a. Erythrocyte   b. Neutrophil
   c. Lymphocyte   d. Platelet
3. Thrombosthenin is a:
   a. Coagulation protein
   b. Contractile protein
   c. Fibrinolytic protein
   d. Regulating protein in platelet production
4. The substance released from platelet during injury to produce vasoconstriction.
   a. Serotonin   b. Histamine
   c. Bradykinin   d. Thrombosthenin
5. Half-life of transfused platelets is:
   a. 4 hours   b. 4 days
   c. 8 days   d. 15 days
6. Life span of platelet in circulation.
   a. 8–12 days   b. 4–6 days
   c. 8–10 hours   d. 2–3 days
7. Smallest of the formed elements in blood.
   a. Erythrocytes   b. Basophils
   c. Small lymphocytes   d. Platelets
8. Presence of abnormal platelets in circulation is referred to as:
   a. Thrombocytopenia
   b. Thrombocytosis
   c. Thrombasthenia
   d. Purpura
9. Spontaneous bleeding occurs when platelet count is less than.
   a. 60,000/mm³ of blood
   b. 30,000/mm³ of blood
   c. 100,000/mm³ of blood
   d. 90,000/mm³ of blood
10. The FALSE statement regarding megakaryocytes is:
    a. They are polyploid cells
    b. They are very large cells
    c. They produce von Willebrand factor
    d. They are normally present in circulation

ANSWERS

1. c   2. d   3. b   4. a   5. b
6. a   7. d   8. c   9. b   10. d

Hemostasis

CHAPTER 18

LEARNING OBJECTIVES

Must know
- Describe the physiological basis of hemostasis (primary and secondary hemostasis)
- Explain bleeding and clotting disorders
- Explain fibrinolytic system
- Discuss the mechanism of action of anticoagulants

Desirable to know
- Enumerate the clotting factors and their sources
- Describe the role of vitamin K in coagulation and the effects of its deficiency

INTRODUCTION

PY2.8: Describe the physiological basis of hemostasis and anticoagulants. Describe bleeding and clotting disorders (hemophilia, purpura).

Hemostasis refers to stoppage of bleeding by physiological processes like clot formation in the walls of damaged blood vessels while maintaining blood in a fluid state within the vascular system. It includes processes like thrombin generation, fibrin clot formation and fibrin clot dissolution. For normal hemostasis, a balance between clot formation and clot dissolution is required so that uncontrolled bleeding or excessive clot formation is prevented. Clotting protects the vasculature from perforating injury and excessive blood loss. Subsequent activation of the fibrinolytic system removes the unwanted fibrin clot, restores blood flow and also helps in tissue repair. Thus hemostasis is an active process which helps in maintaining vascular integrity.

When blood vessels are damaged, the basic mechanisms that occur normally are:
- Vascular spasm
- Platelet plug formation
- Blood coagulation and clot retraction
- Finally, the hole in the vessel is permanently closed by the growth of fibrous tissue into the blood clot

PRIMARY HEMOSTASIS

Primary hemostasis or temporary hemostasis includes vascular spasm and platelet plug formation (**Flowchart 18.1**).

Vascular Spasm

Vessel spasm following injury can last for minutes or even hours depending on the severity of injury. During this time, platelet plugging and blood coagulation can take place. Vascular spasm occurs by the following mechanisms:

Flowchart 18.1: Primary hemostasis: Sequence of events occurring to arrest bleeding immediately following injury to a vessel.

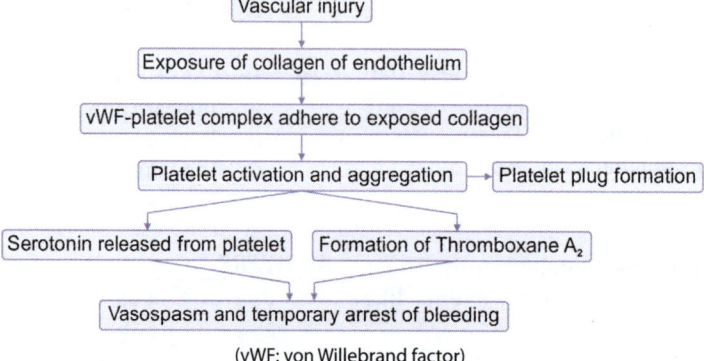

(vWF: von Willebrand factor)

- When smooth muscles of blood vessels are damaged, the circular muscles of the vessel wall contract immediately by a direct action referred to as local **myogenic contraction**.
- **Nervous reflexes**: Pain receptors are stimulated at the site of injury, which causes reflex contraction of the nearby vascular smooth muscle.
- Serotonin and thromboxane A_2 released from activated platelets produces vasoconstriction.
- Thrombin once formed stimulates the endothelium to release endothelin-1 which is a powerful physiological vasoconstrictor.

Platelet Plug Formation

Each day several very small vascular holes develop throughout the body especially in the skin and mucosa and the cuts are often sealed off by the platelet plugs, rather than by blood clots. This is the reason why several bleeding spots referred to as purpura appears in the skin in conditions where the platelet count is very much reduced as in dengue fever.

The properties of platelets like **adhesion, activation and aggregation** help in the formation of temporary hemostatic plug (*refer* Properties of Platelets, Chapter 17). Even though the plug is loose, it can stop blood loss through the wound if the vascular opening is small. Local vasoconstriction and formation of platelet plug lead to temporary arrest of bleeding (*See* **Flowchart 18.1**).

SECONDARY HEMOSTASIS

Secondary hemostasis or permanent hemostasis includes the formation of fibrin from fibrinogen by blood coagulation and clot retraction.

Blood Coagulation or Clotting

The third mechanism in hemostasis is formation of blood clot which begins to develop within 1–2 minutes after injury. The process of coagulation is simultaneously activated along with the activation of platelets. Within 3–6 minutes after rupture of a vessel, the broken end gets filled with clot. **Blood clot** is a semisolid mass composed of platelets and fibrin mesh in which is entrapped red blood cells, leukocytes and serum. After 20 minutes to an hour, the clot retracts further closing the vessel. Within a few hours after the clot is formed, fibroblasts invade the clot, which is promoted by growth factors secreted by the platelets. By about 1–2 weeks, the clot gets organized into fibrous tissue. (*Thrombus is also a blood clot but this term is used only for intravascular clot*)

Coagulation is the conversion of temporary platelet plug into a definitive clot by fibrin. It includes complex cascades of reactions in which, clotting factors activate one another, i.e., a series of **autocatalytic** reactions occur. Once the process is initiated, the reactions act in a positive feedback manner to form a large quantity of product. This is referred to as **enzyme cascade hypothesis**.

The fundamental reaction in clotting is conversion of soluble plasma protein fibrinogen into insoluble fibrin. It involves several substances known as clotting factors synthesized by liver cells or released from platelets or damaged tissues.

Clotting Factors

I : Fibrinogen
II : Prothrombin
III : Thromboplastin or tissue factor
IV : Ca^{2+}
V : Labile factor or proaccerlerin
VI : (This factor is discarded)
VII : Stable factor or proconvertin
VIII : Antihemophilic factor-A
IX : Christmas factor or antihemophilic factor-B
X : Stuart-Prower factor
XI : Plasma thromboplastin antecedent (PTA)
XII : Hageman factor or glass factor or contact factor
XIII : Fibrin stabilizing factor

Other factors involved in coagulation include:
- High molecular weight kininogen (HMW-K)
- Prekallikrein (Pre-Ka)
- Kallikrein (Ka)
- Platelet phospholipid (PL).

The blood clotting factors are mainly plasma proteins and most of these factors are inactive forms of proteolytic enzymes. The clotting factors are designated by Roman numerals. A small letter "a" is added after the Roman numeral to indicate the activated form of the factor. For example, factor VIII is the inactive form and factor VIIIa is the activated form.

Stages of Clotting

There are three stages in clotting:
1. Formation of prothrombinase or prothrombin activator
2. Conversion of prothrombin to thrombin
3. Conversion of soluble fibrinogen to insoluble fibrin.

Formation of Prothrombinase

Prothrombinase is formed in the following ways:
- Extrinsic pathway, which is initiated by tissue thromboplastin
- Intrinsic pathway of coagulation, initiated by platelets
- Common pathway.

Extrinsic Pathway (Tissue Factor Pathway)

Extrinsic pathway of blood coagulation begins with trauma to the vascular wall and surrounding tissues. It occurs only *in vivo*, i.e., within the body and is a **rapid** process. It is completed within **seconds**. The limiting factor is the amount of tissue factor released from the traumatized tissue. More the tissue trauma, more rapid will be the reactions in extrinsic pathway. After injury, the damaged tissue releases tissue thromboplastin (TPL). It activates inactive factor VII to active factor VII (VIIa). Thromboplastin combines with VIIa in the presence of Ca^{2+} and tissue phospholipid to form a complex. This complex converts inactive factor X to active factor X (Xa).

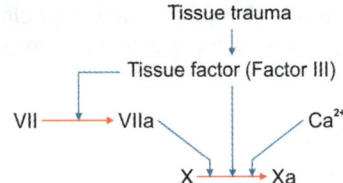

Fig. 18.1: Formation of Xa through extrinsic pathway.

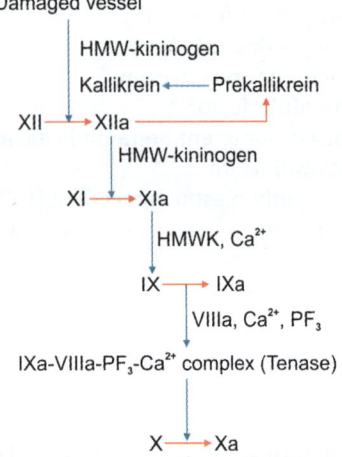

Fig. 18.2: Formation of active factor-X (Xa) by intrinsic pathway.

The steps in extrinsic pathway are as follows:
- Traumatized tissue releases *tissue thromboplastin (factor III)*, which is composed of membrane phospholipids and a lipoprotein complex. Factor III is an integral membrane protein seen in non-vascular cells. This acts as a receptor for factor VII. Tissue factor non-proteolytically activates VII to VIIa.
- Tissue thromboplastin complexes with factor VIIa and calcium ions. This complex proteolytically cleaves the proenzyme, factor *X to form active factor Xa* (**Fig. 18.1**).

Intrinsic Pathway (Contact Activation Pathway)

Intrinsic pathway occurs both *in vivo* and *in vitro*. It begins with trauma to blood cells or exposure of blood to collagen in the injured vessel wall or when blood comes in contact with the membrane of an activated platelet (**Fig. 18.2**). Intrinsic pathway also occurs *in vitro* by exposing blood to electro negatively charged wettable surfaces, such as glass or collagen fibers. It is a **slower process** usually requiring **several minutes** (1-6 minutes).

The steps in intrinsic pathway are:
- Activation of factor XII and release of platelet phospholipids: When there is injury, inactive factor XII comes in contact with collagen and damaged platelets and it is activated to active factor XII (XIIa) in the presence of kallikrein (Ka) and high-molecular-weight kininogen (HMWK). HMWK acts as a cofactor. XIIa converts prekallikrein to kallikrein. Kallikrein accelerates conversion of factor XII to XIIa and a positive feedback sets in. The damaged platelets adhering to the collagen of the vessel wall releases platelet phospholipids (platelet factor 3), which plays an important role in the subsequent reactions of blood clotting.
- XIIa enzymatically activates factor XI to XIa which also requires HMWK and is accelerated by prekallikrein.
- XIa bound to HMWK proteolytically cleaves factor IX and convert it to IXa in the presence of Ca^{2+}.
- Factor VIII is activated to VIIIa when it is separated from von Willebrand factor. VIIIa acts as a cofactor in the next reaction.
- IXa form a complex with VIIIa, platelet factor-3 (PF-3) and Ca^{2+}. This complex known as **tenase** converts factor X to Xa (**Fig. 18.2**). Factor VIII is deficient in patients suffering from classical hemophilia. Thus deficiency of factor VIII or platelets or both will inhibit this step of coagulation leading to bleeding disorders. Xa and thrombin once formed, also cleave VIII to form VIIIa.

> The intrinsic and the extrinsic pathways do not operate independently instead, they are strongly interconnected. For example, factor III, VIIa and Ca^{2+} complex of extrinsic pathway can activate factors IX and XI in the intrinsic pathway. IXa and Xa of intrinsic pathway can activate factor VII of the extrinsic pathway.

Common Pathway

After damage to a blood vessel, clotting occurs by both intrinsic and extrinsic pathways simultaneously. Both the pathways finally converge on a third common pathway (**Fig. 18.3**). Xa combines with tissue phospholipids or platelet phospholipids and factor Va to form a complex called

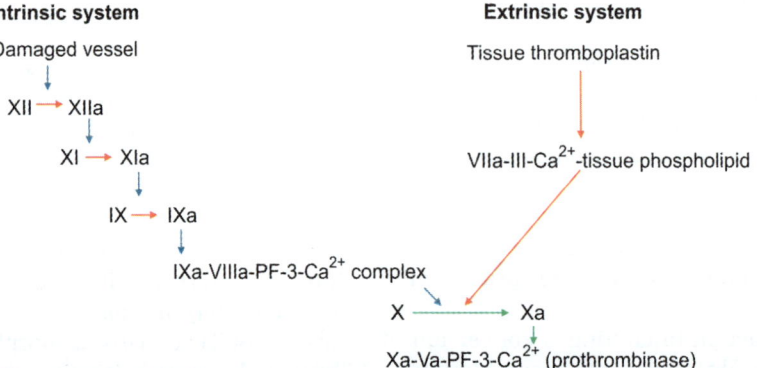

Fig. 18.3: Formation of prothrombinase through intrinsic and extrinsic pathways.

prothrombinase or prothrombin activator. Prothrombin activator in the presence of Ca^{2+} splits prothrombin to thrombin within a few seconds. At first the factor V in the prothrombin activator complex is inactive. But once clotting begins, thrombin converts factor V to active cofactor Va. Thus once thrombin is formed, the clotting process gets accelerated due to the positive feedback effect of thrombin on factor V. The rate limiting step in causing blood coagulation is the formation of prothrombinase.

Conversion of Prothrombin to Thrombin

Prothrombin (clotting factor II) is a plasma protein, an α_2-globulin formed in the liver. Prothrombin requires vitamin K for its normal activation. Therefore, either deficiency of vitamin K or the presence of liver disease that prevents normal prothrombin formation will decrease the prothrombin levels to very low values resulting in bleeding tendency. Prothrombinase, in the presence of Ca^{2+}, converts prothrombin to thrombin. *Thrombin is a proteolytic enzyme.*

$$\text{Prothrombin} \xrightarrow{\text{Prothrombinase, } Ca^{2+}} \text{Thrombin}$$

Conversion of Fibrinogen to Fibrin (Formation of Insoluble Fibrin or Stable Fibrin)

Fibrinogen (clotting factor I) is a high molecular weight plasma protein (MW – 340,000) synthesized in the liver. So, liver diseases can decrease the concentration of plasma fibrinogen leading to bleeding tendency. Thrombin in the presence of Ca^{2+} converts soluble fibrinogen to insoluble fibrin **(Fig. 18.4)**.

* In the first step, fibrinogen is converted to soluble **fibrin monomer** by thrombin which involves the removal of four low-molecular-weight peptides (fibrinopeptides) from each fibrinogen molecule. This step does not require Ca^{2+}.
* Fibrin monomer is composed of α, β and γ chains. By its automatic capability, it spontaneously polymerizes with other fibrin monomer molecules to form **long fibrin fibers** (fibrin polymers) which is a loose mesh or gel of interlacing strands or **reticulum**. It traps blood cells. This clot is weak and can be broken apart with ease because the fibrin threads formed are not cross linked with one another. So the fibrin reticulum should be strengthened and stabilized, which is brought about by fibrin stabilizing factor (F-XIII).
* Thrombin activates factor XIII, to form XIIIa. In the presence of activated fibrin stabilizing factor (XIIIa) and Ca^{2+}, covalent cross-linkages of the α and γ chains of the fibrin polymers are formed between more and more of the fibrin monomer molecules, as well as multiple cross linkages between adjacent fibrin fibers. Thus the loose

mesh of soluble fibrin is converted into a dense, tight aggregate of **stable fibrin or insoluble fibrin**.

Blood cells get entangled or trapped in the fibrin network. The fibrin threads also adhere to damaged surfaces of blood vessels and thus the blood clot becomes adherent to the vascular opening and thereby prevents further blood loss.

Once a clot is formed in a blood vessel, it normally extends into the surrounding blood by initiating a positive feedback to promote more clotting. This positive feedback effect is mainly due to the action of thrombin.

Positive feedback effects of thrombin:
* Thrombin has direct proteolytic effect on prothrombin, thus converting it to more and more thrombin.
* By activating factor V, it accelerates the formation of prothrombinase or prothrombin activator.
* Thrombin also accelerates the action of factors VIII, IX, X, XI and XII which are also responsible for the formation of prothrombin activator. Prothrombinase, in turn, accelerates the production of more thrombin and so on.
* Thrombin activates platelets, which reinforces their aggregation and release of phospholipids.

Functions of Thrombin

Thrombin is unique in its function. It acts both as a pro-coagulant and an anticoagulant.

Pro-coagulant Actions

Thrombin converts:
* Factor XI to XIa
* Factor VIII to VIIIa
* Factor V to Va
* Factor XIII to XIIIa
* Fibrinogen to fibrin.
* Induce platelet aggregation and release of ADP from platelets

Anticoagulant Actions

* Thrombin by binding with thrombomodulin converts inactive protein C to active protein C which is an anticoagulant
* Along with tissue type plasminogen activator (t-PA) converts plasminogen to plasmin

> **APPLIED PHYSIOLOGY**
>
> Clotting should not run out of control. If unchecked, a clot would continue to get larger and larger as a result of positive feedback cycles. However, fibrin has the ability to adsorb and inactivate up to 90% of the thrombin formed from prothrombin. This helps to stop the spread of thrombin into the blood and thus limits the spread of the clot beyond the site of damage.

Clot Retraction

Thrombosthenin is a contractile protein present in the platelets. It has a high molecular weight and is composed of multiple polypeptide subunits. After clot formation, thrombosthenin contracts and the clot shrinks, squeezing out a straw-colored fluid called **serum**. This process is called **clot retraction**. Glycoprotein IIb/ IIIa receptors on platelets

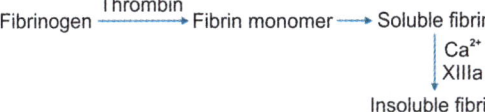

Fig. 18.4: Conversion of soluble fibrinogen to insoluble fibrin.

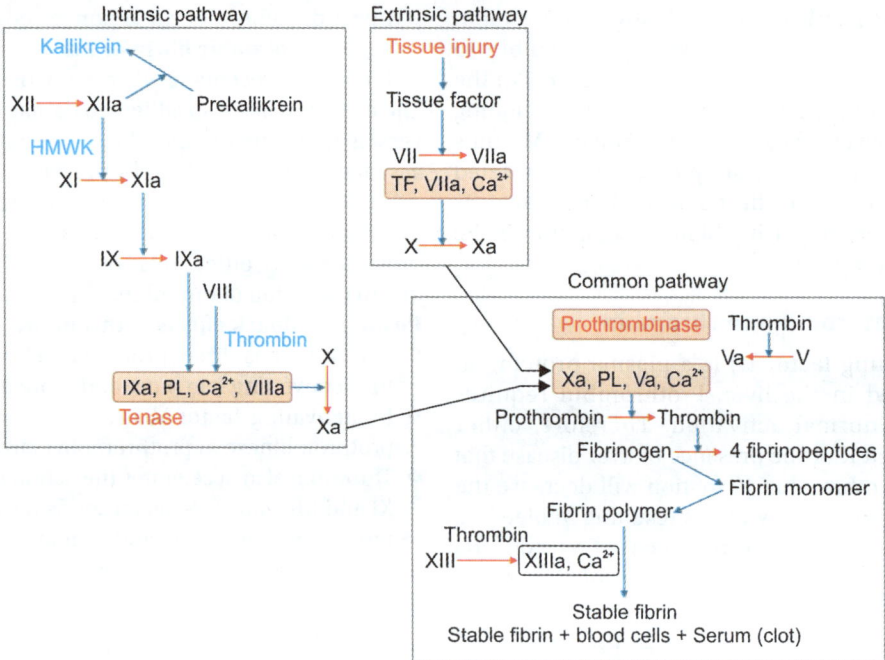

Fig. 18.5: Summary of coagulation of blood.
(PL : phospholipid, TF: tissue factor)

facilitate clot retraction. As the clot retracts, it pulls the edges of the damaged vessel close together. *Serum does not contain factors I, II, V, VIII and XIII. So, serum does not clot.* Serum has higher serotonin content due to breakdown of platelets during clot formation.

1. Normal clotting time: 4–11 min
2. Clot retraction time: 30–60 min.

Summary of coagulation of blood is shown in **Figure 18.5**.

Calcium is needed in all steps of coagulation, *except activation of factors XI, XII and conversion of fibrinogen to fibrin monomer*. So, removal of Ca^{2+} from blood prevents coagulation. In vivo, the calcium ion concentration seldom falls to such low levels to affect blood clotting because such a level is incompatible with life. In vitro, blood can be prevented from clotting by removing Ca^{2+} by deionizing or precipitating the calcium ions.

Role of Vitamin K in Coagulation

Vitamin K is essential for the biosynthesis of functional clotting factors II, VII, IX and X by the liver. In the liver these clotting factors after synthesis will be in the descarboxy form. They become functional only after γ-carboxylation of 9 to 13 NH_2^- terminal glutamic acid residues in them. Reduced form of vitamin K is required for this conversion. Vitamin K acts as a cofactor for the enzyme vitamin K dependent carboxylase that catalyzes the conversion of glutamic acid residues to γ-carboxyglutamic acid residues. Clotting factors **II, VII, IX, X** and anticlotting factors **protein C and protein S** require conversion of a number of glutamic acid residues to γ-carboxyglutamic acid residues before being released into the circulation. Hence these six proteins are said to be **vitamin K-dependent**.

The active form of vitamin K called **vitamin K hydroquinone** carries out the final step of carboxylating glutamate residues. This γ-carboxylation is essential for the ability of the clotting factors to bind Ca^{2+} and to get bound to phospholipid surfaces, which is necessary for the coagulation sequence to proceed. Vitamin K hydroquinone will be converted to **vitamin K epoxide** which is the inactive form of vitamin K. It is converted back to the active form by **vitamin K epoxide reductase** in the presence of NADH. This step is blocked by oral anticoagulants like warfarin (**Fig. 18.6**). Warfarin has structural similarity with vitamin K.

Vitamin K is normally synthesized by the bacterial flora of large intestine. Other sources are green leafy vegetables, cereals, etc. It is absorbed from the small intestine in the presence of bile salts.

Vitamin K Deficiency

Vitamin K deficiency diseases are seen in the following conditions:

❖ In impaired fat absorption, as in obstructive jaundice (vitamin K being a fat-soluble vitamin is not absorbed in the

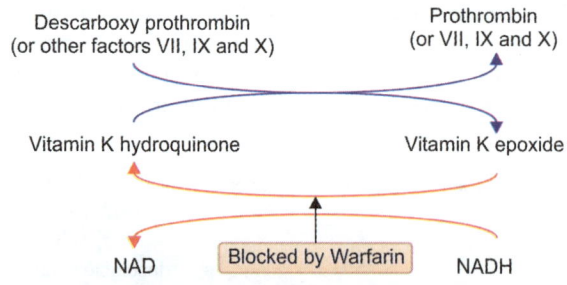

Fig. 18.6: Role of vitamin K in coagulation.

absence of bile salts), there will be uncontrolled bleeding due to the deficiency of vitamin K dependent clotting factors due to vitamin K deficiency.
- Vitamin K deficiency is seen secondary to antibiotic administration where the bacterial flora of the intestine which synthesizes vitamin K are destroyed and is also seen following administration of vitamin K antagonists like warfarin.
- Vitamin K deficiency is also seen in premature infants because the bacterial flora of intestine is not developed and it takes about 1 month for them to develop satisfactorily. Injection of vitamin K causes complete recovery in less than 48 hours.
- In liver disorders like hepatitis, cirrhosis, malignancy, etc., there will be deficiency of bile salts leading to defective fat absorption. But in these conditions, liver function is also impaired and there will be failure of prothrombin synthesis in the liver leading to defective blood clotting. In this case, parenteral administration of vitamin K is ineffective.

Blood does not clot *in vivo* normally and this is due to the following reasons:
- Blood is in constant motion.
- The vascular endothelium is very smooth and prevents platelet adhesion.
- In the blood stream, the anticoagulants normally predominates the procoagulants, so the blood does not coagulate while it is circulating in the blood vessels.
- Liver removes activated clotting factors from blood in times of spontaneous coagulation.
- Presence of natural intravascular anticoagulants, which act by:
  a. Preventing clotting.
  b. Preventing the extension of clot to the surrounding area.
  c. Breaking down any clot that is formed.

FACTORS THAT PREVENT INTRAVASCULAR COAGULATION OR INTRAVASCULAR ANTICOAGULANTS (TABLE 18.1)

- Endothelial surface factors
- Tissue factor pathway inhibitor (TFPI)
- Thrombomodulin
- Antithrombin III and fibrin threads
- Heparin
- α_2 globulin
- Interaction between thromboxane A_2 and prostacyclin
- Role of liver
- Fibrinolytic system

Endothelial Factors

- Smoothness of endothelium prevents platelet adhesion and contact activation of the intrinsic clotting system.
- Surface of endothelium is negatively charged because of the presence of a layer of glycocalyx (mucopolysaccharides adsorbed to the endothelial cell surface), which repels clotting factors and platelets.
- Endothelium produces prostacyclin (PGI_2), which produces vasodilatation and prevents platelet activation.
- Endothelial cells produce a protein called **thrombomodulin**, which combines with thrombin and forms thrombomodulin-thrombin complex, thus inactivating thrombin. This complex also activates protein C which in turn inactivates factors Va and VIIIa.
- Nitric oxide (NO) generated by the endothelial cells from L-arginine inhibits platelet adhesion and aggregation. Thrombin stimulates endothelial cells to produce NO.

Tissue Factor Pathway Inhibitor

Tissue factor pathway inhibitor (TFPI) is a plasma protein that binds with the complex [tissue factor + VIIa + Ca^{2+}] in the extrinsic pathway and blocks the activity of clotting factor VIIa.

Thrombomodulin

All endothelial cells, except those present in cerebral microcirculation, produces **thrombomodulin**, a thrombin binding protein. Thrombin activates factor V and VIII, but when it binds with thrombomodulin, it becomes an anticoagulant. Thrombomodulin-thrombin complex activates protein C, which is a naturally occurring anticoagulant protein. Activated protein C (APC) is a protease. APC along with cofactor protein S, inactivates cofactors Va and VIIIa and also inactivates an inhibitor of tissue plasminogen activator. This increases the rate of formation of plasmin or fibrinolysin from inactive plasminogen **(Flowchart 18.2)**.

Table 18.1: Factors that prevent coagulation of blood.				
Naturally occurring factors that maintain fluidity of blood	**Synthetic anticoagulants**			
Vascular endothelial factors • Smoothness of endothelium • Glycocalyx • Thrombomodulin	**For Laboratory tests** Trisodium citrate	*Acting in vitro* **For storage of blood** Acid-citrate-dextrose (ACD)	**Parenteral** Heparin	*Acting in vivo* **Oral anticoagulants** Warfarin Dicoumarol
	Double oxalate	Citrate phosphate dextrose (CPD)		
Antithrombin III	EDTA	CPD-adenine		
Protein C and protein S	Sodium fluoride			
Heparin	Heparin			
α_2 macroglobulin				

Flowchart 18.2: Extrinsic mechanism of fibrinolysis.

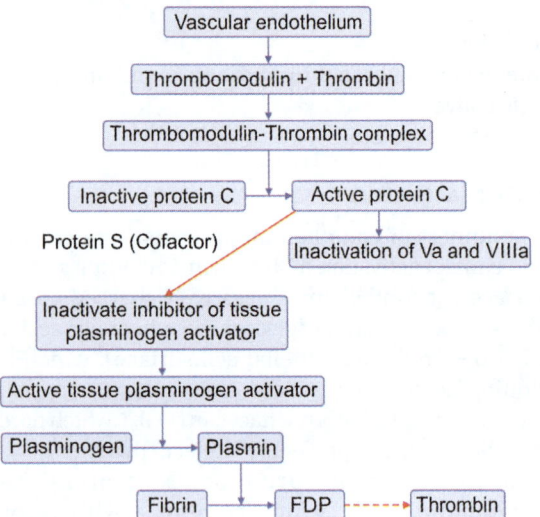

(Va: activated factor V; activated factor VII; FDP: fibrin degradation product; t-PA; tissue type plasminogen activator; dashed line indicate inhibition)

Antithrombin III and Fibrin Threads

Inhibitors of thrombin are antithrombin III and heparin cofactor II. When a clot is formed, 90% of thrombin formed gets adsorbed to the fibrin threads. This prevents excessive spread of clot. The remaining thrombin combines with antithrombin III and is inactivated. Antithrombin III or antithrombin-heparin cofactor, an alpha globulin, is a circulating protease inhibitor secreted by the liver. Antithrombin III binds to serine proteases in the coagulation system thus blocking their action as clotting factors. This binding is facilitated by heparin and the clotting factors inhibited are the active forms of factors IX, X, XI and XII.

Heparin

Heparin is present in basophils and mast cells. It combines with antithrombin III and increases the effectiveness of antithrombin III for removing thrombin 100-1000 fold. The complex of heparin and antithrombin III also inactivates activated factors XII, XI, X and IX. Mast cells are abundant in tissues surrounding the capillaries of lungs and liver. This is because a large quantity of heparin is needed in these areas because many embolic clots are formed in the capillaries of these areas due to the slow movement of venous blood.

α_2-Macroglobulin

α_2-Macroglobulin binds with clotting factors and inactivates them.

Thromboxane A_2 and Prostacyclin

Once platelet gets activated, it activates membrane phospholipid to form thromboxane A_2 and prostacyclin (PGI_2). When TXA_2 stimulate platelet activation, prostacyclin inhibits it. Interaction between thromboxane A_2 and prostacyclin also acts as an intravascular anticlotting mechanism.

Role of Liver

Finally the activated clotting factors are taken up by the Kupffer cells of liver and thus control hemostasis.

FIBRINOLYTIC SYSTEM

Dissolution of clot is referred to as **fibrinolysis**. The active component of fibrinolytic system is **plasmin or fibrinolysin**. Plasmin is formed from its inactive precursor **plasminogen** or profibrinolysin by the action of thrombin and **tissue-type plasminogen activator (t-PA)** and **urokinase-type plasminogen activator (u-PA)**. Plasminogen is converted to active plasmin when t-PA hydrolyses the bond between Arginine 560 and Valine 561. Plasmin is a proteolytic enzyme which resembles trypsin. It lyses fibrin and fibrinogen to form **fibrin degradation products (FDP)**, which inhibits thrombin **(Fig. 18.7 and Flowchart 18.2)**. It also digests other protein coagulants like factor V, VIII, prothrombin and factor XII.

In fibrinolysis there are two types of mechanisms:
1. Intrinsic mechanism
2. Extrinsic mechanism

Intrinsic Mechanism

Whenever there is activation of coagulation pathway, there will be simultaneous activation of the intrinsic fibrinolytic system **(Fig. 18.7)**.

Extrinsic Mechanism

Extrinsic mechanism is the predominant mechanism of fibrinolysis. Vascular endothelium release thrombomodulin which combines with thrombin to form **thrombomodulin-thrombin complex (Flowchart 18.2)**. When thrombin level increases beyond a limit it itself initiate anticlotting mechanism by combining with thrombomodulin. The fibrin degradation products are excreted through urine.

Plasminogen

Human plasminogen is a polypeptide synthesized by the liver. It consists of a 560-amino acid heavy chain and a 241-amino acid light chain. After a clot is formed, the injured tissues and vascular endothelium slowly releases a powerful activator of plasmin called **tissue plasminogen activator (t-PA)** which is a polypeptide. Tissue plasminogen activator or vascular plasminogen activator is a serine protease whose secretion is stimulated by epinephrine,

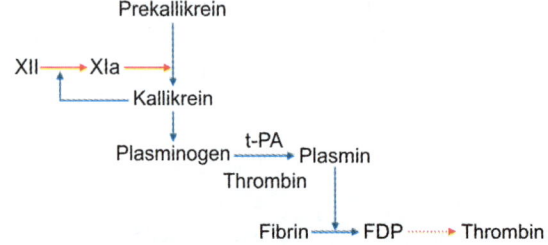

Fig. 18.7: Intrinsic mechanism of fibrinolysis.
(FDP: fibrin degradation product; dashed lines indicate inhibition)

thrombin, serotonin, fibrin, shear stress, vaso-occlusion, etc. Inactive plasminogen is converted to active plasmin when t-PA hydrolyses the bond between arginine and valine. Plasminogen receptors are present on the surfaces of many cells and are plentiful on the endothelial cells. When plasminogen binds to its receptors, plasminogen gets activated to form plasmin. Thus, blood vessel endothelium is provided with a mechanism that prevents clot formation as long as the endothelium is intact. In addition to lysing clots, plasminogen system also plays an important role in cell movement and in ovulation.

Annexins are a group of homologous proteins similar to plasmin, which produce fibrinolysis.

Importance of Fibrinolytic System

- ❖ Normally the clotting system of plasma continuously forms small clots in the tiny peripheral vessels which form a thin layer on the vascular endothelium. Excess formation of clots may occlude these vessels, but this is prevented by the fibrinolytic system.
- ❖ It promotes normal healing process by lysing the clot at the site of injury
- ❖ Helps in the liquefaction of menstrual clot in the uterus and vagina
- ❖ Helps in the liquefaction of sperm in epididymis if ejaculation does not occur
- ❖ Has a role in inflammation. Plasmin can form kinins and thus contribute to the inflammatory process of injury.

> **Human tissue-type plasminogen activator (t-PA)** is now produced by recombinant DNA techniques (Alteplase). It is given to patients soon after the onset of myocardial infarction (MI) and it lyses clots in the coronary arteries. **Streptokinase**, an enzyme produced by *Streptococcus* bacteria and **urokinase**, an enzyme produced by renal cells are also fibrinolytic and are used in the treatment of early MI.

■ FIBRINOLYSIS INHIBITORS

The inhibitors of fibrinolysis is an integral part of the fibrinolytic system in maintaining a state of dynamic equilibrium with the activators.

Plasminogen Activator Inhibitor-1 (PAI-1)

PAI-1 is synthesized by liver, spleen, adipose tissue and endothelial cells. Major fraction in the blood is present in the platelets stored in the alpha granules.

Plasminogen Activator Inhibitor-2 (PAI-2)

PAI-2 is usually seen during the third trimester of pregnancy. The level exceeds that of PAI-1 at this time.

Alpha-2 Antiplasmin

Alpha-2 antiplasmin is synthesized in the liver and kidney. It inactivates plasmin by combining with both lysine binding site and active serine.

> **APPLIED PHYSIOLOGY**
>
> **Hereditary plasminogen deficiency or hypoplasminogenemia:** Type I congenital plasminogen deficiency is inherited in an autosomal recessive pattern. It most often affects the conjunctiva. It presents with conjunctivitis, in which there is accumulation of fibrin which leads to thick, inflamed growths that are yellow, white or red. It may end in blindness if cornea gets affected. These woody or ligneous growths are also seen in the mucous membrane lining the mouth, nasal cavity, gastrointestinal tract and vagina in females.

Tests of Coagulation

1. **Bleeding time:** 1–4 min. Bleeding time is said to be prolonged when it is >8 minutes as in purpura, von Willebrand disease, etc.
2. **Clotting time:** 4–11 min.
3. **Prothrombin time (PT):** It measures the efficiency of extrinsic pathway and the common pathway of coagulation. It gives an indication of the concentration of prothrombin in blood. Oxalated venous blood is mixed with an excess of thromboplastin obtained from tissues. The mixture is then recalcified and the time taken for the formation of clot is measured. Instead of whole blood, plasma of the subject can be used. Prothrombin time is done frequently while treating cases of thrombosis with dicoumarol and fibrinolytic drugs. Normal value is 16 seconds.
4. **International normalized ratio (INR):** The results obtained for prothrombin time varies considerably if there are differences in the activity of tissue factor. INR was devised as a way to standardize measurements of prothrombin time. International sensitivity index (ISI) indicates the activity of the tissue factor of each batch with a standardized sample. ISI varies between 1 and 2. INR is the ratio of the person's prothrombin time to a normal control sample raised to the power of the ISI. The normal range of INR in a healthy person is 0.9-1.3. A high INR indicates a high risk of bleeding, whereas a low INR increases the chance of developing a clot. The INR level in patients on warfarin therapy is maintained between 2 and 3. This test should be done periodically to make sure that the patients are receiving the correct dosage of warfarin needed for them.
5. **Activated partial thromboplastin time (APTT):** It measures the efficiency of the intrinsic and the common coagulation pathways. This test is done by mixing calcium and a contact factor such as silica with oxalated blood and observing the time taken for a clot to form. Normal value is 40 sec.
6. **Platelet count:** 2–4 lakhs/mm^3 of blood.
7. **Clot retraction time:** 30–60 min.

■ ANTICOAGULANTS

More than 50 substances that affect coagulation have been found in blood. Some of them promote coagulation and are called **procoagulants**. **Anticoagulants** are substances, which inhibit coagulation of blood. Under physiological conditions, anticoagulants predominate so that blood does not clot in vivo.

Laboratory Anticoagulants

There are certain criteria for the substances used as anticoagulants in the laboratory.
- Should not alter the size of the cell.
- Should not produce hemolysis.
- Should not disrupt leukocytes.

The anticoagulants used in the laboratory are:
- **Ethylene diamine tetra acetic acid (EDTA)**, 1 mg/mL of blood is used. This is the anticoagulant of choice, since it preserves the cellular components of blood for adequate time. Used for doing ESR, hemocytometry and platelet count.
- **Double oxalate** is a mixture of ammonium and potassium oxalate in the ratio 3:2 (Wintrobe's mixture). The concentration is 2 mg/mL of blood. Ammonium oxalate causes swelling of cells and potassium oxalate causes shrinking of cells. So both are used together to maintain the normal morphology of cells. It is used for doing PCV, ESR, and RBC & WBC count. It is not used for peripheral smear since calcium oxalate is insoluble and will be phagocytosed by neutrophil. Thus the morphology of leukocytes gets distorted.
- **Trisodium citrate**: 3.8% solution of trisodium citrate is used. 0.4 mL of sodium citrate and 1.6 mL of blood is mixed for doing ESR by Westergren's method. For doing PT and APTT, 9 part blood and 1 part sodium citrate solution is used.
- **Sodium fluoride:** It prevents glycolysis by blocking the enzyme phosphorylase in RBC thus preventing loss of glucose. Used in blood sugar estimation.

  The mechanism of action of the above anticoagulants is by removing Ca^{2+}, i.e., they act as **chelating agents**. For example, when sodium citrate is used, Ca^{2+} is precipitated as calcium-sodium citrate, a double salt. Ca^{2+} is necessary in almost all steps of coagulation and hence removal of Ca^{2+} prevents coagulation.
- **Heparin:** One unit of heparin is added to 10 mL of blood. Used for blood gas analysis, osmotic fragility tests etc. Disadvantages are it is costly and it cannot be used for WBC count. It causes clumping of WBC. Since it is highly acidic and may interfere with staining so, cannot be used in peripheral smear examination.
- Acid-citrate-dextrose (ACD) and citrate-phosphate-dextrose-adenine (CPD-A) are used for storing blood in blood bank.

Clinically Used Anticoagulants

- **Heparin**: Heparin is a polysaccharide, which was first isolated from liver and hence the name. It is also present in the granules of basophils and mast cells. Normally, heparin is destroyed by **heparinase**, an enzyme present in liver. Heparin is given in cases of deep vein thrombosis, myocardial infarction, pulmonary embolism, during heart operations in heart-lung machine, during hemodialysis, etc. Heparin potentiates the action of antithrombin III and prevents coagulation by inhibiting factors IX, X, XI and XII. Heparin should be administered intravenously or subcutaneously. Its action lasts for 2 to 4 hours. Clinically low molecular weight fragments of heparin have been produced from unfractionated heparin. It has a longer half-life and produces a more predictable anticoagulant response than unfractionated heparin.

  Antidote for heparin is **protamine sulphate**. The highly basic protein, protamine forms an irreversible complex with heparin and is used clinically to neutralize heparin especially after cardiopulmonary by-pass surgery; carotid endarterectomy etc. 1 mg of protamine neutralizes 100 units of heparin.
- **Vitamin K antagonists**: They are known as oral anticoagulants or **coumarin anticoagulants**. The commonly used one is *warfarin sodium*. It acts indirectly by interfering with the synthesis of vitamin K dependent clotting factors in liver (*refer* **Fig. 18.3**). They act as competitive antagonists of vitamin K and reduce the plasma levels of functional clotting factors. It is used to treat atrial fibrillation, deep vein thrombosis, pulmonary embolism, etc. *Dicoumarol* is another coumarin derivative.
- **Aspirin**: It inhibits the formation of thromboxane A_2 and prevents platelet activation. It is used for prophylaxis of thromboembolism.

Biological Anticoagulants or Natural Anticoagulants

- **Hirudin** obtained from the buccal glands of leech acts as antithrombin and prevents coagulation.
- **Snake venom**, especially cobra venom acts as anticoagulant. Pit viper venom stimulates fibrinolytic system by converting plasminogen to plasmin, which leads to serious internal bleeding.
- Heparin, anti-thrombin and protein C are naturally occurring anticoagulants in humans. **Heparin** is present in the granules of basophils and mast cells. It facilitates the action of antithrombin III, thereby inhibiting the active forms of clotting factors IX, X, XI and XII.
- **Antithrombin** inhibits thrombin and prevents coagulation.
- **Protein C** along with its cofactor *protein S* inactivates clotting factors V and VIII and stimulates the formation of plasmin.

BLEEDING DISORDERS

Bleeding disorders may be due to the following causes:
- Defective clotting
- Vascular defects
- Platelet defects
- Combined defects

Defective Clotting

- **Congenital,** e.g., factor VIII or factor IX deficiency (hemophilia), von Willebrand disease, etc.
- **Acquired,** e.g., disseminated intravascular coagulation (DIC), liver failure, vitamin K deficiency, anticoagulant overdose, etc.

Hemophilia

Hemophilia is a **sex-linked** inherited disease due to an abnormal gene on X-chromosome. In this condition, severe bleeding occurs spontaneously or after minor trauma. There will be subcutaneous and intramuscular hemorrhage, nasal bleeding (hemoptysis), hematuria (blood in urine) and hemorrhage into the joint space, producing severe joint pain. *The clotting time is very much prolonged, but bleeding time is normal.* The primary defect in all types of hemophilia is lack of formation of prothrombinase due to deficiency of certain clotting factors necessary for the formation of prothrombinase. Prothrombinase is necessary for the conversion of prothrombin to thrombin, which in turn converts fibrinogen to fibrin. So in hemophilia, clotting time may be prolonged to 1–12 hours (normal: 5–10 min) and the clot formed will be very soft. Depending on the type of clotting factor that is deficient, hemophilia is of three types:

1. **Hemophilia A** or classic hemophilia (85% of cases) is due to deficiency of clotting factor VIII. This is the most common hereditary coagulation disorder.
2. **Hemophilia B** or Christmas disease (15%) is due to deficiency of factor IX.
3. **Hemophilia C** due to lack of factor XI is much less severe than hemophilia A or B.

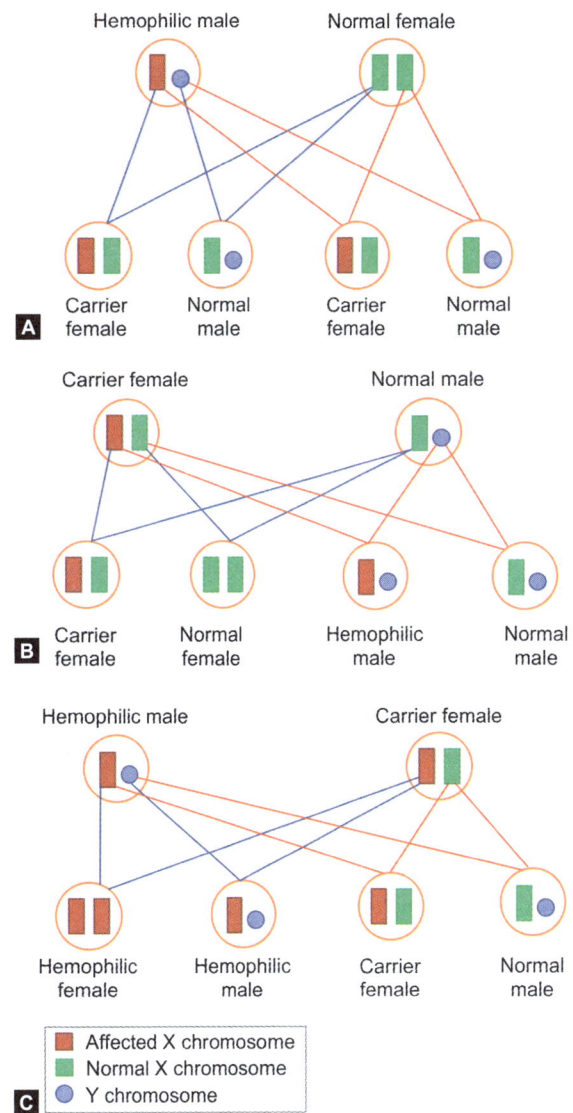

Inheritance of Hemophilia (Figs. 18.8A to C)

Hemophilia A and B occurs primarily among males because these are **sex-linked recessive disorders**. Females usually act as carriers. The defective gene is present in the X chromosome. As it is recessive in character, if a normal homologous gene accompanies one abnormal gene, the disease will not be manifested. Thus, in females if one chromosome is normal, they do not suffer from the disease but act as carriers transmitting the disease to the next generation. Therefore, the sons of a hemophilic man will be normal but the daughters act as carriers. So, this disease is said to skip one generation **(Fig. 18.8A)**.

Females may be affected if a hemophilic man marries a hemophilic carrier female **(Fig. 18.8C)**. Hemophilia A and B can be distinguished by thromboplastin generation test or activated partial thromboplastin time.

Hemophilia C affects both males and females equally and is inherited as **Mendelian dominant**.

Blood tests to confirm hemophilia

Clotting time, activated partial thromboplastin time (APTT), prothrombin time and bleeding time are determined to confirm hemophilia. Clotting time and APTT are prolonged in hemophilia due to deficiency of clotting factor VIII (classic hemophilia or hemophilia-A). Prothrombin time and bleeding time are normal in hemophilia. Factor VIII assay can also be done to assess the severity of the disease.

Treatment

- Cryoprecipitate (fresh frozen plasma) of factor VIII is available and is given intravenously.
- Fresh blood or fresh plasma transfusion is done because factor VIII is destroyed rapidly on storage.
- Factor VIII produced by recombinant DNA techniques can also be used to treat hemophilia
- For Christmas disease, stored blood also can be given because factor IX is not lost during storage.

Figs. 18.8A to C: Inheritance of hemophilia.

Afibrinogenemia

Afibrinogenemia is an inherited disorder, but acquired afibrinogenemia is seen in end-stages of liver disease.

Hypoprothrombinemia

Hypoprothrombinemia may be due to liver disease, vitamin K deficiency, etc.

Vitamin K Deficiency

Vitamin K is required for the synthesis of active clotting factors II, VII, IX and X in the liver. Liver cells contain receptors for vitamin K. Vitamin K deficiency is characterized by prolongation of clotting time and serious hemorrhages. Vitamin K is a fat-soluble vitamin and is absorbed in the small intestine in the presence of bile salts. Vitamin K deficiency is treated by giving vitamin K injection.

Causes of Vitamin K Deficiency

- Absence of bile salts in the intestine as in obstructive jaundice.

- Defective fat absorption as in chronic diarrhea leads to decreased absorption of vitamin K.
- Vitamin K is synthesized in the intestine by certain bacteria. Administration of antibiotics may destroy these bacteria producing defective vitamin K synthesis leading to its deficiency.
- Bleeding due to vitamin K deficiency is common in premature babies.

Protein C Deficiency

Congenital absence of protein C leads to uncontrolled intravascular coagulation and death in infancy.

PURPURA

Purpura is spontaneous hemorrhage into the skin and mucous membrane from capillaries due to abnormalities in blood vessels or platelets. The bleeding is seen as tiny purpuric spots (purple colored patches) and hence the name **(Fig. 18.9)**. *In purpura, bleeding time is prolonged, but clotting time is normal.* It may be due to vascular defects, platelet defects or combined defects.

Vascular Defects

In vascular defects, there may be some abnormality in the integrity of vascular endothelium. It may be due to infections, drugs (aspirin and sulfa drugs), vitamin C deficiency, allergy, vasculitis due to connective tissue disorders, etc. The condition is treated with ACTH or corticosteroids, which reduces the fragility of capillaries.

Platelet Defects

Quantitative defect or thrombocytopenia: In thrombocytopenia, bleeding time is prolonged when platelet count is less than 1 lakh/mm³ of blood, easy bruising occurs when the platelet count is less than 50,000/mm³ and spontaneous bleeding occur when the count is less than 20,000/mm³ of blood.
- *Primary thrombocytopenic purpura or idiopathic thrombocytopenic purpura* (ITP) may be due to autoimmunity (antibodies are produced against platelets) or it may be hereditary or congenital, which usually occurs in children. Splenectomy (removal of spleen) is done in severe cases of primary thrombocytopenic purpura.

  Secondary thrombocytopenic purpura may be due to drugs, infections, bone marrow depression, leukemia and hypersplenism. In hypersplenism, there will be increased destruction of platelets in the spleen.
- **Qualitative defect or thrombasthenic purpura**: Thrombasthenic purpura is due to abnormal platelets in circulation. Here, the platelet count is normal, but there is defect in platelet adhesion and aggregation. This condition can also be due to abnormal functioning of platelets as in leukemia, von Willebrand disease, etc.

Combined Defects

von Willebrand Disease

von Willebrand disease is due to inherited deficiency of von Willebrand factor (vWF) secreted by platelets and damaged vascular endothelium. This deficiency leads to inhibition of platelet adhesion and diminished adherence of platelets to collagen fibers of a damaged vessel. This produces severe bleeding from small injuries.

von Willebrand disease is also known as **pseudohemophilia**. Factor VIII is transported in combination with vWF. Factor VIII gets activated when it is separated from vWF. Thus, vWF is responsible for the survival and maintenance of factor VIII in the plasma. Thus, its deficiency produces secondary deficiency of factor VIII. This results in excessive bleeding, which resembles the bleeding that occurs during platelet dysfunction or hemophilia. So, von Willebrand disease can be included under combined defect.

THROMBOEMBOLIC CONDITIONS IN HUMAN

Thrombosis

Normally, blood does not clot inside the blood vessel. An abnormal clot that develops in the blood vessel is called a **thrombus**. Thrombus may get detached from the vessel wall and will be carried by blood to other areas when it is called an **embolus**. Emboli originating in large arteries and left side of heart may block small arteries in brain, kidney, heart, etc. Emboli arising from large veins and right side of the heart block the pulmonary vessels leading to pulmonary embolism. In embolism, the blood supply to the affected area is cut off leading to **infarction**, e.g., myocardial infarction. The affected area is called an infarct.

Causes of Thrombosis

- Loss of smoothness of endothelium as in atherosclerosis, infection, trauma, etc., initiates clotting.
- Slowness of blood flow as in hypotension, in bed-ridden patients, etc., allows activated clotting factors to accumulate and form clot instead of being washed away. Normally, the activated clotting factors are immediately destroyed when they reach the liver. Sluggish blood flow also causes aggregation of platelets and formation of thrombus.

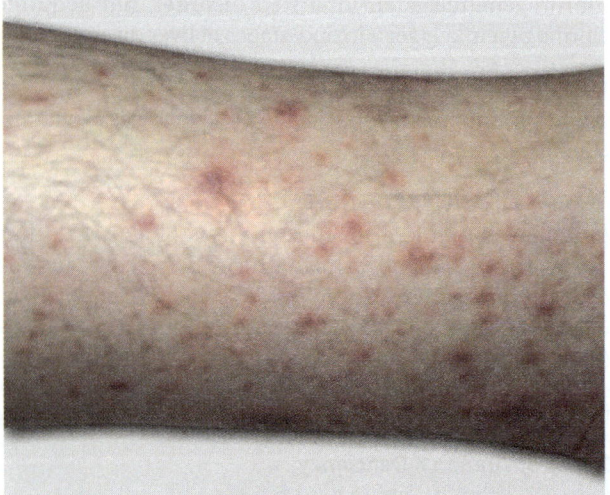

Fig. 18.9: Purpura.

- Defective fibrinolytic system as in mutation of antithrombin III and protein S genes, favor clot formation.
- Congenital absence of protein C can cause thrombosis and death in infancy.
- Venom of certain snakes and poisonous mushrooms contain proteolytic enzymes, which activate clotting factors and enhance intravascular coagulation.

Treatment

Heparin, vitamin K antagonists like warfarin sodium, aspirin, etc., can be used to prevent thromboembolism. Aspirin inhibits the formation of thromboxane A_2, thus preventing activation of platelets and platelet aggregation. Thus, low doses of aspirin administered daily prevent the risk of intravascular coagulation and thromboembolic episodes in high-risk persons. Excess aspirin can produce bleeding.

Disseminated Intravascular Coagulation

Disseminated intravascular coagulation (DIC) is due to the presence of large quantities of traumatized tissues in the body that release **tissue thromboplastin** and initiate coagulation. Numerous small clots are formed, which block peripheral small vessels. This condition is seen in septicemia, abruptio placenta, mismatched blood transfusion, viper and scorpion bite. DIC may be severe and life threatening. *A peculiar feature of DIC is that the patient often begins to* **bleed** *after some time following intravascular coagulation.* This is because many of the clotting factors in the blood are consumed or used up by the widespread clotting. So, for normal hemostasis to occur there is very little clotting factor left. So, *DIC presents with severe bleeding*. Fibrin degradation product (FDP) formed due to lysis of intravascular clots has antihemostatic effect, which further aggravates bleeding.

■ MULTIPLE CHOICE QUESTIONS

1. Which of the following is most characteristic of hemophilia?
   a. Intracranial bleeds b. Hemarthrosis
   c. Petechiae d. Purpura

2. Heparin acts as an anticoagulant by:
   a. Preventing the action of calcium ions
   b. Inhibiting the active form of factor X
   c. Preventing activation of prothrombin to thrombin
   d. Antagonizing vitamin K

3. The clotting factor that is not synthesized in the liver is:
   a. Fibrinogen b. Prothrombin
   c. Factor VIII d. Factor X

4. Arachidonic acid derivatives include all the following, *except*:
   a. Prostaglandins b. Thromboxanes
   c. Leukotrienes d. Serotonin

5. All are vitamin K dependent clotting factors of hepatic origin, *except*:
   a. Factor II b. VII
   c. VIII d. X

6. Not a vitamin K dependent factor:
   a. II b. VII
   c. IX d. XII

7. Activity of factor VIII procoagulant is deficient in:
   a. Hemophilia A
   b. von Willebrand disease
   c. Idiopathic thrombocytopenic purpura
   d. Sickle cell anemia

8. True about hemophilia A are all, *except*:
   a. PTT increased
   b. PT increased
   c. Clotting time increased
   d. Serum level of factor VIII decreased

9. During hemostasis, platelets affect all the coagulation areas, *except*:
   a. Clot retraction
   b. Activation of prothrombinase complex
   c. Vasoconstriction
   d. Conversion of fibrinogen to fibrin

10. All the following clotting factors are synthesized in the liver, *except*:
    a. Factor I b. Factor III
    c. Factor VII d. Factor IX

11. In hemophilia:
    a. Factor VIII is decreased
    b. Factor VII is decreased
    c. Bleeding time is normal
    d. Clotting time is decreased

12. Thromboxane A_2 is released mainly by the:
    a. Platelets b. Vascular endothelium
    c. Liver d. Muscles

13. Thrombosthenin is a:
    a. Coagulation factor
    b. Contractile protein
    c. Thrombosis promoting protein
    d. Regulating platelet protein

14. Which one of the following is released by platelets during hemorrhage to produce vasoconstriction?
    a. Serotonin b. Histamine
    c. Thrombosthenin d. Bradykinin

15. Which of the following is the first to prevent blood loss after rupture of small blood vessel?
    a. Formation of platelet plug
    b. Formation of fibrin threads
    c. Vasoconstriction
    d. Production of hematoma to increase perivascular pressure

16. The best screening test for hemophilia is:
    a. BT b. PT
    c. PTT d. CRT

17. Disseminated intravascular coagulation is seen in:
    a. Hemophilia b. Retained placenta
    c. Thrombocytopenia d. Anemia

18. In vitro coagulation is initiated by factor:
    a. XII b. XI
    c. X d. VII

SECTION 2 — Hematology

19. The source of commercially available heparin is:
    a. Blood
    b. Liver
    c. Animal lung
    d. Spleen
20. Aspirin is given to prevent myocardial infarction because it inhibits the synthesis of:
    a. Thromboxane A$_2$
    b. Prostacyclin
    c. Platelet activating factor
    d. von Willebrand factor
21. In thrombocytopenia, spontaneous bleeding occurs when the platelet count falls below:
    a. 2 lakhs/mm^3
    b. 1.5 lakhs/mm^3
    c. 50,000/mm^3
    d. 20,000/mm^3
22. Bleeding time is the test for:
    a. Platelet activity
    b. Intrinsic mechanism of coagulation
    c. Extrinsic mechanism of coagulation
    d. Both intrinsic and extrinsic mechanism of coagulation
23. The substance released from platelets during injury that produce vasoconstriction is:
    a. Serotonin
    b. Histamine
    c. Thrombosthenin
    d. Bradykinin
24. Pseudohemophilia is:
    a. von Willebrand disease
    b. Christmas disease
    c. Disseminated intravascular coagulation (DIC)
    d. Thrombocytopenic purpura
25. Regarding hemophilia the following statements are correct, *except*:
    a. 25–50% of cases may not give any family history
    b. It is transmitted as a sex linked recessive disorder
    c. Male hemophiliacs pass the trait to half of their sons
    d. Spontaneous bleeding occurs only when the level of factor VIII falls below 5%
26. Serum contains the clotting factor:
    a. Factor VII
    b. Factor VIII
    c. Prothrombin
    d. Factor V
27. Fibrinogen is converted to fibrin by:
    a. Prothrombin
    b. Thrombin
    c. Thromboplastin
    d. Platelet
28. Heparin acts by inhibiting:
    a. Vitamin K synthesis in the liver
    b. Active form of clotting factor VIII
    c. Active form of factor X
    d. Antithrombin III
29. The clotting factor that is lost during storage of blood is:
    a. II
    b. VIII
    c. V
    d. IX
30. Serum does not contain:
    a. Calcium
    b. Factor VII
    c. Factor VIII
    d. Factor XI
31. Clinically used coagulation test during anti-coagulation therapy is:
    a. Clotting time
    b. Bleeding time
    c. Prothrombin time
    d. Clot retraction time
32. Actions of heparin includes all the following, *except*:
    a. Inhibits active forms of clotting factors IX, X, XI, XII
    b. Facilitates the action of antithrombin III
    c. Inhibits thrombin
    d. Activates protein C and protein S
33. Vitamin K is necessary for the synthesis of all the following clotting factors, *except*:
    a. Factor II
    b. Factor VII
    c. Factor X
    d. Factor XI
34. Factor VIII is transported in combination with:
    a. Albumin
    b. von Willebrand factor
    c. Globulin
    d. Transcortin
35. Vitamin K is necessary for the synthesis of functional clotting factors:
    a. II, VIII, IX, X
    b. II, VII, IX, X
    c. I, VII, IX, X
    d. II, IX, X, XII
36. In vitro coagulation is initiated by clotting factor:
    a. VII
    b. XI
    c. XII
    d. X
37. All are true regarding hemophilia-A, *except:*
    a. PT increased
    b. PTT increased
    c. Clotting time is increased
    d. Level of factor VIII in blood decreased
38. Best screening test for hemophilia is:
    a. Bleeding time
    b. Prothrombin time
    c. Clot retraction time
    d. Partial thromboplastin time
39. Aspirin directly inhibits:
    a. Lipoxygenase
    b. Cyclooxygenase
    c. Phospholipase
    d. Prostacyclin synthesis
40. In hemophilia A:
    a. Factor VII is decreased
    b. Bleeding time is increased
    c. Clotting time is increased
    d. Bleeding time is decreased

ANSWERS

1. b	2. b	3. c	4. d	5. c
6. d	7. a	8. b	9. d	10. b
11. a	12. a	13. b	14. a	15. c
16. c	17. b	18. a	19. c	20. a
21. d	22. a	23. a	24. a	25. c
26. a	27. b	28. c	29. b	30. c
31. c	32. d	33. d	34. b	35. b
36. c	37. a	38. d	39. b	40. c

Tissue Fluid and Lymph

CHAPTER 19

LEARNING OBJECTIVES

Must know
- Explain the role of Starling's forces in the formation of tissue fluid
- Explain the functions of lymph
- Discuss the pathophysiology of edema

■ TISSUE FLUID

The fluid, which occupies the intercellular spaces, is called **tissue fluid**. It constitutes the internal environment of the body or **milieu interieur**. Tissue fluid forms 20% of the total body fluid. There is constant exchange of fluid between the different fluid compartments of the body. But, *fluid exchange between intravascular and interstitial compartments occurs only at the level of capillaries*. The other parts of vascular system are impermeable. The capillaries are permeable because a single layer of flattened endothelium lines them.

Tissue fluid is derived from two sources:
1. From blood capillaries
2. From metabolism in tissues.

Functions of Tissue Fluid

There is no direct contact between blood and cells. Tissue fluid acts as the medium for the exchange of substances such as nutrients, CO_2, O_2, metabolic wastes, etc., between the cells and blood.

Formation of Tissue Fluid

Factors affecting the formation of tissue fluid are:
- Filtration and reabsorption
- Permeability of capillaries
- Diffusion
- Metabolic activity of tissues
- Gravity

Filtration and Reabsorption Based on Starling's Forces

Filtration and reabsorption across the capillary wall is the most important mechanism by which tissue fluid is formed. Capillary has an arterial end and a venous end. Diameter of the capillary is about 5 μm at the arterial end and 9 μm at the venous end. Velocity of flow in the capillaries is only 0.5 mm/second. At the arterial end, fluid is filtered out into the tissue spaces, and at the venous end, fluid is reabsorbed into the blood. Ernest Starling, in 1896, put forward the Starling's hypothesis, which states that filtration and reabsorption of fluid across the capillary membrane is determined by the balance of the hydrostatic and oncotic pressures across the capillary wall. As it was first proposed by Sir Ernest Starling, the forces governing the movement of fluid across capillary are referred to as **Starling's forces**. The volume of fluid filtered at any point in the capillary is determined by the Starling forces. These forces are **hydrostatic pressure gradient** and **effective osmotic pressure gradient** (colloid osmotic pressure or oncotic pressure difference) across the capillary wall at that point. Hydrostatic pressure is the pressure exerted by a fluid in a confined space. Hydrostatic pressure in the capillary tends to force fluid and its dissolved substances (except proteins) through the capillary pores into the interstitial spaces. Colloid osmotic pressure tends to cause fluid movement by osmosis from the interstitial spaces into the capillaries.

- Hydrostatic pressure difference (ΔP) across the capillary wall is the difference between the intravascular pressure (capillary hydrostatic pressure) and the extravascular pressure (interstitial fluid hydrostatic pressure). Generally, the capillary hydrostatic pressure falls from approximately 35 mm Hg at the arteriolar end to approximately 15 mm Hg at the venular end of capillary. Interstitial fluid hydrostatic pressure is 1 mm Hg.
- Colloid osmotic pressure difference ($\Delta \pi$) across the capillary wall is the difference between the intravascular colloid osmotic pressure caused by plasma proteins and the extravascular colloid osmotic pressure caused by interstitial proteins and proteoglycans.
- A positive ΔP tends to drive water out of the capillary, whereas, a positive $\Delta \pi$ attracts water into the capillary. Filtration of fluid from the capillary into the tissue space occurs when the net filtration pressure is positive. Conversely, absorption of fluid from the tissue space into

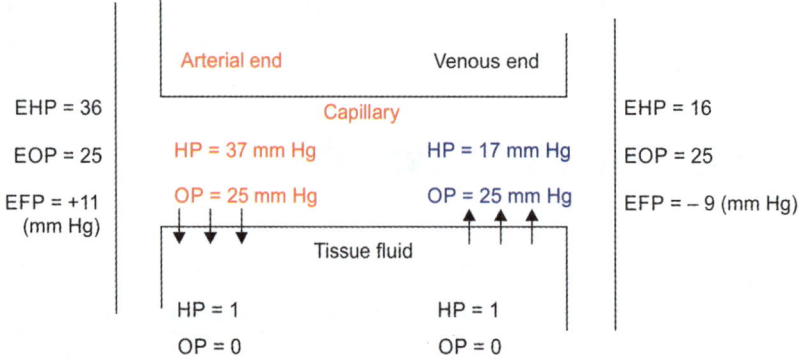

Fig. 19.1: Starling's forces and formation of tissue fluid.

the vascular space occurs when the net filtration pressure is negative.

At the arterial end of capillary, the net filtration pressure (NFP) or effective filtration pressure is positive (+11 mm Hg), and so fluid is filtered out of the capillaries into the tissue space. This 11 mm Hg filtration pressure causes approximately 1/200th of the plasma in the flowing blood to filter out at the arterial end of capillary into the interstitial space each time the blood passes through the capillaries.

But, at the venous end of capillary, the NFP is generally negative (–9 mm Hg) and so fluid is drawn into the capillaries at this end **(Fig. 19.1)**. Most capillary beds filter less than 1% of the fluid entering the arteriolar end of capillary. So, the loss of protein-free fluid does not concentrate plasma proteins at the venular end to the extent to raise colloid osmotic pressure ($\Delta\pi$). The colloid osmotic pressure at the venous end will also be 25 mm Hg. The venous capillaries are more permeable than the arterial capillaries. So less reabsorption pressure is required to cause inward movement of fluid. Thus reabsorption pressure of 9 mm Hg causes about 9/10th of the fluid that has been filtered out to be reabsorbed at the venous ends. The rest enters the lymphatics. But there are certain exceptions to this general rule.

About 24 L of fluid is filtered through the capillaries per day. About 85% (22 L) of filtered fluid is reabsorbed back into the circulation at the venous end of capillary. The rest 15% (2 L) of the filtered fluid is taken up by another system of vessels called lymphatics and returned back to the systemic veins.

The balance of Starling's forces is different in different tissues (exceptions from the general rule)
- Fluid moves out of the entire length of the capillary in renal glomerulus as the glomerular capillary pressure is 60–70 mm Hg.
- In the intestine, fluid moves into the capillary through their entire length.
- Filtration does not occur in the pulmonary capillaries as the pulmonary capillary pressure is only approximately 8 mm Hg. This helps to prevent ultrafiltration and fluid accumulation in the alveolar air spaces.
- In the upright posture, the capillary pressure in the feet is about 100 mm Hg and this is the reason for the occurrence of pedal edema on prolonged standing.
- The retinal capillaries in the eye must also have high capillary hydrostatic pressure because they are in contact with vitreous humor, which has a pressure of approximately 20 mm Hg. If the retinal capillary pressure is less, they will collapse due to high external compressing force.

> *It should be remembered that the capillary hydrostatic pressure in any part depends on the arteriolar diameter and the tone of the pre-capillary sphincter. At rest, most of the capillaries will be collapsed due to increased tone of the pre-capillary sphincter. But during activity, the pre-capillary sphincter relaxes and more blood flows through the capillaries increasing the capillary hydrostatic pressure.*

Permeability of Capillaries

Rate of fluid filtration in tissues is also determined by the number and size of the pores in each capillary as well as the number of capillaries in which blood is flowing. During rest, most of the capillaries remain collapsed. But during activity, more capillaries are recruited and more blood flows through the capillaries and amount of fluid filtered will also be more. During vasodilation, the surface area of the capillaries will be increased and more fluid will be filtered.

Diffusion

Passive transfer of substances across the capillary membrane along their concentration and electrical gradients is called diffusion. Respiratory gases and nutrients are transported by this mechanism. O_2 and nutrients are present in higher concentration in the plasma and so they diffuse into the tissue fluid. CO_2 and waste products whose concentration is higher in tissues move into the capillaries. Lipid soluble substances can pass through the lipid bilayer of the endothelial cells. Water soluble substances like sodium, chloride, glucose etc. pass through the intercellular spaces.

Effect of Gravity

A capillary bed below the level of heart has a higher hydrostatic pressure than a capillary bed at the level of heart.

So, when a person is standing for a long time, venous pressure and thus capillary hydrostatic pressure in the legs increase because of gravity. As a result, more fluid moves into the interstitial space. Normally, the lymphatic system can take up the extra interstitial fluid and return it to the vascular space, thus maintaining proper fluid balance. This requires contractions of the leg muscles to compress the veins and lymphatics so that fluid can be propelled upwards towards the heart. Otherwise, it may lead to edema in the leg.

> **APPLIED PHYSIOLOGY**
> - Left-sided heart failure can lead to pulmonary hypertension and pulmonary edema. In pulmonary hypertension, due to increased hydrostatic pressure in the pulmonary capillaries, more fluid is filtered out into the interstitial space according to Starling's law of tissue fluid formation. This leads to pulmonary edema.
> - Right-sided heart failure can increase pressure inside the large systemic veins leading to increase in the capillary pressure in the lower extremities and abdominal viscera. Fluid transudated from the hepatic and intestinal capillaries may get collected in the peritoneal cavity and the condition is called ascites. There will also be edema in the dependent parts like the legs.
> - In hypoproteinemia as in nephrotic syndrome and protein malnutrition, the plasma colloid osmotic pressure decreases and more fluid will be retained in the interstitial space leading to generalized edema. Hypoproteinemia in liver diseases like cirrhosis liver is due to decreased production of plasma proteins.
> - In dehydration, there is increase in the plasma protein concentration leading to increase in the capillary colloid osmotic pressure and this leads to increased reabsorption of fluid from the interstitial space. This will lead to decreased turgor of the interstitial space. If the skin is pinched and released, it is seen that it is unable to spring back to its normal firm position for some time.

LYMPH

Lymph is a modified tissue fluid, which is transparent, straw colored and faintly alkaline in reaction, drained by the lymphatic vessels. Lymph closely resembles plasma, but there are certain differences (**Table 19.1**). The concentration of electrolytes, urea, glucose, etc., is same in the blood and lymph. The colloidal osmotic pressure of lymph is less than that of plasma. The protein content of interstitial fluid in most of the tissues is about 2 g/dL and the protein content of lymph draining this area is also the same. But the lymph formed in the liver has a protein concentration of 6 g/dL and lymph formed in the intestines has a protein concentration as high as 3–4 g/dL. Since two-thirds (65%) of lymph is formed from the liver and intestine, the lymph in the thoracic duct has a protein concentration of 3–5 g/dL.

Organization of the Lymphatic System

PY5.10: Describe and discuss lymphatic circulation.

The amount of fluid filtered at the arteriolar end of the capillaries into the interstitial fluid exceeds the fluid that is reabsorbed at the venous end of capillary by about 2–4 L/day. The extra fluid and protein remaining in the interstitial space is drained back into the bloodstream by the lymphatics. Thus, the lymphatics return 2–4 liters of interstitial fluid to circulation. This prevents accumulation of fluid in the interstitium and prevents the rise in interstitial fluid pressure, which is normally negative. The amount of lymph entering the lymphatic capillaries from an area is equal to the amount filtered from the arterial ends of capillaries minus the amount reabsorbed at their venous ends.

Lymphatics are present in all tissues, *except central nervous system, bones, cartilage and cornea*. Lymphatics are very abundant in skin, respiratory, genitourinary and gastrointestinal systems. It is a closed system with one-way flow. Lymphatic system begins as a network of fine capillaries termed lymphatic capillaries or **initial lymphatics or terminal lymphatics**. A single layer of flat endothelial cells with no basement membrane or basal lamina lines it. There are no intercellular connections between the cells. The edge of one cell overlaps the edge of the other cell. Thus, it forms a **one-way valve or flap valve or primary lymph valve (Fig. 19.2)**. Interstitial fluid and other diffusible substances push and open the edge of the endothelial cell and enter the lymphatic capillary. Once it has entered the lymphatic capillaries, it cannot escape because the back flow tends to close the pore between the endothelial cells. The lymphatic capillaries are highly permeable to water, proteins, bacteria and viruses. Finally, lymph is drained into the subclavian veins.

Lymphatic capillaries → Small lymph vessels → Large lymph vessels → Thoracic duct (left side) and right lymphatic duct → Right and left subclavian veins.

The large lymphatic vessels or **collecting lymphatics** contain valves called **secondary lymph valves**, which prevent backflow of lymph. It also contains smooth muscle in their walls, which can contract in a peristaltic fashion, propelling the lymph along the lymph vessels. In the course of lymphatic vessels, a number of **lymph nodes** are interposed.

Table 19.1: Differences between lymph and plasma.	
Lymph	**Plasma**
Flows through lymphatic vessels	Flows through blood vessels
Protein content: 2–5 g%	Protein content: 6–8 g%
Coagulation factors are less, so clots slowly	Clots rapidly
WBC count: 1000–2000/ mm³ of lymph; lymphocytes predominate (90%)	WBC count: 4000–11,000/mm³ of blood
Fat content is more especially in the lacteals	Fat content is less

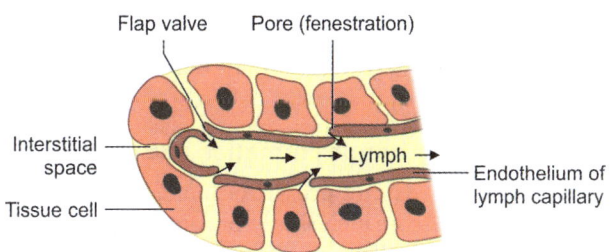

Fig. 19.2: Structure of lymph capillary.

As the lymph vessel reaches the lymph node, it breaks up into a number of fine vessels called **afferent lymphatics**. The lymph flows through the sinuses in the lymph node. Sinuses in the lymph node are lined by highly phagocytic cells called **reticuloendothelial cells**. From the lymph node, the lymph is collected by **efferent lymphatics**. Finally, lymph is drained into the right and left subclavian veins. The central lymphoid organ is thymus.

The pressure in the initial lymphatics is about –1 mm Hg and in the collecting lymphatics it become +1 to +10 mm Hg. In the larger vessels, it goes on increasing.

Mechanism of Movement of Lymph

- **Lymphatic pump**: Rhythmic intermittent contraction of large lymphatic vessels due to the presence of smooth muscle in their walls helps in forward movement of lymph. When a collecting lymphatic become stretched with fluid, the smooth muscle in the wall of the vessel contracts automatically. Also valves exist in all lymph channels which prevent backflow of lymph. Contraction of smooth muscles in the walls of the lymphatic vessels causes peristalsis-like movements and propels lymph from a segment between the valves to the next segment and so on. In large lymph vessels such as the thoracic duct, this lymphatic pump can generate pressures as great as 50–100 mm Hg. Lymphatic pump becomes very active during skeletal muscle contractions. During exercise lymph flow can increase by 10-fold to 30-fold. During resting period, lymph flow is sluggish.
- Transmitted pulsations from arteries adjacent to the lymphatic vessels help in lymph flow.
- Contraction of the neighboring skeletal muscles exerts a massaging effect on the lymph vessels and promotes lymph flow.
- Negative intrathoracic pressure during inspiration helps to suck lymph towards the heart.
- The suction effect of high velocity flow of blood in the veins into which the lymphatics terminate increases drainage of lymph into the bloodstream.
- Movements of parts of the body can increase lymph flow from the area.
- Intestinal movements like peristalsis and movements of villi increases lymph flow from the gastrointestinal tract.

Rate of Flow of Lymph

Rate of lymph flow is much slower than blood. About 100 mL/hour of lymph flows through the thoracic duct at rest. 20 mL flows into the circulation each hour through other lymphatic channels.

Within 24 hours, 2–4 L of lymph is drained into general circulation.

Factors Affecting Lymph Formation and Flow

- **Capillary hydrostatic pressure**: Increase in capillary hydrostatic pressure increases lymph formation.
- Increase in the capillary pressure can be due to increase in venous pressure, which exerts a back pressure to the capillaries. The rate of filtration of fluid in the capillaries is directly proportional to the rise in venous pressure. This is seen in congestive cardiac failure (CCF) and venous obstruction.
- **Plasma colloid osmotic pressure** when increased leads to decreased lymph formation.
- **Interstitial fluid colloid osmotic pressure** when increased leads to increased lymph formation
- **Capillary permeability** when increased causes increased lymph formation. Increase in capillary permeability may be due to:
  - Capillary poisons like histamine, peptone solution, foreign proteins, etc.
  - Increase in local temperature
  - Hypoxia produces vasodilatation and increase in capillary permeability.
- Functional **activity** of organs: When there is increased activity as in exercise, lymph flow from muscles is increased.
- **Pressure gradient** between tissue fluid and lymph vessels. In the tissues, pressure is high (1.9 cm of H_2O) when compared to lymphatic capillaries (1.3 cm of H_2O). Hence, fluid enters the lymphatics through the gaps in the endothelium of lymph vessels. Any factor that increases interstitial fluid pressure also increases lymph flow normally. Such factors include:
  - Increased capillary hydrostatic pressure
  - Decreased colloid plasma osmotic pressure
  - Increased interstitial fluid colloid osmotic pressure
  - Increased capillary permeability.
- **ECF volume**: When there is abnormal retention of salt in the body, water is also retained leading to increase in ECF volume and this cause increased lymph formation.
- **Capillary surface area** when increased leads to increased filtration and increased lymph formation.

Lymphagogue

These are agents, which *increase lymph flow*. For example, histamine, peptones, bacterial toxins, etc., increase lymph formation by increasing capillary permeability. These substances are called lymphagogues.

Functions of Lymph

- Maintenance of the volume and composition of tissue fluid constant by draining away excess tissue fluid and metabolites. Lymphatic system also helps to control interstitial fluid pressure.
- Lymph acts as a special channel that returns proteins to circulation and thus controls the concentration of protein in the interstitial fluid. *The amount of protein returned to circulation by lymph per day is about 25–50% (100–200 g) of the circulating plasma protein.*
- Absorption and transport of long chain fatty acids and cholesterol by the lacteals of intestine.
- *Nutritive function*: Lymph supplies nutrition and O_2 to those areas of the body where blood cannot reach.
- *Defense*: Bacteria and injurious agents are carried by lymph to the lymph nodes and the reticuloendothelial

cells in the lymph node destroy and phagocytose the bacteria.
- Lymphocytes are finally processed and released from the lymph nodes. Lymphocytes enter the circulation through the lymphatics.
- *Immune function*: Antibodies are produced by B-lymphocytes, which are released from lymph nodes.

Of all these functions, *the primary function is to maintain the proper fluid content of the tissues and to return proteins and excess fluid into circulation.*

Lymphadenopathy

The lymph nodes draining areas of infection and inflammation get enlarged during the active phase of the disease process. This is termed as **lymphadenopathy**. In throat infections, submandibular lymphadenopathy is seen. Generalized lymphadenopathy is seen in malignancies like lymphoma, leukemia etc., autoimmune diseases like lupus, rheumatoid arthritis; and systemic viral infections like infectious mononucleosis, HIV, etc.

Edema

Edema is build-up of excess body fluids within tissues. Edema can be **intracellular edema** and **extracellular edema**.

Intracellular Edema

Intracellular edema can be due to hyponatremia, decreased metabolic activity in tissues and inadequate supply of nutrients to the cells. For example, when blood flow to a tissue is decreased very much, there is less delivery of oxygen and nutrients to the tissues. As a result, the cell membrane pumps like Na^+-K^+ pumps fail to function. The Na^+ that leak to the interior of the cell cannot be pumped out of the cell. Increase in the number of osmotically active substances in the cell leads to osmosis of water into the cells. This can increase the intracellular volume to two to three times normal. This intracellular edema can even lead to death of the tissue. Intracellular edema is also seen during inflammation. In inflammation, the cell membrane permeability to sodium and other ions will be increased leading to osmosis of water into the cells.

Extracellular Edema

In certain pathological conditions, there is accumulation of abnormally large amounts of fluid in the tissue spaces. The interstitial fluid tends to accumulate in the dependent parts of the body because of the effect of gravity. Edema is seen in response to diseases of heart, lung, liver or thyroid gland. It is often observed in the feet, ankles, legs and around eyes but it can occur in any areas of the body. Edema occurs due to four reasons:
1. Increase in the hydrostatic pressure of blood leading to increased filtration of fluid from the capillaries
2. Decrease in the oncotic pressure of blood
3. Increase in the capillary permeability
4. Inadequate drainage of interstitial fluid by the lymphatic system

Types of Edema

- **Cardiac edema** is seen in right heart failure. There is increase in venous pressure, which leads to increase in the capillary pressure and there will be increased filtration and accumulation of fluid in the interstitial space.
- Edema due to **venous obstruction**. Thrombosis of veins causes venous obstruction causing back pressure leading to increase in capillary hydrostatic pressure.
- Edema due to renal diseases as in nephrotic syndrome. In **renal diseases**, there is renal damage leading to proteinuria. So, plasma osmotic pressure decreases and more fluid get filtered from capillaries according to Starling's forces.
- **Inflammatory edema** due to infection and inflammation. There is increase in capillary permeability due to vasodilatation produced by toxic substances.
- **Giant edema** or **angioneurotic edema**: This is non-inflammatory edema of sudden onset, usually seen in the hands, face, larynx, etc. It is of allergic origin.
- **Edema** due to **malnutrition** and liver diseases, e.g., cirrhosis liver. There will be generalized edema and is due to decrease in plasma protein and fall in plasma oncotic pressure.
- **Lymphedema** due to chronic lymphatic obstruction draining a part of the body as in filariasis or elephantiasis. Lymphatic drainage also becomes impaired after removal of lymph nodes during surgery or when lymph nodes are obstructed by malignant growths. The edema fluid in lymphedema has high protein content.
- **Heat edema**, which occurs due to excessive temperature, is seen in tropical areas. Increase in temperature produces vasodilatation, thus increasing the surface area and permeability of capillaries leading to edema.
- When edema is gross and generalized, it is referred to as **anasarca** or extreme generalized edema. The patient's whole body, i.e., from head to feet will appear very swollen. It is seen in liver failure, kidney failure, severe allergic reactions, etc.

Other Classifications

- **Localized edema** is seen in inflammatory edema, reduction in lymphatic drainage, etc.
- **Generalized edema** where there is widespread swelling of subcutaneous tissue as in malnutrition, renal diseases, etc.

Depending on whether edema is pitting or not, it is classified into:
- **Non-pitting edema**: Pit is not formed in the edematous area when pressure is applied **(Fig. 19.3A)**. This type is seen in late filariasis (elephantiasis), myxedema, etc., where the swelling is not due to collection of fluid.
- **Pitting edema**: If the skin over an edematous area is pressed by a finger for some time, a small depression is formed **(Fig. 19.3B)**. The pit disappears within 30 sec. This pitting is due to displacement of fluid from the area of pressure. It is usually seen in inflammation, congestive cardiac failure (CCF), renal diseases, etc.

Treatment of edema includes reversing the underlying disorder. General treatments include dietary sodium and

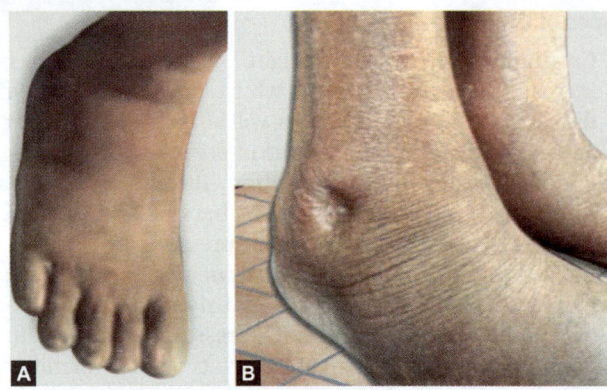

Figs. 19.3A and B: (A) Non-pitting edema in elephantiasis; (B) Pitting edema in congestive cardiac failure (CCF).

fluid restriction and appropriate diuretic therapy. Inflammatory edema can be treated with anti-inflammatory drugs.

MULTIPLE CHOICE QUESTIONS

1. Maximum protein content is seen in the lymph that is drained from:
   a. Intestine
   b. Liver
   c. Skeletal muscle
   d. Spleen

2. The normal 24-hour lymph flow is:
   a. 2-4 L
   b. 100-200 mL
   c. 2-4 mL
   d. 5-6 L

3. Central lymphoid organ is:
   a. Lymph node
   b. Thymus
   c. Spleen
   d. Tonsil

4. Function of lymphatics include all the following, *except*:
   a. Carries protein
   b. Fat absorption
   c. Increases oncotic pressure
   d. Preventive role in infection

5. Lymph flow is increased by all the following factors, *except*:
   a. Massage
   b. Exercise
   c. Decrease in capillary permeability
   d. Venous valve incompetency

6. Select the statement which best characterizes lymph capillaries:
   a. Have smaller diameter than blood capillaries
   b. Less permeable than blood capillaries
   c. Have no endothelial lining
   d. Have a discontinuous basement membrane

7. All the following help in the outward movement of fluid at the arterial end of capillary, *except*:
   a. Increase in plasma colloid oncotic pressure
   b. Increase in capillary hydrostatic pressure
   c. Decrease in plasma oncotic pressure
   d. Increase in interstitial colloid oncotic pressure

8. Lymph normally contains:
   a. RBC
   b. Eosinophil
   c. Lymphocyte
   d. Basophil

9. Rate of lymph flow is:
   a. 10 mL/hr
   b. 20 mL/hr
   c. 50 mL/hr
   d. 120 mL/hr

10. Pitting edema is seen in all the following conditions, *except*:
    a. Renal failure
    b. Myxedema
    c. Congestive cardiac failure
    d. Inflammation

ANSWERS

| 1. b | 2. a | 3. b | 4. c | 5. c |
| 6. d | 7. a | 8. c | 9. d | 10. b |

Blood Volume

CHAPTER 20

LEARNING OBJECTIVES
Must know
- Describe one method for the measurement of blood volume
- Explain the regulation of blood volume

INTRODUCTION

PY1.6: Describe the fluid compartments of the body.

Average **blood volume (BV)** of adults is about 7% of body weight or 5 L in a 70-kg man. Total blood volume is approximately 70 mL/kg body weight in adult female and 80 mL/kg body weight in adult male. In relation to body surface area, the total BV is 3 L/m² body surface area. 85% of blood volume resides in the systemic circulation, 10% in the pulmonary circulation and 5% in the heart chambers.

About 60% of blood is plasma and 40% blood cells. Total red blood cell volume is approximately 28 mL/kg in adult female and 36 mL/kg body weight in adult male.

MEASUREMENT OF BLOOD VOLUME

- Direct method
- Indirect method.

Indirect method includes two stages:
1. Determination of plasma volume
2. Determination of blood cell volume.

Determination of Plasma Volume

Plasma volume can be measured by two methods:
1. Indicator or dye dilution method
2. Radioisotope method.

Dye Dilution Method
Principle
A known quantity of dye is introduced into the body intravenously and the substance is allowed to mix thoroughly with blood. Then a sample of blood is withdrawn and the concentration of the dye is determined by colorimetric method. The plasma volume can be found out using the formula, $V = Q/C$, where V is the volume of plasma, Q is the quantity of dye injected and C the concentration of dye in the blood sample taken.

By this method, we can determine the volume of any fluid compartment like **extracellular fluid (ECF)** volume, total body water, etc.

Characteristics of the Dye
- It should be nontoxic
- It should evenly mix with plasma
- It should not be excreted rapidly, i.e., it should remain in the vascular channels for sufficient length of time
- It should be completely excreted from the body after some time.

The substance used to find out blood volume is **Evans blue (T-1824)**.

Radioactive Method
Albumin tagged with radioactive iodine (^{131}I), i.e., **radioiodinated serum albumin (RISA)** is used. Plasma volume can be found out from the above formula.

Determination of Total Blood Volume

After finding out the plasma volume, the total BV can be determined by dividing it with hematocrit value.

Let the plasma volume determined be 2750 mL and the hematocrit value determined be 45%. The amount of plasma is 55% and the total BV will be:

$$BV = 2750 \div \frac{55}{100} = \frac{2750 \times 100}{55} = 5\,L$$

VARIATIONS IN BLOOD VOLUME

Hypovolemia

Hypovolemia is decrease in BV. Causes are:
- Hemorrhage
- Dehydration due to burns, vomiting, diarrhea, etc
- Hypothyroidism
- Prolonged standing.

Severe hypovolemia leads to circulatory shock and death.

Hypervolemia

Hypervolemia is increase in BV above upper limit. It can be physiological or pathological.

Physiological Hypervolemia

- Pregnancy
- Exercise, high altitude
- Excitement.

Pathological Hypervolemia

- Hyperthyroidism
- Hyperaldosteronism
- Congestive cardiac failure
- Polycythemia vera

REGULATION OF BLOOD VOLUME

Hypothalamus regulates ECF volume and blood volume by acting mainly on kidneys, sweat glands and by inducing thirst. Whenever there is increase in blood volume, there is increased glomerular filtration and increased urine output, which reduces the plasma volume. The renal mechanism is supplemented by hormonal mechanism. Hormones that regulate blood volume (BV) are antidiuretic **hormone (ADH)**, angiotensin II, aldosterone, cortisol and atrial natriuretic peptide (ANP). BV is controlled mainly by two factors:
1. Plasma osmolality
2. Rate of water excretion

Plasma Osmolality (ADH and Thirst Mechanism)

Normal plasma osmolality is 280-295 mOsm/L (average—290 mOsm/L). Na^+ and Cl^- are the predominant osmotically active substances in the plasma. Since changes in Cl^- are mainly secondary to changes in Na^+, the amount of Na^+ in the ECF is the most important determinant of ECF volume. Plasma sodium concentration accounts for 95% of the effective osmotic pressure and therefore it is the primary determinant of ADH secretion. Normal osmolality is maintained by changes in ADH secretion and by thirst mechanism. *The intensity of thirst and ADH secretion is directly proportional to the plasma osmolality*. Significant changes in ADH secretion occur when plasma osmolality is changed as little as 1%. When there is reduction in blood volume, plasma osmolality increases, which stimulates the osmoreceptors located in the anterior hypothalamus. This, in turn increase ADH secretion from the suprachiasmatic nuclei of the hypothalamus. The osmoreceptors are very sensitive and respond to as little as 1% rise in the plasma osmolality. ADH increases water reabsorption from the distal convoluted tubule (DCT) and collecting tubule (CT) and thus increases BV.

The intensity of thirst is directly proportional to the plasma osmolality. Impulses from the osmoreceptors also stimulate the thirst center of hypothalamus and there is increased water intake bringing back the BV to normal. Hyperosmolality, decrease in blood volume and large decrease in blood pressure lead to the sensation of thirst. Decrease in blood volume and low blood pressure also stimulate thirst center via the pathway by which they stimulate ADH release.

Regulation of Blood Volume by Controlling Rate of Water Excretion

Blood volume can also be regulated by controlling water excretion, which in turn, is controlled by the hormones—**antidiuretic hormone (ADH) or arginine vasopressin, angiotensin II, aldosterone and atrial natriuretic peptide**.

- A 10% decrease in effective circulating BV increases ADH secretion. In contrast, an increase in plasma volume inhibits **ADH** secretion. Major stimuli for ADH secretion are plasma hyperosmolality and hypovolemia. A decrease in BV without an alteration in the osmolality of plasma also causes ADH release.

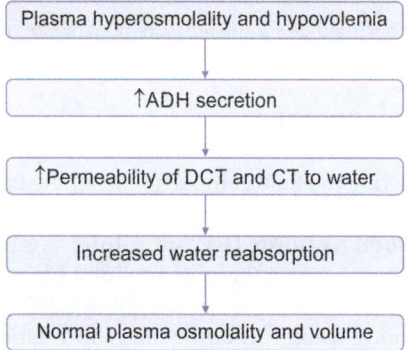

- **Angiotensin II** plays a key role in the body's response to hypovolemia. A decrease in the effective circulating blood volume (hypovolemia) increases renin secretion from juxtaglomerular apparatus of kidney. Renin increases angiotensin II formation (through renin-angiotensin-aldosterone mechanism), which in turn, increases aldosterone secretion, ADH secretion and stimulates thirst mechanism (*refer* **Fig. 55.1**). **Aldosterone** from adrenal cortex increases Na^+ and water reabsorption from the renal tubules and sweat glands leading to increase in BV. An increase in blood volume (hypervolemia) decreases angiotensin II formation, leading to decrease in aldosterone secretion. This produces natriuresis and diuresis leading to reduction in BV.

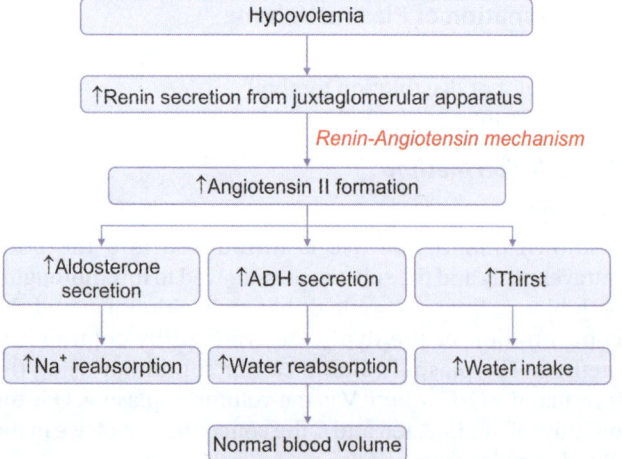

❖ The atrial stretch receptors in the right atrium are stimulated by increase in blood volume leading to increased secretion of **atrial natriuretic peptide** (ANP) by the atrial musculature. In hypovolemia, there is decreased secretion of ANP.
  a. ANP increases urinary excretion of Na⁺ and water, i.e., it produces natriuresis and diuresis in times of hypervolemia.
  b. ANP causes **efferent arteriolar constriction** which leads to increase in glomerular capillary pressure. This leads to increase in GFR and natriuresis (refer glomerulotubular balance).
  c. ANP causes **afferent arteriolar relaxation** which in turn increases hydrostatic pressure in glomerular capillary and increased delivery of NaCl to macula densa (refer tubuloglomerular feedback).
  d. ANP also inhibits renin secretion by kidney and aldosterone secretion by the adrenal gland thereby reducing sodium reabsorption leading to **natriuresis**.
  e. Decreased ADH secretion leads to **diuresis**.

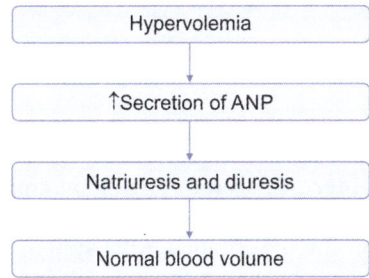

Role of kidneys in regulating effective circulating blood volume
By four pathways kidney plays a role in regulating blood volume:
1. Renin-angiotensin-aldosterone axis
2. Sympathetic nerves
3. Arginine vasopressin or ADH
4. Atrial natriuretic peptide.

All the above factors increase sodium and water reabsorption in times of decreased blood volume bringing back blood volume to normal.

MULTIPLE CHOICE QUESTIONS

1. All the following hormones regulate blood volume, *except*:
   a. Vasopressin
   b. Angiotensin II
   c. Aldosterone
   d. Thyroxine

2. The hormone that produces diuresis:
   a. ADH
   b. Atrial natriuretic peptide
   c. Progesterone
   d. Aldosterone

3. Normal plasma osmolality is:
   a. 290 mOsm/L
   b. 300 mOsm/L
   c. 250 mOsm/L
   d. 280 mOsm/L

4. Maximum sensitivity to osmoreceptors is to change in:
   a. Plasma osmolality
   b. Blood pressure
   c. Blood volume
   d. Oncotic pressure

ANSWERS
1. d   2. b   3. a   4. a

Blood Groups and Blood Transfusion

CHAPTER 21

LEARNING OBJECTIVES

Must know
- Describe the different blood groups
- Discuss the clinical importance of blood grouping
- State Landsteiner's law
- Differentiate between Bombay group and dangerous O group
- Describe the pathophysiology of erythroblastosis fetalis
- Explain blood transfusion reactions

Desirable to know
- Explain the inheritance of ABO blood group system
- Explain the collection and storage of blood in blood banks
- Discuss various blood substitutes
- Discuss preservation injury

■ INTRODUCTION

PY2.9: Describe different blood groups and discuss the clinical importance of blood grouping, blood banking and transfusion.

The blood of different people has different antigenic and immune properties. Antibodies present in the plasma of one blood type will react with the antigen present on the surface of the red blood cells of another blood type. The membranes of red blood cells contain a variety of glycoproteins and glycolipids that act as **blood group antigens**. There are about 342 antigens on the surface of our blood cells. These antigens are called **isoantigens or agglutinogens** (because they cause blood cell agglutination when it comes in contact with its antibody). Most of the red cell antigens are synthesized by the red cells. Some red cell antigens are specific to red cells. Others are also found on other cells of the body. Most of the antigens present on the red cell membrane are weak and does not produce reactions. Based on the presence or absence of various agglutinogens, there are different blood group systems. So far, 35 blood group systems have been recognized in humans. *The two major blood group systems in humans are ABO system and Rh system.* Other minor blood group systems are:
- P system
- MN blood group system
- Lewis, Kell, Kidd, Duffy, Lutheran system, etc. are found in certain families

Knowledge and understanding of blood groups are essential for transfusion therapy.

■ ABO BLOOD GROUP SYSTEM

Karl Landsteiner discovered ABO blood group system **in 1900**. He was awarded Nobel Prize in 1930 for this discovery. Depending on the inheritance, ABO system consists of 4 major blood types based on the presence or absence of A and B antigens (agglutinogens) on the RBC membrane. **Type A (group A)** individuals have A antigen, **blood type B** have B antigen, **type AB** have both antigens and **type O** have no A or B antigen on the RBC membrane. Agglutinogens start appearing by the 6th week of intrauterine life. The adult level is reached at about puberty.

These antigens are also present in the salivary gland, pancreas, liver, kidney, lungs, testis and amniotic fluid. In 80% of individuals, the ABO antigens are soluble in water and will be present in body secretions like tear, saliva, semen, urine etc., and they are known as **secretors**. In the rest, the antigens are insoluble and these individuals are referred to as **non-secretors**. The ability to secrete agglutinogens in body fluids is inherited as Mendelian dominant and is controlled by a pair of allelic secretor genes (**Sese genes**) located on chromosome 19. ABO antigens are absent in the cerebrospinal fluid.

Inheritance of ABO System (Fig. 21.1)

Depending on the inheritance, people may have one agglutinogen of the ABO system or both simultaneously or neither of them on the red blood cell (RBC) membrane. The position of a gene on a chromosome is called its **locus**. Every individual has a locus on each of the paired chromosomes for a gene of the ABO system. ABO blood group genetic locus

Type A individuals have the A antigen, type B have B antigen, type AB have both antigens and type O have neither on their RBC membrane.

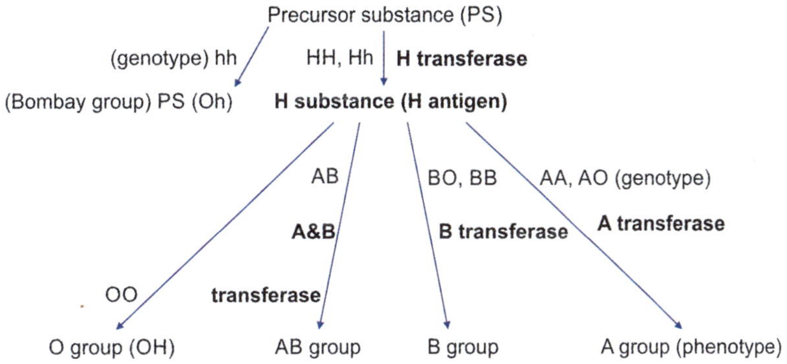

```
                        Precursor substance (PS)
     (genotype) hh   /     HH, Hh  | H transferase
(Bombay group) PS (Oh)     H substance (H antigen)
                           /        |        \
                        AB         BO, BB    AA, AO (genotype)
                        A&B       B transferase   A transferase
              OO     transferase
         O group (OH)   AB group    B group    A group (phenotype)
```

H transferase is fucosyltransferase
A transferase is N-acetylgalactosaminyltransferase
B transferase is D-galactosyltransferase
Glycolipid + fucose = H antigen (HAg)
HAg + N-acetylgalactosamine = A antigen
HAg + galactose = B antigen

Fig. 21.1: Inheritance of ABO blood group system.

has three alleles, i.e., three different forms of the same gene. These three alleles A, B and O determine the blood types. A and B genes are inherited as **Mendelian dominants** and individuals are divided into four major blood types on the basis of this. Genes coding for A and B antigens are dominant and they produce strong antigens on the RBC membrane. Type O allele is functionless and so, it produces no significant type of O agglutinogen on the red cells.

Since a person has only two sets of chromosomes in a pair, only one of the alleles will be present on each of the 2 chromosomes in any individual. Six possible combinations of alleles are possible due to the presence of three different alleles, i.e., OO, OA, OB, AA, BB and AB.

These combinations of alleles are known as **genotypes** and depending on the genes in an allelic pair each person belongs to one of the six genotypes. A person belonging to blood group 'A' (phenotype-A) may have the corresponding 'A' genes on both the loci of the allelic pair, i.e., genotype-AA, a *homozygous individual*; or he may have 'A' gene on one chromosome and 'O' gene on the other one of the homologous pair, i.e., genotype-AO, a *heterozygous individual*. The 'A' gene is described as dominant and the 'O' gene as recessive and so the phenotype will be A. B group individuals have genotype BB or BO and phenotype B.

The genes received by a person from his/her father and mother determine the genotype of the person. The phenotype is determined by the dominant of the two genes. The genotype 'AA' individual can have children all of whom possess 'A' gene ('A' is dominant); while the genotype 'AO' individual may have children, 50% of whom possess 'A' gene and 50% 'O' gene. A person having blood group AB, has 'A' gene on one locus and 'B' gene on the locus of the other chromosome of the pair and the phenotype will be AB since both genes are dominant. O group individuals do not possess either A-gene or B-gene on the paired chromosomes. They have only O gene.

A and B antigens are oligosaccharides that differ in their terminal sugar. The blood group specificity is determined by the terminal sugar. L-fucose is the terminal sugar for H antigen (HAg). N-acetyl galactosamine is the terminal sugar for 'A' antigen and D-galactose for B antigen **(Fig. 21.2)**.

H antigen is formed from a **precursor substance (PS)** which is an oligosaccharide on the cell membrane. It is converted to **HAg** or H substance under the influence of H gene. HAg is under the control of allelic pair of genes, either HH or Hh. H gene is located on chromosome 19 and it encodes for α-(1,2) fucosyl transferase (H-transferase) that adds a terminal fucose to form the H antigen from the precursor substance. "h" gene encodes for a nonfunctional transferase. If the h allele is inherited in a homozygous state (hh), L-fucose molecules are not added to the precursor substance on the red cell membrane and HAg will not be formed. Individuals who lack HAg (hh genotype) is known as the **Bombay phenotype**.

The A and B genes do not encode directly for the antigens but encodes for enzymes that add specific sugars to the HAg on the red cell membrane. Once HAg is formed, under the influence of A or B genes, HAg is converted to A or B antigen. If A gene is present, the person will be of A group; if B gene is present, the person will be of B group; if both A and B genes are present, the person will belong to AB group; and if A or B genes are1 absent, HAg remains as such and the person will be of O blood type.

Individuals with A gene express α-(1,3) **N-acetyl galactosaminyltransferase** (A-transferase) that catalyzes placement of a terminal N-acetylgalactosamine on the H antigen to form 'A' antigen. Those with B gene, express α-(1,3) **galactosyltransferase** (B-transferase) that places a terminal galactose on the H antigen to form B antigen. Type AB individuals have both transferases and forms both A and B antigens. Individuals who are O group do not have A or B transferases and so the H antigen persists.

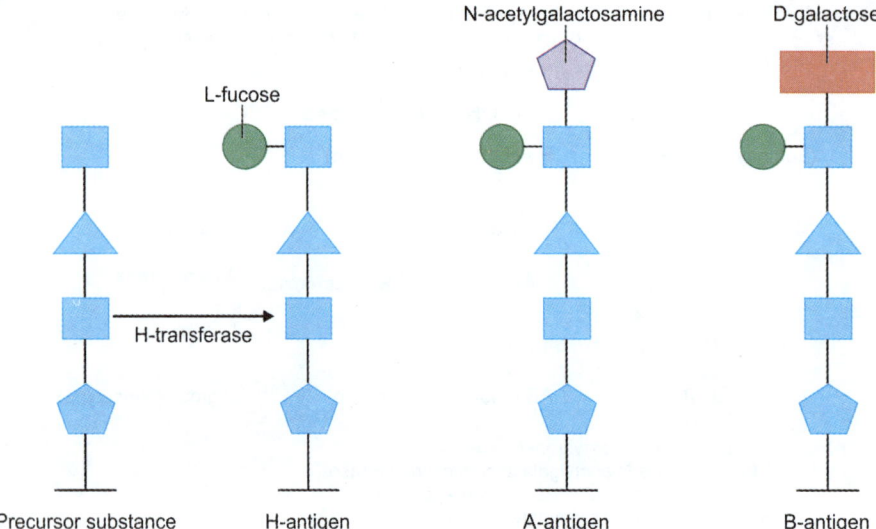

Fig. 21.2: Structure of blood group antigens (ABO system).

So in O group people, an H antigen is present on the RBC membrane.

Bombay Group (hh Phenotype)

The H antigen is the basic antigen present in the human red cells. Some O-group people will lack this H antigen. If the genotype of the person is 'hh', the precursor substance remains as such and H antigen is not formed. Even if the person has genes coding for A or B antigen, these antigens are not formed because H antigen (HAg) is the substrate for A and B antigens. Without the presence of HAg on the red cell membrane, the A and B transferases, even when present, are not able to add the specific sugars that give A and B antigen specificity. They may be genetically A or B or AB group. These people without HAg who are serologically grouped under O group due to the absence of A or B antigens are called **Bombay group or Bombay phenotype**. As A, B or H antigens are absent on the RBC membrane of the Bombay group people, their plasma contains anti-A (α), anti-B (β) and anti-H antibodies (refer Landsteiner's first law). Unlike the true O phenotype which has HAg on the red cells, the Bombay phenotype does not have HAg on their red cells. So, large amount of anti-H antibodies will be present in their plasma. So if they are transfused with O group blood, severe reactions will occur due to the presence of anti-H antibodies. *Due to the presence of all the antibodies in their plasma, these people cannot be transfused with any other blood other than Bombay group.* Bombay phenotype is extremely rare. Children of parent with Bombay phenotype (hh) can have normal A and B antigen expression, if they inherit the dominant H allele from the other parent.

Bombay blood group can be detected using anti-H serum or by reaction with O group cells in cross matching. This blood usually does not cause hemolytic disease of the newborn. Frequency of Bombay phenotype in India—1:13,000.

Agglutinins or Antibodies (Table 21.1)

Antibodies against red cell agglutinogens are called **agglutinins**. Agglutinins are γ globulins produced in the bone marrow and lymph glands. They are predominantly **IgM immunoglobulin molecules** but variable amounts of IgG are also present. Since they are mainly IgM immunoglobulins, ABO antibodies are effective in activating the complement system, which releases proteolytic enzymes that rupture the red cell membrane. So transfusion of ABO incompatible blood produces acute severe hemolytic reactions. The agglutinins of ABO system are **anti-A (α-agglutinin), anti-B (β-agglutinin) and anti-H antibodies**. Anti-H antibody is significant only in Bombay phenotype.

Landsteiner's Laws

I. Landsteiner's **first law** states that—*"If an antigen is present on the RBC membrane, the corresponding antibody will be absent in the plasma."*
II. Landsteiner's **second law** states that—*"If an antigen is absent on the RBC membrane, the corresponding antibody will be present in the plasma."*

Table 21.1: ABO blood group system.					
Genotype	Phenotype	Gene product	Antigen	Antibody	Prevalence (%)
OO	O	Nil	Nil	Anti-A and anti-B	47
OA/AA	A	A transferase	A	Anti-B	41
OB/BB	B	B transferase	B	Anti-A	9
AB	AB	A and B transferase	A and B	Nil	3

This law is not applicable to the Rh system.

Thus, type A blood contains anti-B antibody, type B contains anti-A antibody, AB group contains no antibodies and type O contains both anti-A and anti-B antibodies in plasma.

Antibodies are absent in the plasma of the baby at the time of birth (but some maternal antibodies that are filtered across the placenta may be present in the fetal plasma). The child begins to produce specific antibodies (agglutinins) by 2–8 months after birth and the maximum titer is reached by 8–10 years. After that, the antibody titer begins to decline. Infants develop antibodies against the antigens that are not present in their own cell because of the following reason. Antigens very similar to A and B antigens in the RBC of newborn are common in the intestinal bacteria and those in foods to which newborn babies are exposed. They develop antibodies against these antigens which appear in their blood as anti-A or anti-B agglutinins.

Since newborn infants do not have significant amounts of anti-A or anti-B antibodies in their plasma, pre-transfusion testing is not usually needed for blood transfusions within the first four months of life. But there are exceptions. If other blood group antibodies like anti-D have crossed the placenta of babies born to alloimmunized mothers, then transfusion reaction is likely to occur. As a precaution all transfusions should be done after cross matching.

Determination of blood group is very important before blood transfusion. The donor's and the recipient's blood should be subjected to blood typing and cross matching.

Cross-matching

- Major cross-matching
- Minor cross-matching

In major cross-matching, donor's cell is matched with recipient's serum **(Table 21.2)**.

In minor cross-matching, donor's serum is matched with recipient's cells. This is not of much importance because of the following reasons: (a) the donor's plasma containing the anti-A and anti-B antibodies gets diluted by the much larger volume of plasma of the recipient, (b) the donor's antibodies may get neutralized by the soluble antigens (agglutinogens) found free in the body fluids of the recipient. But in some O group people, there will be a very high titer of anti-A and anti-B antibodies and they are referred to as **dangerous O group**. In this case, minor cross matching becomes significant.

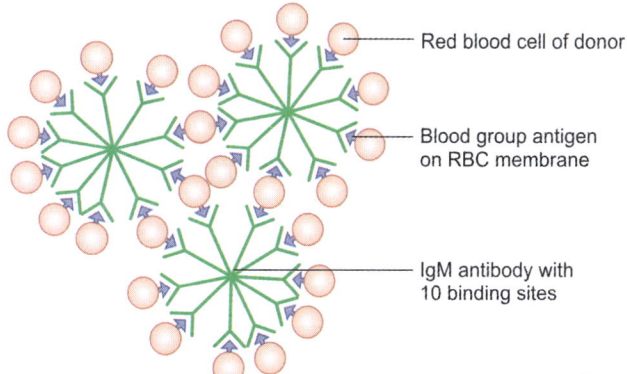

Fig. 21.3: Agglutination of blood cells in incompatible blood transfusion. IgM antibody has 10 binding sites whereas IgG immunoglobulin has only 2 binding sites. Antigen-antibody reaction leading to agglutination of red blood cells with IgM antibody.

From **Table 21.2**, it is seen that *O group is the universal donor (taking into consideration Rh typing also, O-negative individuals should be considered as universal donor) and AB group is the universal recipient*. But, O group blood should also be cross-matched to detect dangerous O group and Bombay group. If such a blood is transfused, severe agglutination reaction may occur. Now, blood transfusion is done only after proper blood typing and cross-matching. This is because, blood contains antigens and antibodies other than those associated with ABO system that can lead on to transfusion reactions. So the terms, universal donor and universal recipient are no longer used.

Agglutination

When incompatible blood samples are mixed outside the body at room temperature, there will be clumping of RBCs, which is visible to the naked eye. This is called **agglutination** and is due to antigen–antibody reaction **(Table 21.2)**. It occurs inside the body during incompatible blood transfusion. The agglutinins attach themselves to the red blood cells having the corresponding agglutinogen during mismatched blood transfusion. IgG type agglutinin has two binding sites and IgM type has 10 binding sites for the agglutinogen **(Fig. 21.3)**. Thus a single agglutinin can attach to two or more red blood cells at the same time, thereby causing the red cells to be bound together by the agglutinin. This clumping of the red cells is referred to as agglutination **(Fig. 21.4)**.

Importance of blood grouping and cross matching:
- To prevent transfusion reactions.
- Blood group is associated with certain diseases. 'O' group people are prone to develop duodenal ulcer. 'A' group people are more susceptible to myocardial infarction, diabetes mellitus, gallstones, carcinoma stomach, pernicious anemia, etc.
- *Medicolegal importance and disputed paternity cases—* in cases of disputed paternity; it can be proved that a particular person is not the father or mother of the child.

Table 21.2: Major cross-matching (recipient's serum against donor's plasma).

Recipient's serum	Donor's cells			
	A	B	AB	O
A group (anti-B antibody)	–	+	+	–
B group (anti-A antibody)	+	–	+	–
AB group (no antibody)	–	–	–	–
O group (α and β Ab)	+	+	+	–

(+ sign denotes agglutination)

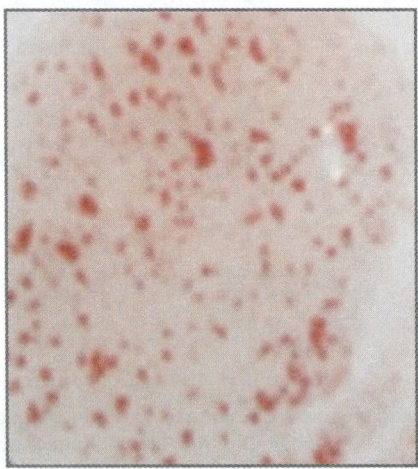

Fig. 21.4: Agglutination of RBCs when incompatible blood samples are mixed.

If the baby is O group, father cannot be AB group. If the baby is AB group, father cannot be O group. If the mother is B or O group and baby A group father cannot be B or O group. If the mother is A or O and baby B, father cannot be A or O. Thus, if the blood types of mother and child are known, typing can prove that the man is not the father, although it cannot prove that he is the father **(Table. 21.3)**. MN blood group system also has medicolegal importance in paternity test. With the use of DNA fingerprinting, the exclusion rate for paternity rises to 100%.

Stain (blood, saliva, semen, etc.) collected from the site of crime helps to identify criminals and victims. In secretors, the blood group antigens will be present in their secretions.

- Useful in the fields of immunology, genetics and anthropology.
- ABO and Rh blood group systems are the most important systems as far as transfusion reactions are concerned. The antibodies of other blood group systems react only at cold temperatures and rarely cause transfusion reaction.
- Blood group O has the lowest vWF antigen level and AB blood group people have the highest levels.

Table 21.3: Possible and impossible blood groups of the baby depending on parents' blood group.

Parent's group	Baby's group possible	Impossible baby's group
A & A	A, O	B, AB
A & B	AB, A, B, O	NIL
A & AB	A, B, AB	O
A & O	A, O	B, AB
B & B	B, O	A, AB
B & AB	B, A, AB	O
B & O	B, O	A, AB
AB & AB	A, AB, B	O
AB & O	A, B	AB, O
O & O	O	A, B, AB

RH SYSTEM

Rh system was first studied by **Landsteiner and Weiner** in 1940 using the blood of **rhesus monkey** and hence the name. This system is composed of 3 allelic pairs, **Dd, Cc and Ee**. There are six common types of Rh antigens designated as C, D, E, c, d and e each of which is called an **Rh factor**. A person who has C antigen does not have 'c' antigen, but a person who do not have C antigen on the RBC membrane always has the 'c' antigen. The same is true for D-d and E-e antigens. Rh factors are present only in the RBC membrane. Unlike the ABO antigens, the antigens of Rh system have not been detected in other tissues. C, D and E are strong antigens and the others are weak antigens. *Individuals having D-antigen or D-agglutinogen are said to be Rh-positive because, D antigen is highly immunogenic.* Rh-negative individuals have no D antigen. 99% of Asians are Rh positive. In Indians, the incidence of Rh-positive is 95%. Unlike the A, B and H antigens which are sugar molecules, Rh antigens are proteins in nature. Now it is known that there are 61 antigens in the Rh system. Rh antibodies are mainly IgG but some amount of IgM is also formed.

Two genes encode the Rh antigens: **RHD and RHCE** located on chromosome-1. RHD encodes for the D antigen, whereas RHCE encodes for the Cc and Ee antigens. The d antigen does not exist; however it is used to indicate the absence of D antigen. Absence of D antigen may be due to the deletion of RHD gene or may be due to an inactive RHD gene. Because of the manner of inheritance of the Rh factors, every person has one of each of the three pairs of antigens.

Genotypes

DcE ⎫		dce ⎫	
DCe ⎬	Rh positive	dCe ⎬	Rh negative
Dce ⎪		dcE ⎪	
DCE ⎭		dCE ⎭	

Unlike ABO system, Rh antibodies are not environmentally stimulated. The D antibodies are not present in the plasma of Rh-negative individuals. They develop antibodies only when Rh-positive cells enter their circulation. This can occur by blood transfusion or entrance of Rh-positive fetal blood into the maternal circulation. Most of the Rh antibodies are IgG, although some may be IgM. IgG immunoglobulins are usually not capable of activating complement.

Rh-positive individuals may be homozygous (DD) or heterozygous (Dd). The three alleles of Rh system are D and d, C and c, E and e. The risk of sensitization to C and E antigens is less than the risk of sensitization to D. So, the blood for transfusion is matched routinely only for D antigen. The other antigens are less immunogenic. However, in some Rh negative individuals, some of the other Rh antigens can cause transfusion reactions, although the reactions are mild. So, proper cross matching of the donor's and the recipient's blood before every blood transfusion is a must.

Differences between ABO blood group system and Rh system are shown in **Table 21.4**.

Table 21.4: Differences between ABO and Rh blood group systems.	
ABO blood group system	**Rh system**
Antigens are present in the cell membrane of most of the tissues	Antigens are present only on red cell membrane
ABO antigens are present in body secretions	Rh antigens not present in body secretions
Only few antigens detected	About 61 Rh antigens have been detected
Antigens are sugar molecules	Antigens are proteins
All antigens are equally antigenic	D-antigen is more antigenic than other Rh antigens
Antibodies (Ab) develop spontaneously	Antibodies develop only when exposed to Rh antigens
Antibodies are predominantly IgM and does not cross the placental barrier	Ab are predominantly IgG and can cross the placental barrier
Acute intravascular hemolysis occur after mismatched transfusion	Delayed hemolysis occur which is usually mild
Severe reaction seen even in the first mismatched transfusion	No immediate reaction occur in un-sensitized person when transfused with Rh-positive blood for the first time
ABO incompatibility not severe in newborn and does not produce hemolytic disease of newborn	Rh incompatibility causes erythroblastosis fetalis or hemolytic disease of newborn (HDN) in the baby born to sensitized mother

Rh Null

Rh null phenotype first described in 1961, occurs when the red cells do not express any of the 61 antigens in the Rh system. They have abnormal RBC membrane, increased fragility and a mild hemolytic state. Rh null blood can be accepted by anyone with a rare blood type in the Rh system. Hence, it is also referred to as **'the golden blood'.**

Hemolytic Disease of Newborn or Erythroblastosis Fetalis

Erythroblastosis fetalis is seen when an Rh-negative mother carries an Rh-positive fetus and is the *most common problem with Rh incompatibility*. Normally, no direct contact occurs between maternal and fetal blood during pregnancy. At the time of delivery, small amount of fetal blood leaks into maternal circulation. These Rh- positive RBCs of fetus stimulate the development of anti-Rh antibodies in the mother's blood during the postpartum period. Most Rh antibodies are IgG, although some may be IgM. During the next pregnancy with Rh-positive baby, the Rh antibodies from the mother cross the placenta and cause agglutination of baby's RBCs. These cells are then hemolyzed by the tissue macrophage system releasing hemoglobin into the blood. The macrophages of the fetus convert the hemoglobin to bilirubin and the baby becomes jaundiced. This is called **hemolytic disease of newborn (HDN)** or **erythroblastosis fetalis**. The baby will be anemic at the time of birth.

In some abnormal cases, fetal-maternal hemorrhage occurs through the placenta during pregnancy and sensitization can occur during pregnancy. In this case, the mother will start to produce anti-Rh antibodies during the course of pregnancy and the first baby will be affected.

Due to increased RBC destruction, there will be increased erythropoiesis. The liver and spleen also take part in erythropoiesis in addition to bone marrow and hence the liver and spleen become greatly enlarged. *Because of the rapid production of red cells, large number of nucleated blast cells (immature RBCs) will be released from the bone marrow into the circulatory system of the baby. It is because of the presence of these nucleated blast red cells, the disease is named* **erythroblastosis fetalis**.

Due to increased hemolysis, in severe cases, the baby may die *in utero* due to severe anemia. If it survives, it may develop anemia, severe jaundice and edema. This condition is called **hydrops fetalis**. Edema is due to hypoproteinemia. Since liver is involved in erythropoiesis, plasma protein synthesis is decreased. Albumin and fibrinogen are synthesized in the liver. The oncotic pressure of blood decreases leading to edema.

Bilirubin rarely crosses the **blood-brain barrier (BBB)**. But unbound, unconjugated bilirubin crosses the BBB in infants. The concentration of unconjugated bilirubin is very high in erythroblastosis fetalis because production of bilirubin is increased due to increased hemolysis and the bilirubin conjugating system is not yet mature in the newborn. So unconjugated bilirubin crosses the BBB and gets deposited in the globus pallidus of basal ganglia leading to a neurological syndrome called **kernicterus**. *Kernicterus is produced when the serum bilirubin is more than 20 mg/ dL in the newborn*. These children will have permanent mental impairment due to damage of neuronal cells because of precipitation of bilirubin in the motor neurons.

The first Rh-positive child born to an Rh-negative mother will be normal. But, *the first child will develop hemolytic disease if the mother had an Rh-positive blood transfusion earlier or had abortion with Rh-positive fetus*. The first baby will also be affected if there had been fetal-maternal hemorrhage during first pregnancy.

In the second pregnancy of a lady who is previously sensitized with Rh-positive cells, if the second baby is Rh-positive, it has a chance to develop HDN. If the second baby is Rh negative, there will be no problem because Rh- negative blood does not have Rh antigens to react with the antibodies. So, even if Rh antibodies cross the placenta and reach the fetus, it is not affected.

Treatment of HDN

❖ *Exchange blood transfusion* is done soon after birth. The baby's blood is replaced with Rh-negative blood. The procedure is repeated several times during the first few weeks of life. This keeps the bilirubin level low and prevents kernicterus and damage to the brain. After 6–8 weeks, the transfused Rh-negative red cells are replaced with the infant's own Rh-positive red cells.

- Jaundice can be treated by *phototherapy* where bilirubin is photoisomerized to lumirubin which can be easily excreted through bile.
- *Drugs like phenobarbitone* is also used to treat HDN.

Prevention of HDN

A single dose of **anti-D serum** usually known as **anti-Rh gamma globulin** (RhOGAM) is administered to the Rh-negative mother within 48 hours of delivery. Rh antibody will immediately destroy the baby's Rh-positive cells in the mother and prevent sensitization. This prevents active antibody formation by the mother and the second baby will be normal. This is an example of **passive immunization**.

A small dose of Rh immunoglobulin, an anti-D antibody is also given prophylactically to Rh-negative mothers starting at 28–30 weeks of gestation assuming that the baby is Rh positive. If the Rh-positive baby's blood reaches the mother's circulation accidentally during pregnancy, the injected antibodies will destroy these RBCs. Usually these antibodies do not cross the placenta. Now fetal Rh typing can be done by amniocentesis or chorionic villus sampling.

Coombs' Test (Antiglobulin Test)

There are two major classes of antibodies that react with red blood cells in humans. One is the **complete or saline antibody** which agglutinates red cells suspended in saline solution. They are usually **IgM.** Second type are antibodies that do not react visibly in saline and are capable of producing agglutination reactions only by special techniques like Coombs test and are called **incomplete antibodies**. They are generally **IgG** antibodies. But they produce delayed hemolytic transfusion reactions. Example of complete antibodies are those that react with antigens of the ABO system (IgM antibodies). Example of incomplete antibodies are those that react with antigens of the Rh system (IgG antibodies).

Rh antibodies are of two types:
1. **Complete type** which agglutinates red blood cells and belong to IgM type.
2. **Incomplete type** which does not produce agglutination but only coat the red blood cells and belong to IgG type. Incomplete type of antibodies can be detected if we have another antibody against this antibody coating. On the basis of this principle, Coombs produced the **antihuman globulin** serum in rabbits by injecting the human antibodies into rabbits. This **antihuman globulin (AHG) reagent** known as **Coombs' reagent** is now successfully used in the detection of incomplete Rh antibody.

Types of Coombs' Test

- Direct test
- Indirect test

Direct or indirect antiglobulin tests are used for the detection of IgG anti-red cell antibodies. These tests involve procedures that diminish the mutually repulsive electrostatic forces between red cells, permitting visible agglutination by IgG antibodies. Such enhancing tests are required for antigens belonging to blood group systems like Rh system.

Direct Coombs' Test

Red blood cells of the patient are washed with low-ionic-strength saline 3–4 times. This is very important because serum proteins will neutralize the Coombs' reagent. Add a drop of 5% red cell suspension in two tubes. To one tube, add a drop of Coombs' reagent and to the other tube add a drop of saline. Mix the contents and after 5 minutes, centrifuge at 1000 revolutions per minute (rpm) for one minute. Shake gently and observe for agglutination. Confirm under the microscope. If there is agglutination, the test is positive (**Fig. 21.5**). In direct Coombs' test, the sensitization of the erythrocytes with the incomplete antibodies take place in vivo as in hemolytic disease of the newborn.

Indirect Coombs' Test

Known O positive red cells are washed with low-ionic-strength saline (LISS) and a drop of 5% red cell suspension is mixed with a drop of the patient's serum. The mixture is kept at 37°C for one hour and centrifuged. If there is agglutination, it signifies the presence of complete antibody or saline type of antibody in patient's serum.

In the absence of agglutination, remove the supernatant, wash the cells 3–4 times with saline and add a drop of Coombs' reagent containing antihuman globulin. Mix and centrifuge gently after three minutes. Shake gently and observe for agglutination to detect indirect Coombs' positive cells. In indirect Coombs' test, sensitization of red cells with the Rh antibody is performed in vitro.

When the serum of the patient containing incomplete anti-Rh antibodies is mixed with Rh positive red cells, the incomplete antibody coats the surface of the red blood cells though they are not agglutinated. When these cells are washed with saline and treated with the Coombs' reagent or antiglobulin serum of rabbit, the cells get agglutinated (**Fig. 21.6**).

Uses of Coombs' Test

- It is used to detect the coating of antibody on the red cells in cases of newborn infants suffering from erythroblastosis fetalis. Here indirect Coombs' test is done.
- Used in autoimmune hemolytic anemia for detecting incomplete antibodies.
- It is used in blood transfusion with incompatible blood. The red cells in such cases are tested for direct Coombs' test.
- Coombs' test is also used for detecting very weak antibodies and also for detecting antibodies against leukocytes and platelets.

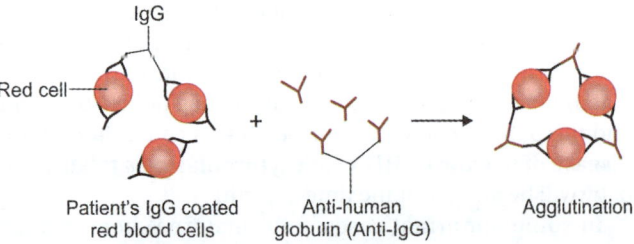

Fig. 21.5: Direct Coombs' test with anti-IgG.

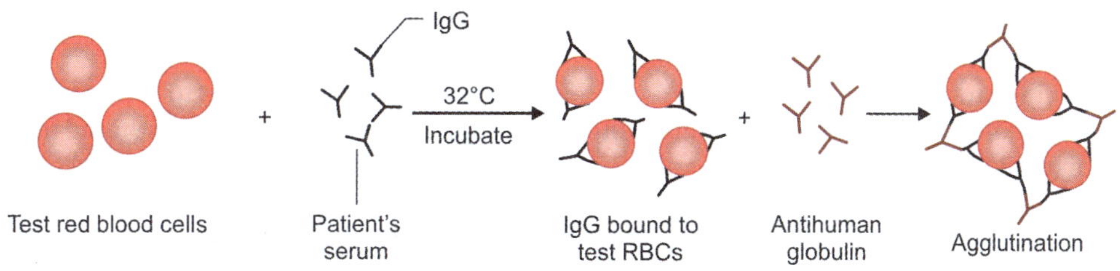

Fig. 21.6: Indirect Coombs' test.

ABO Incompatibility in the Newborn

ABO incompatibility is also detected in the newborn. If the mother is O group, anti-A and anti-B antibodies will be present in the plasma. If baby is A or B group, the anti-A or anti-B antibodies of mother will enter the fetal circulation and destroy fetal RBCs. *ABO incompatibility can occur in the first pregnancy itself.* It is less severe than Rh incompatibility. Usually, antibodies of the ABO system do not cross the placenta because they are large **IgM-type antibodies**. So normally, ABO incompatibility between mother and her fetus rarely produces problems.

The antibodies against ABO antigens usually do produce HDN due to the following reasons:
- The soluble A and B antigens present in the fetal plasma (in case of secretors) can neutralize the antibodies that reach the fetus through the placenta.
- Antigens A and B expressed on other body tissues may also bind the antibodies.
- The alloantibodies against ABO antigens are specific for sugar molecules. They have a weaker binding affinity than antibodies reacting with protein antigens such as the D antigen.

ABO incompatibility can to some extent prevent Rh incompatibility. If the mother is O negative and baby is B positive, the B-positive cells entering the mother's blood will be immediately destroyed by the anti-B antibodies in the mother's blood. So, there is no time for the production of anti-Rh antibodies in the mother.

■ BLOOD TRANSFUSION

Blood transfusion is defined as the transfer of whole blood or blood components into the bloodstream. Blood transfusion is a form of *replacement therapy*. Depending on the requirement, instead of using whole blood, the different components of blood can be used. This avoids the potential hazards from unwanted components. Whole blood means blood containing all the formed elements, plasma and solutes in normal concentration.

The various components of blood are:
- Packed red cells (PRC)
- Platelet concentrate
- Buffy coat
- Plasma
- Cryoprecipitate contains mainly factor VIII and fibrinogen
- Plasma protein solution (PPS)
- Leukoreduced PRCs or washed PRCs.

Indications of Blood Transfusion

- Hemorrhage, e.g., postpartum hemorrhage (PPH), accidents, hematemesis (vomiting of blood), major surgery, etc. whole blood is used.
- *Anemia:* Blood volume will be normal. If whole blood is transfused, it may lead to volume overload. So, packed cell transfusion is advised.
- In hypovolemia due to severe burns, hypoproteinemia, severe dehydration, etc., plasma alone is given.
- Exchange transfusion for newborn with Rh incompatibility.
- Leukemia associated with severe anemia.
- Thrombocytopenia is treated with platelet rich plasma or platelet concentrate.
- *Hemophilia:* Either fresh blood or cryoprecipitate is given. Fresh blood is indicated because factor VIII decreases on storage.
- Circulatory shock, to increase blood volume.
- In CO poisoning, fresh blood transfusion provides a fresh supply of oxyhemoglobin.
- Leukoreduced PRCs or irradiated PRCs (using Cs^{137}) where leukocytes are inactivated can be used to prevent transfusion-related immune modulation (TRIM) during tissue transplantation
- In cases of rare phenotypes like Bombay group, frozen PRC can be used.

Before any blood transfusion, proper blood grouping and cross-matching should be done. The blood should be screened for diseases like AIDS, hepatitis, etc.

Collection and Storage of Blood

Any healthy individual between the age of 18 years and 60 years can donate blood. There should be an interval of 3 months between two successive blood donations. Blood is collected by phlebotomy, i.e., introducing a wide bored needle (16G) into the anterior cubital vein. At a time, about 250–350 mL of blood is collected over a period of 7–10 minutes in appropriate sterile bags containing about 40 mL of a suitable solution. After collection, 3–5 mL of blood is taken for screening HIV, HBsAg, HCV, malaria and syphilis.

The collecting bag should be of standard quality because collection, processing and storage are done with the same bag. The accepted one is PVC bag plasticized with BTHC (butyryl trihexyl citrate) which has minimum interaction with the blood inside. Usually a triple bag is used, i.e., blood is collected in a parent bag and this bag is connected to two other bags for easy processing and component separation.

The solution in the bag used for storage and preservation should maintain the RBCs without much change. The solution should have the following properties:

- It should contain an anticoagulant which is stable and nontoxic. Sodium citrate is usually used.
- It should contain a substance to maintain ATP content of stored blood. ATP content decreases when blood is stored and this will affect the shape of RBC and increases cell fragility leading to hemolysis. Addition of adenine and phosphate to the solution will counteract the loss of ATP and helps in RBC survival.
- It should provide adequate glucose which is the main source of energy for RBCs. So dextrose is added.

The solutions satisfying all these criteria are:

- ACD (acid citrate dextrose) solution, 15 mL/100 mL of blood
- CPD (Citrate phosphate dextrose) solution
- CPD-A (citrate phosphate dextrose-adenine) solution is most commonly used where blood can be stored for 35 days at 4°C. Adenine provides the substrate for adenosine triphosphate (ATP) synthesis. Phosphate buffer maintains the pH of the collected blood and provides a source of phosphate. Dextrose provides the energy source.

Additive solution is added after blood collection. It contains saline, 2.5 times more adenine, more glucose and mannitol (to prevent hemolysis). By using **SAGM solution or Adsol (AS1),** RBCs can be stored for 42 days.

Rejuvenation solution is also added after blood collection. But it cannot be infused. So RBCs should be washed before transfusion. This solution contains pyruvate, inosine, phosphate and adenine. It can maintain ATP and 2,3-DPG levels.

Different components of blood can be separated and stored. Whole blood by slow centrifugation (3000 rpm for 3 minutes) helps to separate RBCs and platelet-rich plasma (PRP). PRP when subjected to high centrifugation (5000 rpm for 5 minutes) helps to separate platelet concentrate and plasma. Platelets and leukocytes will disappear from stored blood after 24-48 hours. So platelet preparation should be made within 24 hours.

Storage

Blood is collected and stored for future use in specialized medical centers called **blood banks**, now referred to as **centers of transfusion medicine**.

- Optimum storage temperature for **whole blood** is 4 ± 2°C. If it is less than 2°C, freezing injury occurs and if it is more than 6°C, bacterial overgrowth occurs. If CPDA solution is used, it can be stored for 35 days and if SAGM is used, it can be stored for 42 days.
- **Platelet-rich plasma (PRP) and platelet concentrate (PC)** when stored at 20–24°C can be used for 5 days. But, it must be agitated continuously in an agitator within the incubator to avoid aggregation.
- **Fresh frozen plasma (FFP)** prepared by freezing plasma at minus 73°C within 8 hours of collection of blood is rich in fibrinogen, protein C and S, antithrombin and albumin. If it is stored at a temperature less than minus 25°C can be used for 1 year.
- Thawing FFP at 4°C helps to separate cryoprecipitate and plasma derivatives. When it is stored at less than 25°C can be used for 1 year.
- Powdered plasma can be stored for 10 years.
- Frozen PRCs is used for storage of rare phenotypes like Bombay group. PRCs treated with glycerol and stored at minus 65°C can be used for 10 years. It should be thawed and deglycerolized before use.
- Heparin is rarely used for storing blood because it alters pH and also causes rapid loss of ATP from blood. Such blood should be used within 48 hours.

Stored blood is not suitable in cases of WBC and platelet deficiency because blood stored for more than 24 hours contains no viable leukocytes and platelets.

Preservation Injury or Storage Lesions

During preservation of blood, certain defects occur in blood collectively called preservation injuries. Loss of red cell viability during storage is known as storage lesion. Survival of transfused RBC is acceptable when at least 75% of transfused RBCs are present in circulation for 24 hours.

Preservation injury includes the following:

- Within the red blood cell, there will be a reduction in ATP.
- Concentration of 2,3-DPG in RBC decrease during storage due to its metabolism by the enzyme phosphatase which is active at acidic pH. pH is decreased in stored blood due to anaerobic metabolism. 2,3-DPG is very important for oxygen delivery by the RBCs. Decrease in 2,3-DPG in RBC, leads to the shift to left of oxygen dissociation curve.
- Hyperkalemia occurs due to leaking out of K^+ from RBC into the plasma. Plasma potassium concentration increases to 20–30 mEq/L in 2 weeks. But potassium overload rarely produce clinical problems unless there is pre-existing hyperkalemia or renal failure.
- Increase in intracellular Na^+ concentration to 30–40 mEq/L, due to decreased activity of Na^+-K^+ pump at low temperature. This leads to increased red cell size due to endosmosis and increased fragility leading to hemolysis.
- Concentration of the coagulation factors decrease on storage, especially factor VIII. So, fresh blood is used to treat hemophilia.
- Decrease in pH due to formation of lactic acid.
- Granulocytes lose their phagocytic and bactericidal properties within 4–6 hours and platelets become nonfunctional within 36–48 hours.
- When stored for several days, red cells become spherical due to metabolic changes and the cell rigidity increases leading to rapid destruction of the transfused RBC in the body of the recipient.
- Citrate toxicity after repeated transfusion rarely leads to hypocalcemia. Ca^{2+} is precipitated as calcium citrate and ionic calcium level falls. (Usually, after administration of citrated blood, citrate is removed from blood by the liver within a few minutes and is polymerized to glucose or

metabolized directly for energy. So it will not produce much consequence).

Autologous Transfusion or Predonation

Autologous transfusion refers to the collection of *patient's own blood* over a 3-weeks period for his requirements for a later date. This can be used for elective surgeries. The resulting anemia can be treated with appropriate iron therapy. About 1–1.5 L of blood is collected 4–6 weeks before elective surgery and is re-infused during the surgery. This method avoids the hazards of disease transmission and immunization and eliminates the risk of transfusion reactions.

Blood Substitutes

Blood substitutes are substances used to substitute blood loss or when there is decrease in blood volume. They are mainly used in cases where blood volume should be corrected to save the patient. Blood substitutes are used in two situations
1. When there is loss of fluid content leading to hemoconcentration as in vomiting, diarrhea, burns, etc.
2. When there is loss of blood as a whole as in acute hemorrhage, surgery, etc.

Substitutes for fluid loss:

Blood substitutes commonly used to replace lost blood volume or used to expand blood volume are non-oxygen carrying solutions or **plasma expanders**. They are of two types: (i) crystalloids, (ii) colloids.

Crystalloids
- Normal saline
- Glucose saline
- 5% Glucose
- Dextrose solution

Colloids
- Albumin solution
- Starch solution
- Dextran solutions

Substitutes used for blood loss or red blood substitutes:

The disadvantages of whole blood transfusion following blood loss are: (1) a cross matching should be done, (2) transmission of deadly diseases like HIV, hepatitis B, etc. The term red blood substitutes refer to oxygen carrying solutions that can both expand blood volume and oxygenate tissues. These solutions contain delivery system for O_2 and are intended to carry out the primary function of red blood cells, i.e., transport of O_2 to the tissues. These solutions should be free of antigen, should be sterile and should have a long shelf life. These include:
- Modified hemoglobin solutions or hemoglobin based products
- Perfluorocarbon-based products

Hemoglobin-based products: Hemoglobin separated from erythrocytes cannot be used because cell free hemoglobin will dissociate to form dimer (hemoglobin is a tetramer consisting of identical dimers; α and β dimers). So its effectiveness as a carrier of O_2 decreases. The associated globin chain will get filtered in the kidney leading to renal failure. The cell free hemoglobin binds with NO and causes vasoconstriction. So hemoglobin should be chemically modified to avoid these problems. The modified forms are:
- Cross link hemoglobin which is produced by cross linking alpha chains at 99th position so that they will not dissociate.
- Polymerized hemoglobin—here hemoglobin molecules are made to polymerize by means of reagents like glutaraldehyde, e.g., polyheme (polymerized human hemoglobin with glutaraldehyde).
- Surface modified hemoglobin where hemoglobin is conjugated with large molecules like dextran.
- Liposome encapsulated hemoglobin—most extensively used liposome to encapsulate hemoglobin is composed of phospholipid in combination with cholesterol and other gangliosides. The problem was when injected they were rapidly coated with opsonins and immunoglobulins and removed by the reticuloendothelial system.

Perfluorocarbon-based products: Perfluorocarbon has the capacity to carry O_2. One product is oxygen-T which is an emulsion of PFC and egg yolk phospholipid. In phase III trials, these products produced stroke in some patients.

Since several side effects are observed during trials, red blood substitutes are not used and are still under trial.

■ COMPLICATIONS OF BLOOD TRANSFUSION

- Non-hemolytic reaction
- Hemolytic reaction

Non-hemolytic Reactions

- If the transfusion set is not sterile, fever may develop due to the presence of pyrogens.
- Transmission of diseases like AIDS, hepatitis, malaria, syphilis, etc.
- Allergic reactions like urticaria, anaphylaxis, etc.
- Circulatory overload leads to heart failure. To prevent this, rate of transfusion should not exceed 1 mL/kg body weight/hour
- Hyperkalemia can cause inhibition of heart.
- **Hemochromatosis** or iron overload is seen in patients on regular blood transfusion. 350 mL of blood that is transfused contains 175 mg of iron.
- Air embolism
- Microembolism like pulmonary embolization leads to **shock lung syndrome**. A filter in the administration set can prevent this.

Hemolytic Reactions

The sequence of events leading to destruction of red cells due to **incompatible transfusion** is included in hemolytic reactions. In an incompatible blood transfusion, iso-antibodies in the recipient's plasma bind to the antigens present on the donor's RBCs and antigen–antibody complexes are formed.
- These complexes activate the complement system leading to hemolysis of the donor's RBCs and release of hemoglobin into the plasma.

- This may lead to circulatory shock, renal failure, jaundice, etc.
- The agglutinated erythrocytes form clumps that may block small blood vessels in the heart, lungs and kidneys.
- When there is massive breakdown of cells due to intravascular hemolysis, large amounts of K^+ are released into the plasma leading to hyperkalemia. This can lead to arrhythmia (**Table 21.5**).

ABO Incompatibility

When the recipient's plasma has agglutinins against the donor's RBC, the donor cells agglutinate and hemolyse. Agglutinins or antibodies belong to IgG or IgM type. IgG has 2 binding sites and IgM has 10 binding sites so that 2–10 RBCs can attach to a single antibody causing the cells to clump (*refer* **Fig. 21.3**). This is **agglutination**. These clumps can block small blood vessels in the circulatory system.

The RBC membrane may rupture releasing free hemoglobin into the plasma. This is **hemolysis**. IgM antibodies are called hemolysins. Plasma bilirubin increases leading to jaundice. There will be renal tubular damage leading to anuria and even death due to **acute renal shutdown**. Renal shutdown is treated by hemodialysis.

Causes of Renal Shutdown

- Renal vasoconstriction caused by toxic substances released due to antigen–antibody reaction.
- Production of toxic substances from the hemolyzed cells often causes circulatory shock. Circulatory shock leads to decrease in blood pressure, which causes a reduction in renal blood flow and decreased urine output.
- If hemoglobin released is high, only little can bind with **haptoglobin**. Rest will be filtered through the glomerulus and hemoglobin precipitates and blocks the renal tubules leading to acute renal shut down.

Rh Incompatibility

If an Rh-negative person is given Rh-positive blood, for the first time there will be no immediate reactions. But anti-Rh antibodies will develop slowly during the next 2–4 weeks due to stimulation of immune system and cause agglutination of the transfused cells that are still in circulation. The maximum concentration of anti-Rh agglutinins is reached about 2–4 months after the transfusion. Thus, a **delayed transfusion reaction** occurs, which is mild. These antibodies remain in blood and on subsequent transfusion of Rh-positive blood into the same person; the transfusion reaction will be immediate and very severe. This is because with multiple exposures to the Rh factor, the Rh negative person becomes strongly sensitized to the Rh factor. The increased formation of anti-Rh antibodies will cause hemolysis of the RBCs in the donated blood.

Erythroblastosis fetalis is seen when an Rh-negative mother carries an Rh-positive fetus and is the *most common problem with Rh incompatibility*.

MULTIPLE CHOICE QUESTIONS

1. ABO blood group antigens are known as:
    a. Duffy factor
    b. Landsteiner factor
    c. Rhesus factor
    d. Lutheran factor

2. The first child of an Rh-negative mother develops symptoms of erythroblastosis fetalis. The reason could be that:
    a. The child happened to be Rh-positive
    b. The child happened to be Rh-negative
    c. The mother had an Rh-positive blood transfusion earlier
    d. The mother had a previous abortion with Rh negative fetus

3. After transfusion of stored blood:
    a. Most of the transfused red cells survive 120 days
    b. The transfused neutrophils survive about 6 days
    c. The transfused platelets survive about 8 days
    d. All the above statements are false

4. If blood transfusion is indicated, fresh blood transfusion is a must in all the following conditions, *except*:
    a. Hemophilia
    b. COPD
    c. CO poisoning
    d. Hemorrhage following accidents

5. All the following are used as anticoagulant in the laboratory, *except*:
    a. EDTA
    b. Sodium chloride
    c. Sodium citrate
    d. Double oxalate

6. In ABO incompatibility between mother and fetus, the class of antibody that is produced in the mother by A or B antigen is mostly:
    a. IgA
    b. IgE
    c. IgG
    d. IgM

7. The following statements regarding agglutinin are true, *except*:
    a. Agglutinins are not present in CSF
    b. Specific agglutinins are present in fetal plasma
    c. The plasma level of agglutinin is maximum by about 10 years of life
    d. Maternal agglutinins may be present in fetal plasma

Table 21.5: Summary of transfusion reactions.

Hemolytic reactions	Non-hemolytic reactions
• Hemoglobinemia • Hemoglobinuria • Disseminated intravascular hemolysis • Circulatory shock • Hyperkalemia • Cardiac arrhythmia	• Transmission of diseases • Iron overload • Cardiorespiratory complications like pulmonary edema and cardiac failure due to hypervolemia • Immunological reactions against WBC, platelets and plasma proteins • Allergic reactions • Fever and chills

8. Although more than 400 blood groups have been identified, the ABO blood group system remains the most important in clinical medicine because:
   a. It was the first blood group system to be discovered
   b. It has four different blood groups: A, B, AB, O(H)
   c. ABO(H) antigens are present in most body tissues and fluids
   d. ABO(H) antibodies are invariably present in plasma when person's RBC lacks the corresponding antigen

9. A 20-year-old female accident victim in casualty urgently needs blood. There is no time to determine her blood group. Emergency transfusion in the patient should be done with:
   a. AB negative whole blood
   b. Positive RBC and colloids/crystalloids
   c. O negative RBC and colloids/crystalloids
   d. O positive packed cell

10. Regarding blood group antibodies, all the following statements are correct, *except*:
    a. At the time of birth, the quantity of agglutinins in plasma is almost zero.
    b. Maximum antibody titer is reached at 8–10 years of age
    c. Development of anti-A and anti-B agglutinins is initiated by group A and B antigens that enter the body in food, bacteria, etc.
    d. Individuals, who genetically lack any antigens in the RBC membrane, have antibodies against the red cell types that they have not inherited

11. True about Rh factor:
    a. Has no naturally occurring antibody
    b. Seen only in humans
    c. Not important for blood transfusion
    d. Obey Landsteiner's second law

12. B positive group people can receive blood from:
    a. Group AB
    b. Group B alone
    c. Group A, B and O
    d. Group O and B

13. The true statement regarding ABO incompatibility is that:
    a. It occurs only in the second pregnancy
    b. It occurs when mother is A and baby O group
    c. It is more common than Rh incompatibility
    d. It occurs when mother is O and baby A

14. The blood group that does not obey Landsteiner's law is:
    a. A blood group
    b. B blood group
    c. O group
    d. Rh blood group

15. An 'O'group child cannot have a parent of group
    a. A
    b. B
    c. AB
    d. O

16. Kernicterus is produced in the newborn when the serum bilirubin is more than:
    a. 3 mg/dL
    b. 20 mg/dL
    c. 2 mg/dL
    d. 8 mg/dL

17. With regard to ABO blood group system, all the following are true, *except*:
    a. A person of group B, has anti-A antibodies in his plasma
    b. In an incompatible blood transfusion, usually the donor cells are lysed
    c. Antibodies to A and B agglutinogens are incomplete antibodies
    d. A severe transfusion reaction is likely to be followed by jaundice

18. Which of the following blood groups can be transfused to a patient in hemorrhagic shock as an emergency measure?
    a. O negative
    b. O positive
    c. AB negative
    d. AB positive

19. Hydroxyethyl starch is a:
    a. Vasodilator
    b. Crystalloid
    c. Plasma expander
    d. Diuretic

20. ABO blood group antigens are:
    a. Carried by sex chromosome
    b. Attached to plasma proteins
    c. Attached to hemoglobin molecule
    d. Found in saliva

21. Stored blood as compared to fresh blood has:
    a. More 2,3-DPG
    b. High extracellular K^+
    c. High extracellular hemoglobin
    d. Increased platelets

22. Aspirin inhibits:
    a. Lipoxygenase
    b. Prostacyclin synthesis
    c. Cyclooxygenase
    d. Phospholipase

23. Father to son inheritance is never seen in case of:
    a. Autosomal dominant inheritance
    b. Autosomal recessive inheritance
    c. X-linked recessive inheritance
    d. Multifactorial inheritance

24. The first child of an Rh-negative mother developed symptoms of erythroblastosis fetalis. The reason could be that:
    a. The child happened to be Rh-positive
    b. The child happened to be Rh-negative
    c. The mother had a previous abortion with Rh-positive fetus
    d. The mother had an Rh-negative blood transfusion earlier

25. Before blood transfusion, it is necessary to match:
    a. Recipient's plasma with donor's cells
    b. Recipient's cells with donor's cells
    c. Recipient's plasma with donor's plasma
    d. Recipient's cells with donor's plasma

26. In Rh negative individuals:
    a. Serum contains anti-Rh antibodies
    b. RBC contains Rh antigen

c. RBC contains D antigen and serum contains no Rh antibody
d. RBC contains no D antigen and serum contains no Rh antibody

27. **Erythroblastosis fetalis in the first pregnancy can be prevented by:**
    a. Exchange transfusion in baby with Rh negative blood
    b. Giving Rh antibodies to the mother immediately after delivery
    c. Immunization of the mother during pregnancy with Rh immunoglobulin
    d. Giving Rh antibody to the baby immediately after birth

28. **The amount of blood collected from a donor at a time is:**
    a. 500 mL   b. 350 mL
    c. 700 mL   d. 150 mL

29. **Glucose is added to stored blood to:**
    a. Prevent hemolysis   b. Provide nutrition
    c. Decrease the pH   d. Increase metabolism

30. **Preservation injury includes all the following, except:**
    a. Decrease in 2, 3 DPG level
    b. Increase in intracellular Na⁺
    c. Hypokalemia
    d. Decrease in pH

ANSWERS

1. b	2. c	3. d	4. d	5. b
6. d	7. b	8. d	9. c	10. d
11. a	12. d	13. d	14. d	15. c
16. b	17. c	18. a	19. c	20. d
21. b	22. c	23. c	24. c	25. a
26. d	27. c	28. b	29. b	30. c

■ NAME THE FOLLOWING/FILL IN THE BLANKS/GIVE THE NORMAL VALUES (HEMATOLOGY)

1. Normal leukocyte count: **4000–11,000 cells/mm³ of blood**.
2. Percentage of neutrophil in the peripheral smear: **60–65%**.
3. **70–80%** of circulating blood lymphocytes is T-lymphocytes and **10–15%** B-lymphocytes.
4. Leukocytes that have the shortest lifespan: **Neutrophils (6–8 days)**.
5. Average production of neutrophils per day: **100 billion**.
6. The process of squeezing of neutrophils through pores of capillaries: **Diapedesis**.
7. The leukocyte that spend minimum period in circulation: **Monocyte (3 days)**.
8. The leukocyte that plays a crucial role in the host's defense against parasites: **Eosinophil**.
9. Basophils function in **type-I hypersensitivity** response.
10. Largest WBC is **monocyte** and smallest WBC is **small lymphocyte**.
11. Cellular immunity is mediated by **T-lymphocyte** and humoral immunity is mediated by **B-lymphocyte**.
12. Most abundant immunoglobulin present in the body: **IgG**.
13. The immunoglobulins present in body secretions like saliva, milk, and tear: **IgA**.
14. ABO antibodies are of which group of immunoglobulin? **IgM**.
15. Increase in WBC count is called **leukocytosis** and decrease in WBC count is **leukopenia**.
16. Dead neutrophils, necrotic tissue and dead bacteria at the site of infection and inflammation form **pus**.
17. Normal platelet count: **2–4 lakhs/mm³ of blood**.
18. Platelets are formed from **megakaryocytes** in bone marrow.
19. Bleeding time is the test for **platelet activity**.
20. In thrombocytopenia spontaneous bleeding occur when the platelet count is less than **20,000/mm³**.
21. Half-life of transfused platelets: **4 days**.
22. The substances released from the endothelium that relax vascular smooth muscles are NO and prostacyclin.
23. The skin surface serves as the first line of defense of the innate immune system.
24. Iron is absorbed from the duodenum in the **ferrous** form and is stored in ferritin in the **ferric** form.
25. Total amount of iron present in the body: **3–5 g**.
26. Best method of hemoglobin estimation in blood: **Cyanmethemoglobin method**.
27. Normal plasma protein content: **6–8 g/dL**.
28. Gamma globulin is produced by **plasma cells** derived from B-lymphocytes.
29. 80% of osmotic pressure of plasma is contributed by **albumin** because of its low molecular weight (69,000) and high blood concentration (3.5–5 g %).
30. Osmotic pressure is determined by the number of particles in solution and not by the mass of the particle
31. Second circulatory system refer to **lymphatics**.
32. Vitamin K dependent factors in blood: **Factors II, VII, IX, X, protein C and protein S**.
33. The clotting factors absent in serum: **I, II, V, VIII and XIII**.
34. Serum has high serotonin content due to breakdown of **platelets** during clotting.
35. Hemophilia A is due to deficiency of clotting **factor VIII** and hemophilia B is due to deficiency of clotting **factor IX**.
36. Prothrombin time (PT) measures efficiency of **extrinsic** pathway of coagulation and the **common** pathway.
37. Partial thromboplastin time (PTT) measures efficiency of **intrinsic and common** pathway.
38. Normal bleeding time: **2–4 minutes**.
39. Normal clotting time: **3–8 minutes**.
40. Normal clot retraction time: **30–60 minutes**.
41. Smallest blood cell: **platelet**.
42. Largest blood cell: **monocyte**.
43. Myeloid:erythroid ratio in the red bone marrow: **3:1**.

CHAPTER 21 — Blood Groups and Blood Transfusion

44. Normal ratio of RBC to WBC in the body: **700:1**.
45. Normal RBC count: **5–5.5 million cells/mm³ of blood**.
46. Normal duration of erythropoiesis: **7 days**.
47. Main site of production of erythropoietin: **kidney**.
48. RBCs can generate ATP only **anaerobically**.
49. Fresh blood refers to blood which is administered within **24 hours**.
50. Reticulocytes are stained by **supravital** staining.
51. Normal reticulocyte count: **0.5–1.5% in human adults**.
52. Life span of plasma cell: **2–3 days**.
53. Life span of platelet: **5–9 days**.
54. Life span of RBC: **120 days**.
55. Cellular target of HIV: **CD4 helper T cell**.
56. Volume of normal RBC (MCV) : **87–90 μm³**.
57. MCV is decreased in **iron deficiency anemia** and increased in **megaloblastic anemia**.
58. The most common form of anemia seen in our country: **iron deficiency anemia**.
59. Most common cause of iron deficiency anemia in children: **hookworm infestation**.
60. Pernicious anemia is due to deficiency of **vitamin B_{12}**.
61. Pyknotic nucleus is present in **late normoblast**.
62. Normally iron in hemoglobin is in the **ferrous** form.
63. Delayed type of hypersensitivity reaction is mediated by **T-lymphocyte**.
64. Inheritance of hemophilia: **X-linked recessive**.
65. In hemolytic jaundice, bilirubin is absent in urine and hence called **acholuric jaundice**.
66. Von Willebrand disease is also known as **pseudohemophilia**.
67. Fibrinogen is converted to fibrin by **thrombin**.
68. Heparin acts by inhibiting active form of **factor X**.
69. Site of absorption of vitamin B_{12} in the intestine: **Terminal ileum**.
70. Hemoglobin appear in the **intermediate normoblast** stage of erythropoiesis.
71. Unbound unconjugated bilirubin crosses the blood-brain barrier to produce **kernicterus**.
72. Kernicterus is produced in the newborn when the serum bilirubin is more than **20 mg/dL**.
73. Normal albumin-globulin ratio in blood: **1.7:1**.
74. Blood groups were discovered by **Karl Landsteiner**.
75. Landsteiner's second law is applicable only to **ABO** system.
76. A person is said to be Rh⁺ if his RBCs contain **D** antigen.
77. Kernicterus is caused due to accumulation of **bilirubin** in brain.
78. Specific gravity of whole blood: **1055–1060**.
79. In hemoglobin S, glutamic acid is replaced by **valine** in the β-chain.
80. In AIDS, there is destruction of **helper T cells**.
81. The active component of fibrinolytic system: **Plasmin or fibrinolysin**.
82. Total blood volume: **80 mL/kg body weight**.
83. The percentage of ECF constituted by blood: **20%**.
84. Oncotic pressure of plasma is contributed mainly by **albumin**.
85. Maximum titer of blood group antibodies is reached by **8 to 10** years of age.

CLINICAL CASE SCENARIO

1. A 50-year-old man who has undergone gastrectomy for carcinoma stomach was admitted with severe pallor, and numbness and paraesthesia of the extremities. On examination, there was loss of fine touch, vibration and position sense in both lower limbs. Blood and bone marrow examination revealed megaloblastic anemia. On treatment with tablets containing vitamin B12 and folic acid there was no improvement and the neurological symptoms worsened.
   a. Explain the cause of anemia in this patient.
   b. Why did the treatment fail?
   c. What is the reason for the worsening of neurological symptoms on treatment?
   d. How will you investigate a case of anemia?

   Ans:
   a. Since there are neurological deficits, the anemia is due to vitamin B12 deficiency (pernicious anemia).

2. A lady in the second trimester of pregnancy comes to the obstetrics OP and gives a history of giving birth to a jaundiced baby in her second delivery. The child died after 3 days. Her first delivery was not in a hospital. The first baby is normal and is Rh positive. On investigation, she was found to be Rh negative and her husband Rh positive.
   a. What was the probable problem in her second pregnancy?
   b. What is the physiological basis of the clinical manifestations in the second baby?
   c. What is the basis of the preventive measures that could have been taken?
   d. What will be the fate of the third baby?

   Ans:
   a. The problem was Rh incompatibility since the first baby was Rh positive and anti-D serum was not administered after the first delivery.

SECTION 2 ⊃ Hematology

3. A 5-year-old boy was brought to the casualty with complaint of pain and swelling in his right knee joint. He gives a history of being kicked on the knee while playing and also gives a history of severe bleeding following tooth extraction. On examination, he had effusion of the right knee joint. Body temperature and pulse rate was normal. On eliciting family history, his mother's brother has history of severe bleeding even on mild trauma and is on treatment.
   a. What can be the probable diagnosis?
   b. How can you explain the family history?
   c. What are the positive investigation findings that would help you to come to a correct diagnosis?
   d. Explain the intrinsic pathway of coagulation.

   Ans:
   a. Hemophilia
   b. Explain X-linked recessive inheritance of hemophilia
   c. Clotting time, activated partial thromboplastin time (APTT), prothrombin time and bleeding time are determined to confirm hemophilia. Clotting time and APTT are prolonged in hemophilia due to deficiency of clotting factor VIII (in classical hemophilia or hemophilia-A). Prothrombin time and bleeding time are normal in hemophilia. Factor VIII assay can also be done to assess the severity of the disease.

4. 35-year-old female complains of tiredness, weakness, palpitation and chest discomfort on exertion. She gives a history of heavy menstrual bleeding for the past 6 months. On examination, there was severe pallor, heart rate 100/min and there was a systolic murmur on auscultation. ECG was normal. Investigations showed:
   Hemoglobin – 6 g%
   RBC count – 3 million/mm³ of blood
   PCV – 35%
   MCV – 76 μm³
   MCH – 25 pg
   MCHC – 17%
   a. What is the probable diagnosis?
   b. What is the physiological basis of tachycardia and murmur?
   c. Write the normal values of the above investigation report.
   d. Explain the steps in erythropoiesis and enumerate the factors affecting it.

   Ans:
   a. Microcytic hypochromic anemia (iron deficiency anemia)
   b. Tachycardia is due to hypoxia. In anemia, viscosity of blood is decreased and this increases velocity of blood flow and produces turbulence. This produces murmur in the heart.

5. Following an accident a man was brought to the casualty with severe bleeding from the wounds. He was immediately given blood transfusion following which he developed rashes, oliguria and hematuria. Answer the following:
   a. Explain the complications of mismatched blood transfusion
   b. What are the precautions to be taken before blood transfusion?
   c. Describe preservation injury
   d. What is autologous blood transfusion?

SECTION 3: CARDIOVASCULAR SYSTEM

Functional Anatomy of the Heart

CHAPTER 22

LEARNING OBJECTIVES

Must know
- Describe the functional anatomy of the heart
- Describe pacemaker tissue and conducting system of heart with the help of a diagram
- Explain the properties of cardiac muscle
- Explain the origin and spread of cardiac impulse

INTRODUCTION

Unicellular organisms meet their metabolic needs by processes like diffusion. But in multicellular organisms, the distance between the external environment and the cells in the interior of the body is very large. So, simple diffusion is inadequate to supply nutrients and oxygen to the cells in the interior and also to eliminate waste materials. Hence they need a circulatory system for the distribution of gases, nutrients and other molecules like hormones necessary for growth and repair. Transfer of substances between plasma and the cells is accomplished by dense networks of capillaries which have a very thin wall. These capillaries offer little resistance to the transfer of substances across their walls.

Cardiovascular system deals with the study of **heart, blood vessels and blood**. Heart acts as the pump which pumps blood into the blood vessels. Blood vessels (arteries and arterioles) help in the distribution of blood throughout the body. Capillaries help in the exchange of substances between blood and tissue fluid. Venules and veins carry blood back into the heart. Blood is the conducting medium in the circulatory system.

The volume of blood in percentage in different parts of vascular system is as follows:
a. **Heart**—7%
b. **Systemic circulation**
   - Veins, venules and venous sinuses—64%
   - Aorta, arteries and arterioles—15%
   - Capillaries—5%
c. **Pulmonary circulation**—9%

Blood flows continuously through the closed circuit of the cardiovascular system due to the following reasons:
- Forward push to the blood in the heart is imparted by the cardiac pump
- Elastic recoil of the stretched arterial wall aids in the forward movement of blood
- Compression of veins by the contraction of skeletal muscles (skeletal muscle pump) helps in the return of blood back to the heart
- Negative intrathoracic pressure during inspiration also aids in venous return to the heart.

The internal environment of the body is the **interstitial fluid**. The composition of this fluid should be maintained within a narrow range. Maintaining a constant internal environment is called homeostasis. The osmolarity, blood chemistry (pH, PO_2, PCO_2), etc., should be kept constant for the proper functioning of the body systems. Cardiovascular system plays a very important role in homeostasis. The circulating body fluid, i.e., blood carries nutrients, O_2, hormones, etc., to the various tissues and remove waste products like CO_2, urea, excess water, etc., to the organs of excretion. Excess heat produced during metabolism is also removed by blood. Blood flow to the tissues should be properly regulated according to the demands. For example, during exercise, the contracting muscles need excess O_2 and glucose. Excess CO_2, lactic acid, heat, etc., produced should be removed to sustain muscle activity. Brain has no capacity to store glucose and it cannot withstand anoxia. So blood flow to the brain must be maintained to ensure consciousness.

The study of the heart and the diseases associated with it is called **cardiology**. Lymphatic system is also included under circulatory system.

Functions of Circulatory System

- Circulatory system helps to **transport** essential substances like O_2 to the tissues, and metabolic by-products like CO_2, water, etc., to the excretory organs.
- Distribution of nutrients for growth and repair
- Distribution of hormones and neurotransmitters to the target tissues
- Circulatory system helps in **homeostasis** by regulating body temperature, body fluid volume, blood chemistry

(PCO_2, PO_2, pH), etc. Helps in heat loss by transmitting heat from the core to the surface of the body
- Aids in hormonal action by transporting hormones from the site of production to the target organs. Hormones play a very important role in homeostasis
- Mediation of inflammatory and host defense mechanism against invading agents
- Heart acting as a pump helps in the movement of the blood throughout the body during life
- Blood vessels carry blood to the various organs and tissues.

To achieve these functions, a *pump* system is present in the circulatory system, which is the heart that pumps blood intermittently into the blood vessels. Large blood vessels like aorta act as *accessory pumps* to make this intermittent flow continuous. Continuous flow through the blood vessels is achieved by:
- Distension of aorta and the large arteries during ventricular contraction or ventricular systole.
- Elastic recoil of the wall of aorta and large arteries during diastole so that blood is pushed forward during ventricular relaxation.

HEART

PY5.1: Describe the functional anatomy of heart including chambers, sounds; and pacemaker tissue and conducting system.

Functional Anatomy of the Heart

Heart is a small, pyramidal, muscular organ situated in the mediastinum obliquely. 2/3 of the heart is to the left and 1/3 to the right of the midline. It has a base, apex and three surfaces—anterior, posterior and inferior surfaces. The apex of the heart is directed anteriorly, inferiorly and to the left. The base is directed posteriorly, superiorly and to the right.

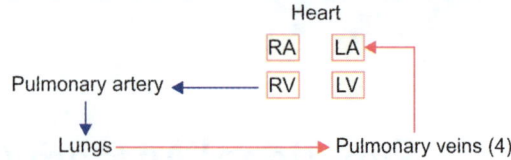

Fig. 22.2: Pulmonary circulation or lesser circulation.
(RA: right atrium; RV: right ventricle; LA: left atrium; LV: left ventricle)

Heart is roughly the size of a clenched fist and weighs about 300–330 g.

Heart is a four-chambered structure composed of two atria and two ventricles. Atria are separated from ventricles by atrioventricular groove which is very evident when viewed from outside. The atria are separated on the inside by interatrial septum and it is seen externally as interatrial groove. There is an oval depression called fossa ovalis in the interatrial septum which is the remnant of foramen ovale, an opening in the septum of fetal heart that closes soon after birth. The ventricles are separated by interventricular septum that is seen externally as interventricular groove.

The right atrium receives blood from three major veins:
- Superior vena cava
- Inferior vena cava
- Coronary sinus.

Left atrium receives blood from lungs through four pulmonary veins **(Fig. 22.1)**.

Heart receives its blood supply from the **coronary arteries**. Coronary arteries branch from the base of ascending aorta and perfuse the heart wall (*refer* coronary circulation).

Heart functions as two separate pumps. Right side of the heart pumps blood into the lungs for the exchange of gases and this component of circulatory system is called **pulmonary circulation or lesser circulation (Fig. 22.2)**. The left side of the heart pumps blood to all other parts of the body and this is referred to as **systemic circulation or greater circulation (Fig. 22.3)**.

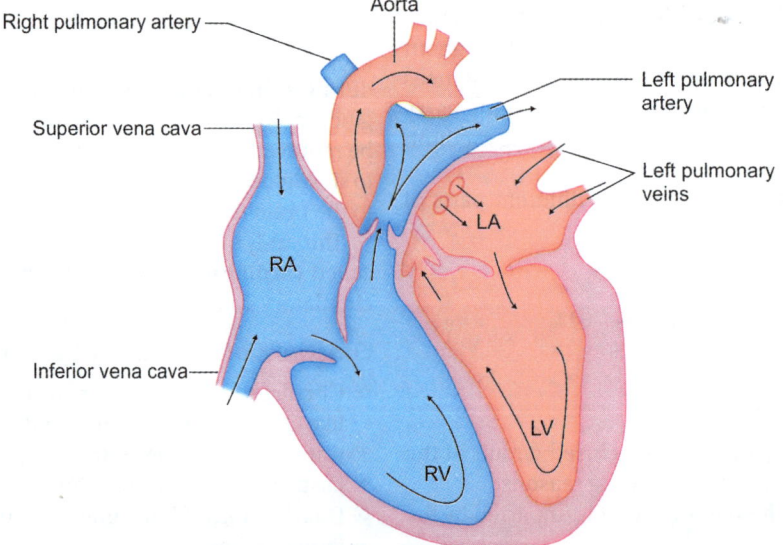

Fig. 22.1: Direction of blood flow through the heart. Arrows denote direction of blood flow.
(RA: right atrium; RV: right ventricle; LA: left atrium; LV: left ventricle)

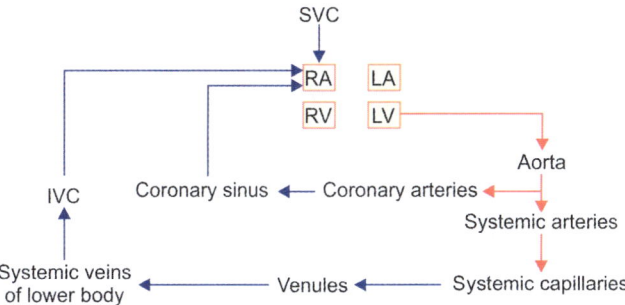

Fig. 22.3: Systemic circulation or greater circulation.
(IVC: inferior vena cava; SVC: superior vena cava; RA: right atrium; LA: left atrium; LV: left ventricle; RV: right ventricle)

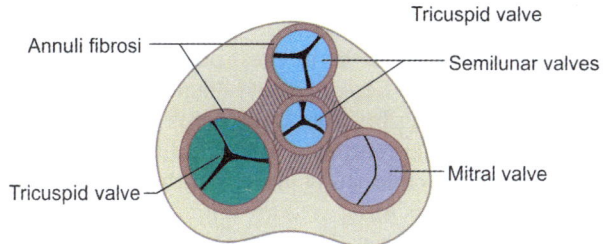

Fig. 22.4: Fibrous skeleton of heart showing the position of different valves.

There is no connection between the right and left halves of the heart. The atrioventricular opening, which is guarded by one-way valves, connects the upper and lower chambers of the heart. They allow blood to flow only in one direction, i.e., from atria to ventricles.

Coverings of Heart

Heart is enveloped in a **fibroserous** covering called **pericardium**. It is a two-layered structure, the outer layer is called the **fibrous pericardium** and the inner double-layered covering is called the **serous pericardium**. The outer layer of serous pericardium is called **parietal layer** and inner layer is called the **visceral layer** of serous pericardium. Between these two layers is a potential space called **pericardial cavity** that contains about 5–15 mL of **pericardial fluid**.

Fibrous pericardium is the superficial, tough, inelastic, dense, irregular connective tissue layer that attaches the heart to the diaphragm. The part of the fibrous pericardium covering the apex of the heart is connected to the central tendon of diaphragm. Towards the base of the heart, fibrous pericardium is attached to the blood vessels and surrounding structures.

Functions of Pericardium

* Pericardium gives a firm *anchorage* to the heart that has no bony connections and maintains its position in the mediastinum.
* As pericardium is attached to the central tendon of diaphragm, it acts as a *fulcrum* for proper cardiac contraction. During contraction, the heart rotates and strikes against the chest wall, which is felt as **apex beat**. *Apex beat is the lowermost and outermost point on the precordium (part of the chest wall overlying the heart) where a definite cardiac pulsation is seen or felt.*
* Pericardial fluid *reduces friction* during cardiac contraction.
* Fibrous pericardium *prevents undue distension* of heart since it is tough and inelastic.

Clinical Importance
Pericarditis

Infection or inflammation of the pericardium is called **pericarditis**. The inflamed pericardial surfaces may rub against each other during cardiac contraction producing a sound called **pericardial rub** that can be heard as a rubbing sound on auscultation. If it results in scarring, cardiac performance may be affected.

When there is increased fluid collection in the pericardial space it is known as **pericardial effusion**. When there is extensive bleeding into the pericardial cavity or if fluid collection is excessive, it causes compression of the heart. This is known as **cardiac tamponade,** which can affect cardiac performance and can even stop the heart.

Fibrous Skeleton of the Heart

The fibrous skeleton of the heart (annuli fibrosi) consists of dense connective tissue rings that surround the valves of the heart. They are interconnected and fuse with one another. Four fibrous rings support the four valves of the heart **(Fig. 22. 4)**.

Functions of the Fibrous Skeleton of Heart

* The heart valves are attached to the fibrous skeleton and the valves are prevented from overstretching when blood passes through them.
* It serves as the point of origin and insertion of cardiac muscle fiber bundles.
* Acts as an electrical insulator between atria and ventricles so that the atria contract a little bit ahead of ventricular contraction.

Musculature of the Heart

The muscles of the heart originate from four fibromuscular connective tissue rings called **annuli fibrosi**, two around atrioventricular orifices, one in the pulmonary orifice and one in the aortic orifice **(Fig. 22.4)**. Those muscles growing up from annuli fibrosi form the atria and arterial trunks. The muscles growing down from the annuli fibrosi form the ventricles. The atrial musculature and ventricular musculature are separate. The only communication for electrical activity between atria and ventricles is through **bundle of His**.

Muscles of the heart are collectively termed **myocardium**. It is three layered and the layers are:
1. Epicardium
2. Myocardium proper
3. Endocardium.

Epicardium

Epicardium is the outermost layer and it blends with the visceral layer of pericardium.

Myocardium Proper

Myocardium proper is the thickest portion of heart. The cardiac muscle fibers are arranged diagonally around the heart in interlacing bundles. This helps in the effective contraction of the ventricles as a whole. The papillary muscles and the conducting system of the heart are also part of myocardium. Atrial walls are thinner than ventricular walls. Left ventricular wall is thicker than right ventricular wall, the ratio being 3:1. Therefore, the cavity of left ventricle is smaller than that of right ventricle. The thickness of the different parts of the heart is:
- Atrial wall—2 mm
- Right ventricular wall—3–4 mm
- Left ventricular wall—8–9 mm.

The left Ventricular Wall is Thicker Because:
- Left ventricle has to pump blood into the systemic circulation which is a high-pressure, high-resistance system. So the left ventricle must work harder than the right ventricle to maintain the same cardiac output as that of right ventricle. So the wall is thicker.
- Left ventricle has to pump blood to a greater distance, i.e., to all parts of the body.

The Right Ventricular Wall is Thin Because:
- The right ventricle has to pump blood into the pulmonary circulation which is a low-pressure, low-resistance, high capacitance system. So, the pressure exerted by the right ventricle need be less and so right ventricular wall is thinner.
- It has to pump blood only to a short distance, i.e., to the lungs.

Endocardium

Endocardium is the innermost layer of the heart and is made up of a layer of endothelium overlying a thin layer of connective tissue and small amount of muscular tissue. The endocardium forms flaps of the valves, valve rings, etc. The layer of **endothelium** forming the innermost lining of the endocardium forms a smooth lining for the chambers of the heart and the valves of the heart. This endothelium is continuous with the endothelial lining of the large blood vessels arising from the heart.

Papillary Muscles of the Heart

Papillary muscles arise from the ventricular myocardium and are attached to the border of atrioventricular valve leaflets (cusps) with the help of **chordae tendineae**, which are cord-like structures originating from papillary muscles **(Fig. 22.5)**.

Valves of the Heart

- Two atrioventricular valves
- Two semilunar valves.

Atrioventricular valves (AV valves) guard the atrioventricular openings. AV valve on the right side is larger than the left and is guarded by 3 cusps or leaflets. So it is called **tricuspid valve**. The left atrioventricular opening is guarded by left AV valve that has only two cusps. It is hence called **bicuspid valve or mitral valve**. Pulmonary arterial opening

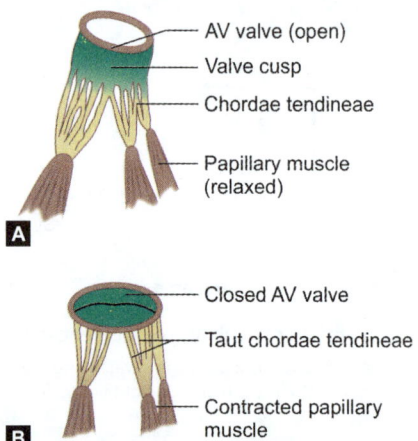

Figs. 22.5A and B: Atrioventricular valves showing papillary muscles and chordae tendineae: (A) Valve open; (B) Valve closed showing taut chordae tendineae.

and aortic openings are guarded by **semilunar valves**. Each consists of 3 cusps **(Fig. 22.4)**. The AV valves as well as the semilunar valves are so arranged that only forward flow of blood open the leaflets, while backward flow of blood will close the valves. Thus, regurgitation of blood is prevented. The valves open and close in response to pressure changes in the chambers as the heart contracts and relaxes.

The AV valves are held in position by **papillary muscles**. These muscles are attached to the edge of the valve leaflets by tough connective tissue strands called **chordae tendineae (Fig. 22.5)**. When the ventricles contract the papillary muscles attached to the ventricles also contract simultaneously.

This helps in proper approximation of the valve leaflets and prevents undue bulging of the AV valves into the atria during ventricular contraction. If there is rupture of chordae tendineae or if there is paralysis of the papillary muscles, the AV valve bulges far backwards into the atria or it gets everted during ventricular contraction leading to **regurgitation** of blood back into the atria producing sounds called cardiac murmurs.

There are no valves at the openings of the great veins into the atria. So when the atria contract, small amount of blood leaks into these veins. This is the reason for the visible jugular venous pulsations when the subject is lying down. However, as the atria contract, it compresses the openings of these veins minimizing the backflow of blood.

Disorders of Heart Valves

Failure of the heart valve to open completely is called **stenosis**, whereas failure of the valve to close completely is called **incompetence** or valvular **insufficiency**. For example, in mitral stenosis, the mitral valve becomes narrow thereby increasing the resistance to blood flow during ventricular diastole leading to turbulence. In mitral insufficiency, the mitral valve fails to close completely leading to regurgitation of blood into the left atrium during ventricular systole. Cause of mitral insufficiency is mitral valve prolapse due to damaged valve or ruptured chordae tendineae. Certain

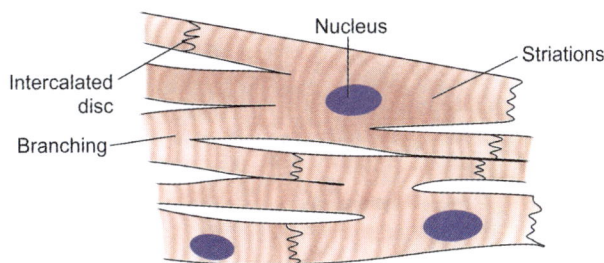

Fig. 22.6: Structure of cardiac muscle.

infectious diseases of heart can destroy the valves. For example, in **rheumatic fever** due to streptococcal infection of throat, the antibodies produced against the bacteria also act as auto-antibodies causing inflammation of connective tissues of joints, heart valves, etc., leading to their damage.

Histology of Cardiac Muscle

The cardiac muscle fibers are cylindrical, striated, highly branched and interdigitated or they are arranged in a latticework. The cardiac muscle fibers are connected in series and parallel with each other. The cell membrane of adjacent cardiac muscle cells is found to be interdigitating, i.e., the junction shows numerous folds which interdigitate. This junction is called **intercalated disc (Fig. 22.6)**.

At each intercalated disc, the cell membranes of adjacent cells fuse with one another forming **gap junctions** that allow free diffusion of ions (There is no continuation of cytoplasm of one cell with another cell). Thus, action potentials can travel easily from one cell to the next cell through the intercalated disc. Also the presence of intercalated discs enables transmission of the force of contraction from one cell to another through the axis of the cell. Because of these two factors, the muscle as a whole can contract as a single unit or it acts as a **functional syncytium** to pump blood out of the heart into the great vessels.

The heart is composed of two syncytia, the **atrial syncytium and ventricular syncytium**. Normally, action potential is not conducted from the atrial muscle to the ventricular muscle directly because they are separated by fibrous tissue. The only path through which action potential can be conducted from atria to ventricles is through the **AV bundle**. This partitioning of the atrial and ventricular musculature allows the atria to contract a short time ahead of ventricular contraction. This is very essential for the effectiveness of ventricular pumping.

■ SPECIALIZED EXCITATORY AND CONDUCTING SYSTEM OF HEART

PY5.4: Describe generation and conduction of cardiac impulse.

Introduction

The heartbeat originates in a specialized conducting system of the heart called **cardiac conducting system or cardiac conduction system**. The peculiarities of the system are:

- ❖ It can generate rhythmical electrical impulses.
- ❖ It can conduct these impulses rapidly throughout the heart to cause rhythmical contraction of the myocardium.
- ❖ The Purkinje system allows all portions of the ventricle to contract simultaneously so that sufficient pressure is created in the ventricles to pump blood into the arterial trunks.
- ❖ By the normal functioning of this system the atria contract about one-sixth of a second ahead of ventricular contraction. This allows adequate filling of the ventricles before ventricular systole.

Components of the Cardiac Conducting System (Fig. 22.7)

- ❖ Sinoatrial node (SA node)
- ❖ Internodal atrial pathways
- ❖ Atrioventricular node (AV node)
- ❖ Bundle of His or atrioventricular bundle (AV bundle)
- ❖ Purkinje fibers.

SA Node

SA node is a small, flattened strip of specialized cardiac muscle situated in the anterosuperior wall of the **right atrium**, immediately below and lateral to the opening of superior vena cava **(Fig. 22.7)**. The fibers of the SA node have no contractile elements and they are smaller than other atrial muscle fibers. But the SA nodal fibers connect directly with atrial muscle fibers so that action potentials from the SA node spread immediately into the atrial wall. So, it is difficult to separate SA node from atrial musculature. SA node develops from structures on the right side of the embryo and so it is supplied by the **right vagus**. It also receives sympathetic innervation from the right cervical sympathetic ganglion (stellate ganglion) through the cardiac nerves.

The SA node is about 15 mm in length, 2 mm wide and 1 mm thick. It contains small rounded cells with few organelles called **P cells**, which are the pacemaker cells of the SA node. The rest of the cells of SA node are called **T cells** or transitional cells. P cells have the property of self-excitation and can spontaneously generate action potentials that rapidly spread throughout the atria. P cells are also present in the rest of the myocardial tissue but in smaller numbers.

Even though, all parts of the conducting system can generate impulses, SA node discharges most rapidly. So depolarization of other parts of the conducting system occurs before they discharge spontaneously. Hence, SA node is considered as the **pacemaker** of heart. If the SA node is not functioning as in **sick sinus syndrome**, the heart rate comes down because some other parts of the conducting system take over the function of SA node. For example, in complete heart block the heart beats at the ventricular rhythm, i.e., about 20–40 beats/min.

Pacemaker Potential

Pacemaker potential is the electrical potential in the SA node. The change in potential from the resting level to the firing level in the pacemaker cell is called **pacemaker potential or prepotential** (*refer* Fig. 9.4). The pacemaker

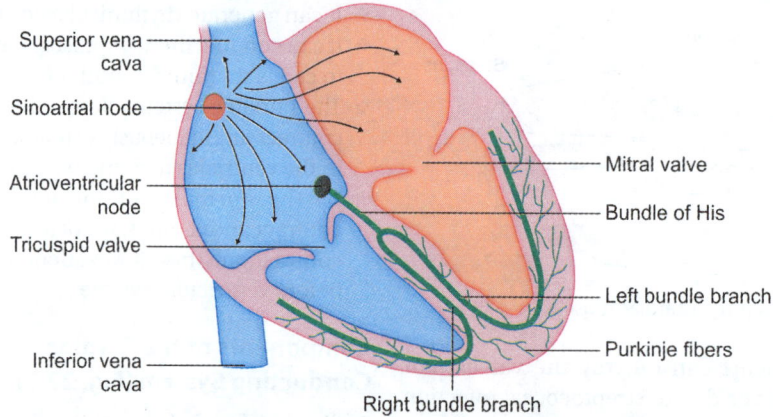

Fig. 22.7: Conducting system of heart.

potential triggers the action potential in the pacemaker cells. Slow diastolic depolarization or pacemaker potential or prepotential is due to three ionic currents:
1. Decrease in K⁺ efflux due to gradually diminishing outward **K⁺ current** (I_k)
2. Inward **Na⁺ current** (I_{Na}) induced by hyperpolarization. This occurs towards the end of repolarization. This current is activated as the membrane potential becomes more negative than -50 mV. Towards the end of action potential, the potassium channels remain open for some more time, temporarily allowing movement of positive charges out of the cell. This leads to excess negativity inside the cell bringing the resting membrane potential down to about -55 to -60 mV at the end of the action potential. This produces a hyperpolarization state. Since the Na⁺ channel is activated following hyperpolarization, it is referred to as **'h' channel**. Because of its unusual or funny activation, it is also called **funny channel** or **'f' channel**. The opening of the funny channels is mediated by cAMP. That is why the funny current channels are now called *hyperpolarization-activated cyclic nucleotide-gated (HCN) channels*. This current, i.e., I_h is mainly responsible for the first part of the prepotential in the pacemaker cell.
3. Inward **Ca²⁺ current** (I_{Ca}) is responsible for the upstroke of the action potential. There are two types of Ca²⁺ channels in the heart, T channel and L channel. Transient Ca²⁺ channel (T-channel) contributes to the prepotential along with Na⁺ (h) channel, whereas long acting channel (L-channel) produces the impulse or action potential. There is also release of Ca²⁺ from sarcoplasmic reticulum (**Ca²⁺ sparks**) during the prepotential. A decrease in the extracellular Ca²⁺ or Ca²⁺ channel blockers diminishes the amplitude of action potential and the slope of the prepotential.

Internodal Atrial Pathways

Since the SA nodal fibers connect directly with surrounding atrial fibers impulses originating in the SA node rapidly spread into the atrial fibers. But conduction is more rapid in some bands of atrial fibers. These bands conduct impulses at a faster rate to the AV node and are called **internodal pathways**. They are:
❖ Anterior internodal tract
❖ Middle internodal tract of Wenckebach
❖ Posterior internodal tract of Thorel.

The anterior internodal tract sends fibers both to the AV node and to the left atrium. The branch going to the left atrium is called **Bachmann's bundle**. The fibers of the internodal tracts conduct impulses at a faster rate because they are a mixture of normal fibers and fast conducting fibers of the Purkinje type **(Fig. 22.7)**.

AV Node

AV node is located in the posterior wall of right atrium immediately behind the tricuspid valve **(Fig. 22.7)**. Since AV node develops from structures on the left side of embryo, parasympathetic supply is through the **left vagus**. **Sympathetic supply is primarily from the left side**. Structure of AV node is similar to SA node but the number of P cells is less and hence rate of impulse production is also less.

Bundle of His takes origin from the AV node. AV node and bundle of His is the only conducting pathway between atria and ventricles. This is because the atrial muscle fibers are separated from the ventricular muscle by a fibrous tissue ring that does not have the property of conduction.

Impulses reaching the AV node are not immediately transmitted to the bundle of His. There is a delay of 0.08–0.1 sec, which is called **AV nodal delay**. This is important because atria gets enough time to empty blood into the ventricles and effective ventricular filling and pumping is made possible. AV nodal delay is shortened by sympathetic stimulation and lengthened by vagal stimulation.

Causes of AV Nodal Delay

❖ AV node is made up of small diameter fibers which have a low conduction velocity.
❖ There are multiple branching systems in the AV node.
❖ Number of gap junctions is less between successive cells in the conducting pathway. So, velocity of conduction is reduced.

Table 22.1: Velocity of conduction of impulse in different parts of the heart.	
Tissue	Conduction velocity (m/s)
SA node	0.05
Internodal pathway	1
AV node	0.05
Bundle of His	1
Purkinje fibers	4
Ventricular muscle	1
Atrial muscle	1

Bundle of His and its Branches

AV node is continuous with the **bundle of His** which is about 15 to 20 mm long. It originates from the ventricular surface of AV node and passes downwards for about 15 mm. Then it gives off a **left bundle branch** and continues as the **right bundle branch** subendocardially on the right side of the interventricular septum. The left bundle branch divides into an **anterior fascicle** and a **posterior fascicle**. All the branches run subendocardially downwards towards the apex of the heart **(Fig. 22.7)**.

Anterior fascicle supplies superior portion of left ventricle and uppermost part of left side of interventricular septum.

Posterior fascicle supplies posterior surface of left ventricle, inferior surface of left ventricle and lower part of left side of interventricular septum. A special characteristic of AV bundle is **one-way conduction** of impulse. It does not conduct impulses from the ventricles back into the atria.

Purkinje Fibers

Purkinje fibers take origin from the terminal divisions of the bundle branches. They are **fast conducting** very large fibers (70–80 μm in diameter) with very few contractile elements and are present subendocardially. Purkinje system has the maximum number of tight junctions. They pierce the myocardium for a short distance from endocardium and blend with the myocardium. So *the direction of impulse conduction is always from endocardium to epicardium*. Since the velocity of conduction of action potential in Purkinje system is about 4–6 times that of ventricular muscle fibers, the cardiac impulse is instantaneously transmitted to the entire ventricular muscle **(Table 22.1)**.

Spread of Cardiac Impulse

Action potential generated in the SA node spreads through the atria and converges on the AV node. Atrial depolarization is completed in about 0.1 sec. In the AV node, there is a delay of about 0.1 sec before the impulse reaches the ventricles. In the interventricular septum, the depolarization wave spreads rapidly through the Purkinje fibers to all parts of ventricles **(Figs. 22.8A to E)**.

First portions of the ventricles to be excited by impulses from the AV node are the interventricular septum (except the basal portion) and the papillary muscles. Normally, depolarization of ventricle starts in the left side of interventricular septum and moves first to the right across the mid-portion of the septum. The depolarization wave then spreads down the septum to the apex of the heart. It then passes along the ventricular walls to the AV groove. *Depolarization is always from endocardial surface to epicardial surface*. Depolarization of papillary muscles occurs when the impulse reaches the middle of interventricular septum. The last parts of the ventricles to be depolarized are:
- Posterobasal portion of left ventricle
- Pulmonary conus
- Uppermost part of interventricular septum.

Ectopic Foci of Cardiac Excitation (Abnormal Pacemakers)

A pacemaker elsewhere than the SA node is called an **ectopic pacemaker**. In abnormal conditions, the AV node,

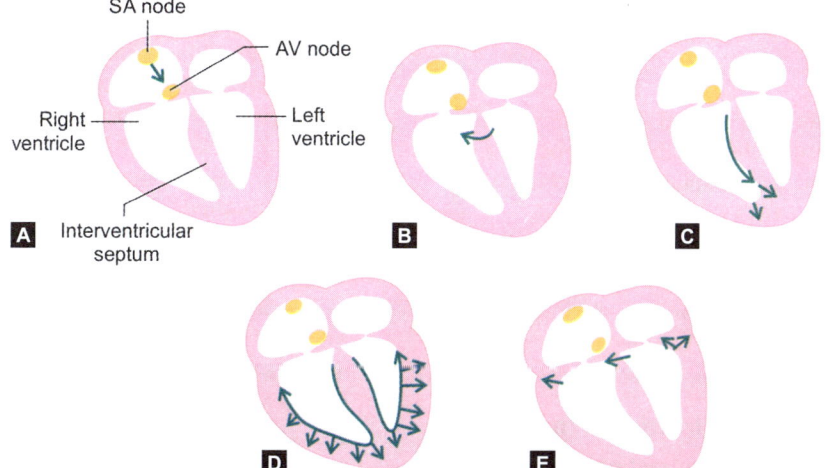

Figs. 22.8A to E: Spread of cardiac impulse: (A) Spread of impulse from SA node to AV node; (B) Activation of interventricular septum from left to right; (C) Activation of anteroseptal region of ventricle; (D) Activation of major portions of ventricular myocardium from endocardial to epicardial surface; (E) Late activation of posterobasal portion of ventricles and uppermost part of interventricular septum.

Purkinje fibers, atrial or the ventricular fibers may discharge spontaneously. The pacemaker of the heart shifts from SA node to the AV node or to the excited Purkinje fibers. If an ectopic focus discharges once, a premature beat occurs before a normal beat and this is called **extrasystole**. If the ectopic focus discharges repetitively at a rate higher than that of SA node, it produces atrial, ventricular or nodal **paroxysmal tachycardia** or atrial flutter depending on the site of the ectopic focus.

PROPERTIES OF CARDIAC MUSCLE

PY5.2: Describe the properties of cardiac muscle including its morphology, electrical, mechanical and metabolic functions.

- Excitability or irritability (Bathmotropism)
- Rhythmicity or automaticity (Chronotropism)
- Conductivity (Dromotropism)
- Contractility (Inotropism)
- Distensibility.

Excitability

Excitability is the property by which a living tissue responds to a stimulus. Cardiac muscle can respond to a stimulus by producing an action potential that leads to muscle contraction either isotonically or isometrically. All-or-none phenomenon is exhibited by cardiac muscle (*refer* action potential in cardiac muscle and its ionic basis in *Section 1*, **Chapter 9**).

Rhythmicity

Rhythmicity is the property of spontaneous discharge of impulses and is exhibited by different parts of the heart.

The rate of impulse production by different parts of the heart is as given further.
- SA node   70–80/min
- AV node   40–60/min
- Atrium   60/min
- Ventricle   20–40/min

SA node controls the rest of the heart because it has the maximum rate of impulse production.

Conductivity

In mammalian heart, there is a special conducting system through which the impulses generated in the SA node spread to the different parts of the heart (explain conducting system of heart).

Contractility

Contractility is the ability to respond to an impulse by contraction. Contractility is mainly exhibited by atrial and ventricular syncytium.

Factors Influencing Force of Contraction of the Heart

Factors that Increase the Force of Contraction:

- Sympathetic stimulation
- Heart rate
- Post-extrasystolic potentiation
- cAMP
- Increase in Ca^{2+}
- Increase in temperature and alkalosis.
- **Sympathetic stimulation** increases the contractility of the myocardium. This inotropic effect is due to norepinephrine released at the sympathetic nerve endings. Epinephrine has a similar effect.
- Myocardial contractility increases as **heart rate** increases.
- The beat following a ventricular extrasystole is stronger than the preceding normal contraction. This is due to increased availability of intracellular calcium. This is **post-extrasystolic potentiation**.
- Substances that increase **cAMP** content of heart are positively inotropic, e.g., xanthines like caffeine and theophylline, hormones like glucagon, etc.

Factors that Decrease the Force of Contraction

- Hypercapnia, hypoxia, acidosis and drugs like barbiturates depress myocardial contractility.
- Contractility of the heart is also reduced in pathological conditions like heart failure and in myocardial infarction where part of myocardium becomes nonfunctional.
- Vagal stimulation.

Distensibility

Distensibility depends on the syncytial nature of myocardium. Venous return during diastole is the cause for distension of the heart within physiological limits. If venous return exceeds a limit, the resistance offered by the heart to stretch increases and the cardiac muscle becomes very stiff and thus prevents over-distension. Fibrous pericardium also prevents over-distension of heart. This is a precaution because over-distension may lead to rupture of the heart.

MULTIPLE CHOICE QUESTIONS

1. **Base of the heart is formed by:**
   a. Right atrium   b. Left atrium
   c. Both atria   d. Left ventricle

2. **Single most important factor in the control of automatic contractility of heart is:**
   a. Myocardial wall thickness
   b. Right atrial volume
   c. SA node pace maker potential
   d. Sympathetic stimulation

3. **The velocity of impulse transmission in heart is maximum in:**
   a. Atrial muscle   b. Purkinje fibers
   c. AV node   d. Ventricular muscle

4. **The discharge frequency of SA node is increased by all the following, *except*:**
   a. Atropine   b. Increase in temperature
   c. Thyroxine   d. Digitalis

5. **Conduction velocity in the Purkinje system is about:**
   a. 1 m/sec   b. 0.02 m/sec
   c. 4 m/sec   d. 0.5 m/sec

6. Stethoscope was invented by:
   a. Harvey
   b. Laennec
   c. Lister
   d. Koch
7. The plateau phase seen in ventricular depolarization is due to opening of:
   a. Fast sodium channels
   b. Fast potassium channels
   c. Slow calcium channels
   d. Slow magnesium channels
8. Maximum conduction velocity is seen in:
   a. SA node
   b. AV node
   c. Internodal pathway
   d. Purkinje fibers
9. Antibodies from maternal circulation enter into fetal circulation by:
   a. Diffusion
   b. Vesicular transport
   c. Pinocytosis
   d. Exocytosis
10. The prepotential in the pacemaker tissue of the heart is primarily due to steady:
    a. Decline in sodium permeability
    b. Decline in potassium permeability
    c. Increase in chloride permeability
    d. Increase in calcium permeability
11. Vagal stimulation causes the following effect on the SA node:
    a. Increase in K$^+$ efflux
    b. Decrease in K$^+$ efflux
    c. Increase in Ca^{2+} efflux
    d. Increase in Ca^{2+} influx
12. The following statements are true regarding SA node, *except*:
    a. Is located at the right border of ascending aorta
    b. It contains specialized nodal cardiac muscle
    c. It is supplied by the atrial branches of right coronary artery
    d. It initiates cardiac conduction
13. SA node acts as pacemaker of the heart because of the fact that it:
    a. Is capable of generating impulses spontaneously
    b. Has rich sympathetic innervation
    c. Has poor cholinergic innervation
    d. Generates impulses at the highest rate
14. Speed of conduction is fastest in:
    a. SA node
    b. AV node
    c. Bundle of His
    d. Purkinje system
15. Least conduction velocity is seen in:
    a. AV node
    b. Bundle of His
    c. Purkinje system
    d. Ventricular myocardial fibers
16. Which of the following is the order of activation after stimulation of Purkinje fiber?
    a. Septum → endocardium → epicardium
    b. Endocardium → septum → epicardium
    c. Epicardium → septum → endocardium
    d. Septum → epicardium → endocardium
17. Repolarization in cardiac muscle fiber proceeds from:
    a. Epicardium to endocardium
    b. Endocardium to epicardium
    c. Left to right
    d. Right to left
18. The cause for post-extrasystolic potentiation is:
    a. Ca^{2+}
    b. b. Na$^+$
    c. K$^+$
    d. Mg^{2+}
19. Repolarization of ventricular muscle:
    a. Occurs last at apex
    b. Begins in septum
    c. Begins in epicardium
    d. Begins at AV node
20. Vagal stimulation can cause all, *except*:
    a. Delayed AV conduction
    b. Increased ventricular contraction
    c. Decreased atrial contraction
    d. Decreased heart rate
21. Conduction velocity is least in:
    a. AV node
    b. Bundle of His
    c. SA node
    d. Purkinje fibers
22. True regarding fibers of AV junction:
    a. Modified muscle fibers
    b. Modified nerve fibers
    c. Highly contractile
    d. Conduct impulse rapidly
23. Parasympathetic stimulation will decrease all the following, *except*:
    a. SA node rhythmicity
    b. Heart rate
    c. AV conduction time
    d. Atrial contractility
24. Plateau phase of cardiac action potential is due to:
    a. Opening of sodium channels
    b. Closing of potassium channels
    c. Opening of slow calcium channels
    d. Closing of sodium channels
25. All the following are true regarding the activity of SA node, *except*:
    a. Initiates impulse at faster rate
    b. Generate impulse spontaneously
    c. Increased by parasympathetic activity
    d. Increased by sympathetic activity
26. Velocity of conduction is fastest through the following part of the heart:
    a. AV node
    b. Bundle of His
    c. Atria
    d. Ventricle

ANSWERS

1. c	2. d	3. b	4. d	5. c
6. b	7. c	8. d	9. b	10. d
11. a	12. a	13. d	14. d	15. a
16. a	17. a	18. a	19. c	20. b
21. a	22. a	23. c	24. c	25. c
26. b				

Recording of Electrical Activity of Heart

CHAPTER 23

LEARNING OBJECTIVES
Must know
- Describe the waves, segments and intervals of electrocardiogram
- Discuss the clinical application of mean electrical axis
- Describe abnormal ECG, arrhythmias, heart block
- Explain the pathophysiology of myocardial infarction

■ ELECTROCARDIOGRAPHY (ECG)

Extracellular recording of the algebraic sum of the action potentials produced by all the cardiac muscle fibers during each heart beat is known as electrocardiography. **Sir William Einthoven** first devised this technique in 1903. He used a very sensitive galvanometer called **string galvanometer**. He is regarded as the **Father of modern ECG** and was awarded Nobel Prize in 1924.

String Galvanometer

String galvanometer consisted of an extremely thin platinum wire or a gold-plated quartz fiber about 5 μm thick suspended in the air gap of a strong horseshoe electromagnet. The electrical current from the heart flowing through the string causes movement of the string perpendicular to the direction of magnetic field. The magnitude of movement was very small but could be magnified several hundred times by an optical projection system for recording on a moving film or paper. A strong beam of light is directed through apertures in the arms of the magnet lying in front and behind the string. The deflections of the string are cast as shadows, which are magnified and brought to a focus upon a photographic surface which is moving vertically at a desired speed in a camera of special design.

Electrocardiograph

The instrument used nowadays is called **electrocardiograph** and the record obtained is **electrocardiogram**. Electrodes are placed on the surface of the body since the electrical activity from the heart spreads to the tissues and body fluids and will be conducted to the surface of the body. The body acts as a **volume conductor** because the body fluids are good conductors. The amplitude will be less when the electrical activity reaches the surface of the body and so it has to be amplified.

Modern instrument consists of three parts:
1. Electrodes
2. Amplifier
3. Recording device

Electrodes

Leads are combination of electrodes which can pick up electrical activity from the surface of the body. There are two types of leads:
I. Bipolar leads
II. Unipolar leads

Bipolar Leads

Here, both the electrodes pick up electrical activity, and potential difference between the two electrodes is recorded.

Bipolar limb leads: bipolar limb leads are also known as **standard limb leads**. These leads were used by Einthoven and he selected three points in the body **(Fig. 23.1)**.
1. Junction between right arm and trunk
2. Junction between left arm and trunk
3. Junction between left foot and trunk.

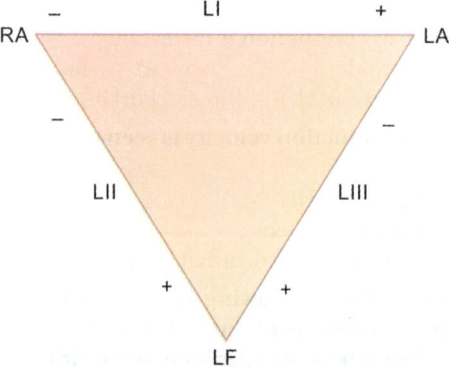

Fig. 23.1: Einthoven's triangle showing standard limb leads LI, LII and LIII. RA, LA and LF show the position of electrodes.
(RA: right arm; LA: left arm; LF: left foot)

When the above three points are joined together, an equilateral triangle is obtained. Heart is assumed to be in the center of this triangle. This is known as **Einthoven's triangle**. There are three standard bipolar limb leads: **lead I, lead II and lead III (Fig. 23.1)**.

1. Lead I connect right arm and left arm with the negative terminal on right arm.
2. Lead II is between right arm and left foot with negative terminal on RA.
3. Lead III is between left arm and left foot with left arm negative.

Lead I – LA+; RA-
Lead II – LF+; RA-
Lead III – LF+; LA-

Einthoven's law
Lead I + Lead III – Lead II = 0
Lead I + Lead III = Lead II

The leads are so arranged that a positive deflection is obtained in all the leads. Otherwise, the equation would have been: Lead I + Lead III + Lead II = 0. This is because in a volume conductor, the sum of the potentials at the points of an equilateral triangle with a current source in the center is zero at all times.

Maximum amplitude is obtained in lead II (L II) and it is the sum of the potentials obtained in L I and L III

Einthoven made another postulate stating that the recording of potential is same if the leads are placed in the distal part of extremities as they are extensions from the body and the electrical activity will be conducted to the distal parts.

Bipolar chest leads: In bipolar chest leads, one electrode is placed on the chest (precordium) and the other electrode on one limb (right arm, left arm or left foot). These leads are represented as CR, CL and CF. The first letter stands for the position of the electrode over the chest and the second letter for the position of the electrode on the limb. Bipolar chest lead is not usually used in clinical practice.

Unipolar Leads

One electrode is kept at **zero potential** and the other electrode is the **active electrode**. Electrode at zero potential is called **indifferent electrode** and the active electrode is called **exploring electrode**. Unipolar recording is better than bipolar recording. An upward deflection is obtained when the active electrode becomes positive relative to the indifferent electrode and a downward deflection is obtained when the active electrode becomes negative. In other words, depolarization wave moving towards an active electrode in a volume conductor produces a positive deflection whereas depolarization moving away from the active electrode produces a negative deflection.

Depending on whether the lead is placed on the chest or limb, it is divided into:
- Unipolar limb leads
- Unipolar chest leads

Unipolar limb leads: One electrode is placed on distal part of one limb and the other electrode should be at zero potential. Exploring electrode or active electrode is placed in the right arm, left arm or left foot. Indifferent electrode is designated as V. So the leads are VR, VL and VF. Indifferent electrode is made by connecting the three limbs, i.e., right arm, left arm and left foot each through a high resistance of 5000Ω to a common terminal **(Figs. 23.2A to C)**. The indifferent electrode is connected to the negative terminal and the active electrode to the positive terminal of the electrocardiograph.

Augmented unipolar limb leads: Nowadays, a modified form of unipolar limb lead is used called **augmented unipolar limb leads (aV)** which gives magnified amplitude. **E Goldberger** introduced this technique. Here, the limb in which exploring electrode is connected is not connected to indifferent electrode. The augmented limb leads are aVR, aVL and aVF which denotes the potentials picked up at the right arm, left arm and left foot **(Figs. 23.3A to C)**.

In augmented unipolar limb leads, the magnification is one and a half times. For example, **aVR = 3/2 VR.**

Unipolar chest leads: Chest lead gives a greater magnitude of potential as the electrode is near the heart. Exploring electrode is placed on the chest and indifferent electrode is formed by connecting right arm (RA), LA and LF each through a high resistance of 5000Ω. Depending on the position of the exploring electrode on the chest, there are 6 unipolar chest leads—V_1 to V_6 **(Figs. 23.4A and B)**.

- V_1 at the fourth right intercostal space (RICS) on the sternal border
- V_2 4th LICS on the left sternal border
- V_3 midway between V_2 and V_4

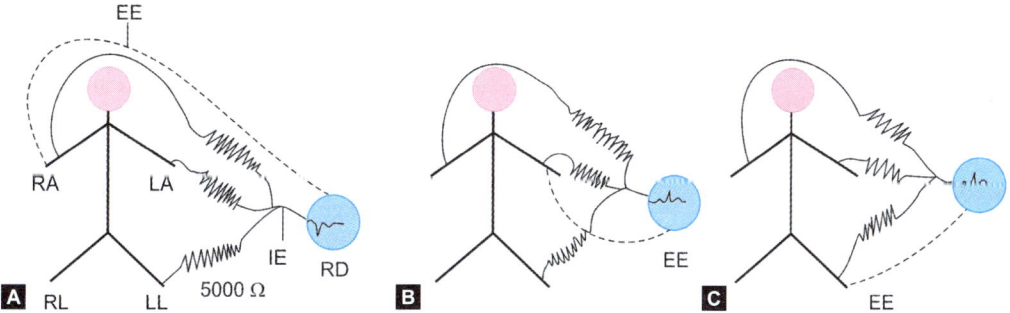

Figs. 23.2A to C: Unipolar limb leads: (A) VR; (B) VL; (C) VF.
(EE: exploring electrode; IE: indifferent electrode; RD: recording device; RA: right arm; LA: left arm; RL: right leg; LL: left leg)

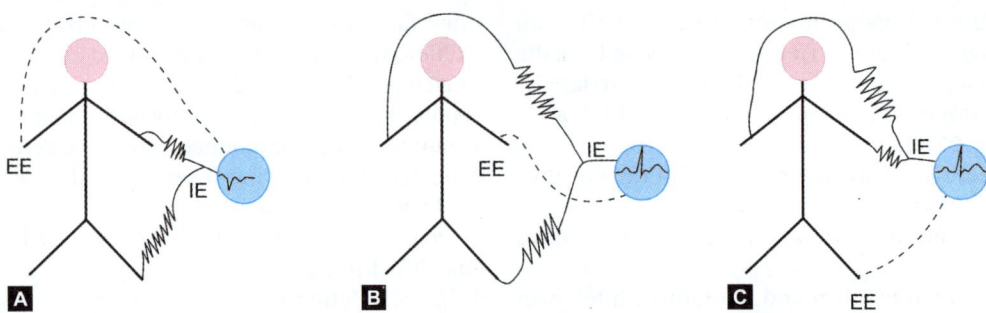

Figs. 23.3A to C: Position of electrodes for augmented unipolar limb leads: (A) aVR; (B) aVL; (C) aVF. The limb in which exploring electrode (EE) is connected is not connected to the indifferent electrode (IE).

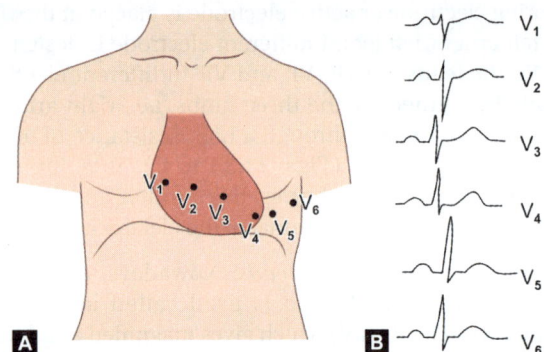

Figs. 23.4A and B: (A) Unipolar chest lead positions; (B) ECG patterns obtained from V_1 to V_6.

- V_4 on the 5th LICS in the mid-clavicular line
- V_5 on the 5th LICS in the anterior axillary line
- V_6 on the 5th LICS in the mid-axillary line.

12 leads are used clinically. They are leads I, II, III, aVR, aVL, aVF, V_1, V_2, V_3, V_4, V_5 and V_6. Other leads used in pathological conditions are **esophageal lead** and **intracardiac lead**.

Esophageal lead is used to record atrial activity. It is nearer to the heart than surface electrode and more information is obtained. The electrode is passed through a nasal catheter and kept at different positions in the esophagus. For example, lead E35 means the lead is placed 35 cm down in the esophagus.

Intracardiac lead is introduced into the chambers of the heart by cardiac catheterization under fluoroscopic observation. For example, the catheter is introduced through the anterior cubital vein into the right atrium. This technique was devised by **Forssmann**. The electrical activity can be directly recorded from the different areas of the heart.

ELECTROCARDIOGRAM (ECG)

PY5.6: Describe abnormal ECG, arrhythmias, heart block and myocardial infarction.

Recording of ECG

Recording of ECG is done with the subject in the supine position. Tie the electrodes on the right arm, left arm and left leg. The chest lead is placed over the precordium. *Earthing is done on the right leg.* Using the lead selector knob in the instrument, the 12 different leads can be selected while recording ECG.

The amplifier present inside the instrument is a **differential amplifier**, i.e., it amplifies only biological signals. Output from the amplifier goes to the recording device. The different types of recording devices are:
- Cathode ray oscilloscope (CRO)
- Paper recording
- Tape recording
- Telemetry.

Recording in CRO

The signal from the amplifier is connected to the Y plate of CRO. This type of recording is used in the **intensive coronary care unit** in cardiac monitors where continuous recording of ECG is shown in the CRO.

Paper Recording

Paper recording is of two types:
1. Ink writing method
2. Heated stylus method.

Heated Stylus Method

Heated stylus method is the most commonly used method. The signal from the amplifier passes through a coil suspended between the two poles of a powerful electromagnet. When the signal passes through the coil, the coil will deflect depending on the nature of the signal. These deflections are written on a paper by means of a stylus attached to the coil. The paper is continuously moving by means of a motor at a speed of 25 mm/sec. This method is called heated stylus method as the stylus gets heated when current passes through it. The paper is a **thermo sensitive** paper which is actually a black paper over which a white thermo sensitive coating is applied. When the heated stylus moves over the paper, the white coating is removed and at these regions a black recording is obtained on a white background.

ECG Paper

ECG is recorded on a special type of paper which is graduated in the X axis and in the Y axis. **X axis** denotes time in seconds and **Y axis** denotes amplitude in mV. In the X axis, 1 sec is

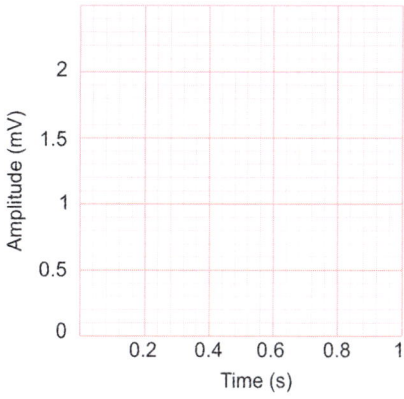

Fig. 23.5: ECG paper (Note: That five large divisions correspond to one second in the X-axis. One second is divided into 5 smaller divisions so that each division corresponds to 0.2 sec. This is again divided into 5 divisions so that the smallest division corresponds to 0.04 sec. In the Y-axis, 10 divisions correspond to 1 mV so that one small division is 0.1 mV).

divided into 5 big squares and each big square is divided into 5 small divisions. In the X axis, as the paper moves at a speed of 25 mm/sec, in every second the stylus moves through 25 small divisions or 5 large squares. Thus in the X axis, one smallest division represents 1/25th of a second or 0.04 sec.

Y axis represents amplitude of the signal and it is calibrated in such a way that one large square represents 0.5 mV. One large square is divided into 5 small divisions so that the smallest division in the Y axis represents 0.1 mV **(Fig. 23.5)**.

Standardization

Standardization is the technique of adjusting the sensitivity of the stylus to give a vertical deflection of ten small divisions in the ECG paper on application of a voltage of 1 millivolt. Thus one small division in the Y axis represents 0.1 mV **(Fig. 23.6)**. Standardization helps in calculating the amplitude of different waves in the ECG.

Tape Recorder Recording

Tape recorder recording of ECG is also called **Holter technique** in which the patient can do his daily activities with simultaneous recording of ECG. The signals are stored in a magnetic tape and can be analyzed at a later date. The effect of exercise can also be recorded by this method.

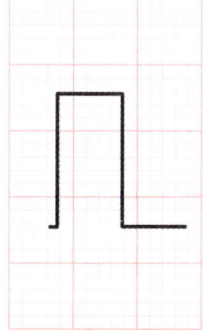

Fig. 23.6: Standardization in the ECG paper so that one small division on the Y-axis represents 0.1 mV.

Telemetry

In telemetry, ECG can be recorded through telephone wires and can be displayed in a computer at a distance. Arrhythmias and other cardiac abnormalities can be assessed in this technique.

■ NORMAL PATTERN OF ECG

In each lead, the normal pattern of ECG is different. *The basic principle is that, when the depolarization wave is passing towards the exploring electrode an upward deflection is obtained, and if the depolarization wave is traveling away from the exploring electrode, a downward deflection is obtained* **(Fig. 23.7)**.

P wave is an upward wave, which is due to **atrial depolarization**. The impulse spreads throughout the atria. It is followed by an isoelectric segment called the **PQ segment** or **PR segment** (if Q wave is absent). This segment is due to AV nodal delay.

QRS complex is due to **ventricular depolarization** **(Table 23.1)**. It consists of an initial downward deflection called Q wave, an upward deflection called R wave and a downward deflection following R wave called S wave. Initial Q wave is due to depolarization of the inter-ventricular septum from left to right. R and S waves are due to depolarization of the ventricle. R wave is the main wave of ventricular depolarization.

During most of the depolarization process of the ventricles, the average direction of current flow is from the base to the apex of the ventricles, with negativity towards the base and positivity towards the apex. The recording device will show a positive deflection when current flows from base to apex. Immediately before depolarization has completed, the average direction of current flow reverses for about 0.01 second, flowing from the ventricular apex towards the base. The last part of the ventricle to become depolarized is the outer walls of the ventricles near the base of the heart. So a small negative S wave is recorded towards the end in the ventricular depolarization wave, i.e., in the QRS complex.

ST segment is an isoelectric segment. It represents the duration from the end of ventricular depolarization to the beginning of ventricular repolarization. It is the time when the ventricular contractile fibers are fully depolarized and it coincides with the plateau phase of ventricular muscle action potential. Junction between the end of S wave and the beginning of ST segment is denoted as the **J point (Fig. 23.8A).**

T wave is an upward deflection, which is due to **ventricular repolarization**. T wave duration is longer since repolarization of ventricles takes a longer time. This is because, ventricular muscle begins to repolarize in some fibers about 0.20 second after the beginning of QRS complex, but in many other fibers, it takes as long as 0.35 second. The amplitude of T wave is less than QRS complex, partly because of its prolonged length. T wave is in the same direction as that of R wave. *This is because direction of ventricular repolarization is opposite to that of ventricular depolarization*. Depolarization of ventricles occurs from endocardial surface to epicardium

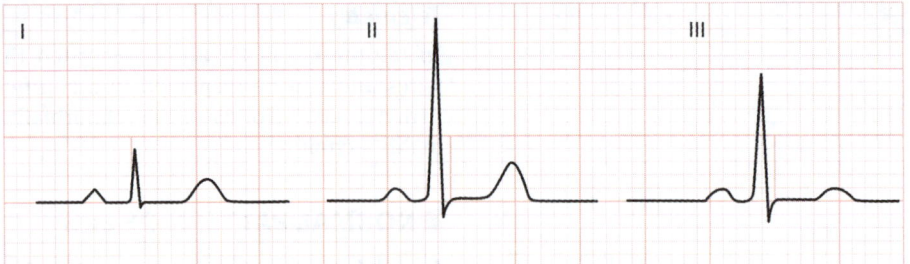

Fig. 23.7: Normal pattern of ECG in LI, LII and LIII.

Table 23.1: Different waves of ECG.

Wave	Cause	Duration (sec)	Amplitude (mV)
P wave	Atrial depolarization	0.08–0.1	0.1–0.3
QRS complex	Ventricular depolarization	0.08–0.1	1–3
T wave	Ventricular repolarization	0.25–0.35	0.2–0.3

and repolarization occurs from epicardium to endocardium. If depolarization and repolarization occur in the same direction, the waves will be in the opposite directions.

U wave if present is seen after the T wave. It is due to delay in the repolarization of papillary muscles. This wave is not usually seen. U wave may be present in hypokalemia **(Fig. 23.8B)**. Recent view is that, the U wave may be due to repolarization of ventricular myocytes with long action potentials.

Ta wave (atrial T wave) is the wave of **atrial repolarization**. The atria repolarize about 0.15 to 0.2 second after termination of P wave. This is approximately when the QRS complex is being recorded in the ECG. So the Ta wave is not seen in normal ECG since the QRS complex masks it. If it is present in ECG, it is seen as a downward deflection at the PQ segment. *Ta wave is seen in atrial tachycardia or sinus tachycardia.*

In the atria, depolarization and repolarization occur in the same direction and so the depolarization and repolarization waves will be in the opposite directions.

■ INTERVALS IN ECG (TABLE 23.2)

PR Interval or PQ Interval

If Q wave is present it is PQ interval, otherwise PR interval. It represents the time between the beginning of P wave and beginning of Q wave or R wave **(Fig. 23.9)**.

PR interval = P wave + PR segment

Due to atrial depolarization and AV nodal delay, ventricular depolarization occurs about 0.16 sec after atrial depolarization. Determination of this interval is important clinically because it gives an idea about AV nodal delay.

ST Interval

ST interval denotes the duration between end of S wave and end of T wave.

ST segment + T wave = ST interval

QT Interval

QT interval represents the time taken for ventricular depolarization and repolarization. It is the duration

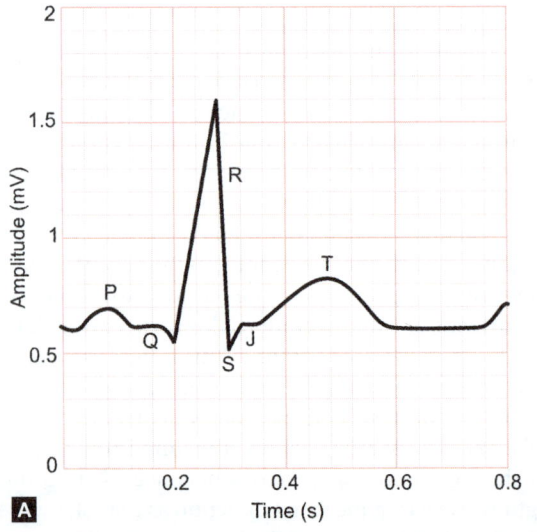
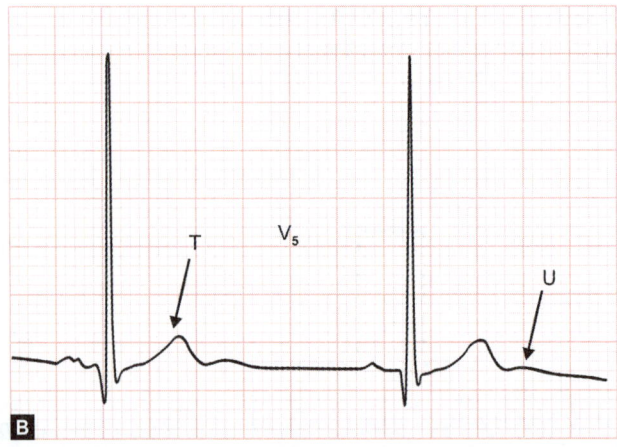

Figs. 23.8A and B: (A) Normal pattern of ECG in lead II; the duration of P wave in the above diagram is 2 × 0.04 = 0.08 sec, amplitude 0.1 mV. QRS complex-duration 3 × 0.04 = 0.12 sec, amplitude of R-1 mV T wave- duration 5 × 0.04 = 0.2 sec, amplitude 2 × 0.1 = 0.2 mV; (B) U wave in ECG.

Table 23.2: Segments and intervals in ECG.

	Cause	Duration
Segments		
PR segment	AV nodal delay	0.04–0.1 sec
ST segment	Interval between ventricular depolarization and repolarization	0.05–0.1 sec
Intervals		
PQ/PR interval	Atrial depolarization + AV nodal delay	0.12–0.2 sec
ST interval	Ventricular repolarization + ST segment	0.3–0.45 sec
QT interval	QRS complex + ST interval	0.4 sec
ST segment	Interval between ventricular depolarization and repolarization	0.05–0.1 sec
PQ/PR interval	Atrial depolarization + AV nodal delay	0.12–0.2 sec
ST interval	Ventricular repolarization + ST segment	0.3–0.45 sec
QT interval	QRS complex + ST interval	0.4 sec

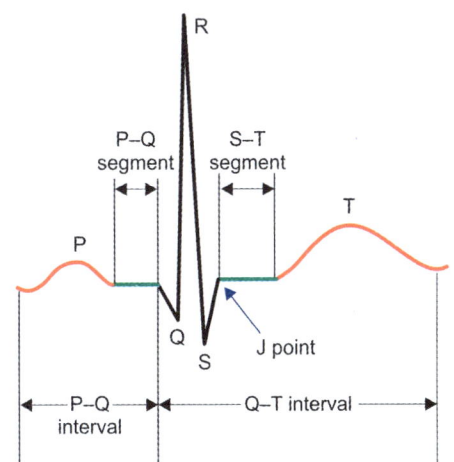

Fig. 23.9: Normal ECG showing different waves, segments, and intervals of a single heartbeat.

between beginning of Q wave and end of T wave (**Fig. 23.9** and **Table 23.2**).

R-R Interval

Interval between two R waves in the ECG pattern obtained is called R-R interval. This helps to find out the heart rate from ECG. If the recording is regular, then heart rate is equal to 60/R-R interval. For example, if R-R interval is 0.8 sec then:
Heart rate = 60/0.8 = 75/min.

If heart rate is irregular, then, count the number of R waves in 10 seconds in one lead and multiply it with 6.

Ventricular Activation Time (VAT) or QR Interval

VAT corresponds to the onset of the QRS complex to the peak of R wave (QR interval). Normal duration is 39.6 ± 0.3 millisecond. VAT in V_5 or V_6 is used as one of the criterion for diagnosing left ventricular hypertrophy. It is also used to assess diastolic dysfunction in early hypertension. In patients with diastolic dysfunction, it may be increased to 46.3 ± 0.4 msec.

PATTERN OF ECG IN OTHER LEADS

Pattern is same in L_I, L_{II} and L_{III} but amplitude is maximal in L_{II}.

In aVR, P, R and T waves are found to be inverted. This is because the exploring electrode is in the right arm and depolarization wave from heart is moving away from the exploring electrode, i.e., to the left (**Fig. 23.10**).

Chest Leads

In V_1, small R and deep S wave are seen. But as the electrode position is changed from V_1 to V_3, S wave becomes smaller and R wave becomes taller. In V_3, R and S waves are of same amplitude. In V_4, V_5 and V_6, R wave is prominent (**Fig. 23.11**). This is because of the principle that if depolarization wave is moving towards exploring electrode then a positive deflection is obtained.

The chest electrode in leads V_1 and V_2 is nearer to the base of the heart and this part is electrically negative during most of the ventricular depolarization process. The QRS complexes in leads V_4, V_5 and V_6 are mainly positive because the chest electrode in these leads is nearer to the apex of the heart which is electrically positive during most of ventricular depolarization.

MEAN ELECTRICAL AXIS

Change in direction of electrical activity is occurring from time to time in the heart. From ordinary bipolar standard limb leads we can calculate the mean electrical axis.

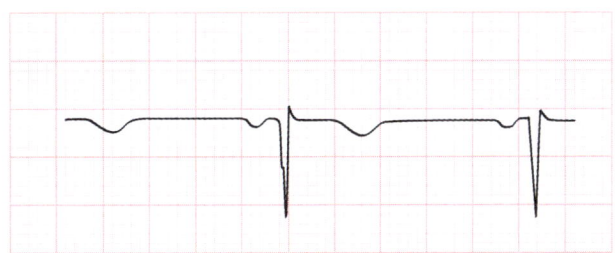

Fig. 23.10: Pattern of ECG in lead aVR.

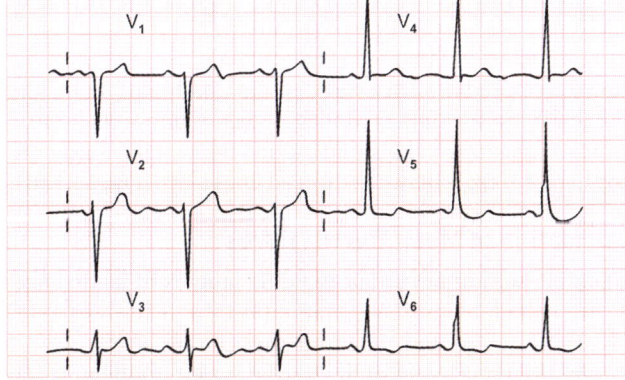

Fig. 23.11: Pattern of ECG recorded in chest leads V_1 to V_6.

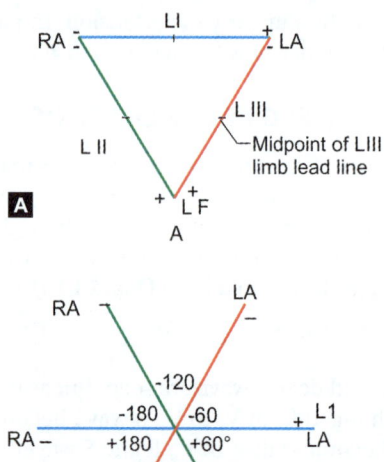

Figs. 23.12A and B: (A) Einthoven's triangle with midpoints of the three bipolar limb lead lines marked; (B) Construction of the triaxial reference system.

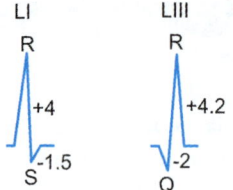

Fig. 23.13: QRS complex in lead I and lead III.

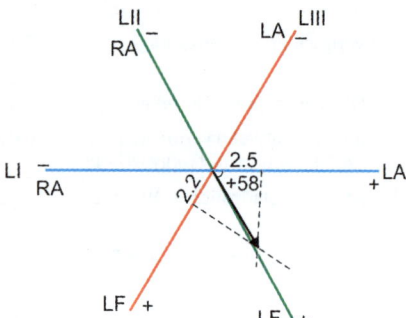

Fig. 23.14: Calculation of mean electrical axis in degree from the triaxial reference system.

Definition

Mean electrical axis is the mean electromotive force which acts in an average direction during any period of electrical activity, i.e., ventricular depolarization or repolarization. Ventricle is taken because electrical activity changes in the ventricle from time to time. Ventricular depolarization phase is taken for calculating mean electrical axis.

QRS complex is taken from bipolar standard limb leads. This QRS complex represents the magnitude and duration of electrical activity but not the direction of spread of electrical activity. To represent the direction, vector quantity known as mean electrical activity is taken. This vector is called **mean QRS vector**.

The mean electrical axis is represented by an arrow, the length of the arrow representing **magnitude** of vector, the spatial position of arrow representing the **direction** and the head of the arrow representing **polarity**, i.e., positivity or negativity.

Mean electrical axis can be calculated using the record of electrical activity from bipolar limb leads using **triaxial reference system** devised by Bayley. To construct the triaxial reference system, the 3 bipolar limb lead lines are selected and midpoints are marked **(Fig. 23.12A)**. The lead lines are then transposed in such a way that their midpoints coincide. The leads are so connected that all values above lead I line indicate negative values and values below lead I line are positive. The angle between the lead lines is 60° **(Fig. 23.12B)**.

Calculation of Mean Electrical Axis

Algebraic sum of potentials in QRS complex in leads I and III are calculated and are marked on the lead lines **(Fig. 23.13)**. Draw perpendicular from these points which meet at a point. Join the center of the triaxial system to the meeting point of the perpendiculars and this line represents the **mean electrical axis**. Length of the line represents the magnitude, the angle from lead I line represents direction and head of the arrow represents polarity **(Fig. 23.14)**.

In adults direction of mean electrical axis is +58° from lead I. It varies with age:
- In infants: +130°
- In children: +52°
- At puberty: +67°
- In adults: +58°

In diseases of the heart there will be a deviation of mean electrical axis either to the right or to the left. Shift of the axis to >110° denotes **right axis deviation** in adults and deviation to > –20° denotes **left axis deviation (Table 23.3)**.

Right axis deviation is seen in:
- Right ventricular hypertrophy
- Right bundle branch block
- Left posterior fascicular hemi block, i.e., block in the posterior fascicle of left bundle branch.

Left axis deviation is seen in:
- Left ventricular hypertrophy
- Left bundle branch block
- Left anterior fascicular hemi block.

Vector Cardiography

The vector showing the instantaneous direction of the electrical activity is known as **instantaneous vector**. The direction of the instantaneous vector changes continuously

Table 23.3: Amplitude of positive R wave and negative S wave in lead I and lead III in axis deviation.		
Mean QRS vector	**Lead I**	**Lead III**
Right axis deviation	Large S wave	Tall R wave
Left axis deviation	Tall R wave	Big S wave

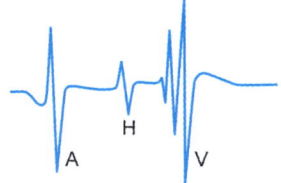

Fig. 23.15: Normal His-bundle electrogram (HBE).

during ventricular depolarization which can be recorded electronically by an instrument called **vector cardiograph**. The record obtained is called **vector cardiogram**. Vector cardiogram can be taken during atrial depolarization, ventricular depolarization and ventricular repolarization. In each case, a **loop** is obtained in the record. The loop is obtained by joining the tips of the arrows representing the instantaneous vectors recorded electronically. The loops obtained are P, QRS and T loop. Different shapes for the loops are obtained in frontal, horizontal and sagittal planes.

His-bundle Electrogram

The electrical activity which is recorded with the electrode placed in the heart chamber close to the tricuspid valve is His-bundle electrogram **(HBE)**. A catheter containing an electrode at its tip is passed through a vein to the right side of heart and placed in a position close to the tricuspid valve. It shows three main deflections. They are an **A deflection** when the AV node is activated, an **H spike** during transmission of impulse through the His bundle and a **V deflection** during ventricular depolarization **(Fig. 23.15)**. Three intervals can be found out using HBE. PA interval represents conduction time from SA node to AV node, AH interval which represents AV nodal conduction time and HV interval which represents conduction in the bundle of His and the bundle branches. The normal values for these intervals are PA, 27 ms; AH, 92 ms; and HV, 43 ms. PA interval is the time from the first appearance of atrial depolarization to the 'A' wave in the HBE.

Stress Electrocardiogram or Stress Test

Stress test like **tread mill test** helps to evaluate the response of heart to the stress of physical exercise in cases of coronary artery narrowing. At rest, blood flow in the narrowed coronary arteries may be adequate to meet the demands of the heart and no changes may be detected in the ECG. But during exercise, the flow may be unable to meet the increased demand for O_2 by the heart that produces ischemic changes in the ECG.

CLINICAL APPLICATION OF ECG

PY5.6: Describe abnormal ECG, arrhythmias, heart block and myocardial infarction.

Heart Rate

After recording ECG, find out the heart rate first and also see whether it is regular. If the heart rate is normal and regular it is called **normal sinus rhythm (NSR),** which is about 70/min. In sinus rhythm, the pacemaker is the SA node. Decrease in heart rate from normal is **bradycardia** and increase is **tachycardia**.

Normal heart rate is 60 to 100 per minute. If the rate is >100/min, the condition is called **sinus tachycardia** as seen in fever, exercise, anxiety, etc. **(Fig. 23.16A)**. If the rate is <60/min, the condition is called **sinus bradycardia** as seen in athletes **(Fig. 23.16B)**. ECG is of normal shape and regular in both sinus tachycardia and sinus bradycardia. Change in the heart rate during different phases of respiration is called **sinus arrhythmia**. Heart rate is increased during inspiration and decreased during expiration.

Cause for Sinus Arrhythmia

During inspiration, impulses passing through the vagus from the stretch receptors in lung inhibit the cardioinhibitory center (CIC) in the medulla oblongata. The tonic vagal discharge coming from the CIC normally keeps the heart rate slow, i.e., at about 70 beats/min. During inspiration, since the CIC is inhibited the heart rate increases slightly from normal.

Abnormalities in the Heart Rate

Arrhythmia

Arrhythmia is the disturbance of the heart rate or cardiac rhythm due to disorders of impulse formation or conduction. Arrhythmias associated with decrease in heart rate are called bradyarrhythmias, e.g., sick sinus syndrome, AV-block, bundle-branch-block, etc. Those associated with increase in heart rate are called tachyarrhythmias, e.g., premature atrial contractions, supraventricular tachycardia, atrial flutter, atrial fibrillation, premature ventricular contraction, ventricular tachycardia, ventricular flutter, ventricular fibrillation, etc. When tachyarrhythmia originates in SA node, it is called sinus tachycardia. Tachyarrhythmias may be due to increased automaticity of ectopic foci or due to re-entry of impulses in closed circuits within the heart.

Atrial Arrhythmia

When the heart rate is more than 160/min, the condition is called **atrial tachycardia**. In **atrial tachycardia**, the atrial

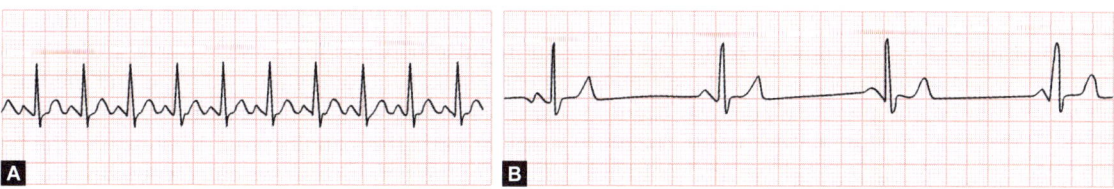

Figs. 23.16A and B: Abnormalities in heart rate: (A) Sinus tachycardia; (B) Sinus bradycardia.

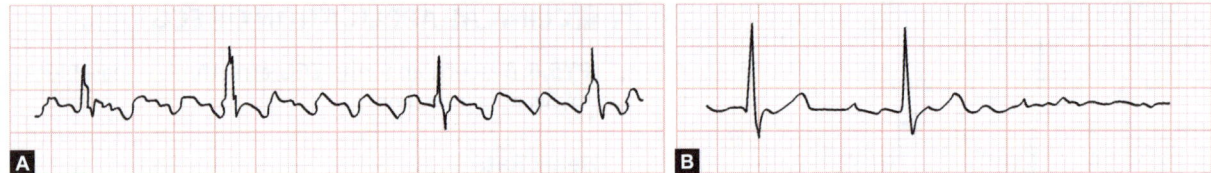

Figs. 23.17A and B: Lead II ECG showing: (A) Atrial flutter; (B) Atrial fibrillation.

rate may increase to about 220/min. This is called paroxysmal atrial tachycardia (PAT). In **atrial flutter**, the atrial rate is 250–350/min. This is associated with AV block because AV node cannot conduct more than 230 impulses per minute because of AV nodal delay **(Fig. 23.17A)**.

In **atrial fibrillation**, the atria beat very rapidly at a rate of 300–500/min in a completely irregular and disorganized fashion. Because of AV nodal delay, the ventricles beat at a completely irregular rate usually 80–160/min **(Fig. 23.17B)**.

Atrial extrasystole or atrial premature beat occurs due to discharge from an independently discharging focus in the atria once. This impulse stimulates the AV node prematurely and the impulse is conducted to the ventricles.

Consequences of atrial arrhythmias: Occasional atrial extrasystole occurs normally in humans and has no clinical significance. In PAT and atrial flutter, the ventricular rate may be so high and the duration of diastole become too short. So, adequate ventricular filling does not occur and end-diastolic volume will be less. This leads to reduction in cardiac output and symptoms of heart failure appear. This can be immediately managed by increasing the vagal discharge to the heart. Digitalis which depresses AV nodal conduction is also used to lower a rapid ventricular rate in atrial fibrillation. Atrial fibrillation predisposes to stroke.

If the SA node is not functioning properly it causes a reduction in heart rate because some other part of the heart takes over the function of pacemaker. It is called **sick sinus syndrome**. In this condition dizziness, hypotension and fainting occur when the rate is very much reduced. This can be corrected using a **pacemaker**.

Ventricular Arrhythmia

Ventricular premature beats originate in an ectopic ventricular focus. These beats in ECG have a bizarrely shaped prolonged QRS complex because of slow spread of impulse. The premature beat is followed by a compensatory pause. This is because, when the normal impulse reaches the ventricle (*refer* **Fig. 23.21**), it will be in the refractory period of the premature impulse. Atrial and ventricular premature beats are not strong enough to produce a pulse at the wrist if they occur early in diastole. This is because the end-diastolic volume is very less in this condition. Ventricular premature beats are common and in the absence of ischemic heart disease is insignificant. If the premature beat occurs late in the relative refractory period of the preceding depolarization, or after full repolarization, the premature depolarization is insignificant. However, if the premature depolarization occurs early in the relative refractory period of the ventricles, conduction of the premature impulse from the site of origin will be slow, and hence re-entry is likely to occur. It may lead to ventricular fibrillation which may be fatal. Thus timing of the premature beat is of great clinical significance.

Paroxysmal ventricular tachycardia is a series of rapid, regular ventricular depolarization due to circus movement. Ventricular tachycardia is more serious than atrial tachycardia because cardiac output is significantly reduced. It is also significant because ventricular fibrillation is an occasional complication of ventricular tachycardia.

Ventricular fibrillation is a condition where the ventricular muscle fibers contract in a totally irregular and ineffective way due to rapid discharge from multiple ventricular ectopic foci or due to a circus movement. The fibrillating ventricle looks like a quivering bag of worms. The fibrillating ventricles cannot pump blood effectively and circulation of blood stops. So it is a medical emergency. If it lasts for more than a few minutes, the condition is fatal. This is the most frequent cause of sudden death in patients with myocardial infarction.

P Wave Abnormalities

- P wave is a positive wave in all leads except aVR.
- Larger P waves indicate atrial enlargement as in mitral stenosis and tricuspid stenosis. In these conditions, atria have to do more work to force blood through the narrowed orifices that leads to atrial hypertrophy.
- P wave is inverted when there is an ectopic focus of impulse production in the atrium.
- Ectopic focus in the atrium may discharge rapidly at a rate of about 150–200/min and this condition is called **atrial tachycardia**.
- When the rate is 200-300/min the condition is **atrial flutter**. Because of AV nodal delay, all these impulses do not reach the ventricle. So the number of QRS complexes will be less than that of the number of P waves. **Saw toothed P wave** in ECG is characteristic of atrial flutter **(Fig. 23.17A)**.
- When the atrial rate is >300/min it is **atrial fibrillation**. Here a definite P wave is not seen **(Fig. 23.17B)**.

PR Interval Abnormalities

If the duration of PR interval is >0.2 sec, it indicates delay in AV nodal conduction. There is disturbance in the conduction of impulse between atria and ventricles. This is known as heart block. In coronary artery disease and rheumatic fever, scar tissue may form in the heart and the impulse takes more time to travel through the atria, AV node and the remaining fibers of the conduction system. Depending on the extent, different degrees of heart block can be classified.

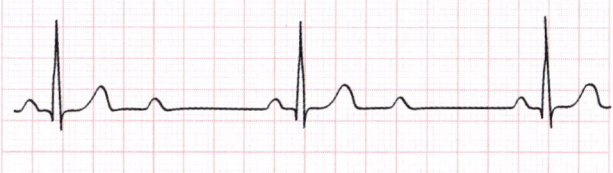

Fig. 23.18: Second degree heart block showing 2:1 block; two P waves are followed by a QRS complex.

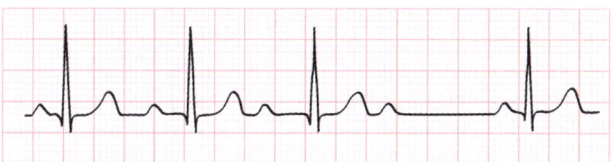

Fig. 23.19: Wenckebach phenomenon. Note the progressive prolongation of PR interval which is followed by a dropped QRS complex (2 P waves can be seen).

- Partial heart block or **first-degree heart block**—Here, all atrial impulses reach the ventricles but the PR interval is prolonged (>0.2 sec)
- **Second-degree block**.

All atrial impulses are not conducted to the ventricle and depending on the severity it may be 2:1 block or 3:1 block. In 2:1 block, two P waves will be followed by a QRS complex (**Fig. 23.18**) and in 3:1 block, 3 P waves will be followed by one QRS complex. Normal AV node has a long refractory period and in adults it cannot conduct more than 230 impulses/min.

In **Wenckebach's phenomenon**, there is progressive prolongation of PR interval with every successive beat and then one QRS complex is dropped (dropped beat), then again normal pattern with prolongation of P-R interval observed (**Fig. 23.19**). The cycle is repeated.

Complete Heart Block or Third-degree Heart Block

When the conduction of impulse from the atria to the ventricles is completely interrupted, the atria and the ventricles beat at different rates. This may be due to diseases of AV node or block in the bundle branch (infranodal block). This produces **third-degree heart block (Fig. 23.20)**. Ventricular rate become 15–20/min (idioventricular rhythm) and this leads to inefficient pumping of heart and fainting attacks due to cerebral ischemia called **Stokes-Adams syndrome**. The condition is treated with artificial pacemakers.

Abnormalities in QRS Complex

- Usual abnormality of QRS complex is increase in its duration, i.e., when the duration is greater than 0.1 sec, the complex will be deformed. This is due to ventricular

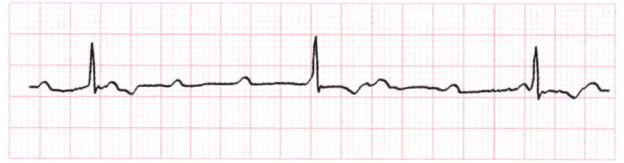

Fig. 23.20: ECG pattern in complete heart block.

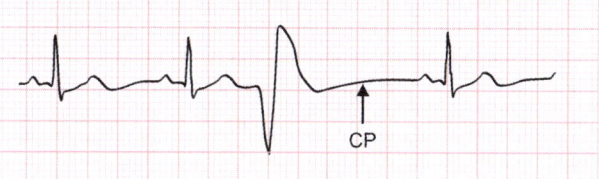

Fig. 23.21: Ventricular ectopic beat followed by compensatory pause (CP).

hypertrophy or bundle branch block. These conditions produce axis deviation as well.
- Changes in the amplitude of QRS complex are also seen. For example, in right axis deviation, S wave is greater than R wave in lead I. In left axis deviation, S wave is greater than R wave in lead III.
- **Ventricular ectopic beat** arises from an ectopic focus in the ventricle and produces a **bizarre-shaped** QRS complex followed by a compensatory pause before the next normal beat (**Fig. 23.21**). When the normal impulse reaches the ventricle the ventricle will be in the absolute refractory period of the premature beat. This is the cause for the compensatory pause.
- **Enlarged Q wave** is seen in myocardial infarction (*refer* Fig. 23.25).

QT Interval Abnormalities

Long QT syndrome

QT interval is the time from the beginning of ventricular depolarization to the end of ventricular repolarization. It may be lengthened by myocardial damage, myocardial ischemia, conduction defects, by certain drugs (omeprazole, antiarrhythmic drugs, antihistamines like diphenhydramine, antidepressants, antibiotics like erythromycin, ciprofloxacin; antifungal drugs like fluconazole and diuretics like furosemide) and by electrolyte abnormalities (K^+ or Mg^{2+} deficiencies). It can also be congenital. It is frequently associated with mutations of voltage gated K^+ channel genes in the heart which may affect the heart's electrical response. The condition is called **long QT syndrome (LQTS)**. It can lead to irregular heart beats, fainting, seizures and cardiac arrest. When QT interval is prolonged, cardiac repolarization is abnormal and the incidence of ventricular arrhythmias increases. The abnormal repolarization can lead to the formation of reentry circuits which may lead to ventricular fibrillation and sudden death.

Ectopic Foci of Impulse Production

Normally, myocardial cells do not discharge spontaneously. In abnormal conditions, the myocardial fibers and the Purkinje fibers may discharge spontaneously. This leads to increased automaticity of the heart. If an ectopic focus discharges once, the result is a beat that occurs before the expected next normal beat and is called **extrasystole** or **premature beat**. It may be atrial, nodal or ventricular beat (**Fig. 23.21**). If the ectopic focus discharges repetitively at a rate higher than that of the SA node it leads to rapid

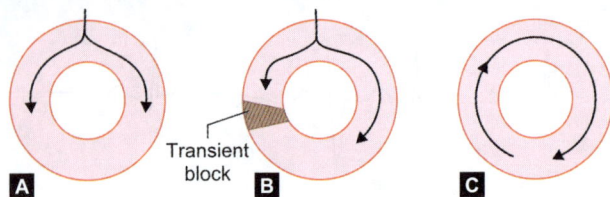

Figs. 23.22A to C: Re-entry or circus movement in a ring of cardiac tissue: (A) Normal spread of impulse; (B) A transient block on one side; (C) Transient block worn off so that the impulse passes this area to produce a circus movement indefinitely.

tachycardia called **paroxysmal tachycardia**, e.g., paroxysmal atrial tachycardia (PAT).

Ventricular tachycardia occurs when there are multiple ectopic foci in the ventricle. Due to ectopic foci and due to circus movement of impulses, **ventricular fibrillation** may occur because of the lack of synchronous contraction of different parts of the ventricle. If fibrillation is not corrected, within a few minutes death occurs.

Ventricular fibrillation is corrected using electronic defibrillators.

Re-entry

A wave of excitation propagates continuously within a closed circuit in the heart. This is called **re-entry** or **circus movement**. Circus movements in turn can cause ventricular fibrillatio. For example, if a transient block is present on one side of the conducting system, the impulse can go down the normal side. If the block immediately disappears, the impulse will be conducted in a retrograde direction in the previously blocked side back to the origin and then descends again establishing a circus movement **(Figs. 23.22A to C)**. Normally, the impulse spreads in both directions and the tissue immediately behind the wave of depolarization will be refractory. This is because a refractory muscle cannot transmit a second impulse. So, re-entry of impulses does not occur and the impulse dies out.

Causes of re-entry of cardiac impulses:
1. Shortening of the refractory period, e.g., drugs like adrenaline decreases refractory period. Here the impulse could continue around and around.
2. Prolongation of the pathway as in dilated heart. In this case, by the time the impulse returns to the stimulated site, the originally stimulated muscle will no longer be refractory and the impulse will continue around the path again and again.
3. Slowing of impulse conduction, e.g., blockage of the Purkinje system, ischemia of cardiac muscle, hyperkalemia, etc. Even if the length of the pathway is normal, if the velocity of conduction becomes decreased, it takes more time for the impulse to reach the stimulated site. By this time, the originally stimulated area will be out of refractory period and the impulse can continue again and again.
4. A temporary block in the pathway.
5. Presence of an alternate pathway with a different conducting velocity.

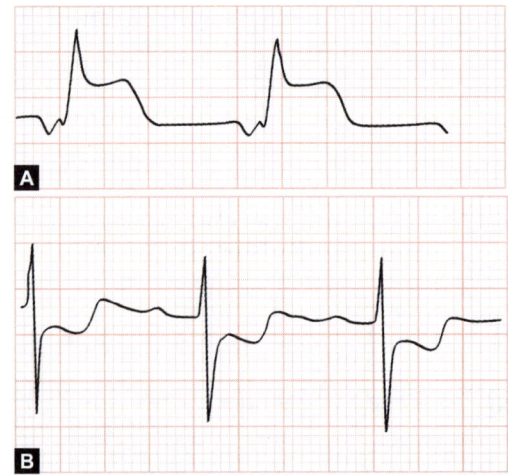

Figs. 23.23A and B: Abnormalities in ST segment: (A) ST elevation; (B) ST depression.

Abnormalities in ST Segment

In myocardial infarction, there will be changes in ST segment. In leads overlying infracted area there will be elevation of ST segment **(Fig. 23.23A)**. In leads placed 180° from the area of infarction there will be depression of ST segment **(Fig. 23.23B)**. ST depression is also seen in hypokalemia and hypoglycemia.

Changes in T Wave

1. T wave inversion **(Fig. 23.24A)** is seen in the following cases:
   - Normally seen in aVR
   - Intake of cold drinks just before taking ECG

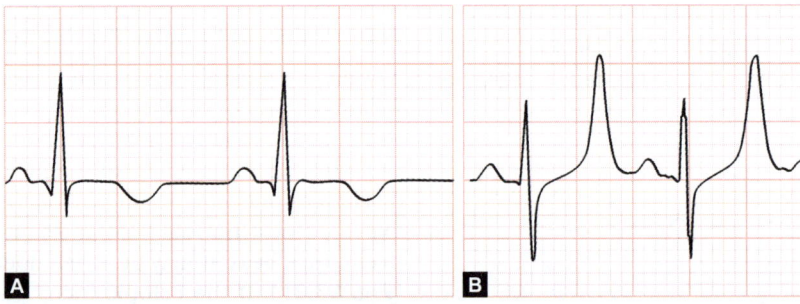

Figs. 23.24A and B: ECG showing changes in T wave: (A) T wave inversion; (B) Tall T wave.

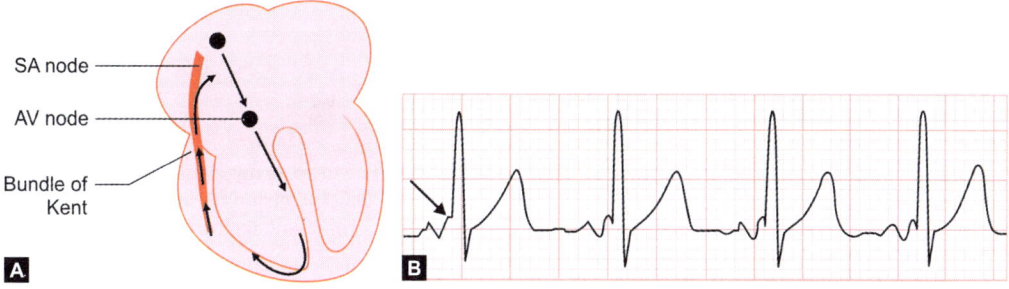

Figs. 23.25 A and B: (A) Wolff-Parkinson-White syndrome where there is an aberrant conducting tissue called bundle of Kent connecting the atria and ventricles. Note the re-entry phenomenon established by the bundle of Kent; (B) Note the delta wave indicated by arrow and shortened PR interval in ECG.

- Emotional states
- Excess smoking
- Following digitalis therapy
- Few hours after myocardial infarction
- Hypokalemia.
2. **Tall T wave (Fig. 23.24B)** is seen in the following conditions:
   - Immediately following myocardial infarction
   - Hyperkalemia.

Wolff-Parkinson-White Syndrome (WPW Syndrome)

WPW syndrome is due to accelerated AV conduction. Normally, the only conducting pathway between the atria and the ventricles is the AV node. People with WPW syndrome have an additional aberrant muscular or nodal tissue called **bundle of Kent** that connects atria and the ventricles **(Fig. 23.25)**.

This conducts impulses more rapidly than the AV node and bundle of His to one ventricle, which becomes excited early. This sets up a circus movement in which the impulse passes from the ventricle back to the atria. This produces paroxysmal atrial tachycardia. ECG shows delta wave in WPW syndrome **(Fig 23.25 B)**.

Classic triad of WPW syndrome includes:
1. Short PR interval
2. Slurring of the ascending limb of QRS complex termed δ-wave
3. Widening of QRS complex.

Myocardial Infarction

Myocardial infarction or heart attack occurs when blood flow decreases or stops to a part of the heart, leading to damage to the heart muscle. Most common cause is coronary artery disease due to atherosclerosis.

Manifestations

Myocardial infarction is usually associated with retrosternal chest pain radiating to the shoulder, arm, back, neck or jaw. Other symptoms include shortness of breath, nausea, vomiting, cold sweat especially in the forehead, tiredness, fainting, etc. Complications include heart failure, heart rate irregularities, cardiogenic shock, cardiac arrest, etc.

Some of the coronary arteries supply the nodal tissue, so a blockage sometimes causes potentially fatal cardiac arrhythmias.

Risk Factors

The risk factors include hypercholesterolemia, low level of high density lipoprotein, hypertension, diabetes mellitus, cigarette smoking, obesity, lack of exercise, collagen vascular diseases like systemic lupus erythematosus, rheumatoid arthritis, spasm of the coronary artery, etc.

Diagnosis

Diagnosis of MI is confirmed by ECG, blood pressure recording, echocardiogram, continuous ECG monitoring, coronary angiography etc. Blood tests for cardiac biomarkers (proteins that are released when cardiac muscle cells are damaged) like **troponin T,** high sensitivity troponin (hs-troponin), **CK-MB** (form of enzyme creatine kinase that is found mostly in the heart muscle cells), etc.

Ionic and ECG Changes in the Infarcted Area in Myocardial Infarction

❖ Abnormally rapid repolarization of the infarcted myocardial cells within seconds of infarction due to accelerated opening of K^+ channels. This lasts for a few minutes.

❖ After about 30 minutes of infarction, the infarcted fibers begin to depolarize more slowly than the surrounding normal fibers.

Rapid repolarization and delayed depolarization make the surface of the infarcted area positive relative to the surrounding normal area. As a result, current of injury flow out of the infarcted area into the surrounding areas. The above changes produce ST segment elevation in the ECG recorded from chest leads overlying the infarcted area.

After some days or weeks, the infarcted area become electrically silent, i.e., it shows no electrical activity. The current of injury stops and ST segment abnormality subsides. But there will be changes in the Q, R and T waves in ECG. There will be increase in the duration and amplitude of Q waves. Q waves appear in leads where they are normally absent. Amplitude of R wave decreases. T wave becomes very tall within the first few hours as a result of local rise

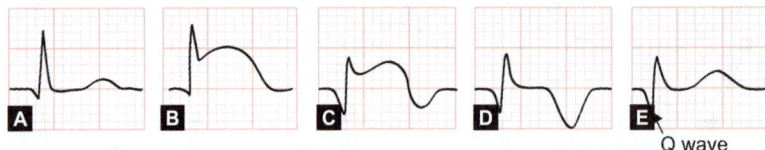

Figs. 23.26A to E: ECG changes in myocardial infarction: (A) Normal ECG pattern; (B) ST elevation in acute myocardial infarction; (C) Prominent Q wave, ST elevation and T wave inversion after a few days of MI; (D) Prominent Q wave and T wave inversion. ST segment comes to isoelectric level after a few weeks; (E) ST segment and T wave came back to normal but Q wave remains prominent even after recovery.

in extracellular K^+ concentration. Later T wave becomes inverted (*refer* **Figs. 23.26A to E**).

If the septum is infarcted, AV block or bundle branch block is seen due to damage to the conducting system. Arrhythmias occur due to re-entry. This is due to damage to the autonomic fibers. Epicardial infarct damages the sympathetic fibers whereas endocardial infarcts damage parasympathetic fibers.

MULTIPLE CHOICE QUESTIONS

1. ECG leads designated as V_1, V_2, etc. refer to:
   a. Unipolar limb leads
   b. Unipolar chest leads
   c. Bipolar limb leads
   d. Bipolar chest leads

2. P-R interval in ECG corresponds to:
   a. Time interval between onset of atrial contraction and onset of ventricular contraction
   b. Time delay in the AV node
   c. SA nodal conduction time
   d. Ventricular depolarization

3. Normal QRS duration is approximately:
   a. 0.2 sec
   b. 0.4-0.6 sec
   c. 0.08-0.1 sec
   d. 1-1.5

4. QRS complex indicates:
   a. Atrial repolarization
   b. Atrial depolarization
   c. Ventricular repolarization
   d. Ventricular depolarization

5. In the normal ECG recorded from lead II, atrial depolarization wave is represented by:
   a. P wave
   b. T wave
   c. U wave
   d. R wave

6. Normal ventricular activation time is:
   a. 0.2-0.4 sec
   b. 0.16-0.2 sec
   c. 2-4 msec
   d. 0.08-0.1 sec

7. Increase in extracellular K^+ concentration produces:
   a. Inverted T wave
   b. ST segment depression
   c. Low voltage ECG waves
   d. Tall peaked T wave

8. If the R-R interval in ECG is 0.6 sec, the heart rate would be:
   a. 60/min
   b. 100/min
   c. 72/min
   d. 120/min

9. In ECG, one small division in X-axis measures:
   a. 0.04 sec
   b. 0.4 sec
   c. 0.02 sec
   d. 0.1 sec

10. All the following statements are true about QRS complex, *except*:
    a. It occurs before ventricular contraction
    b. It corresponds to ventricular contraction
    c. It denotes ventricular depolarization
    d. Increase in Na^+ and Ca^{2+} content is responsible for QRS complex

11. Which part of ECG corresponds to maximum opening of ventricular Na^+ channels?
    a. R wave
    b. Q wave
    c. S wave
    d. T wave

12. Which part of ECG corresponds to maximum opening of ventricular Ca^{2+} channels?
    a. R wave
    b. Q wave
    c. ST segment
    d. T wave

13. PR interval is prolonged in:
    a. Atrial fibrillation
    b. First degree heart block
    c. Ventricular fibrillation
    d. WPW syndrome

14. PR interval is shortened in:
    a. WPW syndrome
    b. First degree heart block
    c. Second degree heart block
    d. Stokes Adams syndrome

15. P waves are absent in:
    a. Atrial flutter
    b. Atrial fibrillation
    c. Atrial extrasystole
    d. Complete heart block

16. In second-degree heart block:
    a. Ventricular ECG complexes are distorted
    b. Ventricular rate is lower than atrial rate
    c. Stroke volume is decreased
    d. Cardiac output is increased

17. The normal AV nodal delay is about:
    a. 0.1 sec
    b. 1 sec
    c. 0.1 millisecond
    d. 1 millisecond

18. What is not true for extrasystole in ventricle is:
    a. Fails to produce radial pulse
    b. Hints at serious heart ailment

c. Associated with abnormal QRS complex
d. Tendency to be followed by a compensatory pause

19. **A decrease in the velocity of impulse conduction through the AV node will usually cause:**
    a. Increase in PQ interval
    b. Decrease in PQ interval
    c. Disappearance of T wave
    d. Increased heart rate

20. **PR interval is prolonged in:**
    a. Myocardial infarction
    b. Atrial flutter
    c. Atrial fibrillation
    d. Heart block

21. **Re-entry is the common cause of the following conditions, *except*:**
    a. Paroxysmal atrial tachycardia
    b. Paroxysmal nodal tachycardia
    c. Atrial flutter
    d. Sinus arrhythmia

22. **Conduction in the AV node is depressed by:**
    a. Na^+ channel blocker
    b. Ca^{2+} channel blocker
    c. Both Na^+ and Ca^{2+} channel blocker
    d. K^+ channel blocker

23. **Bizarre QRS complexes are seen in:**
    a. Paroxysmal atrial tachycardia
    b. Paroxysmal ventricular tachycardia
    c. Atrial extrasystole
    d. Atrial fibrillation

24. **In Wolf-Parkinson-White syndrome, there exists a connection between atria and:**
    a. Bundle of His
    b. Ventricles
    c. AV node
    d. Purkinje fibers

ANSWERS

1. b	2. a	3. c	4. d	5. a
6. b	7. d	8. b	9. a	10. b
11. a	12. c	13. b	14. a	15. b
16. b	17. a	18. b	19. a	20. d
21. d	22. b	23. b	24. b	

Cardiac Cycle

CHAPTER 24

LEARNING OBJECTIVES

Must know
- Discuss the events occurring during the cardiac cycle
- Draw Wigger's diagram
- Draw and label the left ventricular and aortic pressure changes during a cardiac cycle
- Explain different heart sounds
- Discuss the physiological splitting of second heart sound
- Classify and explain the causes of cardiac murmurs

INTRODUCTION

A series of events should occur regularly and systematically in the heart in a particular sequence for accomplishing the proper pumping action of the heart.

Cardiac cycle is defined as the events that occur in the heart cyclically, from the beginning of one heart beat to the beginning of the next beat. Electrical events are followed by mechanical events in this cycle.

Duration of one cardiac cycle when the heart rate is 72/min is 60/72 = 0.8 sec.

PHASES OF CARDIAC CYCLE (FIG. 24.1)

PY5.3: Discuss the events occurring during the cardiac cycle.

Cardiac cycle consists of two phases:
1. **Systole**, which is a period of contraction of the heart.
2. **Diastole**, which is the period of relaxation of the heart.

The duration of various phases of cardiac cycle is as follows when the heart rate is 72/min:
- Atrial systole—0.1 sec
- Atrial diastole—0.7 sec
- Ventricular systole—0.3 sec
- Ventricular diastole—0.5 sec

From **Figure 24.1**, it is clear that atrial systole occurs in the last part of ventricular diastole and all the chambers of the heart are in the relaxed state for a period of 0.4 sec of the cardiac cycle. This period of the heart is called **quiescent period** or silent period or resting period of the heart.

Relation between Electrical and Mechanical Events in Cardiac Cycle

Contraction in the cardiac muscle starts just after depolarization of the muscle. Atrial systole occurs after the P wave of ECG; ventricular systole starts towards the end of R wave and ends after the T wave of ECG (**Fig. 24.2**).

Wigger's Diagram

Events of cardiac cycle can be expressed in a simple diagram called Wigger's diagram. This includes the ECG, pressure and volume changes in the heart and heart sounds. The phases of contraction and relaxation of the heart are named according to the activity of the chambers. Vertical lines separate the successive phases (**Fig. 24.2**).

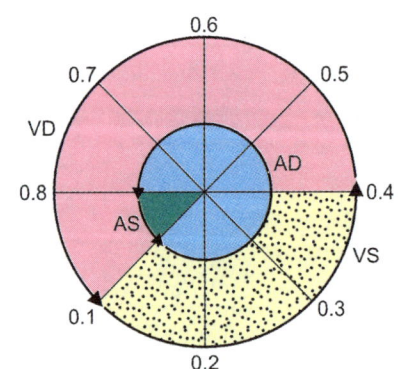

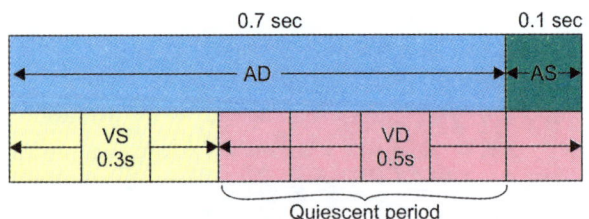

Fig. 24.1: Phases of cardiac cycle.
(AS: atrial systole; AD: atrial diastole; VS: ventricular systole; VD: ventricular diastole)

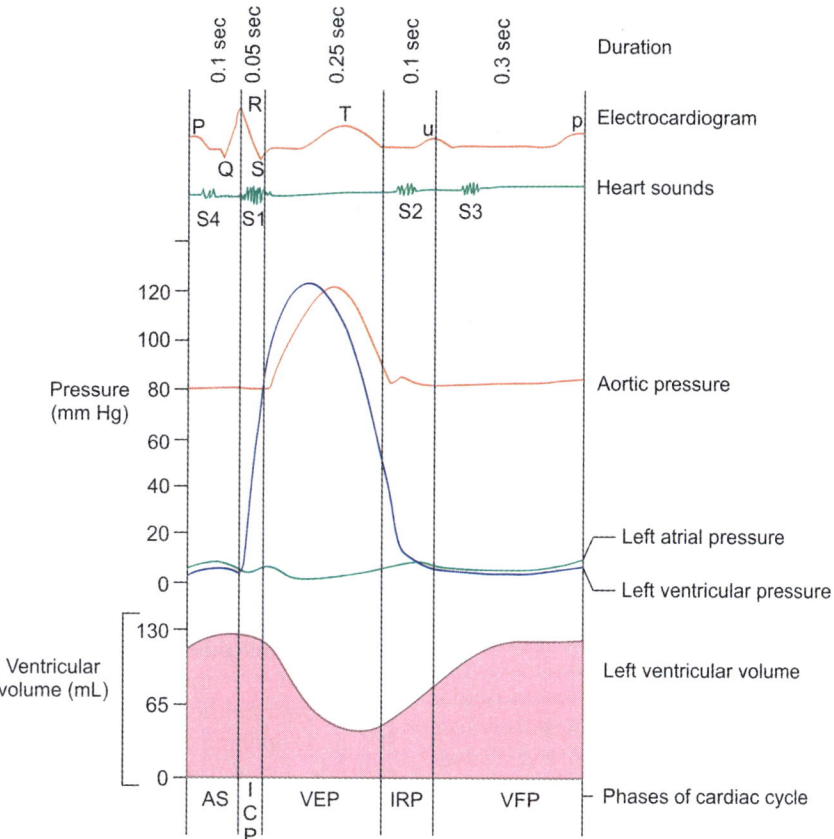

Fig. 24.2: Wigger's diagram showing the correlation between ECG, heart sounds, pressure changes in the left ventricle, left atrium and aorta, and left ventricular volume changes during different phases of a cardiac cycle of duration 0.8 seconds.
(AS: atrial systole; ICP: isometric contraction phase; VEP: ventricular ejection phase; IRP: isometric relaxation phase; VFP: ventricular filling phase)

The different phases of the cardiac cycle according to Wigger's classification are (**Table 24.1**):
- Atrial systole
- Ventricular systole which is subdivided into 3 depending on the type of contraction:
  1. Isovolumetric contraction phase
  2. Maximum ejection phase
  3. Reduced ejection phase
- Ventricular diastole:
  - Protodiastole
  - Isometric relaxation phase
  - Initial rapid filling phase
  - Reduced filling phase or diastasis
  - Last rapid filling phase which corresponds to atrial systole
- Atrial diastole

Atrial Systole

Atrial systole occurs following the impulse generation in the SA node. It occurs in the last part of ventricular diastole, i.e., during the last rapid filling phase. Before atrial systole, 70% of blood from atria has already flowed into the ventricles since the atrioventricular valves (AVV) are already open and the atria and ventricles are in the relaxed state. An additional 30% of blood flows into the ventricles due to atrial contraction (when the heart rate is rapid with short diastole, atrial contraction

Table 24.1: Phases of cardiac cycle.

Event	Phases	Duration (sec)	Position of valves
Atrial systole		0.1	AVV open SLV closed
Ventricular systole	Isometric contraction phase	0.05	AVV and SLV closed
	Maximum ejection phase	0.10	SLV open
	Reduced ejection phase	0.15	SLV open
Ventricular diastole	Protodiastole	0.04	SLV start closing
	Isometric relaxation phase	0.06	SLV and AVV closed
	Initial rapid filling phase	0.1	AVV open, SLV closed
	Reduced filling phase	0.2	AVV open, SLV closed
	Last rapid filling phase	0.1	AVV open, SLV closed
Atrial diastole		0.7	AVV closed, but open towards the end

can contribute to as much as 60% of ventricular inflow). As the atria contract the atrial musculature around the superior vena cava, inferior vena cava and pulmonary veins narrows these orifices and regurgitation of blood into the great veins is prevented to some extent. This mechanical event, i.e., atrial systole corresponds to the P wave of ECG.

Atrial contraction is not of much importance in ventricular filling in the normal resting state. But it gains importance in a slowed heart as in vagal stimulation, in heart block especially 2:1 block, during exercise, etc.

Ventricular Systole

Atrial systole is followed by ventricular systole. Ventricular systole is divided into:
- Isovolumetric or isovolumic contraction phase or isometric contraction phase
- Maximum ejection phase
- Reduced ejection phase.

Isovolumetric Contraction Phase

The AVV are open in the initial part of ventricular systole. When the ventricles start contracting, the intraventricular pressure increases and when it becomes greater than atrial pressure the AVV will close. The semilunar valves are already in the closed state. *So the ventricles become closed* chambers and they contract as closed chambers. Since the ventricles are filled with blood, decrease in the length of the muscle fibers is not possible during this contraction. The contraction in this phase is referred to as **isometric or isovolumetric** contraction since there is no change in the length of the muscle fibers and there is no movement of blood during this period. This causes a sharp rise in the intraventricular pressure since blood is not compressible. The ventricle assumes a spherical shape in this phase.

Maximum Ejection Phase

When the ventricular pressure exceeds aortic and pulmonary arterial pressure, the semilunar valves (SLV) open. When the left ventricular pressure exceeds 80 mmHg and right ventricular pressure exceeds 8 mm Hg, the semilunar valves are pushed open and blood rushes into the great vessels at a very high speed. Since the ventricles are contracting powerfully, the ventricular pressure goes on rising even though blood is being emptied from the ventricles. Simultaneously, pressure in the aorta and pulmonary artery also rises due to ejection of blood into these vessels in spite of peripheral run off of blood. The point at which aortic pressure exceeds the left ventricular pressure denotes the end of maximum ejection phase.

Reduced Ejection Phase

The peripheral run off from the great arteries is not up to the limit and the pressure in the aorta and pulmonary artery goes on rising and so the flow of blood from the ventricle goes on decreasing. This is reduced ejection phase.

Ventricular Diastole

Protodiastole

There is a short interval in which the ventricles have started relaxing and the semilunar valves are not closed. This period is called **protodiastole**. This period ends with the closure of SLV. SLV closes due to backflow of blood in the great arterial trunks because the pressure in the ventricles is less than the pressure in the aorta and pulmonary artery towards the end of ventricular systole. According to some authors, protodiastole is considered as the last part of reduced ejection phase. Because of the controversy, this phase is not mentioned recently.

Isovolumetric Relaxation Phase

Even after ventricular systole, about 40–50 mL of blood remains in the ventricle and both the semilunar valves and the AVV are in the closed state. The ventricles relax as a closed chamber. No change in the volume occurs since it is a closed chamber and hence the phase is referred to as isovolumetric or **isometric relaxation phase**. The intraventricular pressure falls very much. The atria are already filled with blood since atria were in diastole during ventricular systole. The atrial pressure is now greater than ventricular pressure and this force the AVV open. Isovolumetric relaxation phase extends from closure of SLV to the opening of AVV. The efficiency of the cardiac cycle depends on the correct functioning of the valves of the heart.

Initial Rapid Filling Phase

Even though there is no atrial contraction, blood flows rapidly from atria to ventricles passively, i.e., down the pressure gradient. The relaxing ventricle due to decreased pressure actually sucks in blood from the atria. This forms the **initial rapid filling phase**.

Reduced Filling Phase or Diastasis

When ventricle gets filled with blood, the intraventricular pressure rises and this leads to **reduced filling or diastasis**. When the ventricle is fully relaxed, filling is due to venous pressure alone. The atria and the ventricles are now functioning as a single chamber since the AVV are open.

Last Rapid Filling Phase

Towards the end of diastasis, atrial systole occurs which is referred to as the **last rapid filling phase** of ventricular diastole and the next cycle begins. Only 30% of ventricular filling is contributed by atrial systole as already mentioned.

Atrial Diastole

During atrial diastole, atrial muscles relax and blood flows into the atria from the great veins (superior vena cava, inferior vena cava and pulmonary veins). It lasts for about 0.7 sec, i.e., during ventricular systole and up to reduced filling phase of ventricular diastole.

Variation in the Duration of Cardiac Cycle

When the heart rate is increased, duration of cardiac cycle decreases. If it is a slight increase, only the period of diastasis will be affected. But if the rate is high, then the whole of diastole will be affected. Ventricular filling will be reduced very much so that cardiac output will be reduced and symptoms of heart failure develop. Coronary blood flow also becomes inadequate since it occurs during diastole (*refer* phasic variation in coronary blood flow, **Chapter 32, Fig. 32.5**).

In severe tachycardia, i.e., when the heart rate is more than 200/min, the systolic period will also be reduced. The reduced ejection phase is shortened mainly. In normal situations, the highest rate at which ventricles can contract is 230/min because of AV nodal delay. But in disease conditions such as paroxysmal ventricular tachycardia, heart rate increases up to 400/min.

When the heart rate is decreased, the duration of cardiac cycle increases and the diastolic period is mainly affected.

Peculiarities of Cardiac Cycle

- Events occurring on the right and left sides of the heart during a cardiac cycle are asynchronous.
- In the cardiac cycle, right atrial contraction occurs first, but only a very small difference exists.
- Left ventricular musculature contracts first, followed by right ventricular musculature.
- Right ventricular ejection occurs first because the pressure needed is less.
- During expiration, the pulmonary and the aortic valves close at the same time. But during inspiration, the aortic valve closes a little before the pulmonary valve closure. This is because of the lower impedance of the pulmonary vasculature (*refer* physiological splitting, **Fig. 24.5**).
- Myocardium derives its blood supply from the coronary arteries which arise from the base of aorta. During systole, the heart muscle contracts and the coronaries will be compressed. They get filled up with blood only during diastole. Thus the heart musculature is perfused better in diastole and not during systole as is the case in all other areas of the body.

End-diastolic Volume (EDV), End-systolic Volume (ESV) and Ejection Fraction (EF)

The amount of blood present in each ventricle at the end of diastole is **end-diastolic volume**. Normally, EDV is 120–130 mL. After complete ejection, some amount of blood remains in the ventricle. This is **end-systolic volume** which is about 30–50 mL. The difference between EDV and ESV is called **stroke volume**.

Ejection fraction (EF) is the ratio of stroke volume (SV) to the end-diastolic volume (EDV) and it is calculated from the EDV and the end-systolic volume (ESV) as follows:

$$EF = \frac{EDV - ESV}{EDV}$$

Ejection fraction is expressed as percentage of the EDV that is ejected and is normally 60–70%. When there is myocardial depression, the left ventricular ejection fraction is reduced below 55%.

Table 24.2: Pressures in the different chambers of the heart.

Chamber	Systolic pressure (mm Hg)	Diastolic pressure (mm Hg)
Right atrium	5–6	0
Left atrium	7–8	0
Right ventricle	25	0
Left ventricle	120	0
Aorta	120	80
Pulmonary artery	25	8–10

Variations in End-diastolic Volume

- EDV is increased when venous return is increased or when heart rate is decreased.
- ESV is decreased when pumping action of heart is increased. In both the above conditions, stroke volume is increased.

PRESSURE CHANGES DURING CARDIAC CYCLE (TABLE 24.2)

Methods of Measurement of Pressure

In **direct method**, a needle is introduced into the chambers of the heart and it is connected to a manometer. The pressure can be recorded directly and this method is done in experimental animals.

In humans, **cardiac catheterization** is done to record pressure in different chambers of the heart. Catheter is a polythene tube which is introduced through a vein or artery depending on the cavity to be reached. The catheter is connected to a manometer. The position of the catheter can be visualized by fluoroscopic method since the tip of the catheter is coated with a fluorescent material. If the catheter is introduced through the anterior cubital vein, it reaches the right atrium and the right atrial pressure can be recorded. It can also be introduced into the right ventricle through the AVV and from there into the pulmonary artery and the pressures can be recorded. If the catheter is introduced through an artery, it reaches the left side of heart and the pressures in the aorta and left ventricle can be recorded.

It is difficult to measure the left atrial pressure using a direct measuring device because it is difficult to pass a catheter through the heart chambers into the left atrium. But the left atrial pressure can be measured approximately by measuring the **pulmonary wedge pressure**. This is done by inserting a catheter through a peripheral vein into the right atrium and through the right ventricle and the pulmonary artery push the catheter until it wedges tightly in a small branch of the pulmonary artery. The pressure thus measured is called the wedge pressure which is about 5 mm Hg. This indirectly is a measure of the left atrial pressure.

Atrial Pressure Changes

Atrial pressure recording shows three positive waves and two negative waves. Positive waves are **a, c and v waves** and the negative waves are **x and y** descends (**Fig. 24.3**).

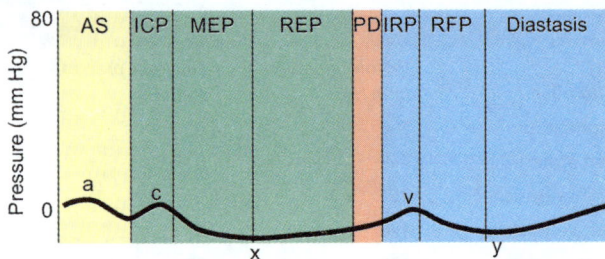

Fig. 24.3: Atrial pressure changes during a cardiac cycle. The positive waves are a, c and v waves and negative waves are x and y descents.

(AS: atrial systole; ICP: isometric contraction phase; MEP: maximum ejection phase; REP: reduced ejection phase; PD: protodiastole; IRP: isometric relaxation phase; RFP: rapid filling phase)

"a" Wave

This positive wave is due to atrial systole. All the fibers are not contracting at the same time. So a smooth curve is obtained. Initially, few fibers start contracting, then more and more fibers contracts to reach the peak of contraction. The AVV remain open in atrial systole.

"c" Wave

After atrial systole, AVV close during the isometric contraction phase of ventricle. The pressure exerted on the AVV is more since the ventricle is contracting as a closed chamber. This leads to a slight bulging of AVV into the atria in spite of the contraction of papillary muscles. This bulging of the AV valves causes a slight increase in the atrial pressure and causes the "c" wave.

"x" Descent

This is a negative wave. During ventricular ejection phase, AV valves are drawn downward along with the atrioventricular ring. This causes a reduction in the pressure of atria causing the "x" descent.

"v" Wave

During atrial diastole, due to increased venous return, there is an increase in the atrial pressure causing the positive "v" wave in the recording. This is seen during the isovolumetric relaxation phase of ventricle.

"y" Descent

Towards the end of isovolumetric relaxation phase of ventricular diastole, the AV valve open and the blood rushes from atria into the ventricles. This causes a fall in the atrial pressure and the "y" descent is recorded in the pressure tracing.

Waves similar to that recorded from the right atrium are obtained in the jugular venous pulse tracing.

Ventricular Pressure Changes

Left Ventricular Pressure Changes (Fig. 24.4)

A small rise in the pressure is seen in the ventricle during atrial systole. At the end of atrial systole, the left ventricular

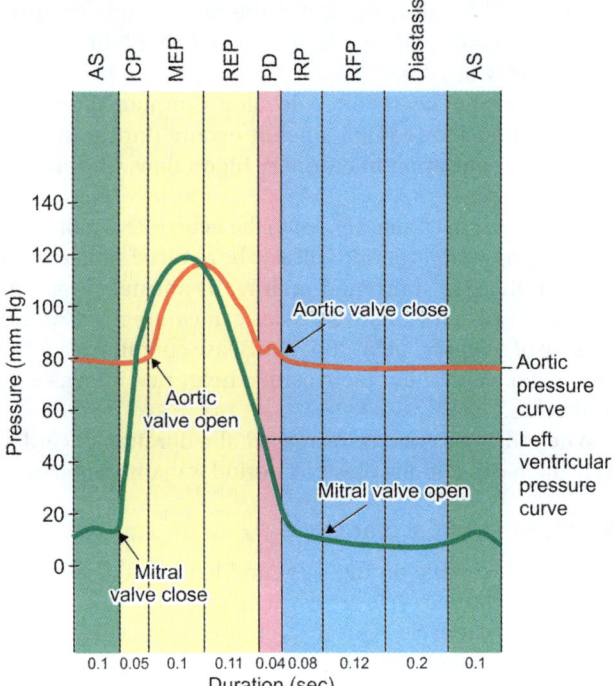

Fig. 24.4: Left ventricular and aortic pressure changes in the phases of cardiac cycle.

(ICP: isometric contraction phase; MEP: maximum ejection phase; REP: reduced ejection phase; PD: protodiastole; IRP: isometric relaxation phase; RFP: rapid filling phase; AS: atrial systole)

pressure is about 2–3 mm Hg. In the isovolumetric contraction phase, the pressure rises and towards the end of this phase, the SLV open. Further contraction in the rapid ejection phase is isotonic and pressure in the ventricle reaches a maximum of 120–130 mm Hg. The pressure in the aorta is also increasing and when the pressure in the aorta is greater than the pressure in the ventricle, the ventricular ejection slows down and the pressure also starts falling because the amount of blood in the ventricle is less.

Towards the end of reduced ejection phase, the ventricular muscle stops contracting. Since the peripheral run off from the aorta does not balance the blood ejected from the ventricle, there is transient backflow of blood from aorta to the left ventricle since the left ventricular pressure is less than that of aortic pressure. This backflow causes approximation of semilunar valves.

In isovolumetric relaxation phase, the left ventricle relaxes without change in volume and there is a rapid fall in left ventricular pressure to very low levels. Now the pressure in the left atrium will be greater than the left ventricular pressure and the AVV open at the end of this phase. Atrial blood rushes into the relaxed ventricle during the filling phase **(Fig. 24.4)**.

Right Ventricular Pressure Changes

Even though left ventricle contracts first, ejection of blood occurs first from the right ventricle. This is because the pressure required to pump blood is less for the right ventricle since the pressure in the pulmonary artery is less.

When compared to left ventricular pressure changes, right ventricular pressure is less in the different phases of cardiac cycle. In isometric contraction phase, the pressure in the right ventricle is 10 mm Hg and in the maximum ejection phase the maximum pressure attained is 20–25 mm Hg.

Right ventricular pressure increases in conditions where there is increased resistance to the flow of blood through the pulmonary capillaries as in pulmonary edema, pulmonary fibrosis, etc. In these conditions there will be pulmonary hypertension.

Aortic Pressure Changes

Since pumping of blood by the ventricle is intermittent, the aortic pressure fluctuates between systolic pressure of 120 mm Hg and diastolic pressure of 80 mm Hg. Diastolic pressure in aorta does not fall to very low levels due to elastic recoil of the vessel wall during diastole. If the aortic pressure falls to very low levels, the tissues especially heart, brain and kidneys will be affected severely.

During **atrial systole**, pressure in the aorta is 80 mm Hg. In the **isometric contraction phase**, the left ventricular pressure increases and when it exceeds 80 mm Hg, the semilunar valves open. In the **maximum ejection phase**, blood is ejected into the aorta and the wall of the aorta stretches due to elasticity and the aortic pressure rises. The blood entering the aorta is more than the blood leaving to the periphery. The aortic pressure rises to about 120 mm Hg. In the **reduced ejection phase**, the amount of blood ejected into the aorta becomes lesser and lesser and the ventricular pressure begins to fall. The peripheral run off into the smaller vessels becomes more and the aortic pressure starts to fall.

In **ventricular diastole**, when the ventricular pressure falls below aortic pressure, backflow of blood causes Eddie currents at the root of the aorta and closes the semilunar valve (SLV). When the semilunar valve closes, an **incisura** is recorded in the aortic pressure curve. Closure of the SLV causes a momentary rise in the aortic pressure because of the sudden cessation to the back flow of blood.

The blood strikes against the SLV causing transient vibrations in the blood column called as **after vibrations** in the recording. The aortic pressure falls throughout ventricular diastole. Due to elastic recoil, blood stored in the distended elastic arteries flows continuously through the peripheral vessels. The aortic pressure falls to 80 mm Hg during diastole (**Fig. 24.4**).

The blood ejected into the aorta sets up a pressure wave which travels along the arteries and causes expansion of the arterial walls. This wave of expansion can be palpated in the peripheral arteries and is known as **pulse**. For example, radial pulse can be palpated at the wrist.

Table 24.4: Volume changes in the heart.

Cavity	Capacity (mL)
Right atrium	160
Right ventricle	140
Left atrium	140
Left ventricle	120

Pressure Changes in the Pulmonary Artery

Pressure changes in the pulmonary artery is almost similar to aortic pressure changes but the systolic pressure is only 25 mm Hg and diastolic pressure 10 mm Hg. **Pulse pressure** is the difference between systolic and diastolic pressure. The pulse pressure is low in the pulmonary artery because of two reasons: (i) compliance is more in the pulmonary circulation, (ii) about half of the blood ejected by the right ventricle runs off from the pulmonary artery to the capillaries and from there into the pulmonary veins and reaches the right atrium at the same time that it is being ejected during systole (**Table 24.3**).

VOLUME CHANGES DURING CARDIAC CYCLE

Regarding the capacities, atrial capacity is slightly greater than that of the corresponding ventricles. The atria mainly act as reservoirs and provide sufficient blood to fill the ventricular cavities (**Table 24.4**). Total diastolic volume of the heart is 540 mL. During systole, about 140 mL is ejected by both ventricles.

Atrial Volume Changes

The flow into the atrium cannot be measured. The degree of atrial filling can be assessed by finding out the flow in the vena cava. This is because the vena cava is continuous with the right atrium without any valves. This flow is described in three phases:
1. During atrial systole, the flow is zero due to the back pressure into the great veins.
2. In ventricular systole, AVV are closed and major part of atrial filling occurs in this phase. The atrioventricular ring moves down during ventricular contraction and so the volume in the atria enlarges and blood rushes from the veins.
3. In ventricular diastole, considerable flow occurs into the atrium.

Ventricular Volume Changes

Study of volume changes in the heart is called **plethysmography** and the instrument used is **cardio-meter**.

Table 24.3: Maximum pressures in aorta, pulmonary artery, ventricles and atria in systole and diastole.

Pressure	Aorta	Pulmonary artery	Left ventricle	Right ventricle	Left atrium	Right atrium
Systolic pressure	120 mm Hg	25 mm Hg	120 mm Hg	25 mm Hg	7–8 mm Hg	4–6 mm Hg
End-diastolic pressure	80 mm Hg	10 mm Hg	5 mm Hg	2–3 mm Hg	2 mm Hg	0–1 mm Hg

During atrial systole, the ventricular volume increases. But the increase in volume depends on the duration of diastole. If ventricular diastole is long, then atrial systole does not contribute much to ventricular filling. During isometric contraction phase there is no change in the volume since all valves are closed. During maximum ejection phase, volume decreases rapidly. During reduced ejection phase decrease in volume is less. The tracing becomes more or less horizontal. During isometric relaxation phase, there is no change in volume. A small rise may be seen in the recording due to entry of blood into the branches of the coronary arteries which were previously compressed during systole. Rapid increase in volume occurs during the rapid filling phase and a slow rise in the reduced filling phase. The rest of the filling is during atrial systole. The amount of blood in the ventricle at the end of each diastole is called **end-diastolic volume** which is approximately 120–130 mL in each ventricle (*refer* **Fig. 24.2**).

HEART SOUNDS (TABLE 24.5)

During different phases of cardiac cycle, the valves should open widely and the closure should be prompt and abrupt. The valves act as diaphragm between low-pressure and high-pressure areas and under normal circumstances it allows blood to flow only in one direction.

Movements of the Valves

Atrioventricular Valve (AVV)

AVV open in early diastole and towards the end of ventricular diastole when the atria contract the AVV are opened widely. Inversion of the valve leaflets into the ventricle is prevented because as the ventricle gets filled with blood there is some back-flow of blood into the atrium. This keeps the valve leaflets in a midposition. In the beginning of isovolumetric contraction phase (ICP), the ventricular pressure increases and the AVV start to close. Towards the end of ICP, the AVV closes completely and tightly to prevent regurgitation of blood back into the atria. This is because the chordae tendineae attached to the valve leaflets become very tense and prevent undue bulging of the valve into the atria.

Semilunar Valves (SLV)

Semilunar valves are guarded by three cusps and when the valve open, a triangular orifice is seen. The working of the aortic semilunar valve is very important because the coronary arteries arise from the root of the aorta. While opening, the valve leaflets should not close the coronary orifice. If it happens, it leads to ischemia and infarction of heart. There are three outpouchings in the valve cusps of aortic valve called **sinuses of Valsalva**. Due to the presence of these outpouchings, the aortic wall and valve leaflets do not approximate to close the coronary orifice.

The SLV opens towards the end of isometric contraction phase. When the aortic and the pulmonary artery pressures exceed the ventricular pressure, the SLV closes. This occurs during protodiastole of cardiac cycle.

Phonocardiography

Phonocardiography is a technique to record the sounds produced by the heart. The sound produced by the heart is picked up by the **phonocardiograph** and can be amplified. This can be recorded by a high-speed recorder. The sites of production of normal heart sounds and also any abnormal sounds can be detected. Sounds are produced in the heart due to vibrations of the valve cusps during closing, due to contractions of the chambers, turbulence of blood flow, etc. Opening of the valve rarely produces sounds. By phonocardiography, four sounds can be recorded from the heart, but by using stethoscope, only two sounds can be heard clearly (**Fig. 24.2**).

First Heart Sound (S_1)

First heart sound is heard in the isometric contraction phase and maximum ejection phase. The sound starts in the ICP and the maximum intensity is heard during the maximum ejection phase and then fades away. *It is due to closure of atrioventricular valve* (AVV). The quality of the sound is **soft and low pitched with long duration**. Its duration is about 0.15 sec and frequency 25–45 Hz. It can be compared to a **LUBB** sound. The sound is heard best in the area of apex beat and this part is called **mitral area**. There are three components for the first sound:

1. **Valvular component** is due to closure of the AVV and the turbulence of blood in the ventricle.
2. **Vascular component** is due to ejection of blood from the ventricle rapidly which produces vibrations in the root of the aorta.
3. **Muscular component** is due to vibrations of the contracting myocardium.

Table 24.5: Heart sounds.

Heart sound	Phase of cardiac cycle	Cause	Characteristics	Duration in sec	Frequency in cps (Hz)	Relation with ECG
First	ICP and MEP	Closure of AVV	Soft, low pitched (LUBB)	0.15 sec	25-45 Hz	Coincides with R wave
Second	End of protodiastole and early IRP	Closure of SLV	Sharp, high pitched (DUBB)	0.11 sec	50 Hz	Summit of T wave
Third	Rapid filling phase	Rush of blood into ventricles	Inaudible or low pitched	0.08 sec	1-6 Hz	Between T and next P wave
Fourth	Atrial systole	Atrial contraction	Inaudible	0.03 sec	1 Hz	Between P wave and Q wave

(ICP: isometric contraction phase; MEP: maximum ejection phase; IRP: isometric relaxation phase; AVV: atrioventricular valve; SLV: semilunar valve; CPS: cycles per second).

In the phonocardiogram, two components can be attributed to the first heart sound, the mitral and the tricuspid component. Mitral component occurs first but cannot be distinguished with a stethoscope.

Second Heart Sound (S₂)

The interval between first and the second heart sound gives the duration of systole. Duration between S_2 and the next S_1 is the diastolic period. S_2 is *due to the closure of semilunar valve* (SLV). The second heart sound is a **high pitched, sharp and short** sound of duration 0.11 sec and frequency 50 Hz. It can be compared to the sound **DUBB**. There are two components for S_2, aortic and pulmonary component (A_2 and P_2) which can be distinguished using a stethoscope.

Closure of SLV occurs at the end of protodiastole. Backward flow of blood causes sudden closure of the SLV causing vibrations in the blood column and blood vessels. It also causes turbulence to the blood flow which also contributes to the sound. The pressure difference across SLV is much more than in the AVV.

Aortic valve close first because the pressure difference is more on the aortic side. Pulmonary vascular resistance is 1/10th that of systemic resistance. So, the right ventricular ejection starts earlier and is completed slightly later than left ventricular ejection. So the pulmonary valve closes after the closure of aortic valve. The splitting of the second sound (aortic and pulmonary components) is normal and is called **physiological splitting (Fig. 24.5)**.

If the person takes a deep inspiration the splitting widens, i.e., A_2 appears earlier and P_2 occurs a little late than normal **(Fig. 24.5)**. This is because of increase in the negativity of intrathoracic pressure and the resulting increase in the venous return to the right atrium. End-diastolic volume in the right ventricle is increased leading to an increase in the ejection period. Thus, P_2 will be a little delayed from normal, i.e., it is postponed. On the left side, increased negativity of intrathoracic pressure causes increase in the volume of left atrium leading to a decrease in the pressure in the left atrium. The pressure gradient becomes less between atrium and ventricle on the left. This leads to decrease in ventricular filling and there will be a reduction in the ventricular ejection time and so, A_2 is preponed than that of normal. During forced expiration, opposite of the above changes occur and the splitting becomes narrow.

Third Heart Sound (S₃)

S_3 is a **diastolic sound** and is heard in early diastole, i.e., during rapid filling phase. Atrial blood flows into the ventricle rapidly in the early part of ventricular diastole and this gives rise to the third heart sound. This sound is normal if recorded in a phonocardiograph but it is not heard normally using a stethoscope. It is audible with a stethoscope in disease conditions like left ventricular failure, cardiomyopathies, aortic and mitral regurgitation, and constrictive pericarditis. It can also be heard under physiological conditions like pregnancy, after exercise, in young healthy adults before the age of 30 years, etc. If S_3 is audible then the rhythm resembles the gentle gallop of a horse and is called **gallop rhythm or triple rhythm**. S_3 is referred to as '**ventricular gallop**'.

Causes of S₃

- Opening of AVV
- Vibrations set up in the ventricular walls due to rush of blood into the ventricles during rapid filling phase. It is heard in the middle part of diastole.

Fourth Heart Sound (S₄)

S_4 is produced by **atrial contraction in the last rapid filling phase** and is a late diastolic sound. It can never be heard using a stethoscope. It is also called '**atrial gallop**'. It can only be recorded and is almost always abnormal. It is a soft low pitched sound of short duration recorded during atrial systole. It immediately precedes the first heart sound which marks the onset of ventricular systole. S_4 if present is a sign of diastolic heart failure. It can be recorded in conditions where the left ventricle is noncompliant like systemic hypertension, severe left ventricular hypertrophy, long standing aortic stenosis, during active myocardial ischemia, etc.

Areas of Auscultation of Heart Sounds

- **Aortic area** in the second right intercostal space close to the sternal border.
- **Pulmonary area** in the second left intercostal space close to the sternal border.
- **Mitral area** at the region of apex beat. Normally, apex beat is felt in the fifth left intercostal space half an inch medial to the mid-clavicular line.
- **Tricuspid area** in the fifth left intercostal space close to the sternal border.

Abnormalities of Heart Sounds

Narrowing of the valvular orifice is called **stenosis**. The narrowing may be due to adherence of valve leaflets preventing free flow of blood through the valve. Sometimes, the edges of the valve cusps may be damaged by disease and when the valves close, tight approximation of valve do not occur. This leads to backflow of blood or regurgitation of blood. This is called **incompetency** of valves. Frequent cause of valvular heart disease is rheumatic fever caused by streptococci. The toxins of the bacteria produce autoimmune response specifically affecting the valves of the heart. As a result, the valve cusps do not move freely and later scarring of valve also occurs. Abnormalities of heart sounds are classified into:

- Variation in the intensity of sound **(Table 24.6)**
- Variation in the splitting of sound
- Abnormal sounds.

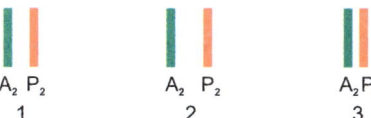

Fig. 24.5: Physiological splitting of second heart sound. 1. In normal inspiration; 2. In deep inspiration; 3. In forced expiration.

(A_2: aortic component P_2: pulmonary component of second heart sound)

Table 24.6: Variation in the intensity of heart sounds.

Sound	Increase in intensity	Decrease in intensity
First heart sound	• Mitral stenosis • Tachycardia • Left ventricular hypertrophy	• Emphysema • Pericardial effusion • Bradycardia • Thick chest wall
Second heart sound	• Systemic hypertension • Pulmonary hypertension	Calcification of aorta

Abnormal changes in the splitting of sound are seen in right bundle branch block and atrial septal defect (ASD). Abnormal heart sounds heard over the precordium are called **murmurs**. When the sound is auscultated over blood vessels, it is called **bruit**. Bruit is heard in hyperdynamic circulation as in hyperthyroidism and in aneurysms.

Murmur

Abnormal sound heard over the heart is called murmur. Murmur is due to **turbulence** created at or near a valve or due to abnormal communication within the heart or between great vessels. Murmurs are heard with the help of a stethoscope or it can even be palpated.

Types of Murmurs

a. Hemic murmur
b. Valvular murmur
c. Fistulous murmur
d. Aneurysmal murmur

❖ **Hemic murmur** is a systolic murmur due to hyper-dynamic circulation as in chronic anemia.
❖ **Valvular murmur** is caused by valvular stenosis or valvular insufficiency which causes turbulence and sound.
❖ **Fistulous murmur** is due to abnormal communication within the heart (atrial septal defect, ventricular septal defect, Fallot's tetralogy, etc.) or abnormal communication between blood vessels as in patent ductus arteriosus where there is flow of blood from aorta into the pulmonary artery through the patent ductus arteriosus.
❖ In **aneurysmal murmur**, aneurysms create turbulence leading to the production of sound. An aneurysm is defined as a pathologic dilatation of a segment of a blood vessel. For example, aortic aneurysm in which atherosclerosis is the most common associated pathological condition.

Another classification of murmurs **(Table 24.7)**:
❖ Systolic murmur
❖ Diastolic murmur
❖ Continuous murmur.

Table 24.7: Causes and classification of murmur.

Systolic murmur	Diastolic murmur	Continuous murmur
• Aortic stenosis • Pulmonary stenosis • Mitral incompetence • Tricuspid incompetence • Anemia • Ventricular septal defect	• Aortic incompetence • Pulmonary incompetence • Mitral stenosis • Tricuspid stenosis	Patent ductus arteriosus (PDA)

MULTIPLE CHOICE QUESTIONS

1. **Atrial systole coincides with ventricular:**
   a. Isometric contraction phase
   b. Isometric relaxation phase
   c. Maximum ejection phase
   d. Reduced filling phase or diastasis

2. **Dicrotic notch on the aortic pressure curve is caused by:**
   a. Closure of mitral valve
   b. Closure of tricuspid valve
   c. Closure of aortic valve
   d. Rapid filling of the left ventricle

3. **Fourth heart sound is caused by:**
   a. Closure of aortic and pulmonary valves
   b. Ventricular filling
   c. Closure of atrioventricular valves
   d. Vibration of the ventricular wall during systole

4. **Heart sound heard immediately before the first heart sound when atrial pressure is high:**
   a. First   b. Second
   c. Third   d. Fourth

5. **Loud, snapping second heart sound is heard in:**
   a. Aortic stenosis
   b. Aortic incompetence
   c. Pulmonary hypertension
   d. Mitral stenosis

6. **Bounding pulse is seen in:**
   a. Aortic stenosis
   b. Aortic incompetence
   c. Mitral incompetence
   d. Mitral stenosis

7. **The record of heart sound is called:**
   a. Electrocardiogram   b. Ballistocardiogram
   c. Phonocardiogram   d. Echocardiogram

8. **'C' wave in atrial pressure tracing corresponds to the following ventricular event:**
   a. Ventricular ejection
   b. Protodiastole
   c. Isometric contraction phase
   d. Isometric relaxation phase

9. **Third heart sound coincides with the following event:**
   a. Isometric contraction phase
   b. Reduced ejection phase
   c. Rapid filling phase
   d. Reduced filling phase

10. **Dicrotic notch in aortic pressure curve is:**
    a. Magnified by aortic regurgitation
    b. Absent in atherosclerosis
    c. Of no diagnostic value
    d. Coincident with second heart sound

11. **The part of ventricle to contract first during ventricular systole is:**
    a. Interventricular septum
    b. Papillary muscles

c. Right ventricle
d. Left ventricle

12. **Splitting of second heart sound is due to:**
    a. Delay in the closure of tricuspid valve
    b. Delay in the closure of mitral valve
    c. Delay in the closure of pulmonary valve
    d. Delay in the closure of aortic valve

13. **Normal end diastolic volume is:**
    a. 70 mL
    b. 100 mL
    c. 130 mL
    d. 160 mL

14. **In normal cardiac cycle:**
    a. Ventricular systole is shorter than atrial systole
    b. End diastolic ventricular volume is 130 mL
    c. Isovolumetric ventricular contraction period is 1.5 sec
    d. Protodiastole is the period after the end of diastole

15. **In cardiac cycle, semilunar valves close at the:**
    a. End of protodiastole
    b. Beginning of protodiastole
    c. End of isometric relaxation phase
    d. End of isometric contraction phase

16. **During the cardiac cycle, opening of aortic valve occurs at the:**
    a. Beginning of systole
    b. End of isovolumetric contraction
    c. End of diastole
    d. End of diastasis

17. **At the end of isometric relaxation phase:**
    a. Atrioventricular valves open
    b. Atrioventricular valves close
    c. Corresponds to peak of C wave in JVP
    d. Corresponds to T wave in ECG

18. **Of the following, which one correlates with isovolumetric contraction phase?**
    a. AV opening and aortic and pulmonary valve closure
    b. AV closure and aortic and pulmonary valve opening
    c. Both valves are closed
    d. Both valves are open

19. **Isovolumetric relaxation phase of cardiac cycle ends with:**
    a. Peak of 'c' venous wave
    b. Opening of AV valve
    c. Closure of semilunar valve
    d. Beginning of T wave

20. **Ventricular filling:**
    a. Produces third heart sound in some healthy persons
    b. Depends mainly on atrial contraction
    c. Begins during isometric ventricular relaxation
    d. Will not occur unless atrial pressure is higher than atmospheric pressure

21. **Cardiac cycle duration in man at rest is:**
    a. 0.4 sec
    b. 0.8 sec
    c. 1.2 sec
    d. 1.6 sec

22. **The second heart sound differs from first heart sound in that:**
    a. Is normally split
    b. Has higher frequency
    c. Duration greater than first sound
    d. Due partly to turbulence set up by valve closure

23. **First heart sound occurs in:**
    a. Isotonic relaxation phase
    b. Isovolumetric contraction phase
    c. Isotonic contraction phase
    d. Isovolumetric relaxation phase

24. **Isovolumetric contraction phase correlates with:**
    a. Opening of AV valves and closure of semilunar valves
    b. Closure of AV valves and opening of semilunar valves
    c. Both valves are closed
    d. Both valves are open

25. **Ventricular gallop refers to presence of:**
    a. Third heart sound
    b. Fourth heart sound
    c. Splitting of second heart sound
    d. Cardiac murmurs

26. **Atrial gallop may be present in:**
    a. Systemic hypertension
    b. Hypotension
    c. Mitral stenosis
    d. Tricuspid stenosis

ANSWERS

1. d	2. c	3. b	4. d	5. c
6. b	7. c	8. c	9. c	10. d
11. a	12. c	13. c	14. b	15. a
16. b	17. a	18. c	19. b	20. a
21. b	22. a	23. b	24. c	25. a
26. a				

Hemodynamics

CHAPTER 25

LEARNING OBJECTIVES

Must know
- Describe and discuss the hemodynamics of circulatory system
- Explain the applications of Law of Laplace in the human body
- Differentiate between laminar and turbulent flow
- Explain the concept of Reynolds number
- Explain Poiseuille's law
- Define critical closing pressure

INTRODUCTION

PY5.7: Describe and discuss hemodynamics of circulatory system.

Hemodynamics means dynamics (motion) of blood. **William Harvey** established that circulation of blood occurs in the body primarily due to the pumping action of heart. Arteries and arterioles by their elastic recoil during diastole push the blood further forwards, acting as accessory pumps. Contraction of skeletal muscles compresses the veins and this favors return of blood to the heart. Sucking of blood into the heart is by the negative intrathoracic pressure during inspiration and also due to the sucking action of the heart during diastole when the chambers relax. Thus blood flows in a continuous circuit throughout life since the circulatory system is a closed system.

Hemodynamics deals with the interrelationship among **pressure, flow and resistance** and also the physical characteristics of blood which influence the flow of blood. It deals with the physical principles applied to the flow of blood through blood vessels, such as vascular geometry, dynamic fluid characteristics of blood and blood pressure (BP).

Study of the flow of water through rigid pipes is called **fluid dynamics**. Unlike water, which is homogenous, blood is a heterogeneous mixture of cells and plasma. Also blood flows through distensible tubes of varying dimensions instead of rigid tubes. Another difference is that blood flow is pulsatile in most parts of the arterial system.

Peculiarities of Different Parts of the Vascular System

Blood vessels are not rigid tubes. They are elastic and the elasticity varies in different segments of the vascular system. In aorta and large arteries, there is large amount of elastic tissue and elasticity is maximal in these vessels. They act as accessory pumps, causing forward propulsion of blood due to elastic recoil and also help in maintaining a pressure gradient. Thus blood continues to flow during diastole.

Arterioles contain less elastic tissue but more smooth muscle. The smooth muscles are innervated mainly by the sympathetic fibers. These vessels can change their caliber or diameter by contraction or relaxation of the smooth muscles. This produces a change in the resistance and thus influences the flow through these vessels. The arterioles are also called **resistance vessels**. Capillaries are thin walled and have fenestrations for exchange of materials across the capillary wall.

Venules and veins are thin walled but highly distensible. They are called **capacitance vessels** because they have the ability to store large amounts of blood.

Cross-sectional area of the different segments of the vascular system varies and the *cross-sectional area of capillaries is 1000 times more than that of aorta* (**Table 25.1**).

Newtonian and Non-Newtonian Fluids

Fluid is a material that flows, e.g., gases and liquids. Blood is a liquid. Sir Isaac Newton studied the relationship between viscosity and shearing force and postulated a formula.

Table 25.1: Total cross-sectional area of vessels and the mean velocity of blood flow.

Vessel	Cross-sectional area in cm^2	Mean velocity in cm/sec
Aorta	4.5	40 (120 in systole and 0 during diastole)
Arteries	20	30 in large arteries and 5 in small arteries
Arterioles	400	0.5
Capillaries	4500	0.05
Venules	4000	0.1
Veins	40	1
Vena cava	18	2

Fluids which obey this law are called **Newtonian fluids**. In a Newtonian fluid, viscosity remains constant with respect to shearing force. Water and plasma are Newtonian fluids.

Blood is thicker than water. Viscosity of blood is 3–4 times more than that of water. Blood is also a non-homogeneous fluid containing a suspension of cells. It is called a **non-Newtonian fluid**. In a non-Newtonian fluid, viscosity is variable with respect to shearing force.

RELATION BETWEEN PRESSURE, FLOW AND RESISTANCE

Velocity is the rate of displacement of a particle of fluid with respect to time and it is expressed in units of distance per unit time, e.g., cm/sec. **Flow** refers to the rate of displacement of a volume of fluid and it is expressed in units of volume per unit time, e.g., cm³/sec. In other words, flow through a tube is defined as the volume of fluid passing through a point in unit time. In a tube with cross-sectional area A, velocity V = Flow (F)/Cross-sectional area (A):

V = F/A

Flow (F) through a blood vessel depends on two main factors:
1. Pressure difference of the blood between the two ends of the vessel is the **effective perfusion pressure (P)**. Blood always flows from areas of high pressure to areas of low pressure or in other words the **pressure gradient (ΔP)** pushes the blood through the vessel.
2. Resistance offered to the flow of blood is called **vascular resistance (R)**. Resistance occurs as a result of friction between the flowing blood and the endothelium of the vessel wall.

ΔP = Mean intraluminal pressure at the arterial end–Mean pressure at the venous end

F = ΔP/R

Blood flow is directly proportional to the pressure difference and inversely proportional to the resistance. This is called **Ohm's law**.

METHODS FOR MEASURING BLOOD FLOW

1. Electromagnetic flow meters
2. Ultrasonic Doppler flow meter
3. Plethysmography
4. Methods based on Fick principle and indicator dilution techniques

Devices used to measure blood flow are called **flow meters**. **Electromagnetic flow meters** depend on the principle that a voltage is generated in a conductor moving through a magnetic field and that the magnitude of the voltage is proportionate to the speed of movement. Since blood is a conductor, if the poles of an electromagnet are placed around the vessel, the voltage across the poles can be measured with an electrode placed on the surface of the vessel which is connected to an electronic recording device.

Another type of flow meter is ultrasonic Doppler flow meter. Ultrasonic waves are sent into a vessel diagonally, and the waves reflected from the blood cells are picked up by a downstream sensor. The frequency of the reflected wave is proportional to the rate of flow towards the sensor because of Doppler effect.

Regional blood flow can be measured by applying **Fick and indicator dilution techniques**. Blood flow to the extremities is determined by **plethysmography**.

LAMINAR FLOW

If pressure is applied to a solid object the whole thing moves. But if pressure is applied to a fluid in a straight tube, the fluid does not move as a whole, but it behaves as if it has several layers or **laminas**. These layers move in concentric circles. This type of flow in which the fluid moves in different laminas is called **laminar flow or streamline flow** which is silent (Fig. 25.1A). The central layer of the fluid moves faster than the outer layers in laminar flow. The frictional force between the vessel wall and the layer is maximal in the outer layer and so it moves very slowly and sometimes it does not move. The velocities of the successive layers from the periphery towards the center of the stream go on increasing. The frictional force is minimal at the center and so, the velocity is greatest at the center of the stream. So the velocity is different in different laminas of the fluid and the velocity at the center is called **axial velocity**. The velocity profile will be a **parabola (Fig. 25.1B)**.

FLOW CONTINUITY EQUATION

The product of velocity and cross-sectional area is a constant. If F is the flow, A, the cross-sectional area and V, the velocity, then $F = A_1V_1 = A_2V_2$, etc. If the vessel becomes narrow, velocity will be more. Velocity is the average linear velocity because velocity is different in different laminae. For example, in the aorta:

F = AV so, V = F/A where F is the cardiac output. The overall blood flow in the circulation is the cardiac output.

Cardiac output = 6000 mL/min = 100 mL/sec

Cross-sectional area of aorta = 4.5 cm²

$$V = \frac{100 \text{ mL/sec}}{4.5 \text{ cm}^2} = 22.2 \text{ cm/sec}$$

In the capillaries, velocity is 0.02 cm/sec (**Fig. 25.2**).

Daniel Bernoulli combined the law of conservation of energy and flow continuity equation and put forward **Bernoulli's principle**: It states that when a constant amount of fluid flows through a tube, sum of its potential energy and the kinetic energy remain constant.

Kinetic energy = 1/2 mv².

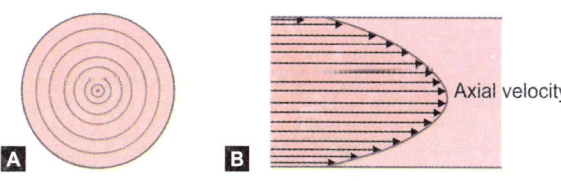

Figs. 25.1A and B: (A) Cross-section of blood vessel showing concentric laminae of blood flowing through the vessels in laminar flow; (B) Parabolic distribution of velocities in laminar flow.

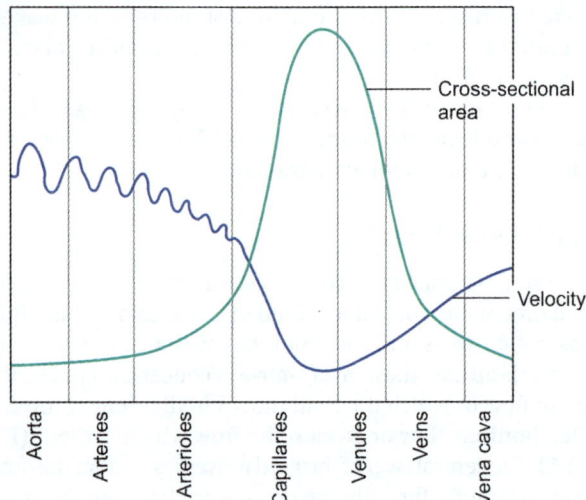

Fig. 25.2: Relationship between velocity of blood flow and cross-sectional area in different segments of vascular system.

CRITICAL VELOCITY

In the course of a blood vessel, if there is narrowing of the vessel the velocity will be increased. Streamline flow occurs at velocities up to a certain velocity called **critical velocity**. When the velocity increases above the critical velocity, the flow becomes turbulent. **Turbulent flow** means that the blood flows crosswise in the vessel as well as along the vessel forming whorls in the blood column called **Eddy currents** (Fig. 25.3). This increases the resistance to the flow of blood since it increases friction of flow in the vessel. *Turbulent flow creates sound whereas streamline flow is silent.* If the blood vessel takes a sharp turn or if the blood vessel becomes narrow due to atherosclerosis or due to spasm of the vessel, the flow becomes turbulent. There is no mixing of the different layers of the blood column in laminar flow. But in turbulent flow, blood flows in different directions in the vessel and there is continuous mixing of blood within the vessel.

At high velocities, the flow of fluid becomes turbulent and does not remain streamlined. The probability of turbulence is also related to the diameter of the vessel, density of blood and viscosity of blood. This relationship was studied by **Osborne Reynolds**. He studied the conditions in which turbulence of flow occurs and found out that:

Velocity (V) of flow ∝ $\dfrac{\text{Viscosity of fluid } (\eta)}{\text{Density of fluid } (\rho) \times \text{Diameter of the vessel (D)}}$
(in cm/sec)

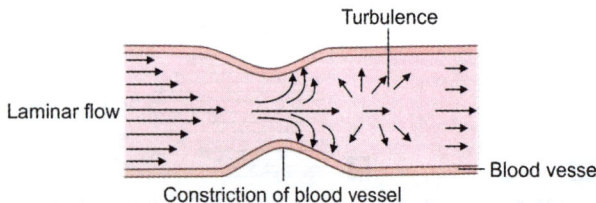

Figs. 25.3: Turbulence in the flow of blood beyond the area of constriction of blood vessel.

$$V \propto \dfrac{\eta}{\rho \times D} \text{ or } V = \text{Re } \eta/\rho D$$

Where, **Re** is a constant called **Reynolds number**.

$$\text{Re} = \dfrac{V\rho D}{\eta} \quad \text{i.e., } \dfrac{\text{Inertial forces}}{\text{Viscous forces}}$$

When Reynolds number is less than 1000, the flow is always laminar. As the value of Re increases, the probability of turbulence also increases. Above an Re value of 2000, turbulent flow occurs even in straight smooth vessels. *When Re is greater than 3000, turbulence is always present in the flow.* If viscosity is more, Re will be less and *vice versa*. Since the viscosity of blood is high normally, the probability of turbulence is less. Viscosity is decreased in conditions, such as fever, anemia, etc. In these conditions, Re is more and there is probability of turbulence. In anemia, since the viscosity is decreased, systolic murmurs are heard while auscultating the heart. *Turbulence of blood flow is responsible for cardiac murmurs and the Korotkoff's sounds* (while recording blood pressure).

Turbulence is always present in the proximal aorta and pulmonary artery because of the following reasons:
- Velocity of flow is high, i.e., the velocity exceeds the critical velocity at the peak of ventricular systole.
- Flow is pulsatile.
- Sudden reduction in the diameter when blood flows from the ventricle to aorta and pulmonary artery.
- When compared to smaller vessels the diameter of aorta and pulmonary artery is large. Reynolds number increases when there is increase in the vessel diameter. In small vessels, due to small diameter, Reynolds number is never high enough to cause turbulence.

Cause of Turbulence When Velocity is increased

Turbulence occurs if velocity of blood flow is increased. When a blood vessel narrows, velocity is increased and Re is also increased as in stenosis of valves, constriction of vessels, etc. When the velocity is increased, the central axial velocity is very high and kinetic energy is also high in the central stream. Potential energy is minimal in the central stream. In the layers closer to the vessel wall, there is maximum potential energy and least kinetic energy.

This sets up a potential energy gradient between the layers closer to the vessel wall and the central layer. So the peripheral layer tends to move inwards. This sets up **Eddy currents or turbulence**. This is only seen when the velocity of the central stream is very much increased as in obstruction to the vessel.

Turbulence is associated with sound. This is the basis of Korotkoff's sounds while recording blood pressure (BP). When the brachial artery is occluded by the BP cuff and when the pressure is released slowly, sounds are heard due to flow of blood through the compressed vessel at high velocity. So, there will be turbulence when the velocity is increased or when viscosity is decreased.

CIRCULATION TIME

Total circulation time is defined as the time which a particle of blood takes to make a complete round around systemic and pulmonary circulation. It is estimated in man by injecting a dye called **fluorescein** into the arm vein on one side. The time taken by the dye to appear in the opposite arm is the circulation time. This can be detected by ultraviolet light, where, fluorescence is produced in the minute vessels of skin of the opposite arm. So the experiment should be conducted in a dark room.

Total circulation time = 21 sec

Similarly, circulation time in different parts can be estimated like **arm-to-face** circulation time. Histamine (0.001 mg) is injected into the arm vein and time at which flushing of face occur is found out. This time is arm-to-face circulation time and this method is applicable only in fair skinned persons. Commonly used method is **arm-to-tongue** circulation time. A bile salt preparation is injected intravenously into the arm vein. Time at which bitter taste first appears in the tongue is noted. This is arm-to-tongue circulation time which is approximately 15 seconds.

Variation in Circulation Time

Increase in circulation time occurs when velocity of blood is decreased as in myxedema, cardiac failure, hypotension, etc.

Circulation time is decreased in exercise, hyperthyroidism, following adrenaline injection, etc.

RESISTANCE TO FLOW OF BLOOD

Resistance is the impediment (hindrance) to blood flow in a vessel.

Flow = P/R or R = P/F

Where P is the mean pressure in the vessel and R the resistance.

Resistance is expressed in **R units** or peripheral resistance unit (**PRU**), which is obtained by dividing pressure in mm Hg by flow in mL/sec. For example, when the mean arterial pressure is 90 mm Hg and left ventricular output is 90 mL/sec, total peripheral resistance is 90 mm Hg/90 mL/sec = 1 R unit.

In the pulmonary system, the mean pulmonary arterial pressure is 14 mm Hg. Therefore, when cardiac output is 90 mL/sec, the total pulmonary vascular resistance will be about 14 mm Hg divided by 90 mL/sec, which is equal to 0.15 R units.

Resistance to flow is influenced by several factors. This was studied by **Jean Louis Poiseuille** using long narrow tubes of uniform radius. Factors which influence the flow through the tubes were studied. He found out that flow (F) is directly proportional to the pressure difference between the ends of the tube (P = PA–PB) and the fourth power of the radius (r) of the tube and inversely proportional to the length of the tube (L) and the viscosity of blood (η) in the tube, provided the tube length exceeded a certain minimum. This is **Poiseuille's law**. Various factors influencing flow were studied and the final equation known as **Poiseuille-Hagen formula** was put forward as follows:

$$F = P \times (\pi/8) \times (1/\eta) \times (r^4/L) \text{ where P is } P_A - P_B$$

$$F = \frac{P\pi r^4}{8L\eta}$$

The relationship between the flow in a long narrow tube, the viscosity of the fluid and the radius of the tube is expressed mathematically in this formula.

From the above formula (Poiseuille-Hagen formula), when the radius is reduced to half, flow will be 1/16. When viscosity is increased, flow will be reduced.

F = P/R or R = P/F

Substituting Poiseuille-Hagen formula for F, $1/R = \dfrac{\pi r^4}{8L\eta}$

or

$$R = \frac{8L\eta}{\pi r^4}$$

Where, $8/\pi$ is a constant. Thus resistance varies with viscosity and the geometry of the tube (L/r4).

Resistance is directly proportional to the length of the tube and inversely proportional to the fourth power of the radius of the tube. This explains the differences in blood flow in the renal cortex and medulla, where blood viscosity, capillary length and capillary diameter all have a role. But flow varies directly with the fourth power of radius. Thus, blood flow and resistance to flow in the body are markedly affected by small changes in the caliber of the vessels. For example, the blood flow through a vessel is doubled when its radius is increased by 20%. When the radius is doubled, resistance is reduced by 6% of its previous value. *This is the reason why variation in the arteriolar diameter causes wide changes in systemic arterial pressure.*

Three conditions have to be met to obey Poiseuille's law. They are:
1. Flow should be laminar or streamline
2. Fluid should have uniform velocity
3. Flow should be continuous

Small vessels obey all the above conditions, i.e., laminar flow occur in small vessels under physiological conditions. Velocity is uniform in small blood vessels and continuous flow is present in capillaries and veins. But in large arteries, such as aorta, flow is pulsatile and not continuous.

Conversion of Pulsatile Flow in Large Arteries into Continuous Flow Beyond Arterioles

Two main factors are responsible:
1. Elasticity of vessel wall
2. Peripheral resistance

Borelli's Experiment

To explain how pulsatile flow in the aorta is converted to continuous flow in the capillaries, an experiment was conducted by **Borelli**. The different steps are:

1. A bulb syringe is taken with a one-way valve on one side. A short tube from one end of the bulb dips into water. When the bulb is pressed and released, water flows out through the long tube on the other end intermittently **(Fig. 25.4)**.
2. Next the long tube was fitted with a nozzle at the free end to increase the resistance or to decrease the diameter. The experiment is performed and it is seen that the flow is again intermittent.
3. The long rigid tube from the bulb is replaced by an elastic tube and again the flow was found to be intermittent.
4. The nozzle was connected to the elastic tube and when the experiment was done it was seen that the flow became continuous. In this case, there was elasticity as well as resistance to outflow. This is compared to the elasticity and peripheral resistance in the small vessels.

In the arterioles, there is elasticity as well as peripheral resistance due to the presence of elastic fibers and smooth muscle fibers. So there is continuous flow beyond arterioles. Pulsatile flow is seen in the capillaries in patients with hyperthyroidism. In these patients, there is arteriolar vasodilatation due to increased metabolism. This decreases the peripheral arteriolar resistance leading to pulsatile flow in the capillaries.

Diastolic pressure is maintained by the property of elasticity and peripheral resistance of blood vessels. Otherwise, there will not be flow during diastole.

Viscosity

Viscosity (η) is the internal friction within the fluid layer. Flowing blood creates a force on the endothelium that is parallel to the long axis of the vessel. This is shearing force or shear stress. Newton expressed viscosity as the ratio of the shearing force applied, to the shearing strain rate. Shearing force is the force applied for unit area or F/A where, A is the area between two adjacent layers in the fluid. Shear strain rate is the velocity gradient of the fluid expressed as $\Delta V/\Delta X$ where V is the velocity and X the area between two adjacent layers of the fluid. In other words, shear rate is the rate at which the axial velocity increases from the vessel wall towards the lumen. Unit of viscosity is **dynes sec/cm^2 or poise**.

$$\eta = \frac{F/A}{\Delta V/\Delta X}$$

Those fluids which have constant viscosity, irrespective of fluid velocity are called **Newtonian fluids** and fluids in which viscosity varies with fluid velocity are called **non-Newtonian fluids**. Plasma is considered to be a Newtonian fluid but whole blood is a non-Newtonian fluid because it is a suspension of cells in plasma. Plasma is about 1.8 times as viscous as water and whole blood is 3–4 times as viscous as water.

Factors Influencing Viscosity of Blood

❖ **Hematocrit**: It is the percentage of the volume of blood occupied by red blood cells. The viscosity increases with increase in hematocrit value. For example, viscosity is high in polycythemia-vera and at high altitudes. Hematocrit value influences viscosity especially in large vessels. In large vessels, increase in hematocrit causes appreciable increase in viscosity. But in vessels smaller than 100 μm in diameter, such as arterioles, capillaries and venules, the viscosity change per unit change in hematocrit is much less. This is due to differences in the nature of flow through the small vessels.

❖ **Body temperature**: Increase in **temperature** decreases viscosity.

❖ **Plasma protein**: When plasma protein concentration is increased, viscosity is also increased.

❖ **Shape of RBC**: When there is an alteration in the shape of RBC, viscosity will be increased. For example, in hereditary spherocytosis, viscosity is increased because the cells are abnormally rigid.

❖ **Velocity of blood flow**: When the velocity is decreased, there is increase in viscosity. This is due to increased tendency for Rouleaux formation. When the velocity is decreased, the cells tend to stick to the wall of the vessels causing blockage and increase in frictional force and an apparent increase in viscosity.

Fahraeus-Lindqvist Effect and Plasma Skimming

Even though the velocity of fluid is slow in the capillaries, the viscosity is not much increased. This is because of the effect

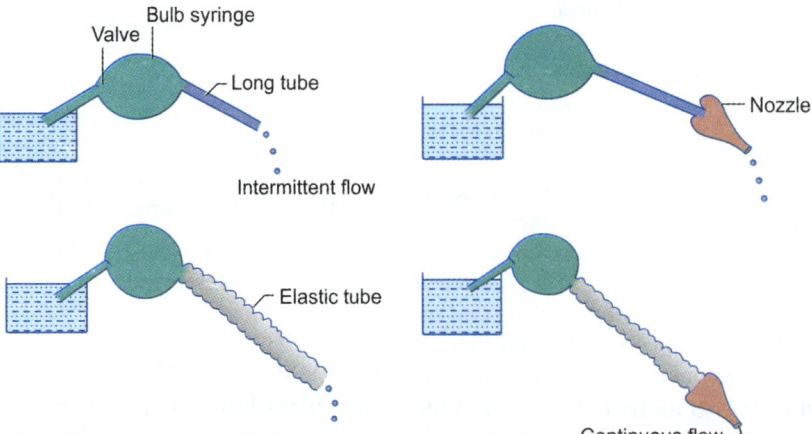

Fig. 25.4: Borelli's experiment to prove that elasticity and resistance are responsible for the conversion of intermittent flow to continuous flow.

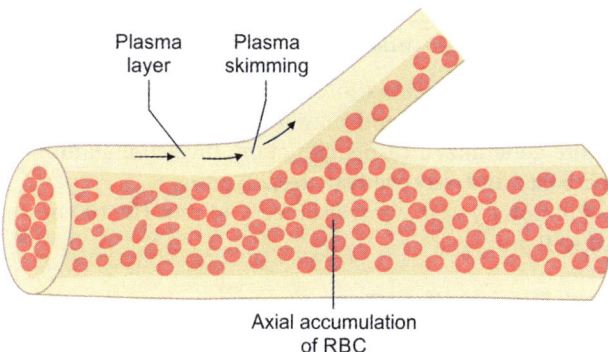

Fig. 25.5: Plasma skimming.

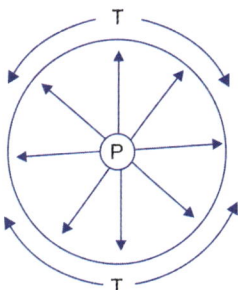

Fig. 25.6: Relation between distending pressure (P) and wall tension (T) in a hollow spherical organ.

called Fahraeus-Lindqvist effect. Blood in vessels smaller than 0.5 mm in diameter show a decrease in viscosity because the red blood cells tend to align themselves in the central axial stream in an orderly pattern. In the small blood vessels, there are factors which increase viscosity and which decrease viscosity. If a branch arises at right angles to the vessel, cell-poor blood flows through the branch. This is called plasma skimming (**Fig. 25.5**). In the capillaries, hematocrit value is less than that of total blood hematocrit value because of plasma skimming. Thus, there is a reduction in the viscosity of blood flowing through small vessels, such as capillaries and the viscosity is more or less uniform in these vessels.

Geometry of the Tube (L/r4) and Critical Closing Pressure

Radius (r) of the tube is a very important factor in regulating blood flow. If radius is decreased, resistance will be increased which leads to a reduction in the flow. It is the distensibility of the blood vessel that causes deviation of pressure-flow relationship in vivo. Distensibility depends on neural and chemical factors which affect the radius of the tube. Arterioles are the main sites of peripheral resistance in the vascular system. There are three important factors which affect the diameter of the vessel:
1. Hydrostatic pressure which tends to distend the tube.
2. Elastic tension in the vessel wall and smooth muscle tone tend to decrease the lumen diameter. There is a resting sympathetic tone in the blood vessel.
3. Tissue pressure, i.e., the vessels is surrounded by tissues that exert a small but definite pressure on the vessels.

When the hydrostatic pressure is decreased, at a particular stage, the other three forces oppose the tendency for the vessel to remain open and the vessel wall closes. The pressure at which blood vessel closes is known as **critical closing pressure (CCP)**. For flow to occur, there should be certain amount of pressure especially in the capillaries. When the intraluminal pressure falls below the tissue pressure, the vessel collapses.

Law of Laplace

Law of Laplace states that the **tension** (T) in the wall of a cylinder is equal to the product of the **transmural pressure** (P) and the **radius** of the tube (r) divided by the **wall thickness**. The transmural pressure is the pressure inside and outside the cylinder. When a blood vessel is taken, the tissue pressure is low and is negligible. So in a blood vessel, the transmural pressure is equal to the intraluminal pressure. In thin-walled vessels like capillaries, thickness of the wall is negligible and it is also ignored. In thin-walled viscus, P = T divided by the two principal radii of curvature of the viscus (**Fig. 25.6**). Thus, $P = T/r_1 + T/r_2 = T(1/r_1 + 1/r_2)$. In a cylinder, such as blood vessel one radius of curvature is infinite, so $P = T/r$. In the case of a sphere, $r_1 = r_2$, so $P = 2T/r$

Application of Law of Laplace in CVS

- **Critical closing pressure** can be explained by this law. From the above equation $P = T/r$, when pressure decreases, the stretching pressure in the vessel wall, i.e., tension also decreases. This causes a decrease in the radius. When r is less, T is also less. This becomes a vicious cycle. When the pressure in a small blood vessel is reduced, a point is reached at which no blood flows through the vessel even though the intraluminal pressure is not zero. This is because when the intraluminal pressure falls below the tissue pressure, the pressure exerted by the tissues on the blood vessels causes the vessel to collapse. The pressure at which the flow ceases is called **critical closing pressure** (Fig. 25.7). This is the reason why most of the capillaries in the inactive tissues are collapsed. The pressure in these capillaries is low because precapillary sphincters are constricted at rest.
- The reason why capillaries do not rupture even though thin walled can be explained based on the equation $P = T/r$. Capillaries are small in diameter and r is small. The internal pressure in the capillary is about 25 mm Hg. Capillaries can withstand this high pressure without rupturing because they have a very small radius (r). Even though the wall tension is low, the small value of 'r' in the denominator helps the capillaries to withstand the very high P. The tension to be exerted on the wall needs to be very less to balance the distending pressure because of the small radius. In the aorta tension in the wall is 170,000 dynes/cm, whereas in the capillaries, tension in the wall is only 16 dynes/cm.
- **Application of law of Laplace in dilated diseased heart**: The law of Laplace puts the dilated heart at a disadvantage.

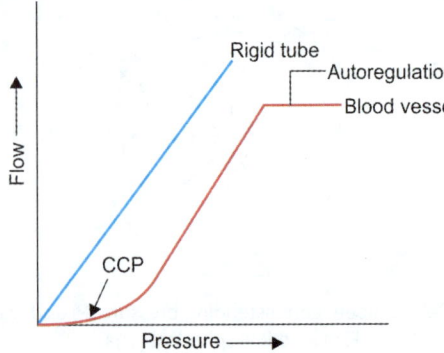

Fig. 25.7: Relation of pressure to flow in a rigid tube and blood vessel. In the blood vessel, flow is maintained at a constant rate by autoregulation which occurs only within a particular range of pressure. Below that pressure, autoregulation fails and the flow decreases and stop before the pressure reaches zero value. The pressure at which flow stops is critical closing pressure.

When the radius of the cardiac chamber increases, the tension to be developed in the wall must go up proportionately if the intraventricular pressure is to be maintained within normal limits. So, the force of contraction should be increased and the dilated heart must do more work to maintain the cardiac output. Cardiac failure may result due to reduced O_2 supply because O_2 demand is more when more work has to be done.

Application of Law of Laplace in Other Parts of the Body

- In accordance with the law of Laplace, the lower the functional residual capacity of lungs, the more difficult it is to inflate it. This is because the radii of the alveoli will be small when the FRC is less. So, more pressure is required to inflate them.
- Based on $P = 2T/r$, the greater the gastric filling, the lower is the pressure that causes gastric emptying. This helps in proper digestion.
- In the urinary bladder as the bladder gets filled with urine, the detrusor muscle tension (T) does not increase due to the property of plasticity of smooth muscles. There is also corresponding increase in the radius (r) of the bladder. This prevents rise of intravesical pressure (P) even if the bladder fills up to greater volumes. So the feeling of fullness occurs only when the intravesical volume exceeds the physiological limit.

Measurement of Resistance

Resistance can be found out by measuring flow and pressure.
Flow (F) = Pressure/Resistance or P/R
R = P/F

Total peripheral vascular resistance (TPVR)

$$= \frac{P_{SA} - P_{SV}}{\text{Cardiac output (6 L/min)}}$$

$P_{SA} - P_{SV}$ is the pressure difference between an artery and vein in the periphery.

$$TPVR = \frac{100 \text{ mm Hg}}{100 \text{ mL/sec}} = 1 \text{ R unit (resistance unit)}$$

The value increases in conditions of vasoconstriction or in hypertension and may increase up to 4 R units in severe generalized vasoconstriction. In vasodilatation, it is decreased and may even fall to 0.2 R units.

Pulmonary vascular resistance = 14 mm Hg/100 mL/sec = 0.14 R unit

Work Done by the Heart

Heart has to perform two types of work:
1. To pump blood from heart to blood vessels (potential energy)
2. To impart certain amount of energy to blood for its forward movement (kinetic energy)

Total work = Potential energy (PE) + Kinetic energy (KE)
PE = Pressure × Volume
KE = ½ mv^2, where v is the velocity of blood and m is the mass.

Blood pressure is defined as the lateral pressure exerted on the wall of the blood vessel and it depends on kinetic energy.

TESTS TO ASSESS CARDIAC FUNCTION

Investigations involving direct cardiac catheterization are the standard methods for assessing cardiovascular functions. But these invasive procedures have catheter-induced vascular and cardiac complications. The non-invasive techniques permit study of cardiac patients reliably and in a reproducible way without ill effects.

Noninvasive Techniques

- Electrocardiogram
  - Standard ECG
  - Holter monitoring
  - Vector cardiogram
  - Treadmill test (exercise-stress testing)
- Chest X-ray
- Echocardiogram
  - Standard echocardiogram
  - Doppler study
    - Color Doppler
    - Pulsed wave Doppler
    - Continuous wave Doppler
  - Trans-esophageal echo
- CT scan
  - Conventional CT scan
  - Single photon emission CT scan (SPECT)
- Positron emission tomography (PET) scan
- Magnetic resonance imaging (MRI) scan
- Radionuclide imaging

ECG is useful for diagnosing cardiac arrhythmias, myocardial infarction, heart blocks, etc. (*refer* Chapter 23 for details).

Treadmill test can diagnose angina and coronary artery disease. It also helps to determine safe level of exercise in cardiac patients. It is a follow up to assess improvement in coronary artery circulation in patients with myocardial infarction. In this test, ECG, heart rate, respiration, and blood pressure are recorded during exercise.

Echocardiography

In echocardiography, cardiac function is monitored using ultrasonic waves.

2D Echocardiography

In 2D echo imaging is done from multiple acoustic windows with different transducer rotations. Images of heart and great vessels can be displayed in real time and in various planes.

Uses of 2D echo

- To assess cardiac chamber sizes by electronic calipers. Mainly systolic and diastolic dimensions of left ventricle are measured.
- Regional wall motion abnormalities can be assessed
- Useful in diagnosing left ventricular hypertrophy
- Helps in assessing valve abnormalities related to leaflet thickness, mobility, calcification, etc.
- Helps to detect valve stenosis, severity of stenosis by measuring valve orifice, regurgitation, etc.
- Pericardial effusion can be visualized as a black echo lucent ovoid structure surrounding the heart. Echo-guided pericardiocentesis can be done.
- Used in visualizing intracardiac mass. It is seen as echo dense structure in cardiac chambers.
- Aortic diseases involving proximal aorta and arch of aorta can be visualized.

Doppler Echo

Principle is based on ultrasound waves reflecting off moving RBCs to assess the velocity of blood flow across valves, in cardiac chambers and great vessels. A piezoelectric probe works both as a transmitter of ultrasonic waves as well as a receiver of the reflected waves from different parts of the heart. The reflected waves are displayed against time on a monitor. It gives information like morphology of the heart, valves and also helps to determine ejection fraction and cardiac output.

Color flow Doppler displays blood velocities in real time superimposed on a 2D echo image. Blood velocities are color coded and colors indicate the direction of blood flow. Blue towards transducer, red away from the transducer and green indicates turbulent flow. Regurgitant lesions and shunts can be assessed by color Doppler.

Pulsed wave Doppler measures the blood velocity in a specific location in a 2D image and displays the velocities in a spectral pattern using time as X-axis.

Continuous wave Doppler can measure high blood velocities. It can be used to assess intracardiac pressure and severity of stenosis.

Tissue Doppler measures velocity of myocardial movements.

Uses of Doppler echo

- Velocity of blood flow across a stenotic valve can be assessed.
- Can detect valve regurgitation by seeing the high velocity jet in the proximal chamber.
- Intracardiac pressures can be calculated from the peak velocity signal of a regurgitant lesion.
- Cardiac output can be calculated by the formula

Stroke volume = outflow area × velocity × time in seconds of left ventricular outflow tract.

Cardiac output = stroke volume × heart rate

- Help to assess congenital stenotic or regurgitant valve lesions

Trans-esophageal Echo

Uses

- For the diagnosis of aortic diseases
- To detect masses in atria
- Helps to define the source of embolism
- Helps to detect vegetation in infective endocarditis
- Used for the evaluation of mitral valve prosthesis
- Used in emergency situations, such as pericardial tamponade, acute valvular regurgitation due to papillary muscle dysfunction.

SPECT Scan

SPECT scan (single photon emission CT scan) evaluates coronary circulation and working of the heart. SPECT scan is presented as cross-sectional slices and so can provide true 3D information. It helps to image myocardial perfusion for the diagnosis of ischemic heart disease. Imaging can point out areas of myocardium receiving less blood supply.

PET Scan

PET scan is very accurate in detecting areas of low blood flow. It can detect dead cells as well as living viable heart cells which can be saved. Used to detect coronary artery disease (CAD), myocardial infarction, etc. PET scans generally have a higher sensitivity and specificity for detecting viable myocardium and identifying CAD. It can also be used to detect calcium deposition in an atherosclerotic plaque and can also detect myocarditis. It is also useful in assessing the benefit of angioplasty, stenting or coronary artery bypass grafting.

MRI Scan

The patient is placed in a high strength magnetic field. The hydrogen nuclei (protons) behave, such as miniature spinning magnets and align parallel to external magnetic field with a rotation (precession) frequency proportional to the magnetic field. When an RF wave with frequency identical to the precession frequency is applied by a coil over a body region, the magnetic moment will be flipped at an angle to the magnetic field (excitation). After excitation, the magnetic moment gradually returns to baseline emitting RF signals which are captured by the receiver coils and used to create the final image. Intravenous gadolinium containing paramagnetic contrast media can be used to increase the signal intensity or brightness in the area of interest. MRI with contrast can study tissue perfusion and viability.

The velocity of blood flow and cross-sectional area over time can be measured and the valvular regurgitant fractions, shunt ratios, etc., can be measured.

Uses of MRI in assessing cardiac function
- Assess myocardial viability and perfusion
- Assess right and left ventricular volumes and mass and systolic function
- To detect congenital heart disease and shunt ratio calculation
- Helps in the evaluation of valvular, pericardial and aortic diseases
- To detect myopathies of heart

MULTIPLE CHOICE QUESTIONS

1. **All the following occur as blood flows through the systemic capillaries, *except*:**
   a. Its hematocrit increases
   b. Hemoglobin dissociation curve shifts to the left
   c. Protein content increases
   d. Red blood cells increase in size

2. **When radius of resistance vessel is increased which of the following is increased?**
   a. Systolic blood pressure
   b. Diastolic blood pressure
   c. Viscosity of blood
   d. Capillary blood flow

3. **When viscosity of blood is increased which of the following is increased?**
   a. Mean blood pressure
   b. Radius of resistance vessel
   c. Central venous pressure
   d. Capillary blood flow

4. **The velocity of blood flow:**
   a. Falls to zero in the descending aorta during diastole
   b. Is higher in the capillaries than in the arterioles
   c. Is higher in the veins than in the venules
   d. Is higher in the veins than in the arteries

5. **Laminar flow is directly proportional to:**
   a. Density
   b. Radius
   c. Viscosity
   d. Velocity

6. **In anemia, turbulent flow occur due to:**
   a. Decrease in viscosity
   b. Decrease in velocity
   c. Decrease in Reynolds number
   d. Decrease in plasma proteins

7. **Rate of flow is directly proportional to:**
   a. Length of the tube
   b. Radius of the tube
   c. Density
   d. Viscosity

8. **Poiseuille-Hagen formula is used to find out:**
   a. Reynolds number
   b. Rate of flow through a tube
   c. Velocity of flow
   d. Resistance to flow

9. **Highest velocity is seen in:**
   a. Capillaries
   b. Small arteries
   c. Arterioles
   d. Aorta

10. **Of the following, the velocity of blood is maximum in the:**
    a. Large veins
    b. Small veins
    c. Venules
    d. Capillaries

11. **Maximum velocity of blood is seen in the:**
    a. Aorta
    b. Artery
    c. Arteriole
    d. Capillary

12. **Mean velocity of blood in the aorta is:**
    a. 4 cm/sec
    b. 40 cm/sec
    c. 20 cm/sec
    d. 30 cm/sec

13. **Linear velocity of blood at normal cardiac output in the aorta is:**
    a. 32 cm/sec
    b. 64 cm/sec
    c. 8 cm/sec
    d. 50 cm/sec

14. **Turbulent blood flow is produced by:**
    a. Decreased velocity of circulation
    b. Decreased cardiac output
    c. Decreased hematocrit
    d. Decreased heart rate

15. **Velocity of blood flow is inversely proportional to:**
    a. Viscosity
    b. Flow
    c. Cross-sectional area
    d. Length

16. **Blood flow through a vessel varies directly with:**
    a. Resistance
    b. Viscosity
    c. Pressure difference between the ends
    d. Length of vessel

17. **The resistance of a blood vessel is 16 PRU. Doubling the vessel diameter would change the resistance to:**
    a. 1 PRU
    b. 2 PRU
    c. 8 PRU
    d. 12 PRU

18. **Calculate peripheral resistance if cardiac output is 5.4 L/min and mean arterial pressure 90 mm Hg**
    a. 11
    b. 12
    c. 14
    d. 16

19. **Viscosity of blood is:**
    a. Same as ECF
    b. 10 times that of urine
    c. 5 to 6 times more than that of water
    d. 5 to 6 times less than that of water

20. **Bernoulli principle states that:**
    a. Flow velocity is inversely related to pressure in a vessel
    b. Measure of blood flow
    c. Sum of kinetic energy of flow and pressure energy is constant
    d. All of the above are correct

ANSWERS

1. b	2. d	3. a	4. c	5. c
6. a	7. b	8. b	9. d	10. a
11. a	12. b	13. a	14. c	15. c
16. c	17. a	18. d	19. c	20. c

Heart Rate

CHAPTER 26

LEARNING OBJECTIVES

Must know
- Describe the innervation of heart with the help of diagrams
- Describe the cardiovascular reflexes
- Describe the factors affecting heart rate
- Explain the regulation of heart rate
- Describe sinoaortic reflex and its significance

Desirable to know
- Explain sympathovagal balance and heart rate variability

INTRODUCTION

PY5.8: Describe and discuss local and systemic cardiovascular regulatory mechanisms.
PY5.9: Describe the factors affecting heart rate, regulation of cardiac output and blood pressure.

The pacemaker of heart, i.e., the sinoatrial node generates impulses and the conducting tissue conducts impulses to the different parts of the heart. If the pacemaker is out of order, the rest of the heart can generate impulses at a lower rate. Normally, in humans, heart rate is kept constant. Heart rate varies depending on the body surface area and depending on the species. For example, in elephant, heart rate is 25/min; in rabbit, 200/min; and in rat, 300/min.

Normal heart rate in adult—60–100/min
In well-trained athletes—60/min due to increased vagal tone
In newborn—120–130/min

Variation in Heart Rate

Increase in heart rate from normal is called **tachycardia**. Decrease in heart rate is called **bradycardia (Table 26.1)**.

FACTORS AFFECTING HEART RATE

- Neural factors
- Chemical factors
- Physical factors
- Age and sex.

Neural Factors

Innervation of Heart

Heart is supplied by sympathetic and parasympathetic divisions of the nervous system **(Fig. 26.1)**.

Table 26.1: Variations in heart rate.

	Physiological	Pathological
Tachycardia	• Infancy • Excitement, anger • Exercise • Extreme pain • Inspiration • Increased temperature • High altitude	• Fever (10 beats rise for 1°F) • Hyperthyroidism • Cardiac arrhythmias
Bradycardia	• Sleep • Expiration • Well-trained athletes	• Raised intracranial tension • Hypothyroidism • Heart block

Neural regulation of heart rate is important because it responds within seconds.

Sympathetic Innervation

The sympathetic fibers that supply the heart arise from **intermediolateral horn cells** of T_1 to T_5 segments of spinal cord. T_2 and T_3 segments send maximum number of fibers to the heart. These form the preganglionic neurons. These fibers synapse in the sympathetic ganglion and the unmyelinated postganglionic fibers form three groups, **superior, middle and inferior cardiac nerves**. Maximum number of fibers to the heart comes through middle cardiac nerve arising from the stellate ganglion. On the way to the heart they combine with parasympathetic fibers and together form the **deep and superficial cardiac plexus**, which supply the heart.

Sympathetic fibers supply the whole of the heart, i.e., the nodal tissues, atrial and ventricular musculature. Since SA node originates from the right side of the heart, the sympathetic fibers coming from the right side supply SA node. Sympathetic fibers from the left side supply the AV node.

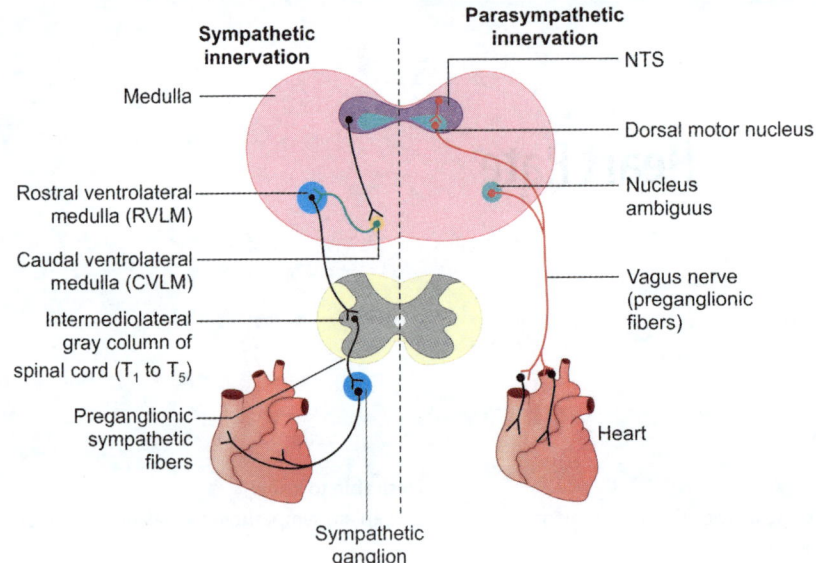

Fig. 26.1: Innervation of heart. Sympathetic innervation is shown on the left side and parasympathetic innervation on the right side.
(NTS: nucleus of the tractus solitarius)

The postganglionic fibers release **norepinephrine** as the neurotransmitter.

Effects of Sympathetic Stimulation on Heart

- Positive chronotropic effect (increase in heart rate)
- Positive dromotropic effect (increase in conductivity)
- Positive bathmotropic effect (increase in excitability)
- Positive inotropic effect (increase in force of contraction)

Mechanism of Action of Sympathetic Fibers on Heart

Norepinephrine exerts its effect on the body via two types of receptors, **and receptors**. The effects vary depending on the type of receptor stimulated. In the heart, norepinephrine produces its effect via β-**receptors**. Stimulation of β-receptors of the nodal tissue decreases K^+ permeability. The potential does not come to the normal resting level during repolarization. The slope of the pre-potential become steep and the heart rate is increased due to increase in rhythmicity **(Fig. 26.2)**. It is the slope of the prepotential that determines the heart rate. Norepinephrine secreted by the sympathetic endings binds to the $β_1$ receptors leading to increase in the intracellular cAMP levels. This facilitates the opening of L-Ca^{2+} channels, increasing I Ca^{2+} and the rapidity of the depolarization phase of the action potential. There is decrease in the refractory period of myocardium. There is also increase in the force of contraction of heart. Since there is increase in heart rate, sympathetic center in the spinal cord is also called **cardio-acceleratory center**.

The neurons of the cardioaccelerator center are under higher influences from cerebral cortex and medulla oblongata. A constant stream of impulses passes through the sympathetic fibers to the heart under the control of higher centers, which is called **sympathetic tone**. Sympathetic tone to the heart is insignificant in human, but the sympathetic

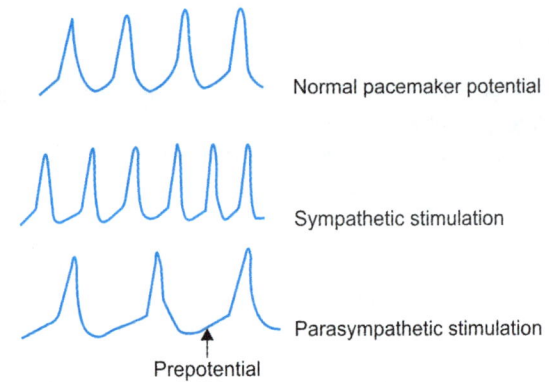

Fig. 26.2: Effect of sympathetic and parasympathetic stimulation on the pacemaker potential.

tone to the blood vessels is very important in maintaining normal blood pressure. *Parasympathetic tone to the blood vessels is negligible.*

Parasympathetic Innervation of Heart

Parasympathetic fibers supplying the heart originate in the **dorsal nucleus of vagus** in the medulla, which is referred to as **cardioinhibitory center (CIC)**. Parasympathetic fibers also originate from the **nucleus of tractus solitarius and nucleus ambiguus (Fig. 26.1)**. Preganglionic myelinated fibers are very long and they reach the heart through the right and the left vagus. The ganglion is close to the heart and the fibers mix with the sympathetic fibers to form the superficial and deep cardiac plexus. Postganglionic unmyelinated parasympathetic fibers supply the SA node, AV node and atrial musculature. *Ventricle is devoid of parasympathetic efferent supply.* Right vagus supplies SA node and left vagus supplies AV node. *Parasympathetic tone or vagal tone is prominent in the human heart.* In well-trained athletes, the vagal tone is high under normal resting conditions and the heart rate will be 50–60/min.

Mechanism of Action of Parasympathetic Fibers

Parasympathetic stimulation has an inhibitory effect on heart, i.e., they depress the SA node and decrease heart rate. There is also increase in the refractory period of cardiac muscle. Neurotransmitter at the postganglionic ending is **acetylcholine**. The resting membrane potential of the SA node is brought to hyperpolarizing level, i.e., to about −80 to −85 mV due to increase in K^+ permeability. The acetylcholine released at the nerve endings via the βγ subunit of a G protein open a special set of K^+ channels. This action is mediated through M_2 muscarinic receptors. In addition, activation of the M_2 receptors decreases cAMP in the cells, and this slows the opening of Ca^{2+} channels. As a result, the slope of the pre-potential become less steep and the heart rate decreases **(Fig. 26.2)**. Rate of conduction of impulse as well as force of contraction of heart is also decreased. *Heart rate is kept constant by vagal tone. Sympathetics come into action only in times of emergencies.* If there is strong stimulation of vagus, it leads to vagal inhibition. The heart stops in diastole. After some time, the ventricle starts beating at its own rhythm, which is called **vagal escape**. The ventricular rhythm is called **idioventricular rhythm**.

If the vagal supply to the heart is cut, the heart rate increases to 150–180/min due to the over activity of sympathetics. The same effect is seen when a parasympatholytic drug is given.

If both the sympathetic supply and parasympathetic supply to the heart are cut, the heart rate comes to about 100/min. This proves that the balancing action between the sympathetic and the parasympathetic systems is responsible for maintaining the heart rate at normal level. Noradrenergic sympathetic fibers are epicardial, whereas the vagal cholinergic fibers are endocardial. Connections exist between the sympathetic and the parasympathetic innervation for the heart, which is responsible for the reciprocal inhibitory effects of the two innervations. Thus, acetylcholine acts pre-synaptically to reduce norepinephrine release from the sympathetic nerves, and neuropeptide-Y released from noradrenergic endings may inhibit the release of acetylcholine.

Central Influences on Heart Rate

There are four levels at which neurons are present that control the functioning of the heart.
1. Spinal cord
2. Medulla oblongata
3. Hypothalamus
4. Cerebral cortex.

Spinal Cord Level

The lateral horn cells in the thoracic segments (T_1–T_5) of the spinal cord form the **spinal cardioacceleratory center**. Even though these neurons are under the control of higher centers, they can spontaneously generate impulses if the higher control is cut off. For example, in spinal animals, changes in heart rate are observed in response to distension of bladder. Here, there is no higher control since the spinal cord is transectioned.

Medulla Oblongata and Hypothalamus

In the **reticular formation of medulla**, many vital centers are present that control cardiac function called cardiac centers. These centers control the lateral horn cells of spinal cord.

Hypothalamus is the center for autonomic functions. Rostral hypothalamus contains neurons which produce parasympathetic effect and caudal hypothalamus contains the center for sympathetic effects.

Cerebral Cortex

Stimulation of certain areas of the cortex like premotor area and motor area produces an increase in arterial blood pressure with intense constriction of cutaneous, splanchnic and renal vessels and dilatation in skeletal muscles. Cerebral cortex is the highest center that controls cardiovascular functions to a certain extent. There are descending tracts to the vasomotor center from the limbic cortex that relay in the hypothalamus. These fibers are responsible for the rise in blood pressure and tachycardia seen during sexual excitement and anger. Another example is the cardiovascular changes associated with flight and fright response.

Medullary Centers

Reticular formation of medulla contains the vital cardiovascular centers which are the prime centers concerned with neural control of circulation. The medullary centers exert their effect almost entirely through the autonomic nervous system (ANS). The medullary centers are:
❖ Cardioinhibitory center (parasympathetic center)
❖ Vasomotor center (sympathetic center).

Cardioinhibitory Center

Cardioinhibitory center (CIC) is a group of neurons constituted by **dorsal motor nucleus of vagus, nucleus tractus solitarius (NTS) and nucleus ambiguus (Fig. 26.3)**. There is a constant discharge of impulses from the CIC through the vagus which influences the activity of the heart. Continuous stream of impulses from the CIC to the heart is responsible for **vagal tone** which is very prominent in humans.

Vasomotor Center

Vasomotor center (VMC) or medullary sympathetic center—VMC consists of groups of neurons situated bilaterally in the reticular formation of medulla in the floor of the fourth ventricle. The cell bodies of these neurons are located in the **rostral ventrolateral medulla (RVLM)**. These neurons send impulses through the sympathetic fibers to the blood vessels and heart and influence the caliber of blood vessels and heart rate. The axons of the VMC go to the lateral horn cells of spinal cord and influence the discharge through the sympathetic fibers **(Fig. 26.3)**. The excitatory neurotransmitter at the axonal endings of VMC neurons is **glutamate**.

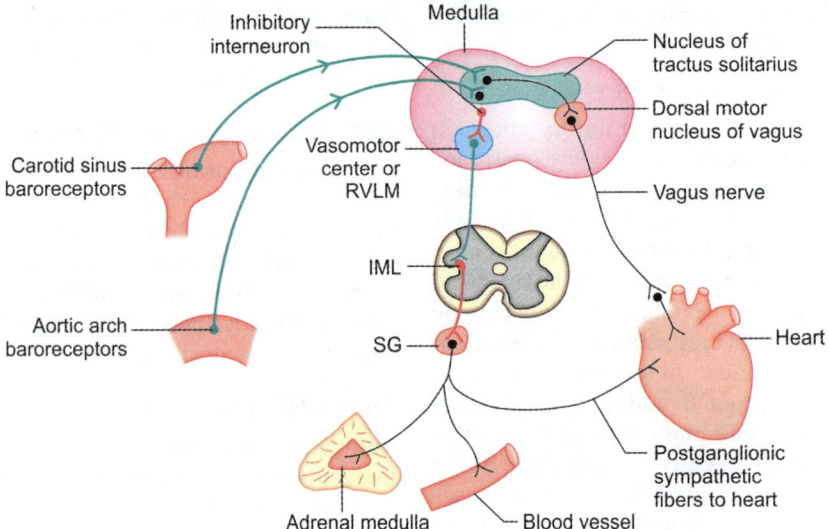

Fig. 26.3: Innervation of heart and pathway for sinoaortic reflex or baroreceptor reflex.
(IML: intermediolateral horn cells; SG: sympathetic ganglion)

The neurons of VMC show inherent tonic activity, i.e., they discharge rhythmically to excite the sympathetic preganglionic neurons in the intermediolateral horn (IML) cells of spinal cord of thoracolumbar area. This sympathetic tone maintains the blood vessels in a partial state of contraction called **sympathetic vasoconstrictor tone**.

Effects of Stimulation of VMC

- Vasoconstriction and increase in blood pressure
- Venoconstriction and increased venous return to heart
- Increase in heart rate
- Increase in the force of myocardial contraction.

Summary

CIC when stimulated leads to a reduction in heart rate since the vagus is inhibitory to the heart. When the VMC is stimulated, due to sympathetic stimulation, there is increase in heart rate and increase in blood pressure as a result of vasoconstriction and increase in peripheral resistance. In short, the CIC sends impulses through vagus to the heart and is responsible for the vagal tone of heart and the VMC sends impulses to the spinal cord neurons in the lateral horn and is responsible for the sympathetic vasoconstrictor tone of blood vessels.

AFFERENTS TO THE CARDIAC CENTERS

- Afferents from baroreceptors
- Parts of central nervous system
- Chemoreceptors and respiratory system
- Receptors within the heart and great blood vessels
- Miscellaneous afferents.

Afferents from Baroreceptors

Location of Baroreceptors

- Carotid sinus
- Aortic arch
- Walls of atria
- Pulmonary vascular bed
- Left ventricular wall.

Baroreceptors

Baroreceptors are receptors that respond to stretch. Stretch of the vessel wall or chambers of the heart stimulates the **baroreceptors**. Since increase in pressure in the vascular tree causes stretch of the vessel, baroreceptors are also called **pressoreceptors**. Baroreceptors are present in the root of the internal carotid artery just above the bifurcation of the common carotid artery. **Carotid sinus** is the dilated part of the root of the internal carotid artery that contains the baroreceptors. Baroreceptors are also present in the arch of aorta, called **aortic arch baroreceptors**. In the right atrium, the baroreceptors are concentrated around the openings of superior and inferior vena cava. In the **left atrium**, baroreceptors are found around the openings of pulmonary veins. They are also present in the wall of left ventricle.

Structure and Innervation of Baroreceptors

In the blood vessels, baroreceptors are situated in the tunica adventitia. Baroreceptors are endings of myelinated nerve fibers which have knobby endings which are highly branched, intertwined and coiled. They respond to stretch of the vessel wall and the degree of firing varies depending on the degree of stretch.

Twigs of nerve fibers from carotid sinus pass through glossopharyngeal nerve (IX cranial nerve) and reach the nucleus tractus solitarius in the medulla. The twig of fibers emerging from the carotid sinus that joins the glossopharyngeal nerve is called **carotid sinus nerve or Hering's nerve**. From the aortic arch receptors, the afferent fibers pass through the vagus nerve and reach the nucleus tractus solitarius. The nerve fibers arising from the carotid sinus and aortic arch receptors are also called **buffer nerves** or sinoaortic nerves. Nucleus tractus solitarius (NTS) is the medullary relay station for the cardio-respiratory afferents, i.e., it receives afferents from both baroreceptors and chemoreceptors. The excitatory transmitter released by the afferent fibers in the NTS is **glutamate.** The NTS sends excitatory impulses directly to the CIC and indirectly through inhibitory interneurons to the VMC. The inhibitory neurotransmitter is **gamma amino butyric acid (GABA).** The part of medulla which contains the inhibitory interneurons to RVLM (VMC) is called caudal ventrolateral medulla (CVLM). Thus, when NTS is stimulated, the VMC is inhibited via inhibitory interneurons and the CIC is stimulated **(Fig. 26.3)**. The net effect is decrease in sympathetic tone and increase in vagal tone. The heart rate decreases.

Mechanism of Action of Baroreceptors

The baroreceptors are active even under resting conditions and the effect of baroreceptor stimulation is inhibition of VMC. The impulses from the baroreceptors also reach the CIC. The effect of baroreceptors on VMC is through inhibitory interneurons that release inhibitory transmitters like GABA. The effect of buffer nerves on CIC is direct and it causes stimulation of CIC causing a slight increase in vagal tone and decrease in heart rate.

Sinoaortic Reflex or Baroreceptor Reflex

When the blood pressure is increased very much, i.e., in times of **hypertension,** body tries to decrease the blood pressure by different mechanisms. When there is increase in BP, there is increased stretch of the vessel wall which leads to increase in the degree of firing through the buffer nerves. There is inhibition of VMC, and the sympathetic discharge is very much decreased leading to vasodilatation and decrease in peripheral resistance. This leads to a reduction in the blood pressure. At the same time the baroreceptor stimulation causes pronounced stimulation of CIC and reflex bradycardia occurs. Reduction in the heart rate reduces cardiac output which also reduces blood pressure. This is known as **sinoaortic reflex** mechanism where there is *a fall in BP and reflex bradycardia* **(Flowchart 26.1)**. When the blood pressure comes back to normal level, the baroreceptor reflex disappears. This is an example of negative feedback mechanism.

When pulse pressure, mean pressure and sustained pressure are taken into consideration, the baroreceptors respond to all these factors but better to changes in pulse pressure and less to sustained pressure. This is because in sustained pressure, the baroreceptors get adapted and the response to that pressure becomes less.

When there is a fall in blood pressure, i.e., in times of **hypotension**, there is no stretch on the vessel wall and there will be no stimulation of baroreceptors. Even the normal stream of impulses coming through the buffer nerves cease. Thus there is no inhibition of VMC and no stimulation of CIC, which leads to an increase in the blood pressure due to increased sympathetic tone to blood vessels and an increase in heart rate because there is no stimulation of CIC. Here there is *reflex increase in BP and reflex tachycardia*.

Marey's Law

Marey's law states that heart rate is inversely proportional to blood pressure (BP). Whenever BP is increased, there will be reflex bradycardia and whenever BP falls there will be reflex tachycardia. *Reverse of this law is not possible,* i.e., when heart rate increases there will be no fall in BP.

Afferents from Other Parts of CNS

Afferents from cerebral cortex and hypothalamus Changes in heart rate are observed in relation to emotional states like anxiety, anger, etc. This is due to discharge from cerebral cortex particularly the **limbic cortex via hypothalamus** to the medullary cardiac centers.

Flowchart 26.1: Schematic representation of the pathway for sinoaortic reflex or baroreceptor reflex mechanism when there is an increase in blood pressure (plus and minus signs denote stimulation and inhibition respectively).

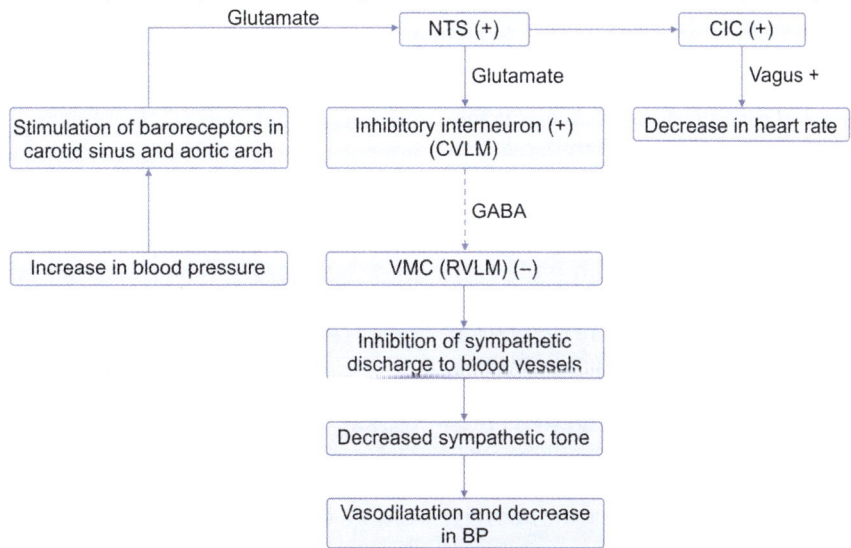

Respiratory Afferents

Change in heart rate observed during respiration is called **sinus arrhythmia**. Inspiration produces increase in heart rate and expiration produces decrease in heart rate. The explanations for sinus arrhythmia are the following:

- There is irradiation of inhibitory signals from the inspiratory center to the cardiac centers leading to inhibition of CIC producing an increase in the heart rate. Neuronal activity in the inspiratory center in the medulla oblongata, in addition to initiating inspiration also sends inhibitory impulses to nucleus of tractus solitarius and the CIC. Since the CIC is inhibited, there is inhibition of cardiac vagal discharge leading to the increase in heart rate even during normal inspiration.
- In deep inspiration, inhibitory impulses from the lungs pass through the vagal afferents to the inspiratory center (Hering Breuer reflex) as well as to the nucleus tractus solitarius (NTS). When NTS is inhibited, there is no stimulation of CIC and this leads to an increase in the heart rate. In forced expiration, reverse occurs and the CIC is stimulated leading to decrease in the heart rate.
- In inspiration there is decrease in the intrathoracic pressure which produces increase in the venous return and increased right atrial filling. The atrial stretch receptors are stimulated and through Bainbridge reflex, there is increase in heart rate (refer Bainbridge reflex).
- In forced inspiration, there is a reduction in blood pressure due to decreased left ventricular output. Through baroreceptor reflex there will be an increase in heart rate.

Afferents from Chemoreceptors

Chemoreceptors send impulses through the afferent fibers passing through glossopharyngeal and vagus nerves. Increase in PCO_2, decrease in PO_2 and decrease in the pH stimulate the chemoreceptors. Impulses from chemoreceptors reach the respiratory and cardiac centers in the medulla and produces variation in blood pressure, heart rate and respiratory rate. Experiments have proved that the cardiovascular neurons respond to changes in blood chemistry as well as to signals coming from respiratory center to the cardiac center.

The cardiac response to chemoreceptor stimulation is the net result of primary and secondary reflex mechanisms. When the peripheral chemoreceptors are stimulated, the **primary effect** is stimulation of medullary vagal center, which leads to decrease in heart rate. The **secondary effects** are mediated by the respiratory system. Stimulation of peripheral chemoreceptors in the carotid body and aortic body increases the rate and depth of respiration. There will be hypocapnia due to hyperventilation and increased stretch of lungs, which initiates the Herring-Breuer reflex. Both these effects inhibit the medullary vagal center. Small increase in respiration inhibits the vagal center slightly and so there is only slight increase in heart rate. Severe hyperventilation will increase the heart rate. *Very little variation in heart rate is seen on peripheral chemoreceptor stimulation since the primary and the secondary effects neutralize each other.*

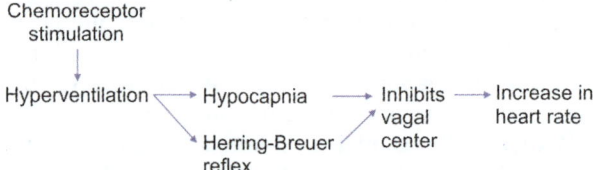

Direct Effects of Hypoxia, Hypercapnia and Acidosis on Cardiac Centers

Central Nervous System Ischemic Response

When blood flow to brain is decreased, it causes cerebral ischemia. There will be hypoxia, hypercapnia and lactic acid accumulation in the brain due to decreased blood flow. This stimulates the VMC (RVLM) as well as the cardioinhibitory center at the same time by a direct action. This leads to increase in blood pressure and decrease in the heart rate. This response is called **CNS ischemic response** and this response can elevate the mean arterial pressure to as high as 250 mm Hg. When vasoconstriction is severe, the peripheral vessels become totally occluded. Due to renal vasoconstriction, there may be renal shutdown and oliguria or anuria. But CNS ischemic response operates only when the mean arterial BP falls below 60 mm Hg.

Cushing Reflex or Cushing Reaction

Cushing reflex is a special type of CNS ischemic response. The cause is **increase in the intracranial tension**. For example, a tumor in the brain exerts pressure effects on the nearby structures and at the same time increases the intracranial pressure. When the intracranial tension rises to reach the arterial pressure, it compresses the whole brain as well as the arteries of the brain. When blood flow to the VMC is decreased, it suffers from ischemia. Hypercapnia, hypoxia and acidosis occur in the region of VMC. This leads to cerebral ischemia and initiates **CNS ischemic response**. The VMC is stimulated leading to vasoconstriction and increase in blood pressure. When the arterial pressure becomes more than the intracranial pressure, blood flows through the vessels of brain to relieve ischemia. Cushing reflex is important in that it protects the vital centers of brain from the damages caused by brain ischemia. There is simultaneous stimulation of cardioinhibitory center by sinoaortic reflex mechanism and thus, *reflex hypertension is associated with bradycardia*. This response seen in raised intracranial tension is called **Cushing reflex (Flowchart 26.2)**.

Afferents from Receptors in Heart and Great Blood Vessels

Atrial and Ventricular Baroreceptors

The atrial walls contain atrial baroreceptors type A and type B. Type A baroreceptors discharge primarily during atrial

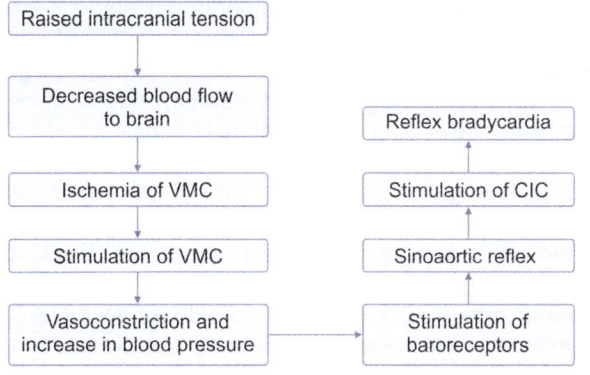

Flowchart 26.2: Mechanism of Cushing reflex.

systole and type B discharge when there is distension of atria during late diastole, i.e., at the peak of atrial filling. When there is stretch to the atrial wall, the atrial baroreceptors get stimulated and they start discharging impulses. The effect is inhibition of the CIC leading to tachycardia and inhibition of VMC leading to hypotension. Another reason for increase in heart rate is that when the right atrium gets stretched it stretches the SA node, which gets stimulated leading to a direct increase in heart rate.

When the left ventricular and pulmonary baroreceptors are stimulated the effect is bradycardia and hypotension. No stretch receptors are found in the right ventricle.

Bainbridge Reflex

Rapid infusion of blood or saline into a heart with bradycardia produces reflex tachycardia and hypotension.

In bradycardia, atrial filling is increased due to increased venous return and the atrial baroreceptors get stimulated leading to tachycardia **(Flowchart 26.3)**. This reflex is obtained only if the initial heart rate is slow; it does not operate if the initial heart rate is high. Mechanism is stimulation of type B atrial stretch receptors. This reflex is abolished by bilateral vagotomy. This proves that it is a true reflex and not a local response to stretch. This reflex is not present in transplanted heart.

Bezold-Jarisch Reflex or Coronary Chemoreflex

When a substance called **veratridine** is injected into the left coronary artery, the effects produced are reflex apnea followed by rapid breathing, hypotension and bradycardia. The drug reaches the left ventricle and the receptors present in the left ventricular wall, which are C-fiber endings gets stimulated. The afferent fibers go through the vagus nerve. This reflex is called Bezold-Jarisch reflex. This reflex is abolished by bilateral vagotomy. During myocardial infarction, when blood supply to the area is cut off, toxic substances similar to veratridine are liberated from the infarcted tissue, which stimulate the ventricular receptors leading to apnea, hypotension and bradycardia.

A similar reflex called **pulmonary chemoreflex** is obtained when substances like serotonin, veratridine, etc., are injected into the pulmonary artery. The receptors are C fiber endings.

Miscellaneous Afferents

Other afferents that produce changes in heart rate are:
- Pain produces variations in the heart rate. Superficial pain produces tachycardia and rise in blood pressure, whereas deep pain produces bradycardia and fall in blood pressure. Superficial pain carried by unmyelinated C fibers sends collaterals to the RVLM (VMC) and increases sympathetic discharge leading to increase in heart rate and blood pressure. Whereas, pain arising from deep body tissues which is severe and excruciating carried by thin myelinated fibers sends collaterals to the CVLM of medulla leading to inhibition of VMC producing bradycardia and decrease in blood pressure due to vasodilatation.
- Pressure on the outer canthus of eyeball produces hypotension and bradycardia referred to as the **oculocardiac reflex**.
- Pressure on the carotid sinus from outside produces reflex bradycardia and hypotension and may lead to fainting attacks.
- Manipulation of viscera during abdominal surgery produces reflex hypotension and bradycardia.

Sometimes anesthetic accidents occur when the respiratory passages are irritated with endotracheal tube and anesthetic gases. There will be hypotension and bradycardia.

■ CHEMICAL FACTORS AFFECTING HEART RATE

The chemical factors that affect heart rate are:
- Catecholamines
- Thyroxine
- PCO_2
- Hypoxia
- Lactic acid
- Drugs

Catecholamines released from adrenal medulla and from the sympathetic nerve endings increase rhythmicity and contractility of the heart. In stress conditions associated with flight, fright and fight reactions, catecholamines are liberated to overcome the emergency situation. Norepinephrine is a net vasoconstrictor that causes increase in the mean arterial pressure. This produces reflex bradycardia via the sinoaortic mechanism. The net effect of epinephrine on blood vessels

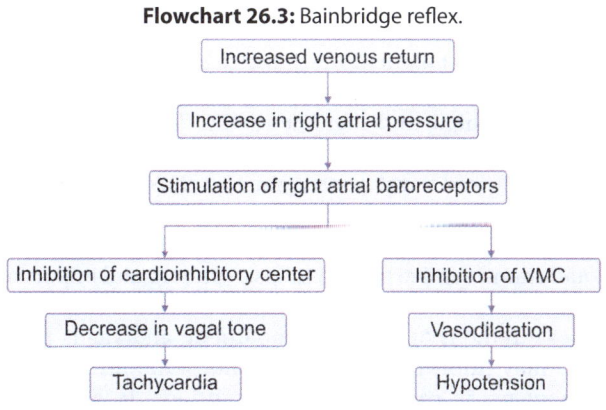

Flowchart 26.3: Bainbridge reflex.

is vasodilatation. Hence, the mean arterial pressure is not raised and reflex bradycardia is not seen with epinephrine.

Increased level of **thyroid hormones** in hyperthyroidism increases the activity of heart causing tachycardia. In hypothyroidism there is decrease in heart rate.

Hypercapnia (increase in PCO_2) decreases heart rate and hypocapnia increases heart rate.

Hypoxia in the initial stages increases heart rate. When the degree of hypoxia becomes severe, heart rate becomes irregular and arrhythmias occur.

Lactic acidosis and all conditions that increase H^+ concentration in blood decrease heart rate.

Parasympatholytic **drugs** like atropine increase heart rate. Parasympathomimetic drugs like pilocarpine decrease heart rate. Nicotine increases heart rate. Digitalis depresses nodal tissue and exerts an effect like that of vagal stimulation.

PHYSICAL FACTORS

When there is an increase in body **temperature** as in increased metabolic activity, fever, etc., heart rate is increased (tachycardia). For every 1°F rise in body temperature, the heart rate increases by 10 beats. Experimentally this can be proved in animals by applying warmth on SA node, when increase in heart rate is observed.

Muscular exercise increases heart rate. Even the thought of exercise increases heart rate through impulses coming from cortex. In well-trained athletes, heart rate is less due to increase in vagal tone by constant training. Increase in heart rate during exercise is due to the following reasons:
- ❖ Stimulation of sympathetic system
- ❖ Decrease in vagal tone
- ❖ Increased release of thyroxine and catecholamines into the circulation
- ❖ Hypoxia, hypercapnia and acidosis that occur during exercise causes stimulation of peripheral chemoreceptors, which lead to increase in heart rate due to hyperventilation (secondary effect of chemoreceptor stimulation on heart is pronounced during exercise).

AGE AND SEX

At birth, the heart rate is 130-140 beats/min. It decreases as age advances and in adults heart rate is 70-80/min. But in old age heart rate is high and it is around 100/min.

Heart rate is slightly higher in females when compared to males because the resting sympathetic tone to the heart is more in females. In the reproductive age group, after ovulation there is a slight increase in body temperature (0.5°C) due to the thermogenic action of progesterone. This also increases the heart rate in females.

REGULATION OF HEART RATE

Neural Regulation

- ❖ *Role of cardiac centers and cardiac innervation (effects of sympathetic and parasympathetic supply to the heart)*: Efferent fibers from the VMC project to thoracolumbar preganglionic sympathetic neurons. Preganglionic fibers to the heart relay in the superior, middle and inferior cervical ganglia. The post-ganglionic sympathetic fibers, which release norepinephrine as the neurotransmitter, supply the whole heart. Stimulation of these fibers produces increase in heart rate by opening L-calcium channels.

  Dorsal motor nucleus (DMN) of vagus (part of nucleus ambiguus) gives rise to parasympathetic cardiac efferent fibers that supply the atria, SA node and AV node. Stimulation of DMN reduces heart rate. Hence it is also known as cardioinhibitory center (CIC). The parasympathetic efferent fibers release acetylcholine (ACh) that increases the permeability of SA node to K^+ producing K^+ efflux and hyperpolarization. This leads to decrease in heart rate.

- ❖ *Role of afferents to the cardiac centers (VMC and CIC)*:
  - Afferents from baroreceptors (explain baroreceptor reflex)
  - From parts of central nervous system (change in heart rate in emotional states)
  - From chemoreceptors (chemoreceptor reflex) and respiratory system (sinus arrhythmia)
  - From receptors within the heart and great blood vessels (cardiac reflexes - Bainbridge reflex, Bezold-Jarisch reflex).
- ❖ *Role of other reflexes*:
  - CNS ischemic response
  - Cushing reflex.

Chemical Regulation

Chemical factors affecting heart rate (Page 249).

REGULATION OF TRANSPLANTED HEART

The functions in a transplanted heart are regulated by hormonal factors because the heart is devoid of nerve supply. The blood supply is normal in the transplanted heart. Another factor by which transplanted heart is controlled is by the operation of Frank-Starling law. Frank-Starling law states that the force of contraction of heart is directly proportional to the end diastolic volume within physiological limits. During exercise there is a slight inrease in heart rate due to the action of circulating catecholamines.

SYMPATHOVAGAL BALANCE

Sympathovagal balance is the balance between sympathetic and parasympathetic activity of the individual at any given time. Sympathetic and vagal neural outflows are opposing neural mechanisms. Instantaneous balance between sympathetic and vagal nerve activities can be obtained by finding the ratio between R-R interval in ECG and respiratory frequencies. This ratio or the sympathovagal balance, which is a totally non-invasive means, helps to understand important autonomic interrelations in humans.

Measurement of human sympathetic and vagus nerve traffic may inform physiological and pathophysiological mechanisms in cardiovascular conditions. It is used for prediction, diagnosis, management and prevention of many cardiovascular dysfunctions.

Sympathetic and vagal nerve activities change reciprocally. For example, if face is immersed in cold water, there will be simultaneous increase in muscle sympathetic nerve activity and bradycardia. This bradycardia can be prevented by vagotomy or by giving large dose of atropine.

HEART RATE VARIABILITY

Heart rate variability (HRV) analysis is used to assess the state of sympathovagal balance of the individual. HRV is the cardiac beat-to-beat variation, i.e., variation in cardiac cycle length. This variation may be due to several causes like respiratory sinus arrhythmia, circadian rhythm, exercise, etc.

HRV depends on the rate of discharge from the SA node. The balance between vagal activity and sympathetic activity determines SA nodal activity at any particular time. Vagal activity slows it while sympathetic activity accelerates it. Sinus arrhythmia is primarily due to alteration in vagal tone in inspiration and expiration. HRV is mainly influenced by vagal nerve activity. HRV analysis can be used for determining the individual's susceptibility to develop autonomic dysfunctions like hypertension.

MULTIPLE CHOICE QUESTIONS

1. **Carotid sinus massage stops supraventricular tachycardia by:**
   a. Decreasing sympathetic discharge to SA node
   b. Increasing vagal discharge to SA node
   c. Decreasing sympathetic discharge to the conducting tissue between atria and ventricles
   d. Increasing vagal discharge to the conducting tissue between atria and ventricles

2. **Vagal tone decreases heart rate by acting through:**
   a. M_2 receptors on SA node
   b. M_1 receptors
   c. Nicotinic receptors
   d. M_2 receptors on AV node

3. **Baroreceptor stimulation produces:**
   a. Decreased heart rate and BP
   b. Increased heart rate and BP
   c. Increased cardiac contractility
   d. Decreased cardiac contractility

4. **Sympathetic stimulation causes all the following, *except*:**
   a. Increase in heart rate
   b. Increase in blood pressure
   c. Increase in total peripheral resistance
   d. Increase in venous capacitance

5. **Pressure on the carotid sinus causes:**
   a. Hyperpnea   b. Reflex bradycardia
   c. Tachycardia   d. Dyspnea

6. **Receptors for sinoaortic reflex are located in:**
   a. Carotid body   b. Aortic body
   c. Carotid sinus d. Large veins

7. **Bainbridge reflex is characterized by:**
   a. Hypotension, bradycardia and apnea
   b. Hypertension, bradycardia and apnea
   c. Hypertension, tachycardia and apnea
   d. Hypotension and tachycardia

8. **Factors decreasing heart rate includes all the following, *except*:**
   a. Hypervolemia
   b. Raised intracranial tension
   c. Stokes Adams syndrome
   d. Inspiration

9. **Tachycardia is produced by:**
   a. Deep expiration
   b. Increased intracranial tension
   c. Hypoxia
   d. Increased baroreceptor activity

10. **For edema to be detected in tissues the interstitial fluid volume should increase above:**
    a. 30%   b. 5%
    c. 10%   d. 50%

11. **Which of the following is *NOT* synthesized mostly in the liver?**
    a. α_2 macroglobulin
    b. Angiotensinogen
    c. Angiotensin II converting enzyme
    d. Fibrinogen

12. **Following adrenalin injection the heart rate:**
    a. Increase because increase in BP stimulates baroreceptors
    b. Increase because adrenalin has a direct chronotropic effect on heart
    c. Increase because of decreased tonic para-sympathetic discharge to heart
    d. Decrease because of increased tonic para-sympathetic discharge to heart

13. **Angiotensin II act by activating:**
    a. Protein kinase A
    b. Guanylyl cyclase
    c. Phospholipase C
    d. Phospholipase A_2

14. **The only organ where hypoxia produces vaso-constriction is:**
    a. Heart   b. Lung
    c. Brain   d. Skeletal muscle

15. **Stimulation of baroreceptors in carotid sinus produces:**
    a. Tachycardia   b. Bradycardia
    c. Hyperventilation d. Increase in BP

16. **Carotid body contains:**
    a. Chemoreceptors   b. Baroreceptors
    c. Osmoreceptors   d. Thermoreceptors

17. **All the following are increased in the heart by adrenalin, *except*:**
    a. Automaticity   b. Conduction velocity
    c. Refractory period d. Contractility

18. The heart rate is NOT increased by:
    a. Atropine
    b. Acetyl choline
    c. Adrenaline
    d. Increased sympathetic activity
19. Norepinephrine increases heart rate by all the following, *except:*
    a. Increasing intracellular cAMP in SA node
    b. Opening long acting Ca^{2+} channels
    c. Increasing the slope of prepotential
    d. Increasing K^+ efflux
20. Baroreceptor stimulation leads to all the following, *except:*
    a. Bradycardia
    b. Hypotension
    c. Respiratory stimulation
    d. Increase in vagal tone
21. Hypoxia may produce:
    a. Rise in BP
    b. Fall in BP
    c. Fall followed by rise in BP
    d. No change
22. Tachycardia at the onset of exercise is due to stimulation of:
    a. Chemoreceptors
    b. Baroreceptors
    c. Stretch receptors
    d. Joint proprioceptors
23. Vagus inhibits pace maker potential by all, *except:*
    a. Hyperpolarization
    b. Prepotential slope becomes more steep
    c. Stabilizing resting membrane potential
    d. Increase K^+ permeability
24. Baroreceptors mainly act through:
    a. Sympathetic system
    b. Parasympathetic system
    c. Cerebral cortex
    d. Blood volume
25. In athletes, bradycardia is because of:
    a. Decreased sympathetic tone
    b. Increased vagal tone
    c. Increased cardiac output
    d. Low venous return
26. Heart rate is maximal in:
    a. Fetus
    b. Newborn
    c. Adults
    d. Old age
27. Carotid sinus afferents pass through:
    a. IX cranial nerve
    b. X cranial nerve
    c. V cranial nerve
    d. VII cranial nerve
28. Carotid sinus stimulation result in:
    a. Decreased vagal activity
    b. Increased heart rate
    c. Decreased sympathetic discharge to heart
    d. Increased vasomotor tone
29. Sympathetic vasoconstrictor tone is diminished due to increased activity of:
    a. Carotid sinus baroreceptor
    b. Carotid body chemoreceptor
    c. Pain receptor
    d. Medullary chemoreceptor
30. Vagal stimulation can cause all, *except*:
    a. Decreased heart rate
    b. Delayed AV conduction
    c. Increased ventricular contraction
    d. Decreased atrial contraction
31. Stimulation of baroreceptor leads to:
    a. Increase in BP and heart rate
    b. Decrease in BP and heart rate
    c. Increased intracranial tension
    d. Decreased in BP and increase in heart rate
32. Carotid baroreceptor is most sensitive to:
    a. Systolic BP
    b. Diastolic BP
    c. Mean blood pressured.
    d. Stroke volume
33. In cerebral ischemia, systemic blood pressure rises due to:
    a. Monro-Kellie doctrine
    b. Cushing reflex
    c. Autoregulation
    d. Bainbridge reflex
34. Bradycardia in athletes is due to:
    a. Decreased sympathetic tone
    b. Increased vagal tone
    c. High cardiac output
    d. Low venous return
35. Heart rate is maximum in:
    a. Newborn
    b. Fetus
    c. Adults
    d. Old age
36. Maximum heart rate per minute with exercise is:
    a. 120
    b. 140
    c. 160
    d. 200
37. Right and left vagal nerves respectively go to:
    a. AV node, SA node
    b. SA node, AV node
    c. SA node, bundle of His
    d. AV node, bundle of His
38. Baroreceptors mainly act through:
    a. Parasympathetic system
    b. Sympathetic system
    c. Cerebral cortex
    d. Blood volume

ANSWERS

1. d	2. a	3. a	4. d	5. b
6. c	7. d	8. d	9. c	10. a
11. c	12. b	13. c	14. b	15. b
16. a	17. c	18. b	19. d	20. c
21. a	22. d	23. b	24. a	25. b
26. a	27. a	28. c	29. a	30. c
31. b	32. c	33. b	34. b	35. b
36. d	37. b	38. b		

Cardiac Output

CHAPTER 27

LEARNING OBJECTIVES

Must know
- Define cardiac output and stroke volume
- Describe the regulation of cardiac output
- Explain end-diastolic volume and the factors affecting it
- Describe the different methods used to measure cardiac output
- Discuss the regulation of cardiac output in transplanted heart

■ INTRODUCTION

PY5.9: Describe the factors affecting heart rate, regulation of cardiac output and blood pressure.

The output per ventricle per beat is called **stroke volume or stroke output or systolic discharge**. The amount of blood pumped out of the heart per beat is about 70 mL from each ventricle in a resting man of average size in the supine position. Output per ventricle per minute is **cardiac output or minute volume**. In the resting supine position, it averages about 5 L/min.

A man at rest in the supine position has the following values normally:
- **End-diastolic volume (EDV)** = 120–140 mL
- **End-systolic volume (ESV)** = 50–70 mL
- **Stroke volume (SV)** = EDV−ESV = 70 mL
- **Cardiac output** = SV × HR (heart rate) = 70 mL × 72/ min = 5 L/min
- **Ejection fraction:** SV/EDV × 100 = 60–65% (Percentage of EDV that is ejected with each heart beat is called ejection fraction. It is a measure of ventricular contractility)

The 5 L of blood ejected from the left ventricle is distributed to the body in 1 minute through the systemic circulation. The entire cardiac output, i.e. 5 L goes into the pulmonary circulation from the right side of heart. There is slight difference in the output from both sides of the heart. The right ventricular output is a little less than that of left ventricular output (Chapter 36 page 350).

Output from the left ventricle into the aorta occurs at high pressure since the systemic circulation is a high-pressure system. Only 1/6 of systemic pressure is present in the pulmonary system. So resistance against pumping is very less since it is a low-pressure system.

Distribution of Cardiac Output

Seventy-five per cent of cardiac output is distributed to the vital organs and the rest 25% to skeletal muscles, other organs and skin **(Table 27.1)**.

■ MEASUREMENT OF CARDIAC OUTPUT

- Direct method
- Indirect methods
  - Fick method
  - Indicator dilution method
  - Doppler combined with echocardiography.

Direct Method

In the direct method, cardiac output can be measured with an **electromagnetic flow meter** placed in the ascending aorta. This method can be performed only in experimental animals.

Indirect Method

Fick's Method

Fick's principle states that the amount of substance taken up by an organ or by the whole body per unit time is equal to the

Table 27.1: Distribution of cardiac output at rest.

Organ	Distribution (mL/min)	% of Cardiac output	Blood flow in mL/100 g of tissue
Liver	1500	27	80–90
Kidneys	1250	22	350–400
Brain	750	13.5	50–55
Skeletal muscle	750	13.5	2–4
Skin	450	8	8–12
Heart	250	5	70–80
Other regions	550	11	

arteriovenous concentration difference (A-V difference) of the substance times the blood flow. From this law the blood flow can be calculated by the formula:

Amount of substance taken up by the body in unit time
= (A-V concentration difference) × (Blood flow).

So, blood flow = Amount of substance taken up ÷ A-V concentration difference.

The above principle can be applied to determine cardiac output by measuring the amount of O_2 consumed by the body in a given period and dividing this value by the A-V concentration difference of O_2 across the lungs. Because systemic arterial blood has the same O_2 content in all parts of the body, the arterial concentration can be determined in a sample obtained from any peripheral artery. A sample of venous blood from the pulmonary artery is obtained by cardiac catheterization. The oxygen consumption per minute is determined with the help of a spirometer. From the above values, cardiac output can be calculated by the formula:

$$\text{Cardiac output} = \frac{O_2 \text{ consumption in mL/min}}{\text{Arterial } O_2 - \text{Venous } O_2 \text{ (mL/L)}}$$

$$= \frac{250 \text{ mL/min}}{(190 \text{ mL/L}) - (140 \text{ mL/L})}$$

$$= \frac{250 \text{ mL/min}}{50 \text{ mL/L}} = 5 \text{ L/min}$$

Indicator Dilution Technique

A known amount of substance (a dye or a radioactive isotope) is injected into an arm vein and the concentration of the indicator in serial samples of arterial blood is determined. The dye commonly used is **Evans blue**.

Criteria for the Indicator Used

- The concentration of the substance can be accurately measured.
- It should not leave circulation during the test.
- It should give the maximum concentration in the first circulation itself.
- Should not produce hemolysis, i.e., it should be nontoxic.
- Should not affect hemodynamics.

The cardiac output is equal to the amount of indicator injected divided by its average concentration in arterial blood after a single circulation through the heart. The concentration of the dye in each sample is analyzed by photoelectric method. The log of the indicator concentration in mg/L in the serial arterial samples is plotted against time in seconds in a semi log paper. It is seen that the concentration of the indicator rises, falls and then rises again as the indicator recirculates. It takes about 6 sec for the indicator to first appear in the circulation.

This is called **appearance time**. It reaches a peak in 10-12 sec. It falls and again rises. The initial decline in concentration is extrapolated to the abscissa. This gives the **disappearance time**. Difference between appearance time

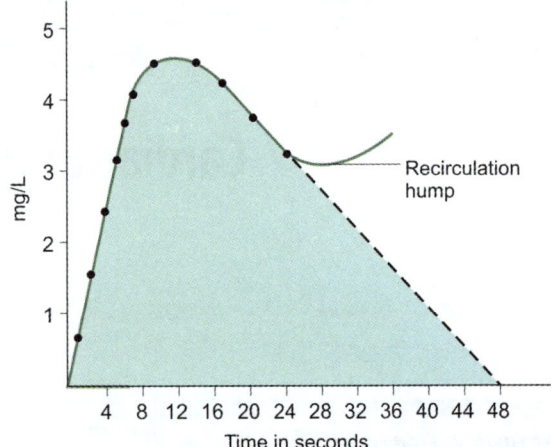

Fig. 27.1: Determination of cardiac output by dye dilution method.

and disappearance time gives the **passage time**, i.e., the time for the first passage of the indicator through the circulation (**Fig. 27.1**). Average concentration of dye is determined from the area under the curve. The cardiac output for that period is calculated and then converted to output per minute. This method is called **Hamilton's method**.

For example, if the amount of dye injected (A) is 5 mg, average concentration of dye (C) is 1.6 mg/L and the passage time (T), 34 sec, then, flow/minute or cardiac output can be calculated from the formula:

$$CO = \frac{A \times 60}{C \times T} = \frac{5 \times 60}{1.6 \times 34} = 6 \text{ L}$$

Thermodilution Method

In this method the indicator used is **cold saline**. A definite volume of cold saline whose temperature is accurately measured is injected into the right atrium through one side of a double lumen catheter. The temperature change in the blood is recorded in the pulmonary artery using a thermistor in the other side of the catheter, which is long. The temperature change recorded by the **thermistor** is inversely proportional to the amount of blood flowing through the pulmonary artery.

Since the volume of saline injected and the exact difference of temperature between the two spots are known, the flow of blood in between these two spots in a specified period of time can be found out. Thus, flow of blood per minute or cardiac output can be found out. Saline is harmless and repeated determinations can be made.

Doppler Technique Combined with Echocardiography

Echocardiography is a non-invasive technique to assess cardiac function. In echocardiography, pulses of ultrasonic waves at a frequency of 2.25 MHz are emitted from a **transducer**. The transducer also functions as a receiver to detect waves reflected back from various parts of the heart. Reflections occur whenever acoustic impedance changes and a recording of the echoes displayed against time on an oscilloscope provides a record of the movements of ventricular wall, thickness of the walls, diameter of the heart chambers, movement of septum and valves during the cardiac cycle. When combined with Doppler techniques, echocardiography can be used to measure velocity and volume of flow through the valves.

Uses of Echocardiography

- When combined with Doppler techniques, echocardiography can be used to determine cardiac output.
- Volume of flow and velocity of blood flow can be measured.
- Congenital heart diseases like atrial septal defect (ASD), ventricular septal defect (VSD), patent ductus arteriosus (PDA), etc., can be detected.
- Two-dimensional echocardiography helps to detect diseases of valves and blood vessels.
- Ejection fraction can be determined by finding out the end-diastolic volume and end-systolic volume.

VARIATIONS IN CARDIAC OUTPUT

Physiological Variation

- *Age*: Cardiac output increases from infancy to adulthood.
- *Sex*: Value is less in females than in males.
- *Body surface area*: **Cardiac index** is CO/min/m² body surface area and is approximately 3.4 L/min/m² (2.8–4.2 L).
- *Sleep*: In deep sleep, cardiac output is minimal, and it gradually increases during the waking hours.
- *Emotional excitement*: 30% increase in cardiac output is observed.
- *Environmental temperature*: Very high temperature increases cardiac output.
- *Exercise*: Depends on the type of exercise, whether isotonic or isometric, or on the severity of exercise and it also depends on previous training. In severe exercise, cardiac output (CO) can increase from 5 L/min to 30–35 L/min.
- Cardiac output increases by about 30% during digestion, i.e., after meals.
- It is increased in pregnancy since body demand is more. There is increase in blood volume during pregnancy.
- At high altitudes, CO is increased due to polycythemia and increase in blood volume.
- *Posture*: Cardiac output is maximal in the lying down posture and minimum in the standing posture. This is because when the person assumes erect posture, there is pooling of blood in the lower extremities leading to a reduction in venous return and decrease in the end-diastolic volume. This causes decrease in the force of contraction and decrease in stroke volume and cardiac output.

Pathological Variation of Cardiac Output

1. **Pathological increase** is seen in hyperthyroidism, fever, etc.
2. **Pathological decrease** is seen in hypothyroidism, fibrillation, hypovolemia (e.g., hemorrhage), myocardial infarction, heart failure, acidosis, etc.

CARDIAC RESERVE

Cardiac reserve refers to the maximum increase in cardiac output above normal and is expressed in percentage. In a healthy adult it is 300–400% and in athletes it is 500–600%. A measure of the cardiac reserve can help predict the likelihood of heart failure if suspected.

In persons with severe cardiac failure there will be no cardiac reserve. Any factor that prevents the heart from pumping blood effectively will decrease the cardiac reserve. The factors can be myocardial infarction, cardiomyopathy, vitamin B deficiency, valvular heart disease, etc. A diagnosis of low cardiac reserve can be made by asking the subject to exercise on a treadmill or by walking up and down the steps. Exercise tolerance is assessed by measuring the maximum heart rate attained after a standard exercise test, and the time required for the heart rate to return to normal. ECG and blood pressure will be monitored continuously during the test. Exercise tolerance is an excellent indicator of cardiac reserve.

FACTORS AFFECTING CARDIAC OUTPUT

- Heart rate
- Stroke volume

REGULATION OF CARDIAC OUTPUT

Regulation of cardiac output includes all factors that regulate stroke volume and heart rate since *cardiac output is the product of heart rate and stroke volume*. So, variation in cardiac output is produced by factors that affect stroke volume or heart rate or both. Four factors mainly affect cardiac output: heart rate, contractility, preload and after load of the heart. The force of contraction of the heart depends on its preloading and its after loading. After load and preload are determined both by peripheral circulation and the heart. Preload is the degree to which the myocardium is stretched before it contracts and after load is the resistance against which blood is expelled from the heart.

REGULATION OF STROKE VOLUME

Stroke volume is regulated mainly by two mechanisms:

1. **Heterometric regulation** includes factors affecting ventricular performance or the factors that regulate cardiac output as a result of changes in the initial cardiac muscle fiber length. It mainly includes end-diastolic volume. **End-diastolic volume** is the preload acting on the heart and **aortic impedance or arterial resistance** is the afterload on the heart. The preload is the degree to which the cardiac muscle is stretched before it contracts. Afterload is the resistance against which the ventricles have to pump the blood. *Heterometric regulation is independent of cardiac innervation.*
2. **Homometric regulation** includes factors that produce changes in contractility independent of resting cardiac muscle fiber length. It includes neural and chemical factors.

Heterometric Regulation of Stroke Volume

End-diastolic Volume

The amount of blood in each ventricle at the end of diastole is end-diastolic volume. End-diastolic volume (EDV) is the **preload**, i.e., the load that operates in the heart before the beginning of contraction. **Frank-Starling law** states that the force of contraction of the heart is directly proportional to the end-diastolic volume *within physiological limits*. When the EDV increases, the stroke volume also increases due to increase in the force of contraction. The length of the cardiac muscle fiber to which it shows maximum force of contraction is called **optimum length**. Length beyond which the cardiac muscle fiber ruptures on stretch is called **point of imminent rupture**.

Factors affecting End-diastolic Volume

- **Venous return:**
  - Skeletal muscle pump or muscular activity
  - Venous tone
  - Intrathoracic pressure
  - Posture and gravity
  - Blood volume
  - Positive abdominal pressure
  - Pressure gradient.
- **Ventricular filling:**
  - Atrial contraction
  - Intrapericardial pressure
  - Myocardial compliance
  - Blood volume.

Factors Affecting Venous Return or Factors that Keep the Blood Flowing in the Veins

- **Skeletal muscle pump:** When there is movement or muscular activity, there is more contraction of skeletal muscles leading to the compression of blood vessels especially veins leading to increase in venous return. In bed-ridden patients, movement is minimal and the skeletal muscle pump is not working. This leads to pooling of blood and decrease in venous return. Pooling of blood also leads to venous thrombosis and embolism. So such patients are advised to move their limbs frequently.

  Limb veins have valves that ensure one-way flow. When muscle squeezes blood through the vein during muscle contraction this blood cannot go back when the muscle relax because of the presence of one-way valves along the course of the vein. That is why incompetent valves may lead to varicose vein in the legs.
- **Venous tone:** The walls of veins contain smooth muscles which play an important role in propelling blood back to the heart rather than determining venous pressure. Large veins act as blood reservoirs by accommodating large volumes of blood when blood volume is increased. In times of need like hypovolemia, they contract, increasing venous return and cardiac output.
- **Suction forces which draw blood towards the atria:**
  - Negative intrathoracic pressure especially during inspiration exerts a sucking effect on the great veins leading to increased venous return. This is referred to as **respiratory pump**.
  - Rapid blood flow from atria to ventricles during early diastole creates a suction force which draws blood towards atria.
- **Posture and gravity:** Venous return is decreased in standing posture due to pooling of blood in the lower extremities and is maximal in the lying down posture.
- **Blood volume:** Decrease in the blood volume decreases venous return and thus decrease cardiac output. In pregnancy, there is increase in blood volume and increase in venous return and cardiac output.
- **Positive intra-abdominal pressure:** Positive abdominal pressure also squeezes the abdominal veins promoting venous blood flow.
- **Pressure gradient produced by left ventricular contraction:** The left ventricular pump generates a systolic pressure of 120 mm Hg in the aorta. The pressure drops to 10 mm Hg in small veins, about 5 mm Hg in large veins and to almost 0 mm Hg in the right atrium. This pressure gradient favors blood flow from vein to right atrium.

Factors Affecting Ventricular Filling

- **Atrial contraction:** About 70% of ventricular filling occurs passively. The rest is contributed by atrial contraction. This is insignificant under normal conditions. But it becomes important when there is increase in heart rate.
- **Intrapericardial pressure:** When there is increase in intrapericardial pressure as in pericardial effusion, pericarditis, etc., there is a limit to the extent of distension of the chambers of heart. This leads to reduced filling and decrease in end-diastolic volume. According to Starling's law, force of contraction will be reduced leading to decrease in stroke volume and cardiac output.
- **Myocardial compliance:** Compliance is the ability of an organ to distend. Myocardial infarction leads to scarring and fibrosis of myocardium which affects the distensibility of heart because of increased ventricular stiffness. As a result, the EDV will be reduced leading to decrease in stroke volume.
- **Blood volume:** When blood volume is decreased, ventricular filling will be reduced due to decrease in venous return. This leads to decrease in stroke volume.

Aortic Impedance

Since aortic pressure is 7 times greater than pulmonary artery pressure, the stroke work of left ventricle is 7 times the stroke work of right ventricle. The aortic resistance offered to the outflow of blood when the ventricle contract is aortic impedance. It is the hydrostatic pressure of the blood in the aorta which opposes ventricular ejection. Thus it acts as a load against ventricular shortening. This is the **afterload**, i.e., the load acting on the heart after it begins to contract. It is the resistance against which ventricles pump the blood. If the resistance offered is high, as in systemic hypertension, the force of cardiac contraction should be increased to overcome this afterload. This is the reason for left ventricular hypertrophy in long-standing systemic hypertension.

Table 27.2: Factors involved in the homometric regulation of cardiac output.

Neural factors	Chemical factors
• Sympathetics	• Blood chemistry
• Parasympathetics	• Catecholamines, glucagon, thyroxine
• Higher centers	• Xanthenes, quinidine
• Spinal cord	• Procainamide, digitalis
• Medulla	• Propranolol, calcium
• Hypothalamus	• Ca^{2+} channel blockers
• Cortex	

Thus peripheral resistance has an important role in determining aortic impedance. In aortic stenosis where aortic impedance is high, intraventricular pressure must be increased to force blood through the stenotic valve. If the ventricular pressure is not adequate then there will be a reduction in stroke volume and cardiac output. In aortic insufficiency, regurgitation of blood produces an increase in the end-diastolic volume which produces an increase in stroke volume with little change in aortic impedance.

Homometric Regulation of Stroke Volume

Those factors operating from outside on the heart are included under homometric regulation of cardiac output (Table 27.2). The increased myocardial contractility occurs without any increase in the initial muscle length. Increase in the force of contraction increases stroke volume. The factors involved in homometric regulation are:

Neural Factors

Sympathetic stimulation increases force of cardiac contraction due to the positive inotropic effect of norepinephrine liberated at the sympathetic nerve endings. Inhibition of sympathetic activity decreases the force of cardiac contraction. Sympathetic stimulation not only increases the force of contraction but also increases heart rate. Since cardiac output is the product of stroke volume and heart rate, sympathetic stimulation leads to a marked increase in cardiac output. In exercise, sympathetic stimulation causes a 200–300% increase in heart rate and 50–60% increase in stroke volume leading to manifold increase in cardiac output.

Parasympathetic stimulation has negative inotropic effect but the reduction in the force of contraction is not significant because ventricles are devoid of parasympathetic supply.

Chemical Factors

- **Hypercapnia, hypoxia and acidosis** produce negative inotropic effect by decreasing the formation of cAMP.
- **Catecholamines** exert positive inotropic effect by acting on cardiac $β_1$ adrenergic receptors. Activation of $β_1$ receptors leads to activation of adenylyl cyclase. The resulting increase in cAMP increases intracellular Ca^{2+} concentration and increases myocardial contractility.
- **Xanthines** like caffeine and theophylline exert positive inotropic effect by inhibiting the breakdown of cAMP.
- **Glucagon** exerts positive inotropic effect by increasing the formation of cAMP.
- **Digitalis** increases cardiac contractility by inhibiting Na^+-K^+ ATPase in the myocardial cell. The resulting increase in intracellular Na^+ increases the availability of Ca^{2+} in the cell (*refer* Fig. 5.6)

REGULATION OF HEART RATE

- Neural factors
- Chemical factors
- Physical factors

NEURAL FACTORS

Autonomic Control

Heart is supplied by sympathetic and parasympathetic divisions of the nervous system (Chapter 26, Fig. 26.1). Neural regulation of heart rate is important because it responds within seconds. Sympathetic stimulation produces a positive chronotropic effect (increase in heart rate). **Norepinephrine** is the neurotransmitter. In the heart, norepinephrine produces its effect via **β-receptors**.

Parasympathetic preganglionic myelinated fibers reach the heart through the right and the left vagus. Parasympathetics have an inhibitory effect on heart, i.e., they depress the SA node and decrease heart rate. Neurotransmitter at the postganglionic ending is **acetylcholine**. Heart rate is kept constant by vagal tone (for details *refer* Chapter 26).

Central Influences on Heart Rate (*Refer* Chapter 26)

Chemical Factors (*refer* Chapter 26)

The chemical factors that affect heart rate are:
- Catecholamines
- Thyroxine
- PCO_2
- Hypoxia
- Acidosis
- Drugs.

PHYSICAL FACTORS REGULATING HEART RATE

When there is an increase in body temperature as in increased metabolic activity, heart rate is increased. Muscular exercise increases heart rate.

Regulation of Cardiac Output in Transplanted Heart

Normally during exercise, there is increased sympathetic discharge so that myocardial contractility and heart rate are increased and there is increase in cardiac output. But transplanted heart is devoid of cardiac innervation.

However, patients with transplanted heart are able to increase their cardiac output during exercise through the operation of **Frank-Starling mechanism**. During exercise there is increase in venous return and ventricular end-diastolic volume increases and the cardiac muscle contracts

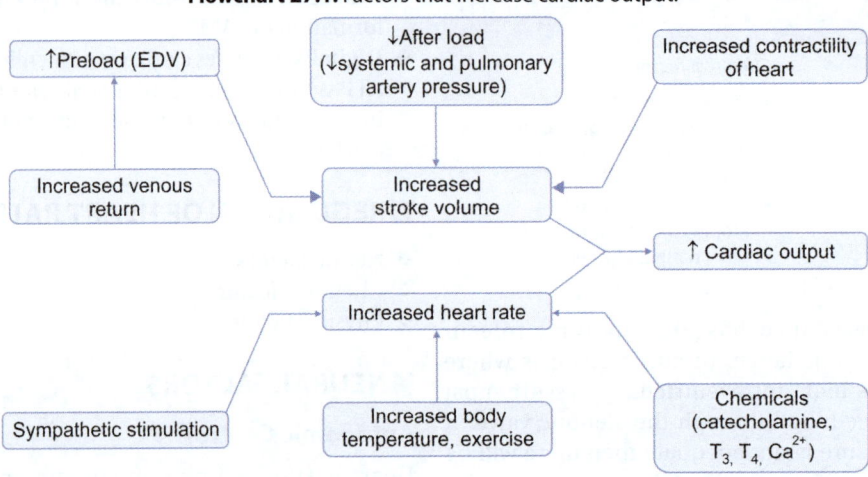

Flowchart 27.1: Factors that increase cardiac output.

more forcefully. Increase in venous return is due to the action of **skeletal muscle pump and respiratory pump**. In addition, there is vasodilatation in the muscle leading to decrease in peripheral resistance and thus the afterload **(aortic impedance) is decreased**. Thus there is marked increase in cardiac output in transplanted heart.

Factors that increase cardiac output are summarized in Flowchart 27.1.

MULTIPLE CHOICE QUESTIONS

1. **All the following statements are true regarding exercise, *except*:**
   a. The stroke volume remains almost unchanged in isometric exercise
   b. In isotonic exercise, there is appreciable increase in stroke volume
   c. In isotonic exercise, the venous return decreases remarkably
   d. In isotonic exercise, the cardiac output may increase to as high as 35 L/min

2. **Increase in cardiac output during exercise is due to:**
   a. Increased heart rate
   b. Decreased heart rate
   c. Increased total peripheral resistance
   d. Increased blood pressure

3. **The average blood flow in normal adult is:**
   a. 75 mL/100 g/min
   b. 54 mL/100 g/min
   c. 250 mL/100 g/min
   d. 2000 mL/100 g/min

4. **Cardiac index ratio is determined by:**
   a. Cardiac output and surface area
   b. Stroke volume and surface area
   c. Surface area only
   d. Peripheral resistance

5. **Cardiac output can be determined by all, *except*:**
   a. Fick's principle
   b. V/Q ratio
   c. Echocardiography
   d. Thermodilution method

6. **Volume determining preload is:**
   a. End-diastolic volume of ventricles
   b. End-systolic volume
   c. Volume of blood in aorta
   d. Ventricular ejection volume

7. **Cardiac output in liter per minute divided by heart rate equals:**
   a. Cardiac efficiency
   b. Cardiac index
   c. Stroke volume
   d. Mean arterial pressure

8. **A man consumes 1.5 L of O_2/min. his arterial PO_2 is 190 mL/L and O_2 content of mixed venous blood is 140 mL/L. Find out his cardiac output:**
   a. 3 L/min
   b. 15 L/min
   c. 30 L/min
   d. 60 L/min

9. **In a person with cardiac output 5 L/min and body surface area 1.7 m², what will be the cardiac index?**
   a. 3 L/min/m²
   b. 4 L/min/m²
   c. 5 L/min/m²
   d. 25 L/min/m²

10. **Cardiac index is defined as:**
    a. Stroke volume per square meter body surface area
    b. Cardiac output per unit body surface area
    c. Systolic pressure per square meter body surface area
    d. End-diastolic volume

11. **Cardiac index in a normal person is:**
    a. 2.1 L/min/m² body surface area
    b. 3.2 L/min/m² body surface area
    c. 4.6 L/min/m² body surface area
    d. 5.9 L/min/m² body surface area

12. **Basal cardiac output in an adult is approximately:**
    a. 7.5 liters
    b. 5 liters
    c. 12 liters
    d. 10 liters
13. **The work performed by the left ventricle is greater than that performed by the right ventricle because:**
    a. Contraction of left ventricle is slower
    b. Left ventricular wall is thicker
    c. Stroke volume is greater
    d. After load is greater on the left ventricle
14. **Starling's law of heart:**
    a. Explains the increase in cardiac output that occur when venous return is increased
    b. Explains the increase in cardiac output when sympathetic nerves to heart are stimulated
    c. Explains the increase in heart rate in exercise
    d. Does not operate during exercise
15. **Preload on myocardium depends on:**
    a. Stroke volume
    b. Aortic pressure
    c. End-diastolic volume
    d. Peripheral resistance
16. **Capacitance vessels are:**
    a. Large arteries
    b. Small arteries
    c. Arterioles
    d. Veins
17. **Increased level of circulating epinephrine produces all the following effects, *except*:**
    a. Increased thermogenesis
    b. Increased blood flow to skeletal muscle
    c. Tachycardia
    d. Increased total peripheral resistance
18. **Preload of the heart is determined by:**
    a. End-diastolic volume
    b. End-systolic volume
    c. Ejection volume
    d. Peripheral vascular resistance
19. **Exercise increases cardiac output by:**
    a. Vasodilatation
    b. Increasing heart rate
    c. Increasing blood pressure
    d. Decreasing peripheral resistance
20. **Cardiac output:**
    a. Increases in arrhythmia
    b. Decreases during sympathetic stimulation
    c. Is equal to the stroke volume times the heart rate
    d. Remains the same during exercise
21. **Cardiac output in a normal new born baby in mL/kg/min is:**
    a. 350
    b. 150
    c. 40
    d. 80
22. **Preload of the heart is determined by:**
    a. End-diastolic volume
    b. Ejection systolic volume
    c. End-systolic volume
    d. Systolic vascular resistance
23. **Direct Fick method of measuring cardiac output requires estimation of:**
    a. O_2 content of arterial blood
    b. O_2 consumption per unit time
    c. O_2 content of blood from right ventricle
    d. All of the above
24. **All the following factors increase cardiac output, *except*:**
    a. Late pregnancy
    b. Adrenaline
    c. Food intake
    d. Sitting from lying posture
25. **Which of the following is true about ventricular filling?**
    a. Atrial contraction mainly contributes
    b. Maximum during isometric ventricular relaxation
    c. Filling pressure is important for cardiac output
    d. Inotropic state of myocardium limits cardiac output
26. **Ejection fraction of the ventricle refers to the ratio of:**
    a. Amount of blood received/amount of blood ejected
    b. Stroke volume/end-diastolic volume
    c. End-systolic volume/end-diastolic volume
    d. Stroke volume/end-systolic volume
27. **Ejection fraction increases with increase in:**
    a. End-systolic volume
    b. End-diastolic volume
    c. Peripheral vascular resistance
    d. Venodilation
28. **All the following factors normally increase the length of the ventricular cardiac muscle fibers, *except*:**
    a. Increased venous tone
    b. Increased total blood volume
    c. Increased negative intrathoracic pressure
    d. Lying to standing change in posture
29. **A shift from lying down to erect posture is associated with all the following cardiovascular adjustments, *except*:**
    a. Rise in central venous pressure
    b. Rise in heart rate
    c. Decrease in cardiac output
    d. Decrease in stroke volume
30. **Increase in cardiac output during exercise is due to:**
    a. Increased heart rate
    b. Decreased heart rate
    c. Increased total peripheral resistance
    d. Increased blood pressure
31. **Increase in cardiac output in exercise is due to:**
    a. Decrease in peripheral resistance
    b. Increase in blood pressure
    c. Increase in heart rate
    d. Increase in peripheral resistance

SECTION 3 → Cardiovascular System

32. **The following may be the cause for right ventricular hypertrophy:**
    a. Aortic stenosis
    b. Pulmonary stenosis
    c. Athletic training
    d. Mitral stenosis

33. **All are increased during exercise, *except*:**
    a. Cardiac out put
    b. Venous return
    c. Coronary blood flow
    d. Peripheral vascular resistance

34. **Left ventricular systole corresponds to:**
    a. Atrial diastole
    b. Atrial systole
    c. T wave of ECG
    d. P wave of ECG

35. **All the following hormones affect myocardial performance, *except*:**
    a. Growth hormone
    b. Thyroxine
    c. Insulin
    d. Cortisol

36. **In a patient with transplanted heart, which of these are the reasons for the increased cardiac output during exercise?**
    a. Re-innervation of transplanted heart
    b. Intrinsic mechanism
    c. Epinephrine from medulla
    d. Frank-Starling mechanism

ANSWERS

1. c	2. a	3. a	4. a	5. b
6. a	7. c	8. c	9. a	10. b
11. b	12. b	13. d	14. a	15. c
16. d	17. d	18. a	19. b	20. c
21. a	22. a	23. d	24. d	25. c
26. b	27. b	28. d	29. a	30. a
31. c	32. b	33. d	34. a	35. a
36. c				

Vascular System and Arterial Blood Pressure

CHAPTER 28

LEARNING OBJECTIVES

Must know
- Define blood pressure and give the normal value for different age groups
- Explain the regulation of blood pressure
- Describe the pathophysiology of circulatory shock, heart failure and syncope
- Explain the determinants of arterial blood pressure
- Explain the regulation of peripheral resistance

■ VASCULAR SYSTEM

PY5.8: Describe and discuss local and systemic cardiovascular regulatory mechanisms.

Introduction

The term **artery** is used to describe vessels that are leaving the heart and the term **vein** is applied to vessels that return blood to the heart. Arteries are elastic, muscular tubes that divide to form arterioles and finally form microscopic capillary network. Venules conduct blood from capillary network, join together to form veins which carry blood back to the heart.

Development of Blood Vessels

Blood vessel formation starts by 15–16 days of development in the mesoderm of yolk sac, chorion and the connecting stalk. Blood vessels develop from mesenchymal cells called **angioblasts**. These cells aggregate to form isolated masses of cells called **blood islands**. Spaces appear in the islands which form the lumen of the blood vessel. The angioblasts lining these spaces give rise to the endothelium of blood vessels. Angioblasts around the endothelium form tunica media and tunica externa of larger vessels. Fusion of the blood islands forms an extensive network of blood vessels throughout the embryo. **Angiogenesis** means formation of new blood vessels.

Functions of Arteries

- Conduct blood to tissues.
- Serve as a high-pressure reservoir during systole. The blood volume contained in the arteries is called the **stressed volume**. The elastic nature of the arteries prevents blood pressure from increasing abnormally in ventricular systole. It also allows continuous blood flow in spite of intermittent pumping of heart, i.e., blood flow is maintained even during diastole. This is due to elastic recoil of large arteries and the resistance offered by the resistance vessels.
- Blood flow to the tissues is controlled by the degree of contraction or dilation of the small arteries and arterioles, i.e., the resistance vessels. This is achieved by the smooth muscle of these vessels. Normal arterial and venous pressures are shown in **Table 28.1**

Functions of Veins

- Veins function as a low-pressure system and a large reservoir of blood. The blood volume contained in the veins is called **unstressed volume**.
- Veins can constrict (venoconstriction) and propel blood forwards by means of venous pump towards the heart.
- The check valves present in series along the veins ensure that blood flows only in one direction, i.e., towards the heart. Backflow is prevented by these valves (*refer* Fig. 28.1).
- The vena cava which is the largest vein returns impure blood back to the heart.

Vascular system of systemic circulation is divided into:
1. Aorta and its branches which form the **distributing system**.
2. Arterioles, capillaries and venules form the **exchange system**.
3. Venous channels form the **collecting system**.

Table 28.1: Normal average arterial and venous pressures.

Vessel	Pressure (mm Hg)
Arterial pressure in adults	120/80
Arterial pressure at birth	80/60
Mean arterial pressure	95
Small veins	10
End of vena cava	0

Structure of Blood Vessels

The wall of blood vessels (except capillaries) consists of three layers, **tunica intima**, **tunica media** and **tunica adventitia**. These layers are well-developed in the arteries, but in the veins, these layers are less well-demarcated and the tunica media is thinner, with few smooth muscle cells. Large blood vessels, such as aorta and vena cavae are supplied by a network of small blood vessels called **vasa vasorum** (meaning: the vessels of the vessels). The wall of capillaries consists of only a single layer of endothelial cells resting on a basement membrane.

Tunica Intima

Tunica intima consists of endothelium resting on the connective tissue layer, the **internal elastic lamina** consisting of dense elastic matrix. The endothelium is one-cell thick and the cells are sealed to each other by tight junctions in many tissues. The endothelium completely lines the inside of the vascular system including the lymphatics. It regulates vascular permeability, blood clotting and immune function. Normally it is very smooth since it is in contact with blood so that blood flows through the vessels with very little friction. But in atherosclerosis, cholesterol gets deposited in the sub-intimal layer and endothelium becomes rough.

Types of Endothelium

1. *Continuous type* found in blood-brain barrier is impermeable to large molecules.
2. *Fenestrated type* found in liver, endocrine glands and kidney contain numerous holes or fenestrae which allow molecules to cross.
3. *Discontinuous type* found in spleen allows red blood cells to pass out.

Tunica Media

Tunica media is the middle, main part of the vascular wall. In muscular arteries this layer contains **elastin** and **vascular smooth muscle** arranged in a circular layer. Vascular smooth muscle is a combination of visceral smooth muscle and multiunit smooth muscle. In large arteries, elastic tissue predominates, whereas in arterioles, smooth muscle predominates. When the smooth muscle contracts, it causes narrowing of the lumen referred to as **vasoconstriction**. Veins contain more elastin and less smooth muscle. Tunica media is limited by external elastic lamina. Nerve bundles infiltrate the tunica media and the vascular smooth muscle is under the control of sympathetic nervous system. The vascular smooth muscles are in a state of partial contraction called the **vasomotor tone** which is regulated by sympathetic fibers. Sympathetic endings release **norepinephrine** at their endings in the vascular smooth muscle and cause vasoconstriction. The action is mediated via α-receptors. Vasomotor tone is also controlled by higher centers, hormones and chemicals. Thus the middle layer profoundly influences blood flow.

Tunica Adventitia

Tunica adventitia is the outer layer composed of connective tissue. It contains elastin and collagen. This layer provides flexibility, strength and stability to blood vessels.

Classification of Blood Vessels

- Windkessel vessels
- Resistance vessels
- Sphincter vessels
- Exchange vessels
- Capacitance vessels
- Shunt vessels.

Windkessel Vessels

Windkessel vessels (distensible vessels) are large vessels that contain large amount of elastic fibers and lesser amount of smooth muscle fibers. These vessels can distend due to elasticity during systole and can recoil back during diastole. Examples are **aorta and its large branches**. Since these vessels are elastic, during systole, they are stretched to accommodate the extra blood. The forward flow becomes continuous because of the elastic recoil of these vessels during diastole. This recoil effect is called **Windkessel effect** and the vessels are called windkessel vessels. Windkessel is the German word for an elastic reservoir.

Resistance Vessels

Resistance vessels are **small arteries and arterioles** which contain more of smooth muscle fibers and less of elastic fibers. Since smooth muscles are arranged circularly around the vessel, their contraction produces vasoconstriction and their relaxation produces vasodilation. Vasoactive substances and the sympathetic supply to the blood vessel decide the caliber of the vessel and thereby the diastolic blood pressure.

Sphincter Vessels

Sphincter vessels are **met-arterioles and pre-capillary sphincters**. Contraction of pre-capillary sphincter regulates blood flow through capillaries. During rest, many of the capillaries remain closed by the contraction of met-arterioles and precapillary sphincters. During activity, such as exercise the met-arteriole and the pre-capillary sphincter will dilate and more capillaries are opened up, which is called **recruitment** of closed capillaries. Now, more blood flows through the capillaries. Thus these vessels along with resistance vessels are the main sites of peripheral resistance which regulates blood flow through a circuit. Small variations in the tone of these vessels can effectively alter blood flow, tissue perfusion and hydrostatic pressure.

Exchange Vessels

Exchange vessels are the **capillaries** which is about 1 μm thick. Diameter of the capillary is about 6–7 μm. Tunica media and tunica adventitia are absent in the capillaries. Tunica intima has a single layer of endothelial cells so that

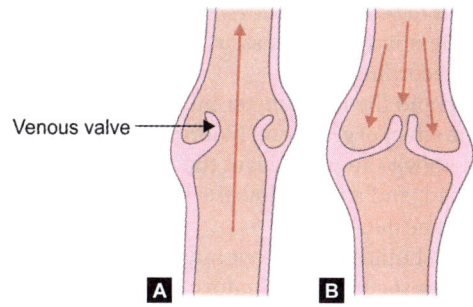

Figs. 28.1A and B: Mechanism of action of venous valves: (A) Valves open when blood flows towards the heart; (B) Valves close when blood flows in the opposite direction.

filtration and reabsorption can occur effectively between blood and interstitial fluid. Capillaries are devoid of nerve supply. The factors that affect the tone of the pre-capillary sphincters regulate the blood flow in the capillaries.

Capacitance Vessels

Capacitance vessels are thin walled and highly distensible because they contain more of elastic tissue and little smooth muscle. So, they can accommodate large amount of blood, e.g., **veins**. Even if there is increase in the blood volume there is not much change in the pressure in the veins. But in the arterial system increase in blood volume causes increase in the arterial pressure. Capacitance vessels can undergo severe constriction in times of need and can thus maintain cardiac output. The smooth muscles of these vessels are supplied by autonomic nervous system. Since these vessels can change the capacity of the vascular system to accommodate blood, they are called **capacitance vessels**. Valves are present in the course of the veins particularly those of the limbs. This prevents back flow of blood and thus helps to direct blood flow towards the heart (**Figs. 28.1A and B**).

Shunt Vessels

Shunt vessels or **thoroughfare vessels** are communications between met-arterioles and venules, i.e., they are **arteriovenous anastomotic channels or shunts**. These vessels bypass the capillary circulation (*refer* **Fig. 32.1**). These shunts are seen in exposed areas, such as hands and feet, earlobes, lips etc. These vessels play an important role in thermoregulation. They also play a role in diverting blood to active tissues in times of need.

■ ARTERIAL BLOOD PRESSURE

PY5.9: Describe the factors affecting heart rate, regulation of cardiac output and blood pressure.

Definition

Arterial blood pressure is defined as the lateral thrust or lateral pressure exerted on the walls of the blood vessels by the contained blood. Blood pressure is expressed as systolic pressure/diastolic pressure in terms of mm of Hg. Normal average blood pressure in a healthy adult is about **120/70 mm Hg**.

When the left ventricle contracts, it forces blood into the already full systemic arteries. This creates a pressure that drives blood through the systemic circulation. Instead of pumping a continuous stream, the heart pumps intermittently. As a result, the arterial pressure rises during systole and falls during diastole. In a cardiac cycle, during ventricular systole, the pressure in the aorta and the large arteries rises to a peak value of about 120 mm Hg and is referred to as the **systolic blood pressure**. During ventricular diastole, the pressure falls to a minimum value of 70 mm Hg (average value) which is called the **diastolic blood pressure** (*refer* **Table 28.1**).

Difference between systolic and diastolic pressure is called the **pulse pressure** which is about 50 mm Hg in an adult in the resting state.

Mean arterial pressure is the average pressure throughout the cardiac cycle.

Mean arterial pressure = Diastolic pressure + 1/3 Pulse pressure = 70 + 16 = 86 mm Hg.

The mean arterial pressure determines the average rate of blood flow through the systemic vessels and thereby tissue perfusion.

The pressure falls to half of this pressure in the arterioles and to one-fourth in the capillaries because the resistance to flow is high in the small arteries and arterioles (**Fig. 28.2**). The mean pressure at the end of arterioles is 30–38 mm Hg. The pulse pressure is only 5 mm Hg at the ends of arterioles. The pressure drop will be still more in cases of vasoconstriction.

Normal Range of Blood Pressure

1. Systolic pressure—100–140 mm Hg
2. Diastolic pressure—60–90 mm Hg

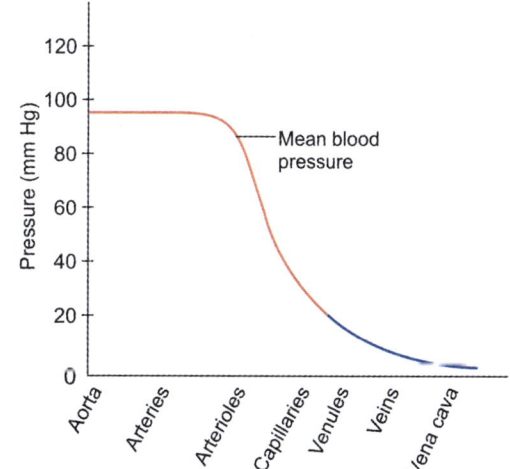

Fig. 28.2: Mean blood pressure in the different parts of the vascular system.

MEASUREMENT OF ARTERIAL BLOOD PRESSURE

- Direct method
- Indirect method.
  - Palpatory method
  - Auscultatory method

Direct Method

In **direct method**, a cannula is inserted into an artery and the pressure in the artery can be measured by connecting the cannula to a mercury manometer. By this method, **end arterial pressure** can also be determined. Direct method can be employed only in experimental animals.

Indirect Method

Palpatory Method

An inflatable cuff called **Riva-Rocci cuff** attached to a mercury manometer called **sphygmomanometer** is wrapped around the upper arm. The cuff is inflated until the radial pulse disappears. Slowly deflate the cuff and note the cuff pressure at which the radial pulse first reappears. The pressure now recorded gives an approximate idea about the systolic blood pressure. Deflate the cuff completely. This method is the **palpatory method** for determining blood pressure (BP) and it is usually 2-5 mm Hg lower than that obtained by the auscultatory method.

Auscultatory Method

The arterial blood pressure in humans is routinely measured by the auscultatory method. After the palpatory method, inflate the cuff to a pressure 5-10 mm Hg more than the systolic value obtained by the palpatory method. Place a stethoscope over the **brachial artery** at the elbow and slowly deflate the cuff. No sound is heard initially. At a point at which the systolic pressure in the brachial artery is just above the cuff pressure, a **tapping sound** is heard through the stethoscope. The cuff pressure at which the sound is first heard is taken as the systolic pressure. The tapping sound is heard because; a spurt of blood passes through the compressed artery with each heart beat causing turbulence in the blood flow. The cuff pressure is lowered further and the sound becomes **louder, dull, muffled and finally disappears**. The cuff pressure at which the sound disappears is taken as the diastolic pressure. The sounds heard while recording blood pressure are called **Korotkoff's sounds**, named after a Russian scientist. The cause for the Korotkoff's sounds is turbulence to the flow of blood in the brachial artery. Streamline flow in the unconstricted (normal patent) artery is silent but when the artery is narrowed, the velocity of flow through the constriction exceeds **critical velocity** and the flow becomes **turbulent**, producing sound.

Other instruments used to record BP, such as aneroid manometers, electronic devices, etc., should be periodically calibrated with the mercury manometer.

Precautions to be taken while recording BP:

- The patient is allowed to sit in a quiet room for 5 minutes before recording BP.
- The cuff and the manometer must be at the heart level so that the effect of gravity on blood pressure can be avoided. If it is above the heart level the pressure is found to be increased, and if it is below the heart level the pressure is found to be decreased.
- The cuff should not be kept inflated in the arm for some time after recording palpatory BP because it produces a generalized reflex vasoconstriction giving a false high value in the auscultatory method. It also produces much discomfort to the patient because of reduced blood flow to the limb.
- When blood pressure is recorded in a person for the first time, pressure in both arms should be recorded to rule out any vascular obstruction.
- In obese individuals, accurate pressure can be obtained by using a cuff that is wider than the standard arm cuff. Larger cuffs are required for people with arm circumference more than 32 cm and vice versa. Using a cuff of smaller size than required, gives higher values of BP. Brachial arterial pressure gives high readings because there is more tissue between the cuff and the artery in obese people. The standard bladder of the cuff is 12 to 13 cm wide and 35 cm long. Smaller and larger bladders are available.
- Palpatory method should be first employed before doing auscultatory method to **avoid auscultatory gap** (silent gap). When the cuff pressure is lowered, the Korotkoff's sounds sometimes disappear at pressures well above diastolic pressure and then reappear at lower pressures. This is auscultatory gap and is usually seen in people with high blood pressure. If palpatory method is not done in such subjects a false pressure will be recorded. For example, if the cuff pressure is raised only up to the auscultatory gap the systolic pressure will be taken as the manometer reading at which the sound reappears after the auscultatory gap. This gives a false low value for the systolic pressure. Auscultatory gap can also be avoided by inflating the cuff till the radial pulse disappears.
- At least two measurements made 1 to 2 minutes apart are taken and the average value is recorded as the blood pressure.
- In the first visit blood pressure in both hands should be recorded and the higher value should be taken as reference.

VARIATIONS IN BLOOD PRESSURE

Physiological Variation

- **Age**: The systolic as well as the diastolic pressure increases with advancing age but the rise in systolic pressure is more pronounced. Systolic pressure increases up to about 80 years, whereas diastolic pressure increases only up to the age of 50 years. In the elderly, diastolic blood pressure may fall. This causes widening of pulse pressure with advancing age.

In newborn, systolic pressure is only 30-60 mm Hg, in children it is 105 mm Hg, in adults it is 120 mm Hg and in old age it becomes 140 mm Hg.

- ❖ **Sex**: As compared to men of the same age, females have a lower BP up to menopause.
- ❖ **Diurnal variation**: BP is minimal in the early morning and maximum in the evening.
- ❖ **Built**: Obese people have a high BP.
- ❖ **Digestion**: During digestion, there is a slight increase in systolic BP.
- ❖ **Sleep**: During quiet restful sleep, there is a fall in BP by about 10-20 mm Hg. This fall is absent in hypertension.
- ❖ **Emotional state**: BP may increase or decrease depending on the type of emotion. For example, in anxiety there is increase in cardiac output and peripheral resistance and hence there is increase in BP. Frustration, depression, etc. produce a fall in BP.
- ❖ **Muscular exercise** increases BP temporarily. Systolic BP increases in all types of exercise because there is increase in cardiac output. In severe exercise, the diastolic BP falls due to vasodilatation and fall in peripheral resistance.
- ❖ **Posture and gravity**: In the standing posture, diastolic BP is high, whereas in the lying down posture, systolic BP is high. The pressure in any vessel below the heart level is higher than that in any vessel above the heart level due to the effect of gravity. In an adult man in the standing posture, the mean arterial pressure at heart level is 100 mm Hg, that in a large artery of head it is about 62 mm Hg and pressure in a large artery in the foot is 180 mm Hg.
- ❖ **Phases of respiration**: During inspiration, there is a slight increase in BP and during expiration slight fall in BP.
- ❖ **Climate**: Exposure to cold increases both systolic and diastolic blood pressure due to vasoconstriction and increased sympathetic activity. Exposure to warmth decreases both systolic and diastolic BP due to vasodilatation.
- ❖ **White coat hypertension or isolated clinic hypertension**: This refers to the condition in which blood pressure is persistently elevated in the clinic and normal out of the clinic. It is seen in 13% of individuals.

Pathological Variation

Hypertension

A sustained elevation of the systemic arterial BP above the normal range is termed as **systemic hypertension**. In adults, elevation of systolic blood pressure **above 140 mm Hg** and diastolic BP **above 90 mm Hg** is considered as hypertension. A prolonged high BP may result in serious consequences. *Serial recording of BP should be done before establishing as hypertension*. Elevation of blood pressure without an evident organic cause is called **primary or essential hypertension**. If the cause is known, it is called **secondary hypertension**. Classification of blood pressure is given in **Table 28.2**.

Pulmonary hypertension is increase in the pressure in the pulmonary artery and this is independent of the pressure in the systemic arteries.

Table 28.2: Classification of blood pressure.

	Systolic pressure (mm Hg)	Diastolic pressure (mm Hg)
Normal	120–129	80–84
High normal	130–139	85–89
Grade 1 hypertension	140–159	90–99
Grade 2 hypertension	160–179	100–109
Grade 3 hypertension	≥180	≥110
Isolated systolic hypertension	≥140	< 90

Consequences of Sustained High BP

- ❖ High pressure makes the heart do extra work and subjects the arterial system to undue strain leading to cardiac failure.
- ❖ Enlargement of the heart due to hypertrophy especially left ventricular hypertrophy due to increased aortic impedance.
- ❖ Atherosclerosis and myocardial infarction.
- ❖ Rupture or thrombosis of cerebral vessels leading to stroke and even death.
- ❖ Renal failure occurs due to changes occurring in the renal arteries.
- ❖ Retinopathy due to changes occurring in the retinal vessels
- ❖ Congestive cardiac failure
- ❖ Arrhythmias

Types of Hypertension

1. Malignant hypertension
2. Primary or essential hypertension
3. Secondary hypertension

Malignant Hypertension

If chronic hypertension is left untreated, necrotic arteriolar lesions develop in different parts, such as retina, brain, kidney, etc., leading to papilledema, cerebral symptoms and renal failure. This is malignant hypertension and the arterial BP increases up to or above 260/150 mm Hg.

Primary Hypertension

Primary hypertension is the type of hypertension seen in 88% of hypertensive and the arterial BP is persistently more than 150/90 mm Hg. The *exact cause is not known*. Environmental factors play a significant role in the pathogenesis of hypertension and are more common in women. Peripheral resistance is found to be increased. The condition is treated with α-adrenergic blockers, β-blockers, Ca^{2+} channel blockers, angiotensin converting enzyme (ACE) inhibitors, etc.

Secondary Hypertension

In secondary hypertension, the cause is known. The various types are:

a. **Neurogenic hypertension**: Bilateral lesions of nucleus tractus solitarius (NTS) cause severe hypertension where the blood pressure will be about 300/200 mm Hg. This is called neurogenic hypertension. This can be experimentally produced by cutting the baroreceptor afferents to NTS coming through carotid sinus nerve (a branch of IX cranial nerve) and vagus.

b. **Renal hypertension**: Nephritis, renal artery stenosis, etc. cause hypertension. The hypertension that follows constriction of the renal artery or compression of the kidney is called renal hypertension. This is due to increased plasma renin activity and decreased excretion of Na$^+$ (*refer* Goldblatt hypertension, Chapter 55).
c. **Endocrine disorders** such as, *pheochromocytoma* secrete large amounts of catecholamines. In *thyrotoxicosis*, increase in cardiac output increases systolic blood pressure. *Cushing syndrome, acromegaly, primary hyperaldosteronism and metabolic syndrome* are also associated with hypertension.
d. **Pill hypertension**: Oral contraceptive pills contain large doses of estrogen which causes retention of fluid and electrolytes and also increases formation of angiotensin II which in turn increases blood pressure.
e. Epithelial sodium channel (ENaC) gene mutation leads to excess renal Na$^+$ retention leading to hypertension called **Liddle's syndrome**.
f. **Severe polycythemia** increases blood viscosity, which increases peripheral resistance leading to hypertension.
g. **Toxemia** of pregnancy is characterized by hypertension.

Hypotension

A persistent reduction in the arterial BP is known as hypotension. A reduction in the systolic pressure **below 100 mm Hg** and diastolic **below 60 mm Hg** is hypotension. Sudden hypotension will cause loss of consciousness called **fainting or syncope**. Hypotension is due to an inadequate cardiac output or a decrease in the peripheral resistance or a decrease in the blood volume or a combination of these (for details *refer* circulatory shock Page 272).

Postural hypotension: As a result of prolonged standing as in parades, venous return is reduced due to pooling of blood in the lower limbs which leads to a reduction in cardiac output and hypotension called postural hypotension or **orthostatic hypotension**. In orthostatic hypotension there should be a fall in BP by at least 30 mm Hg systolic and 15 mm Hg diastolic within 3 minutes of standing from a previous 3 minute interval in the recumbent position.

DETERMINANTS OF ARTERIAL BLOOD PRESSURE

1. Cardiac output
2. Blood volume
3. Peripheral resistance
4. Viscosity of blood
5. Elasticity of vessel wall

Factors 1 and 2 determine systolic BP and the other factors determine diastolic BP.

Cardiac Output

Pumping action of heart is the main factor for controlling cardiac output. During ventricular systole, when blood is pumped into the already full arterial system, it cannot escape at once into the periphery in the same amount as it enters the aorta. This leads to distension of the large arteries and the pressure in these vessels rises until the outflow balances the inflow. The arterial blood pressure depends on the rate at which blood enters the arterial system and the rate at which it leaves the arterial system into the capillaries and veins. Thus blood pressure depends on cardiac output. Increase in cardiac output due to increase in heart rate or stroke volume or both will increase the systemic arterial BP.

Blood Volume

The arterial wall is elastic and distensible. Certain degree of stretching must occur before a considerable pressure is created. Actually the arterial system is overfilled with the normally circulating blood. The greater the overfilling due to increased blood volume, greater will be the arterial pressure. Thus the arterial pressure depends on blood volume. In cases of decreased blood volume as in persistent diarrhea, vomiting, hemorrhage, etc., the blood volume is decreased and so the blood pressure also falls.

Peripheral Resistance

The rate of outflow from the arterial system depends upon the peripheral resistance. The peripheral resistance depends on the caliber of small arteries, mainly the arterioles, and to a small extent the capillaries. Up to small arteries, the vessels are highly elastic, but arterioles are less distensible and the lumen diameter is also less. So they offer the maximum resistance. The smooth muscles of the arterioles are in a state of partial constriction and this exerts resistance to the outflow of blood from the arterial system. Greater part of peripheral resistance is offered by vessels of skeletal muscles and splanchnic vessels. So the state of constriction or dilatation of these vessels determines the diastolic BP to a large extent.

In severe exercise, there is dilatation of the skeletal muscle blood vessels due to the accumulation of metabolites and also due to stimulation of the sympathetic cholinergic fibers innervating the skeletal muscle blood vessels. This is the *reason for a fall in the diastolic pressure in exercise*.

Viscosity of Blood

Peripheral resistance also depends on the viscosity of blood. Greater the viscosity greater will be the pressure required to force blood through the blood vessel in a given time. If the pressure gradient is kept constant, the greater the viscosity the longer will be the time required by the blood to traverse the vessel. Viscosity of blood affects blood pressure at the arteriolar level and the diastolic pressure is mainly affected. For example, in polycythemia, leukemia, etc., the viscosity is increased and there is an increase in the diastolic pressure.

Elasticity of the Vessel Wall

Elasticity of the vessel wall and peripheral resistance together maintain the normal arterial blood pressure. When the ventricle forces blood into the already full aorta, the blood cannot flow out into the peripheral vessels in the same amount due to peripheral resistance. Since the vessel wall is elastic and distensible in nature, it gets distended. The distended arterial wall can accommodate some amount of blood and the blood pressure is prevented from rising to high values. The distensibility of the vessel wall determines the systolic pressure. During diastole, no blood flows into the arterial system from the ventricles. The distended arterial wall now recoils and rebounds on the contained blood. Thus the elastic recoil acts as a subsidiary pump to force blood onwards along the peripheral vessels. This elastic recoil prevents the fall of BP to zero during diastole and it is maintained at about 70–80 mm Hg. For elastic recoil to occur, a prior distension of the vessel should be there. But for distension to occur, peripheral resistance is necessary. Thus, the *elasticity of the vessel wall and peripheral resistance act together to maintain the diastolic BP*. Elasticity of the vessel wall also affects the systolic pressure.

REGULATION OF PERIPHERAL RESISTANCE

Peripheral resistance is contributed by small arterioles and to a small extent the capillaries. The arteriolar smooth muscles are in a partially contracted state and this contributes an inherent **vascular tone** to the arterioles. This is the cause for peripheral resistance and its value depends on the caliber of the vessels. The vascular tone can be altered by nervous factors, physical factors and chemical factors.

Regulation of peripheral resistance is divided into:
1. Neural factors
2. Reflex regulation
3. Hormonal factors
4. Non-hormonal factors
5. Local factors

Neural Factors

Control of vascular tone is called **vasomotor control**. Blood vessels are supplied by vasoconstrictor and vasodilator fibers. Both sets of fibers together constitute vasomotor nerves.

Vasoconstrictor Fibers

Most important is the **sympathetic vasoconstrictor fibers** which arise from thoracolumbar outflow of autonomic nervous system. They arise from a group of neurons in the lateral horn of the gray matter of spinal cord from T_1 to L_2 segments. The neurons in the lateral horn are the preganglionic neurons. The preganglionic fibers (myelinated) emerge out of the spinal cord through the ventral root, enter the white rami communicantes and enter the paravertebral sympathetic chain and relay in the sympathetic ganglion. The postganglionic fibers (unmyelinated) enter the spinal nerve through the gray rami communicantes and supply the blood vessels (*refer* Fig. 94.1).

Since the sympathetic fibers release norepinephrine at their endings they are called **adrenergic fibers**. Action of sympathetic vasoconstrictor fibers is to produce vasoconstriction, thereby increasing the peripheral resistance and diastolic BP. *Thus, peripheral resistance is controlled by the sympathetics*. The action of sympathetic vasoconstrictor fibers is not pronounced in the cerebral and coronary blood vessels.

Here, the vasomotor effect is mainly by the action of local factors such as metabolites. The postganglionic sympathetic fibers, supply all blood vessels except capillaries and small venules. Capillary dilatation is affected by local factors.

Sympathetic Tone

The tonic discharge through the sympathetic fibers maintains the blood vessels in a partially contracted state and this is called **sympathetic tone**. The normal physiological rate of discharge through these nerves is 1–2 impulses/sec but may come to 10/sec with maximal physiological excitation. This is held in check by the neurons in the vasomotor center (VMC) in medulla. The neurons in the VMC control the spinal sympathetic neurons. VMC is located bilaterally in the reticular formation of medulla and lower part of pons. It consists of three areas:

1. A vasoconstrictor area, called rostral ventrolateral medulla (RVLM) contains neurons whose axons are distributed to the preganglionic vasoconstrictor sympathetic neurons of spinal cord.
2. A vasodilator area in the lower part of medulla. The fibers from the neurons in this area project to the vasoconstrictor area and inhibit the vasomotor activity of this area leading to vasodilatation. The existence of the vasodilator area is now controversial. Equivalent of this area is caudal ventrolateral medulla (CVLM) which inhibits the RVLM.
3. A sensory area located in the nucleus tractus solitarius in the lower pons and medulla. This area receives sensory nerve impulses from the baroreceptors through vagus and glossopharyngeal nerve. The output from this area controls the activities of both vasoconstrictor and vasodilator areas of VMC. An example is sino-aortic reflex which controls arterial blood pressure.

When the sympathetic nerve is cut, the blood vessels dilate. This shows that in most of the tissues, vasodilatation is produced by inhibition of the sympathetic discharge. But in skeletal muscles, vasodilatation is produced by activating the vasodilator fibers.

The degree of discharge through the sympathetic fibers is also influenced by spinal neurons in addition to control by the VMC.

Higher Control of Vasomotor Center (VMC)

Stimulation of **motor cortex** excites the VMC by impulses coming through the hypothalamus to the constrictor area of VMC and causes increase in BP. Afferents to VMC also come from **limbic cortex** and this pathway is responsible for the change in BP during emotional states. For example, there is an increase in BP and heart rate in sexual excitement and during anger. Stimulation of the cingulate gyrus, a part of limbic system, produces a fall in BP due to vasodilatation. Acute pain produces a rise in BP due to the afferents coming to the VMC from reticular formation. But excruciating and prolonged pain produce fall in BP and even fainting.

Sympathetic Vasodilator Fibers

Some **sympathetic fibers** supplying the blood vessels especially of the **skeletal muscles** release acetylcholine at

Flowchart 28.1: Sympathetic vasodilator system.

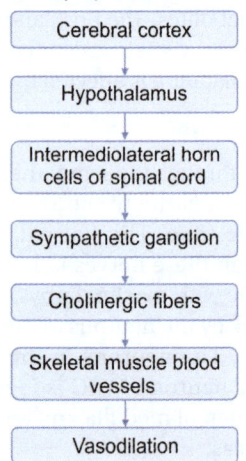

their endings. Acetylcholine produces vasodilatation by acting on M_3 muscarinic receptors on blood vessels. Mechanism is by releasing nitric oxide (NO) or endothelium derived relaxing factor (EDRF). Sympathetic cholinergic fibers do not exhibit tonic discharge because they have no connection with the VMC. The sympathetic cholinergic fibers originate from the cerebral cortex and relay in the **anterior hypothalamus**. From here, fibers pass through the mesencephalon and reach the spinal cord lateral horn cells. They have no relay in the medulla. They are known as **sympathetic cholinergic fibers** (Flowchart 28.1 and Fig. 28.3).

Discharge through these fibers occurs during exercise. Skeletal muscle blood vessels also have adrenergic supply (action on α-receptors of muscle blood vessels and produces vasoconstriction) and exhibit the resting sympathetic tone. *Baroreceptor afferents do not affect the vasodilator cholinergic transmission.*

Sympathetic vasodilator fibers fire during exercise and also during certain intense emotional conditions, such as fear, which is the cause for fainting attacks in times of fear. This is because of the activation of muscle vasodilator system leading to a rapid fall in arterial pressure. This leads to decreased blood flow to the brain and causes loss of consciousness. This is called **fainting or syncope**. If there is simultaneous stimulation of vagal cardioinhibitory center, the heart rate decreases markedly and the condition is called **vasovagal syncope**.

Parasympathetic vasodilator fibers come through the craniosacral outflow and supply the blood vessels of salivary glands, gastrointestinal glands, tongue, external genitalia, anal canal, etc. They are not tonically active under normal circumstances. Parasympathetic stimulation releases **acetylcholine** at their endings which causes vasodilatation. Parasympathetic fibers also liberate kallikreins which lead to the production of **bradykinin** which is a powerful vasodilator. Effect is more in the glands and gastrointestinal tract. Parasympathetic vasodilator system does not have a significant role in regulating peripheral resistance.

Axon Reflex

According to **Bell-Magendie law**, all the afferents from sensory receptors in the periphery pass only through the dorsal root of spinal cord and efferent fibers pass only through the ventral root. There are a few exceptions to this law where the forward conduction dies off and **antidromic** (in the reverse direction) conduction occurs. An example is **axon reflex (Fig. 28.4)**. Stimulation of the skin in a particular area produces cutaneous vasodilatation in the adjacent area. Axon reflex is not a true reflex; it is a **local reflex**. Since there is no center in the reflex, it is also called a **pseudoreflex**. The afferent fiber gives collaterals to the blood vessels supplying the area adjacent to the area that is stimulated. When the skin is stimulated, there is vasodilatation in the adjacent area because the impulses traverse in the reverse direction through collaterals and cause vasodilatation. The transmitters released at the collateral endings are substance P, acetylcholine, ATP, histamine-like substances, etc. Stimuli for axon reflex include trauma, cooling, frostbite, heating, etc. The **flare** reaction seen in triple response is due to axon reflex elicited by the mechanical stimulus. Axon reflex does not contribute to systemic control of circulation.

Reflex Mechanisms

- Baroreceptor reflex
- Chemoreceptor reflex
- Bainbridge reflex
- Bezold-Jarisch reflex
- Cushing reflex
- CNS ischemic response
- Skeletal muscle tone
- Venous tone

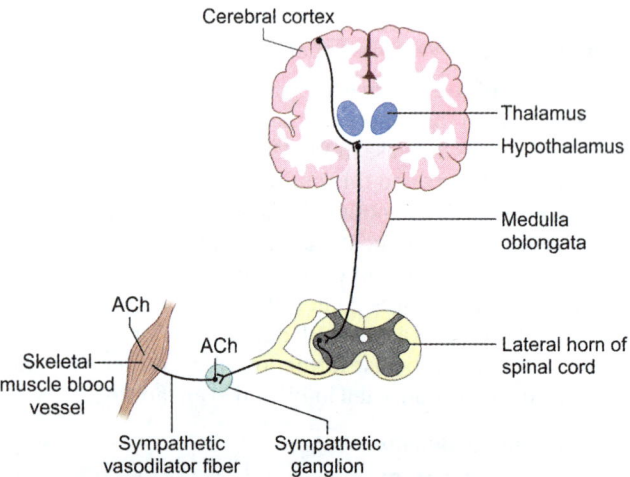

Fig. 28.3: Pathway of sympathetic vasodilator system.

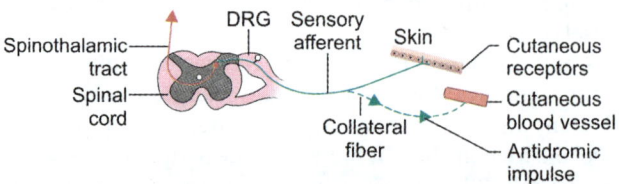

Fig. 28.4: Pathway for axon reflex (it is a pseudoreflex because the impulse does not reach the spinal cord).

Baroreceptor Reflex or Sino-aortic Reflex

When there is stretch of the blood vessel wall, baroreceptors located in the carotid sinus and aortic arch get stimulated. There is a continuous stream of impulses from baroreceptors to the blood vessels through the vasomotor center (VMC). Depending on the degree of stretch, the rate of impulses increases causing change in the vasomotor tone and thereby adjusting blood pressure. Baroreceptor mechanism is an instantaneously acting mechanism and is short lived due to the property of adaptation. *Baroreceptor mechanism is the most important mechanism for the short- term regulation of blood pressure in the range of 50–200 mm Hg.* In chronic hypertension, the baroreceptor mechanism becomes reset to maintain an elevated rather than a normal blood pressure. So this reflex is important only in short-term regulation of blood pressure.

When there is increase in BP, there is increased stretch of the vessel wall which leads to increase in the degree of firing through the buffer nerves from the baroreceptors. There is inhibition of VMC, and the sympathetic discharge is very much decreased leading to vasodilatation and decrease in peripheral resistance. This leads to a reduction in the blood pressure. At the same time the baroreceptor stimulation causes pronounced stimulation of cardioinhibitory center (CIC) and reflex bradycardia occurs. This is known as **sino-aortic reflex** mechanism where there is *a fall in BP and reflex bradycardia* (*refer* **Fig. 26.3**).

When there is a fall in blood pressure, i.e., in times of **hypotension**, there is no stretch on the vessel wall and there will be no stimulation of baroreceptors. Even the normal stream of impulses coming through the buffer nerves cease. Thus there is no inhibition of VMC and no stimulation of CIC, which leads to an increase in the blood pressure due to increased sympathetic tone to blood vessels and an increase in heart rate because there is no stimulation of CIC. Here, there is *reflex increase in BP and reflex tachycardia*.

Chemoreceptor Mechanism

Chemoreceptor mechanisms involve changes in blood chemistry affecting the VMC. When the mean arterial BP falls to 30–40 mm Hg, this mechanism is important to increase BP.

Bezold-Jarisch Reflex

When veratridine is injected into the left coronary, the effects are reflex apnea, hypotension and bradycardia. Receptors are present in the left ventricular wall.

Cushing Reflex

In **Cushing reflex**, there is hypertension with bradycardia in raised intracranial tension (*refer* **Fig 26.5**).

CNS Ischemic Response

Central nervous system (CNS) ischemic response operates when the mean arterial BP falls below 60 mm Hg. The blood flow to the VMC is decreased to cause CNS ischemia. This leads to accumulation of CO_2 and other metabolites in the area of VMC and causes excitation of VMC neurons. This leads to strong sympathetic stimulation leading to generalized vasoconstriction and increase in peripheral resistance and increase in BP.

Venous Tone

Venous tone affects venous return and thereby cardiac output and blood pressure.

Skeletal Muscle Tone

When there is skeletal muscle contraction the veins are compressed leading to increase in venous return and cardiac output, thereby increasing BP.

Hormonal Regulation of Peripheral Resistance

1. Epinephrine and norepinephrine
2. Vasopressin
3. Renin-angiotensin-aldosterone mechanism

Epinephrine and Norepinephrine

Epinephrine and norepinephrine produce varying effects on cardiovascular system. They exert their effect via α **and β receptors**. Cardiac acceleration by epinephrine is via β-receptor stimulation. On blood vessels, β-receptor stimulation produces vasodilatation and this effect is seen in the skeletal muscle blood vessels. The main action of epinephrine is through β-receptors. Epinephrine produces vasoconstriction via β-receptors in the blood vessels of skin and mucous membrane. *Epinephrine is a net vasodilator* because the skeletal muscle blood vessels outnumber the others and hence reduces diastolic BP. The pulse pressure is widened because there is increase in systolic pressure due to **increase in heart rate and cardiac output**. There is no reflex bradycardia since the mean pressure is not increased. **Norepinephrine** mainly acts on β-receptors and causes constriction of the blood vessels of skin, mucous membrane and skeletal muscles. It has very slight β-effect on blood vessels and heart. *Norepinephrine is a net vasoconstrictor*. It causes increase in both systolic and diastolic BP. So there is an increase in the mean blood pressure and administration of norepinephrine produces **reflex bradycardia**. This is due to the operation of sino-aortic mechanism. So the cardiac output is decreased.

Vasopressin

Vasopressin is a posterior pituitary hormone and it has vasopressive action on blood vessels only in times of hypotension. It acts on kidney and increases the reabsorption of water from the renal tubules and thus increases blood volume and blood pressure. It also potentiates the vasoconstrictor effect of catecholamines on blood vessels.

Renin-Angiotensin-Aldosterone Mechanism

Renin-angiotensin-aldosterone mechanism (*refer* Chapter 55, **Fig. 55.1**).

Non-hormonal Factors

Capillary Fluid Shift Mechanism

Whenever there is a rise in the pressure in the blood vessels, pressure in the capillaries also increases. As systemic arterial pressure increases, capillary hydrostatic pressure which is one of the driving forces in filtration of fluid across capillary is increased and fluid escapes from the capillaries into the interstitium, thereby decreasing the capillary pressure (*refer* Starling's forces).

Stress Relaxation Mechanism

With rise in systemic BP, the venous reservoirs will dilate and accommodate large volumes of blood which leads to a reduction in the blood volume in the systemic side and decrease in BP. This is called **stress relaxation mechanism**. In times of hypotension, the veins undergo constriction diverting blood to the systemic side. There is increase in blood volume on the arterial side and increase in BP.

Local Mechanisms

Autoregulation

Autoregulation is the ability of certain tissues to maintain a constant tissue perfusion pressure in spite of wide fluctuation of the pressure in the systemic side. This mechanism fails at extremes of systemic pressure and tissue perfusion fails. Autoregulation is exhibited by organs, such as **brain, kidney, heart, skeletal muscle, mesentery and liver**.

Theories to explain autoregulation

- Myogenic theory
- Tissue perfusion theory
- Metabolic theory

Myogenic Theory

It is the inherent property of the smooth muscle to contract when stretched. When there is increase in BP, the vessel wall is stretched which leads to immediate vasoconstriction and increase in the resistance to flow of blood. So, less blood flows to the organ. When there is a fall in BP, no stretch to the vessel wall, so no constriction and more blood flows. Thus, tissue perfusion is maintained constant.

Table 28.3: Local vasoconstrictors and vasodilators of blood vessels.

Local vasoconstrictors	Vasodilators
Serotonin	Histamine, adenosine (in cardiac muscle)
Calcium	Prostacyclin
Decrease in temperature	Lactic acid and increase in H^+
Norepinephrine	Increase in temperature
Increase in PO_2 and pH	Hypoxia and hypercapnia
Decrease in PCO_2	Cations, such as K^+, Na^+, Mg^{2+}
Thromboxane A_2	Bradykinin, NO or EDRF

(EDRF: endothelium derived relaxing factor)

Tissue Perfusion Theory

When there is increase in BP, the hydrostatic pressure in the capillaries increases and more fluid escapes from the capillaries into the interstitium. This fluid exerts pressure on the capillaries from outside and compresses the capillaries leading to decreased flow and decrease in the perfusion pressure.

Metabolic Theory

When arterial pressure increases, there is increase in the blood flow through the organ and the local metabolites are washed off. These metabolites, such as lactic acid, CO_2, etc. produce vasodilatation if they accumulate in the tissue.

When the metabolites are washed off it leads to vasoconstriction and increased resistance. Thus the blood flow and perfusion pressure of the tissue are brought back to normal. This is the mechanism by which local metabolites cause autoregulation.

Vasoconstrictors and Vasodilators

Vasoconstrictors and vasodilators is shown in **Table 28.3**.

REGULATION OF BLOOD PRESSURE (FLOWCHART 28.2)

In humans, there are several cardiovascular regulatory mechanisms to control blood pressure. Both local and systemic mechanisms are there.

Regulation of blood pressure is discussed under the following headings:

Flowchart 28.2: Regulation of blood pressure.

Regulation of blood pressure

- **Short-term regulation**
  Neural factors—vasoconstrictor (adrenergic) and vasodilator (cholinergic) systems
  Reflex mechanisms
  1. Baroreceptor reflex
  2. Chemoreceptor reflex
  3. CNS ischemic response

- **Intermediate and long-term regulation**
  1. Capillary fluid shift mechanism
  2. Stress relaxation and reverse stress relaxation mechanisms
  3. Epinephrine, norepinephrine and ADH
  4. Renin-angiotensin-aldosterone mechanism
  5. Autoregulation
  6. Local vasoconstrictors and dilators

Flowchart 28.3: Long-term regulation of decreased blood pressure due to hypovolemia.

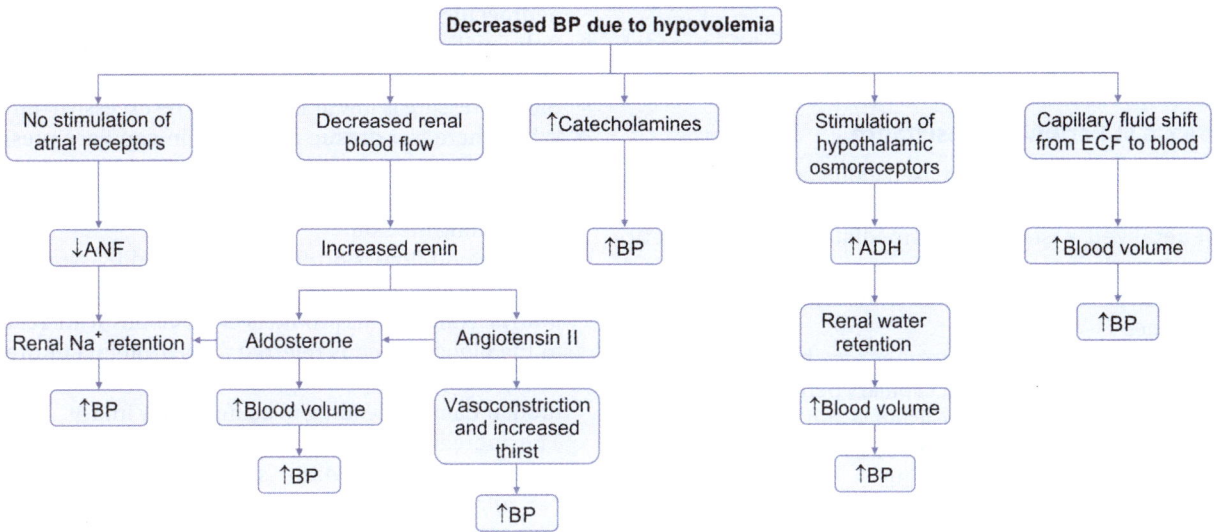

- **Short-term regulation** includes neural factors, baroreceptor reflex (sino-aortic reflex), CNS ischemic response and chemoreceptor reflex. These short-term mechanisms can act only for a few hours because of the following reasons:
  - Baroreceptor adaptation and CVS adaptation
  - Autoregulation (long-term regulatory mechanisms come into play and nullify the effect of short-term system)
- **Intermediate-term and long-term regulation** includes non-hormonal factors, hormonal factors and local mechanisms (*refer* regulation of peripheral resistance). Long-term mechanism regulates blood pressure by adjusting the body fluid volume. The long-term regulatory mechanisms that operate when there is a fall in BP due to hypovolemia are shown in **Flowchart 28.3**. The reverse occurs when there is a rise in BP.

FACTORS AFFECTING BLOOD PRESSURE

Arterial blood pressure is determined by cardiac output and peripheral resistance. Blood pressure is the product of cardiac output and peripheral resistance. Variation in any of these factors will alter blood pressure. For example, if there is an increase in peripheral resistance with normal cardiac output, the blood pressure increases. If there is a reduction in cardiac output with normal peripheral resistance then there will be a reduction in blood pressure. So, regulation of cardiac output and peripheral resistance is very important in the regulation of BP. Systolic BP is mainly regulated by cardiac output and diastolic BP depends on peripheral resistance. All factors affecting cardiac output and peripheral resistance affect blood pressure.

FACTORS AFFECTING CARDIAC OUTPUT

Increased Cardiac Output

- Increase in blood volume increases venous return and leads to increase in stroke volume and cardiac output. Increase in cardiac output increases blood pressure.
- Exercise increases stroke volume and heart rate and thereby increase cardiac output and systolic BP.
- Emotional excitement increase cardiac output due to increased sympatho-adrenal activity. This increases systolic as well as diastolic blood pressure.

Decreased Cardiac Output

- **Posture:** When a person stands up from lying down posture, there is decrease in cardiac output and BP. This is due to pooling of venous blood in the lower limbs due to gravity. But it soon comes back to normal due to the operation of baroreceptor reflex.
- Decrease in blood volume decreases cardiac output, which causes a fall in blood pressure. If there is loss of more than 30% of blood volume as in hemorrhage, the compensatory mechanisms fail leading to fatal fall in BP.
- Pericardial effusion produces cardiac compression leading to decrease in cardiac output and BP.
- Myocardial infarction reduces myocardial contractility and decreases cardiac output and BP. BP also decreases due to liberation of certain metabolites by the ischemic myocardium.
- Intense pain produces generalized vasodilatation and fall in cardiac output and BP.

FACTORS AFFECTING PERIPHERAL RESISTANCE

Increase in Peripheral Resistance

- **Chemoreceptor reflex:** Decrease in PO_2, increase in PCO_2 and decrease in pH of blood lead to direct stimulation of vasomotor center leading to vasoconstriction and increase in peripheral resistance and blood pressure (BP).
- **Baroreceptor reflex:** When baroreceptors are not stimulated as in decrease in blood volume, there is vasoconstriction and increase in BP (sino-aortic mechanism).
- **Renin-angiotensin mechanism:** Renal hypoxia stimulates renin secretion which in turn increases formation of angiotensin II. Angiotensin II is a powerful vasoconstrictor which increases peripheral resistance and BP.

- Stimulation of pain fibers if not intense, reflexly increases peripheral resistance and BP.
- Increase in viscosity of blood as in polycythemia increases peripheral resistance and BP.

Decrease in Peripheral Resistance

- If the blood volume is decreased more than 30% it leads to fall in peripheral resistance leading to shock.
- Generalized vasodilatation mediated by sympathetic cholinergic vasodilator fibers decrease peripheral resistance. This leads to a fall in BP leading to vasovagal syncope.
- Anaphylaxis, crush syndrome, etc. lead to systemic vasodilation and increased capillary permeability leading to decrease in peripheral resistance and decrease in BP.
- Decrease in the viscosity of blood as in anemia decreases the peripheral resistance and BP.

CIRCULATORY SHOCK

PY5.11: Describe the pathophysiology of shock, syncope and heart failure.

Introduction

Circulatory shock is a clinical syndrome in which perfusion of body tissues is inadequate to meet normal metabolic demands. The tissues are damaged due to decreased blood flow, decreased availability of O_2 and nutrients and inadequate removal of cellular waste products.

Any condition that can cause decrease in blood volume, inadequate venous return to the heart, reduction in cardiac output or a fall in peripheral resistance may initiate circulatory shock. The inadequate perfusion of tissues leads to increased **anaerobic glycolysis** with the production of large amounts of lactic acid and the condition is called **lactic acidosis**. This is characteristic of all forms of shock. Normal lactic acid level is 1 mmol/L. In lactic acidosis it will be >9 mmol/L. Lactic acidosis depresses the myocardium, decreases peripheral vascular responsiveness to catecholamines and may even lead to coma.

Rarely, shock occurs not due to failure of circulation but due to inability of vital organs to make use of the blood supply.

The cardinal feature of shock is a disparity between the circulating blood volume and the available blood space or the capacity of the circulatory system. So, in shock there is either decrease in blood volume or increase in the capacity of cardiovascular space. Hemorrhage and extravasation of blood into the tissues are examples of decrease in blood volume. Capillary dilatation due to histamine as in anaphylaxis or due to snake venom is an example of increase in cardiovascular space.

Clinical Picture

- Patient looks pale, gray or cyanotic.
- Respiration is rapid and shallow.
- Patient shows mental dullness, restlessness and decreased sensibility.
- Skin is cold and moist in hypovolemic shock and warm in neurogenic shock.
- Pulse will be rapid and thready (thready pulse is a manifestation of feeble pulse pressure).
- Blood pressure is low and there will be excessive thirst.
- When there is a drastic reduction in capillary pressure, there will be increased reabsorption of fluid from the tissue spaces leading to loosening of the skin and can be detected by pinching the skin.
- Renal blood flow is profoundly reduced by sympathetic constriction of afferent arteriole and the patient develops **anuria**. Nitrogenous products of metabolism are retained in the blood, which is referred to as azotemia or uremia. If hypotension is prolonged, there may be severe renal tubular damage, leading to acute kidney injury.

The increased sympathetic discharge contributes to survival in the immediate stages following bleeding. *Never apply warmth to a patient in circulatory shock* because, hypothalamic responses to warming abolishes sympathetic vasoconstriction and it increases the severity of shock.

End Stages of Circulatory Shock

When shock reaches a critical state, the myocardium, walls of blood vessels, vasomotor center and other parts of circulatory system begin to deteriorate, decreasing the cardiac output and it becomes a vicious cycle, i.e., the severity of shock increases, leading to further reduction in tissue perfusion leading to death eventually.

Causes of Circulatory Shock (Table 28.4)

Circulatory shock can be due to the following four causes:
1. Due to inadequate volume of blood to fill the vascular system (hypovolemic shock)

Table 28.4: Types of shock and their causes.

Type of shock	Conditions
Hypovolemic shock	• Hemorrhage • Trauma • Surgery • Burns • Loss of fluid and electrolytes associated with vomiting or diarrhea
Distributive or low resistance shock	• Fainting (neurogenic shock) • Anaphylaxis • Sepsis with increased capillary permeability and loss of fluid into tissues
Cardiogenic shock	• Myocardial infarction • Heart failure • Ventricular arrhythmia
Obstructive shock	• Tension pneumothorax • Pulmonary embolism • Cardiac tumor • Pericardial tamponade

2. Due to increased size of vascular system produced by vasodilation in the presence of normal blood volume (distributive, vasogenic or low-resistance shock)
3. Due to inadequate output of the heart as a result of myocardial abnormalities (cardiogenic shock)
4. Due to inadequate cardiac output as a result of obstruction of blood flow in the lungs or heart (obstructive shock)

Classification and Pathophysiology of Shock

- Cardiogenic shock
- Hypovolemic shock or cold shock:
    - Hemorrhagic shock
    - Traumatic shock
    - Burns
    - Surgical or wound shock
    - Shock due to fluid and electrolyte loss
- Neurogenic shock, low-resistance shock or warm shock
- Septic shock due to septicemia
- Anaphylactic shock
- Addisonian crisis
- Obstructive shock

Cardiogenic Shock

A diseased heart that produces a gross reduction in cardiac output as in myocardial infarction leads to cardiogenic shock. In this condition, the pumping function of the heart is impaired to the point that blood flow to the tissues is no longer adequate to meet the resting metabolic demands. The blood volume will be normal. About 7% of patients with myocardial infarction presents with fainting attack. Here, the hypotension is due to **Bezold-Jarisch reflex** produced by serotonin and other substances released by the ischemic myocardium.

Cardiogenic shock can also be caused by diseases, such as ventricular fibrillation and end stages of congestive cardiac failure (CCF) that severely compromise normal ventricular function. There will be congestion of lungs and viscera in addition to the symptoms of hypovolemic shock. The heart fails to put out all the venous blood returned to it. Hence, cardiogenic shock is also known as **congested shock**.

Hypovolemic Shock or Cold Shock

Hemorrhagic Shock

Hemorrhage is the most important cause of hypovolemic shock. There will be reduction in venous return leading to a fall in cardiac output and blood pressure. The severity of shock depends on the rapidity of blood loss. When there is gradual removal of blood, compensatory mechanisms come into play. Plasma protein losses are replaced by hepatic synthesis over a period of 3–4 days. Erythropoietin secretion is increased and red cell mass is restored to normal in 4–8 weeks.

Traumatic Shock

Traumatic shock occurs when there is severe damage to muscle or bone. This is the type of shock seen in battle casualties and automobile accident victims. Frank bleeding into the injured area is the cause for shock. If it is a crush injury there will be no external bleeding and the amount of blood lost from the blood vessels cannot be assessed. For example, the thigh muscles can accommodate about 1 L of extravasated blood with an increase in the diameter of the thigh of only 1 cm. In severe muscle crushing, myoglobin leaks into circulation and gets precipitated in renal tubules causing renal shutdown and anuria. This condition due to myoglobinuria is called **crush syndrome**. Severe pain will inhibit vasomotor center leading to vasodilatation and hypotension. When the crushed muscles are once again perfused with blood, free radicals are generated, which cause further tissue destruction referred to as **reperfusion-induced injury**.

Burn Shock

Loss of plasma from the burned surface can cause shock due to hypovolemia. The hematocrit increases producing severe hemoconcentration. When third degree burns cover more than 75% of the body, the mortality rate is close to 100%.

Surgical or Wound Shock

Surgical shock is due to a combination of external hemorrhage, bleeding into the injured tissues and dehydration.

Shock Due to Fluid and Electrolyte Loss

Severe vomiting or diarrhea as in cholera can lead to excessive loss of fluid and electrolytes causing drastic reduction in circulating blood volume. This leads to hypovolemic shock.

Neurogenic Shock or Vasogenic Shock

Neurogenic shock is a type of distributive shock. Here, the blood volume is normal but the capacity of circulatory system is increased due to extensive vasodilatation. The normal amount of blood becomes inadequate to fill the circulatory system. There will be sudden loss of sympathetic autonomic activity that results in vasodilation and pooling of blood in the veins. The resulting decrease in venous return reduces cardiac output drastically leading to fainting attack or **syncope**. Vasodilatation causes the skin to be warm rather than cold and clammy. Causes of neurogenic shock are:
a. Deep general anesthesia depressing vasomotor center
b. Severe brain and spinal cord injuries
c. Endotoxin shock due to endotoxins
d. High fever and severe pain
e. Drugs that block sympathetic discharge or its effects on blood vessels

Septic Shock

Septic shock is seen in septicemia. Bacterial lipopolysaccharide produced by gram negative organisms is the main cause of septic shock. It is a combination of hypovolemic shock and cardiogenic shock. Hypovolemia is due to loss of plasma into tissues. Toxins produced in the body depress the myocardium and decreases myocardial performance. This condition is associated with excess production of nitric oxide (NO) which produces generalized vasodilatation.

In most patients with septic shock, the syndrome of **disseminated intravascular coagulation** (DIC) sets in. Features of septic shock are:
- High fever
- Severe vasodilatation and sludging of blood
- Development of micro clots due to release of thromboplastic substances
- Oliguria due to inadequate renal perfusion and due to the direct toxic effect on kidneys.
- Respiratory failure is a frequent cause of death in septic shock. The respiratory lesions are collectively called **shock lung syndrome or adult respiratory distress syndrome**. The lungs will be airless, congested, hemorrhagic and edematous.

Anaphylactic Shock

Anaphylactic shock is another form of distributive shock, which is due to administration of protein materials after initial sensitization. The first dose acts as antigen and produces antibodies. The antigen–antibody reaction releases large quantities of histamine. Histamine increases capillary permeability and also produces widespread dilatation of capillaries and arterioles. The condition becomes worse in patients with fever because the blood vessels are already dilated. Blood pressure falls because the size of the vascular system exceeds the amount of blood in it even though blood volume is normal.

Addisonian Crisis

Addisonian crisis is a severe form of shock characterized by adrenocortical insufficiency, hypotension and fluid and electrolyte loss. This is an acute exacerbation of adrenocortical deficiency as a result of stress. The symptoms of Addison's disease become intensified in times of stress. Severe hypotension develops and the resulting hypovolemic shock is fatal if untreated.

Obstructive Shock

The picture in obstructive shock is almost same as that of cardiogenic or congested shock. It occurs in massive pulmonary embolism, tension pneumothorax with obstruction to great veins and in cardiac tamponade (bleeding into the pericardium with external pressure on the heart decreasing the compliance of the heart). Pulsus paradoxus occurs in cardiac tamponade. Normally blood pressure falls about 5 mm Hg during inspiration. In pulsus paradoxus, this response is exaggerated, and BP falls 10 mm Hg or more.

Vasogenic, distributive or low-resistance shock includes neurogenic shock, anaphylactic shock, septic shock and acute adrenocortical insufficiency.

Stages of Shock

(Wigger's classification)
1. Initial or developing stage
2. Non-progressive stage or compensatory stage
3. Progressive stage
4. Irreversible stage or refractory shock

Initial Stage
In the initial stage, the circulating blood volume is decreased to a lesser extent not sufficient to cause serious symptoms.

Compensatory Stage
In this stage, the compensatory mechanism will revert the effects of shock, provided the cause does not become worse. The sympathetic reflexes and other mechanisms operate to tide over the situation. This stage is divided into:
1. Immediate compensatory mechanisms
2. Delayed mechanisms

Immediate or Rapid Compensatory Mechanisms
- *Baroreceptor reflexes*: In shock, there is no stimulation of arterial baroreceptors and so, sympathetic output is increased leading to vasoconstriction and reflex tachycardia (*refer* sino-aortic mechanism).
- Venoconstriction increases venous return.
- *Vasoconstriction*: Vasoconstriction occurs mainly in the skin and viscera diverting blood to the vital organs. The blood vessels of brain and heart are spared. The coronaries dilate due to increased myocardial metabolism secondary to increase in heart rate.
- Contraction of spleen increases blood volume to a lesser extent in humans.
- *Release of catecholamines*: Hemorrhage is a potent stimulus for adrenal medulla. Moreover, discharge from sympathetic noradrenergic neurons increases and hence circulating norepinephrine is also increased. This stimulates the reticular formation. The restlessness shown by some patients in shock is due to stimulation of reticular formation. Restlessness causes increased pumping of venous blood.
- *Chemoreceptor stimulation*: In shock, stagnant hypoxia is seen which stimulates peripheral chemoreceptors. This stimulates respiration. There is also stimulation of vasomotor center leading to vasoconstriction and increase in blood pressure.
- Increased secretion of renin which in turn increases angiotensin II leading to increase in blood pressure
- Increased secretion of vasopressin and aldosterone also occurs in circulatory shock. Both these hormones cause retention of Na^+ and water, thus increasing blood pressure.

Delayed Compensatory Mechanisms
- Shift of fluid from interstitial space to intravascular space since there is a reduction in capillary pressure. Up to 1 L of fluid per hour may reenter the circulation in this way.
- When ECF volume is decreased, hypothalamus is stimulated increasing thirst.
- Increased production of angiotensin II increases aldosterone secretion leading to increased reabsorption of salt and water by kidneys.
- If plasma proteins are decreased as in hemorrhagic shock, there will be increased hepatic synthesis of plasma proteins especially albumin.
- There will be increased erythropoiesis due to increased secretion of erythropoietin. Reticulocyte count reaches a peak within 10 days.

- There is increase in 2,3-DPG in red cells shifting O_2 dissociation curve to right.

Progressive Stage

When the shock is severe, various **positive feedback mechanisms** cause further and further reduction in cardiac output. The chief mechanisms are:

- **Cardiac depression**: Decrease in coronary blood flow and toxic substances can depress the myocardium
- Fall in BP →↓ Cardiac output →↓ Coronary blood flow
  ↑ ↓
  Decreased cardiac output ← Myocardial depression
- **Failure of vasomotor center**: Though the vasomotor center tries to bring back blood pressure and cardiac output back to normal, there occurs a stage when vasomotor center suffers from severe ischemia leading to its depression.
- **Thrombosis of minute vessels due to sludged blood**: In shock, blood flow becomes sluggish, but tissue metabolism continues. The acidity of blood increases due to accumulation of lactic acid and carbonic acid. Small blood clots form minute plugs in small vessels. The tendency for cells to stick together makes blood flow difficult. Hence the term, **sludged blood**.
- **Increased capillary permeability**: In hypoxia, the capillary permeability increases and fluid transudates into the tissues. This leads to decrease in blood volume and cardiac output.
- **Release of toxins by ischemic tissues**: Substances, such as histamine, serotonin and tissue enzymes are released from damaged tissues. Diminished blood flow to the intestine causes increased absorption of **endotoxins** from the intestine. Endotoxin is a toxin released from gram-negative bacteria in the intestine. Endotoxin causes vascular dilatation, increased cellular metabolism and cardiac depression.
- **Generalized cellular deterioration**:
  - The organ commonly affected is the liver. There will be depression of its metabolic and detoxification process.
  - A complication of shock that has very high mortality rate is pulmonary damage with production of acute respiratory distress syndrome. There will be pulmonary edema. Death is usually due to **shock lung syndrome** where there is capillary endothelial cell damage and damage to alveolar epithelial cells with the release of cytokines.
  - Myocardial depression is another feature of cellular deterioration.
  - Renal failure is also seen.
  - At the cellular level:
    - Na^+-K^+ pump is inhibited leading to increase in intracellular sodium and hyperkalemia.
    - Mitochondrial activity is depressed.
    - Lysosomes cause autodigestion due to release of hydrolytic enzymes into the cytoplasm.
    - Cellular metabolism of glucose is depressed.

Irreversible Stage or Refractory Stage

When shock has progressed to a certain stage, the patient will not show any response to transfusion therapy or vasopressor drugs. Even if the blood volume is returned to normal, cardiac output remains depressed. This stage is called stage of irreversible shock or refractory shock. The main factor responsible for irreversible shock is depletion of high-energy phosphate compounds especially in the liver and heart. Severe cerebral ischemia leads to depression of vasomotor center and cardiac areas of brain leading to bradycardia and vasodilatation. The pulse rate and blood pressure fall and the patient dies.

Treatment of Shock

General Measures

- Early diagnosis of circulatory shock is very important.
- Complete bed rest with foot end of the bed elevated to increase venous return.
- Pulse, BP, respiration and urine output should be monitored.
- A venous cannula is introduced into the jugular vein to monitor central venous pressure. It should be kept at 10–14 cm water.
- Metabolic acidosis is corrected by giving 50–100 mEq of sodium bicarbonate as a 7.5% solution.
- Use sedatives and antidepressants as less as possible.
- **Avoid heating the patient**. If heat is applied the patient sweats and more water will be lost from the body which may aggravate the shock. The patient can be covered with a blanket.

Specific Treatment Aimed at Correcting the Cause

- In hemorrhagic, traumatic and surgical shock, rapid blood transfusion should be done with compatible blood.
- In burn shock and other forms of shock where there is hemoconcentration, plasma and plasma expanders, such as dextran can be used. In burn shock, Ringer lactate solution should also be given in large doses.
- Blood pressure can be maintained by noradrenaline. Dopamine can also be given intravenously in traumatic and cardiogenic shock to increase blood pressure.
- In anaphylactic shock, antihistamines should be given. Intramuscular injection of 1/1000 adrenaline corrects hypotension and bronchospasm. Intravenous hydrocortisone is also beneficial.
- High doses of antibiotics should be given in septic shock.
- In cardiogenic shock, inotropic agents are used to improve cardiac contractility.

CARDIAC FAILURE OR HEART FAILURE

Cardiac failure is the condition in which heart fails to pump blood adequately to all parts of the body to meet the needs of the body. It may be left ventricular failure or right ventricular failure or both. Congestive cardiac failure is heart failure associated with accumulation of fluid in lungs and other tissues. When the heart fails, the cardiac output falls, the venous pressure rise or both occurs. In cardiac failure, more blood remains in the heart chambers since heart is not able to effectively pump blood into the aorta or pulmonary artery.

Left heart failure: Left heart failure leads to elevated pulmonary arterial pressure, pulmonary congestion and pulmonary edema. This is due to increased back pressure in the pulmonary veins. The pulmonary blood pressure rises leading to congestion and pulmonary edema.

Right heart failure: If it is right heart failure, the systemic venous pressure increases leading to generalized edema especially in the feet, legs, abdomen, etc. Collection of fluid in the peritoneal cavity is called ascites which is a feature of cardiac failure. The jugular venous pressure is raised (due to increased right atrial pressure) and there will be hepatomegaly. There will be increase in the size of the heart due to dilatation in the early stages and hypertrophy in the late stages.

High output failure: The inadequate cardiac output in heart failure may be relative rather than absolute. When there is a large arteriovenous fistula, in conditions, such as thyrotoxicosis, thiamine deficiency etc. the cardiac output may be elevated but it will be inadequate to meet the needs of the tissues. This is high output failure.

Heart failure can also be classified as systolic failure and diastolic failure.

In **systolic failure**, stroke volume is reduced due to weak ventricular contraction. The end-systolic volume will be increased and ejection fraction falls from 65% to as low as 20%. There will be cardiac hypertrophy and cardiac remodeling. There will be increased sympathetic discharge and increased secretion of renin and aldosterone as a compensatory mechanism.

In **diastolic failure**, the elasticity of the myocardium is reduced and so diastolic filling is reduced. This leads to inadequate stroke volume and cardiac output.

Pathophysiology of Heart Failure

The right heart failure may be primary as in chronic lung disease or it may be secondary to left heart failure. In left heart failure, there will be elevation of pressures in the pulmonary circulation with secondary right heart failure. Severe heart failure can produce fatigue, weakened pulse, peripheral vasoconstriction with cyanosis of the extremities and decreased flow through the organs including the kidneys. Elevation of the left atrial pressure and pulmonary venous pressure due to left ventricular failure produces pulmonary congestion and shortness of breath. If the increase in pressure is high, there will be leakage of fluid into the interstitium of lung and the alveoli leading to pulmonary edema.

In right ventricular failure, which may be primary or secondary, the venous pressure in the systemic veins becomes elevated. If the elevation is severe, leakage of fluid out of the capillaries can occur, leading to fluid accumulation in the extravascular spaces leading to edema in the dependent portions of the body, such as legs, enlargement of liver, ascites etc. This stage of cardiac failure is called **congestive cardiac failure** (CCF).

Causes of Cardiac Failure

❖ Coronary artery disease or ischemic heart disease where there is decreased contractility of the myocardium due to diminished coronary blood flow caused by blockage of the coronary blood vessels. This is the most common cause for heart failure.
❖ Defective heart valves, e.g., mitral stenosis leads to left heart failure and causes high pressure in the left atrium and in the pulmonary circulation. It also produces secondary failure of the right ventricle
❖ Severe hypertension
❖ Viral myocarditis and cardiomyopathies
❖ Hyperthyroidism (high output failure)
❖ Long-standing complete heart block with a very slow heart rate and large stroke volume can lead to cardiac enlargement and eventual heart failure
❖ In chronic lung disease (e.g., COPD), right heart failure is seen
❖ Thiamine deficiency impairs production of adenosine triphosphate, leading to accumulation of adenosine. Thiamine serves as an important cofactor in body metabolism and energy production. Thiamine deficiency may contribute to myocardial weakness by limiting the energy available for contraction. Thiamine deficiency mainly affects cardiovascular and nervous systems. Heart failure due to thiamine deficiency is called cardiac beriberi. This is usually seen in chronic alcoholics.

Immediate Effects of Acute Cardiac Failure

In acute myocardial infarction (MI), the pumping action of the heart is suddenly reduced leading to decrease in cardiac output and accumulation of blood in the veins leading to increase in venous pressure. If the block on the coronary vessel is complete and severe there will be sudden death. The normal cardiac output at rest is 5 L/min. In acute myocardial infarction, cardiac output becomes greatly reduced to less than 2 L/min within a few seconds (**Fig. 28.5**). This may be associated with fainting. At the same time the right atrial pressure will be about 4 mm Hg because the venous blood returning to the heart will get collected in the atria.

Compensatory Mechanisms of Heart Failure or Compensated Heart Failure

Autonomic Compensations

Within a few seconds of MI, sympathetic nervous system gets stimulated and sympathetic nervous reflexes come into play. Since the blood pressure is very low due to decreased cardiac output, the baroreceptor reflex is activated to increase blood pressure. The chemoreceptor reflex, CNS ischemic response etc. also operate to compensate for the decrease in blood pressure. Sympathetic stimulation increases the force of contraction of the normal muscles of the heart and the cardiac output will be increased 2 fold. It comes to about 4 L/min but the right atrial pressure will be 5 mm Hg (**Fig. 28.5**). Sympathetic stimulation also increases venous return to heart by increasing the tone of the blood vessels especially veins. This also leads to increase in cardiac output.

After about 30 seconds the cardiac output may return to adequate levels to sustain the person provided he remains quiet. But the chest pain persists.

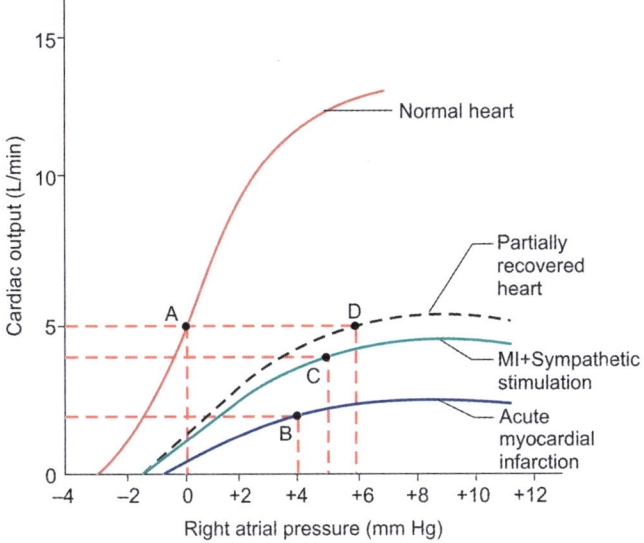

Fig. 28.5: Changes in the cardiac output curve after acute myocardial infarction.

Point A: Normal cardiac output (5 L/min) and right atrial pressure zero.
Point B: In acute myocardial infarction before compensation. Cardiac output: 2 L/min; right atrial pressure: +4 mm Hg
Point C: Compensation by sympathetic stimulation cardiac output: 4.2 L/min; right atrial pressure: +5 mm Hg.
Point D: Cardiac output curve after partial recovery where cardiac output is 5 L/min and right atrial pressure increased to 6 mm Hg.

Late effects of cardiac failure which was compensated by sympathetic stimulation
1. Renal compensation: Retention of fluid by the kidneys
2. Recovery of the heart over a period of weeks to months and increase in cardiac size

Renal Compensation

Decrease in cardiac output depresses renal function. The urine output will be low as long as cardiac output and BP remain low. Normal urine output occurs only when cardiac output and BP return to normal level. There will be increased secretion of renin and aldosterone and thus Na$^+$ and water are retained. These are the initial compensatory responses.

Moderate fluid retention in cardiac failure is of some benefit. Moderate increase in blood volume helps to increase venous return. This increased venous return can compensate for the heart's diminished pumping ability as long as the person is at rest. After a week or so after MI, due to fluid retention and increased venous return the right atrial pressure increases to about 6 mm Hg **(Fig. 28.5)**. The cardiac output may increase to 5 L/min. When cardiac output becomes normal, renal function also returns to normal and no further fluid retention occurs. The patient will have normal cardiovascular dynamics as long as he is in complete rest. When the heart recovers, the sympathetic stimulation also comes to normal levels and features, such as tachycardia, pallor, cold skin, etc., disappear. This stage is called **compensated heart failure**.

Increased Cardiac Size

Initially, there is acute dilation due to increased venous return. According to Frank Starling law of heart, force of contraction of the heart increases when there is increase in the end diastolic volume. In chronic heart failure, heart enlargement is associated with some degree of hypertrophy. In chest X-ray, the heart is found to be enlarged. The ventricular enlargement helps to maintain the stroke volume.

Severe Cardiac Failure or Decompensated Heart Failure

If the cardiac output is too low, blood flow to the kidney is affected and it becomes unable to excrete salt and water equal to the intake. So fluid retention continues and this leads to increased work load on the already damaged heart and severe edema develops throughout the body which can even lead to death. Filtration of fluid into the lungs leads to pulmonary edema. Thus moderate fluid retention in cardiac failure is beneficial whereas extreme excess of fluid makes the condition worse. This condition is called **decompensated heart failure**. Here the heart is unable to pump sufficient blood to make the kidneys function normally **(Flowchart 28.4)**.

Treatment of Heart Failure

Treatment is aimed at
    a. Improving cardiac contractility
    b. Relieving the symptoms
    c. Decreasing the load on the heart
❖ Angiotensin converting enzyme inhibitors (ACE inhibitors) or angiotensin receptor (AT1) blockers is now the treatment of choice for heart failure. ACE inhibitors decrease angiotensin II and aldosterone levels. Thus blood pressure

Flowchart 28.4: Steps leading to decompensated heart failure.

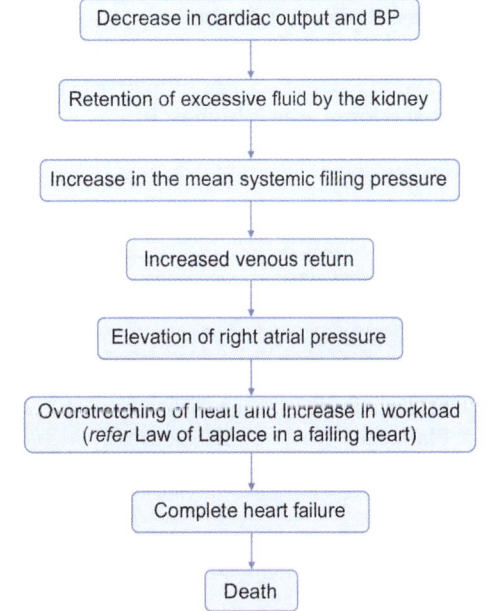

is decreased and after load against which the heart pumps is decreased. Renin-angiotensin system is present in the walls of the blood vessels of heart. Angiotensin II is a significant growth factor in the heart and blood vessels. ACE inhibitors may inhibit the growth effects of angiotensin II in the heart and this may also be the reason for the benefits of ACE inhibitors in heart failure.
- Aldosterone receptors blockers
- Positive inotropic drugs, such as digitalis increase intracellular Ca^{2+} in the myocardial cells.
- Diuretics are given to decrease fluid overload which in turn reduce edema
- Beta adrenergic blockers decrease heart rate and blood pressure
- Vasodilators, such as nitroglycerin help to reduce venous tone and venous return to the heart and thereby decrease the preload
- Specific treatment on the causes of heart failure, e.g., heart block can be treated by implanting pacemakers, severe hypertension is treated by appropriate antihypertensive drugs and severe coronary artery disease can be treated by angioplasty or bypass-grafting of the coronary arteries.

MULTIPLE CHOICE QUESTIONS

1. **Nitric oxide is inactivated by:**
   a. Phosphodiesterase
   b. Cyclo-oxygenase
   c. Amino peptidase
   d. MAO

2. **Sildenafil (viagra) given to produce penile erection produces transient inability to distinguish between blue and green. The reason is that it:**
   a. Dilates arteries of penis and retina
   b. Constricts arteries of penis and retina
   c. Inhibits phosphodiesterases in penis and retina
   d. Inhibits production of cGMP in penis and retina

3. **Windkessel effect is seen in:**
   a. Large arteries
   b. Small arteries
   c. Arterioles
   d. Metarterioles

4. **Cross-sectional area is highest in:**
   a. Arteries
   b. Arterioles
   c. Capillaries
   d. Venules

5. **NO act by activating:**
   a. Protein kinase A
   b. Guanylyl cyclase
   c. Phospholipase C
   d. Phospholipase A_2

6. **Nitric oxide (NO) is produced in:**
   a. Endothelium
   b. Plasma
   c. Platelets
   d. Serum

7. **Which of the following is referred to as Windkessel vessel?**
   a. Capillary
   b. Arteriole
   c. Vein
   d. Aorta

8. **Choose a vasoconstrictor substance from the following:**
   a. Norepinephrine
   b. Bradykinin
   c. Histamine
   d. Nitric oxide

9. **Mean arterial pressure is:**
   a. Systolic pressure + (diastolic pressure)/2
   b. Systolic pressure + 1/3 pulse pressure
   c. Diastolic pressure + (systolic pressure)/2
   d. Diastolic pressure + 1/3 pulse pressure

10. **Blood pressure is defined as the product of:**
    a. Systolic pressure x pulse rate
    b. Diastolic pressure x pulse rate
    c. Pulse pressure x pulse rate
    d. Cardiac output x peripheral resistance

11. **Spuriously high BP is seen in all, *except*:**
    a. Auscultatory gap
    b. Small cuff
    c. Thick calcified vessels
    d. Obesity

12. **A loss of 0.5 liter of blood in 30 minutes leads to:**
    a. Increase in heart rate and decrease in BP
    b. Slight increase in heart rate and normal BP
    c. Decrease in heart rate and BP
    d. Prominent increase in heart rate

13. **Blood pressure is increased by the following:**
    a. Prostacyclin
    b. NO synthase inhibitor
    c. Endothelin inhibitor
    d. Angiotensin converting enzyme inhibitor

14. **The basis of Korotkoff's sound is due to:**
    a. AV valve closure
    b. Aortic valve closure
    c. Arterial expansion
    d. Arterial turbulence

15. **If the blood pressure of an adult man is 130/70 mm Hg, his mean arterial pressure will be:**
    a. 130 mm Hg
    b. 60 mm Hg
    c. 100 mm Hg
    d. 90 mm Hg

16. **The relationship between heart rate and blood pressure is called:**
    a. Bainbridge reflex
    b. Frank-Starling law
    c. Marey's law
    d. Sino-aortic reflex

17. **The reflex that is initiated by baroreceptors in the right atrium and venae cavae due to increase in venous pressure is:**
    a. Sino-aortic reflex
    b. Bezold Jarisch reflex
    c. Hering-Breuer reflex
    d. Bainbridge reflex

18. **Angiotensin converting enzyme is produced by:**
    a. Lungs
    b. Liver
    c. Spleen
    d. Kidney

19. **All the following increase blood pressure, *except*:**
    a. Nor epinephrine
    b. Calcitriol
    c. ADH
    d. ANP

20. All the following are features of shock, *except*:
    a. Tachycardia
    b. Thready pulse
    c. Alkalosis
    d. Sweating
21. **Digoxin acts by inhibiting:**
    a. Ca channel
    b. Na-K ATPase
    c. K channel
    d. Adenylyl cyclase
22. Nitric oxide is synthesized in the body from the amino acid:
    a. Histidine
    b. Arginine
    c. Tryptophan
    d. Glutamate
23. Catecholamines acting on α-adrenergic receptors:
    a. Increase the contractility of cardiac muscle
    b. Increase rate of discharge from SA node
    c. Dilate blood vessels in skeletal muscles
    d. Constrict coronary arteries by a direct action
24. Which of the following is not increased in isotonic exercise?
    a. Reticulocyte count
    b. Stroke volume
    c. Heart rate
    d. Total peripheral resistance
25. **Vasopressin secretion is increased by:**
    a. Decreased pressure in the right ventricle
    b. Decreased pressure in the right atrium
    c. Increased pressure in aorta
    d. Increased pressure in right atrium
26. All the following drugs are slow Ca^{2+} channel blockers, *except*:
    a. Nifedipine
    b. Diltiazem
    c. Digitalis
    d. Verapamil
27. The circulating level of circulating angiotensinogen is increased by all the following hormones, *except*:
    a. Glucocorticoids
    b. Thyroid hormones
    c. Angiotensin II
    d. Atrial natriuretic peptide
28. The best method to access the adequacy of replacement of fluid in a case of circulatory shock is:
    a. Decrease in thirst
    b. Increase in PaO_2
    c. Increase in urine output
    d. Increase in blood pressure
29. **Blood supply during exercise is increased in:**
    a. Cutaneous circulation
    b. Hepatosplanchnic circulation
    c. Renal circulation
    d. Coronary circulation
30. **Carotid sinus baroreceptor is most sensitive to:**
    a. Mean blood pressure
    b. Diastolic blood pressure
    c. Systolic blood pressure
    d. Pulse pressure
31. **Stimulation of baroreceptor leads to:**
    a. Increase in BP and heart rate
    b. Decrease in BP and heart rate
    c. Increased intracranial tension
    d. Decreased intracranial tension
32. The first reactive change to occur after hemorrhage is:
    a. Vasoconstriction
    b. Tachycardia
    c. Raised cortisol
    d. Raised adrenaline
33. **Anaphylaxis is mediated by all, *except*:**
    a. Serotonin
    b. Bradykinin
    c. Prostaglandin
    d. Anaphylatoxin
34. Tachycardia in hypertension is caused by stimulation of:
    a. Alpha 1 receptor
    b. Alpha 2 receptor
    c. Beta 1 receptor
    d. Beta 2 receptor
35. Essential hypertension is generally associated with an early increase in:
    a. Oxygen use
    b. Coronary flow
    c. Cardiac work
    d. Cardiac output
36. Hypovolemic shock is characterized by all of the following, *except*:
    a. Cold and clammy skin
    b. Intense thirst
    c. Tachycardia
    d. Inhibition of respiration
37. Pulse pressure in a particular vessel is determined chiefly by:
    a. Distance from heart
    b. Fractional characteristics of lumen
    c. Distensibility
    d. Cross sectional area
38. **Maximum heart rate that can occur with exercise:**
    a. 120
    b. 140
    c. 160
    d. 200
39. **Major part of total peripheral resistance is due to:**
    a. Medium and small arteries
    b. Venules
    c. Capillaries
    d. Arterioles
40. Sympathetic vasoconstrictor tone is diminished in response due to increased activity of:
    a. Carotid body chemoreceptors
    b. Carotid sinus pressure receptors
    c. Pain receptors
    d. Medullary chemoreceptors

41. All the following cause vasodilatation, *except*:
    a. Mg^{2+}
    b. K^+
    c. Ca^{2+}
    d. Kinins

42. Most potent stimulus for vasoconstriction is:
    a. Cerebral hypoxia
    b. Renal perfusion
    c. Cardiac perfusion
    d. Skeletal muscle perfusion

43. True regarding capillaries:
    a. Contains 5% of total blood volume
    b. Contains 10% of total blood volume
    c. Velocity of blood flow is maximum
    d. Offers maximum resistance to blood flow

44. Blood pressure is defined as the product of:
    a. Systolic pressure x pulse rate
    b. Cardiac output x peripheral resistance
    c. Diastolic pressure x pulse rate
    d. Pulse pressure x pulse rate

45. Pressure on carotid sinus causes:
    a. Hyperpnea
    b. Dyspnea
    c. Tachycardia
    d. Reflex bradycardia

46. Not true about capillaries:
    a. Greatest cross-sectional area
    b. Contains less blood than veins
    c. Contains 25% of blood volume
    d. Have single layer of cells bounding the lumen

47. Velocity of blood flow is highest in:
    a. Large veins
    b. Small veins
    c. Capillaries
    d. Venules

48. SI unit of blood pressure is:
    a. Torr
    b. mm Hg
    c. Barr
    d. kPa

49. If during blood pressure measurement, muffled sound does not disappear with return of mercury to zero, the conclusion is:
    a. Aortic stenosis
    b. Zero diastolic pressure
    c. Low hematocrit
    d. Patent ductus arteriosus

50. Left ventricular failure may be associated with:
    a. No breathlessness in lying position
    b. Presystolic murmur over heart
    c. Rise in lung compliance
    d. Decrease in ventricular end diastolic pressure

51. Which one structural feature is common to all blood capillaries?
    a. Presence of intracellular fenestrations in endothelial cells
    b. Absence of intracellular fenestrations in endothelial cells
    c. A continuous basement membrane
    d. Remain patent in healthy subjects

52. Autoregulation is seen in:
    a. Liver
    b. Muscle
    c. Kidney
    d. All of the above

53. Maximum surface area in the circulatory system is seen in:
    a. Veins
    b. Arteries
    c. Arterioles
    d. Capillaries

54. 40% loss of blood volume in a patient is managed by:
    a. Cardiac stimulants
    b. Intracardiac adrenaline
    c. Vasopressor agents
    d. Saline infusion

55. Most permeable capillaries are seen in:
    a. Posterior pituitary
    b. Liver
    c. Kidney
    d. Small intestine

56. Capillaries with tight junction are found in:
    a. Brain
    b. Skin
    c. Kidney
    d. Muscle

57. Arteriolar dilation is caused by all, *except*:
    a. Decrease in adrenergic discharge
    b. Substance P
    c. Histamine
    d. Serotonin

58. Which of the following is true regarding systemic veins?
    a. Contains 5% of blood volume
    b. Contains 12% of blood volume
    c. Contains 18% of blood volume
    d. Contains 54% of blood volume

ANSWERS

1. a	2. c	3. a	4. c	5. b
6. a	7. d	8. a	9. d	10. d
11. a	12. b	13. b	14. d	15. d
16. c	17. d	18. a	19. d	20. c
21. b	22. b	23. d	24. d	25. b
26. c	27. d	28. c	29. d	30. a
31. b	32. a	33. a	34. c	35. c
36. d	37. c	38. d	39. d	40. b
41. c	42. a	43. a	44. b	45. d
46. c	47. a	48. d	49. c	50. b
51. c	52. d	53. d	54. d	55. d
56. a	57. d	58. d		

Arterial and Venous Pulse

CHAPTER 29

LEARNING OBJECTIVES
Must know
- Draw and explain arterial pulse wave
- Explain jugular venous pulse

ARTERIAL PULSE

PY5.12: Record blood pressure and pulse at rest and in different grades of exercise and postures in a volunteer or simulated environment.
PY5.16: Record Arterial pulse tracing using finger plethysmography in a volunteer or simulated environment.

Definition
The expansile wave of local distension and rise in pressure, as blood is ejected from the left ventricle into the already full aorta, transmitted through the blood column and vessel walls of the arterial tree throughout its length is called **arterial pulse**.

When blood is ejected into the already full aorta during ventricular systole, initially the peripheral run off will not be equal to the amount of blood entering the aorta. So there is local distension of the aortic wall due to increase in pressure in the root of aorta. Soon there is peripheral run off and the distended part recoils followed by distension of the next part of the vessel and thus the distension wave is transmitted to the periphery along the arterial wall and this wave is felt as pulse.

Velocity of Pulse Wave
- In aorta: 3–5 m/sec
- In small arterioles: 15–35 m/sec.

Factors Deciding the Velocity of Pulse Wave
- Compliance of vessel wall: Greater the compliance lesser is the velocity of pulse wave.
- Age: Velocity of pulse wave increases as age advances.
- Total cross-sectional area: As cross-sectional area increases, velocity also increases. The total cross-sectional area of the peripheral arteries is more than that of aorta and so, velocity of the pulse wave is more in the smaller arteries. *Pulse waves are obtained only up to the smallest arteries.*

It is not present in the arterioles. This is called **damping of the pulse**. Causes for this damping are:
- When flow become less and less, the distension of the vessel wall also decreases.
- The arterioles offer very high resistance to the flow of blood when compared to the arteries. So distension is minimal and is not expressed outwards.

Recording of Arterial Pulse
Pulse is recorded by **sphygmography** and the apparatus is **sphygmograph**. When pulse is recorded from a central artery it is called **central pulse tracing** and if recorded from a peripheral artery like brachial artery it is called **peripheral pulse tracing**.

Peripheral Pulse Tracing
Peripheral pulse tracing consists of an upstroke, peak and a down-stroke. Upstroke is called **anacrotic limb**, down-stroke **catacrotic limb** and the notch seen in the down-stroke is called **dicrotic notch**. Anacrotic limb is due to ejection of blood from the ventricle during systole. The factors affecting the height of anacrotic limb are:
- Stroke volume
- Duration of cardiac cycle
- Diastolic pressure
- Distensibility of the vessel wall.

Catacrotic limb is due to diastole and elastic recoil of vessel wall.

Dicrotic notch is due to backflow of blood in the aorta at the beginning of diastole and it corresponds to the incisura of aortic pressure curve **(Fig. 29.1)**. It marks the end of ventricular systole.

Central Pulse Tracing
A special type of small metal cup is placed on the supraclavicular fossa and pulse tracing from the **subclavian artery** is obtained. The central pulse tracing is almost similar to peripheral pulse tracing. But before the anacrotic limb there

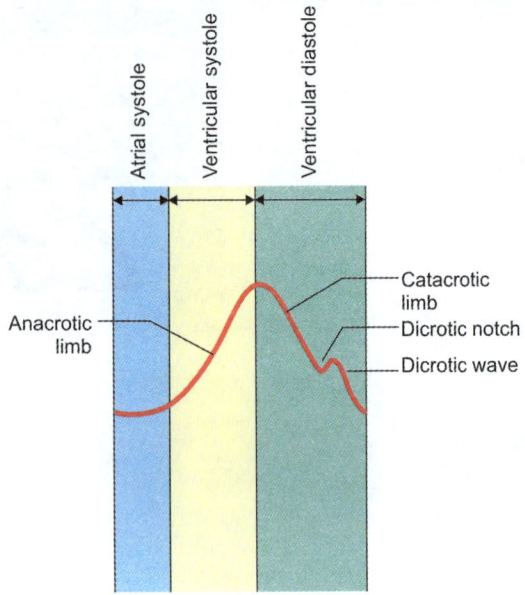

Fig. 29.1: Arterial pulse tracing.

is an irregular deflection followed by a prominent anacrotic limb and after the dicrotic notch also irregular vibrations are seen. The movements of the atrial walls during atrial systole and ventricular wall during isometric contraction phase produce the first deflection. After the dicrotic notch, the deflections are due to vibrations of the aortic valve and also due to vibrations of the blood column. Interval from the dicrotic notch to next anacrotic limb is called **dicrotic run off period**.

Examination of Peripheral Pulse

Pulse is usually examined by feeling the radial artery at the wrist. The other arteries that can be palpated are femoral artery, dorsalis pedis and carotid arteries.

The following aspects should be included while examining the pulse:

- **Pulse rate**: Count the number of pulses felt per minute. In an adult, the normal pulse rate ranges from 60 to 100 per minute (average about 72/min.)
- **Volume** of pulse: It represents the amplitude of pulse or the stroke volume.
- **Character** of pulse: It denotes the rhythm and force of the pulse.
  - **Rhythm** of pulse: Note whether the pulse is regular or irregular. If irregular, see whether it is regularly irregular or irregularly irregular. Regularly irregular pulse is seen in second degree heart block. Irregularly irregular pulse is obtained in atrial fibrillation,
  - **Force** refers to the pressure of the pulse as it expands the artery. It is expressed as full or thready. A full pulse feels as if a strong wave has passed under the finger tips. A thready pulse feels weak.
- **Condition of the vessel wall**: Feel the blood vessel after emptying the blood from a small segment of the radial artery and see whether the vessel can be palpated by moving the finger over the artery. The vessel wall becomes palpable if the vessel is thickened due to atherosclerosis or due to old age.
- **All peripheral pulses** like femoral, posterior tibial, dorsalis pedis should be examined
- Look for **radio-femoral delay**

Abnormalities of Arterial Pulse

- **Rate**: Increase in the pulse rate denotes tachycardia and decrease in the pulse rate denotes bradycardia.
- **Volume** and force of pulse
  - Rapid and thready pulse (small, weak pulse) occurs in hypotension or circulatory shock. Normal pulse pressure is 30–40 mm Hg. In thready pulse the pulse feels weak and small and the pulse pressure is very much diminished. This is seen in severe heart failure, hypovolemia and severe aortic stenosis.
  - Increase in the volume of pulse is seen in exercise and ventricular hypertrophy. Here the pulse pressure is increased and the pulse feels strong and bounding.
- **Rhythm** of pulse: Irregular pulse is seen in ectopic beats, atrial fibrillation and other arrhythmias.
- Other abnormal pulses (Fig. 29.2)
  - **Pulsus alternans**: There is a beat to beat alternation in pulse size and intensity. Here alternating strong and weak beats are felt but the rhythm is basically regular. It is indicative of left ventricular systolic impairment (left sided heart failure).
  - **Water hammer pulse** or collapsing pulse or large bounding pulse where the pulse is bounding and forceful, rapidly increasing and subsequently collapsing seen in aortic insufficiency, anemia, hyperthyroidism etc. The pulse pressure is increased. Causes are increased stroke volume, decreased peripheral resistance, or both.

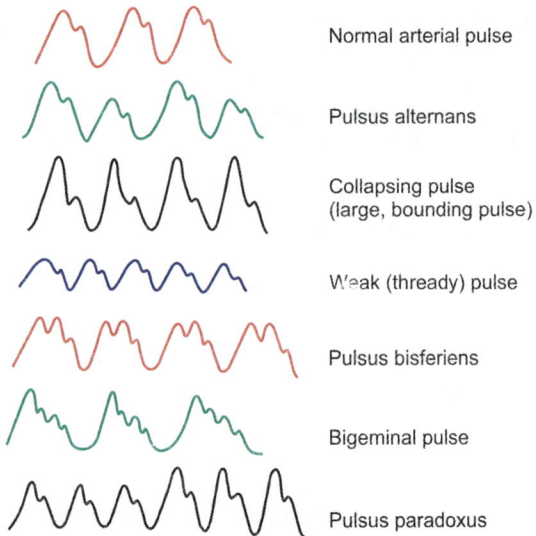

Fig. 29.2: Abnormal arterial pulses.

- **Bisferiens pulse** is an arterial pulse with a double systolic peak. It is seen in aortic regurgitation.
- **Pulsus bigeminus** is characterized by groups of two heart beats close together followed by a longer pause. This is a disorder of rhythm and is caused by a normal beat alternating with a premature contraction. The stroke volume of the premature beat is less and so the second pulse is weaker than the first and sometimes may not be palpable. It is seen in digitalis toxicity, myocardial infarction, electrolyte imbalance, hypothyroidism, etc.
- **Pulsus paradoxus** where the pulse disappears in deep inspiration seen in pericardial effusion, cardiac tamponade and in exacerbations of chronic obstructive pulmonary disease. There is a palpable decrease in the amplitude of the pulse in quiet inspiration **(Fig. 29.2)**. The systolic pressure decreases by more than 10 mm Hg during inspiration.

JUGULAR VENOUS PULSE

Central venous pressure is the pressure in the right atrium. Factors affecting central venous pressure are:
- **The effectiveness of the right atrium at pumping blood into the right ventricle.**
- **The amount of blood returning to the heart, i.e., the venous return.**
- Right ventricular function.

Pressure in the atria can be roughly detected by observing the great veins. Certain veins are in direct communication with the superior vena cava in the neck. Right atrial pressure changes can be visualized in the neck veins by observing the jugular venous pulse (JVP). Any pressure change in the right atrium can be detected in the jugular veins.

The fluctuation in the right atrial pressure during the cardiac cycle is transmitted backwards into the jugular veins since there is no valve guarding the opening of superior vena cava into the right atrium. **Internal jugular vein** is usually observed. External jugular vein contains valves in its course, which may interrupt the pressure changes and hence it is not observed. Another reason is that the external jugular vein passes through tense fascia under the clavicle and is subjected to compression.

Since the jugular vein reflects right atrial pressure the **jugular pulse tracing** also has the same waves as that of atrial pressure changes, i.e., positive waves a, c, v and x and y descents **(Fig. 29.3)**. The perpendicular level at which pulsation is obtained over the jugular vein depends on the hydrostatic pressure in the right atrium. Normally, it corresponds to manubrium sterni (sternal angle) in the erect posture. So it is not visible in the erect posture. When the person is reclined at an angle of 45°, the pulsation cannot be seen above the clavicle. If the pulsation is seen above the clavicle at this angle, then there is increase in the right atrial pressure and it indicates some pathology. The JVP is measured in centimeters vertically from the sternal angle to the upper level of the venous pulse. Normal JVP is 3 cm

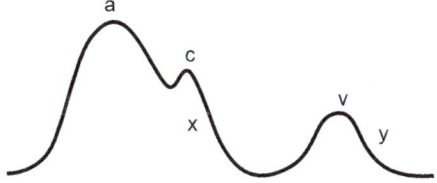

Fig. 29.3: Jugular venous pulse tracing.

above the sternal angle. The normal upper limit is 4 cm. The right atrium is 5 cm below the sternal angle. So to obtain the right atrial pressure, add 5 to the value obtained by the above measurement. Thus the jugular venous pressure (central venous pressure) comes to 5 + 3 = 8 mm Hg. Normal range is 6–8 mm Hg.

Causes of "a" Wave

During atrial systole, some amount of blood regurgitates into the superior vena cava (SVC) since there is no valve at the junction of SVC and right atrium. This causes a slight increase in the pressure in the SVC.

During atrial systole, the opening of the SVC becomes closed at the atrial side due to contraction of atrial musculature and this causes accumulation of blood in the terminal part of SVC, which also causes a slight increase in pressure in the SVC. This is because venous return is continuing but blood is not being emptied into the atrium.

Cause of "c" Wave

In the isometric contraction phase of ventricle, there is slight bulging of the tricuspid valve into the right atrium producing a slight increase in pressure. This rise is reflected into the SVC.

"x" Descent

Causes of x descent are:
- During ventricular ejection, the atrioventricular (AV) ring is pulled down, which decreases the pressure in the atrium by increasing the volume.
- Another reason is increase in the negativity of mediastinum because of discharge of blood from the heart.

Differences between venous pulse and arterial pulse are given in **Table 29.1**.

Table 29.1: Differences between venous pulse and arterial pulse in the neck.	
Jugular venous pulse	Arterial pulse in neck
Can be seen and there is an upper limit, cannot be felt	Cannot be seen clearly but can be palpated
The upper level falls during inspiration	No change with respiration
JVP can be abolished by applying pressure at the root of the neck	Cannot be abolished by applying pressure
JVP rises when pressure is applied over the abdomen	No change

(JVP: jugular venous pulse)

"v" Wave

Atrial filling continues during ventricular systole with the AV valve closed. This causes an increase in the atrial pressure and pressure in the SVC producing the positive "v" wave.

"y" Descent

At the end of isometric relaxation phase, the AV valves open and blood flows from atria to ventricles decreasing the atrial pressure. This produces the "y" descent in the JVP tracing.

Alterations in Jugular Venous Pulse

- **Prominent "a"** wave is seen in any condition that decreases emptying of blood into the right ventricle as in tricuspid stenosis.
- **Prominent "c"** wave is seen in tricuspid incompetency where blood is regurgitated into the atria during ventricular contraction.
- **"a" wave is absent** in atrial fibrillation. In complete heart block, the "a" wave is asynchronous with the radial pulse.
- **Cannon waves** are giant "a" waves seen when atria contract against a closed AV valve which may be due to conduction defects as in complete heart block.
- Jugular venous pulse is raised in right heart failure or congestive heart failure.

MULTIPLE CHOICE QUESTIONS

1. What is not true for jugular venous pulse pressure?
   a. Pressure typically raised in right ventricular failure
   b. Pressure typically raised in partial obstruction of superior vena cava
   c. Commonly not visible with normal heart
   d. Pulsations exaggerated in tricuspid incompetence

2. Shape of arterial pulse is influenced by:
   a. Viscosity of blood
   b. Velocity of blood
   c. Arterial wall expansion
   d. Cross sectional area of artery

3. The arterial pulse pressure in the femoral artery is:
   a. Less than the pulse pressure in the upper aorta
   b. Less than 20 mm Hg
   c. Greater than the pulse pressure in upper aorta
   d. Equal to the pressure in the upper aorta

4. Not true of 'a' wave of venous pulsation in neck:
   a. Exaggerated in tricuspid stenosis
   b. Occurs just after pulsation in carotid artery
   c. Abolished in atrial fibrillation
   d. Exaggerated in complete heart block when P wave falls between QRS and T waves

5. Feature of JVP in atrial fibrillation:
   a. 'c' wave absent
   b. 'a' wave absent
   c. x-descent abnormal
   d. 'v' wave absent

6. 'c' wave in JVP is due to:
   a. Downward movement of AV valves during maximum ejection phase
   b. Rise in atrial pressure before tricuspid valve opens in protodiastole
   c. Bulging of tricuspid valve into the atrium during isometric contraction phase
   d. Atrial systole

7. Prominent 'v' wave in JVP suggest:
   a. Atrial flutter
   b. Tricuspid incompetence
   c. Pulmonary hypertension
   d. Systemic hypertension

8. Water hammer pulse occurs in:
   a. Aortic insufficiency
   b. Mitral stenosis
   c. Tricuspid stenosis
   d. Mitral regurgitation

9. True regarding jugular venous pulse:
   a. Can be felt
   b. The upper level falls during inspiration
   c. 'a' wave becomes prominent in mitral stenosis
   d. Cannot be abolished by applying pressure

10. Dicrotic notch in arterial pulse tracing is due to:
    a. Vibrations of the aortic valve cusps
    b. Flow of blood into the aorta
    c. Opening of the aortic valve
    d. End of ventricular diastole

ANSWERS

| 1. c | 2. c | 3. c | 4. b | 5. b |
| 6. c | 7. b | 8. a | 9. b | 10. a |

Cardiovascular Adjustments in Exercise

CHAPTER 30

LEARNING OBJECTIVES

Must know
- Explain the cardiovascular adjustments in exercise
- Mention the changes in the body following training

■ INTRODUCTION

> **PY11.4:** Describe and discuss cardiorespiratory and metabolic adjustments during exercise; physical training effects.

The most important factor in exercise is to deliver the required O_2 and nutrients to the exercising muscles. Due to large mass of skeletal muscles in the body, during exercise it requires large amounts of blood flow. For this, the muscle blood flow should increase very much. During exercise in between each contraction, the blood flow increases as much as 30 fold. In **intermittent contraction**, the muscle blood flow decreases during each contraction because the contracting muscle compresses the intramuscular blood vessels. But in **tonic contraction**, there will be rapid muscle fatigue due to lack of O_2 and nutrients as a result of sustained contraction.

At rest, the skeletal muscle blood flow is 2–4 mL/100 g/min. But during maximal exercise, the flow increases to 90 mL/100 g/min. This occurs by the following mechanisms:
- Stimulation of sympathetic nervous system
- Increase in arterial pressure
- Increase in cardiac output
- Local factors.

■ INCREASE IN SYMPATHETIC DISCHARGE

Blood flow to the muscle increases at or even before the start of exercise and this is a neurally mediated response. Impulses coming through the sympathetic vasodilator system may be involved. At the onset of exercise, signals are transmitted from brain to muscles as well as to the vasomotor center to initiate mass sympathetic discharge. Once exercise has started, increase in flow is due to local mechanisms. The effects of increased sympathetic discharge are increase in heart rate and force of contraction of heart. The maximum heart rate that can be attained is 210/min. Increase in heart rate is seen even before the start of exercise. This is because of increased impulses coming from the hypothalamus and limbic system to the sympathetic neurons even at the thought of exercise. Other causes of tachycardia in exercise are:
- Peripheral reflexes originating from muscle spindle and receptors of tendons and joints.
- Hormonal factors, such as adrenaline, noradrenaline, thyroxin, etc., released during exercise increase heart rate.
- Bainbridge reflex operating in the heart due to increased venous return in exercise. This is due to stimulation of SA node in the right atrium. When the atrium is stretched by increased venous return, the SA node is also stretched which stimulates the sinoatrial (SA) node.
- Increase in the temperature of the myocardium during exercise directly increases the rhythmicity of the pacemaker.

Increased sympathetic discharge also lead to the following effects:
- Peripheral vasoconstriction *except in the arterioles of muscles* which are supplied by the sympathetic vasodilator system. There is constriction of the vascular beds of skin and splanchnic area so that more blood is made available to perfuse the exercising muscles. Due to stimulation of sympathetic vasodilator system and also due to the vasodilator effects of local metabolites there is an increase of 2 L/min of extra blood flow to the muscle. *Vasoconstriction is also not seen in the coronary and cerebral vessels* during exercise because they have poor sympathetic vasoconstrictor innervation.
- Sympathetic stimulation causes contraction of veins which diverts blood to the arterial side so that arterial blood volume is increased.

■ INCREASE IN ARTERIAL PRESSURE

Arterial pressure is increased due to increase in heart rate and stroke volume. Systolic blood pressure is increased in all types of exercise. Diastolic pressure depends on peripheral resistance. Usually vasodilatation in the skeletal muscles balances the vasoconstriction in other tissues so that diastolic BP is not changed much. Pulse pressure and mean blood pressure are increased.

Mechanisms responsible for the increase in stroke volume are:

- Intrinsic autoregulation is by **Frank-Starling mechanism**. Increased venous return due to skeletal muscle pump and thoracic pump in exercise increases venous return which in turn increases end-diastolic volume and stroke volume.
- Extrinsic regulation is by neural mechanism. Here, increase in the force of contraction is by sympathetic stimulation without any increase in the initial muscle length.

INCREASE IN CARDIAC OUTPUT

During exercise, the cardiac output increases from 5.5 L/min to 20–30 L/min depending on the severity of exercise. In an untrained person, the cardiac output increases by about 4-fold whereas in a well-trained athlete, the increase is about 6-fold. Increase in cardiac output is mainly due to increase in heart rate. Additional factors are increase in stroke volume and increase in venous return. Venous return is facilitated by the contraction of the exercising muscles.

LOCAL MECHANISMS

In exercise, depending on the severity, muscle blood flow is increased 10 to 100-fold. Local mechanisms that increase muscle blood flow during exercise include the following factors that produce vasodilatation:

- Decrease in tissue PO_2 and increase in tissue PCO_2.
- Accumulation of K^+, lactic acid, adenosine, H^+ and other vasodilator metabolites.
- Increase in tissue temperature due to muscular activity further dilates the vessels.

Due to the above effects there is dilatation of arterioles and pre-capillary sphincter and there is 10 to 100-fold increase in the number of open capillaries. At rest, 2/3rd of the capillaries remain closed.

EFFECT OF TRAINING

- Cardiac hypertrophy by about 40%.
- Increase in the force of contraction of heart.
- Decrease in the heart rate due to increased vagal tone.
- Increase in stroke volume at rest due to increase in the force of contraction.
- Since heart rate is decreased and stroke volume increased, there is no change in the cardiac output at rest.
- During exercise, the stroke volume increases by 50% and the heart rate increases by 270%. So, increase in cardiac output is mainly due to increase in heart rate.
- Increase in **VO_2 max**, which is the maximum amount of O_2 that can be consumed by a person while doing severe exercise. VO_2 max in an adult is 3 L/min and in a trained athlete, it may be as high as 5 L/min. Increase in VO_2 max depends on the degree to which cardiac output can increase and not by the ventilatory capacity or oxygen diffusion capacity of the lungs.

MULTIPLE CHOICE QUESTIONS

1. **At rest, the skeletal muscle blood flow is:**
   a. 10–15 mL/100 g/min
   b. 2–4 mL/100 g/min
   c. 25–30 mL/100 g/min
   d. 8–10 mL/100 g/min

2. **True statement regarding isometric exercise:**
   a. Stroke volume changes relatively little
   b. Systolic pressure increases and diastolic pressure decreases
   c. Net fall in peripheral vascular resistance due to vasodilation in the exercising muscle
   d. Decrease in heart rate

3. **Venous return during exercise is primarily increased due to the following factors, *except*:**
   a. By the activity of muscle
   b. By the thoracic pump
   c. Due to increase in cardiac output
   d. By noradrenergically mediated venoconstriction

4. **During isotonic exercise, in between contraction, blood flow to the muscle is increased by about:**
   a. 5 fold
   b. 10 fold
   c. 15 fold
   d. 30 fold

5. **The following statements regarding exercise are true, *except*:**
   a. In isometric contraction, there is increase in the total peripheral resistance
   b. Increase in cardiac output during isotonic exercise is proportional to the increase in O_2 consumption
   c. The maximum heart rate achieved during exercise increases with age
   d. Trained athletes have larger hearts

6. **During exercise, blood supply to the splanchnic area is decreased due to:**
   a. Vasoconstriction with decreased blood flow
   b. Vasodilation with decreased blood flow
   c. Decreased parasympathetic activity
   d. Decreased sympathetic activity

7. **During exercise, blood flow is increased in:**
   a. Cutaneous circulation
   b. Coronary circulation
   c. Renal circulation
   d. Hepato-splanchnic circulation

8. **In cardiac muscle, V_{max} is used as a measure of:**
   a. Excitability
   b. Contractility
   c. Rhythmicity
   d. Conductivity

9. **In which of the following areas, change of blood flow during exercise is least?**
   a. Brain
   b. Heart
   c. Skeletal muscle
   d. Gastrointestinal tract

10. **All are increased during exercise, *Except*:**
    a. Cardiac output
    b. Venous return
    c. Coronary blood flow
    d. Peripheral vascular resistance

11. **Tachycardia at the onset of exercise is caused by stimulation of:**
    a. Chemoreceptors   b. Baroreceptors
    c. Joint proprioceptors d. Muscle spindle

12. **VO_2 max in a trained athlete comes to about:**
    a. 500 mL/min   b. 5 L/min
    c. 3 L/min   d. 750 mL/min

ANSWERS

1. b	2. a	3. c	4. d	5. c
6. a	7. b	8. b	9. a	10. d
11. c	12. b			

Effect of Acceleratory Forces on Circulatory System

CHAPTER 31

LEARNING OBJECTIVES
Must know
- Explain the effect of gravity on the circulatory system
- Explain the effects of positive g and negative g in the body
- Differentiate between black out and red out when exposed to acceleratory forces

INTRODUCTION

In aviation, there are rapid changes in the velocity and direction of motion. At the beginning of flight simple **linear acceleration** occurs. At the end of flight **deceleration** occurs, and when the vehicle takes a turn, the body is subjected to **centrifugal acceleration**.

Acceleratory force is normally designated by **"g."** 1 g is the **force of gravity** on the earth's surface. When a person is sitting on the earth's surface, the force with which he is pressing against his seat is due to force of gravity and is equal to his weight. The intensity of this force is +1 g, which is equal to the force of gravity. If the force applied on the seat during acceleration is four times his weight, the force acting on the seat is +4 g. On the contrary, if the person is held down by his seat belt during motion, negative g is applied to his body. If the force with which the belt holds him down is equal to his body weight, the force acting is minus 1 g (–1 g).

EFFECTS OF POSITIVE "G" ON CIRCULATORY SYSTEM

Positive g is the force due to acceleration acting in the long-axis of the body from **head-to-foot** when the person is in the erect posture. Since blood is mobile, gravitational forces translocate it. When a person is subjected to positive g, blood moves towards the lower part of the body depending on the position of the body. If the person is standing and exposed to positive g, blood gets pooled in the lower limbs and the pressure of the veins of legs especially feet becomes very much increased. The increase will be less if the person is in the sitting posture. Because of pooling of blood in the lower extremities, **venous return and cardiac output is reduced**. Immediately after the exposure to positive g, systolic and diastolic pressure falls very much for the first few seconds of acceleration and if the force is less than +3 g, there will be activation of baroreceptor reflex and the blood pressure rises. Acceleration greater than +5 g causes **black out** of vision in about 5 seconds followed by unconsciousness due to severe brain ischemia. If it continues, the person may die.

EFFECTS OF NEGATIVE "G"

Negative g is the force due to acceleration acting in the long-axis of the body from **foot-to-head direction**. When the aircraft goes through outside loops, the body is subjected to negative acceleratory forces. This causes increase in cardiac output and cerebral arterial pressure. Due to translocation of blood towards the upper part of the body, especially head, there will be **hyperemia** of head leading to **cerebral edema**. This leads to **ecchymosis** around eyes, severe **throbbing headache** and **mental confusion**. Sometimes, the pressure in the cerebral blood vessels reaches 300–400 mm Hg and this causes small vessels on the surface of the head to rupture. Subconjunctival hemorrhages are also seen. The intracranial vessels have a less tendency to rupture even though there is increase in the blood pressure of brain. This is because along with translocation of blood, cerebrospinal fluid (CSF) is also translocated towards brain increasing the CSF pressure. This pressure from outside exerted by the CSF acts as a cushioning buffer preventing intracerebral vascular rupture. Since the eyes are outside the cranium, when the body is exposed to strong negative g, sometimes transient blindness occurs due to hemorrhages in the eye and this is called **red out**.

EFFECT OF GRAVITY ON CIRCULATORY SYSTEM

In the standing posture, due to the effect of gravity on blood, the mean arterial blood pressure in the feet becomes 180–200 mm Hg and venous pressure 85–90 mm Hg. Arterial pressure at head level in this position becomes 60–75 mm Hg and venous pressure zero. The rise in venous pressure in the feet is due to pooling of 300–500 mL of blood in the veins of lower extremities. Blood also moves from the capillaries to the interstitial spaces of lower extremities due to increase in capillary hydrostatic pressure in the lower parts. As a result, venous return is decreased which leads to a reduction in cardiac output. If the cerebral blood flow decreases to less than 60% of normal, symptoms of cerebral ischemia develop and consciousness may be lost. This is seen in prolonged standing in some individuals. *Fainting is a protective mechanism because falling to the horizontal position restores venous return, cardiac output and cerebral blood flow to adequate levels.*

■ COMPENSATORY CARDIOVASCULAR ADJUSTMENTS IN PROLONGED STANDING

A drop in the mean arterial pressure in the upper part of the body leads to a drop in the pressure in the carotid sinus and aortic arch. The **baroreceptor reflex** mechanism operates and there will be an increase in heart rate, which leads to increase in cardiac output. There is also increase in renin secretion and renin-angiotensin-aldosterone mechanism operates leading to arteriolar constriction and increase in BP. In the brain, cerebral ischemic response operates due to increase in PCO_2, decrease in PO_2 and pH in the brain tissue. This response protects the brain, and cerebral blood flow declines only by 20% on standing.

■ EFFECTS OF ZERO GRAVITY IN THE BODY (WEIGHTLESSNESS)

Cardiovascular function can be maintained (to some extent) for up to 14 months of weightlessness. The effects of zero gravity on the body are:

❖ Flaccidity and atrophy of skeletal muscles occur because muscular effort to move objects is very much reduced in space since they are weightless.
❖ Postural hypotension on returning to earth is seen. This is because baroreceptor mechanism takes time to readapt.
❖ Decrease in plasma volume due to diuresis.
❖ Demineralization of bone leading to increased Ca^{2+} excretion and increased risk of fracture.
❖ Decrease in RBC count.
❖ Psychological problems.

(Details of weightlessness are given in Chapter 40)

■ MULTIPLE CHOICE QUESTIONS

1. **True statement regarding the effect of gravity in the body:**
   a. The pressure in any vessel below the heart level is decreased
   b. The venous pressure at the head level in the standing posture becomes zero
   c. The magnitude of the gravitational effect is 7 mm Hg/cm of vertical distance above or below the heart
   d. Gravity does not affect venous pressure

2. **Compensatory cardiovascular adjustment during prolonged standing is due to:**
   a. Operation of baroreceptor mechanism
   b. Decrease in the activity of renin-angiotensin mechanism
   c. Arteriolar dilation
   d. Inhibition of cerebral ischemic response

3. **Red out occurs:**
   a. When exposed to positive g
   b. When exposed to negative g
   c. On prolonged standing
   d. Due to decreased blood flow to the brain

4. **Weightlessness results in:**
   a. Decreased cardiac output
   b. Diminished gut motility
   c. Hypotension
   d. Osteoporosis

5. **When an aviator is subjected to negative 'g':**
   a. Hydrostatic pressure in lower limb increases
   b. Black-out occurs
   c. Cardiac output decreases
   d. Cerebral arterial pressure rises

ANSWERS

1. b 2. a 3. b 4. d 5. d

Circulation through Special Regions

CHAPTER 32

LEARNING OBJECTIVES
- Describe capillary circulation, coronary, cerebral, cutaneous, fetal and splanchnic circulation
- Enumerate the special features of coronary circulation
- Explain the physiology of triple response
- Explain the regulation of coronary blood flow
- Discuss the consequences of inadequate coronary blood flow
- Describe the functional anatomy of cerebral circulation
- Describe the measurement of cerebral circulation
- Explain the regulation of cerebral circulation.

■ CAPILLARY CIRCULATION

PY5.10: Describe and discuss regional circulation including microcirculation, lymphatic circulation, coronary, cerebral, capillary, skin, fetal, pulmonary and splanchnic circulation (Lymphatic circulation is discussed in chapter 19 and Pulmonary circulation in chapter 36)

Capillaries are microscopic blood vessels, 8 to 10 μm in diameter and they connect arterioles to venules. Capillaries are also referred to as **microvascular bed**. Blood reaches the capillary through arterioles and leaves the capillary through venules. The flow of blood from arterioles to venules through capillaries is called **microcirculation**. Density of the capillaries determines the vascularity of an organ. Body tissues with high metabolic activity like muscles, liver, kidney, lungs and nervous system have extensive capillary networks. Areas where activity is lower like tendons and ligaments have fewer capillaries. Few tissues like cornea, lens, epiphyseal cartilage, etc. are avascular, i.e., devoid of blood supply.

Normally, two-third of the capillaries remain collapsed in the resting state i.e., when the metabolic needs are low. In times of increased need like excess activity as in exercise, more and more capillaries become patent. This is called **recruitment** of closed capillaries. The total surface area of the capillaries comes to about 6300 m^2. The cells of the different tissues are in close proximity to the capillaries so that easy diffusion of substances can occur between the cells and blood in the capillary. So capillaries are called **exchange vessels**.

■ STRUCTURAL ORGANIZATION OF CAPILLARIES

Arterioles divide into **met-arterioles** (met means beyond), which have a very thin layer of smooth muscle. Met-arterioles divide to form **capillaries**. The capillaries are connected to **venules** and venules join to form **veins**. Sometimes met-arterioles may be connected directly to venules by way of **thoroughfare channels** and true capillaries arise as anastomosing side branches from them **(Fig. 32.1)**. The thoroughfare channels serve as low-resistance pathway to the flow of blood when the pre-capillary sphincters are constricted. These channels thus bypass the capillary bed and sustain blood flow through a region when the capillaries are collapsed.

The part of the met-arteriole that joins the capillary is surrounded by circular smooth muscle fibers and this part is called **pre-capillary sphincter**. The sympathetic vasoconstrictor fibers supply the met-arterioles and the pre-capillary sphincter. When these nerve fibers are stimulated, it causes constriction of the pre-capillary sphincter leading to decreased blood flow through the capillary.

Smooth muscles are absent in the capillaries. A single layer of endothelial cells resting on a basement membrane lines the capillaries. Between adjacent cells there is a gap about 70-100 nm wide filled with an amorphous material. Molecules of size less than 40 nm can pass through the capillary pore with ease. Usually macromolecules cross the capillary endothelial cells by **transcytosis** (*refer* 'transcytosis'). From the capillaries, O_2 and nutrients enter the interstitial space and CO_2 and other waste products formed in the cells enter the blood in the capillaries.

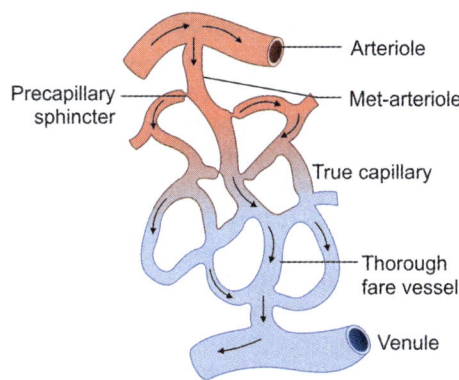

Fig. 32.1: Capillary circulation.

Classification of Capillaries

1. Continuous or non-fenestrated capillaries
2. Fenestrated capillaries
3. Discontinuous capillaries

Continuous Capillaries

The endothelial cells are arranged without gap in between them, e.g., skin, blood-brain barrier, etc. These capillaries with tight junctions allow only very small molecules to pass through.

Fenestrated Capillaries

There are gaps in between the endothelial cells ranging from 70 to 100 nm in diameter which are lined by a basement membrane, e.g., capillaries of intestinal villi, renal glomeruli, choroid plexus of the ventricles of brain, ciliary process of eyes and endocrine glands.

Discontinuous Type

Very wide clefts are present between the endothelial cells in discontinuous type of capillaries. Basement membrane is incomplete or absent. Almost all substances present in plasma can cross these gaps. For example, in the liver **sinusoids** even proteins can escape out. Newly formed blood cells enter the blood stream through the sinusoids of red bone marrow. Spleen, anterior pituitary and parathyroid glands also have sinusoids.

Capillary Pressure

At any time, 5% of the total circulating blood is in the capillaries. In the resting state, most of the capillaries remain collapsed. *Blood flows from met-arterioles into the venules through the thoroughfare vessels or shunt vessels bypassing the capillaries at rest* **(Fig. 32.1)**. During activity, the met-arterioles and the pre-capillary sphincters dilate and the intra-capillary pressure rises. The vasodilatation is mainly due to the release of vasodilator metabolites released from the active tissues like lactic acid, K^+, etc. During exercise, vasodilatation of the skeletal muscle blood vessels is due to stimulation of sympathetic cholinergic fibers innervating the skeletal muscle blood vessels in addition to local metabolites.

This overcomes the critical closing pressure in the capillaries, and blood flows through the capillaries.

At rest, the interstitial fluid pressure around the capillary will be more than the hydrostatic pressure in the capillaries. This pressure from outside causes most of the capillaries to collapse in the resting state. This pressure is called **critical closing pressure** (*refer* **Fig. 25.7**). When there is sympathetic stimulation, there will be decreased blood flow through the capillaries due to constriction of the pre-capillary sphincters supplied by sympathetic adrenergic fibers.

The capillary pressure varies in different parts of the body and at different times. For example, the capillary pressure in the nail bed at the arteriolar end of capillary is 30 mm Hg whereas at the venous end it is only 15 mm Hg. The capillary pressure is very low in the pulmonary capillaries whereas it is very high in the glomerulus of kidney. *Since the cross-sectional area of capillaries is very large, velocity of blood flow is less in the capillaries, i.e., 0.07 cm/sec.*

Normally, capillaries can withstand high hydrostatic pressures. But in conditions where capillary fragility is increased as in viral infections like dengue fever, small hemorrhages occur in the capillary producing hemorrhagic purplish spots in the skin referred to as **purpura** (*refer* **Fig. 18.9**).

Mechanism of Transport of Substances Across Capillary Wall

- Vesicular transport
- Diffusion
- Filtration

Vesicular Transport

Small vesicles are present in the cytoplasm of the endothelial cells lining the capillaries. These vesicles fuse with the inner and outer membranes of the cell, discharging their contents into the cell or out of the cell. Sometimes they coalesce with each other forming a continuous channel from the inside to the outside of the cell called **pinocytic channel or vesicular channel**.

Diffusion

O_2, glucose, etc., are present in higher concentration in the blood than in the interstitial fluid and hence they diffuse into the interstitial space, and CO_2, urea, etc., which are present in higher concentration in the interstitial space will diffuse into the blood. Lipid-soluble substances can pass easily across the capillary wall.

Filtration

The rate of filtration depends on the balance between the **Starling's forces**, i.e., the hydrostatic pressure gradient and osmotic pressure gradient (*refer* Starling's forces; Chapter 19). The amount of fluid filtered across the capillary wall every minute is equal to the total plasma volume. An equal volume of fluid enters the capillaries and lymphatics each minute.

Table 32.1: Regulation of capillary circulation.	
Vasoconstrictors	**Vasodilators**
• Catecholamines, vasopressin • Decrease in temperature (cold) • Sympathetic (adrenergic) stimulation	• Hypoxia, acidosis, hypercapnia • Histamine, bradykinin, and acetylcholine • Increase in temperature, extreme cold • Sympathetic cholinergic stimulation

Functions of Capillaries
- Diffusion
- Filtration
- Absorption

Regulation of Capillary Circulation (Table 32.1)
- **Local factors** like acidosis, hypoxia, hypercapnia, histamine, etc., produce vasodilatation.
- **Hormonal factors** usually produce vasoconstriction.
- **Mechanical factors** include temperature, pressure, etc.
- **Neural factors** like stimulation of autonomic nervous system produce varying effects.

CUTANEOUS CIRCULATION

Circulation through the **skin** is cutaneous circulation and it serves two functions:
1. It is necessary for the metabolic needs of the skin.
2. Blood flow through the skin helps to regulate body temperature.

Types of Vessels in the Skin
- Vessels, which provide nutrition to the skin and help in metabolic activities, like arterioles, capillaries and venules.
- Vessels that help in temperature regulation by conduction of heat include:
  - **Subcutaneous venous plexus**, which are seen parallel to the skin surface. The color of the skin depends on the amount of blood in the subcutaneous plexus. The color may be pale if blood flow is decreased, reddish if the flow is high and bluish if the amount of reduced hemoglobin is high.
  - **Arteriovenous anastomoses**, which are direct communications between arteries and veins (*refer* **Fig. 58.1**). They are present mainly in the **hands, lips, nose, ears**, etc. These vessels that contain smooth muscles are richly supplied by sympathetic vasoconstrictor fibers, which release norepinephrine at their endings. *This is the reason why cyanosis is mainly seen in these regions when exposed to cold climate.* There will be strong sympathetic stimulation when the body is exposed to extreme cold.

Measurement of Cutaneous Blood Flow
- Continuous temperature recording
- Colorimetry
- Clearance rate of radioactive substances

Regulation of Cutaneous Blood Flow
- **Nervous factors**: The center for temperature regulation is located in the **pre-optic** region of **anterior hypothalamus**. This center controls blood flow through the skin in relation to changes in body temperature by producing vasoconstriction or vasodilatation. The skin blood vessels are extremely sensitive to catecholamines. *The cutaneous vessels do not have parasympathetic supply.*
- **Hormonal control**: Cutaneous vasoconstriction is produced by catecholamines, vasopressin, angiotensin II, etc.
- **Chemical factors** like histamine, bradykinin, acetyl choline, acidosis, hypercapnia and hypoxia produce vasodilatation.
- **Physical factors** like increase in temperature cause vasodilatation, and cold produces vasoconstriction. But extreme cold produces vasodilatation.

Cutaneous Vascular Responses
- White reaction
- Triple response
- Dermographism
- Axon reflex
- Reactive hyperemia
- Responses to cold.

Vascular Responses to Mechanical Stimuli
- White reaction
- Triple response

White Reaction
When the skin is lightly stroked with a blunt pointed object, it produces a pale or white line along the line of stroke within 15–20 sec and the line becomes prominent in 1 min. It then gradually fades in about 3–5 min time. The reason for this reaction is contraction of the precapillary sphincter due to mechanical stimulus so that, less blood flows into the capillaries producing the pale color. *No nervous mechanism is involved in white reaction.*

Triple Response
Triple response has three components:
1. Red reaction
2. Flare
3. Wheal

Red reaction: If the skin is stroked strongly with a pointed object, instead of the white reaction a red line appears along the line of stroke in 3–15 sec. The color reaches a peak in ½–1 min, gradually fades and disappears by about 3–5 min. This reaction is called red reaction or red line. This reaction also *does not involve any nervous mechanism.* This is due to the direct effect of the strong mechanical stimulus causing cutaneous vasodilatation. Even after cutting of the cutaneous nerve or degeneration of the cutaneous nerve, the red reaction persists.

Flare: If the cutaneous stroke is a bit stronger than above, the redness of the red band spreads over a variable extent for a width of about 1–10 mm surrounding the stroke

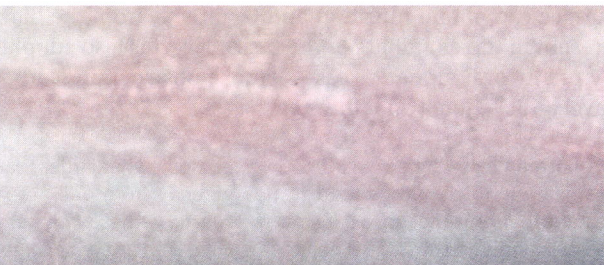

Fig. 32.2: Flare reaction on the skin.

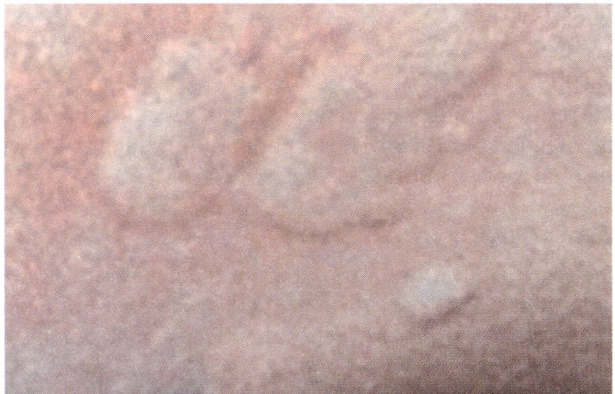

Fig. 32.3: Wheal reaction on the skin.

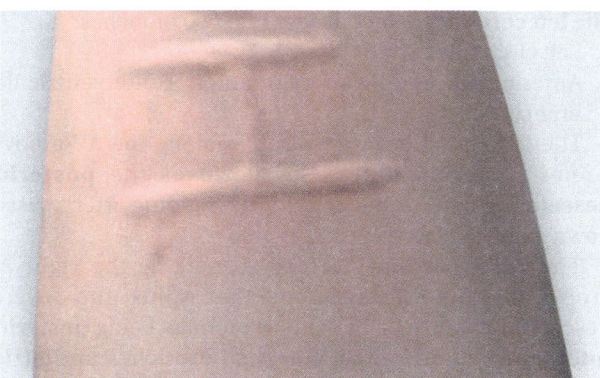

Fig. 32.4: Dermographism.

(Fig. 32.2). This is called the spreading **flush or flare**. This is also associated with a local rise in temperature. This reaction is due to a *local neuronal mechanism called* **axon reflex**. The transmitter released is substance P. This reaction is absent in locally anesthetized skin and in denervated skin (*refer* Axon reflex; **Fig. 28.4**).

Wheal: If the stroke is very strong, the skin along the line of stroke becomes blanched and raised to a height of 1–2 mm. It persists for about 1–3 min or sometimes hours. This reaction is called wheal reaction (**Fig. 32.3**). This is due to increased permeability and transudation of fluid from the capillaries. The local edema is due to chemical substances like histamine, bradykinin etc., released from mast cells at the site of injury.

The three part response which consists of red reaction, flare and wheal is called the triple response and is part of the normal reaction to injury or allergy. Wheal and flare reaction is often made use of in testing for allergies to determine which allergens trigger a reaction in a patient.

Dermographism

In sensitive individuals, if something is written on the skin with a blunt object, areas of raised skin follows the line of letters and the letters can be read clearly for some time (**Fig. 32.4**). This is due to **exaggerated wheal response**.

Reactive Hyperemia

When a blood vessel is occluded, the cutaneous arterioles below the level of occlusion dilate. When the circulation is re-established, blood flowing into the dilated vessels makes the skin red. This is reactive hyperemia. The arteriolar dilatation is due to the local effect of hypoxia.

Cutaneous Response to Cold

During exposure to cold, there is widespread cutaneous vasoconstriction. However, prolonged exposure to extreme cold produces vasodilatation of cutaneous vessels due to axon reflex. Severe cold also promotes formation of plasma kinins which also produce vasodilatation.

■ CORONARY CIRCULATION

Introduction

Even though the heart is filled with blood, nutrients and O_2 cannot diffuse from the blood present in the heart chambers to supply all the layers of the heart wall. So the myocardium is supplied by coronary arteries and the blood flow through the heart is referred to as **coronary circulation**. In addition, human heart cannot withstand anaerobic conditions because normal myocardial metabolism is aerobic. Even under resting conditions, myocardium extracts about 75% of O_2 delivered via the coronary circulation. An increase in myocardial metabolism should be accompanied by a corresponding increase in coronary blood flow. So, any reduction in the blood flow seriously affects the myocardium.

Functional Anatomy of Coronary Vessels

Heart is supplied by the **right and the left coronary arteries** which arise from the base or root of the aorta, i.e., from the sinuses of Valsalva (**Table 32.2**).

Table 32.2: Parts supplied by right and left coronary arteries.	
Right coronary	*Left coronary*
• Right atrium • Posterior portion of interventricular septum • Right ventricle • Posterior part of left ventricle	• Anterior and lateral portions of left ventricle • Anterior portion of interventricular septum • Left atrium

The **left coronary artery** divides into two branches:
1. Left circumflex artery
2. Anterior descending artery or anterior interventricular branch

The left circumflex artery passes along the AV groove, comes posterior and passes down as the **posterior descending artery**. The anterior descending artery passes down along the interventricular groove.

The right coronary artery goes along the right AV groove for some distance and then splits into several descending branches, the important ones being **posterior interventricular branch, marginal branches and atrial branch** that supply the right atrium. The arteries break up into arterioles and then to capillaries.

All the descending branches pass subendocardially towards the apex of the heart. At the apex the branches pierce the myocardium. The blood flow in both the coronaries is same in 30% of individuals. The flow through the right coronary is more in 50% of individuals and in 20%, the left coronary has a greater flow.

Venous Drainage of the Heart

Venous blood is drained from the heart through two systems:
1. Superficial system
2. Deep system

The **superficial system** drains the left ventricle and ends in the **coronary sinus and anterior cardiac veins** which open into the right atrium. A vascular sinus is a thin-walled vein that has no smooth muscle on its wall.

The **deep system** drains the rest of the heart and has three components.
i. **Arteriosinusoidal vessels**: They originate from an arteriole and resemble a sinus. They empty into the heart chambers.
ii. **Arterioluminal vessels**: They are special vessels opening into the heart chambers. They do not resemble capillaries or sinuses.
iii. **Thebesian veins**: They are small vessels that arise from capillaries or small veins and empty directly into the ventricles.

Collaterals and Anastomosis of Heart

The union of the branches of two or more arteries which supply the same region of the body is called an anastomosis (singular). Anastomoses (plural) between arteries provide alternative routes for blood to reach a tissue or organ.

The anastomoses between coronary arterioles and extra-cardiac arterioles are minimal. *Extracardiac anastomosis* includes anastomoses between branches of coronary arteries and between branches of vessels lying near the heart like intrathoracic arteries, bronchial arteries and vasa vasora of aorta and pulmonary artery. The *intercoronary arteriolar anastomoses*, i.e., between branches of the right and the left coronary arteries are also very minimal. So the coronaries are functionally regarded as **end arteries**. In humans, occlusion to a branch of the coronary artery leads to death of the part supplied by the occluded vessel. Even though heart is filled with blood, only the inner 75-100 μm of the endocardial surface can obtain nutrition and O_2 directly from the blood present in the chambers of the heart. Heart is also supplied by plenty of lymphatic vessels whose obstruction leads to myocardial edema and fibrosis.

> **Collateral vessels** are small blood vessels somewhat larger than capillaries which allow blood to flow directly from one artery to another. In times of occlusion to an artery, these collateral vessels undergo substantial enlargement. So if an artery becomes occluded, and if there are collateral channels, they can allow arterial blood to enter the blocked artery beyond the site of obstruction. This prevents ischemia and infarction of the area supplied by the blocked vessel.

Coronary Blood Flow

The resting coronary blood flow is about 250 mL/min (70-80 mL of blood per 100 g of heart per minute) which is 4-5% of the total cardiac output.

Myocardial Oxygen Demand

The O_2 consumption of the heart at rest is about 7-8 mL/100 g/min, i.e., at rest, 70-80% of O_2 is extracted from each unit of coronary blood which is the highest of all organs. O_2 consumption of the whole body at rest is 250 mL/min, of this 25 mL/min, i.e., 10% of the total O_2 consumption is by the left ventricle. Since O_2 extraction by the myocardium is very high, the venous blood from the myocardium is only 25% saturated with O_2. This is the maximum possible extraction ratio. *So, the only way to increase the O2 supply to the heart is by increasing the blood flow since the increased demand for O2 cannot be met by increased extraction.*

■ MEASUREMENT OF CORONARY BLOOD FLOW

Indirect Method

Kety's Method

Coronary blood flow is measured based on **modified Fick's principle** using N_2O. This method is known as Kety's method. The blood flow can be measured from:
- The amount of substance removed from each mL of blood as it flows through the organ.
- The total quantity of substance removed by the organ in a given period of time.

Procedure: The subject is asked to breathe a known concentration of **N_2O (15%)** for 10 min. During inhalation of gas, serial arterial blood samples are collected from any peripheral artery and by cardiac catheterization, venous samples are drawn from the coronary sinus at 1 min intervals. The concentration of N_2O in both of these samples is plotted against time in minutes. The heights of the two curves differ and the difference is measured, which is the arteriovenous concentration difference. Another method to find out arteriovenous concentration difference is by noting the AV concentration difference for each minute for a period of 10 min and the average is taken. This denotes the quantity of

N$_2$O taken up by from heart from each mL of blood as it passes through the heart. Quantity of N$_2$O consumed by the heart is obtained by multiplying the quantity of N$_2$O in the venous blood by the partial pressure coefficient of N$_2$O. From these data, the blood flow can be calculated using the formula:

$$\text{Blood flow} = \frac{\text{Quantity of substance taken up}}{\text{Arteriovenous concentration difference}}$$

Radionuclide technique: Recently, a number of techniques using radionuclides have been used to measure coronary blood flow. Radionuclides are injected intravenously. After 10 min, the amount of tracer taken up by the myocardial cells can be detected with the help of **gamma scintillation camera** placed over the chest. Distribution of the radioactive tracers in the heart is directly proportional to myocardial blood flow. It helps to measure regional blood flow in the heart and also helps to detect areas of ischemia and infarction due to their low uptake of the tracer. The substance usually used is **thallium-201 (^{201}Tl)**.

Technetium-99 (^{99}Tc) combined with **stannous pyrophosphate** forms technetium-stannous pyrophosphate which has selected affinity for infarcted tissue. So the areas of infarction stand out as **hot spots** on the gamma camera due to high radioactivity.

Coronary angiography: In this method, a radiopaque dye is introduced into the coronary circulation together with radioactive xenon (^{133}Xe). Serial X-ray pictures are taken and any obstruction to the flow of blood can be detected. After that, X-rays are replaced by gamma camera. Radioactivity from different regions is measured and this gives a detailed analysis of regional coronary blood flow.

Direct Method

Electromagnetic flow meter technique is employed in animals to measure the phasic flow and coronary flow per minute.

Factors Influencing Coronary Blood Flow

- Phases of cardiac cycle
- Heart rate
- Aortic pressure
- Temperature and exercise.

Variation of Coronary Blood Flow in Different Phases of Cardiac Cycle

The coronary vessels originating from the coronary sinuses at the root of the aorta pass along the epicardial surface and their branches pass through the myocardium to form sub-endocardial plexus to perfuse the myocardium. So during systole, these arterial branches are compressed and prevent perfusion of myocardium. So, coronary perfusion occurs more during diastole rather than during systole i.e., *the coronary blood flow during systole is different from that of diastole*. With the onset of isometric contraction phase, there is a sharp reduction in the flow through the left coronary artery. Towards the end of this phase the flow even stops, i.e., it comes to zero value (**Fig. 32.5**). During systole, the pressure

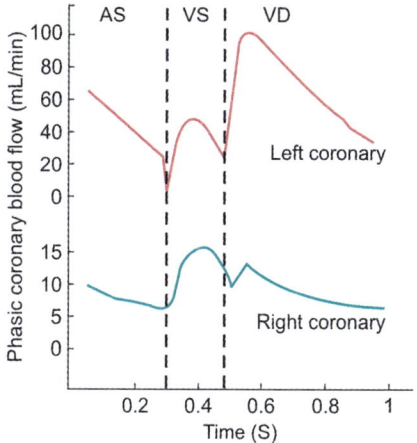

Fig. 32.5: Blood flow in the left and right coronary during various phases of the cardiac cycle.
(AS: atrial systole; VS: ventricular systole; VD: ventricular diastole)

in the sub-endocardial layer of the heart becomes as great as the ventricular pressure.

The pressure in the outer layers of the heart is less when compared to this. Therefore, the sub-endocardial vessels are compressed to a very great extent in systole.

The flow never comes to zero in the right coronary artery since the right ventricular pressure is not as high as the left ventricular pressure. This is because lower pressures are sufficient to perfuse the pulmonary circulation. But the flow through the right coronary artery during ventricular systole is also significantly reduced.

At the onset of ejection phase, the aortic pressure rises and the flow through the coronaries rises rapidly to reach a peak shortly before the peak of aortic pressure curve. The flow then falls slightly and then again rises with the closure of semilunar valve. During systole, the intramural pressure is very high in the left ventricle than in the right ventricle. So the left coronary flow is maximally affected.

During diastole, greater flow occurs in the coronaries due to the reduction in the intramural pressure (**Fig. 32.5**). The sub-endocardial capillary plexus is very great and so the flow through the sub-endocardial portions of the heart is very great during ventricular diastole.

Applied physiology: In patients with **aortic stenosis**, the pressure in the left ventricle must be much greater than that of aorta to eject the blood through the stenosed valve. So the force of contraction should be more and the coronary vessels get severely compressed during ventricular systole. Hence, patients with **aortic stenosis** are particularly prone to develop symptoms of **myocardial ischemia.** The reasons are greater compression of the myocardium and increased demand for O$_2$ for the myocardium to pump blood through the stenotic valve.

Effect of heart rate: Tachycardia shortens diastole and the coronary flow is reduced. The coronary flow will be increased in bradycardia.

Effect of mean aortic pressure: Aortic pressure also decides coronary blood flow because mean aortic pressure is the driving force for the flow into the coronary arteries. A fall in the mean arterial pressure as in circulatory shock decreases coronary flow. If the pressure changes are not extreme, i.e., within physiological limits, the coronary flow will be maintained by autoregulation. When the blood flow decreases, there will be hypoxia in the cardiac muscle which induces vasodilatation and thus increases the flow by autoregulation.

Temperature and exercise: Increase in **temperature** increases coronary blood flow by increasing myocardial metabolism, and hypothermia decreases coronary flow. During exercise, coronary flow is increased by about 4 times due to sympathetic stimulation and increased metabolism in the heart.

Regulation of Coronary Blood Flow

- Chemical factors
- Physical factors
- Hormonal factors
- Neural factors
- Autoregulation.

Chemical Factors

- The coronary blood flow and myocardial O_2 consumption are closely and directly related. In times of hypoxia, the coronary blood flow is increased. Products of metabolism like CO_2, H^+, K^+, *lactic acid, adenosine, bradykinin, prostaglandins, adenine nucleotides*, etc. produce coronary vasodilatation. **Adenosine** seems to be the main physiological regulator of coronary blood flow. It is also the major factor that produces coronary vasodilatation in hypoxic states.
- *Endothelium derived relaxing factor (EDRF)* is released from the endothelium by the action of calcitonin gene-related peptide (CGRP) and substance-P is released from the cardiac nerves. Both produce vasodilatation. EDRF produces maximal dilatation of epicardial coronary arteries.
- Hypoxia also acts directly to produce coronary arteriolar vasodilatation.
- Drugs like *nitrates* produce coronary vasodilatation. **Nitroglycerine** is the drug used to relieve pain in angina pectoris.

Physical Factors

- Arterial blood pressure
- Peripheral resistance
- Heart rate
- Phases of cardiac cycle.

When arterial BP is increased, coronary blood flow also increases. There is a decrease in the blood flow when there is an increase in the coronary resistance. During diastole, the flow increases, and during systole, the flow decreases. In times of tachycardia, the blood flow decreases due to reduction in the diastolic period. Coronary blood flow increases during diastole and decreases during systole which is called phasic coronary flow.

Hormonal Regulation

- *Thyroxine* increases coronary blood flow. This is because thyroxine increases metabolic rate of myocardium which increases O_2 demand. The hypoxia produces vasodilatation.
- *Catecholamines* increase coronary blood flow. This is because epinephrine combines with $β_2$ receptors and causes vasodilatation. With norepinephrine, increased flow is secondary to increase in the metabolic rate. The direct effect of norepinephrine is vasoconstriction by acting on α-receptors.
- *Angiotensin* increases vascular resistance and decreases blood flow.
- *Acetylcholine and histamine* cause vasodilatation and thus increase blood flow.

Neural Regulation

Coronary blood vessels are supplied by sympathetic and parasympathetic divisions of autonomic nervous system. When sympathetics to the heart are stimulated, the blood flow through the coronaries increases. This is secondary to increase in heart rate and increased metabolic activity of the heart which produces vasodilatation. Moreover, the coronary vessels contain more number of beta receptors than alpha receptors (stimulation of beta receptors produces vasodilation). The neurotransmitter released at the nerve ending is norepinephrine.

The parasympathetic supply (vagal supply) to the coronary vessels is minimal and hence *parasympathetic stimulation has very little effect on coronary blood flow*. But, parasympathetic stimulation decreases heart rate and force of contraction of heart and thus can indirectly reduce coronary blood flow. But when heart rate is reduced, diastolic period is prolonged and so coronary flow is not much affected. This is because most of the coronary blood flow occurs during diastole.

Reflex control—when the pressure in the carotid sinus is increased, the sinus nerve is stimulated which in turn inhibits the vasomotor center producing vasodilatation. When the carotid body chemoreceptors are stimulated, it also results in reflex coronary vasodilatation.

Autoregulation

Autoregulation refers to the ability of an organ to maintain a relatively constant blood flow over a wide range of arterial blood pressure. The coronary circulation has the intrinsic capacity to adjust its resistance to maintain a constant blood flow, despite changes in arterial perfusion pressure within a **range of 60–140 mm Hg**. Autoregulation is due to local metabolic factors especially **hypoxia** and accumulation of **adenosine**.

Adenosine is released from cardiac muscle fibers due to increased breakdown of adenine nucleotides in hypoxic states. The coronary flow is decreased when the mean arterial pressure falls below 60 mm Hg because autoregulation fails below this pressure.

Special Features of Coronary Circulation

- Myocardium is the only tissue that generates its **own perfusion pressure**. Coronary perfusion pressure refers

to the pressure gradient that is responsible for coronary and thus myocardial perfusion to meet myocardial O_2 demand. In the left ventricle, it is the difference between the diastolic aortic pressure and left ventricular end diastolic pressure. Coronary perfusion pressure = (Aortic diastolic pressure)− (Left ventricular-diastolic pressure)
- ❖ Coronary perfusion pressure becomes reduced in heart failure and coronary artery disease like myocardial infarction. Minimum coronary perfusion pressure required is 15 mm Hg. Coronary perfusion pressure is based on diastolic pressure because the left ventricular myocardium gets perfused only during diastole.
- ❖ Myocardium is the only tissue that is perfused more during diastole. Since the coronary vessels are distributed in the walls of the heart, they are subjected to compression during systole of the heart. So unlike other organs of the body, there is greater blood flow during diastole than during systole in the heart. In the left ventricle, 80% of coronary blood flow occurs during diastole and the remaining 20% occur during systole. Right ventricular perfusion occurs in systole as well as diastole since the right ventricular pressure is far lower than the pressure exerted by the left ventricle. It is also perfused more during diastole. This is called **phasic coronary blood flow** (variation in coronary blood flow in different phases of cardiac cycle).
- ❖ Myocardium is an aerobic tissue, i.e., it cannot withstand anaerobic conditions.
- ❖ Resting O_2 extraction by the myocardium is very high, i.e., 75%. This is the maximum possible extraction ratio. Therefore, the only way to increase O_2 supply to the myocardium is to increase the coronary blood flow by increasing coronary perfusion pressure or by producing coronary vasodilation. If coronary perfusion is inadequate, myocardial ischemia and infarction result. Therefore, coronary blood flow increases when metabolism of the myocardium is increased as in exercise to meet the increased O_2 demand. Coronary blood flow can be increased 4 to 5 folds during exercise.
- ❖ The coronary flow is principally regulated by metabolic factors which override nervous influences. Blood flow increases when metabolism of the myocardium is increased as in exercise which produces increase in heart rate and force of contraction. Coronary vasodilatation occurs because of metabolic products like adenosine, K^+, H^+, CO_2, etc. Increase in blood flow due to the vasodilator effects of metabolites is known as **reactive hyperemia**.
- ❖ Myocardium has a high capillary density. There is approximately one capillary for each myocardial fiber.
- ❖ Heart has very poor collateral circulation, so, more prone for ischemic attacks. The coronary arteries are referred to as end arteries. Anastomoses between the coronary vessels are quite small and hence sudden occlusion of a coronary artery results in a localized area of myocardial ischemia or infarction.
- ❖ Exhibits autoregulation, the coronary blood flow remains unchanged between mean arterial pressures of 60 and 140 mm Hg. Coronary vasoconstriction and vasodilation are responsible for the autoregulation of coronary flow. The autoregulation seems to be metabolically mediated with adenosine as its main mediator.
- ❖ The coronary circulation has one of the shortest circulation times in the body, being about 8 sec.
- ❖ Major source of energy supply in the heart is free fatty acid. 1/3rd of energy is derived from the metabolism of fat. It can also utilize substrates like glucose, pyruvate, lactate, ketone bodies and amino acids for energy.

Defects of Coronary Circulation

- ❖ Coronary circulation lacks functional anastomosis between major branches, i.e., coronary arteries are end arteries. When an artery is blocked, the area supplied by that vessel suffers from ischemia.
- ❖ O_2 extraction from the blood is very high (75–80%) and so arteriovenous oxygen concentration difference is very high in the heart even at rest.
- ❖ Blood flow is periodically interrupted during stages of cardiac cycle.
- ❖ Coronaries are more prone to degenerative changes. All these features make its dysfunction a common cause of death.

Coronary Artery Disease

Coronary artery disease (CAD) is the buildup of plaque (atherosclerosis) in the arteries supplying the heart. Plaque leads to narrowing or blockage of the coronary arteries that may result in a heart attack. Coronary artery disease is also known as coronary heart disease or ischemic heart disease (IHD).

Coronary arteries are end arteries, which perfuse their own exclusive capillary bed. So when the blood flow through a coronary artery is decreased, the part of the myocardium it supplies suffers from hypoxia. **"P" factor** released from the ischemic tissue due to hypoxia accumulates and results in chest pain during exertion, called **angina pectoris**. **Adenosine** formed by the degradation of ATP in the ischemic tissue also contributes to the anginal pain. The pain is usually felt in the chest behind the sternum towards the left side and it typically radiates to the ulnar border of the left arm. But the pain can also radiate to the neck, jaw, back or abdomen.

If the ischemia is severe and prolonged, irreversible changes occur in the myocardium resulting in **myocardial infarction (MI)**. The infarcted area generates ectopic impulses that can lead to ventricular fibrillation. Coronary artery disease is a major threat to life and is the leading cause of death in developed countries. Common causes are thrombosis or thromboembolism and death is mainly due to ventricular fibrillation.

Causes of Myocardial Infarction

When there is more than 75% obstruction of the coronary arteries, there will be infarction or cell death of the myocardium which is referred to as myocardial infarction. The causes are:
- ❖ Atherosclerosis and spasm of the coronary vessel at the site of lesion

- Platelet aggregation and thrombus formation at the site of atherosclerosis
- Stress induces coronary artery spasm
- Dyslipidemia is a very important cause for MI
- Increased circulating level of C-reactive protein, antiphospholipid antibody, homocysteine, etc. are strongly correlated with MI.

Diagnosis of Coronary Artery Disease

Clinical presentation: The patient complains of severe chest pain over the precordium with or without radiation to the ulnar border of left arm. In right coronary obstruction there will be referred pain in the lower jaw and neck. Patients suffering from chronic diabetes mellitus may not have pain during acute MI (silent attack). There will be associated symptoms like fatigue, excessive sweating, nausea, etc. in MI. The patient will be relieved of chest pain when sublingual nitroglycerin or sorbitrates are given. This is because these drugs produce both arterial and venous dilation and thus decreases both preload (end-diastolic volume decrease due to decreased venous return which in turn is due to venodilation and peripheral pooling of blood) and after load (peripheral resistance and aortic impedance) on the heart. This decreases myocardial O_2 consumption and demand. The relief of pain on taking these drugs is diagnostic of MI.

- **ECG changes**: There will be typical ECG changes which may help in diagnosing and locating areas of infarction. In acute infarction, there will be ST-segment elevation in the ECG leads overlying the infarcted area (**Fig. 32.6B**). This is referred to as **STEMI** (ST-elevation myocardial infarction). ST-segment depression is seen in leads placed opposite to the area of infarction. MI where ST-elevation is absent is referred to as **NSTEMI (non-ST elevation myocardial infarction) (Figs. 32.6A and B)**. Another finding in MI is T wave inversion and prominent Q wave.
- **Changes in the level of enzymes specific for heart** in the blood: The damaged myocardial tissue releases isoenzymes like *serum glutamate-O-methyl transferase (SGOT), creatine phosphokinase (CPK), lactate dehydrogenase (LDH)*, etc., and the blood level of these enzymes will be elevated in MI. The most specific diagnostic blood test is the increased concentration of *CPK-MB,* the cardiac isoenzyme of CPK. *Troponin T and troponin I* are proteins released when there is damage to the cardiac muscle as in MI. Troponins are normally not detectable in the blood. Most patients who had an MI have increased troponin levels within 6 hours. Positive TROP T test is an indication of myocardial damage even if the patient shows normal ECG.
- **Coronary angiography**: By cardiac catheterization, a contrast dye containing iodine is injected into the coronary arteries and serial X-ray pictures are taken (**Fig. 32.7**). The pictures show the site and extent of obstruction in the coronary vessels.

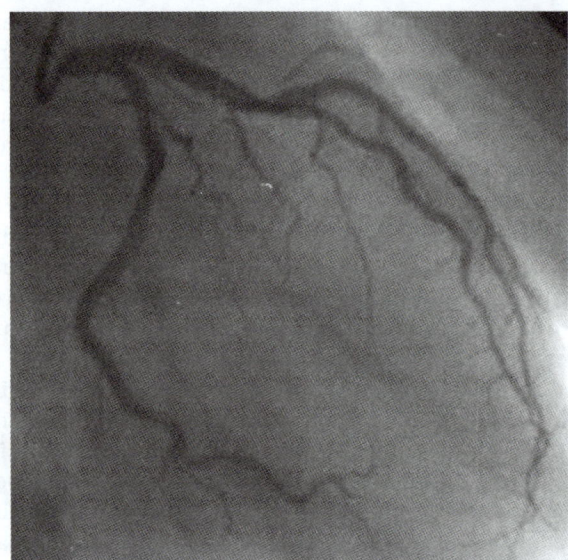

Fig. 32.7: Angiogram showing normal left coronary artery and its branches.

Risk Factors for Coronary Artery Disease (CAD)

- **Age**: As age advances, there is increased risk of CAD
- **Genetic predisposition**: Those people having positive family history of ischemic heart disease or cerebrovascular accident occurring at a relatively younger age among close relatives are at a higher risk.
- **Personality**: Aggressive and competitive individuals are more prone to develop myocardial infarction.
- **Sex**: Prevalence is less in women in the reproductive age group.
- **Cigarette smoking**: Smokers are at a higher risk
- **Hyperlipidemia**: Increased serum cholesterol > 250 mg/dL, high LDL cholesterol and low HDL cholesterol are at a higher risk.
- **Hypertension**: Hypertensives with high cholesterol level are at a higher risk.
- **Diabetes mellitus**: Diabetes and hypercholesterolemia interact strongly in the genesis of ischemic heart disease.
- **Exercise**: Sedentary persons are at a higher risk than those having regular physical exercise.
- **Other risk factors**: Increased levels of homocysteine, c-reactive protein (CRP), plasma fibrinogen and fibrin D-dimer and lipoprotein-α have higher risk to develop atherosclerosis and ischemic heart disease.

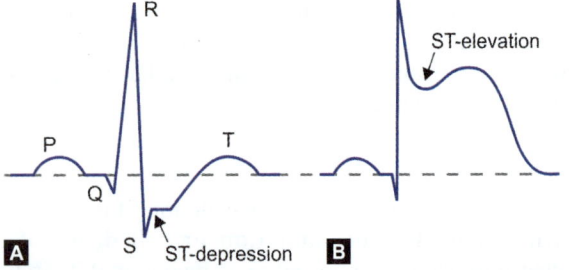

Figs. 32.6A and B: Myocardial infarction ECG changes in (A) NSTEMI (Non-ST-elevation myocardial infarction); (B) STEMI (ST-segment elevation myocardial infarction).

Treatment of Myocardial Infarction

The aim of *medical management* is to reduce the cardiac work load, thereby reducing the myocardial O_2 demand. This is achieved by controlling heart rate using β-blockers and by reducing after load and preload on the heart by using vasodilators like angiotensin converting enzyme (ACE) inhibitors, Ca^{2+} channel blockers and nitrates. Administration of folic acid and vitamin B_{12} is also useful to prevent MI. It is seen that there is strong correlation with increased plasma level of homocysteine and myocardial infarction. Homocysteine produces damage to the endothelium of blood vessels leading to platelet aggregation and atherosclerosis. Folic acid and vitamin B_{12} convert homocysteine to methionine which is nontoxic.

Surgical intervention is required only when there is more than 75% reduction in vessel diameter. This is done by a **bypass surgery** in which the occluded vessel is bypassed using an autograft. **Coronary artery bypass grafting (CABG)** is a surgical procedure in which a blood vessel from another part of the body is grafted to a coronary artery to bypass the area of blockage. A piece of the grafted blood vessel is sutured between the aorta and the unblocked portion of the coronary artery. Another method is **percutaneous transluminal coronary angioplasty (PTCA)** along with lysis of the clot by intracoronary injection of **streptokinase** which stimulates the fibrinolytic system. Streptokinase facilitates conversion of plasminogen to plasmin which leads to fibrinolysis and also prevents further progress of infarction.

This treatment is most valuable if done within the first few hours of pain in MI. By PTCA, a stent which is a spring coil made of stainless steel can be permanently placed in the area of occlusion inside the artery to keep the artery patent. After PTCA, the patient should be given antiplatelet drugs and low dose of aspirin to prevent platelet aggregation at the region of angioplasty. Aspirin acts by inhibiting cyclo-oxygenase and thus prevents formation of thromboxane A_2 (TxA_2). TxA_2 produces vasoconstriction and platelet aggregation.

Reperfusion Damage

After a block to a vessel supplying the myocardium, reperfusion may occur and this further damages the myocardium and is called **reperfusion damage**. Most of the damage is due to the formation of super oxide free- radicals (O_2^-). A **free-radical** is an electrically charged atom or group of atoms with an unpaired electron in its outermost shell. O_2^- is formed by the addition of an electron to an oxygen molecule. The unpaired electron makes the free radicals unstable, highly reactive and destructive to nearby molecules causing cellular damage and cell death. Normally the body produces enzymes like **superoxide dismutase and catalase** that counter the effects of free radicals by converting them to less reactive substances. Nutrients like vitamin E, vitamin C, β-carotene, selenium, etc., are **antioxidants** that inactivate and remove oxygen free radicals. Other diseases associated with oxygen derived free radicals are cancer, atherosclerosis, diabetes mellitus, Alzheimer's disease, rheumatoid arthritis, etc.

CEREBRAL CIRCULATION

Introduction

The brain, especially the cerebral cortex, is extremely sensitive to hypoxia and occlusion of its blood supply produces unconsciousness within a short period of 10 sec. Brain is one of the actively metabolizing tissues and it depends on glucose for its energy requirements. 90% of energy comes from glucose and insulin is not necessary for most of the brain cells to utilize glucose.

Storage of glucose in the brain tissue is almost negligible and hence, when the circulation to the brain is interrupted, it may lead to brain death and coma due to lack of O_2 and glucose. *Hypoglycemia can cause irreversible damage to the brain especially cerebral cortex.* This is very important in diabetics who are frequently exposed to sub-lethal hypoglycemia.

O_2 **consumption** by the whole brain is 50 mL/min which is about 20% of the total resting O_2 consumption. The O_2 consumption of gray matter is much more than the white matter. The gray matter has a high density of capillary network since the O_2 demand is high. The brain can withstand hypoglycemia for longer periods than hypoxia. The vegetative parts of brainstem are more resistant to hypoxia than the cerebral cortex. So, in cases of prolonged hypoxia to the brain as in cardiac arrest, there will be permanent intellectual deficiencies with normal vegetative functions.

Normal cerebral blood flow is **750 mL/min**, i.e., approximately 15% of resting cardiac output. The weight of the brain is 1500 g and therefore the cerebral blood flow is **50 mL/100 g of brain tissue/min**. A reduction in cerebral blood flow below 30 mL/100 g/min for about 5 sec results in fainting.

Functional Anatomy

Blood flow to the brain is through a pair of **internal carotid arteries** and a pair of **vertebral arteries**. The two vertebral arteries enter the brain through the posterior aspect and the two internal carotid arteries enter through the anterior aspect of brain. At the base of the brain the two vertebral arteries join to form the **basilar artery**. The basilar artery divides into two posterior cerebral arteries. The internal carotid artery divides into anterior and middle cerebral arteries near the optic chiasma. The anterior, middle and posterior cerebral arteries of both sides are united by communicating vessels to form a vascular ring at the base of the brain around the optic chiasma called **circle of Willis** (described by Thomas Willis in 1664). The circle of Willis gives rise to 6 large arteries that supply the brain **(Fig. 32.8)**. It is seen that substances injected into one carotid artery are distributed almost exclusively on the cerebral hemisphere of that side showing that the anastomosis in the circle of Willis does not allow significant crossing of blood to the opposite side. This is because the blood pressure is approximately equal in the two carotid arteries so that there is no pressure gradient between them. Precapillary anastomoses between cerebral arterioles are present in human beings. But they are not sufficient to render

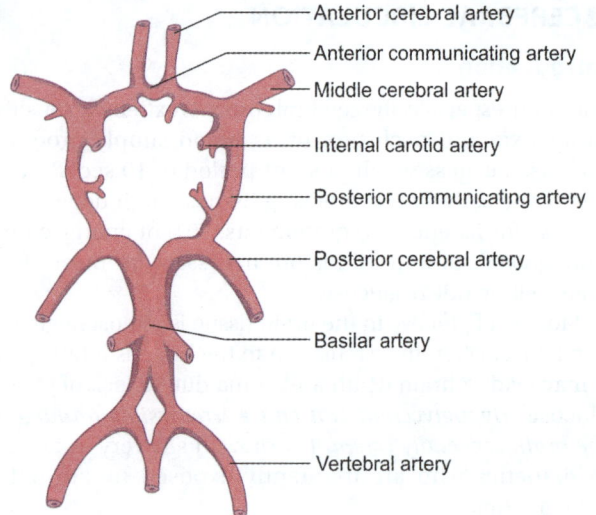

Fig. 32.8: The circle of Willis (arterial supply of the brain).

blood supply to prevent infarction. So, occlusion of internal carotid artery of one side produces symptoms of ischemia and even infarction if the occlusion is prolonged.

Venous blood is drained from the brain by the **deep veins and dural sinuses** that empty into the **internal jugular veins**. A small amount is drained into the **ophthalmic and pterygoid venous plexuses**.

Carotid Angiogram

A radiopaque dye is introduced into one of the carotid arteries followed by serial X-ray pictures of the brain **(Fig. 32.9)**. The distribution of the dye to the different areas of brain is studied. If the dye is not detected in any area, it suggests occlusion of a particular vessel. Thus the site of obstruction can be detected.

Innervation of Cerebral Vessels

Brain blood vessels have both **sympathetic and parasympathetic supply**. The sympathetic supply to the meningeal vessels is through the **cervical sympathetic ganglia**. Sympathetic fibers to the brain tissue proper have their adrenergic neurons in the brainstem. Parasympathetic cholinergic fibers from the facial nerve reach the brain through the **greater superficial petrosal nerve**. Stimulation of sympathetic fibers causes vasoconstriction and parasympathetic fibers produce vasodilatation in the brain.

Sensory nerve endings are found in the distal arteries of brain and they have their cell bodies in the **trigeminal ganglia**. The neurotransmitters are substance-P, CGRP, VIP, etc. These nerves are responsible for the production of pain on touching or pulling the cerebral vessels and in times of severe vasodilatation of cerebral vessels.

Measurement of Cerebral Blood Flow

1. Direct method
2. Indirect method

Cerebral blood flow can be measured directly in experimental animals using **electromagnetic flow meters**.

In human beings, indirect method known as **Kety's method** is employed where N_2O is used.

Indirect Method

Kety's Method

Principle: Kety's Method is based on Fick principle. Nitrous oxide (N_2O) is selectively taken up by the brain tissue. The N_2O concentration of brain will be equilibrated with the N_2O concentration of blood in 9–11 min. So, after this period, the N_2O concentration of cerebral venous blood will be same as N_2O concentration of brain tissue. Thus, N_2O concentration of 100 g of venous blood from brain will be equal to N_2O content of 100 g of brain tissue.

Blood flow to 100 g of brain tissue/min =

$$\frac{N_2O \text{ in 100 g of venous blood from brain}}{\text{Mean arteriovenous concentration difference of } N_2O}$$

Procedure: 15% N_2O is inhaled. Arterial and venous samples are collected separately at 1 min intervals for 10 min. Arterial sample is collected from any peripheral artery. Venous sample is taken from the jugular bulb. After 10 min, the last sample is taken and the various samples are analyzed for the N_2O content separately. Arteriovenous concentration difference is calculated. The mean arteriovenous concentration difference is calculated from a graph plotted with volume% of N_2O on the Y axis and time in minutes of inhalation on the X axis. The last sample from the jugular bulb gives the venous concentration in 100 g. From this the blood flow through 100 g of tissue can be calculated. The total blood flow to the brain can be calculated by multiplying it with the weight of the brain. But this method does not give an idea about regional blood flow and a normal value is obtained even in infarction due to block to a vessel.

For example, if the flow is 54 mL/100 g/min and average weight of brain is 1400 g then,

$$\text{Blood flow to the brain} = \frac{54 \times 1400}{100} = 756 \text{ mL/min}$$

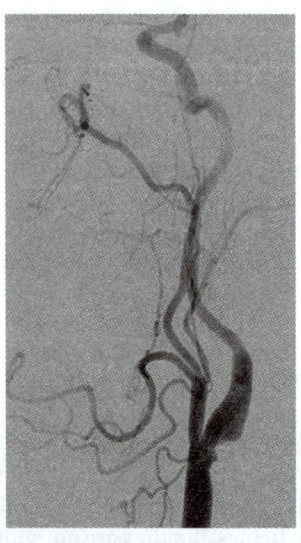

Fig. 32.9: Carotid angiogram.

Measurement of Regional Blood Flow to Brain

A radioactive gas like ^{133}**Xe** is dissolved in saline and injected into one of the internal carotid artery. The appearance of the gas and its clearance in various regions are monitored by a battery of 254 scintillation detectors placed over the scalp. Each detector will scan about 1 cm^2 of the brain surface. The output from the detectors is processed in a computer and displayed on a color television screen. The intensity of the color corresponds to the amount of radioactivity picked up by that particular counter, which in turn depends on the blood flow to the area. This is a simple and accurate procedure. Also, the regional blood flow to the cortex during various mental and physical activities can be studied. But the blood flow to the cerebral cortex alone can be measured and radioactivity from the deeper parts cannot be found out by this method.

Average Values of Blood Flow to Brain

- Hemisphere flow at rest = 48 mL/100 g/min
- Gray matter = 69 mL/100 g/min
- White matter = 28 mL/100 g/min

In experimental animals it is seen that blood flow is highest in the **inferior colliculus** where the flow is 1.8 mL/g/min when compared to the blood flow to the spinal cord white matter which is only 0.14 mL/g/min. *Blood flow to the gray matter is 6 times more than that of white matter.*

Cerebral Vascular Resistance

Cerebral vascular resistance is the sum of all factors opposing the blood flow to the brain. It is found that the cerebral vascular resistance for the whole brain is 7.2 R units.

Factors Affecting Cerebral Blood Flow

- Arterial pressure at the brain level
- Venous pressure at the brain level
- Intracranial pressure
- Viscosity of blood
- State of cerebral arterioles, whether constricted or dilated
- **Arterial pressure** at the brain level is closely related to the mean arterial pressure. Flow increases with increase in arterial pressure.
- **Changes in the venous pressure** have profound influence on cerebral blood flow. When the venous pressure is increased at the brain level, the cerebral blood flow is found to be reduced. This reduction in flow is due to two mechanisms:
  - High venous pressure decreases the pressure gradient (arterial pressure minus venous pressure) necessary for flow. This decreases the effective perfusion pressure and hence the flow.
  - When the venous pressure is increased, there will be venous pooling in the brain causing an increase in the intracranial pressure. The increase in intracranial pressure compresses the cerebral vessels and decreases the cerebral blood flow.

Advantage of the effect of venous pressure in the effective perfusion pressure:
In times of head-ward acceleration with the person in the sitting or standing posture, as the person moves away from the earth, pooling of blood occurs in the lower extremities. The arterial pressure at the brain level decreases and so there will be a corresponding decrease in the venous pressure. So, the **effective perfusion pressure** is not much affected and the brain will be perfused normally.

In movements towards the earth in sitting posture, there will be pooling of blood in the upper parts of the body. So, arterial pressure at the brain level increases with a corresponding increase in the venous pressure. Here also the pressure gradient is not much affected. Otherwise, rupture of the cerebral capillaries may occur due to very high pressure in the cerebral vessels.

- **Intracranial pressure**: Intracranial pressure is the pressure in the cranial cavity especially in the subarachnoid space and the ventricles of brain. The brain, spinal cord, cerebrospinal fluid and the cerebral vessels are encased in a bony case. Weight of the brain tissue comes to about 1400 g; volume of blood is about 75 mL and that of CSF is 75 mL. Brain tissue and CSF are incompressible. So, at any time the volume of brain, blood and spinal fluid in the cranium should be a constant since the brain case is rigid. This is known as **Monro-Kellie doctrine**.

Whenever there is increase in the intracranial pressure, the cerebral vessels get compressed. The body tries to maintain the intracranial pressure by changing the blood flow to brain. This is achieved by compressing the vessels when there is a rise in the intracranial pressure, thereby decreasing the flow. When the intracranial pressure exceeds 33 mm Hg, over a short period of time, cerebral blood flow is decreased due to decrease in the cerebral perfusion pressure. The resulting ischemia stimulates the vasomotor center which causes constriction of the systemic vessels due to increased sympathetic discharge. The systemic blood pressure is increased and the cerebral perfusion pressure will be increased correspondingly and this prevents ischemia to a certain extent. At the same time, there is stimulation of cardioinhibitory center producing reflex bradycardia. This reflex is called **Cushing reflex** and this reflex helps to maintain cerebral blood flow constant despite the increase in intracranial pressure. But this mechanism has a limit and if the intracranial tension rises very high, the systemic blood pressure cannot rise correspondingly and the cerebral blood flow falls to very low levels which produce serious symptoms.

- **Viscosity**: As the viscosity of blood increases, the cerebral vascular resistance increases. Thus, the blood flow to brain decreases in conditions like polycythemia where there is marked increase in viscosity. In anemia there is decrease in viscosity and the flow is increased.
- **State of cerebral arterioles**: The caliber of the vessels is controlled by the structural peculiarities of the cerebral vessels, nerve supply to the vessels, local metabolism and autoregulation of blood flow.

- The cerebral blood vessels contain more elastic tissue and less smooth muscle.
- The vessels are innervated by noradrenergic vasoconstrictor fibers mainly. When the systemic blood pressure is elevated markedly, there will be increased sympathetic noradrenergic discharge leading to constriction of cerebral vessels. This can prevent the increase in blood flow due to rise in the systemic BP.
- Changes in blood chemistry affect cerebral blood flow. Arterial hypercapnia produces cerebral vasodilatation and increases the flow. Hypocapnia causes vasoconstriction of cerebral vessels and this is the cause for the cerebral symptoms seen in voluntary hyperventilation when CO_2 is washed off. Increase in H^+ concentration causes vasodilatation of cerebral vessels due to a direct effect. Hypoxia also produces vasodilatation. Ammonia is very toxic to neurons. Neurological symptoms in hepatic coma are due to effect of ammonia on neurons of brain.
- The range of autoregulation of cerebral blood flow is 60–140 mm Hg mean arterial pressure. Within this range of mean arterial blood pressure, cerebral blood flow is maintained constant. Increase in the pressure results in active vasoconstriction of cerebral arterioles and a decrease in the pressure produces vasodilatation. This is the **myogenic hypothesis of cerebral autoregulation**. Pressures below 60 mm Hg causes syncope (fainting) while pressures above 140 mm Hg cause disruption of the blood-brain barrier and cerebral edema.

Special Features of Cerebral Circulation

❖ The brain accounts only 2% of the body weight but its blood flow represents 15% of the resting cardiac output.
❖ Functionally circle of Willis formed by the branches of right and left internal carotid arteries and the two vertebral arteries is not adequate for collateral circulation in the brain. So, unilateral arterial blockade leads to ischemia on the affected side.
❖ CNS is highly sensitive to changes in extracellular environment. The blood-brain barrier prevents many substances especially toxic substances from entering the brain interstitial tissue from the cerebral blood vessels.
❖ Cerebral blood flow shows autoregulation between 60 to 140 mm Hg perfusion pressures. Increase in the mean arterial blood pressure results in vasoconstriction of the cerebral arterioles so that there is no increase in cerebral blood flow, i.e., the cerebral blood flow is kept constant. A decrease in the pressure produces vasodilatation.
❖ When the mean arterial pressure falls below 60 mm Hg, the blood flow to the brain is decreased leading to cerebral ischemia. There will be a direct stimulation of vasomotor center and cardioinhibitory center leading to increase in blood pressure and bradycardia. This is called CNS ischemic response.
❖ All metabolic reactions in the brain are aerobic and it constantly maintains an extremely high metabolic rate. Brain uses 20% of the total O_2 consumed. Whenever there is a reduction in blood flow to the brain since brain cannot withstand O_2 lack, symptoms of hypoxia like dizziness, fainting, etc. develop. Anoxia lasting for even 5 sec leads to unconsciousness. Interruption of blood flow for 3–4 min leads to irreversible damage to the brain tissue.
❖ Brain is also vulnerable to hypoglycemia as glucose is the chief source of energy for the brain. Reduction in cerebral blood flow leads to glucose deficiency in the brain.
❖ Even though cerebral circulation is affected by gravity, the effective perfusion pressure is not much affected and the brain will get adequate perfusion. This is because, whenever there is increase or decrease in the arterial pressure at the brain level due to gravitational forces, there will be a corresponding increase or decrease in the venous pressure in the brain. So the effective perfusion pressure will not be altered. Otherwise the cerebral capillaries will rupture due to high pressure in the cerebral vessels.
❖ According to Monro-Kellie doctrine, whenever there is increase in the intracranial pressure, the cerebral vessels get compressed and cerebral blood flow decreases. This is because the brain case is rigid and the brain tissue and CSF are incompressible. But this reduction within a limit is overcome by the operation of Cushing reflex where there will be an increase in systemic blood pressure and bradycardia.
❖ There is regional variation in blood flow to the brain. The blood flow to the grey matter is approximately 70 mL/100g/min, whereas in the white matter it is only 28 mL/100g/min. The activity in the neuronal circuits of brain determines the regional pattern of cerebral blood flow. There is a rapid increase in blood flow in those areas of the brain involved in a particular physical or mental activity. For example, reading increases blood flow in the occipital and temporal areas of the brain. Changes in blood flow to different areas of brain also occur in disorders of brain. During epileptic attacks, blood flow in the epileptic foci is found to be increased. In Alzheimer's disease, there is early reduction in the metabolism and blood flow in the superior parietal region and frontal cortex.

Regulation of Cerebral Blood Flow

❖ Autoregulation mediated by local pH changes principally control cerebral blood flow.
❖ Neural regulation: Parasympathetic stimulation causes release of acetyl choline, NO and vasoactive intestinal polypeptide which produce vasodilatation of cerebral vessels. Sympathetic adrenergic nerves supplying cerebral vessels release norepinephrine and neuropeptide Y (NPY) which causes localized vasoconstriction and decrease cerebral blood flow.
❖ Sleep induces cerebral vasodilatation and there is slight increase in cerebral blood flow
❖ Cerebral vasodilators include NO, VIP, ACh, K^+, increased $PaCO_2$, decreased PaO_2, and increased H^+.
❖ Cerebral vasoconstrictors include increased HCO_3^-, norepinephrine, NPY, decreased $PaCO_2$, and increased PaO_2 (arterial partial pressure of oxygen).

❖ Astrocytes are neuroglial cells that surround blood vessels of central nervous system. Increased neuronal activity especially stimulation of excitatory glutaminergic neurons leads to increase in the calcium ion concentration in the foot processes of astrocytes. This leads to release of vasoactive metabolites from astrocytes like nitric oxide, metabolites of arachidonic acid, potassium ions and adenosine which produce vasodilatation of nearby arterioles.

Stroke

Sudden increase in blood pressure can result in rupture of cerebral blood vessels. Hemorrhage occurs which compress the local brain tissue. Atherosclerotic plaques or embolus can block the cerebral vessels and lead to ischemia. The cells in the ischemic area die. Both hemorrhage and block leads to the condition called **stroke** characterized by sudden attack of paralysis. The affected brain area determines the neurological effects of stroke. One of the most common causes of stroke is blockage of the middle cerebral artery that supplies the mid-portion of one cerebral hemisphere. If the left artery is blocked, it leads to spastic paralysis of most of the muscles of the right side of the body. Speech may also be affected because the Wernicke's area and the Broca's area are located in the left hemisphere in majority of individuals. If the block is in an artery that supplies the midbrain, it can block nerve conduction in the major pathways between the brain and spinal cord, causing both sensory and motor abnormalities.

SPLANCHNIC CIRCULATION

Splanchnic circulation consists of blood supply to the **gastrointestinal tract, liver, pancreas and spleen**. The splanchnic organs receive 25% of cardiac output, i.e., about 1500 mL/min. The splanchnic organs are supplied by the **celiac artery, inferior and superior mesenteric arteries** all being branches of aorta. The celiac artery supplies blood to stomach, spleen and pancreas and the inferior and superior mesenteric arteries supply the small intestine and large intestine.

Arterial blood delivers O_2 and nutrients to the splanchnic organs and the splanchnic venous blood carries away metabolic by-products like CO_2. The venous blood also carries nutrients that have been absorbed from the intestinal lumen through the portal vein to the liver.

Splanchnic circulation also functions as a major blood reservoir. The spleen and the large splanchnic veins can accommodate large volumes of blood and can divert this blood when there is a reduction in central venous pressure and cardiac output. In times of need like severe exercise, hemorrhage, etc., splanchnic blood flow may be less than one-fourth of its normal value.

In splanchnic circulation, **autoregulation** occurs in the intestine and liver, but not in the stomach.
❖ **Vasoconstrictors** of splanchnic vessels: Epinephrine, norepinephrine and angiotensin.
❖ **Vasodilators** of splanchnic vessels: ACh, histamine, serotonin, ATP, ADP, AMP, CO_2.

INTESTINAL MICROCIRCULATION

Intestinal blood flow in the resting state is **30 mL/min/100 g tissue**. Vasoconstriction of intestinal vessels can decrease the flow to 8 mL/min/100 g and vasodilatation can increase the flow to 200–250 mL/100 g/min.

Small arteries penetrate through the muscular layer of intestinal wall and branch extensively in the sub-mucosal layer and form a capillary bed. Some sub-mucosal arteries carry blood to the mucosa and to each intestinal villus where they form dense capillary networks. Veins from the villus join the veins from the mucosa and the muscular layer and join with the veins from the stomach, pancreas and spleen to form the **hepatic portal vein**.

Counter Current Exchange Mechanism in the Intestinal Villus

In the intestinal villus, the incoming arteriole passes up the center of the villus. At the tip of the villus the arteriole breaks up into numerous capillaries that carry blood back to the base of the villus where they empty into the venules. Thus the vessels carrying blood into and out of the villus lie close together in parallel paths. This **counter current blood flow** allows permeable substances like water to diffuse from the arterioles and capillaries to the venules and Na to diffuse from the venules into the arteriole before the arterial blood reaches the tip of the villus. Thus, the blood reaching the tip of the villus will have a high osmolarity, i.e., 2–3 times the normal plasma osmolarity. This facilitates absorption of more water from the intestinal fluid into the capillaries at the tip of the villus.

Much of the oxygen in the blood of the arterioles in the villi diffuses out directly into the adjacent venules and very little oxygen reaches the tip of the villi. As much as 80% of oxygen may take this short circuit route. Under normal conditions, this is not harmful to the villi. But in disease conditions like circulatory shock, the oxygen deficiency at the tips of the villi becomes so great that the villi suffer from ischemia and may disintegrate. The villi become blunted leading to diminished absorptive capacity.

Factors Affecting Intestinal Blood Flow

❖ Metabolic factors
❖ Hormonal factors
❖ Neural factors

Metabolic Factors

In times of increased metabolism, there will be hypoxia and accumulation of CO_2, H^+ and adenosine. All these factors cause vasodilatation and increases intestinal blood flow. When metabolism is decreased, the reverse operates. The vasodilatation is due to local release of histamine, prostaglandin and gastrointestinal hormones. Intestinal blood flow exhibits autoregulation. It is the intrinsic property of intestinal tissue and does not depend on neural or humoral factors. Whenever there is decrease in intestinal flow as in conditions of low arterial pressure or when the metabolic rate of intestinal tissue is high, there will be intestinal hypoxia and accumulation of vasodilator metabolites in the intestinal wall. This leads to arteriolar dilatation and increase in blood flow to meet the demands.

Hormonal Factors

Cholecystokinin and neurotensin selectively cause vasodilatation in the digestive organs. Secretin causes vasodilatation, but does not have the selective property. Gastrin, glucagon, substance-P, GIP, somatostatin, etc., produce vasodilatation. Neurohumoral agents that produce vasodilatation include VIP, substance-P, endorphins, etc. Circulating catecholamines, angiotensin-II, vasopressin, etc., cause vasoconstriction and decrease in the intestinal blood flow.

Neural Regulation

Sympathetic stimulation produces vasoconstriction and decrease in the flow. Postganglionic sympathetic neurons are present in the celiac, superior and inferior mesenteric ganglia. Sympathetic neurons innervate all the intestinal blood vessels except capillaries. The neurotransmitter is norepinephrine. Norepinephrine causes vasoconstriction by acting on the α-adrenergic receptors on the vascular smooth muscle. β-Adrenergic stimulation causes vasodilatation by relaxing the vascular smooth muscle. This effect is minimal in the intestine since the number of β-receptors is less in the intestinal vascular smooth muscle.

Preganglionic **parasympathetic** fibers to the intestine come through **vagus and pelvic nerves**. The post ganglionic neurons are present in the intestinal wall. The effect of parasympathetic stimulation on blood flow is indirect. Parasympathetic stimulation causes increase in intestinal motility, secretion and metabolism. The increased metabolism results in increased intestinal blood flow due to the vasodilator action of the metabolites.

HEPATIC PORTAL CIRCULATION

Liver is supplied by two groups of vessels:
1. **Hepatic artery**, a branch of aorta which carries arterial blood to liver.
2. **Hepatic portal vein** brings venous blood from spleen, pancreas, gall bladder, stomach and intestine *except rectum and anal canal*.

A **portal vein** is one that carries blood from one capillary network to another capillary network. *Other portal systems in the body include the hypothalamo-hypophyseal portal system in the brain and glomerular-peritubular capillary arrangement in the kidney.* Hepatic portal vein delivers blood into the sinusoids of liver. All the substances absorbed from the gut reach the liver and liver stores some of them and modifies others before they enter the general circulation. For example, liver converts glucose to glycogen which is stored in the liver. This prevents hyperglycemia after a meal. Liver also detoxifies harmful substances and destroys bacteria by phagocytosis. This is achieved by cells called **Kupffer cells** which belong to the reticuloendothelial system.

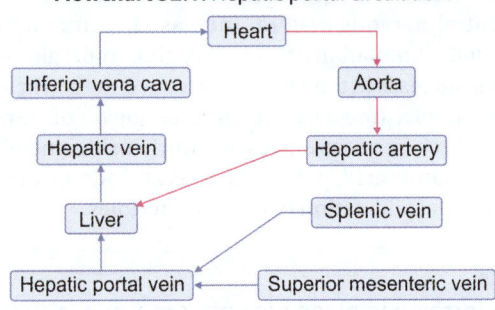

Flowchart 32.1: Hepatic portal circulation.

Liver also receives oxygenated blood via the hepatic artery which is a branch of aorta. The oxygenated blood mixes with the deoxygenated blood in the sinusoids. Blood leaves the sinusoids through the hepatic veins which drain into the inferior vena cava **(Flowchart 32.1)**.

Hepatic blood flow is about 1500 mL/min of which 1200 mL/min is via the portal vein and 300 mL/min via hepatic artery. Thus 1/3 of cardiac output flows through the liver.

Portal Hypertension

The pressure in the portal vein is 10 mm Hg, which is slightly above the vena caval pressure. Normally, both will be almost the same because the liver offers very little resistance to blood flow. According to **Ohm's law** for portal blood flow through the liver:
- Portal venous pressure – Vena caval pressure = (Portal blood flow) × (Hepatic vascular resistance)
- From the above equation, portal venous pressure will be increased when there is increase in vena caval pressure or increase in the resistance to blood flow through the liver. When portal venous pressure rises above normal the condition is called **portal hypertension**. Increased hepatic vascular resistance is the most common cause of portal hypertension. The most common cause of high hepatic resistance is **cirrhosis of liver** in which the liver tissue becomes fibrosed. The causes for cirrhosis liver are chronic alcoholism, chronic hepatitis, etc.

Complications of Portal Hypertension

When the portal pressure rises above 25 mm Hg, the splanchnic veins distend and rupture. The veins in the lower esophagus and stomach are most susceptible and bleeding occurs into the esophagus and stomach. The swollen esophageal veins are called **esophageal varices** which can be visualized by endoscopy **(Fig. 32.10)** and by barium swallow.

Another complication is **ascites** which is excessive accumulation of free fluid in the peritoneal cavity. This is because portal hypertension leads to pooling of blood in the splanchnic capillaries. This leads to increase in the hydrostatic pressure in the capillaries and fluid is filtered out into the interstitial spaces leading to edema. The high interstitial pressure squeezes fluid out of the tissues into the peritoneum leading to ascites.

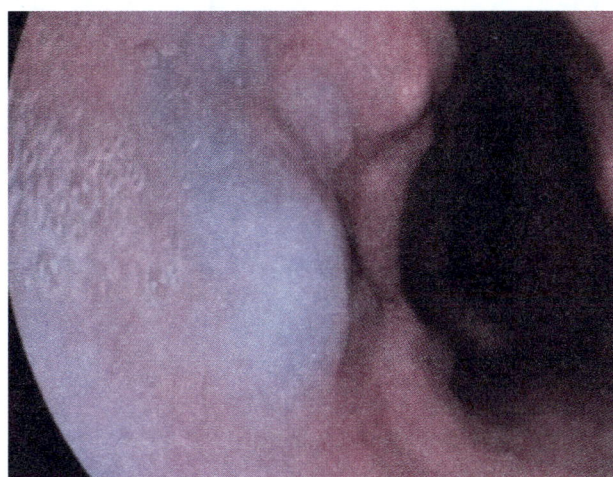

Fig. 32.10: Esophageal varices as seen in endoscopy.
Courtesy: Dr Anil Sundaram.

FETAL CIRCULATION

Circulatory system of fetus during the intrauterine life is different from that after birth. This is because, in the fetal life, circulation to lungs, kidney and gastrointestinal system does not function fully until birth. The fetus obtains O_2 and nutrients from the maternal blood and eliminates CO_2 and other waste products into the maternal blood.

The exchange of materials between fetal and maternal circulation occurs through the placenta. The placenta is attached to the fetus by the umbilical cord. Normally there is no direct mixing of maternal and fetal blood. Exchange of materials between fetal and maternal circulation occurs by diffusion through the capillary walls.

Blood passes from the fetus to the placenta through **two umbilical arteries,** which are branches of internal iliac arteries (branches of abdominal aorta). The umbilical arteries on reaching the placenta branch into an extensive capillary network. These capillaries absorb O_2 and nutrients from the maternal blood and eliminate CO_2 and other waste materials into the maternal blood. The oxygenated blood from the placenta returns to the fetus through a **single umbilical vein**. The blood in the umbilical vein is 80% saturated with O_2. The umbilical vein on reaching the liver of the fetus, divides into two branches. One small branch joins the hepatic portal vein to enter the liver sinusoids. The other branch through which most of the blood flows is called **ductus venosus** and it drains directly into the inferior vena cava **(Flowchart 32.2)**.

The deoxygenated blood returning from the lower regions of the body gets mixed with the oxygenated blood coming through the ductus venosus in the inferior vena cava (IVC). The O_2 saturation of the blood in the IVC is 67%. The IVC opens into the right atrium. Deoxygenated blood that is drained from the upper parts of the fetus enters the right atrium through the superior vena cava.

In the fetal life, the right and the left atria are connected by an opening called **foramen ovale** present in the inter-atrial septum. This opening is guarded by a valve on the left atrial side, which allows blood to flow from right to left atrium, but not in the reverse direction. So, one-third of blood reaching the right atrium bypasses the right ventricle and enters the left atrium through foramen ovale. The rest two-third of blood reaches the right ventricle and is pumped into the pulmonary artery. Very little blood enters the non-functioning fetal lung because of the high resistance offered by the collapsed lung to the flow of blood. There is a connection between the pulmonary trunk and the aorta called **ductus arteriosus**. The pressure in the pulmonary trunk is higher than that of aorta and hence the blood from the pulmonary trunk enters the aorta. Thus the blood from right ventricle bypasses the fetal lung. The blood in the aorta that is pumped from the left ventricle is 60% saturated with O_2 and is carried to all fetal tissues through the systemic circulation. Even though the O_2 saturation is very less in the fetal blood, the fetus does not suffer hypoxic damage because the fetal RBC contains fetal hemoglobin (HbF). HbF has a very high affinity for O_2 and the oxygen dissociation curve is shifted to the left in the case of HbF. The abdominal aorta divides into right and left common iliac arteries. Common iliac artery divides to form internal and external iliac arteries. The umbilical artery is a branch of internal iliac artery. Thus there are two umbilical arteries, one from each side, which enters the umbilical cord to reach the placenta for the exchange of materials. Since the placenta serves the functions of lungs, kidneys and gut, these organs start functioning only after birth.

Changes in the Fetal Circulation after Birth

After birth, the lungs, kidneys and digestive functions begin and so certain changes occur in the fetal circulation. When the umbilical cord is cut, the blood flow through the umbilical artery ceases and it gets filled with connective tissue. The part of the **umbilical artery** in the baby becomes fibrous cords called **medial umbilical ligaments**. It takes 2–3 months for the complete closure of umbilical arteries.

The part of the abdominal wall to which umbilical cord was attached forms the **umbilicus** of the baby.

The **umbilical vein** collapses and remains as **ligamentum teres or round ligament** which attaches umbilicus to the liver.

The **ductus venosus** collapses and forms **ligamentum venosum** which is seen on the inferior surface of liver.

The **foramen ovale** closes to form **fossa ovalis** which is seen as a depression in the interatrial septum. It takes 1 year for the permanent closure of foramen ovale. Explanation is, when the child takes the first breath, the lungs expand and the pulmonary vascular resistance falls to less than 20% of the fetal pulmonary vascular resistance. As a result, the amount of blood entering the left atrium through the pulmonary veins increases and this in turn increase the left atrial pressure. This causes blood to enter from the left atrium to the right atrium. This helps to close the foramen ovale by pushing the valve that guards it against the interatrial septum.

After birth the systemic arterial resistance increases. 55% of the blood flows through the placenta before birth. When the umbilical cord is cut, this blood flows into the systemic vessels of the baby, which approximately doubles the

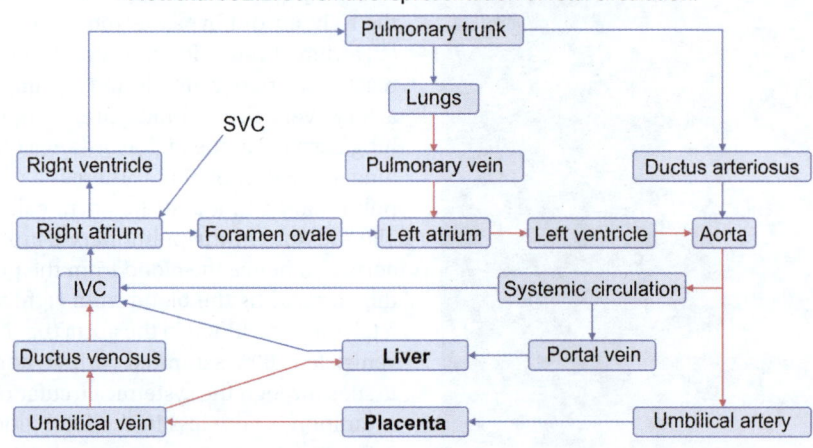

Flowchart 32.2: Schematic representation of fetal circulation.

systemic vascular resistance after birth. This increases the aortic pressure as well as the pressure in the left ventricle and left atrium.

The **ductus arteriosus** closes by vasoconstriction and becomes **ligamentum arteriosum**. This is because no blood passes through the ductus arteriosus since the aortic pressure becomes more than the pulmonary arterial pressure. Another reason is that there is a reduction in the prostaglandin availability in the ductus arteriosus after birth due to inhibition of cyclooxygenase enzyme necessary for the synthesis of prostaglandin in the ductus arteriosus.

If the ductus arteriosus fails to close, administration of indomethacin, a drug which blocks the synthesis of prostaglandin often leads to its closure.

MULTIPLE CHOICE QUESTIONS

1. **Renal blood flow is:**
   a. 250 mL/min
   b. 800 mL/min
   c. 1260 mL/min
   d. 1500 mL/min

2. **Blood supply of liver in mL/min is:**
   a. 800
   b. 1200
   c. 1500
   d. 1800

3. **O_2 consumption of whole human brain is about:**
   a. 29 mL/min
   b. 35 mL/min
   c. 49 mL/min
   d. 61 mL/min

4. **The organ with maximum O_2 consumption per minute is:**
   a. Liver
   b. Brain
   c. Skeletal muscle
   d. Heart

5. **Next to liver the organ that has the maximum O_2 consumption is:**
   a. Heart
   b. Brain
   c. Skeletal muscle
   d. Kidney

6. **O_2 consumption of the liver is:**
   a. 51 mL/min
   b. 20 mL/min
   c. 25 mL/min
   d. 30 mL/min

7. **Blood flow in mL/100 g/min is maximal in:**
   a. Kidney
   b. Liver
   c. Heart
   d. Skin

8. **Arteriolar dilatation is produced by all the following, *except*:**
   a. Decrease in adrenergic discharge
   b. Histamine
   c. Substance P
   d. Serotonin

9. **Coronary blood flow stops during:**
   a. Protodiastole
   b. End of diastole
   c. Isometric relaxation
   d. Isovolumetric contraction

10. **The average coronary blood flow in human being at rest is:**
    a. 4–5 % of cardiac output
    b. 5–10 % of cardiac output
    c. 10–15 % of cardiac output
    d. 15–20 % of cardiac output

11. **Capillaries with tight junctions allowing the passage of only small molecules are found in:**
    a. Brain
    b. Skin
    c. Kidney
    d. Muscle

12. **Blood brain barrier is maximally permeable to:**
    a. Sodium
    b. Potassium
    c. Chloride
    d. Carbon dioxide

13. **For cerebral blood flow to be doubled, PCO_2 should be:**
    a. 40 mm Hg
    b. 80 mm Hg
    c. 100 mm Hg
    d. 200 mm Hg

14. **In which of the following part is change of blood flow least during exercise:**
    a. Brain
    b. Heart
    c. Skeletal muscle
    d. GIT

15. **Vascular distensibility is least for the following vascular segment:**
    a. Pulmonary artery
    b. Systemic artery
    c. Systemic vein
    d. Pulmonary vein

16. Most permeable capillaries are present in:
    a. Posterior pituitary
    b. Liver
    c. Kidney
    d. Small intestine
17. Maximum surface area is present in:
    a. Capillary   b. Arteriole
    c. Artery   d. Vein
18. Maximum peripheral resistance is seen in:
    a. Capillary   b. Vein
    c. Aorta   d. Arterioles
19. Respiratory quotient of cerebral tissue is:
    a. 0.75-0.95   b. 0.95-0.99
    c. 1-1.1   d. 1.1-1.2
20. Maximum surface area in the circulatory system is seen in:
    a. Arteries   b. Veins
    c. Arterioles   d. Capillaries
21. The vasodilatation produced by carbon dioxide is maximum in one of the following:
    a. Kidney   b. Brain
    c. Liver   d. Heart
22. Up to what systolic pressure is the brain capable of autoregulation?
    a. 65 mm Hg   b. 55 mm Hg
    c. 45 mm Hg   d. 75 mm Hg
23. The first event in atherosclerosis is damage to:
    a. Endothelium
    b. Tunica media
    c. Tunica adventitia
    d. Smooth muscle fibers
24. Most important factor determining closure of ductus arteriosus is:
    a. Prostaglandins
    b. Oxygen tension
    c. Pulmonary pressure
    d. Systemic pressure
25. Fenestrations are seen in:
    a. Endothelium
    b. Internal elastic lamina
    c. External elastic lamina
    d. Tunica media
26. The percentage of total blood volume contained in the liver at normal resting conditions is:
    a. 15%   b. 2%
    c. 5%   d. 30%
27. Decreased perfusion of the coronary arteries is seen in:
    a. Aortic stenosis
    b. Aortic incompetence
    c. Pulmonary hypertension
    d. Mitral stenosis
28. The chief site of peripheral resistance is:
    a. Veins   b. Capillaries
    c. Arteries   d. Arterioles
29. Vasoconstriction in vivo is caused by all the following, *except*:
    a. Angiotensin II
    b. Endothelin I
    c. Norepinephrine
    d. Substance P
30. All the following produce vasodilatation in vivo, *except*:
    a. NO   b. VIP
    c. Bradykinin   d. Endothelin I
31. The prostaglandin that produces vasoconstriction is:
    a. PGF^2 b. PGE$^2\alpha$
    c. PGI$_2$ d. PGD$_2$
32. Maximum sympathetic innervation to veins is seen in:
    a. Splanchnic veins
    b. Hepatic vein
    c. Cutaneous veins
    d. Skeletal muscle veins
33. Aortic pressure is more than pulmonary artery pressure by:
    a. 5 times   b. 7 times
    c. 10 times   d. 2 times
34. The largest volume of blood in the circulatory system is contained in:
    a. Veins   b. Arteries
    c. Arterioles   d. Capillaries
35. Ductus arteriosus is a temporary connection between:
    a. Right atrium and left atrium
    b. Right ventricle and left ventricle
    c. Pulmonary trunk and superior vena cava
    d. Aorta and pulmonary trunk
36. Tetralogy of Fallot includes the following defects, *except*:
    a. Ventricular septal defect
    b. Pulmonary valve stenosis
    c. Right ventricular hypertrophy
    d. Coarctation of aorta
37. The condition that cause a 'blue baby' is:
    a. Tetralogy of Fallot
    b. Patent ductus arteriosus
    c. Atrial septal defect
    d. Ventricular septal defect
38. Risk factors in heart disease include all the following, *except*:
    a. High LDL cholesterol
    b. High HDL cholesterol
    c. Obesity
    d. High blood pressure
39. The percentage of the total blood volume that is present in the veins and venules at rest is:
    a. 15%   b. 60%
    c. 30%   d. 8%

40. The flare that occur in triple response is due to:
    a. Arteriolar dilation
    b. Capillary dilation
    c. Venous dilation
    d. Increased capillary permeability

41. Most important factor determining closure of ductus arteriosus is:
    a. Prostaglandin
    b. Oxygen tension
    c. Pulmonary blood pressure
    d. Systemic blood pressure

42. In an adult, the normal cerebral blood flow per minute is approximately:
    a. 250 mL
    b. 500 mL
    c. 750 mL
    d. 1200 mL

43. Which of the following is NOT correct regarding capillaries?
    a. Greatest cross sectional area
    b. Contains 25% of blood
    c. Contains less blood than veins
    d. Lined by a single layer of cells

44. Which of the following statements is true about capillaries?:
    a. Contains 5% of total blood volume
    b. Contains 25% of total blood volume
    c. Velocity of blood flow is maximum
    d. Offer maximum resistance to blood flow

45. All are true regarding capillaries, *except*:
    a. Have large total cross sectional area
    b. Contain larger quantity of blood than veins
    c. Site of gaseous exchange
    d. Lined by endothelium

46. Distribution of blood flow is mainly regulated by:
    a. Arteries
    b. Arterioles
    c. Capillaries
    d. Venules

47. Which of the following mediate pre-capillary sphincter relaxation?
    a. Sympathetic stimulation
    b. Catecholamines
    c. Local hormones
    d. Capillary filling

48. True about blood flow in various organs:
    a. Liver > kidney > brain > heart
    b. Liver > brain > kidney > heart
    c. Kidney > brain > heart > liver
    d. Liver > heart > brain > kidney

49. Local control of blood flow is seen in all, *except*:
    a. Skin
    b. Muscle
    c. Splanchnic vessels
    d. Cerebrum

50. Which one of the following is the correct statement regarding coronary blood flow?
    a. Coronary blood flow is directly related to perfusion pressure and inversely related to resistance
    b. Coronary blood flow is inversely related to perfusion pressure and directly related to resistance
    c. Coronary blood flow is inversely related to both pressure and resistance
    d. Coronary blood flow is directly related to perfusion pressure and also to resistance

51. True about pulmonary circulation:
    a. It receives 30% of cardiac output
    b. Hypoxia causes vasoconstriction
    c. Blood volume in the lung is 70 ml
    d. Pulmonary capillaries contain most of the blood volume in lung

52. True regarding vascularity of lung is:
    a. Hypoxia causes vasodilatation
    b. Pulmonary vascular resistance is half of systemic vascular resistance
    c. Perfusion is more at the apex of lung than at the base
    d. Distended pulmonary veins in the lower lobe

53. Pulmonary vascular resistance when compared to systemic vascular resistance is:
    a. 1/7th of systemic vascular resistance
    b. 1/2 of systemic vascular resistance
    c. 1/3rd of systemic vascular resistance
    d. 1/4th of systemic vascular resistance

54. The percentage of total blood volume present in the lungs:
    a. 9%
    b. 25%
    c. 20%
    d. 30%

55. Maximum blood supply to the liver is by:
    a. Portal vein
    b. Hepatic artery
    c. Splenic artery
    d. Mesenteric artery

56. The percentage of blood reaching the liver through the portal vein is:
    a. 50%
    b. 80%
    c. 10%
    d. 20%

57. Blood supply of liver through hepatic artery is:
    a. 50%
    b. 80%
    c. 10%
    d. 20%

58. Wedged hepatic venous pressure represents pressure in:
    a. Main portal vein
    b. Main hepatic vein
    c. Sinusoids
    d. Central vein radicles

59. Effectiveness of blood brain barrier is by:
    a. Tight endothelial junction
    b. Microglial cells
    c. Thick basement membrane
    d. Tight arrangement of astrocytes

60. Protein filtration across cerebral capillaries is limited by:
    a. Fibrous tissue
    b. Foot process of astrocytes
    c. Low blood pressure
    d. High CSF pressure

61. Blood supply in the splanchnic vessels decrease due to:
    a. Venodilation with normal blood flow
    b. Venodilation with increased blood flow
    c. Venoconstriction with decreased blood flow
    d. Venodilation with decreased blood flow

62. Normal hepatic blood flow per minute is:
    a. 50 mL/100 g of liver tissue
    b. 100 mL/100 g of liver tissue
    c. 200 mL/100 g of liver tissue
    d. 300 mL/100 g of liver tissue

63. In brain ischemia, systemic blood pressure rises due to:
    a. Monro-Kellie doctrine
    b. Cushing reflex
    c. Autoregulation
    d. White reaction

64. The following occurs when an aviator is subjected to negative G:
    a. The hydrostatic pressure in the veins of lower limbs increases
    b. The cardiac output decreases
    c. Black out occurs
    d. Cerebral arterial pressure rises

65. Major blood reservoirs in the body include all the following, *except*:
    a. Thoracic vena cava
    b. Liver sinuses
    c. Venous plexus of skin
    d. Venous sinuses of spleen

66. Blood flow through the left coronary artery:
    a. Regulated by sympathetic vasodilator nerves
    b. Increase when myocardial hypoxia is present
    c. Greater during early systole
    d. Decreased in reflex response to fall in blood pressure

67. For each 10 degree fall in temperature, cerebral blood flow falls by:
    a. 1%
    b. 2%
    c. 4%
    d. 7%

68. Occlusion of common carotid artery on both sides leads to:
    a. Increase in heart rate and BP
    b. Increase in BP and decrease in heart rate
    c. Decrease in heart rate and BP
    d. No effect on BP and heart rate

69. Myocardial O_2 demand is:
    a. Inversely proportional to heart rate
    b. Directly proportional to heart rate
    c. Increased by digitalis
    d. Not related to heart rate

70. O_2 consumption of the human brain is:
    a. 1 mL/100 g/min
    b. 1.5 mL/100 g/min
    c. 3.5 mL/100 g/min
    d. 5 mL/100 g/min

71. Regional arterial resistance of mesentery and renal vessels is reduced by:
    a. Dopamine
    b. Noradrenaline
    c. Dobutamine
    d. Isoprenaline

72. Blood flow through left coronary artery:
    a. Is regulated by sympathetic vasodilator nerves
    b. Greater during early systole
    c. Increases when myocardial hypoxia is present
    d. Decreased in reflex response to fall in blood pressure

73. The average coronary blood flow in a man at rest is how much % of cardiac output?
    a. 4 – 5%
    b. 5 – 10%
    c. 10 – 15%
    d. 15 – 20%

74. Average coronary blood flow at rest:
    a. 200 – 250 mL/min
    b. 500 – 700 mL/min
    c. 100 – 150 mL/min
    d. 750 – 800 mL/min

75. After birth, umbilical vein becomes:
    a. Medial umbilical ligament
    b. Ligamentum teres
    c. Ligamentum venosum
    d. Ligamentum arteriosum

76. Cerebral blood flow is usually measured using:
    a. Electromagnetic flow meter
    b. Dye dilution method
    c. Ultrasonography
    d. Kety's method

ANSWERS

1. c	2. c	3. c	4. a	5. c
6. a	7. a	8. d	9. d	10. a
11. a	12. d	13. b	14. a	15. b
16. d	17. a	18. d	19. b	20. d
21. b	22. a	23. a	24. b	25. a
26. a	27. a	28. d	29. d	30. d
31. a	32. a	33. b	34. a	35. d
36. d	37. a	38. b	39. b	40. a
41. b	42. c	43. b	44. a	45. b
46. b	47. c	48. a	49. a	50. a
51. b	52. d	53. a	54. a	55. a
56. b	57. d	58. c	59. a	60. b
61. c	62. a	63. b	64. d	65. a
66. b	67. c	68. a	69. b	70. c
71. a	72. c	73. a	74. d	75. b
76. d				

FILL IN THE BLANKS/GIVE THE NORMAL VALUE/NAME THE FOLLOWING (CARDIOVASCULAR SYSTEM)

1. SA node is located at the junction of superior vena cava with right atrium
2. AV node is located in the right postero-inferior region of interatrial septum near the opening of coronary sinus
3. The only conducting pathway between atria and ventricles: **AV node and bundle of His**
4. Innervation to the SA node: **Right vagus and right sympathetics**
5. Innervation of AV node –Left vagus and left sympathetics
6. Cardiac pace maker: **SA node**
7. Normal heart rate in humans: **60–100 beats/min**
8. Increase in heart rate is called tachycardia and decrease in heart rate is called bradycardia
9. Alteration of heart rate in different phases of respiration: **Sinus arrhythmia**
10. In athletes, bradycardia is because of increased vagal tone
11. Marey's law states that heart rate is inversely proportional to blood pressure
12. Normal AV nodal delay: **0.1 sec**
13. Plateau phase of cardiac action potential is due to opening of slow Ca^{2+} channels and K^+ channels
14. The last parts of the heart to be depolarized: **Postero-basal portion of left ventricle, pulmonary conus and uppermost portion of interventricular septum**
15. RMP of myocardial cells: **minus 90 mV**
16. Conduction velocity in the Purkinje fibers: **4 m/sec**
17. Depolarization of ventricle proceeds from endocardium to epicardium
18. AV valves open towards the end of isovolumetric relaxation phase of cardiac cycle.
19. AV valves close at the beginning of isometric contraction phase
20. Semilunar valves open towards the end of isovolumetric contraction phase
21. Semilunar valves close at the beginning of isovolumetric relaxation phase
22. Duration of cardiac cycle at rest when the heart rate is 72/min: **0.8 second**
23. In ECG, one small division in X-axis measures 0.04 sec and one small division in the Y-axis denotes 0.1 mV
24. A condition where PR interval is shortened: **WPW syndrome**
25. P waves are absent in atrial fibrillation
26. Inverted T wave suggests myocardial infarction
27. Tall peaked T wave is seen in hyperkalemia
28. A condition that produces low voltage ECG: **Hypothyroidism**
29. The cause for extra systolic potentiation is increased availability of Ca^{2+}
30. Normal end diastolic volume: **130 mL**
31. The amount of blood ejected by each ventricle in one minute - Cardiac output
32. Normal cardiac output at rest: **5 L/min**
33. The amount of blood pumped out of each ventricle per beat: **Stroke volume**
34. Normal stroke volume at rest: **70 ml/beat**
35. Cardiac index is cardiac output divided by body surface area
36. Normal cardiac index: **3.2 L/min/m²**
37. The average coronary blood flow in human being at rest: **4-5% of cardiac output**
38. Preload on myocardium depends on end diastolic volume and after load depends on peripheral resistance
39. Stimulation of baroreceptors leads to inhibition of vasomotor center and stimulation of cardioinhibitory center
40. Baroreceptors fire maximally at mean blood pressure of 150 mm Hg
41. Pressure on the carotid sinus cause reflex bradycardia
42. Hypoxia, hypercapnia and acidosis stimulate peripheral chemoreceptors
43. Normal systolic blood pressure: **100-140 mm Hg**
44. Normal diastolic blood pressure: **60-90 mm Hg**
45. Pulse pressure is the difference between systolic and diastolic blood pressure
46. Mean arterial pressure is diastolic pressure + 1/3rd pulse pressure
47. The organ with maximum O_2 consumption at rest: **Liver (51 mL/min)**
48. O_2 consumption of human brain: **3.3 mL/100 g/min**
49. Capillaries have maximal cross sectional area of 4500 cm² and aorta has minimum cross sectional area, i.e., 4.5 cm²
50. Minimum velocity in circulation is seen in capillaries
51. Velocity of blood is maximal in aorta
52. In anemia, turbulent flow occur due to decrease in viscosity
53. Flow is almost always turbulent if Re is > 3000
54. The opening of aorta and pulmonary artery are guarded by semilunar valves
55. Closure of A-V valves produces the first heart sound whereas closure of semilunar valves produces the second heart sound
56. Stethoscope was invented by Laennec
57. The record of heart sound is called phonocardiogram
58. Nitric oxide is synthesized from arginine by the enzyme NO synthase in endothelial cells
59. The only organ where hypoxia produces vasoconstriction: **Lung**
60. Maximum resistance to blood flow is exerted by arterioles
61. Veins and venules are referred to as capacitance vessels
62. Capillaries are called exchange vessels
63. Normal hepatic blood flow per minute: **50 mL/100 g of liver tissue/min**
64. Normal cerebral blood flow in an adult: **750 mL/min or 50-60 mL/100 g/min**
65. Cerebral O_2 consumption: **45 mL/min or 3.3 mL/100g/min**

66. Mean velocity of blood in the aorta: **40 cm/sec**
67. Cardiac muscle cannot be tetanized because of long absolute refractory period (200 ms)
68. The law which states that, greater the end diastolic volume (preload) within physiological limits, greater will be the force of contraction of heart: **Frank-Starling's law**
69. Collapsing pulse is seen in aortic regurgitation
70. JVP reflects right atrial pressure
71. Prominent "a" wave in JVP is seen in tricuspid stenosis
72. Prominent "c" wave in JVP is seen in AV valve incompetency
73. "a" wave in JVP is absent in atrial fibrillation
74. Giant 'a' waves are seen in complete heart block
75. The mean pressure in the pulmonary circulation: **15 mm Hg**
76. Mean pressure in the systemic circulation: **90 mm Hg**
77. Both ventilation and perfusion are more in the lower lobes of lung in the erect posture
78. The first reaction to occur in the body following hemorrhage: **Vasoconstriction**
79. Digoxin acts by inhibiting Na^+-K^+ ATPase in cardiac muscle
80. Vagal stimulation decreases heart rate by acting through M_2 receptors on SA node
81. The tissues which exhibit autoregulation: **Kidney, mesentery, skeletal muscle, brain, liver and myocardium**
82. Epinephrine produces vasoconstriction in all areas except in skeletal muscle and liver
83. Local metabolites that causes vasodilatation and increase in coronary blood flow: **Adenosine, K^+, H^+ and CO^2**

CLINICAL CASE SCENARIO

1. A man was brought to the casualty with severe bleeding following a road accident. On examination he had rapid thready pulse, respiratory rate 30/min, systolic blood pressure 84 mm Hg and pale cold skin. Answer the following:
   a. What can be the probable condition specifying the type?
   b. What are the compensatory mechanisms occurring in the body in this condition?
   c. What is the immediate management?
   Diagnosis – Hemorrhagic shock

2. A 40-year-old man presented with retrosternal pain during exertion and the pain was proportional to the amount of exertion. He was relieved of pain on taking rest. He also experienced pain in the medial aspect of left arm during exertion. On examination, BP was 140/90 mm Hg, heart rate – 70/min, no murmur, no cyanosis and no anemia. On investigation:

   ECG showed ST elevation. Cardiac index – 3.2 L/min, ejection fraction – 65%
   a. Define cardiac index, ejection fraction and blood pressure, giving the normal values.
   b. What are the reasons for the pain felt in the two areas in this patient?
   c. Explain the short-term and long-term regulation of blood pressure.

SECTION 4: RESPIRATORY SYSTEM

Structure and Functions of Respiratory System

CHAPTER 33

LEARNING OBJECTIVES
- Describe the non-respiratory functions of lungs.
- Describe the functional anatomy of tracheobronchial tree.
- Enumerate the functions of pleural fluid.

INTRODUCTION

Life begins and ends with breathing. Living organisms need a constant supply of energy because of the continuous expenditure of energy by the body. Energy is obtained by oxidation of food substances and this energy is stored in the form of high-energy phosphate compounds, such as adenosine triphosphate (ATP), creatine phosphate, etc. The products of oxidation are CO_2 and H_2O. The main function of respiratory system is to provide O_2 to the tissues and remove CO_2 produced in the tissues.

The body can store only about 1500 mL of O_2 at a time. This can maintain life only for 5 minutes. Myocardium and brain are very much dependent on O_2 for their functioning. Cessation of blood flow to cerebral cortex results in loss of function within 5 sec, loss of consciousness in 10–20 sec and irreversible changes in 3–5 minutes. Once the neurons are damaged they cannot regenerate.

Pulmonologist is a physician specialized to treat pulmonary diseases.

DEFINITION

Respiration is defined as the complex physiological process by which living organisms exchange O_2 and CO_2 between the organism and the environment. Or in other words, the collective process of absorption of O_2 from the environment and oxidation of food materials in the cells with the release of water, CO_2 and energy and elimination of CO_2 into the environment is called respiration.

Respiration occurs by simple diffusion in unicellular organisms **(Fig. 33.1)**, through skin and lungs in frogs, through gills in aquatic animals, through air tubes in insects and through lungs in higher animals.

Respiration in man includes three processes:
1. External respiration or pulmonary ventilation
2. Transport of gases in blood
3. Internal respiration

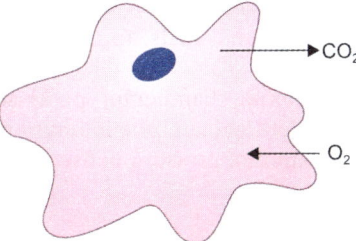

Fig. 33.1: Exchange of gases (respiration) in unicellular organisms.

The exchange of O_2 and CO_2 between the blood in the pulmonary capillaries and the alveolar air is termed **external respiration**.

The exchange of gases between the cells and extracellular fluid and the utilization of O_2 and production of CO_2 by the cells is known as **internal respiration** or **oxidative phosphorylation**.

FUNCTIONS OF THE RESPIRATORY TRACT

Nasal Cavity

- **Air conditioning function:** The nasal mucosa is moist, highly vascular and ciliated. These features are responsible for the air conditioning function of nose, i.e., warming, humidification and filtration of inhaled air. Due to large cross-sectional area, the nose has the capacity to modify temperature and water vapor content of inspired air.
    - Warming of inhaled cold air is important so that gas exchange occurs in the alveoli at body temperature. Otherwise, if cold air reaches the alveoli, the pulmonary capillary blood surrounding the alveoli will become cooler than the body temperature. This affects the solubility of gases.
    - Moisturizing the inhaled air is important to prevent the alveoli from becoming desiccated. Moisture is added to the inhaled air by the capillaries and the mucus lining the mucosa of the respiratory tract. When the air reaches

the alveoli the vapor pressure becomes 47 mm Hg. Oxygen and carbon dioxide cannot diffuse through dry membrane.
- Cooling the airway by inhaling cold air causes bronchoconstriction.
- The nasal cavity also removes some of the pollutants present in air. Fine particles in the air called **aerosols,** which are greater than 5 µm in size are filtered by the hair and cilia present in the nasal cavity. They are expelled out by **sneezing reflex**. In mouth breathing, warming, moisturizing and filtering function become less efficient.

❖ **Olfactory function:** Olfactory stimuli are received by the olfactory epithelium of the nasal cavity which contains olfactory receptors.

❖ Large hollow resonating chambers of the nose called paranasal sinuses modify **speech** sounds.

Pharynx

❖ Nasopharynx carries air from nose to pharynx. Oropharynx is the common passage for food and air.
❖ Pharynx houses the tonsils and thus plays a role in immunity.
❖ Provides a resonating chamber for speech sounds.
❖ Opening of the eustachian tube into nasopharynx helps in the equalization of pressure between middle ear and pharynx.

Larynx

❖ Larynx helps in the production of sound with the help of vocal cords.
❖ Closure of glottis by approximation of vocal cords during swallowing, vomiting, etc., helps to prevent entry of food into the trachea. This is also brought about by horizontal deflection of the epiglottis.

Respiratory Function of the Airways

Airways conduct atmospheric air to alveoli and help in gas exchange so as to maintain normal CO_2 and O_2 levels in the body. Lungs synthesize surfactant, collagen and elastin necessary for proper expansion of lungs. Collagen and elastin form the structural framework of the lung.

Before reaching the alveoli, inhaled air is warmed by blood in the capillaries of the respiratory tract. This is significant because cold air increases airflow resistance and also causes bronchospasm. This is of great importance in patients suffering from bronchial asthma. Inhaled air is also humidified, i.e., saturated with water vapor, by mucus secreted by the goblet cells lining the respiratory tract and the vapor pressure becomes 47 mm Hg at a body temperature of 37°C.

Non-respiratory Functions of Lungs

❖ **Protective function:**
- Numerous mucus-secreting goblet cells are interspersed in the lining mucosa of the respiratory tract, which secrete sticky mucus. Particles less than 5 µm in size enter the lung and adhere to the mucus. This will be expelled out by cough reflex triggered by airway irritation and also by the escalator action of cilia. This type of transport is called **mucociliary transport**. The cilia beat upwards towards the pharynx and this action is not influenced by nervous mechanism. The O_2 content in the air influences the activity of cilia. Ciliary activity moves the superficial mucous lining layer continuously towards the pharynx from deep within the lung. In a congenital disease called **Kartagener's syndrome**, the motility of the cilia is defective leading to collection of secretions in the lung, called **bronchiectasis**. It also leads to sinusitis. A similar condition is produced by cigarette smoke that contains ciliotoxins that damage the cilia.
- The neutrophils, lymphocytes and alveolar macrophages present in the alveoli defend against bacteria and viruses.
- Plasma cells present in the lungs synthesize secretory immunoglobulins, such as IgA for its own defense. IgA is present in the bronchial mucus.

❖ **Acid-base balance:** Lungs play an important role in maintaining the body pH by regulating the CO_2 content of blood.

❖ **Anticoagulant function and filtration of blood:** Lungs contain mast cells that contain **heparin,** which is an anticoagulant. Small emboli present in blood are removed from the pulmonary circulation before they reach the brain and other vital organs. If these emboli reach the systemic circulation, they may get lodged in small vessels and occlude them especially in organs, such as heart that has very poor collateral circulation.

❖ **Regulation of blood pressure:** The endothelial cells of the pulmonary capillaries secrete an enzyme called **angiotensin converting enzyme (ACE)** which converts angiotensin I to active angiotensin II which is a potent vasoconstrictor. This will increase blood pressure.

❖ **Temperature regulation:** Some amount of heat is lost from the body during expiration.

❖ **Regulation of blood volume:** Lungs act as a storage organ for blood since pulmonary circulation is a low- pressure system and the vessels are highly distensible. About 300 mL of blood from lungs can be diverted to the systemic circulation in times of need as in circulatory shock.

❖ **Endocrine function:** Lungs synthesize hormones, such as prostaglandins (PGs), serotonin, histamine, etc., with the help of **amine precursor uptake and decarboxylation (APUD) cells** present in the lung. PGE_2 helps to constrict the patent ductus arteriosus in the postnatal period. In asthma or anaphylaxis, lungs release substances, such as histamine, bradykinin, prostaglandin, slow reacting substance, etc., into circulation, which are responsible for the reactions of anaphylaxis.

❖ **Degradation of substances:** Bradykinin, norepinephrine, serotonin, PGE1, PGE2 and PGF2 are degraded and removed by the lungs.

- The rhythmic movement of the diaphragm and chest wall during breathing produces rhythmic alteration of pressure in the abdomen and chest cavity. This helps to suck blood from the lower part of the body and abdomen to the heart there by increasing venous return.

FUNCTIONAL ANATOMY OF THE RESPIRATORY SYSTEM

PY6.1: Describe the functional anatomy of respiratory tract.

Respiratory system is composed of:
- A gas-exchanging organ, the lungs
- A pump that ventilates the lungs which consists of chest wall and respiratory muscles
- Centers in the brain that control respiration
- Tracts and nerves that connect brain to the respiratory muscles

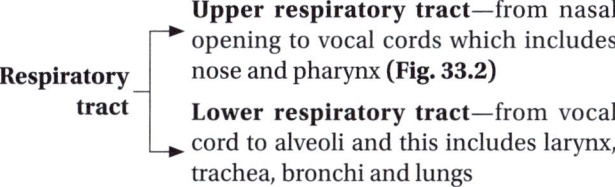

Lining Epithelium of the Respiratory Tract

- *Mucous membrane of nose*: Lined by ciliated columnar epithelium containing scattered goblet cells.
- *Pharynx*: Nasopharynx is lined by ciliated columnar epithelium with goblet cells. Oropharynx is lined by stratified squamous epithelium.
- *Larynx*: Upper part of larynx and vocal cords are lined by stratified squamous epithelium. Lower part is lined by ciliated columnar epithelium.
- *Trachea and bronchi*: Lined by **pseudostratified ciliated columnar epithelium**, which contain mucous and serous glands. Ciliary action helps to remove particulate matter. An optimum amount of mucus of correct thickness (5 µm) and optimum viscosity is essential for proper ciliary function. Plenty of mucus-secreting goblet cells are seen interspersed between the ciliated cells.
- *Bronchioles*: Lined by non-ciliated cuboidal epithelium that is devoid of glands. *Smooth muscles are absent from respiratory bronchiole onwards and only a single layer of lining cells is seen.* In the bronchioles, the goblet cells are replaced by another type of secretory cell, the **Clara cell,** which secrete proteins, such as surfactant apoproteins SP-A, SP-B, SP-C and SP-D, lipids, glycoproteins and modulators of inflammation.
- *Alveoli*: Lined by simple **squamous** epithelium.

Tracheobronchial Tree

The air that is inspired is distributed to the alveoli by way of trachea, bronchi and bronchioles (**Fig. 33.3**).

Trachea

Trachea is a hollow tubular structure 11 cm in length and 1.5 cm in diameter, placed anterior to the esophagus. It is kept permanently open by C-shaped cartilages on its wall, which are deficient posteriorly.

In between the cartilages, there are fibro-elastic tissue and smooth muscle fibers. Mucus secreted by mucous glands in

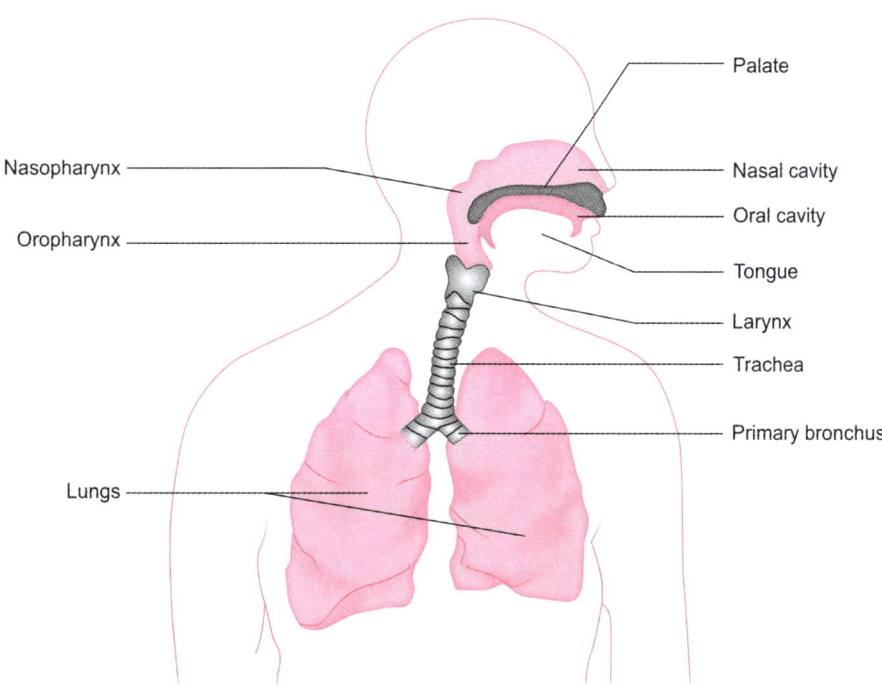

Fig. 33.2: Structure of respiratory system.

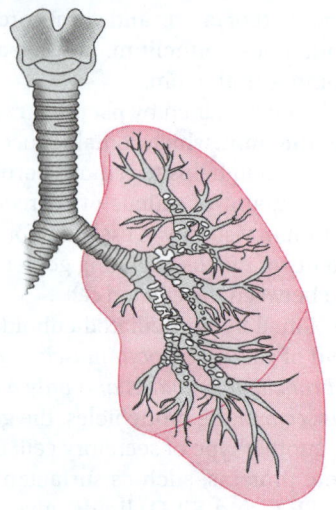

Fig. 33.3: Tracheobronchial tree.

the mucous membrane of trachea moistens the surface and facilitates ciliary action.

Trachea divides into two main bronchi or **primary bronchi**. Each main bronchus divides into **secondary or lobar bronchi**, 3 on the right and 2 on the left side. Each secondary bronchus divides to form **tertiary** or segmental bronchi, 10 on the right side and 8 on the left side. Bronchi also have cartilage plates in their walls to keep them patent. The cartilage is important for preventing airway collapse, which is especially a problem during expiration.

Cartilage-free airways are called bronchioles. Since they lack cartilage, bronchioles can maintain a patent lumen only by maintaining a more negative pressure outside than the pressure inside. Thus, bronchioles are especially susceptible to collapse during expiration.

Tertiary bronchi divide to form **bronchioles,** which in turn divide to form **terminal bronchiole** with a diameter of 1 mm or less. Terminal bronchiole divides to form **respiratory bronchiole** with a diameter of 0.5 mm. *Cilia are absent from respiratory bronchioles.* Each respiratory bronchiole divides to form 5–6 dilated sacs called **alveolar sacs**. Each alveolar sac is studded with pouches called **alveoli (Fig. 33.4)**.

These multiple divisions greatly increase the total cross-sectional area of the airways from 2.5 cm^2 in the trachea to 11,800 cm^2 in the alveoli.

Weibel's Model

Weibel numbered each generation of the tracheobronchial tree from generation zero to 22. From trachea to alveoli there are about **23 generations** of division. Trachea is considered as generation zero. Up to terminal bronchiole, there are 16 generations. This part is called **conducting zone or anatomical dead space** because up to this part, no exchange of gases occurs **(Fig. 33.4)**. It includes the air present in the respiratory passage from nose and lips down to the terminal bronchiole.

Next 7 generations, i.e., from respiratory bronchiole to alveoli is called **respiratory zone** or **gas exchanging zone**

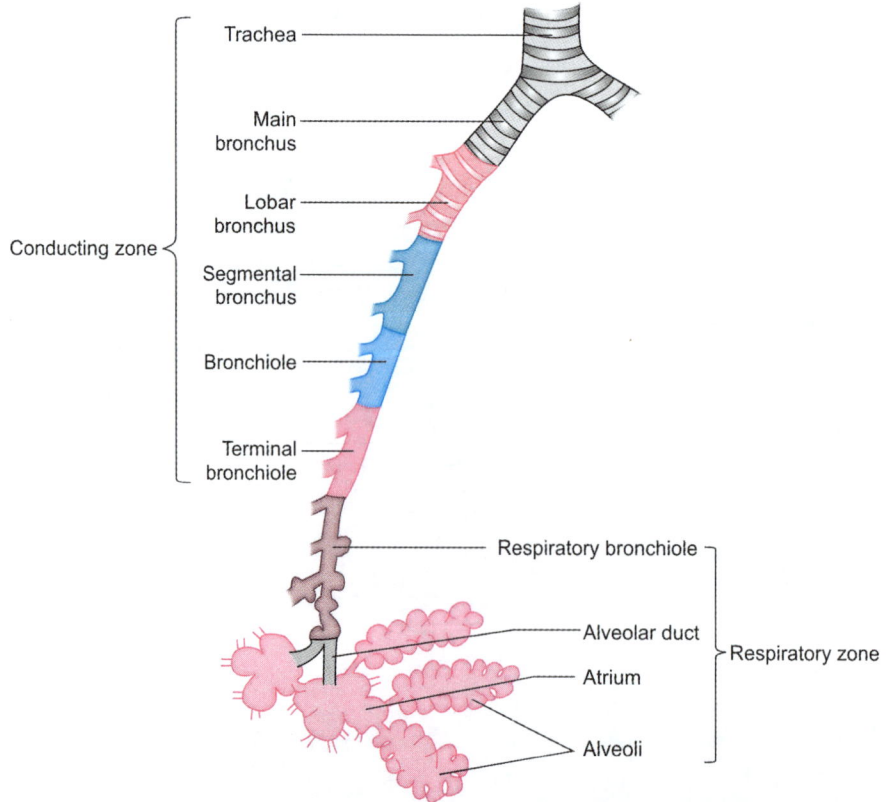

Fig. 33.4: Tracheobronchial tree showing divisions of the airways.

or **physiological unit of lung** or **primary lobule of lung** or **respiratory unit of lung**. From respiratory bronchioles onwards, few alveoli are found on the walls so that some exchange of gases occurs from the 17th generation.

Bronchial Tone

Glands are absent from the epithelium of bronchioles but their walls contain more smooth muscles. Maximum amount of smooth muscle is found in terminal bronchiole relative to the thickness of the wall. Constriction and dilation of the bronchi and bronchioles is due to the presence of these smooth muscles in their walls. Due to the presence of smooth muscles in the bronchial walls, the bronchi dilate during inspiration and constrict during expiration. The airway epithelial cells secrete **epithelium-derived relaxing factors** (suggested to be prostaglandin E_2 and CO) that causes relaxation of airway smooth muscles. This inhibitory factor counteracts activation of the airway smooth muscle by bronchoconstrictor substances. Reduced release of these epithelium-derived relaxing factors may explain in part the bronchial hyper-reactivity seen secondary to epithelial damage.

Receptors present in bronchial smooth muscles, which influence bronchial tone:
- M_3 muscarinic acetylcholine receptors, stimulation of which, produce bronchoconstriction and increase in bronchial tone
- β_2 adrenergic receptor stimulation produces bronchodilation and decreases bronchial tone (**Table 33.1**)
- Stimulation of vasoactive intestinal polypeptide (VIP) receptors produce bronchodilation
- Histamine and leukotriene receptor stimulation produce bronchoconstriction

Importance of Bronchial Smooth Muscle

- Bronchial smooth muscle maintains an even distribution of ventilation.
- Bronchial muscles protect the airway during coughing.
- It is responsible for the bronchial tone.
- A circadian rhythm in bronchial tone is observed, maximum constriction of bronchial muscles occur at 6:00 am and maximum dilation at 6:00 pm. So asthma attacks are more severe in early morning.
- Cooling the airway causes bronchoconstriction. *Exercise triggers asthmatic attacks because it lowers airway temperature due to increased ventilation.*

Table 33.1: Bronchoconstrictors and dilators.

Bronchoconstrictors	Bronchodilators
Substance P	Vasoactive intestinal polypeptide (VIP)
Adenosine	
Leukotrienes	β_2-adrenergic agonists like salbutamol
Interleukins	
Cold air	Glucocorticoids
Aspirin	Nitric oxide
IgE	Carbon monoxide
α-adrenergic agonists	PGE_2

Alveoli

The alveolus is the fundamental unit of gas exchange.
- Total number of alveoli in both lungs: 300–480 million
- Diameter of a single alveolus: 0.075–0.3 mm (apical alveoli are larger than basal alveoli in the erect posture)
- Total weight of alveolar tissue: 250 g
- Total surface area of alveoli of both lungs: 50–100 m² (~70 m²).

Both the diameter and the surface area of the alveoli depend on the degree of lung inflation. Small holes called **pores of Kohn** connect the adjacent alveoli. The function of these pores, which are surrounded by capillaries, is unknown.

Cells in the Alveolar Epithelium

Alveolar epithelium is of simple **squamous** type. Mainly two types of epithelial cells line the alveoli:
1. Type I cells
2. Type II cells or granular pneumocytes

Type I cells are flat, thin cells with numerous cytoplasmic extensions and cover about 95% of the alveolar surface. Gas exchange takes place across these cells. They also help to remove liquid from the alveolar surface by actively pumping sodium and water from the alveolar surface into the interstitium.

Type II cells are large, cuboidal secretory cells containing lamellated inclusion bodies, which produce and store **surfactant**. These cells are seen between type I cells. They secrete surfactant whose function is to decrease surface tension in the alveoli. Type II cells also help in the repair of alveoli. After an injury, type I cells slough and degenerate, whereas type II cells proliferate and line the alveolar space.

In addition to the above cells, alveoli also contain:
- Pulmonary alveolar macrophages (PAMs) and dendritic cells
- Mast cells
- Neutrophils, lymphocytes, plasma cells
- Fibroblasts
- Amine precursor uptake and decarboxylation cells (APUD cells)

Pulmonary alveolar macrophages (PAMs) are derived from monocytes of blood. They phagocytose particles less than 5 μm reaching the alveolus, such as dust particles or microorganisms. When these cells engulf carbon and dust particles they are called **dust cells**. Dust cells are common in smoker's lungs. When they engulf red blood cells in congestive cardiac failure (CCF) they are called **heart failure cells**, which produce brick red sputum. Alveolar macrophages are also involved in the phagocytosis of apoptotic and necrotic cells. Coughing eliminates them. PAMs and dendritic cells are mononuclear phagocytic cells.

Neutrophils phagocytose bacteria and produce inflammatory changes.

Lymphocytes act against both bacteria and viruses. Plasma cells derived from B-lymphocytes secretes IgA which helps in immunity.

Mast cells contain histamine, 5 hydroxytryptamine, leukotrienes, prostaglandins, thromboxane and platelet activating factor that participate in allergic reactions and produce bronchospasm.

APUD cells produce certain hormones, such as prostaglandin.

INNERVATION OF LUNGS

The walls of the bronchi and bronchioles are innervated by the **autonomic nervous system** (ANS). **Sympathetic fibers** release **norepinephrine** at their endings and the effect of sympathetic stimulation depends on the type of receptors stimulated. β_2 adrenergic receptors predominate in the lungs. The overall effects of sympathetic stimulation are bronchodilation, decreased bronchial secretion and vasoconstriction.

Parasympathetic innervation to lung is through **vagus** and the neurotransmitter is **acetylcholine**.
- Receptors—M_3 muscarinic acetylcholine receptors.
- Effects—bronchoconstriction, vasodilation and increased mucus secretion.

There is, in addition, a **non-cholinergic, non-adrenergic** innervation of the bronchioles that produces **bronchodilation**. Vasoactive intestinal polypeptide **(VIP)** is the mediator responsible for the dilation. Most of the patients suffering from bronchial asthma have deficiency of VIP.

BRONCHOSCOPY

A flexible fiberoptic bronchoscope can reach up to the second or third division of bronchi and is used to visualize the trachea, bronchi and their branches, aspirate secretions, remove obstructions and obtain biopsy material.

BRONCHOGRAPHY

The technique of visualizing the bronchial tree using radiopaque dye is called bronchography. The record obtained is **bronchogram** (**Fig. 33.5**).

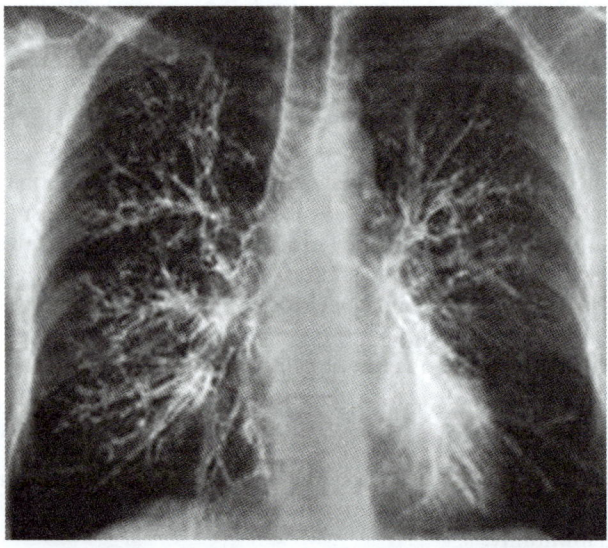

Fig. 33.5: Bronchogram.

PLEURA

In the embryo, each lung invaginates into a separate pleural sac, which reflects over the surface of the lung. Thus, a double-layered serous membrane called **pleura** covers the lung. The layer, which is closely covering the lung, is the **visceral pleura** and the layer that is reflected back at the root of the lungs on to the surface of diaphragm and thoracic cage is the **parietal pleura**. There is a potential space between the two pleural layers called **pleural cavity**, which contains about 2 to 5 mL of mucoid pleural fluid (**Fig. 33.6**). Pleural fluid, which is an ultrafiltrate of plasma, is secreted by the blood vessels of the parietal pleura. Excess pleural fluid is pumped away or absorbed by capillaries of visceral pleura and by the lymphatics.

Functions of Pleural Fluid
- Pleural fluid keeps the two pleural layers together.
- Acts as a lubricant and helps in the sliding movement between the two layers.
- It is essential for the proper expansion and contraction of the lungs.

Pleural Effusion

Accumulation of significant quantity of fluid in the pleural cavity is called pleural effusion. Depending on the nature of the fluid if it is:
- Watery— hydrothorax
- Pus—pyothorax
- Blood—hemothorax
- Lymph—chylothorax

Causes of Pleural Effusion
- Blockage to lymphatics or rupture of lymphatics leads to chylothorax
- Increase in pulmonary capillary pressure leads to excessive transudation of fluid into the pleural cavity as in cardiac failure

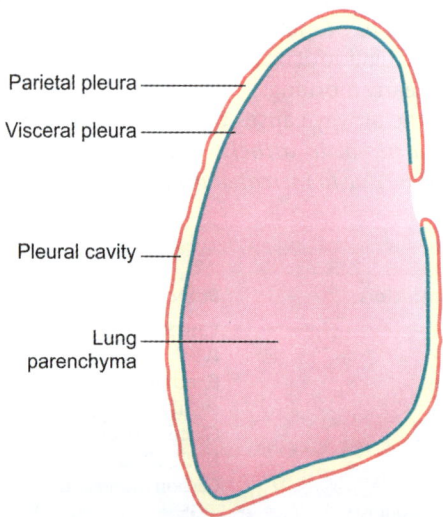

Fig. 33.6: Pleural anatomy.

- ❖ Reduced plasma colloid osmotic pressure as in hypoproteinemia
- ❖ Infection or inflammation of the pleura leads to damage to capillary membrane and transudation of proteinaceous fluid into the pleural cavity.

Pneumothorax

Presence of air in the pleural space is called pneumothorax. This leads to collapse of lung on the affected side because of elastic recoil of lung. **Figure 33.7** shows right-sided pneumothorax. The negative intrapleural pressure that keeps the lungs distended is lost in pneumothorax.

Causes of Pneumothorax
- ❖ Rupture of lung
- ❖ Injury to pleura or chest wall

Types of Pneumothorax
- ❖ Open pneumothorax
- ❖ Tension pneumothorax
- ❖ Closed pneumothorax

Open Pneumothorax

If the communication between the pleural space and the exterior remains open, more air moves in and out of the pleural space with each breath. This is open pneumothorax. The intrapleural pressure on the affected side will be atmospheric. There will be respiratory distress due to hypoxia, hypercapnia and activation of pulmonary deflation receptors (J receptors). Little air enters the intact lung because the resistance to airflow into the pleural cavity on the affected side is less than to the intact lung.

Tension Pneumothorax

If there is a flap of tissue over the hole in the pleura that acts as a one-way valve permitting air to enter the pleural space during inspiration but preventing its exit during expiration, the pressure in the pleural space rises above atmospheric pressure. This is tension pneumothorax and is a medical emergency. The condition is fatal if the pneumothorax is not decompressed by removing the air.

Closed Pneumothorax

If the hole through which air enters the pleural space gets sealed off, the condition is called closed pneumothorax. It does not produce much respiratory distress and the gas in the pleural space gets absorbed into blood within 1–2 weeks.

BLOOD SUPPLY TO LUNGS

Lungs receive blood from **pulmonary vessels and bronchial vessels**.

Pulmonary Circulation

Pulmonary artery carries deoxygenated blood to the lungs from the right ventricle and supplies bronchioles, alveoli and visceral pleura. It divides repeatedly to form capillaries that form a dense network around alveoli.

So, dense is the network that blood forms a continuous sheet in the alveolar wall. Oxygen from alveoli diffuses into these capillaries and CO_2 is removed from blood. They form venules and veins and finally form pulmonary veins 4 in number carrying pure blood into the left atrium (*refer* **Chapter 36**, Pulmonary Circulation).

Bronchial Circulation

Bronchial vessels nourish trachea, bronchi and parietal pleura. Bronchial artery is a branch of descending aorta and contains pure blood. Impure blood is carried by bronchial veins, which drain into azygos vein, which in turn opens into the right atrium. The bronchial veins may also anastomose with the pulmonary veins and so there is a slight mixing of impure blood from the bronchial veins with the pure blood coming from the lungs in the pulmonary veins.

Due to mixing of blood, the left atrium receives more blood than the right atrium and therefore *the left ventricular output is about 1–2% greater than the right ventricular output.*

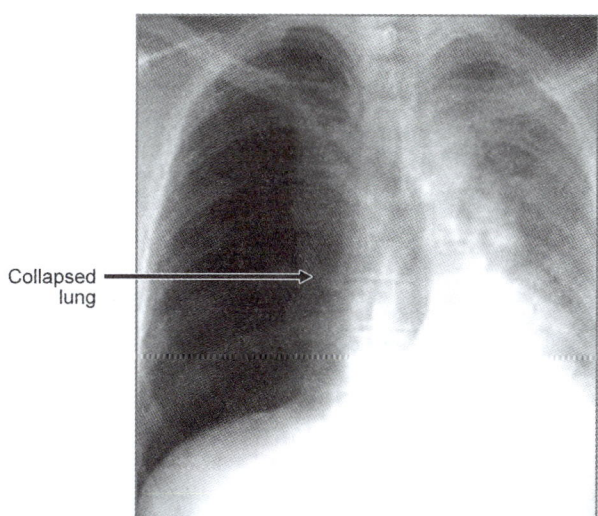

Fig. 33.7: Pneumothorax of right side.

MULTIPLE CHOICE QUESTIONS

1. **Particle size which can easily reach the alveoli is:**
   a. 0.5–3 µm
   b. 3–5 µm
   c. 5–10 µm
   d. 10–15 µm

2. **Alveoli are lined by:**
   a. Simple squamous epithelium
   b. Ciliated columnar epithelium
   c. Cuboidal epithelium
   d. Stratified squamous epithelium

3. **Which of the following is the best known metabolic function of the lung?**
   a. Inactivation of serotonin
   b. Conversion of angiotensin-I to angiotensin-II
   c. Inactivation of bradykinin
   d. Metabolism of basic drugs by cytochrome P-450 system

4. Bronchial muscle relaxation occur due to stimulation of the following receptors:
   a. H_1 receptors
   b. J-receptors
   c. Alpha adrenergic receptors
   d. β_2 adrenergic receptors

5. In the tracheobronchial tree, cilia are absent from the:
   a. Respiratory bronchiole
   b. Terminal bronchiole
   c. Alveolar duct
   d. Alveolar sac

6. The pleural fluid is formed from:
   a. Parietal pleura
   b. Visceral pleura
   c. Alveoli
   d. Lung interstitial fluid

7. Alpha-1 antitrypsin (AAT) is secreted by:
   a. Liver
   b. Lung
   c. Spleen
   d. Kidney

8. The quantity of fluid in the pleural cavity normally is about:
   a. 2 mL
   b. 5 mL
   c. 10 mL
   d. 20 mL

9. Resistance to airflow in the lung is maximal in the:
   a. Trachea and larger bronchi
   b. Smaller bronchi
   c. Bronchioles
   d. Alveolar duct

10. The number of alveoli in man is about:
    a. 50 million
    b. 100 million
    c. 300 million
    d. 500 million

11. Maximum resistance of airway is due to:
    a. Trachea
    b. Medium sized airway
    c. Respiratory bronchiole
    d. Terminal bronchiole

12. Irreversible damage to neurons occur if exposed to significant hypoxia for:
    a. 15 sec
    b. 30 sec
    c. 2 min
    d. 8 min

13. Surfactant is produced by:
    a. Type I pneumocytes
    b. Type II pneumocytes
    c. Macrophages
    d. Endothelial cells

ANSWERS

1. a	2. a	3. b	4. d	5. a
6. a	7. a	8. a	9. a	10. c
11. a	12. d	13. b		

Mechanics of Ventilation

CHAPTER 34

LEARNING OBJECTIVES
- Describe the mechanism of normal respiration
- Explain the differences between intrapleural and intrapulmonary pressures
- Explain the functions of surfactant
- Discuss the factors that keep the alveoli dry
- Explain the application of Law of Laplace in lung
- Describe the deleterious effects of cigarette smoking

INTRODUCTION

Movements of the thorax, inflation and deflation of lungs and flow of air into and out of the lungs constitute **ventilation**. Taking in of air is **inspiration** and giving out of air is **expiration**.

PATTERNS OF BREATHING

- **Eupnea:** Normal breathing is called **eupneic breathing**. Normal respiratory rate is 12–16/min.
- **Tachypnea:** Increase in the rate of respiration is called tachypnea, e.g., in exercise, fever, anxiety, etc.
- **Apnea:** Arrest of respiration is called apnea, e.g., deglutition apnea, adrenaline apnea, sleep apnea, etc.
- **Sighs:** Larger than normal breaths occurring normally are sighs. They prevent alveolar collapse.
- **Yawn:** Exaggerated sigh.
- **Kussmaul breathing:** Deep, rapid breathing seen in metabolic acidosis, e.g., diabetic ketoacidosis.
- **Cheyne-Stokes breathing:** Cycles of gradual increase in tidal volume followed by decrease in tidal volume followed by a period of apnea.
- **Dyspnea:** Difficulty in breathing or shortness of breath associated with marked awareness of the effort of respiration is called dyspnea, e.g., bronchial asthma.
- **Orthopnea:** Dyspnea in the lying down posture and getting considerable relief in the erect posture is called orthopnea, e.g., mitral stenosis, left-sided heart failure, etc.
- **Gasping:** Brief inspiratory efforts followed by long periods of expiration. Seen in patients with brainstem lesion or cardiac arrest.
- **Apneusis:** Prolonged inspiration separated by brief expiration.

BOUNDARIES OF THE THORACIC CAGE

- Behind and laterally—Vertebral column and ribs
- In front and laterally—Sternum and ribs
- In the lower part—Diaphragm
- Upper part—Upper ribs and tissues of the neck
  Heart, lungs and great vessels occupy the thoracic cavity.

MUSCLES OF RESPIRATION

Muscles of Inspiration

- *Normal quiet inspiration*: Diaphragm and external intercostal muscles (**primary muscles** of inspiration).
- *In forced inspiration* as in exercise, asthma, etc., **accessory muscles or secondary muscles** of inspiration act which are sternocleidomastoid, pectoralis, elevators of scapula, scalenes, serratus anterior and alae nasi.
  - Scalenes lift the first two ribs.
  - Sternocleidomastoids lift the sternum outwards, contributing to pump-handle effect
  - Neck muscles elevate the pectoral girdle increasing the cross sectional area of the thorax and back muscles extend the back increasing the vertical dimension of the thoracic cage.
  - Alae nasi help to open the nostrils widely.

Muscles of Expiration

No muscles are actively involved in normal quiet expiration. So, there are no primary muscles of expiration.

Expiration during quiet breathing is passive in the sense that no muscles, which decrease intrathoracic volume contract. However, there is some contraction of the inspiratory muscles in the early part of expiration. This contraction exerts a braking action on the recoil forces and slows expiration. The inspiratory muscles that have contracted relax in normal expiration. But in pathological conditions such as emphysema, expiration becomes an active process due to loss of elasticity of lung.

In forced expiration, muscles of the anterior abdominal wall (internal and external oblique, recto-abdominal and transverse abdominal muscles), internal intercostal muscles and latissimus dorsi (**accessory muscles of expiration**) contract and make intrapleural pressure more positive. Contraction of the abdominal muscles increases intra-abdominal pressure and forces the diaphragm upwards into the thoracic cavity, decreasing the vertical dimension of thoracic cage. Contraction of internal intercostal muscles reduces the anteroposterior and transverse diameters of the thorax.

■ MECHANISM OF VENTILATION OF LUNGS

PY6.2: Describe the mechanics of normal respiration, pressure changes during ventilation, lung volume and capacities, alveolar surface tension, compliance, airway resistance, ventilation, V/P ratio, diffusion capacity of lungs.

The lung and chest wall are elastic structures. When the inspiratory muscles contract, the thoracic cage moves out and parietal pleura, which is closely adherent to the thoracic cage also moves out. This draws along with it the visceral pleura which is adherent to the lungs. The visceral pleura and the parietal pleura function as a single unit because of the presence of pleural fluid in between them. Due to the dragging force exerted by the visceral pleura and also due to elastic property of lung, the lungs expand. The inside volume is increased and the alveolar pressure becomes sub-atmospheric. As a result, air from outside is sucked into the lungs. This is **inspiration**. The contraction of the inspiratory muscles lasts for about 2–3 seconds.

Then the contracted muscles relax and the lungs retract due to elastic recoil, thereby creating a pressure more than atmospheric pressure in the alveoli and air is driven out. This is **expiration**.

In normal quiet breathing, inspiration is an active process and expiration is passive.

■ MOVEMENTS OF THE THORACIC CAGE

During inspiration, dimensions of the thoracic cage increase in three ways:
❖ Increase in vertical dimension
❖ Increase in anteroposterior dimension
❖ Increase in transverse dimension

Mechanism of Increase in Vertical Dimension

Increase in vertical dimension is mainly brought about by contraction of the **diaphragm,** which is a dome-shaped musculotendinous sheet that separates thoracic cavity from abdominal cavity. In normal quiet inspiration when diaphragm contracts, it moves downwards like a piston for about 1.5–3 cm (**Fig. 34.1A**). In forceful inspiration, vertical dimension is increased by 7–10 cm. *75% of air entry during inspiration is by the activity of diaphragm.* In diaphragmatic paralysis, respiration is seriously impaired. Diaphragm is supplied by phrenic nerve whose root value is C3, C4 and C5.

Applied Aspect

Transection of the spinal cord above the third cervical segment is fatal without artificial respiration because it causes paralysis of all respiratory muscles. But transection below the 5th cervical segment leaves the phrenic nerves that innervate the diaphragm intact and its activity is adequate to maintain life.

Mechanism of Increase in Anteroposterior and Transverse Diameter

Increase in the anteroposterior and transverse diameter of the thorax is by the contraction of **external intercostal muscles**, which originate from the lower border of upper rib and inserted into the upper border of lower rib. The fibers are directed downwards, forwards and medially.

Each rib is connected posteriorly to vertebral column and anteriorly to sternum. The posterior joint is hinged, i.e., it is movable. The lower ribs are more obliquely placed than the upper ribs. During inspiration, the external intercostal muscles contract and the upper ribs become more horizontal. Sternum is thrust upwards and forwards, i.e., it moves away from the vertebral column like a water pump handle. Thus, the anteroposterior dimension of the thoracic cage is increased. This movement is referred to as **water pump- handle effect** (**Fig. 34.1B**).

The lower ribs (7, 8, 9 and 10) in addition to moving upwards also swing outwards, thereby increasing the antero-posterior and transverse dimension of the thoracic cage. This movement is called **bucket handle movement** (**Fig. 34.1C**).

If the contribution by the diaphragm is more in inspiration, then the breathing is called **abdominal** type of **breathing**. If external intercostal muscle action predominates, it is called **thoracic or costal breathing**.

Types of Breathing

❖ Abdominothoracic in men.
❖ Thoracoabdominal in women.
❖ Abdominal in children and in injury to the chest wall. In infants, the ribs are more horizontal than oblique, so movement of the thorax is less visible.
❖ Thoracic type is seen in conditions like severe ascites (collection of fluid in the peritoneal cavity) where the movement of diaphragm is restricted.

■ BREATH SOUNDS

Cause of Breath Sounds

Breath sounds are produced due to passage of air through respiratory passages. Breath sounds have intensity and quality.

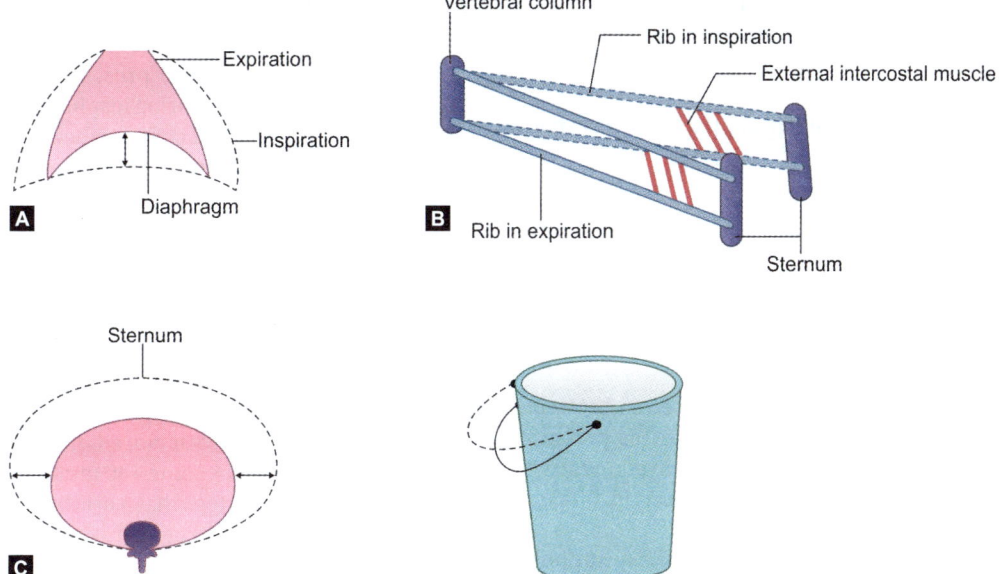

Figs. 34.1A to C: Movements of the thoracic cage in inspiration: (A) Increase in vertical dimension by contraction of diaphragm; (B) Increase in anteroposterior dimension (pump-handle movement); (C) Increase in the transverse dimension (bucket-handle movement).

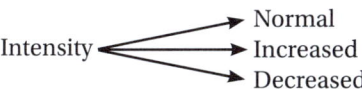

Depending on the quality of sound, breath sounds are of two types:
1. Vesicular breath sounds
2. Bronchial breath sounds

Breath sounds are produced by turbulent flow of air through trachea and larger bronchi.

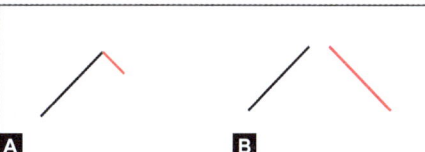

Figs. 34.2A and B: Difference in the duration of inspiration and expiration on auscultation in (A) Vesicular breath sound; (B) Bronchial breath sound.

Vesicular Breath Sounds

Vesicular breath sound is heard when auscultated in the lower regions of lungs. The sound of air passing through the airways is attenuated and filtered by normal lung parenchyma. The lung parenchyma, which is air filled, filters off the higher frequency components (≥200 Hz) and this changes the character of the breath sound to vesicular which is a **fine, low-pitched rustling sound**. There is no distinct pause between end of inspiration and beginning of expiration. Expiratory phase when auscultated with a stethoscope is 1/3rd of inspiration (**Fig. 34.2A**).

When the filtering effect is lost, the sounds are directly transmitted to the chest wall and breath sound becomes bronchial sound over the affected areas. This occurs in consolidation of lung, collapse, fibrosis, etc.

Bronchial Breath Sounds

Bronchial breath sound is heard when auscultated over larger air passages like trachea and bronchi. It is **harsh and coarse** in character and there is a definite pause in between inspiration and expiration. Inspiratory and expiratory phases are equally heard with a stethoscope (**Fig. 34.2B**).

Added Sounds or Adventitious Sounds

Adventitious sounds are abnormal sounds that arise in the pleura or in the lungs. Adventitious sounds may be continuous or interrupted.

Continuous adventitious sounds include:
- Stridor
- Wheezes (rhonchi)

Stridor occurs in laryngeal and bronchial obstruction. It can be due to an object blocking the airway, vocal cord paralysis, tumors in the upper airway, etc.

Wheezes arise from narrowed air passages. They are dry, musical, wheezing sounds which are heard in conditions like asthma, bronchitis, etc.

Interrupted adventitious sounds include:
- Crackles (crepitation)
- Pleural rub

Crackles are moist, crackling or bubbling sounds. It may be due to the presence of secretion or exudates in the air passages or due to sudden opening of closed small airways, e.g., pulmonary edema, respiratory infections, etc.

Pleural rub is a rubbing sound produced by rubbing of inflamed pleural surfaces, e.g., pleural inflammation as in pleurisy.

PRESSURE CHANGES DURING RESPIRATORY CYCLE

Respiratory pressures are of three types:
1. Intrathoracic/intrapleural pressure
2. Intrapulmonary/intra-alveolar pressure
3. Transpulmonary pressure/transmural pressure

Intrapleural Pressure

Intrapleural pressure is the pressure developed in between the two layers of pleura. In normal breathing, this pressure is *always sub-atmospheric*, i.e., it is always negative. Atmospheric pressure, which is equal to 760 mm Hg, is taken as zero atmospheres.

Normal intrapleural pressure at the end of expiration = –2.5 to –3 mm Hg or 757 to 757.5 mm Hg

Intrapleural pressure is same as intrathoracic pressure, i.e., the pressure everywhere in the thorax except in the lumens of blood vessels, lymphatics or airways. Thus, intraesophageal pressure is same as that of intrapleural pressure.

Causes of Negative Intrapleural Pressure

- The natural tendency of lungs is always to recoil inwards because of its elasticity and surface tension in the alveoli. The tendency of thoracic cage is to expand or recoil outwards. These two forces are equal in intensity and act in opposite directions against a closed space so that the pressure in the space becomes less than barometric pressure, i.e., the intrapleural space becomes a relative vacuum (**Fig. 34.3**).
- Negative intrapleural pressure is also caused by the more rapid absorption rate of pleural fluid by pulmonary capillaries and also by the lymphatics. The pressure in the capillaries of visceral pleura is low, i.e., about 8 mm Hg because they belong to pulmonary circulatory system.

Measurement of Intrapleural Pressure

- By introducing a needle into the pleural space and connecting it to a manometer.
- By introducing a catheter, whose tip contains a thin-walled balloon, into the esophagus and connecting it to a manometer. The **intraesophageal pressure** will be same as intrapleural pressure because the negativity of intrapleural pressure makes the mediastinal pressure negative, which in turn makes the intraesophageal pressure negative.

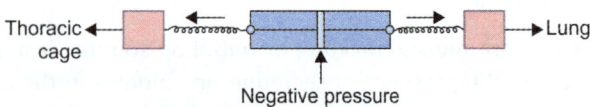

Fig. 34.3: Diagrammatic representation of the development of negative intrapleural pressure in the pleural cavity.

Variations in Intrapleural Pressure

- *During different phases of respiration*: At the end of expiration, the intrapleural pressure is –2.5 mm Hg in normal quiet breathing. During inspiration, thoracic cavity expands and intrapleural pressure becomes –6 to –8 mm Hg. During expiration, muscles are relaxed and intrapleural pressure becomes less negative and towards the end of expiration, it becomes –2.5 to –3 mm Hg (**Fig. 34.4**).

  In forced inspiration, intrapleural pressure becomes –12 to –18 mm Hg and in forced expiration, it becomes a positive pressure.

  In **Muller's maneuver**, i.e., forced inspiration with closed glottis as if sucking fluid with a straw, the intrapleural pressure become –40 mm Hg. In **Valsalva's maneuver**, i.e., forced expiration with closed glottis as in straining, intrapleural pressure become +40 mm Hg.

- *Regional variation*: Regional variation in intrapleural pressure is due to the effect of gravity and posture. When the subject is in the standing posture, the negativity is greatest near the apex of lung and progressively falls along the longitudinal axis to its lowest value near the base of the lung.
  - Near the apex it is more negative, i.e., –6 mm Hg
  - Near the base it is about –1 mm Hg.
  - In the middle of the lung it is –2.5 mm Hg.

The reasons for the apex-to-base gradient in intrapleural pressure are **gravity and posture**. When the subject stands on the ground, gravity pulls the lungs downward and away from the apex of the thoracic cage. This force creates a greater vacuum at the apex. Gravity also pushes the bases of the lungs into the lower part of the thoracic cavity reducing the vacuum at the base. In the outer space, the pressure gradient from apex to base will be absent because of the absence of gravitational field.

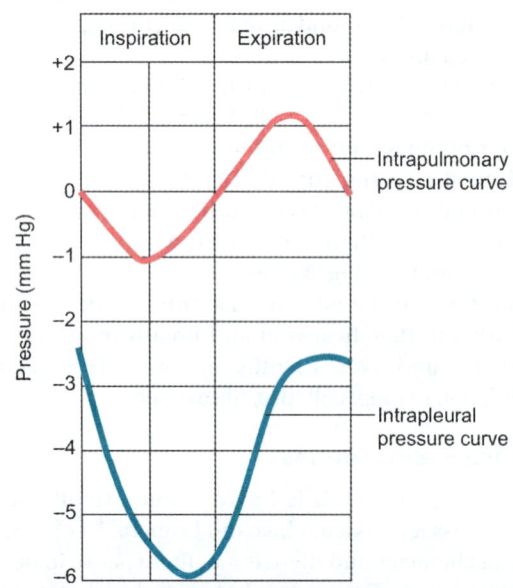

Fig. 34.4: Intrapulmonary and intrapleural pressure tracing in normal quiet inspiration and expiration.

Importance of Negative Intrapleural Pressure

- Negative intrapleural pressure increases venous return. During inspiration, the increased negativity in the mediastinum helps to suck blood from periphery towards great veins and to the heart.
- Maintains alveolar stability.
- Keeps the airways open.
- Prevents collapse of lung, i.e., keeps lungs in an expanded position. If the chest wall is opened, the negative intrapleural pressure is lost and the lungs collapse.

Effects of Positive Intrapleural Pressure

Positive intrapleural pressure compresses the great vessels in the thoracic cavity and decreases venous return to heart, which in turn decreases cardiac output. This produces cerebral ischemia leading to loss of consciousness. *This is the reason for the syncopial attacks following continuous severe bouts of cough especially in old people and in cardiac patients.*

Intrapulmonary Pressure

Pressure developed inside the alveoli is intrapulmonary pressure. As alveoli are in connection with the atmosphere, at the end of normal expiration, the intrapulmonary pressure is equal to atmospheric pressure, i.e., zero.

During normal breathing in inspiration, it becomes negative and at mid-inspiration, becomes –1 to –2 mm Hg. As more and more air enters the lungs, the negativity decreases and at the end of inspiration, the intrapulmonary pressure becomes zero or atmospheric.

During quiet expiration, it becomes more positive and at mid-expiration, it becomes +1 to +2 mm Hg and towards the end of expiration again the pressure becomes same as that of atmospheric pressure (**Fig. 34.4**).

In forced inspiration, i.e., in **Muller's maneuver**, it becomes –80 mm Hg and in forced expiration, i.e., **Valsalva's maneuver**, it becomes +100 mm Hg.

Transpulmonary/Transmural Pressure

The pressure difference across the lung, i.e., the pressure difference between the alveolar pressure and pleural pressure, is called transpulmonary pressure.

Transpulmonary pressure = Intrapulmonary pressure – Intrapleural pressure

Importance of Transmural Pressure

- It is necessary for the expansion of lung.
- It gives a measure of the elastic recoil of lung.
- An increase in transpulmonary pressure causes greater stretching of lung and more will be the lung volume, i.e., transpulmonary pressure decides the lung volume.

Transpulmonary pressure is increased during inspiration and decreased during expiration.

The different values of transpulmonary pressures at the end of normal expiration in different parts of the lung are as follows:

At the apex of the lung: 0 – (–6) = 6 mm Hg
At the base of the lung: 0 – (–1) = 1 mm Hg
In the middle of the lung: 0 – (–2.5) = 2.5 mm Hg

Since the transmural pressure is more at the apex than at the base, during first part of inspiration more of inspired air goes to the apex than to the base of the lung.

Since the transmural pressure is less at the base of the lung, the lung is less expanded at the base. The transmural pressure again decreases at the end of forced expiration leading to the closure of the airways at the base.

■ ELASTIC BEHAVIOR OF LUNGS OR REASONS FOR RECOIL OF LUNG

- Tissue elasticity
- Surface tension of alveolar fluid

Tissue Elasticity

Lung parenchyma contains large quantity of elastic fibers arranged in a peculiar pattern. The geometric arrangement of elastin fibers in lung can be compared to nylon stocking elasticity. This elasticity contributes to 1/3rd of elastic recoil tendency of lung.

Surface Tension

Surface tension phenomenon in lungs contributes to 2/3 of recoil tendency of lung. The alveolar wall is lined by epithelial cells, which secrete alveolar fluid. Inside the alveolus there is air. The interphase is between air and alveolar fluid and the surface tension exerted between air and alveolar fluid is very high ~60 dynes/cm. So, there is a tendency to reduce the size of the alveolus due to intermolecular attraction. But the surface tension in the lung is decreased to 5–30 dynes/cm due to the presence of surfactant in between the alveolar fluid and air in the alveolus.

■ SURFACTANT

Introduction

Surfactant is a surface tension lowering agent present in the alveolus between the alveolar fluid and air. It is secreted by **type II alveolar epithelial cells,** which contain lamellar bodies.

Pulmonary surfactant is a complex mixture of **lipid and protein**. Approximately 90% of surfactant is made up of lipids. Proteins constitute remaining 10%. It also contains Ca^{2+} and carbohydrate in very small quantity. The phospholipid in surfactant is **dipalmitoyl lecithin** or dipalmitoylphosphatidyl-choline. The surfactant proteins are albumin, secretory immunoglobulin A (IgA), and 4 apoproteins, namely—SP-A, SP-B, SP-C and SP-D. Surfactant forms a monomolecular layer inside the alveolus.

The lipid component reaches the type-II cells from the bloodstream. The apoproteins are synthesized in the type-II cells itself. The final assembly occurs in the lamellar bodies in the type II cells. Secretion of surfactant occurs by exocytosis.

Functions of Surfactant

- Surface tension accounts for most of the elastic recoil in normal lungs. Surfactant **decreases surface tension** 6 times. Distending pressure of each alveolus lined by surfactant is only 3 mm Hg. If the alveolus was lined by water the distending pressure may be as high as 15 mm Hg (18 cm of water).
  Surface tension of alveolar fluid – 50 dynes/cm Surface tension of surfactant – 5–30 dynes/cm
- Surfactant maintains **alveolar stability** and helps in even distribution of ventilation among alveoli. Surfactant prevents over-distension or collapse (atelectasis) of alveoli. Thus, it helps to keep alveolar size relatively uniform during the respiratory cycle.
  Surface tension in the alveolus is inversely proportional to the number of surfactant molecules per unit area. When there is increase in the diameter of the alveolus, as in inspiration, the number of surfactant molecules per unit area decreases and the surface tension increases and this prevents over distension of lung.
  When there is decrease in the diameter of alveoli, as in expiration, the surfactant molecules come closer and number of surfactant molecules per unit area increases and surface tension decreases, and this prevents collapse of lung during expiration. Surfactant thus maintains alveolar stability (**Fig. 34.5**).
- Surfactant prevents pulmonary edema and keeps the **alveoli dry**. Collection of fluid in the alveoli is called **pulmonary edema**. If surfactant was not present in the alveoli, the unopposed surface tension in the alveoli will produce a 20 mm Hg force favoring transudation of fluid from the interstitium and pulmonary capillary blood into the alveoli leading to pulmonary edema. This is prevented by surfactant by decreasing surface tension.
- In newborn infants, surfactant prevents **hyaline membrane disease or infant respiratory distress syndrome (IRDS)**. At the time of birth, the alveoli of the fetus are filled with fluid and the lung is completely collapsed. When the umbilical cord is cut, fetus develops hypoxia and violent inspiratory effort produces very high negativity in the mediastinum and the lungs try to expand. Surfactant should be there for proper expansion of lung.

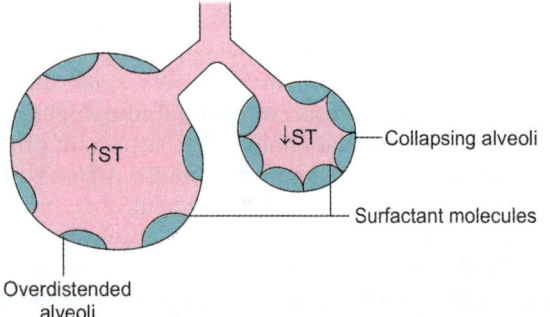

Fig. 34.5: Mechanism of prevention of overdistension and collapse of alveoli. Note the distribution of surfactant molecules in large and small alveoli affecting surface tension.

Due to stretching of capillaries when the lungs expand, there is a sharp fall in the pulmonary capillary pressure and the colloidal osmotic pressure will be more. So, alveolar fluid enters the pulmonary capillaries due to Starling's forces and the fetal alveoli become dry. In the fetus, development of surfactant is completed only by 31–32 weeks of intrauterine life. If birth occurs prematurely, the lung maturity is not complete because it lacks sufficient levels of surfactant and the lungs fail to expand and may lead to the death of the baby. This is **neonatal or infant respiratory distress syndrome** (NRDS/IRDS). Prenatal estimation of lecithin:sphingomyelin ratio in amniotic fluid is useful to predict the chances of developing respiratory distress syndrome (RDS). If L: S ratio is less than 1.5, the risk is high. If L: S ratio is more than 2, the risk of RDS is minimal.

The condition is treated using synthetic surfactant or bovine surfactant preparation available for use by inhalation. This decreases the severity of IRDS. Steroid is also of much benefit because glucocorticoids increase the synthesis of surfactant. Immediately before the birth of the baby, there is a surge in maternal glucocorticoid secretion, which trigger the synthesis, maturation and secretion of surfactant in the baby's lungs. This is another reason for the development of IRDS in premature babies.

In adults, deficiency of surfactant is a cause for **adult respiratory distress syndrome (ARDS)**. Causes of surfactant deficiency include chronic cigarette smoking, long-term inhalation of 100% O_2, occlusion of a main bronchus or one pulmonary artery, etc.

- Surfactant increases the **compliance** of lungs by decreasing the surface tension, making it far easier to inflate the lungs.
- It reduces the **work** of breathing by decreasing the elastic recoil of lung.
- Protective function—Surfactant proteins, SP-A and SP-D stimulate phagocytosis and chemotaxis and form part of innate immunity. Both act as opsonins and coat bacteria, viruses, mycobacteria and fungi to enhance phagocytosis by the macrophages present in the alveoli.
- Surfactant secretion is regulated by the feedback control exerted by SP-A.
- SP-B and SP-C increase the rate at which surfactant enters the air-water interface and then spreads to form a surface film. Congenital absence of SP-B leads to infant respiratory distress syndrome (IRDS), which is fatal. The baby can be rescued only by lung transplantation.

Factors Affecting Surfactant Production

Factors Increasing Surfactant Production

- **Nervous factors**: Vagus stimulates type II cells and increases the production of surfactant. Cutting vagal supply to the lungs leads to the development of pulmonary edema due to surfactant deficiency.
- **Hormonal factors**
  - Thyroid hormone stimulates type II cells. Surfactant production is decreased in hypothyroidism.
  - Glucocorticoid hormones stimulate production and maturation of surfactant. Towards the later stages

of pregnancy, glucocorticoid levels are high in the fetus and mother, and the lung of fetus is rich in glucocorticoid receptors.

Other factors:
- Hyperinflation of lung as in exercise, sighing, yawning, etc.
- β-adrenergic agonists.

Factors Decreasing Surfactant Production
- Smoking
- Hypoxia
- Oxygen toxicity
- Occlusion of a main bronchus or one pulmonary artery
- Hyperinsulinemia (children born to mothers with uncontrolled diabetes mellitus will suffer from IRDS due to surfactant deficiency. The hyperglycemia in the fetus will stimulate the pancreas to secrete more insulin. This excess insulin will inhibit surfactant production leading to IRDS).

APPLICATION OF LAW OF LAPLACE IN LUNG

Law of Laplace

Laplace's Law states that the **distending pressure** P, in the case of a distensible spherical organ is equal to 2T/R, where, T is the **surface tension** and R the **radius** of the organ. P is the pressure required to keep the alveoli inflated. P will be high when T is high or R is less.

In the lung, all the alveoli will have a constant size due to the presence of surfactant. Whenever the diameter of the alveoli changes, surfactant causes appropriate changes in the surface tension so that pressure in the alveoli is maintained constant.

According to Law of Laplace
- During expiration, the radius of the alveolus is reduced and if surface tension is not simultaneously reduced it will exceed the distending pressure and lead to collapse of lung. But due to the presence of surfactant, surface tension is suitably altered during the phases of respiration and collapse or over-distension is prevented.
- If there is no surfactant, air flows from smaller alveoli to larger ones so that smaller ones become smaller and larger ones become larger and finally collapse of smaller alveoli occurs (**Fig. 34.6**).

ALVEOLAR STABILITY

Alveolar stability depends on three important factors:
1. Interdependence
2. Negative intrapleural pressure
3. Surfactant

Interdependence

As the adjacent alveoli are supported by each other, it is difficult for an alveolus to contract on its own without contraction of other alveoli. This mutual support offered to lung units by those surrounding them is termed interdependence.

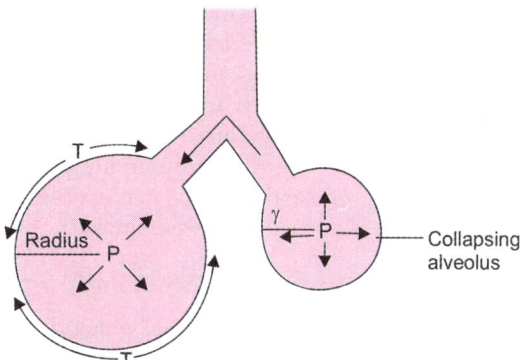

Fig. 34.6: Mechanism of collapse of smaller alveoli and over distension of larger alveoli if surfactant is absent. As the pressure increased in the smaller alveolus air moves from the smaller ones to larger ones so that larger alveoli become still larger.

Intrapleural Pressure

Negative or sub-atmospheric intrapleural pressure prevents collapse of alveoli and help in maintaining alveolar stability.

Surfactant

Surfactant maintains **alveolar stability** and helps in even distribution of ventilation. Surfactant prevents overdistension or collapse (atelectasis) of alveoli (refer functions of surfactant).

Factors that Keep the Alveoli Dry
- Surfactant prevents the collection of fluid in the alveoli by decreasing surface tension.
- The colloidal osmotic pressure of pulmonary capillary blood is more (25 mm Hg) than capillary hydrostatic pressure (10 mm Hg). This is because pulmonary circulation is a low-pressure system. This inward directed pressure gradient of about 15 mm Hg favors reabsorption of fluid from the alveoli according to Starling's forces and thus alveoli are kept dry. When pulmonary capillary hydrostatic pressure becomes more than 25 mm Hg, as in left ventricular failure or in mitral stenosis, there is increase in the backpressure and increase in pulmonary capillary pressure leading to fluid collection in the alveoli.

EFFECTS OF CIGARETTE SMOKING

Smoking is one of the biggest causes of preventable deaths worldwide. It is the second commonest cause of cerebrovascular disease, the first being high blood pressure. Smokers are prone for chronic inflammatory processes due to generation of free radicals and this high level of oxidative stress promotes atherosclerosis and cardiovascular diseases. Smoking alters several hematological parameters like increase in plasma fibrinogen levels. Fibrinogen is an acute phase reactant in the pathogenesis of atherosclerosis and thrombosis. Increase in fibrinogen increases blood viscosity. Cigarette smoke contains around 43 known carcinogens and about 400 known toxins. Nicotine, tar, carbon monoxide, formaldehyde, ammonia, methane, hydrogen cyanide, arsenic, DDT, cadmium, etc., are present in cigarette smoke. The "side stream" smoke, which arises from the burning tip of the cigarette, is more dangerous as it contains relatively higher concentrations of toxic components than "main stream" smoke (the smoke that directly enters the mouth). Side stream smoke is inhaled by passive smokers.

Deleterious Effects of Cigarette Smoking

- Tobacco smoke contains **ciliotoxins,** which destroy the cilia. Inhibition of ciliary activity leads to accumulation of secretions in the lung leading to chronic bronchitis and bronchiectasis. In this case, only coughing can remove the mucus and dust particles from the airways. This is the reason why *smokers often cough.*
- Carbon monoxide in smoke is injurious and decreases the O_2 carrying capacity of blood.
- Cigarette smoke contains very fine particles, <0.3 µm in size, which reaches the alveoli and cause **fibrosis** of lung.
- Smoke decrease surfactant secretion.
- Smoke destroys lung tissue, especially the inter-alveolar septa, causing a decrease in the surface area for gas exchange. This is due to accumulation of large quantities of elastases released by macrophages in lung, which destroy the lung tissue. Normally, these elastases are destroyed by α_1 **antitrypsin**. α_1-antitrypsin (AAT) is secreted by liver and released into circulation. Cigarette smoke inactivates α_1-antitrypsin leading to accumulation of elastases in large quantity leading to **emphysema**. All the above-mentioned factors impair oxygenation of blood in the lungs.
- Smoking leads to lung **cancer**. Carcinogens in cigarette smoke include tar, polynuclear hydrocarbons, nitrosamines, etc.
- Smoking produces coronary heart disease like angina, coronary thrombosis, etc.
- Cigarette smoke contains high concentration of various **free radicals** that are extremely reactive, leading to damage of almost all biological macromolecules. For example, it causes damage to cell membrane, polysaccharide depolymerization and DNA breaks leading to inhibition of protein and enzyme synthesis. All these lead to cell death or mutation and carcinogenesis.
- Chronic tobacco smoking lead to **tobacco amblyopia** (scotoma) caused by cyanide in tobacco smoke. It also leads to optic atrophy, psychosis, headache, vertigo, etc.
- Inhalation of cigarette smoke by pregnant ladies (either active or passive smoking) leads to fetal abnormalities and sudden infant death syndrome **(SIDS)**. SIDS is more common in newborns whose mothers smoked during pregnancy.
- Nicotine is the main addictive substance identified in cigarette smoke. Chronic smokers try to maintain the nicotine levels in their brain. In regular smokers, withdrawal symptoms and mood alterations are commonly observed on ceasing smoking.

- Nonsmokers exposed to passive smoke have a 25–30% rise in the risk of developing coronary vascular disease. About 28% of these are children.
- Cigarette smoke incapacitates alveolar macrophages.
- Noxious agents in cigarette smoke irritate the mucous linings of the respiratory tract, resulting in excess mucus production. This may partially obstruct the airways due to lack of ciliary action.

MULTIPLE CHOICE QUESTIONS

1. The intrapleural pressure is negative both during inspiration and expiration because:
   a. Intrapulmonary pressure is always negative
   b. Thoracic cage and lungs are elastic structures
   c. Transpulmonary pressure determines the negativity
   d. Surfactant prevents the collapse of lung

2. The following statements are true of intrapleural pressure, *except*:
   a. It is about –3 mm Hg at the start of inspiration
   b. It becomes +2 mm Hg at the end of normal expiration
   c. It is a measure of elastic recoil of lung
   d. Blood flow to left atrium is facilitated by negative intrapleural pressure

3. Surfactant is essential for:
   a. Keeping the alveoli moist
   b. Preventing the collapse of alveoli
   c. Diffusion of gases
   d. Maintaining alveolar PO_2

4. Surfactant acts by decreasing:
   a. Intrapleural pressure
   b. Intrathoracic pressure
   c. Surface tension
   d. Pleural fluid secretion

5. Lung alveoli are lined by all, *except*:
   a. Type I pneumocytes
   b. Type II pneumocytes
   c. Alveolar macrophages
   d. Endothelial cells

6. Surfactant is produced by:
   a. Type I pneumocytes
   b. Type II pneumocytes
   c. Alveolar macrophages
   d. Endothelial cells

7. Surfactant is made up of:
   a. Fibrin
   b. Mucoprotein
   c. Phospholipids
   d. Fibrinogen

8. The correct statement regarding pulmonary surfactant is:
   a. It is made of mucin
   b. Secreted by type I pneumocyte
   c. Maintain alveolar integrity
   d. Under electron microscopy, eosinophilic nodules are found

9. **Hyaline membrane contains:**
    a. Albumin b. Fibrin
    c. Globulin d. Leukocytes
10. **All the following statements regarding pulmonary surfactant are correct, *except*:**
    a. Secreted from 28th week of gestation
    b. In hyaline membrane disease deficiency occurs
    c. Therapeutic application seen
    d. It is made of mucin
11. **Surfactant production in fetal lungs starts at:**
    a. 28 weeks b. 32 weeks
    c. 34 weeks d. 36 weeks
12. **Alveolar surfactant is secreted by:**
    a. Pulmonary alveolar macrophages
    b. Granular pneumocytes type II
    c. Type I alveolar epithelial cells
    d. APUD cells in lung
13. **All statements regarding surfactant are true, *except*:**
    a. It is a lipoprotein
    b. It is produced by type II alveolar cells
    c. It is inhibited by cortisol in fetus
    d. Surfactant production is completed only by 8th month of intrauterine life
14. **False statement about intrapleural pressure is that:**
    a. It becomes more negative in Muller's maneuver
    b. It is negative due to elastic recoil of lung
    c. It is less negative than intra-alveolar pressure
    d. It is positive at mid-expiration
15. **The elastic recoil tendency of lungs is promoted by all the following, *except*:**
    a. Elastic fibers in alveolar wall
    b. Collagen fibers in the alveolar wall
    c. Surfactant lining the alveoli
    d. Alveolar surface tension
16. **All the following are true of the action of external intercostal muscle except that it brings about:**
    a. Active expiration
    b. Decrease in intrapleural pressure
    c. Elevation of ribs
    d. Forward thrust of sternum
17. **All the following may lead to respiratory distress syndrome in new born, *except*:**
    a. Prematurity
    b. Glucocorticoid deficiency
    c. Maternal diabetes mellitus
    d. Hyperthyroidism
18. **The following are muscles of inspiration, *except*:**
    a. External intercostal muscle
    b. Internal intercostal muscle
    c. Pectoralis major
    d. Sternocleidomastoid
19. **Alveoli are lined by:**
    a. Simple squamous epithelium
    b. Ciliated columnar epithelium
    c. Cuboidal epithelium
    d. Stratified squamous epithelium
20. **The following statements are true of surfactant, *except*:**
    a. It is a mixture of lipids and proteins
    b. It causes alveolar collapse
    c. It is decreased in hyaline membrane disease
    d. It prevents pulmonary edema
21. **During initial part of inspiration all the following are present, *except*:**
    a. Intrapulmonary pressure falls
    b. Intrathoracic pressure rises
    c. Intra-abdominal pressure rises
    d. Partial pressure of oxygen in the dead space increases
22. **The period of gestation in weeks from which surfactant system becomes functional:**
    a. 24 b. 28
    c. 32 d. 34
23. **The intrapleural pressure at the end of deep inspiration is:**
    a. –4 mm Hg b. +4 mm Hg
    c. –18 mm Hg d. +18 mm Hg
24. **Effort during normal respiration is done due to:**
    a. Lung elasticity
    b. Respiratory air passages
    c. Alveolar air spaces
    d. Creating negative pleural pressure
25. **During the initial part of inspiration, which of the following does not occur?**
    a. Intrapulmonary pressure falls
    b. Intrathoracic pressure rises
    c. Intra-abdominal pressure rises
    d. The partial pressure of O_2 in the dead space rises
26. **Surfactant lining the lung alveoli:**
    a. Increase the surface tension of alveolar fluid
    b. Decrease the compliance of lungs
    c. Has increasingly more effect when the lungs are more inflated
    d. Is decreased when pulmonary blood flow is interrupted
27. **Type II pulmonary epithelial cells secrete:**
    a. Mucus b. Heparin
    c. Surfactant d. Polypeptides
28. **In normal adult, the alveoli are kept dry because of:**
    a. Residual volume
    b. Surfactant
    c. Hydrostatic pressure
    d. Tidal volume
29. **In cigarette smoking surfactant is:**
    a. Increased
    b. Decreased
    c. Unaltered
    d. Increase followed by decrease

30. Smoking causes all the following, *except*:
    a. Increase in ciliary motility
    b. Cellular hyperplasia
    c. Increased mucus secretion
    d. Decrease in surfactant

31. Pulmonary surfactant reduces the following, *except*:
    a. The filtration forces from pulmonary capillaries
    b. The surface tension in the lungs
    c. Transpulmonary pressure
    d. Alveolar radius

32. Muscle of expiration is:
    a. Diaphragm
    b. Internal intercostal
    c. External intercostal
    d. Sternocleidomastoid

33. All the following may lead to respiratory distress syndrome in new born, *except*:
    a. Prematurity
    b. Glucocorticoid deficiency
    c. Maternal diabetes mellitus
    d. Hyperthyroidism

34. The value of intrapleural pressure in normal quiet respiration is:
    a. 2–6 mm Hg below atmospheric pressure
    b. 2–6 mm Hg above atmospheric pressure
    c. 1 mm Hg above atmospheric pressure
    d. 1 mm Hg below atmospheric pressure

35. The part of the lung that does not take part in gas exchange is:
    a. Terminal bronchiole
    b. Respiratory bronchiole
    c. Alveolar duct
    d. Atrium

36. The most important muscle of inspiration is:
    a. Diaphragm
    b. External intercostal
    c. Serratus anterior
    d. Sternocleidomastoid

37. Surfactant is present in amniotic fluid at:
    a. 34 weeks
    b. 32 weeks
    c. 28 weeks
    d. 36 weeks

38. The muscle that actively contract during normal quiet expiration:
    a. Internal intercostal muscle
    b. Abdominal muscles
    c. Sternocleidomastoid
    d. No muscles actively contract

ANSWERS

1. b	2. b	3. b	4. c	5. d
6. b	7. c	8. c	9. b	10. d
11. a	12. b	13. c	14. d	15. c
16. a	17. d	18. b	19. a	20. b
21. b	22. c	23. c	24. d	25. b
26. d	27. c	28. b	29. b	30. a
31. a	32. b	33. d	34. a	35. a
36. a	37. c	38. d		

Methods of Study of Respiratory Movements

CHAPTER 35

LEARNING OBJECTIVES
- Describe the lung volumes and capacities
- Draw and label a normal spirogram
- Explain the significance of timed vital capacity
- Differentiate between anatomical and physiological dead space
- Explain compliance of lungs

INTRODUCTION

PY6.2: Describe the mechanics of normal respiration, pressure changes during ventilation, lung volume and capacities, alveolar surface tension, compliance, airway resistance, ventilation, V/P ratio, diffusion capacity of lungs.

Respiratory volumes and capacities are an important aspect of pulmonary function testing because they can provide information about the physical condition of the lungs. The lung volumes vary depending on the depth of respiration, gender, age, body size and in certain respiratory diseases. Taller people, people living at high altitudes, athletes and singers have larger lung volumes. Shorter people and obese individuals have smaller volumes. Exposure to polluted air affects FVC and FEV_1 even in healthy individuals. Lung capacity can be expanded by flexibility exercises like yoga, breathing exercises and physical activity.

There are different techniques to measure lung volumes and capacities. Spirometry is one of the primary pulmonary function tests used to assess the health of the respiratory system by the pulmonologists. It is also used for follow up. There are direct methods and indirect methods to study respiratory movements. Direct methods are usually carried out in experimental animals.

DIRECT TECHNIQUE TO STUDY RESPIRATORY MOVEMENTS

The respiratory movements can be directly studied by cannulating the trachea.

INDIRECT TECHNIQUES

- Stethography
- Fluoroscopy
- Spirometry

Stethography or Pneumography

Stethography is the process of recording the respiratory movements in man indirectly. The instrument is called stethograph and the recording obtained is called stethogram. A corrugated rubber tube covered with canvas, closed at both ends is tied around thoracic cage of the individual at the level of nipple. To the cavity of the stethograph is connected a pressure tubing and this tube is connected to a Marey's tambour which has a cup-shaped structure covered with a thin diaphragm and a tube. The pressure tubing is connected to the tubular portion. Over the diaphragm of the Marey's tambour is placed a movable lever.

During inspiration, the corrugated rubber tube elongates and pressure is decreased and the thin diaphragm moves downwards and an upstroke is recorded. In expiration, diaphragm moves up and a down stroke is recorded. Now these movements can be recorded in a physiograph using appropriate transducers.

Fluoroscopy

Chest fluoroscopy is an imaging test that uses X-rays to look at how well the lungs, diaphragm and other parts of the chest are working. It is used for the evaluation of pulmonary function for clinical purposes. A fluoroscope consists of a fluorescent screen and an X-ray beam passing through the body. Continuous images are displayed on a monitor. Since this procedure uses X-ray technology, there is some radiation exposure. So the standard method used to assess lung volumes and capacities is spirometry.

Spirometry

- *Technique*: Spirometry
- *Device*: Spirometer
- *Record*: Spirogram
- Hutchinson devised spirometer in 1846.

Two types of spirometers are:
1. Dry type or bellow type
2. Wet type or water filled type

Procedure of Wet Type

The subject is asked to breathe normally through a mouth piece connected to the spirometer and the volume of air that is taken in or given out with each normal breath is recorded on the graduated paper provided in the spirometer. The subject is then asked to inhale maximally and then to exhale rapidly and completely into the mouthpiece. It should be taken care that the subject's nose is clipped properly so that he breathes only through the mouthpiece (**Fig. 35.1**).

Using spirometer, we can determine the volume of air taken in, given out, etc., at various stages of respiration.

A graph is recorded on a graph paper with time on the X-axis and volume in mL on the Y-axis. *During inspiration, an upstroke is recorded, and during expiration, a down stroke is recorded.*

Vitalograph is a portable and easy-to-use instrument used to measure forced expiratory volume in one second (FEV_1) and forced vital capacity (FVC). It provides accurate and effective monitoring of lung function for conditions like COPD, cystic fibrosis, etc.

LUNG VOLUMES AND CAPACITIES

Lung volumes and capacities are divided into:
❖ Static lung volumes and capacities
❖ Dynamic lung volumes and capacities

Static Lung Volumes and Capacities (Fig. 35.2)

Lung Volumes

❖ Tidal volume (TV)
❖ Inspiratory reserve volume (IRV)
❖ Expiratory reserve volume (ERV)
❖ Residual volume (RV)

Lung Capacities

❖ Vital capacity (VC)
❖ Inspiratory capacity (IC)
❖ Functional residual capacity (FRC)
❖ Total lung capacity (TLC)
❖ Closing volume and closing capacity (CV)

Dynamic Lung Volumes

❖ Maximum voluntary ventilation (MVV)
❖ Forced expiratory volume or timed vital capacity (FEV or TVC)
❖ Maximum mid-expiratory flow rate (MMEFR)
❖ Peak expiratory flow rate (PEFR)

Static Lung Volumes

Static lung volumes are lung volumes which do not overlap and whose values do not change with time. (The lung capacities are various combinations of the four primary lung volumes: TV, IRV, ERV, and RV)

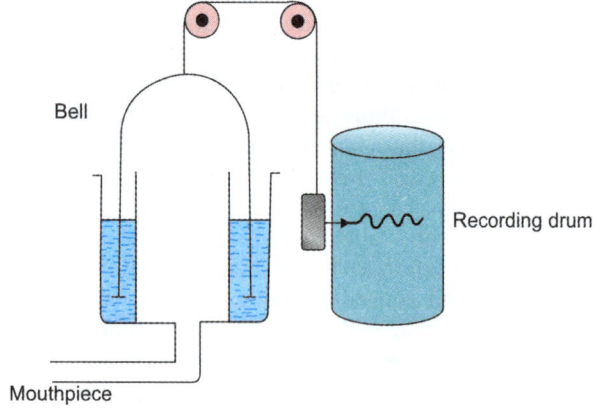

Fig. 35.1: Spirometer (wet type).

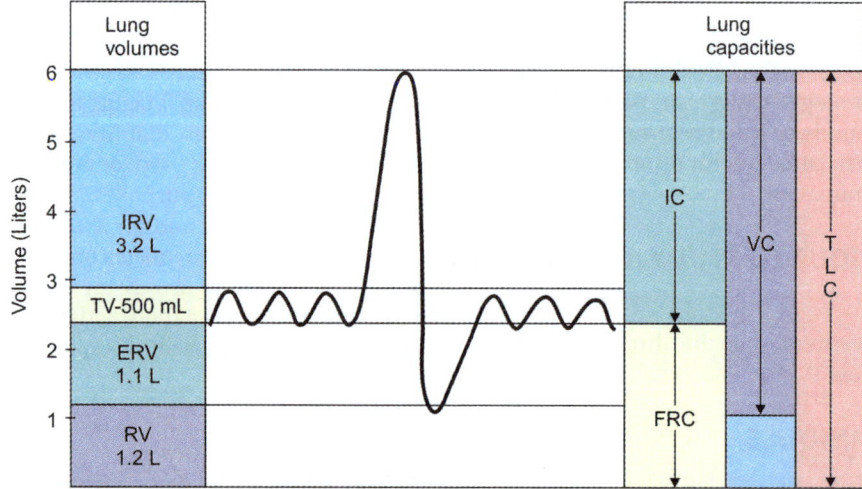

Fig. 35.2: Spirogram.

(TV: tidal volume; IRV: inspiratory reserve volume; IC: inspiratory capacity; FRC: functional residual capacity; VC: vital capacity; TLC: total lung capacity; ERV: expiratory reserve volume; RV: residual volume)

Tidal Volume

Volume of air inspired or expired during each normal breath is tidal volume. Normal values:
Newborn—15-20 mL
Males—600 mL
Females—450 mL

Inspiratory Reserve Volume

Extra volume of air that can be inspired over and above the normal tidal volume by taking a deep inspiration is called inspiratory reserve volume.

Normal Value—3–3.2 L

The magnitude of the IRV depends on the following factors:
- The greater the lung volume after inspiration, the smaller will be the IRV
- Decrease in compliance decreases IRV
- If the respiratory muscles are weak, the IRV will be less
- Pain associated with inspiration decreases IRV
- Skeletal disorders like joint stiffness due to arthritis, kyphoscoliosis, etc., decrease IRV
- IRV is less in the lying down posture than in the erect standing posture

Expiratory Reserve Volume

Extra volume of air that can be expired by forceful expiration after the end of a normal expiration is expiratory reserve volume. In addition to the above-mentioned factors, it also depends on the strength of abdominal muscles.

Normal value—1.1 L

Residual Volume

The volume of air remaining in the lungs even after the most forceful expiration is residual volume. This volume cannot be measured by spirometry.

Normal value—1.2 L

The residual volume can be removed from the lungs only by surgery or by collapsing the lungs. It is much greater in emphysema.

Functions of Residual Volume

- RV acts as a **buffer** in between breaths to aerate the pulmonary capillary blood. If the RV was not there, the composition of blood leaving the lungs would oscillate widely with a high PO_2 at the peak of inspiration and a very low PO_2 at the end of expiration.
- **Medicolegal importance**: To detect whether the baby was stillborn (born dead) or born alive. If the baby has taken the first breath, **minimal air volume** will be there and lungs float in water. Some amount of air remains in the lungs even after collapse of lung because proximal airways collapse before the distal airways, trapping air. The resulting minimal air volume is about 10% of the total lung capacity. If the baby was stillborn, lungs will be solid because they contain no air and sink down.
- RV prevents the lungs from collapsing at very low lung volumes. If an airway collapses, unusually high pressure is needed to re-inflate it, which requires very high energy-expenditure.

Minimal Volume

Opening the thoracic cavity allows the intrapleural pressure to equal the atmospheric pressure forcing out some of the residual volume. Even though the lungs are collapsed, the lung volume is not zero because the proximal airways collapse before the distal ones trapping air. The air remaining is called **minimal air volume**. Minimal volume is approximately 10% of TLC, i.e., ~500 mL.

Lung Capacities

Lung capacities are combinations of specific lung volumes.

Inspiratory Capacity

The volume of air that can be inspired by a forceful effort after a normal expiration is inspiratory capacity.

$$IC = TV + IRV = 0.5 + 3 = 3.5 \text{ L}$$

Functional Residual Capacity

Volume of air remaining in the lungs after a normal expiration is functional residual capacity. This is also called resting volume of lungs.

$$FRC = ERV + RV = 1.1 + 1.2 = 2.3 \text{ L}$$

Importance of FRC

- This gas helps in the continuous exchange of gases between lungs and blood in between two breaths.
- It prevents marked rise or fall in concentration of blood O_2 and CO_2 levels in between breaths.
- If FRC is increased, it means that lungs are hyperinflated as in emphysema, partial obstruction to airways, old age, etc.

Total Lung Capacity

Volume of air in the lungs after a maximum inspiration is the total lung capacity. It is the sum of all the four lung volumes. It includes the air in the nasopharynx, trachea, smaller airways, and alveoli.

$$TLC = TV + IRV + ERV + RV = 6 \text{ L}$$

Total lung capacity is decreased in:
- Pulmonary edema
- Pneumothorax
- Pulmonary congestion
- Lung tumors

Vital Capacity

The volume of air that can be expired rapidly and forcefully after a maximum inspiration is called vital capacity.

$$VC = IRV + TV + ERV = 3 + 0.5 + 1.1 = 4.6 \text{ L}$$

Vital capacity is frequently measured clinically as an index of pulmonary function since it can be measured using simple spirometer.

Factors Affecting Vital Capacity

- Age—vital capacity is maximal in young adults.
- Sex—VC is more in males than in females. (All lung volumes and capacities are about 20-25% less in women than in men) Males—4.8 L Females—3.2 L
- Build and physical training—VC will be more in well-built individuals and in athletes.
- Height—VC varies with height In males—height in cm × 25 mL
  In females—height in cm × 20 mL Athletes—height in cm × 29 mL
- Body surface area—VC can be calculated from body surface area
  In males—2.6 L/m² body surface area
  In females—2.1 L/m² body surface area
  In athletes—2.8 L/m² body surface area
  Vital index: Vital capacity related to the body surface area is called vital index.

$$\text{Vital index} = \frac{\text{Vital capacity}}{\text{Body surface area}}$$

$$= \frac{4.6\,L}{1.8\,m^2} = 2.6\,L/m^2 \text{ body surface area}$$

- Posture—VC is maximal when the person is seated in a slightly reclined posture. VC is decreased in lying down and standing posture.
- Other factors affecting VC are:
  - Strength or power of the respiratory muscles
  - Airway resistance
  - Compliance of lung
  - Elasticity of lungs

Variations in Vital Capacity

Physiological decrease: In pregnancy due to inability of diaphragm to move down satisfactorily, there will be a reduction in VC.

Pathological decrease:
- Neurological diseases affecting muscles of respiration like neuritis, poliomyelitis, etc.
- Diseases of muscles like myasthenia gravis.
- Deformities of thoracic cage like kyphosis, scoliosis, etc.
- Diseases of lung like emphysema, fibrosis, pneumonia, tuberculosis, etc.
- Diseases of pleura like pleural effusion, pneumothorax, etc.
- Diseases of heart like congestive cardiac failure (CCF), pericardial effusion, etc.
- Diseases of abdominal cavity like ascites, large tumors, etc. Ascites is collection of fluid in the peritoneal cavity.

Importance of Vital Capacity

- Vital capacity has prognostic value during treatment of a respiratory problem. In patients with pulmonary disease, the physician periodically monitors VC to follow the progress of the disease. If the vital capacity increases with treatment it means that the patient is responding to the treatment.
- We can assess the progress of a chronic disease like emphysema. If there is a rapid reduction in vital capacity it means that the disease is rapidly progressing and the mortality is higher.
- VC is used for assessing physical fitness (sportsmen, health checkups in schools, recruitment in police, etc.).
- Total lung capacity can be calculated from vital capacity.
  - 15–34 years $\quad \dfrac{VC}{0.8} = TLC$
  - 35–50 years $\quad \dfrac{VC}{0.75}$
  - 50–70 years $\quad \dfrac{VC}{0.65}$

TLC, FRC and RV cannot be measured using an ordinary spirometer since RV cannot be expelled out.

Measurement of RV, FRC, and TLC

The methods are:
- N_2 wash out method
- Closed circuit helium dilution method
- Plethysmography

In **closed circuit helium (He) dilution method**, ask the subject to breathe 10% He from a spirometer of known volume from the end of maximum expiration for 7–10 minutes. Now the He concentration in the spirometer and lung becomes the same. He is insoluble and inert and so does not enter blood.

Let the initial volume of spirometer be V_1
Initial concentration of He in spirometer C_1
Amount of He in spirometer = $C_1 V_1$
Initial volume of air in the lungs—V_2
Initial concentration of He in the lungs—0
Final concentration of He in lungs or spirometer—C_2
Final amount of He in lungs and spirometer = $C_2 (V_1 + V_2)$

$C_2 (V_1 + V_2) = C_1 V_1$
$C_2 V_1 + C_2 V_2 = C_1 V_1$
$C_2 V_2 = C_1 V_1 - C_2 V_1 = V_1 (C_1 - C_2)$

$$V_2 = \frac{V_1 (C_1 - C_2)}{C_2}$$

Here, V_2 is the initial volume of air in the lung, which is the **residual volume** because the subject breathed He from the end of maximum expiration, i.e., only the residual volume is remaining in the lungs at the beginning of the procedure.

We can find out FRC if the experiment is started at the end of normal expiration when the functional residual volume will be present in the lungs. TLC can be calculated if the experiment is started at the end of maximum inspiration.

Dynamic Lung Volumes and Capacities

Dynamic lung volumes quantify time rate of gas flow along respiratory tree.

Significance

- Dynamic volumes and capacities have greatest application in conditions with impaired expiratory flow like emphysema, bronchial asthma, etc.
  - Helps in clinical evaluation of dyspnea and pulmonary disability.

Maximum Ventilatory Volume or Maximum Voluntary Ventilation or Maximum Breathing Capacity (MBC)

Maximum volume of air that can be moved into or out of the lungs in 1 minute by maximum voluntary effort is called MVV. It is the maximum volume of air that can be breathed rapidly and deeply for 1 minute.

Normal value in healthy adult is 125–170 L/min.

Drawback of the technique is that it produces giddiness and visual blackout due to washing out of CO_2.

MVV is decreased in emphysema and asthma.

Forced Expiratory Volume or Timed Vital Capacity

Forced vital capacity (FVC) is the largest volume of air that can be expired forcefully after a maximal inspiratory effort. Timed vital capacity is the fraction of forced vital capacity that is expired during the first second (FEV_1), during the first 2 seconds (FEV_2) and during the first 3 seconds (FEV_3) of forced expiration. For example, TVC_1 or FEV_1 is the fraction of vital capacity that is expired in the first second of forced expiration (**Fig. 35.3**). If the amount of air that is expired in the first second of forced expiration after a maximum inspiration is 3.3 L and that expired in the first two seconds is 3.7 L, then TVC_1 or FEV_1 = 3.3 L and TVC_2 or FEV_2 = 3.7 L, respectively. A maximal expiratory effort is made during this maneuver.

TVC_1%

TVC_1% is the fraction of vital capacity expelled at the end of first second of forced expiration expressed in percentage.

$$TVC_1\% = \frac{TVC_1}{FVC} \times 100$$

If TVC_1 is 3.32 L and vital capacity 4 L then

$$TVC_1\% = \frac{3.32}{4} \times 100 = 83\%$$

TVC_2% = 93%
TVC_3% = 97%

These are the values recorded from a normal healthy person using spirometer. It takes about 4 seconds to expel the whole of the vital capacity.

Importance of TVC or FEV

- FEV_1 is a valuable measurement for monitoring a variety of pulmonary disorders and the effectiveness of treatment.
- In the early stages of many chronic diseases like emphysema, the VC may remain within normal limits but the TVC shows abnormality. So, it helps in the early detection of diseases like emphysema.
- TVC is a very important index to differentiate between obstructive and restrictive diseases. Restrictive diseases are diseases that restrict the movement of either thoracic cage or lungs like kyphosis, scoliosis, fibrosis of lung, etc. In restrictive diseases, the total vital capacity will be reduced, but TVC will be normal (**Fig. 35.3**). Obstructive diseases are due to obstruction of airways like bronchial asthma.

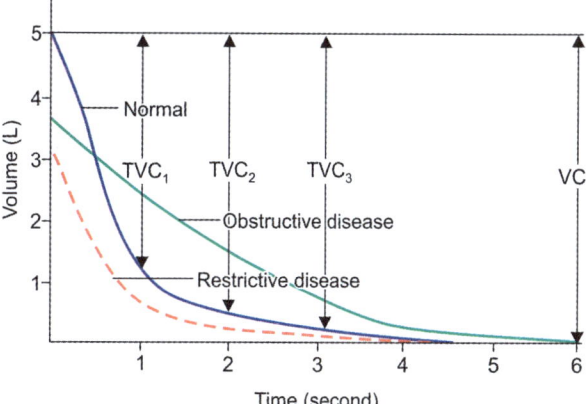

Fig. 35.3: Timed vital capacity (TVC) in a normal subject, in obstructive lung disease and in restrictive disease.

In obstructive diseases, total vital capacity may be reduced or sometimes normal, but TVC_1% is reduced very much. *If TVC_1% is reduced to 40%, the person will develop dyspnea.*

Peak Expiratory Flow Rate

This is the flow rate at the peak of forced vital capacity. It is measured using **Wright's peak expiratory flow meter** and electronic spirometer.

Normal value—400–600 L/min

The value depends on the caliber of large airways and strength of respiratory muscles.

Maximum Mid-expiratory Flow Rate or Forced Expiratory Flow Rate (FEF 25–75%)

The average rate of airflow during the middle two quarters (middle ½) of the volume segment of forced vital capacity (i.e., from 25 to 75% of the volume) is maximum mid expiratory flow rate. It helps to assess small airway function.

Normal value—200–400 L/min.

Various lung disorders can be diagnosed by comparing the obtained values of lung volumes and capacities with the normal predicted value depending on sex, age, height, etc.

■ PULMONARY VENTILATION AND ALVEOLAR VENTILATION

Ventilation is the cyclic process by which there is mass movement of air in and out of the lungs through nasal passages or mouth. Ventilation is divided into two:
1. Pulmonary ventilation
2. Alveolar ventilation

Pulmonary Ventilation or Respiratory Minute Volume (RMV) or Minute Ventilation

Pulmonary ventilation is the amount of air that is taken in or given out during quiet normal respiration for 1 minute.
Pulmonary ventilation = Tidal volume × Respiratory rate
= 500 × 12 = 6 L/min

Breathing Reserve

Breathing reserve indicates the reserve capacity of the lungs.
Breathing reserve = Maximum breathing capacity (MBC) – Pulmonary ventilation (PV)
= 170 L/min – 6 L/min = 164 L/min

Dyspneic Index

$$\text{Dyspneic index} = \frac{(\text{MBC} - \text{PV})}{\text{MBC}} \times 100$$

$$= \frac{164}{170} \times 100 = 97\%$$

When dyspneic index is <70%, there will be symptoms and signs of dyspnea.

Alveolar Ventilation

Alveolar ventilation is the volume of fresh air entering the respiratory zone in 1 minute. The physiologically significant part of pulmonary ventilation is alveolar ventilation because it represents the amount of fresh air available for gas exchange.

Even though tidal volume is about 500 mL, only 350 mL takes part in gaseous exchange. The rest 150 mL present in the conducting zone or respiratory dead space does not take part in gas exchange.

Alveolar ventilation = (TV–RDS) × Respiratory rate (RR)
= (500 – 150 mL) 12/min
= 350 × 12 = 4.2 L/min
So wasted ventilation = RR × Dead space air
= 12/min × 150 mL = 1800 mL/min

■ RESPIRATORY DEAD SPACE

*The portion of tidal volume that does not take part in gas exchange is **respiratory dead space (RDS)**.* It is divided into:
- Anatomical dead space
- Physiological dead space

In normal subjects both are nearly the same. But in patients with lung disease the physiological dead space will be larger due to inequality of blood flow and ventilation in the lungs.

Anatomical Dead Space

Anatomical dead space (ADS) is the volume of air in the respiratory passage from nose to the terminal bronchiole (conducting zone) which does not take part in gas exchange. Normal value is 150 mL and it is approximately equal to the body weight in pounds.

Physiological Dead Space

Physiological dead space is the volume of air in the respiratory system that is not equilibrating with blood. It includes anatomical dead space plus the volume of air in the alveoli which does not take part in gas exchange.
Physiological dead space = Anatomical dead space + Alveolar dead space

Alveolar dead space is the air in the non-functional alveoli, i.e., in the under-perfused or non-perfused alveoli and over ventilated alveoli. Non-perfused alveoli do not receive pulmonary capillary blood and the air in these alveoli contributes to the alveolar dead space, e.g., pulmonary embolism. The volume of air that ventilates alveoli in excess of the volume required to oxygenate the blood in the pulmonary capillaries contributes to over-ventilation. This air also contributes to alveolar dead space.

Normally alveolar dead space air is about 5–10 mL.

Increase in physiological dead space is seen in pulmonary embolism and in emphysema as seen in chronic obstructive pulmonary disease (COPD). In emphysema, there is loss of elasticity of lung which decreases elastic recoil leading to hyperinflation of lung. This leads to increase in alveolar dead space.

Variations in Dead Space

- *Age:* As age advances, there is increase in anatomical dead space (ADS) due to loss of elasticity of respiratory system. In old age, anatomical dead space increases to 200 mL from 150 mL.
- *Sex:* In females ADS is less than in males due to decrease in body size. In adult female, ADS is only 100 mL.
- *Posture:* ADS is decreased in lying down posture.
- *Phases of respiration:* In inspiration there is increase in dead space, and in expiration there is decrease in ADS volume.
- *Position of neck:* Dead space is less when neck is fully flexed and chin depressed than when neck is fully extended.
- *Body weight:* ADS in adults in mL is approximately equal to the weight of the subject in pounds.
- In bronchoconstriction, ADS is decreased.
- Tracheostomy decreases ADS.
- Emphysema and exercise increase dead space volume.
- Physiological dead space is increased in COPD and pulmonary embolism.

Methods of Determination of Dead Space

Anatomical Dead Space

Single Breath Method or Fowler's Method

Principle

A gas analyzer known as **nitrogen meter** is used. Flow rate and concentration of N_2 in inspired air and expired air are obtained.

Procedure

At mid inspiration, the subject is asked to take a deep breath of pure O_2 and then to breathe out slowly and evenly into a N_2 meter. The N_2 meter analyses the volume flow rate and concentration of N_2. A graph is plotted with N_2 concentration in percentage on the Y-axis and volume of expired air on the X-axis (**Fig. 35.4**).

Four phases are seen in the graph (**Fig. 35.4**):
1. Phase I—the initial gas exhaled is the gas that filled the dead space and contains no N_2.
2. Phase II—this part contains a mixture of dead space air and alveolar air.
3. Phase III—pure alveolar air come out and a plateau phase is seen called alveolar plateau.
4. Phase IV—during this phase, the N_2 content of expired air increases and the graph goes up.

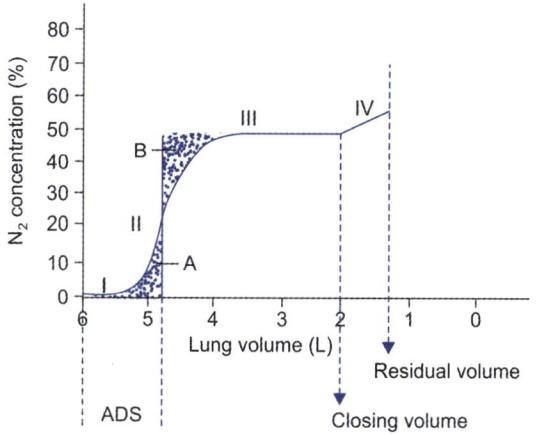

Fig. 35.4: Single-breath N_2 curve for the determination of anatomical dead space (ADS).

The gas in the upper portion of the lung is richer in N_2 than the gas in the lower dependent portions because the alveoli in the upper portions are more distended at the start of inspiration of O_2, and the N_2 in them is less diluted with O_2.

The dead space volume is found out by drawing a vertical line in phase II of the above graph such that area A is equal to area B. The dead space air is the volume exhaled from peak of inspiration up to the vertical line in phase II. This point is the demarcating point between the gas exchange zone and conducting zone. So the above experiment determines only the anatomical dead space.

Closing Volume

Closing volume is the lung volume above residual volume at which airways in the lower dependent parts of the lung begin to close off because of the lesser transmural pressure in these areas. The intrapleural pressure is more negative at the apex than at the base.

In normal young adults, closing volume is 10% of vital capacity.
In old age, it becomes 40% of vital capacity.
Closing volume is more in smokers.

Physiological Dead Space Using Bohr's Equation Principle

Volume of expired air is equal to the sum of dead space air and alveolar air.
Nitrogen or carbon dioxide is taken.

$$V_D = \frac{V_E (PaCO_2 - P_ECO_2)}{PaCO_2}$$

V_D – Dead space volume
V_E – Volume of expired air which is equal to tidal volume
P_ECO_2 – Partial pressure of CO_2 in expired air
$PaCO_2$ – Partial pressure of CO_2 in arterial blood

Sample Calculations

❖ Calculate alveolar ventilation from the given data:
 Wasted ventilation—2250 mL
 Respiratory rate—15/min
 Tidal volume—450 mL
Ans:
 Dead space volume = $\frac{2250}{15}$ = 150 mL
 Alveolar ventilation = (TV–RDS) RR
  = (450–150) 15
  = 300 mL × 15/min
  = 4500 mL/min

❖ Calculate the dead space from the following data:
 Respiratory rate-12/min
 Pulmonary ventilation-6 L/min
 $PaCO_2$ - 40 mm Hg
 $PECO_2$ - 28 mm Hg
Ans:
 TV = $\frac{6000}{12}$ = 500 mL
 VD = $500 \frac{(40-28)}{40}$ = 150 mL

COMPLIANCE (PRESSURE–VOLUME RELATIONSHIP)

❖ Static compliance
❖ Specific compliance

Static Compliance

Static compliance is defined as the change in lung volume per unit change in airway pressure. Compliance is a measure of the distensibility or the ease with which the lungs and thoracic wall can be expanded. The stiffer the lung, the less will be the compliance.

Compliance = $\frac{\Delta V}{\Delta P}$

Total compliance is the compliance of thorax and lungs together.

Total compliance = 0.13 L/cm of water, i.e., for every centimeter of water pressure change, the lungs and thorax expand by 0.13 L. This means that, to inspire a normal tidal volume of 500 mL, the intrapleural pressure must fall by about 4 cm H_2O.

When the compliance of thorax and lungs are taken separately, the value will be more than total compliance. At FRC, compliance of thorax alone is 0.22 L/cm of water and that of lungs alone is also 0.22 L/cm of water.

Measurement of Compliance

Total Compliance

Procedure: Nose is clipped and after maximum expiration, the subject is asked to inspire 50 mL of air from the spirometer through a mouth piece. Close the valve in the mouth piece in front of the manometer and allow the respiratory muscles to relax. The intrapulmonary pressure is measured. Repeat the procedure for every 50 mL increments (**Fig. 35.5**).

Plot a graph with volume on the Y-axis and pressure on the X-axis. This is the **relaxation pressure curve** of the total

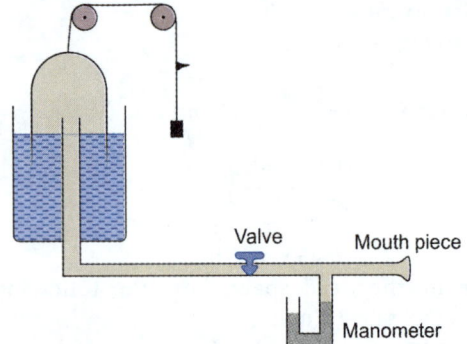

Fig. 35.5: Adjustment of spirometer to record relaxation pressure curve.

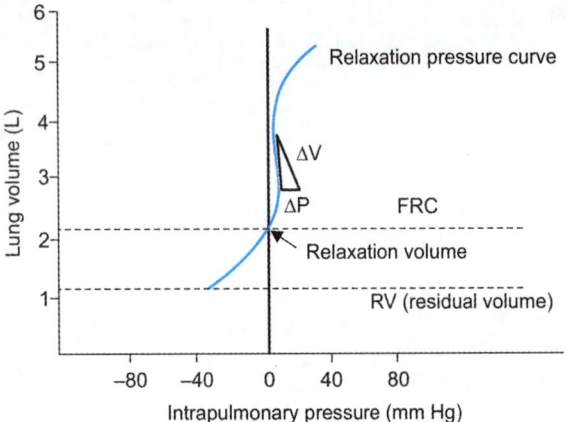

Fig. 35.6: Relation between intrapulmonary pressure and volume.

respiratory system. Compliance is measured in the pressure range where the relaxation pressure curve is steepest.

Relaxation volume: In the graph shown in **Figure 35.6**, pressure is zero at a volume which corresponds to FRC. This is **relaxation volume**. Pressure is positive at volumes greater than FRC and pressure is negative at volumes lesser than FRC.

Compliance of Lung Alone

Volume changes are plotted against transpulmonary pressure changes, i.e., intraesophageal pressure changes are recorded during inspiration and expiration. Lung is an elastic organ. The compliance of lungs varies inversely with lung volume. At FRC, lungs are normally very compliant.

To produce same volume more pressure is required in inspiration than in expiration. For the same pressure, inspiratory compliance curve lags behind expiratory curve and hence a **hysteresis loop** is obtained (**Fig. 35.7**). Slope of AB gives lung compliance. The difference between the pressure-volume curve for inflation and the curve for deflation is called hysteresis.

Compliance of Chest Wall

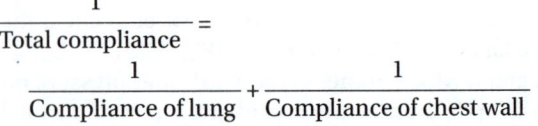

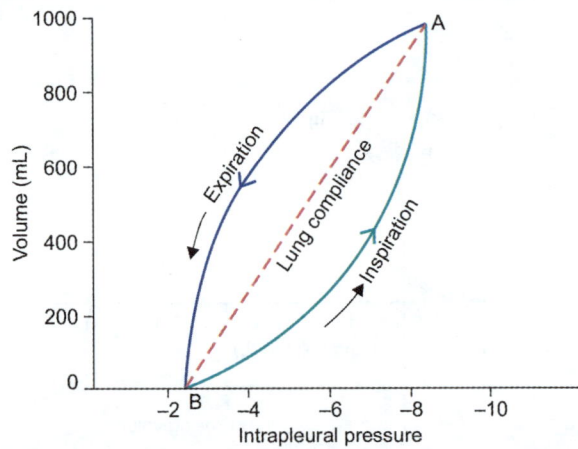

Fig. 35.7: Hysteresis loop. Change in volume per unit change in intrapleural pressure. Dashed line AB represents lung compliance.

$$\frac{1}{0.13} = \frac{1}{0.22} = \frac{1}{C}$$

$$\frac{1}{C} = \frac{1}{0.13} - \frac{1}{0.22}$$

$$= 0.2 \text{ L/cm of water}$$

Factors Affecting Compliance

- **Lung volume:** An individual with only one lung has ½ the DV for a given DP. Lung compliance is volume dependent.
- **Phases of respiration:** Compliance is slightly greater when measured during deflation than when measured during inflation.

Variations in Lung Compliance

Total compliance is decreased in:
- Restrictive diseases of the thorax like kyphosis, scoliosis, etc.
- Fibrosis of respiratory muscles
- Obesity

Lung compliance is decreased in diseases of lung like:
- Pulmonary edema
- Pleural effusion
- Atelectasis or collapse of lung
- Surfactant deficiency
- Pneumothorax
- Lobectomy of lung

Compliance is increased in conditions due to loss of elasticity as in:
- Old age
- Emphysema, where there is destruction of alveolar septal tissue

Specific Compliance

Compliance of a lung depends on its size. Since compliance varies with lung volume, specific compliance is usually measured. Specific compliance is the compliance per unit volume of lung

$$\text{Compliance} = \frac{\text{Lung volume}}{\text{Pressure}}$$

$$\text{Specific compliance} = \frac{\text{Lung compliance}}{\text{Lung volume}}$$

For example, the lung compliance was calculated to be 0.2 L/cm of water in a person. In this case if the person inhaled 1 L of air, the specific compliance will be 0.2/1 = 0.2.

If the compliance of the same person is calculated after removing one lung it will be 0.1 L/cm of water because the volume of air inhaled now will only be 0.5 L. But if the specific compliance is calculated in the same person it will be 0.1/0.5 = 0.2. This shows that the distensibility of the remaining lung is normal as in the initial case and lung volume is not interfering with the compliance value.

■ WORK OF BREATHING

Work is required to move the lungs and chest wall. Work is done only in inspiration and forced expiration. No work is done in normal quiet expiration.

$$\begin{aligned}\text{Work} &= \text{Force} \times \text{Displacement} \\ &= \text{Pressure} \times \text{Volume}\end{aligned}$$

During inspiration, all dimensions of thorax increase and certain amount of work has to be done by the respiratory muscles to overcome three factors. Work done is divided into three:
1. Compliance work or elastic work (65%)
2. Tissue resistance work (7%)
3. Airway resistance work (28%)

Compliance Work
Compliance work is done to overcome elastic resistance, i.e., work done in stretching the elastic tissues of chest wall and lungs (**Fig. 35.8**).

Tissue Resistance Work
Tissue resistance work is done to overcome inelastic tissue resistance or viscous resistance, i.e., in moving inelastic tissues.

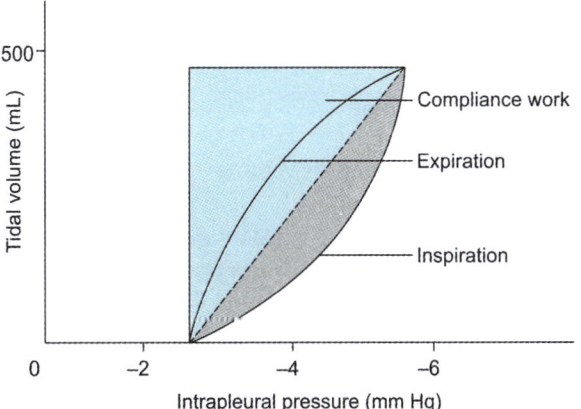

Fig. 35.8: Pressure and volume changes during quiet inspiration and expiration. Shaded area represents work done to overcome airway resistance and tissue resistance.

Airway Resistance Work
Airway resistance work is done to overcome frictional force of air moving through the respiratory passages.

Total work done in quiet breathing = 0.3–0.8 kg-m/min.
Work done is increased in:
❖ Exercise
❖ Labored breathing
❖ Obstruction to airflow as in bronchial asthma
❖ Pulmonary fibrosis and other lung diseases where compliance is decreased
❖ Congestive cardiac failure (CCF) associated with dyspnea and orthopnea

■ MULTIPLE CHOICE QUESTIONS

1. **Which among the following lung capacity is maximal?**
   a. IRV
   b. ERV
   c. IRV + ERV
   d. VC

2. **N_2 wash out method directly measures:**
   a. Total lung capacity
   b. Residual volume
   c. Functional residual capacity
   d. Dead space volume

3. **All the following tend to increase in old age, *except*:**
   a. Residual volume
   b. Systolic BP
   c. Pulse pressure
   d. Vital capacity

4. **Tidal volume is calculated by:**
   a. Inspiratory capacity minus inspiratory reserve volume
   b. Total lung capacity minus reserve volumes
   c. Functional residual capacity minus residual volume
   d. Vital capacity minus expiratory reserve volume

5. **Total lung capacity depends on:**
   a. Size of airway
   b. Closing volume
   c. Lung compliance
   d. Residual volume

6. **Functional residual capacity is:**
   a. Volume remaining after forced expiration
   b. Tidal volume + volume inspired forcefully
   c. Volume remaining after normal expiration
   d. Tidal volume + volume expired by forced expiration

7. **Volume of air taken in or given out during normal respiration is referred to as:**
   a. Inspiratory reserve volume
   b. Tidal volume
   c. Vital capacity
   d. Inspiratory capacity

8. **Functional residual capacity of lung is defined as:**
   a. Volume expired after normal expiration
   b. Volume remaining after forced expiration
   c. ERV + RV
   d. Tidal volume + volume inspired forcefully

9. Which of the following is used to measure the resistance to small airways?
   a. Vital capacity
   b. FEV_1
   c. Maximum mid expiratory flow rate
   d. Closing volume

10. Total alveolar ventilation volume is:
    a. 1.5 L/min
    b. 3.5 L/min
    c. 5 L/min
    d. 4.2 L/min

11. Calculate the alveolar ventilation per minute of a patient with respiratory rate 14/min, tidal volume 500 mL, dead space 150 mL and vital capacity 7000 mL.
    a. 4900 mL
    b. 2000 mL
    c. 7700 mL
    d. 7000 mL

12. Bohr's equation is applied to determine:
    a. Anatomical dead space
    b. Physiological dead space
    c. Residual volume
    d. Total lung capacity

13. Pulmonary function abnormalities in interstitial lung diseases include all the following, *except*:
    a. Reduced vital capacity
    b. Reduced FEV_1/FVC ratio
    c. Reduced diffusion capacity
    d. Reduced total lung capacity

14. Set of data which correctly defines restrictive lung disease is:
    a. Increased FRC, increased compliance of lung tissue
    b. Increased FEV_1/FVC, decreased compliance of lung tissue
    c. Decreased FEV_1/FVC, decreased compliance of lung tissue
    d. Increased TLC, decreased RV

15. In upper airway obstruction, all the following changes are seen, *except*:
    a. Decreased maximum breathing capacity
    b. Decreased residual volume
    c. Decreased FEV
    d. Decreased vital capacity

16. Pulmonary function change seen in emphysema is:
    a. Increased TLC
    b. Decreased RV
    c. Increased FEV_1
    d. Increased vital capacity

17. Which of the following tends to decrease with increasing age?
    a. Vital capacity
    b. Systolic BP
    c. Pulse pressure
    d. Residual volume

18. More resistance during expiration is due to:
    a. Increased compression of airway
    b. Due to change from linear to turbulent flow
    c. Saturation with moisture
    d. Increased rate of flow during expiration

19. Alveolar ventilation per minute is equal to:
    a. The volume of fresh air entering the alveoli per minute
    b. Total volume of air entering the respiratory tract per minute
    c. Product of tidal volume and respiratory rate per minute
    d. Maximum breathing capacity minus respiratory minute volume

20. Breathing reserve is equal to:
    a. The volume of fresh air entering the alveoli per minute
    b. Total volume of air entering the respiratory tract per minute
    c. Product of tidal volume and respiratory rate per minute
    d. Maximum breathing capacity minus respiratory minute volume

21. Pulmonary ventilation is equal to:
    a. The volume of fresh air entering the alveoli per minute
    b. Total volume of air entering the respiratory tract per breath
    c. Product of tidal volume and respiratory rate per minute
    d. Maximum breathing capacity minus respiratory minute volume

22. The tidal volume in an adult male at rest is:
    a. 0.5 L
    b. 1.2 L
    c. 2.5 L
    d. 4.2 L

23. Tidal volume is equal to:
    a. Pulmonary ventilation/respiratory rate
    b. Maximum breathing capacity/respiratory rate
    c. Alveolar ventilation/respiratory rate
    d. Pulmonary ventilation/dead space volume

24. Spirometer measures all the following, *except*:
    a. Tidal volume
    b. Vital capacity
    c. Expiratory reserve volume
    d. Functional residual capacity

25. Routine Spirometry measures all the following, *except*:
    a. Tidal volume
    b. Vital capacity
    c. Forced expiratory volume
    d. Residual volume

26. Dyspneic index is: (MVV-maximum voluntary ventilation; RMV-respiratory minute volume):
    a. MVV/RMV × 100
    b. MVV-RMV/MVV × 100
    c. RMV/MVV × 100
    d. MVV/RMV × 100

27. Dyspnea is felt when dyspneic index is:
    a. Less than 70%
    b. Less than 50%
    c. Less than 40%
    d. Less than 90%

28. Vital capacity is a measure of:
    a. Tidal volume + inspiratory reserve volume
    b. Tidal volume + inspiratory reserve volume + expiratory reserve volume
    c. Total lung capacity
    d. Expiratory reserve volume + residual volume
29. Normal value of $FEV_1\%$ in adult male is:
    a. 80%   b. 95%
    c. 65%   d. 50%
30. In COPD, all are affected, *except*:
    a. FEV
    b. Ratio of FEV to vital capacity
    c. FVC
    d. None
31. Respiratory minute volume in a normal person:
    a. 1.2 L/min   b. 2.1 L/min
    c. 4.2 L/min   d. 6 L/min
32. Normal functional residual capacity is:
    a. 0.05 L   b. 1.5 L
    c. 2.2 L   d. 4 L
33. Closing volume of lung determines:
    a. Distensibility of lung
    b. Residual volume
    c. Small airway resistance
    d. Dead space
34. The alveolar ventilation in an individual with tidal volume 600 mL, dead space volume 150 mL and respiratory rate 15/min is:
    a. 2.5 L/min   b. 4 L/min
    c. 6.75 L/min d. 9 L/min
35. The most important substance controlling alveolar ventilation is:
    a. Oxygen   b. Carbon dioxide
    c. 2–3-BPG   d. HCO_3
36. Vital capacity is:
    a. Tidal volume + expiratory reserve volume
    b. Tidal volume + inspiratory reserve volume
    c. Inspiratory reserve volume + expiratory reserve volume
    d. Tidal volume + inspiratory reserve volume + expiratory reserve volume
37. Compliance of lung is decreased in all the conditions, *except*:
    a. Fibrosis of lung   b. Emphysema
    c. Pulmonary edema   d. Kyphosis
38. In a normal adult, the ratio of physiological and anatomical dead space is:
    a. 2:1   b. 1:3
    c. 3:1   d. 1:1
39. Total vital capacity is decreased but timed vital capacity is normal in:
    a. Bronchial asthma   b. Scoliosis
    c. Chronic bronchitis d. COPD
40. The instrument used for measuring the vital capacity and FEV is:
    a. Wright peak flow meter
    b. Vitalograph
    c. Stethograph
    d. Carlens' catheter
41. Work done in quiet breathing is:
    a. 0.1 kg-m/min   b. 0.2 kg-m/min
    c. 0.5 kg-m/min   d. 2.5 kg-m/min
42. Total lung capacity in an adult is:
    a. 3–4 L   b. 5–6 L
    c. 6–7 L   d. 7–8 L
43. A person is having normal lung compliance and increased airway resistance, the most economical way of breathing for him:
    a. Rapid and deep   b. Rapid and shallow
    c. Slow and deep   d. Slow and shallow
44. Anatomical dead space is the:
    a. Volume of air in the conducting passages of the respiratory tract
    b. Air that ventilates non-perfused alveoli
    c. Volume of air present in the lungs after maximum expiration
    d. Air present in over-ventilated alveoli
45. True statement regarding pulmonary ventilation is:
    a. PaO_2 is maximum at the apex
    b. V/Q is maximum at the base
    c. Ventilation per unit lung volume is maximum at the apex
    d. Blood circulation is minimum at the base
46. Residual volume can be measured by:
    a. Drinker's respirator
    b. Tonometer
    c. Helium dilution method
    d. Dye dilution method
47. If the tidal volume is 600 mL, dead space volume 150 mL and respiratory rate 15/min the alveolar ventilation will be:
    a. 2.5 L/min   b. 4 L/min
    c. 6.75 L/min d. 9 L/min
48. Breathing reserve is equal to:
    a. Sum of total lung capacity and maximum breathing capacity
    b. Difference between maximum breathing capacity and respiratory minute volume
    c. Sum of tidal volume and respiratory minute volume
    d. Difference between respiratory minute volume and tidal volume
49. Volume of air remaining in the lungs at the end of maximum expiration is:
    a. Functional residual capacity
    b. Expiratory reserve volume

c. Residual volume
d. Inspiratory reserve volume

50. **Site of maximum airway resistance is:**
   a. Alveoli
   b. Terminal bronchiole
   c. Tertiary bronchi
   d. Trachea

51. **Which of the following lung volumes cannot be measured by a simple spirometer?**
   a. Vital capacity
   b. Inspiratory capacity
   c. Tidal volume
   d. Functional residual volume

52. **Anatomical dead space is greater in:**
   a. Supine position vs. sitting posture
   b. Women vs. men
   c. Old age vs. young adults
   d. Maximum expiration vs. inspiration

53. **All are true of FEV_1% except that:**
   a. It is normally 80%
   b. It can be measured using a spirometer
   c. It may be normal in restrictive lung disease
   d. It is increased in obstructive lung disease

54. **The functional residual capacity in the lungs of a healthy adult male of average size is:**
   a. About 1200 mL
   b. Becomes smaller if air flow resistance increases
   c. The volume at which some airways normally begin to close during expiration
   d. Can be estimated by helium dilution method

55. **Maximum voluntary ventilation is:**
   a. 20-50 L/min
   b. 50-75 L/min
   c. 75-125 L/min
   d. 125-170 L/min

56. **In normal adult, VD/VT (dead space : tidal volume) ratio is:**
   a. 20
   b. 0.35
   c. 40
   d. 50

57. **Regarding pulmonary function test, all are true, except:**
   a. Compliance decreases in interstitial lung disease
   b. Compliance is total lung distensibility
   c. Total lung capacity increases in emphysema
   d. FEV_1 is the forced expiratory rate in one minute

58. **Restrictive lung disease shows:**
   a. Increased FEV_1/FVC; decreased compliance of lung tissue
   b. Decreased FEV_1/FVC; decreased compliance of lung tissue
   c. Increased FRC; increased compliance of lung
   d. Increased TLC; decreased RV

59. **Most important substance controlling alveolar ventilation is:**
   a. O_2
   b. CO_2
   c. Water vapor
   d. N_2

60. **Compliance of thorax and lungs together is:**
   a. 0.22 L/cm of water
   b. 2 L/cm of water
   c. 0.13 L/cm of water
   d. 0.3 L/cm of water

61. **Alveolar-arterial O_2 tension gradient increases in all, except:**
   a. Hypoventilation
   b. Right to left shunt
   c. Ventilation-perfusion abnormality
   d. Diffusion defect

ANSWERS

1. d	2. d	3. d	4. a	5. c
6. c	7. b	8. c	9. c	10. d
11. a	12. b	13. b	14. b	15. b
16. a	17. a	18. a	19. a	20. d
21. c	22. a	23. a	24. d	25. d
26. b	27. a	28. b	29. a	30. d
31. d	32. c	33. c	34. c	35. b
36. d	37. b	38. d	39. b	40. b
41. c	42. b	43. c	44. a	45. a
46. c	47. c	48. b	49. c	50. d
51. d	52. c	53. d	54. d	55. d
56. b	57. d	58. a	59. b	60. c
61. a				

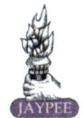

TOP DOC BANE WOHI
JISKA GUIDE HO SAHI

diginerve
A Jaypee Initiative

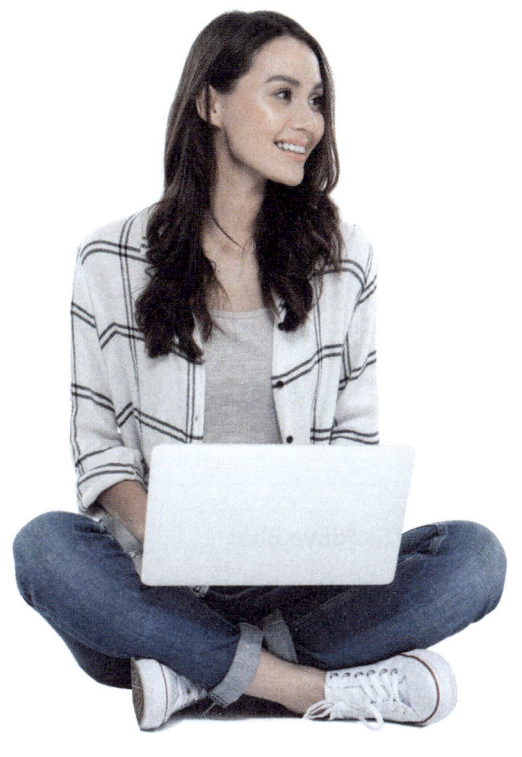

YOUR GUIDE AT EVERY STEP

Expert Knowledge Anytime, Anywhere

SCAN QR CODE
FOR MORE DETAILS

WHY CHOOSE US

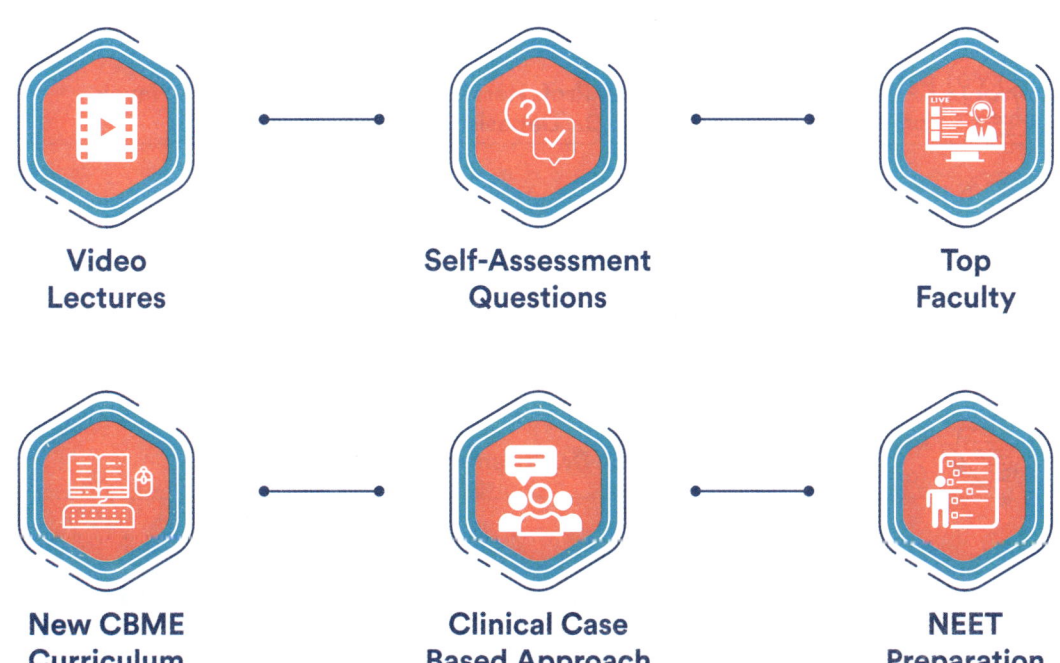

- Video Lectures
- Self-Assessment Questions
- Top Faculty
- New CBME Curriculum
- Clinical Case Based Approach
- NEET Preparation

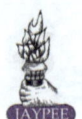

TOP DOC BANE WOHI | JISKA GUIDE HO SAHI

diginerve — A Jaypee Initiative

Video Lectures | Notes | Self-Assessment

UnderGrad Courses Available

 Community Medicine for UnderGrads — by Dr. Bratati Banerjee

 Forensic Medicine & Toxicology for UnderGrads — by Dr. Gautam Biswas

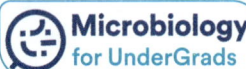 **Medicine** for UnderGrads — by Dr. Archith Boloor

 Microbiology for UnderGrads — by Dr. Apurba S Sastry, Dr. Sandhya Bhat & Dr. Deepashree R

 OBGYN for UnderGrads — by Dr. K. Srinivas

 Ophthalmology for UnderGrads — by Dr. Parul Ichhpujani & Dr. Talvir Sidhu

 Orthopaedics for UnderGrads — by Dr. Vivek Pandey

 Pathology for UnderGrads — by Prof. Harsh Mohan, Prof. Ramadas Nayak & Dr. Debasis Gochhait

 Pediatrics for UnderGrads — by Dr. Santosh Soans & Dr. Soundarya M

 Pharmacology for UnderGrads — by Dr. Sandeep Kaushal & Dr. Nirmal George

Surgery for UnderGrads — by Dr. Sriram Bhat M (SRB)

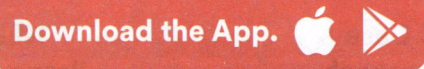
Download the App.

*T&C Apply

Contact:
+91 8800 418 418
marketing@diginerve.com

Pulmonary Circulation

CHAPTER 36

LEARNING OBJECTIVES
- Explain the features of pulmonary circulation
- Describe the regional variation in ventilation-perfusion ratio
- Explain the clinical significance of ventilation-perfusion ratio
- Define physiological and pathological shunt
- Describe the factors regulating pulmonary circulation

INTRODUCTION

PY5.10: Describe and discuss pulmonary circulation.

Pulmonary circulation carries deoxygenated blood from right ventricle to the alveoli and returns oxygenated blood from alveoli to left atrium. The pulmonary artery arising from the right ventricle divides into right and left branches **(Flowchart 36.1)**. Each branch enters the corresponding lung along with primary bronchus. Inside the lung it divides into small vessels up to capillaries with multiple anastomoses.

Features of Pulmonary Circulation

- Lung is the only organ receiving the entire cardiac output. Thus the lungs accommodate a blood flow that is almost equal to that accommodated by all the other organs of the body.
- Distance of pulmonary vessels from the heart when compared to systemic circulation is less. Still, in an upright subject, due to the effect of gravity regional perfusion is greater near the base of the lung than at the apex.
- The pulmonary arteries are thin walled (it is 30% as thick as the wall of the aorta) and contain very little smooth muscles and elastic tissue and have larger diameter.
- Pulmonary capillaries are larger than systemic capillaries and denser with multiple anastomoses so that each alveolus seems to sit in a **capillary basket**. There are approximately 500–1000 pulmonary capillaries per alveolus.
- The pulmonary veins are highly distensible and act as a blood reservoir. The pulmonary blood volume increases by 400 mL as the person lies down and this is *the reason for the reduction in vital capacity in lying down posture and the cause for orthopnea in cardiac failure.*
- Since the pulmonary vessels are highly distensible, pulmonary circulation is a *low-pressure, low-resistance, high capacitance system with high compliance.* So all the blood contained in the right ventricle can be pumped into this system. Causes for the low resistance are:
    - Pulmonary blood vessels are shorter, thinner and wider than systemic vessels
    - The number of pulmonary arterioles is very high
    - The pulmonary arterioles are less muscular and their resting tone is low
- Blood vessels of lung consist of two sets originating from two different sources, performing different functions.
    - From **pulmonary artery** belonging to pulmonary circulation and contain deoxygenated blood and the function is gas exchange.
    - From **bronchial arteries** arising from aorta belonging to systemic circulation and contains oxygenated blood. Function is to supply nutrition to respiratory tree up to terminal bronchiole.
- Pulmonary blood flow is influenced by intrathoracic pressure.
- Pulmonary circulation acts as a filter that prevents emboli from reaching the systemic circulation due to the presence of fibrinolytic system in lung.

Flowchart 36.1: Schematic representation of pulmonary circulation.

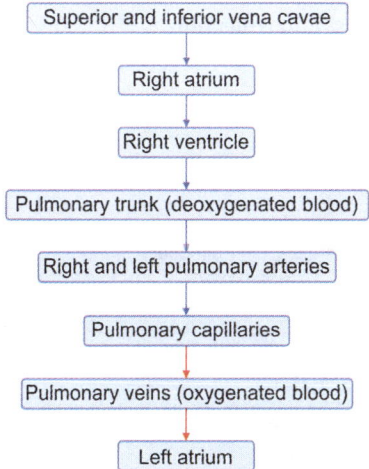

- The pulmonary arteries are the only postnatal arteries that carry deoxygenated blood, and pulmonary veins are the only postnatal veins that carry oxygenated blood.
- Lymphatic channels are abundant in lungs that help to keep alveoli dry and maintain negative intrapleural pressure.
- **Angiotensin converting enzyme** (**ACE**) produced by endothelial cells of pulmonary vasculature helps in the conversion of angiotensin I to angiotensin II which has a major role in maintaining blood pressure.
- **Physiological shunt**—**Shunt** is defined as any mechanism by which blood that has not been oxygenated in the lungs is added to systemic circulation. In the lung there is anastomosis between capillaries of pulmonary vessels and bronchial vessels. So, some bronchial venous blood (impure blood) enters pulmonary veins (pure blood) bypassing the right ventricle and returns to the left side of heart. This constitutes 2% of blood in systemic circulation (**Fig. 36.1**).
- **Pathological shunt** in lungs—Blood coming from areas of lung with low ventilation-perfusion ratio also contributes to the shunt in abnormal situations, i.e., blood that is drained from non-ventilated gas-exchanging units of lung.
- The effects of changes in PO_2, PCO_2 and pH on pulmonary vascular resistance are opposite to those observed in the systemic circulation. Hypoxia, hypercapnia and low interstitial pH produce pulmonary vasoconstriction. The effect of PO_2 in the alveolar air adjacent to the pulmonary capillary affects pulmonary vascular resistance more than the PO_2 in the lumen of arterioles and venules. Thus, pulmonary arterioles constrict in areas where alveolar PO_2 decrease diverting blood to well-ventilated areas. This helps to decrease pathological shunt. The low PO_2 acts directly on the pulmonary vascular smooth muscle cells, i.e., vasoconstriction is not mediated by nervous or hormonal mechanism.
- The volume of blood in the pulmonary vessels at any one time is about 450 mL, i.e., 9% of the total blood volume. Of this approximately 70 mL is present in the pulmonary capillaries. Rest is present in the pulmonary arteries and veins.

Causes for Reduction in Arterial PO_2

- Physiological shunt in the lung.
- Some amount of coronary venous blood, which is drained from the heart, enters the left ventricle through the **thebesian veins**. This constitutes 0.5% of blood in systemic circulation.
- Right-to-left shunts (septal defects) in patients with cyanotic congenital heart disease contribute to reduction in arterial PO_2. This occurs when there is increase in pressure in the right side of heart as in pulmonary hypertension. Otherwise, the shunt is only from left to right since the pressure in the left side of heart is more.

Reasons

- *Right ventricular output is a little less than that of left ventricular output.*
    - This is due to two reasons: (a) Part of bronchial blood flow enters pulmonary capillaries and veins bypassing the right ventricle due to anastomosis between the bronchial capillaries and pulmonary vessels; (b) Some amount of venous blood flows from coronary veins to left side of heart through thebesian veins.
- *The blood in the systemic arteries has a PO_2 about 2 mm Hg less than that of blood that is in equilibrium with alveolar air and the saturation of hemoglobin is 0.5% less.* Reason is physiologic shunt (explain).

PULMONARY BLOOD PRESSURE

The entire pulmonary vascular system is a distensible low-pressure system. Pulmonary arterial blood pressure is *very low* when compared to systemic arterial blood pressure.

Pulmonary pressure = 24/9 mm Hg
Systemic blood pressure = 120/80 mm Hg

The pulmonary capillary pressure is about 10 mm Hg, whereas in the systemic capillary it is 30 mm Hg. Pulmonary capillary oncotic pressure is 25 mm Hg. According to Starling's forces, the inward directed pressure gradient of about 15 mm Hg keeps the alveoli free of fluid. When the pulmonary capillary pressure becomes more than 25 mm Hg, it leads to **pulmonary edema**, e.g., mitral stenosis.

Factors that Keep the Alveoli Dry

- The inward-directed pressure gradient of 15 mm Hg in the pulmonary capillaries.
- Surfactant lining the alveoli decreases the surface tension and prevents fluid collection.

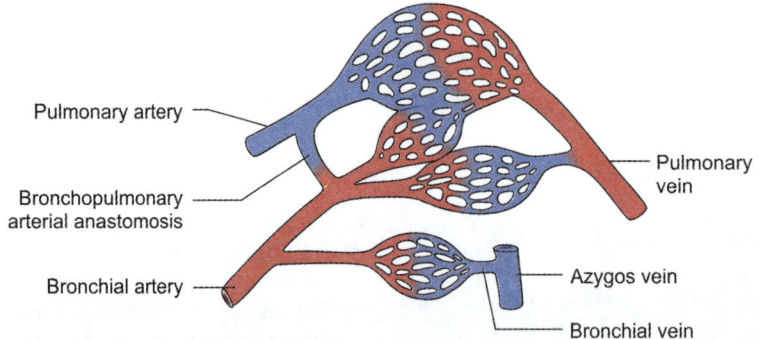

Fig. 36.1: Physiological shunt in pulmonary circulation.

- ❖ Negative pulmonary interstitial fluid pressure (-8 mm Hg) sucks any fluid that collects in the alveoli. This is drained away by the pulmonary capillaries and the lymphatics.
- ❖ Lung is richly supplied with lymphatic vessels which rapidly drain away excess fluid. Lymph flow can be increased as much as 10-fold under pathologic conditions where there is fluid accumulation in the interstitium.

Pulmonary Edema

When there is increase in the pulmonary interstitial fluid pressure to a positive value there will be sudden filling of pulmonary interstitial spaces and alveoli with large amounts of fluid. This condition is called pulmonary edema.

Causes

- ❖ Left heart failure or mitral valve disease leads to increase in pulmonary venous pressure and pulmonary capillary pressure.
- ❖ Damage to pulmonary capillary membrane as in infections like pneumonia; SO_2, Cl_2 gas poisoning, etc. This leads to leakage of fluid out of the capillaries into the interstitial space and alveoli.
- ❖ Obstruction to lymphatic drainage from lungs.

Pulmonary Hypertension

Sustained elevation of pulmonary arterial pressure is called pulmonary hypertension. Most important causes are chronic hypoxia and systemic lupus erythematosus (SLE). If the condition is not treated, the increased right ventricular afterload leads to right heart failure and death.

■ MEASUREMENT OF PULMONARY BLOOD FLOW

Since the whole of cardiac output goes through lungs, pulmonary blood flow can be obtained from **Fick's principle or indicator dilution technique** (refer measurement of cardiac output in cardiovascular system).

Factors Influencing Pulmonary Blood Flow or Regulation of Pulmonary Blood Flow

- ❖ **Cardiac output**: Since pulmonary blood flow is directly proportional to cardiac output, any factor that alters cardiac output affects pulmonary perfusion like venous return, force of contraction, etc.
- ❖ **Pulmonary vascular resistance**: Pulmonary perfusion is inversely proportional to pulmonary vascular resistance.
- ❖ **Nervous factors**
  - Sympathetic stimulation especially of the cervical sympathetic ganglia reduces pulmonary blood flow by as much as 30% by producing pulmonary vasoconstriction.
  - Parasympathetic stimulation produces vasodilatation leading to decreased pulmonary vascular resistance and increased pulmonary perfusion.
- ❖ **Chemical factors**: Hypoxia, hypercapnia and acidosis produce vasoconstriction and increase pulmonary arterial pressure. *In all other areas other than lung, hypoxia produces vasodilation.* This is the reason for the development of pulmonary hypertension in patients with chronic obstructive pulmonary disease (COPD). Chronic generalized hypoxia of lung leads to prolonged vasoconstriction and produces histological changes in the pulmonary vasculature leading to increased pulmonary vascular resistance.
- ❖ **Effect of gravity**: Gravity has a remarkable effect on pulmonary circulation. In the erect posture, there is a relatively marked pressure gradient in the pulmonary arteries from the top to the bottom of the lungs because of the effect of gravity. This results in a linear increase in pulmonary blood flow from the apex to the base of the lung.
- ❖ **Hormonal factors (Table 36.1)**
  - *Pulmonary arteriolar vasoconstrictors:* Angiotensin II, epinephrine, norepinephrine, PGF_2-α, etc.
  - *Vasodilators:* Acetylcholine, NO, etc.
  - *Constrictors of pulmonary venules*: Serotonin.
- ❖ **Phases of respiration**
  - In inspiration there is pulmonary vasodilation and increased pulmonary perfusion.
  - In expiration there will be vasoconstriction and increased pulmonary vascular resistance leading to decreased perfusion.

■ REGIONAL VARIATION IN DISTRIBUTION OF VENTILATION AND PERFUSION

Ventilation

Inhaled air is not distributed equally to all regions of the lung. In erect posture this is due to the effect of gravity on

Table 36.1: Factors affecting smooth muscles in the pulmonary arteries and veins in regulating pulmonary blood flow.	
Agents	**Response**
Autonomic transmitters and receptors involved	
Noradrenaline $α_1$	Contraction
Noradrenaline $α_2$, $β_2$	Relaxation
Acetylcholine M_3	Relaxation
Vasoactive intestinal polypeptide (VIP)	Relaxation
Calcitonin gene related peptide (CGRP)	Relaxation
Hormonal factors	
Adenosine A_1	Contraction
Adenosine A_2	Relaxation
Angiotensin II	Contraction
Atrial natriuretic peptide (ANP)	Relaxation
Bradykinin	Relaxation
Endothelin ET_A	Contraction
Endothelin ET_B	Relaxation
Histamine	Relaxation
Serotonin 5-HT_1	Contraction
Prostacyclin (PGI_2)	Relaxation
Thromboxane	Contraction
Vasopressin	Relaxation

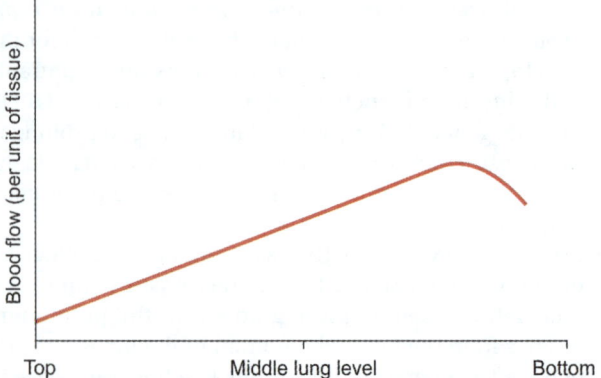

Fig. 36.2: Blood flow at different levels in the lung at rest in the standing posture.

intrapleural pressure. Pleural pressure is more negative at the apex and less negative at the base.

At functional residual capacity (FRC), more negative intrapleural pressure at the apex causes greater expansion of the apical alveoli in the erect posture and has a larger resting volume and less compliance than at the base. At high lung volumes, the lung becomes stiffer, i.e., it becomes less compliant. In contrast, the lower zone of the lung has a lower resting volume because the alveoli are of small size initially, the compliance is more at low lung volumes and this area expands more readily during inspiration. So, the lower zone of the lung is ventilated better than the apex during inspiration.

Perfusion

The apex of the lung is well above the level of the heart and the base of lung is below the level of heart. *Gravity plays an important role in perfusion of the lung*. In the erect posture there is a linear increase in blood flow from the top to the bottom of the lung **(Fig. 36.2)**.

Besides gravity, hypoxic pulmonary vasoconstriction also regulates blood flow. It is not the reduction in PO_2 of the blood in the pulmonary arterioles and venules that cause vasoconstriction of pulmonary vessels. It is the PO_2 in the alveolar air adjacent to the vessel that leads to pulmonary vasoconstriction. The smooth muscle cells of pulmonary arterioles are very sensitive to alveolar PO_2. As alveolar PO_2 falls in a particular area, there is arteriolar constriction in that area and redistribution of blood flow occurs to regions of higher alveolar PO_2. But if there is generalized alveolar hypoxia it leads to pulmonary hypertension.

■ EFFECT OF GRAVITY IN PULMONARY CIRCULATION

In an upright subject, due to the effect of gravity regional perfusion is greater near the base of the lung than at the apex. The upper portions of the lungs are well above the level of heart and the middle portion at the level of heart and the basal portion below it. Alveoli at the apex of the lung are approximately 20 cm above the level of left atrium. A pressure difference of 23 mm Hg exists in the pulmonary vessels between the apex and the base of the lung, of which about 15 mm Hg is above the heart level and 8 mm Hg below the heart level. The pulmonary arterial systolic pressure at the level of heart is 25 mm Hg. That means, the pulmonary arterial pressure in the apex of the lung in a standing person is about 15 mm Hg less than the pulmonary arterial pressure at the level of the heart and the pressure in the lowest part of the lung is about 8 mm Hg greater than that at the level of the heart. Thus at the upper part of lung, the pulmonary arterial pressure is 10 mm Hg and at the lower part, 33 mm Hg. This pressure difference affects the blood flow through the different areas of the lungs.

The alveolar air pressure is normally close to the atmospheric pressure at the functional residual capacity, i.e., 0 atmospheres. The pressure in the capillaries at the apex of the lungs is only a little more than the pressure in the alveoli. So when the alveolar pressure becomes greater than the capillary blood pressure, the capillaries surrounding the alveoli (alveolar capillaries) gets compressed and there will be no blood flow. (Extra-alveolar capillaries feed or drain the alveolar capillaries.)

Alveolar capillaries include the capillaries that are surrounded by alveoli. The capillaries surrounding the alveoli are kept distended by the blood pressure inside them but simultaneously are compressed by the alveolar air pressure on their outside. Depending on this factor, 3 zones can occur in the lungs with regard to pulmonary blood flow.

Zone 1

In zone 1, the alveolar air pressure will be always greater than the pulmonary capillary pressure in that area of the lung. So no blood flow occurs in the pulmonary capillaries in that area throughout the cardiac cycle. No gas exchange occurs in the affected alveoli and the air in them becomes part of physiological dead space or alveolar dead space. Under normal conditions this situation does not occur in the lungs. Zone 1 blood flow occurs in the apex of the lung in the following situations:
❖ When the pulmonary systolic arterial pressure is very low as in severe blood loss
❖ When the alveolar air pressure is too high as in case of breathing against positive air pressure so that the intra-alveolar air pressure is almost 10 mm Hg greater than normal and the pulmonary systolic pressure normal

Zone 2

In zone 2 areas of the lungs, blood flow through the pulmonary capillaries surrounding the alveoli occurs intermittently. In the upper part of the lungs, the alveoli are larger and less compliant and so ventilation is less at the apex than at the base. In the upright posture, since the upper portions of the lungs are well above the level of heart, blood flow is also less than the base due to hydrostatic pressure. Flow occurs during systole when the pulmonary arterial pressure is maximal and the pulmonary capillary pressure greater than the alveolar air pressure. At the apex during systole, the pulmonary arterial pressure is 10 mm Hg (it is 15 mm Hg less than at the level of the heart which is 25 mm Hg). But in diastole, the pulmonary arterial pressure at the level of heart is only 8 mm Hg. This pressure is not enough to push blood to the apex of the lung in diastole. It will be less than alveolar air pressure and no flow occurs during diastole in the pulmonary alveolar capillary. Normally zone 2 blood flow is seen in the upper part of the lungs. Thus, **intermittent or pulsatile flow of blood** occurs during the phases of cardiac cycle at the upper part of the lungs **(Fig. 36.3)**. The pulmonary capillary bed is one of the few capillaries in which flow is pulsatile. In systole, in zone 2, alveolar capillary pressure > alveolar air pressure > pulmonary venous pressure. During diastole, alveolar air pressure > alveolar capillary pressure > pulmonary venous pressure.

Zone 3

From about 10 cm above the level of heart to the bottom of the lungs the pulmonary artery pressure during systole and diastole remains greater than the alveolar air pressure. Therefore continuous flow occurs through the alveolar capillaries in the lower part of the lungs **(Fig. 36.3)**. In zone 3, venous pressure exceeds alveolar pressure, and flow is determined by the arteriovenous pressure difference. The increase in blood flow in zone 3 occurs by distension of vessels and also by recruitment of previously closed vessels. In zone 3, alveolar capillary pressure > pulmonary venous pressure > alveolar air pressure.

The resistance in the alveolar vessels depends on the transmural pressure gradient and lung volume. Increase in lung volume or decrease in the intrapulmonary blood pressure compress the alveolar vessels and increase their resistance. The resistance of the extra-alveolar vessels depends on intrapleural pressure and lung volume. Increased negative value of intrapleural pressure and higher lung volumes tend to dilate them. At the extreme base of the lung, the alveolar vessels behave as in zone 3. But the resistance in the extra-alveolar vessels increases because the intrapleural pressure is least negative at the extreme base. The extra-alveolar pulmonary vessels are kept dilated mainly by the negative intrapleural pressure. So the distending forces acting on the extra-alveolar blood vessels decrease and the resistance increases. So, blood flow through these vessels decrease. Since these extra-alveolar vessels feed or drain alveolar vessels, blood flow through the lung decrease from its peak as we approach the extreme base of the lungs as shown in **Figure 36.2**.

■ RELATIONSHIP BETWEEN PULMONARY ARTERY PRESSURE AND PULMONARY VENOUS PRESSURE IN PULMONARY CAPILLARY BLOOD FLOW

In the middle portion of the lungs, the pulmonary arterial pressure and the capillary pressure exceed the alveolar air pressure during the phases of cardiac cycle. But the pressure in the pulmonary venules may be lower than the alveolar air pressure. This leads to narrowing down of the capillary bed near the venous end. Under this condition, the pulmonary capillary blood flow is determined by the difference between pulmonary arterial pressure and alveolar air pressure rather than the difference between pulmonary arterial pressure and pulmonary venous pressure. Beyond the constriction, blood falls into the pulmonary veins which are compliant. This is called the **waterfall effect**.

Towards the base of the lungs, the compression of the capillaries produced by alveolar air pressure decreases and pulmonary flow increases as the pulmonary arterial pressure increases towards the base of the lungs. So at the base of the lungs, alveolar air pressure is lower than the pressure in the pulmonary circulation and blood flow is determined by the arterial-venous pressure difference and flow is continuous throughout the cardiac cycle.

But when a person is lying down, blood flow through the pulmonary capillaries will be continuous during systole and diastole in all parts of the lungs. This is because all parts of the lungs will be almost at the level of heart in lying down posture.

In exercise, where the pulmonary arterial pressure is high, both the lung apices and the lower parts of the lungs have continuous blood flow throughout the cardiac cycle.

Mechanism of Hypoxic Pulmonary Vasoconstriction

Hypoxic pulmonary vasoconstriction occurs locally, i.e., only in the area of alveolar hypoxia.
- ❖ Hypoxia may cause release of vasoactive substances from the pulmonary parenchyma or mast cells like histamine, serotonin, prostaglandins, etc.
- ❖ Decreased release of vasodilator substances such as nitric oxide may lead to vasoconstriction.
- ❖ Recent studies suggest that hypoxia act directly on pulmonary vascular smooth muscle cells which contains potassium channels which open when it is oxidized and close when it is reduced. Hypoxia inhibits outward

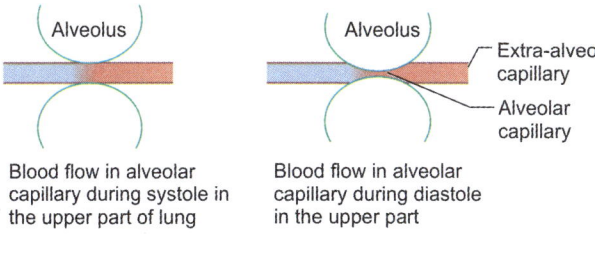
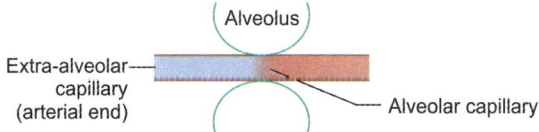

Fig. 36.3: Effect of gravity in pulmonary circulation in the standing posture in the upper and lower parts of the lung.

potassium current, which causes depolarization of pulmonary vascular smooth muscle cells, allowing calcium to enter the cells. This causes them to contract.

VENTILATION-PERFUSION RATIO

PY6.2: Describe the mechanics of normal respiration, pressure changes during ventilation, lung volume and capacities, alveolar surface tension, compliance, airway resistance, ventilation, V/P ratio, diffusion capacity of lungs.

Ventilation-perfusion ratio is the ratio between alveolar ventilation in 1 minute and pulmonary perfusion in 1 minute. For proper O_2 and CO_2 exchange in the lungs, ventilation and perfusion must be matched. Resting alveolar ventilation is 4 L/min, while pulmonary blood flow which is equal to cardiac output is 5 L/min.

Ventilation-perfusion ratio is designated as:

$$V_A/Q = \frac{4 \text{ L/min}}{5 \text{ L/min}} = 0.8 \text{ at the middle of the lung}$$

At the apex of the lung, $V_A/Q = 3$
At the base of the lung, $V_A/Q = 0.6$

Ventilation and perfusion are not uniformly distributed throughout the lung. Both are preferentially distributed to the dependent regions of the lungs at rest.

In the upright posture, ventilation and perfusion are less at the apex and more towards the base. In lying down posture, the posterior part of lung is well ventilated and perfused than the anterior part. This gravity-dependent reduction in flow is more marked with perfusion than with ventilation, or in other words, the gravity-dependent reduction in perfusion is more marked at the apex than reduction for ventilation. Hence, the ratio of ventilation to perfusion is highest at the apex and lowest at the base in upright posture.

Clinical Importance of VA/Q

If one lung is not functioning, the patient is advised to lie on the side in which the lung is functioning so that this lung will be well ventilated and perfused.

Pulmonary tuberculosis affects apex of the lung first because of the following reasons:

- ❖ This is because reduction in perfusion is more than reduction in ventilation at the apex of the lung. So, more O_2 is available at the apex of lung. This provides a favorable environment for the growth of tubercle bacilli which are aerobic bacteria.
- ❖ Another reason is poor perfusion at the apex. Antibodies in the blood do not reach the apex satisfactorily. So, apex of the lung is more vulnerable to bacterial attack.

Importance of Ventilation-perfusion Ratio

- ❖ V_A/Q is important in determining the gas concentration in the alveoli.
- ❖ Effectiveness of gas exchange through the alveolar-capillary membrane is determined by V_A/Q.
- ❖ VA/Q helps to assess whether there is imbalance between alveolar ventilation and alveolar blood flow.

Measurement of Ventilation and Perfusion in Different Parts of the Lung

Even if total alveolar ventilation and total pulmonary blood flow are normal, in many lung diseases, some areas of the lung are well ventilated but have almost no blood flow, whereas other areas may have normal blood flow but little or no ventilation. In both these conditions gas exchange through the respiratory membrane in the affected part is seriously impaired. If a large part of the lung is involved, the person may suffer from severe respiratory distress. So, regional measurement of ventilation and perfusion is also important.

Measurement of Ventilation

The subject inhales a breath of **radioactive xenon** gas ^{133}Xe. When it enters the lung, it penetrates the chest wall and can be measured by placing scintillation counters over appropriate areas of the thorax. In this way the volume of inhaled radioactive xenon going to various regions of the lung can be determined. It is seen that ventilation per unit volume is greater near the base of the lung and progressively lesser towards the top in the erect posture. This difference disappears in the supine position. In the supine position, the posterior part of lung is more ventilated than the anterior part.

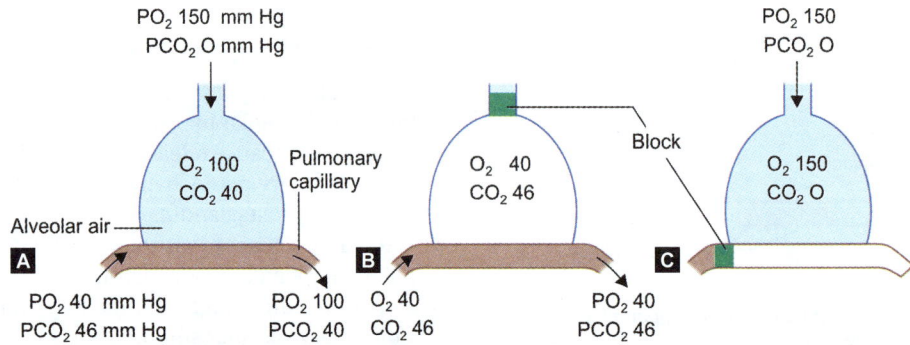

Figs. 36.4A to C: Effect of alterations of ventilation; perfusion ratio (V_A/Q) on the PO_2 and PCO_2 in a lung unit: (A) Normal ventilation and perfusion V_A/Q—Normal; (B) Perfusion without ventilation V_A/Q—Zero; (C) Ventilation without perfusion V_A/Q—Infinity.

When the subject lies on his side (lateral position), it is seen that the dependent lung is better ventilated.

Measurement of Distribution of Blood Flow

Radioactive xenon gas is dissolved in saline and injected into the superior vena cava or any peripheral vein. When it reaches the pulmonary capillaries, the distribution of radioactivity is measured by a radiation camera mounted behind the chest.

In the upright posture, blood flow seems to decrease linearly from bottom to top of lungs, reaching very low values at the apex. This distribution of radioactivity is affected by change in posture.

Assessment of Ventilation-perfusion Uniformity

- Measurement of dead space. If physiological dead space is increased, VA/Q will be greater than normal.
- Continuous monitoring of CO_2 content of expired air.
- Radioisotope method—a breath of 133Xe is taken. Chest is monitored with a radiation camera. This help to assess ventilation.
- Intravenous injection of saline solution of 133Xe into superior vena cava and measuring the distribution of radioactivity helps to assess regional blood flow.

Abnormalities in VA/Q

When the alveolar ventilation and blood flow are normal for the same alveolus then V_A/Q of that alveolus is said to be normal. When the ventilation is zero and perfusion of the alveolus is normal then V_A/Q is zero. When there is adequate ventilation but zero perfusion, V_A/Q is infinity. At a ratio of either zero or infinity, there is no exchange of gases through the respiratory membrane of the affected alveolus (**Figs. 36.4A to C**).

- *Ventilation without perfusion (alveolar dead space)*: V_A/Q is greater than normal or infinity, e.g., pulmonary embolism, pulmonary hypertension.
- *Perfusion without ventilation*: This produces a shunt where impure blood passes to systemic circulation without coming in contact with alveolar air. V_A/Q will be < normal or zero, e.g., consolidation of lung, fibrosis, atelectasis or collapse, pulmonary edema and bronchial obstruction as in chronic obstructive pulmonary disease (COPD).

MULTIPLE CHOICE QUESTIONS

1. The partial pressure of oxygen in the blood is decided by:
   a. Oxygen content of arterial blood
   b. Amount of oxygen dissolved in plasma
   c. Oxygen content of venous blood
   d. Amount of hemoglobin in blood

2. High oxygen tension in alveoli is due to:
   a. Right to left shunt
   b. Ventilation perfusion mismatch
   c. Bronchial asthma
   d. Inappropriate gas exchange

3. Ventilation perfusion ratio is maximum at:
   a. Apex of lung
   b. Base of lung
   c. Posterior lobe of lung
   d. Middle of the lung

4. Not a stimulus for pulmonary vasoconstriction:
   a. Hypoxemia   b. Hypercapnia
   c. PGI_2 d. Thromboxane

5. Apex of lung is more prone for pulmonary tuberculosis because, at the apex:
   a. Alveolar PCO_2 is high
   b. Alveolar PO_2 is low
   c. Ventilation is high
   d. Ventilation perfusion ratio is high

6. Pulmonary wedge pressure corresponds to:
   a. Right atrial pressure
   b. Right ventricular pressure
   c. Left atrial pressure
   d. Left ventricular pressure

7. Rise in pulmonary arterial pressure is caused by:
   a. Hypoxia   b. Acidosis
   c. Alkalosis   d. Decrease in 2,3-BPG

8. Following acute left ventricular failure, pulmonary edema begins to appear when the left atrial pressure approaches:
   a. 15 mm Hg   b. 20 mm Hg
   c. 30 mm Hg   d. 50 mm Hg

9. The alveolar PO_2 in the apex of vertical lung is high because in this part:
   a. Compliance is more during inspiration
   b. Blood flow is high
   c. Ventilation-perfusion ratio is high
   d. Intrapleural pressure is less negative

10. True statement regarding lung vascularity is:
    a. Pulmonary vascular resistance is half of the systemic vascular resistance
    b. Hypoxia causes vasodilation
    c. Pulmonary veins are distended in the lower lobe
    d. Perfusion is more in the apical lobe than at the base

11. In ventilation without perfusion, VA/Q will be:
    a. Infinity   b. Zero
    c. 0.8   d. 3

12. In conditions of perfusion without ventilation, VA/Q will be:
    a. 0.6   b. 0.8
    c. Infinity   d. Zero

13. Difference of pulmonary circulation from systemic circulation is:
    a. Blood volume in lung is about 450 mL
    b. Hypoxia causes vasodilation
    c. Has high capillary pressure
    d. High basal vasoconstrictor tone

14. Alveoli are kept dry due to the following causes, *except*:
    a. Low pulmonary capillary pressure
    b. Decreased lymphatic drainage in the lungs
    c. Negative interstitial fluid pressure
    d. Decreased alveolar surface tension
15. Normal ventilation-perfusion ratio at the apex of lung is:
    a. 0.6
    b. 0.8
    c. 3
    d. 6
16. The normal pulmonary systolic arterial pressure is:
    a. 10 mm Hg
    b. 35 mm Hg
    c. 0 mm Hg
    d. 25 mm Hg

ANSWERS

1. b	2. b	3. a	4. c	5. d
6. c	7. a	8. c	9. c	10. c
11. a	12. d	13. a	14. b	15. c
16. d				

Pulmonary Gas Exchange

CHAPTER 37

LEARNING OBJECTIVES
- Explain diffusion capacity of lungs
- Discuss respiratory quotient
- Explain with the help of a diagram the structure of respiratory membrane and the factors affecting diffusion of gases across it

INTRODUCTION

PY6.2: Describe the mechanics of normal respiration, pressure changes during ventilation, lung volume and capacities, alveolar surface tension, compliance, airway resistance, ventilation, V/P ratio, diffusion capacity of lungs.

The structure of the respiratory system is uniquely suited for the transport of O_2 into the body and CO_2 out of the body. O_2 continuously diffuse out of the gases in the alveoli into the bloodstream, and CO_2 continuously diffuses into the alveoli from the blood. Still the composition of alveolar gas is kept constant by various mechanisms which are explained below.

PARTIAL PRESSURE OF GASES

According to **Dalton's law**, each gas in a mixture of gases exerts its own pressure as if all the other gases were not present. Atmospheric pressure is the sum of the pressures of all the gases present in air like O_2, CO_2, N_2, water vapor and several other gases. In a mixture of gases, the pressure exerted by any one gas is its **partial pressure** and is equal to the total pressure multiplied by the fraction of the total amount of gas, which it represents. Total pressure is the barometric pressure at that height.

Barometric pressure at sea level is 760 mm Hg. The percentage of O_2 in air is 20.8%.

So, partial pressure of O_2 (PO_2) in air is calculated by:

$$PO_2 = \frac{20.8 \times 760}{100} = 158 \text{ mm Hg}$$

The partial pressure of gases is important in the movement of gases, especially O_2 and CO_2, across the respiratory membrane and between blood and body cells. During diffusion across a permeable membrane, each gas diffuses from an area where its partial pressure is greater to an area where its partial pressure is less (**Fig. 37.1**).

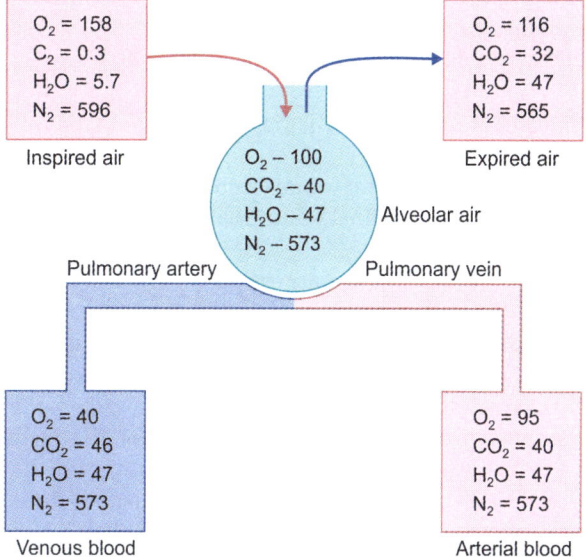

Fig. 37.1: Partial pressure of gases in mm Hg in the inspired air, alveolar air, venous blood, arterial blood and expired air. H_2O denotes water vapor.

TECHNIQUES OF COLLECTION OF ALVEOLAR AIR OR SAMPLING OF ALVEOLAR AIR

- **Haldane–Priestly method**
  Principle: Expired gas is a mixture of dead space and alveolar air. The initial portion will be dead space air and latter portion contains alveolar air. The last 10 mL of expired air is collected in a sampling tube and analyzed using a gas analyzer.
  Apparatus: Haldane's alveolar air tube is used. It is a long tube made of rubber or plastic, about 1 m long and 2.5 cm diameter. A mouthpiece is connected to one end and close to the mouthpiece is a side tube and through it, a sampling tube is connected.

Procedure: Ask the subject to breathe rapidly and forcefully into the Haldane's tube. Because of the force of expiration, the initial portion of air goes straight, and latter portion goes to the side sampling tube. This gas is then analyzed.

- **Two-bag technique**: The subject is asked to breathe out through the mouthpiece. The initial part of expired air enters bag II because bag I is closed. Then bag I is opened and bag II closed so that latter part of air is collected in bag I. This is alveolar air.
- **Continuous sampling technique**: Mouthpiece is connected to devices with automatic inspiratory and expiratory valves. In expiration, 10 mL of end expiratory air is collected in a side bag and analyzed.

METHODS OF ANALYSIS OF THE COLLECTED ALVEOLAR GAS

- **Haldane's gas analyzer**: Alveolar air contains O_2 and CO_2. The concentration of each gas can be calculated using **KOH and pyrogallol**. Air is passed through KOH. Let the initial volume of air be X.
  After passing through KOH let the volume be Y.

$$\text{Concentration of } CO_2 = \frac{(X-Y) \times 100}{X}$$

Now pass the air having volume Y through pyrogallol, which absorbs O_2. Let the final volume be Z.

$$\text{Concentration of } O_2 = \frac{(Y-Z) \times 100}{X}$$

- **Infrared CO_2 analyzer**: Amount of infrared rays absorbed is proportional to the quantity of CO_2 in the alveolar air.
- **Paramagnetic O_2 analyzer**: Between the poles of two magnets, an evacuated metallic sphere is kept. The quantity of O_2 is proportional to the distance through which the sphere is displaced when the alveolar air is passed through the sphere.
- Other methods are by using:
  - Polarographic electrodes for CO_2 estimation
  - N_2 analyzer
  - Mass spectrometer
  - Gas chromatography.

REASONS FOR THE DIFFERENCE IN THE COMPOSITION OF ATMOSPHERIC AIR AND ALVEOLAR AIR (TABLE. 37.1)

- Partial replacement of alveolar air by atmospheric air with each breath.
  Constant absorption of O_2 from alveoli to pulmonary capillaries.
- Diffusion of CO_2 from pulmonary capillaries to alveoli.
- Humidification of atmospheric air as it passes through the respiratory passages leads to dilution of gases. Water in the respiratory passage is evaporated and the atmospheric air entering the respiratory passage gets saturated with water vapor. Vapor pressure is the pressure exerted by water molecules to escape from a surface. At 37°C, vapor pressure is 47 mm Hg.

Table 37.1: Composition of gases in the inspired air and alveolar air.

Gas	Inspired air	Alveolar air
O_2	20.8%	13.2%
CO_2	0.04%	5.2%
Water vapor	0.8%	6.2%
N_2	78%	75.4%

Mechanisms by which Composition of Alveolar Air is Kept Constant

- By proper ventilation and perfusion of lung. O_2 continuously diffuses out of the alveoli into the bloodstream, and CO_2 continuously diffuses into the alveoli from blood. Inspired air mixes with alveolar air, replacing the O_2 and diluting the CO_2.
- Because of the functional residual capacity of about 2 L at the end of expiration, 350 mL of inspired air or expired air has little effect on PO_2 and PCO_2 of alveolar air and alveolar gas composition remains constant (only 350 mL of air reaches the gas exchange zone). The large volume of the functional residual air dilutes the small volume of tidal air reaching the alveoli (about 350 mL) during each inspiration. The tidal air is thus unable to cause any sudden and wide fluctuation in the temperature and the composition of the air inside the lungs. This small change in the composition of the air in the lungs is further made insignificant by the continuous absorption of oxygen and addition of carbon dioxide from the pulmonary capillaries. The alveolar air therefore possesses a composition that is relatively constant.
- Central and peripheral control mechanisms also operate to maintain alveolar gas composition constant.

MECHANISM OF GAS EXCHANGE AT LUNG LEVEL (EXTERNAL RESPIRATION)

Conditions Necessary for Proper Gas Exchange

For proper gas exchange between alveoli and the bloodstream, certain conditions must be satisfied:
- The lungs must be sufficiently large. If the surface area of alveoli is reduced as in emphysema or in surgical resection of lung, the surface area of the respiratory membrane is decreased and sufficient gas exchange does not occur.
- Alveolar ventilation must be adequate to replenish O_2 and wash out CO_2 from the alveoli.
- Pulmonary circulation must be sufficient in quantity, and ventilation and perfusion must be to the same alveoli, i.e., VA/Q must be normal (0.8).

Structure of Blood-Gas Barrier or Respiratory Membrane

The exchange of respiratory gases between the lungs and blood takes place by diffusion across the alveolar and

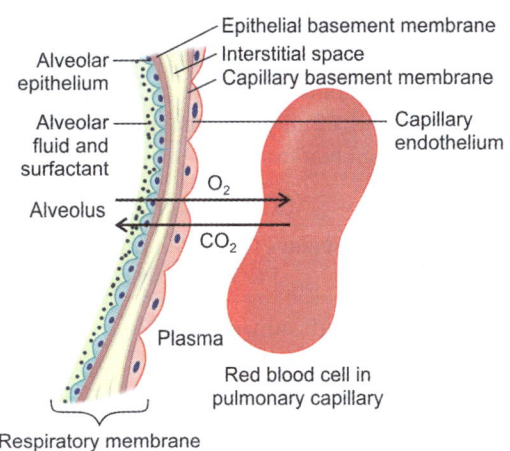

Fig. 37.2: Structure of respiratory membrane.

capillary walls. These layers are collectively called **alveolar-capillary membrane or respiratory membrane** (Fig. 37.2).

Factors Affecting Diffusion of Gases across the Respiratory Membrane

- Thickness of the respiratory membrane
- Surface area of the respiratory membrane
- Pressure gradient of gases across the respiratory membrane
- Solubility of the gas
- Molecular weight of the gas
- Diffusion coefficient of gases.

Thickness of Respiratory Membrane

- Thickness of respiratory membrane — 0.5 mm
- Diameter of pulmonary capillary — 8 mm
- Diameter of RBC — 7.2 mm.

So, red blood cells are squeezed through pulmonary capillary and so they are in close contact with respiratory membrane. These factors allow rapid diffusion of gases across the respiratory membrane from alveoli to red blood cells. *Rate of diffusion of gases is inversely proportional to thickness of respiratory membrane.*

For example, rate of diffusion of gases is decreased in fibrosis of lung, pulmonary edema, etc., because the thickness of the membrane is increased.

Surface Area of Respiratory Membrane

Rate of diffusion is directly proportional to the surface area of respiratory membrane. Normal surface area is 70 m^2. Surface area is decreased in emphysema, in chronic smokers and in surgical resection of lung. In emphysema, there is destruction of alveolar walls, thereby reducing the total surface area to 1/3rd to 1/4th normal.

Partial Pressure Difference of Gases

Greater the partial pressure gradient more will be the rate of diffusion.

Alveolar PO_2 = 100 mm Hg

Pulmonary capillary PO_2 = 40 mm Hg

Partial pressure gradient for O_2 across the membrane is 100–40 = 60 mm Hg

Alveolar PCO_2 = 40 mm Hg

Pulmonary capillary PCO_2 = 46 mm Hg

Partial pressure gradient for CO_2 across the respiratory membrane is 46–40 = 6 mm Hg

Gases diffuse from a region of higher partial pressure to a region of lower partial pressure across the membrane until the pressure of the gases on the two sides become equal.

Solubility of the Gas

The amount of gas that moves through a membrane is directly proportional to the solubility of the gas in the membrane. Although the partial pressure difference for CO_2 across the respiratory membrane is only 6 mm Hg, it is much more soluble than O_2 and diffuses with ease. Even though the molecular weight of O_2 is less than that of CO_2, CO_2 diffuses 20 times more rapidly than O_2 across the alveolar-capillary membrane. This is because the solubility of CO_2 is 24 times greater than the solubility of O_2 in the membrane.

Molecular Weight of the Gas

Rate of diffusion is inversely proportional to the square root of the molecular weight of the gas.

Diffusion Coefficient of Gases

Diffusion coefficient is the rate of diffusion of a gas through a given area for a given distance for a given pressure gradient in unit time.

Or the diffusion coefficient of a gas is the volume of gas in mL which diffuses through 1 cm^2 of a membrane in 1 minute when there is a pressure difference of 1 mm Hg across the membrane. The diffusion coefficient is directly proportional to the solubility of gas in the membrane and inversely proportional to the square root of molecular weight.

Assuming that the diffusion coefficient for oxygen is 1, the relative diffusion coefficients for different gases of the body are as follows:

O_2 = 1
CO_2 = 20
N_2 = 0.5
CO = 0.8
He = 0.9

The diffusion coefficient of CO_2 is 20 times more than that of O_2.

The relation between rate of diffusion of a gas and the factors affecting it can be expressed by the formula

$$D \alpha \frac{\Delta P \times A \times S}{d \times \sqrt{MW}}$$

D → Rate of diffusion of the gas
DP → Pressure gradient
A → Surface area
S → Solubility of the gas
d → Thickness of the respiratory membrane
MW → Molecular weight of the gas

Diffusing Capacity of Lungs for O_2 and CO_2

Diffusing capacity (DC) is the volume of gas in mL that is transported across the respiratory membrane in 1 minute for 1 mm Hg partial pressure gradient.

$$DO_2 = \frac{A \times dO_2}{t}$$

- $DO_2 \rightarrow$ Diffusing capacity for O_2
- $A \rightarrow$ Total area of respiratory membrane
- $t \rightarrow$ Thickness of the membrane
- $dO_2 \rightarrow$ Diffusion coefficient

Diffusing capacity for O_2 = 20 mL/min/mm Hg

Diffusing capacity for CO_2 = 400 mL/min/mm Hg

Diffusing capacity for CO_2 is 20 times that of O_2. Even though the pressure gradient for CO_2 across the respiratory membrane is only 6 mm Hg, it is adequate for CO_2 transfer because of its high diffusing capacity and diffusion coefficient. It is for the same reason that *diffusion defects causes hypoxemia but not CO_2 retention*.

Variations in Diffusing Capacity

Diffusing capacity is increased in exercise. In severe exercise, diffusing capacity of O_2 become 65 mL/min/mm Hg and that of CO_2 becomes 1400 mL/min/mm Hg. This increase is due to the following reasons:
- Opening up of closed capillaries (recruitment of capillaries)
- Vasodilatation
- Stretching of alveolar membrane decreases the thickness of the respiratory membrane, thereby increasing diffusion rate.

Diffusing capacity is decreased in pulmonary edema, pulmonary fibrosis, sarcoidosis, etc.

Measurement of Diffusing Capacity

$$\text{Diffusing capacity of } O_2 = \frac{O_2 \text{ consumption/min}}{\text{Pulmonary alveolar } PO_2 - \text{Pulmonary capillary } PO_2}$$

Since it is difficult to find out the mean PO_2 of pulmonary capillary blood, diffusing capacity of carbon monoxide is estimated.

DC for O_2 = DC for CO × 1.23

The subject is asked to inhale a mixture of 0.2% CO in the inspired air to maintain a steady concentration of CO in alveolar air. Hemoglobin has affinity for O_2 and CO. When this affinity is compared, affinity of hemoglobin for CO is about 210 times more than that for O_2.

$$\text{DC for CO} = \frac{\text{CO consumption/min}}{\text{Alveolar PCO} - \text{Pulmonary capillary PCO (initially zero)}}$$

= 17 mL/min/mm Hg

DC for O_2 = DC for CO × 1.23

= 17 × 1.23 = 20.9 mL/min/mm Hg

This technique was devised by Bohr in 1909 and later modified by Mary Krogh.

INTERNAL RESPIRATION

Diffusion at Tissue Level

Diffusion of O_2

Partial pressure of O_2 in the arterial blood is 95 mm Hg and PO_2 of tissues is 40 mm Hg because of continuous metabolic activity. A pressure gradient of 55 mm Hg exists between blood and tissues so that O_2 can easily diffuse into the tissues (**Fig. 37.3**).

- O_2 content of arterial blood → 19.8 mL/100 mL of blood
- O_2 content of venous blood → 15 mL/100 mL of blood
- Cardiac output → 5000 mL

So, when 100 mL of blood passes through the tissue 4.8 mL (~5 mL) of O_2 diffuses into the tissues.

Therefore, **O_2 consumption** by the body =

$$\frac{5 \times 5000}{100} = 250 \text{ mL/min}$$

Diffusion of CO_2

Due to continuous metabolic activity, CO_2 is produced constantly in the tissues and so partial pressure of CO_2 in the cells is about 46 mm Hg. PCO_2 of arterial blood is 40 mm Hg. A pressure gradient of 6 mm Hg is responsible for the diffusion of CO_2 from tissues to blood (**Fig. 37.3**).

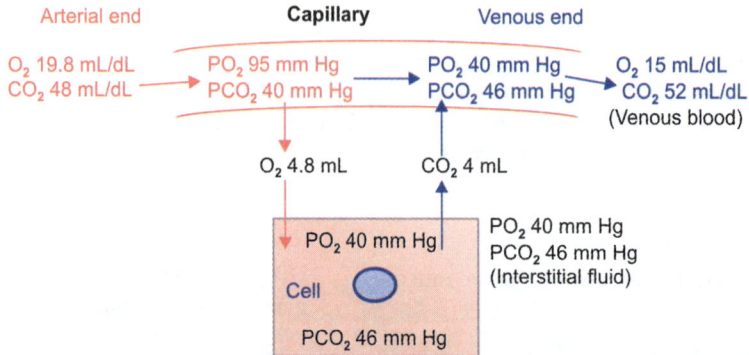

Fig. 37.3: Diffusion of O_2 and CO_2 at tissue level.

CO_2 content of arterial blood – 48 mL/100 mL of blood CO_2 content of venous blood – 52 mL/100 mL of blood

So, the diffusion of CO_2 from tissues to the blood is 4 mL/100 mL of blood, i.e., when 100 mL of blood passes through tissues, 4 mL of CO_2 enters the bloodstream (**Fig. 37.3**).

So CO_2 output/min $= \dfrac{4 \times 5000}{100} = 200$ mL/min

■ RESPIRATORY QUOTIENT OR RESPIRATORY EXCHANGE RATIO

Respiratory quotient (RQ) is the ratio between CO_2 output and O_2 consumption by the body.

$$RQ = \dfrac{200 \text{ mL}}{250 \text{ mL}} = 0.8$$

During exercise, RQ increases to 1.5–2. But during the recovery phase, it decreases to 0.5 due to O_2 debt. RQ depends on the type of food consumed. RQ of various foods are:

Carbohydrate → 1
Fat → 0.7
Protein → 0.8

The reason for the difference in RQ is that when carbohydrate is utilized by the body, for every molecule of O_2 consumed one molecule of CO_2 is formed. So, RQ is one. When fat (e.g., palmitic acid) is utilized, O_2 reacts with fat and a large portion of O_2 combines with hydrogen ions to form water instead of CO_2. So, CO_2 output is less and RQ is less.

For carbohydrates:
$C_6H_{12}O_6 + 6O_2 \longrightarrow 6CO_2 + 6H_2O$
Glucose

$RQ = \dfrac{6CO_2}{6O_2} = 1$

For fats:
$C_{15}H_{31}COOH + 23O_2 \longrightarrow 16CO_2 + 16H_2O$
Palmitic acid

$RQ = \dfrac{16CO_2}{23O_2} = 0.7$

■ MULTIPLE CHOICE QUESTIONS

1. **Normal alveolar PO_2 is:**
   a. 100 mm Hg
   b. 110 mm Hg
   c. 150 mm Hg
   d. 40 mm Hg

2. **Respiratory acidosis is characterized by:**
   a. Decrease in PCO_2 and decrease in pH
   b. Increase in PCO_2 and increase in pH
   c. Increase in PCO_2 and decrease in pH
   d. Decrease in PCO_2 and increase in pH

3. **As blood passes through the capillaries in the lungs:**
   a. Blood PCO_2 increases
   b. Blood PO_2 decreases
   c. Plasma chloride increases
   d. Plasma bicarbonate increases

4. **Normal quiet breathing is called:**
   a. Apnea
   b. Eupnea
   c. Hyperpnea
   d. Orthopnea

5. **Difficulty in breathing is called:**
   a. Apnea
   b. Eupnea
   c. Hyperpnea
   d. Dyspnea

6. **Partial pressure of O_2 in arterial blood in mm Hg is:**
   a. 40
   b. 46
   c. 95
   d. 100

7. **Diffusing capacity for O_2 in the lung normally is:**
   a. 21 mL/min/mm Hg
   b. 19.5 mL/min/mm Hg
   c. 14.5 mL/min/mm Hg
   d. 5 mL/min/mm Hg

8. **Under normal resting conditions, the amount of O_2 released into the tissues when 100 mL of blood passes through the tissue is:**
   a. 250 mL
   b. 15 mL
   c. 20 mL
   d. 5 mL

9. **The amount of CO_2 that enters the blood when 100 mL of blood passes through the tissue under normal resting condition is:**
   a. 4 mL
   b. 46 mL
   c. 200 mL
   d. 20 mL

10. **Normal oxygen consumption under resting condition is:**
    a. 200 mL
    b. 250 mL
    c. 5 L
    d. 5 mL

11. **Orthopnea means:**
    a. Temporary cessation of breathing
    b. Breathlessness on exertion
    c. Difficulty in breathing in the recumbent position
    d. Stimulation of respiration following exercise

12. **Diffusion across the respiratory membrane may be affected by all the factors, *except*:**
    a. Area of the membrane
    b. Thickness of the membrane
    c. Molecular weight of the gas
    d. Pulmonary capillary pressure

13. **The strongest direct stimulus to the respiratory center to increase ventilation is:**
    a. Increase in PCO_2 of arterial blood
    b. Increase in the PCO_2 of venous blood
    c. Decrease in PO_2 of arterial blood
    d. Fall in pH of arterial blood

14. **Arterial blood analysis of a child done at sea level gives the following results: pH 7.41, PaO_2 100 mm Hg, $PaCO_2$ 40 mm Hg. The child is being ventilated with 80% O_2. What is the (A-a) PO_2?**
    a. 570.4 mm Hg
    b. 520.4 mm Hg
    c. 470.4 mm Hg
    d. 420.4 mm Hg

15. **Respiratory quotient during exercise is:**
    a. 0.6–0.8
    b. 1.5–2
    c. 3–4
    d. 2.5–3
16. **Weightlessness result in:**
    a. Decreased cardiac output
    b. Hypotension
    c. Increased gut motility
    d. Osteoporosis
17. **Alveolar-arterial O_2 tension gradient increases in all, except:**
    a. Hypoventilation
    b. Right to left shunt
    c. Diffusion defect
    d. Ventilation perfusion abnormality
    Ans. (a)
18. **Alveolar hypoventilation is present in all, except:**
    a. Bulbar poliomyelitis a. COPD
    b. Kyphoscoliosis   c. Lobar pneumonia
19. **Addition of glucose to stored blood is to:**
    a. Prevent hemolysis
    b. Provide nutrition
    c. Increase hemoglobin content
    d. Increase 2-3-DPG
20. **Destruction of lung tissue and defective gas exchange causes all, except:**
    a. Prominent P wave in ECG
    b. Decreased cerebral blood circulation
    c. Increased red cell count
    d. Pulmonary hypertension
21. **The diffusing capacity of CO_2 when compared to that of O_2 is:**
    a. 20 times
    b. 10 times
    c. 5 times
    d. 2 times
22. **An increase in ventilation occurs in all the following situations, except:**
    a. Fall in plasma bicarbonate
    b. Sleep
    c. Fall in the pH of CSF
    d. Rise in blood adrenaline level
23. **Increase in thickness of the respiratory membrane occurs in:**
    a. Emphysema
    b. Bronchial asthma
    c. Pulmonary artery thrombosis
    d. Pulmonary edema
24. **Hematocrit of venous blood is:**
    a. 3% greater than arterial blood
    b. 3% less than arterial blood
    c. 3 times greater than arterial blood
    d. 3 times less than arterial blood
25. **Respiratory acidosis can cause:**
    a. Decreased PCO_2 and decreased pH
    b. Right to left shunt
    c. Diffusion defect
    d. Ventilation perfusion abnormality
26. **Normal respiratory quotient in an adult at rest is:**
    a. 0.6
    b. 1.5
    c. 0.8
    d. 2
27. **Partial pressure of oxygen in venous blood is:**
    a. 100 mm Hg
    b. 40 mm Hg
    c. 46 mm Hg
    d. 97 mm Hg
28. **Partial pressure of CO_2 in venous blood is:**
    a. 60 mmHg
    b. 40 mm Hg
    c. 37 mm Hg
    d. 46 mm Hg
29. **Which of the following diffuses freely from plasma to extracellular fluid?**
    a. CO_2
    b. H_2O
    c. Glucose
    d. Proteins

ANSWERS

1. a	2. c	2. d	4. b	5. d
6. c	7. a	8. d	9. a	10. b
11. c	12. d	13. a	14. d	15. b
16. d	17. a	18. d	19. d	20. b
21. a	22. b	23. d	24. a	25. a
26. c	27. b	28. d	29. a	

Transport of Gases

CHAPTER 38

LEARNING OBJECTIVES
- Describe the mechanisms of transport of oxygen in blood.
- Explain with the help of a diagram oxygen-hemoglobin dissociation curve.
- Enumerate the factors affecting ODC
- Describe the methods of transport of CO_2 in blood.
- Explain Bohr effect and Haldane effect

INTRODUCTION

PY6.3: Describe and discuss the transport of respiratory gases: Oxygen and carbon dioxide.

Transport of O_2 and CO_2 in the body depends on both the respiratory system and the cardiovascular system. Diffusion of gases occurs from higher partial pressures to lower partial pressures. As a result, O_2 from the alveoli diffuses into the deoxygenated blood in the pulmonary vasculature and CO_2 leaves the pulmonary vasculature into the alveoli where it is expired. The CO_2 formed in the tissues is carried to the alveoli and O_2 from the alveoli is carried to the tissues by the cardiovascular system **(Fig. 38.1)**. About 99% of O_2 entering the blood combines with hemoglobin and about 94.5% of CO_2 entering the blood from the tissues undergo a series of reversible chemical reactions that convert it into other compounds. These processes increase the O_2-carrying capacity of arterial blood 70-fold and the CO_2 content of venous blood 17-fold.

TRANSPORT OF OXYGEN

Oxygen (O_2) is transported from lungs to metabolically active tissues by the cardiovascular system. O_2 delivery to a particular tissue depends on the following factors:
- Amount of O_2 entering the lungs
- Adequacy of pulmonary gas exchange
- Blood flow to the tissue
- Capacity of the blood to carry O_2
- Capacity of the tissues to extract O_2 from blood

Blood flow to the tissue depends on:
- Degree of constriction of vascular bed in the tissue
- Cardiac output

Amount of O_2 in the blood depends on:
- Amount of dissolved O_2
- Amount of hemoglobin in blood
- Affinity of hemoglobin for O_2

Forms in which O_2 is Transported in Blood

- **Soluble form**: About 3% of O_2 is transported in the dissolved form, i.e., 100 mL of pure blood contains 0.3 mL of O_2 dissolved in plasma. Venous blood contains 0.12 mL of dissolved O_2 in 100 mL. *The volume of dissolved O_2, although very less, is of great functional importance for; it is the gas in solution alone that exerts the partial pressure.* It is the PO_2 of blood that determines the quantity of O_2 that will combine with hemoglobin.
- In combination **with hemoglobin** (97%): The amount of O_2 dissolved in blood is very little to meet the metabolic demands of the body. Since the amount of dissolved O_2 in blood is only 0.3 mL/100 mL of blood, the amount of O_2 that can be delivered to the tissues in one minute will be only 15 mL/minute. But at rest an adult human consumes

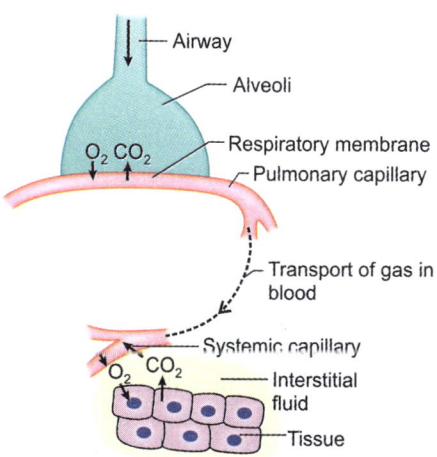

Fig. 38.1: Steps in the transport of gases.

O_2 at a rate of ~250 mL/min. So the O_2 content of blood should be increased and this is achieved by hemoglobin within the erythrocytes.

Reaction of Hemoglobin and O_2 or Oxygenation of Hemoglobin

Hemoglobin is a protein made up of 4 heme subunits. Iron is present in the ferrous form in the center of each heme subunit. Under normal conditions, hemoglobin reversibly binds approximately 97% of O_2 that diffuses from the alveolar air spaces to the pulmonary capillary blood. This greatly increases the O_2 carrying capacity of blood.

Oxygenation of Hemoglobin

Oxygenation of hemoglobin is the loose and reversible combination of O_2 with ferrous ion in the hemoglobin molecule. *No oxidation reaction takes place,* only oxygenation of iron occurs which is only a physical combination.

Even after combination of O_2 with iron, iron remains in the ferrous form, i.e., it is not oxidized to ferric form. That is why the combination of O_2 with hemoglobin is called oxygenation and not oxidation.

Advantages of Oxygenation

- Hemoglobin accepts O_2 readily when partial pressure of O_2 in blood is more to form the loose compound **oxyhemoglobin**.
- Oxyhemoglobin releases O_2 readily whenever the partial pressure of O_2 in the blood is less, forming deoxygenated hemoglobin or **reduced hemoglobin**.

Heme-heme Interaction

One molecule of hemoglobin can combine with 4 molecules of O_2. Hemoglobin molecule is represented as Hb_4 and when it reacts with 4 molecules of O_2 it forms Hb_4O_8.

$Hb_4 + O_2 \leftrightarrow Hb_4O_2$

$Hb_4O_2 + O_2 \leftrightarrow Hb_4O_4$

$Hb_4O_4 + O_2 \leftrightarrow Hb_4O_6$

$Hb_4O_6 + O_2 \leftrightarrow Hb_4O_8$

Combination of the first heme in the hemoglobin molecule with one molecule of O_2 increases the affinity of second heme subunit in that hemoglobin molecule for the next molecule of O_2 and so on. This is known as **heme-heme interaction**. The reaction is rapid and is completed within 0.01 sec.

In the tissues these reactions are reversed releasing O_2. Deoxygenation of Hb_4O_8 is also very rapid.

There are two configuration states for hemoglobin: T or **tense state** and R or **relaxed state**. Change from tense state to relaxed state increases the O_2 affinity of hemoglobin 500 fold.

Change from tense to relaxed state is due to the release of bonds holding globin units and it occurs 108 times in the life of a red blood cell.

In pure blood, 19.5 mL of O_2 is bound to hemoglobin per 100 mL of blood. In impure blood, 15 mL of O_2 is bound to hemoglobin per 100 mL of blood.

Oxygen Carrying Capacity of Hemoglobin

Oxygen carrying capacity of hemoglobin is the amount of O_2 contained in 100 mL of blood in combination with hemoglobin when all the hemoglobin is fully saturated with O_2. About 97% of O_2 in blood combines with hemoglobin and the presence of hemoglobin increases the O_2 carrying capacity of blood 70-fold. When fully saturated each gram of hemoglobin can combine with 1.34 mL of O_2. Hemoglobin concentration is ~ 15 g/dL of blood. So, 100 mL of blood contain 15 × 1.34 = 20.1 mL of O_2 bound to hemoglobin when hemoglobin is 100% saturated with O_2.

Oxygen Content

Amount of O_2 normally present in 100 mL of arterial blood. It is the sum of the amount of O_2 in solution and the amount of O_2 in combination with hemoglobin.

Oxygen content = 0.3 + 19.5 = 19.8 mL/100 mL of blood. Because of **physiological shunt**, the hemoglobin in the systemic arterial blood is only 97% saturated. Even though the theoretical value is 20.1 mL/100 mL, the actual value is only 19.5 mL/100 mL of arterial blood. At rest, hemoglobin in the venous blood is 75% saturated and the total O_2 content in venous blood is 15 mL/100 mL of blood. Thus, at rest tissues remove 4.8 mL of O_2 from each 100 mL of blood passing through them. Thus, 250 mL of O_2 is transported to tissues from blood in 1 min at rest. This is O_2 **consumption**.

Percentage Saturation of Hemoglobin

$$\% \text{ Saturation} = \frac{O_2 \text{ bound to Hb}}{O_2 \text{ capacity of Hb}} \times 100$$

$$= \frac{19.5 \text{ mL}}{20.1 \text{ mL}} \times 100 = 97\%$$

Oxygen Dissociation Curve of Hemoglobin (ODC)

Principle

Blood samples are exposed to varying O_2 tensions in tonometers and O_2 content is determined. Finally, PO_2 is so adjusted that hemoglobin is fully saturated with O_2 and O_2 capacity is determined. For each PO_2, the % saturation is found out.

Procedure

Ten **tonometers** are filled, each with a known quantity of blood having known hemoglobin concentration. The blood in each tonometer is exposed to O_2 at different partial pressures at a constant temperature. Then the blood in each tonometer is analyzed to measure the % saturation of hemoglobin with O_2 **(Table 38.1)**. The partial pressure of O_2 and % saturation are plotted to get the oxygen dissociation curve (ODC) for hemoglobin. The graph is plotted with PO_2 on the X axis and % saturation on the Y axis.

The ODC of hemoglobin is **sigmoid shaped** or S-shaped because when the partial pressure of O_2 is more, hemoglobin accepts O_2 and when partial pressure of O_2 is less, hemoglobin

Table 38.1: PO_2 and % saturation of Hb in the ten tonometers.

PO_2 (mm Hg)	% saturation of hemoglobin
10	13.5
20	35
30	57
40	75
50	83.5
60	89
70	92.7
80	94.5
90	96.5
100	100

releases O_2. This is due to heme-heme interaction or T-R interconversion. It denotes easy binding of hemoglobin with O_2 when PO_2 is high, which occurs at lung level in the body. It also denotes increased dissociation of O_2 from oxyhemoglobin where PO_2 is low, i.e., at tissue level in the body.

The graph has three parts or phases (**Fig. 38.2**):
1. Flat top
2. Steep fall
3. Flat bottom

Flat Top

When PO_2 falls from 100 mm Hg to 60 mm Hg, there is not much change in the % saturation of hemoglobin. Even at a PO_2 of 60 mm Hg, hemoglobin is 90% saturated and this is sufficient for normal activities. This is a protective measure for a person going to high altitude. Up to 60 mm Hg, he does not develop hypoxic symptoms.

Steep Fall (Dissociation Phase)

Below PO_2 of 60 mm Hg, there is a marked reduction in % saturation and the curve becomes steep. In this phase there is wide variation in % saturation with minute change in PO_2 and O_2 is released readily from hemoglobin. This is the **tissue phase**. In the tissues, PO_2 is only 40 mm Hg and so oxyhemoglobin releases O_2 rapidly and tissues can extract large quantities of O_2.

Flat Bottom

At very low levels of PO_2, dissociation of oxyhemoglobin becomes difficult. For a person with chronic lung disease this is a safety measure. *There will be symptoms of hypoxia at lower PO_2 and adequate measures can be taken.*

Factors Affecting ODC

Shift to Right of ODC (Fig. 38.3)

Shift to right indicates easy dissociation of O_2 from hemoglobin. Here, a higher PO_2 is required for hemoglobin to bind a given amount of O_2, i.e., the affinity of O_2 for hemoglobin is decreased.

P50: This is an index used to indicate the affinity of hemoglobin for O_2. P_{50} is the PO_2 at which hemoglobin is half saturated with O_2 (*See* **Fig. 38.2**).

Normal P_{50} – 25 mm Hg

Higher the P_{50} lower is the affinity of hemoglobin for O_2, i.e., dissociation is favored. In shift to right, P_{50} is increased. Here, more PO_2 is required to half saturate hemoglobin with O_2, i.e., when P_{50} is increased, the affinity of hemoglobin for O_2 is less.

Factors Causing Shift to Right

- Increase in PCO_2
- Decrease in PO_2
- Increase in H^+ concentration (decrease in pH)
- Increase in temperature
- Increase in 2,3-DPG (diphosphoglycerate) or 2,3-BPG (bisphosphoglycerate)

All the above factors are increased when tissue metabolism is increased as in exercise. 2,3-DPG is seen in plenty in the RBC. The concentration of 2,3 DPG in the RBC is about the

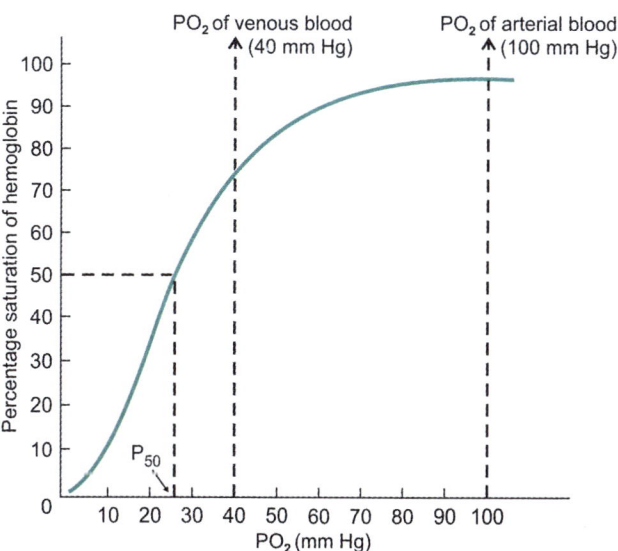

Fig. 38.2: Oxygen-hemoglobin dissociation curve (ODC). P_{50} is the PO_2 at which hemoglobin is half saturated with O_2. Normal P_{50} is 25 mm Hg.

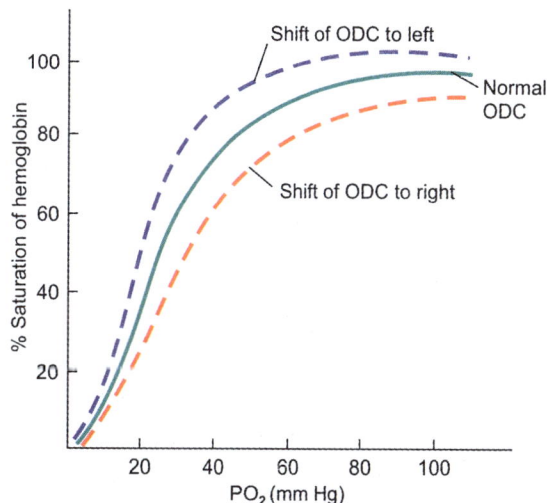

Fig. 38.3: Shift of oxygen-hemoglobin dissociation curve.

same as that of hemoglobin. It is a product of glycolysis via **Embden-Meyerhof pathway**. It is a highly charged anion that binds to the β-chain of deoxyhemoglobin. An increase in 2,3-DPG causes liberation of more O_2 and ODC is shifted to the right.

More O_2 becomes available to the tissues.
$$HbO_2 + 2,3\text{-DPG} \leftrightarrow Hb\text{-}2,3\text{-DPG} + O_2$$

2,3-DPG is increased in:
- Exercise
- Hypoxic conditions as in chronic lung disease, anemia, at high altitude, etc. Hypoxia increases glycolysis in RBC
- Hormones such as thyroid hormones, androgen, growth hormone, etc.
- Alkalosis

Bohr Effect

The decrease in the O_2 affinity of hemoglobin when the pH of blood falls due to increase in PCO_2 is called **Bohr Effect**. There is unloading of O_2 from hemoglobin. The O_2 dissociation curve shifts to the right and P_{50} rises. This is because deoxyhemoglobin binds H^+ more actively, than oxyhemoglobin. Greater the CO_2 tension in the tissue greater will be the O_2 release.

$$HbO_2 + CO_2 \leftrightarrow HbCO_2 + O_2$$
$$HbO_2 + H_+ \leftrightarrow HbH^+ + O_2$$

All factors that shift ODC to the right influence Bohr effect.

Shift to Left of ODC

Affinity of hemoglobin for O_2 is more and P_{50} is decreased in shift to left. A lower PO_2 is required for hemoglobin to bind a given amount of O_2.

Factors Causing Shift to Left

- Decrease in PCO_2
- Decrease in H+ concentration (alkalosis)
- Decrease in temperature
- Decrease in 2,3-DPG
- Fetal hemoglobin

2,3-DPG is decreased in acidosis and in stored blood. In acidosis there is inhibition of red cell glycolysis and 2,3-DPG falls.

Ability of blood stored with **acid citrate dextrose (ACD)** as anticoagulant, to release O₂ to the tissues is less. This decrease is less if blood is stored in citrate-phosphate-dextrose (CPD) solution rather than ACD. This is a form of **preservation injury** due to ACD. The 2,3-DPG level falls and ODC shifts to left. *This is the reason why stored blood is not safe to be transfused to a hypoxic patient.*

In fetal hemoglobin (HbF) instead of β chains, there are γ chains. 2,3 DPG cannot combine with γ chains. So, there is a shift to left of ODC, i.e., affinity of hemoglobin for O_2 is more and the P50 is reduced. Significance of this is that:
- It helps in the movement of O_2 from maternal blood to fetal blood because affinity of fetal hemoglobin for O_2 is more.
- Release of O_2 to the fetal tissues is less since HbF has more affinity for O_2. So, tissues suffer from hypoxia, which in turn stimulates erythropoietin secretion. *This is the reason for the high RBC count in fetus.*

Coefficient of Utilization

Coefficient of utilization is the percentage of O_2 utilized, out of the amount which is made available to the tissues in arterial blood.

$$\text{Coefficient of utilization} = \frac{O_2 \text{ taken up by the tissue}}{O_2 \text{ content of arterial blood}} \times 100$$

$$\text{Normal value} = \frac{5}{19.8} \times 100 = 25\%$$

In severe exercise, the coefficient of utilization in skeletal muscle will be as high as 90%. Here, 80–90% of O_2 in arterial blood reaching the muscle is utilized by the muscle because the tissue PO_2 may fall to zero.

Myoglobin

Myoglobin is an iron-containing pigment in muscle, especially skeletal muscle. Only one heme unit is present in myoglobin and so one molecule of myoglobin can combine with only one molecule of O_2. Myoglobin does not show Bohr effect. Myoglobin has a lower P_{50} than adult hemoglobin **(Table 38.2)**. *The ODC for myoglobin is a rectangular hyperbola.* The curve is to the left of hemoglobin curve. So it takes up O_2 from hemoglobin and releases O_2 only at very low PO_2 values, i.e., below 5 mm Hg **(Fig. 38.4)**.

In exercise when there is sustained muscle contraction due to compression of blood vessels, blood flow is cut off and PO_2 in the muscle becomes zero or very low and the muscle

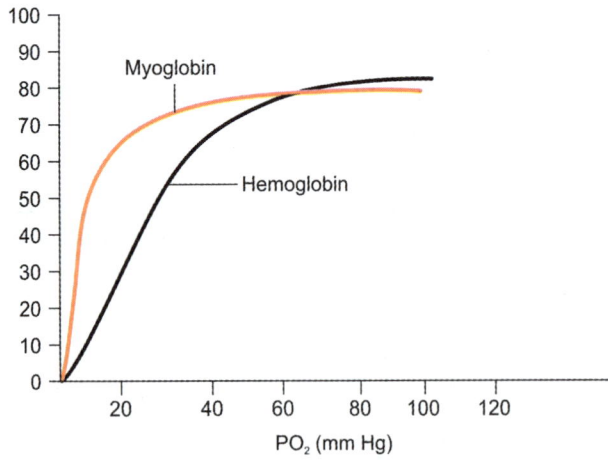

Fig. 38.4: Oxygen dissociation curves for hemoglobin (sigmoid curve) and myoglobin (rectangular hyperbola).

Table 38.2: Differences between hemoglobin and myoglobin.	
Hemoglobin	**Myoglobin**
Present in red blood cells	Present in muscles, especially skeletal muscle
Contains 4 heme subunits	Contains only one heme subunit
Combines with 4 molecules of O_2	Combines with only one molecule of O_2
Shows Bohr effect	Does not show Bohr effect
P_{50}—25 mm Hg	P_{50}—5 mm Hg
ODC—sigmoid-shaped	ODC—rectangular hyperbola

utilizes O_2 in myoglobin. Thus, myoglobin acts as a temporary storehouse of O_2 in the muscle. A man of average size can store about 1.5 L of O_2 in his myoglobin at rest.

CARBON DIOXIDE TRANSPORT

Carbon dioxide entering the blood undergoes a series of reversible chemical reactions and forms different compounds. These reactions of CO_2 increase the blood CO_2 content 17-fold. In the blood, CO_2 is transported in three forms:

1. Dissolved form	–	10%
2. As carbamino compounds	–	20%
3. In the form of bicarbonate	–	70%

Dissolved Form

About 10% of CO_2 in the blood is in the dissolved form, i.e., 2.5 mL of CO_2 is dissolved in 100 mL of arterial blood. Solubility of CO_2 in blood is 20 times that of O_2 and so there is more CO_2 than O_2 in simple solution.

As Carbamino Compounds

About 20% of CO_2 in blood is transported in combination with the amino group of plasma proteins and hemoglobin. CO_2 combines with hemoglobin to form **carbaminohemoglobin** and with plasma proteins to form **carbaminoprotein**.

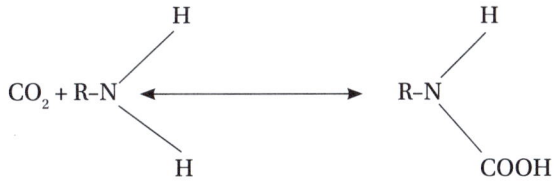

As HCO_3^-

Changes at the Tissue Level

Since the PCO_2 in the tissue is high, CO_2 diffuses from tissues into the plasma. From there it enters the RBC which contains plenty of carbonic anhydrase (CA). In blood, 70% of CO_2 is transported as HCO_3^-. In RBC, the following reaction takes place:

$$CO_2 + H_2O \xrightarrow{CA} H_2CO_3 \longleftrightarrow H^+ + HCO_3^-$$

About 70% of HCO_3^- formed in the RBC enters the plasma and combines with Na^+ to form $NaHCO_3$. Rest of the HCO_3^- inside the RBC combines with K^+ to form $KHCO_3$.

H^+ is buffered by hemoglobin, thus maintaining acid-base balance.

Reduced hemoglobin has more affinity for CO_2 and is a good proton acceptor, i.e., it is a strong buffer. This occurs at tissue level. When HCO_3^- diffuses from RBC to plasma, in order to maintain electrical neutrality, Cl^- ions enter RBC. This is called **chloride shift or Hamberger phenomenon**. For each CO_2 molecule added to the RBC, there is an increase of one osmotically active particle, either HCO_3^- or Cl^- in the RBC. As the osmotically active substances in the RBC increase, water enters the RBC. This is called **water shift**. *This is the reason for the larger size of RBCs in venous blood than in arterial blood and also for the increased fragility of red blood cells in venous blood* (Fig. 38.5).

Reasons for the 3% Increase in the Hematocrit Value in Venous Blood

❖ Water shift and chloride shift (explain).
❖ Small amount of fluid in the arterial blood returns to circulation through the lymphatics rather than through the veins. So, the amount of plasma in venous blood will be less than that in arterial blood.

Changes Occurring at Lung Level

In the lungs, PO_2 is high and hemoglobin combines with O_2 and releases H^+.

$$HHb + O_2 \longrightarrow HbO_2 + H^+$$

Oxyhemoglobin is a good proton donor and a poor buffer. H^+ combines with HCO_3^- to form H_2CO_3 which dissociates to form H_2O and CO_2. CO_2 diffuses into the alveoli. HCO_3^- from plasma enters RBC in exchange for Cl^-. Water also diffuses out of RBC along with Cl^-. This is called **reverse Cl^- and water shift** (Fig. 38.6).

Carbon Dioxide Dissociation Curve (CDC)

A graph is plotted with PCO_2 on the X-axis and CO_2 content on the Y-axis for venous and arterial blood. CO_2 dissociation curve will be at a higher level for venous blood than for arterial blood. Point A in the graph denotes that in the arterial blood at a PCO_2 of 40 mm Hg, CO_2 content is 48 mL/100 mL of blood. Point B denotes that in the venous blood at a PCO_2

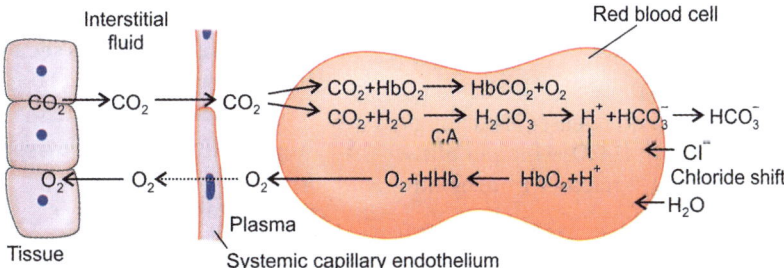

Fig. 38.5: Events occurring in gas exchange at the tissue level.
(CA: carbonic anhydrase; HbO_2: oxyhemoglobin; HHb: reduced hemoglobin; $HbCO_2$: carbaminohemoglobin)

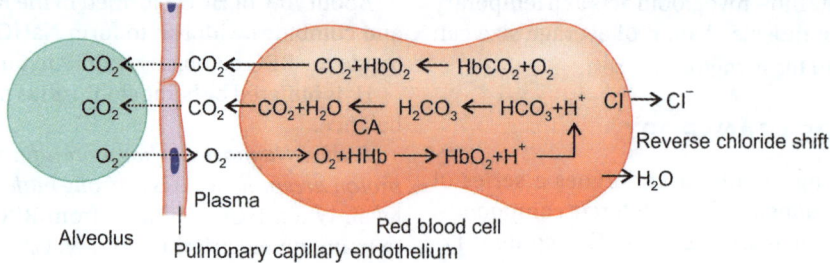

Fig. 38.6: Events occurring at the lung level. Chloride and water leaves the RBC at the lung level. This is reverse water and chloride shift.

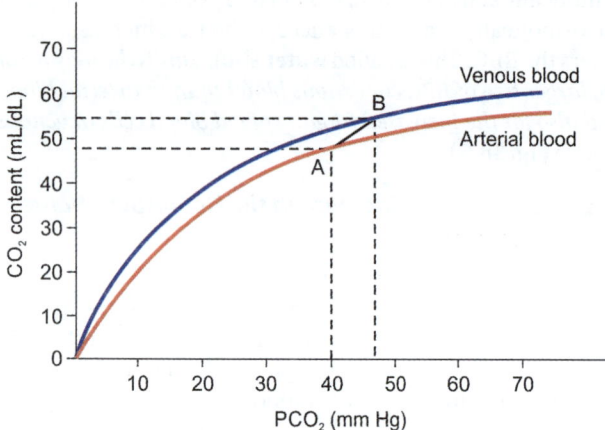

Fig. 38.7: Carbon dioxide dissociation curve for arterial and venous blood to demonstrate Haldane effect.

of 46 mm Hg, CO_2 content is 52 mL/100 mL of blood. The line joining A and B is called *physiological dissociation curve for CO_2* (Fig. 38.7).

Haldane Effect or Role of O_2-Hb Reaction in CO_2 Transport

Deoxygenated hemoglobin binds more CO_2 than oxyhemoglobin and forms carbamino-hemoglobin and CDC shifts to left. Whenever hemoglobin is oxygenated, it displaces CO_2 from its combination and CDC shifts to right. This was first detected by Haldane and is known as **Haldane effect or CDH effect** (Christiansen, Douglas, Haldane effect).

Causes of Haldane Effect

- Deoxyhemoglobin has more affinity for CO_2 and so there is increased pickup of CO_2 from tissues.
- Oxyhemoglobin has less affinity for CO_2 and so CO_2 is released from blood to alveoli in the lungs.
- Reduced hemoglobin is a weaker acid and a strong buffer and binds more H^+ at tissue level.

$$Hb + H^+ \longrightarrow HHb$$

- Oxyhemoglobin is a stronger acid and releases H+ at lung level. H+ binds with HCO_3^- to form H_2CO_3 which in turn splits to form CO_2 and H_2O, and CO_2 is released from blood to alveoli.

$$HHb + O_2 \longrightarrow HbO_2 + H^+$$
$$HCO_3^- + H^+ \longrightarrow H_2CO_3 \longrightarrow CO_2 + H_2O$$

Importance of CDH Effect

- Haldane effect doubles the amount of CO_2 released from blood into the lungs and doubles the pickup of CO_2 from the tissues. If Haldane effect was not there, at the lung level the CO_2 content of blood would have fallen only to 50 volume%. But due to Haldane effect CO_2 content falls to 48 volume%. Thus, 4 mL of CO_2 is removed by lungs when 100 mL of blood passes through the lungs.
- Haldane effect increases the uptake of O_2 by blood in the lungs.

Changes Occurring in Exercise

In exercise there is increased metabolism leading to increased CO_2 production and increased O_2 uptake by the tissues.

- Pressure gradient for CO_2 at tissue level increases and more CO_2 diffuses into blood.
- Capillary dilatation in exercise due to metabolites increases capillary surface area which increases diffusion of gases.
- O_2 uptake in tissues is increased in exercise leading to increase in the concentration of reduced hemoglobin leading to increased production of carbaminohemoglobin and HHb.
- *Bohr effect*: Due to decrease in pH and increase in PCO_2, ODC shifts to right. Greater the CO_2 tension in the tissue, greater will be the amount of O_2 released from hemoglobin. In other words, increased PCO_2 lowers the affinity of hemoglobin for O_2 and more O_2 will be released from oxyhemoglobin.

MULTIPLE CHOICE QUESTIONS

1. **The affinity of O_2 for hemoglobin decreases with fall in pH. This is called:**
   a. Bain bridge effect
   b. Bohr effect
   c. Haldane effect
   d. Herring effect

2. **Shift to right of ODC is seen in:**
   a. Increased $PaCO_2$
   b. Decreased $PaCO_2$
   c. Increased pH
   d. Increased PO_2

3. **Right shift of oxygen dissociation curve occurs in all, *except*:**
   a. Blood transfusion
   b. Shock
   c. Respiratory distress syndrome
   d. Congestive cardiac failure

CHAPTER 38 → Transport of Gases

4. Myoglobin binds with:
   a. 1 mole of oxygen per mL
   b. 2 mole of oxygen per mL
   c. 3 mole of oxygen per mL
   d. 4 mole of oxygen per mL
5. H$^+$ is more bound to:
   a. Deoxygenated hemoglobin
   b. Oxygenated hemoglobin
   c. Carbonmonoxy hemoglobin
   d. Not related to oxygenation
6. Oxygen affinity decreases in:
   a. Hypoxia   b. Hypothermia
   c. HbF   d. Increase in pH
7. Oxygen dissociation curve is shifted to the right in all the following, *except*:
   a. Fall in pH   b. Rise in temperature
   c. Increase in 2-3-BPG d. Fetal hemoglobin
8. In Bohr effect:
   a. O$_2$ dissociation increases in hypoxia
   b. O$_2$ dissociation decreases in hypoxia
   c. O$_2$ dissociation increase with increase in temperature
   d. O$_2$ dissociation increases with fall in pH
9. Which of the following diffuses freely from plasma to extracellular space?
   a. CO$_2$ b. Water
   c. Glucose   d. Proteins
10. Role of 2-3-BPG in hemoglobin:
    a. Unloading O$_2$ to tissues
    b. Increased affinity for O$_2$
    c. Buffering capacity
    d. Osmotic fragility
11. In anemia, the concentration of 2,3-BPG is:
    a. Decreased
    b. Increased
    c. Not changed
    d. May be decreased or increased
12. Decreased O$_2$ affinity of hemoglobin in blood with decreased pH:
    a. Haldane effect   b. Double Haldane effect
    c. Bohr effect   d. Double Bohr effect
13. PCO$_2$ is maximum in:
    a. Interstitial fluid   b. Venous blood
    c. Intracellular fluid d. Lymph
14. PCO$_2$ of venous blood is:
    a. 40 mm Hg   b. 0.3 mm Hg
    c. 46 mm Hg   d. 100 mm Hg
15. PCO$_2$ of arterial blood is:
    a. 40 mm Hg   b. 0.3 mm Hg
    c. 46 mm Hg   d. 100 mm Hg
16. PCO$_2$ of intracellular fluid is:
    a. 40 mm Hg   b. 50 mm Hg
    c. 46 mm Hg   d. 0.3 mm Hg
17. O$_2$ carrying capacity of blood with hemoglobin content of 15 g/100 mL is:
    a. 14 mL/100 mL   b. 19.5 mL/100 mL
    c. 20.1 mL/100 mL   d. 15.2 mL/100 mL
18. The percentage of total CO$_2$ transported in combination with hemoglobin is:
    a. 13%   b. 30%
    c. 20%   d. 7%
19. Sigmoid shape of oxygen-hemoglobin dissociation curve is due to the fact that as the combination of oxygen with hemoglobin molecule proceeds, there is:
    a. Decreased affinity of heme subunits for oxygen
    b. Oxidation of hemoglobin molecule
    c. Increased affinity of heme subunits for oxygen
    d. Decreased affinity of hemoglobin for H$^+$
20. The term, Hamberger phenomenon refers to:
    a. Movement of chloride out of RBC
    b. Movement of chloride into RBC
    c. Movement of carbon dioxide into RBC
    d. Movement of bicarbonate into RBC
21. Maximum CO$_2$ is transported in venous blood:
    a. Dissolved in plasma
    b. Bound to plasma proteins
    c. Bound to hemoglobin
    d. As HCO$_3^-$
22. Oxygen dissociation curve of hemoglobin shows that:
    a. O$_2$ saturation of hemoglobin is 100% at PO$_2$ 80 mm Hg
    b. % saturation of hemoglobin is almost the same between PO$_2$ 100 and 70 mm Hg
    c. O$_2$ is rapidly released from hemoglobin at a PO$_2$ of 100 mm Hg
    d. At the normal PO$_2$ of arterial blood, hemoglobin is almost 75% saturated
23. Chloride shift during CO$_2$ transport causes:
    a. Split of HCO$_3$
    b. Formation of carbonic acid
    c. Increase in hematocrit
    d. Formation of carbamino compound
24. Shift of oxygen dissociation curve to the right occurs in:
    a. Acidosis
    b. Decrease in 2-3 BPG
    c. Decrease in temperature
    d. Decrease in PCO$_2$
25. Impairment of CO$_2$ diffusion is rarely a clinical problem because:
    a. PCO$_2$ level is not so high as that of O$_2$
    b. The pulmonary diffusion capacity for CO$_2$ is much higher than that of O$_2$
    c. Hypercapnia is not so harmful as that of hypoxia
    d. All of the above

26. Oxygen dissociation curve shift to left in all the following conditions, *except*:
    a. Alkalosis
    b. Acidosis
    c. Decrease in 2,3 BPG
    d. Decrease in temperature
27. In Bohr effect:
    a. Oxygen dissociation increases in hypoxia
    b. Oxygen dissociation decreases in hypoxia
    c. Oxygen dissociation increase with increase in temperature
    d. Affinity of hemoglobin for oxygen increases
28. The most important factor in the transport of CO_2 as bicarbonate in blood is:
    a. Affinity of CO_2 for hemoglobin
    b. Basic nature of bicarbonate
    c. Increased solubility of CO_2 in plasma
    d. Presence of plenty of carbonic anhydrase in RBC
29. Effect of changes in PCO_2 on oxygen dissociation curve is denoted by:
    a. Dalton's law
    b. Boyle's law
    c. Bohr effect
    d. Haldane effect
30. During exercise, increase in O_2 delivery to muscles is because of all, *except*:
    a. Oxygen dissociation curve shifts to left
    b. Increased stroke volume
    c. Increased extraction of O_2 from blood
    d. Increased blood flow to muscles
31. Oxygen dissociation curve (ODC) shifts to right in all, *except*:
    a. Diabetic ketoacidosis
    b. Blood transfusion
    c. High altitude
    d. Anemia
32. Which compound shifts ODC to the right?
    a. 1-phosphoglycerate
    b. 2,3 DPG
    c. 1,3 DPG
    d. Glyceraldehyde
33. ODC shifts to right in:
    a. Hypothermia
    b. Hypercapnia
    c. Fetal hemoglobin
    d. Hypothermia
34. ODC is shifted to the right in all, *except*:
    a. Hypercapnia
    b. Rise in temperature
    c. Raised 2,3 DPG level
    d. Metabolic alkalosis
35. True about hemoglobin dissociation curve is:
    a. Acidosis shifts ODC to right
    b. Increase in CO_2 shifts the curve to left
    c. Hypoxia shifts curve to left
    d. 2,3 DPG has no effect on the curve
36. The important feature of 2-3 diphosphoglycerate include:
    a. Higher concentration in adult blood than fetal blood
    b. Contribution to Bohr effect
    c. Increases affinity of O_2 to hemoglobin
    d. Associated with fetal blood to promote oxygenation
37. All the following factors influence hemoglobin dissociation curve, *except*:
    a. Chloride ion concentration
    b. CO_2 tension
    c. Temperature
    d. 2-3 DPG level
38. An increase in which of the parameters will shift the ODC to the left?
    a. Temperature
    b. Partial pressure of CO_2
    c. 2-3 DPG concentration
    d. Oxygen affinity of hemoglobin
39. Oxygen affinity is increased by all the following, *except*:
    a. Alkalosis
    b. Hypoxia
    c. Increased HbF
    d. ypothermia
40. Oxygen delivery to the tissues is decreased by:
    a. Increase in hemoglobin
    b. Increased PaO_2
    c. Increased $PaCO_2$
    d. Increased pH
41. The factor responsible for the left shift of ODC:
    a. Increase in 2-DPG in RBC
    b. Fall in temperature
    c. Fall in pH
    d. Increased level of CO_2 in blood
42. The sigmoid nature of ODC is because of:
    a. Binding of one molecule of O_2 increases the affinity for the next O_2 molecule
    b. Alpha chain has more affinity for O_2 than beta chain
    c. Beta chain has more affinity for O_2 than alpha chain
    d. Hemoglobin is acidic in nature
43. Hamberger phenomenon means:
    a. Movement of chloride out of red blood cells
    b. Movement of chloride into erythrocytes
    c. Movement of CO_2 into erythrocytes
    d. Movement of O_2 into the interstitial space
44. The highest PCO_2 is generally found in:
    a. Intracellular fluid
    b. Interstitial fluid
    c. Arterial blood
    d. Venous blood
45. Dissociation of oxyhemoglobin is greater for declining PO_2 values in the range of:
    a. 100–80 mm Hg.
    b. 80–60 mm Hg
    c. 40–20 mm Hg
    d. 20–0 mm Hg
46. The normal value of P_{50} on the oxyhemoglobin dissociation curve in an adult is:
    a. 1.8 kPa
    b. 2.7 kPa
    c. 3.6 kPa
    d. 4.5 kPa

47. The concentration of O_2 in blood is calculated to be 0.0025 mL/mL of blood. Considering atmospheric pressure as 760 mm Hg, calculate the O_2 tension in the blood.
   a. 40 mm Hg
   b. 60 mm Hg
   c. 80 mm Hg
   d. 100 mm Hg

48. Arterial blood O_2 in mL of O_2 per deciliter is:
   a. 12.1
   b. 19.8
   c. 15.6
   d. 27.8

49. The normal value of PO_2 in a healthy man is:
   a. 45 mm Hg
   b. 110 mm Hg
   c. 90 mm Hg
   d. 60 mm Hg

50. Percentage of O_2 carried in chemical combination:
   a. 97%
   b. 3%
   c. 66%
   d. 33%

51. Arterial CO_2 level is:
   a. 40 mm Hg
   b. 37 mm Hg
   c. 45 mm Hg
   d. 60 mm Hg

52. CO_2 is transported in combination with hemoglobin as:
   a. Carboxyhemoglobin
   b. Carbamino hemoglobin
   c. Meth hemoglobin
   d. Reduced hemoglobin

53. Hemoglobin is responsible for carrying:
   a. Oxygen
   b. H⁺
   c. Carbon monoxide
   d. All of the above

54. CO_2 is transported in arterial blood mainly as:
   a. Dissolved CO_2
   b. Carbaminohemoglobin
   c. Carbonic acid
   d. Bicarbonate

55. Oxygen dissociation curve shifts to the right in all *except*:
   a. High altitude
   b. Diabetic ketoacidosis
   c. Anemia
   d. Blood transfusion

56. Hemoglobin unlike myoglobin shows:
   a. Sigmoid curve of oxygen dissociation
   b. Hill's coefficient of one
   c. Parabolic curve for oxygen dissociation
   d. None of the above

57. Hemoglobin dissociation curve is influenced by all *except*:
   a. CO_2 tension
   b. Temperature
   c. 2, 3-DPG level
   d. Chloride concentration

ANSWERS

1. b	2. a	3. a	4. a	5. a
6. a	7. d	8. d	9. a	10. a
11. b	12. c	13. c	14. c	15. a
16. b	17. c	18. a	19. c	20. b
21. d	22. b	23. c	24. a	25. b
26. b	27. a	28. d	29. c	30. a
31. b	32. b	33. b	34. d	35. a
36. a	37. a	38. d	39. b	40. d
41. b	42. a	43. b	44. a	45. b
46. c	47. c	48. b	49. c	50. a
51. a	52. b	53. d	54. d	55. d
56. a	57. d			

Regulation of Respiration

CHAPTER 39

LEARNING OBJECTIVES
- Draw the neural centers of respiration
- Describe the neural regulation of respiration including reflex regulation
- Describe the chemical regulation of respiration
- Explain the mechanism of action of central chemoreceptors
- Explain the pathophysiology of periodic breathing
- Classify the different types of hypoxia and explain the features of each type
- Explain the pathophysiology of asphyxia and cyanosis

■ INTRODUCTION

The main function of the respiratory system is to maintain PCO_2, PO_2 and pH of arterial blood constant by adjusting ventilation.

Spontaneous respiration is produced by rhythmic discharges from the brain to the motor neurons that innervate the respiratory muscles. This discharge is regulated by arterial PO_2, PCO_2 and H^+ concentration.

Respiration is regulated by two mechanisms—**neural control and chemical control**.

NEURAL CONTROL OF RESPIRATION
- Voluntary control
- Automatic control
- Reflex control

■ VOLUNTARY CONTROL

Respiration is a spontaneous (reflex) process. But to some extent it can be controlled voluntarily because most of the muscles concerned with respiration are voluntary muscles. The center for voluntary control is the **motor cortex** which sends impulses through the corticospinal tract to the respiratory motor neurons.

Voluntary hyperventilation and voluntary apnea are possible. The point at which breathing can no longer be voluntarily inhibited is called **breaking point**. Normally it is 40 seconds. This is because during apnea there is increase in PCO_2, decrease in PO_2 and increase in H^+ concentration. This will stimulate respiration.

In conditions like bulbar poliomyelitis, tumors of brainstem, etc., automatic control will be lost and voluntary control alone will be present. This is because impulses arising from brainstem control automatic respiration. This condition is known as **Ondine's curse**.

■ AUTOMATIC CONTROL

The automatic system for control of respiration is located in the **pons and medulla (Fig. 39.1)**. The respiratory centers are located bilaterally. The nerve fibers mediating inspiration converge on phrenic motor neurons (C3, 4, 5) and external intercostal neurons in spinal cord. The fibers concerned with expiration converge on the motor neurons in the spinal cord controlling the muscles of expiration, mainly internal intercostal muscles.

The motor neurons to expiratory muscles are inhibited when those supplying the inspiratory muscles are active and vice versa through **reciprocal innervation**. Exception to reciprocal innervation is a small amount of activity in phrenic axons in the early part of expiration. This is to put a brake to the lung's elastic recoil and make expiration smooth and not spasmodic.

Medullary Centers (Fig. 39.1)

Rhythmic respiration is initiated by a small group of pacemaker cells in the **pre-Botzinger complex** on both sides of medulla, between nucleus ambiguus and lateral reticular nucleus. These neurons can discharge rhythmically and are responsible for the rhythmicity of respiration. The cells in the pre-Botzinger complex contain opioid receptors and opioids inhibit respiration. Depression of respiration is a side effect of opioids which are given to relieve pain.

In addition to pre-Botzinger complex, medulla also contains **dorsal respiratory group (DRG) and ventral respiratory group (VRG)** of neurons.

Dorsal respiratory group of neurons (DRG) is located in and near the nucleus of tractus solitarius (NTS).

Respiratory portion of NTS is located ventrolateral to the tractus solitarius. These NTS neurons, as well as some immediately adjacent neurons in the dorsal medulla, make up the DRG. DRG is made up of I (inspiratory) neurons which

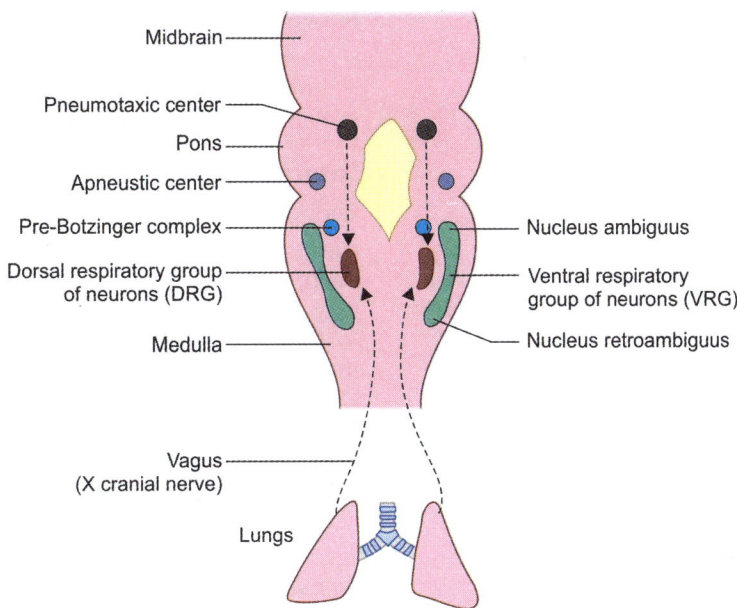

Fig. 39.1: Medullary and pontine respiratory centers. Note the inhibitory effect of vagal afferent fibers from the stretch receptors of lungs on the inspiratory center (DRG).

are controlled by the pacemaker cells in the pre- Botzinger complex. They are active during inspiration. They also receive impulses from lungs, chemoreceptors and baroreceptors through vagus and glossopharyngeal nerve.

Ventral respiratory group of neurons (VRG) is located in the ventrolateral part of medulla. It extends through **nucleus ambiguus and nucleus retroambigualis**. VRG is made up of 'E' (expiratory) neurons mainly, but some 'I' neurons are also present in its mid-portion. 'E' neurons inhibit 'I' neurons in expiration through reciprocal inhibition. 'E' neurons and 'I' neurons are connected by interneurons.

Inspiratory Ramp Signal

The pattern of action potentials produced by the respiratory center is called inspiratory ramp signal (IRS). Initially there is a latent period, then the intensity of action potentials increases and then decreases followed by a latent period. The cycle is repeated 12-13 times per minute and normally the duration of one cycle is 4-5 seconds. The impulses pass to the inspiratory muscles and produce inspiration **(Fig. 39.2)**.

Pontine Centers

Although the rhythmic discharge of medullary respiratory neurons is spontaneous, it is modified by neurons in the pons and afferents coming from receptors in airways and lungs through vagus. In the upper part of pons, there is a pair of respiratory centers called **pneumotaxic center**. Neurons of this center are located in the **nucleus parabrachialis medialis** and the **Kolliker-Fuse nucleus (Fig. 39.1)**.

Pneumotaxic center has inhibitory effect on 'I' neurons. When this area is stimulated, I neurons are inhibited and duration of inspiratory ramp signal is reduced. Rate of respiration will be increased and filling volume will be decreased, i.e., respiration becomes shallow and rapid.

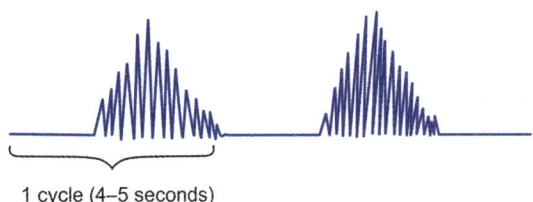

Fig. 39.2: Pattern of inspiratory ramp signal (IRS).

When pneumotaxic center is damaged, respiration becomes slower and tidal volume will be increased, and if vagi are also simultaneously cut, it leads to apneusis, i.e., prolonged inspiratory spasms that resembles breath holding.

The inspiratory spasm following mid-pontine section and bilateral vagotomy may be only a manifestation of decerebrate rigidity of inspiratory muscles. This is due to the over activity of the bulbar facilitatory area or due to imbalance of inputs to medullary centers. It may not be due to the unopposed activity of apneustic center as previously believed.

Previously it was believed that the lower part of pons contained another set of neurons called **apneustic center**. It was thought to have an excitatory effect on 'I' neurons, and stimulation of apneustic center increased the duration of IRS producing sustained contraction of inspiratory muscles with expiratory gasps in between. This is called **apneusis**. The existence of this center is yet to be proved.

Vagal Influences on Respiration

Stretch of the lungs during inspiration stimulates stretch receptors in lung which generate impulses in afferent pulmonary vagal fibers. These impulses inhibit 'I' neurons and produce expiration **(Fig. 39.1 and Flowchart 3.1)**.

The switch-off mechanism coming from pneumotaxic center and vagus are the key factors which determine the rate and rhythm of respiration.

Flowchart 39.1: Effect of vagus on respiration.

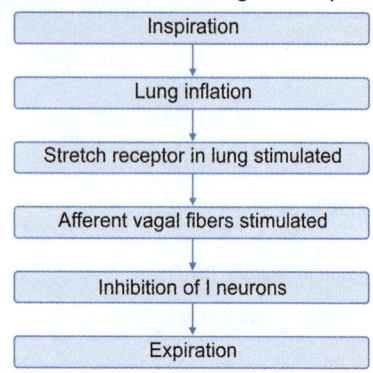

Methods of Study of the Activity of Respiratory Centers

- Stimulation studies
- Ablation studies
- Electroneuronography

Ablation Studies

In experimental animals, brainstem is cut at different levels and respiratory movements are recorded (**Fig. 39.3**).
- Section above pons—Normal breathing is recorded since respiratory centers are intact.
- Just below pneumotaxic center or mid-pontine section. Vagus intact—Rate of respiration decreases and depth increases.
- After vagotomy—Apneusis
- Section at the junction of pons and medulla— Irregular breathing due to absence of impulses coming from pons.
- Section below medulla—No respiration.

REFLEX CONTROL OF RESPIRATION

Receptors are classified into two types:
1. Receptors inside respiratory system
2. Receptors outside respiratory system

Receptors inside Respiratory System

- Stretch receptors
- J-receptors
- Pulmonary irritant receptors

Stretch Receptors

Hering-Breuer Reflexes

Hering-Breuer Inflation Reflex: When there is increase in the tidal volume to more than 1 L, the stretch receptors of lung are stimulated to a greater extent and there is increase in the rate of afferent impulses passing through the vagus to the inspiratory center. Vagus is inhibitory to the inspiratory center and this leads to inhibition of inspiratory muscles and there will be increase in the expiration time. This brings back the lung volume back to normal. This reflex is called **Hering-Breuer inflation reflex**.

This reflex operates only when the tidal volume exceeds 1–1.5 L as in exercise and this reflex prevents over inflation of lung and may help to minimize the work of breathing. It is also important in the control of breathing in babies.

- Stimulus—Distention of lung which stimulates stretch receptors of lung.
- Receptors—Stretch receptors in the airway smooth muscle, i.e., trachea, bronchi and bronchioles.
- Afferent limb—Vagus.
- Center—Inspiratory center in medulla.
- Effect—Inhibition of inspiratory center and switching off of inspiratory ramp signal (IRS) leading to expiration. Lung volume is thus brought back to normal (**Fig. 39.4**).

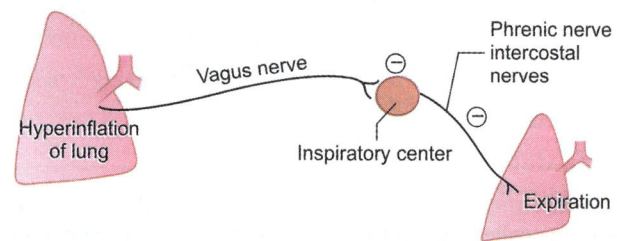

Fig. 39.4: Hering-Breuer inflation reflex.

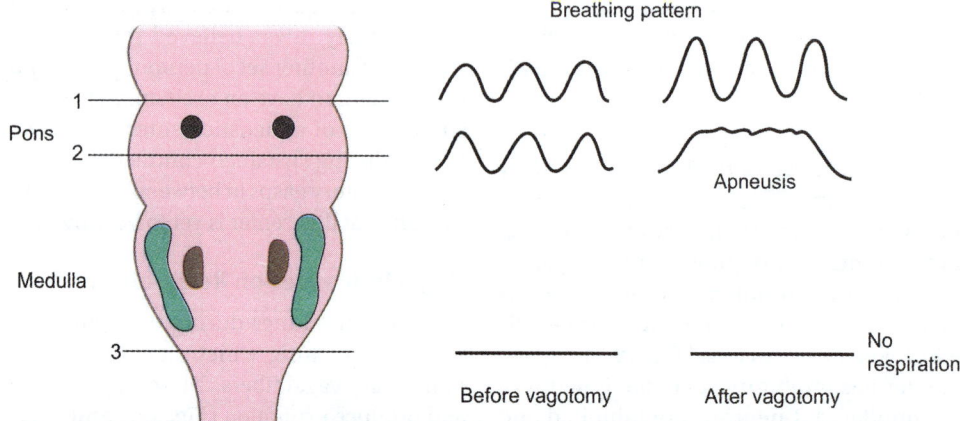

Fig. 39.3: Ablation studies at different levels of brainstem to demonstrate the activity of respiratory centers: (1) Lesion at the junction of midbrain and pons; (2) Below the level of pneumotaxic center; (3) Below the medullary centers.

Hering-Breuer Deflation Reflex

Hering-Breuer deflation reflex operates when there is excessive deflation of lungs. Extreme deflation of the lung occurs in collapse of lungs, pneumothorax, sucking of air from trachea, etc. Here, there is stimulation of inspiration to bring back the lung volume to normal. This is **Hering-Breuer deflation reflex**.

Two theories are there to explain this reflex:
1. In severe deflation of lung, there is no stimulation of stretch receptors of lung and so, no inhibitory impulses pass through vagus from lung to the inspiratory center. The inspiratory ramp signal (IRS) will be prolonged leading to increase in filling volume and lung size is brought back to normal.
2. **J-reflex or pulmonary chemoreflex:** According to this view, stretch receptors are not involved; instead, J receptors or **juxtapulmonary capillary receptors** are involved. J receptors are non-myelinated vagal nerve endings (C fibers) in alveoli which are in close proximity to pulmonary capillaries (hence the name juxtapulmonary capillary receptors). These receptors are stimulated in pulmonary embolism, pulmonary congestion, pulmonary edema, congestive cardiac failure, etc. They do not function during normal quiet respiration.

The effects of stimulation of J receptors are:
- Hypotension
- Bradycardia
- Tachypnea (rapid shallow breathing)
- Intense stimulation causes apnea
- Dyspnea due to bronchospasm
- Increased mucus secretion in the airways
- Weakness of skeletal muscles.

This is **pulmonary chemoreflex or J-reflex**. This reflex is similar to coronary chemoreflex or Bezold-Jarisch reflex. J receptors are responsible for hyperventilation in patients affected by pulmonary congestion and left heart failure.

Hering-Breuer reflexes are abolished by vagotomy.

Importance of Hering-Breuer Reflexes
- Hering-Breuer inflation reflex prevents excessive inflation of lungs. It decides the filling volume of lungs especially in conditions of hyperinflation as in exercise.
- It functions as an important feedback mechanism and may contribute to the rhythmicity of respiration in newborn babies.
- The Hering-Breuer deflation reflex may be very important in helping to actively maintain infants' functional residual capacities. This is because the inward recoil of their lungs is considerably greater than the outward recoil of their chest walls. Thus, atelectasis is prevented.

Pulmonary Irritant Receptors

Irritant receptors are found in between airway epithelial cells. They are stimulated by smoke, dust, cold air, irritant gases like SO_2 and chemicals like histamine. Stimulation of these receptors produces:
- Bronchoconstriction
- Hyperventilation
- Cough, sneezing, etc.

Significance of Pulmonary Irritant Receptors

Pulmonary irritant receptors help to remove noxious agents from tracheobronchial tree. Bronchospasm is also beneficial as it prevents further entry of noxious agents into the alveoli.

Cough Reflex

Cough reflex is a protective reflex. Stimulation of irritant receptors of larynx, trachea and bigger bronchi produces cough. Coughing begins with a deep inspiration followed by forced expiration against a closed glottis. The glottis is suddenly opened and air is expelled at very high velocity, i.e., there is explosive outflow of air. There is a great rise in intrapleural pressure during coughing. Excessive cough may lead to alveolar rupture, visual blackout, fainting attack, herniation, etc.

Sneezing Reflex

Stimulation of irritant receptors of nasal cavity and upper airway produces sneezing. Mechanism is similar to coughing, but with a continuously open glottis.

Receptors outside Respiratory System

- Those receptors which stimulate respiration:
    - Proprioceptors
    - Nociceptors
    - Thermoreceptors

    Emotional stimuli from hypothalamus and limbic system also stimulates respiration.
- Those receptors which inhibit respiration:
    - Baroreceptors
    - Visceroceptors

Receptors that Stimulate Respiration

Proprioceptors

Proprioceptors are receptors in muscles, tendons, joints, etc. Stimulation of these receptors reflexly stimulates I neurons. This helps to increase ventilation at the start of exercise even before changes in PCO_2, PO_2 and H^+ concentration occur.

Nociceptors

Nociceptors are pain receptors. Somatic pain generally causes hyperpnea; visceral pain generally causes apnea or decreased ventilation.

Chemoreceptors

Acidosis and hypoxia stimulate the chemoreceptors. Hypotension or shock produces hyperventilation due to stimulation of chemoreceptors.

Thermoreceptors

Thermoreceptors present in the hypothalamus are stimulated when there is increase in body temperature as in fever, exercise, etc. They send impulses to respiratory center and produce increase in the rate of respiration.

Emotional Stimuli

Emotional stimuli produce impulses from hypothalamus, limbic system, etc., which stimulate the respiratory center. Thus emotional stimuli alter respiration as in crying, laughing, sighing, etc. Hyperventilation also occurs during panic attacks in patients with depression.

Others

Stretching the anal sphincter increases respiratory rate and is employed to stimulate respiration in a person who has stopped breathing.

Hyperventilation occurs in pregnancy and liver cirrhosis due to increased progesterone.

Receptors which Inhibit Respiration

Baroreceptors

Increase in blood pressure stimulates baroreceptors leading to inhibition of respiration. Injection of adrenaline produce an increase in blood pressure, which in turn stimulates baroreceptors producing apnea called **adrenaline apnea**.

Visceroceptors

In visceral reflexes like vomiting, swallowing, etc., there is reflex inhibition of respiration. For example, **deglutition apnea** occurs during swallowing to prevent entry of food into respiratory passages.

CHEMICAL REGULATION OF RESPIRATION

■ INTRODUCTION

Chemical control of breathing is aimed at maintaining the PO_2 and PCO_2 of arterial blood at about 95 mm Hg and 40 mm Hg, respectively. Changes in blood chemistry (PCO_2, PO_2 and pH) acts on respiratory center and ventilation is adjusted to bring the blood chemistry back to normal. Changes in PCO_2, PO_2 and pH of blood act on the respiratory center through a set of receptors called **chemoreceptors**.

■ CHEMORECEPTORS

Chemoreceptors are receptors that respond to changes in the chemical composition of blood or any fluid around it.

Chemoreceptors are classified into two types depending on their location:
1. Central chemoreceptors
2. Peripheral chemoreceptors

The response to hypoxia is mediated entirely by peripheral chemoreceptors while the response to hypercapnia and acidosis is mediated mainly (75%) by central chemoreceptors and partly (25%) by peripheral chemoreceptors.

Central Chemoreceptors

Central chemoreceptors are a set of neurons located 200– 400 micrometer below the ventral surface of medulla oblongata on both sides near the exit of IX and X cranial nerves **(Fig. 39.5)**.

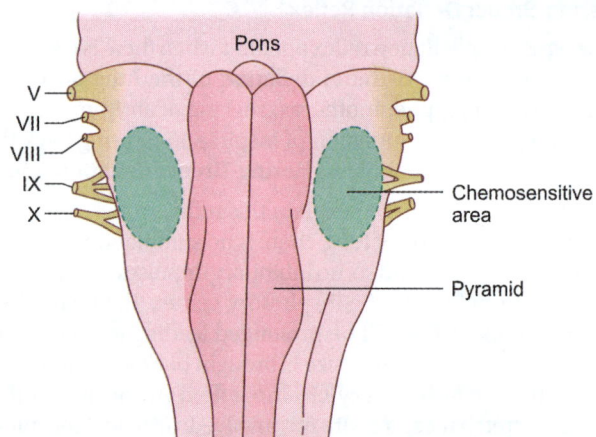

Fig. 39.5: Location of central chemoreceptor on the ventral surface of medulla oblongata.

Neurons in this **chemosensitive area** can sense changes in H^+ concentration especially in the brain interstitial fluid. Central chemoreceptors are surrounded by brain extracellular fluid.

The blood-brain barrier and blood-CSF barrier can be crossed by CO_2 very easily since it is lipid soluble but not so by H^+. Another reason is that increase in blood PCO_2 produces cerebral vasodilation, which enhances diffusion of CO_2 into cerebrospinal fluid (CSF) and brain interstitial fluid. So, *increase in H^+ concentration of blood does not stimulate central chemoreceptors since it cannot cross the above barriers.*

Whenever there is hypercapnia (increase in PCO_2), CO_2 enters the brain tissue and CSF, and it is hydrated to form H_2CO_3. This splits to form H^+ and HCO_3^-. *Increase in H^+ in the brain interstitial fluid is the only direct stimulant of central chemoreceptors. CO_2 has only indirect action by forming H^+* **(Fig. 39.6).**

Stimuli from central chemoreceptors go to the inspiratory center and stimulate respiration. Increase in H^+ has only acute action on central chemoreceptors, i.e., central chemoreceptors respond only to abrupt changes in blood PCO_2. So, change in blood PCO_2 has only a potent acute effect on controlling ventilation and only a weak chronic effect due to adaptation. *If the PCO_2 of brain interstitial fluid and CSF is persistently high, the action of H^+ on central chemoreceptors stops.*

Reason: Normally, CSF has fewer buffers than blood and so increase in H^+ in CSF has more action on central chemoreceptors. But if hypercapnia is prolonged, HCO_3^- diffuses into CSF and neutralizes the H^+, and pH in the CSF will no longer be acidic but becomes alkaline. Thus, CO_2 level in blood regulates ventilation by its effect on the pH of CSF and brain interstitial fluid. Acidic pH is necessary for the stimulation of central chemoreceptors.

The resulting hyperventilation reduces blood PCO_2 to normal. Central chemoreceptors are inhibited by anesthesia, cyanide poisoning and during deep sleep.

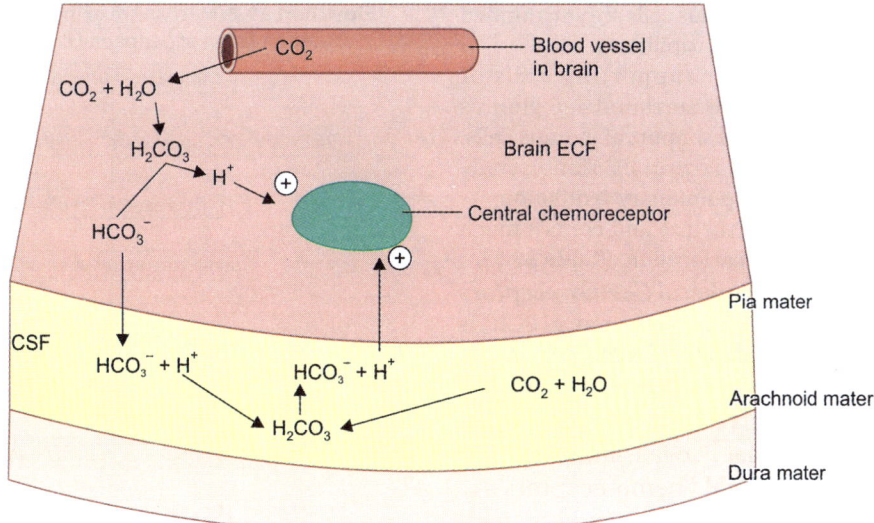

Fig. 39.6: Mechanism of stimulation of central chemoreceptors by hydrogen ions.

Central chemoreceptors are not stimulated by hypoxia rather, they are depressed by hypoxia.

Peripheral Chemoreceptors

Peripheral chemoreceptors (PCR) are situated in the **carotid body and aortic body**. These are neurovascular structures. Another name for aortic and carotid body is **glomus**. Their function as chemoreceptors was first provided by Corneille Heymans, for which he was awarded the 1938 Nobel Prize for Physiology/ Medicine.

Location of PCR

Carotid bodies are located at the bifurcation of common carotid artery and aortic bodies are scattered along the underside of the aortic arch **(Fig. 39.7)**. Carotid body is important in humans. It has a very high blood flow, i.e., 20 mL/g/min (0.04 mL/min). Carotid body weighs about 2 mg and blood flow, normalized for weight, is 40 times than that of brain and 4 times that of kidney. They also have a very high metabolic rate, 2–3 fold greater than that of brain.

Innervation of Peripheral Chemoreceptor

Carotid body is supplied by **sinus nerve**, a branch of IX cranial nerve. It is also called **Hering's nerve**. Sensory impulses from carotid body are carried through this nerve.

Aortic body is supplied by **aortic nerve**, a branch of vagus. Sinus nerve and aortic nerve are together referred to as **sinoaortic nerve**.

Structure of Carotid Body

Carotid body is composed of two types of cells surrounded by fenestrated sinusoidal capillaries **(Fig. 39.8)**.
1. **Type I cell or Glomus cell**: Type I cells are 10 μm in diameter, roughly spherical and occur in clusters. Embryologically, the glomus cell is neuroectodermal in origin. They resemble adrenal medullary chromaffin cells with dense granules containing **dopamine**. They are in close approximation to cup-like endings of afferent nerve

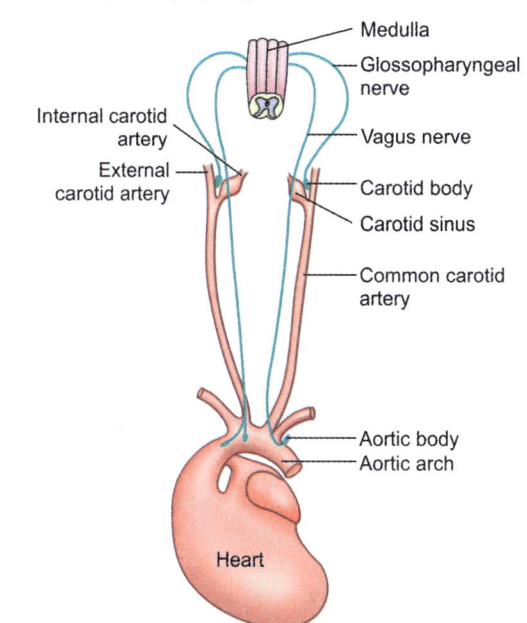

Fig. 39.7: Location of peripheral chemoreceptors in the carotid and aortic bodies.

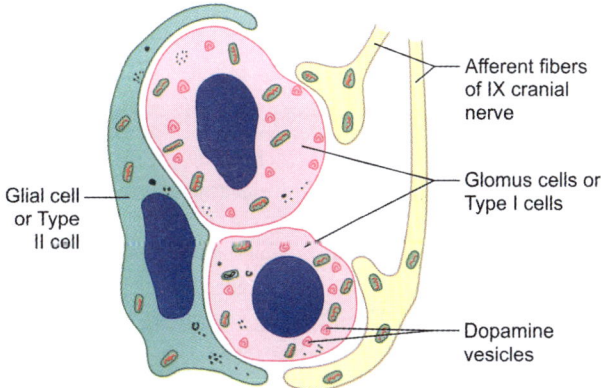

Fig. 39.8: Microscopic structure of carotid body.

fibers of IX cranial nerve. The glomus cells are surrounded by a dense network of fenestrated capillaries.

2. **Type II cells or glial cells or supporting cells or sustentacular cells**: These cells surround 4–6 glomus cells. Function is protection and support of glomus cells. **C Heymans** was awarded Nobel Prize in 1938 for his study on the role of carotid bodies in pulmonary ventilation.

Aortic bodies have a similar structure and are not much studied because of their anatomical location. **(Table 39.1).**

Mechanism of Action of Peripheral Chemoreceptors

Major function of the peripheral chemoreceptors (PCR) is to sense hypoxia in the arterial blood and signal cells in the medulla to increase ventilation. Reduction in the partial pressure of O_2 (PO_2) in arterial blood is the most potent stimulus for PCR. If the arterial PO_2 falls from 100 mm Hg to 50 mm Hg, the peripheral chemoreceptors are strongly stimulated. They are also stimulated by high PCO_2 and low pH of arterial blood but to a lesser extent than hypoxia.

Type I glomus cells are excited by hypoxia and dopamine is released from the vesicles. Dopamine stimulates the afferent nerve endings bearing **dopamine (D_2) receptors** on them. Impulses pass through the afferent nerves, which makes its first synapse on the neurons of nucleus of tractus solitarius (part of DRG).

Type I glomus cells have O_2-sensitive K^+ channels. At low arterial PO_2, these K^+ channels close producing accumulation of K^+ and depolarization of the glomus cells. Depolarization of the glomus cell opens up the L-type Ca^{2+} channels in the glomus cell membrane leading to an increase in Ca^{++} influx. The Ca^{2+} influx triggers the release of dopamine as a neurotransmitter, which excites the afferent nerve endings and an impulse is transmitted along the afferent fibers to the respiratory center **(Flowchart 39.2).**

The inspiratory center is stimulated and there is increase in the rate and depth of respiration. This brings the blood PO_2 back to normal. In the absence of PCR, severe hypoxemia depresses respiration by a direct inhibitory action on respiratory center. (The direct effect of hypoxia on respiratory center is depression.)

Baroreceptor stimulation inhibits respiration whereas chemoreceptor stimulation stimulates respiration. Chemoreceptors are of great importance in the regulation of respiration.

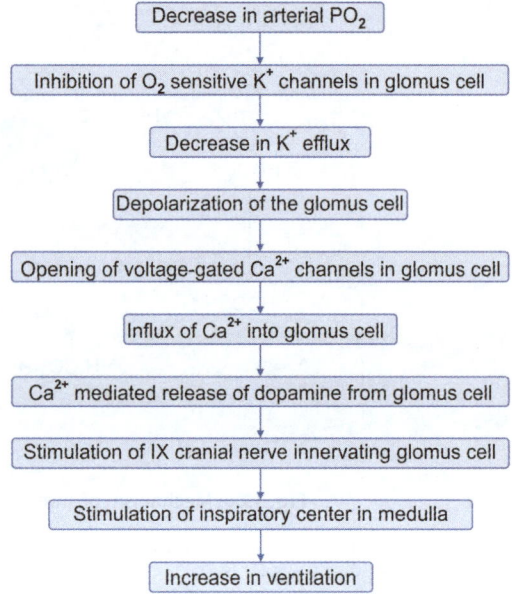

Flowchart 39.2: Mechanism of increase in ventilation by stimulation of peripheral chemoreceptors.

Factors Stimulating Peripheral Chemoreceptors

❖ Low arterial PO_2, high PCO_2 and low pH.
❖ Vascular stasis as in circulatory shock (stagnant hypoxia).
❖ Drugs like cyanide, nicotine, small doses of adrenaline, lobeline (a drug that inhibits dopamine release), etc.
❖ Increase in plasma K^+ levels as in exercise. This is one reason for exercise-induced hyperventilation.

The peripheral chemoreceptors (PCR) utilize the dissolved O_2 in blood for their metabolic demands because the blood supply to PCR is so large. So they respond only to a reduction in the dissolved O_2 in blood. So *in anemic hypoxia as in anemia, carbon monoxide poisoning, etc., where PaO_2 is normal, there is no stimulation of respiration through PCR.* But in stagnant hypoxia as in circulatory shock, PCR are stimulated since PaO_2 is decreased. Summary of the factors that influence the respiratory center is shown in **Figure 39.9**.

Ventilatory Responses to CO_2

Ventilatory Responses to Increased PCO_2

Increase in tissue metabolism increases arterial PCO_2. This will stimulate central chemoreceptors leading to an increase in ventilation. CO_2 is eliminated until arterial PCO_2 falls to normal limits. This feedback mechanism keeps CO_2 production and excretion in balance.

Similar effect is seen when a gas mixture containing CO_2 is inhaled. There is a linear relationship between respiratory minute volume and PCO_2 up to a certain limit. If PCO_2 of inspired air is increased to 50%, ventilation is increased 10 fold **(Table 39.2).**

When PCO_2 of inspired air is close to alveolar PCO_2, elimination of CO_2 becomes difficult. When CO_2 in inspired air is 7% the alveolar and arterial PCO_2

Table 39.1: Differences between carotid body and aortic body.

Carotid body	Aortic body
Located near the bifurcation of the common carotid artery	Located in the arch of aorta
Supplied by the IX cranial nerve	Supplied by the X cranial nerve
Seven times more effective than aortic bodies in stimulating respiration	Less effective
Increases both rate and depth of respiration	Increases only the rate of respiration

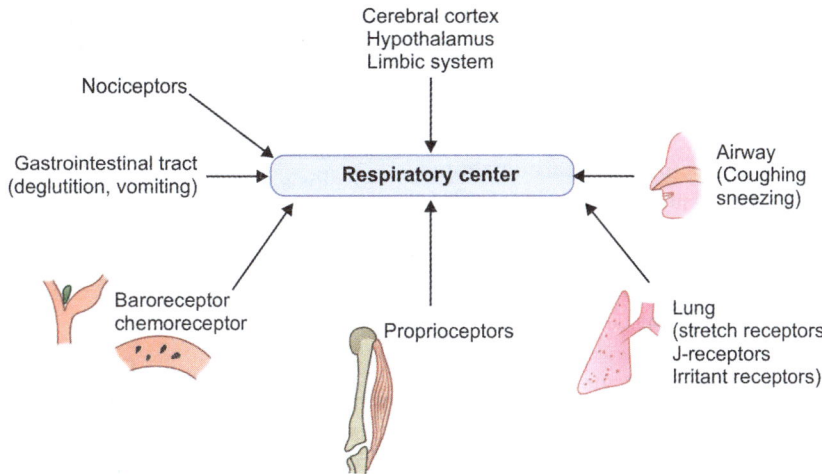

Fig. 39.9: Summary of the impulses from different parts of the body which influences the respiratory center.

Table 39.2: Relationship between PCO_2 of inspired air and respiratory minute volume (RMV).

Inspired air CO_2 (%)	Tidal volume (mL)	Respiratory rate	Respiratory minute volume (L/min)
0.04	450	16	7
2	560	16	9
4	820	17	14
5	1300	20	26

increases leading to hypercapnia. This depresses the respiratory center leading to **CO_2 narcosis** characterized by headache, confusion, tremor, muscular rigidity, coma, etc. Further increase in CO_2 leads to death.

Narcotics, anesthetics and endorphins profoundly depress the ventilatory response to CO_2. A depressed response to CO_2 during sleep may be involved in central sleep apnea.

Ventilatory Responses to Decreased PCO_2

When alveolar PCO_2 is decreased to 30 mm Hg or if a person hyperventilates voluntarily, CO_2 is washed off leading to a reduction in arterial PCO_2. This causes depression of respiratory center leading to **apnea**. When there is arrest of respiration, CO_2 accumulates leading to increase in arterial PCO_2. During apnea there will be a decrease in arterial PO_2. Both these factors stimulate respiration.

Hyperventilation → ↓$PaCO_2$ → Depression of respiratory center
↓
Stimulation of respiratory center ← ↑$PaCO_2$ ← Apnea
↓PaO_2

$PaCO_2$—Arterial PCO_2
PaO_2—Arterial PO_2

Effect of Hypoxia on Respiration

When PO_2 of inspired air is decreased below 60 mm Hg, there is an increase in respiratory minute volume (RMV) due to stimulation of respiration. Between 60 mm Hg and 100 mm Hg PaO_2 (alveolar PO_2), there is not much stimulation of respiration because of **counterbalancing inhibitory effects**. They are:
1. Decrease in arterial H^+ concentration
2. Decrease in arterial PCO_2

Reduced hemoglobin is a weaker acid and a stronger buffer than oxyhemoglobin. Since reduced hemoglobin buffers H^+ to form HHb there is a slight decrease in the H^+ concentration of arterial blood when the PaO_2 falls and hemoglobin becomes less saturated with O_2. This fall in H inhibits respiration.

Hypoxia causes increased ventilation which washes off CO_2 leading to a decrease in arterial PCO_2 and this in turn inhibits respiration. Therefore, a small reduction in arterial PO_2 has not much effect on ventilation.

Hypoxia → ↑Ventilation → ↓$PaCO_2$ → Inhibit respiratory center

Effect of H⁺ Concentration on Respiration (Table 39.3)

Acidosis

Acidosis is defined as a condition in which there is addition of acid or removal of alkali from the system. Acidosis may be metabolic acidosis or respiratory acidosis. Metabolic acidosis is due to addition of acid or removal of bases. Respiratory acidosis is due to retention of CO_2 due to hypoventilation.

Acidosis produces hyperventilation by stimulation of peripheral chemoreceptors. Hyperventilation decreases

Table 39.3: Causes of acidosis and alkalosis.

Condition	Abnormality
Respiratory acidosis	Increase in $PaCO_2$
Respiratory alkalosis	Decrease in $PaCO_2$
Metabolic acidosis	Decrease in HCO_3^-
Metabolic alkalosis	Increase in HCO_3^-

($PaCO_2$: Arterial PCO_2; PaO_2: Arterial PO_2)

alveolar PCO_2 and thus produces a compensatory fall in blood H^+ concentration.

Metabolic Acidosis

Causes of metabolic acidosis
- Diabetes mellitus: There is impaired fat and carbohydrate metabolism leading to increased production of ketoacids-like acetoacetic acid.
- Renal failure: There is inadequate renal excretion of acid metabolites leading to accumulation of these metabolites.
- Severe exercise leads to lactic acidosis.
- Starvation leads to ketoacidosis.
- Loss of bases from ECF as in diarrhea leads to acidosis.
- Anemia severe enough to increase tissue anaerobic metabolism causes metabolic acidosis.

When acids stronger than HHb and other buffer acids are added to blood, metabolic acidosis is produced. The H^+ added is buffered and the reduced hemoglobin, protein (A) and HCO_3^- level in plasma drop. The H_2CO_3 formed is converted to H_2O and CO_2, and CO_2 is rapidly excreted through lungs. The rise in plasma H^+ stimulates respiration and PCO_2 is reduced. This is the respiratory compensation in acidosis.

The renal compensatory mechanisms bring about the excretion of the extra H^+ and return the pH to normal. Urine buffer systems are HCO_3^-, HPO_4^{2-} and NH buffer systems.

Kussmaul's breathing refers to extremely deep rapid breathing seen in metabolic acidosis like diabetic ketoacidosis.

Respiratory Acidosis

Hypoventilation that is not secondary to a fall in plasma H^+ concentration causes respiratory acidosis.

$\downarrow$ Pulmonary ventilation $\rightarrow \uparrow PCO_2 \rightarrow \uparrow H_2CO_3 \rightarrow \uparrow H^+$

Causes of respiratory acidosis
- Respiratory center depression
- Obstruction to respiratory passage
- Fibrosis of lung
- Emphysema.

Alkalosis

Alkalosis is defined as the condition in which bases are added or acids are removed excessively from the system. Alkalosis may be metabolic or respiratory in origin. When the arterial plasma pH is above 7.4, the resulting condition is alkalosis. Alkalosis may be produced by a decrease in arterial PCO_2 or an increase in plasma HCO_3^-.

Metabolic Alkalosis

The primary abnormality is an increase in plasma HCO_3^- leading to an increase in pH.

Causes
- Vomiting, where there is increased loss of gastric acid
- Loop diuretics and thiazides, which cause excretion of large volumes of acidic urine
- Cushing's syndrome
- Primary hyperaldosteronism
- Hypokalemia

In hypokalemia, H^+ shifts into the intracellular compartment. In addition, the renal loss of H^+ is also increased in hypokalemia and this lead to alkalosis. In Cushing syndrome and in hyperaldosteronism, there is hypokalemia.

Respiratory Compensation
In alkalosis there is depression of respiratory center which increases the PCO_2 of blood, thus increasing the H ion concentration and pH is brought back to normal.

$\downarrow H^+ \rightarrow$ Depression of respiratory center $\rightarrow$ Hypoventilation
$\downarrow$
$\uparrow PCO_2 \rightarrow \uparrow H^+$

But there is a limiting factor to this compensation. When there is hypoventilation there will be a reduction in arterial PO_2 which stimulates peripheral chemoreceptors leading to increase in ventilation.

Hypoventilation $\rightarrow \downarrow PaO_2 \rightarrow$ Stimulation of PCR $\rightarrow \uparrow$ Ventilation

Respiratory Alkalosis

Hyperventilation that is not secondary to a rise in arterial H^+ concentration produces a drop in arterial PCO_2, which in turn lowers H^+ below normal leading to respiratory alkalosis.

$\uparrow$ Pulmonary ventilation $\rightarrow$ Elimination of more CO_2 from the body $\rightarrow \downarrow PaCO_2$
$\downarrow$
$\downarrow H^+ \leftarrow \downarrow H_2CO_3$
(Alkalosis)

Causes of Respiratory Alkalosis
a. Voluntary hyperventilation
b. High altitude

- 50% increase in $PaCO_2$ produces 10-fold increase in ventilation.
- Decrease of pH from 7.4 to 7 causes 3–4-fold increase in ventilation.
- Decrease of PaO_2 from 100 to 40 mm Hg increases ventilation 1.5 fold.

This shows that the most potent stimulus to increase ventilation is increase in $PaCO_2$.

INTERACTION OF CHEMICAL FACTORS IN REGULATION OF RESPIRATION

Interaction of CO_2 and O_2

- *When alveolar PCO_2 is kept constant and PO_2 reduced*
  - If PCO_2 in alveolar air is adjusted to 4–5 mm Hg above normal and if PO_2 is decreased from 100 to 60 mm Hg, there is marked increase in ventilation.
  - If alveolar PCO_2 is kept 5 mm Hg lower than normal and if PO_2 is decreased from 100 to 60 mm Hg, there is not much increase in ventilation. Below 60 mm Hg, there is marked increase in ventilation **(Fig. 39.10)**.
    This experiment shows that when alveolar PCO_2 is increased, the person will be more sensitive to hypoxia.
- *When alveolar PO_2 is kept constant and $PaCO_2$ increased*
  The ventilatory response is recorded on a graph by increasing alveolar PCO_2 with alveolar PO_2 kept constant.

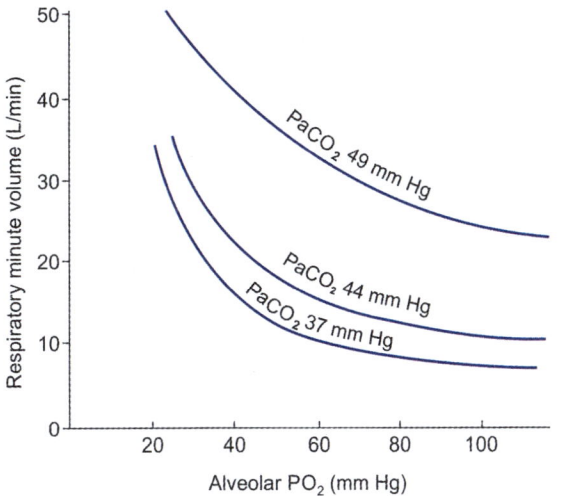

Fig. 39.10: Interaction of CO_2 and O_2 when alveolar PCO_2 is kept constant.

Three curves are plotted with alveolar PO_2 equal to 100 mm Hg, 55 mm Hg and 40 mm Hg. It is seen that the slope of the curve is increased when alveolar PO_2 is less. This proves that hypoxia makes the individual more sensitive to increase in PCO_2.

Effect of H⁺ on CO_2 Response

The above experiment is repeated and two families of curves are plotted with pH 7.4 and 7.3. When pH is reduced, CO_2 response curve shifts to left, i.e., the same amount of respiratory stimulation is produced by lower arterial PCO_2 levels when pH is reduced **(Fig. 39.11)**.

Effect of Hormones on Respiration

- Progesterone stimulates ventilation by acting on medullary respiratory centers. So ventilation is increased in pregnancy and during the secretory phase of menstrual cycle.
- Progesterone increases body temperature which in turn stimulates ventilation.

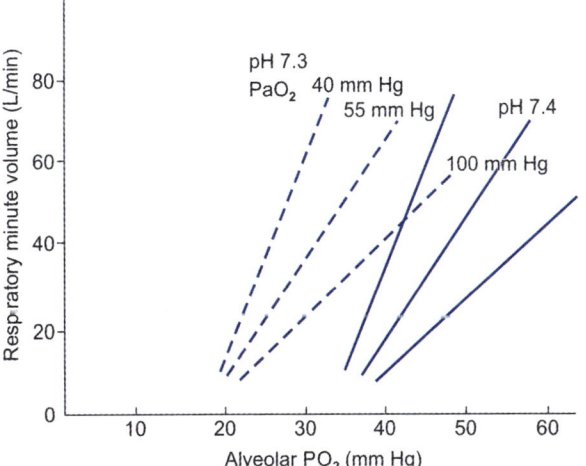

Fig. 39.11: Effect of pH on carbon dioxide response curve.

- Thyroxine, catecholamines and cortisol also stimulate respiration.

ABNORMALITIES IN REGULATION OF RESPIRATION

- **Respiratory center depression**
  Causes:
  - Old age
  - Thrombosis, hemorrhage, etc., in the brain
  - Anesthetics
- **Periodic breathing**
  Periodic breathing consists of alternate waxing and waning of respiration or alternate hyperventilation and apnea. It may be normal or abnormal.

Types of periodic breathing are:
- Voluntary hyperventilation
- Cheyne-Stokes respiration
- Biot's breathing
- Sleep apnea

Voluntary Hyperventilation

Hyperventilation in normal subjects is followed by a period of apnea, which in turn is followed by a few shallow breaths and then by another period of apnea followed again by a few breaths. This is a type of periodic breathing. The cycles last for some time before normal breathing is resumed **(Fig. 39.12)**.

Explanation for the Periodicity in Voluntary Hyperventilation

The different phases in voluntary hyperventilation are:
- *Apnea:* Decrease in arterial PCO_2 due to hyperventilation.
- *Shallow breaths:* Decrease in PO_2 due to apnea leads leading to increase in $PaCO_2$, followed by increased to stimulation of peripheral chemoreceptors which stimulate respiration.
- *Again apnea:* PCR stimulation corrects hypoxia leading to increase in PO_2, i.e., hypoxic stimulus is eliminated.
- *Normal breathing:* Arterial PCO_2 comes back to normal.

Voluntary hyperventilation → Washing off of CO_2 →
↓ Arterial PCO_2
↓
Stimulation ← ↑ $PaCO_2$ ← Apnea ← Respiratory center
of respiration ↓ PO_2 depression

Cheyne-Stokes Respiration

Cheyne-Stokes respiration is a type of periodic breathing which is seen in both physiological and pathological conditions. In this type, **regular** alternating periods of

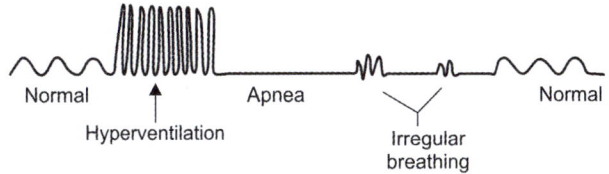

Fig. 39.12: Pattern of respiration in voluntary hyperventilation.

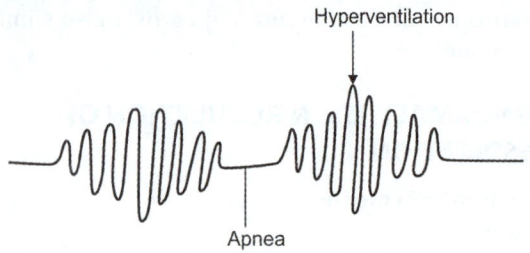

Fig. 39.13: Cheyne-Stokes breathing in which two periods of apnea are separated by an increase and a smooth decrease in tidal volume.

hyperventilation and apnea are seen. The change over from one to the other occurs gradually **(Fig. 39.13)**.

Physiological Conditions
- Deep sleep
- Infants
- High altitude
- Prolonged hyperventilation

Pathological Causes of Cheyne-Stokes Breathing
- Congestive cardiac failure (CCF)
- Morphine poisoning
- Raised intracranial tension
- Uremia

Theories Explaining Cheyne-Stokes Breathing
- The respiratory center over-responds to CO_2 leading to hyperventilation followed by apnea. The cycle is repeated regularly.

$$CO_2 \rightarrow \text{Hyperventilation} \rightarrow \downarrow PaCO_2 \rightarrow \text{Apnea}$$
$$\text{Hyperventilation} \leftarrow \uparrow PaCO_2$$

Prolongation of lung-to-brain circulation time as in congestive cardiac failure. Here it takes more time for changes in arterial gas tension to affect the respiratory center. If this person hyperventilates there will be a decrease in $PaCO_2$ and when this blood reaches the brain there will be marked reduction in $PaCO_2$, and respiratory center will be depressed leading to apnea. During apnea there is accumulation of CO_2 leading to increase in $PaCO_2$, followed by increased ventilation.

Biot's Breathing

Biot's breathing was first described in patients with meningitis by Biot in 1876. This type of breathing is always pathological. It consists of **irregular** periods of apnea and hyperventilation. The changes are abrupt **(Fig. 39.14)**.

It is seen in:
- Meningitis
- Medullary lesions

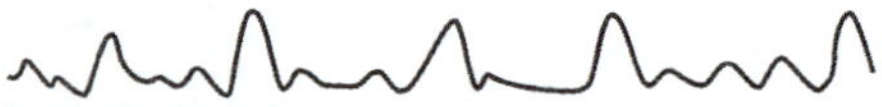

Fig. 39.14: Biot's respiration.

Sleep Apnea

The respiratory control mechanism is less effective during sleep and brief periods of apnea occur in normal sleeping adults. During sleep there is decreased sensitivity to decrease in PCO_2. Because of this decreased sensitivity, PCO_2 may fall during sleep, which may lead to apnea.

Sometimes, it produces **sleep apnea syndrome**, i.e., when it occurs repeatedly the patient wakes up frequently and the loss of sleep causes headache, tiredness, confusions and poor performance during daytime.

In normal adults, sleep apnea occurs during rapid eye movement (REM) sleep when, muscles are most hypotonic. Sleep apnea is said to be significant if more than 5 apneic episodes occur per hour of sleep or more than 30 apneic episodes during a night and breathing ceases for more than 10 seconds during each episode. Sleep apnea is diagnosed by **polysomnographic studies** during sleep.

Causes of Sleep Apnea
- Elderly
- Alcoholics
- Hypnotics which produce respiratory depression
- *Acromegaly:* Causes are prolapse of enlarged tongue and thickening of the tissues of the larynx.

Sleep apnea can be relieved to some extent by advising the subjects not to sleep on their backs.

Theories to Explain Sleep Apnea
Central Cause
Decrease in PCO_2 is the main cause for sleep apnea especially during REM sleep. The respiratory center is less sensitive to hypocapnia which causes further decrease in PCO_2 followed by apnea.

Obstructive Sleep Apnea
Sleep apnea may be caused by obstruction of airway during inspiration. Two causes are known:
1. Pharyngeal muscles relax during sleep especially REM sleep, leading to respiratory obstruction.
2. Failure of genioglossus muscle of tongue to contract during inspiration, and tongue falls back and obstructs the airway.

Symptoms of Sleep Apnea
- Loud snoring
- Morning headache
- Fatigue
- Daytime sleepiness
- Apneic episodes during sleep

Complications of Sleep Apnea
- Pulmonary hypertension
- Heart failure
- Myocardial infarction
- Stroke
- Increased incidence of motor vehicle accidents

Sudden Infant Death Syndrome

Sudden infant death syndrome (SIDS) may be a form of sleep apnea when, the apneic spells are so much prolonged leading to death. Healthy babies are found dead in their cribs in this disorder.

Causes
- Prolonged sleep apnea
- Prematurity
- Cardiac arrhythmias
- Babies of mothers who smoked during pregnancy
- Increased β-endorphin level in CSF and serum
  - *Normal endorphin level in CSF:* <15 pg/mL
  - *In serum:* 100 pg/mL

Hypercapnia

Hypercapnia is retention of CO_2 in the body, i.e., there is an increase in the concentration of CO_2 in blood than normal. Hypercapnia initially stimulates respiration, but retention of larger amounts of CO_2 produces depression of CNS and leads to **CO_2 narcosis**, which is characterized by:
- Confusion, headache, tremor
- Paresthesia (altered sensation), muscular rigidity
- Coma with respiratory depression
- Finally death

There will be respiratory acidosis and plasma HCO_3^- may exceed 40 mEq/L (normal value is 24 mEq/L). Urine becomes acidic.

Causes of Hypercapnia
- Ventilation-perfusion inequality
- Inadequate alveolar ventilation as in pump failure, e.g., fatigue, respiratory center depression, mechanical defects, paralysis of respiratory muscles, obstruction to airway, etc.
- Hypercapnia is exacerbated when CO_2 production is increased as in fever (13% increase in CO_2 production for each 1°C rise in body temperature.); high carbohydrate diet increases CO_2 production because of increase in RQ. *Hypercapnia is rarely a problem in pulmonary fibrosis because CO_2 is 20 times more soluble than O_2 and diffuses with ease through the thickened membrane.*

Hypocapnia

Decrease in the concentration of CO_2 in arterial blood below normal is called hypocapnia. The arterial PCO_2 falls from 40 mm Hg to as low as 15 mm Hg. Hypocapnia occurs due to hyperventilation especially in neurotic patients. The alveolar PO_2 rises to 120–140 mm Hg.

Effects of Hypocapnia
Cerebral blood flow may be reduced by 30% or more because of the direct constrictor effect of hypocapnia on cerebral vessels. Cerebral ischemia produces headache, dizziness, visual blackouts, paresthesia, etc. Tetany may also be seen in this condition. Even though hypocapnia has a direct constrictor effect on many blood vessels, it does not increase blood pressure because it depresses vasomotor center. Urine becomes alkaline.

Reason for Tetany in Hyperventilation
In hyperventilation, there will be respiratory alkalosis and urine becomes alkaline and the plasma ionic calcium level falls. Plasma calcium is partly bound to protein especially albumin and the rest is ionized calcium (Ca^{2+}) and calcium in complex with bicarbonate and citrate. It is the free, ionized Ca^{2+} that is biologically active. It is necessary for blood coagulation, muscle contraction, normal nerve function, etc. Ca^{2+} is necessary for stabilizing the nerve and muscle membranes.

When the total serum calcium level is less than 9 mg/dL or when the ionized calcium level is less than 4.5 mg/dL, it is referred to as hypocalcemia. A low ionic calcium level has an excitatory effect on nerve and muscle cells. It leads to hypocalcemic tetany (increased contraction of muscles) which is due to increased activity of motor nerve fibers. Hypocalcemic tetany is characterized by spasms of skeletal muscles especially muscles of extremities, larynx, etc. **Carpopedal spasm and Chvostek's sign** are manifestations of hypocalcemic tetany (*refer* 'calcium homeostasis').

Mechanism by which Blood pH Affects Ionic Calcium Level (Ca^{2+})

In hyperventilation there is increase in plasma pH due to decrease in H^+ concentration. Even though the total plasma calcium level is normal, the ionic calcium level falls and bound form increases. This is because plasma proteins are more ionized when pH is high, providing more protein anion to bind with Ca^{2+}.

Normally, a portion of both H^+ and Ca^{2+} in blood are bound to serum albumin. Albumin is a good buffer (proton donor) and when blood becomes alkaline, bound H^+ dissociates from albumin freeing up the albumin to bind with more Ca^{2+}. This decreases the freely ionized portion of total serum calcium. For every 0.1 increase in pH, ionized calcium level decreases by about 0.05 mmol/L. Decrease in extracellular ionic calcium increases the excitability of nerve and muscle cells leading to tetany.

Asphyxia

Asphyxia is a condition where **acute hypoxia and hypercapnia** occur together.

Cause of asphyxia is obstruction to respiratory passage as in:
- Strangulation
- Choking
- Drowning, where there is reflex laryngeal spasm
- Hypocalcemic tetany with severe laryngospasm

Stages of Asphyxia
- Stage of exaggerated breathing
- Stage of convulsions
- Stage of coma

Stage of Exaggerated Breathing

Initially there is strong stimulation of respiration with violent respiratory efforts which ends in loss of consciousness due to severe hypoxia.

Stage of Convulsions

There will be increase in blood pressure, heart rate, acidosis and convulsions. This is due to increased secretion of catecholamines. It is associated with micturition and defecation. The patient can be revived at this stage by artificial respiration.

Stage of Coma

If artificial respiration is not started, respiratory movements become sluggish and gasping in nature and the person goes into coma state. Death occurs due to respiratory center depression and cardiac arrest within 5–6 minutes.

Hiccup

Hiccup is spasmodic contraction of the diaphragm and other inspiratory muscles that produces an inspiration during which there is sudden closure of glottis. Sudden glottic closure is responsible for the characteristic sensation and sound. Function of hiccup is unknown. They respond to measures that increase arterial PCO_2 like breath holding. Hiccup also occurs in the fetus in utero.

Yawning

Yawning is an "infectious" respiratory act!!! Yawning is involuntary deep inspiration whose significance is uncertain. It also occurs in the fetus in utero. Under-ventilated alveoli have a tendency to collapse. Yawning opens these alveoli and prevents their collapse or atelectasis. It also increases venous return to heart because of increase in negative intrapleural pressure.

■ HYPOXIA

> **PY6.6:** Describe and discuss the pathophysiology of dyspnea, hypoxia, cyanosis, asphyxia; drowning, periodic breathing.

Hypoxia is defined as O_2 deficiency at the tissue level. This term should not be mistaken for anoxia which means absence of O_2. Anoxia is not possible in the body during life.

Hypoxia is classified into four types depending on the following factors:
- PO_2 of arterial blood
- O_2 carrying capacity of blood
- Rate of blood flow to the tissues
- Utilization of O_2 by the tissues

Types of Hypoxia

- Hypoxic hypoxia or hypoxemia
- Anemic hypoxia
- Stagnant or ischemic or circulatory or hypokinetic hypoxia
- Histotoxic hypoxia

Hypoxic Hypoxia

Hypoxic hypoxia is a condition in which the PO_2 of arterial blood is reduced. O_2 content and O_2 saturation are decreased. The underlying problem is ventilation-perfusion mismatch. This type is the most common form of hypoxia seen clinically.

Causes

- Decreased PO_2 of inspired air, which occurs:
  - At high altitude
  - Breathing gas mixture with low PO_2
  - Breathing in closed spaces
- Hypoventilation or decreased pulmonary ventilation:
  - Obstruction of respiratory passages in bronchial asthma or foreign body aspiration
  - Paralysis of respiratory muscles as in poliomyelitis
  - Respiratory center depression by drugs like morphine
  - Bony deformities as in kyphosis and scoliosis
  - Pneumothorax
- Cardiac disorders:
  Cyanotic congenital heart disease like interatrial septal defect, where there is right-to-left shunt in which large amounts of blood are shunted from the venous to the arterial side of the circulation
- Alveolar capillary diffusion block and ventilation-perfusion imbalance
  - Collapse of lung
  - Pulmonary congestion
  - Pulmonary fibrosis
  - Pneumonia
  - Pulmonary edema
  - Emphysema

Hypoxic hypoxia is a problem in normal individuals at high altitudes.

Anemic Hypoxia

In anemic hypoxia, arterial PO_2 is normal but the amount of hemoglobin available to carry O_2 is reduced.

Causes

- Anemia
- Carbon monoxide poisoning
- Chemicals like nitrates, chloride and ferricyanide which convert hemoglobin to methemoglobin. (When iron in hemoglobin is oxidized to ferric form it is called **methemoglobin.**)

CO Poisoning

Normally, small amounts of CO are formed in the body which acts as chemical messenger in the brain and other parts of the body. In large amounts, CO is poisonous. CO poisoning is included under anemic hypoxia because the amount of hemoglobin that can carry O_2 is reduced.

Sources of CO
- By incomplete combustion of carbon
- CO is a constituent of coal gas
- From exhausts of gasoline engines which contain 6% or more of CO
- A smoker may have 5-8% COHb in the blood

CO is toxic because it reacts with hemoglobin to form **carbonmonoxyhemoglobin or carboxyhemoglobin (COHb)**. COHb cannot take up O_2. So when CO combines with hemoglobin, the amount of hemoglobin available to combine with O_2 is reduced. Moreover, COHb releases CO very slowly. 15% of inhaled CO combines with myoglobin.

The affinity of hemoglobin for CO is 210 times its affinity for O_2. Further, the ODC shifts to left decreasing the amount of O_2 released. This is why an anemic person with 50% of normal amount of HbO_2 can do moderate work, but an individual whose HbO_2 is reduced to 50% due to formation of COHb cannot. When hemoglobin saturation with CO is 70-80%, death occurs.

Signs and Symptoms of CO Poisoning
- Acute symptoms:
  - Headache
  - Nausea
  - Loss of consciousness
  - **Cherry red** discoloration of skin, mucous membrane and nail bed **(Fig. 39.15)**
- Chronic symptoms:
  - Progressive brain damage
  - Mental changes

Fatal dose: >0.1% in inspired air

Lethal blood level: 60-80% of COHb in blood

Diagnosis: COHb level in blood can be measured by **spectrophotometry**.

Treatment of CO Poisoning
- Termination of exposure and restriction of physical activity. Otherwise, it leads to extensive cerebral demyelination.
- Adequate ventilation by artificial respiration preferably by:
  - Hyperbaric oxygenation which increases the dissociation of COHb
  - Using carbogen inhalation. Carbogen is a mixture of 5% CO_2 and 95% O_2. The CO_2 will stimulate the respiratory center.

Stagnant Hypoxia or Ischemic hypoxia

In stagnant hypoxia, blood flow to the tissue is reduced so that adequate O_2 is not delivered to the tissues. PaO_2 and hemoglobin content are normal.

Causes of Stagnant Hypoxia
Generalized
- Congestive cardiac failure (CCF)
- Shock
- Polycythemia

Localized
- Thrombosis
- Embolism
- Vascular spasm (Raynaud's phenomenon)

Kidney, heart, liver and brain are damaged in severe circulatory shock and congestive cardiac failure (CCF). If hypotension is prolonged, it damages the lung leading to **shock lung syndrome**.

Histotoxic Hypoxia

Inability of tissues to utilize O_2 is called histotoxic hypoxia. Here there is inhibition of tissue oxidative process. The amount of O_2 delivered to the tissues is adequate but tissues cannot extract this O_2. Powerful stimulation of peripheral chemoreceptors occur in cyanide poisoning because O_2 utilization is prevented at the tissue level.

Causes of Histotoxic Hypoxia
- Cyanide poisoning
- Sulfide poisoning

Cyanide Poisoning

Cyanide inactivates **cytochrome oxidase** and other enzymes in tissues, and tissue oxidation is affected which leads to quick death. Acute poisoning affects central nervous system and cardiovascular system. The person experiences overall weakness, nausea, confusion, headache, difficulty in breathing, seizures, loss of consciousness and cardiac arrest. Cyanosis is a late feature in cyanide poisoning.

- *Sources of Cyanide*
  - *Industry:* Plastic, synthetic rubber, electroplating, photographic processing.
  - Laboratories
  - *Pest control:* HCN gas used in ship
  - *Biological:* Bitter almond, seeds of apricot, peach, plum, pear, apple, etc.
  - *Medical:* Sodium nitroprusside, the antihypertensive drug produces cyanide as a metabolite.
  - Chronic exposure to tobacco smoke.
- *Absorption and Metabolism of Cyanide*

Cyanide is absorbed through all routes including intact skin. It is metabolized by the enzyme **rhodanase** in liver and kidney to thiocyanate and excreted through urine.

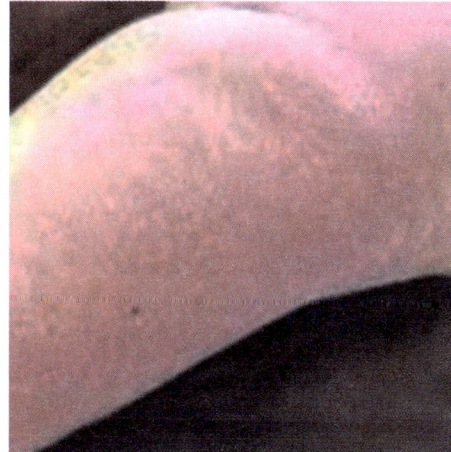

Fig. 39.15: CO poisoning (Note the cherry-red discoloration of skin).

Cyanide poisoning is diagnosed by the **Lee-Jones test**. There will also be the odor of **bitter almond** in the breath.

Fatal dose:

HCN: 50 mg

NaCN: 200–300 mg

- Treatment
  - Methylene blue or nitrites are used in cyanide poisoning. These convert hemoglobin to methemoglobin, which then reacts with cyanide to form cyanmethemoglobin, which is a nontoxic compound. Methemoglobin has increased affinity for cyanide, and is therefore useful in the treatment of cyanide poisoning. Nitrites can be used to oxidize hemoglobin to methemoglobin, which can then bind cyanide. This restores cytochrome oxidase's ability to function normally.
  - Sodium thiosulfate when given, converts cyanide to thiocyanate which can be excreted by the kidneys.
  - Hyperbaric oxygenation may also be useful along with the above treatment.
  - Vitamin B_{12}

Clinical Features of Hypoxia

Severe Hypoxia of Sudden Onset

A sudden drop in the inspired PO_2 to less than 20 mm Hg leads to loss of consciousness in 10–20 seconds and death in 4–5 minutes. In all types of hypoxia, brain is affected first.

Hypoxia of Gradual Onset

- Dyspnea
- Drowsiness
- Headache
- Disorientation
- Anorexia or loss of appetite
- Nausea and vomiting
- Tachycardia
- Pulmonary and systemic hypertension

O_2 Therapy

> **PY6.5:** Describe and discuss the principles of artificial respiration, oxygen therapy, acclimatization and decompression sickness.

Before O_2 therapy, the physiological basis of hypoxia should be considered. Administration of O_2-rich gas mixture is of limited value in stagnant hypoxia, anemic hypoxia and hypoxia due to heart disease with right-to-left shunt. In other forms of hypoxic hypoxia, O_2 therapy is of great benefit.

O_2 therapy alone is of no use in histotoxic hypoxia. O_2 therapy must be started with care in patients with hypercapnia who are in severe pulmonary failure. The reason is that very high PCO_2 depresses the respiratory center. These patients breathe only because of hypoxic drive by stimulation of peripheral chemoreceptors. When O_2 is administered, this hypoxic drive is lost and breathing stops and it becomes a vicious cycle.

O_2 Toxicity

While O_2 is necessary for life, it is also toxic when present in excess. The toxicity of O_2 is due to the production of **superoxide anion (O_2^-)** which is a free radical and H_2O_2. Hyperbaric oxygen therapy is the most common cause for O_2 toxicity. When 80–100% O_2 is administered for 8 hours there will be irritation of respiratory passage, nasal congestion and coughing.

Infants treated with O_2 for IRDS develop **bronchopulmonary dysplasia** characterized by lung cysts and densities. Another complication is **retrolental fibroplasia** that is, fibrous tissue formation behind the lens, which leads to serious visual defects. There will be spasm of central artery of retina due to high PO_2 leading to degeneration of retina and **blindness**.

O_2 toxicity can be prevented by decreasing the concentration of O_2 in the gas mixture to 20% or less. If the subject shows symptoms of toxicity, decrease the pressure at which O_2 is administered.

Symptoms of O_2 Toxicity

Symptoms of toxicity depend on the pressure at which O_2 is given. They are:

- Muscle twitching
- Dizziness
- Pulmonary edema leading to dyspnea
- Convulsions and coma when pressure is increased to 6 atmospheres

Mechanism of O_2 Toxicity

Metabolic rate is increased in tissues and the temperature increases very much which affects the cellular enzymes and damage of tissues occurs. Brain is predominantly affected. Cerebral vasoconstriction decreases cerebral blood flow.

Hyperbaric O_2 Therapy

100% O_2 is administered at high pressure (3 atmospheres) in hyperbaric O_2 therapy. Its main aim is to increase the amount of dissolved O_2 in plasma. This is the most common cause for O_2 **toxicity**. When 100% O_2 is administered at 3 atmosphere pressure, the amount of dissolved O_2 in arterial blood will increase to 6 mL/100 mL. The needs of the tissue can be met with this dissolved O_2 in case of severe CO poisoning.

Indications for Hyperbaric O_2 Therapy

- CO poisoning
- Gas gangrene, which is produced by anaerobic bacteria. They cannot survive in excess of O_2
- Decompression sickness
- Air embolism
- Organophosphorus poisoning
- Histotoxic hypoxia

Complications of Hyperbaric O_2 Therapy

- Cerebral gas embolism
- Rupture of tympanic membrane
- Visual defects
- O_2 toxicity (*refer* O_2 toxicity)

Contraindications
- Asthma and emphysema
- High fever, viral infections, chronic sinusitis
- Pregnancy

CYANOSIS

Cyanosis is bluish discoloration of skin and mucous membrane when the amount of **reduced hemoglobin** in capillary blood is >5 g/100 mL of blood. Usually cyanosis is noticed in areas where skin is thin like fingertips, ear lobe, tip of nose, nail bed, mucous membrane, etc.

Cyanosis is classified into three types:
1. Central cyanosis
2. Peripheral cyanosis
3. Mixed type

Central Cyanosis

Central cyanosis results from imperfect oxygenation of blood at the level of lung or heart, e.g., lung diseases, congenital cyanotic heart disease, heart failure, etc. Here cyanosis is generalized and cyanosed extremities are warm due to peripheral vasodilatation. Pulse is bounding. It characteristically affects the tongue and lips (Fig. 39.16).

Peripheral Cyanosis

Peripheral cyanosis is due to excessive reduction of oxyhemoglobin in capillaries when blood flow is slow. It is seen in conditions that produce stagnant hypoxia, e.g., venous obstruction, exposure to cold, circulatory shock, etc. (Fig. 39.17). The cyanosed extremities are cold and tongue is unaffected. Pulse is thready.

Mixed Type

Both central and peripheral cyanosis occurs together as in heart failure.

Cyanosis is not seen in anemic hypoxia. This is because hemoglobin concentration is already less in anemia and hence the amount of reduced hemoglobin will be <5 g%. For cyanosis to occur, it should be >5 g%.

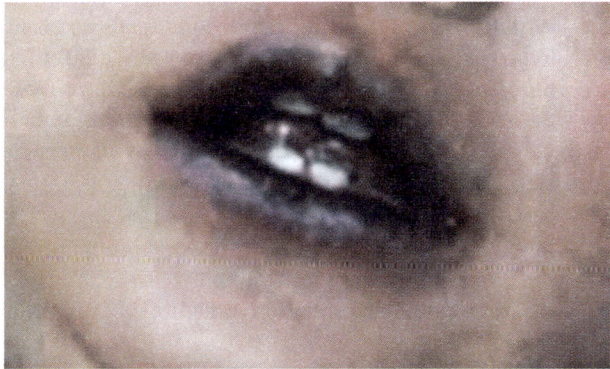

Fig. 39.16: Central cyanosis (Note the bluish discoloration of lips and tongue).

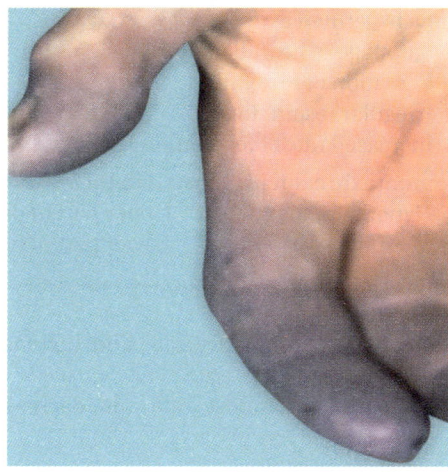

Fig. 39.17: Peripheral cyanosis.

Bluish discoloration of skin and mucous membrane will be produced by drugs like **phenacetin** due to **methemoglobinemia**. This may be mistaken for cyanosis, but here the patient will be cyanosed but not breathless.

MULTIPLE CHOICE QUESTIONS

1. **Respiration stops in the last stage of expiration, in forced expiration because of:**
   a. Respiratory muscle fatigue
   b. Collapse of alveoli
   c. Dynamic compression of airways
   d. Breaking effect of inspiratory muscles

2. **Cheyne-Stokes breathing is produced due to:**
   a. CO_2 retention
   b. Increased CO_2 sensitivity
   c. Hypoxia
   d. Acidosis

3. **Hering-Breuer inflation reflex is mediated by:**
   a. Pulmonary stretch receptor
   b. Bronchial stretch receptor
   c. J receptor
   d. Chest wall proprioceptors

4. **Inflation of lungs induces further inflation is explained by:**
   a. Hering-Breuer inflation reflex
   b. Hering-Breuer deflation reflex
   c. Head's paradoxical reflex
   d. J-reflex

5. **Carbon dioxide retention is most likely to occur in:**
   a. Ventilatory failure   b. Pulmonary fibrosis
   c. Hyperventilation   d. CO poisoning

6. **All the following cause hyperventilation, *except*:**
   a. Decreased pH in CSF
   b. Decreased plasma HCO_3^-
   c. CO poisoning
   d. Increased adrenergic levels

7. Apnea is defined as:
   a. Stoppage of heart beat
   b. Cessation of respiration
   c. Irregular respiration
   d. Increased rate of respiration

8. Pneumotaxic center is located in the:
   a. Hypothalamus   b. Upper part of pons
   c. Medulla   d. Lower part of pons

9. Bilateral vagotomy leads to:
   a. Apneustic breathing
   b. Decreased respiratory rate and increased tidal volume
   c. Increased respiratory rate and decreased tidal volume
   d. Periodic breathing

10. Chemoreceptors are seen in the following areas, *except*:
    a. Carotid sinus   b. Aortic body
    c. Medulla oblongata   d. Carotid body

11. Breathing stops upon destruction of:
    a. Medulla oblongata
    b. Cerebellum
    c. Pneumotaxic center
    d. Carotid and aortic bodies

12. The following statements regarding Hering-Breuer inflation reflex are true, *except*:
    a. The reflex is initiated by stimulation of stretch receptors of lung
    b. The reflex inhibits inspiration
    c. The afferent impulses mediating the reflex is transmitted through glossopharyngeal nerve
    d. The reflex help to prevent over inflation of lung

13. The main respiratory control neurons are located in:
    a. Pneumotaxic center
    b. *Pre-Bötzinger* complex
    c. Ventral respiratory group
    d. Dorsal respiratory group

14. The neurons may get irreversibly damaged if exposed to significant hypoxia for:
    a. 6 minutes   b. 2 minutes
    c. 30 seconds   d. 15 seconds

15. Patient with anemia tends to have all the following, *except*:
    a. Compensatory increase in cardiac output
    b. Increased incidence of heart murmurs
    c. Pallor of mucous membrane
    d. A low PO_2 in arterial blood

16. What is the useful function of nitrogen in the body?
    a. Prevents atelectasis
    b. Decrease rate of combustion
    c. Delays alveolar collapse
    d. All of the above

17. Hypoxia is characterized by:
    a. Low arterial PO_2
    b. Intense chemoreceptor response
    c. Favorable response to 100% O_2
    d. All of the above

18. Hypoxia produces vasoconstriction in:
    a. Muscles   b. Lungs
    c. Liver   d. Spleen

19. In a normal adult, 24 hours production of CO is about:
    a. 150 µmol/day   b. 290 µmol/day
    c. 330 µmol/day   d. 430 µmol/day

20. Hyperbaric oxygenation is useful in all, *except*:
    a. Congenital heart disease
    b. Gas gangrene
    c. Carbon monoxide poisoning
    d. Nitrogen toxicity

21. Arterial blood gas analysis in CO poisoning shows:
    a. PO_2 less, O_2 saturation normal
    b. PO_2 normal, O_2 saturation less with normal or slightly decreased PCO_2
    c. PO_2 less, O_5 saturation normal
    d. $PO2$ less, O_2 saturation decreased

22. Which of the following variants of hypoxia does not stimulate peripheral chemoreceptors?
    a. Hypoxic hypoxia   b. Anemic hypoxia
    c. Stagnant hypoxia   d. Histotoxic hypoxia

23. Anemic hypoxia is due to:
    a. Decreased PO_2 of arterial blood
    b. Increased PO_2 in arterial blood
    c. Increased PCO_2 in arterial blood
    d. Decreased O_2 content in arterial blood

24. Which is the best parameter for analysis of hypoxic hypoxia?
    a. Arterial PO_2 b. Arterial PCO_2
    c. Venous PO_2 d. A-V difference

25. Condition where severe hypoxemia occurs without cyanosis:
    a. Bronchial asthma   b. High altitude
    c. Anemia   d. Interstitial lung disease

26. Which of the following conditions leads to tissue hypoxia without alteration of oxygen content of blood?
    a. CO poisoning   b. Methemoglobinemia
    c. Cyanide poisoning   d. Respiratory acidosis

27. With reference to hypoxia, all the following statements are correct, *except*:
    a. When it is severe, causes stimulation of sympathetic nervous system
    b. It leads to accumulation of hydrogen and lactate ions
    c. It causes decrease in cerebral blood flow
    d. If it is chronic, causes rightward shift of oxygen hemoglobin dissociation curve

28. Tachycardia is caused by hypoxia due to:
    a. Reflexly through peripheral chemoreceptors
    b. Diffuse vasodilatation
    c. Through central chemoreceptor
    d. Secondarily after hyperventilation
29. Which of the following areas is most prone to hypoxic injury?
    a. Thalamus   b. Hippocampus
    c. Caudate nucleus   d. Cerebellum
30. Which of the following does not stimulate peripheral chemoreceptors?
    a. Hypoxia
    b. Hypocapnia
    c. Acidosis
    d. Low perfusion pressure
31. Peripheral chemoreceptors are stimulated maximally by:
    a. Cyanide   b. Anemia
    c. Hypocapnia   d. Alkalosis
32. Death due to cyanide poisoning results from which of the following types of hypoxia?
    a. Hypoxic hypoxia   b. Anemic hypoxia
    c. Stagnant hypoxia   d. Histotoxic hypoxia
33. Arterial PO_2 is reduced in:
    a. Anemia
    b. Cyanide poisoning
    c. Pulmonary hypoventilation
    d. CO poisoning
34. Oxygen therapy is not effective in:
    a. Hypoxic hypoxia   b. Anemic hypoxia
    c. Ischemic hypoxia   d. Histotoxic hypoxia
35. CO_2 retention is seen in all the following conditions, *except*:
    a. Carbon monoxide poisoning
    b. Lung failure
    c. Drowning
    d. Ventilatory failure
36. Hyperbaric oxygen is dangerous because it:
    a. Decreases displacement of O_2 from hemoglobin
    b. Decreases respiratory drive
    c. Causes enzyme damage
    d. Is toxic to tissues
37. Administration of pure O_2 to hypoxic patient is dangerous because:
    a. Apnea occurs due to hypostimulation of peripheral chemoreceptors
    b. Pulmonary edema occurs
    c. Decrease 2,3-DPG
    d. Produce convulsions
38. Hyperbaric oxygen therapy is useful in the following conditions, *except*:
    a. High altitude
    b. Cyanide poisoning
    c. Severe anemia
    d. Congestive cardiac failure
39. Arterial hypoxemia is a consequence of:
    a. Low hemoglobin concentration
    b. Carbon monoxide poisoning
    c. Hyperventilation
    d. Living at high altitude
40. The type of hypoxia produced due to diffusion defects in lungs:
    a. Hypoxic hypoxia   b. Anemic hypoxia
    c. Stagnant hypoxia   d. Histotoxic hypoxia
41. Cyanosis is produced when the blood level of:
    a. Reduced hemoglobin is more than 5 g%
    b. Reduced hemoglobin is more than 5 mg%
    c. Hemoglobin content is less than 9 g%
    d. Bilirubin is more than 2 mg%
42. Central cyanosis is seen if:
    a. Methemoglobin is 0.5 g/dL
    b. O_2 saturation is less than 85%
    c. O_2 saturation is less than 94%
    d. Hemoglobin 4 g%
43. In which of the following a reduction in arterial oxygen tension occurs?
    a. Anemia   b. CO poisoning
    c. Moderate exercise   d. Hypoventilation
44. Anemic hypoxia occurs in:
    a. Cyanide poisoning
    b. CO poisoning
    c. Carbon dioxide toxicity
    d. Vascular stasis
45. Oxygen therapy is of minimum use in:
    a. Hypoxic hypoxia   b. Anemic hypoxia
    c. Stagnant hypoxia   d. Histotoxic hypoxia
46. Cyanosis is seen when the concentration of:
    a. Deoxygenated hemoglobin increases above 5 g%
    b. Oxygenated hemoglobin increases
    c. Deoxygenated hemoglobin increases above 5 mg%
    d. Deoxygenated hemoglobin increases above 2–8 mg%
47. There is no stimulation of peripheral chemoreceptors in:
    a. Collapse of lung
    b. Hypoxic hypoxia
    c. Carbon monoxide poisoning
    d. Right to left shunt
48. Hypoxic hypoxia occurs in all of the following conditions, *except*:
    a. Congenital cyanotic heart disease
    b. Pulmonary fibrosis
    c. High altitude
    d. CO poisoning
49. Anemic hypoxia occurs in:
    a. Cyanide poisoning
    b. Arteriovenous shunt
    c. CO poisoning
    d. High altitude

50. Oxygen therapy is most effective in:
    a. Anemic hypoxia
    b. Hypoxic hypoxia
    c. Histotoxic hypoxia
    d. Stagnant hypoxia

51. Which type of hypoxia occur in cyanide poisoning:
    a. Histotoxic hypoxia
    b. Stagnant hypoxia
    c. Hypoxic hypoxia
    d. Anemic hypoxia

52. In anemic hypoxia:
    a. O_2 carrying capacity of blood is normal
    b. O_2 content of arterial blood is normal
    c. Oxygen tension of arterial blood is reduced
    d. Peripheral chemoreceptors are not stimulated

53. Most common type of hypoxia is:
    a. Hypoxic hypoxia
    b. Anemic hypoxia
    c. Stagnant hypoxia
    d. Histotoxic hypoxia

54. Apnea following voluntary hyperventilation is due to:
    a. Rise in PO_2 of arterial blood
    b. Fall in PCO_2 of arterial blood
    c. Rise in H^+ concentration of arterial blood
    d. Fall in PO_2 of arterial blood

55. J receptor stimulation produces:
    a. Apnea
    b. Tachypnea
    c. Tachycardia
    d. Hypertension

56. Rhythmic respiration continues *except* when?
    a. Bilateral vagotomy is done
    b. Bilateral vagotomy and mid-pontine section is done
    c. Brain stem transected above the level of pons
    d. Brain stem transected at the middle of pons

57. Respiratory centers are situated in:
    a. Medulla
    b. Pons
    c. Cerebral cortex
    d. Medulla and pons

58. Hering-Breuer inflation reflex:
    a. Is mediated by slowly adapting receptors
    b. Increases the duration of inspiration
    c. Operates at normal lung volumes
    d. Mediated by glossopharyngeal nerves

59. CO_2 affects respiratory center via:
    a. CSF H^+ concentration
    b. Carotid body
    c. Inflation and deflation receptors
    d. Aortic body

60. Hypercarbia (hypercapnia) is characterized by:
    a. Miosis
    b. Cold extremities
    c. Bradycardia
    d. Hypertension

61. Acute hypoxia and hypercapnia occur together in:
    a. Asthma
    b. Emphysema
    c. Asphyxia
    d. Hyperventilation

62. Cyanosis does not occur in:
    a. Hypoxic hypoxia
    b. Anemic hypoxia
    c. Stagnant hypoxia
    d. Histotoxic hypoxia

63. Hering-Breuer reflex is mediated by:
    a. Pulmonary stretch receptor
    b. Bronchial stretch receptor
    c. J receptor
    d. Chest wall proprioceptor

64. The following statements regarding cyanosis is true, *except*:
    a. Central cyanosis occurs due to defective oxygenation of arterial blood
    b. There is excess of reduced hemoglobin in peripheral blood
    c. Inhalation of O_2 clears the cyanosis in respiratory diseases
    d. Cyanosis is an important sign in anemia

65. Which of the following discharge spontaneously during quiet breathing?
    a. Inspiratory neurons
    b. Expiratory neurons
    c. Pneumotaxic center neurons
    d. Motor neurons supplying diaphragm

66. What will be the effect on respiration if a transection is made between pons and medulla?
    a. Apnea
    b. Irregular and gasping
    c. No effect
    d. Slow and deep

67. True regarding respiratory center is:
    a. Directly stimulated by fall in PaO_2
    b. Inhibited during swallowing
    c. Connected with cardiac center
    d. Situated in midbrain

68. J-receptors are situated in:
    a. Heart
    b. Blood vessels
    c. Alveolar interstitium
    d. Carotid body

69. Blood flow in the carotid body in mL/100 g of tissue is:
    a. 500
    b. 1000
    c. 2000
    d. 4000

70. When CO_2 in the inspired air increases beyond 10% at atmospheric pressure all the following occur, *except*:
    a. Depression of CNS
    b. Increased ventilation
    c. Diminished sensory acuity
    d. Confusion, coma and death

71. Most potent respiratory stimulant is:
    a. Oxygen
    b. Carbon dioxide
    c. K^+
    d. H^+

72. What is NOT true of respiratory center?
    a. Situated in the medulla and pons
    b. Sends out regular bursts of impulses to expiratory muscles during quiet respiration
    c. Sends out regular bursts of impulses to inspiratory muscles during quiet respiration
    d. Is inhibited during swallowing and vomiting

73. Normal O_2 tension with decreased O_2 carrying capacity is seen in:
    a. Histotoxic hypoxia
    b. Stagnant hypoxia
    c. Anemic hypoxia
    d. Hypoxic hypoxia

74. **Hyperventilation is caused by all, *except*:**
    a. Decreased pH in CSF
    b. Decreased plasma HCO_3^-
    c. Increased adrenergic level
    d. CO poisoning

75. **Hypoxic hypoxia is caused by all of the following, *except*:**
    a. Inadequate respiratory movements
    b. High altitude
    c. Cyanide poisoning
    d. Respiratory obstruction

76. **A reduction in arterial O_2 tension occurs in:**
    a. Anemia
    b. CO poisoning
    c. Moderate exercise
    d. Hypoventilation

77. **The mechanism by which hyperventilation may cause muscle spasm:**
    a. Decrease in Ca^{2+} level
    b. Decreased CO_2
    c. Decreased potassium
    d. Decreased sodium

78. **Hypoxia causes vasoconstriction in:**
    a. Muscle
    b. Lung
    c. Liver
    d. Spleen

79. **In Bohr effect:**
    a. O_2 dissociation increases in hypoxia
    b. O_2 dissociation decreases in hypoxia
    c. O_2 dissociation increases with elevated temperature
    d. O_2 dissociation increases with low pH

80. **When CO_2 in inspired air exceeds 10% at atmospheric pressure, the following may occur, *except*:**
    a. Depression of central nervous system
    b. Diminished sensory acuity
    c. Hyperventilation
    d. Confusion, coma and death

ANSWERS

1. c	2. b	3. a	4. c	5. a
6. c	7. b	8. b	9. c	10. a
11. a	12. c	13. b	14. a	15. d
16. d	17. d	18. b	19. d	20. a
21. b	22. b	23. d	24. a	25. c
26. c	27. c	28. b	29. b	30. b
31. a	32. d	33. c	34. d	35. a
36. d	37. a	38. c	39. d	40. a
41. a	42. b	43. d	44. b	45. d
46. a	47. c	48. d	49. c	50. b
51. a	52. d	53. a	54. b	55. b
56. b	57. d	58. a	59. a	60. d
61. c	62. b	63. a	64. d	65. a
66. b	67. b	68. c	69. c	70. b
71. b	72. b	73. c	74. d	75. c
76. d	77. a	78. b	79. d	80. c

Environmental Physiology

CHAPTER 40

LEARNING OBJECTIVES

Must know
- Describe the pathophysiology of acute mountain sickness
- Explain the physiology of acclimatization at high altitude
- Describe the physiology of deep sea diving
- Explain decompression sickness

Desirable to know
- Explain the physiological effects of weightlessness
- Explain the effects of ionizing radiation in the body

HIGH ALTITUDE PHYSIOLOGY

PY6.4: Describe and discuss the physiology of high altitude and deep sea diving.

Height of more than 10,000 feet above sea level is referred to as high altitude. Study of high altitude physiology is important in:
- Mountaineering
- Aviation
- Space flight.

Effects of high altitude on the body are due to:
- Hypoxic hypoxia as a result of decreased barometric pressure
- Physical factors like temperature, ultraviolet radiation, ionizing radiation, etc.
- Acceleratory forces on the body (*refer* **Chapter 31**).

EFFECTS OF BAROMETRIC PRESSURE ON RESPIRATORY SYSTEM

EFFECTS OF DECREASED BAROMETRIC PRESSURE

Effects of Hypoxia

As a person ascends to high altitude, the composition of air stays the same, but the total barometric pressure falls because the total barometric pressure at any altitude is proportional to the weight of the air above it. As the barometric pressure decreases at high altitude, the atmospheric PO_2 decreases proportionately. *Hypoxic hypoxia is a problem in normal individuals going to high altitude.* As the inspired air passes through the airways, it is normally warmed to body temperature and completely humidified. So, the partial pressure exerted by the water vapor entering the alveoli is fixed at 47 mm Hg at any altitude.

The effects of hypoxia at high altitude depend on the physical fitness, duration of stay, previous training, rapidity of ascent, etc. As the person ascends, there is marked reduction in alveolar PO_2 and arterial PO_2. Percentage saturation is decreased and hypoxic symptoms are produced. Fall in PCO_2 is gradual.

Up to a height of 8,000 feet, there is no increase in pulmonary ventilation because the percentage saturation at 8000 feet is 93%. At a height of 10,000–20,000 feet, there is increase in ventilation because of hypoxic stimulation of peripheral chemoreceptors. As one ascends higher, the alveolar PCO_2 falls very much because of hyperventilation. This leads to respiratory alkalosis.

At a height of 23,000 feet, the percentage saturation is decreased to 50% and there will be loss of consciousness and coma. We can delay this up to a height of 47,000 feet by inspiring pure O_2. Above 50,000 feet, coma cannot be prevented even by breathing 100% O_2. But, it is possible to ascend to any altitude, even in the interplanetary space, if an artificial atmosphere is created around the person. The person should be in a pressurized suit or cabin supplied with O_2 and a system to remove CO_2.

Acute Mountain Sickness

If a person ascends rapidly to altitudes above 8,300 feet and does physical activity, he may become acutely sick and may die if O_2 is not given or if he is not removed to a low altitude. This is acute mountain sickness characterized by cerebral edema and pulmonary edema. The alveolar PCO_2 falls at greater altitudes because hypoxic stimulation of the arterial chemoreceptors increases alveolar ventilation. This leads to removal of more CO_2.

Hypocapnia is a strong cerebral vasoconstrictor. Hypoxic stimulation of arterial chemoreceptors causes hypocapnia and respiratory alkalosis. Most of the CNS symptoms of acute mountain sickness could be attributed to these factors.

But the direct effect of hypoxia in the cerebral vessels is vasodilation. This finally leads to cerebral hyperperfusion and edema with increase in intracranial pressure. This leads to increased sympathetic stimulation producing pulmonary edema due to pulmonary hypertension.

Acute Cerebral Edema

Acute cerebral edema is due to local vasodilation of the cerebral blood vessels caused by hypoxia. There will be transudation of fluid into the brain tissue leading to **high altitude cerebral edema**. In severe cases, if cerebral autoregulation fails, the brain swelling becomes severe which leads to coma and death due to herniation of brain through the tentorium. The symptoms are due to a combination of hypoxemia and respiratory alkalosis.

Symptoms

- Headache, irritability, disorientation, ataxia and insomnia
- Breathlessness
- Nausea and vomiting
- Convulsions, coma and even death.

Cerebral edema can be reduced by giving large doses of glucocorticoids. Carbonic anhydrase inhibitor acetazolamide is also given which decreases cerebrospinal fluid (CSF) production, increases HCO_3^- excretion in urine and increases arterial PCO_2. The resulting metabolic acidosis stimulates ventilation. Being a diuretic, acetazolamide prevents fluid retention and edema. It also inhibits pulmonary vasoconstriction and thus prevents pulmonary hypertension. It is given for a few days before ascending to high altitude and helps to prevent acute mountain sickness.

Acute Pulmonary Edema

Severe hypoxia causes pulmonary arterioles to constrict leading to increase in pulmonary vascular resistance and pulmonary hypertension. This leads to exudation of fluid into the interstitial space and alveoli due to increase in capillary pressure producing **high altitude pulmonary edema**. Pulmonary edema responds to **rest** and **hyperbaric O_2 therapy**. **Nifedipine**, a Ca^{2+} channel blocker, lowers pulmonary artery pressure and is of benefit.

Acute mountain sickness can be prevented by slow ascent and by avoiding physical exertion for the first few days of high altitude exposure.

At 63,000 feet, the barometric pressure is only 47 mm Hg and the body fluids boil at body temperature. This does not happen because the person would be dead of hypoxia before the steam could cause death.

In a pressurized cabin supplied with O_2 and a system to remove CO_2, a person can ascend to any altitude.

Chronic Mountain Sickness or Monge's Disease

If a person stays at high altitude for a long time, initially he may get acclimatized but later he fails. This is chronic mountain sickness.

The effects are:
- Polycythemia, which increases viscosity of blood leading to decreased tissue blood flow.
- Pulmonary hypertension due to pulmonary vasoconstriction as a result of pulmonary hypoxia.
- Right ventricular hypertrophy due to pulmonary hypertension.
- Fall in peripheral arterial pressure since less blood is ejected by the left ventricle. Due to pulmonary hypertension, less blood is returned to the left atrium.
- Congestive cardiac failure (CCF) due to pulmonary hypertension.
- Death often follows unless the person is removed to a lower altitude.

Acclimatization at High Altitude or Physiological Adjustments to Hypoxia

Acclimatization refers to a number of compensatory mechanisms that operate over a period of time to increase altitude tolerance.

The compensatory mechanisms include:
- **Increase in pulmonary ventilation**: Within 2–5 days at high altitude, pulmonary ventilation increases by about 5 times normal due to hypoxic stimulation of peripheral chemoreceptors. After a few days, the increase in ventilation declines slowly but it takes years for it to come to the initial level.
- **Increase in RBC count and hemoglobin content**: Hypoxia stimulates erythropoietin secretion, and increase in RBC count is seen within 2–3 days of stay. The subjects will be polycythemic. Blood volume will be increased by 20–30%. PCV will be 60–65%; hemoglobin content will be 20–22 g%.
- **Increase in 2,3-DPG**: Due to increase in 2,3-DPG as a result of alkalosis, there will be decreased affinity of hemoglobin for O_2 and this makes more O_2 available to the tissues. Hypoxia also increases the synthesis of 2,3-DPG in the red blood cells. There will be increased unloading of O_2 to the tissues, i.e., the oxygen dissociation curve shifts to the right.
- **Increased vascularity of tissues**: Cardiac output is increased by 20–30% and blood flow to the vital organs will be increased. There will be opening up of closed capillaries.
- **Increase in diffusing capacity**: Diffusing capacity at lung level is increased 3-fold. Due to increase in ventilation and increase in pulmonary blood flow, there is increase in surface area and decrease in thickness of respiratory membrane.
- **Increased extraction of O_2 at tissue level.** This is by:
  - Increase in the number of mitochondria
  - Increase in tissue content of cytochrome oxidase
  - Increased capillarity of tissues
  - Increase in myoglobin
- Renal compensation: Renal compensation for respiratory alkalosis begins within a day. Renal excretion of HCO_3^- is increased and hydrogen ions are conserved and thus prevent alkalosis.

- **CO_2 dissociation curve** shifts to the left for any given arterial PCO_2, i.e., for any given arterial PCO_2, the ventilatory response is greater than normal after several days of stay at high altitude.
- **Resolution of cerebral edema:** Intracranial tension falls and resolution of cerebral edema occurs due to increased reabsorption of cerebrospinal fluid, autoregulation of cerebral blood flow and sympathetically mediated cerebral vasoconstriction. The cerebral vessels produce less nitric oxide, which is the mediator of cerebral vasodilatation in response to hypoxia.

Natural Acclimatization of Inhabitants at High Altitude (18,000 feet)

In persons living at high altitude, acclimatization occurs from birth onwards. They have:
- Barrel shaped chest due to increase in functional residual capacity
- Polycythemia due to increased erythropoiesis in response to hypoxia
- Hypertrophy of right side of heart due to pulmonary hypertension and increased viscosity of blood
- Shift of oxygen dissociation curve (ODC) to the right
- Work capacity of skeletal muscle and cardiac muscle is increased.

FACTORS OTHER THAN BAROMETRIC PRESSURE AT HIGH ALTITUDE

1. Temperature
2. Humidity
3. Solar and ultraviolet radiation
4. Ionizing radiation.

Effect of Temperature

Temperature falls with increasing altitude at a rate of about 1°C for every 150 meters. In high mountains such as Mt Everest, the average temperature near the summit is about minus 40°C. Cold injury is common in the mountains. The core temperature will fall over days or weeks. **Hypothermia** is defined as lowering of the central core temperature below 35°C. When the core temperature goes below 32°C, it is called **severe hypothermia.** The subject has altered mental function, loss of memory, somnolence (increased sleepiness), slurred speech and ataxia. There will be loss of consciousness when the core temperature falls to 30°C and there will be violent shivering. When the core temperature falls below 30°C, ventricular fibrillation may occur. In profound hypothermia, pupils do not react to light and other reflexes will be absent. Pulmonary edema develops when the temperature falls to 22°C. At 20°C, heart stops beating and the subject appear dead. External cardiac massage should be given and the subject should be warmed.

In hypothermia, there is shift of body fluids from the intravascular to the interstitial compartment causing edema. This leads to hypovolemia and fall in blood pressure.

Effect of Humidity

The absolute humidity at high altitude will be very low and this leads to dehydration. There is increase in insensible water loss through respiratory passage due to increase in ventilation at high altitude. Plenty of fluid intake will prevent dehydration.

Effect of Solar and Ultraviolet Radiation

At high altitude, the thinner atmosphere absorbs less of the sun's rays, especially those of short wave length in the near ultraviolet region of the spectrum. Another factor is that the air at high altitude is so dry that there is not enough water vapor in the atmosphere to absorb solar radiation. Prolonged exposure to sunlight may lead to the development of skin cancer.

Ultraviolet light comes under the wavelength range of 1500–5000°A. UV light of wavelength 2800–3000°A is absorbed practically completely in the stratum corneum of the skin. Light of wavelength 5000°A may penetrate into the underlying subcutaneous tissues.

Maximum lethal effect is produced by UV light of wavelength 2650°A. For example, the sunburn produced on prolonged exposure to high intensity sunlight is due to the effect of UV rays. The symptoms associated with sunburn are reddening (erythema), peeling of external layers of skin, pain, blistering and appearance of pigmentation. The reddening of skin is due to dilation of the blood vessels of skin, which in turn is due to liberation of substances like histamine from the tissues. The outer layer of the skin finally dies and is sloughed off. If the damage is extensive, enough fluid pockets accumulate in the epidermal layers and form blisters. After a few days, erythema disappears and a brownish color takes its place, which is called **tanning**. It is due to the formation of brown pigments in the skin.

Damage to the eye (**photophthalmia**) is an inflammation to the cornea quite similar to the origin and effects of sunburn. Eye damage due to looking directly into the sun includes loss of sight in the area of the image of the sun in the eye and is due to the "burning glass" action of the optical system of the eye.

Ionizing Radiation

The intensity of cosmic radiation increases at high altitude because there is less of the earth's atmosphere to absorb the rays as they enter from space. Ionizing radiation produces irreversible as well as reversible effects on the skin. (*Refer* the heading "Diseases due to Ionizing Radiation" in this chapter).

EFFECTS OF INCREASED BAROMETRIC PRESSURE

Deep sea divers, people working in mines, those who dig underwater tunnels in **caissons**, which are chambers in which these people work where the pressure is high to keep

out the water, etc., are exposed to high barometric pressure. The increased pressure creates two problems:
1. Compression effect on the body and internal organs
2. Decrease in the volume of gas.

The barometric pressure increases by one atmosphere for every 33 feet of depth in sea water. According to **Boyle's law**, volume of a gas is inversely proportional to pressure. The tissues of the body are composed mainly of water and are therefore incompressible, but gases are compressible and follow Boyle's law. As the pressure increases, the air gets compressed into smaller and smaller volumes. So, as the atmospheric pressure is increased there is a tendency for lungs to collapse and air should be provided at high pressure to prevent collapse. This exposes the blood in the lungs to very high alveolar gas pressure. This condition is called **hyperbarism**.

As the total pressure increases, the partial pressure of the constituent gases in body fluids also increases according to Dalton's law. As the partial pressure of gases increases, the amount of gases dissolved in the tissues of the body increase according to Henry's law. Inspired air contains mainly N_2, O_2 and CO_2. At high barometric pressure, there are side effects of increased concentration of the above gases in the body. Increased PO_2 can cause **oxygen toxicity** (*refer* oxygen toxicity in Chapter 39).

Effects of Increase in N_2 or Nitrogen Narcosis or Raptures of the Deep

Narcosis means unconsciousness or stupor produced by drugs like anesthetics. **Stupor** is lethargy with suppression of sensations and feelings. N_2 readily dissolves in the fat of body, especially in the membranes of neurons. This alters ionic conductance through the membrane and reduces neuronal excitability. N_2 at high pressure produces this effect and is called **nitrogen narcosis**. Euphoria is seen in N_2 narcosis and so it is also known as **raptures of the deep**. Rapture means being uplifted into the air or a feeling of intense pleasure or joy.

About 80% (4/5th) of atmospheric air is N_2. Being an inert gas, it does not produce any adverse effect on the functions of the body at normal atmospheric pressure. When a person breathes pressurized air (as in the depths of the sea) the narcotic effects of N_2 start. At high barometric pressures, N_2 gets dissolved in body fluids and acts as an anesthetic agent.

At 4–5 atmospheres (at depths of 30–40 m in the ocean), if the diver is breathing 80% N_2, symptoms are similar to alcohol intoxication. It includes euphoria (a feeling of intense happiness), decreased mental performance, etc. At 8–9 atmospheres, the person becomes unconscious. The problem of N_2 narcosis can be avoided by breathing O_2-**He mixture**.

Advantages of Helium over N_2

❖ Helium is less dense than N_2. It is the second lighter gas. Density of He is 1/7th that of N_2. So, He decreases airway resistance and work of breathing.
❖ It is less soluble in body fluids. Helium has only 1/5th the solubility of N_2.

❖ It has less narcotic effect. Pressurized helium produces much less intellectual impairment than pressurized N_2.

High Pressure Nervous Syndrome

But during deep dives with O_2-He mixture, when the barometric pressure is very high, i.e., more than 500 feet, Helium produces **high pressure nervous syndrome (HPNS) or high pressure neurological syndrome**. The effects and the severity of the effects depend on the rate of descent, the depth and the percentage of Helium. The symptoms are tremor, ataxia, nausea, vomiting, dizziness, myoclonic jerking, somnolence, EEG changes, visual disturbance, and decreased mental performance. The cause for HPNS is that the inert gases act as anesthetics at increased pressure. They become lipid soluble and get dissolved in nerve membranes leading to the above symptoms. HPNS was also found to be caused by the high pressure itself and the speed of compression also plays a role. Small amounts of N_2 or H_2 added to the inspired gas mixture help to suppress the neurological effects.

Decompression Sickness or Dysbarism or Diver's Paralysis or Bends or Caisson Disease

> **PY6.5:** Describe and discuss the principles of artificial respiration, oxygen therapy, acclimatization and decompression sickness.

Decompression sickness is the disorder that occurs when a person returns rapidly to atmospheric pressure after exposure to high barometric pressure as in deep sea. It occurs only if the diver is breathing pressurized air. If the diving is done using breath holding, decompression sickness will not occur even if the ascent is rapid. (A caisson is a watertight enclosure inside which under water construction work is done. The pressure in the caisson is increased to keep out the water.)

In deep-sea divers, due to increased barometric pressure all the gases, especially N_2, get dissolved in body fluids and in the body fat. As long as the person remains in deep sea, N_2 remains in solution and does not cause many problems. As the diver who is breathing 80% N_2, rapidly ascends from the dive, the alveolar PN_2 falls. The N_2 is decompressed and escapes from the tissues at a faster rate. Being a gas, it forms bubbles while escaping rapidly in the tissues and in the blood causing symptoms of **decompression sickness**. The bubbles may block blood flow producing air embolism leading to ischemia and tissue death.

Depending on the sites of bubble formation and size of bubbles, symptoms vary:
❖ Bubbles in and around joints lead to severe joint pain called **bends**.
❖ Bubbles in the myelin sheath of sensory fibers cause sensory impairment, numbness, paresthesia and itching.
❖ Bubbles in the motor fibers produce temporary paralysis, respiratory failure, etc.
❖ Bubbles in muscle produce muscle cramps associated with severe pain.

- Bubbles in brain and spinal cord lead to sensory and motor impairment.
- Bubbles in pulmonary capillaries lead to pulmonary edema and dyspnea referred to as **chokes**.
- Bubbles in coronary arteries lead to myocardial damage and may cause myocardial infarction due to arterial gas embolism. Bubbles may also be carried to the cerebral vessels, which may lead to stroke.

Treatment and Prevention of Decompression Sickness

- While returning to sea level, the ascent should be very slow with short stay at regular intervals. This allows N_2 to diffuse into the blood without forming bubbles, and it diffuses into the lungs along the partial pressure gradient.
- If affected by decompression sickness, immediate recompression in a **recompression chamber (hyperbaric chamber)** is done. This should be followed by very slow decompression.
- O_2- He mixtures can be provided for divers.
- Hyperbaric O_2 therapy is also useful in treating decompression sickness.
- Deep sea divers and underwater tunnel workers can use **SCUBA** (**S**elf-**c**ontained **U**nderwater **B**reathing **A**pparatus). The disadvantage is that the person can remain in the depth only for a limited time.

Decompression sickness also occurs in:
- Escape from submerged submarines
- Ascent in an unpressurized cabin of airplane.

Explosive decompression occurs when an aircraft flying at a great height gets suddenly depressurized. Death is due to fatal air embolism.

Effects of Increase in O_2 at High Barometric Pressure

The harmful effect of breathing O_2 is proportionate to the PO_2. If 100% O_2 is inspired at high barometric pressure, it produces symptoms of **O_2 toxicity**. This can be prevented by decreasing the concentration of O_2 in the gas mixture to 20% or less.

Effects of Increased CO_2

Alveolar PCO_2 up to 80 mm Hg does not produce many side effects. Respiratory minute volume will be increased 8–10-fold. When the PCO_2 become >80 mm Hg, it leads to **CO_2 narcosis** (*refer* 'Hypercapnia,' Chapter 39).

BAROTRAUMA

Barotrauma occurs in unventilated areas of the body that cannot equilibrate with the ambient pressure when the barometric pressure increases or decreases. It can affect the middle ear if the Eustachian tube is blocked, the sinuses, lungs, cavities of teeth, etc.

The barotrauma of descent is called **squeeze**. Effects are severe earache since the pressure in the middle ear cannot equilibrate with the outside pressure; toothache, pulmonary congestion, edema or hemorrhage.

The barotrauma of ascent can occur if gases are trapped in areas of the body and begin to expand when the diver ascends. If the diver does not exhale during the ascent, expanding pulmonary gas may over distend and burst the lung. This may result in hemorrhage, pneumothorax or air embolism. Gases trapped in the gastrointestinal tract may cause abdominal discomfort. Barotrauma of ears, sinuses and teeth may also occur on rapid ascent from great depths.

SPACE PHYSIOLOGY

WEIGHTLESSNESS IN SPACE

Introduction

Weightlessness or zero gravity or microgravity is the strangest problem man faces in an orbiting spacecraft. He floats in the spacecraft if not supported by the seat belt. Weightlessness may be experienced during periods of free fall as when diving off a diving board. Another example is, when a stationary elevator accelerates downwards, the person experiences a decrease or even total absence of weight briefly.

Weightlessness may be defined as the condition produced when the resultant of all forces acting on a body is zero, i.e., when the force of inertia is exactly equal and opposite to that of gravity. The term "zero gravity" and "weightlessness" means the same. Weightlessness denotes a psychophysiological condition, whereas zero gravity denotes a physical condition.

Since there is no atmosphere in the outer space, an artificial atmosphere and climate must be provided in the spacecraft. In the modern space shuttle, gases present in atmospheric air are used with four times nitrogen as much as oxygen and a total pressure of 760 mm Hg. High concentration of N_2 prevents the development of local patches of lung atelectasis that often occur when pure O_2 is used for breathing. This is because O_2 will be absorbed rapidly from areas where small bronchi are temporarily blocked by mucus plugs.

The force of gravity decreases as one goes away from the earth in inverse proportion to the square of the distance from the earth's center. When a person ascends 4,000 miles from the earth's surface, his weight will be only 1/4 of what is on the ground. The weight will be 1/100th of what was on the ground if he goes 36,000 miles up.

Short periods of weightlessness present no physiological problems. It creates mechanical problems, which can be overcome by adequate design and by training and experience. In longer flights, basic biological alterations may occur and should be compensated. By proper designing and training, weightlessness may prove to be an enjoyable and stimulating experience.

Physiological Effects of Weightlessness

Almost all the physiological changes occurring during weightlessness are the same as those encountered in chronic bed ridden patients and can be cured by taking proper exercise.

Effects on Cardiovascular System

- Heart rate increases initially but soon comes back to normal
- Blood volume decreases

- Red cell mass decreases
- Maximum cardiac output decreases
- Blood pressure and electrocardiogram show no significant changes
- When the stay is prolonged, cardiovascular deconditioning happens leading to orthostatic hypotension after returning to earth. This is because of impaired baroreceptor reflexes and decreased blood volume.

On Respiratory System
- Initially, there is increase in ventilation but returns to normal rapidly.
- In the absence of convection, mixing and diffusion of gas is impaired. Exhaled water vapor and CO_2 would remain in front of the face suffocating the person. So, forced air circulation is essential to replace natural convection for respiration during weightlessness.

Effects on Muscular System
About 1/3rd of our total energy production is spent in overcoming the force of gravity by the contraction of skeletal muscles. Weightlessness reduces the muscular efforts required to perform physical tasks and to control posture. So on prolonged exposure to weightlessness, disuse atrophy of skeletal and cardiac muscle occur. In skeletal muscle, there is decrease in fiber length and diameter. Sarcomere volume and number of mitochondria decrease. All these are due to disuse of muscle. Muscle atrophy is accompanied by increased urinary excretion of N_2 and phosphorus and there will be negative nitrogen balance.

Effects on Skeletal System
- The most important and serious effect of microgravity is the demineralization of bone which is unpreventable.
- Bone loss seems to be regional, with greater losses from trabecular than from cortical bones.
- There is increased urinary excretion of calcium, which increases the risk of calcium nephropathy.
- Plasma level of parathormone is found to be elevated.
- Disuse is the main cause for demineralization and there is increased risk of fracture after return to normal gravity. Demineralization can be prevented to some extent if artificial gravity is provided. Strengthening exercises are also advised during the stay. Studies have shown that astronauts on space flights lose as much as 1% of their bone mass each month even though they continue to exercise.

Effects on Vestibular System
- Most important disturbance encountered in weightlessness is motion sickness. It is due to rapid head movements and labyrinthine edema due to the preceding acceleration. After 3 days, most astronauts can move their heads without discomfort. Physiologically space sickness is probably due to absent or incorrect otolithic information. Drugs like hyoscine are effective in the treatment and prevention of this condition.
- Righting reflexes are affected.
- During weightlessness, some experience postural and visual illusions, which appear to be related to the function of otoliths.

Effect on Vision
Weightlessness does not produce any change in the weight of the optical components of the eye or in the intraocular pressure. Vision will be the main intact and fully functioning sensory response.

Psychological Changes
The subjective sensation experienced during weightlessness depends on the emotional attitude of the subject as well as on his training. For majority of astronauts, the experience is pleasant, a sensation of floating, slight amusement, relaxation, wellbeing and comfort. Some complained of frustrations due to lack of accustomed physical activity and a state of somnolence. Elimination of body wastes, eating, and personal hygiene all pose problems leading to frustration.

Sleep
Rapid eye movement (REM) sleep increases during sleep period in weightlessness but later return to normal due to adaptation.

Immunity
In short duration flights, humoral and cellular immunity is normal. But in long duration flights, T cell response is depressed.

Fluid Shift in Weightlessness
In the absence of gravity, about 2 L of fluid moves from legs to upper parts of the body which occurs very rapidly, i.e., within 3-6 hours and is reversible. Both intravascular and extravascular fluids are involved. Face becomes puffy and upper body veins are engorged. Fluid shift leads to hemoconcentration and increase in hematocrit value. There is lowering of venous pressure in the lower parts of the body. Kidneys excrete more of sodium and water.

Weight Loss
Due to fluid loss and disuse atrophy, there will be weight loss, which starts from first day and continues for 10–15 days.

Anthropometric Changes
Due to lack of gravitational load, the thoracolumbar spine straightens and there is increase in height. This causes decrease in the girth of abdomen and chest. Thus, the space suit fitted on earth becomes too small and difficult to zip up.

Metabolic Changes
- Glucose metabolism is decreased.
- Liver glycogen increases by 50-100%.
- Glycogen content in skeletal muscle also increases.
- The mitochondrial size decreases and there is decrease in myosin ATPase activity.
- There is loss of cell mass, negative nitrogen balance and increased renal loss of nitrogen and phosphorus.

Other Problems

Weightlessness affects mainly the ingestion of food. Food will not adhere to the eating utensil. When the astronaut tries to drink water, the fluid leaves the container as an amoeboid mass and causes choking. Liquids no longer flow, but break up into small globules. Plastic squeeze bottles can be used.

DISEASES DUE TO IONIZING RADIATION

Sources of Radiation

Environmental Sources

- Cosmic radiation
- From the ground
- Through inhalation (Radon)
- Through ingested materials.

Man Made Sources

- From X-ray equipment
- Nuclear weapons
- Radioactive medications.
  Radiation is measured in Roentgens (R) in an ionization chamber.

Biologic Effects of Radiation

- Double strand breaks in DNA to kill the cell.
- About 80% of cell is water and the following reaction occur

  Ionizing radiation + $H_2O \rightarrow H_2O^+ + e^-$

  $H_2O^+ + H_2O \rightarrow H_3O + OH^-$ (radical)
- Mutations may lead to cancerous growths many years after exposure to radiation.
- Chromosomal aberrations occur in cells irradiated in the G1 phase of the cell cycle.
- Chromosome breaks occur when cells are irradiated and the broken ends of chromosomes can combine with the broken ends of different chromosomes.

Factors Affecting the Clinical Manifestation of Irradiation

- Total dose
- Dose per fraction
- Volume of organs irradiated (field size)
- Length of time taken to deliver the dose.

Effects on Different Tissues

Effects on Skin

The effects are classified into:
- Reversible changes
- Conditioned reversible changes
- Irreversible changes
- Rare skin manifestations.

Skin manifestations depend on radiation dose, the quanta absorbed into the skin, field size, constitutional factors like type of skin, skin color, hair color, etc.

Reversible Changes

- Roentgen erythema
- Epilation of hair
- Suppression of sebaceous gland function.

In Roentgen erythema, following a dose of ionizing radiation, the skin shows a series of episodes of reddening called **erythema**. Initially (early erythema), there will be a pale pink color due to release of amines from the injured tissues which produces dilatation of capillaries and arterioles. If the exposed dose is high, by the 8th day, the skin color becomes red to violet and pigmentation appears on the 20th day (second erythema).

In epilation of hair, the hair of scalp and beard gets easily epilated. The germinal layers of hair follicle are sensitive to ionizing radiation causing hair to enter the resting stage of growth. Hair falls off in 2 weeks and grows after 2-3 months. As the pigment cells are vulnerable to ionizing radiation, the new hair will be white. Higher doses may cause permanent destruction of hair follicles. There will also be suppression of sebaceous gland function.

Conditioned Reversible Changes

Pigmentation of irradiated skin lasts from weeks to months. Since the pigmented skin reacts to further exposure with a greater sensitivity, it is classified as conditioned reversible effect.

Irreversible Changes

- Acute radiation dermatitis
- Chronic radiation dermatitis
- Radiation cancer.

Acute radiation dermatitis (Fig. 40.1): After exposure of the skin to doses of 1000 R or more, skin becomes purple in color

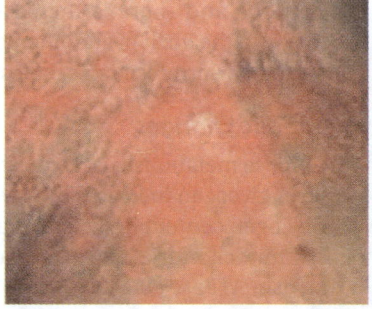 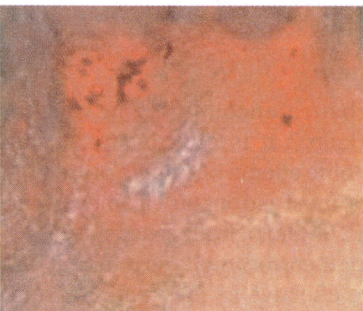

Fig. 40.1: Acute radiation dermatitis.

and it deepens. This is followed by formation of large blisters with serous exudate.

The bullae bursts and secondary pyogenic infection occur. Later it heals with deeply pigmented atrophic scars.

Very high dose produces Roentgen ulcers in 6–8 weeks. It can be treated using lukewarm compresses, antibiotics, steroid creams and analgesics. Full thickness graft after wide excision is the surgical treatment.

Chronic radiation dermatitis: If the skin is exposed to repeated small doses of ionizing radiation for long periods, hands, feet and face are affected. On the hands, there will be flattening of epidermal ridges of fingers, thickening of creases, atrophy of sebaceous and sweat glands and appearance of warty lesions. In the face, there is deepening of skin furrows, skin becomes diffusely thickened and keratosis appears.

Radiation cancer: Radiation cancer is a common complication of exposure to smaller doses of radiation over longer periods. The latent period between exposure and carcinoma is long varying from 7 to 12 years. The tumors are multiple and metastasize in 25% of cases. Healing is poor and recurrence is common. Tumors include squamous cell carcinoma of hands, feet and face; basal cell carcinoma, sarcomas and malignant melanomas. Most cases of radiation cancer are seen in those patients treated for acne and for epilation of hair using radiation. Topical therapy with 5-fluorouracil is the treatment of choice.

Rare Skin Manifestation

It includes skin eruptions like urticaria or maculopapular rashes.

Effects on Other Tissues

Effects on Central Nervous System

Central nervous system (CNS) has been described as relatively resistant to radiation-induced changes. Transient demyelination of spinal cord, infarction and necrosis may be seen. Dementia, dysarthria and rarely transverse myelitis occur if combined with chemotherapy.

Bone marrow: Aplasia, pancytopenia

Liver: Acute and chronic hepatitis

Stomach: Perforation, hemorrhage, ulcers

Intestine: Ulcer, perforation, hemorrhage

Heart: Pericarditis, pancarditis

Lung: Acute and chronic pneumonitis

Kidney: Acute and chronic nephrosclerosis

Fetus: Death.

■ MULTIPLE CHOICE QUESTIONS

1. **On the summit of Mt Everest where the barometric pressure is about 250 mm Hg, partial pressure of O_2 (PO_2) will be about:**
   a. 0.1 mm Hg b. 0.5 mm Hg
   c. 50 mm Hg d. 5 mm Hg

2. **A person goes to the mountains. When he reaches about 5,000 feet. he develops dyspnea. Which of the following correctly explains for the symptoms?**
   a. CNS depression
   b. CO_2 wash out
   c. Increased work of breathing
   d. Increased blood flow to the pulmonary tissues

3. **All the following are seen in high altitude climbers, *except*:**
   a. Hyperventilation   b. Decreased $PaCO_2$
   c. Pulmonary edema   d. Bradycardia

4. **In high altitude mountain sickness, feature of pulmonary edema is:**
   a. Decreased pulmonary capillary permeability
   b. Increased pulmonary capillary pressure
   c. Increased left atrial pressure
   d. Increased left ventricular back pressure

5. **Compensatory mechanisms involved in acclimatization to high altitude includes all the following, *except*:**
   a. Hyperventilation
   b. Respiratory stimulation
   c. Respiratory acidosis
   d. Respiratory alkalosis

6. **Deep sea diving is associated with:**
   a. Dysbarism
   b. Respiratory distress syndrome
   c. Acclimatization
   d. Hemothorax

7. **Changes during acclimatization to high altitude include all the following, *except*:**
   a. Increased sensitivity of respiratory center to CO_2
   b. Increase in RBC count
   c. Increase in heart rate
   d. Excretion of more acidic urine

8. **Acclimatization include all the following, *except*:**
   a. Bradycardia
   b. Hyperventilation
   c. Increase in 2,3 BPG
   d. Increase in erythropoietin

9. **During acclimatization at high altitude all the following take place, *except*:**
   a. Increase in minute ventilation
   b. Increase in the sensitivity of central chemoreceptors
   c. Increase in the sensitivity of carotid body to hypoxia
   d. Shift in the ODC to the left

10. **Pathological changes in Caisson disease are due to:**
    a. N_2 b. O_2
    c. CO_2 d. CO

11. **Decompression sickness is due to:**
    a. Increased partial pressure of N_2 in the alveolar air
    b. Bubbling of CO_2 in tissues and blood
    c. Bubbling of N_2 in tissues and blood
    d. Decreased partial pressure of O_2 in the inspired air

12. Earliest change at high altitude is:
    a. Hyperventilation
    b. Decrease in work capacity
    c. Drowsiness
    d. Polycythemia
13. When the atmospheric pressure is halved, which of the following is NOT likely to develop?
    a. An increase in pulmonary ventilation
    b. A fall in arterial PO_2
    c. A rise in arterial pH
    d. A rise in cerebral blood flow
14. Which of the following does not occur in high altitude acclimatization?
    a. Reticulocytosis
    b. Increased serum erythropoietin
    c. Increased serum cortisol
    d. Increased blood glucose
15. Which of the following is seen at high altitude?
    a. Respiratory alkalosis   b. Metabolic alkalosis
    c. Respiratory acidosis   d. Metabolic acidosis
16. A person who ascends to 12,000 feet develops acute breathlessness due to:
    a. Increased pulmonary blood flow
    b. Carbon dioxide wash out
    c. Decreased hypoxic stimulation of respiration
    d. Mechanical interference of thorax
17. Dysbarism is caused by:
    a. Escape of nitrogen from solution in blood and fatty tissues
    b. Liberation of CO_2 from myelin sheath during sudden decompression
    c. Development of acute hypoxia
    d. Collapse of alveoli
18. Decompression sickness occurs in:
    a. Diver
    b. Pilot
    c. Diver and pilot
    d. Mountaineer and astronaut
19. All the following are seen in high altitude climbers, *except*:
    a. Hyperventilation
    b. Pulmonary edema
    c. Decreased $PaCO_2$
    d. Bradycardia
20. Compensatory mechanism involved in acclimatization to high altitude:
    a. Hypoventilation   b. Respiratory alkalosis
    c. Respiratory acidosis d. Respiratory depression
21. Causes for high pressure nervous syndrome includes all the following, *except*:
    a. Rapid descent
    b. Very high pressure
    c. O_2 toxicity
    d. Descent to more than 500 feet
22. Fatal dose of radiation is:
    a. 1 rad   b. 5 rad
    c. 50 rad   d. 500 rad
23. Which of the following has maximum ionizing power?
    a. Alpha-rays   b. Beta-rays
    c. Ultraviolet-rays d. Infrared-rays
24. Which among the following has maximum ionizing power?
    a. Neutron   b. Proton
    c. X-rays   d. Alpha-rays
25. Radioactivity was discovered by:
    a. Madam Curie   b. Pierre Curie
    c. Roentgen   d. Henri Becquerel
26. X-rays were discovered by:
    a. Madam Curie   b. Pierre Curie
    c. Roentgen   d. Henry Becquerel
27. The major cause of death in radiation poisoning is:
    a. Septicemia
    b. Hemorrhage
    c. Coronary artery disease
    d. Hypothermia
28. Which of the following is most sensitive to radiation?
    a. Stem cell   b. Skin
    c. Lymphocyte   d. Bone

ANSWERS

1. c	2. b	3. d	4. b	5. c
6. a	7. d	8. a	9. d	10. a
11. c	12. a	13. d	14. d	15. a
16. b	17. a	18. c	19. d	20. b
21. c	22. d	23. a	24. d	25. d
26. c	27. a	28. a		

Respiratory Adjustments in Exercise

CHAPTER 41

LEARNING OBJECTIVES
- Discuss the cardiorespiratory and metabolic adjustments in exercise and compare it with that of the resting state
- Explain the effects of physical training
- iscuss oxygen debt and its causes

INTRODUCTION

PY11.4: Describe and discuss cardiorespiratory and metabolic adjustments during exercise; physical training effects (Cardiovascular adjustments in exercise are given in Chapter 30).

Many cardiorespiratory adjustments must operate in an integrated manner in exercise. The exercising muscles require extra O_2. Excess CO_2 and heat liberated in the muscle should be removed. There is increase in muscle blood flow and increased extraction of O_2 by the muscles. Increase in ventilation provides extra O_2 and eliminates heat and excess CO_2.

There are three types of exercise based on the amount of O_2 utilized, change in pulse rate and the work done:
1. Mild exercise
2. Moderate exercise
3. Severe exercise

In **mild exercise**, no cardiorespiratory adjustments are needed, e.g., slow walking.

Moderate exercise is less severe and can be continued for a long time, e.g., steady running.

Severe exercise can be kept up only for a short time and maximum cardiorespiratory adjustments occur in this type of exercise. The person will be totally exhausted at the end of exercise, e.g., fast running, heavy weight lifting, etc.

Need for Exercise
- To make body fit
- Psychological satisfaction
- Competitions

Effects of Exercise

The active tissues need extra O_2, and excess CO_2 and heat are liberated during exercise. Circulatory adjustments increase muscle blood flow and there is increased extraction of O_2 by the muscles and more of CO_2 enters the blood. In exercise, cardiac output increases from 5 L/min to as much as 20–35 L/min. Respiratory adjustments provides extra O_2 and eliminate more CO_2 and some of the heat.

Changes in Ventilation

There is an abrupt increase in ventilation with the onset of exercise followed by a brief pause, and then there is a gradual increase in ventilation (**Fig. 41.1**). The increase in ventilation is proportionate to the increase in O_2 consumption and CO_2 output. The O_2 consumption increases from 250 mL/min to as high as 4000 mL/min. For 1 L of O_2 to be consumed, ventilation should be increased to 25 L/min. CO_2 output increases from 200 mL/min to as much as 8000 mL/min.

Since CO_2 output is more, respiratory quotient comes to 1.5–1.7.

In moderate exercise, there is an increase in the depth of breathing. In severe exercise, there is an increase in the depth as well as rate of respiration.

The abrupt increase in ventilation at the start of exercise is due to psychic stimuli and afferent impulses from proprioceptors of muscles, tendons and joints going to the respiratory center causing an increase in ventilation.

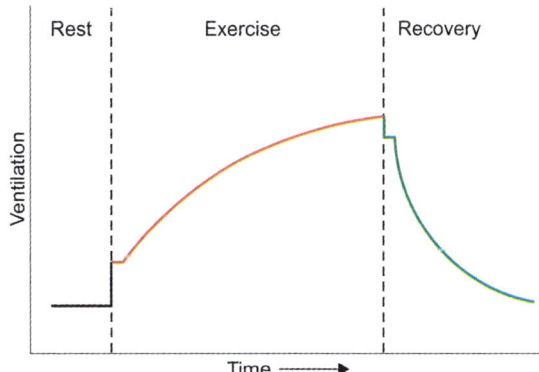

Fig. 41.1: Changes in ventilation in exercise.

Gradual increase in ventilation is due to:
- Increase in PCO_2 due to increased metabolism and increased sensitivity of respiratory center to CO_2.
- Decreased PO_2 due to increased O_2 utilization and stimulation of peripheral chemoreceptors (PCR).
- Decreased pH due to increased production of lactic acid through anaerobic metabolism.
- Increase in body temperature.
- Increased plasma K^+ which stimulates PCR.
- Increased sympathetic stimulation leading to increased secretion of catecholamines. It produces vasoconstriction and stimulation of PCR leading to increase in ventilation.
- Irradiation of impulses from the motor cortex or hypothalamus to respiratory center.

Changes in Diffusion

Cardiac output is increased in exercise. The pulmonary blood flow increases from 5 L/min to 25 L/min. Thus, pulmonary vascularity is increased. Pulmonary vascular system can act as blood reservoir without much change in pressure. Only 1/3rd of pulmonary vasculature is open at rest. The remaining 2/3rd is opened during exercise. This is known as **recruitment of closed capillaries**.

There is also stretching of respiratory membrane due to increase in ventilation. So, the thickness of the respiratory membrane is decreased and surface area is increased, which favors diffusion of gases.

In exercising muscle, more O_2 is utilized and hence mixed venous blood coming from muscles contains only 3–7 mL of O_2/100 mL of blood (normally it is 15 mL/100 mL of blood). Thus the alveolo-capillary gradient for O_2 becomes very high. The PO_2 of blood in pulmonary capillaries fall from 40 mm Hg to 25 mm Hg. So, more O_2 enters the blood from lungs.

Due to vasodilation and increased cardiac output, there is increased vascularity at tissue level and more O_2 is extracted by the tissues. Vascularity at the tissue level is increased due to increase in cardiac output and opening up of closed capillaries. Blood flow is slow due to vasodilation and so, there is more time for diffusion of gases. Vasodilation is due to the effect of metabolites produced during exercise on blood vessels.

The ODC is shifted to the right due to hypercapnia, hypoxia, acidosis, increase in temperature and increase in 2,3-DPG.

Changes in Metabolism

Carbohydrate Metabolism
- Aerobic glycolysis
- Anaerobic glycolysis

Glucose in the blood stream enters cells where it is degraded through a series of chemical reactions to pyruvate. When adequate O_2 is present, pyruvate enters the **citric acid cycle** and is metabolized to CO_2 and H_2O. This process is called **aerobic glycolysis**.

$$\text{Glucose} + 2\text{ ATP} \xrightarrow{O_2} 6CO_2 + 6H_2O + 40 \text{ ATP}$$
$$(C_6H_{12}O_6)$$

If O_2 supply is insufficient, the pyruvate formed from glucose is reduced to lactate. It does not require the presence of O_2. This process is called **anaerobic glycolysis**.

In severe exercise, aerobic glycolysis alone is not sufficient to provide energy. So, anaerobic glycolysis occurs where pyruvic acid is converted to lactic acid. Lactic acid enters the blood and decreases pH. The enzymes are inactivated when there is severe acidosis and so anaerobic glycolysis can continue only for a short time.

The maximum metabolic rate reached during exercise is often said to be 10 times the basal metabolic rate (BMR). Normal BMR is 2000 kcal/day. Trained athletes can increase their metabolic rate as much as 20 fold. During severe exercise, metabolic rate of muscles rises to as much as 100 fold.

VO_2 Max (Maximal O_2 Consumption)

VO_2 max is the rate of O_2 usage under maximal aerobic metabolism.

Normal value:
- In males—38–45 mL/kg body weight/min
- In females—29–30 mL/kg body weight/min

VO_2 max can be increased by constant training. VO_2 max is the product of maximal cardiac output and maximal O_2 extraction by tissues. Both these increase with training. In trained athletes, VO_2 max comes to about 75–80 mL/kg/min. It is used as an index to test a sportsman's endurance. VO_2 max detects the ability of cardiorespiratory and muscular system for adjustments in exercise.

Recovery Phase of Exercise

When exercise is stopped, there is an abrupt decrease in ventilation followed by a pause and then a gradual decline to pre-exercise levels.

O_2 Debt

O_2 debt is the extra amount of O_2 consumed during the recovery period of exercise in excess of the resting O_2 consumption. The increase in ventilation continues for as long as 90 min after exercise, i.e., until O_2 debt is repaid. This increase in ventilation is due to lactic acidosis which decreases pH. It is not due to increased PCO_2 or hypoxia because PCO_2 and PO_2 are normal at the stoppage of exercise.

Calculation of O_2 debt: Find out the resting O_2 consumption for 30 min; let it be A. Then find out post-exercise period O_2 consumption; let it be B.

$$O_2 \text{ debt} = B - A.$$

O_2 debt is needed to:
- Resynthesize the high-energy phosphate compounds utilized during exercise, like ATP and phosphoryl creatine.
- Remove or wash off the metabolites, especially lactic acid. 80% of lactic acid is converted to glycogen, and 20% is metabolized to CO_2 and H_2O during recovery period.
- Replace O_2 that has come from myoglobin.

During recovery, respiratory quotient (RQ) falls to 0.5 because O_2 debt is being repaid and more O_2 is being consumed.

Changes in trained athletes:
- O_2 debt falls.
- VO_2 max increases to 70–80 mL/kg/min from 45 mL/kg/min.
- When lactate level is 70 mg/100 mL of blood, the person stops exercise. This is the **breaking point in exercise**. Breaking point can be increased to 110 mg/100 mL of blood by training.
  Normal blood lactate level is 20 mg/100 mL of blood at rest.
- Hypertrophy of left ventricle and skeletal muscles.
- Bradycardia due to increased vagal tone.

FATIGUE

Fatigue is subjective sensation of heaviness or hardness of work. It depends on the amount of work done and the amount of O_2 consumed.

Causes of Fatigue
- Lactic acidosis.
- Cerebral hypoxia.
- Depletion of muscle glycogen.
- Pain in the muscles due to stimulation of pain nerve endings in muscles by P factor produced in exercising muscles, especially in sustained contraction. Intermittent contractions wash off the P factor.
- Dyspnea and the uncomfortable sensations produced by activation of J receptors in the lungs.
- Heaviness of muscles due to accumulation of interstitial fluid leads to fatigue.

MULTIPLE CHOICE QUESTIONS

1. **Oxygen debt refers to the extra amount of oxygen consumed:**
   a. At the beginning of exercise
   b. During muscular exercise
   c. After exercise is over
   d. At the thought of exercise

2. **The abrupt increase in ventilation that occurs at the onset of exercise is due to:**
   a. Rise in CO_2 tension
   b. Rise in body temperature
   c. Impulses from proprioceptors
   d. Rise in H⁺ concentration in blood

3. **Increased oxygen supply to muscle during exercise is due to:**
   a. Shift to left of oxygen dissociation curve
   b. Rise in pH of blood
   c. Increase in oxygen tension gradient between muscle and blood
   d. Decrease in 2,3 BPG concentration in blood

4. **In strenuous exercise PO_2 in venous blood falls from:**
   a. 40 to 15 mm Hg   b. 60 to 35 mm Hg
   c. 20 to 10 mm Hg   d. 35 to 0 mm Hg

5. **In moderate exercise, stimulation of respiration is due to:**
   a. Stimulation of J-receptor
   b. Stimulation of lung receptor
   c. Joint proprioception receptor
   d. Stimulation of medullary center

6. **VO_2 max in trained athletes:**
   a. 40–45 mL/kg/min
   b. 70–80 mL/kg/min
   c. 20–30 mL/kg/min
   d. 90–95 mL/kg/min

7. **Causes of fatigue in exercise is due to the following, *except*:**
   a. Lactic acidosis
   b. Stimulation of proprioceptors
   c. Cerebral hypoxia
   d. Accumulation of interstitial fluid in muscle

8. **Normal breaking point in exercise is:**
   a. 120 mg/100 mL of lactate
   b. 50 mg/100 mL of lactate
   c. 60 mg/100 mL of lactate
   d. 70 mg/100 mL of lactate

9. **Breaking point in exercise in trained athletes:**
   a. 110 mg/100 mL of lactate
   b. 90 mg/100 mL of lactate
   c. 70 mg/100 mL of lactate
   d. 80 mg/100 mL of lactate

10. **Normal BMR is:**
    a. 20,000 kcal/day   b. 2000 kcal/day
    c. 200 kcal/day   d. 1000 kcal/day

11. **In severe exercise, CO_2 output increases from 200 mL/min to:**
    a. 8000 mL/min.   b. 4000 mL/min
    c. 5000 mL/min   d. 3000 mL/min

ANSWERS

1. c 2. c 3. c 4. a 5. c
6. b 7. b 8. d 9. a 10. b
11. a

Artificial Respiration and Cardiopulmonary Resuscitation

CHAPTER 42

LEARNING OBJECTIVES
Must know
- Describe the principles of artificial respiration
- Explain the technique of mouth to mouth resuscitation

Desirable to know
- Describe the methods of cardiopulmonary resuscitation

INTRODUCTION

> **PY6.5:** Describe and discuss the principles of artificial respiration, oxygen therapy, acclimatization and decompression sickness.

Respiratory arrest may occur as a result of drowning, suffocation, electrocution, myocardial infarction, etc. Vital organs like brain and heart should be supplied with oxygen within 2–3 minutes. Otherwise respiratory arrest leads to death. So artificial respiration should be given as a life-saving measure. In an emergency, outside the hospital, manual methods of artificial respiration prove valuable. In the meantime, the patient can be shifted to a hospital where ventilators are available especially when artificial respiration has to be maintained for a long time.

Indications for Artificial Respiration
- In conditions of sudden cessation of breathing as in:
  - Drowning
  - Carbon monoxide poisoning
  - Electric shock
  - Anesthetic accidents
  - Severe myocardial infarction
- In cases of gradually progressing respiratory failure due to paralysis of respiratory muscles, e.g., poliomyelitis, diphtheria, etc.

In any method of artificial respiration, **promptness** in starting treatment is of first importance. Cells of heart and brain are very susceptible to O_2 lack. If the blood is not oxygenated, within minutes, heart will stop beating and irreversible damage occurs to the brain. *Prompt, proper and prolonged application of artificial respiration may save a life.*

In all methods of artificial respiration, it should be ensured that the airway is free. Clean the mouth and pull out the tongue. When a person is unconscious there is a tendency for the tongue to fall back causing obstruction to the airway. Clothes should be loosened. If the person is in a state of severe shock, he should be kept warm if possible. He can be covered with a blanket.

Methods of Artificial Respiration
- Manual method (done by hand)
- Mechanical method (done by machines).

Manual Methods
- Mouth-to-mouth method
- Holger-Nielsen method
- Schafer method
- Silvester method
- Eve's rocking method.

Mouth-to-mouth method: Mouth-to-mouth method is **superior** to all other methods. It is reported to be *the only manual method capable of producing adequate ventilation.*

The patient is placed in the supine position with the neck extended and jaw elevated. The rescuer should place one hand behind the neck of the subject. This will eliminate the obstruction of the airway due to falling back of tongue. The rescuer takes a deep inspiration and places his mouth over the subject's mouth and expires into the subject's mouth. While doing this, the nostrils of the subject should be closed. *Expiration should be forceful so that it consists of two times the tidal volume.* Thus, the subject's lungs are inflated and the expansion of the chest can be seen. The rescuer then removes his mouth from that of the subject to allow the subject to expire passively by elastic recoil of lung. The procedure is repeated about 12–20 times per minute. *If the subject is a small baby, the rescuer should only blow a* **mouthful** *of air into the mouth of the baby.* If he does a forceful expiration, the lungs of the baby would burst.

If the patient is in the hospital then the effectiveness and ease of performance of this type of resuscitation can be improved by using an anesthesia mask or an oropharyngeal airway or an endotracheal tube.

Holger-Nielsen method (arm lift–back pressure method): Clean the mouth and pull out the tongue. The victim is placed in prone position, i.e., on his abdomen. His arms are folded and kept at right angles to the trunk and face is turned sideways with the cheek resting on his hands. The operator kneels in front of him near the head. Then he places his hands spread out on the victim's back and sways forwards applying pressure over the back by putting his weight on his hands. The elbows should be straight. This movement compresses the chest and causes expiration.

Then the rescuer holds the victim's arms above the elbows and draws them forwards. Raise the arms until slight tension is felt. Then draw the arms slightly towards the operator. This position causes expansion of chest and inspiration takes place. The operator then swings forward again and repeats first phase. This **double movement** is repeated 12 times/minute.

Schafer's method: The victim is laid in the prone position and the operator kneels at his side at about the level of his hips. Then he places his hands flat on the loin with the thumb nearly touching and parallel to the spine and fingers spread out on each side of the body over the lower ribs.

The operator leans forward over the victim keeping his arm straight. Thus the operator throws the weight of his body over the victim and applies pressure over the abdomen and lower part of the chest. This movement drives out air from the lungs causing expiration. After 2 sec, the operator releases the pressure by swinging his body backwards without lifting his hands. The technique is repeated about 12 times per minute.

Mechanical Method

Drinker's method: Drinker's method involves the use of an air-tight tank called **Tank respirator** or Drinker's respirator **(Fig. 42.1)** into which the patient is placed with head outside. Alternate negative and positive pressures are obtained in the tank by means of electrically driven pump and the effect is to produce movements of the chest wall resembling those of normal inspiration and expiration. The negative pressure pulls on chest wall and causes inspiration. The positive pressure compresses the chest and produces expiration. This method is used for patients with paralysis of respiratory muscles like poliomyelitis or in patients with severe respiratory failure where artificial respiration has to be continued for long periods.

Now, **ventilators** are used from which pulses of air or mixtures of respiratory gases are delivered after intubating the patient.

CARDIOPULMONARY RESUSCITATION

PY11.14: Demonstrate basic life support in a simulated environment.

Cardiopulmonary resuscitation is performed in patients whose hearts have stopped beating or are fibrillating and breathing has also stopped immediately. Causes are myocardial infarction, electrocution (including lightning), drowning, etc. Palpate the carotid pulse for at least 10 seconds not to miss weak pulses. Then if the heart is not beating, give external cardiac massage.

Technique

The rescuer places the heel of one hand on the lower sternum of the subject about 3 cm above the xiphoid process and the heel of the other hand on top of the first. Pressure is applied straight down, depressing the sternum 4–5 cm towards the spine. The procedure is repeated 80–100 times/min. Someone else should assess the adequacy of compression by palpating the carotid pulse.

At the same time mouth-to-mouth breathing should also be performed at a rate of one ventilation to five chest compressions (ratio 1:5). Thus cardiac output and perfusion of coronaries can be maintained by closed-chest cardiac massage. Artificial respiration maintains PO_2 of arterial blood adequate.

Ventricular fibrillation can be stopped and converted to normal sinus rhythm by means of electric shocks using electronic defibrillators. They should be used as rapidly as possible. It is a major determinant of survival in cardiac arrest due to ventricular fibrillation. In the meantime, cardiopulmonary resuscitation should be performed to maintain coronary perfusion and blood oxygen tension. At the same time, adrenaline and sodium bicarbonate can be administered intravenously. If possible, endotracheal intubation should be done as soon as possible to administer 100% oxygen. If the patient can be revived, the underlying cause should be treated.

MULTIPLE CHOICE QUESTIONS

1. **The best method of artificial respiration for infants is:**
    a. Mouth-to-mouth breathing expiring twice the tidal volume

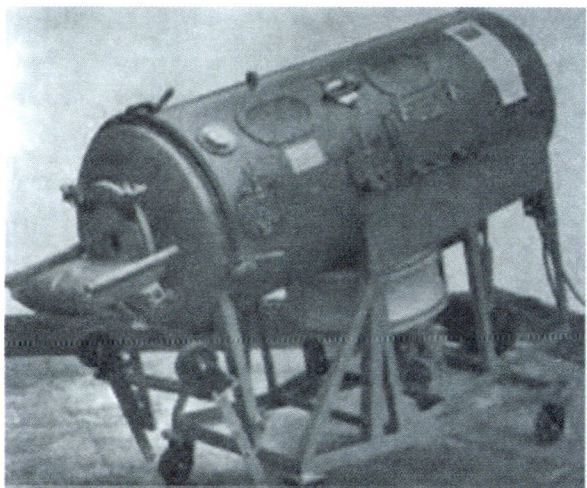

Fig. 42.1: Tank respirator.

    b. Mouth-to-mouth method expiring a mouthful of air
    c. Holger-Nielsen method
    d. Drinker's method

2. The fraction of inspired air in mouth-to-mouth respiration is:
    a. 0.16
    b. 0.19
    c. 0.21
    d. 0.26

3. Mouth-to-mouth respiration provides an O_2 concentration of:
    a. 16%
    b. 20%
    c. 22%
    d. 24%

ANSWERS

1. b   2. a   3. a

Pulmonary Function Tests

CHAPTER 43

LEARNING OBJECTIVE
- Describe the principles of artificial respiration

■ INTRODUCTION

PY6.7: Describe and discuss lung function tests and their clinical significance.

Pulmonary function tests (PFTs) are noninvasive tests to assess the functioning of the lungs. The tests measure lung volumes, capacities, rate of airflow and gas exchange. It also helps to differentiate between obstructive and restrictive lung diseases. Normal PFT values vary from person to person. So the result is compared with the average of normal persons of the same age, height, sex, etc. PFT is also done routinely in healthy individuals as part of routine physical examination.

Uses of PFT

- Helps in the objective assessment of lung performance.
- Helps in the diagnosis of respiratory diseases in patients complaining of breathlessness.
- Helps to assess the progress of a respiratory disease.
- Useful for monitoring the efficiency of treatment.
- Helps to evaluate the respiratory fitness before general anesthesia and surgery, especially in cases of thoracic surgery with lung resection.

Classification of PFT

- Tests to assess ventilation
- Ventilation and perfusion
- Diffusion
- Pulmonary blood flow and pulmonary pressure
- Miscellaneous tests.

Tests to Assess Ventilation

- Lung volumes and capacities
- **Tests for mechanical factors:**
  - Timed vital capacity (TVC)
  - Maximum voluntary ventilation (MVV)
  - Maximum mid expiratory flow rate (MMEFR)
  - Peak expiratory flow rate (PEFR)
  - Closing volume.

Tests to Assess Distribution of Ventilation and Perfusion

- N_2 wash out method
- Radioisotope imaging.

Albumin labeled with **technetium-99** is given intravenously and gamma camera pictures are taken. This helps to diagnose pulmonary embolism. Distribution of ventilation can be studied by inhalation of radioactive gas **krypton-81**.

Tests to Assess Diffusion

- Diffusing capacity of O_2 is measured using carbon monoxide as marker gas. Diffusing capacity of CO multiplied by 1.23 gives the diffusing capacity of O_2. It is reduced in pulmonary fibrosis, sarcoidosis, etc.
- Determination of PO_2, PCO_2 and pH of blood by arterial blood sampling. $PaCO_2$ (partial pressure of CO_2 in arterial blood) is directly related to the level of alveolar ventilation. Normal $PaCO_2$ is 35–45 mm Hg. $PaCO_2$ is increased when alveolar ventilation is reduced as in chronic obstructive pulmonary disease (COPD), emphysema, sedative drug overdose, etc. In this case, there will also be a reduction in PaO_2 and pH.
  Decrease in $PaCO_2$ is seen when there is increased alveolar ventilation as in metabolic acidosis, anxiety, etc.
- Ventilation-perfusion ratio.

Tests to Assess Perfusion and Pulmonary Pressure

Pulmonary blood flow is determined by applying Fick's principle. Using a special catheter, pulmonary artery pressure can be measured directly.

Miscellaneous Tests

- **Plain X-ray chest:** PA view and lateral view help to diagnose pleural effusion, pneumothorax, pneumonia, sarcoidosis, etc.
- CT scan helps to detect lung malignancy.
- Biopsies can be taken using fiberoptic bronchoscopy.
- Bronchography

- Ultrasound scan (USS) helps to detect pleural effusion and tumors.
- Magnetic resonance imaging (MRI)
- **Immunological tests:**
  - **Skin prick test** is done in patients with asthma who have type I hypersensitivity to certain allergens. IgE levels are often raised in patients with asthma.
  - **Manteaux test** to diagnose tuberculosis.
- VO_2 Max (maximal O_2 uptake): **VO_2** is the amount of O_2 a person consumes in 1 minute. It is normally 250 mL/min. **VO_2 max** is the maximal amount of O_2 consumed by a person during physical activity. In highly trained athletes, VO_2 max may be 3000 mL/min or even more than that. VO_2 max is decreased in emphysema, pulmonary edema and anemia. Determination of VO_2 max is now routinely done in sportsmen.

MULTIPLE CHOICE QUESTIONS

1. **Regarding pulmonary function test, all are true, except:**
   a. Total lung volume increases in emphysema
   b. Compliance decreases in interstitial lung disease
   c. Compliance is total lung distensibility
   d. FEV_1 is forced expiratory rate at one minute

2. **Destruction of lung tissue and defective gaseous exchange causes all, except:**
   a. Increase in red cell number
   b. Pulmonary hypertension
   c. Prominent P wave
   d. Decreased cerebral blood circulation

3. **Pulmonary hypertension in emphysema is:**
   a. Secondary to hypoxia
   b. Due to hypertrophy of right ventricle
   c. Due to mitral stenosis
   d. Due to polycythemia

ANSWERS

1. d   2. d   3. a

FILL IN THE BLANKS/GIVE THE NORMAL VALUE/NAME THE FOLLOWING

1. About **70%** of CO_2 is transported in the form of bicarbonate ions from tissues to lungs.
2. Percentage of CO_2 transported in blood in the dissolved form: **7%**.
3. Hematocrit of venous blood is 3% greater than that of arterial blood due to **chloride and water shift**.
4. pH of venous blood: **7.36**.
5. pH of arterial blood is: **7.4**.
6. Hemoglobin can bind **4 molecules** of O_2.
7. Myoglobin can bind **one molecule** of O_2.
8. **P_{50}** is the PO_2 at which hemoglobin is half (50%) saturated with O_2.
9. Normal P50: **25 mm Hg**.
10. 2,3 DPG is found in **red blood cells**.
11. Normal 2,3 DPG level: **15 µmol/g of hemoglobin**.
12. Fetal blood and stored blood have high affinity for O_2 because of low **2,3 DPG**.
13. Physiological dead space is the sum of **anatomical dead space** and **alveolar dead space**.
14. Under-perfused and over-ventilated alveoli contribute to **alveolar dead space**.
15. Physiological dead space can be measured by **Bohr's method** and anatomical dead space by **Fowler's method**.
16. PO_2 of arterial blood: **100 mm Hg**.
17. PO_2 of mixed venous blood: **40 mm Hg**.
18. O_2 content of arterial blood: **19 mL/dL**.
19. Oxygen content of venous blood: **14 mL/dL**.
20. Percentage saturation of hemoglobin of arterial **blood: 97%**.
21. Percentage saturation of venous blood: **75%**.
22. PO_2 of atmospheric air: **159 mm Hg**.
23. PO_2 of alveolar air: **104 mm Hg**.
24. PO_2 of tissue fluid: **40 mm Hg**.
25. PCO_2 of arterial blood: **40 mm Hg**.
26. PCO_2 of venous blood: **46 mm Hg**.
27. Diffusion of CO_2 from blood to alveoli is **4 mL**/100 mL of blood.
28. PCO_2 of alveoli: **40 mm Hg**.
29. Percentage of O_2 transported in combination with hemoglobin: **97%**.
30. Percentage of oxygen transported in dissolved state: **3%**.
31. One gram of hemoglobin combines with **1.34 mL** of O_2.
32. One gram of hemoglobin contains **3.34 mg** of iron in it.
33. Arterial blood contains **19.8 mL** of O_2/dL.
34. Venous blood contains **15.2 mL** of O_2/dL.
35. Normal respiratory quotient: **0.8**.
36. The amount of air present in the lungs after maximal expiration - **residual volume** (1.2 L).
37. Spirometry cannot be used to measure **total lung capacity, residual volume** and **functional residual capacity**.
38. Respiratory minute volume at rest: **6L/min**.
39. Alveolar ventilation: **4.2 L/min**.
40. Maximal voluntary ventilation: **125–170 L/min**.
41. Normal—TVC 1% or FEV 1%: **83%**.
42. Work of breathing at rest: **0.5 kg-m/min**.
43. **Compliance** is change in lung volume per unit change in airway pressure (V/P).
44. A condition where there is increase in lung compliance: **emphysema**
45. Obstruction to small airways is best measured by **maximal mid expiratory flow rate** (25–75% of vital capacity).
46. The major site of increased resistance to airflow during expiration in COPD is airways less than **2 mm** in diameter.
47. Normal intrapleural pressure at the end of normal expiration is **2.5 mm Hg**.

48. Normal intrapulmonary pressure at the end of normal expiration is **0 mm Hg (equal to atmospheric pressure)**.
49. The ratio of pulmonary ventilation to pulmonary blood flow is **ventilation perfusion ratio**.
50. Apex of the lung is more prone for pulmonary tuberculosis because of the **high ventilation-perfusion ratio** at the apex.
51. Reduction in PO_2 of arterial blood is the most potent stimulant for the **peripheral chemoreceptors** to stimulate respiration.
52. In anemia and CO poisoning, since arterial PO_2 is normal **peripheral chemoreceptors** are not stimulated.
53. CO has **210** times more affinity for hemoglobin than O_2.
54. **Cyanosis** is bluish discoloration of skin and mucous membrane due to increased quantity of reduced hemoglobin in blood (it should be more than 5 g/dL).
55. **Cyanosis** is not seen in severe anemia since the total concentration of hemoglobin is reduced.
56. **Hippocampus** in brain is most vulnerable to hypoxic ischemia.
57. **Kussmal's respiration** is rapid and deep breathing seen in diabetic ketoacidosis and uremia.
58. Periodic breathing in which respiration is regularly irregular: **Cheyne-Stokes respiration**.
59. Periodic breathing in which breathing is irregularly irregular: **Biot's breathing**.
60. Increased PCO_2 of blood is referred to as **hypercapnia**.
61. **Hyperventilation** leads to hypocapnia and respiratory alkalosis.
62. The center for automatic control of respiration is located in the **medulla oblongata** and **pons**.
63. The pacemaker cells responsible for rhythmic discharges are in the **pre-Botzinger complex** in medulla.
64. Central chemoreceptors are located in the **medulla**.
65. Peripheral chemoreceptors are located in the **carotid body** and **aortic bodies**.
66. Blood flow to peripheral chemoreceptors: **2000 mL/100 g of tissue/min**.
67. Surfactant is secreted by **type II alveolar pneumocytes**.
68. The main component of surfactant: **dipalmitoylphosphatidylcholine**
69. Surfactant deficiency in premature infants results in **infant respiratory distress syndrome**.
70. Surfactant in the lungs of fetus begins to be secreted at **28 weeks**.
71. Acute mountain sickness is characterized by **pulmonary edema** and **cerebral edema**.
72. The condition that occurs when a person returns rapidly to normal atmospheric pressure after exposure to high barometric pressure is known as **caisson disease or bends or diver's paralysis**.
73. The most effective method of artificial respiration outside a hospital is **mouth to mouth method**.
74. Types of hypoxia: **hypoxic hypoxia, anemic hypoxia, stagnant hypoxia and histotoxic hypoxia**.
75. O_2 administration is of greatest value in **hypoxic hypoxia** and least for **histotoxic hypoxia**.
76. The first change at high altitude in response to hypoxia is hyperventilation.
77. J receptors in the lungs are situated in the alveolar interstitium close to the pulmonary capillaries.
78. Name two hypoxic conditions where arterial O_2 tension remains unaltered: **anemia and CO poisoning**
79. The most common complication of hyperbaric O_2 therapy: **oxygen toxicity**.
80. Tissue hypoxia without alteration in the O_2 content in blood occurs in **cyanide poisoning**.
81. Binding of one molecule of O_2 to hemoglobin increasing the affinity of hemoglobin for the next O_2 molecule is known as **heme-heme interaction**.
82. Percentage of O_2 in the atmospheric air: **20%**
83. The amount of air present in the lung after forceful inspiration: **total lung capacity**.
84. The lung volume that cannot be measured using routine spirometry: **residual volume**

CLINICAL CASE SCENARIO

1. **A 50-year-old man was brought to the casualty with difficulty in breathing and restlessness. He gave a past history of similar episodes several times. On examination:**
   Severely dyspneic
   Auscultation of chest revealed rhonchi and crepitations
   Tongue, lips and nail bed showed cyanosis
   Heart rate – 110/min
   Arterial gas analysis – Po_2 – 55 mm Hg; Pco_2 – 41 mm Hg
   FEV_1% - 50%
   1. What is the probable condition?
   2. Describe the mechanisms of CO_2 transport in the body
   3. Explain timed vital capacity and its significance
   4. Give the normal Po_2 and Pco_2 of arterial blood. Why there is no significant increase in Pco_2 in the above case?

   Ans:
   1. Bronchial asthma/obstructive airway disease

SECTION 5 GASTROINTESTINAL SYSTEM

Introduction to Digestive System

CHAPTER 44

LEARNING OBJECTIVES
- Describe the structure and functions of the digestive system
- Explain enteric nervous system
- Explain the mechanism of secretion from the cells of the digestive glands
- Describe the gut-brain axis

INTRODUCTION

PY4.1: Describe the structure and functions of digestive system.

The food we consume is mainly in the form of macromolecules and these have to be digested to their component monomers. The gastrointestinal system helps in nutrient acquisition and assimilation into the body. The nutrients and water are absorbed in a controlled manner across a single layer of columnar epithelial cells lining the gastrointestinal tract. Gastrointestinal functions are regulated in an integrated manner by the endocrine, paracrine and neurocrine mechanisms. The peculiarities of gastrointestinal system are:
- It is functionally continuous with the external environment
- It has a well-developed immune system
- The intestinal circulation is unique in that the major portion of its venous outflow does not return directly to the heart, but reaches the liver via the portal vein.

The gastrointestinal system (GIS) consists of the alimentary canal which is a continuous tube that extends from mouth to anus and the associated glands that empty their contents into the alimentary canal like salivary glands, liver and pancreas **(Fig. 44.1)**. The gastrointestinal tract or the alimentary canal consists of a series of hollow organs which are separated from each other by specialized sphincters. The sphincters include upper and lower esophageal sphincters, the pyloric sphincter, ileocecal valve, and the inner and outer anal sphincters.

The mouth and oropharynx help in grinding, lubricating, initiating carbohydrate and fat digestion and propelling food into the esophagus. Esophagus conducts food to the stomach. Stomach temporarily stores food and initiates digestion. The small intestine (duodenum, jejunum and ileum) completes digestion and is the primary site of absorption. The large intestine (cecum and colon) also absorbs electrolytes and water and stores fecal matter before expulsion from the body. The meal is mixed with the secretions produced by the

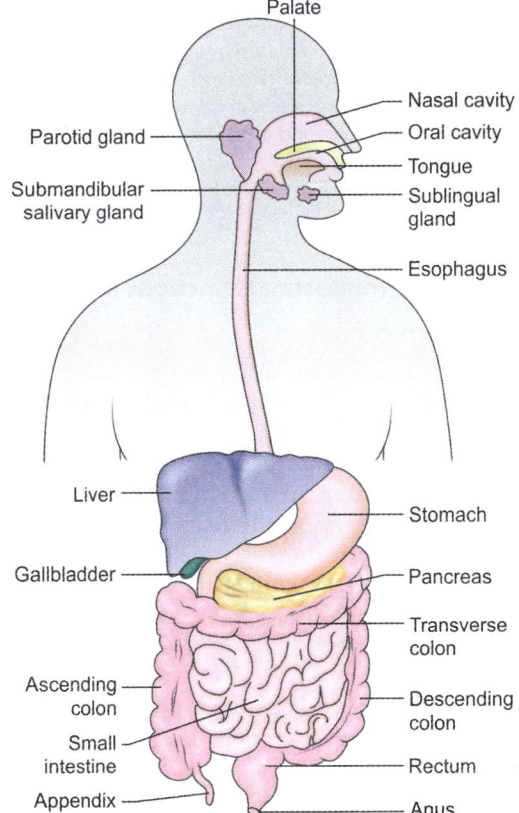

Fig. 44.1: Parts of the gastrointestinal system.

gastrointestinal tract as well as by the associated glands that drain into it for proper digestion.

FUNCTIONS OF GASTROINTESTINAL SYSTEM

- Nutritive function
- Endocrine function
- Role in immunity

The functions of GIS are to take in nutrients and water into the body and to eliminate wastes by the processes of **motility, secretion, digestion, absorption and excretion**. These processes can occur only if there is proper regulation of the above functions by the control systems of the body, like endocrine, neural and paracrine systems.

Many hormones are produced by specialized cells of GIT called amine precursor uptake and decarboxylation (**APUD**) **cells**, e.g., gastrin produced by G cells of pyloric antrum, secretin and cholecystokinin secreted by specialized cells of duodenum, etc.

Gastrointestinal tract is an important part of body's immune system. Intestine has very well-developed innate and adaptive immune systems. There are more lymphocytes in the wall of the intestine than in the blood. Humoral antibodies secreted by the gut mucosa and the cellular immune system within the gut mucosa have an important role in protecting the body against microorganisms entering the gut, and foreign bodies which are antigenic. **IgA** of gut is resistant to digestion by intestinal enzymes.

> The absorptive surface of alimentary canal is not absolutely necessary for life. It can be replaced by intravenous administration of water, electrolytes and nutrients including vitamins and trace elements. Removal of pancreas can be tolerated with exogenous administration of insulin and pancreatic enzymes. *But, removal of liver is fatal because, its metabolic and excretory functions cannot be replaced.* Now liver can be transplanted with great success.

Control of Gastrointestinal Functions in General

Endocrine Control

In this control mechanism, a stimulus causes secretion of a hormone that travels through the blood stream to interact with a target tissue to cause a response. For example, fatty acids in the duodenum cause release of cholecystokinin (CCK), a hormone from the endocrine cells in the duodenal mucosa. CCK enters the blood stream and reaches pancreas where CCK receptors are present and causes secretion of pancreatic juice rich in fat-digesting enzymes. Endocrine cells secrete hormones from their basolateral surface into the adjacent capillary.

Neural Control

In the GIT, there are a variety of neural receptors that detect both chemical and mechanical stimuli. The information may be transmitted to the target tissue through nerves and may involve only the enteric nervous system (ENS). For example, peristalsis in the esophagus moves a bolus of food from pharynx to stomach. Here the reflex arc is localized to the GIT. In some other situations, the sensory information from the GIT may be processed in the central nervous system, e.g., vagovagal reflex.

Paracrine Control

The paracrine responses are those where the hormone or chemical signal released by a cell acts as a local mediator only on cells in its **immediate vicinity**. The action is confined to the vicinity of its release because the transmitter is rapidly degraded, taken up or diluted, e.g., histamine stimulated HCl secretion from the parietal cells in gastric mucosa. The histamine-containing cells are present in close proximity to the parietal cells. *The transmission of message is said to be paracrine when it is through the intercellular space.*

DIGESTION

Digestion is defined as the process of breaking down naturally occurring, highly complex foodstuffs which are chemically inert and less soluble in water into smaller units in the GIT, which can be easily absorbed by the intestinal mucosa. Food mixes with saliva during mastication and it passes through the pharynx and esophagus during deglutition and reaches the stomach, which acts as a temporary reservoir of food. First stage of digestion occurs in the stomach. Partially digested food enters small intestine where digestion is completed. Most of the essential nutrients are absorbed here and unwanted residue passes into the large intestine and is expelled out during defecation. Types of digestion are:
1. Mechanical digestion
2. Chemical digestion

Mechanical Digestion

It is carried out by muscular activity by which food is broken down to smaller units. It may be:
- Voluntary as in chewing
- Involuntary, as the contraction of stomach breaks down solid chunks of food into smaller pieces.

Chemical Digestion

- Food is mixed with digestive juices as it passes along the GIT and various enzymes act on the complex food converting it into simple absorbable units.
- Almost 8 L of digestive juices are secreted in man in 24 hours, but most of this is reabsorbed in the intestine.

Functional Anatomy of Alimentary Canal

Alimentary canal is a long tubular system extending from **mouth to anus** which measures about **9 m** in length (**Fig. 44.1**). Different parts of the GIT have different structures adapted for specific functions like passage of food (esophagus), storage of food (stomach), digestion and absorption (small intestine), storage and excretion of unwanted materials (large intestine).

General Structure and Histology of GIT

Organization of structure that makes the intestinal wall is same throughout the alimentary canal. The wall of the gut is made up of four layers (**Fig. 44.2**):
1. **Mucosa**
    - Epithelial lining
    - Lamina propria
    - Muscularis mucosa or muscularis interna
2. **Submucosa**
3. **Muscular layer or muscularis externa**

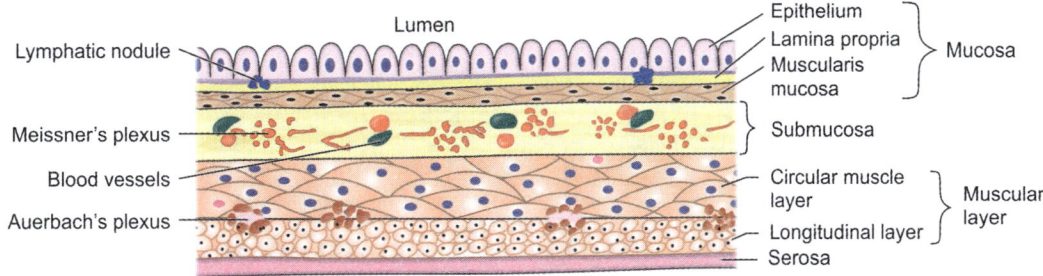

Fig. 44.2: Structure of gastrointestinal tract showing different layers; Mucosa is thrown into folds called villi in the small intestine (not shown in this figure).

- Inner circular layer
- Outer longitudinal layer
- In stomach, an additional oblique layer is seen

4. **Serosa or adventitia**

Mucosa

The mucosal surface of the GIT maintains the barrier between the host and the harmful pathogens, toxins and carcinogenic substances in the lumen. This is achieved by the intact mucosal surface and the extensive population of immune cells in the mucosa. Due to the presence of intense number of immune cells in the mucosa, the mucosa is vulnerable to numerous inflammatory conditions. The mucous membrane contains the gastrointestinal glands.

Epithelium

The **epithelium** of the mucosa is thrown into folds to increase surface area. Gastrointestinal epithelium is one of the most rapidly dividing tissues in the body. There is **rapid turnover** of the cells epithelial layer, and there is complete turnover of epithelium every 24–72 hours. This reduces the exposure time and thus decreases the risk of malignancy produced by mutagens present in the luminal contents. But, the disadvantage is that due to this high proliferative potential, neoplastic disorder is very common in the GIT. Function of the epithelial lining depends on the location. Major functions of the epithelium are:

- Protection
- Absorption
- Secretion

Lamina Propria and Muscularis Mucosa

Lamina propria contains loose connective tissue, numerous glands, lymphatics, small blood vessels and nerves. **Muscularis mucosa** is present from esophagus and it consists of a thin layer of smooth muscle fibers.

Submucosa

Submucosa contains connective tissue, blood vessels, lymphatics and nerve plexus called **Meissner's plexus**. *Glands are absent in submucosa except in the duodenum where Brunner's glands are present in the submucosa.*

Muscular Layer

The function of muscular layer is mixing and propulsion of food. It is made up of thick layer of smooth muscle fibers arranged in two layers, inner **circular layer** and outer **longitudinal layer**. In the stomach, an additional **oblique layer** of muscles is seen. When the circular layer of muscles in the gut contract the lumen of the intestine obliterate. At the areas of sphincters, the circular muscle fibers get thickened. The function of the muscular layer is mixing and propulsion of food. In between the circular and longitudinal layer of muscles lie the **myenteric plexus or Auerbach's plexus of nerves (Fig. 44.2)**.

Serosa

Serosa is the outermost layer formed by **visceral peritoneum**. Blood vessels, lymph vessels, etc., reach the gut through the mesentery which is continuous with the serosa. *The serosal layer is absent in the esophagus and the lower end of rectum, and incompletely encloses the duodenum.* Serosa is a binding and protective layer. It helps in the attachment of gut to the surrounding structures.

> The **muscles** of GIT are not fully constituted by smooth muscles or involuntary muscles. **Striated muscle** makes up the walls of the pharynx, proximal 1/3rd of esophagus and the external anal sphincter. These muscles are supplied by **somatic nerves** and are under voluntary control.

■ INNERVATION OF GUT

There are two sets of nerves in the GIT **(Figs. 44.3A to C)**:
1. Intrinsic or enteric nervous system
2. Extrinsic or autonomic nervous system (ANS)

Enteric Nervous System

The enteric nervous system (ENS) is a collection of nerve plexuses that surround the gastrointestinal tract. It lies entirely in the wall of the gut beginning in the esophagus and extending all the way to the anus. The system contains about 100 million sensory neurons, interneurons and motor neurons and is considered as a part of central nervous system (CNS) that is concerned with the regulation of gastrointestinal function. ENS receives input from the sympathetic and parasympathetic divisions of the autonomic nervous system (ANS) which modulates the activity of the ENS. ENS consists mainly of two plexuses:
1. Auerbach's or myenteric plexus
2. Meissner's or submucosal plexus

The **myenteric plexus** consists of a linear chain of interconnecting neurons that extends the entire length of

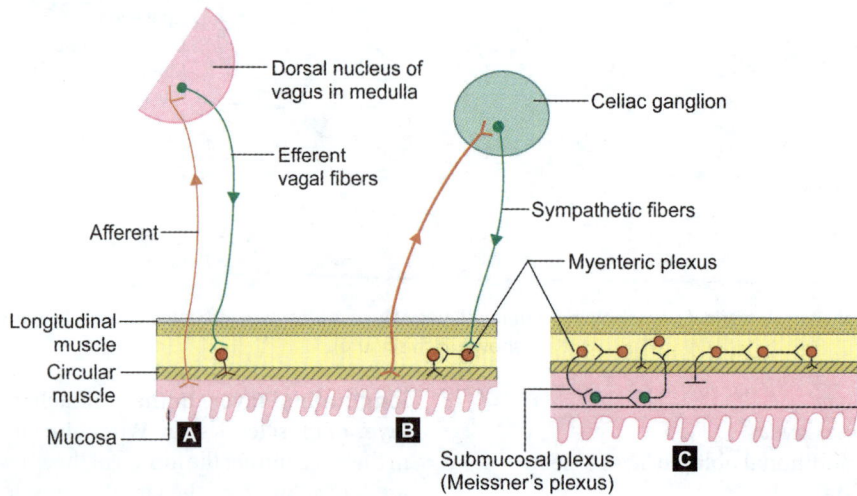

Figs. 44.3A to C: Innervation of gut: (A) Extrinsic innervation through vagus (long reflex); (B) Extrinsic innervation through sympathetic chain (short reflex); (C) Intrinsic or enteric nervous system (local reflex).

the GIT. Because this plexus extends all the way along the intestinal wall and since it *lies between the longitudinal and circular layers* of intestinal smooth muscle, it is concerned mainly with controlling muscle activity along the length of the gut. The **Meissner's plexus** lies in the submucosa and is mainly concerned with controlling functions within the inner wall of each minute segment of intestine.

These two plexuses are interconnected with each other **(Fig. 44.3A to C)**. ENS consists of both sensory and motor nerve fibers and associated ganglia which produce a **local reflex or short reflex**. The sensory receptors are **osmoreceptors, thermoreceptors, mechanoreceptors and chemoreceptors** present in the wall of the gut. Motor fibers supply the exocrine glands of the mucous membrane of GIT, muscular layer and gut endocrine cells called amine precursor uptake and decarboxylation (APUD) cells.

ENS is capable of functioning absolutely independently. ENS can function in the total absence of the extrinsic innervation. But, it is strongly influenced by the extrinsic nervous system. It is derived from the neural crest cells. ENS is referred to as the **brain of the gut** or the **little brain** because it can integrate sensory information and effect complex motor response independent of central nervous system (CNS). ENS is responsible for coordinating much of the secretory activity and motility of GIT through intrinsic pathways called **short loop reflexes or local reflexes (Fig. 44.4)**. In myenteric and Meissner's plexus, the axons branch profusely so that stimulation of one region of the gut produces a widespread response in the GIT.

The cell bodies of the intrinsic nerves of the gut lie in the ganglia of ENS. The substances secreted by the neurons in the ENS include **acetylcholine, norepinephrine, NO, CO,** **serotonin, GABA, VIP, substance P, CCK, somatostatin, neurotensin, leuenkephalin, metencephalin, gastrin releasing peptide, prostaglandin, ATP, dopamine, bombesin, etc.**

NO is a major mediator of smooth muscle relaxation in the GIT. Vasoactive intestinal polypeptide (VIP) containing neurons occur throughout alimentary canal, salivary glands and pancreas. Distension of gut results in release of VIP. VIP causes relaxation of smooth muscles in front of the peristaltic wave and relaxation of sphincters.

Some of the substances secreted by the neurons of ENS act as **synaptic transmitters**; others diffuse into the ECF and act in a **paracrine** manner and still others enter the bloodstream becoming **hormones**. Some of the neurons of myenteric plexus are excitatory and some are inhibitory **(Table 44.1)**.

In a congenital disease called **Hirschsprung's disease**, there is absence of ENS in parts of large intestine. Here, peristaltic movement of large intestine will be absent.

Functions of ENS

Auerbach's plexus or myenteric plexus innervates the longitudinal and circular smooth muscle fibers of gut and is mainly concerned with motor control. It is concerned with control of gastrointestinal movement, i.e., peristaltic activity.

Effects of Myenteric Plexus Stimulation

❖ Increase in the tone of gut wall.
❖ Increase in the intensity and rate of the rhythmical contractions.
❖ Increase in the velocity of conduction of excitatory waves along the gut wall.
❖ Increase in peristalsis.

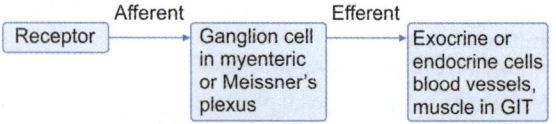

Fig. 44.4: Local enteric reflex.

Table 44.1: Neurotransmitters of myenteric plexus.	
Excitatory	**Inhibitory**
Acetylcholine	VIP, norepinephrine
Serotonin	Neurotensin
Substance P	Encephalin

- Relaxation of pyloric sphincter, ileocecal sphincter and internal anal sphincter. Some of the neurons of myenteric plexus are inhibitory. Their endings release an inhibitory transmitter, possibly vasoactive intestinal polypeptide which inhibits the intestinal sphincter muscles leading to their relaxation.

Meissner's plexus innervates glandular epithelium, intestinal endocrine cells and submucosal blood vessels. It is concerned with the control of secretion from both exocrine and endocrine glands of gut and regulation of local blood flow.

Extrinsic Innervation of Gut

Extrinsic innervation is from the autonomic nervous system (ANS), i.e., sympathetic and parasympathetic nervous system.

Parasympathetic Supply

Parasympathetic supply is through **craniosacral outflow**. Cranial supply is through **glossopharyngeal, facial and vagus nerves**. Glossopharyngeal nerve supplies muscles of pharynx and upper esophageal sphincter. Facial nerve and glossopharyngeal supply the salivary glands. Vagus supplies esophagus, stomach, small intestine, proximal colon, liver and pancreas. Sacral outflow is through **pelvic nerve** ($S_{2,3,4}$) and it supplies distal colon and rectum. These fibers function in defecation reflex. Parasympathetic fibers are **cholinergic**.

Vagus is a mixed nerve which contains 90% **sensory** fibers (somatic and visceral afferents) and the rest constituted by general and special visceral efferent fibers. The parasympathetic efferent fibers constitute less than 10% of vagal fibers. Sensory fibers carry information from the gut to the CNS where it is processed.

Vagal efferents contain:
- Somatic motor fibers to the striated muscles of the proximal esophagus.
- Preganglionic parasympathetic fibers which end on the cholinergic nerve cells of the myenteric and Meissner's plexus. Since the preganglionic parasympathetic fibers terminate on the ganglia of ENS, *functions of parasympathetic system on the gut are implemented through the ENS*.
- Postganglionic sympathetic fibers from the cervical sympathetic ganglia.

Effects of Parasympathetic Stimulation

- Smooth muscle contraction of GIT and increase in motility and tone, except in pyloric, ileocecal and internal anal sphincters.
- Parasympathetic stimulation causes relaxation of these sphincters.
- Increased secretion from salivary glands, stomach, pancreas and small intestine.

Sensory neurons in the vagal nuclei (nucleus tractus solitarius) help in the processing of sensory information from the gut, reaching the CNS. This leads to an alteration in the vagal output reaching the ENS from CNS through vagal efferents. This reflex is referred to as **vagovagal reflex or long loop reflex (Fig. 44.3A)**. Here, the afferent and efferent fibers go through the vagus, e.g., distension of the stomach leads to increased gastric juice secretion through this reflex.
- Stimulus – Stretch of gut wall
- Receptor – Stretch receptors
- Afferent – Vagus
- Center– Vagal nuclei in brainstem
- Efferent – Through vagus
- Effect – Increase in gastric juice secretion due to release of gastrin from G cells which stimulates gastric glands

Sympathetic Supply

Sympathetic fibers to the gut originate from the lateral horn cells of T_5 to L_2 segments of spinal cord, synapse in the **celiac and mesenteric ganglia** and postganglionic fibers reach the gut through **splanchnic nerves**. The sympathetic fibers are **adrenergic** since the neurotransmitter released is **norepinephrine**. Norepinephrine relaxes the GIT musculature by hyperpolarizing the smooth muscle membrane. The sympathetic fibers reaching the gut are postganglionic and they terminate:
- On the postganglionic cholinergic parasympathetic nerve endings. Here, the norepinephrine released by the sympathetic endings inhibits acetylcholine secretion by the parasympathetic fibers by presynaptic inhibition, i.e., the α_2 presynaptic receptors in the postganglionic parasympathetic endings are stimulated. This effect is seen in the sphincters of GIT.
- Directly on the intestinal smooth muscle cells.
- Still others innervate intestinal blood vessels and produce vasoconstriction. The intestinal blood vessels have a dual innervation. They have an extrinsic noradrenergic innervation and an intrinsic innervation by nerve fibers of the enteric nervous system. VIP and NO are among the mediators in the intrinsic innervation and these are responsible for the hyperemia (increased blood flow) seen in the gut during digestion of food.

Effects of Sympathetic Stimulation on Gut

- Inhibition of motility and tone of the gut by:
  - A direct action that inhibits the smooth muscles of gut.
  - Indirect action by inhibiting the neurons of ENS.
- Contraction of sphincters.
- Decrease in the blood flow and decreased secretion from the stomach and intestine.

GUT-BRAIN AXIS

PY4.6: Describe the gut-brain axis.

The **gut brain axis (GBA)** is the biochemical communication network that links the enteric and the central nervous system (CNS) through neuroendocrine and metabolic pathways. It consists of bidirectional communication between the CNS and the enteric nervous system, linking emotional and cognitive centers of the brain with peripheral intestinal functions. It is sometimes used to refer to the role of the gut flora where it is referred to as **microbiota-gut-brain axis (MGBA)**. Microbiota refers to the microbe population in a specific ecosystem, such as those populations found in the gut microbiota or skin microbiota. MGBA includes signaling from gut- microbiota to brain and from brain to gut-microbiota by means of neural, endocrine, immune and humoral links. Irritable bowel syndrome is considered as an example of the disruption of these complex relationships.

This complex communication system ensures the proper maintenance of gastrointestinal homeostasis and is likely to have multiple effects on the affect, motivation and higher cognitive functions. The role of gut-brain axis is to monitor and integrate gut functions as well as to link emotional and cognitive centers of the brain with peripheral intestinal functions and mechanisms such as immune activation, intestinal permeability, enteric reflex, and entero-endocrine signaling. It involves neuro-immuno- endocrine mediators.

The bidirectional communication network includes the central nervous system, neuroendocrine and neuro- immune systems including the autonomic nervous system, the enteric nervous system, and the hypothalamic pituitary adrenal axis, vagus nerve and gut microbiota. Cephalic phase of digestion is an example of gut-brain interactions where gastric and pancreatic secretions increase in response to smell and sight of food. The sympathetic and parasympathetic divisions of the ANS drive both afferent signals, arising from the lumen transmitted through the enteric, spinal and vagal pathways to the CNS, and efferent signals from the CNS to the intestinal wall.

In the gut, there are approximately 10^{14} micro-organisms. 75% of the gut microbiota is comprised of the bacterial phyla Firmicutes and Bacteroidetes.

Disruption to the microbiome is associated with allergies, autoimmune diseases, metabolic disorders and neuropsychiatric disorders. Microbiota can influence ENS activity by producing molecules that can act as local neurotransmitters, such as GABA, serotonin, melatonin, histamine and acetyl-choline and by generating a biologically active form of catecholamines in the lumen of the gut. Lactobacilli also utilize nitrate and nitrite to generate nitric oxide. Gut bacteria produce neurochemicals that the brain uses to regulate mental processes such as learning, memory, and mood. For example, gut bacteria manufactures about 90% of the body's supply of serotonin, which influences mood and gastrointestinal activity. Serotonin plays a vital role in the communication between gut and brain, as well as in the proper functioning of the gut.

Gut microbiome affect mood by producing neurotransmitters such as dopamine, norepinephrine, acetyl choline and GABA, which have important role in mood, anxiety, concentration, reward and motivation. Thus gut microbiome is related to various states of mental health. There is bidirectional communication between gut and brain. Mood disorders are prevalent in patients with irritable bowel syndrome. Depression may be caused by dysfunctional gut-brain-immune system interactions.

Galanin released from the entero-endocrine cells of gut stimulates the activity of the central branch of hypothalamus-pituitary-adrenal (HPA) axis and cause release of corticotropin releasing hormone (CRH) and adrenocorticotropic hormone (ACTH). This enhances glucocorticoid secretion from the adrenal cortex. Galanin directly act on the adrenal cortical cells and increase cortisol secretion and norepinephrine release from the adrenal medulla. **Ghrelin** also stimulate secretion of ACTH and cortisol and is involved in the modulation of the HPA axis response to stress.

Gut microbiota interact with the gut-brain axis by the following mechanisms:

- **Interaction through the vagus nerve:** Information from the intestine is carried by the vagus nerve to the brain stem, hypothalamus and limbic system involved in the regulation of emotions. Efferents from the limbic system during stress influence the autonomic activity of the gut.
- **Interaction through gut hormone signaling:** Bacterial products stimulate the entero-endocrine cells of the gut to produce neuropeptides such as peptide YY, neuropeptide Y, cholecystokinin, glucagon like polypeptide 1 and GLP-2 and substance P. These substances enter the blood stream and can influence the enteric nervous system.
- **Role in tryptophan metabolism:** 95% of serotonin is produced by gut mucosal enterochromaffin cell. It is involved in the regulation of gastrointestinal secretion, motility and pain perception. In the brain serotonin plays a role in regulating mood and cognition. Gut microbiota also plays a role in tryptophan metabolism which is the precursor of serotonin.
- **Interaction with the immune system:** The microbiota also influences mucosal immune activation. The gut associated lymphoid tissue comprises 70% of the body's immune system. The immune system is intimately connected to the gut microbiome and the nervous system and thus act as a mediator of the gut's effects on the brain and the brain's effect on the gut. Stress and stress hormones such as cortisol can have a negative impact on the gut microbiome. Patients with psychiatric disorders have different population of gut micobiomes when compared to microbes in healthy individuals.
- **By altering intestinal permeability:** Chronic stress has been shown to alter intestinal permeability which is associated with a low grade inflammation of the gut. This is functionally linked to psychiatric disorders such as depression. It is due to increase in the circulating level of bacterial endotoxins called lipopolysaccharides. Microbiota also produces neuroactive substances that lead to neuropsychiatric disorders like schizophrenia, autism, anxiety and depression. Irritable bowel syndrome is now considered a microbiome-GBA disorder.
- **Role of microbial metabolites:** The microbial community of gut has important metabolic and physiological functions for the host and contributes to its homeostasis during life. Species of Lactobacillus and Bifidobacterium produce gamma amino butyric acid (GABA) which is the main inhibitory transmitter in the brain. Candida, Escherichia and enterococcus produce the neurotransmitter serotonin while some *Bacillus* species produce dopamine.

One of the main product of gut bacterial metabolism are short chain fatty acids, such as butyric acid, propionic acid and acetic acid, that can stimulate the sympathetic nervous system, mucosal serotonin release and can influence memory and learning process. Neuroactive substances produced by gut microbiome like butyrate has been shown to reduce anxiety and depression. So to conclude, the gut bacteria should be good and adequate for good quality life, better mental health and a sharper brain.

Electrical Responses of Smooth Muscle

The smooth muscles of GIT shows spontaneous rhythmic fluctuations in membrane potential ranging between –65 and –45 mV *except in the esophagus and the proximal portion of stomach*. This is called **basic electrical rhythm (BER)**. BER is initiated in the stellate muscle-like **pacemaker cells** in the gut wall called **interstitial cells of Cajal**. BER is also called slow wave pattern. Slow wave is due to waxing and waning of the activity of Na⁺ pump. They are slow, undulating changes in resting membrane potential. BER by itself rarely causes muscle contraction (except stomach) as BER waves are not action potentials. When the slow wave potential becomes less and less negative, spike potentials are superimposed on the BER waves to increase muscle tension. *The spike potentials are true action potentials.* So, BER waves are called **pacemaker waves (Fig. 44.5)**. The depolarizing phase of each spike is due to Ca^{2+} influx and repolarization due to K^+ efflux. The function of BER is to coordinate peristaltic and other motor activities of the gut.

Rate of BER Varies in Different Parts of GIT

Stomach – 4/min
Duodenum – 12/min
Distal ileum – 8/min
Cecum – 9/min
Sigmoid colon – 16/min

Stretch is a stimulus for visceral smooth muscle. When stretched, more spike potentials become superimposed on the BER waves. **Acetylcholine** increases the number of spikes and the tension in the smooth muscle. **Epinephrine and norepinephrine** decrease the number of spikes and muscle tension.

Short bursts of spikes cause phasic motor activity; longer bursts cause tonic muscle contraction. Tonic contraction occurs at sphincters, whereas phasic activity occurs in between sphincters.

Gastrointestinal Glands

Types of gastrointestinal glands (structural classification):
- **Simple mucous** glands or goblet cells
- **Crypts of Lieberkuhn** of small intestine – glands formed by invagination of epithelium (pits).
- **Deep tubular glands** – gastric glands and upper duodenal glands.
- **Complex glands** or mixed glands, e.g., salivary gland, pancreas, liver.

Goblet cells extrude their mucus directly onto their epithelial surface to act as a lubricant and to protect the surfaces from excoriation and digestion.

Small intestine is lined by pits that represent invaginations of the epithelium into the submucosa called **crypts of Lieberkuhn**, which contain specialized secretory cells.

In the stomach and upper duodenum are found **deep tubular glands**, e.g., gastric glands.

Complex glands like salivary glands, pancreas and liver provide secretions for digestion and emulsification of food. They lie outside the walls of the alimentary canal.

Salivary glands and pancreas are compound acinous glands which contain millions of acini lined with secreting glandular cells. *Complex glands are drained by a system of ducts that finally empty into the alimentary canal.*

Functional Classification of Exocrine Glands

Functional classification is based on the mechanism by which secretion is released from the gland:
- Merocrine glands
- Apocrine glands
- Holocrine glands

Merocrine glands release their secretions by exocytosis or emeiocytosis **(Fig. 44.6)**, e.g., salivary glands, pancreas. **Apocrine** glands accumulate their secretory products at the apex of the cell. Then the apex of the cell pinches off from the rest of the cell to release the secretion. The remaining part of the cell repeats the process. Apocrine glands are not present in humans. In **holocrine** glands, the secretory cells accumulate the secretory products in their cytoplasm. As the cell matures, the cell is sloughed off and is replaced by new cells by mitosis from the underlying cells. For example,

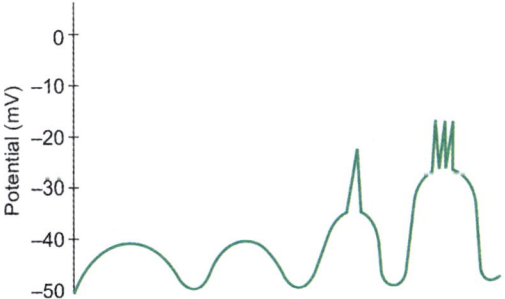

Fig. 44.5: Basic electrical rhythm or pacemaker waves recorded from smooth muscles.

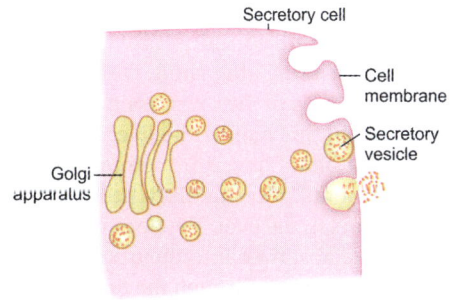

Fig. 44.6: Mechanism of secretion by emeiocytosis in a secretory cell.

the epithelial cells of small intestine containing digestive enzymes slough off into the lumen of the intestine; they break apart and release enzymes that digest nutrients in the chyme. Sebaceous gland is also a holocrine gland.

Basic Mechanism of Secretion from the Glands

The stimuli that cause secretion from the glands are:
- Tactile stimuli
- Chemical irritation
- Distension of gut wall

The presence of food in a particular segment of GIT causes the glands of that region and of adjacent regions to secrete moderate-to-large quantities of digestive juices. Part of this local effect results from direct contact stimulation of the surface glandular cells with food and in addition, epithelial stimulation also activates ENS leading to increased secretion.

Mechanism of Secretion

The nutrients needed for the formation of the secretion diffuse or are actively transported from the capillary into the base of the glandular cell. There are a number of mitochondria at the base of the cell which provide energy for the synthesis of ATP. Energy from ATP is used for the synthesis of organic substances from the nutrients. Synthesis of secretion, especially proteins, occurs in the rough endoplasmic reticulum.

The secretory materials are transported through the tubules of endoplasmic reticulum to the vesicles of Golgi complex. Here, the secretions are modified and concentrated. When the vesicle reaches a diameter of 1–2 μm, it separates as an independent secretory vesicle into the cytoplasm and is stored in the apical portion of the secretory cell. Each vesicle contains a number of granules called **zymogen granules**.

When an appropriate neurohumoral stimulus reaches the cell, the Ca^{2+} channels on the membrane open and Ca^{2+} enters the cell from ECF. The Ca^{2+}, in turn, causes the vesicles to move towards the apical membrane of the cell. The secretory vesicles fuse with the cell membrane and the membrane breaks open emptying their contents to the exterior. This process is called exocytosis or **emeiocytosis or reverse pinocytosis (Fig. 44.6)**.

Gastrointestinal Blood Flow

Blood vessels of gastrointestinal system form part of **splanchnic circulation**. It includes blood flow through gut, spleen, pancreas and liver. The **portal vein** carries venous blood from these regions into the liver.

Portal venous blood contains most of the non-fat, water-soluble nutrients absorbed from the gut. The reticuloendothelial cells of liver remove bacteria and other harmful agents from this blood. The liver cells also absorb nutrients from the blood and store temporarily ½ to ¾ of all absorbed nutrients. Intermediary processing of these nutrients also occurs in the liver. The non- water soluble, fat-based nutrients are absorbed into the intestinal lymphatics and reach the blood stream through the thoracic duct.

After a meal, the motor, secretory and absorptive activity in the gut increases and blood flow to the gut increases as much as 8-fold during the next 1 hr. The reasons are:

- Several vasodilator substances are released from the mucosa of the intestinal tract during digestion like NO, CCK, VIP, gastrin, secretin, etc.
- The gastrointestinal glands release kinins like kallidin and bradykinin, which are powerful vasodilators.
- During increased metabolism, the O_2 concentration in the gut decreases, producing local hypoxia. This causes release of adenosine which is a well-known vasodilator.

Nervous Factors Controlling Gastrointestinal Blood Flow

Stimulation of sympathetic fibers to the gut causes vasoconstriction and decreased splanchnic blood flow. It is unsettled whether the blood vessels of the gut have cholinergic innervation (For details of intestinal blood flow, *refer* Chapter 32).

MULTIPLE CHOICE QUESTIONS

1. **All are true of myenteric reflex, *except*:**
   a. Distension of intestine elicits the reflex
   b. Extrinsic innervation should be intact
   c. Efferent neurons are in the myenteric plexus
   d. Substance P is a mediator

2. **Major mediator of smooth muscle relaxation in the gut:**
   a. Nitric oxide   b. Acetylcholine
   c. Norepinephrine   d. Serotonin

3. **Stimulation of myenteric plexus causes:**
   a. Increased secretion from intestinal glands
   b. Relaxation of sphincters of gut
   c. Decrease in the tone of gut wall
   d. Decrease in peristalsis

4. **The following statements are true regarding gastrointestinal tract, *except*:**
   a. There are more number of lymphocytes in the intestinal wall than in the blood
   b. IgA of gut is resistant to digestion by intestinal enzymes
   c. Hormones secreted by gastrointestinal tract are produced by APUD cells
   d. Submucosa contains myenteric plexus

5. **Peyer's patches are present in:**
   a. Stomach   b. Duodenum
   c. Jejunum   d. Ileum

6. **Rate of basic electrical rhythm is maximum in:**
   a. Stomach   b. Duodenum
   c. Jejunum   d. Sigmoid colon

7. **Stimulation of sympathetic nerve to the gut produces:**
   a. Increase in motility of the gut
   b. Increase in blood flow to the gut
   c. Contraction of sphincters
   d. Increased secretion from the glands

ANSWERS

1. b   2. a   3. b   4. d   5. d
6. d   7. c

Salivary Glands and Esophagus

CHAPTER 45

LEARNING OBJECTIVES
- Describe the composition of saliva and its functions
- Explain the histology of the salivary glands and the mechanism of secretion of saliva
- Explain the innervation of salivary glands and the regulation of secretion of saliva

INTRODUCTION

Saliva is the first digestive juice that comes in contact with food. There are 3 pairs of major salivary glands (**Fig. 45.1**):
1. Parotid gland
2. Submandibular or submaxillary gland
3. Sublingual gland

In addition, there are small **buccal glands** distributed all over the oral and pharyngeal cavity. The salivary glands secrete saliva continuously to keep the mouth moist. Saliva is a colorless, odorless, slimy fluid.

FUNCTIONAL ANATOMY

Parotid Gland
- It is the largest salivary gland weighing about 25–30 g.
- **Location:** Side of the face just below and in front of the ear.
- Duct draining the gland is **Stensen's duct**, which emerges from the anterior border of the gland near its upper end. It passes across the surface of the masseter muscle and when it reaches the anterior border of the muscle it takes a sharp turn medially, pierces the buccal pad of fat, buccinator muscle and mucosa of cheek to open into the oral cavity. *Stensen's duct opens at a point opposite the crown of the second upper molar tooth on the cheek.*

Submandibular Gland
- **Weight:** 8–10 g
- **Location:** In the submandibular triangle
- **Duct: Wharton's duct** which opens in the floor of the mouth on either side of the frenulum of tongue.

Sublingual Gland
- **Location:** Beneath the tongue under the mucous membrane of oral cavity.
- **Duct:** Drained by 5-15 small ducts opening into the floor of the mouth called **ducts of Rivinus and Bartholin**.

HISTOLOGY OF SALIVARY GLAND

Salivary glands are exocrine glands, i.e., the secretion is conveyed by ducts. Histologically, salivary glands are **racemose** glands because they appear like clusters of grapes. They are composed of groups of cells known as **acini** or secretory end piece. The cells lining the acinus are called **end piece cells**. The acini are classified into three main groups depending on the cell type contained in the end piece (**Fig. 45.2**):
1. Serous acini
2. Mucous acini
3. Seromucinous or mixed acini

These can be differentiated by their staining characteristics and nuclear appearance. Glands containing predominantly serous cells in the end pieces are called **serous glands**, e.g., parotid gland.

Those containing predominantly mucous cells are **mucous glands**, e.g., sublingual gland.

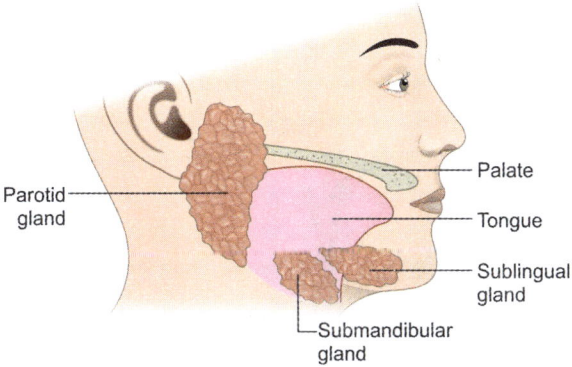

Fig. 45.1: Location of salivary gland.

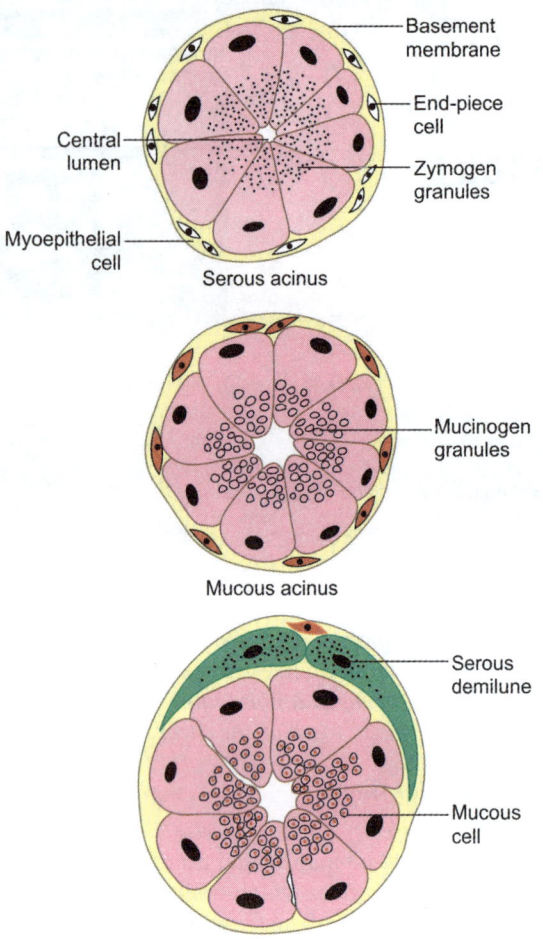

Fig. 45.2: Microscopic structure of acini.

Table 45.1: Ratio of cells in different salivary glands.		
Gland	Serous: Mucous cells	% of total saliva
Parotid	4:1	20
Sublingual	1:4	5
Submandibular	1:1	70

Glands containing both serous and mucous elements are called **mixed glands**, e.g., submandibular gland **(Table 45.1)**.

Serous Acini

Serous acini are composed of predominantly serous cells which are large pyramidal cells with apex towards the center and base towards periphery enclosed by a basement membrane. The cells contain apically located secretory granules called **zymogen granules** which are **small, dark and opaque**. These granules stain **acidophilic** and contain **amylase** and mucopolysaccharide. The number of zymogen granules depends on the secretory activity of the cell, being less numerous after a meal and reaches a peak just before meals. Secretion is **thin and watery**.

Mucous Acini

Mucous acini are also lined by pyramidal cells containing apical granules which are larger and **translucent**. The cytoplasm contains numerous droplets of **mucinogen** which is the precursor of mucin. Mucous acini have a larger lumen than the serous acini. Secretion is **thick and viscous**.

Seromucinous Acini or Mixed Acini

Seromucinous acini contain both serous and mucous cells. The mucous cells are placed near the lumen and the serous cells are displaced towards the periphery of the acinus and appear as crescent-shaped aggregation of cells. These serous cells are dark staining and appear to cap the mucous elements of the acinus and are called **serous demilunes or demilunes of Heidenhain or Gianuzzi**. These demilunes drain into the lumen of the acinus through a duct which passes between the mucous cells.

Between the basement membrane and the glandular cells are scattered **myoepithelial cells** which are contractile in nature and compress the acinus to expel its contents into the central lumen **(Fig. 45.2)**.

The acini are drained by small ductules called **intercalated ducts**. A number of intercalated ducts join to form **intralobular duct**. A number of intralobular ducts join to form **interlobular ducts**. The interlobular ducts finally join to form **major duct** of the gland which opens into the oral cavity **(Fig. 45.3)**. Myoepithelial cells also surround the ductules.

Sialography

Salivary ducts can be visualized by the technique called **sialography**. A radiopaque substance is introduced through a cannula into the opening of the duct of the salivary gland to be visualized. X-rays are taken which clearly show the duct system **(Fig. 45.4)**. Any growth, block, dilatations, etc., in the gland can be detected.

BLOOD SUPPLY

Salivary glands are supplied by branches of external carotid artery:

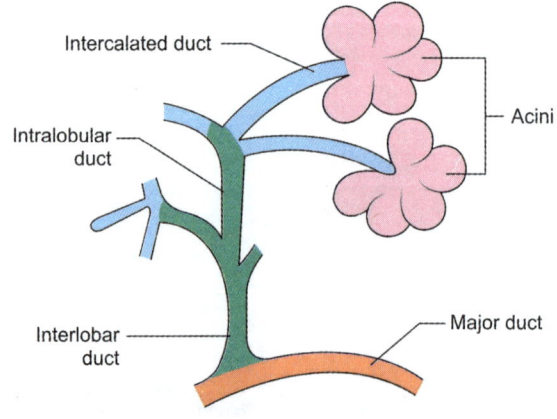

Fig. 45.3: Duct system of salivary gland.

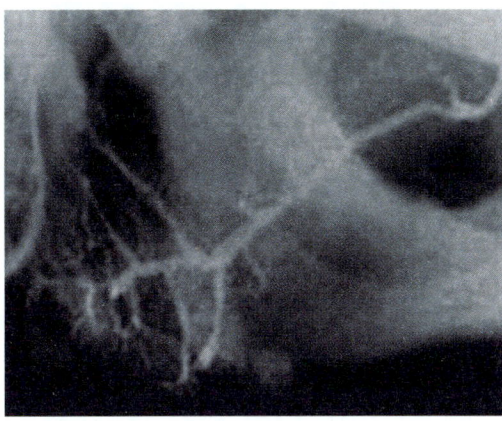

Fig. 45.4: Sialogram of parotid gland.

- Parotid gland is supplied by **posterior auricular artery**.
- Submandibular gland by **facial artery** and its submental branch.
- Sublingual gland is supplied by **sublingual artery**.

INNERVATION OF SALIVARY GLANDS

Salivary gland is exclusively under nervous control. Salivary glands are innervated by both sympathetic and parasympathetic divisions of ANS.

Parasympathetic supply is more important and its stimulation causes:
- Profuse secretion of watery saliva with a relatively low content of organic material.
- Vasodilatation in the gland due to local release of vasoactive intestinal polypeptide (VIP).

Sympathetic stimulation causes:
- Secretion of small amounts of saliva rich in organic constituents, especially from submandibular glands.
- Vasoconstriction

Parasympathetic Supply

Cell bodies of the parasympathetic fibers are located in the brainstem. Groups of neurons called **salivary nuclei** are seen in the lower part of pons and upper part of medulla. These constitute the bulbar salivary centers which are:
- Superior salivary nucleus in the anterior part
- Inferior salivary nucleus in the posterior part

Parasympathetic Supply to Submaxillary and Sublingual Gland

Course of the Parasympathetic Efferent Fibers

Parasympathetic fibers to the submandibular and sublingual glands take origin from **superior salivatory nucleus**. They course through **nervus intermedius of Wrisberg** and join the **facial nerve**. Fibers leave the facial nerve through chorda tympani branch and join the lingual branch of **trigeminal nerve**. The preganglionic fibers synapse in the **submandibular ganglion**. The postganglionic fibers innervate the submandibular and sublingual glands (**Fig. 45.5A**).

The parasympathetic afferent fibers arise from the taste buds of anterior 2/3rd of tongue and pass through nervus intermedius of Wrisberg and reach superior salivatory nucleus. This forms a simple reflex arc.

Parasympathetic Supply to Parotid Gland

Afferent fibers originate from the posterior 1/3rd of tongue and pass through the glossopharyngeal nerve to **inferior salivatory nucleus**.

Efferent fibers from inferior salivatory nucleus, initially pass through the glossopharyngeal nerve, then separate from it and reach the **tympanic plexus**. From this plexus originate the **tympanic nerve** and **lesser superficial petrosal nerve** which synapse in the otic ganglion. Postganglionic fibers from the otic ganglion travel in the **auriculotemporal branch** of the trigeminal nerve to innervate the parotid glands (**Fig. 45.5B**).

Sympathetic Supply to the Salivary Glands

Sympathetic supply to the salivary glands arises from the lateral horn cells of the 1st and 2nd thoracic spinal segments. The fibers leave the spinal cord and synapse in the superior **cervical ganglion**. Postganglionic fibers travel along the external carotid artery to reach the salivary glands (**Fig. 45.6**).

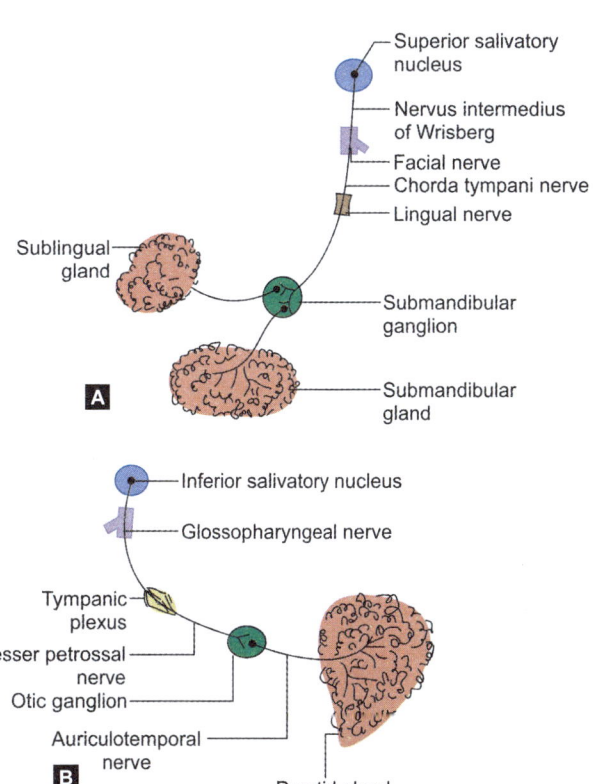

Figs. 45.5A and B: Parasympathetic supply to: (A) Sublingual and submandibular salivary gland; (B) Parotid.

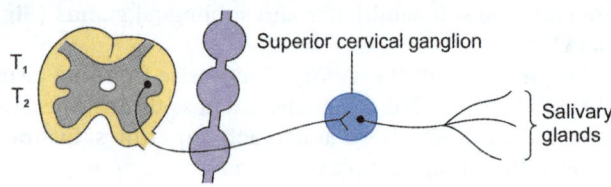

Fig. 45.6: Sympathetic supply to salivary glands.

COMPOSITION OF SALIVA

PY4.2: Describe the composition, mechanism of secretion, functions, and regulation of saliva, gastric, pancreatic, intestinal juices and bile secretion.

The composition of saliva depends on the type of salivary gland, the stimulus and the rate of flow of saliva.
- **Rate of secretion**—1.5 L/day or 1 mL/min
- **pH of saliva**—6–8
- **Specific gravity**—1.002–1.009
- **Viscosity**
  - Sublingual secretion—13.4
  - Submandibular secretion—3.4
  - Parotid secretion—1.5

Variation in the viscosity is due to the variation in the amount of mucin present in saliva. Saliva is usually **hypotonic** to plasma, but when flow rate is high it becomes isotonic.

Composition of a mixed salivary secretion is as follows:
- Water—99.5%
- Solids (inorganic and organic)—0.5%
- Certain gases

Inorganic Constituents

HCO_3^-, H_2CO_3, PO_4^{3-}, Na^+, K^+, Ca^{2+}, Mg^{2+}, Cl^-, thiocyanate ions, etc.

Organic Constituents

- Mucin
- Ptyalin or α-amylase
- Lingual lipase
- Lysozyme
- Kallikrein
- Blood group substances
- IgA
- Urea, creatinine
- Parotin
- Nerve growth factor
- Lactoferrin
- Proline-rich protein

Mucin is a specialized glycoprotein secreted especially from the sublingual gland which lubricates food and protects oral mucosa. It is responsible for the viscosity and buffering property of saliva.

Amylase is the starch-splitting enzyme in saliva which acts mainly on **cooked starch**. Cl^- is essential for its activation. Thiocyanate acts as a coenzyme to activate ptyalin in the absence of NaCl. *Amylase has no action on cellulose.*

Lingual lipase is the fat-splitting enzyme produced by glands of tongue called **Ebner's glands**. It is active in the stomach and can digest 30% of dietary triglyceride.

Lysozyme is an enzyme present in saliva which causes lysis of the walls of the bacteria present in mouth, i.e., it has **bactericidal** action. People with dry mouth due to absence of saliva have a tendency to develop infections of the oral cavity.

Kallikrein is an enzyme that acts on $α_2$-globulin in the interstitial fluid to form a vasodilator substance called kallidin or bradykinin. Parasympathetic stimulation results in vasodilatation due to increased secretion of kallikrein and VIP.

Blood group antigens are present in the saliva of **secretors**. Immunoglobulins, such as **IgA and IgM** are present in saliva. They may act against various bacteria in the oral cavity.

Parotin is a local hormone secreted by parotid and submaxillary gland. It helps in deposition of calcium in the teeth and acts on mesenchymal tissues to promote their growth and development.

Nerve growth factor helps in the growth of sympathetic ganglia.

Lactoferrin binds iron and is bacteriostatic.

Proline-rich protein is the glycoprotein of parotid salivary secretion. It binds Ca^{2+} and toxic tannins and protects tooth enamel.

Importance of HCO_3^- and H_2CO_3 Ratio in Saliva

Ratio of HCO_3^- and H_2CO_3 in saliva is very important. The pH of saliva depends on the ratio of H_2CO_3 and $NaHCO_3$. In conditions where blood PCO_2 is high, the pH of saliva falls because the salivary H_2CO_3 increases. This mobilizes Ca^{2+} from teeth, reducing the size and thickness of teeth. When pH rises due to reduction in CO_2 in saliva, Ca^{2+} precipitates in the teeth, called **tartar.** This condition is seen in mouth breathing.

FUNCTIONS OF SALIVA

- **Moistening and cleansing** function—saliva keeps the oral and pharyngeal mucosa moist and gives a feeling of comfort. A constant flow of saliva has a cleansing effect on the mouth and teeth and helps in oral hygiene and prevents dental caries.
- Saliva has **antibacterial activity** due to the presence of proteolytic enzymes, such as lysozyme which kills viruses and bacteria. Lysozyme aids the thiocyanate ions present in saliva to enter the bacteria where these ions become bactericidal. Saliva also contains antibodies, such as immunoglobulin A, which can destroy oral bacteria. Patients with **xerostomia** (deficient salivation) have a higher than normal incidence of dental caries.
- Saliva helps in **mastication, swallowing and speech** due to the presence of mucin which acts as a lubricant. This facilitates movement of lips and tongue. Constant salivation in between meals gives a feeling of comfort.

Flowchart 45.1: Steps in the digestion of starch by salivary amylase.

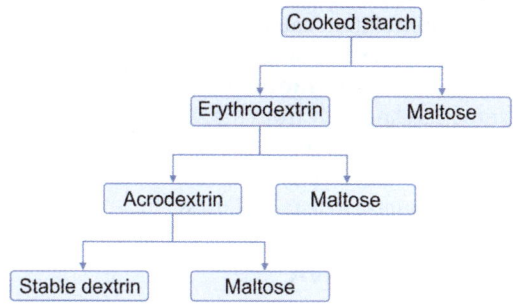

- **Excretory function**—substances, such as lead, mercury, thiocyanate, alkaloids, such as morphine, drugs, such as streptomycin, viruses of rabies, mumps, poliomyelitis, etc., are excreted through saliva especially in people who are in the habit of spitting saliva.
- **Digestive function**—amylase or ptyalin present in saliva acts on cooked starch, converting it into disaccharide **maltose**. It has no action on uncooked raw starch. This is because it cannot break the insoluble cellulose covering of the starch granules. Cooking disrupts this covering. The digestive function of saliva can be studied by treating boiled starch with saliva at 37°C and adding iodine to it. Iodine stains different carbohydrates formed during digestion of starch (**Flowchart 45.1**).

Food stays in the mouth only for a very short period. The partially digested food reaches the stomach. *Salivary digestion is completed in the stomach.* The pH of stomach is 1–2. The pH of the interior of the bolus of food is 7. So, the action of salivary amylase continues in the interior of the bolus but not on the exterior for some time.
- **Buffering action**—HCO_3^-, PO_4^{3-} and mucin are the 3 buffering systems of saliva which maintains the pH of saliva at about 7. At this pH, saliva is saturated with Ca^{2+}, and therefore Ca^{2+} does not diffuse from teeth to saliva. When the pH goes below 5.5, Ca^{2+} of the teeth go into solution leading to tooth decay. Buffers present in saliva neutralize the acid regurgitated into the esophagus due to **reflux** from the stomach and thus prevent heartburn due to esophagitis.
- Saliva acts as a **solvent** for the molecules that stimulate taste buds and thus helps in the appreciation of taste.
- Saliva helps in **water balance**. In times of dehydration, salivary secretion is suppressed and there is drying up of mouth and pharynx. Dryness of the mouth evokes the sensation of thirst. Drinking of water restores fluid balance. Thus, salivation plays a part in the maintenance of water balance of the body.
- **Temperature regulation**—salivation helps to dispose excess heat by panting in animals, such as dogs where sweat glands are absent.

MECHANISM OF SECRETION OF SALIVA

Saliva is secreted in two stages (**Fig. 45.7**):
1. Primary secretion from the acini
2. Modification of the primary secretion in the ductal system

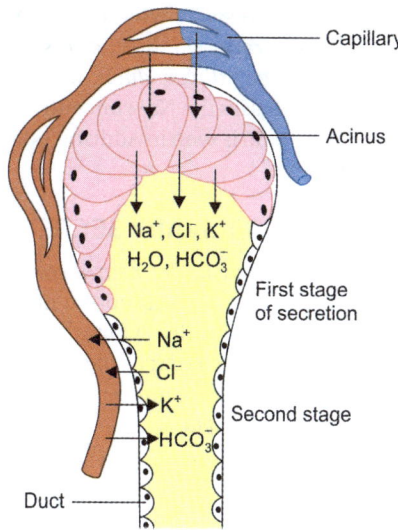

Fig. 45.7: Stages of salivary secretion.

Primary Secretion

Primary secretion is formed from the acini. Substances diffuse or are actively transported from the capillaries to the acinar cells. This solution is isotonic with plasma having concentrations of Na^+, K^+, Cl^- and HCO close to that of plasma (**Fig. 45.7**).

Second Stage

As the primary secretion reaches the ductal system especially the intercalated ducts, the composition is modified by reabsorbing Na^+ and Cl^- and secreting K^+ and HCO_3^-. There is active reabsorption of Na^+ and to maintain electrical gradient, Cl^- is reabsorbed through Cl^--HCO_3^- exchanger (**Fig. 45.8**). The ducts are relatively impermeable to water and saliva becomes **hypotonic** and alkaline, with a high content of K^+ and HCO_3^-, and a low content of Na^+ and Cl^-.

When salivary flow is rapid, there is less time for ionic composition to change in the ducts and the primary secretion increases 20 times. So, saliva contains more Na^+ and Cl^-, and

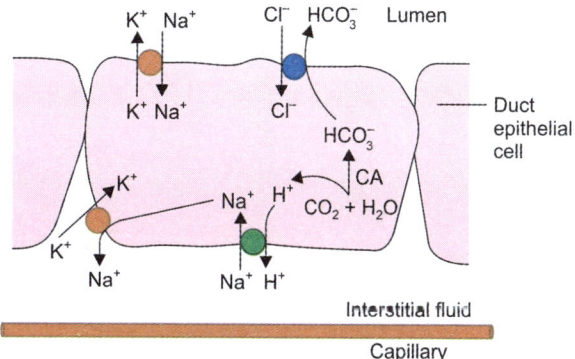

Fig. 45.8: Modification of salivary secretion from the acini in the duct. K^+ and HCO_3^- are secreted into the lumen and Na^+ and Cl^- are reabsorbed.

(CA: carbonic anhydrase)

less of K⁺ and HCO₃⁻, and saliva will be almost isotonic to that of plasma. *Aldosterone, the hormone secreted by the adrenal cortex acts on the salivary ducts.* It increases the K⁺ concentration and decreases the Na⁺ concentration of saliva. A high salivary Na⁺/K⁺ ratio is seen in Addison's disease where aldosterone is deficient.

■ REGULATION OF SALIVARY SECRETION

Salivary secretion is *entirely under neural control*, with the parasympathetic branch of the autonomic nervous system playing the most prominent role. Sympathetic stimulation slightly increases the organic content of saliva but has little influence on volume. *No hormonal regulation of salivary secretion has been demonstrated.*

Basal Secretion

Saliva is being continuously secreted. Continuous secretion of saliva in the absence of any stimulus is called **spontaneous secretion** or resting secretion or basal secretion of saliva. This secretion keeps the mucous membrane of mouth and pharynx always moist. Exact mechanism of continuous secretion is not clearly known. But it is suggested that there is continuous secretion of minute quantities of acetylcholine by the nerve endings which causes continuous secretion of saliva. Basal secretion decreases during sleep and increases during mastication and sexual excitement.

Parasympathetic Stimulation

- Stimulation of parasympathetic fibers to the salivary gland causes **profuse** (abundant) secretion of **watery saliva** with a relatively low content of organic material.
- Duct cells increase HCO⁻ secretion
- Contraction of myoepithelial cells to increase the flow of saliva
- Along with acetylcholine, a co-transmitter is also released at the postganglionic parasympathetic nerve endings, called **VIP**, which along with **kallikrein** produces **vasodilatation** and increased blood flow in the gland. Kallikrein is produced from acinar cells. Atropine and other anticholinergic drugs reduce salivary secretion **(Flowchart 45.2)**.

Sympathetic Stimulation

Sympathetic stimulation causes
- **Vasoconstriction** and decreased blood flow to the glands
- Secretion of **small amounts** of saliva rich in organic constituents especially from the submandibular gland
- Increased protein secretion for enzyme synthesis.

A dry mouth is an important characteristic feature of sympathetic response to fear and stress.

■ NATURE OF SALIVA

The nature of saliva secreted depends on the type of substance present in the mouth. Rough objects inhibit salivation. Of the primary tastes, sour taste stimulates maximum secretion of saliva.
- **Edible and smooth** substance produces viscous saliva rich in mucin and enzyme.
- **Inedible dry powder** or sand in mouth produces thin watery saliva.
- **Acidic substances** in mouth produce saliva rich in amino acid.

■ SALIVARY REFLEXES

Secretion of saliva depends on two different reflex mechanisms:
1. Conditioned reflexes
2. Unconditioned reflexes

Conditioned Reflex

In humans, sight, smell and even thought of food causes salivation. This conditioned reflex occurs only when there is previous experience or training. This is an **acquired reflex**. In conditioned reflex, *the afferent limb of the reflex starts from the higher centers to end in the salivary centers.*

An experiment was done by a Russian Physiologist, **Ivan Pavlov**, on dogs. He gave certain lessons to dogs. Dogs were conditioned to salivate at the sound of a bell. Here bell is the **conditioned stimulus**. Instead of bell, colored lights, whistle, etc. can be used. The salivatory center also receives inputs from the cortex, amygdala, hypothalamus, olfactory

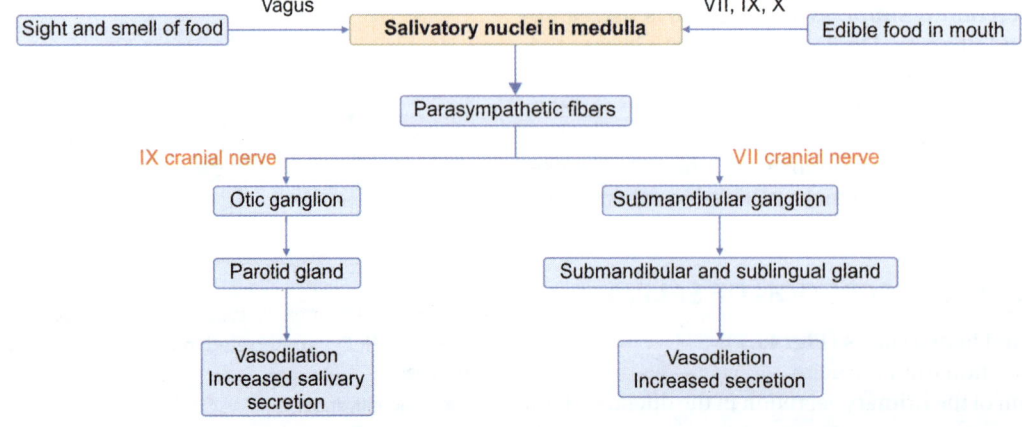

Flowchart 45.2: Regulation of salivary secretion by the parasympathetic nervous system.

areas, etc., accounting for the conditioned reflex described by Pavlov. It is said that intrinsic connections occur between centers of special nerve of special senses and pathway that produce salivation.

Unconditioned Reflex

Substances placed in the mouth produce a reflex salivation with a latent period of 2–3 sec and it depends quantitatively and qualitatively on the type of food ingested. This is unconditioned reflex and is present **from birth** onwards. Salivation is also produced by reflexes originating in the esophagus, stomach and upper small intestine when irritating food materials are ingested. The increased salivary secretion will dilute the irritating substance or neutralize it.

Gustatory Salivary Reflex

When food is ingested, large quantities of saliva are poured into the mouth due to the activation of afferent pathways going to the salivatory centers. Dryness of oral mucosa also stimulates the pathway. Receptors are present in the taste buds and there are also **tactile and mechanoreceptors** in the oral and pharyngeal mucosa. Center is the salivatory center in medulla and the effector organ is the salivary gland. The most edible and palatable food is the most potent stimulus for salivary secretion. Mere movement of tongue on palate and cheek produces salivation due to stimulation of receptors that produce reflex salivation.

Unconditioned reflex is brought about through salivary centers located in the medulla. This area is in close proximity to the vomiting center and the respiratory center in medulla. Cross connections between these centers and salivary center exist. So, when a person is nauseated or in the early phase of vomiting, there is increased salivation and a catch in the respiration.

> In unconditioned salivary reflex, the afferent limb starts from the receptors in the oral cavity or upper GIT, whereas in conditioned reflex the afferent limb starts from the higher centers to end in the salivary center.

Masticatory Salivary Reflex

Mastication reflexly evokes salivation. The approximation of the teeth of the upper and lower jaws on an object is the stimulus for this reflex. Receptors are the mechanoreceptors in the periodontal membrane, in the oral and pharyngeal mucosa and tongue.

Esophago-salivary Reflex

Stimulation of esophageal mucosa and distension of esophagus by the bolus of food reflexly brings about salivation. This is due to stimulation of vagal afferent fibers at the gastric end of esophagus.

Gastro-salivary Reflex

Stimulation of stomach by food causes reflex secretion of saliva. This is gastro-salivary reflex.

DISTURBANCES OF SALIVARY SECRETION

Mumps

Inflammatory enlargement of salivary glands due to viral infection (paramyxovirus) is mumps. Parotid gland is mainly affected, but submandibular gland may also be involved. It affects mainly children of school age and young adults. **Orchitis** occurs in one in four males who develop mumps after puberty and if it is bilateral, **sterility** may result.

Temporary Cessation of Salivation

- Dry mouth is frequently seen in patients with high fever, dehydration, in emotional states, such as anxiety, fear, etc.
- Bell's palsy—here, there is paralysis of terminal part of facial nerve and there is temporary cessation of salivation on the affected side.
- Block of salivary duct by calculus (stone) or tumors. Presence of stone in the salivary duct is called **sialolithiasis**.
- Administration of parasympatholytic drugs, such as atropine, antihistamines, etc.

Permanent Cessation of Salivation or Aptyalism

- Absence of salivary gland, congenital absence or surgical removal of gland.
- Due to damage or atrophy of salivary gland when head and neck tumors are irradiated.
- Permanent damage of salivary gland occurs in **Sjogren's syndrome**, an autoimmune disorder.
- Congenital aplasia or hypoplasia of salivary gland.

The above disorders lead to dryness of mouth known as **xerostomia**, difficulty in speech and swallowing. It also produces dental caries and disturbances of taste.

Hypersalivation or Sialorrhea

Drooling of saliva due to excessive salivation is known as sialorrhea. It occurs in:
- Pregnancy
- During epileptic attacks or seizures
- Treatment with cholinergic, adrenergic or histamine, such as drugs in mental disorders
- Lack of swallowing results in pooling of saliva in the mouth. This is often seen in neuromuscular disorders, such as Parkinson's disease, cerebral palsy, motor neuron disease, etc.
- Administration of iodides and mercury salts
- Inflammation and growth in the oral and pharyngeal mucosa
- Constant irritation of oral mucosa by decayed tooth or ill-fitting dentures
- Cancer of stomach and esophagus
- Treatment with anticholinesterases as in myasthenia gravis, Alzheimer's disease, etc.

Chorda Tympani Syndrome

Trauma or surgical procedures may damage the chorda tympani nerve. The regenerating fibers may sometimes be misdirected and join the nerve fibers innervating the sweat glands in the submental region. As a result, when food is taken, there will be increased sweating in the submental region on the affected side. This is called **chorda tympani syndrome**.

Paralytic Salivary Secretion

This was first demonstrated by **Claude Bernard** in 1864. He cut the chorda tympani branch of submaxillary gland. Gradually, the gland hypertrophied and began to secrete a thin, turbid juice which was not abolished by atropine. The flow of juice increased and reached a maximum by 7th-8th day and remained at this level for 3 weeks. Then it declined gradually and disappeared around 6th week. This is called **paralytic secretion**. It increases with sympathetic stimulation.

Reason

Paralytic secretion is due to hypersensitivity of the end piece cells or acinar cells towards sympathetic stimulation or adrenaline. This is an example of **denervation hypersensitivity**.

ESOPHAGUS

Introduction

Esophagus is a hollow muscular tube which conducts food from pharynx to stomach. It passes behind the trachea and the heart and in front of the vertebral column. It passes through the diaphragm to reach the stomach.

Esophagus starts at the level of **6th cervical vertebra** and the lower margin of cricopharyngeus muscle. It ends in the cardia of stomach and the gastroesophageal junction is at the level of 10th thoracic vertebra. Esophagus is about 24 cm long and 2 cm wide. Parts are **cervical esophagus, thoracic esophagus and abdominal esophagus**.

The musculature of upper 1/3rd of esophagus is striated and that of the lower part is made of smooth muscles. The longitudinal muscle coat of the esophagus continues as the outer longitudinal muscle layer of stomach. There is a moderate thickening of the circular and longitudinal muscles in the lower end of esophagus. This lower 2-5 cm of the esophagus, half lying in the thorax and half in the abdomen, functions as a sphincter. It is a physiological sphincter and not an anatomical sphincter and it is referred to as **inferior esophageal sphincter or lower esophageal sphincter or gastroesophageal sphincter**.

Function of Lower Esophageal Sphincter (LES)

It is believed that this sphincter prevents regurgitation of acidic gastric contents into the esophagus. It remains closed and relaxes only during swallowing. The intrathoracic pressure is low when compared to the high intra-abdominal pressure. So, there is a tendency for the gastric contents to regurgitate into the esophagus. The tonic contraction of the lower esophageal sphincter at rest is **myogenic**.

Upper Esophageal Sphincter

In addition to the lower esophageal sphincter, there is a physiological sphincter in the upper part of esophagus called **upper esophageal sphincter** which remains normally contracted in between meals. It is formed of cricopharyngeus and inferior pharyngeal constrictor muscle and is under voluntary control. Otherwise, air may be forced into the esophagus during inspiration since the resting pressure in the esophagus is 5-10 mm Hg less than that in the pharynx. It also prevents food and secretions from entering the trachea. The resting contraction of the upper esophageal sphincter is **neurogenic**. It is supplied by glossopharyngeal and vagus nerves. There is continuous firing of the somatic nerves innervating this area and the neurotransmitter is **acetylcholine**. Prior to swallowing, the upper sphincter relaxes.

Factors that Prevent Regurgitation of Gastric Contents into Esophagus

- Inferior esophageal sphincter
- Angulation of esophagus as it passes through the diaphragm.
- A rosette like formation of loose gastric mucosa at the cardia.
- Diaphragmatic crus which surround the lower esophageal sphincter.

Histology

The mucosa of esophagus is smooth and pale in color. It is lined by **stratified squamous epithelium**. Two types of glands are seen in the esophagus:
1. **Simple mucous glands** which are distributed throughout the entire length of the tube.
2. **Compound mucous glands,** also known as **cardiac glands** because they are identical with the cardiac glands of stomach. They are found at both ends of the esophagus. The mucus secreted by the upper glands prevents mucosal excoriation by the food entering the esophagus while the glands in the lower end protect the esophageal wall from digestion by gastric juices that often reflux from the stomach back into the lower esophagus. **Peptic ulcer** at times may occur at the gastric end of esophagus leading to **heartburns**. Disordered lower esophageal sphincter tone is a major cause of **esophageal reflux**, presenting as heartburn.

Innervation of Esophagus

- Intrinsic innervation of esophagus is by the enteric nervous system (**ENS**).
- Extrinsic is through ANS, **parasympathetic supply** through **vagus** and **sympathetic** from T_4 to T_6 segments of spinal cord. Sympathetic fibers also pass through vagus.

Functions of Esophagus

- Transport of food bolus from mouth to the stomach, achieved by peristaltic contractions of the esophagus.

- Prevention of retrograde flow of gastrointestinal contents by the two esophageal sphincters which remain closed in between swallows. The upper esophageal sphincter remains closed by the elastic properties of its wall and by tonic contraction of the cricopharyngeus and inferior constrictor of pharynx. This is due to continuous excitation of neurons which innervate these muscles. Lower esophageal sphincter remains closed because of its intrinsic myogenic tone.

MULTIPLE CHOICE QUESTIONS

1. Highest concentration of K^+ is seen in:
   a. Saliva
   b. Gastric juice
   c. Bile
   d. Pancreatic secretion

2. The proportion of total salivary secretion contributed by the submandibular glands is:
   a. 25% b. 5%
   c. 75% d. 90%

3. For salivary secretion to occur by conditioned reflex:
   a. Food should be placed in the mouth
   b. Previous experience with the food evoking the secretion is not necessary
   c. Synapses between taste center and salivary nuclei should be intact
   d. Parasympathetic innervation of the salivary gland should be intact

4. The gland which contribute maximum volume of salivary juice is:
   a. Parotid gland b. Submandibular gland
   c. Sublingual gland d. Buccal glands

5. Excessive salivation is known as:
   a. Sialorrhea b. Xerostomia
   c. Aptyalism d. Sialolithiasis

6. Secretion that is exclusively under neural control is:
   a. Pancreatic juice b. Saliva
   c. Gastric juice d. Bile

7. All are true of the parasympathetic fibers innervating the parotid gland, *except*:
   a. They arise from inferior salivary nucleus
   b. They traverse the IX cranial nerve
   c. Stimulation increases the rate of secretion
   d. Acetylcholine is the transmitter at the endings

8. Dryness of mouth is called:
   a. Xerostomia b. Xerophthalmia
   c. Sialorrhea d. Sialolithiasis

9. Lower esophageal sphincter:
   a. Has no tonic activity
   b. Has a tone provided by the sympathetic system
   c. Relaxes on increasing abdominal pressure
   d. Relaxes ahead of the peristaltic wave

10. In the gastrointestinal tract serosal layer is absent in the:
    a. Esophagus b. Jejunum
    c. Ileum d. Colon

11. BER is exhibited by all the following areas of gut, *except*:
    a. Duodenum b. Jejunum
    c. Colon d. Esophagus

ANSWERS

1. a 2. c 3. d 4. b 5. a
6. b 7. b 8. a 9. d 10. a
11. d

Stomach

CHAPTER 46

LEARNING OBJECTIVES
- Explain the functions of stomach
- Describe the composition and functions of gastric juice
- Draw and explain the mechanism of secretion of HCl by the parietal cells
- Explain the regulation of gastric acid secretion
- Discuss the pathophysiology of acid-peptic disease (peptic ulcer) and its management
- Discuss the pathophysiology of vomiting and gastro-esophageal reflux disease

INTRODUCTION

Stomach is a muscular hollow organ located on the left side of the upper abdomen. It is located between the esophagus and the small intestine. Food is stored in the stomach after it is properly chewed in the mouth and swallowed through the esophagus. In the stomach, food is mixed with acid, mucus and pepsin. Food is churned by the stomach through muscular contraction of the wall reducing the volume of the bolus which is a mass of chewed up food. After partial digestion, food is released at a controlled, steady rate into the duodenum through the pyloric sphincter where further digestion occurs. The food that leaves the stomach is called chyme.

FUNCTIONS OF STOMACH

- **Storage function:** Stomach acts as a reservoir for the ingested food which is mixed with saliva. This is due to the property of **receptive relaxation** mediated by vagus. Maximum capacity of stomach is 1.5 L.
- **Mechanical function:** The digestive secretions of stomach aided by mechanical activity of the gastric musculature convert food into a homogenous semi-fluid mass, **the chyme**. Larger particles of food are broken down into smaller particles by the strong contractions of the stomach.
- Stomach regulates the passage of chyme into the small intestine. Food is released at a controlled, steady rate into the duodenum to avoid the rapid delivery of highly acidic or hyperosmolar substances into the small intestine so that, proper digestion and absorption occur.
- **Digestive function:** Salivary digestion is completed in the stomach. The enzymes of gastric juice like pepsin help in further digestion of food.
- **Protective function:** HCl present in gastric juice destroys microorganisms present in food.
- **Hemopoietic function:** Intrinsic factor in the gastric juice is necessary for the absorption of vitamin B_{12}, a maturation factor for erythropoiesis, whose deficiency leads to *pernicious anemia*. HCl is necessary for the proper absorption of iron, the deficiency of which leads to *iron deficiency anemia*. HCl converts ferric form of iron to the ferrous form which is the absorbable form of iron.

FUNCTIONAL ANATOMY OF STOMACH

In humans the stomach is divided into four portions **(Fig. 46.1)**:
1. Cardia or cardiac area
2. Fundus
3. Body or corpus
4. Pyloric area which consists of three parts:

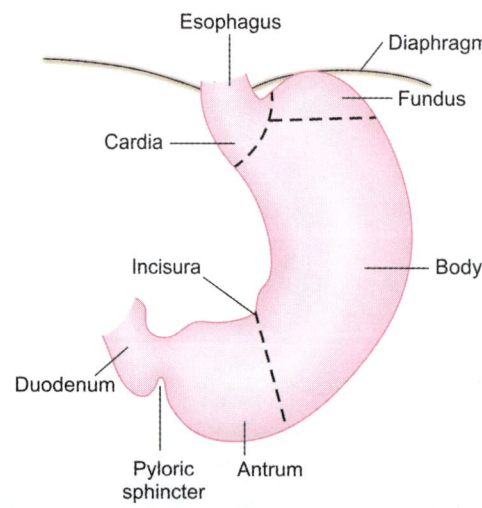

Fig. 46.1: Parts of stomach.

a. Pyloric antrum
b. Pyloric canal
c. Pyloric sphincter or pylorus

The **cardiac area** is located just distal to the entry of esophagus and the circular muscle layer is thickened to form the **cardiac sphincter**. **Fundus** is the dome-shaped portion of the stomach that extends above the level of cardia.

The **body** of the stomach is the **largest** portion occupying about 80% of the entire stomach. The **pyloric area** is divided into pyloric antrum, a narrow pyloric canal and pylorus which open into the duodenum. At the pylorus, the circular muscle fibers are considerably thickened to form the **pyloric sphincter**.

The mucous membrane of stomach is **red and velvety** (**Fig. 46.8**). Blood flow to the gastric mucosa is very high. When the stomach is empty, the gastric mucosa is thrown into a number of longitudinal folds called **rugae**. These are obliterated when stomach is full.

The muscular coat of stomach is made up of three layers. They are **circular, longitudinal and an oblique layer**. The oblique layer extends from the cardia along the lesser curvature as a fan-like structure to the pyloric area. It is seen inner to the circular layer and is an incomplete coat and towards its termination it is attached to the circular muscle fibers. Purpose of this layer is to regulate the size of the lesser curvature.

HISTOLOGY

The **gastric epithelium** is composed of a single layer of columnar cells called **surface mucous cells** which secrete thick, visible or insoluble, viscid mucus about 1–2 mm in thickness. This lines the mucous membrane and protects it from acids and enzymes in the gastric juice.

The gastric epithelial surface shows a number of small openings called **gastric pits** or **gastric foveolae** (sing: foveolus). About 3–7 gastric glands open into a single gastric pit (**Fig. 46.2**). The glands of the stomach are tubular glands and are of three kinds. They are:
1. Cardiac glands
2. Oxyntic/fundic/parietal glands
3. Pyloric glands

Cardiac Glands

The cardiac glands are found in the cardiac area and are **coiled** glands lined by mucous cells and scattered endocrine cells. The mucous cells secrete alkaline mucus.

Oxyntic or Parietal or Fundic Glands

Oxyntic glands are found in the fundus and over the greater part of the body of the stomach. These glands are fairly **long and straight** (tubular) and each gland is divided into three areas:
1. Isthmus containing surface mucous cells and parietal cells.
2. Neck containing mucous neck cells and parietal cells.
3. Base containing chief cells and some parietal cells.

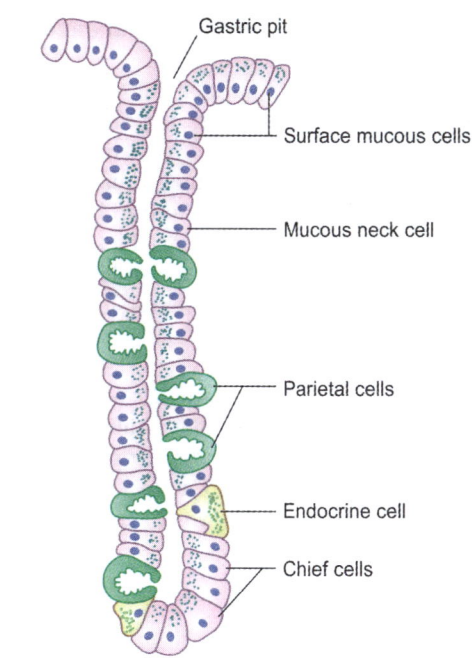

Fig. 46.2: Structure of gastric gland in the fundus of stomach.

Table 46.1: Cell types in the oxyntic glands and their secretions.	
Cell type	**Secretions**
Chief cells	Pepsinogens, lipase, rennin
Parietal (oxyntic) cells	HCl, intrinsic factor of castle
Mucous cells	Mucus
Endocrine cells or APUD cells	Hormones like gastrin, somatostatin, VIP, etc.
Enterochromaffin-like cells	Histamine, serotonin

Oxyntic gland is lined by four types of cells (**Fig. 46.2 and Table 46.1**):
1. Chief cells or zymogen cells or peptic cells.
2. Parietal cells or oxyntic cells.
3. Mucous cells which includes mucous neck cells and surface mucous cells.
4. Endocrine cells or APUD cells.

Peptic Cells or Chief Cells

Chief cells contain abundant endoplasmic reticulum and apical zymogen granules which are **basophilic**. These cells produce **pepsinogen, rennin, gelatinase and collagenase**.

Parietal Cells

Parietal cells are seen towards the periphery of the gland. Each cell is pyramidal or triangular in shape, relatively large and the basal side bulges into the lamina propria and is **acidophilic** due to large number of densely packed mitochondria. The mitochondria supply energy to drive the apical H^+-K^+ ATPase or proton pump, that moves H^+ out of the parietal cell against a concentration gradient of more than a million-fold. The parietal cell also contains small amounts of endoplasmic reticulum involved in the synthesis of intrinsic factor.

Electron microscopy of a parietal cell shows a number of intracellular secretory canaliculi. The microvilli of these canaliculi are long, numerous and face the lumen of the stomach. They increase the surface area of the apical membrane. H$^+$-K$^+$ATPase or proton pump involved in the final step of H$^+$ secretion is located on the cell membrane of these canaliculi. Intrinsic factor is also localized on this membrane. Since the parietal cells are situated deeper in the gland, they are drained by intercellular canaliculi into the lumen of the gland.

The peripheral location of the parietal cells gives a beaded appearance to the oxyntic glands after staining. One-third of cells of oxyntic glands are parietal cells. Parietal cells produce **HCl, H$_2$O and intrinsic factor of Castle**. Oxyntic cells also release a hormone called **ghrelin** which increases appetite.

Mucous Cells

Mucous Neck Cells

Mucous neck cells produce **soluble mucus** and are present in the neck region as well as the base of the gland. These cells also secrete some pepsinogen.

The mucous neck cells show high degree of mitosis and after maturation they move upwards towards the isthmus to line the gastric pit as well as to form the surface columnar epithelium on the luminal surface of stomach. Others travel downwards into the glands and differentiate into parietal and peptic cells. The mucosal cells of stomach are replaced within about 5 days. A gastrin inhibitory substance is present in the soluble mucus, called gastrone.

Surface Mucous Cells

The surface mucous cells secrete **insoluble mucus** or **visible mucus** and **HCO$_3$**$^-$. The mucous cells absorb carbohydrate from blood stream and process them into special glycoproteins called **mucins**. When hydrated, mucins form mucus. Gastric mucus is extruded by exocytosis, apical expulsion and cell exfoliation. Gastric mucin consists of coiled threads and they become filled with large volumes of water, some lipid and protein on the luminal surface. It is viscous and has elastic properties. This mucus forms a **flexible gel** that coats the mucosa. Mucus acts as a lubricant for food particles in their passage throughout the gut.

Enteroendocrine Cells or Amine Precursor Uptake and Decarboxylation (APUD) Cells and ECL Cells

More than 15 types of enteroendocrine cells which secrete hormones have been identified in the mucosa of stomach, small intestine and colon. Some of these cells produce only one hormone like G cells which secrete gastrin, S cells which secrete secretin, etc. The cells that secrete serotonin or histamine are called enterochromaffin-like cells (ECL cells).

APUD cells are endocrine-paracrine cells present at the base of the gastric glands. They produce **somatostatin, glucagon, etc**. Enterochromaffin-like cells lie in close proximity to the parietal cells and secrete **histamine and serotonin**.

Pyloric Glands

The pyloric glands located in the pyloric region are short and **tortuous** glands lined by mucous cells, **argentaffin cells** (enterochromaffin cells) and **G cells**. Argentaffin cells are stained by silver stains and produce **serotonin**. G cells produce **gastrin**, a gastrointestinal hormone. **Somatostatin**-containing cells are also seen and these endocrine-paracrine cells are in close proximity to G cells, chief cells, etc., and exert a local paracrine inhibitory effect on these cells.

■ GASTRIC MUCOSAL BARRIER

Gastric mucosal barrier protects the gastric mucosa from auto-digestion by the acid-pepsin mixture present in the gastric lumen. Factors contributing to the gastric mucosal barrier are the following:

The surface mucous cells secrete **visible mucus and HCO$_3$**$^-$. This HCO$_3$$^-$ is trapped in the mucus gel and this layer is 0.1–0.2 mm thick. It coats the gastric epithelial surface, and the pH at the surface of the epithelial cells becomes 6–7. This layer of mucus is referred to as **unstirred layer** or mucus-HCO$_3$$^-$ barrier. This layer offers a barrier between the acid-pepsin mixture and the epithelium so that the epithelium is not directly exposed to the acid. HCl secreted by the parietal cells in the gastric glands crosses this barrier in finger-like channels, leaving the rest of the gel layer intact. The space between the gel and the surface epithelium contains HCO$_3$$^-$ and therefore the pH immediately adjacent to the surface epithelial cell is neutral, while pH within the gastric lumen is 1–2 (**Fig. 46.3**). So, the pH of acid-pepsin mixture rises more and more as it come nearer and nearer the epithelium. The proteolytic ability of pepsin becomes ineffective at pH above 5.

The gel thickness is increased by prostaglandin E and decreased by non-steroidal anti-inflammatory drugs (NSAIDs) like aspirin.

❖ The surface membranes of the mucosal cells and the **tight junctions** between the cells are also part of the mucosal barrier that protects the gastric epithelium from damage. Substances that tend to disrupt the barrier and cause gastric irritation include alcohol, vinegar, aspirin, bile salts, other NSAID, etc.

❖ **Prostaglandins**, especially PGE$_2$ and PGI$_2$, have a cytoprotective action on gastric mucosa. Prostaglandin stimulates secretion of mucus and HCO$_3$$^-$. It also causes vigorous protein synthesis and thus helps in cell renewal. Aspirin and related drugs inhibit prostaglandin synthesis.

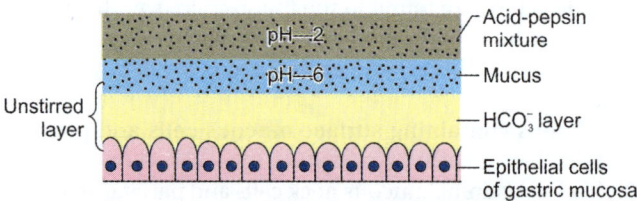

Fig. 46.3: Mucosal barrier of stomach.

- The duodenal mucosa also serves as a protective barrier from acid and peptic damage as well as ingested toxic substances to the duodenum especially the first part of duodenum which is exposed to highly acidic chyme.
- Resistance of the gastric mucosa to auto digestion is also provided by the presence of acid-resistant **trefoil peptides** in the mucosa. It has a three-loop structure and the loops are held together by disulfide bonds and so it looks like a 3-leaf clover. These peptides are also found in the rest of GIT, hypothalamus, pituitary and in rapidly proliferating tissues. Deficiency of trefoil peptides leads to histologically abnormal gastric and intestinal mucosa and high incidence of benign as well as malignant mucosal tumors.
- The gastric mucus also contains blood group substances in secretors which protect the mucosa from acid-pepsin mixture.

INNERVATION OF STOMACH

Parasympathetic Innervation

- **Receptors** are in the mucosa, submucosa and deeper layers of stomach.
- **Afferent:** Vagus
- **Center:** Dorsal nucleus of vagus in the floor of 4th ventricle.
- **Efferent and effectors:** Preganglionic fibers come through the right and left vagus, ganglia are present in the Auerbach's plexus (part of enteric nervous system) and short postganglionic fibers reach the glandular cells and smooth muscles of stomach. Thus, the action of parasympathetic stimulation is through ENS.

Parasympathetic stimulation causes increased secretion and increased motility of stomach.

Sympathetic Innervation

- **Receptors** are present in the wall of stomach.
- **Afferent** fibers pass through the posterior nerve roots in spinal cord without synapsing in the sympathetic ganglia. Pain sensation from stomach is carried by sympathetic afferent fibers.
- **Center** is the lateral horn cells of T_5–T_{10} segments of spinal cord.
- **Efferent** preganglionic fibers emerge in the anterior spinal nerve roots and reach the ganglia of thoracic sympathetic chain. Some of the fibers synapse here and most of the fibers synapse in the ganglia of **celiac plexus**. Post-ganglionic fibers enter the stomach along its arterial supply.

Sympathetic stimulation causes decreased secretion and decreased motility of stomach.

GASTRIC JUICE

> **PY4.2:** Describe the composition, mechanism of secretion, functions, and regulation of saliva, gastric, pancreatic, intestinal juices and bile secretion.

Gastric juice is a combination of secretion from gastric glands and surface epithelial cells.

Table 46.2: Composition of gastric juice.

Inorganic constituents	Organic constituents
HCl	• Pepsinogen I, II, III • Rennin or chymosin, gastric lipase
Na^+, K^+, Ca^{2+}, Mg^{2+}	• Gelatinase, amylase, urease, carbonic anhydrase • Intrinsic factor of Castle
PO_4^{3-}, SO_4^{2-}, HCO_3^-	• Blood group substances in secretors • Lysozyme, carbonic anhydrase • Soluble and visible mucus

- Rate of secretion: 1.5–2.5 L/day
- pH: 1–2
- Specific gravity: 1.002–1.009
- Composition: 99.5% water, 0.5% solids (inorganic and organic—**Table 46.2**).

Pepsinogens I, II, III

Pepsinogen is the inactive proenzyme or precursor of **pepsin** which is the principal proteolytic enzyme of gastric juice. It is produced by chief cells of gastric gland and stored in the zymogen granules in the inactive state.

In the presence of acids, especially HCl, or at pH values <2, pepsinogens are converted to active pepsins and further activation is autocatalytic, i.e., pepsin in turn can activate pepsinogen.

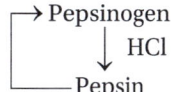

Pepsinogen I is secreted by chief cells of fundic glands and the other types are secreted by other gastric glands and also by the Brunner's glands of duodenum. Some amount of pepsinogen I is absorbed into the blood stream and is excreted through urine as **uropepsinogen**.

The optimal pH for the action of pepsin is around 2 (1.6–3.2). Pepsin becomes inactive due to denaturation at pH of 5 or more and also at high temperature.

Action of Pepsin

Pepsin is a proteolytic enzyme and it acts on peptide linkages between aromatic and aliphatic amino acids.

$$\text{Protein} \xrightarrow{\text{Pepsin}} \text{Proteoses, peptones, polypeptides}$$

Rennin or Chymosin

Rennin is a milk clotting (curdling) enzyme present in the gastric juice of young animals, but is probably absent in humans. *In humans, digestion of milk is done by pepsin.* Rennin has an optimum pH of 6–6.5 and requires Ca^{2+} for its action.

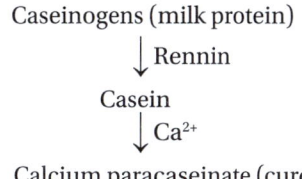

Gastric Lipase

Gastric lipase is a **tributerase** which acts mainly on **butter fat**. It acts on triglycerides converting it into fatty acid and glycerol. Optimum pH is 4–5 and is inactivated at pH less than 3.5. Compared to pancreatic lipase, *it is a very weak lipase*.

Gelatinase helps to liquefy some of the proteoglycans in meat.

Gastric amylase plays a minor role in the digestion of starch.

Intrinsic Factor of Castle

Intrinsic factor of Castle is produced by the **parietal cells**. It is a glycoprotein necessary for the absorption of cyanocobalamin or **vitamin B_{12}** from the ileum. Deficiency of B_{12} leads to a specific megaloblastic anemia called **pernicious anemia** characterized by the appearance in the blood stream of large immature red cell precursors called **megaloblasts**. There is also associated deterioration of certain sensory pathways in the central nervous system referred to as **subacute combined degeneration**.

There are two vitamin B_{12} binding proteins secreted by cells of GIT, intrinsic factor of Castle and **haptocorrin**. Haptocorrin is a glycoprotein produced by gastrointestinal cells and by the salivary gland, and it has higher affinity for B_{12} than intrinsic factor. Haptocorrin is also called **R-protein** (rapidly migrating glycoproteins during electrophoresis).

In the small intestine, R-protein-vitamin B_{12} complex is cleaved by pancreatic proteases and thus all vitamin B_{12} is effectively transferred to intrinsic factor (IF) to facilitate absorption of B_{12} in the terminal ileum.

The IF-B_{12} complex binds to specific receptors in the ileum and is absorbed by endocytosis. Vitamin B_{12} is transferred from IF to **transcobalamin II**, another B_{12} binding protein that transports cyanocobalamin in plasma.

In totally gastrectomized patients, in patients with gastric atrophy and chronic gastritis there will be deficiency of intrinsic factor leading to pernicious anemia. The condition is treated with parenteral administration (injections) of vitamin B_{12}. Oral administration is ineffective due to the absence of intrinsic factor.

Autoimmune destruction of parietal cells produces not only **achlorhydria** *due to lack of acid secretion but also pernicious anemia due to vitamin B_{12} deficiency.*

Blood Group Substances

In secretors, gastric juice contains agglutinogens found in the RBC membrane. They act against digestion of gastric and duodenal mucous membrane by the acid-pepsin mixture and thus contribute to gastric mucosal barrier.

Carbonic Anhydrase

Carbonic anhydrase is present in small amounts in gastric juice. Its presence is due to disintegration of desquamated cells, especially parietal cells, which contain a large concentration of carbonic anhydrase concerned with the formation of HCl.

HCO_3^-

Bicarbonates are secreted by the surface epithelial cells of stomach. HCO_3^- is present in the unstirred layer of mucus as well as in between the unstirred layer and surface epithelial cells. Thus, a pH gradient is established that ranges from pH 1–2 at the luminal side to pH 6–7 at the surface of epithelial cells. The HCO_3^- neutralizes the acidity and protects the gastric epithelium from damage. The proteolytic ability of pepsin is lost at pH more than 5.

Mechanism of Secretion of HCO_3^-

- By Cl^-/HCO_3^- antiport mechanism. This active transport of HCO_3^- into the lumen in exchange for Cl^- is stimulated by glucagon and inhibited by furosemide.
- By active transport of HCO_3^- which is Cl independent and is stimulated by prostaglandin and cAMP
- Through paracellular route.

HCl

HCl is secreted by the parietal cells into the intracellular canaliculi.

Functions of HCl in Stomach

- HCl converts inactive pepsinogen to active pepsin. It provides necessary pH for the action of pepsin to start protein digestion.
- It kills many ingested bacteria.
- Due to the presence of HCl, gastric chyme is acidic in nature and when this acid chyme enters the small intestine it stimulates release of gastrointestinal hormones like secretin, cholecystokinin-pancreozymin (CCK-PZ), etc., which help in further digestion of food. These enzymes stimulate the flow of bile and pancreatic juice.
- HCl is necessary for the absorption of iron from intestine. Dietary iron is in the ferric form and the absorbable form is **ferrous form**. HCl converts ferric form to ferrous form and thus helps in iron absorption. This is accomplished by dissolving the dietary iron and permitting it to form soluble complexes with ascorbic acid that help in the reduction of iron to ferrous form. This is the reason for the *occurrence of iron deficiency anemia as a frequent complication of partial gastrectomy.*

Mechanism of Secretion of HCl

Parietal cell secretion is an isotonic solution of pure HCl (**0.17N HCl**) that contains 150 mEq of Cl^- and 150 mEq of H^+ per liter. Since the acid is formed in the **intracellular canaliculi**, the pH of the cytoplasm of parietal cell is 7–7.2, whereas that of pure parietal cell secretion in the intracellular canaliculi is 0.87. Since HCl is not formed in the cytoplasm, the parietal cell is not damaged due to very high acidity.

The parietal cells are polarized with an apical membrane facing the lumen of gastric glands and a basolateral membrane in contact with the interstitial fluid. Intracellular canaliculi extend from the apical surface into the cell and it contains **H^+-K^+ ATPase** and **chloride channels** on their walls. At rest, the cell also contains abundant **tubulovesicular structures** in the cytoplasm with H^+-K^+ ATPase molecules in their walls. When the cells are stimulated, the tubulovesicular structures move to the apical membrane and fuse with it inserting more number of H^+-K^+ ATPase molecules into the membrane. This forms numerous microvilli that project into the lumen of the canaliculi. The canalicular lumen contains extracellular fluid (ECF). There are also Cl^--HCO_3^- exchangers and Na^+-K^+ ATPases in the basolateral membrane of parietal cells.

When the parietal cell is stimulated, there is hydration of CO_2 in the cell catalyzed by the enzyme **carbonic anhydrase** to form H_2CO_3. Carbonic anhydrase is present abundantly in the parietal cell cytoplasm. H_2CO_3 dissociates to form H^+ and HCO_3^-. The HCO_3^- is extruded into the interstitium by an **antiport** mechanism in the basolateral membrane of parietal cell. This antiporter exchanges HCO_3^- for Cl^- which is the most abundant anion in the interstitial fluid **(Fig. 46.4)**. The HCO_3^- enters the blood in the capillaries and combines with Na^+ to form $NaHCO_3$. This raises the pH of blood leaving the stomach. This **alkaline tide** of HCO_3^-- rich blood flowing through the surface capillaries in the gastric mucosa provides a last line of defense against acid mediated mucosal injury.

The H^+ formed by the dissociation of H_2CO_3 is pumped out into the canaliculi in exchange for K^+ by H^+-K^+ ATPase and the energy for this is provided by the hydrolysis of ATP. Tight junctions between the mucosal cells normally keep the H^+ within the gastric lumen and prevent back diffusion of H^+ into the gastric mucosa. Back diffusion of H^+ usually occurs in gastritis where the mucosal barrier is disrupted.

Cl^- is also extruded into the canaliculi from the cytoplasm of the cell down its electrochemical gradient through channels that are activated by cAMP in the apical membrane. The H^+ and Cl^- present in the canaliculi combine to form HCl and is secreted into the lumen of the gland.

The events can be summarized as follows.
- CO_2 combines with H_2O in the presence of carbonic anhydrase in the parietal cell cytoplasm to form H_2CO_3.
- H_2CO_3 dissociates to form H^+ and HCO_3^-.
- H^+ passes into the canaliculi in exchange for K^+ by H^+-K^+ ATPase (proton pump).
- HCO_3^- moves into the interstitial space in exchange for Cl^- which enters the parietal cell.
- Cl^- is extruded into the canaliculi through Cl^- channels passively.
- The H^+ and Cl^- in the canaliculi combine to form HCl in the canaliculi of the parietal cell.

Respiratory quotient of stomach and postprandial alkaline tide: *Stomach is the only organ that has a **negative respiratory quotient (RQ)***, i.e., the amount of CO_2 in arterial blood is greater than the amount of CO_2 in gastric venous blood. Normal RQ in other organs is 0.8 because CO_2 is being added to the venous blood that is draining the tissue. So, the venous blood contains more CO_2 than the arterial blood that is reaching the tissue. Whereas, in parietal cell, the CO_2 formed due to cell metabolism is being utilized for the formation of H_2CO_3. It is not released into the venous blood as in the case of other organs. In addition, the CO_2 from the venous blood diffuses into the parietal cell when the amount of HCl production has to be increased.

After a meal, the gastric acid secretion is elevated and for one HCl formed in the parietal cell, one HCO_3^- reaches the blood. This raises the pH of systemic blood or the blood becomes alkaline after a meal. To bring back the pH of blood to normal, excess HCO_3^- is excreted through urine. *This is the explanation for passing alkaline urine after a heavy meal.* This phenomenon is known as **postprandial alkaline tide**.

Factors Affecting HCl Secretion (Table 46.3) or Regulation of Gastric Acid Secretion

Factors Stimulating Acid Secretion
- Nervous factors
  - Vagus through long vago-vagal reflex
  - Local autonomic reflexes mediated via the ENS (short reflexes)
- Hormonal factors
  - Gastrin
  - Histamine
- Miscellaneous factors

Nervous factors: All the secretory nerves ending on the glandular cells release **acetylcholine** at their nerve endings except those innervating the G cells of the pyloric glands. Here there is an interneuron which secretes **gastrin releasing peptide (GRP) or bombesin** as the neurotransmitter. GRP stimulates the release of gastrin from G cells.

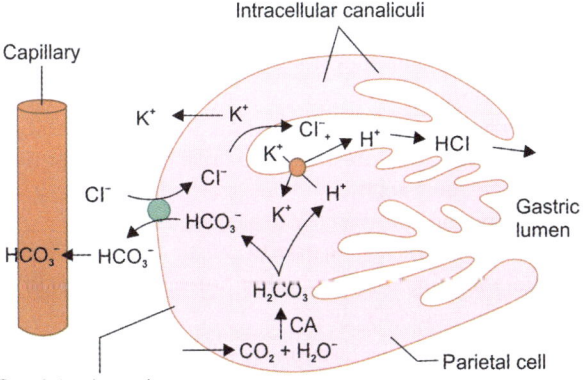

Fig. 46.4: Mechanism of HCl secretion by parietal cell in the stomach.

Table 46.3: Factors affecting HCl secretion.	
Factors stimulating acid secretion	*Factors inhibiting acid secretion*
• Parasympathetic stimulation	• Sympathetic stimulation
• Gastrin, histamine, acetylcholine	• Secretin, CCK-PZ, somatostatin, GIP, VIP, enterogastrones, chalone, PG_E
• Hypoglycemia	• Hyperglycemia
• Amino acids, caffeine, alcohol, steroids, calcium salts, NSAID like aspirin, etc.	• Emotional states like fear, depression, etc.
• Anxiety, hostility, anger, frustration	• Nausea

Vagus $\xrightarrow{ACh}$ Interneuron $\xrightarrow{GRP}$ G cells ⟶ Gastrin
Increased HCl secretion ⟵ Parietal cell stimulation ⟵

Acetylcholine stimulates all the cells of the gastric glands. Acetylcholine acts via M_3 **muscarinic receptors** on the glandular cell membrane and these receptors increase intracellular free Ca^{2+} **(Fig. 46.5)**.

Vagus stimulates HCl secretion through **long vago-vagal reflexes** that are transmitted from the gastric mucosa all the way to the brainstem and then back to stomach through vagus nerve.

Local reflexes mediated by enteric nervous system (ENS) are short reflexes that originate locally and are transmitted through the ENS.

❖ Stimuli responsible for local reflexes:
- Distension of stomach
- Tactile stimuli
- Chemical stimuli especially amino acids, peptides and acids.

❖ Efferents in both types of reflexes (short and long reflexes) stimulate acid secretion by:
- Directly stimulating the oxyntic cells.
- Indirectly by stimulating gastrin release from the antral glands.

Hormonal factors: The main hormones that stimulate gastric acid secretion are **gastrin and histamine (Fig. 46.5)**.

❖ **Gastrin:** Gastrin is produced by **G cells** in the antral portion of the gastric mucosa. Gastrin secreted by the G cells is absorbed into the blood stream and carried to the oxyntic glands where it stimulates the parietal cells strongly to secrete HCl as much as 8 times the basal secretion. Small amounts of HCl, in turn, stimulate the enteric reflex mechanism to cause further secretion of HCl. But, *excess HCl decreases gastrin secretion by a feedback mechanism.* Gastrin acts via **gastrin receptors** present in the basolateral membrane of the parietal cell. Gastrin exerts its effect by increasing intracellular Ca^{2+} **(Fig. 46.5)**.

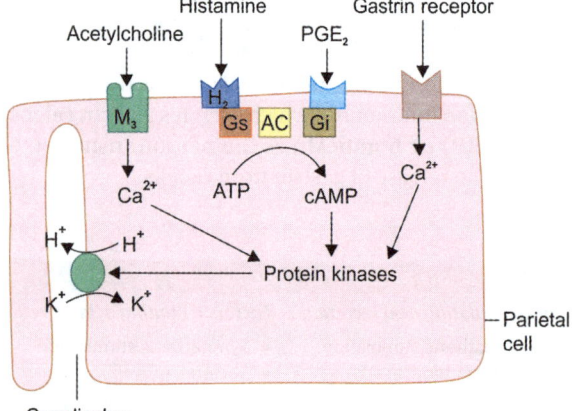

Fig. 46.5: Regulation of gastric acid secretion by the parietal cell. Histamine acts via Gs which increases adenylyl cyclase activity. PGE_2 acts via Gi to decrease adenylyl cyclase (AC) activity thereby inhibiting gastric acid secretion. Acetylcholine and gastrin stimulate acid secretion by increasing intracellular Ca^{2+}.

❖ **Histamine:** Histamine is produced by certain cells in the gastric mucosa that resemble mast cells called **enterochromaffin-like cells (ECL cells)**. Histamine secretion by ECL cells is stimulated by gastrin, and this is the principal way in which gastrin stimulates H^+ secretion in the parietal cell. Histamine binds to H_2 **receptors** on the basolateral surface of the parietal cell membrane and these receptors activate **adenylate cyclase or adenylyl cyclase** and increase intracellular **cAMP via Gs** (stimulatory G protein). Histamine, in turn, augments the H^+ secretory effect of gastrin and acetylcholine in the parietal cell. ECL cells are the predominant endocrine cell type present in the acid-secreting portion of stomach.

Gastrin, histamine and acetyl choline are the three agonists of the parietal cells. They act synergistically. Each binds to distinct receptors on the basolateral membrane of the parietal cell. Gastrin and acetylcholine promote secretion by increasing free calcium concentration in the cytoplasm. Histamine acts by increasing intracellular cAMP level.

There is a **multiplicative effect** of acetylcholine, gastrin and histamine in stimulating acid secretion in the parietal cells. If the three receptors are stimulated simultaneously, copious amounts of acid are secreted than when each receptor functions alone, e.g., if the action of histamine is blocked by cimetidine, an H_2 receptor blocker, neither acetylcholine nor gastrin can then cause significant increase in acid secretion. Thus, *histamine is a necessary* **cofactor** *for significant acid secretion in the stomach.*

Miscellaneous factors:
❖ **Hypoglycemia** acts via vagal efferents to stimulate gastric acid secretion.
❖ Various emotions also have strong influences on gastric juice secretion. Anxiety, hostility, anger, frustration, etc., stimulate acid secretion. This is the reason for the increased frequency of peptic ulcer in chronically anxious business executives.
❖ Substances like amino acids, caffeine, alcohol, calcium salts and drugs like cortisol also stimulate gastric acid secretion.
❖ Thought of food, distension of the stomach and protein ingestion also stimulates acid secretion.

Factors Inhibiting Acid Secretion

Acid secretion by stomach is also controlled by mechanisms that inhibit acid secretion. These mechanisms may be neural or chemical and may originate from the stomach itself or from proximal parts of small intestine. Some of the inhibitory influences are extra-intestinal and arise from higher neural centers. They may act by:

❖ Inhibiting the parietal cells directly.
❖ Inhibiting the release of gastrin.
❖ Stimulating the release of other hormones which in turn inhibit the parietal cells.

1. **PGE** inhibits acid secretion by activating Gi (inhibitory G protein) on the parietal cell membrane. Gi inhibits adenylyl cyclase activity, thereby decreasing intracellular cAMP **(Fig. 46.5)**. There is incidence of ulcers in patients

taking anti-inflammatory drugs like aspirin that inhibit prostaglandin synthesis.
2. There is also a **feedback inhibition** of gastric glands by **excess HCl** in the stomach. Reduction in the intragastric pH to 3 produces partial inhibition of gastrin release and reduction of pH to 1.5 or less, completely blocks the release of gastrin in response to almost all stimuli. The gastrin mechanism for stimulating gastric acid secretion becomes blocked by two mechanisms:
   a. Blocking the secretion of gastrin by G cells by a direct effect.
   b. By an inhibitory nervous reflex that inhibits gastrin secretion.

   Excess H⁺ causes release of an inhibitory chemical messenger, **chalone** that inhibits parietal cell activity directly.
3. **Hormones** *like GIP, VIP, somatostatin, etc., inhibit gastric acid secretion.* **Somatostatin**-containing endocrine-paracrine cells (D cells) have long cytoplasmic extensions that contain somatostatin. They terminate in close proximity to effector cells such as G cells, chief cells and parietal cells. It exerts a local paracrine inhibitory effect via these cellular extensions and is the most important factor responsible for the acid-induced feedback control inhibition of gastrin release. D cells are present in the antral mucosa.
4. **Intestinal factors** like **enterogastric reflex** also cause inhibition of gastric secretion.
5. **Duodenal hormones** like **secretin and CCK-PZ** also inhibit gastric acid secretion.
6. **Sympathetic stimulation** causes decrease in gastric secretion indirectly by decreasing the blood flow to the mucosa.
7. **Emotional states** like fear and depression decrease gastric secretion. Sensations of **nausea** are associated with reduced acid output. These central neural factors originating from limbic system, hypothalamic and cortical level reduce gastric acid secretion by reducing the normal tonic stimulation of vagus or by over activity of sympathetic nerves to stomach.
8. Hyperglycemia, hypertonic fluids or fat in the duodenum inhibit gastric acid secretion.

PHASES OF GASTRIC JUICE SECRETION

❖ Inter-digestive phase or basal secretion
❖ Cephalic or psychic phase
❖ Gastric phase
❖ Intestinal phase

Interdigestive Phase or Basal Secretion

Basal secretion occurs in the absence of environmental and gastrointestinal stimulation. It is approximately 10% of maximal acid secretion in humans and the basal secretion occurs in between meals. A **circadian rhythm** of basal acid secretion is seen. Minimum acid secretion is seen in the morning and maximum in the evening. Rate of secretion is less than 50 mL/day. It contains more of mucus and less of pepsin and HCl.

Tonic **vagal** parasympathetic stimulation as well as small amounts of circulating **gastrin** contributes to the basal secretion. When there are strong emotional stimuli, it exceeds 50 mL and contains more of HCl and pepsin. This is believed to be one of the factors in the development of peptic ulcer. In patients with duodenal ulcers, the amount of acid secretion in the inter-digestive phase is found to be high.

The gastric acid secretory response to a meal can be divided into three phases—cephalic phase, gastric phase and intestinal phase, named according to the areas of stimulus arousal. These phases overlap.

Cephalic Phase or Psychic Phase

Sight, smell, thought or taste of appetizing food causes an increase in gastric juice secretion. This is the cephalic phase of gastric secretion which occurs even before food enters the stomach. This is a **conditioned reflex** established in the early life of the individual. *If the subject dislikes the food cephalic phase will be absent.* This secretion is also referred to as **appetite juice or ignition juice** which accounts for about 20% of the gastric juice secretion associated with food intake.

Cephalic phase was experimentally demonstrated by **Pavlov** using a technique called **sham feeding** (false feeding) in dogs. The esophagus was divided transversely and both cut ends were brought out through an opening in the neck. The food ingested by the animal escapes from the upper segment of the esophagus without reaching the stomach. But, the animal experiences all the pleasures of eating. Fresh gastric juice can be collected by introducing a catheter through the lower segment into the stomach. It was observed that there was an increase in the gastric juice secretion even though food did not reach the stomach.

Neurogenic signals that produce the cephalic phase arise from the centers of special senses in the **cortex** or in the appetite centers of **amygdala** or **hypothalamus** and reach the dorsal motor nuclei of vagus. Efferent fibers come through vagus and this phase is basically under neural control. This phase is abolished by vagotomy or by parasympatholytic drugs like atropine.

The vagal efferents from the brainstem to the stomach increase gastric acid and pepsinogen secretion by two mechanisms:
1. Directly stimulating the oxyntic glands.
2. Indirectly by increasing the release of gastrin from G cells of pyloric glands.

Resection of gastric antrum, which is the principal source of gastrin, reduces the acid secretion to sham feeding by 50%. This proves that a portion of sham-induced acid secretory response is mediated through gastrin.

Gastric Phase of Gastric Juice Secretion

Entry of food into the stomach increases gastric juice secretion that continues for several hours, i.e., as long as food remains in the stomach. This phase accounts for about 70% of total gastric juice secretion or 2/3rd of gastric juice secretion and comes to about 500–800 mL/day. *Gastric phase is mediated by neural and hormonal mechanisms.*

Neural Mechanism
Distension of stomach wall by the bulk of food stimulates stretch receptors in the stomach wall and increases gastric juice secretion by two reflexes:
1. Short intramural or local enteric reflex
2. Long vago-vagal reflex

Short Intramural or Local Enteric Reflex
The reflex arc is situated inside the gastric wall. Fibers from the receptors reach the **Meissner's or Auerbach's plexus** and synapse in the ganglion cells in the plexus. The postganglionic fibers innervate the chief cells, mucous cells, parietal cells, G cells, etc., and increase their secretion.

Long Vago-vagal Reflex
From the receptors, impulses pass through the vagus to the brainstem (dorsal motor nucleus of vagus) and efferent fibers also pass through the vagus nerve to reach the ganglion cells of enteric nervous system (ENS). The postganglionic fibers innervate different cells of gastric glands to increase gastric juice secretion.

Hormonal or Chemical Regulation
Chemical factors present in partially digested food like **amino acids, polypeptides,** etc., as well as mechanical distension of pyloric antrum by food, evoke gastric acid secretion even in the absence of vagal stimulation. This is due to release of a hormone called **gastrin** produced by G cells, which enters circulation and influences the secretion of gastric glands.

> Chemicals that increase gastric juice secretion are called **secretagogues**, which include amino acids, peptides, alcohol, caffeine, etc.

The local effect of gastrin secretion can be blocked by applying a local anesthetic like **cocaine** to the antral mucosa. But the release of gastrin by reflex mechanisms persists. This reflex can be blocked by administration of ganglion blocking agents like **hexamethonium**.

■ GASTRIN
Gastrin is a polypeptide hormone produced by **G cells** of the pyloric glands. G cells belong to the group of amine precursor uptake and decarboxylation **(APUD) cells** which are of neural crest origin. Intestinal gastrin is produced by the proximal glands of duodenum. Gastrin was discovered by **Edkins in 1906**. Gastrin is also found in:
- Pancreatic islets in fetal life
- Anterior and intermediate lobes of pituitary gland
- Hypothalamus, medulla oblongata
- Vagus and sciatic nerves

Morphology of G Cell
G cells are **flask shaped** with a broad base containing numerous gastrin granules and a narrow apex that reaches the mucosal surface. Microvilli project from the apical end into the lumen of the gland. Receptors mediating gastrin responses to changes in gastric contents are present on the microvilli. The G cells also contain **epinephrine and serotonin** as they belong to APUD cells.

A second type of gastrin-producing cell, the **TG cell**, is found throughout the stomach and small intestine and it contains only G_{34} and lacks G_{17}. G_{17} is the principal form of gastrin with respect to gastric acid secretion.

Chemistry of Gastrin
Gastrin is synthesized from **preprogastrin** which is processed into fragments of various sizes. Three main fragments are:
1. G_{34}–Big gastrin present predominantly in blood
2. G_{17}–Little gastrin present in tissues
3. G_{14}–Minigastrin present in blood and tissues

There is also a large form which contains more than 45 amino acid residues called **big-big gastrin**.

These forms differ in their NH_2 terminal extensions. The COOH terminal amino acid sequences are identical. Full biological activity of gastrin is retained in the COOH terminal or C-terminal (tetra-peptide in the C terminal residue).

The tyrosine in the 6th position from the COOH terminal may be present as either a sulfated or non-sulfated residue. Both are of equal potency.

Synthetic analogue of gastrin is **pentagastrin** with 5 amino acids. Gastrins are inactivated primarily in the kidney and small intestine.

Functions of Gastrin
- Gastrin stimulates parietal cells to secrete **acid** and **intrinsic factor** of Castle. Gastric juice secreted due to vagal stimulation is rich in acid and pepsin but *gastrin- induced juice is rich in acid but poor in pepsinogen.*
- Stimulates chief cells to secrete pepsinogen to a lesser extent.
- Trophic action, i.e., stimulates the growth of mucosa of stomach, small intestine and large intestine.
- Increases tone of stomach and upper small intestine. Gastrin also increases gastric motility especially antral motor activity.
- Causes contraction of gastroesophageal sphincter.
- Increases insulin, glucagon and calcitonin secretion. Calcitonin, in turn, by a negative feedback mechanism, inhibits gastrin secretion.
- Increases Brunner's gland secretion, small intestinal juice, pancreatic secretion and bile.
- Gastrin stimulates secretion of histamine from enterochromaffin-like cells (ECL cells). ECL cells have numerous gastrin receptors on their membrane.

Factors Affecting Gastrin Secretion (Table 46.4)
Factors that Increase Gastrin Secretion
- Luminal factors: Presence of amino acids particularly, phenylalanine and tryptophan, peptides, calcium-rich foods like milk, etc., in the gastric lumen stimulate the G cells to release gastrin.

Table 46.4: Factors affecting gastrin secretion.	
Increase in gastrin secretion	Decrease in gastrin secretion
• Presence of amino acids, peptides, calcium in gastric lumen • Short and long reflexes • Catecholamines, GRP, I/V calcium • Achlorhydria	• Hyperchlorhydria produce negative feedback inhibition of gastrin secretion • Secretin, GIP, VIP, calcitonin, somatostatin • Some prostaglandins like PGE • Vagotomy • Hyperglycemia

❖ Nervous factors: Nervous factors are mediated by cephalic stimulation of vagus and distension of stomach through short and long reflexes.
❖ Catecholamines, gastrin releasing peptide (GRP), intravenous calcium, etc., increase gastrin secretion.
❖ In pernicious anemia, where parietal cells of stomach are damaged, gastrin secretion is chronically elevated due to lack of negative feedback inhibition by acid.

Factors which Decrease Gastrin Secretion

❖ Luminal factors like increased acid in stomach especially in the antral region (pH <2.5) inhibit gastrin secretion. This is partly by a direct action of acid on G cells by feedback inhibition and partly due to the release of an inhibitor like **somatostatin**. Somatostatin is a potent inhibitor of gastrin secretion.
❖ Somatostatin is secreted by D cell which is a gut endocrine cell belonging to APUD group. Paracrine release of somatostatin in the gastric antrum is stimulated by low luminal pH.
❖ Other factors that decrease gastrin secretion include PGE, secretin, GIP, VIP, calcitonin, vagotomy and hyperglycemia.

Effect of Vagotomy on Gastric Secretion

After vagotomy, no gastric juice secretion occurs during the cephalic phase. Gastric phase secretion is also decreased. If resection of antral mucosa is done along with vagotomy there is loss of cephalic and gastric phase secretion of acid to a great extent. During digestion, there is interdependence of neural and humoral mechanisms, each potentiating the other.

Gastrinomas

Gastrinomas are gastrin secreting **tumors** occurring mainly in the pancreas but is also seen in the stomach and duodenum.

Achalasia Cardia

The term achalasia is derived from the Greek word meaning absence of relaxation. The lower end of esophagus becomes massively dilated (megaesophagus) due to accumulation of food in the esophagus **(Figs. 46.6A and B)**. This is because there is incomplete relaxation of the sphincter on swallowing. In this condition, the myenteric plexus is usually deficient at the distal 2/3rd of the esophagus including the lower esophageal sphincter (LES). There is selective loss of intramural inhibitory neurons that regulate the LES, the neurotransmitters for which are VIP and NO. The condition is treated by physical distension of the LES with a pneumatic-bag dilator or by cutting the LES (esophageal Heller myotomy). In achalasia cardia, the smooth muscle of the LES is found to be *hypersensitive to gastrin*.

Intestinal Phase

Factors that Stimulate Gastric Juice Secretion in the Intestinal Phase

Presence of partially digested food and mechanical distension of intestine elicits acid secretion in the stomach. It is mediated through **intestinal gastrin** secreted by G cells in the mucosa of small intestine. Amount of secretion is less than that of cephalic and gastric phase. It takes a latent period of 2–3 hours and once started lasts for 8–10 hours. It constitutes about 10% of total gastric juice secretion.

The **secretagogues** of the intestinal phase of gastric secretion are peptides and amino acids, especially phenylalanine and tryptophan.

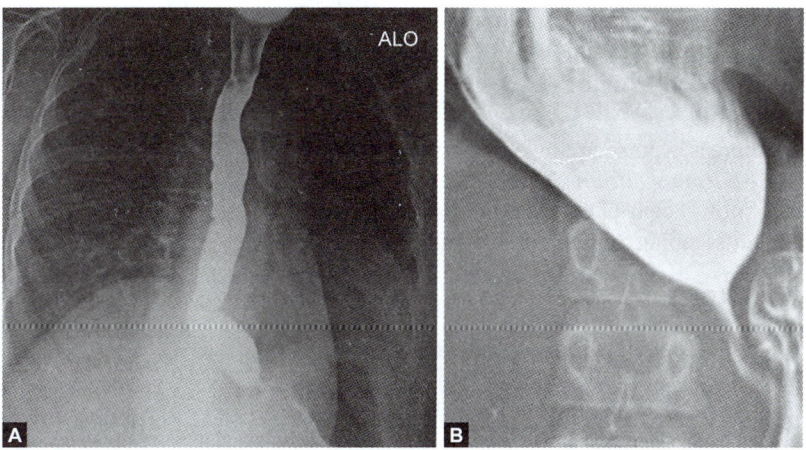

Figs. 46.6A and B: Achalasia cardia: (A) Early stage; (B) Late stage with typical bird beak appearance.
Courtesy: Dr Anil Sundaram.

Some are of the opinion that intestinal phase operates independently of gastrin release. A substantial proportion of the response to intestinal amino acid is likely secondary to their absorption and entry into circulation.

Factors that Inhibit Gastric Juice Secretion in the Intestinal Phase

❖ Too much acidity of gastric chyme, too much fat in gastric chyme and hypertonic gastric chyme can inhibit gastric secretion via neural and hormonal mechanisms.
❖ There are a number of humoral agents that inhibit gastric acid secretion in the intestinal phase, released from the small intestine and colon referred to as **enterogastrones**. Inhibition of gastric acid secretion due to the presence of acid chyme in the duodenum is mediated by **secretin** secreted from the **S cells** of duodenal mucosa. *S cells are endocrine cells. Secretin increases pepsinogen secretion even though it inhibits acid secretion.*

Luminal fatty acids, especially those with 10 or more carbon atoms, are the most effective inhibitors of gastric acid secretion in intestinal phase. The humoral agents (enterogastrones) responsible for fat-induced inhibition of acid secretion include **GIP, VIP, CCK-PZ, neurotensin, glucagon, peptide YY**, etc. *The most important enterogastrone is neurotensin*. It is released by fat in the distal small intestine and inhibits gastric acid secretion. It is a very potent inhibitor in the innervated stomach. Following vagotomy, the inhibitory effect of neurotensin is abolished.

> Gastric acid secretion is increased after the removal of large parts of the small intestine. This is due to removal of the source of hormones (enterogastrones) that inhibit acid secretion.

ABNORMALITIES OF GASTRIC SECRETORY FUNCTION

❖ Hyposecretion
❖ Hypersecretion

Hyposecretion or Hypochlorhydria

Failure of gastric acid secretion occurs in pernicious anemia, gastric atrophy, gastric ulcer, gastric carcinoma, etc.

Hypersecretion of Gastric Acid

Common conditions where there is hypersecretion of acid are *duodenal ulcer and Zollinger-Ellison syndrome*. In Zollinger-Ellison syndrome, tumors of non-β cells of pancreatic islets produce gastrin in large amounts leading to hyperchlorhydria.

Peptic Ulcer or Acid Peptic Disease (APD)

> **PY4.9:** Discuss the physiology aspects of: peptic ulcer, gastroesophageal reflux disease, vomiting, diarrhea, constipation, adynamic ileus, Hirschsprung's disease.

Peptic ulcer or **APD** refers to a group of ulcerative disorders of upper GIT which is exposed to acid-pepsin mixture. Most common sites are **lower end of esophagus, lesser curvature of stomach and first part of duodenum.** Major forms are gastric ulcer, duodenal ulcer and ulcer associated with Zollinger-Ellison syndrome. *An ulcer is a **crater-like** lesion in the mucous membrane* **(Fig. 46.7)**. The appearance of normal gastric mucosa is shown in **Figure 46.8**. Increased acid production or decreased mucosal defenses predispose to APD.

Factors Affecting the Integrity of Gastric Mucosa

Resistance to ulceration depends on the balance between aggressive factors and factors that comprise mucosal resistance to ulceration **(Table 46.5)**.

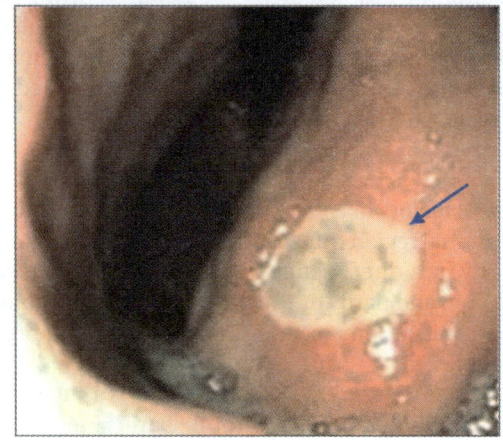

Fig. 46.7: Gastric ulcer.
Courtesy: Dr Anil Sundaram, Surgeon.

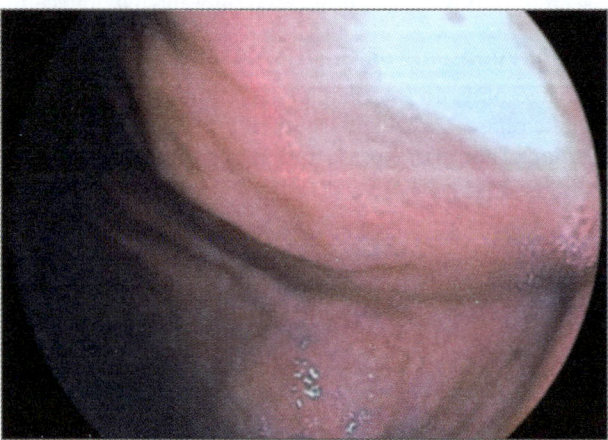

Fig. 46.8: Normal gastric mucosa.
Courtesy: Dr Anil Sundaram, Surgeon.

Table 46.5: Factors affecting integrity of gastric mucosa.	
Aggressive factors	**Mucosal barrier**
Acid, pepsin	• Gastric mucus, HCO_3^- • Tight junctions between epithelial cells • Prostaglandin, high mucosal blood flow • Trefoil peptides

(PG: prostaglandin)

Gastric Mucus

Gastric mucus forms a protective gel lining the gastric mucosa and forms a barrier between gastric epithelium and acid-pepsin mixture protecting the epithelium from the mixture. The gel thickness is increased by prostaglandins (PG) and decreased by non-steroidal anti-inflammatory drugs (NSAIDs) like aspirin. Mucus also contains blood group substances which protect the mucosa from damage.

HCO_3^-

HCO_3^- secreted by the gastric epithelium is trapped in the mucus gel and is also present in the space between epithelium and gel so that the pH immediately adjacent to epithelium is neutral, whereas luminal pH is 1–2. HCO_3^- secretion is stimulated by Ca^{2+}, PG and cholinergic agents and inhibited by aspirin, alcohol, etc.

Intercellular Tight Junctions

The intercellular tight junctions between gastric epithelial cells form part of mucosal barrier. It prevents back diffusion of H^+ from lumen into submucosa. This barrier is disrupted by aspirin, bile acids, alcohol, etc.

Prostaglandin

Prostaglandin (PG) stimulates secretion of mucus and HCO_3^- by gastric and duodenal mucosa, increases mucosal blood flow and also promotes epithelial cell repair and renewal following mucosal injury. PG increases protein synthesis in the epithelial cells. PG synthesis is inhibited by aspirin and related drugs.

Blood flow to mucosa is very high. When there is a reduction in blood flow it leads to ulceration.

Trefoil peptides in the mucosa are acid resistant and also prevent auto-digestion of gastric mucosa and promote healing of mucosal lesions (*refer* 'Mucosal barrier section' for details).

Causes of Peptic Ulcer

Peptic ulcer occurs as a result of breakdown of mucosal barrier by irritation or auto-digestion.

* Stress situations like anxiety, anger, frustrations, etc., cause increase in HCl secretion and produce stress ulcers.
* Increase in gastric acidity due to increase in parietal cell mass, hypersecretion of gastrin and increased vagal tone.
* Reflux of gastric contents into the esophagus causes esophagitis and esophageal ulcer **(Fig. 46.9)**.
* Gastric colonization with **Helicobacter pylori** is reported in 90–95% of patients with duodenal ulcer and 60–70% of patients with gastric ulcer. *H. pylori* are spiral, gram-negative bacteria with multiple flagella and reside in the mucous gel causing inflammation of gastric mucosa referred to as **gastritis**. Gastritis causes disruption of mucosal barrier leading to ulceration especially of duodenal mucosa. The organism does not invade tissues.

H. pylori produce an enzyme **urease** which splits urea into NH_3 and CO_2. This NH_3 damages the mucous layer of stomach. The bacteria also produce **catalase** which protects the organism from the phagocytic activity of macrophages. The organism also affects apoptosis in the GIT.

* Drugs like steroids, NSAID, etc., cause irritation of gastric mucosa leading to ulceration.
* Endocrine disorders: Cushing's syndrome, insulinoma, hyperparathyroidism, gastrinomas, etc., produce ulcer.
* Malnutrition, smoking, irregular meal habits, spicy and caffeine-rich foods, impaired mucosal blood flow, etc., produce ulcers. These are predisposing factors.
* Duodenal ulcers occur as a result of decreased alkalinity of small intestinal secretions like pancreatic juice, bile and secretion from Brunner's gland. Smoking decreases HCO_3^- secretion by pancreas.
* Genetic predisposition: "O" blood group individuals and non-secretors are more prone to develop duodenal ulcers.

Differences between duodenal ulcer and gastric ulcer are given in **Table 46.6**.

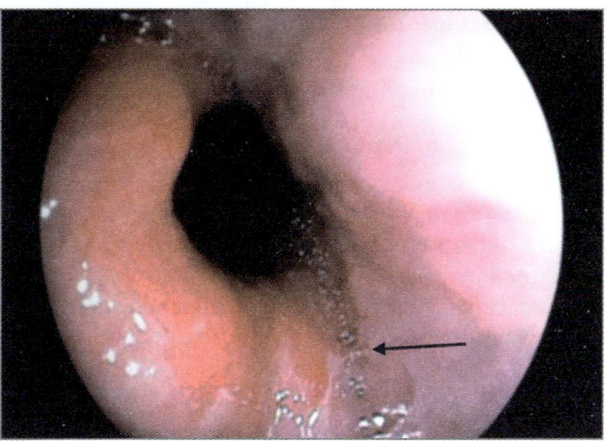

Fig. 46.9: Esophagitis as a result of reflux of acidic gastric contents into the esophagus.
Courtesy: Dr Anil Sundaram, Surgeon.

Table 46.6: Differences between duodenal and gastric ulcer.

Duodenal ulcer	Gastric ulcer
More frequent, 6–15% of population affected	Less frequent
Equal incidence in male and female	Incidence more in males
Incidence between 20–50 years	Affects individuals >40 years
Hyperacidity and rapid gastric emptying. No back diffusion of H^+. Decreased secretion of mucus and HCO^- by duodenal mucosa	Hypoacidity due to back diffusion of H^+ and gastric emptying is delayed
Increased appetite	Anorexia (loss of appetite) and weight loss are present
Pain relieved by food intake	Pain aggravated by food intake
Genetic predisposition present	No genetic predisposition
Small and superficial ulcers	Large and deep seated ulcers
Hemorrhage and perforation less common	Hemorrhage and perforation common if left untreated
Mortality less	Mortality high
Non-secretors are affected	
Greater gastric acid secretory response to gastrin and the negative feedback on gastrin secretion by acid is less	

Signs and Symptoms of Peptic Ulcer

Epigastric pain and tenderness, heartburn, etc., are the common signs and symptoms of peptic ulcer.

Complications of Peptic Ulcer

- Hemorrhage and perforation at the ulcer site may lead to circulatory shock.
- When ulcers are present in the pyloric area, gastric obstruction results.
- Hyperacidity leads to inactivation of pancreatic enzymes especially lipase leading to steatorrhea and weight loss.

Investigations and Diagnosis

- Barium meal study: **50% BaSO$_4$** is given orally and X-ray pictures are taken at intervals. The ulcers can be visualized.
- Endoscopy and biopsy: A flexible fiber optic tube is introduced into the GIT and esophagus, stomach and duodenum can be visualized. Biopsy can also be taken for histological examination.
- Basal acid estimation
- Fractional test meal helps to differentiate between achlorhydria, hypochlorhydria and hyperchlorhydria.
- Pentagastrin test (6 mg pentagastrin given subcutaneously) and histamine test (0.5 mg histamine given subcutaneously) are done if achlorhydria is suspected. Gastric samples are aspirated and analyzed for free acidity and combined acidity. If there is no free acid present in the samples it is called true achlorhydria.
- Serum gastrin level is detected in gastrinomas.
- Estimation of antibodies against *Helicobacter pylori*.
- Plain X-ray abdomen is taken to diagnose perforation. If there is perforation, air will be present beneath the diaphragm.
- Relief of epigastric pain by food intake and antacids strongly suggests duodenal ulcer.

Management of Peptic Ulcer

Principles of management are:
- Neutralization of gastric acid
- Inhibition of acid secretion
- Enhancement of mucosal resistance
- Relieve pain and accelerate ulcer healing

Medical Management

- Gastric acid can be neutralized by giving antacids like Al(OH)$_2$, CaCO$_3$, Mg(OH)$_2$, etc.
- Acid secretion can be inhibited by:
  - **H$_2$ receptor blockers** like cimetidine, ranitidine, famotidine, etc., which decrease basal acid secretion by 80% and meal-induced secretion by 70%.
  - **Anticholinergic agents** like atropine, pirenzepine, etc. block the effect of acetylcholine on M$_1$-muscarinic receptors on parietal cell membrane and decrease acid secretion and also decrease gastric emptying.
  - **Omeprazole** inhibits H$^+$-K$^+$ pump and thus decreases acid secretion. It binds to the proton pump irreversibly inactivating the pump. It completely blocks basal and stimulated acid secretion. It is given once daily because it has a longer duration of action.
- Mucosal resistance can be enhanced by:
  - PGE$_1$, PGE$_2$ and PGE$_1$ analog **misoprostol** increase mucosal resistance by increasing mucus and HCO$_3$ secretion, increasing mucosal blood flow and by preventing back diffusion of H$^+$.
  - Coating agents like **sucralfate** (a basic aluminum salt of sucrose octasulfate), **colloidal bismuth compounds**, etc., enhance mucosal resistance and also aid in ulcer healing. Coating agents bind to the ulcer bed for about 12 hours, thereby increasing the resistance of the mucosa to acid. It prevents back diffusion of H$^+$ to the base of the ulcer. It also binds bile acids and pepsin. Colloidal bismuth compounds when given in combination with appropriate antibiotics eradicate *H. pylori*.
- Pain can be relieved by giving **sedatives**. Stress ulcers respond well to sedatives and **Yoga**. Patient is advised to take **small frequent feeds** so that, food dilutes the gastric juice. **Avoid** cigarette smoking and foods that aggravate symptoms, like alcohol, spicy foods, coffee, etc.

Surgical Management of APD

Surgery is done in patients who do not respond to medical management. Surgery includes **partial gastrectomy or vagotomy** and in 20% of cases both the procedures are done simultaneously. In gastrinomas, surgical removal of tumor that secretes gastrin is done.

Gastroesophageal Reflux Disease (GERD)

GERD occurs when the gastric acid frequently regurgitates into the esophagus. It is a chronic condition. The acid irritates the mucosa of the esophagus leading to its inflammation. Esophagitis occurs when the refluxed gastric acid and pepsin cause necrosis of the esophageal mucosa causing erosions and ulcers **(Fig. 46.9)**.

Causes

- Abnormal relaxation of lower esophageal sphincter or weakening of the sphincter causes reflux of gastric contents.
- Another cause is hiatus hernia.
- Very fatty and fried foods, alcohol, too much coffee, drugs like aspirin may also lead to reflux.

Symptoms

- Burning pain in the chest that usually occur after taking food and worsens on lying down especially at night. Difficulty in swallowing (dysphagia), regurgitation of sour contents into the throat and a sensation of a lump in the throat.
- Chronic cough and laryngitis also can occur if the reflux is severe.
- If not treated, leads to narrowing of esophagus (esophageal stricture) due to scar formation. This leads to dysphagia.
- There is an increased risk of cancer of esophagus (**esophageal adenocarcinoma**) in long standing ulcers. Esophageal ulcers can be visualized by endoscopy and biopsy can be taken to rule out carcinoma.
- Bleeding from the ulcers is also common.

Treatment is same as that for peptic ulcer.

Dumping Syndrome

Dumping syndrome is a condition seen after partial or total gastrectomy. It is characterized by dizziness and sweating following meals.

The causes are:
- Rapid entry of hypertonic meals into the intestine following gastrectomy. This causes movement of water into the gut lumen that causes reduction in plasma volume and significant reduction in cardiac output. This is responsible for the symptoms seen in **early dumping syndrome** which occur within half an hour of food intake.
- Direct entry of carbohydrates into the small intestine leads to rapid digestion and absorption of carbohydrates. The resulting hyperglycemia causes increased secretion of insulin leading to **reactive hypoglycemia**. This is **late dumping syndrome** which occurs 2 hours after a meal. In normal individuals, gastric emptying occurs slowly at a controlled rate preventing dumping syndrome.

Zollinger-Ellison Syndrome

Zollinger-Ellison syndrome is seen in patients with **gastrinomas**. In most cases the tumors are seen in the pancreas but, it may also be seen in the stomach and duodenum. The increased level of gastrin causes prolonged hypersecretion of HCl leading to the formation of severe ulcers.

MULTIPLE CHOICE QUESTIONS

1. Optimal activity of pepsin occurs at a pH of:
   a. 5
   b. 6
   c. 4.5
   d. Less than 4

2. Post-prandial alkaline tide in urine occurs due to:
   a. Increase in blood glucose level
   b. Increase in insulin level
   c. Increased gastric acid secretion
   d. Increased H$^+$ secretion in renal tubule

3. Intrinsic factor is secreted from:
   a. Chief cells
   b. Oxyntic cells
   c. Argentaffin cells
   d. Mucus secreting cells

4. Factors responsible for causing diarrhea after vagotomy are all, *except*:
   a. Reduced gastric emptying
   b. Hypoacidity in duodenum leading to bacterial overgrowth
   c. Irregular peristalsis
   d. Fat malabsorption

5. Factors stimulating gastric acid secretion includes all the following, *except*:
   a. Vagal stimulation
   b. Gastrin
   c. Histamine
   d. Secretin

6. Gastric emptying is delayed by all the following, *except*:
   a. Fat in duodenum
   b. High acidity in pyloric antrum
   c. Distension of duodenum
   d. Products of carbohydrate digestion in pyloric antrum

7. Mucus and HCO$_3^-$ secretion in the stomach is increased by:
   a. Prostaglandin
   b. NSAIDs
   c. Fat
   d. Protein

8. All the following are functions of stomach, *except*:
   a. Accommodation of ingested food
   b. Secretion of HCl for protein digestion
   c. Absorption of water and electrolytes
   d. Absorption of products of protein digestion

9. Gastric emptying is delayed by all the following, *except*:
   a. Fatty meal
   b. Hyperosmolarity of duodenal contents
   c. Increased secretion of secretin and cholecystokinin
   d. Carbohydrate rich meal

10. Receptive relaxation of the stomach is due to:
    a. Vago-vagal reflex
    b. Enterogastric reflex
    c. Distension of stomach
    d. Gastrin

11. Total gastrectomy leads to all the following, *except*:
    a. Iron deficiency anemia
    b. Pernicious anemia
    c. Dumping syndrome
    d. Protein indigestion

12. Stress ulcer in stomach is mainly due to increase in the:
    a. Basal acid secretion
    b. Cephalic phase secretion
    c. Gastric phase secretion
    d. Intestinal phase secretion of acid

13. Commonest cause of peptic ulcer is:
    a. Administration of NSAIDs
    b. Disruption of mucosal barrier
    c. Infection with *H. pylori*
    d. Increased secretion of gastric juice

14. Hydrogen ions in the gastric juice come from:
    a. Dissociation of lactic acid in the parietal cell
    b. Dissociation of carbonic acid in the parietal cell
    c. Passive transport of H$^+$ from the parietal cell
    d. Dissociation of HCl in the parietal cell

15. Achalasia cardia leads to:
    a. Peptic ulcer
    b. Dysphagia
    c. Indigestion
    d. Constipation

16. Gastric secretion is:
    a. Inhibited by curare
    b. Stimulated by noradrenaline
    c. Increased by stomach distension
    d. Stimulated by an increase in tonic activity

17. The gastric phase of gastric juice secretion is brought about by:
    a. Neural factors
    b. Hormonal factors
    c. Gastric distension
    d. Presence of proteins in the stomach
18. Gastric secretion is stimulated by all the following, *except*:
    a. Secretin
    b. Gastric distension
    c. Gastrin
    d. Vagal stimulation
19. Cephalic phase of gastric secretion is mediated by:
    a. Neurohormones
    b. Parasympathetics
    c. Sympathetics
    d. Gastrin
20. The normal basal acid output is:
    a. 1–2 mmol/hr
    b. 5–10 mmol/hr
    c. 10–15 mmol/hr
    d. 20–25 mmol/hr
21. Pepsinogen is activated by:
    a. Enterokinase
    b. Low pH
    c. Trypsin
    d. Chymotrypsin
22. Normal gastric juice contain all, *except*:
    a. Na^+
    b. K^+
    c. Ca^{2+}
    d. Mg^{2+}
23. All the following statements are correct regarding acid secretion in stomach, *except*:
    a. Gastrin increases acid secretion
    b. Secretin decreases acid secretion
    c. Total acid secretion reflects functional parietal cell mass
    d. Somatostatin increases acid secretion
24. HCl secretion in the stomach is stimulated by:
    a. Secretin
    b. Histamine
    c. Somatostatin
    d. VIP
25. Which of the following is true about gastric emptying?
    a. Decreased by cholecystokinin
    b. Decreased by gastrin
    c. Increased by secretin
    d. Increased by GIP
26. Physiological gastrectomy is:
    a. Ligate all major arteries
    b. Antrectomy
    c. Upper 1/3 of stomach resected
    d. Ligation of 4 out of 5 arteries
27. Pacemaker of GIT is located in:
    a. Cardiac end of stomach
    b. Pyloric end of stomach
    c. Fundus of stomach
    d. Long muscle of small intestine
28. pH of gastric juice is:
    a. 2
    b. 4
    c. 6
    d. 0.5
29. A patient with gastrinomas (gastrin secreting tumor) is most likely to develop:
    a. Duodenal ulcer
    b. Indigestion
    c. Protein malabsorption
    d. Diarrhea
30. Gastric emptying is facilitated by all the following, *except*:
    a. Carbohydrate meal
    b. Fatty meal
    c. Protein diet
    d. Liquid diet
31. HCl of gastric juice is secreted by:
    a. Chief cells
    b. Neck cells
    c. Enterochromaffin cells
    d. Parietal cells
32. Gastric juice includes all the following, *except*:
    a. HCl
    b. Pepsin
    c. Trypsin
    d. Mucus
33. The property of the smooth muscle which enables it to change its length greatly, without marked changes in tension is:
    a. Plasticity
    b. Rhythmicity
    c. Distensibility
    d. Dual innervation
34. Stomach can accommodate sufficient quantities of food without significant increase in pressure due to:
    a. Peristalsis
    b. Receptive relaxation
    c. Gastroileal reflex
    d. Gastrocolic reflex
35. The pacemaker cells in the gut responsible for basic electrical rhythm (BER) is called:
    a. Interstitial cells of Cajal
    b. Pre-Botzinger complex
    c. P cells
    d. T cells
36. Iron deficiency anemia usually follows gastrectomy because:
    a. Gastric acid converts ferrous ion to ferric ion
    b. Iron is absorbed from the stomach
    c. Stomach produces intrinsic factor
    d. Gastric acid converts ferric ion to ferrous form
37. The gas present in the stomach is mainly due to:
    a. Digestion of protein
    b. Aerophagia
    c. Digestion of carbohydrate
    d. Fermentation
38. Entrance of food into the larynx during swallowing is prevented by all the following, *except*:
    a. Arrest of breathing
    b. Forward movement of epiglottis
    c. Closure of glottis
    d. Elevation of larynx

39. **All are true of myenteric reflex, *except*:**
    a. Distension of intestine elicit the reflex
    b. Extrinsic innervation should be intact
    c. Efferent neurons are in the myenteric plexus
    d. Substance P is a mediator

40. **A patient with achalasia has a defect in the following:**
    a. Expression of neuronal NO synthase at the lower esophageal sphincter
    b. Esophageal peristalsis
    c. Acetylcholine receptors
    d. Substance P release

41. **Omeprazole acts by inhibiting:**
    a. H^+-K^+ ATPase
    b. ACh receptors
    c. Histamine receptors
    d. Na^+-K^+ ATPase

42. **Heart burn can be relieved by all the following, *except*:**
    a. Vagotomy
    b. Antacids
    c. High protein diet
    d. Cimetidine

43. **Neurotransmitter that causes relaxation of the lower esophageal sphincter is:**
    a. GRP
    b. ACh
    c. NO
    d. Substance P

44. **Approximate length of the alimentary canal in an adult is:**
    a. 12 meters
    b. 9 meters
    c. 5 meters
    d. 6 meters

45. **Vomiting center is located in the:**
    a. Cerebral cortex
    b. Reticular formation of medulla
    c. Hypothalamus
    d. Spinal cord

46. **Afferent impulses which initiate the second stage of swallowing arise from:**
    a. Taste receptors of tongue
    b. Cerebral cortex
    c. Neurons of swallowing center
    d. Pressure receptors of pharynx

47. **Post-prandial alkaline tide of urine is due to the entrance into the blood of:**
    a. OH^- ions during gastric juice secretion
    b. HCO_3^- during gastric juice secretion
    c. HCO_3^- during pancreatic juice secretion
    d. HCO_3^- from renal tubular fluid

48. **Vagotomy for peptic ulcer helps in healing by reducing HCl secretion during:**
    a. Cephalic phase alone
    b. Gastric phase alone
    c. Cephalic and gastric phase
    d. Intestinal and gastric phase

49. **Vomiting center lies in close relation to:**
    a. Salivatory nuclei
    b. Respiratory center
    c. Vasomotor center
    d. All of the above

50. **Vomiting in motion sickness is due to:**
    a. Impulses arising from gastrointestinal tract
    b. Direct stimulation of vomiting center
    c. Stimulation of chemoreceptor trigger zone
    d. Excessive stimulation of semicircular canal

ANSWERS

1. d	2. c	3. b	4. a	5. d
6. d	7. a	8. d	9. d	10. a
11. d	12. a	13. b	14. b	15. b
16. c	17. b	18. a	19. b	20. a
21. b	22. c	23. d	24. b	25. a
26. a	27. c	28. a	29. a	30. b
31. d	32. c	33. a	34. b	35. a
36. d	37. b	38. b	39. b	40. a
41. b	42. c	43. c	44. b	45. b
46. d	47. b	48. c	49. d	50. d

Exocrine Pancreas

CHAPTER 47

LEARNING OBJECTIVES
- Describe the composition and mechanism of secretion of pancreatic juice
- Explain the functions of pancreatic juice
- Explain the regulation of secretion of pancreatic juice
- Discuss the pathophysiology of pancreatitis
- Describe pancreatic exocrine function tests

INTRODUCTION

PY4.2: Describe the composition, mechanism of secretion, functions, and regulation of saliva, gastric, pancreatic, intestinal juices and bile secretion.

Pancreas is both an **exocrine and endocrine** secretory organ. Exocrine part secretes pancreatic juice and the endocrine part secretes hormones. Pancreas is 4–6 inches long and it extends transversely across the abdomen from the concavity of duodenum to the spleen. It is a **retroperitoneal** organ.

Exocrine part of pancreas is a large compound **racemose** gland and the structure is similar to salivary gland. **Islets of Langerhans** form the endocrine part. Exocrine pancreas is drained by the **duct of Wirsung** which joins with the common bile duct to form a dilated portion called **ampulla of Vater** (Fig. 47.1) which opens into the second part of duodenum on the duodenal papilla. The opening is guarded by a sphincter called **sphincter of Oddi**. An accessory pancreatic duct called **duct of Santorini** may also be present in some individuals which drains parts of exocrine pancreas. It opens into the duodenum more proximally.

INNERVATION

Pancreas is supplied by sympathetics and parasympathetics. **Sympathetics** supply mainly the blood vessels of pancreas and the fibers come through **splanchnic nerve**. **Parasympathetic fibers** supply acinar cells and smooth muscles of ducts and the fibers come through **vagus**.

COMPOSITION OF PANCREATIC JUICE

In man, pure pancreatic juice can be collected using a **fiberoptic catheter** introduced into the pancreatic duct under direct vision.

Pancreatic juice is a colorless, clear, watery, alkaline fluid which is **isotonic** with plasma.
- Rate of secretion: 2–2.5 L/day
- pH: 8–8.4
- Specific gravity: 1.007–1.042

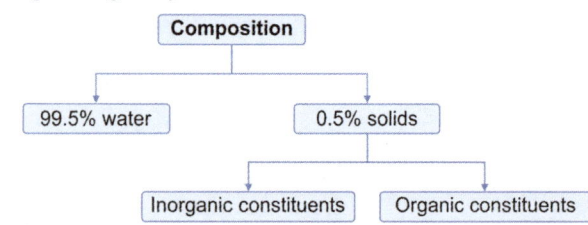

Inorganic Constituents

H_2O, Na^+, K^+, Ca^{2+}, Mg^{2+}, HCO_3^-, Cl^-, SO_4^{2-}, HPO_4^{2-}, etc.

Organic Constituents

- Enzymes: Trypsinogen, chymotrypsinogen A and B, procarboxypeptidase A_1 and A_2, proelastase, amylase,

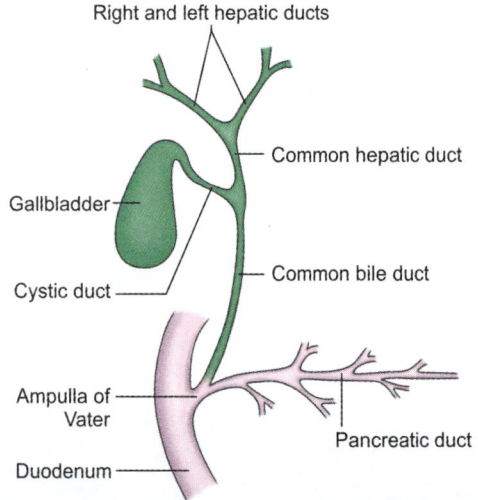

Fig. 47.1: Hepatopancreatic duct system.

lipase, cholesterol esterase, phospholipase, colipase, RNAse, DNAse, etc.
- ❖ Trypsin inhibitor
- ❖ Albumin, globulin (immunoglobulins), kallikrein, mucoproteins, lysosomal enzyme, alkaline phosphatase, etc.

Enzymes are produced by acinar cells and HCO_3^- is secreted by ductal epithelial cells which contain abundant carbonic anhydrase. *HCO_3^- content in pancreatic juice comes to about 113 mEq/L while it is 24 mEq/L in plasma.* Concentration of Na^+, K^+ and Ca^{2+} is same as that of plasma. Concentration of HCO_3^- varies directly with the rate of flow of pancreatic juice, whereas concentration of Cl^- in the juice varies inversely with the rate of flow. So the sum of Cl^- and HCO_3^- remains constant and comes to about 154 mEq/L. As Cl^- concentration increases HCO_3^- concentration decreases and vice versa. HCO_3^- neutralizes acid chyme reaching the duodenum from the stomach.

Protein-splitting Enzymes

Protein-splitting enzymes are trypsinogen, chymotrypsinogen A and B, procarboxypeptidase and proelastase. These enzymes are the inactive forms and are activated only after they are secreted into the intestinal tract. Optimum pH for enzyme action is 8–9.

- ❖ **Trypsinogen**: It is the inactive proenzyme of **trypsin** and is activated only in the intestine that too in the presence of **enteropeptidase or enterokinase**, an enzyme secreted by duodenal mucosa. Deficiency of enterokinase leads to protein malnutrition.

$$\text{Trypsinogen} \xrightarrow[\text{Trypsin}]{\text{Enterokinase, Ca}^{2+}} \text{Trypsin}$$

Once trypsin is formed, it can further activate trypsinogen to trypsin by autocatalytic reaction.

Actions of trypsin:
- Trypsin converts proteins to **proteoses and polypeptides**. Trypsin cleaves peptide bond that occupies an internal position and hence referred to as **endopeptidase**. Endopeptidases split proteins into peptides of various sizes but do not release individual amino acids.
- It coagulates blood.
- At a pH of 8–9, trypsin curdles milk.
- Activates chymotrypsinogen, procarboxypeptidase, collagenase and proelastase into their active forms.
- Activates phospholipase-A_2 which converts fatty acids to lysolecithin. Lysolecithin damages the cell membrane.
- **Autocatalytic** action, i.e., it catalyzes the conversion of more trypsinogen to active trypsin.

Trypsin inhibitor is synthesized and stored in the same acinar cells that secrete trypsin. It prevents activation of trypsinogen to trypsin both inside the cell and in the duct. It also inactivates trypsin formed in the pancreas by forming a relatively stable complex with the enzyme.

Since trypsin activates other enzymes, trypsin inhibitor pancreatic indirectly prevents their activation also. When there is damage to pancreas or block to the duct, pancreatic juice become pooled in the gland and the effect of trypsin inhibitor is overpowered. This causes auto-digestion of the gland leading to **acute pancreatitis** and has to be treated as a medical emergency. Mortality rate in acute pancreatitis is 20%.

- ❖ **Chymotrypsinogen A and B** are also **endopeptidases** which are activated to chymotrypsin by trypsin. It coagulates milk but not blood. Trypsin and chymotrypsin do not release individual amino acids.
- ❖ **Procarboxypeptidase** is an **exopeptidase** because it splits off end amino acids from polypeptide chain. It is also activated by trypsin and enterokinase to the active form, **carboxypeptidase**. It contains **zinc** in its molecular structure.
- ❖ **Proelastase** activated by trypsin to **elastase**, acts on elastin and some other proteins and hydrolyses peptide linkages.

Fat-splitting Enzymes

- ❖ **Colipase** acts as a **cofactor** for pancreatic lipase. It exposes the active site of pancreatic lipase and thus helps in the activation of pancreatic lipase.
- ❖ **Pancreatic lipase** causes hydrolysis of emulsified fat in the presence of bile salts. *Pancreatic lipase is the most potent lipase and the products of fat hydrolysis are fatty acid and monoglycerides. Colipase acts as the cofactor.*
- ❖ Cholesteryl ester hydrolase converts cholesteryl esters to cholesterol.
- ❖ **Prophospholipase-A_2** is activated to phospholipase-A_2 by trypsin. It acts on phospholipids to form lysolecithin and lysocephalin. Lysolecithin damages cell membrane. In acute pancreatitis, there is activation of phospholipase leading to the formation of lysolecithin from lecithin. This causes disruption of pancreatic tissue and necrosis of surrounding fat (pancreatitis).
- ❖ **Bile salt–activated lipase** catalyzes the hydrolysis of cholesterol esters, esters of fat-soluble vitamins and phospholipids, as well as triglycerides.

Carbohydrate-splitting Enzyme

Pancreatic amylase is the carbohydrate-splitting enzyme similar to salivary amylase, but acts both on **cooked** and **uncooked starch**. It also acts on related polysaccharides like amylopectins, glycogen, dextrins, etc., but it has *no action on cellulose*. Normally, small amounts of pancreatic amylase leak into circulation. In acute pancreatitis, circulating level of amylase increases markedly. It will be present in urine also and *estimation of urinary amylase is a good indicator of pancreatic activity.*

Nucleic Acid–splitting Enzymes

Ribonuclease and deoxyribonuclease hydrolyse nucleic acids releasing nucleotides. They are **endonucleases**.

MECHANISM OF SECRETION OF PANCREATIC JUICE

Mechanism of secretion of enzymes is same as that of secretion of salivary amylase, i.e., by **emeiocytosis** (Chapter 44, **Fig. 44. 6**).

Mechanism of Secretion of Electrolytes by Duct Cells

HCO_3^- is formed in the duct cells by the hydration of CO_2 in the presence of carbonic anhydrase. HCO_3^- reaches the duct lumen in exchange for Cl- with the help of HCO_3^--Cl- exchanger. Na+, K+, Cl- and H_2O reach the lumen by paracellular route (**Fig. 47.2**).

REGULATION OF SECRETION OF PANCREATIC JUICE

The secretions of the exocrine pancreas are regulated by neural and hormonal mechanisms.
- Neural regulation
- Humoral regulation

Neural Regulation

Stimulation of **sympathetics** causes vasoconstriction and decreased secretion from pancreas. Stimulation of **vagus** (parasympathetic) causes vasodilatation and secretion of small amount of pancreatic juice rich in enzymes. Vagal stimulation increases pancreatic juice secretion by releasing **acetylcholine and VIP**. Acinar cells have muscarinic receptors as well as receptors for VIP. Acetylcholine acts on the acinar cells by activation of phospholipase C. The effect is blocked by atropine.

Cephalic phase of pancreatic juice secretion comes to about 15–20% of the secretion. Sight or smell or thought of food increases pancreatic juice secretion and it is mediated by vagus. It does not occur after vagotomy. Gastric phase of pancreatic juice secretion is mainly mediated by vagus and is called *gastropancreatic reflex*. Part of this secretion is mediated by gastrin.

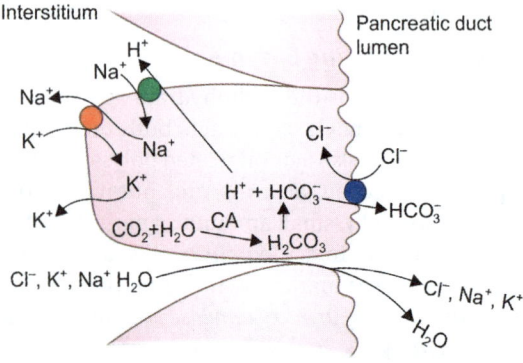

Fig. 47.2: Mechanism of secretion of HCO_3^- and H_2O by pancreatic duct cells.

Hormonal Control

Secretion of pancreatic juice is primarily under hormonal control. The main hormones involved are **secretin and cholecystokinin-pancreozymin (CCK-PZ)**. CCK and secretin are secreted into the blood and they reach the pancreas through circulation and cause secretion of pancreatic juice. Intestinal phase of pancreatic juice secretion is responsible for about 75% of pancreatic juice secretion and is due to release of secretin and CCK-PZ.

Secretin is the first hormone identified and was isolated by **Bayliss and Starling in 1902**. It is a polypeptide hormone secreted by the endocrine cells (**S cells**) present in the duodenal mucosa. Stimuli for the secretion of secretin are products of protein digestion and acidic chyme in the duodenum. *Acid in the duodenum is the most potent stimulus for secretin secretion. Secretin causes copious secretion of watery pancreatic juice rich in HCO_3^- but poor in enzymes.* The effect is on the pancreatic duct cells and is due to increase in intracellular cAMP.

CCK-PZ is a hormone secreted by **I cells** of duodenal mucosa and jejunum. The stimuli for the secretion of CCK are products of protein and fat digestion especially fatty acid and monoglycerides in the duodenum. *CCK causes secretion of thick, viscous pancreatic juice rich in enzymes but small in volume.* The action is mediated by phospholipase C. It acts on acinar cells and causes release of zymogen granules. CCK also augments the action of secretin (**Table 47.1**).

Insulin has long-term effects on the regulation of synthesis of digestive enzymes by exocrine pancreas. The venous blood draining the islet cells passes to the acinar cells before returning to systemic circulation. This arrangement exposes the acinar cells to a high concentration of islet hormones.

Table 47.1: Actions of secretin and cholecystokinin.

Secretin	Cholecystokinin
Acts on pancreatic duct cells and action is mediated via cAMP	Acts on pancreatic acinar cells and the action is mediated by phospholipase C
Causes copious secretion of very alkaline pancreatic juice, poor in enzymes	Increases the release of zymogen granules and produces pancreatic juice rich in enzyme but low in volume
Stimulates bile secretion rich in HCO_3^-	Causes gallbladder contraction
Inhibits gastric acid secretion	Causes contraction of pyloric sphincter and relaxation of sphincter of Oddi
Causes contraction of pyloric sphincter and delays gastric emptying	Increases the motility of small intestine and colon
Increases insulin secretion and augments the action of CCK	Increases enterokinase activity
	Has a trophic effect on pancreas
	Increases glucagon secretion and augments action of secretin

Pancreatic juice secretion is inhibited by:
- Sympathetic stimulation
- Peptide hormones, such as pancreatic polypeptide, glucagon, somatostatin, encephalin, adrenaline, noradrenaline, etc.

PHASES OF PANCREATIC JUICE SECRETION

The three phases of pancreatic juice secretion are:
1. Cephalic phase
2. Gastric phase
3. Intestinal phase

Cephalic Phase

Sight, smell and taste of food increase pancreatic juice secretion rich in enzymes and this response is mediated through **vagus**. This cephalic phase is responsible for 15–20% of the secretion.

Gastric Phase of Pancreatic Juice Secretion

Presence of food in the stomach increases pancreatic juice secretion and this gastric phase contributes to 5–10% of the secretion. This occurs by two mechanisms:
- Mediated by gastrin
- Presence of food leads to distension of stomach which in turn causes **gastropancreatic reflex**. This reflex is mediated through vagus.

Intestinal Phase

Intestinal phase is the important phase of pancreatic juice secretion and is responsible for 75% of pancreatic secretion. Presence of acidic chyme in the duodenum causes release of **secretin** which increases pancreatic juice rich in HCO_3^- and H_2O. Products of protein and fat digestion in the duodenum release **CCK** which releases pancreatic juice rich in enzymes. Food in the intestine elicits another reflex mediated by vagus called **enteropancreatic reflex**, which increases pancreatic juice secretion.

Applied Physiology

The two most common conditions that cause decrease in pancreatic juice secretion are **chronic pancreatitis** and **pancreatic carcinoma**. In non-tropical **sprue** or intestinal mucosal disease there is defective secretion of secretin and CCK-PZ. In **cystic fibrosis of pancreas,** the acini are replaced by fibrous tissue and there will be lack of pancreatic juice. Carcinoma of the head of pancreas may obstruct the bile duct and produce obstructive jaundice.

Pancreatic lipase is the most potent lipase. So, the most common effect of pancreatic insufficiency is **steatorrhea** due to impaired fat digestion. Normal excretion of fat through stools is 5–7 g/day. In steatorrhea it will be more than 50 g/day. There will be weight loss and symptoms of deficiency of fat-soluble vitamins. If the endocrine part of pancreas is affected it leads to **diabetes mellitus**.

Pancreatitis

Pancreatitis is inflammation of pancreatic acini. It may be **acute pancreatitis or chronic pancreatitis**.

Causes

- Most common cause is **alcoholism**.
- Block in major pancreatic duct or accessory duct by gallstones or growths like carcinoma head of pancreas
- Regurgitation of bile into pancreatic duct
- Inactivation of trypsin inhibitor
- Infections, drugs, poisons like scorpion venom
- Vasculitis, e.g., systemic lupus erythematosus (SLE)

Acute pancreatitis is a medical emergency. Here, pancreatic enzymes get activated within the gland due to pooling of secretion within the gland. This leads to **auto-digestion** of the gland. **Serum amylase** level is very much increased (10–20 times normal) in acute pancreatitis. **Serum lipase** level is elevated about 72 hours after the onset of symptoms and forms a better diagnostic test for pancreatitis.

Effects of Total Pancreatectomy

- Endocrine disturbances - diabetes mellitus due to lack of insulin.
- Digestive disturbances due to lack of exocrine secretion:
  - Impaired fat digestion due to lack of pancreatic lipase.
  - Impaired protein digestion due to lack of protein splitting enzymes.
  - Steatorrhea and increased frequency of stools.

Pancreatic Function Tests

> **PY4.8:** Describe and discuss gastric function tests, pancreatic exocrine function tests and liver function tests.

- Fecal fat estimation (Normal 5 to 7g/day)
- Estimation of serum and urinary amylase and serum lipase (Serum amylase: 40 to 140 units/L; Serum lipase: 0 to 160 units/L; Urinary amylase: 2.6 to 21.2 International units/hour [IU/hour])
- **Secretin-pancreozymin test**: Secretin and pancreozymin (CCK) are injected intravenously and the pancreatic juice is collected and analyzed for volume, HCO_3^- content and enzymes.
- **Endoscopic retrograde cholangiopancreatography (ERCP)**: Using a fiber optic duodenoscope, the pancreatic duct is cannulated and a radiopaque dye is injected into the duct system. X-ray pictures are taken and growths, strictures, dilatations, etc., can be visualized. It is the best imaging procedure for assessing the severity and extent of ductal changes **(Fig. 47.3)**.
- Ultrasonography (USS)
- X-ray abdomen reveals pancreatic calcification in chronic pancreatitis.
- **Computed axial tomography (CAT scan)** can reveal calcifications and cystic areas not noted on plain X-ray and ultrasound scan (USS).

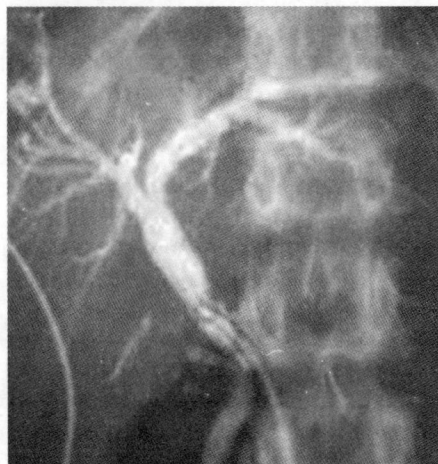

Fig. 47.3: Endoscopic retrograde cholangiopancreatography (ERCP).

MULTIPLE CHOICE QUESTIONS

1. Most common cause of chronic pancreatitis is:
   a. Alcohol consumption
   b. Gallstone
   c. Increased blood cholesterol
   d. Trauma

2. Pancreatic juice contains all the following enzymes, *except*:
   a. Lipase
   b. Amylase
   c. Trypsin
   d. Enterokinase

3. The carbohydrate splitting enzyme that act both on cooked and uncooked starch is:
   a. Salivary amylase
   b. Pancreatic amylase
   c. Gastric amylase
   d. Intestinal amylase

4. Highest pH is seen in:
   a. Gastric juice
   b. Gallbladder bile
   c. Pancreatic juice
   d. Small intestinal juice

5. All the following increases enzyme secretion from pancreas, *except*:
   a. Secretin
   b. Cholecystokinin
   c. Vagal stimulation
   d. Products of fat digestion in duodenum

6. Enterokinase deficiency leads to:
   a. Pancreatitis
   b. Decreased glucose absorption
   c. Decreased protein digestion
   d. Gastritis

7. Test of pancreatic exocrine function include administration of:
   a. Sodium tetraiodophenolphthalein
   b. Histamine
   c. Pentagastrin
   d. Glucose

8. Total pancreatectomy leads to all the following conditions, *except*:
   a. Weight gain
   b. Hyperglycemia
   c. Metabolic acidosis
   d. Steatorrhea

9. Trypsin inhibitor is normally present in:
   a. Pancreatic acinar cells
   b. Duodenal mucosa
   c. Bile
   d. Centroacinar cells

10. Pancreatic juice contains all the following, *except*:
    a. Amylase
    b. Lipase
    c. Secretin
    d. Trypsin

11. Major pancreatic duct is known as:
    a. Stensen's duct
    b. Duct of Wirsung
    c. Duct of Santorini
    d. Bartholin's duct

12. Which of the following has the highest pH?
    a. Saliva
    b. Gastric juice
    c. Pancreatic juice
    d. Hepatic bile

13. The mechanism that protects normal pancreas from autodigestion is:
    a. Secretion of HCO_3^-
    b. Protease inhibitors present in plasma
    c. Proteolytic enzymes secreted in inactive forms
    d. The resistance of pancreatic cells

14. Pancreatic secretion contain all, *except*:
    a. Trypsin
    b. Lipase
    c. Enteropeptidase
    d. Amylase

ANSWERS

1. a	2. d	3. b	4. c	5. a
6. c	7. b	8. a	9. a	10. c
11. b	12. c	13. c	14. c	

Liver and Biliary System

CHAPTER 48

LEARNING OBJECTIVES
- Describe the structure and functions of liver
- Discuss the composition of hepatic and gallbladder bile
- Describe the structure and functions of gallbladder
- Differentiate the different types of jaundice
- Discuss the various liver function tests

INTRODUCTION

PY4.7: Describe and discuss the structure and functions of liver and gallbladder.

Liver is a vital organ essential for life and removal of the liver is fatal. *It is the largest gland in the body.* It weighs about 1400–1600 g in adult male. Liver cells are called **hepatocytes**. The liver is organized into many lobes and each lobe is made up of a number of **lobules**. In the lobules, hepatocytes are arranged in different plates in circular rows around a **central vein**. The plates are one-cell thick. Blood entering the liver through the portal vein flows through **sinusoids** in between the rows of liver cells and is drained into the central vein of each lobule. There is only one layer of hepatocytes between sinusoids. Blood from the hepatic artery also enters the sinusoids **(Figs. 48.1A and B)**. The substances produced by the liver cells, and waste products like CO_2 are discharged into the sinusoids. The endothelium of the sinusoids has large fenestrations, and plasma is in close contact with the liver cells. Liver receives about 1000 mL of blood per minute from portal vein and 500 mL/min from the hepatic artery. Numerous macrophages called **Kupffer cells** are present in the endothelium lining the sinusoids. They belong to the reticuloendothelial system.

The central veins coalesce to form the **hepatic vein** that drains into the inferior vena cava. At the periphery of each lobule are present a branch of hepatic artery, a branch of portal vein and a bile duct forming a triad called **portal triad (Fig. 48.2)**.

FUNCTIONS OF LIVER

- Formation and secretion of bile.
- Storage of carbohydrate, fat, vitamin A, vitamin B, folic acid, and iron. The liver cells absorb from the blood and store temporarily ½ to ¾ of all absorbed nutrients. Intermediary processing of these nutrients also occurs in the liver.
- Synthesis of plasma proteins, clotting factors, heparin, blood group substances, etc.
  - All the plasma proteins except gamma globulins are synthesized by the liver. Serum albumin is synthesized only in the liver.

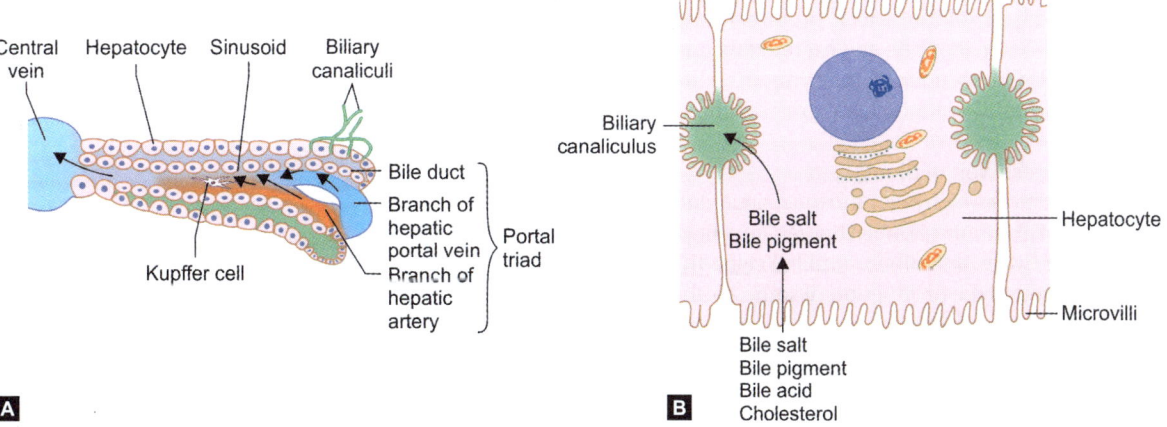

Figs. 48.1A and B: (A) Histology of a liver lobule; (B) A single hepatocyte showing bile canaliculi.

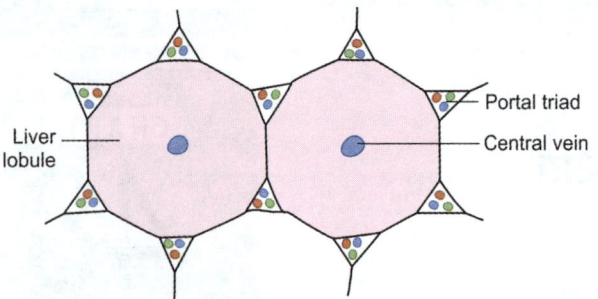

Fig. 48.2: Structural organization of liver showing two liver lobules each containing central vein. The periphery of lobules contain portal triad (bile duct, portal vein and hepatic artery branches).

- Clotting factors synthesized in the liver are factors II, V, VII, VIII, IX, X, XI and XII.
- Coagulation inhibitors like protein C and protein S are also synthesized in the liver.
- Acute phase proteins, steroid binding and other hormone binding proteins, C_3, C_5 and C_6 components of the complement system are also synthesized in the liver.

❖ Reduction and conjugation of adrenal and gonadal steroid hormones, peptide hormones, etc., occurs in the liver. Hormones like thyroxine, insulin, glucagon, parathormone, growth hormone, glucocorticoids, estrogen and testosterone are metabolized in the liver.

❖ Detoxification of drugs, toxins, etc. Fat-soluble harmful substances are converted into water-soluble substances by the liver and are excreted through bile or urine. This occurs by the action of enzymes like cytochromes located in the smooth endoplasmic reticulum of liver. Drugs like sulphonamides, penicillin, ampicillin, etc., are excreted by liver.

❖ Excretion of substances like toxins, heavy metals like copper, lead, arsenic, bismuth; bile pigments, cholesterol, alkaline phosphatase and metabolic end products through bile. Bile also excretes bacteria (typhoid) and viruses (yellow fever). Bile is the only route by which the body can dispose cholesterol as such or after conversion to bile acids. Bile is an essential excretory route for substances which cannot be eliminated in urine, like unconjugated bilirubin, cholesterol, etc. Lipid soluble waste products that cannot enter urine are secreted into bile and excreted through feces.

❖ Liver has hemopoietic function in intrauterine life.
❖ Reticuloendothelial cells of liver are the sites of RBC destruction.
❖ Liver acts as a reservoir of blood.
❖ **Kupffer cells** of liver which belong to the reticuloendothelial system helps in immunity. Foreign bodies are phagocytosed and destroyed by the reticuloendothelial cells. These cells are also involved in the production of some antibodies.
❖ Metabolic functions of liver:
  - On carbohydrate metabolism:
    ♦ Gluconeogenesis
    ♦ Glycogen synthesis
    ♦ Glycogenolysis
  - On protein and nucleic acid metabolism:
    ♦ Deamination of amino acid
    ♦ Synthesis of urea from ammonia ($CO_2 + 2NH_3 \rightarrow NH_2\text{-}CO\text{-}NH_2 + H_2O$)
    ♦ Synthesis of amino acid from fatty acid
    ♦ Purine and pyrimidine metabolism
  - On fat metabolism:
    ♦ Storage of fat
    ♦ Formation of ketone bodies
    ♦ Formation of phospholipids
    ♦ Synthesis of 25-hydroxycholecalciferol

❖ Liver is the organ where heat is produced maximally in the body.

BILIARY SYSTEM

> **PY4.2:** Describe the composition, mechanism of secretion, functions, and regulation of saliva, gastric, pancreatic, intestinal juices and bile secretion.

The biliary system begins in the **biliary canaliculi** which are a network of spaces between hepatocytes. Bile secreted by the hepatic cells is drained into small biliary canaliculi which join to form larger ducts. These ducts join to form **right and left hepatic ducts**. These two join to form **common hepatic duct** which joins with the **cystic duct** to form **common bile duct** which joins the pancreatic duct and opens on the **duodenal papilla**. The opening is guarded by **sphincter of Oddi** (*refer Chapter 47, Fig. 47.1*).

When the sphincter of Oddi is contracted, bile is diverted into the gallbladder. Bile is stored and concentrated in the gallbladder during the interdigestive phase. Bile secreted by liver is termed **hepatic bile** and bile that is concentrated and modified during storage in the gallbladder is termed **gallbladder bile**. The composition of both is different **(Table 48.1)**.

Bile

Bile is a golden yellow, greenish fluid which is a secretory, as well as excretory product of liver. It is continuously secreted by the hepatic cells into the biliary canaliculi.

Bile is an essential excretory route for substances which cannot be eliminated in urine like unconjugated bilirubin, cholesterol, etc.

Rate of secretion: 500–1000 mL/day pH: 7.5–8.5

Table 48.1: Differences between hepatic bile and gallbladder bile.

	Hepatic bile	Gallbladder bile
Color	Golden yellow	Greenish brown
Water content	97%	89%
Solids	2–4%	10–12%
Bile salt	10–20 mmol/L	50–200 mmol/L
pH	7.6–8.6	7–7.4
Viscosity	Less viscous	More viscous due to secretion of mucus

Composition of Hepatic Bile

Water: 97%
Solids: 3% → Organic: 60% of the solids
→ Inorganic: 40%

Organic constituents:
Bile salts: 0.7% Bile pigment: 0.2%
Cholesterol: 0.04–0.08%
Lecithin: 0.1–0.8%
Fatty acid: 0.15%
Fat: 1%
Alkaline phosphatase in minute quantity

Inorganic constituents:
Salts of Na^+, K^+, Ca^{2+}, HCO_3^-, Cl^-, etc.

Mechanism of Secretion of Bile

Bile is secreted in two stages by the liver.
- In the **first stage**, hepatocytes secrete bile containing large amounts of bile acids, cholesterol and other organic constituents into minute biliary canaliculi.
- In the **second stage**, while passing through the bile ducts, a second portion of secretion is added to the initial secretion. This additional secretion is a watery solution of sodium and bicarbonate ions secreted by the secretory epithelial cells lining the biliary ducts. This second secretion is stimulated by **secretin** which increases the HCO_3^- content of bile.

Bile Salts

Bile salts are sodium and potassium salts of bile acids conjugated with glycine or taurine. Hepatic cells secrete primary bile acids, **cholic acid and chenodeoxycholic acid** which are synthesized from cholesterol. In the colon, bacteria convert cholic acid to **deoxycholic acid** and chenodeoxycholic acid to **lithocholic acid**. Small quantities of **ursodeoxycholic acid** are formed from chenodeoxycholic acid. Because they are formed by bacterial action, they are called secondary bile acids.

Bile acids exert a negative feedback effect on further conversion of cholesterol to bile acids. Primary bile acids conjugate with taurine or glycine to form **taurocholic acid and glycocholic acid**. These form salts with sodium and potassium to form **sodium taurocholate, sodium glycocholate, and potassium taurocholate and potassium glycocholate**. These are the bile salts.

- **Primary bile acids**: Cholic acid and chenodeoxycholic acid formed in the hepatocytes.
- **Secondary bile acids**: Deoxycholic acid, lithocholic acid and ursodeoxycholic acid are formed in the colon.

Rate of bile salt synthesis is 0.2–0.4 g/day. 95% of bile salts are reabsorbed in the terminal ileum by an extremely efficient Na^+-bile salt cotransport system which enters the portal circulation. They reach the liver and are re-excreted into bile. *The circular route of bile salts from intestine to the liver and then through bile back to the intestine is called **enterohepatic circulation** of bile salts.*

About 5% of bile salts that reach the colon are converted to **secondary bile salts**. In the colon, by the action of bacterial enzymes, primary bile acid is converted to secondary bile acids which are **deoxycholic acid and lithocholic acid and ursodeoxycholic acid (Flowchart 48.1)**. Because they are formed by bacterial action they are called secondary bile acids. Deoxycholate is reabsorbed, but lithocholate is excreted since it is water insoluble. Total bile salt pool in the body is 3.5 g. This can recycle 2 times during a meal and 6–8 times per day.

> Substances that undergo enterohepatic circulation are bile salts, bile pigments, adrenocortical and other steroid hormones and a number of drugs.

Properties and Functions of Bile Salts

- **Hydrotropic effect** of bile salts helps in digestion and absorption of fat.
  Bile salts are **amphipathic**, i.e., one side of bile salt is hydrophilic whereas the other side is hydrophobic.
  Due to this property, bile salt combines with fatty acids, cholesterol and fat-soluble vitamins to form water-soluble compounds and this helps in easy digestion and absorption of fat.
- *Bile salts decrease surface tension* of lipids: Lipids are insoluble in water due to high surface tension. Bile salts reduce surface tension of lipids due to their detergent action so that lipids become water soluble. In association with monoglycerides and phospholipids, bile salts are responsible for **emulsification** of fat. Emulsification is the process by which large fat globules are broken down into small droplets thus increasing the surface area available for

Flowchart 48.1: Formation of primary and secondary bile salts.

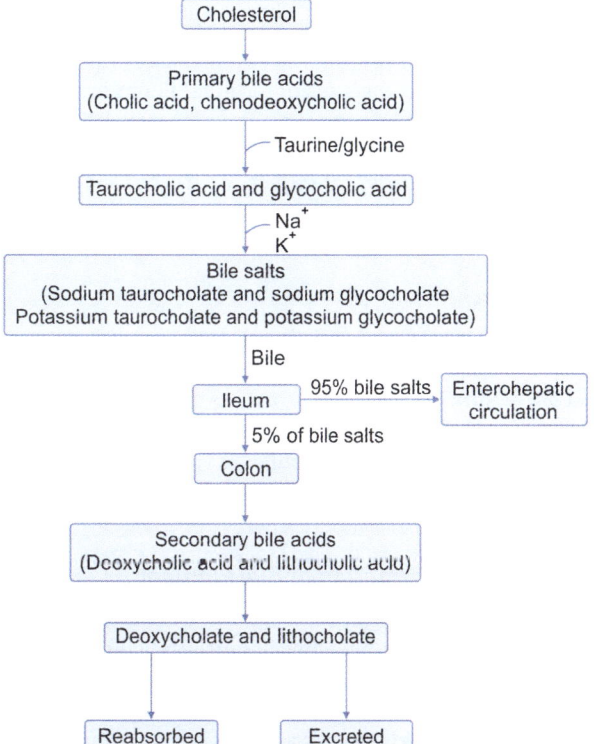

lipase action. This helps in easy digestion and absorption of fat.
- *Micelle formation*: At low concentration, bile salts remain in molecular solution. As the concentration of bile salts increases and when it reaches a critical level, the bile salts form molecular aggregates or cylindrical discs with a hydrophilic surface facing out and a hydrophobic surface facing in. These aggregates are called **micelles**. Critical concentration of micelle formation is called **critical micelle concentration**. Lipids like cholesterol, phospholipids, monoglycerides, etc., collect in the micelle and micelle plays an important role in keeping lipids in solution. Thus it helps in easy absorption of fatty acids, monoglycerides, cholesterol and other lipids by intestinal mucosa (*refer* **Chapter 52, Fig. 52.2**).
- Activates intestinal lipase.
- Antiseptic and **detergent action**: Bile salt is a natural detergent and inhibits growth of bacteria in the intestine.
- **Choleretic effect**, i.e., ingestion of an excess of bile salt increases secretion of bile from the liver to several 100 mL/day.
- Acts as a **laxative** by stimulating peristaltic movements of intestine. Most of the synthetic purgatives contain bile salt preparation.
- Decreases blood cholesterol by inhibiting the synthesis of cholesterol in the liver and increasing the excretion of cholesterol through bile.
- Bile salts keep cholesterol and lecithin in solution and prevent the occurrence of gallstones.
- Bile salts act as **cholagogues** indirectly by stimulating the secretion of CCK which causes gallbladder contraction.

Importance of Bile Salts

When bile is absent in the intestine, up to 50% of ingested fat appears in the feces. There is also severe malabsorption of fat-soluble vitamins. In diseases of terminal ileum or following resection of terminal ileum, enterohepatic circulation of bile salts is interrupted and this leads to **steatorrhea**. *Steatorrhea is excessive excretion of fat in feces characterized by bulky, frothy, foul smelling stools.* Liver cannot increase the rate of bile salt production to compensate for the loss.

Bile Pigment

Bile pigment gives characteristic color to bile and it constitute 15–20% of total solids in bile. The bile pigments are **bilirubin and biliverdin**. Biliverdin is the oxidative product of bilirubin. The golden yellow color of bile is due to the presence of glucuronides of the bile pigments.

Normal plasma bile pigment—0.2–0.8 mg/100 mL of blood.

Mechanism of Formation of Bile Pigment

Most of the bilirubin in the body is formed in the tissues by the breakdown of hemoglobin especially in the reticuloendothelial system. In circulation, bilirubin is bound to albumin. When it reaches liver, bilirubin dissociates from the bound form, and free bilirubin enters liver cells and gets bound to cytoplasmic proteins. The smooth endoplasmic reticulum of liver cells contains the enzyme **glucuronyl transferase**, which helps in the conjugation of bilirubin with glucuronic acid. Each bilirubin molecule reacts with two molecules of glucuronic acid to form **bilirubin diglucuronide**. This compound is more water soluble than free bilirubin and is transported into biliary canaliculi. A small amount of bilirubin diglucuronide escapes into the blood and is excreted through urine. So, the total plasma bilirubin includes **free bilirubin** as well as **conjugated bilirubin** (*refer* Chapter 13, Fig. 13.9).

Bilirubin diglucuronide reaching the intestine through bile is acted upon by intestinal bacteria to form unconjugated bilirubin and **urobilinogen**. Some of the bile pigment and urobilinogen is reabsorbed into the portal circulation and reaches the liver. This undergoes **enterohepatic circulation**. Small amount of urobilinogen enters the general circulation and is excreted through urine. *Conjugated bilirubin does not undergo enterohepatic circulation because intestinal mucosa is impermeable to conjugated bilirubin.* The rest of urobilinogen in the intestine is excreted through feces as stercobilinogen.

■ JAUNDICE OR ICTERUS

PY2.5: Describe different types of anaemias and Jaundice.

Jaundice is yellowish discoloration of skin, sclera and mucous membrane when, total plasma bile pigment (free + conjugated bilirubin) level goes **above 2 mg/100 mL** of blood. This condition is also called **icterus**. Sclera is affected because bilirubin binds with elastic fibers (**Fig. 48.3**).

Yellowish discoloration is also seen in **carotinemia** where carotene is not converted to vitamin A as in hypothyroidism. This condition can be distinguished from hyperbilirubinemia by the absence of discoloration of sclera in carotinemia.

Types of Jaundice (Table 48.2)
- Prehepatic jaundice or hemolytic jaundice.
- Hepatic jaundice or hepatocellular jaundice.
- Posthepatic jaundice or obstructive jaundice or cholestatic jaundice.

Prehepatic Jaundice

Prehepatic jaundice is due to excess production of bilirubin as in hemolytic anemia. The amount of bilirubin in blood is more than the healthy liver can conjugate and excrete. Unconjugated bilirubin is insoluble in water and so cannot be excreted in urine. This is because it is bound to albumin

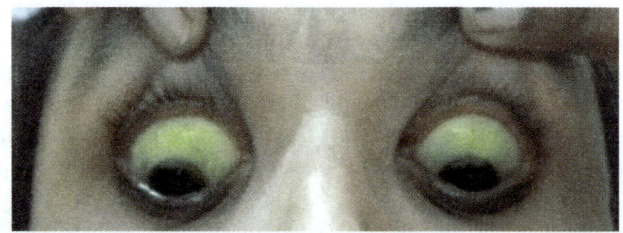

Fig. 48.3: Jaundice (note the yellowish discoloration of sclera).

Table 48.2: Different types of jaundice.

	Prehepatic	Hepatic	Posthepatic
Cause	Increased RBC destruction	Liver damage, e.g., hepatitis	Bile flow obstruction
Type of bilirubin in blood	Unconjugated	Both conjugated and unconjugated	Conjugated
Bilirubin in urine	Absent	Present	Increased
Urobilinogen in urine	Increased	Decreased	Absent
Stercobilinogen in feces	Increased	Decreased	Absent
Color of feces	Dark brown	Pale	Clay or very pale in color
Serum alkaline phosphatase	Normal	Increased	Marked increase
Anemia	Hemolytic anemia	No anemia	No anemia
Blood coagulation	Normal	Prolonged only if liver damage is severe	Prolonged due to vitamin K deficiency

and cannot be filtered. Because of the absence of bilirubin in urine, hemolytic jaundice is also called **acholuric jaundice**.

Hepatic Jaundice

Hepatic jaundice is due to diseases of liver. It can be due to:
❖ Decreased uptake of bilirubin by liver.
❖ Decreased conjugation of bilirubin.
❖ Decreased secretion of conjugated bilirubin into canaliculi.

In hepatic jaundice, the type of hyperbilirubinemia depends on the extent of liver damage. If the damage is mild, the free bilirubin level as well as conjugated bilirubin level in plasma increase leading to both unconjugated and conjugated hyperbilirubinemia. If the liver function is markedly impaired, then there will be unconjugated hyperbilirubinemia and the stool will be pale in color. Most common cause of hepatic jaundice is **cirrhosis** of liver where the liver dysfunction is due to degeneration of hepatic cells due to inflammation and damage.

Posthepatic Jaundice

Posthepatic jaundice is due to bile duct obstruction. The intrahepatic pressure rises and bilirubin diglucuronide regurgitates into blood leading to conjugated hyperbilirubinemia. Conjugated bilirubin is water soluble and it is excreted through urine and the urine will be deep yellow in color. Since bile is not reaching the intestine, urobilinogen is not formed and it will be absent in urine which is diagnostic of obstructive jaundice. Since stercobilinogen is absent in stools, stool will be clay colored **(Table 48.2)**.

Biliary tract obstruction causes two defects:
1. Deficiency of bile acids in the small intestine causes lipid malabsorption along with deficiency of fat-soluble vitamins especially vitamin K which will be manifested as bleeding.
2. Retention of bile in the liver leads to regurgitation of bile acids, bilirubin and cholesterol into the bloodstream. If obstruction is prolonged, it causes destruction of hepatocytes, scarring and fibrosis of liver leading to portal hypertension and death.

REGULATION OF BILIARY SECRETION

❖ Neural regulation through vagus
❖ Hormonal regulation through secretin, CCK and somatostatin.

Neural Regulation

Neural regulation is through **vagus** which increases bile secretion and bile flow. Vagal stimulation also causes gallbladder contraction and relaxation of sphincter of Oddi. Acetylcholine (ACh) is a choleretic as well as a cholagogue. The vagal effect on bile secretion is abolished by atropine, a parasympatholytic drug.

Hormonal Regulation

Bile secretion is more during day time than at night. When food enters mouth, sphincter of Oddi relaxes and releases bile into duodenum. Fatty acids and amino acids in the duodenum release CCK from the duodenum, which causes gallbladder contraction and relaxation of sphincter of Oddi. Substances that cause contraction of gallbladder are called cholagogues, e.g., CCK, calcium, ACh, etc. Substances that increase secretion of bile from liver are called choleretics. Bile salts and bile acids are the most important physiologic choleretics. **Hydrocholeretics** are substances that increase water and HCO_3^- content of bile like secretin, dehydrocholic acid and high-protein diet. **Somatostatin** inhibits water and HCO_3^- secretion by duct cells.

GALLBLADDER

PY4.7: Describe and discuss the structure and functions of liver and gallbladder.

Gallbladder is a thin-walled sac which stores, concentrates, acidifies and discharges bile (*refer* **Fig. 47.1**). The mucous membrane of gallbladder is extensively folded to increase the surface area. Capacity of gallbladder is 60 mL.

Functions of Gallbladder

❖ **Storage of bile**: In between meals, the sphincter of Oddi is closed and bile is diverted into the gallbladder from hepatic duct through cystic duct. During overnight fasting, half of hepatic bile enters gallbladder and is stored there.
❖ **Concentration of bile**: Gallbladder mucosa absorbs water, Na^+, Cl^- and HCO_3^-, but not bile salt, bile pigment, cholesterol, lecithin, calcium, etc. About 1000 mL of bile is secreted by the liver per day, but the capacity of gallbladder is only 60 mL. Bile is concentrated in the gallbladder under

normal conditions by about 5 fold. But it can concentrate bile to a maximum of 20 fold.
- **Increases the viscosity of bile:** The gallbladder mucosa secretes mucus, thereby increasing the viscosity of bile. This mucus acts as a lubricant for the chyme in the intestine.
- **Acidification of bile** or reduction in the alkalinity of bile. This occurs by two mechanisms:
  - Reabsorption of HCO_3^- from bile.
  - Gallbladder mucosa reabsorbs Na^+ in exchange for H^+. This H^+ combines with HCO_3^- to form H_2CO_3 decreasing the pH of bile.
- **Equalization of pressure in the biliary system:** This is accomplished by reabsorption of water. This can be proved by clamping the cystic duct and common bile duct. It is seen that the pressure in the biliary system rises to about 250-320 mm of bile within 30 minutes and secretion of bile stops. If the ligature in the cystic duct is removed, the pressure falls down to about 100 mm of bile.

Contraction of Gallbladder

In the interdigestive phase, when the pressure in the biliary system comes to about 50-70 mm of bile, bile flows into the gallbladder and is stored there. When the pressure in the gallbladder increases to 70-100 mm of bile, it contracts and releases bile into the duodenum. Flow of bile into the duodenum is not continuous but occurs in **spurts**.

Gallbladder contraction is controlled by **neural and hormonal factors**.
- Conditioned reflex in biliary secretion is mediated through **vagus**.
- Substances that cause contraction of gallbladder are called **cholagogues**. **CCK** causes contraction of gallbladder and relaxation of sphincter of Oddi.
- **Atropine and morphine** inhibit gallbladder contraction.
- **Histamine and adrenaline** increase bile secretion and stimulate gallbladder contraction

Applied Physiology

Cholecystectomy is surgical removal of gallbladder. These patients maintain good health due to slow discharge of bile into the duodenum. In the long run, their bile duct becomes dilated so that it can accommodate more bile. They should avoid foods with high fat content.

Cholelithiasis

Presence of **stones** in the gallbladder is known as cholelithiasis. It is common in fatty, fertile, females in the forties. Three types of gallstones are seen:
1. Calcium bilirubinate stones.
2. Cholesterol stones (80–85%).
3. Mixed stones containing 90% cholesterol, calcium bilirubinate, calcium phosphate, calcium carbonate, calcium sulfate, etc.

Causes of Formation of Gallstones

- Stasis of bile due to defective gallbladder contraction or due to obstruction of bile flow from the gallbladder.
- When bile is supersaturated with cholesterol, it forms small crystals and these fuses to form cholesterol stones.
- Too much concentration of bile due to increased water reabsorption by gallbladder mucosa. The concentration of cholesterol, bile pigments and calcium become high leading to their precipitation.
- High cholesterol-lecithin ratio leads to the formation of gallstones. Cholesterol is insoluble in bile and it is held in solution by forming micelles with lecithin. When cholesterol-lecithin ratio becomes high, cholesterol precipitates forming stones.
- Damage or infection of gallbladder epithelium leads to inflammation (cholangitis) which alters the absorptive characteristics of gallbladder mucosa.

Treatment of Gallstones

- Oral administration of bile acids such as chenodeoxycholic acid dissolves gallstones.
- Cholecystectomy.

INVESTIGATIONS OF LIVER AND GALLBLADDER [LIVER FUNCTION TESTS (LFT)]

> **PY4.8:** Describe and discuss gastric function tests, pancreatic exocrine function tests and liver function tests.

Biochemical Liver Function Tests

- **Serum and urinary bilirubin estimation:** Normal serum bilirubin is 0.2–0.8 mg/dL. Serum bilirubin levels are elevated in all types of jaundice.
  Bilirubin and bile salts are normally absent in urine. When serum bilirubin exceeds 2 mg% bilirubin appears in urine and it denotes liver dysfunction.
  Presence of bilirubin in urine indicates conjugated hyperbilirubinemia as in biliary obstruction. Bilirubin is absent in urine in hemolytic jaundice due to unconjugated hyperbilirubinemia.
- Urine urobilinogen excretion is less than 4 mg/day normally. It is increased in hemolytic jaundice and absent in obstructive jaundice.
- **Fecal fat estimation:** Fecal fat normally comes to about 5–6 g/day on an average fat intake of 100 g/day. It is increased in hepatic insufficiency leading to steatorrhea.
- **Fecal stercobilinogen estimation:** Normally it is 20–250 mg/day. In liver damage it is decreased.
- Estimation of serum alkaline phosphatase, serum glutamic-oxaloacetic transaminase (SGOT) or aspartate aminotransferase (AST), serum glutamic pyruvic transaminase (SGPT), etc. Serum alkaline phosphatase (normal: 20–100 IU/L) moderately increases in liver cell damage and markedly increases in bile duct obstruction up to about 1000 IU/L. Both SGOT and SGPT are increased from a normal value of 10–40 units/L to about 100–400 units/L in liver insufficiency. Increase in SGPT is more specific for liver insufficiency than increase in SGOT.

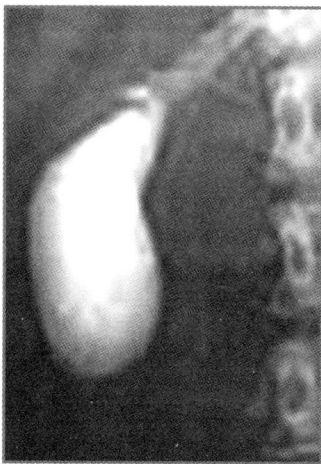

Fig. 48.4: Normal appearance of gallbladder in oral cholecystography.

❖ **Plasma protein estimation:** In hepatic insufficiency, total plasma protein concentration is decreased. Serum albumin decreases and there is a relative increase in serum globulin. This leads to reversal of albumin-globulin ratio (normal A/G ratio is 1.7:1). Serum fibrinogen and prothrombin levels decrease in liver insufficiency. Prothrombin time (normal: 11–16 sec) is increased in hepatic insufficiency. **Liver biopsy** is done for histopathological studies.

Gallbladder and liver can be visualized by:

❖ **Ultrasonography** and **computed tomography** help in visualizing gallbladder and detecting gallstones. Liver cysts and liver abscess can also be detected.

❖ **Nuclear cholescintigraphy or isotope scan:** Technetium-99m-labelled derivative of iminodiacetic acid is given intravenously, and using gamma camera, gallbladder and bile duct can be visualized. The size and shape of the liver and primary and secondary tumors of the liver, liver cysts, etc., can be visualized.

❖ **Oral cholecystography:** Telepaque (sodium tetraiodophenolphthalein), an iodine-containing dye is given orally to the subject at night. The dye is taken up by the liver and is excreted through bile. After overnight fasting, X-ray pictures are taken, and gallbladder can be visualized and any defect can be detected **(Fig. 48.4)**. To see if the gallbladder is capable of normal contraction, give a fatty meal and again take X-ray pictures. If the size of the gallbladder has decreased to 1/3rd the normal size within 30 min, gallbladder contraction is normal.

❖ **Intravenous cholangiography:** The dye is given intravenously and X-ray pictures are taken.

❖ **ERCP (Endoscopic retrograde cholangiopancreatography)** (*refer* **Fig. 47.3**).

MULTIPLE CHOICE QUESTIONS

1. **Bile is formed in the liver at a rate of:**
   a. 20 mL/hr
   b. 40 mL/hr
   c. 80 mL/hr
   d. 100 mL/hr

2. **Liver is the only organ which normally:**
   a. Synthesize heparin
   b. Synthesize urea
   c. Degrades hemoglobin
   d. Convert glucose to glycogen

3. **Fat in the duodenum:**
   a. Stimulates gallbladder contraction
   b. Inhibits gallbladder contraction
   c. Inhibits CCK secretion
   d. Releases secretin

4. **CCK-PZ causes all the following, *except*:**
   a. Gallbladder contraction
   b. Pancreatic enzyme secretion
   c. Increased gastrin secretion
   d. Decrease lower esophageal sphincter tone

5. **Gallbladder contraction is stimulated by:**
   a. Gastrin
   b. Secretin
   c. Vagus
   d. Cholecystokinin

6. **Most important stimulant for bile secretion is:**
   a. Cholecystokinin
   b. Secretin
   c. Bile acid
   d. Bile salt

7. **Maximum contraction of gallbladder is seen with:**
   a. CCK
   b. Secretin
   c. Gastrin
   d. Enterogastrone

8. **Bilirubin is derived from:**
   a. Myoglobin
   b. Amino acid
   c. Muscle
   d. Cholesterol

9. **Function of hepatic stellate cells (Ito cells) is:**
   a. Formation of sinusoids
   b. Vitamin-A storage
   c. Increases blood perfusion
   d. Phagocytosis

10. **Bile acid has a detergent action due to:**
    a. Formation of soap
    b. Formation of zwitterion
    c. Amphipathic nature of bile acid
    d. Formation of medium chain triglyceride

11. **Bilirubin is formed from hemoglobin in the:**
    a. Parenchymal cells of liver
    b. Intestine
    c. Kidney
    d. Reticuloendothelial cells

12. **Normal bilirubin content of plasma is:**
    a. 0.2–0.8 g/dL
    b. 2 mg/dL
    c. 0.2–0.8 mg/dL
    d. 2 g/dL

13. **In the body heat is produced maximally in the:**
    a. Heart
    b. Liver
    c. Skeletal muscle
    d. Skin

14. **The characteristic color of feces is due to the presence of:**
    a. Stercobilin
    b. Urobilin
    c. Bilirubin
    d. Urobilinogen

15. Which of the following is diagnostic of obstructive jaundice?
    a. Increased plasma alkaline phosphatase level
    b. Indirect Vandenberg test positive
    c. Low plasma protein levels
    d. Absence of bile pigment in urine

16. Cholelithiasis means:
    a. Stones in gallbladder
    b. Removal of gallbladder
    c. Absence of gallbladder
    d. Obstruction of cystic duct

17. In common bile duct obstruction, the following are present, *except*:
    a. Bleeding tendency
    b. Increased urinary urobilinogen
    c. Increased serum bilirubin
    d. Steatorrhea

18. Sepsis secondary to translocation of intestinal bacteria is prevented by the following cell type:
    a. Hepatocyte
    b. Stellate cell
    c. Plasma cell
    d. Kupffer cell

19. Following are functions of bile salts, *except* that they:
    a. Emulsify fat
    b. Form chylomicrons
    c. Increase bile secretion
    d. Hydrolyze fat

20. Normal function of adult liver include all the following, *except*:
    a. Conversion of amino acid to glucose
    b. Production of erythrocytes
    c. Synthesis of albumin
    d. Inactivation of drugs and hormones

21. Functions of gallbladder include all the following, *except*:
    a. Increasing the alkalinity of bile
    b. Absorption of water
    c. Absorption of bicarbonate
    d. Reduction of pressure in the biliary system

22. Unconjugated bilirubin does not appear in urine because:
    a. Of its high molecular weight
    b. It is bound to albumin
    c. It is reabsorbed from renal tubules
    d. It is removed by liver

23. The hormone that causes gallbladder contraction is:
    a. Secretin
    b. Gastrin
    c. GIP
    d. Cholecystokinin

24. After complete hepatectomy (removal of liver), there will be a rise in the blood level of:
    a. Estrogens
    b. Glucose
    c. Conjugated bilirubin
    d. Fibrinogen

25. Bile salt is maximally absorbed in:
    a. Duodenum
    b. Jejunum
    c. Ileum
    d. Colon

ANSWERS

1. a	2. b	3. a	4. c	5. d
6. d	7. a	8. a	9. b	10. c
11. d	12. c	13. b	14. a	15. a
16. a	17. b	18. d	19. d	20. b
21. a	22. b	23. d	24. a	25. c

Small Intestine

CHAPTER 49

LEARNING OBJECTIVES
- Draw and explain the structure of a villus of small intestine
- Explain the composition and functions of small intestinal juice

FUNCTIONAL ANATOMY

Small intestine extends from pyloric sphincter to the ileocecal valve.
- **Diameter:** 3 cm
- **Length:** 300 cm during life and 700 cm after death. This is because the smooth muscle of the small intestine is in a state of tonic contraction during life and this tone is lost after death.

PARTS OF SMALL INTESTINE

- **Duodenum** is the first part of small intestine which is C shaped and is about 30 cm in length. The first portion of duodenum is called **duodenal cap or bulb**. Duodenum is referred to as the **hypophysis of abdomen** as it secretes a number of hormones, such as CCK, secretin, etc.
- **Jejunum** is the second part which constitutes about 40% of small intestine beyond duodenum. At the **ligament of Treitz**, duodenum becomes jejunum.
- **Ileum** forms the rest 60% of small intestine which ends in the colon at the ileocecal valve.

Mucosa of small intestine is thrown into a number of valve-like folds called **valvulae conniventes** which contain a number of finger-like projections called **villi** whose free edges contain **microvilli**. The microvilli make up the **brush border** of small intestinal mucosa. The adjacent epithelial cells of the small intestinal mucosa are connected by *tight junctions*.

There are about 20–40 villi per square millimeter of mucosa. Each villus is about 0.5–1 mm long lined by a single layer of columnar epithelial cells called **enterocytes**. Smooth muscles of the submucosa run longitudinally up each villus to its tip. The core of the villus contains a network of capillaries, nerve fibers and lymphatic vessel called **lacteal (Fig. 49.1)**. The epithelial cells of the villi contain numerous microvilli forming the brush border. The microvilli are lined by a dense glycocalyx that protects the cells from the effects of digestive enzymes. Digestive enzymes of small intestine are actually

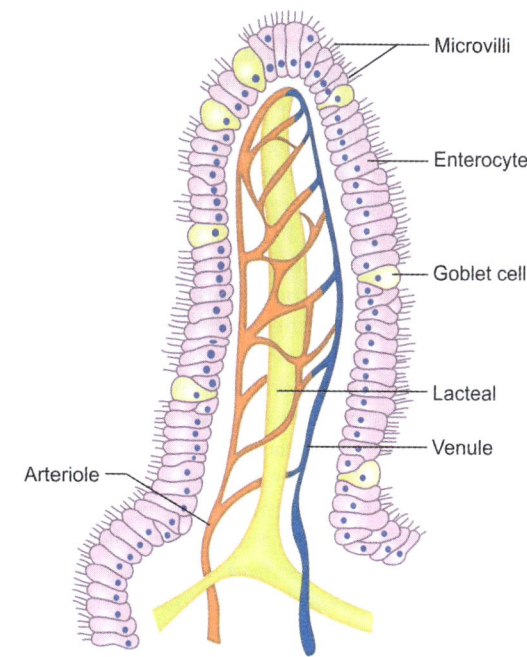

Fig. 49.1: Structure of a villus of small intestine.

part of the brush border existing as membrane bound proteins. They are called **brush-border hydrolases** involved in the final steps of digestion of nutrients. The absorptive surface of small intestine is increased 600 times by the villi and microvilli. Total surface area of small intestine comes to about 200 m².

The venous blood from the villus which contains the absorbed nutrients reaches the portal vein and enters the liver. The lymphatic channels join together and finally open into the thoracic duct which empties into the venous system.

Between the villi are infoldings known as crypts. Stem cells that give rise to both crypt and villus epithelial cells reside towards the base of the crypts and are responsible for renewing the epithelium frequently. The newly formed cells migrate out on to the villi and are finally shed. There are also collections of aggregated lymphatic nodules called **Peyer's patches** in the small intestinal mucosa especially in the ileum. The epithelium over the Peyer's patches contain specialized cells called **M cells (microfold cells or membranous cells)**. They are antigen presenting cells involved in IgA-mediated secretory immunity. They transport antigens from the lumen of intestine to the cells of the immune system, thereby initiating an immune response.

Small Intestinal Glands

Crypts of Lieberkuhn

Crypts of Lieberkuhn are simple tubular glands lined by columnar epithelial cells. Different kinds of cells lining the gland are **enterocytes** which contain digestive enzymes, **Paneth cell, goblet cell and argentaffin cells**.

The enterocytes of the small intestine are formed from undifferentiated cells in the crypts of Lieberkuhn. These cells divide mitotically and migrate up to the tips of the villi, from where they are sloughed off into the intestinal lumen in large numbers forming part of small intestinal juice. This type of secretion of enzymes is known as **holocrine secretion**. About 17 billion cells are shed per day and they are replaced by rapid mitosis in the deeper part of the small intestinal glands or crypts. The amount of protein secreted through these cells into the small intestine comes to about 30 g/day. The microvilli of the epithelial cells covering the villi contain the enzymes involved in the final digestion of food materials. **Argentaffin** or **enterochromaffin cells** of the small intestinal gland secrete **serotonin**.

Crypts of Lieberkuhn also contain **Paneth cells and goblet cells**. Goblet cells secrete mucus and are most numerous in the terminal ileum. Paneth cells are endocrine cells that secrete **defensins** which are naturally occurring peptide antibiotics that protect the mucous cells from microbes. Paneth cells also secrete lysozyme, immunoglobulin, growth factors and **guanylin**. Guanylin binds to guanylyl cyclase and increases the concentration of intracellular cGMP. The cGMP, in turn, increases the secretion of Cl^- into the intestinal lumen.

> Pathogenic *E. coli* produce **enterotoxins,** whose structure is similar to guanylin and the combination of the toxin with guanylin receptors leads to severe diarrhea due to increased secretion of water and Cl^- into the intestinal lumen.

Brunner's Glands

Brunner's glands are small, coiled compound tubuloalveolar glands present in the submucosa of the duodenum. They secrete **alkaline mucus** which protects the duodenal mucosa from the acid chyme coming from stomach. The pH of Brunner's gland secretion varies from 8.2 to 9.3. This mucus and the mucus secreted by the goblet cells, in addition to protecting the mucosa also lubricate the intestinal contents and holds immunoglobulins in place.

SMALL INTESTINAL JUICE OR SUCCUS ENTERICUS

> **PY4.2:** Describe the composition, mechanism of secretion, functions, and regulation of saliva, gastric, pancreatic, intestinal juices and bile secretion.

In human beings, small intestinal juice is collected using a multiluminal tube called **Miller-Abbot's tube**.
Rate of secretion—1–2 L/day
pH—6.5–9
Composition → Water 98.4%
Solids 1.6% → Inorganic constituents
→ Organic constituents

Inorganic constituents: Na^+, K^+, Cl^-, PO_4^{3-}, SO_4^{2-}, HCO_3^-, etc.
Organic constituents: Shed enterocytes containing digestive enzymes, albumin, globulin, mucus, etc.

Enzymes

- The digestive enzymes of small intestine are called **brush border hydrolases** since they are actually part of the brush border, being membrane-bound proteins. The type of secretion is said to be holocrine since the epithelial cells containing the enzymes are shed into the secretion.
- **Protein-splitting enzymes** are enterokinase, aminopeptidase, carboxypeptidase, tetrapeptidase, dipeptidases, etc., which convert peptones and polypeptides to amino acids.
- **Nucleases** are nucleotidase and nucleosidase which convert nucleic acids into purine and pyrimidine bases.
- **Carbohydrate-splitting enzymes** are:
  - **Maltase** converts maltose to glucose.
  - **Lactase** converts lactose to galactose and glucose.
  - **Sucrase** converts sucrose to glucose and fructose.
  - **α-Dextrinase** converts dextrin to glucose.
  - **Trehalase** converts trehalose to glucose.
- **Lipase** converts triglyceride to fatty acids.
- **Enterokinase** or enteropeptidase activates trypsinogen to trypsin.

FUNCTIONS OF SMALL INTESTINE

- **Mechanical function**: Mixing or segmentation contractions in the small intestine help in mixing the chyme coming from stomach into the intestine with pancreatic juice, bile and intestinal juice for proper digestion.
- **Digestive function**: End stages of digestion occur in the small intestine.
- **Absorptive function**: Final products of digestion, vitamins, minerals, water, etc., are absorbed in the small intestine. The villi and microvilli are responsible for absorption.
- **Endocrine function**: A large number of hormones are secreted by the APUD cells present in the small intestine that regulates gastrointestinal function. **Enterogastrones, secretin and CCK** control the secretory activity of pancreas, small intestine and also control gastrointestinal

movements. Enterogastrones inhibit gastric secretion and gastric motility in the intestinal phase of gastric juice secretion. Other hormones secreted by the intestine are **GIP, VIP** (*refer* Chapter 46), **glicentin, somatostatin, motilin, substance-P,** etc.

- **Activation** of trypsinogen occurs by **enterokinase** secreted by small intestinal mucosa.
- **Water balance**: Amount of juice presented to the small intestine comes to about 9 L. Out of this, 2 L is from dietary sources and 7 L from gastrointestinal juices. But only 1–2 L of fluid reaches the colon. Rest is reabsorbed in the small intestine.
- **Mucus** secreted by the Brunner's gland and goblet cells protects intestinal mucosa and prevents intestinal ulcer. Mucus also binds certain bacteria and immunoglobulins.
- **Hemopoietic function**: Vitamin B_{12} is absorbed from small intestine in the presence of intrinsic factor. Deficient absorption of B_{12} leads to pernicious anemia.

REGULATION OF SMALL INTESTINAL SECRETION

- Neural regulation
  - Local reflexes
  - Parasympathetic through vagus
  - Sympathetics
- Hormonal regulation

Neural Regulation

Contact of chyme with small intestinal mucosa and stretch of the intestinal wall increases small intestinal secretion through a **local reflex**. Local reflexes form the most important means of regulation of intestinal secretions. **Parasympathetic** stimulation through vagus increases small intestinal secretion and produces vasodilatation in the gland. Vagal stimulation also increases Brunner's gland secretion. *Sympathetic* stimulation has no effect on small intestinal secretion. It produces vasoconstriction in the gland. But, if sympathectomy is done, there is increased secretion called **paralytic secretion**. This may be due to vasodilatation or due to unopposed action of parasympathetics.

Hormonal Regulation

In hormonal regulation, secretin, gastrin, CCK, glucagon, VIP and calcitonin increase secretion of small intestinal juice. Secretin also increases secretion from Brunner's gland. **Enterocrinin** specifically increases secretion from small intestinal glands.

MULTIPLE CHOICE QUESTIONS

1. The secretion of Brunner's gland differs from that of crypts of Lieberkuhn in that:
   a. It contains the enzyme which activates trypsinogen
   b. It is alkaline in nature
   c. It does not contain mucus
   d. Its rate of secretion is not altered by tactile stimuli

2. Highest basic electric rhythm (BER) is seen in:
   a. Stomach
   b. Jejunum
   c. Sigmoid colon
   d. Ileum

3. The following movements are exhibited by the small intestine, *except*:
   a. Peristalsis
   b. Segmentation contractions
   c. Tonic contractions
   d. Mass action contraction

4. In adynamic ileus there is:
   a. Decrease in the peristaltic activity in small intestine
   b. Increase in peristaltic activity in small intestine
   c. Mass action contraction
   d. Decreased noradrenergic discharge in splanchnic nerves

5. Cholera causes diarrhea by:
   a. Increasing K^+ secretion into the colon
   b. Increasing Na^+–K^+ cotransport in the intestine
   c. Inhibiting K^+ absorption from the intestine
   d. Increasing Cl^- secretion into the intestinal lumen

6. Chyme is propelled forward in small intestine by:
   a. Segmentation
   b. Haustrations
   c. Migratory motor complexes
   d. Peristalsis

7. All the following are secreted in the proenzyme form, *except*:
   a. Trypsin
   b. Chymotrypsin
   c. Pepsin
   d. Ribonuclease

8. Enterogastric reflex is caused by all, *except*:
   a. Distension of duodenum
   b. Alkaline pH in duodenum
   c. Increased osmolality of chyme
   d. b and c

9. Small intestinal peristalsis is controlled by:
   a. Myenteric plexus
   b. Meissner's plexus
   c. Vagus nerve
   d. Sympathetic system

10. Which of the following does not stimulate enterogastric reflex?
    a. Products of protein digestion in the duodenum
    b. Duodenal distension
    c. H^+ bathing duodenal mucosa
    d. Hormones

11. Enterogastric reflex is stimulated by all, *except*:
    a. Alkaline content of small intestine
    b. Hyperosmolarity of chyme
    c. Distension of duodenum
    d. Products of protein and fat digestion in intestine

12. All are true about peristalsis in the intestine, *except*:
    a. Induced by motilin
    b. Relaxation occur proximal to food bolus
    c. Chemical mediators are involved
    d. Occurs in the forward direction
13. Weak anti-peristaltic movement is normally seen in:
    a. Colon
    b. Jejunum
    c. Duodenum
    d. Esophagus
14. The symptoms of dumping syndrome are caused in part by:
    a. Increased secretion of glucagon
    b. Increased secretion of CCK
    c. Hypoglycemia
    d. Hyperglycemia
15. The following are true of resting salivary secretion, *except*:
    a. The regulation of salivary secretion is exclusively neural
    b. In healthy individuals, 1-1.5 liter of saliva is secreted per day
    c. The pH of saliva is about 8
    d. About 99.5% of saliva is water
16. Lower esophageal sphincter:
    a. Has no tonic activity
    b. Has a resting tone provided by the sympathetic nervous system
    c. Relaxes on increasing abdominal pressure
    d. Relaxes ahead of the peristaltic wave
17. The only part in the gastrointestinal tract where glands are present in the submucosa:
    a. Stomach
    b. Duodenum
    c. Jejunum
    d. Ileum
18. The following statements regarding BER is true, *except*:
    a. They are action potentials
    b. They can produce muscle contraction in the stomach
    c. They are initiated in the pace maker cells in the gut wall
    d. They are not present in the esophagus
19. Hypophysis of abdomen is:
    a. Stomach
    b. Jejunum
    c. Duodenum
    d. Ileum
20. Function of peritoneum are all, *except*:
    a. Visceral lubrication
    b. Hormone release
    c. Pain sensitive
    d. Phagocytosis
21. The following secretion is isotonic to plasma:
    a. Gastric juice
    b. Gallbladder bile
    c. Pancreatic juice
    d. Small intestinal juice
22. Which of the following enzyme is secreted by the intestine?
    a. Trypsin
    b. Elastase
    c. Dipeptidase
    d. Phospholipase A_2
23. Which of the following is true regarding Brunner's gland?
    a. Secrete enzymes
    b. Secretes water
    c. Secretes electrolytes
    d. Secrete mucus to protect intestine from acid
24. Which of the following is the function of M cells in intestine?
    a. Antigen presenting cells
    b. Meissner's plexus cell
    c. Mucus secreting cells
    d. Hormone secreting cells

ANSWERS

1. b	2. b	3. d	4. a	5. d
6. d	7. d	8. a	9. a	10. d
11. a	12. b	13. a	14. c	15. c
16. d	17. b	18. a	19. c	20. b
21. d	22. c	23. d	24. a	

Large Intestine

CHAPTER 50

LEARNING OBJECTIVES
- Explain the functions of large intestine
- Discuss the physiological role of dietary fiber in health

INTRODUCTION

PY4.2: Describe the composition, mechanism of secretion, functions, and regulation of saliva, gastric, pancreatic, intestinal juices and bile secretion.

Large intestine extends from ileocecal valve to anus and is about 100 cm in length during life and 150 cm at autopsy (due to loss of smooth muscle tone after death). Mucosa of large intestine is smooth with *no villi*. The longitudinal muscle fibers of muscularis externa in the colon are collected into three longitudinal bundles, the **teniae coli**. These bands are shorter than the rest of the colon. So, the wall of the colon forms outpouchings called **haustrae** between the teniae coli. Colonic glands are lined by columnar epithelial cells and large number of goblet cells which secrete mucus. Secretion of large intestine is thick, viscous and alkaline with a pH around 8.

Ileocecal valve marks the point where ileum ends in colon or cecum **(Fig. 50.1)**. This portion of ileum projects slightly into the cecum and the muscular coat is thickened to form the **ileocecal sphincter**. This sphincter normally remains slightly constricted and slows down the emptying of ileal contents into the colon. This gives sufficient time for digestion to be completed in small intestine. Increase in colonic pressure squeezes the valve shut and this prevents reflux of colonic contents into the ileum. Increase in ileal pressure opens the valve. Sympathetic stimulation increases the tone of sphincter, whereas gastrin relaxes the ileocecal valve (in the case of cardiac sphincter gastrin causes contraction of the sphincter). When food leaves the stomach, the cecum relaxes and ileocecal valve opens allowing the passage of chyme into the colon. This reflex is called **gastroileal reflex** and is mediated through vagus.

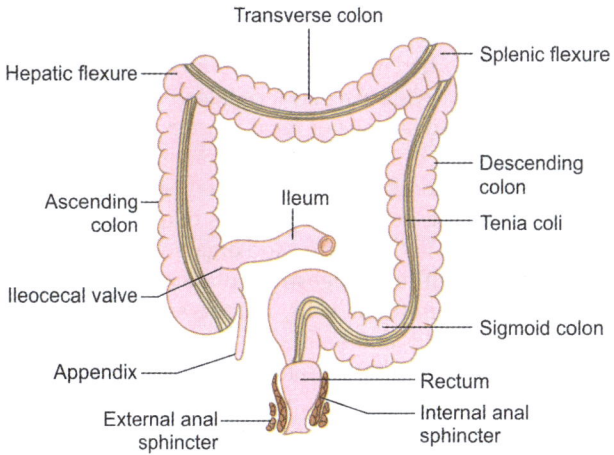

Fig. 50.1: Parts of large intestine (colon).

Ascending colon extends upwards from the cecum along the right side of the abdomen up to the liver. At the hepatic flexure, it bends to the left to form the **transverse colon** to reach the left splenic flexure. **Descending colon** extends from the left splenic flexure to the pelvic inlet below. **Sigmoid colon** begins at the pelvic inlet and joins the **rectum** in front of the sacrum. Rectum descends and leaves the pelvis by piercing the pelvic floor. Here, it becomes the **anal canal** in the perineum. Anal canal opens to the exterior through the **anus** which is guarded by two sphincters internal and external anal sphincters.

Appendix is a worm-shaped structure that arises from the medial side of cecum and is involved in immunity. In human beings, it is a vestigial organ.

Functions of Large Intestine

- **Lubrication** of fecal matter by mucus secreted by large intestinal glands. Mucus and HCO_3^- neutralize acid formed by bacterial flora of intestine. Mucus also protects the large-intestinal mucous membrane from mechanical injury especially when the fecal matter is hard.

- **Absorption:** Large intestine absorbs water, electrolytes, vitamins, short chain fatty acids, glucose; certain drugs, such as steroids, sedatives and anesthetics. **Aldosterone** increases sodium reabsorption in the colon. Drugs are given as an **enema** especially in children. Most of the absorption occurs in the proximal half of large intestine referred to as **absorptive colon**. It absorbs 90% of fluid entering it. Large intestine can absorb about 5–7 L of fluid and electrolytes per day. Na$^+$–glucose co-transporters are absent in the colon. So, its absorptive capacity is considerably less when compared to that of the small intestine which is 12 L/day. The distal half of the large intestine is called **storage colon**.
- **Synthesis of vitamins:** Even though jejunum and ileum contain bacteria, colon contains large numbers of bacteria. Some of these bacteria synthesize vitamins, such as B-complex, vitamin K, folic acid, etc., and these vitamins are absorbed from the colon in significant amounts.
- The **colonic bacteria** form short chain fatty acids, such as acetate, propionate, butyrate, etc., from materials that escape digestion in the upper GIT. These short chain fatty acids are absorbed in the large intestine. Certain bacteria in the intestine can even digest cellulose.
- **Formation and storage of fecal matter:** Large intestine converts 1–2 L of isotonic chyme that enters the colon each day into about 200–250 mL of semisolid feces which is stored in the pelvic colon. Feces contains inorganic materials like Ca^{2+}, PO$_4$, etc., and organic materials, such as cellulose, other indigestible plant fibers, bacteria, desquamated mucosal cells, mucus, small amounts of digestive enzymes and water.
- Fermentation of carbohydrates leads to the formation of gases, such as CO_2, H_2, H_2S, CH_4, etc., which contributes to flatus and decarboxylation and deamination of proteins and amino acids lead to the formation of indole, skatole, mercaptan, H_2S, etc., which contributes to the odor of feces.
- **Excretory function:** Large intestine excretes heavy metals, such as Hg, Pb, Bi, Ar, etc., through the feces.
- Lymphatic nodules are present in the mucosa of the proximal parts of large intestine. Plasma cells produced from the B lymphocytes secrete IgA and IgM which coat the mucosa and prevent entry of pathogenic organisms. The T cells also produce NO which kills microorganisms.

Intestinal Bacteria

Bacteria in the GIT are of three types: **pathogens, symbionts and commensals**. At birth, intestine is sterile, but the bacterial flora becomes established early in life. Large intestine contains harmless bacteria, such as *E. coli, lactobacilli, Enterobacter aerogenes*, etc. as well as harmful bacteria, such as various types of cocci, gas gangrene bacilli, etc. The harmful bacteria can cause serious disease in tissues outside the colon.

Organic acids formed from carbohydrates by bacteria are responsible for the slightly acidic reaction of the stools. Amines, such as indole and skatole, and sulfides produced by colonic bacteria contribute to the odor of feces. Brown color of feces is due to pigments formed from bile pigments by the action of colonic bacteria. In obstructive jaundice, stool is white colored (**acholic stools**) due to the absence of bile pigments because bile fails to enter the intestine. The colonic bacteria convert cholic acid and chenodeoxycholic acid (primary bile acids) into deoxycholic acid and lithocholic acid (secondary bile acids).

Advantages of Intestinal Bacteria

- Some intestinal bacteria synthesize **vitamin K**, a number of **B complex vitamins and folic acid**. Beneficial bacteria of gut are referred to as **probiotics**.
- Short chain fatty acids produced by intestinal flora are absorbed in the colon. Some of the short chain fatty acids have a trophic effect on colonic mucosa.
- Non-pathogenic strains of *Salmonella* bacteria block steps that initiate inflammation.
- Certain intestinal flora lower plasma LDL and cholesterol levels.
- Some colonic bacteria can even digest cellulose. (*Refer* gut microbiota; Chapter 44)

Harmful Effects of Intestinal Flora

- Useful substances, such as ascorbic acid, cyanocobalamin, choline, etc., are utilized by some bacteria of intestine.
- *Overgrowth of bacteria in the small intestinal lumen is harmful.* It occurs when there is stasis of the intestinal contents. The effects are macrocytic anemia, steatorrhea and other metabolic abnormalities. It is seen in blind loop syndrome, diverticulitis and disorders of small intestinal motility.
- Colonic bacteria also produce ammonia, which is absorbed by blood and is normally detoxified quickly in the liver. But in liver dysfunction, hyperammonemia results leading to hepatic encephalopathy.
- Normally, the intestinal flora is confined to the lumen of the intestine. They do not invade the rest of the body. When a person is exposed to ionizing radiation, the body defenses that prevent this invasion break-down. This leads to severe **septicemia** if adequate measures are not taken. Septicemia is the major cause of death in **radiation poisoning**.

DIETARY FIBER

PY4.3: Explain role of dietary fiber.

Dietary fiber also known as roughage includes all ingested food that reaches the large intestine in an unchanged state. They are of two types, soluble and insoluble fiber. It includes **cellulose, hemicelluloses, lignin, gums, algal polysaccharides, pectins, oligosaccharides, beta-glucans,** etc., present in the vegetables in the diet. Requirement of dietary fiber is 20 to 30 g/day and is very important for keeping the gut healthy. For people over 70 years, fiber requirement decreases. Most fiber containing foods are also good sources of vitamins, minerals, and antioxidants, which offer many health benefits.

Advantages of Dietary Fiber

- **Insoluble dietary fiber** does not dissolve in water and passes through the GIT almost intact. Thus it adds bulk to the stool, preventing constipation. It does not provide calories. Good sources of insoluble fiber are fruits, nuts, vegetables, whole grain foods.
- **Soluble fiber** absorbs water, forming a gel like substance in the digestive tract. It helps to lower cholesterol and help to regulate blood sugar level. Fiber can help slow down the body's absorption of sugar, helping to prevent sugar spikes after meals. Good sources of soluble fiber are beans, fruits, oats, nuts and vegetables. Soluble fiber provides some calories to the individual.
- Dietary fiber also encourages healthy gut microbiota.
- In the human digestive tract, the dietary fibers are not digested and hence reach the large intestine in an unchanged state. Thus, it increases the bulk of stool and initiates defecation reflex due to distension of the wall of large intestine and prevents constipation. In constipation, bulk laxatives are given, which contain substances, such as pectin which increase the volume of colon, thereby stimulating defecation.
- People who live on a diet containing large amounts of dietary fiber have a low incidence of gastroesophageal reflux disease (GERD), cancer of colon and rectum, diverticulitis, hemorrhoids, type-2 diabetes mellitus, coronary artery disease, etc. It prevents heart disease mainly by reducing total cholesterol and low density lipoprotein (LDL) cholesterol which is a major risk of heart disease. Dietary fiber decreases cholesterol absorption by binding to cholesterol.
- Helps to decrease body weight. High fiber foods give a sensation of fullness for longer periods which prevents over eating and hunger in between meals. Thus they can adhere to their dietary caloric restriction.
- Many toxic substances produced in the colon that are carcinogenic get bound to dietary fiber and their absorption is prevented. Another mechanism is that the frequency of stool is increased and so the harmful substances remain in the intestine for a short time. If the amount of dietary fiber is less, the bulk of stool will be less, leading to inhibition of bowel movements and constipation.

Disadvantages

- Eating too much fiber (more than 70 g/day) can cause cramping, bloating, gas, and constipation.
- Fiber also binds with certain nutrients and carries them out of the body.
- Eating a high fiber diet may interfere with the absorption and effectiveness of some medications.
- At-least 8 glasses of fluid should be taken each day when consuming a high fiber diet. Otherwise constipation may result.

■ MULTIPLE CHOICE QUESTIONS

1. **Gastrocolic reflex is related to:**
   a. Mass peristalsis
   b. Segmental movement
   c. Pendular movement
   d. Inhibition of colon

2. **While doing sigmoidoscopy, if the rectum is inflated with gas, increased peristalsis is seen in:**
   a. Whole colon   b. Proximal colon
   c. Distal colon   d. Whole intestine

3. **While doing sigmoidoscopy, if the rectum is inflated with gas increased peristalsis is seen in:**
   a. Whole colon
   b. Whole intestine
   c. Proximal colon
   d. Distal colon

4. **Distal colon includes the following:**
   a. Descending colon, sigmoid colon and rectum
   b. Sigmoid colon and rectum
   c. Descending colon and sigmoid colon
   d. Sigmoid colon

5. **Part of the intestine devoid of villi is:**
   a. Large intestine   b. Jejunum
   c. Ileum   d. Duodenum

6. **Defecation following a meal in infants is due to:**
   a. Gastrocolic reflex
   b. Gastroileal reflex
   c. Enterogastric reflex
   d. Gastropancreatic reflex

7. **The type of movement seen characteristically in the large intestine is:**
   a. Segmentation contraction
   b. Peristalsis
   c. Mass action contraction
   d. Peristaltic rushes

8. **Longest transit time in GIT is seen in:**
   a. Stomach   b. Jejunum
   c. Ileum   d. Colon

9. **True about high roughage in diet is:**
   a. Decreases stool transit time
   b. Increase stool transit time
   c. Normalize stool transit
   d. No effect on stool transit time

10. **Following constitute dietary fiber, *except*:**
    a. Pectin   b. Cellulose
    c. Hemicelluloses d. Riboflavin

11. **Dietary fiber contains:**
    a. Collagen   b. Pectin
    c. Proteoglycans   d. Starch

12. **Probiotics is the name given to:**
    a. Invasive bacteria of gut
    b. Beneficial bacteria of gut
    c. Substances given to increase the efficacy of antibiotics
    d. Vitamins given along with antibiotics
13. **Colonic bacteria, on digestion of dietary fibers, produce:**
    a. Free radicals b. Sucrose
    c. Butyrate d. Glycerol
14. **Short chain fatty acids produced by bacteria are absorbed maximally in:**
    a. Duodenum b. Jejunum
    c. Ileum d. Colon

ANSWERS

1. a	2. c	3. d	4. a	5. a
6. a	7. c	8. d	9. a	10. d
11. b	12. b	13. c	14. d	

Movements of Gastrointestinal Tract

CHAPTER 51

LEARNING OBJECTIVES
- Explain different phases of deglutition
- Describe the physiology of vomiting
- Describe the movements exhibited by the stomach
- Discuss the types of small intestinal movements
- Describe defecation reflex with the help of a diagram
- Discuss diarrhea, constipation, adynamic ileus and Hirschsprung's disease

INTRODUCTION

PY4.3: Describe GIT movements, regulation and functions. Describe defecation reflex. Explain role of dietary fiber.

The movement of food through the gastrointestinal tract (GIT) requires coordinated contraction and relaxation of the different muscle layers of the GIT. At the junctions between different parts of GIT, muscular sphincters mainly made up of circular muscle fibers control the movement of food between adjacent segments. For example, contraction and relaxation of the pyloric sphincter present at the junction between pylorus and duodenum control the rate of emptying of acidic chyme from stomach into the duodenum.

There are two types of sphincters, **anatomical sphincter and physiological sphincter**. In anatomical sphincter, the circular and longitudinal muscles are thickened and there is increased resting tone as in pyloric sphincter. In physiological sphincter, there is no increase in the thickness of musculature and the muscle is normally in continuous contraction at rest. It relaxes only when a peristaltic wave reaches the sphincter as in the case of lower esophageal sphincter.

TYPES OF MOVEMENTS

The different types of movements exhibited by the GIT are:
- Mastication or chewing
- Swallowing or deglutition
- Gastric movements
- Small intestinal movements
- Movements of large intestine
- Abnormal movements

Mastication or Chewing

Cutting the food substances into small particles and grinding them into a soft bolus is known as mastication. Mastication is the first mechanical process to which food is subjected to.

Chewing is a rhythmic movement brought about by lips, tongue and jaws along with teeth. Lower jaw can move in all planes and it can rotate. Movement of jaw is affected by contraction of the muscles of mastication which are innervated by 5th cranial nerve except buccinator which is innervated by 7th cranial nerve. The muscles of mastication are **masseter, temporalis, pterygoids, and buccinators**. All muscles involved in the act of mastication are voluntary muscles and are the strongest muscles in the body. A crushing force of 50–80 kg can be generated on the molars during chewing.

Mastication is a voluntary as well as a reflex act. The movements during mastication are closure and opening of mouth; rotational movement of jaw, protraction and retraction of jaw. The center for mastication is in the **medulla and cerebral cortex**. Chewing reflex is influenced by higher centers, e.g., stimulation of hypothalamus, reticular formation, amygdala and cerebral cortex near the sensory areas of taste causes movements similar to mastication.

Aim of Mastication

- Primary function of mastication is to facilitate **deglutition** or swallowing by reducing the size of food particles and lubricating them with saliva.
- Helps in **digestion**—chewing increases salivary, gastric and pancreatic secretion of cephalic phase. Surface area of food particles is increased by chewing so that digestive enzymes can act more effectively.
- Chewing helps in the appreciation of **taste** and gives the pleasure of eating.

Disturbances of Chewing

- Absence of teeth leads to indigestion.
- Paralysis of facial nerve leads to collection of food between teeth and cheek.
- Inability to chew is an early sign of myasthenia gravis.

Deglutition or Swallowing

Food after mastication is carried to the stomach by a complex coordinated movement of muscles of mouth, pharynx and esophagus. This process is called **deglutition**. Swallowing is initiated when the food bolus comes into contact with the pressure receptors in the pharynx. It is a complex reflex involving the **swallowing center in medulla**, the glossopharyngeal nerve and superior laryngeal branch of vagus. Deglutition is divided into three stages:
1. Oral or voluntary or buccal stage
2. Pharyngeal stage
3. Esophageal stage

Oral Stage

Before swallowing, food is made into a **bolus**, by the action of tongue against hard palate and cheek. Bolus is brought to the posterodorsal aspect of tongue and it is known as the **preparatory position (Fig. 51.1B)**. Tongue is raised and touches the hard palate. There is depression of posterior part of tongue. By strong contraction of **hyoglossus muscle**, the bolus of food is carried to the oropharynx. Afferent and efferent fibers pass through 5th, 9th and 10th cranial nerves, and the center is the swallowing center in lower **pons and medulla**.

Disturbances of oral stage

Dysphagia means difficulty in swallowing. In the 1st stage, dysphagia is due to:
- Inflammation of mouth and pharynx
- Cleft lip and cleft palate
- Paralysis of tongue
- Aptyalism (deficiency in secretion of saliva)
- Lesions of swallowing center

Odynophagia means painful swallowing. This is different from dysphagia. Odynophagia may occur in pharyngitis, tonsillitis, ulcers of mouth, esophageal cancer, candida infection of mouth and throat, gastroesophageal reflux disease associated with heart burn and following radiation therapy in the neck region.

Pharyngeal Stage (Fig. 51.2)

Duration of this second stage of deglutition is less than 2 sec. This stage is initiated when food comes in contact with the posterior aspect of tongue, soft palate, anterior and posterior pillars of fauces, tonsils and posterior pharyngeal wall. This stimulates sensory receptors located in these areas and initiates a reflex stimulation of pharyngeal wall. A series of automatic pharyngeal muscle contraction follows and food is propelled down the oropharynx. Once food is in the oropharynx, there are *four possible outlets for the exit of food*. They are:
- It can move back into the mouth
- Into the nasopharynx
- Into the larynx
- Into the esophagus

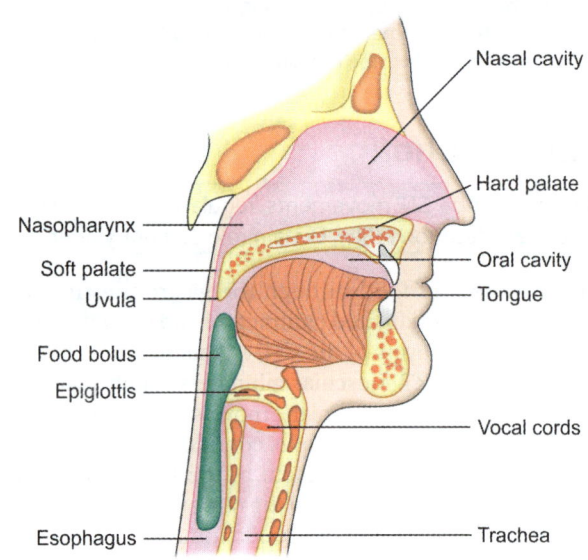

Fig. 51.2: Pharyngeal stage (second stage) of deglutition; Note the epiglottis closing the laryngeal opening, approximation of soft palate against the posterior pharyngeal wall and approximation of vocal cords.

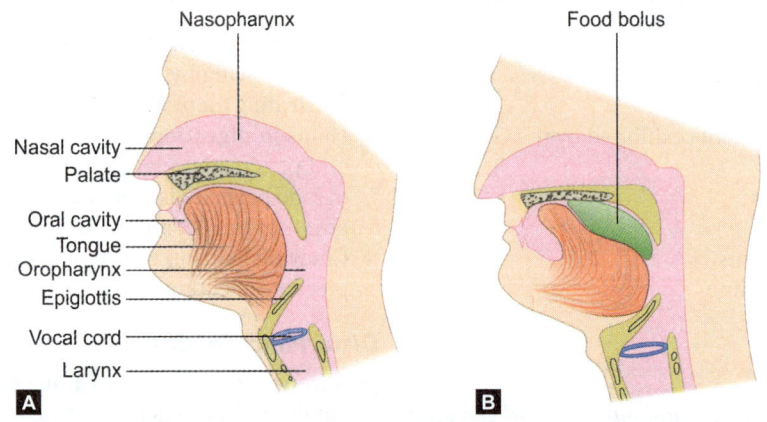

Figs. 51.1A and B: (A) Normal anatomy of oropharynx; (B) Oral stage of deglutition.

Swallowing reflex should be well coordinated so that, food enters only into the esophagus. Entry of food back into the mouth is prevented by approximation of tongue against the roof of mouth. Food is prevented from entering the nasopharynx by pressing the soft palate against the posterior pharyngeal wall, thus sealing off the opening (**Fig. 51.2**).

Food is prevented from entering the respiratory passage by the following mechanisms:
- **Deglutition apnea**—swallowing center specifically inhibits respiratory center in medulla during swallowing leading to arrest of respiration.
- By the tight approximation of vocal cords, the laryngeal opening is closed.
- There is horizontal deflection of **epiglottis** during swallowing so that it covers the laryngeal opening. This is accomplished by the backward movement of tongue and forward and upward movement of larynx.

If food enters the respiratory passage, there will be cough, severe choking and if the bolus is large it may even lead to death due to asphyxia.

Contraction of **superior constrictor** muscle of pharynx initiates **peristaltic wave** which moves the bolus through the pharynx into the esophagus by relaxing the **upper esophageal sphincter**. This sphincter remains strongly contracted in between swallows to prevent air from entering esophagus during inspiration. *Afferent fibers go through 5th, 9th, 10th and 12th cranial nerves in the second stage.*

Disturbances of pharyngeal stage

- Pharyngitis, tonsillitis, diphtheria
- Carcinoma of pharynx
- Myasthenia gravis
- Bulbar poliomyelitis
- Tetanus, rabies
- Cranial nerve neuritis

When there is paralysis of muscles of palate or pharynx, there will be regurgitation of food into the nasal cavity, or aspiration of food into larynx and lungs during swallowing.

Esophageal Stage of Deglutition

Esophagus conducts food from pharynx to stomach by peristalsis. It exhibits two types of peristaltic movements:
1. First degree peristalsis or primary peristalsis
2. Second degree peristalsis or secondary peristalsis

Peristalsis that is initiated by swallowing is called **primary peristalsis**, whereas that elicited by distension of the esophagus is called **secondary peristalsis**.

First degree or primary peristalsis is a continuation of the peristaltic wave that begins in pharynx and spreads into the esophagus during pharyngeal stage of swallowing. A wave takes about 8–10 sec to pass from pharynx to stomach and food is swept down the esophagus at a speed of 4 cm/sec. During peristalsis, a ring of contraction occurs proximal to the bolus of food. The portion distal to the bolus relaxes to accommodate the food and this is called **receptive relaxation**.

Second degree peristaltic waves result from distension of esophagus with food and its purpose is to move all the food that has entered the esophagus into the stomach. These second degree waves are initiated partly by **enteric nervous system** and partly by **long vagovagal reflex**.

In the upright position, liquids and semisolid foods fall by gravity to lower esophagus ahead of peristaltic wave. Lower 3–5 cm of esophagus is tonically active and is called **lower esophageal sphincter (LES)**. When peristaltic wave reaches the lower esophageal sphincter, it relaxes allowing food to enter the stomach. This relaxation is mediated via neurons that release **NO and vasoactive intestinal polypeptide (VIP)**. Tonic spasm of lower esophageal sphincter in between meals prevents reflux of gastric contents into the esophagus and protects esophagus from ulceration.

Disturbances of esophageal stage

- **Diffuse spasm** of esophagus due to hypersensitivity of nerve plexus to stimuli. Patient complains of retrosternal pain due to spasm of esophagus.
- **Achalasia cardia** or **cardiospasm:** In this condition, food accumulates in the lower end of esophagus and this area becomes greatly distended. It is associated with difficulty in swallowing (dysphagia). Liquids pass the lower esophageal sphincter with ease but solids do not (**Figs. 51.3A and B**). *Causes of cardiospasm are*:
  - Tonic spasm of lower esophageal sphincter due to gastrinomas.
  - Due to deficiency of VIP and NO there will be incomplete relaxation of lower esophageal sphincter.
  - Defects in enteric nervous system produce weak esophageal peristalsis leading to incomplete relaxation of lower esophageal sphincter.
- The condition is diagnosed by barium swallow. The patient is asked to swallow 25% barium sulfate and X-ray pictures are taken. The lower end of esophagus is found to be severely distended. Treatment is mechanical dilatation of sphincter or myotomy. Injection of botulinum toxin locally is also beneficial.
- **Chalasia** or **lower esophageal incompetence** or **gastroesophageal reflux disease (GERD):** There is reflux of gastric contents into the esophagus leading to esophageal ulceration, esophagitis, scarring and stricture of esophagus. The patient complains of heartburn. This condition is treated by inhibiting gastric acid secretion with

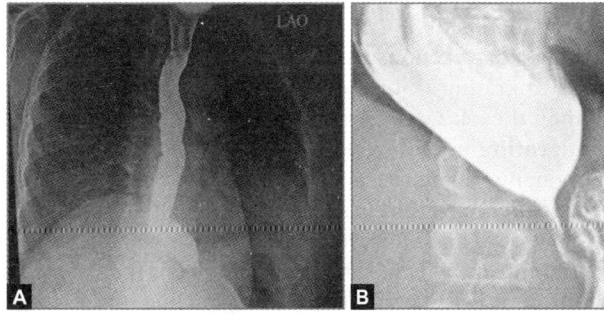

Figs. 51.3A and B: (A) Achalasia cardia; (B) Typical bird beak appearance in severe achalasia cardia.
Courtesy: Dr Anil Sundaram, Surgeon.

H_2 receptor blockers or omeprazole. Surgical treatment is **fundoplication**. Here, a portion of the fundus of stomach is wrapped around the lower esophagus so that the lower esophageal sphincter is inside a short tunnel of stomach. *In pregnancy, high circulating level of progesterone causes LES incompetency producing heart burn.*

- **Carcinoma** of esophagus and inflammation leads to dysphagia and odynophagia.
- **Aerophagia**: Swallowing of air is called aerophagia. Some air is swallowed during eating and drinking. Total number of swallows per day is about 600 (200 during eating and drinking, and 400 in between meals). Some people, especially nervous individuals swallow large amount of air, and is called aerophagia. Some of this air is regurgitated and is called **belching**. Some amount is absorbed in the GIT and the rest reaches colon and is expelled as **flatus**. The smell is largely due to sulfides. About 500–1500 mL of gas is produced in the GIT per day. In some people, excess gas in the intestine causes abdominal discomfort, cramps and rumbling noises called **borborygmi sounds**.

Control of deglutition

First stage is initiated voluntarily but further it is reflex in nature. Second and third stages are involuntary. Receptors are present in mucous membrane around the entrance of oropharynx. Afferent fibers carried by 5, 9, 10 cranial nerves, center is the swallowing center in the **nucleus tractus solitarius and nucleus ambiguus**. Efferent fibers pass through 5, 7, 10 and 12th cranial nerves which supply muscles of deglutition.

GASTRIC MOVEMENTS

Types of Gastric Movements

- Movement of empty stomach
- Gastric filling movement
- Gastric mixing movement
- Gastric emptying movement
- Abnormal movements

Movements of Empty Stomach

Contraction of stomach when it has been empty for several hours is known as **hunger contraction**. Hunger contraction is associated with the sensation of hunger and it immediately stops on food intake.

Hunger contractions are powerful rhythmical contraction waves migrating from the body of stomach to the distal ileum and each wave is called **migrating motor complex** or **migrating myoelectrical complex (MMC)**. It has two components: an electrical and a muscular component. The **electrical component** is spike potential superimposed on the slow wave or BER wave. It is a wave of depolarization of smooth muscle which starts in the stomach. The **muscular component** is the contraction wave starting in the empty stomach. This wave sweeps forwards till it reaches the end of the ileum. This whole wave which sweeps down until it reaches the end of ileum is called MMC. MMC migrate at a rate of 5 cm/min and occur at intervals of 90 min. MMCs are initiated by motilin, a gastrointestinal hormone secreted by the enterochromaffin cells in the stomach and intestine. Function of MMC is to clear the stomach and small intestine of luminal contents in preparation for the next meal. When food is ingested, there is suppression of motilin release and MMCs stop immediately with return to normal pattern of activity.

When the contractions become extremely strong, they fuse and cause tetanic contraction that lasts for 2–3 min. During these contractions, the person experiences pain called **hunger pangs**. It usually occurs after 12–24 hours of starvation and maximum intensity is seen in 3–4 days.

Functions of Hunger Contractions

- These contractions clear the stomach and small intestine of luminal contents in preparation for the next meal.
- It also increases pancreatic, biliary and gastric secretions.

Gastric Filling Movements

As the esophageal peristaltic wave reaches the stomach, due to **receptive relaxation** the fundus and proximal portion of the body of stomach relax to accommodate the food with little increase in pressure. This is due to the property of **plasticity** of the smooth muscle of stomach. Receptive relaxation is a **vagovagal reflex** and the neurotransmitter is **NO**.

Solid food first occupies the greater curvature and fundus of stomach. Then, it is deposited in the lesser curvature and finally near the cardiac orifice. When liquids are swallowed, they remain in the lesser curvature and flow towards the pyloric area. A completely relaxed stomach can accommodate about 1.5 L of food.

Gastric Mixing and Emptying Movements

As the stomach is filled with food, initially there is no rise in pressure. When it exceeds a certain limit there is increase in the tone of gastric musculature and strong gastric peristaltic waves appear due to basic electrical rhythm (BER).

BER waves start from the pacemaker cells situated in the middle of the greater curvature of stomach.

In the beginning, a ring of contraction of the circular muscle layer develops near the middle of the body of stomach and sweeps towards pylorus **(Fig. 51.4)**. These occur at a frequency of **3/min**. At a time, 3 waves are seen in the stomach and the time taken for one wave to traverse the stomach is 1 min. The contraction ring deepens as it

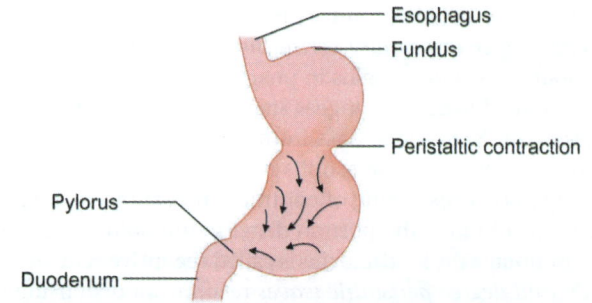

Fig. 51.4: Peristaltic contraction begin in the middle of stomach and pushes the food towards pylorus.

moves towards the pylorus. These constrictor rings play an important role in grinding and mixing the food with gastric juice and also help to propel food forwards.

As these rings reach the pyloric antrum, strong peristaltic waves appear called **peristaltic constrictor rings or antral systole**. These powerful waves force the antral contents under high pressure towards the pylorus. The pyloric opening is small and only a few mL of chyme is expelled into the duodenum with each peristaltic wave. The rest is pushed back into the body of stomach, called **retropulsion**. This movement is important in the mixing of food with gastric juice, grinding of solid food and sieving mechanism of stomach. Only solid particles which are <2 mm in diameter escape the stomach. Pumping action of antrum is known as **pyloric pump**.

Normally, duodenal contents do not regurgitate into the stomach because the pressure exerted by antrum is greater than duodenal pressure. In addition, secretin and CCK increase the tone of pyloric sphincter.

The rate at which stomach empties its contents into the duodenum depends on the type of food ingested. Food rich in carbohydrates leaves the stomach in a few hours. Protein-rich food leaves more slowly and slowest for fat.

Regulation of gastric emptying or factors affecting gastric emptying
a. Gastric factors
b. Duodenal factors
c. Other factors

❖ *Gastric factors*
- **Volume** of gastric contents—distension of stomach stimulates stretch receptors which initiates vagovagal reflex and local myenteric reflex which relaxes the pyloric sphincter and promotes gastric emptying.
- **Consistency** of gastric contents—liquids leave the stomach rapidly. Solids move out of stomach only after being converted into a semifluid mass called chyme.
- Chemical **composition** of food—food rich in carbohydrate leaves the stomach in a few hours. Protein- rich food leaves more slowly and fat is the slowest.
- **pH** of gastric content—highly acidic content leave the stomach slowly.
- **Osmolality** of gastric contents—isotonic gastric contents leave the stomach rapidly than contents hypotonic or hypertonic to blood.
- **Hormonal** factor—distension of stomach and presence of protein in stomach release gastrin from antral mucosa which promotes pyloric pumping.

❖ *Duodenal Factors*
Duodenal factors are inhibitory to gastric emptying.
- **Enterogastric reflex**—distension of duodenum, presence of products of protein digestion and increased acidity in duodenum inhibit gastric emptying by enterogastric reflex. This reflex inhibits antral peristalsis and increases the tone of pyloric sphincter. This occurs by the following mechanisms:
  - Inhibitory impulses pass directly from duodenum to stomach through ENS.
  - Impulses pass to the sympathetic ganglia and through inhibitory sympathetic fibers reach the stomach and inhibit gastric emptying.
- **Hormonal feedback**—presence of acidic, hyperosmolar and fatty chyme in the duodenum releases **secretin, CCK and GIP** from intestinal mucosa, which contracts the pyloric sphincter and delay gastric emptying.

❖ *Other factors*
- Excitement and parasympathetic stimulation increase gastric emptying.
- Fear, grief, vagotomy and sympathetic stimulation decrease gastric emptying. Sympathetic stimulation causes relaxation of the stomach.

Normal gastric emptying time is 2–5 hours.

Gastroparesis

Delayed gastric emptying is known as **gastroparesis**, e.g., after vagotomy, in diabetes mellitus, etc. In diabetes mellitus, there will be autonomic neuropathy which leads to loss of vagal control of pyloric sphincter. This leads to tonic contraction of pyloric sphincter and gastric outlet obstruction, the condition being known as **gastroparesis diabeticorum**.

Abnormal Movements of Stomach

PY4.9: Discuss the physiology aspects of: peptic ulcer, gastroesophageal reflux disease, vomiting, diarrhea, constipation, adynamic ileus, Hirschsprung's disease.

Vomiting

Vomiting also known as emesis is an uncontrollable reflex by which upper gastrointestinal tract expels its contents forcefully through the mouth. Recurrent vomiting may be caused by underlying medical conditions. Frequent vomiting may lead to dehydration and electrolyte imbalance, which can be life-threatening if left untreated. Other complications include aspiration into the respiratory tract which may lead to aspiration pneumonia, erosions and small tears in the esophageal mucosa, destruction of tooth enamel due to acid in the vomit.

❖ *Causes*
- Food poisoning and indigestion
- Eating too much food or drinking too much alcohol
- Anesthesia, chemotherapy
- Migraine
- Gag reflex due to irritation of throat
- Presence of irritating substances in the stomach
- Intestinal obstruction due to growths or due to spasms.
- Inflammatory conditions, such as gastritis, appendicitis, etc.
- Diseases of organs, such as uterus, kidney, CVS, vestibular apparatus, etc.
- Psychic vomiting due to nauseating smell, sickening sight, taste, etc.
- Vomiting associated with pregnancy due to stimulation of vomiting center by certain metabolites.

- Air sickness, sea sickness, etc., due to stimulation of vestibular apparatus.
- **Central vomiting** due to drugs, such as morphine, digitalis, etc., and brainstem lesions, meningeal irritation. Here, vomiting is projectile and is due to stimulation of the **chemoreceptor trigger zone** on the lateral wall of 4th ventricle.

Vomiting is a reflex activity. The pathway for vomiting reflex is as follows:

- ❖ **Stimulus**—irritation of mucosa of upper GIT.
- ❖ **Afferent** fibers travel through vagus and sympathetics from stomach, other viscera of abdomen and organs, such as heart. Afferents from vestibular nuclei mediate nausea and vomiting of motion sickness.
- ❖ **Center**—is **reticular formation** at the level of olivary nucleus close to respiratory center, salivary center and vasomotor center. So, vomiting is associated with changes in respiration, salivation and vasomotor changes.
- ❖ **Efferent** fibers pass along phrenic nerve, vagus and sympathetic fibers from the vomiting center. Impulses also go through spinal nerves to abdominal muscles and through cranial nerves (5, 7, 9, 10 and 12th cranial nerves) to muscles of pharynx, palate, etc.

Mechanism of vomiting

- Vomiting starts with the sensation of nausea and increased salivation. **Retching** is physical movement of vomiting without carrying the vomitus out. This is due to incoordinated spasmodic contraction of respiratory muscles. Simultaneously, there is relaxation and distension of stomach. Forceful spasmodic contraction of duodenum due to **reverse peristalsis**, releases its contents into the relaxed stomach. Both the esophageal sphincters relax. Contraction of abdominal muscles squeezes the gastric contents into the esophagus and into the mouth. The throat relaxes completely for the free passage of vomitus. During vomiting, respiration is inhibited in mid inspiration and glottis is closed to prevent aspiration into trachea. Nasal regurgitation is also prevented by elevation of soft palate.
- Prolonged and severe vomiting may cause electrolyte imbalance due to loss of H$^+$ and K$^+$, i.e., it produces **metabolic alkalosis and hypokalemia**.

Complications of Gastrectomy

Total or partial gastrectomy (removal of stomach) is done in carcinoma of stomach or in gastric ulcers. The effects of gastrectomy are:

- ❖ **Pernicious anemia** due to lack of intrinsic factor.
- ❖ **Iron deficiency anemia** due to deficiency of HCl. HCl is necessary for the conversion of ferric ion to ferrous ion which is the absorbable form of iron.
- ❖ The patient has to take small, frequent feeds to maintain nutrition due to lack of reservoir function of stomach.
- ❖ **Dumping syndrome**—if large amount of food is taken at a time after gastrectomy, the hyperosmolar food reaches the intestine rapidly. This hyperosmolar food draws fluid from plasma into the intestinal lumen leading to intestinal distension and hypovolemia within half an hour of food intake. This causes symptoms, such as sweating, palpitation (awareness of one's own heart beat), flushing, etc., and this condition is known as dumping syndrome.
- ❖ **Reactive hypoglycemia**—if a carbohydrate-rich meal is taken by the patient, there will be rapid absorption of glucose from intestine leading to a **temporary hyperglycemia** initially. This stimulates insulin secretion in large amounts from the pancreas which leads to reactive hypoglycemia. The symptoms are similar to hypoglycemic attacks, such as sweating, dizziness, confusion, weakness, loss of consciousness, etc. This occurs two hours after a meal and is also referred to as **late dumping syndrome**.

MOVEMENTS OF SMALL INTESTINE

Such as stomach, small intestine also has BER which originate in the pacemaker cells located in the circular muscle layer near the myenteric plexus in the second part of duodenum. Movements of small intestine are:

- ❖ MMC
- ❖ Segmentation contraction or mixing contraction
- ❖ Tonic contractions
- ❖ Peristalsis

All these movements require an intact myenteric plexus and they mix, churn and propel the intestinal contents. Two patterns of motility occur in the intestine, one during fasting and other during feeding.

Migrating Motor Complex (MMC)

Occurs during fasting and it starts in the stomach. This movement keeps the GIT clear of bacteria, undigested material, desquamated cells and secretions. The MMC appears to be under the control of the gut hormone **motilin**.

Segmentation Contractions

These are **concentric** ring-like contractions of circular muscles that appear at regular intervals along the small intestine, dividing the lumen of the intestine into segments.

The stimulus is distension of a portion of small intestine with chyme and the receptors are **stretch receptors** of the wall of the small intestine. The length of one contraction is about 1 cm so that, each set of contractions divide the intestine into spaced segments. These contractions disappear and are replaced by another set of ring contractions in segments between the previous contractions, i.e., areas of relaxation becomes areas of constriction and vice versa. It is associated with an increase in intraluminal pressure **(Fig. 51.5A)**.

The frequency of segmentation contraction is determined by the basic electrical rhythm (BER). Normally, it is **10–12/min**. Segmentation contraction is independent of extrinsic innervation.

Tonic Contractions

These are prolonged contractions that isolate one segment of intestine from another. The length of small intestine is less during life due to this tonic contraction.

Functions of Segmentation and Tonic Contractions

- Help in thorough **mixing** of food with digestive juices.
- Assist in active **absorption** by continuously bringing newer portions of food in contact with intestinal mucosa.
- Have a **massaging** effect on blood vessels and lymphatics of intestinal wall.
- These movements increase transit time in small intestine so that chyme remains in contact with enterocytes for a longer time and favors absorption.

Peristalsis

Peristalsis is a type of movement in the GIT first described by **Bayliss and Starling**. Peristalsis is a reflex propulsive movement of GIT that is initiated when the gut wall is stretched by the contents of the lumen. It occurs in all parts of the GIT from esophagus to rectum **(Fig. 51.5B)**. Peristalsis helps to move the chyme forward towards the large intestine. Such movements are also seen in hollow tubes, such as ureter, fallopian tube, etc.

Local stretch releases **serotonin** which activates the sensory fibers of the myenteric plexus, which causes a deep circular contraction of the gut proximal to the stimulus and an area of relaxation in front of the stimulus called **receptive relaxation**. The contraction ring passes along the intestine to the colon at a rate varying from 2 to 25 cm/sec. This response to stretch is known as **myenteric reflex or peristaltic reflex**.

The time taken by chyme to pass from pylorus to ileocecal valve is 3-5 hours.

Mechanism of Peristalsis

Local stretch releases serotonin which activates sensory neurons, which in turn stimulate the myenteric plexus. Cholinergic neurons in the myenteric plexus passing in a retrograde direction, release **acetylcholine** and **substance P** which cause smooth muscle contraction at a point proximal to the stimulus. Cholinergic fibers passing in an anterograde direction activate neurons which release **NO, VIP,** etc., producing smooth muscle relaxation ahead of the stimulus.

The contraction ring passes along the small intestine to the colon in an oral to caudal direction propelling the chyme forwards a few inches. The peristaltic reflex and the anal ward direction of movement of peristaltic wave is called **law of intestine**.

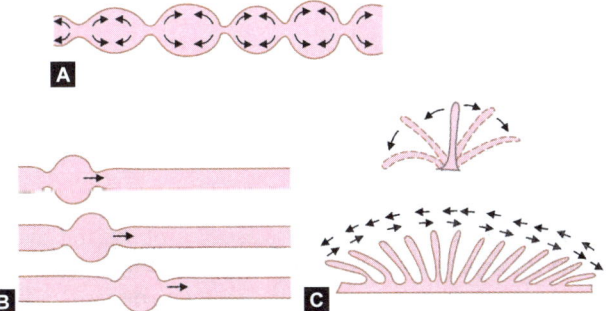

Figs. 51.5A to C: Movements exhibited by small intestine: (A) Segmentation contraction; (B) Peristalsis; (C) Lashing movement of villi.

Peristalsis is an example of integrated activity of the enteric nervous system (ENS). Peristaltic waves are superimposed on segmentation contraction. Peristalsis produces audible sounds called **bowel sounds** which can be studied by means of a stethoscope.

Factors Influencing Peristalsis

Stimulating Factors

- Stretch of gut wall.
- **Gastroenteric or gastroileal reflex**—distension of stomach sends impulses through the myenteric plexus from the stomach down along the wall of small intestine and intensifies peristaltic contraction
- Irritation of gut epithelium
- Parasympathetic stimulation
- Hormones, such as gastrin, CCK, insulin, serotonin, etc., increase peristalsis.

Inhibiting Factors

- Sympathetic stimulation
- Hormones, such as secretin, glucagon, etc.

Movements of Intestinal Villi

Small intestine is lined by numerous villi and these villi exhibits two types of movements **(Fig. 51.5C)**:
1. Lashing movement or swaying movement
2. Lengthening and shortening movement

These movements of villi enhance mucosal blood flow and lymph flow, stir the luminal contents and accelerate absorption of nutrients. Fine extensions of the smooth muscle of the submucosa run longitudinally up each villus to its tip. Contractions of these smooth muscles help in the movements of the villi. Vagal stimulation, local reflex and the hormone **villikinin** increase movements of villi, whereas sympathetic stimulation inhibits it. An intact submucosal plexus is essential for normal movements of villi.

Diseases of Small Intestine

Adynamic Ileus or Paralytic Ileus

Adynamic ileus is seen following abdominal operations. It may be due to direct irritation of intestine or due to peritoneal irritation. There is increased discharge of **noradrenergic** fibers leading to reflex inhibition of intestinal motility. This leads to distension of intestine with gas and fluid. The condition is painless and is diagnosed by auscultating the abdomen. *Bowel sounds will be absent.* Intestinal peristalsis returns within 6-8 hours after the surgery.

Intestinal Obstruction

Localized obstruction of small intestine may be due to spasm, growths and worms or due to adhesions. It causes severe pain called **intestinal colic**. The segment of intestine above the point of obstruction dilates and become filled with fluid and gas. Very intense peristaltic waves called **peristaltic rushes** occur when the intestine is obstructed. When the local pressure rises, blood vessels become compressed leading to ischemia of intestine. This is a medical emergency. Peristaltic rushes are also present in severe diarrhea.

Malabsorption Syndrome

Major function of small intestine is digestion and absorption of food. Removal of a short segment of small intestine does not cause severe symptoms. This is due to compensatory hypertrophy and hyperplasia of the remaining mucosa. If more than 50% of small intestine is removed, it leads to **malnutrition** and **emaciation**. Malabsorption is also seen in a condition called **sprue**. Effect varies with the cause and type of food that is not absorbed. If it is protein, it leads to body wasting, hypoproteinemia and edema. If it is fat, it leads to steatorrhea and vitamin deficiency especially vitamin K leading to bleeding disorders.

Irritable Bowel Syndrome

Irritable bowel syndrome occurs due to disordered small intestinal motility. Individuals complain of alternating constipation, diarrhea and abdominal pain. No structural problem or underlying disease can be identified in these subjects.

MOVEMENTS OF LARGE INTESTINE

Movements of colon are very sluggish. Large intestine exhibits the following type of contractions:
- Segmentation contraction
- Peristalsis
- Mass action contraction

Segmentation contraction and peristalsis

Segmentation contraction and peristalsis are very similar to those occurring in the small intestine. Segmentation contraction mixes the contents of colon and facilitates absorption. Peristaltic waves propel the contents towards rectum.

Mass Action Contraction or Mass Peristalsis

This type of contraction occurs only in colon in which there is simultaneous contraction of smooth muscle over large areas. It occurs frequently in transverse and descending colon. Usually, these strong peristaltic waves begin at about the middle of the transverse colon and quickly drive the contents of the colon forward into the rectum. Rectal distension initiates defecation reflex.

Conditions where Mass Movement is Seen

- **Gastrocolic and duodenocolic reflexes** where, there is distension of stomach and duodenum.
- Constant irritation of large intestine as in ulcerative colitis
- Strong parasympathetic stimulation

Transit Time in the Gastrointestinal Tract

First part of a test meal reaches cecum in 4 hours. All undigested particles enter colon in 8 hours and reach pelvic colon in 12 hours. 70% of undigested matter is expelled in 72 hours, but it takes more than a week for the total removal of all undigested matter from GIT.

DEFECATION

Act of expelling fecal matter is called **defecation**. By means of mass action contraction, fecal matter is propelled for- wards and stored in pelvic colon, not in the rectum. Internal and external anal sphincters prevent continuous dribbling of feces because normally they are in a state of tonic contraction.

Internal anal sphincter is a layer of smooth muscle immediately inside the anus. It relaxes when rectum is distended, and sympathetics are excitatory to internal anal sphincter and parasympathetics inhibitory.

External anal sphincter is a layer of voluntary muscle innervated by **pudendal nerve**. Due to peristalsis, rectum gets filled with fecal matter and there is reflex contraction of rectum. When rectal pressure reaches about 18 mm of Hg, a desire to defecate occurs. When this pressure reaches 55 mm Hg, both internal and external anal sphincters relax and feces will be expelled out. Defecation is a spinal reflex that can be voluntarily initiated by relaxing the external anal sphincter and contracting the abdominal muscles (straining).

Defecation reflex can be voluntarily inhibited by contracting the external anal sphincter.

Defecation Reflex (Fig. 51.6)

- **Stimulus**: Distension of rectum
- **Receptors**: Mechanoreceptors of rectum
- **Afferent and efferent** fibers:
  - Some afferent fibers pass to the myenteric plexus and efferent impulses initiate peristaltic waves by local myenteric reflex. This propels the fecal matter forwards and relaxes the sphincters. This is a very weak reflex and is called **internal defecation reflex**.
  - Afferent impulses pass to upper sacral segments and from there, efferent fibers pass through parasympathetic pelvic nerve which intensify peristalsis and relax the sphincters. This is **parasympathetic defecation reflex**.

Distension of the stomach can cause reflex contraction of rectum and a desire to defecate. This is called **gastrocolic reflex**. That is why defecation after meals is a rule in children. In adults, social and cultural factors play an important role in defecation.

Abnormalities of Defecation

- Constipation
- Diarrhea or watery stools
- Hirschsprung's disease (aganglionic megacolon)

Constipation

> **PY4.9:** Discuss the physiology aspects of: peptic ulcer, gastroesophageal reflux disease, vomiting, diarrhea, constipation, adynamic ileus, Hirschsprung's disease.

Constipation refers to infrequent or difficult defecation due to decreased motility of intestine. The feces will be dry and

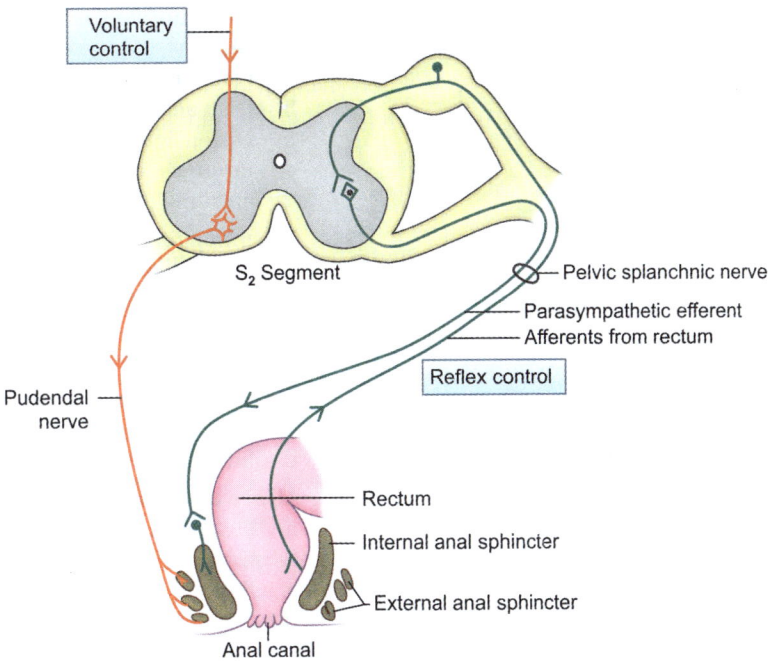

Fig. 51.6: Defecation reflex.

hard because of excessive water reabsorption as feces remain in the colon for a longer time.

Causes
- Dehydration
- Decrease in dietary fiber
- Neglecting call for stools
- Malfunctions of large intestine
- Diseases, such as hypothyroidism
- Drugs which have constipation as a side effect, such as Ca^{2+} channel blockers.

Symptoms of Constipation
Headache, irritability, anorexia, abdominal distension, discomfort, etc.

Treatment
Treatment depends on the cause. Laxatives, such as milk of magnesia, increasing the fiber content of diet, exercise, increased fluid intake, etc., relieve constipation.

Diarrhea
Increase in the frequency, volume and fluid content of stool due to increased intestinal motility, increased secretion of water and electrolytes into the lumen and decreased absorption from the intestine is called **diarrhea**.

Diarrhea is seen in typhoid fever, cholera, gastroenteritis, rotaviral infections, indigestion, etc. Severe diarrhea is caused by certain strains of *E. coli* that produce toxins which increases secretion of water and Na^+ into the small intestine. In **cholera**, modification of G-protein by the cholera toxin results in uncontrolled chloride channel activation in the crypts of small intestine. The result is loss of huge amounts of chloride ions. Along with chloride, sodium and water is also lost leading to rapid dehydration and death. Severe diarrhea leads to dehydration, hypovolemia, electrolyte imbalance especially hypokalemia, shock and cardiovascular collapse. The condition is treated according to the cause.

Hirschsprung's Disease or Adynamic Colon
Hirschsprung's disease is due to congenital absence of the ganglion cells in both the myenteric and Meissner's plexus in a particular segment of distal colon especially in the pelvic rectal junction. It is also known as **aganglionic megacolon**. This is due to failure of migration of neural crest cells during development and is due to the **lack of endothelin B receptor** in the affected segment.

Endothelins are necessary for the normal migration of neural crest cells. Due to absence of peristalsis in the affected segment, feces pass this region with difficulty, and the affected children defecate once in 3 weeks.

Symptoms
The symptoms associated with this disease are constipation, abdominal distension, discomfort, anorexia and lassitude.

Treatment
Surgical removal of the part of large intestine without ganglia and anastomosing the distal and proximal cut ends.

MULTIPLE CHOICE QUESTIONS

1. The involuntary phase of swallowing is:
   a. Oral phase
   b. Oral and pharyngeal phase
   c. Oral and esophageal phase
   d. Pharyngeal and esophageal phase

2. During swallowing, food is prevented from entering the trachea by the following mechanisms, *except*:
   a. Approximation of vocal cords
   b. Deglutition apnea
   c. Vertical deflection of epiglottis
   d. Forward and upward movement of larynx

3. Swallowing center is located in:
   a. Midbrain   b. Pons
   c. Medulla   d. Hypothalamus

4. Relaxation of cardiac sphincter is inhibited by:
   a. Gastrin
   b. Acetylcholine
   c. Nitric oxide
   d. Vasoactive intestinal polypeptide

5. Gastric emptying is increased by:
   a. Hyperosmolarity of duodenal chyme
   b. Presence of protein and fat in the duodenum
   c. Presence of increased fat in the stomach
   d. Decreased secretion of cholecystokinin

6. Peristaltic waves of stomach originate in the:
   a. Cardia of stomach   b. Fundus of stomach
   c. Body   d. Pylorus

7. Vomiting center is located in the:
   a. Chemoreceptor trigger zone
   b. Stomach
   c. Midbrain
   d. Cerebral cortex

8. The potent stimulus for peristalsis is:
   a. Distension
   b. Sympathetic stimulation
   c. Gastrin
   d. Acidic chyme

9. The following movements are exhibited by small intestine, *except*:
   a. Segmentation contraction
   b. Mass action contraction
   c. Peristalsis
   d. Movements of villi

10. A disease condition where a segment of large intestine is devoid of myenteric plexus:
    a. Celiac disease
    b. Irritable bowel syndrome
    c. Tropical sprue
    d. Hirschsprungs disease

11. Defecation follows a meal in children due to:
    a. Gastroileal reflex
    b. Gastrocolic reflex
    c. Enterogastric reflex
    d. Increased secretion of bile

12. Longest transit time is seen in:
    a. Colon   b. Stomach
    c. jejunum   d. Ileum

13. Gastric emptying is delayed in all the following, *except*:
    a. Fat in duodenum
    b. High acidity in pyloric antrum
    c. Distension of duodenum
    d. Products of carbohydrate digestion in pyloric antrum

14. Receptive relaxation of the stomach is due to:
    a. Vago-vagal reflex
    b. Enterogastric reflex
    c. Distension of stomach
    d. Gastrin

15. Achalasia cardia leads to:
    a. Peptic ulcer   b. Dysphagia
    c. Indgestion   d. Constipation

16. All are true of myenteric reflex, *except*:
    a. Distension of intestine elicits the reflex
    b. Extrinsic innervation should be intact
    c. Efferent neurons are in the myenteric plexus
    d. Substance P is a mediator

17. Afferent impulses which initiate the second stage of swallowing arise from:
    a. Taste receptor of tongue
    b. Cerebral cortex
    c. Swallowing center
    d. Pressure receptors of pharynx

18. Migrating motor complex is triggered by:
    a. Motilin   b. Nitric oxide
    c. CCK   d. Secretin

19. Vomiting center lie in close relation to:
    a. Salivatory nuclei   b. Respiratory center
    c. Vasomotor center   d. All of the above

20. Gastric emptying is facilitated by all the following, *except*:
    a. Carbohydrate meal   b. Fatty meal
    c. Protein diet   d. Liquid diet

21. Chyme in small intestine is propelled forward by:
    a. Haustration movements
    b. Segmentation
    c. MMC
    d. Peristalsis

22. Antiperistalsis is normally seen in:
    a. Colon   b. Jejunum
    c. Duodenum   d. Ileum

23. True about gastric emptying:
    a. Decreased by CCK   b. Increased by secretin
    c. Decreased by gastrin d. Increased by GIP

ANSWERS

1. d	2. c	3. c	4. a	5. d
6. b	7. a	8. a	9. b	10. d
11. b	12. a	13. d	14. a	15. b
16. b	17. d	18. a	19. d	20. b
21. d	22. c	23. a		

Digestion and Absorption of Food

CHAPTER 52

LEARNING OBJECTIVES
- Describe the physiology of the digestion and absorption of carbohydrates and comment on its abnormalities
- Describe the steps in the digestion and absorption of fat and the role of bile acids in this process
- Discuss the pathophysiology of steatorrhea
- Explain the mechanism of absorption of vitamins and minerals

INTRODUCTION

PY4.4: Describe the physiology of digestion and absorption of nutrients.

A balanced diet should include adequate calories, protein, fat, minerals, vitamins and sufficient water. Essential amino acids cannot be synthesized in the body and must be obtained from dietary protein. A daily good quality protein intake of 1 g/kg body weight is necessary to provide the **essential amino acids** which include **lysine, histidine, valine, leucine, isoleucine, phenyl alanine, tryptophan, threonine and methionine.** Animal proteins like egg, meat, fish, etc., contain these amino acids. A diet low in saturated fat and that containing the essential fatty acids is desirable. Fat supplies 9.3 kcal/g of energy. Carbohydrates present in diet supplies more than 50% of calories in most diets. A moderately built man needs about 2800 kcal/day to maintain his weight. Of this approximately 50% come from carbohydrates, 15% from protein and 35% from fat.

Digestion of food is an orderly process involving the action of various enzymes aided by HCl and bile. Intestine absorbs nutrients, minerals, trace elements, vitamins, electrolytes, bile acids, water, etc. Enzymes from the salivary gland and lingual gland digest carbohydrates and fats, gastric enzymes act on protein and fat, pancreatic enzymes act on carbohydrate, protein, lipid and nucleic acids. The enzymes present in the brush border of the enterocytes complete the digestive process.

Most of the absorption occurs in the proximal 1/3rd of small intestine but bile salts, bile acids and vitamin B_{12} are absorbed in the terminal ileum. A complex meal will be fully digested and absorbed in 3–5 hours. Efficient digestion and absorption requires the coordination of gastric emptying, small intestinal mixing and propulsion, secretion of bile and pancreatic juice.

Monosaccharides, amino acids, electrolytes, minerals and water-soluble vitamins enter portal blood and reach the liver. Lipids including cholesterol esters and fat-soluble vitamins are converted to chylomicrons in the enterocytes and this enters the intestinal lymphatics. From there it is discharged into the subclavian vein through the thoracic duct. Total surface area available for absorption in the gut is about 400 m².

Substances pass from the lumen of GIT into the enterocytes and from the basal and lateral cell membranes of the enterocytes into the interstitial fluid. Substances then enter the blood and lymph by simple diffusion, facilitated diffusion, osmosis, solvent drag, active transport, secondary active transport and endocytosis.

DIGESTION AND ABSORPTION OF CARBOHYDRATES

Principal carbohydrates in the diet are:
- Polysaccharides like starch (amylopectin).
- Disaccharides like lactose and sucrose
- Monosaccharides like fructose and glucose
- Pentose, glycogen, alcohol, pectin, dextrin, etc.

Amylopectin is one of the two components of starch, the other being amylose. Amylopectin molecules are huge, water soluble, branched polymers of glucose, each containing between one and two million residues of D-glucose monomers. **Amylose** is water insoluble, unbranched chains of glucose molecules, which is more resistant to digestion than amylopectin. Amylose acts as a prebiotic which is fermented by gut microflora. Prebiotics supply good gut microflora which promotes health. Amylose is a non-fiber type of prebiotic good for boosting immunity, preventing cancer, obesity and heart ailments.

Digestion of carbohydrates starts in the mouth by the action of α-**amylase or ptyalin**. Optimum pH for the action of salivary amylase is 6.7, and it converts cooked starch into maltose. Amylase is more effective in the presence of chloride ions. When the food bolus reaches the stomach, amylase acts in the interior of the bolus for some time. Thus, salivary digestion of starch is completed in the stomach. When the food gets mixed with gastric juice, the action of amylase is inhibited due to the low pH.

In the small intestine, **pancreatic amylase** acts both on *cooked and uncooked starch* converting it into maltose. Action is promoted by alkaline medium and presence of bile salts. As the food passes forwards, it is acted upon by **sucrase, maltase, lactase, trehalase,** etc., present in small intestinal juice converting them into glucose, fructose, galactose, etc. Some amount of glucose reaches large intestine unabsorbed, which is acted upon by bacterial flora releasing CO_2 and other products. Within the large intestine, dietary fiber is digested to some extent by the enzymes cellulases and hemicellulases of microbial origin by a process called fermentation. Fermentation does not yield monosaccharides that can be absorbed. Its chief products are short chain volatile fatty acids, which are readily absorbed by the large intestine. These fatty acids are utilized for energy and lipid synthesis.

Summary of Carbohydrate Digestion

Cooked starch $\xrightarrow{\text{Salivary amylase}}$ Maltose, maltotriose and α-limit dextrins

Cooked and uncooked starch $\xrightarrow{\text{Pancreatic amylase}}$ Maltose, maltotriose and α-limit dextrins

Maltose $\xrightarrow{\text{Maltase}}$ Glucose

Lactose $\xrightarrow{\text{Lactase}}$ Galactose and glucose

Sucrose $\xrightarrow{\text{Sucrase}}$ Fructose and glucose

Maltotriose, α-dextrin $\xrightarrow{\text{α-dextrinase}}$ Glucose

Trehalose $\xrightarrow{\text{Trehalase}}$ Glucose

About 80% of carbohydrate is absorbed in the form of glucose and the main site of absorption is the **jejunum**. Some amount of pentose, dextrose, etc., is also absorbed. Glucose is absorbed from the lumen with the help of a co-transporter or symporter present on the microvilli of enterocytes called **sodium dependent glucose transporters (SGLT-1)**. (SGLT-2 is responsible for glucose transport out of the renal tubules.) SGLT-1 can transport glucose into the cell only if sodium is attached to the carrier. Along with sodium, one molecule of glucose is transported into the cell by **symport**. So, transport of glucose depends on the concentration of sodium inside the enterocytes. The energy for the transport of glucose into the enterocyte from the lumen is provided indirectly by the active transport of Na^+ out of the cell into the lateral intercellular space by Na^+-K^+ pump. This leads to a reduction in the concentration of sodium in the enterocyte and more sodium is absorbed into the cell along with glucose. Thus, glucose is transported into the cell by **secondary active transport**. On entering the cell, glucose becomes phosphorylated and this reaction traps glucose within the cell since the transporter cannot transport phosphorylated glucose back into the lumen. This also establishes a concentration gradient for the absorption of more glucose into the cell.

From the cell, sodium is pumped actively by sodium pump present in the basolateral membrane of the cell into the lateral intercellular space. Glucose is transported by **facilitated diffusion** with the help of **glucose transporter (GLUT-2)** in the basal surface of the enterocyte into the interstitial space (**Fig. 52.1**).

The same mechanism transports galactose, but fructose utilizes a different mechanism. SGLT-1 also transports galactose. Fructose is absorbed by facilitated diffusion by GLUT-5 and its absorption is independent of Na^+. Fructose is transported out of the enterocytes into the interstitium by GLUT-2. Some fructose is also converted to glucose in the mucosal cells. Pentoses are absorbed by simple diffusion. *Insulin has very little effect on the intestinal transport of sugars.* The same is applicable for the reabsorption of glucose from the proximal convoluted tubule of kidney. Thyroxine increases glucose absorption from the intestine. Maximum rate of glucose absorption from the intestine is about 120 g/hr. The drug **phlorizin** inhibits transport of glucose across various cell membranes.

Defective Carbohydrate Digestion and Absorption

❖ In **pancreatic insufficiency**, starch maldigestion is severe due to the deficiency of amylase.
❖ **Disaccharidase deficiency** as in celiac sprue, characterized by loss of villi leads to carbohydrate malabsorption. It leads to belching, diarrhea, flatulence, distension, abdominal cramps, etc., following ingestion of sugars.
❖ **Lactase deficiency** is a common condition and it leads to **lactose intolerance**. Lactose is the sugar present in milk. When milk or milk-based products are ingested, diarrhea occurs due to increase in the number of osmotically active particles in the intestinal lumen (osmotic load), causing an increase in the volume of intestinal contents. Flatulence and distension is due to production of CO_2 and H_2 by the

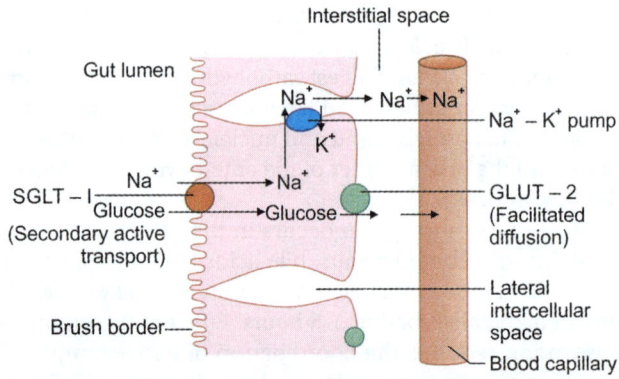

Fig. 52.1: Mechanism of glucose absorption across intestinal epithelial cell.

fermentation action of anaerobic colonic bacteria on lactose present in the colon.
- When SGLT-1 is congenitally defective, the resulting glucose and galactose malabsorption causes severe diarrhea that may lead to death unless glucose and galactose are removed from the diet.

DIGESTION AND ABSORPTION OF PROTEINS AND NUCLEIC ACIDS

Protein Digestion and Absorption

Sources of intestinal protein are:
- Dietary protein—50%
- Enzymes of digestive juices—25%
- Desquamated epithelial cells—25%

Protein digestion starts in the stomach by the action of pepsin-HCl mix. Optimum pH is 1.6–3.2. **Pepsin** hydrolyses proteins into polypeptides of varying sizes and **gelatinase** liquefies gelatine. **Rennin** acts on milk protein converting it into calcium paracaseinate. In the small intestine, the polypeptides are further digested by pancreatic enzymes, **trypsin, chymotrypsin and elastases**, which are endopeptidases, into smaller peptides. These endopeptidases are secreted as inactive proenzymes. The formation of the active endopeptidases occurs only in the intestine secondary to the action of brush border hydrolase, **enterokinase**. **Carboxypeptidase**, which is an exopeptidase, releases some free amino acids. Further digestion of proteins occurs by the action of **amino peptidases, carboxypeptidases** and **dipeptidases** present in the small intestinal juice and in the brush border of the intestinal mucosal cells. The final products of protein digestion are amino acids. Some dipeptides and tripeptides are actively transported into the enterocytes and are hydrolyzed by intracellular peptidases into amino acids. Thus the final digestion of proteins occurs in the intestinal lumen, the brush border and in the cytoplasm of the enterocytes.

Summary of Protein Digestion

Proteins and polypeptides $\xrightarrow{\text{HCl, pepsin}}$ Proteoses, peptones and amino acids

Proteins and polypeptides $\xrightarrow{\text{Enterokinase, trypsin}}$ Smaller peptides

Proteins and PP $\xrightarrow{\text{Chymotrypsin}}$ Smaller peptides

Proteins and PP $\xrightarrow{\text{Carboxypeptidase}}$ Peptides and amino acids

Polypeptides $\xrightarrow{\text{Aminopeptidase}}$ Amino acids

Polypeptides $\xrightarrow{\text{Carboxypeptidase}}$ Amino acids

Dipeptides $\xrightarrow{\text{Dipeptidase}}$ Two amino acids

Absorption of Proteins

Absorption of **amino acids** is rapid in the duodenum and jejunum but slow in the ileum. Maximum absorption occurs in the proximal jejunum. L-isomers are absorbed more rapidly than D-isomers. Seven different transport systems are responsible for the transport of amino acids into the enterocyte. Five of these systems **co-transport** Na⁺ and amino acid in a manner similar to the co-transport of glucose. Transport is independent of Na⁺ in the other two systems. Dipeptides and tripeptides are transported into the enterocyte by a system that requires H⁺ instead of Na⁺. From the enterocytes, amino acids are transported into the interstitial space by 5 transport systems present in the basolateral borders of the enterocytes. From the interstitial space the amino acids diffuse into the portal blood. Significant amount of small peptides also enter the portal blood. 2–5% of protein reaches the colon and is acted upon by colonic bacteria.

In **infants**, moderate amounts of undigested proteins are also absorbed from the intestine by **pinocytosis**, e.g., colostrum contains secretory immunoglobulin, IgA which is absorbed from the intestine of the infant by endocytosis and subsequent exocytosis, and it provides passive immunity to the baby against infections. This type of transport across cell is called **transcytosis**.

In adults, certain proteins that enter the circulation stimulate the production of antibodies against the protein causing allergic symptoms due to antigen-antibody reaction. *Absorption of proteins from the intestine is a common cause for the occurrence of allergic symptoms after eating foods like crustaceans, molluscs, certain fishes, etc.* The incidence of **food allergy** in children is about 8% and this is because the child's intestine absorbs larger peptides leading to antigen-antibody reactions.

Disturbances of Protein Digestion and Absorption

- In a congenital condition called **Hartnup disease**, there is defective transport of neutral amino acids in the intestine and renal tubules.
- A congenital defect in the transport of basic amino acids causes **cystinuria**.
- Enterokinase deficiency occurs as a congenital abnormality and leads to protein malnutrition.

Digestion and Absorption of Nucleic Acids

Nucleoproteins are acted upon by gastric juice forming nucleic acid and protein. Nucleic acid is acted upon by **nucleases** of pancreatic juice to form nucleotides. Nucleotide is converted to nucleoside and phosphate by **nucleotidase** present in the brush border of small intestine. Nucleoside is acted upon by **nucleosidase** to form pentose, purine and pyrimidine bases.

Pentose is absorbed from the intestine by **passive** diffusion and purine and pyrimidine bases by **active transport**.

Digestion and Absorption of Fat

60–150 g of lipid is ingested per day. Out of this, 90% is triacylglycerol, cholesterol, cholesterol esters, phospholipid and free fatty acids. Fat-soluble vitamins constitute the rest.

Fat is first acted upon by **lingual lipase** secreted by Ebner's glands on the dorsal surface of the tongue, which can digest as much as 30% of dietary triglyceride to free fatty acids.

Gastric lipase is not of much importance and it acts only on butter fat. Most of the fat digestion occurs in the duodenum by the action of the most potent lipase, **pancreatic lipase**, and the products are free fatty acids and 2-monoacylglycerol. It acts on fat that is emulsified by bile salts. The activity of pancreatic lipase is facilitated by **colipase** which is a protein secreted in the pancreatic juice in an inactive form. Colipase is activated by trypsin. A **bile salt activated lipase** or **cholesterol esterase** is also present in pancreatic juice. Unlike pancreatic lipase, bile salt activated lipase catalyzes the hydrolysis of cholesterol esters, esters of fat-soluble vitamins, phospholipids and triglycerides.

Fats can cross the unstirred layer and reach the mucosal cell surface only after emulsification by the detergent action of bile salts, lecithin and monoglycerides. When the concentration of bile acids in the intestine is high after ingestion of a meal, the **critical micellar concentration** will be reached and bile salts and lipids interact spontaneously to form **micelles** with lecithin. These cylindrical aggregates take up fatty acids, monoglycerides, fat-soluble vitamins and cholesterol in their hydrophobic centers to form mixed micelles **(Fig. 52.2)**. Fats, which are relatively insoluble, are made soluble by the formation of mixed micelles. The micelles move through the **unstirred layer** to the brush border of mucosal cells.

At the brush border, the lipids diffuse out of the micelles and by the action of certain carrier proteins, lipids enter the enterocytes by **diffusion**. Bile salts stay back in the intestinal lumen. Inside the cells, lipids are rapidly esterified to maintain a concentration gradient for the absorption of more lipids from intestinal lumen.

The fate of fatty acids in the enterocytes depends on their size. *Fatty acids with less than 10-12 carbon atoms are water-soluble and are actively transported as free fatty acids into the portal blood.* They circulate as **unesterified or free fatty acids**. Fatty acids containing more than 10-12 carbon atoms are insoluble and are re-esterified in the enterocyte to **triglycerides**. Cholesterol is also re-esterified to form cholesterol esters. Triglycerides and cholesterol esters are coated with a layer of protein, cholesterol and phospholipids to form **chylomicrons** in the smooth endoplasmic reticulum. They are further processed in the Golgi apparatus. Carbohydrate molecules are added to the protein of chylomicrons, and the chylomicrons are extruded into the interstitial space by **exocytosis**. The lining of the chylomicrons by β-lipoprotein is essential for the exocytosis of chylomicrons into the interstitium from the enterocyte.

They enter the lymphatics (lacteals) of intestinal villi. From here through the thoracic duct chylomicrons enter the venous blood. *It is due to the presence of chylomicrons that the plasma has a milky appearance after a heavy fatty meal.*

95% or more of the ingested fat is absorbed. Absorption of long-chain fatty acids is greatest in the upper parts of small intestine. The fatty acids reaching the colon are acted upon by colonic bacteria to form short chain fatty acids like acetate (60%), propionate (25%) and butyrate (15%). These short chain fatty acids are absorbed in the colon. Short chain fatty acids are also formed by fermentation of complex carbohydrates, dietary fiber, etc., by the action of colonic bacteria. They are absorbed by specific transporters present in colonic epithelial cells. The small chain fatty acids exert a trophic effect on colonic epithelial cells and also helps to prevent inflammation. *Less than 5% of fat is excreted through feces.*

Cholesterol is absorbed from the small intestine if bile and pancreatic juice are present. *Non-absorbable plant sterols such as those found in soya beans reduce the absorption of cholesterol.*

Steatorrhea

Steatorrhea is a condition where there is increased amount of fat in stools. Causes are:

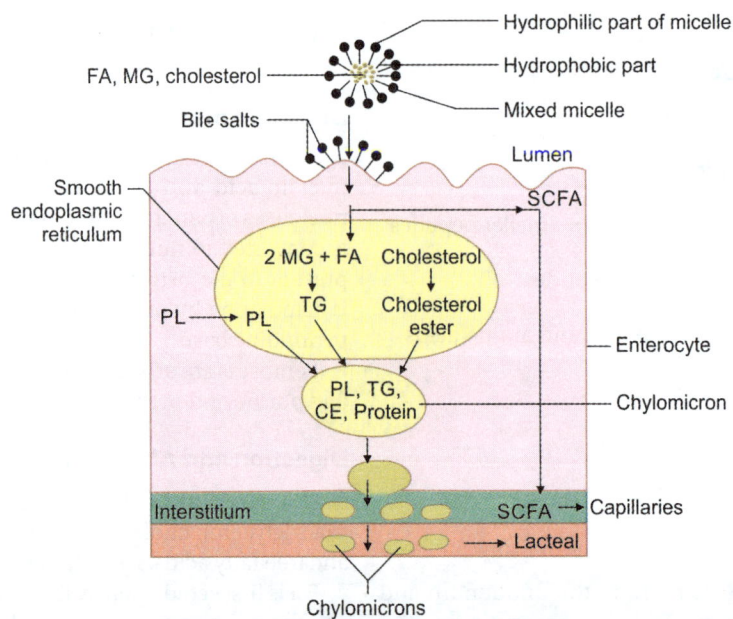

Fig. 52.2: Steps of fat absorption in intestine.
(FA: fatty acid; MG: monoglyceride; TG: triglyceride; PL: phospholipid; CE: cholesterol ester; SCFA: short-chain fatty acid)

- In deficiency of pancreatic lipase as in diseases of pancreas or after pancreatectomy, there will be impaired digestion and absorption of fat leading to steatorrhea. Here, the stools are **fatty (greasy) and bulky** because the amount of fat in stool is very high.
- In some cases, hypersecretion of acid as in gastrinomas leads to steatorrhea because high acidity inhibits the activity of lipase.
- Deficiency of HCO_3^- in the intestine increases the acidity of chyme. Increased acidity inhibits pancreatic lipase and also causes precipitation of bile salts.
- In obstructive jaundice, steatorrhea is due to the deficiency of bile salts in the duodenum when emulsification of lipids does not occur. The stool will be fatty, bulky and clay colored.
- Defective absorption of bile salts in the distal ileum also causes steatorrhea. For example, when more than 50% of small intestine is resected or bypassed, digestion and absorption of fat and absorption of bile salts and bile acids are so compromised leading to severe steatorrhea and malnutrition.

Absorption of Water and Electrolytes

Water is absorbed from the stomach, small intestine and large intestine by diffusion, obeying the laws of **osmosis**. Of the 9 L of fluid in the GIT from dietary sources and from digestive juices, 8800 mL is reabsorbed and only 200 mL is excreted through feces daily. *Maximum water reabsorption occurs in the jejunum which is approximately 5500 mL.* Absorption in the small intestine shares common features with fluid and electrolyte uptake by the proximal renal tubule. Absorption in the colon resembles that in the distal renal tubule in that both have **aldosterone-sensitive sodium transporters**.

Ions

Sodium

Na^+ is reabsorbed by co-transport (**symport**) with glucose in the small intestine. The transporter transports Na^+ only if glucose and Na^+ are bound to the transporter. Thus, the presence of glucose in the intestinal lumen facilitates reabsorption of sodium. This is the physiological basis of treating Na^+ and water loss in diarrhea with **oral rehydration solution (ORS)** which contains both Na^+ and glucose. Some Na^+ diffuses into or out of the small intestine depending on the concentration gradient. Due to the presence of Na^+-K^+ pump in the basolateral membrane of the enterocytes, Na^+ is actively pumped into the lateral intercellular space and this provides energy for the secondary active transport of glucose and amino acids into the enterocyte along with Na^+. Reabsorption of sodium in the colon is regulated by **aldosterone**.

Potassium, Chloride and Bicarbonate

K^+ diffuses through intestinal epithelium and is mainly secreted into the lumen. Chronic diarrhea can lead to severe hypokalemia. Cl^- is absorbed along with Na^+ to maintain electrical neutrality. Cl^- normally enters the enterocytes via Na^+-K^+-$2Cl^-$ **co-transporters**. In ileum and colon, Cl^- is reabsorbed in exchange for HCO_3^-. HCO_3^- is actively absorbed in jejunum, while in ileum it is secreted into the lumen.

Absorption of Vitamins and Minerals

Vitamins

Vitamins are referred to as organic dietary constituents necessary for life, health and growth which cannot be synthesized in the body in adequate amounts. Vitamins do not supply energy. Most vitamins have important functions in intermediary metabolism or special metabolism. Fat soluble vitamins (vitamins A, D, E and K) are absorbed along with dietary fat. In pancreatic insufficiency and in obstructive jaundice, absorption of fat-soluble vitamins is deficient even if their intake is adequate. Most vitamins are absorbed in the upper small intestine but vitamin B_{12} is absorbed in the ileum. For the absorption of vitamin B_{12}, intrinsic factor secreted by parietal cells of stomach is necessary.

Except vitamin B_{12} and folate, all water-soluble vitamins utilize sodium co-transporters for their absorption. Absorption of water-soluble vitamins is rapid. Fat soluble vitamins are absorbed only in the presence of bile salts since their absorption depends on micellar formation.

Large doses of fat-soluble vitamins are toxic. Hypervitaminosis A is characterized by anorexia, headache, irritability, bone pain, etc. Hypervitaminosis D is associated with weight loss, calcification of soft tissues and acute kidney injury. Hypervitaminosis K is characterized by gastrointestinal disturbances, and anemia. Large doses of water soluble vitamins are less likely to produce problems because they can be easily cleared from the body. Mega doses of pyridoxine (vitamin B_6) produce peripheral neuropathy.

Minerals

For the maintenance of health a number of minerals should be present in the diet. A variety of trace elements should be included in the diet. Trace elements are elements found in tissues in minute amounts. The trace elements essential for life include **arsenic, chromium, cobalt, copper, fluorine, iodine, iron, manganese, molybdenum, nickel, selenium, silicon, vanadium and zinc**. Deficiency of iron leads to microcytic, hypochromic anemia; cobalt is part of vitamin B_{12} and deficiency of B_{12} leads to megaloblastic anemia; iodine deficiency causes goiter; zinc deficiency leads to skin ulcers, decreased immunity and hypogonadal dwarfism; copper deficiency leads to anemia; chromium deficiency causes insulin resistance; fluorine deficiency leads to dental caries. Some minerals will be toxic when present in the body in excess. For example iron over load leads to hemochromatosis, copper excess leads to Wilson disease, etc.

Calcium

About 30–80% of Ca^{2+} ingested is actively absorbed in the duodenum and jejunum. **Calcitriol** (1,25-dihydroxycholecalciferol), the active form of vitamin D increases the absorption of Ca^{2+} from the intestine. Proteins also increase Ca^{2+} absorption but phosphates and oxalates inhibit Ca^{2+}

absorption. This is because phosphates and oxalates form insoluble salts with Ca^{2+} in the intestine. Ca^{2+} absorption is adjusted to body needs, i.e., absorption is increased in the presence of Ca^{2+} deficiency and vice versa.

Iron

The amount of iron absorbed from the intestine comes to about 3–6% of the amount ingested. Phosphates, oxalates and phytic acid in food inhibit iron absorption by forming insoluble salts. Dietary iron is in the ferric form. It has to be reduced to **ferrous form** for absorption from the intestine. Reduction of ferric ion to ferrous form is done by the ferric reductase activity of the iron transporter in the brush border of enterocytes in the presence of HCl produced in the stomach. This is the reason for the development of iron deficiency anemia in partial gastrectomy.

Iron is absorbed by an active process in the upper small intestine especially in the **duodenum**. Ferrous ion is transported into the enterocytes by the apical membrane iron transporter called **divalent metal transporter-1 (DMT1)**. Some of the iron is stored in **ferritin** in the enterocyte and the rest is transported out of the enterocyte by a basolateral transporter called **ferroportin-1**. A protein called **hephaestin** associated with ferroportin-1 facilitates basolateral transport of iron. In the plasma, ferrous form is converted to ferric form and gets bound to the iron transport protein, **transferrin**. Normally, transferrin is 35% saturated with iron. Ferritin molecules in lysosomal membranes in the tissues may aggregate in deposits that contain as much as 50% iron. These deposits are called **hemosiderin**.

Total body iron in a healthy adult comes to about 4–5 g.
  Normal plasma iron level
  In male – 110 µg/dL
  In female – 130 µg/dL
70% of iron in the body is in hemoglobin, 5% in myoglobin, 20% in ferritin and hemosiderin, and the rest in intracellular enzymes like cytochrome oxidase, catalase, peroxidase, etc.

Regulation of iron absorption

Intestinal absorption of iron is regulated by three factors:
1. Dietary intake of iron
2. Amount of iron stored in the body
3. Rate of erythropoiesis in the bone marrow

Iron deficiency leads to **anemia**. Iron overload causes hemosiderin to accumulate in tissues leading to **hemosiderosis**. Large amounts of hemosiderin can damage the tissues and cause **hemochromatosis** which is a common genetic disorder. Hemochromatosis is characterized by pigmentation of skin, destruction of pancreas leading to a type of diabetes called **bronze diabetes**, cirrhosis of liver, hepatic carcinoma, atrophy of gonads, etc. hemochromatosis may be hereditary or acquired. Acquired hemochromatosis occurs in iron overload due to chronic destruction of red blood cells, repeated blood transfusion, and disturbances in iron-regulating systems. Repeated withdrawal of blood helps to increase the life expectancy in hereditary hemochromatosis.

■ VITAMINS

The important vitamins, their sources, functions and deficiency states are given in **Table 52.1**.

Table 52.1: Important vitamins, their sources, functions and deficiency states.

Vitamin	Dietary sources	Actions	Deficiency
Thiamin (Vitamin B_1)	Liver, whole cereals and grains	Cofactor in decarboxylation reactions	Beri-beri, neuritis
Riboflavin (Vitamin B_2)	Liver, milk	Constituent of flavoproteins	Glossitis, cheilosis
Niacin (Vitamin B_3)	Yeast, meat, liver	Constituent of NAD^+ and $NADP^+$	Pellagra
Pantothenic acid (Vitamin B_5)	Egg, liver, yeast	Constituent of CoA	Dermatitis, enteritis, alopecia, adrenal insufficiency
Pyridoxine (Vitamin B_6)	Yeast, meat, liver	Converted in the body into pyridoxal phosphate and pyridoxamine phosphate	Convulsions, hyperirritability
Biotin (Vitamin B_7)	Egg yolk, liver, tomato	Catalyzes CO_2 fixation in fatty acid synthesis	Dermatitis, enteritis
Folic acid and related compounds (B_9)	Green leafy vegetables	Coenzymes in methylating reactions	Sprue, anemia. Neural tube defects in children born to mothers who are folate deficient
Cyanocobalamin (Vitamin B_{12})	Liver, meat, egg, milk	Coenzyme in amino acid metabolism. Stimulates erythropoiesis	Pernicious anemia
Vitamin C	Citrus fruits, green leafy vegetables	Free radical scavenger	Scurvy
Vitamin D	Fish liver	Increase intestinal absorption of calcium and phosphate	Rickets
Vitamin E	Milk, egg, meat, green leafy vegetables	Antioxidant	Ataxia and other signs of spinocerebellar dysfunction
Vitamin K	Green leafy vegetables	Catalyze γ-carboxylation of glutamic acid residues on various proteins concerned with clotting. Vitamin K dependent clotting factors are 2, 7, 9 and 10	Hemorrhage due to defective clotting

MULTIPLE CHOICE QUESTIONS

1. The amount of water absorbed in the intestine in a day is:
   a. 5 liter
   b. 1 liter
   c. 10 liters
   d. 8 liters

2. Maximum absorption of short chain fatty acids produced by bacteria occurs in:
   a. Stomach
   b. Duodenum
   c. Ileum
   d. Colon

3. Ileum is the principal site for the absorption of the following:
   a. Glucose
   b. Iron
   c. Bile salts
   d. Vitamin K

4. The substances that undergo enterohepatic circulation include all, *except*:
   a. Primary bile acids
   b. Secondary bile acids
   c. Bile salts
   d. Stercobilin

5. Maximum water reabsorption occur in the:
   a. Duodenum
   b. Jejunum
   c. Ileum
   d. Colon

6. All the following are necessary for the digestion of dietary fat, *except*:
   a. Bile pigment
   b. Bile salt
   c. Pancreatic lipase
   d. Colipase

7. True about fat absorption:
   a. Fat in stool more than 6 g/day indicate malabsorption
   b. Sudan III test best for screening malabsorption
   c. Major fat absorption occur in the proximal intestine
   d. Steatorrhea means stool fat more than 10 g/day

8. Vitamin B_{12} is absorbed in:
   a. Duodenum
   b. Jejunum
   c. Ileum
   d. Stomach

9. Iron absorption is increased by:
   a. Fiber diet
   b. Vitamin C
   c. Phosphate
   d. Phytic acid

10. Fat is maximally absorbed in:
    a. Ileum
    b. Colon
    c. Stomach
    d. Jejunum

11. The final sugars in intestinal chyme are:
    a. Glucose and fructose
    b. Ribose and mannose
    c. Ribose and xylulose
    d. Xylulose and fructose

12. The only sugar normally absorbed in the intestine against a concentration gradient is:
    a. Glucose
    b. Xylose
    c. Mannose
    d. Ribose

13. Chymotrypsinogen is activated to chymotrypsin by:
    a. Pepsin
    b. Trypsin
    c. Fatty acids
    d. Bile salts

14. Surgical removal of about 90% of ileum and jejunum tends to cause all, *except*:
    a. Steatorrhea
    b. Demineralization of bones
    c. A fall in the extracellular fluid volume of circulation
    d. Anemia

15. Which of the following is the fastest to be absorbed from the stomach?
    a. Carbohydrate
    b. Protein
    c. Fat
    d. Alcohol

16. Which of the following is absorbed in the colon?
    a. Iron
    b. Electrolytes
    c. Bile salts
    d. Proteins

17. Which of the following is absorbed in the proximal intestine?
    a. Iron
    b. Bile salts
    c. Vitamin B_{12}
    d. b and c

18. Maximum absorption of bile salt occurs in:
    a. Duodenum
    b. Jejunum
    c. Ileum
    d. Colon

19. Intestinal absorption is faster for:
    a. Hexoses
    b. Disaccharides
    c. Oligosaccharides
    d. Polysaccharides

20. Glucose is converted to glucose-6-phosphate in the cell by:
    a. Pyruvate kinase
    b. Hexokinase
    c. Pyruvate carboxylase
    d. Isomerase

21. Function of large intestine includes all the following, *except*:
    a. Absorption of steroids
    b. Synthesis of vitamins
    c. Absorption of iron
    d. Production of urobilinogen

22. Ca^{2+} absorption in the intestine is increased by:
    a. Hypercalcemia
    b. Oxalates in the diet
    c. 1,25-dihydroxycholecalciferol
    d. Increased Na^+ reabsorption

23. Mucosal transfer of iron in the GIT is by:
    a. Transferrin
    b. Apoferritin
    c. Ferritin
    d. Apotransferrin

24. Maltase is present in:
    a. Gastric juice
    b. Saliva
    c. Bile
    d. Shed epithelial cells of small intestine

25. Urobilinogen is:
    a. Formed in the liver
    b. Not present in urine normally
    c. Present in urine in obstructive jaundice
    d. Formed in the intestine

26. **The following is absorbed from the large intestine:**
    a. Water and certain drugs
    b. Amino acids and glucose
    c. Iron
    d. Vitamin B_{12}

27. **Lactase deficiency leads to:**
    a. Constipation
    b. Dysphagia
    c. Diarrhea
    d. Steatorrhea

28. **Man is unable to digest:**
    a. Dextrin
    b. Glycogen
    c. Lactose
    d. Cellulose

29. **The rate of absorption of glucose from the intestine is not influenced by:**
    a. Activity of amylolytic enzymes
    b. Sodium concentration in the intestinal lumen
    c. Insulin
    d. Activity of sodium potassium pump in the mucosal cells

30. **Impaired exocrine pancreatic function affects mainly the digestion of:**
    a. Starch
    b. Protein
    c. Fat
    d. Nucleoproteins

31. **Colonic bacteria on digestion of dietary fibers produce:**
    a. Free radicals
    b. Glycerol
    c. Butyrate
    d. Sucrose

32. **True regarding action of alpha-amylase:**
    a. Breaks glucose from carbohydrate end
    b. Cleaves only at α 1-4 glycosidic bond
    c. Cleaves only at α 1-6
    d. b and c

33. **In the following food items, which one has the highest glycemic index?**
    a. Corn-flakes
    b. Brown rice
    c. Ice-cream
    d. Whole wheat bread

34. **The major part of water is absorbed by:**
    a. Active transport
    b. Passive diffusion along osmotic gradient
    c. Pinocytosis
    d. Facilitated diffusion

35. **The symptoms in dumping syndrome following gastrectomy may be due to:**
    a. Deficiency of gastric acid
    b. Deficiency of intrinsic factor
    c. Inadequate digestion of protein
    d. Rapid absorption of glucose from jejunum

36. **Absorption of fat is impaired in all the following conditions, *except*:**
    a. Obstructive jaundice
    b. Hemolytic jaundice
    c. Pancreatic insufficiency
    d. Ileal resection

37. **Steatorrhea occurs due to impaired digestion of:**
    a. Fat
    b. Protein
    c. Carbohydrate
    d. Protein and carbohydrate

38. **Iron is absorbed almost entirely in:**
    a. Duodenum
    b. Jejunum
    c. Upper ileum
    d. Lower ileum

39. **Calcium absorption in the small intestine is increased by:**
    a. Hypercalcemia
    b. Oxalates in the diet
    c. Increased iron absorption
    d. Calcitriol

40. **Complex polysaccharides are converted to glucose and absorbed by the help of:**
    a. Sucrase
    b. Enterokinase
    c. Carboxypeptidase
    d. Chymotrypsin

41. **Chief carrier of exogenous (dietary) triglyceride is:**
    a. Chylomicrons
    b. VLDL
    c. LDL
    d. HDL

42. **Chief carrier of endogenous triglyceride synthesized in the liver is:**
    a. Chylomicrons
    b. VLDL
    c. LDL
    d. HDL

44. **Oral rehydration mixture contains glucose and sodium because both of them:**
    a. Are needed to maintain plasma osmolarity
    b. Are prominent energy source of the body
    c. Facilitate the transport of each other from the intestinal mucosa to blood
    d. Are required for the activation of Na^+-K^+ ATPase

ANSWERS

1. d	2. d	3. c	4. d	5. b
6. a	7. d	8. c	9. b	10. d
11. a	12. a	13. b	14. c	15. d
16. b	17. a	18. c	19. a	20. b
21. b	22. c	23. c	24. b	25. d
26. d	27. a	28. c	29. d	30. c
31. c	32. c	33. b	34. a	35. b
36. d	37. b	38. a	39. a	40. d
41. a	42. a	43. b	44. c	

Gastrointestinal Hormones

CHAPTER 53

LEARNING OBJECTIVES
- Describe the source of gastrointestinal hormones, their regulation and functions
- Explain the physiological role of incretins

INTRODUCTION

PY4.5: Describe the source of GIT hormones, their regulation and functions.

Regulation of secretion and motility of gastrointestinal tract (GIT) is by nervous and hormonal factors. The endocrine cells that secrete gastrointestinal hormones are seen scattered in the epithelium of the GIT. For example, G cells that secrete gastrin are present in the pyloric antrum, and the S cells that secrete secretin are scattered in the duodenal mucosa. These cells mainly belong to the group called **amine precursor uptake and decarboxylation (APUD) cells**. Another important feature of gastrointestinal hormones is that most of the hormones act in more than one target tissue. For example, secretin acts on both exocrine pancreas and in the liver. Similarly, one gastrointestinal gland responds to more than one hormone. Endocrine cells release their secretions into the base of the epithelium and are absorbed into the blood stream. Through the blood stream they reach the concerned gastrointestinal glands. So *the hormones are not present in the glandular secretions*. Some of the hormones act in a paracrine manner.

AMINE PRECURSOR UPTAKE AND DECARBOXYLATION (APUD) CELLS

A.G.E Pearse (initials) coined the term APUD cell in 1969. These cells constitute a component of diffuse neuroendocrine system, which are histologically identified by their staining behavior. They form a group of unrelated endocrine cells scattered throughout the body. They may also be specialized neurons. There are more than 40 types of APUD cells, which secrete low molecular weight polypeptide hormones or neurotransmitters. They are seen in plenty in the gastrointestinal tract and pancreas. The cells are not clustered together but spread as single cells throughout the intestinal tract.

The APUD cells contain high content of the enzyme, **amino acid decarboxylase**, which convert precursors to amines. Hormones secreted by these cells include somatostatin, motilin, cholecystokinin, secretin, neurotensin, vasoactive intestinal polypeptide, enteric glucagon, incretins, gastrin, serotonin, etc.

APUD cells are also seen in the urogenital tract, airway epithelium, pineal gland, adrenals, thyroid gland (C cells), adenohypophysis, hypothalamus, carotid body, skin and sympathetic ganglia. Neurotransmitters secreted by APUD cells include epinephrine, norepinephrine, dopamine, serotonin, encephalin, somatostatin, substance P, neurotensin, etc. These act in a paracrine, endocrine and neurocrine manner on neighboring and distant cells.

Apudoma commonly known as **neuroendocrine tumor** is a tumor that arises from APUD cells. For example, gastrinomas, VIPoma, insulinoma and somatostatinoma of pancreas; pheochromocytoma of adrenal medulla are apudomas. **Carcinoid tumors** secrete serotonin, histamine and vasoactive substances causing symptoms, such as flushing and diarrhea (carcinoid syndrome).

INCRETINS

Incretins are a group of gastrointestinal hormones that cause an increase in the amount of insulin released from the beta cells of the islets of Langerhans after food intake, even before blood glucose levels become elevated. *Incretins and insulin both tend to suppress appetite and reduce further intake of food*. They also slow the rate of absorption of nutrients into the blood stream by reducing gastric emptying. Incretins also inhibit glucagon release from the alpha cells of the islets of Langerhans. The action of glucagon is to increase blood glucose level. Stimulus for incretin secretion is absorbable carbohydrate and lipid load of GIT. The presence of incretins in the gut mucosa gives signals to the beta cells of the islets before nutrients are being absorbed. This helps the beta cells to amplify their response to glucose. Thus, incretins prime the beta cells and thus magnify insulin release following meal-induced increases in blood glucose.

The two main incretins are **glucagon-like peptide-I (GLP-I) and glucose-dependent insulinotropic polypeptide (GIP)**. Previously, GIP was referred to as **gastric inhibitory peptide**. Plasma half-life of GLP-I and GIP is only a few minutes. Both are rapidly inactivated by the enzyme **dipeptidyl peptidase-4 (DPP-4)** and are excreted by the kidneys. The entire GLP-I molecule has no effect on insulin levels. Only one specific sequence of GLP-I [GLP-I (7-36) amide] has **insulinotropic** effect. Fat is a more potent stimulator of GIP secretion than carbohydrate in humans.

The insulin secreting response of incretins known as the incretin effects, accounts for at least 50% of the total insulin secreted after oral glucose.

GLUCAGON-LIKE PEPTIDE-I (GLP-I)

GLP-I is a peptide hormone belonging to glucagon-secretin superfamily. It is the most important incretin, which is released from endocrine cells (L cells) in the distal ileum and colon. Intestinal L cells generate two peptides from pro-glucagon, GLP1 and GLP2. Both are glucagon-like but have weak activity when compared to glucagon. GLP1 is the most potent incretin to stimulate insulin secretion. GLP-2 is not an incretin and its function is not known.

Stimulus for secretion of GLP-1 is orally administered absorbable carbohydrate and lipids. The receptors for GLP-I (type II G-protein coupled receptor) are present in α and β cells of pancreatic islets, nervous system, heart, kidney, lung and gastrointestinal tract. The effect of incretins in areas other than pancreas is unsettled. Action in the β cells of endocrine pancreas is through cAMP. There is activation of protein kinase-A which opens L-type calcium channels in the β cells. Increased intracellular calcium mobilizes insulin granules leading to exocytosis.

Actions of GLP-I

❖ Increases glucose-induced insulin secretion from β cells
❖ Increases insulin biosynthesis by stimulating all steps involved in insulin biosynthesis
❖ Decreases glucagon secretion
❖ Decreases gastric emptying
❖ Decreases body weight by decreasing appetite
❖ Stimulates β cell proliferation and differentiation
❖ Exert anti-apoptotic effect on β cells and increase the life span of existing β cells.

GLUCOSE-DEPENDENT INSULINOTROPIC POLYPEPTIDE (GIP)

GIP is produced by **K cells** in proximal small intestine (duodenum) in response to oral glucose. It was the first incretin to be isolated and properties characterized in 1973. Type-II G-protein coupled receptor for GIP is present only in the pancreatic β cell. Mechanism of action is same as that of GLP-I. GIP has no effect on appetite and gastric motility. Actions are:
❖ Increases glucose dependent insulin secretion
❖ Decreases secretion of glucagon

Physiologically both GLP-I and GIP are equally important even though the concentration of GIP is 10 fold higher than that of GLP-I. Together they act in an additive manner.

Clinical Application

In type 2 diabetes mellitus, there is impaired secretion of GLP-I but the action is normal. Secretion of GIP is normal but there is loss of function in diabetes. Type II diabetes patients are usually resistant to the action of incretins. Even very high levels of GIP did not decrease blood glucose level in type II diabetes mellitus. But GLP-I is still insulinotropic in type II diabetes mellitus. GLP-I could increase insulin secretion and normalize blood glucose in type II diabetes mellitus when given intravenously. This led to the development of compounds that activate the GLP-I receptor inorder to improve insulin secretion. Two types of drugs have been developed:
1. Incretin mimetic or incretin agonist
2. Incretin enhancing DPP-4 inhibitors

Incretin mimetic, **exenatide**, can be used as an adjuvant along with metformin and sulfonylurea in treating type-II diabetes. It is a potent agonist at GLP-I receptor. Actions are same as that of GLP-I. It also preserves and restores beta cell function by inhibiting apoptosis. The drug has to be administered subcutaneously twice daily.

Dipeptidyl peptidase-4 (DPP-4) inhibitors (gliptins) delay the metabolism of incretins there by prolonging the half-life of incretins, both GLP-I and GIP. DPP-4 is an enzyme that destroys incretins. DPP-4 inhibitors increase endogenous blood levels of active incretins thus leading to prolonged action of incretin. These can be administered orally as a single dose. The drugs include **vildagliptin, saxagliptin and sitagliptin.** This can be given to patients with type II diabetes mellitus who have not responded to drugs, such as metformin and sulfonylureas. It also reduces appetite and helps in weight loss.

A brief summary of the various gastrointestinal hormones is given in **Table 53.1**.

CHAPTER 53 — Gastrointestinal Hormones

Table 53.1: Different gastrointestinal hormones and their actions.

Hormone	Site	Chemistry and stimuli	Functions
Gastrin	G cells, TG cells and pancreatic islets in fetal life	• 34 amino acids • Distension, peptides, amino acids, vagal discharge, hypercalcemia, epinephrine	• Increase secretion of pepsin, HCl, insulin • Trophic effect on gastric mucosa • Increase gastrointestinal motility • Contraction of cardiac sphincter
CCK-PZ	Duodenum, nerves in distal ileum and colon, neurons in brain	• 39 amino acids • Peptides, amino acids, fatty acids >10 carbon atoms	• Increase secretion of pancreatic juice rich in enzymes, glucagon and enterokinase • Contraction of gallbladder • Contraction of pyloric sphincter • Inhibit gastric emptying • Trophic effect on pancreas • Increase motility of small intestine and colon • Augments action of secretin
Secretin	S cells of upper small intestine	• 27 amino acids • Protein and acid in upper small intestine	• Increase secretion of watery, alkaline pancreatic juice • Decrease gastric acid secretion • Contraction of pyloric sphincter • Augment actions of CCK
VIP	APUD cells, nerves of GIT, brain, ANS, blood	28 amino acids	• Increases intestinal secretion of electrolytes and water, pancreatic HCO_3^- • Decrease gastric secretion • Decrease gastric motility • Relaxation of intestinal smooth muscle including sphincters
GIP	K cells of duodenum, jejunum, nerves of GIT	• 42 amino acids • Glucose and fat in duodenum	• Stimulate pancreatic secretion • Inhibit gastric secretion and motility • Increase insulin secretion
Motilin	Enterochromaffin cells of stomach, small intestine and colon	22 amino acids	• Increase gastrointestinal motility • Increase gastric acid secretion • Antibiotic erythromycin binds to motilin receptors and cause diarrhea, which is a side effect of this antibiotic
Bombesin	Stomach	Tetradecapeptide	• Increase intestinal and pancreatic secretion • Decrease gastric acid secretion
Substance-P	APUD cells of GIT and nerve cells	11 amino acids	Increase small intestinal motility
GRP	Vagal nerve endings terminating on G cells	27 amino acids	Vagally mediated increase in gastric juice secretion through gastrin
Somatostatin	D cells of GIT and pancreas	• SS14 and SS28 • Acid in the lumen	• Decrease secretion of gastrin, secretin, VIP, GIP, motilin • Inhibit gastric secretion and motility, pancreatic secretion and gallbladder contraction • Decrease absorption of glucose, amino acids and triglycerides
Glucagon	A cells in stomach and duodenum	29 amino acids	Increase blood glucose level. It is responsible for hyperglycemia after pancreatectomy
Glicentin	L cells in the lower GIT	Derivative of glucagon processed in the L cells	Stimulates insulin secretion and increase glucose utilization
Guanylin	Paneth cells of intestinal mucosa	15 amino acids	Increases intracellular cGMP leading to increased secretion of Cl^- into the intestinal lumen
Ghrelin	Stomach	28 amino acid	Stimulate growth hormone secretion, increases food intake by stimulating arcuate nucleus
Peptide YY	Jejunum	Stimulated by fat	Inhibit gastric acid secretion and motility, inhibit food intake
Neurotensin	Neurons and cells of ileum	• 13 amino acids • Stimulated by fatty acids	Inhibits gastrointestinal motility and increases ileal blood flow

MULTIPLE CHOICE QUESTIONS

1. Gastric secretion is inhibited by:
   a. Histamine
   b. Somatostatin
   c. Acetylcholine
   d. Gastrin

2. Following are gastrointestinal hormones, *except*:
   a. CCK-PZ
   b. GIP
   c. Motilin
   d. Chymotrypsin

3. Pancreatic juice rich in water and electrolytes and poor in enzymes is secreted in response to:
   a. Pancreozymin
   b. Fat
   c. Secretin
   d. Proteins

4. Best stimulus for CCK secretion is:
   a. Acid
   b. Protein
   c. Bile
   d. Fat

5. Action of gastrin includes:
   a. Decrease gastric motility
   b. Increases the tone of lower esophageal sphincter
   c. Decreases the tone of lower esophageal sphincter
   d. Decreases pepsin secretion

6. Gastrin level is increased in blood in all the following conditions, *except*:
   a. Hyperchlorhydria not due to gastrinoma
   b. Pernicious anemia
   c. Gastrinomas
   d. Carcinoma stomach

7. The gastrin inhibitory substance present in soluble mucus of stomach is called:
   a. Somatostatin
   b. HCO_3^-
   c. Gastrone
   d. Prostaglandin

8. The credit of discovering the first hormone goes to:
   a. Bayliss and Starling
   b. Banting and Best
   c. Claude Bernard
   d. WB Cannon

9. The first hormone to be isolated is:
   a. Insulin
   b. Secretin
   c. Glucagon
   d. Gastrin

10. The stimulus for the release of gastrin includes:
    a. Acid in the pyloric antrum
    b. Products of fat digestion in the antrum
    c. Distension of the duodenum
    d. Products of protein digestion in the antrum

11. Migrating motor complex (MMC) is triggered by which of the following?
    a. Motilin
    b. NO
    c. CCK
    d. Secretin

12. The gastrin inhibitory substance present in the soluble mucus of stomach is:
    a. Gastrone
    b. Enterogastrone
    c. Enterokinase
    d. Inhibin

13. Regarding CCK-PZ, all are true, *except*:
    a. Increase pepsinogen secretion
    b. Delays gastric emptying
    c. Causes gallbladder contraction
    d. Increase pancreatic juice secretion

14. CCK-PZ stimulates the release of:
    a. Pancreatic juice rich in bicarbonate
    b. Gastric juice
    c. Pancreatic juice rich in enzymes
    d. bile from liver

15. True about secretin is:
    a. Increase HCO_3 rich pancreatic fluid
    b. Increased gastrin secretion
    c. Gastric hypermotility
    d. Increase enzyme rich pancreatic fluid

16. Secretin does not cause:
    a. Bicarbonate secretion
    b. Augments action of CCK
    c. Contraction of pyloric sphincter
    d. Increase in gastric secretion

17. Most potent stimulus for secretin is:
    a. Dilatation of intestine
    b. Acid chyme
    c. Protein
    d. Fat

18. The duodenum secretes hormone, CCK which has the following effects, *except*:
    a. Increases gastric motility
    b. Causes gallbladder contraction
    c. Relaxes sphincter of Oddi
    d. Leads to meager flow of pancreatic juice rich in enzymes

19. Stimulus for gastric emptying:
    a. Secretin
    b. CCK
    c. Gastrin
    d. Enterogastrone

20. Which of the following inhibits gastric secretion?
    a. Secretin
    b. High gastric pH
    c. Insulin
    d. Calcium

21. Actions of cholecystokinin include all the following, *except*:
    a. Contraction of gallbladder
    b. Secretion of pancreatic juice rich in enzymes
    c. Increases enterokinase activity
    d. Augments secretion of gastrin

22. Gastrin is produced by:
    a. Pancreas
    b. Gastric antral cells
    c. Pituitary
    d. All of the above

23. Gastrin regulates gastric acid secretion at:
    a. Gastric cardia
    b. Antrum
    c. Pyloric canal
    d. First part of duodenum

ANSWERS

1. b	2. d	3. c	4. b	5. b
6. a	7. c	8. a	9. b	10. d
11. a	12. a	13. a	14. c	15. a
16. d	17. b	18. a	19. c	20. a
21. d	22. d	23. b		

FILL IN THE BLANKS/NAME THE FOLLOWING/GIVE THE NORMAL VALUE (GASTROINTESTINAL SYSTEM)

1. Parotid gland is drained by **Stenson's duct**, submandibular by **Wharton's duct** and sublingual by ducts of Rivinus.
2. Amount of saliva secreted per day: **1000–1500 mL**.
3. Percentage of total salivary secretion contributed by submandibular gland: **70%**.
4. Deficient salivation is termed **xerostomia**.
5. There is receptive relaxation of **lower esophageal sphincter** ahead of the peristaltic wave during swallowing.
6. The transmitters that cause relaxation of lower esophageal sphincter: **NO and VIP**.
7. Amount of gastric juice secreted per day: **2500 mL**.
8. Parietal cells or oxyntic cells of stomach secrete HCl and **intrinsic factor of Castle**.
9. Gastrin is a hormone secreted by antral G cells in response to the neurotransmitter, **gastrin releasing peptide**.
10. The most potent amino acids that directly stimulate G cells are **phenylalanine and tryptophan**.
11. Name a hormone that decreases gastric acid secretion: **Secretin**.
12. Name the three agonists of the parietal cell which increases acid secretion: **gastrin, histamine (via H2 receptor) and acetyl choline (via M3 receptor)**.
13. A substance that disrupts gastric mucosal barrier: **aspirin**.
14. Dizziness and sweating following meals after gastrectomy is due to **dumping syndrome**.
15. pH of saliva: **7**.
16. pH of gastric juice: **1.2–1.3**.
17. pH of intestinal juice: **8**.
18. The hormone that stimulates secretion of pancreatic juice rich in HCO_3^- and water: **Secretin**.
19. CCK secreted by I cells in the upper intestine increases secretion of pancreatic juice rich in **enzymes**.
20. The hormone that causes gallbladder contraction and relaxation of sphincter of Oddi: **CCK**.
21. Amount of bile secreted per day: **500 mL**.
22. The bile pigments which are responsible for the golden yellow color of bile: bilirubin and biliverdin.
23. Bile acids are synthesized from **cholesterol**.
24. Name the primary bile acids formed in the liver: **Cholic acid and chenodeoxycholic acid**.
25. Secondary bile acids formed in the intestine by bacterial action: **Deoxycholic acid, lithocholic acid and ursodeoxycholic acid**.
26. Name the bile salts: **Sodium taurocholate, sodium glycocholate, potassium taurocholate and potassium glycocholate**.
27. Bile salts form **micelles** at a critical concentration.
28. About 90–95% of bile salts are absorbed from the **terminal ileum**.
29. The normal rate of bile salt synthesis: **0.2–0.4 g/day**.
30. Substances that increase secretion of bile: **choleretics**.
31. Give two examples of choleretics: **Bile salts, secretin**.
32. Substances that cause gallbladder contraction are called **cholagogues**.
33. The sources of bilirubin in the body: hemoglobin (70–80%), cytochrome P450 and myoglobin.
34. Rate of bilirubin production per day: **250–350 mg**.
35. One gram of hemoglobin produces **35 mg** of bilirubin.
36. Bile salts decrease surface tension of lipids because of their **amphipathic** nature.
37. Major pancreatic duct is called **duct of Wirsung** and the accessory pancreatic duct is called **duct of Santorini**.
38. Amount of pancreatic juice secreted per day: **1500 mL**.
39. The hormone that acts on pancreatic ducts and increase the volume of pancreatic juice rich in water and HCO_3^-: **Secretin**.
40. The hormone that acts on acinar cells and produce pancreatic juice rich in enzymes: **CCK**.
41. Name the digestive enzymes that increase in blood in acute pancreatitis: **Amylase and lipase**.
42. Rate of BER is maximum in the **sigmoid colon (16/min)**.
43. The basic reflex operating in peristalsis: **Myenteric reflex**.
44. Very intense peristaltic waves seen in intestinal obstruction: **peristaltic rushes**.
45. **Migrating motor complexes** are seen in the gut during fasting.
46. The hormone that increases Na^+ reabsorption in the distal colon via ENaC: **Aldosterone**.
47. Maximum water reabsorption occurs in the **jejunum** (5500 mL/day).
48. The cAMP concentration in the intestinal epithelial cells is increased in **cholera**.
49. The most potent lipase in the intestine: **pancreatic lipase**.
50. Lingual lipase is secreted by **Ebner's** glands of tongue.
51. Short chain fatty acids are absorbed from the **colon**.
52. Fat content in stool more than **6 g/day** indicate fat malabsorption.
53. Steatorrhea is defined as fat in stool more than **7 g/day**.
54. Site of absorption of vitamin B_{12} in the intestine: **Ileum**.
55. Iron is absorbed from the duodenum in the **ferrous** form.
56. Two substances that decrease iron absorption in the intestine: **Phytates and phosphates**.
57. **Dietary fiber** is defined as all ingested food that reaches the large intestine in an essentially unchanged form.
58. The segment of the intestine that has the longest transit time: **Colon**.
59. Congenital absence of myenteric plexus in a segment of large intestine causes **Hirschsprung's disease**.
60. Glycemic index of glucose: **100**.
61. The primary members of gastrin family: **Gastrin and CCK**.

SECTION 5 → Gastrointestinal System

CLINICAL CASE SCENARIO

1. A 50-year-old male business executive came to the casualty with complaint of severe epigastric pain and vomiting blood. He gave a history of taking 1 g of aspirin that day for headache. He is a chronic smoker and consumes alcohol occasionally. He is on treatment for peptic ulcer for the past 3 years. Answer the following questions:
    1. What are the factors contributing to gastric mucosal barrier?
    2. Explain the mechanism of secretion of HCl in the stomach and its regulation.
    3. What is the role of aspirin and smoking in the development of peptic ulcer?

2. A 60-year-old man complains of abdominal pain, yellowish discoloration of skin and sclera, severe itching, loss of appetite and passing deep yellow urine and large quantities of pale-colored greasy stools for the past few days. The following investigations were done:
    Serum bilirubin – 16 mg%
    Total protein – 7 g/dL of blood
    Urine routine:
    Bilirubin +++
    Bile salts ++
    Urobilinogen – absent
    Van den Bergh test – direct positive
    1. What can be the probable condition?
    2. What is the reason for the absence of urobilinogen in urine and bulky white-colored stool?
    3. Explain the digestion and absorption of fat in the body.

    Ans.
    1. Obstructive jaundice

3. A 40-year-old chronic alcoholic complains of severe pain in the upper abdomen on the left side. He gives a history of passing bulky, greasy stools and increased frequency of stools for the past few days. Investigations showed marked increase in serum amylase and lipase level and fat content in stool was more than 200 g/day. Urine examination for bile salt, bile pigment and urobilinogen was found to be normal.
    a. What is the probable diagnosis?
    b. What is the physiological basis of the symptoms?
    c. Give the composition and functions of the secretion of the affected organ.
    d. Write a note on the regulation of secretion from the organ.

    Ans.
    a. Pancreatitis

SECTION 6 RENAL PHYSIOLOGY

Functional Anatomy of Kidney

CHAPTER 54

LEARNING OBJECTIVES
- Describe the structure and functions of kidney
- Describe the structure and functions of juxtaglomerular apparatus
- Explain the physiological role of renin-angiotensin system

INTRODUCTION

A human waste product is any substance which has no function in the body, e.g., CO_2, ammonia, urea, uric acid, excess ions like Na^+, Cl^-, SO_4^{2-}, HPO_4^{2-}, H^+, etc., excess water, undigested materials and heat. These are removed by:
- Body buffers which bind excess hydrogen ions.
- Blood helps in the transport of waste materials to the excretory organs.
- Liver changes toxic substances to less toxic ones, e.g., ammonia is converted to less toxic urea in the liver. Bile secreted by the liver is the route of excretion of many waste products, such as bile pigments, heavy metals, etc.
- Lung is the route of excretion of CO_2, heat and water vapor.
- Sweat glands remove water, heat, salts, urea, etc.
- Gastrointestinal tract eliminates solid undigested food, heat, salts, etc.
- Kidneys eliminate excess water, NH_3, urea, bilirubin, uric acid, toxins, H^+, other ions, heat, etc.

The major function of the urinary system is to help maintain **homeostasis** by controlling the composition, volume and pressure of blood within normal limits. Kidney plays a relatively minor part in the homeostasis of substances like Ca^{2+}, Mg^{2+} and glucose which are regulated primarily through hormones.

The branch of medicine that deals with the structure, function, and diseases of the kidney is known as **nephrology**. The branch that deals with urinary tract and male reproductive system is called **urology**.

KIDNEY

PY7.1: Describe structure and function of kidney.

Kidneys are paired, reddish, bean shaped, **retroperitoneal** organs in the abdominal cavity located between the last thoracic and third lumbar vertebrae on either side of the vertebral column.

Functions of Kidney

- **Excretory function:** The most important function of kidney is formation and excretion of urine. Products of protein and nucleic acid metabolism, such as urea, uric acid, SO_4^{2-}, PO_4^{3-} and creatinine are effectively eliminated from the body by the kidneys. Metabolism of carbohydrate and fat produces only CO_2 and water. So in kidney dysfunction, only protein restriction is advised.
- **Acid-base balance:** Kidney controls blood pH by its various buffer systems. Acids like H_2SO_4 and H_3PO_4 which are products of protein metabolism can be removed from the body only by the kidneys.
- Regulation of **blood volume and composition** of body fluids (blood and interstitial fluid). Normal blood osmolarity is 290 mOsm/L. Control of body fluid osmolarity is important for maintaining the normal cell volume in all the tissues of the body.
- Regulation of **blood pressure** by secreting renin. Renin activates renin-angiotensin-aldosterone pathway causing an increase in blood volume and blood pressure. 80% of angiotensin converting enzyme (ACE) is produced by lungs and 20% by the kidneys.
- **Metabolic function:** Kidney performs *gluconeogenesis*, i.e., synthesis of glucose from amino acid, lactic acid, glycerol, etc., during periods of prolonged fasting.
- **Endocrine function:**
  - Kidney regulates Ca^{2+} homeostasis and bone metabolism by activating 25-hydroxycholecalciferol to *1, 25 dihydroxycholecalciferol* (calcitriol or vitamin D_3) the active form of vitamin D in the proximal tubule cells. This hormone acts on intestine, kidneys and bone and controls Ca^{2+} and phosphorus metabolism. It is important for the development and maintenance of bone structure.
  - Fibroblast like cells in the interstitium of the cortex and outer medulla synthesize *erythropoietin* in response to local hypoxia and regulate erythropoiesis. In chronic

renal failure, the deficiency of erythropoietin leads to severe anemia.

- Through *renin* secretion kidney helps in the long-term regulation of blood pressure.
- Kidney also secretes hormones, such as *prostaglandin E2, prostacyclin (PGI2) and kinins*, such as bradykinin that control circulation within the kidney. These substances are generally vasodilators and play an important role when renal blood flow is compromised.
- Tubule cells also secrete angiotensin, bradykinin, etc. into the lumen which can modulate nephron function.

❖ Regulation of **electrolyte and water balance**: Kidneys regulate the concentration of inorganic ions in the body like Na^+, K^+, Cl^-, HCO_3^-, H^+, Ca^{2+}, PO_4^{3-}, etc. For this purpose, the excretion of these ions must be equal to their intake. Thus, kidneys regulate water and electrolyte balance, and also blood and extracellular fluid (ECF) volume.

❖ Kidneys synthesize metabolic substrate, such as **L-arginine**, which is the precursor of NO.

Functional Anatomy of Kidney

Adult kidney is about 4–5 inches long, 2–3 inches wide and 1 inch thick. Renal **hilus** is a deep vertical fissure on the center of the concave border of each kidney. Renal vein, renal artery, ureter, nerves and lymphatics enter and exit the kidney through the hilus.

The right kidney is located at a lower level than the left kidney. Upper pole of right kidney lies against the 12th rib and that of left kidney between the 11th and 12th ribs.

Weight of two kidneys together is 300 g, i.e., 0.4% of body weight.

Longitudinal Section of Kidney (Frontal Section)

Frontal section of kidney reveals two distinct regions: (i) superficial (outer) reddish area called **renal cortex**, (ii) a deep reddish brown region called **renal medulla**. Cortex and medulla together form **renal parenchyma**.

Within the medulla, are 8–18 cone-shaped structures called **renal pyramids** or medullary pyramids. The base of each pyramid faces the renal cortex and its apex called **renal papilla** points towards the center of the kidney. Striations are seen in the renal pyramids due to the presence of straight tubules of the nephron, such as loop of Henle and collecting duct and blood vessels, such as vasa recta. The portion of the renal cortex that extends between renal pyramids is called **renal column or column of Bertin (Fig. 54.1)**. One renal pyramid and its bounding renal columns constitute a renal lobule.

Renal papilla opens into a cup-like structure called **minor calyx** (8–18 in number). Minor calyces join together to form **major calyx** (2–3 in number). The major calyces open into a large funnel-shaped cavity called **renal pelvis** which opens into the **ureter**. Ureters from both kidneys open into the **urinary bladder** which in turn opens to the outside through the **urethra**. *The structures from the minor calyces to the urethra are collectively called the **urinary tract**.*

Nerve Supply of Kidney

Kidney receives its innervation from the **renal plexus** of the sympathetic division of autonomic nervous system. The kidneys lack parasympathetic innervation. The sympathetic fibers supply efferent and afferent arterioles, proximal and distal tubules and juxtaglomerular cells. Nerves accompany renal artery and they are **vasomotor nerves** which regulate blood flow through the kidney by regulating the diameter of the arterioles. At rest, there appears to be a little sympathetic tone to the kidneys. The varicosities of the sympathetic fibers release **norepinephrine and dopamine** near the smooth muscle cells of the vasculature and near the proximal tubules.

Effects of Sympathetic Stimulation to the Kidney

❖ Norepinephrine causes vasoconstriction
❖ Catecholamines strongly enhance Na^+ reabsorption by proximal tubule cells

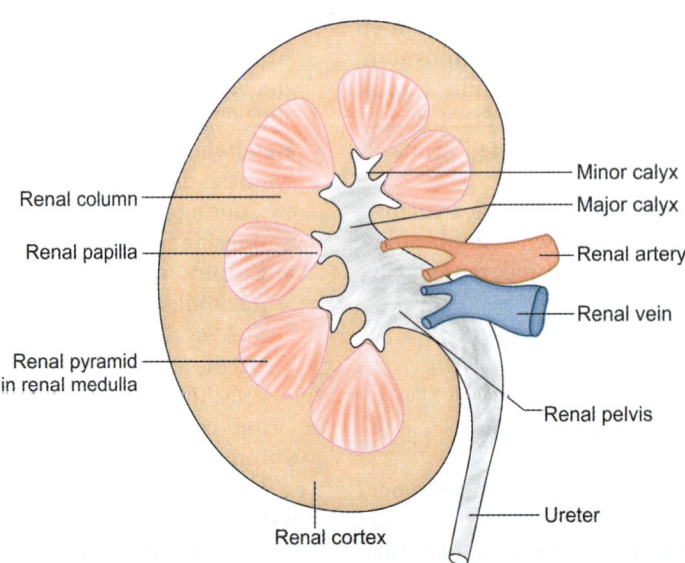

Fig. 54.1: Longitudinal section of left kidney.

- ❖ Granular cells of the juxtaglomerular apparatus (JGA) are densely innervated by sympathetic fibers. Increased sympathetic activity stimulates renin secretion.

Renal nerves also contain **afferent or sensory fibers**. A few myelinated fibers conduct **baroreceptor** and **chemoreceptor** impulses that originate in the kidney. Increased perfusion pressure in the afferent arteriole stimulates renal baroreceptors. Renal ischemia and changes in the ionic composition (mainly high K^+ and H^+ concentration) of the interstitial fluid stimulate chemoreceptors located in the renal pelvis. **Nociceptive (pain) afferents** mediate pain sensation from the kidneys and lie parallel to the sympathetic fibers. They enter spinal cord through the lower thoracic and upper lumbar dorsal roots.

Functions of Renal Nerves

Stimulation of renal sympathetic nerves increase renin secretion by a direct action of norepinephrine on β_1-adrenergic receptors on the juxtaglomerular cells and increases Na^+ reabsorption. The proximal and distal tubule and thick ascending limb of loop of Henle are richly innervated. Strong stimulation produces vasoconstriction and decreased glomerular filtration rate (GFR) and renal blood flow. This effect is mediated by β_1-adrenergic receptors.

Renorenal Reflex

Increase in ureteral pressure in one kidney leads to a decrease in the efferent nerve activity to contralateral kidney, and this decrease helps to increase its excretion of sodium and water. This is **renorenal reflex** mediated by renal afferents.

Nephron

Nephron is the structural and functional unit of the kidney. Each kidney has approximately 1.3 million nephrons.

Functions of Nephron
- ❖ Glomerular filtration
- ❖ Tubular reabsorption
- ❖ Tubular secretion

By performing these functions, nephron maintains homeostasis of blood.

Parts of Nephron

Each nephron consists of two portions (**Fig. 54.2**):
- ❖ A renal corpuscle where plasma is filtered.
- ❖ A renal tubule through which the filtered fluid passes.

Renal Corpuscle or Malpighian Corpuscle

Renal corpuscles lie in the renal cortex. Each corpuscle has two components:
1. The glomerulus which is a capillary network.
2. Bowman's capsule or glomerular capsule which is a double-walled epithelial cup which surrounds the glomerulus.

Glomerulus

Glomerulus is a tuft of capillaries about 200 mm in diameter, situated in the invagination of Bowman's capsule. Blood

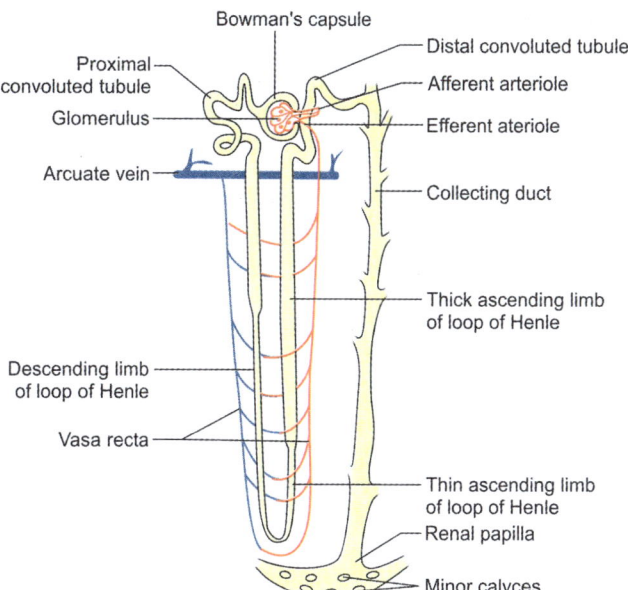

Fig. 54.2: Structure of juxtamedullary nephron and its blood supply (note the arrangement of vasa recta).

enters the glomerulus through the **afferent arteriole** and it divides into a highly branched anastomotic network which join together to form **efferent arteriole** which leaves the glomerulus. *Diameter of efferent arteriole is less than that of afferent arteriole.*

Mesangial cells are stellate-shaped contractile cells which surround the glomerular capillaries. They are located inside the glomerulus in between the glomerular capillaries and are a type of specialized vascular smooth muscle cells. They are similar to pericytes, which are found in the walls of all capillaries in the body. Mesangial cells provide structural support for the glomerular capillaries, exhibit phagocytosis by taking up immune complexes, secrete hormones, such as prostaglandins, cytokines, etc., and also secrete extracellular matrix in the glomerulus. The primary function of mesangial cell is to remove residues and aggregated protein from the basement membrane which is essential for proper filtration. Since they have the capacity to contract, they can influence glomerular filtration rate by regulating blood flow through the glomerulus. Contraction of mesangial cells is associated with contraction of the basement membrane of the endothelium of the glomerular capillaries. This causes a decrease in the surface area of the basement membrane and thus a decreased glomerular filtration rate.

Mesangial cells located outside the glomerulus are called **extraglomerular mesangial cells or lacis cells**. They are present in the juxtaglomerular apparatus in between afferent and efferent arterioles.

Bowman's Capsule

Bowman's capsule is the expanded blind end of the renal tubule invaginated by the glomerulus, thus forming a double-layered cup-shaped structure. The inner membrane which adheres closely to the glomerular capillary endothelium is called **visceral layer**, and the outer layer formed of simple squamous epithelium is called **parietal layer**. The capillary wall and the visceral layer of Bowman's capsule together form the endothelial-capsular membrane or filtration membrane or **glomerular membrane** which acts as a filter **(Fig. 54.3)**.

Structure of the Filtering Membrane (Fig. 54.3)

Glomerular membrane is a three-layered membrane of thickness 0.1 micrometer. The layers are:
- Capillary endothelium
- Basement membrane of glomerulus
- Visceral layer of Bowman's capsule

Capillary Endothelium or Lamina Fenestra

Capillary endothelium is made up of a single layer of endothelial cells, which has large fenestrations or pores of diameter 50–100 nm. These pores prevent filtration of blood cells. A layer of negatively charged **glycocalyx** overlies the luminal surface of the endothelial cells. This layer plays a role in preventing leakage of large negatively charged macromolecules.

Basement Membrane

The **basement membrane** of the glomerulus is acellular and it is located between the endothelial cells and podocyte foot processes. It is made up of fibrils in a glycoprotein matrix and contains hydrated channels approximately 6 nm wide which prevents filtration of larger proteins. This is because the basement membrane is mainly made up of negatively charged proteoglycans like **chondroitin sulfate proteoglycan and heparin sulfate proteoglycans (HSPGs)** which repel the anions. HSPG is particularly important in imparting selectivity to the glomerular basement membrane as it restricts large, negatively charges solutes. Loss of the negative charge on the basement membrane even without any structural damage to the membrane is enough to produce albuminuria.

Visceral Epithelium of Bowman's Capsule

The **visceral epithelium** is composed of specialized epithelial cells called **podocytes**. Extending from each podocyte are thousands of foot-like structures called **pedicels or pseudopodia**. These pedicels interdigitate and cover the glomerular capillary except for spaces between them called **filtration slits (Fig. 54.3)**. The filtration slits are 4 to 14 nm wide and are covered by a thin membrane called **slit membrane** which prevents filtration of medium-sized proteins. Glycoproteins with negative charges cover the podocyte and the slit membrane. The integral membrane proteins in the podocytes, such as **nephrin** and **podocin** also contribute to the slit membrane. Genetic defects in any of these integral proteins make the filtration barrier leaky, leading to albuminuria as in congenital nephrotic syndrome.

The glomerular membrane permits free passage of neutral substances up to 4 nm in diameter. They prevent filtration of substances greater than 8 nm. *Total area of glomerular capillary endothelium across which filtration occurs is 0.8 m².*

Renal Tubule

Renal tubule consists of:
- Proximal tubule
    - Proximal convoluted tubule (PCT)
    - Proximal straight tubule (PST)
- Loop of Henle (LH)
- Distal convoluted tubule (DCT)
- Collecting duct
- Papillary duct or duct of Bellini

Renal corpuscle, PCT and DCT lie in the renal cortex. Loop of Henle extends into the renal medulla, makes a hairpin turn and then returns to the renal cortex. In a nephron, the loop of Henle connects PCT and DCT. The first portion of loop of Henle dips into the renal medulla and is called **descending limb** of loop of Henle. It then bends in a U shape and returns to the renal cortex as **ascending limb** of loop of Henle. The distal convoluted tubule begins at the macula densa.

The DCT of several nephrons empty into a single collecting duct. Collecting ducts unite to form large papillary duct which opens at the apex of the renal pyramid into minor calyx. A single papillary duct or duct of Bellini collects urine from approximately 2800 nephrons. The collecting duct and papillary duct extend from renal cortex through renal medulla to renal pelvis. There are about 30 papillary ducts per renal papilla **(Fig. 54.2)**.

> PCT is 15 mm long, DCT 5 mm long and collecting duct 20 mm long. Total length of the nephron including the collecting duct ranges from 45 to 65 mm. The length of loop of Henle depends on the type of nephron. It is longer in juxtamedullary nephron.

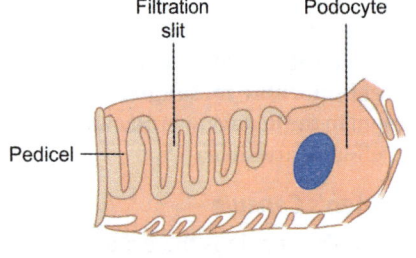
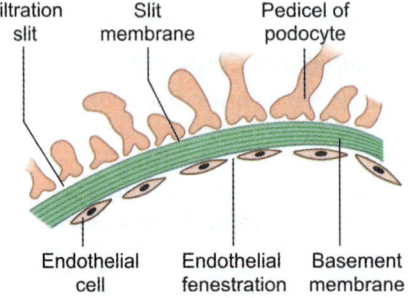

Fig. 54.3: Structure of filtration membrane (Endothelial-capsular membrane).

Types of Nephron (Fig. 54.4)

- Cortical nephron
- Juxtamedullary nephron

Cortical nephrons are located superficially in the renal cortex. The glomerulus of the **juxtamedullary nephron** is located near the cortico-medullary junction. They have long tubules that loop through the inner medulla reaching up to the papilla. These nephrons help in concentration of urine by building up an extremely high osmolarity in the renal medulla. The differences between cortical and juxtamedullary nephron is given in **Table 54.1**.

Histology of Renal Tubule

Each segment of the nephron is made up of cells which are suited to perform specific transport functions **(Fig. 54.5)**.

Proximal Convoluted Tubule

PCT is lined by **cuboidal epithelium** with numerous apical microvilli which give a brush border appearance. The basolateral membrane of the cell is highly folded and this area contains plenty of mitochondria. Leaky tight junctions are present between the apical surfaces of adjacent cells. 65% of water and 100% of some solutes, such as glucose and amino acids in the filtrate are absorbed in the PCT. Organic acids, bases, such as drugs and drug metabolites, and NH_3 are secreted in the PCT.

Descending Limb and Thin Ascending Limb

They are lined by simple **squamous epithelium**. Thin ascending limb is absent in the cortical nephrons.

Thick Ascending Limb

This part is lined by **cuboidal** to low columnar epithelium with numerous mitochondria in the basolateral surface.

DCT and Collecting Duct

They are lined by **cuboidal** epithelium with few microvilli. Two types of cells are present in DCT and collecting tubule:

1. **Principal cells** which make two-thirds of the cells of the collecting duct respond to ADH and aldosterone. These cells reabsorb Na^+ and Cl^- and secrete K^+.
2. **Intercalated cells** one type (α-intercalated cell) secretes hydrogen ions and reabsorbs K^+ and another type (β-intercalated cells) secretes HCO_3^-.

Papillary Duct

Papillary duct is lined by tall simple **columnar epithelium**.

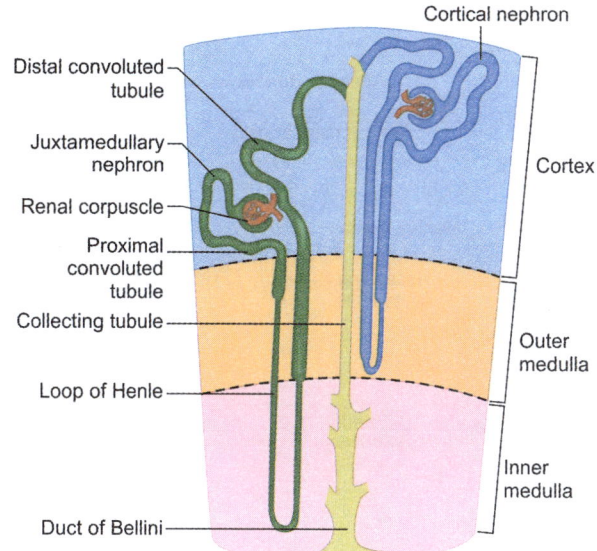

Fig. 54.4: Juxtamedullary nephron (left) and cortical nephron (right).

Table 54.1: Differences between cortical and juxtamedullary nephron.	
Cortical nephron	**Juxtamedullary nephron**
• Constitute 80–85% of nephrons • Has short loop of Henle that penetrates only into the superficial region of medulla • Glomerulus located in the superficial region of cortex • Receive blood supply from peritubular capillaries arising from efferent arteriole • Ascending limb of loop of Henle uniform, no thin part • No role in the concentrating or diluting mechanism of urine	• Constitute 15–20% of nephrons • Long loop of Henle that stretch through the medulla almost to the renal papilla • Glomerulus in the deeper part of cortex close to renal medulla • Receive blood supply from peritubular capillaries as well as from vasa recta that arise from efferent arteriole • Ascending limb of loop of Henle consists of two portions, a thin ascending limb followed by a thick ascending limb • Enable the kidney to excrete very dilute or very concentrated urine

Juxtaglomerular Apparatus (Fig 54.6)

> **PY7.2:** Describe the structure and functions of juxta-glomerular apparatus and the role of renin-angiotensin system.

The juxtaglomerular apparatus is located at the angle of the afferent and efferent arterioles where it comes in contact with

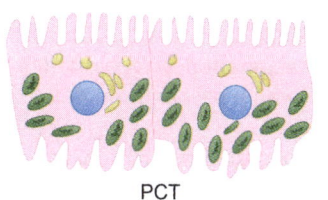
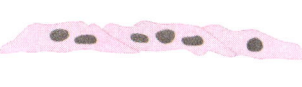
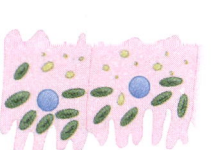
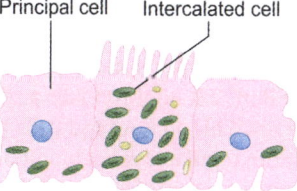

Fig. 54.5: Histology of different segments of nephron.

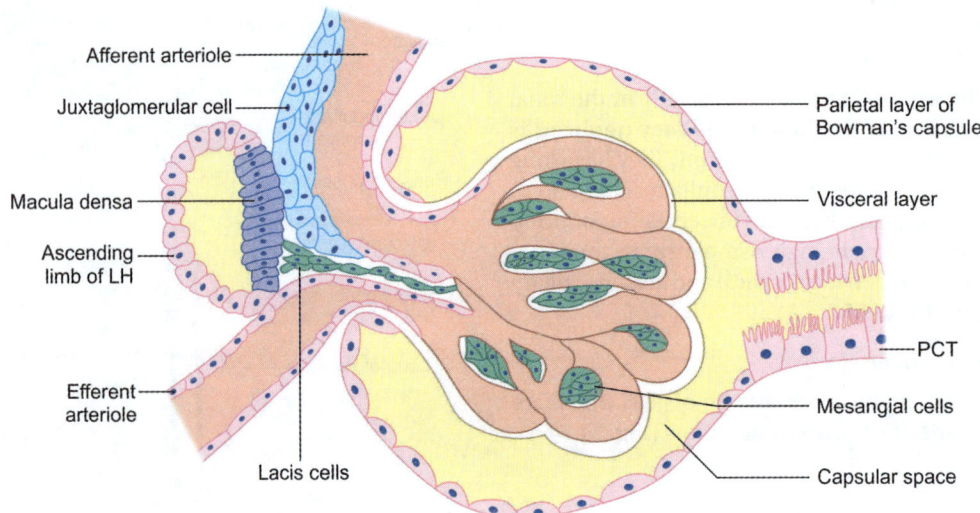

Fig. 54.6: Structure of renal corpuscle and juxtaglomerular apparatus (JGA).

the cortical part of the thick ascending limb of loop of Henle or the first part of DCT.

In each nephron, the ascending limb of loop of Henle makes contact with the afferent arteriole of its own renal corpuscle. The cells of the renal tubule in this region are tall and crowded together and that part is known as **macula densa (Fig. 54.6)**. The macula densa cells monitor the Na^+ and Cl^- concentration of fluid in the tubular lumen. The distal convoluted tubule starts at the macula densa.

Next to macula densa, the wall of afferent arteriole contains modified smooth muscle fibers of tunica media, called **juxtaglomerular cells or granular cells or epithelioid cells**. These cells produce, store and release renin. The large granules in the juxtaglomerular cells store **renin**. Granular cells are densely innervated by sympathetic nerve terminals and they release renin in response to sympathetic discharge. Renin is a hormone as well as an enzyme. It hydrolyses angiotensinogen to angiotensin I.

Between the afferent and efferent arterioles in this area are present **lacis cells** or extraglomerular mesangial cells which are derived from smooth muscle cells. Lacis cells also contain renin. The exact function of lacis cells is unclear. *Juxtaglomerular cells, lacis cells or extraglomerular mesangial cells and macula densa cells together constitute juxtaglomerular apparatus (JGA)*.

Functions of Juxtaglomerular Apparatus

- Macula densa cells sense the amount of fluid and NaCl reaching it and adjust the glomerular filtration rate by tubuloglomerular feedback. When the amount of fluid and NaCl reaching a nephron's macula densa increases, the GFR of that nephron falls and vice versa (*refer* 'regulation of renal blood flow and GFR').
- Renin regulates renal blood flow and filtration rate.
- Renin also indirectly modulates sodium balance and systemic blood pressure through renin-angiotensin-aldosterone axis. When there is a decrease in the pressure of the renal artery the baroreceptors in the afferent arterioles senses the decreased stretch in the arteriolar wall. This stimulates the neighboring granular cells to secrete renin into the general circulation. This is important in the long-term control of systemic arterial pressure.

Secretory Cells in the Kidney

- Juxtaglomerular cells or the granular cells secrete renin.
- Type-I medullary interstitial cells present in the interstitial tissue of medulla secrete prostaglandin, predominantly PGE_2. PGE_2 is also secreted by cells in the collecting duct.
- PGI_2 and other prostaglandins and kinins are secreted by the arterioles and glomeruli. These substances are generally vasodilators and may play a protective role when renal blood flow is decreased.
- Cortical and outer medullary interstitial peritubular fibroblast-like cells secrete erythropoietin in response to local tissue hypoxia. Erythropoietin stimulates the development of red blood cells by its action on hematopoietic stem cells in the bone marrow.
- Tubule cells also secrete bradykinin, cAMP, and ATP into the lumen, which can modulate nephron function.
- Proximal tubule cells convert circulating 25-hydroxyvitamin D to active metabolite 1, 25-dihydroxy vitamin D. This hormone controls calcium and phosphorus metabolism by acting on intestines, kidneys and bone.

Blood Supply of Kidney

The kidneys receive 20–25% of the cardiac output through **renal arteries**, i.e., 1.2–1.3 L of blood/min.

Within the kidney, the renal artery divides into several **segmental arteries**. Each segmental artery divides into several **interlobar arteries**, which passes through the renal columns **(Fig. 54.7)**.

When it reaches the corticomedullary junction, interlobar artery arches between the medulla and cortex and now they are referred to as **arcuate arteries**. The arcuate artery

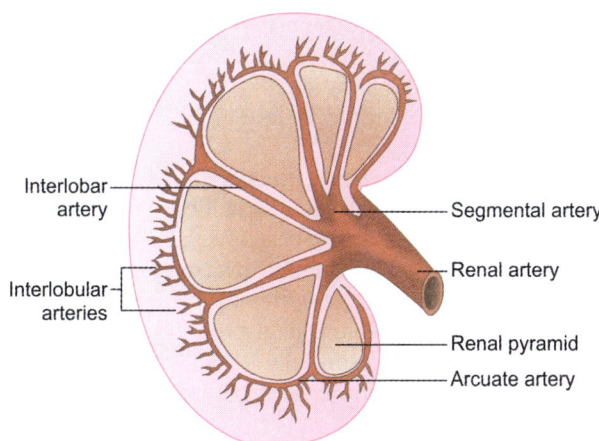

Fig. 54.7: Arterial blood supply to the kidney.

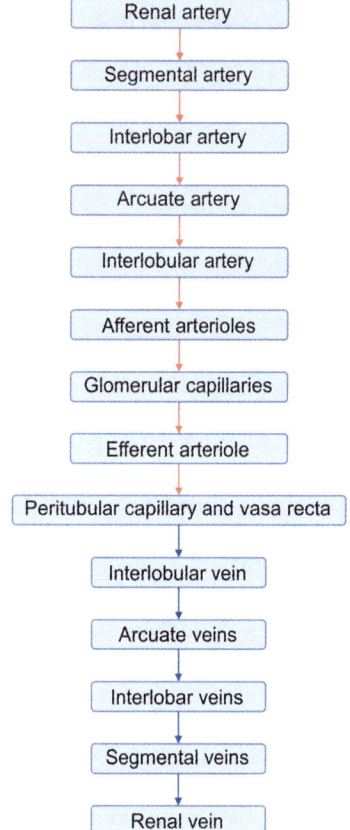

Flowchart 54.1: Blood supply of kidney; red arrow indicates pure blood and blue indicates deoxygenated blood.

gives rise to a series of **interlobular arteries** (cortical radial arteries) which enter renal cortex and give off branches called **afferent arterioles**.

Each nephron receives one afferent arteriole which divides to form a ball-shaped capillary network called **glomerulus**. The glomerular capillaries then reunite to form an **efferent arteriole (Fig. 54.7)**. Unique feature of glomerulus is that it forms a **portal system**, i.e., it begins and ends in arterioles (usually capillaries begin in arterioles but ends in venules).

Fate of efferent arteriole depends on the type of nephron. In cortical nephron, efferent arteriole divides to form a dense network of capillaries which surround the tubular portion of the nephron in renal cortex. This is referred to as **peritubular capillaries**. The peritubular capillaries have two main functions.
1. These vessels deliver oxygen and nutrients to the epithelial cells.
2. They are responsible for taking up from the interstitial space the fluid and the solutes that the renal tubules reabsorb. Glomerular filtration concentrates the plasma proteins and thereby increases the oncotic pressure of blood entering the peritubular capillary network to approximately 35 mm Hg. The efferent arteriolar resistance decreases the intravascular hydrostatic pressure in the peritubular capillaries to ~20 mm Hg. Interstitial oncotic pressure is 4 to 8 mm Hg and hydrostatic pressure 6 to 10 mm Hg. The effect is a large net reabsorptive pressure of about 17 mm Hg at the beginning of the peritubular capillaries. Towards the venular end of the peritubular capillaries the Starling forces fall from 17 mm Hg to 12 mm Hg which is also in favor of absorption. Thus, there is reabsorption along the entire length of the peritubular capillary.

In juxtamedullary nephron, long loop-shaped capillaries called **vasa recta** arise from efferent arteriole which lies parallel to and close to the loop of Henle and this arrangement has a major role in concentrating urine. Peritubular capillaries are also present in juxtamedullary nephron in addition to vasa recta but it is less dense than in the cortical nephron.

Venous Drainage

The vessels of the venous system run parallel to the arterial vessels. The peritubular capillaries reunite to form **peritubular venules** which in turn unite to form **interlobular veins**. The interlobular veins also receive blood from vasa recta. Then the blood drains through the **arcuate veins** to **interlobar veins** and on to the **segmental veins**. Blood leaves the kidney through a single **renal vein** that exits from the kidney at the renal hilum **(Flowchart 54.1)**.

Measurement of Renal Blood Flow

- By using electromagnetic flow meters
- By using Fick's principle

Fick's Principle

Amount of substance taken up or removed by an organ in unit time is equal to the product of arteriovenous concentration difference of the substance and blood flow through the organ. Since the kidney filters only plasma, only plasma flow through the kidney can be calculated using Fick's principle.

Plasma flow through the kidney =

$$\frac{\text{Amount of substance removed by the kidney in unit time}}{\text{Arteriovenous concentration difference of the substance in renal artery and vein}}$$

Criteria for the Substance to be used to Measure Renal Plasma Flow

- It should not affect renal blood flow.
- Concentration of the substance can be measured in arterial and renal venous plasma.
- The substance should not be produced or stored or metabolized in the body.
- It should be completely eliminated during a single circulation through the body.

The substances used are:
- Paraaminohippuric acid (PAH)
- Diodrast

Technique

Paraaminohippuric acid (PAH) is infused intravenously and its urine and plasma concentrations are measured. 90% of PAH in arterial blood is removed in a single circulation through the kidney by glomerular filtration and tubular secretion. So, renal venous PAH level is negligible and is not taken into consideration.

So, renal plasma flow =

$$\frac{\text{Urinary PAH} \times \text{Urine flow rate (V)}}{\text{Plasma PAH}}$$

$$\text{or} = \frac{\text{UPAH} \times \text{V}}{\text{PPAH}}$$

Peripheral venous plasma can be taken because its PAH concentration is same as the PAH concentration in the renal artery. The value obtained from the above formula is called **effective renal plasma flow (ERPF)** because the level of PAH in the renal venous plasma was not measured. ERPF is also known as **clearance** of PAH. ERPF can be converted to total renal plasma flow by using a correction factor. Since only 90% of PAH is removed by the kidney in a single circulation, actual renal plasma flow is obtained by dividing ERPF with extraction ratio.

$$\text{Extraction ratio} = \frac{90}{100} = 0.9$$

If the ERPF obtained is 630 mL/min, then actual renal plasma flow will be:

$$\frac{630 \text{ mL/min}}{0.9} = 700 \text{ mL/min}$$

From renal plasma flow, renal blood flow can be calculated by determining the hematocrit value. If the hematocrit value is obtained as 45%, then

$$\text{Renal blood flow} = \frac{700 \times 100}{100 - 45} = 1273 \text{ mL/min}$$

Special Features of Renal Circulation

- Pressure in the glomerular capillary is very high, i.e., 50 mm Hg when the mean systemic arterial pressure is 100 mm Hg. This is very high when compared to the pressure in the capillaries elsewhere in the body which is only 30 mm Hg. This is because the diameter of the afferent arteriole is more than that of efferent arteriole. This high capillary pressure helps in glomerular filtration.
- Blood flow to the kidney is very high, i.e., 200–300 mL/100 g/min.
- The O_2 consumption per 100 g of renal tissue is 5 mL/min (heart—8 mL/min). Oxygen extraction by the kidney is low, i.e., 1.5 mL/100 mL of blood because the blood flow to the kidney is so high relative to its oxygen need. (Heart consumes about 12 mL of O_2 when 100 mL of blood passes through it.) 80% of renal O_2 consumption is for the active reabsorption of ions especially Na^+ and solutes. The renal O_2 consumption is directly proportional to the amount of sodium reabsorbed.
- Renal blood flow exhibits **autoregulation** which means that renal blood flow is maintained constant even though there is wide variation in systemic blood pressure. Autoregulation in kidney is seen between 70 and 170 mm Hg mean arterial pressure.
- Blood flow to the renal medulla is less than that of cortex. About 90% of total renal blood flow perfuses the cortex and only 10% perfuse the medulla (9% goes to the outer medulla and 1% goes to the inner medulla). This is the cause for increased susceptibility of renal medulla to hypoxic injury in disease states of kidney. The causes for the reduction in medullary blood flow are:
    - Increase in the resistance to flow of blood in the medulla because of increased length of vasa recta (vascular resistance is proportional to the length of the vessel according to Poiseuille-Hagen formula).
    - The viscosity of medullary blood is high due to loss of large amounts of water into the hyper-osmolar interstitium.
- Blood traverses two arterioles and two capillary networks before entering the venous system.
- The peritubular capillaries form a low-pressure bed with a pressure of 8–10 mm Hg. This low pressure helps in renal tubular reabsorption.

Regional Blood Flow to the Kidney

- Renal cortex—4–5 mL/g/min
- Outer medulla—1.5 mL/g/min
- Inner medulla—0.2 mL/g/min

Regulation of Renal Blood Flow

Renal blood flow is regulated by two mechanisms:
1. Intrinsic mechanism or autoregulation.
2. Extrinsic mechanism which includes neural, hormonal and chemical factors.

Autoregulation (Intrinsic Mechanism)

Autoregulation is the capacity of a tissue to regulate its own blood flow in spite of variations in systemic arterial blood pressure. Autoregulation is seen in skeletal muscle, kidney, heart and brain.

At a pressure range between **90–220 mm Hg** systolic blood pressure (or between 70 and 170 mm Hg mean arterial pressure), the renal vascular resistance varies with the pressure so that, renal blood flow is maintained constant. Normal mean arterial blood pressure (diastolic pressure + 1/3 pulse pressure) is 93 mm Hg. Autoregulation is seen between **70–170 mm Hg mean arterial pressure**.

Autoregulation is not dependent on nerves because it is present in denervated kidney as well.

Theories of Autoregulation
- Myogenic theory
- Tubuloglomerular feedback
- Hormonal mechanism

Myogenic Theory
It is the intrinsic property of the arteriolar smooth muscle to contract when it is stretched. So, when more blood passes through the afferent arteriole to the glomerulus, the wall of the afferent arteriole is stretched and hence it contracts reducing the blood flow. The stretch of the vessel opens stretch-activated cation channels in vascular smooth muscle. The resultant depolarization leads to an influx of Ca^{2+} that stimulates contraction. This intrinsic response is blocked by drugs which paralyze vascular smooth muscles like papaverine, procaine, cyanide, etc.

Tubuloglomerular Feedback
When more blood flows through the afferent arteriole, the glomerular filtration rate in that nephron increases. So more fluid, Na^+ and Cl^- will be present at the region of macula densa. The Na^+ and Cl^- enter the macula densa cells via the $Na^+/K^+/2Cl^-$ cotransporter in their apical membranes. Adenosine is formed in the macula densa. This adenosine causes increased entry of Ca^{2+} into the vascular smooth muscle of afferent arterioles. This causes afferent arteriolar vasoconstriction, decrease in glomerular blood flow and decrease in glomerular filtration rate.'

Summary of Tubuloglomerular Feedback
- An increase in arterial pressure leads to increase in glomerular capillary pressure, renal plasma flow and GFR.
- Increased GFR leads to increased delivery of Na^+, Cl^- and fluid to the macula densa cells of the JGA.
- Via the apical $Na^+/K^+/2Cl^-$ cotransporter of the macula densa cells these ions enter and the concentration of these ions increases in the macula densa cells.
- This leads to depolarization which activates a basolateral cation channel, which allows Ca^{2+} to enter the macula densa cells.
- Increase in calcium ion concentration in the macula densa leads to the release of paracrine agents, such as adenosine produced from the breakdown of ATP.
- Adenosine binds to the A_1 adenosine receptors on the smooth muscle cells of the nearby afferent arteriole.
- Afferent arteriolar constriction increases resistance to blood flow leading to a decrease in the GFR thus counteracting the initial increase in GFR.

Hormonal Mechanism or Juxtaglomerular Hypothesis
A fall in the systemic blood pressure or a decrease in the effective circulating blood volume leads to a fall in the perfusion pressure in the renal artery. This stimulates release of **renin** and production of angiotensin II. Angiotensin II causes efferent arteriolar constriction more than afferent arteriolar constriction leading to increase in renal perfusion pressure and the renal blood flow will be maintained constant (*refer* **renin-angiotensin-aldosterone mechanism**, Chapter 55, Flowchart 55.1). The release of renin following a decrease in circulating volume occurs in three ways:

1. Decrease in systemic blood pressure stimulates the sympathetic system. The granular cells of JGA which are richly supplied by sympathetic fibers are stimulated and releases renin. Beta adrenergic blocking drugs inhibit renin release.
2. Decreased NaCl concentration at the macula densa stimulates renin release. A decrease in the effective circulating volume leads to a decrease in the amount of NaCl reaching the macula densa which in turn stimulates renin secretion.
3. Decrease in the renal perfusion pressure is sensed by the granular cells in the afferent arteriole due to decreased stretch of the smooth muscles of afferent arterioles. The granular cells contain stretch receptors which sense the decreased distension of afferent arteriole associated with low effective circulating volume. The decreased stretch lowers calcium ion concentration in the granular cells which increases renin release. Conversely, increased distension inhibits renin release. (This is in contrast to most Ca^{2+} activated secretory processes. Usually increase in Ca^{2+} increases secretion.)

Extrinsic Mechanism
Neural Factors
Sympathetic stimulation causes constriction of afferent arteriole leading to a decrease in blood flow to the glomerular capillaries and decrease in filtration pressure. Sympathetic stimulation is usually followed by a rise in systemic blood pressure. But the renal blood flow is maintained constant.

Hormonal and Chemical Factors (Table 54.2)
Angiotensin II constricts both afferent and efferent arterioles but efferent arteriole is more sensitive to angiotensin II and hence constriction of efferent arteriole predominates.

Table 54.2: Constrictors and dilators of renal vessels.

Renal vasoconstrictors	Vasodilators
Angiotensin II	Dopamine
Norepinephrine	Acetylcholine
Vasopressin (ADH)	Bradykinin
Serotonin	Prostaglandin I_2 and E_2
Hypoxia	Nitric oxide
Endothelin	Glucocorticoids

- **Norepinephrine** causes vasoconstriction mainly of afferent arterioles.
- **Endothelin** is a potent vasoconstrictor secreted by endothelial cells of renal vessels, mesangial cells, etc. It causes constriction of afferent and efferent arterioles and decreases GFR and renal blood flow. Usually endothelin secretion is increased in renal diseases associated with diabetes mellitus.
- **Prostaglandins** do not affect renal blood flow in normal healthy conditions. During pathological conditions like hemorrhage, prostaglandin I_2 and E_2 are produced within the kidney and increase renal blood flow without changing GFR. The action of prostaglandin is antagonistic to the vasoconstrictor effects of sympathetic stimulation and angiotensin II. This effect of prostaglandin prevents renal ischemia.
- **Nitric oxide** is a vasodilator of renal blood vessels, both afferent and efferent arterioles. NO production is increased in pathological conditions like diabetes mellitus and hypertension.
- **Bradykinin** acts by stimulating the release of NO and prostaglandins. It increases renal blood flow and GFR.
- **Dopamine** increases renal blood flow by inhibiting renin secretion. It produces vasoconstriction in other parts of the body, whereas in kidney it produces vasodilatation, thereby maintaining renal blood flow. *So, dopamine infusion is given in circulatory shock in order to increase the blood pressure by producing generalized vasoconstriction.* At the same time in the kidney, it produces vasodilatation and thus prevents renal ischemia. Dopamine also produces natriuresis.
- **Glucocorticoids** increase renal blood flow and GFR.

MULTIPLE CHOICE QUESTIONS

1. According to myogenic hypothesis of renal auto-regulation, the afferent arterioles contract in response to stretch induced by:
   a. NO release
   b. Noradrenaline release
   c. Opening of Ca^{2+} channels
   d. Adenosine release

2. The prostaglandin increasing renal blood flow is:
   a. PGI_2
   b. PGF_2
   c. PGE_2
   d. $PGF_{1\alpha}$

3. Prostaglandins causing renal vasodilatation are:
   a. PGI_2, PGE_2
   b. $PGF_{1\alpha}$, PGF_2
   c. TXA_2, PGF_2
   d. TXA_2, $PGF_{1\alpha}$

4. Renal plasma flow can be measured by determining the clearance of:
   a. PAH
   b. Inulin
   c. Urea
   d. Creatinine

5. Capillary pressure in the renal glomeruli is:
   a. 45 mm Hg
   b. 30
   c. 25
   d. 20

6. The percentage of cardiac output that is distributed to the two kidneys at rest in an adult male weighing 70 kg is:
   a. 5%
   b. 25%
   c. 2%
   d. 10%

7. Blood pressure in the glomerular capillary is:
   a. 30 mm Hg
   b. 25 mm Hg
   c. 90 mm Hg
   d. 50 mm Hg

8. Weight of each kidney in adult male is about:
   a. 150 g
   b. 400 g
   c. 100 g
   d. 50 g

9. Total surface area of all the glomerular capillaries across which filtration occurs in the two kidneys is:
   a. $1.7 m^2$
   b. $70 m^2$
   c. $45 m^2$
   d. $2.5 m^2$

10. The filtering membrane of the Malpighian corpuscle consists of all the following, *except*:
    a. Endothelial cells
    b. Basement membrane
    c. Mesangial cells
    d. Epithelial cells

11. Collecting tubules from different nephrons join to form:
    a. Duct of Bellini
    b. Duct of Santorini
    c. Duct of Rivinus
    d. Duct of Wirsung

12. Erythropoietin is secreted by:
    a. Juxtaglomerular cells of kidney
    b. Mesangial cells
    c. Interstitial cells of peritubular capillary bed
    d. Macula densa cells

13. All the following statements regarding renal circulation are correct, *except*:
    a. Renal blood flow is decreased during exercise
    b. About 25–30% of cardiac output passes through the two kidneys in one minute at rest
    c. Renal circulation is a portal system
    d. Hypoxia, hypercapnia and acidosis increase renal blood flow

14. All the following hormones increase renal blood flow and GFR, *except*:
    a. Bradykinin
    b. Angiotensin II
    c. NO
    d. ANP

15. All the following hormones decrease renal blood flow and GFR, *except*:
    a. Norepinephrine
    b. Angiotensin II
    c. NO
    d. Endothelin
16. Which of the following is not formed by the kidney?
    a. Erythropoietin
    b. Renin
    c. Calcitriol
    d. Aldosterone
17. Which of the following is not a part of juxtaglomerular apparatus?
    a. Macula densa
    b. Lacis cell
    c. Afferent arteriole
    d. Efferent arteriole
18. The following produce renal vasodilatation:
    a. Dopamine
    b. Adrenaline
    c. Noradrenaline
    d. Acetylcholine
19. Erythropoietin level is increased by:
    a. Decrease in PO_2
    b. Decrease in PCO_2
    c. Decrease in hemoglobin
    d. Decrease in pH
20. Erythropoietin is secreted by all, *except*:
    a. Hemangioblastoma
    b. Hepatoma
    c. Renal cell carcinoma
    d. Adrenocortical tumors
21. What is true about renin?
    a. It helps to convert angiotensinogen to angiotensin-I
    b. Secreted by PCT
    c. Increase in GFR causes increased secretion of renin
    d. Increase in plasma sodium and water increases renin secretion

ANSWERS

1. c	2. a	3. a	4. a	5. a
6. b	7. d	8. a	9. a	10. c
11. a	12. c	13. d	14. b	15. c
16. d	17. d	18. a	19. a	20. d
21. a				

Mechanism of Formation of Urine

CHAPTER 55

LEARNING OBJECTIVES
- Describe the mechanism of formation of urine involving the processes of filtration, tubular reabsorption and secretion
- Explain the mechanisms involved in the formation of concentrated and dilute urine
- Explain the mechanisms involved in the reabsorption of glucose, sodium and water from the filtrate
- Discuss the factors affecting sodium reabsorption
- Differentiate between tubuloglomerular feedback and glomerulotubular balance
- Describe and discuss the significance of renal clearance
- Describe the renal regulation of fluid and electrolytes and acid-base balance
- Explain artificial kidney, dialysis and renal transplantation

■ INTRODUCTION

The mechanism of formation of urine includes:
- Glomerular filtration
- Tubular reabsorption
- Tubular secretion
- Concentration and acidification of urine

■ GLOMERULAR FILTRATION

PY7.3: Describe the mechanism of urine formation involving processes of filtration, tubular reabsorption and secretion; concentrating and diluting mechanism.

Filtration that occurs in the glomeruli is the same as the filtration of plasma across the capillaries in other vascular beds. The only difference is that the rate of filtration that occurs in the glomeruli exceeds that in all the other capillaries because of greater Starling forces [net filtration pressure (NFP)] and higher capillary permeability. This is very essential for the blood to be cleared per unit time of certain solutes and excess water. A high blood flow and a high glomerular filtration rate (GFR) help the kidneys to eliminate harmful materials originating from metabolism like urea, rapidly from the body. This helps to maintain homeostasis.

Glomerular filtration occurs across the **glomerular membrane** into the Bowman's capsule. Mechanism is similar to tissue fluid formation, i.e., it is governed by **Starling forces** of capillary exchange. The amount of any substance that is filtered is the product of the GFR and plasma level of the substance. Since the pressure in the glomerular capillary is very high, water and solutes which are <4 nm are forced through the glomerular membrane into the capsular space. This fluid is called **glomerular filtrate** which is an **ultrafiltrate** of plasma. It is mostly protein free and only low molecular weight proteins whose size is smaller than that of albumin are present in the filtrate. The electrolyte composition of the filtrate is identical to that of plasma. About 180 L of filtrate enter the capsular space each day. Out of this, 178–179 L returns to circulation by tubular reabsorption. Only 1–2 L is excreted as urine.

Factors Favoring Filtration

- The glomerular membrane is thin and porous. Glomerular capillaries are 50 times more permeable than capillaries elsewhere in the body. The glomerular filtrate contains all the materials present in blood except formed elements and most plasma proteins. So it is referred to as ultrafiltrate.
- Glomerular capillaries present a large surface area. The total surface area of the renal capillaries is approximately 12 m^2.
- Glomerular capillary blood pressure is high. This is because efferent arteriole is smaller in diameter than afferent arteriole. So there is high resistance to the outflow of blood from the glomerulus. Since the plasma is filtered out from the glomerular capillary, the blood in the efferent arteriole becomes very viscous and this also contributes to the increased resistance to flow. Thus, the pressure in the glomerular capillary becomes very high.
- The Starling forces are in equilibrium toward the efferent arteriolar end of the glomerular capillaries. Fluid is filtered out from the afferent arteriolar side of the glomerular capillaries under a net filtration pressure (NFP) of 10 mm Hg while there is no reabsorption or filtration force at the efferent arteriolar end. So fluid is not reabsorbed from the efferent arteriolar end of glomerulus.

- As the blood moves towards the efferent arteriolar end of the glomerulus, the oncotic pressure of the blood progressively rises due to continuous filtration of protein free plasma. At a point before the end of glomerular capillary, the forces favoring and opposing filtration may balance each other. So no further filtration occurs from this point of the glomerulus. The system is said to be in **filtration equilibrium**.

GLOMERULAR FILTRATION RATE

Glomerular filtration rate is defined as the amount of filtrate formed in all the nephrons of both kidneys in 1 minute. It is normally **125 mL/min or 180 L/day**.

Factors Influencing GFR
- Net filtration pressure
- Permeability of glomerular membrane
- Surface area of filtering membrane
- Age

Net Filtration Pressure

Filtration across the glomerular membrane depends on three main pressures: one that promotes filtration and two that oppose filtration.

1. **Glomerular blood hydrostatic pressure (GBHP)**: This pressure promotes filtration. Hydrostatic pressure is the force that a fluid under pressure exerts against the walls of its container.
2. **Capsular hydrostatic pressure (CHP)** opposes filtration.
3. **Blood colloidal osmotic pressure (BCOP)** opposes filtration. Osmotic pressure is the pressure required to prevent the net movement of water into a solution containing solutes when the solutions are separated by a semipermeable membrane like plasma membrane. The greater the solute concentration greater will be the osmotic pressure.
   - GBHP is normally 55–60 mm Hg and this forms the driving force. GBHP is taken as 55 mm Hg.
   - CHP is the pressure in the Bowman's capsular space, and it constitutes the back pressure that opposes filtration. It is 15 mm Hg.
   - BCOP is due to the presence of plasma proteins, mainly albumin, and this force opposes filtration. The blood entering the glomerular capillaries has a BCOP of 25 mm Hg but the blood leaving the glomerular capillary has an osmotic pressure of 35 mm Hg. So the average BCOP in the glomerular capillary is taken as 30 mm Hg.
   - The tubular colloid osmotic pressure (TCOP) is negligible and is taken as zero because the ultrafiltrate is protein free.

Net filtration pressure
= (GBHP + TCOP) − (CHP + BCOP)
= (55 + 0) − (15 + 30) = 55 − 45 = 10 mm Hg

Thus, a pressure of 10 mm Hg causes plasma to be filtered from the glomerulus into the capsular space.

GFR = NFP × K_f, where K_f is the **ultrafiltration coefficient** which is equal to 12.5 mL/min/mm Hg.

GFR = 10 mm Hg × 12.5 mL/min/mm Hg = 125 mL/min.

K_f is the product of intrinsic permeability of glomerular capillary and glomerular surface area available for filtration.

Thus, GFR can be altered by changing K_f or by changing one of the Starling forces.

- Increase in K_f increases GFR. Some drugs and hormones that dilate the glomerular arterioles increase K_f.
- Decrease in K_f decreases GFR. Drugs and hormones which constrict the glomerular arterioles decrease K_f. Destruction of renal glomeruli decrease the surface area of the filtering membrane, and this in turn decreases K_f. Any of the following factors that affect Starling forces changes the GFR:
- A rise in systemic blood pressure increases capillary hydrostatic pressure and therefore increases GFR.
- Increase in the hydrostatic pressure in the Bowman's capsule as seen in ureteric obstruction decreases GFR.
- Increase in plasma oncotic pressure as in dehydration decreases GFR.
- Decrease in plasma oncotic pressure as in hypoproteinemia increases GFR.

Permeability of the Glomerular Membrane

Glomerular filtration occurs across four layers in the glomerular membrane:
1. The layer of glycocalyx overlying the endothelial cells
2. Endothelial cells
3. The glomerular basement membrane
4. Epithelial podocytes

Layers 1, 3 and 4 contain negatively charged proteoglycans like heparin sulfate proteoglycan which repel negatively charged particles. The junctions between adjacent podocytes which forms the filtration slits are the predominant barrier to filtration of macromolecules.

Permeability of the glomerular capillary is 50 times that of other capillaries. The glomerular membrane restricts the filtration of molecules on the basis of their size, molecular weight and charge. Neutral substances with diameter less than 4 nm and molecular weight less than 5,500 Da are freely filtered, e.g., water, urea, glucose and inulin. The concentration of these substances in the filtrate will be the same as in plasma. Substances having molecular weight greater than 70,000 Daltons and diameter more than 8 nm will not be filtered. Substances having diameter between 4 and 8 nm are filtered depending on their charge. Filtration of cationic substances is greater than that of neutral substances and anionic substances.

Even though the molecular diameter of albumin is 7 nm, it is not filtered by the glomerular membrane due to its negative charge. This is the reason why albumin is absent in urine. But if the glomerular membrane is damaged as in **glomerulonephritis and nephrotic syndrome,** the negative charges on the filtration barrier are reduced and large amount of albumin appears in urine. Presence of albumin in urine is called **albuminuria or proteinuria**.

The increased synthesis of albumin by the liver cannot compensate for the severe albuminuria, and **hypoproteinemia** results. This leads to a fall in the colloidal osmotic pressure of plasma, leading to increase in GFR due to increase in the NFP. There is also a decrease in blood volume and **interstitial edema**. Since the osmotic pressure of plasma is less, more fluid is filtered from the capillary and less amount is reabsorbed at the venous end of capillary. So more fluid remains in the interstitial space and this is the reason for generalized edema in nephrotic syndrome.

Surface Area of the Filtering Membrane

Effective area available for filtration is decreased when mesangial cells contract by the action of **angiotensin II** and **thromboxane A_2**. **Mesangial cells** are contractile cells present in between the capillaries of the glomerulus. They provide support for the glomerular capillaries and are mainly *responsible for the development of glomerulonephritis in* pathological conditions.

Age

After the age of 30, there is a progressive decline in GFR but this does not affect the excretory function of kidney.

Measurement of GFR

> **PY7.4:** Describe and discuss the significance and implication of renal clearance.

- Direct method
- Indirect method

Direct method is by the micropuncture technique.
Indirect method is by clearance measurements.

Clearance of a substance is the volume of plasma cleared of the substance by the kidney in unit time, i.e., in 1 minutes. Measurement of the renal clearance of various substances helps to evaluate the ability of kidneys to handle solutes and water.

Clearance of a substance

$$= \frac{\text{(Concentration of the substance in urine)} \times \text{(Volume flow rate)}}{\text{Concentration of substance in plasma}}$$

$$= \frac{UV}{P}$$

Clearance of a substance is equal to GFR if there is no net tubular secretion or reabsorption, e.g., inulin.

Clearance of a substance will be greater than GFR if there is net tubular secretion. Greater volume of plasma will be cleared of the substance in unit time because in addition to glomerular filtration it is also secreted by the tubules, e.g., PAH.

Clearance of a substance will be less than GFR if there is net tubular reabsorption, i.e., a smaller volume of plasma will be cleared of the substance because some amount of it is being reabsorbed by the tubular cells, e.g., urea.

Clearance of a substance will be zero if the substance is completely reabsorbed from the renal tubules, e.g., glucose up to a transport maximum of 375 mg/min.

Criteria of the Substance Used for Measurement of GFR

- Should be freely filtered by the glomerular membrane.
- Should not be reabsorbed or secreted by the renal tubule.
- Should not be metabolized, stored or synthesized in the body.
- Should not be protein bound.
- Should not affect GFR.
- Should not be toxic, i.e., it should be physiologically inert with no effect on renal function.
- The concentration of the substance can be measured in plasma and urine.

The substances usually used are:
- **Inulin**, a polymer of fructose with molecular weight 5,000 Da. Inulin is the usually used glomerular marker for measuring GFR
- **Mannitol**
- **Vitamin B_{12}** labeled with radioactive cobalt

Inulin Clearance

Procedure: Inulin is given intravenously till a constant arterial level is reached. Plasma and urine samples are collected and the concentration of inulin in these samples is found out.

Amount of inulin in glomerular filtrate = Amount of inulin in plasma = Amount of inulin in urine.

GFR = Plasma clearance of inulin

The amount of inulin filtered per minute = the amount of inulin excreted per minute since it is not reabsorbed or secreted.

The amount of inulin filtered per minute = GFR × Plasma inulin

The amount of inulin excreted per minute = Urinary inulin × Urine volume per minute (U_{in} is urinary inulin concentration, P_{in} the plasma inulin concentration and V the urine flow rate.)

$$GFR = \frac{U_{in} \times V}{P_{in}}$$

By substituting the normal values,

$$GFR = \frac{29 \times 1.1}{0.25} = 128 \text{ mL/min}$$

Filtration Fraction

The ratio of GFR to renal plasma flow is called filtration fraction, or the fraction of plasma in the afferent arterioles of the kidney that become glomerular filtrate is called **filtration fraction**. The normal value is 0.16–0.2.

When it is expressed in percentage, normal value is 16–20%.

Filtration fraction

$$= \frac{\text{Glomerular filtrate formed per minute}}{\text{Renal plasma flow per minute}} \times 100$$

$$= \frac{130}{650} \times 100 = 20\%$$

Glomerular Ultrafiltration Coefficient

Glomerular ultrafiltration coefficient, K_f, is the GFR of both kidneys per mm Hg filtration pressure. *K_f is the product of glomerular capillary permeability and the effective filtration surface area.*

Thus, $K_f = 15.5$ mL/min/m²/mm Hg × 0.8 m² = 12.5 mL/min/mm Hg.

If normal GFR is taken as 125 mL/min and NFP 10 mm Hg, K_f can be calculated as follows:

GFR = K_f × NFP.

So, K_f = GFR/NFP = $\dfrac{125 \text{ mL/min}}{10 \text{ mm Hg}}$

= 12.5 mL/min/mm Hg

K_f of glomerular capillary is 800 times more than the K_f of extra renal capillaries. This is because of the presence of numerous fenestrae in the glomerular capillary endothelium.

K_f is decreased in the following conditions:
- K_f is decreased in diseases which cause thickening of the filtering membrane or that which decrease its surface area due to destruction of glomerular capillary.
- The effective surface area of the glomerular membrane is regulated physiologically by the mesangial cells which are contractile and can constrict adjacent capillaries. Mesangial cell contraction by hormones and other endogenous substances also decrease K_f.

Regulation of GFR
- Autoregulation
- Hormonal regulation
- Neural regulation

Autoregulation

Myogenic Hypothesis

A rise in systemic blood pressure increases capillary hydrostatic pressure and therefore increases GFR. The afferent arterioles constrict in response to increased blood pressure. Arteriolar constriction restores GFR to normal levels. The stretching of the arterioles by increased pressure leads to opening of stretch-sensitive Ca^{2+} channels on the arteriolar smooth muscle cells, resulting in Ca^{2+} influx and contraction of the smooth muscle cells of the afferent arteriole. This is the **myogenic hypothesis of autoregulation**. The ultimate purpose of renal autoregulation is to hold the GFR constant.

Tubuloglomerular Feedback

Signals from the renal tubule in each nephron exert a feedback mechanism to affect filtration in its own glomerulus. As the rate of flow of the filtrate through the ascending limb of loop of Henle and first part of the distal tubule increases, glomerular filtration in the same nephron decreases. Conversely, a decrease in flow increases the GFR in the same nephron. This process of autoregulation is called **tubuloglomerular feedback**.

When more fluid reaches the distal tubule, there will be increased amount of Na^+ and Cl^- in it. This is sensed by **macula densa**. Na^+ and Cl^- enter the macula densa cells via the Na^+-K^+-$2Cl^-$ cotransporter in their apical membranes. The increased intracellular Na^+ causes increased activity of Na^+-K^+ pump leading to increased ATP hydrolysis. This causes more adenosine to be secreted from the basal membrane of the macula densa cells. Adenosine acts via adenosine A_1 receptors on the vascular smooth muscle cells leading to increased entry of Ca^{2+} into the vascular smooth muscle of afferent arteriole by opening up Ca^{2+} channels of the smooth muscles. This leads to afferent arteriolar vasoconstriction and a resultant decrease in GFR (*refer* autoregulation of renal blood flow). The amount of fluid delivered to the distal tubule is maintained constant by tubuloglomerular feedback.

Hormonal Regulation
- Renin-angiotensin-aldosterone mechanism
- Atrial natriuretic peptide (ANP).

Renin-Angiotensin System in Regulation of GFR

When there is a reduction in the GFR, the juxtaglomerular cells of juxtaglomerular apparatus are stimulated to secrete **renin**. Renin converts angiotensinogen to angiotensin I. **Angiotensin converting enzyme (ACE)** produced by the lungs converts angiotensin I to angiotensin II [for the actions of angiotensin II, **(Flowchart 55.1)**]. **Angiotensin II** increases the glomerular hydrostatic pressure, which in turn increases the GFR.

Atrial Natriuretic Peptide
- ANP is a hormone secreted by the cells of atria.
- *Action*: Diuresis and natriuresis (increased water and sodium excretion).
- *Stimulus*: Stretching of atria as in increase in blood volume.
- *Receptors*: Stretch receptors.
- *Effects*:
  - Permeability of glomerular membrane is increased.
  - Dilatation of afferent arteriole
  - Suppression of antidiuretic hormone (ADH) secretion
  - Decrease in aldosterone and renin secretion.
- *Importance of ANP*: In patients with hypertension and renal failure administration of ANP is of great benefit since it increases GFR, decreases water retention and edema and thus decreases blood pressure.

Neural Regulation
- Moderate sympathetic stimulation causes constriction of both afferent and efferent arteriole and so, GFR remains unaltered. With maximum sympathetic stimulation as in exercise, hemorrhage, stress (fight and flight response), etc., vasoconstriction of afferent arteriole predominates leading to decrease in GFR.
- Sympathetic stimulation also causes release of adrenaline from adrenal medulla which also causes vasoconstriction of afferent arteriole and decreased hydrostatic pressure in glomerulus, leading to decrease in GFR.

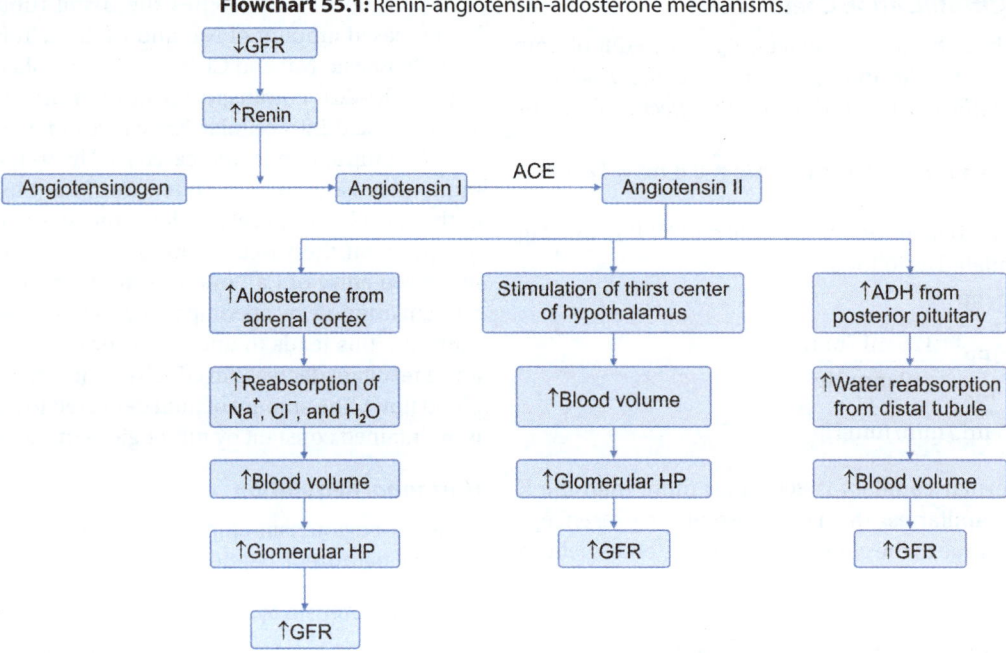

Flowchart 55.1: Renin-angiotensin-aldosterone mechanisms.

(GFR: glomerular filtration rate; ADH: antidiuretic hormone; ACE: angiotensin converting enzyme; HP: hydrostatic pressure)

Renal Tubular Functions

Renal tubular functions include:
- Tubular reabsorption
- Tubular secretion
- Concentration of urine
- Acidification of urine.

Tubular functions modify the glomerular filtrate so that urine contains only waste materials. Renal tubular functions are studied by:
- Micropuncture technique
- Stop flow technique

Micropuncture Technique

This procedure helps in the study of cellular functions in different segments of the nephron. The technique involves the puncture of individual nephrons on the surface of an exposed kidney with **micropipettes** and the withdrawal of tubular fluid for quantitative and qualitative analysis. The disadvantage is that the micropipette should have a tip diameter of <20 mm and only a few nanoliters of fluid can be collected for analysis.

Stop Flow Technique

The ureter of one kidney is exposed and catheterized. The catheter is clamped for a few minutes. During this time the pressure in the nephron increases and glomerular filtration is reduced due to back pressure. The concentration of fluid in the various segments of the nephron gets modified depending on the transport mechanisms operating in each segment. When the clamp is released, the columns of fluid moving out are collected as samples coming from different segments and each sample is analyzed. This method is technically easier than micropuncture technique in experimental animals.

Tubular Reabsorption

PY7.5: Describe the renal regulation of fluid and electrolytes and acid-base balance.

The amount of any substance that is filtered is the product of GFR and the plasma level of the substance. As the filtrate passes through the renal tubules, about 99% of it is reabsorbed and only 1% leaves the body as urine. Solutes are reabsorbed by **active and passive** processes. Water accompanies solute reabsorption by **osmosis**. Small proteins and some peptide hormones are reabsorbed in the proximal tubules by **endocytosis**.

Rate of reabsorption is maximal in the proximal tubule because of large surface area due to the presence of microvilli (brush border). Proximal tubule reabsorbs 100% of glucose and amino acid, 80–90% of HCO_3^-, 65% of water, Na^+ and K^+, 50% of Cl^- and urea. *Creatinine is not reabsorbed by the renal tubules.*

Reabsorption occurs mainly by four mechanisms:
1. **Passive diffusion:** Water, urea, Cl^-, etc.
2. **Facilitated diffusion:** Glucose, amino acids.
3. **Active transport:** Na^+ by way of ion channels, exchangers, cotransporters and pumps.
4. **Leakage** through paracellular pathway, i.e., through leaky tight junctions. Water and electrolytes, especially Mg^{2+} and Cl^-, are absorbed through this route.

Transport Maximum

The maximal rate at which a substance can be reabsorbed by renal transport systems is called **transport maximum** for that substance. Transport maximum is seen only for substances transported by means of **transporters** (transport proteins). At higher concentrations of the substance, the transport mechanism gets saturated and there will be no increase in the amount of substance transported, e.g., transport maximum for glucose (TmG) is 375 mg/min, i.e., renal tubules can reabsorb glucose at a maximum rate of 375 mg/min. If glucose is present in excess of this level, it will be lost through urine.

Renal Threshold

Substances having tubular maximum value have a threshold level in plasma. Below the threshold level the substance is completely reabsorbed and does not appear in urine. When the concentration of substance increases above threshold level, the excess amount is not reabsorbed and it appears in urine. **Renal threshold** is the plasma level of the substance at which, the substance first appears in urine, e.g., renal threshold for glucose is 180 mg/100 mL of blood, i.e., glucose is completely reabsorbed from the tubular fluid if its concentration in blood is below 180 mg%. If it is >180 mg%, glucose appears in urine.

Glomerulotubular Balance

An increase in GFR causes an increase in the reabsorption of solutes and water primarily in the proximal tubule, so that the percentage of solute reabsorbed in the proximal tubule is held constant. This process is called **glomerulo- tubular balance** and it is particularly prominent for Na^+. This process prevents spontaneous fluctuations in GFR from causing marked changes in Na^+ excretion.

- ❖ The most important factor responsible for this process is the oncotic pressure in the peritubular capillaries. When GFR is high, there is a relatively large increase in the oncotic pressure of the plasma leaving the glomeruli via the efferent arteriole. As a result the blood in the peritubular capillaries surrounding the nephron has a high oncotic pressure since it arises from the efferent arteriole. The large net absorptive pressure favors increased absorption along the entire length of the peritubular capillary from the interstitium. This in turn increases the reabsorption of Na^+ and water from the tubule.
- ❖ It has been observed that increased flow along the proximal tubule without any peritubular effects leads to an increase in reabsorption of fluid, Na, glucose and other Na^+-coupled solutes.
- ❖ Luminal factors also contribute to glomerulotubular balance. Increased flow may cause increased bending of the microvilli on the apical membrane of proximal tubular cells. This produces some signals that causes increased fluid and solute reabsorption.
- ❖ Humoral factors also contribute to glomerulotubular balance. Angiotensin II is secreted by proximal tubular cells and some amount is filtered in the glomeruli. This hormone increases sodium reabsorption in the proximal convoluted tubule (PCT).

Sodium Reabsorption (Table 55.1)

Sodium is filtered in large amounts, but it is actively transported from all parts of the tubule except the descending thin limb of loop of Henle. Normally about 99% of the filtered Na^+ is reabsorbed. When sodium intake is increased, natriuresis occurs. When extracellular fluid (ECF) volume is reduced as in vomiting or diarrhea, a decrease in sodium excretion occurs. Thus, urinary Na^+ excretion ranges from less than 1 mEq/day on a low salt diet to 400 mEq/day when the dietary Na^+ intake is high.

Sodium Reabsorption in the Proximal Tubule

- ❖ Passive transport
- ❖ Active transport

Passive transport: In passive transport, the transport across the membrane occurs without the expenditure of energy. The concentration of Na^+ inside the proximal tubular cell is low and the interior of the cell is negatively charged. So, along the electrochemical gradient, Na^+ diffuses into the cell from the tubular fluid. A transport protein is usually involved which acts as cotransporter and the mechanism is **symport**. The cotransporter may be Na^+- glucose cotransporter or Na^+-amino acid cotransporter. In Na^+-glucose symport mechanism, the carrier protein simultaneously binds with one ion of sodium and one molecule of glucose, and sodium and glucose enter the cells. Instead of glucose, the cotransported material can be amino acid **(Fig. 55.1)**. The transport of sodium occurs by facilitated diffusion, but the transport of glucose and amino acid occurs by secondary active transport.

Cl^-**-driven** Na^+ **transport:** This transport occurs through the leaky tight junctions of the proximal tubular epithelium. Cl^- diffuses passively and Na^+ accompanies Cl^- to maintain the electrical gradient.

Active transport: In active transport, the transport occurs with the expenditure of energy.

Na^+**-**H^+ **exchange mechanism:** Na^+-H^+ exchanger is a carrier protein present on the brush border that transports one Na^+ into the cell in exchange for one H^+ ion that is transported into the tubular lumen. The mechanism is **antiport** and it requires energy. Normally, about 60% of filtered sodium

Table 55.1: Sodium transport in different segments of the nephron.

Segment	Transporter	% reabsorbed
PCT	Na^+-H^+ exchanger	60
	Na^+-glucose cotransporter (CT)	
	Na^+-amino acid CT	
Thick ascending limb	Na^+-$2Cl^-$-K^+ CT	30
	Na^+-H^+ exchanger	
DCT	Na^+-Cl^- CT	7
Collecting duct	ENaC	3

(ENaC: epithelial sodium channel; PCT: proximal convoluted tubule; DCT: distal convoluted tubule)

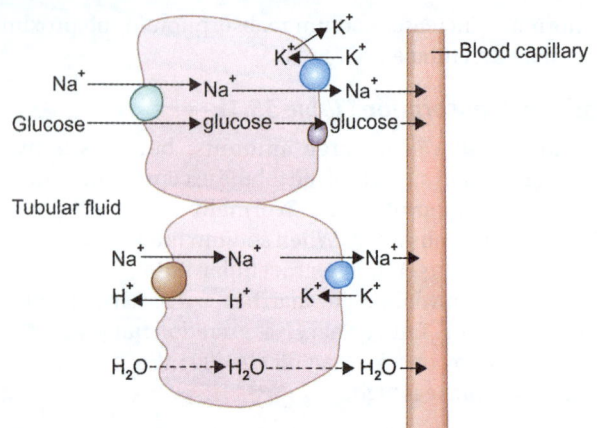

Fig. 55.1: Transport mechanisms for the reabsorption of sodium and glucose in the proximal tubule of nephron.

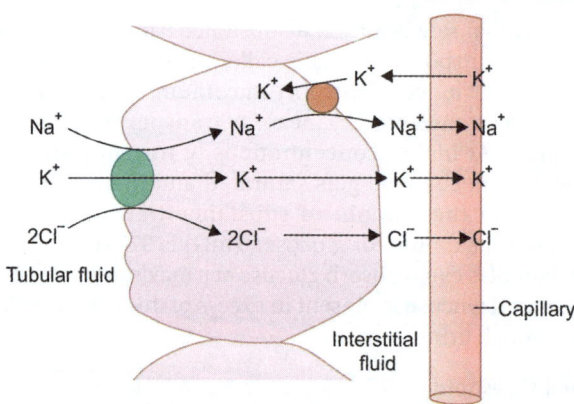

Fig. 55.2: Reabsorption of sodium in the thick ascending limb of loop of Henle.

is reabsorbed in the proximal tubule, primarily by Na^+H^+ antiport mechanism (**Fig. 55.1**).

Sodium Reabsorption in the Loop of Henle

Descending limb of loop of Henle is impermeable to solutes.

Na⁺ Reabsorption in the Ascending Limb

In the thin part of ascending limb of loop of Henle it is Cl^--driven Na^+ transport. Cl^- diffuses into the cell and Na^+ follows passively.

In the thick part of ascending limb, it is carrier-mediated Na^+ transport. The carrier protein is Na^+-$2Cl^-$-K^+ transporter. 30% of Na^+ is absorbed via Na^+-$2Cl^-$-K^+ cotransporter (**Fig. 55.2**).

Sodium Reabsorption in the Distal Convoluted Tubule

Na^+ is reabsorbed by **Na^+-Cl^- cotransporter** in the DCT. 7% of Na^+ is reabsorbed in the distal convoluted tubule (DCT).

Sodium Reabsorption in the Collecting Tubule

About 3% of Na^+ is reabsorbed via ENaC (epithelial Na^+ channel) in the collecting ducts and this is the portion that is regulated by **aldosterone** in the production of homeostatic adjustments in Na^+ balance (**Fig. 55.4A**).

Fate of Na⁺ Inside the Tubular Cell

Na^+-K^+ATPase is present in the basolateral membrane of the tubular epithelium. This pumps sodium actively from the tubular cell into the lateral intercellular space and the peritubular space and pumps in K^+ from the interstitial space into the cell. This decreases intracellular sodium producing a gradient for the further reabsorption of sodium from the tubular lumen by facilitated diffusion. The Na^+ in the interstitial and lateral intercellular space enters the peritubular capillaries (**Fig. 55.1**).

The movement of Na^+ from the lateral intercellular space and interstitial space into the peritubular capillary is essentially passive. Low hydrostatic pressure and high colloid osmotic pressure of peritubular capillaries help in the movement of water and Na^+ into the peritubular capillaries.

The osmotic pressure of blood in the peritubular capillaries is high because fluid has been filtered across the glomerulus into the renal tubule leading to an increase in the concentration of plasma proteins. The movement of water from the basolateral spaces into the peritubular capillaries drags with it Na^+. Hence factors that increase water reabsorption into the peritubular capillaries like decreased hydrostatic pressure and increased oncotic pressure also enhance Na^+ reabsorption.

Importance of Na⁺ Reabsorption

❖ Na^+ is the most abundant cation in the ECF and because sodium salts account for over 90% of osmotically active solute in the plasma and interstitial fluid, the amount of Na^+ in the body is the prime determinant of ECF volume. When there is hyponatremia, there will be a fall in the ECF volume followed by a fall in the blood pressure.

❖ Reabsorption of Na^+ promotes the reabsorption of water and other solutes from the filtrate. Water is reabsorbed by osmosis from the renal tubules into the peritubular space. As water leaves the filtrate, the concentration of the remaining solutes in the filtrate increases. This creates a concentration difference for substances like K^+, Cl^-, HCO_3^-, urea, etc., and these will be absorbed by simple diffusion into the tubular cell and from there into the peritubular capillaries. Thus, the reabsorption of Na^+ and Cl^- plays a major role in body electrolyte and water homeostasis.

❖ Solutes like glucose and amino acids are reabsorbed along with Na^+ by secondary active transport in the proximal tubule.

Factors Affecting Na⁺ Reabsorption

❖ GFR and glomerulotubular balance
❖ Neural factors
❖ Hormonal factors:
  ▪ Renin-angiotensin-aldosterone mechanism
  ▪ ANP
❖ Starling forces
❖ Drugs

GFR and glomerulotubular balance: Increase in GFR increases tubular reabsorption of solutes and water in the proximal tubule. A constant fraction of the filtered load is reabsorbed which is called **load-dependent reabsorption or glomerulotubular balance**. The % of solute reabsorbed is held constant.

If the filtered load of Na⁺ is increased, an increased amount of Na⁺ will be reabsorbed so that the fraction reabsorbed remains nearly constant. It occurs because the tubular Na⁺ reabsorption is flow limited. 2/3rd of filtered Na⁺ is reabsorbed from the proximal tubule, e.g., if GFR is increased from 125 mL/min to 150 mL/min, the absolute rate of proximal tubular reabsorption also increases from 81 mL/min (65% of GFR) to 98 mL/min (65% of GFR). The rate of reabsorption increases as the filtered load increases so that the % of GFR reabsorbed in the proximal tubule remains constant, i.e., at about 65%.

Thus, it is clear that Na⁺ excretion cannot be regulated by changes in GFR alone.

Mechanism of glomerulotubular balance
- When GFR increases, the oncotic pressure in the peritubular capillaries increases since proteins are not filtered. The capillary is freely permeable to Na⁺ and water. So there is increase in the reabsorption of Na⁺ and water from the interstitial space according to Starling forces. This in turn increases the reabsorption of Na⁺ from the tubular lumen.
- The surface area of the proximal tubule is very high because of microvilli in the brush border epithelium, which increases reabsorption of Na⁺ and water.
- Presence of leaky tight junctions in the proximal tubule helps in the leakage of substances (proximal tubule is 90 times more permeable than the gallbladder epithelium).

Significance of glomerulotubular balance: Glomerulotubular balance helps to prevent overloading of the distal tubular segments when GFR increases.

Neural factors: Sympathetic stimulation of kidney directly stimulates Na⁺ reabsorption in the proximal tubule and also stimulates renin secretion. Renal sympathetic nerves are stimulated when there is a decrease in ECF volume.

An increase in plasma volume stimulates the baroreceptors and decrease sympathetic tone, thereby inhibiting Na⁺ reabsorption and renin secretion. Thus, Na⁺ and water excretion is increased and blood volume is brought back to normal.

Hormonal factors:
- ***Renin-angiotensin-aldosterone mechanism:*** This mechanism operates when plasma Na⁺ decreases and plasma K⁺ increases. Angiotensin II directly stimulates Na⁺ reabsorption in the proximal tubule. It also stimulates aldosterone secretion from the adrenal cortex, which in turn increases Na⁺ reabsorption in the distal tubule **(Flowchart 55.2)**.

An increase in the plasma volume decreases renin secretion from juxtaglomerular apparatus and thus decreases formation of angiotensin II, thereby inhibiting Na⁺ reabsorption in proximal tubule. Decreased angiotensin II also decreases aldosterone secretion and decreases Na⁺ reabsorption in the distal tubule **(Flowchart 55.2)**.

Actions of aldosterone:
- Aldosterone increases the permeability of luminal membrane to Na⁺. It increases reabsorption of Na⁺ in association with secretion of K⁺ and H⁺. It also increases Na⁺ reabsorption with Cl⁻.
- Aldosterone act primarily in the collecting ducts to increase the number of active epithelial sodium channels (ENaCs) in this part.
- Stimulates Na⁺-K⁺ ATPase in the basolateral membrane so that intracellular Na⁺ is decreased in the renal tubular cell and more Na⁺ is reabsorbed from the tubule.

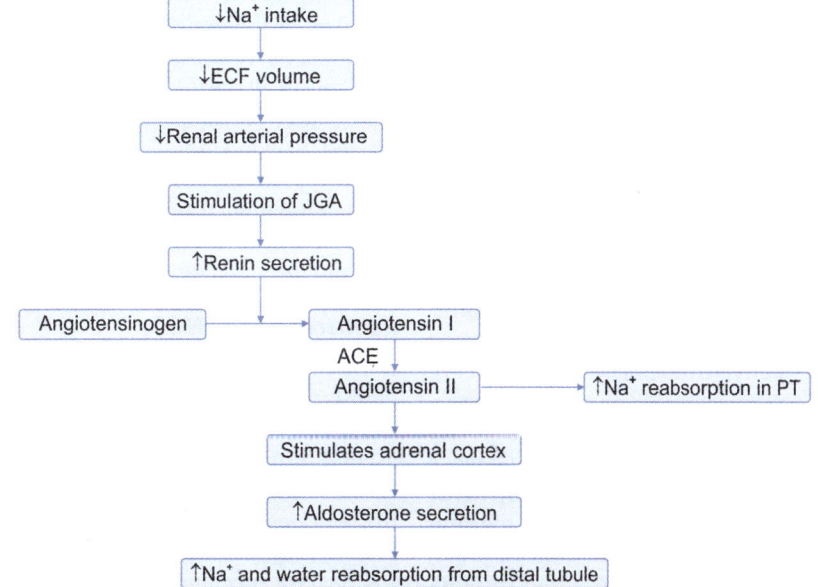

Flowchart 55.2: Regulation of sodium reabsorption from renal tubules by renin-angiotensin-aldosterone mechanism.

(PT: proximal tubule; ECF: extracellular fluid; ACE: angiotensin converting enzyme; JGA: juxtaglomerular apparatus)

- **Atrial natriuretic peptide**: An increase in plasma volume increases secretion of ANP from the atrium and the stimulus is atrial stretch.

  Actions of ANP:
  - Dilates afferent arteriole.
  - Relaxes mesangial cells so that surface area for filtration is increased. Both these factors increase GFR.
  - Inhibits Na$^+$ reabsorption in collecting duct by decreasing aldosterone secretion by a direct action on adrenal cortex.
  - Inhibits renin secretion.
  - Inhibition of renal sympathetics.
  - ANP increase intracellular cGMP and this inhibits transport of sodium ions via ENaC.

- *Other humoral effects*:
  - Prostaglandin E$_2$ (PGE$_2$) causes natriuresis by inhibiting Na-K ATPase
  - Endothelin and interleukin-1 cause natriuresis by increasing the formation of PGE$_2$.

Starling forces: According to Starling's principle, an increase in peritubular capillary hydrostatic pressure or a decrease in peritubular capillary oncotic pressure will retard the reabsorption of fluid into the capillaries. The hydrostatic pressure of interstitial space is increased and this decreases reabsorption of water and solutes from the tubular lumen especially from the proximal tubule. This leads to increased excretion of Na$^+$ and water.

Drugs:
- **Xanthines** like caffeine and theophylline decrease tubular reabsorption of Na$^+$ and increase GFR.
- **Carbonic anhydrase inhibitors** like acetazolamide (Diamox) decrease H$^+$ secretion, thereby increasing Na$^+$ and K$^+$ excretion.
- **Thiazides** inhibit Na$^+$-Cl$^-$ cotransporter in the distal tubule and increase Na$^+$ excretion.
- **Loop diuretics** like furosemide (Lasix) inhibit Na$^+$-K$^+$- 2Cl$^-$ cotransporter in the thick ascending limb of loop of Henle and increase Na$^+$ excretion.
- **K$^+$ sparing diuretics** like spironolactone (Aldactone), triamterene, amiloride, etc., inhibit Na$^+$-K$^+$ exchange in the collecting duct by inhibiting actions of aldosterone (spironolactone) or inhibiting ENaC (amiloride).

Glucose Reabsorption

The amount of any substance that is filtered is the product of GFR and plasma level of the substance. Glucose is filtered at a rate of about 100 mg/min (80 mg/dL of plasma × 125 mL/min). Normally, 100% of the filtered glucose is reabsorbed in the PCT by **secondary active transport** (*refer* **Chapter 5, Fig. 5.7A**).

Glucose is reabsorbed along with Na$^+$ by a symporter called **SGLT-2** present in the luminal membrane. Glucose can be reabsorbed completely from the filtrate only up to the **tubular maximum for glucose (TmG)** which is 375 mg/min in men and 300 mg/min in women. When the concentration of glucose exceeds TmG, then it will be excreted through urine. The condition is known as **glucosuria or glycosuria**.

Once inside the tubular epithelial cell, Na$^+$ is pumped out of the cell by Na$^+$-K$^+$ pump present in the basolateral membrane of the cell and glucose is transported into the interstitial fluid by **GLUT-2** by **facilitated diffusion**. From the interstitium glucose enters the peritubular capillaries by **simple diffusion**. Rate of transport of D-glucose is greater than that of L-glucose.

Glucose transport in the kidney is inhibited by plant glucoside **Phlorizin** which competes with D-glucose for binding to the carrier.

Splay

Renal threshold for glucose is the plasma glucose level at which glucose first appears in urine.

$$\text{Renal threshold} = \text{TmG/GFR} \times 100 = \frac{375 \text{ mg/min}}{125 \text{ mL/min}} \times 100$$

$$= 300 \text{ mg/100 mL of blood}$$

Thus, glucose would be expected to appear in urine when the arterial concentration of glucose exceeds 300 mg/dL, which corresponds to a venous glucose concentration of about 200 mg/dL. This is the theoretical value. However, the actual measured renal threshold is about 200 mg/dL of arterial blood and 180 mg/100 mL of venous blood. This is because the calculated value represents the average value of 2 million nephrons. The actual value is less than that of the predicted value because the TmG is not the same in all the renal tubules. A nephron can have a TmG that is either higher or lower than the average of 375 mg/min. Some of the nephrons with lower TmG excrete glucose into urine before others have reached their transport maximum. These nephrons with lower TmG leak glucose into urine at plasma glucose levels below the calculated threshold. This discrepancy shows up graphically as the **splay**.

If a graph is plotted with plasma glucose on the *x*-axis and the amount of glucose reabsorbed on the *y*-axis, the actual curve appears to be rounded and deviated considerably from the ideal or theoretical curve. This deviation is called **splay**. The ideal curve shown in the diagram would be obtained if the TmG in all the tubules was identical and if all the glucose molecules were removed from each tubule when the amount filtered in all the tubules was below TmG (**Fig. 55.3**).

- Glucose first appears in urine when plasma glucose is more than the renal threshold.
- *Glucose clearance is zero at plasma glucose levels below the renal threshold for glucose.*

Reabsorption of HCO$_3^-$

More than 99.99% of filtered HCO$_3^-$ is reabsorbed from the glomerular filtrate. Kidney reabsorb approximately 80% of the filtered HCO$_3^-$ from the proximal tubule, 10% from the ascending limb of loop of Henle and the remaining 10% from the DCT and collecting duct. The amount of HCO$_3^-$ lost in urine depends on the pH of urine. Normally only 0.01% of filtered HCO$_3^-$ is excreted.

The basic mechanism of HCO$_3^-$ reabsorption is the same in all segments of the nephron. It is not the same HCO$_3^-$ molecule

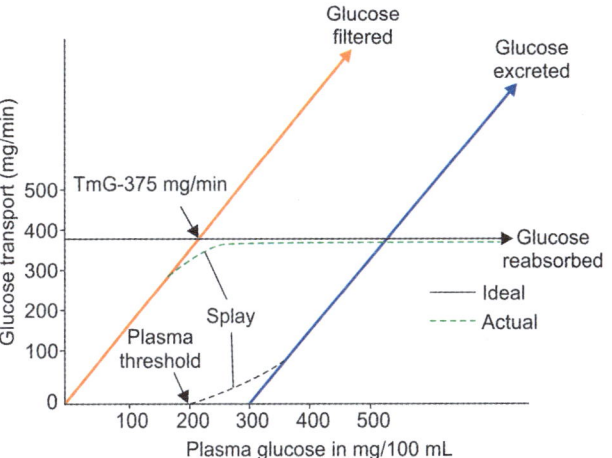

Fig. 55.3: Relation between plasma glucose level and amount of glucose reabsorbed.
(TmG: transport maximum for glucose)

Table 55.2: Percentage of substances reabsorbed in the renal tubules.	
Substance	**% Reabsorbed**
Na$^+$	99.4
K$^+$	93.3
Cl$^-$	99.2
HCO$_3^-$	100
Urea	53
Creatinine	0
Uric acid	98
Glucose	100
Amino acids	100
Water	99.4

that is filtered reaches the peritubular capillaries. H$^+$ secreted into the lumen from the tubular cells titrate the filtered HCO$_3^-$ to form CO$_2$ and H$_2$O in the presence of carbonic anhydrase (CA). This is a slow reaction.

$$H^+ + HCO_3^- \xrightarrow{CA} H_2CO_3 \longrightarrow H_2O + CO_2$$

Another reaction which is much faster is splitting of HCO$_3^-$ to CO$_2$ and OH$^-$. The secreted H$^+$ neutralizes this OH$^-$ to form H$_2$O in the tubular fluid.

$$HCO_3^- \rightarrow CO_2 + OH^-$$
$$H^+ + OH^- \rightarrow H_2O$$

The apical membranes of the H$^+$ secreting cells in the tubule are highly permeable to CO$_2$. The CO$_2$ and H$_2$O produced in the tubular lumen diffuse into the tubular cell. Inside the cell, CO$_2$ and H$_2$O react to form H$_2$CO$_3$ which splits to form H$^+$ and HCO$_3^-$ in the presence of carbonic anhydrase. Finally H$^+$ is secreted into the tubular lumen and HCO$_3^-$ pass out into the interstitium through the basolateral membrane of the tubular cell. This HCO$_3^-$ diffuses into the blood in the peritubular capillaries. The HCO$_3^-$ that disappears from the tubular lumen and the HCO$_3^-$ that reach the blood is not the same molecule. Thus each HCO$_3^-$ that is filtered indirectly reaches the blood. The largest fraction of H$^+$ secreted into the tubular lumen is titrated by HCO$_3^-$.

Reabsorption of Amino Acids

Filtered amino acids are completely reabsorbed in the proximal tubule by secondary active transport with the help of sodium–amino acid symporter (**Table 55.2**). Once inside the cell, amino acid is transported to the peritubular space by **simple diffusion or facilitated diffusion**.

Reabsorption of Uric Acid

The tubular transport of uric acid is confined to the proximal tubule and involves both reabsorption and secretion. 98% of filtered uric acid is reabsorbed by the renal tubules. *80% of uric acid in urine is due to tubular secretion.*

Normal plasma uric acid concentration: 3–6 mg/100 mL
Normal uric acid excretion: 1 g/day

Increase in the plasma uric acid may be due to:
- Decreased excretion, e.g., treatment with thiazide diuretics which act on distal tubules.
- Increased production of uric acid, e.g., leukemia, pneumonia, etc., due to increased breakdown of uric acid-rich white blood cells.

Reabsorption of uric acid by the renal tubules can be inhibited by drugs like **probenecid, phenylbutazone,** etc., and thus, renal excretion of uric acid can be increased. These drugs are used in the treatment of gout. **Gout** includes a group of disorders like arthritis, renal stones, etc., due to hyperuricemia.

Other drugs used in the treatment of gout include:
- **Colchicine** which inhibits uric acid crystal phagocytosis by WBC and decrease joint manifestations.
- **Allopurinol**, which inhibits xanthine oxidase, acts by decreasing uric acid production.

Cl$^-$ Reabsorption

- By passive diffusion along with Na$^+$ into the cell.
- Cl$^-$ diffuses passively through the leaky tight junctions in the proximal tubule.

Ca^{2+} Reabsorption

About 45% of plasma calcium is bound to plasma proteins and therefore does not get filtered into the tubules. 99% of filtered free Ca^{2+} is reabsorbed by the nephron. 1% is excreted through urine. Urinary Ca^{2+} excretion is 200 mg/day. 80% of Ca^{2+} is reabsorbed passively and 20% by facilitated diffusion with the help of a carrier protein called calbindin in the renal tubule. From the cell, Ca^{2+} reaches the interstitial space with the help of a Ca^{2+} pump (Ca^{2+}-Mg^{2+} ATPase), which is an active process. Ca^{2+} reabsorption is regulated by **parathormone, calcitonin and calcitriol**. Calcitonin increases urinary excretion of calcium and phosphate ions. Calcitriol increases the synthesis of calbindin and thereby increases Ca^{2+} reabsorption. It also stimulates the activity of Ca^{2+}- Mg^{2+} ATPase. Parathormone and calcitriol increase reabsorption of Ca^{2+} by the ascending limb of loop of Henle and distal tubule.

Normal plasma Ca^{2+} level is 9–11 mg/100 mL.

Phosphate Reabsorption

About 90% of filtered inorganic phosphate (Pi) is reabsorbed by renal tubules. About 10% is excreted through urine. Urinary Pi is an important buffer for the maintenance of acid-base balance. Parathormone inhibits phosphate reabsorption by the proximal tubule. Growth hormone increases reabsorption of phosphate from the proximal tubule. Calcitriol promotes the reabsorption of both Ca^{2+} and phosphates.

Normal plasma inorganic phosphate level is 4 mg/100 mL.

K^+ Reabsorption

Whole of the filtered load of K^+ is reabsorbed from the renal tubules. About 2 g of K^+ is excreted per day and this is due to the secretion of K^+ by the renal tubules. Distal tubules secrete K^+ in exchange for Na^+ under the influence of aldosterone.

Urea Reabsorption

Urea is filtered freely into the glomerular filtrate. About half of the filtered urea is reabsorbed passively in the proximal tubule. In the medullary collecting duct, a large amount of urea is reabsorbed into the interstitium using a special urea transport protein. The synthesis of this protein is stimulated by ADH. Nearly 50% of the medullary hyperosmolarity is attributable to urea. Urea is also secreted into the tubular lumen from the medullary interstitium in the thin ascending limb of loop of Henle and the proximal straight tubule.

The amount of urea excreted depends on the amount of urea formed, which in turn depends on the amount of protein ingested. Urea is the breakdown product of protein metabolism.

Normal blood urea = 20–40 mg/100 mL of blood.
Amount excreted = 25 g/day.

Increase in the blood urea level is known as **uremia or azotemia**.

Factors Determining Urea Reabsorption

- When urine flow rate is increased, there is increased excretion of urea.
- When water reabsorption is increased, more urea is reabsorbed and urinary urea content decrease.
- Urea reabsorption, like that of water is affected by ADH. In the absence of ADH, urea reabsorption decreases and with it, the medullary hyperosmolarity also decreases.

If urinary output is 2 mL/min urea clearance will be 75 mL/min. This is **maximum urea clearance**.

$$\text{Urea clearance} = \frac{UV}{P} = 75 \text{ mL/min}$$

Water Reabsorption

Of the 180 L of glomerular filtrate formed per day, only 1–1.5 L is excreted as urine. The rest is reabsorbed by the renal tubular cells.

% of water reabsorbed in the different segments of the nephron (Figs. 55.4A and B).

- Proximal tubule: 65%
- Loop of Henle: 15%

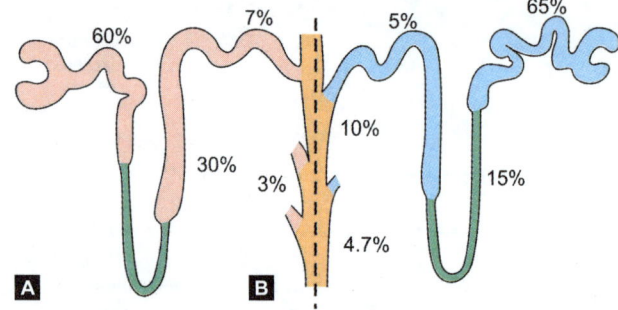

Figs. 55.4A and B: (A) Reabsorption of sodium; (B) Water in different segments of nephron.

- Distal convoluted tubule: 5%
- Collecting tubule:
  - Cortical collecting tubule: 10%
  - Medullary collecting tubule: 4.7%

Obligatory Water Reabsorption

About 85% of water reabsorption occurs by **osmosis**, together with the reabsorption of solutes such as Na^+, Cl^- and glucose. This is termed **obligatory** (compulsory, not optional) **water reabsorption** because water is obliged to follow the solutes. 65% of obligatory water reabsorption occurs in the PCT and 20% of the obligatory reabsorption occurs in the distal tubules. The bulk of water reabsorption occur secondary to the active reabsorption of Na^+ in the tubules. Solutes reabsorbed accumulate in the peritubular and lateral intercellular spaces leading to an increase in the tonicity of this area. So, water moves from tubular lumen to these areas by osmosis through two routes:
1. Transcellular route
2. Pericellular route

Proximal tubule: Aquaporin-1 is localized to both the apical and the basolateral membrane of the proximal tubular cells. This allows water to move rapidly out of the tubule along the osmotic gradients set up by the active transport of solutes. At the end of the proximal tubule, 60–70% of the filtered solute and 60–70% of the filtered water have been removed from the filtrate.

Loop of Henle: The descending limb of loop of Henle is permeable to water due to the presence of aquaporin-1 in the apical and basolateral membranes. 15% of filtered water is reabsorbed in the descending limb. *The ascending limb is impermeable to water.*

Distal convoluted tubule: The first part of the distal tubule is relatively impermeable to water. 5% of water is reabsorbed from the middle part of the DCT.

The increase in hydrostatic pressure in the peritubular space drives water and solutes into the peritubular capillaries which has a high osmotic pressure. The capillaries are freely permeable to water and solutes.

Facultative Water Reabsorption

Water reabsorption in the collecting duct: The remaining 15% of water reaching the distal nephron may/may not be reabsorbed depending on the body water balance. It is called **facultative (optional) water reabsorption**. It occurs in the distal nephron, i.e., the last part of DCT and collecting tubule under the influence of **ADH or vasopressin,** which controls the permeability of the collecting tubule to water.

Vasopressin binds to V_2 receptors present on the epithelial principal cells of the collecting tubule. The binding activates adenylyl cyclase increasing the level of cyclic adenosine monophosphate (cAMP) in the cytoplasm, which then stimulates protein kinase A. It leads to rapid insertion of vesicles containing **aquaporin-2** present in the cytoplasm of principal cells into their luminal membrane. Aquaporins are water channels. More water will enter the principal cells. Aquaporins 3 and 4 are present in the basolateral plasma membrane of the principal cells and they are responsible for the high water permeability of the basolateral membrane. Thus water reaches the peritubular space from where it is absorbed by the capillaries (vasa recta or peritubular capillaries). In this manner, 10% of the filtered water is removed from the cortical collecting duct and 4.7% of water is removed from the medullary collecting duct producing a concentrated urine. Thus, 99.7% of filtered water is reabsorbed from the tubule normally. The osmolality of urine may reach 1,400 mOsm/kg of water.

In the absence of vasopressin or ADH, the collecting tubule is relatively impermeable to water and therefore only 2% of filtered water is reabsorbed from this part. This 2% of water is reabsorbed along with the salt that is pumped out of the collecting duct fluid. As much as 13% of the filtered water will be excreted in the absence of ADH. The urine flow may reach 15 mL/minute or more. The urine osmolality may become as low as 30 mOsm/kg of water. Thus homeostasis is maintained by this portion of renal water reabsorption.

A negative feedback system regulates ADH-stimulated water reabsorption. When osmotic pressure of blood is high as in dehydration, osmoreceptors in the hypothalamus are stimulated. They send impulses to the **supraoptic and paraventricular nuclei** of hypothalamus and also to the posterior pituitary gland leading to the release of **ADH** into the bloodstream. ADH acts on the collecting duct causing increased reabsorption of water from the distal tubule bringing the blood osmotic pressure back to normal.

Aquaporins: Diffusion of water across cell membrane depends on protein water channels called **aquaporins**. There are different types of aquaporins in humans like aquaporin-1 (AQP1), AQP2, AQP3, AQP4, AQP5 and AQP9. Till date 13 aquaporins have been cloned.

Most of the aquaporins are found in the kidneys (aquaporin-1 to 4). They are also found in liver, lungs, spleen, salivary and lacrimal glands. Aquaporin-1 is localized in the proximal tubule. Aquaporin-2, AQP3 and AQP4 are present in the principal cells of the collecting ducts. Apical AQP2 is the basis of ADH-regulated water permeability. Unlike other aquaporins, aquaporin-2 is stored in vesicles in the cytoplasm of **principal cells**. These aquaporins get inserted on the cell membrane of collecting duct only in the presence of ADH. The effect is mediated via V_2 **receptors**. AQP3 and AQP4 are present in the basolateral membrane of principal cells and they provide the pathway for water movement into the peritubular fluid.

Diabetes insipidus is a condition caused by ADH deficiency where the urine becomes hypotonic to plasma and urine volume is increased (*refer* **Chapter 63**. Posterior pituitary).

In **nephrogenic diabetes insipidus**, the collecting ducts fail to respond to ADH. This can be due to mutation of the gene coding for V_2 receptors, making the receptors unresponsive or may be due to mutation of the gene for aquaporin-2.

Normal osmolality of urine is 1,200 mOsm/kg of water. It varies with urine flow rate.

In diabetes insipidus, it becomes 30 mOsm/kg of water.

Water Intoxication

Normal urine flow rate is 2 mL/min. Maximum urine flow that can be achieved is 16 mL/min. If water is ingested at a higher rate than this, swelling of the cells become severe due to hypotonic ECF. This leads to symptoms of water intoxication like convulsions, coma, etc., due to swelling of cells in the brain that may even lead to death.

Tubular Secretion

Tubular secretion is the movement of materials from blood into the tubular fluid, i.e., tubular secretion removes materials from blood into the renal tubules across the renal tubular cells. Secreted substances include H^+, K^+, NH_3, creatinine, steroids, drugs like penicillin, salicylates, etc.

K^+ Secretion

Normally, almost all the K^+ that is filtered is reabsorbed by the renal tubules. Constancy of total body potassium is achieved when the daily intestinal absorption of K^+ equals its daily urinary excretion. To maintain K^+ homeostasis (concentration of K^+ in body fluids constant), DCT and collecting duct secrete variable amounts of K^+. The rate of K^+ secretion is proportionate to the rate of flow of tubular fluid through the distal portions of the nephron because with rapid flow there is less opportunity for the tubular K^+ concentration to rise to a value that stops further secretion of K^+. So, when urine flow rate is increased there will be increased secretion of K^+. However, rapid losses of large amounts of K^+ can cause serious hypokalemia.

> Total body K^+ content is about 4,500 mmol. 95% of K^+ is present within cells, mostly muscle cells, with smaller quantities in hepatocytes and blood cells. Normal serum K^+ level ranges from 3.5 to 5.3 mmol/L. Even a small leakage of intracellular K^+ drastically raises the plasma K^+ levels leading to hyperkalemia which has lethal consequences like cardiac arrhythmias.

Regulation of K^+ Secretion

- ❖ Aldosterone increases K^+ secretion by increasing reabsorption of Na^+ from the distal tubule. Glucocorticoid also increases K^+ excretion.
- ❖ When plasma K^+ concentration increases, K^+ secretion also increases.

- In the distal tubules, Na⁺ is reabsorbed and K⁺ secreted into the tubular lumen. When the concentration of Na⁺ in the DCT is high, there will be increased Na⁺ reabsorption by the principal cells, and K⁺ will be secreted into the lumen in exchange for Na⁺. This is because, reabsorption of Na⁺ lowers the potential difference across the tubular cell and there will be passive movement of K⁺ out of the cell. It is also secreted by an antiport mechanism in exchange for Na⁺.
- When urine flow rate is increased, K⁺ secretion is also increased because the tubular K⁺ concentration is low. When flow rate is increased, there is less opportunity for the tubular K⁺ concentration to rise to a value that stops further secretion of K⁺. So in conditions of increased urine flow that occurs with extracellular volume expansion, osmotic diuresis, administration of diuretics like acetazolamide, furosemide, etc. leads to increased K⁺ excretion. On the contrary, when luminal flow is low, the movement of K⁺ from cell to lumen causes luminal K⁺ concentration to rise, which opposes further K⁺ diffusion from the cell and limits total K⁺ secretion.
- When H⁺ ion secretion is increased in the renal tubules K⁺ secretion is decreased due to competition with Na⁺ for the carrier protein. This is seen in acidosis.
- If H⁺ secretion is increased, K⁺ excretion will decrease as K⁺ is reabsorbed in the collecting duct cells in exchange for H⁺ via the H⁺-K⁺ ATPase.

Importance of K⁺ Secretion

The amount of K⁺ secreted is approximately equal to the K⁺ intake and K⁺ balance is thus maintained in the body. High plasma K⁺ referred to as **hyperkalemia** is a serious situation and it may even cause **cardiac arrest**. It occurs only in cases of impaired renal function and adrenocortical insufficiency.

Normal K⁺ excretion = 2–3 g/day.

Hypokalemia

Decrease in plasma K⁺ is known as hypokalemia and is a common condition.

Causes of hypokalemia:
- Excessive loss of K⁺ from the body as in severe vomiting, diarrhea, polyuria, etc.
- Decreased dietary intake of K⁺
- Hyperaldosteronism
- Cushing's disease
- Drugs like:
  - Steroids increase K⁺ excretion
  - Insulin shifts K⁺ intracellularly
  - Loop diuretics inhibit Na⁺-K⁺-2Cl⁻ cotransporter
  - Carbonic anhydrase inhibitors.

H⁺ Secretion

H⁺ secretion occurs by two mechanisms in the proximal and distal tubules:

1. *By secondary active transport*: Extrusion of Na⁺ into the lateral intercellular space by Na⁺-K⁺ ATPase decreases intracellular Na⁺, and Na⁺ enters the cell from the tubular lumen in exchange for H⁺ (antiport). Thus, for each H⁺ secreted, one Na⁺ and one HCO_3^- enter the interstitial fluid (**Fig. 55.5**).
2. *By aldosterone*: Aldosterone acts on H⁺-K⁺ ATPase and increases the secretion of H⁺ by the intercalated cells.

NH₃ Secretion

In the tubular cell, the following reactions occur:

$$\text{Glutamine} \xrightarrow{\text{Glutaminase}} \text{Glutamate} + NH_3$$

$$\text{Glutamate} \xrightarrow{\text{Glutamic dehydrogenase}} \alpha\text{-ketoglutarate} + NH_3$$

$$NH_4^+ \longleftrightarrow NH_3 + H^+$$

The NH_3 formed inside the tubular cell is secreted into the tubular fluid and is converted to NH_4^+, thus maintaining the concentration gradient for the diffusion of more NH_3 into urine. This is called **non-ionic diffusion**. Drugs like salicylates are also secreted by non-ionic diffusion (**Fig. 55.8**).

Renal Regulation of Urine Volume and Osmolarity

Concentration and Dilution of Urine

Even though the fluid intake varies, the total volume of body fluid remains constant. This is accomplished by the ability of the kidney to regulate the rate of loss of water through urine. Urine osmolarity can vary from 50 to 1,200 mOsm/L of water and the corresponding urine volume varies from 18 to 0.5 L/day. When fluid intake is high, large volume of dilute urine is produced (**diuresis**), and when fluid intake is low or water loss from the body is high as in heavy sweating, vomiting, diarrhea, etc., a small volume of highly concentrated urine is formed (**antidiuresis**).

Kidney is the major route of elimination of water from the body since other routes of water loss, like sweating, through respiratory passages, gastrointestinal tract, etc., are not under regulation. Another important function of kidney is to conserve water in times of hypotension or hyperosmolarity. While conserving water, wastes and excess ions should be eliminated. This occurs by the influence of ADH on distal nephron. ADH can conserve water only if an

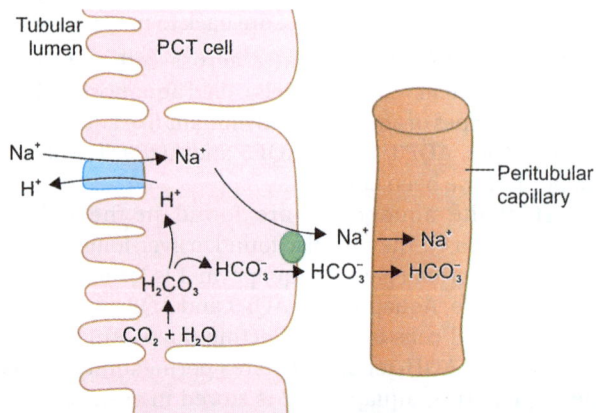

Fig. 55.5: Secretion of H⁺ by Na⁺-H⁺ antiporter in the proximal convoluted tubule (PCT).

osmotic gradient of solutes is present in the interstitial fluid of renal medulla. This is because water can move across the tubular epithelium only passively, i.e., along the osmotic gradient. So, a hyperosmotic environment is generated in the interstitial fluid of renal medulla. The solute concentration in the interstitial fluid increases from 300 mOsm/L in the renal cortex to 1,200 mOsm/L in the deeper parts of renal medulla. The major solutes contributing to this high osmolarity are **NaCl and urea**. The part of the nephron that plays a major role in maintaining this osmotic gradient is the thick ascending limb of loop of Henle.

Factors Responsible for the Production and Maintenance of Osmotic Gradient in the Renal Medulla

Counter Current System

- Differences in the water and solute permeability in different segments of the nephron, especially in the loop of Henle is responsible for the production of osmotic gradient (**countercurrent multiplier system**).
- **Countercurrent exchange mechanism** operating in the vasa recta is responsible for the maintenance of the medullary osmotic gradient.

Differences in water and solute permeability (countercurrent multiplier system): Since the PCT is freely permeable to water and solute, the fluid leaving the PCT is isotonic to that of plasma. *The descending limb of loop of Henle is permeable to water but not to solutes.* So, water is reabsorbed by osmosis from tubular fluid into the interstitial space. As a result, the fluid in the tubular lumen becomes more and more concentrated as it reaches the hairpin bend of loop of Henle. The greater the length of loop of Henle, greater will be the osmolarity at the hairpin bend (**Fig. 55.6**).

The thin ascending limb is relatively impermeable to water, but permeable to Na$^+$ and Cl$^-$. *The thick ascending limb of loop of Henle is impermeable to water, but permeable to solutes.* The cells here have symporters that actively reabsorb Na$^+$, K$^+$ and 2Cl$^-$ from the tubular fluid. From the tubular cells, these ions reach the interstitial fluid. The reabsorbed ions become concentrated in the interstitial fluid of medulla contributing to the osmotic gradient. So, the osmolarity of fluid in the tubular lumen drops to about 150 mOsm/L when it enters the DCT. DCT is also not very permeable to water.

In the collecting duct, the **principal cells** become highly permeable to water under the influence of ADH and the tubular fluid becomes more and more concentrated.

The action of ADH on collecting duct is mediated via V_2 receptors present on the basolateral membrane of the principal cells. Binding of ADH to V_2 receptors activates **adenylyl cyclase** and this causes insertion of **aquaporins** (water channels) into the luminal membrane of the collecting duct. Thus, water reabsorption occurs along an osmotic gradient from the lumen of collecting duct to the hypertonic medullary interstitium. The major stimulus for ADH secretion is hypertonicity of plasma. The effective osmolarity of plasma is determined by the plasma Na$^+$ concentration since it is the major ECF solute.

Role of Urea in the Establishment of Hyperosmolar Medullary Interstitium

When water is reabsorbed from the collecting duct under the influence of ADH, the concentration of urea in the tubular fluid becomes high and so, urea diffuses from the tubular

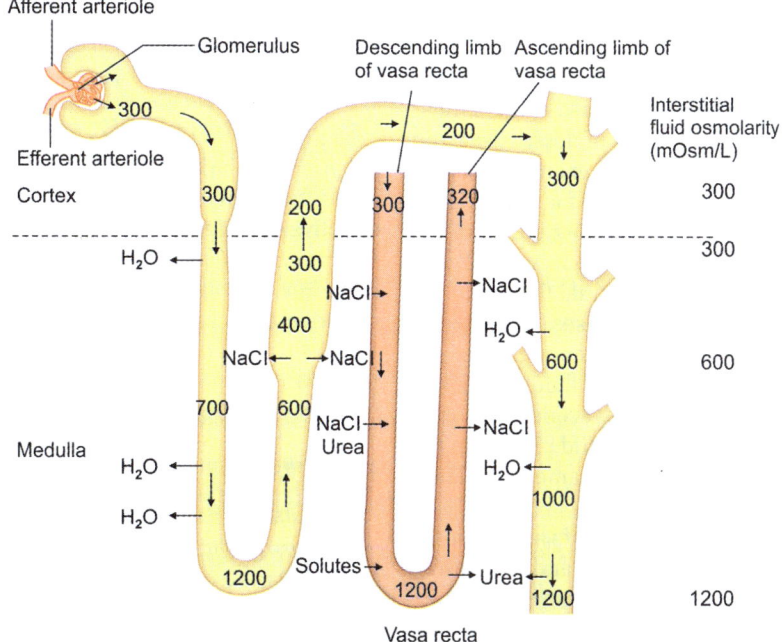

Fig. 55.6: Mechanism of concentration of urine; Loop of Henle and collecting duct form countercurrent multiplier system and vasa recta forms the countercurrent exchanger. Numbers denote osmolarity expressed in mOsm/L of water. Note the increase in medullary interstitial osmotic gradient towards inner medulla.

lumen into the interstitial fluid, increasing the osmolarity of medullary interstitium. Urea is transported by facilitated diffusion, and is mediated by urea transporters.

As urea accumulates in the interstitial fluid, some of it diffuses into the tubular fluid in the descending and thin ascending limb of loop of Henle. The constant transfer of urea between the different segments of the renal tubule and interstitial fluid in medulla is called **urea recycling**.

Thus, reabsorption of water from the tubular fluid of renal medulla increases urea concentration of the interstitial fluid. This increase in urea in the interstitium, in turn, promotes further water reabsorption from collecting tubule and thus urine becomes highly concentrated.

The amount of urea in the medullary interstitium varies with the amount of urea filtered and this depends on the dietary intake of protein. Therefore, a high protein diet increases the ability of kidney to concentrate urine.

Mechanism of Excretion of Dilute Urine

When plasma osmolarity is low, i.e., in hypervolemia or when plasma Na+ concentration is <135 mmol/L, ADH secretion does not occur and the plasma ADH falls to almost zero level. So, the reabsorption of water from the collecting duct is inhibited because it is impermeable to water in the absence of ADH. But, the reabsorption of NaCl continues. So, the fluid in the collecting duct becomes progressively hypo-osmotic with low concentration of NaCl and urea. The volume of urine excreted can be as much as 18 L/day and the osmolarity of urine will be approximately 50 mOsm/L of water.

Countercurrent Exchange Mechanism

A **countercurrent system** is a system in which the inflow runs parallel to, counter to and in close proximity to the outflow for some distance. This is seen in the loop of Henle and vasa recta in the renal medulla.

The osmotic gradient in the medullary interstitium will be lost if solutes and urea are washed off by vasa recta. Similar to loop of Henle, vasa recta also consists of descending and ascending limbs that are parallel to each other and to the loop of Henle. Blood entering the vasa recta has an osmolarity of 300 mOsm/L. As it flows in the descending part into the renal medulla the interstitial fluid is highly concentrated, and Na+, Cl- and urea diffuse from the interstitial fluid into the blood, and the osmolarity of blood increases. Since blood flow is sluggish in the vasa recta, there is enough time for diffusion of solutes to occur among tubular fluid, interstitial fluid and blood. Thus, the fluids in the descending limb of loop of Henle, medullary interstitial fluid and plasma in the descending limb of vasa recta attain the same osmolarity (**Fig. 55.6**).

As blood flows into the ascending limb of vasa recta the interstitial fluid becomes less concentrated and as a result, ions and urea diffuse from blood into the interstitial fluid, and water diffuses from interstitial fluid into blood in vasa recta. *Thus, vasa recta prevent washing off of solutes from medullary interstitium*. Thus, in vasa recta solutes diffuse out into the medullary interstitium in the ascending limb and solutes diffuse into the vasa recta in the descending limb. But, water diffuses into the vessels in the ascending limb and out of the vessel in the descending limb. Thus, the solutes, especially urea and NaCl, recirculate in the medulla, and water bypasses it. Thus, the hypertonicity of medullary interstitium is maintained.

Counter current mechanism is a passive process in vasa recta because vasa recta are freely permeable to solutes and water.

Counter current mechanism operates both in the loop of Henle and vasa recta in the renal medulla. Since the medullary osmotic gradient is produced by loop of Henle it is called **counter current multiplier system (Fig. 55.6)**. Vasa recta are referred to as **counter current exchanger** because the medullary osmotic gradient is maintained by the functioning of vasa recta (**Fig. 55.6**).

> It is the countercurrent multiplier that makes the renal medulla hyperosmotic. The fluid leaving the proximal tubule is isosmotic to body fluids. The tubular fluid becomes hyperosmolar for the first time in the descending limb of loop of Henle. In the thick ascending limb, the tubular fluid becomes iso-osmolar. In the collecting tubule, the fluid again becomes hyperosmolar a second time in the presence of ADH. The maximum possible osmolarity of the tubular fluid is 1,200 mOsm/L.

Importance of Diluting and Concentrating Mechanisms of Kidney

If there is a reduction in plasma osmolarity (**hypo-osmolarity**), water enters the cells and leads to cell swelling especially of the brain cells, leading to symptoms like nausea, headache, confusion, coma, etc.

When there is **hyperosmolarity**, water is lost from the cells and the cells shrink. This is also manifested by neurological symptoms like weakness, seizures, coma and even death.

Osmotic Control of ADH Secretion

In hyperosmolarity, the **osmoreceptors** in the hypothalamus sense the change due to shrinking of osmoreceptors. Only **effective osmoles** like NaCl can stimulate the osmoreceptors. *Increase in ineffective osmoles like urea and glucose does not stimulate the osmoreceptors*. The osmoreceptors are very sensitive and can sense changes in osmolarity as small as 1%. The osmoreceptors send impulses to the supraoptic and paraventricular nuclei of hypothalamus, and ADH secretion is increased (**Table 55.3**).

Table 55.3: Factors affecting antidiuretic hormone (ADH) secretion.	
Stimulants of ADH secretion	**Inhibitors**
Hyperosmolarity of body fluids	Hypo-osmolarity of body fluids
Decreased blood volume and BP	Increase in blood volume and BP
Nausea	Atrial natriuretic peptide
Angiotensin II	
Nicotine	Alcohol

In hypo-osmolarity, osmoreceptors of hypothalamus swell and no excitatory signals are sent to increase ADH secretion. The ½ life of ADH in the blood is very less and it is rapidly broken down in plasma, and the plasma level of ADH becomes negligible or zero. This leads to increased water excretion or diuresis, bringing the body fluid osmolarity back to normal.

Hemodynamic Control of ADH Secretion

A decrease in blood volume and blood pressure stimulates ADH secretion mediated via **baroreceptors** or stretch receptors. **Low-pressure receptors** are present in the left atrium and pulmonary vessels and they respond to changes in blood volume. **High-pressure receptors** are present in the carotid sinus and aortic arch and they respond to changes in arterial blood pressure. Signals from the baroreceptors reach the brainstem through IX and X cranial nerves. From the brainstem, impulses reach the supraoptic and paraventricular nuclei of hypothalamus. When there is baroreceptor stimulation ADH secretion is inhibited. If there is no stimulation of baroreceptors as in hypovolemia and hypotension, ADH secretion is stimulated. The sensitivity of baroreceptors to changes in blood pressure and blood volume is less than that of osmoreceptors. A reduction in 5–10% of blood volume and blood pressure is necessary to stimulate ADH secretion. ADH also has vasoconstrictor action mediated via V_1 receptors located in the blood vessels. So ADH is also called **arginine vasopressin (AVP)** as it increases blood pressure.

Abnormalities of ADH Secretion

- **Neurogenic diabetes insipidus or Pituitary diabetes insipidus or Central diabetes insipidus:** This condition is due to inadequate release of ADH from posterior pituitary. This results in excretion of large volumes of dilute urine (polyuria) and increased intake of water due to excessive thirst (polydipsia). The hyperosmolarity of body fluids stimulates the thirst center in the hypothalamus. The average osmotic threshold for thirst is approximately 295 mOsm/L. NaCl is the most effective osmole which can stimulate the thirst center.
- **Syndrome of inappropriate ADH secretion (SIADH):** Here, the plasma ADH level is high. There is retention of body water due to excessive reabsorption of water by the distal nephron. If water intake is not restricted it leads to hypo-osmolarity.
- **Nephrogenic diabetes insipidus:** In nephrogenic diabetes insipidus, the ADH level in blood is normal, but the collecting ducts do not respond normally to ADH. So, they cannot concentrate urine, which leads to polyuria and polydipsia. The condition is mainly due to metabolic disorders like hypercalcemia or due to drugs like lithium. Rarely is it inherited, in which condition it may be due to mutation of the genes coding for V_2 receptors or aquaporin-2.

> **Goldblatt hypertension or renal hypertension**
>
> **Harry Goldblatt** a pathologist noted a characteristic narrowing of the renal blood vessels in patients who have died of hypertension. He suggested that decreased blood flow and oxygen supply to the kidney, i.e., renal ischemia led to the hypertension. He did experiments in dogs in 1934 by clamping the major renal arteries in dogs. Partial constriction of both renal arteries resulted in a persistent rise in blood pressure in the absence of overt renal failure indicating that hypertension resulted specifically from kidney ischemia. This experiment led to the isolation of renin. Later it was discovered that angiotensin II is responsible for the hypertension. This led to the production of ACE inhibitors to decrease blood pressure in patients with high circulating levels of renin.
>
> In unilaterally nephrectomized animals, Goldblatt produced hypertension experimentally by placing a clip around the renal artery of the remaining kidney. The clip is so adjusted that there is no complete obstruction to blood flow. There is only a reduction of the perfusion pressure distal to the obstruction. Increase in blood pressure following obstruction of blood flow to this kidney is referred to as **one-kidney Goldblatt hypertension**. This is an animal model of hypertension which resembles renal hypertension but is produced in experimental animals by decreasing the blood flow to one kidney. Renal ischemia leads to increased renin secretion which in turn causes increased angiotensin II formation leading to increased BP. Within minutes of clamping the renal artery there will be increase in systemic arterial blood pressure. This increase in pressure maintains the renal perfusion. This early rise in pressure is due to the vasoconstriction by angiotensin II. It is seen that the circulating renin and angiotensin levels come back to normal after 5–7 days, but the systemic arterial pressure remains high. The later phase of the hypertension is the result of aldosterone released which in turn leads to retention of salt and water.
>
> Unilateral partial clamping of the renal artery in a healthy animal also produces hypertension. This is referred to as **two kidney Goldblatt hypertension.** Here the clamped kidney increases renin secretion. This causes increase in the level of angiotensin II and aldosterone in blood. So the clamped and the non-clamped kidney retain salt and water. In both types of Goldblatt hypertension, administration of ACE inhibitors can lower arterial blood pressure.
>
> **Renal hypertension** can occur similarly in conditions like renin secreting tumors of the juxtaglomerular apparatus, stenosis or atheromatous narrowing of renal artery, etc.

Renal Regulation of Acid-base Balance

> **PY7.5:** Describe the renal regulation of fluid and electrolytes and acid-base balance.

The kidneys and the lungs are mainly responsible for regulating the acid-base balance in the body. The largest source of **volatile acid** in the body is CO_2 which is formed during oxidation of carbohydrate, fat and most amino acids. The lungs excrete this CO_2 by diffusion across the respiratory membrane preventing the CO_2 from forming H^+. If this CO_2 accumulates in the body, it forms H_2CO_3 which splits to form H^+ and HCO_3^-. This H^+ leads to acidosis.

Metabolism also generates **non-volatile acids** that the lungs cannot remove. Metabolism also generates non-volatile bases which form HCO_3^-.

There is a net production of approximately 70 mmol of non-volatile acids per day. The kidneys handle this acid load by excreting approximately 70 mmol of H⁺ per day into the urine and simultaneously transporting 70 mmol of HCO_3^- per day into the blood. This HCO_3^- neutralizes the daily load of 70 mmol of non-volatile acid. If this does not happen, the H⁺ reacts with HCO_3^- present in blood leading to depletion of HCO_3^- in the body. This leads to drastic reduction in the pH and may lead to death due to severe acidosis. This is what happens in renal failure where there will be severe acidosis due to acid retention.

Normal body functions can occur only within a narrow range of pH because many metabolic functions in the body are highly sensitive to pH. A pH of 6.8–7.8 in the ECF is compatible with life. The pH of body fluids is maintained within this range by the coordinated function of lungs and kidneys. Normal body pH is taken as 7.4. Acid is any substance that increases the H⁺ concentration and alkali is any substance that removes H⁺ from body fluids. When the body pH changes, kidney excretes acidic or alkaline urine, thus maintaining the pH of ECF constant. The kidneys must excrete acids in the amount equivalent to the production of non-volatile acids in the body. Lung is the major excretory route of volatile acids. Kidneys should also reabsorb the filtered plasma bicarbonate and thus prevent the loss of bicarbonate in the urine to maintain the pH of body fluids. The pH of urine in humans varies from 4.5 to 8 depending on the rate of acid secretion.

Sources of Acids in the Body

- Dietary sources
- Cellular metabolism.

The excess acid must be excreted from the body at a rate equal to its addition. If excretion of acid is reduced, it leads to **acidosis**. Usually, aerobic metabolism of carbohydrates and fats produces large quantity of CO_2 which forms **volatile acid** carbonic acid, and it is effectively removed by lungs. But metabolism of cysteine, methionine, and other sulfur-containing amino acids produces H_2SO_4. Metabolism of lysine, arginine and histidine produces HCl. These are non-volatile acids. A non-vegetarian diet produces large amount of **non-volatile acids** than a vegetarian diet.

In cases of diseases like diabetes mellitus, where there is insulin deficiency, metabolism of carbohydrate produces ketoacids like β-hydroxy butyric acid. In hypoxia, anaerobic metabolism leads to production of lactic acid. Non-volatile acids like $H_2PO_4^-$, H_2SO_4, β-OH butyric acid, acetoacetic acid, lactic acid, etc., are eliminated by the kidneys. Usually in circulation itself these strong acids are buffered by buffers in blood like $NaHCO_3$.

$$H_2SO_4 + 2NaHCO_3 \rightarrow Na_2SO_4 + 2CO_2 + 2H_2O$$
$$HCl + NaHCO_3 \rightarrow NaCl + CO_2 + H_2O$$

The kidneys must excrete these acid salts to maintain normal body pH. Also, the HCO_3^- that has been used up for buffering H⁺ should be replaced. This replacement occurs by the formation of new HCO_3^- in the kidney. These functions are effectively performed by kidneys.

Renal Handling of H⁺

H⁺ is secreted into the tubular fluid in the proximal tubule, the thick ascending limb and the collecting duct by three mechanisms: (1) H⁺-Na⁺ antiport, (2) H⁺-K⁺ antiport and (3) primary active H⁺ transport. In the proximal tubules the Na⁺-H⁺ exchanger secretes H⁺ into the tubular lumen in exchange for Na⁺. In the distal tubules and collecting ducts, H⁺ secretion is relatively independent of Na⁺ in the tubular lumen. Here, most H⁺ is secreted by an ATP-driven proton pump. Aldosterone acts on this pump to increase distal H⁺ secretion. Some of the H⁺ is secreted by H⁺-K⁺ ATPase where H⁺ is secreted in exchange for K⁺ (**Table 55.4**).

H⁺ secretion makes the tubular fluid more acidic. A low blood pH, as occurs in acidosis increases H⁺ secretion. The H⁺ secreted into the tubule is removed by the urinary buffers present in the tubular fluid so that more acid can be secreted into the tubular lumen.

The H⁺ is produced in the tubular cell through the following reaction:

$$CO_2 + H_2O \xleftrightarrow{\text{Carbonic anhydrase}} H_2CO_3 \longleftrightarrow H^+ + HCO_3^-$$

The HCO_3^- leaves the basolateral membrane of the tubular cell through a HCO_3^--Cl^- antiporter into the interstitium from where it is absorbed into the peritubular capillaries. The reabsorption of HCO_3^- is very important for acid-base balance, as loss of a single HCO_3^- in the urine would be equivalent of adding one H⁺ to the blood. Causes of acidosis are given in (**Table 55.5**).

Table 55.4: Factors affecting H⁺ secretion.

	Increased H⁺ secretion	Decreased H⁺ secretion
1.	Decrease in intracellular pH	Increase in intracellular pH
2.	Increase in intracellular PCO_2	Decrease in intracellular PCO_2
3.	Increase in the filtered load of HCO_3^-	Decrease in the filtered load of HCO_3^-
4.	Decrease in principal extracellular fluid (ECF) volume	Increase in ECF volume
5.	Increase in aldosterone	Decrease in aldosterone
6.	Hypokalemia	Hyperkalemia
7.	Increase in carbonic anhydrase	Carbonic anhydrase inhibitors like acetazolamide (Diamox)

Table 55.5: Causes of acidosis.

Metabolic acidosis	Respiratory acidosis
- Diabetic ketoacidosis - Diarrhea (loss of alkali) - Renal failure - Lactic acidosis - Aspirin in large doses - Starvation	- Hypoventilation (depression of respiratory center) - Pulmonary edema

Urinary Buffers

There are three mechanisms by which H^+ in the tubular fluid is buffered by the kidney:
1. HCO_3^- buffer system
2. HPO_4^{2-} buffer system
3. NH_3 mechanism

HCO_3^- Buffer System

The HCO_3^- buffer system differs from other buffer systems because it is regulated by both lungs and kidneys, and hence is the most important buffer system. A decrease in the plasma level of HCO_3^- is called **metabolic acidosis**, whereas an increase in plasma PCO_2 is termed **respiratory acidosis**. The lungs control changes in PCO_2 whereas kidneys are responsible for regulating the concentration of HCO_3^- in plasma.

HCO_3^- buffer system operates mainly in the **proximal tubule**. The concentration of HCO_3^- in the glomerular filtrate is 24–26 mEq/L. Therefore, in the proximal tubule most of the secreted H^+ reacts with HCO_3^-. The epithelial cells secrete H^+ into the tubular lumen in exchange for Na^+ by secondary active transport mechanism. H^+ is formed within the cell by the following reaction:

$$H_2O + CO_2 \xleftrightarrow{\text{Carbonic anhydrase}} H_2CO_3$$
$$H_2CO_3 \longleftrightarrow HCO_3^- + H^+$$

Carbonic anhydrase is present in the cytoplasm and brush border of proximal tubular epithelium and this facilitates the formation of H_2CO_3 in the tubular cell. The H^+ is secreted into the tubular lumen and HCO_3^- enters circulation. The H^+ in the lumen reacts with HCO_3^- present in the tubular fluid to form H_2CO_3, which splits to form H_2O and CO_2. Thus, when one HCO_3^- is lost through urine, one HCO_3^- enters circulation even though it is not the same HCO_3 that is present in the tubular fluid. About 4,500 mEq of HCO_3^- are filtered and reabsorbed each day.

When there is excess H^+ formation in the renal tubules, excess of HCO_3^- will enter the plasma. The excess of HCO_3^- that enters the plasma is called **new HCO_3^-**. So, the blood leaving the kidney through the renal vein has a higher concentration of HCO_3^- than blood entering the kidney through the renal artery.

Normal plasma HCO_3^- level is 24–26 mEq/L. The plasma HCO_3^- level cannot go above a value of 28 mEq/L. Normally, all the H^+ present in the proximal tubule is buffered by HCO_3^-. When the plasma HCO_3^- level goes above 28 mEq/L, which is the renal threshold for HCO_3^-, HCO_3^- appears in urine and urine becomes alkaline.

The pH of PCT cannot go below 6.9 and the pH of distal tubule cannot go below 4.5. This is called **limiting pH of urine**. So, the minimum pH of urine is approximately 4.5. Once limiting pH is reached, further secretion of H^+ stops if the H^+ in the lumen is not removed. If the excess H^+ in urine reacts with HCO_3^-, the plasma HCO_3^- level will go above 28 mEq/L. To prevent this, excess H^+ in the tubular fluid reacts with HPO_4^{2-} and NH_3. This permits more acid to be secreted into the tubular lumen and the plasma pH will be brought back to normal. Also, most of the filtered HCO_3^- will be absorbed when the filtrate reaches the collecting duct.

In the PCT, H^+ is secreted by two mechanisms:
1. By secondary active transport utilizing Na^+-H^+ antiporter.
2. By active transport using H^+ATPase **(Fig. 55.7)**.

In the collecting duct, H^+ secretion occurs via the intercalated cells with the help of H^+-K^+ ATPase, which secretes one H^+ in exchange for one K^+ which is reabsorbed.

Phosphate Buffer System

The kidney cannot eliminate the 70 mmol of non-volatile acids produced per day by excreting them in urine. This is because the lowest urinary pH possible is approximately 4.5. This is overcome by binding the H^+ to buffers that the kidney filter and synthesize. The kidney filters buffers like phosphate, urate and creatinine. Phosphate is the most important non-volatile filtered buffer. The other major urinary buffer is NH_3/NH_4^+ which the tubular cell synthesizes. On an average diet, approximately 40% of non-volatile acids produced by the metabolic reactions are excreted as **titrable acid** by the phosphate system. The PO_4 excreted through urine is derived from the diet. Main site of action of this buffer system is the **distal tubules and collecting duct**. This is because it is here that the phosphate that escapes proximal reabsorption is greatly concentrated by the reabsorption of water. The distal tubule contains alkaline phosphate which forms acid PO_4 in combination with H^+. Urine is normally acidic due to the presence of acid PO_4 **(Fig. 55.7)**.

$$H^+ + HPO_4^{2-} \rightarrow H_2PO_4^-$$

Excreted acid PO_4 is known as **titrable acidity**. Other acids contributing to titrable acidity are β-OH butyric acid, uric acid, creatinine, acetoacetic acid, and lactic acid. Titrable acidity is the amount of alkali needed to raise the pH of urine to 7.4. The amount of alkali added is equal to the H^+ titrated by the HPO_4^{2-} buffer system. Titrable acidity does not account for HCO_3^- and NH_3 buffer system. Thus titrable acidity measures only a fraction of the acid secreted, since it does not account for the H_2CO_3 that has been converted to H_2O and CO_2.

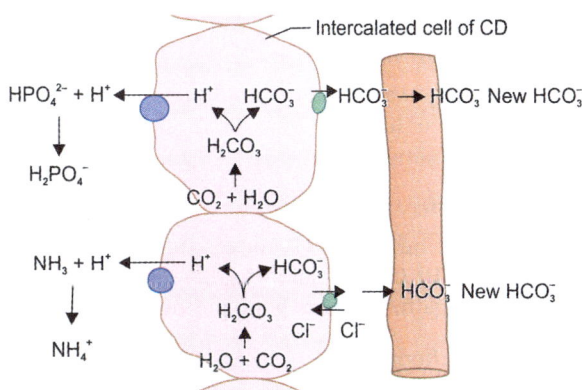

Fig. 55.7: Formation of new HCO_3^- by phosphate and ammonia buffer systems.

NH₃ Mechanism

NH$_3$ is produced in the kidneys by the metabolism of amino acid glutamine. This mechanism operates both in the proximal tubule and in the distal tubules. 60% of non-volatile acid is excreted as NH$_4^+$.

$$\text{Glutamine} \xrightarrow{\text{Glutaminase}} \text{Glutamate} + NH_4^+$$

$$\text{Glutamate} \xrightarrow{\text{Glutamate dehydrogenase}} \alpha\text{-ketoglutarate} + NH_4^+$$

Since NH$_3$ is lipid soluble, it freely passes through the tubular membrane. In the tubular fluid, it reacts with H$^+$ to form NH$_4^+$. NH$_4^+$ does not enter the cell since it is polarized; instead, it forms NH$_4$Cl or (NH$_4$)$_2$SO$_4$ and is excreted through urine. Trapping of NH$_4^+$ in the tubular lumen is called **non-ionic diffusion or diffusion trapping**. The process by which NH$_3$ is secreted into urine and then changed to NH$^+$, maintaining the concentration gradient for the diffusion of more NH$_3$ is called non-ionic diffusion (**Fig. 55.7**). In acidosis, there is increased formation of NH$_4^+$ in urine. Since the amount of phosphate buffer filtered at the glomerulus cannot be increased, urinary excretion of acid via the phosphate buffer system is limited. The production of NH$_4^+$ by the renal tubules is the only way the kidneys can remove the excess of non-volatile acid produced in the body. Of the new HCO$_3^-$ that the kidney generates, 60% is due to NH$_4^+$ excretion.

New HCO$_3^-$ means the HCO$_3^-$ that is generated in the kidney by forming titrable acids which include H$^+$ bound to phosphate, creatinine and urate; and H$^+$ bound to NH$_3$.

Net urinary acid excretion = (H$^+$ bound to phosphate, creatinine, urate in urine + H$^+$ bound to NH$_3$) – Excretion of filtered HCO$_3^-$.

In case of alkalosis, as in conditions like ingesting alkali or by vomiting (loss of HCl or gain in NaHCO$_3$), the kidney responds by decreasing net acid excretion that is, by reducing the excretion rate of titrable acid and NH$_4^+$. This leads to a decrease in the production of new HCO$_3^-$. In extreme alkalosis, the excretion of urinary HCO$_3^-$ also increases and net acid excretion becomes negative. In this case, the amount of HCO$_3^-$ in the renal vein will be less than the HCO$_3^-$ in the renal arteries.

Compensatory Responses of the Body in Acid-base Disturbances

- Intracellular and extracellular buffering
- Changes in ventilation
- Renal adjustments

Intracellular Buffering

In intracellular buffering, H$^+$ moves into the cell and it combines with HCO$_3^-$, PO$_4$ and histidine group of proteins. Reduced hemoglobin is a very good proton acceptor.

Extracellular Buffering

The HCO$_3^-$ buffer system is the principal ECF buffer. Approximately 70 mmol of non-volatile acid is produced per day in the body. It is removed in three steps:

1. HCO$_3^-$ neutralizes most of the H$^+$ load in the ECF. As a result HCO$_3^-$ decreases by an amount that is equal to the H$^+$ it consumes.

$$H^+ + HCO_3^- \rightarrow H_2CO_3 \rightarrow H_2O + CO_2$$

Non-HCO$_3^-$ buffers (B$^-$) in the blood neutralize most of the remaining H$^+$ in the blood. Thus non-HCO$_3^-$ buffer concentration also decrease in the blood by an amount equal to the H$^+$ it consumes. Plasma proteins also have a role in buffering excess H$^+$ in the ECF.

$$B^- + H^+ \rightarrow BH$$

2. The lungs excrete the CO$_2$ formed by the HCO$_3^-$ buffers.
3. The kidneys secrete about 4,390 mmol of H$^+$ per day into the renal tubular lumen. Kidney uses 98% of this H$^+$ to replace filtered HCO$_3^-$. The rest of the total secreted H$^+$, i.e., 70 mmol/day are used to generate new HCO$_3^-$ by the kidney. The kidneys create new HCO$_3^-$ at a rate equal to the rate of H$^+$ production to regenerate the HCO$_3^-$ and B$^-$ used up by the H$^+$ in the ECF. This is accomplished by the phosphate and ammonia buffer systems in the kidney. Thus 70 mmol of HCO$_3^-$ leaves the renal veins in excess to that which is present in the renal arteries. This excess HCO$_3^-$ forms the **new HCO$_3^-$**. Most of this new HCO$_3^-$ replenishes the HCO$_3^-$ consumed during the neutralization of non-volatile acids in the ECF. Thus, the ECF HCO$_3^-$ concentration is maintained at 24–26 mmol. The rest of the new HCO$_3^-$ regenerates the non-HCO$_3^-$ buffers.

$$HCO_3^- + BH \rightarrow B^- + CO_2 + H_2O$$

The lungs excrete this CO$_2$. Thus by generating new HCO$_3^-$ the kidneys maintain constant levels of both HCO$_3^-$ and non-HCO$_3^-$ buffers in the ECF.

Changes in Ventilation

Changes in PCO$_2$ alter blood pH. When PCO$_2$ increases, it leads to respiratory acidosis. Chemoreceptors in the medulla sense changes in PCO$_2$ and H$^+$ concentration, and alter the rate of respiration. In metabolic acidosis, there is increase in H$^+$ concentration which increases ventilation and brings back the PCO$_2$ to normal. In diabetic ketosis where there is metabolic acidosis, the patient develops deep and rapid breathing known as **Kussmaul breathing**.

Renal Mechanism

When there is acidosis, the kidneys excrete more acid mainly by the increased synthesis and excretion of NH$^+$. The secretion of H$^+$ by the nephron is stimulated and more of new HCO$_3^-$ is generated because of increased excretion of H$^+$. This **new HCO$_3^-$** increases the plasma HCO$_3^-$ level, thereby increasing the buffering capacity of blood. Of the new HCO$_3^-$ that the kidney generates, 60% is due to NH$_4^+$ excretion.

Opposite of the above mechanisms occurs in alkalosis.

Effects of Disturbances in pH in the Body

- Acidosis produce hyperventilation called Kussmaul breathing by stimulating central chemoreceptors. Alkalosis depresses ventilation.

- Acidosis shifts oxygen dissociation curve to the right and alkalosis shifts oxygen hemoglobin dissociation curve (ODC) to the left.
- Acidosis depresses cardiac contractility by a direct effect.
- Acidosis causes vasodilatation of peripheral vessels due to a direct effect on smooth muscles.
- Serum potassium levels rise in acidosis. In metabolic alkalosis there is hypokalemia. Acidosis increases plasma ionic calcium levels. Alkalosis decreases plasma Ca^{2+} leading to tetany as a result of neuronal hyperexcitability.
- Acidosis produces CNS depression resulting in lethargy, stupor and even coma. Alkalosis increases neuronal excitability manifested as mental confusion, paresthesia and seizures.

Anion Gap

According to the law of neutrality, the concentration of cations and anions in plasma must be equal. Therefore, there is no real anion gap in the plasma. Only certain anions and cations are routinely measured in the laboratory. The cation normally measured is Na^+ and the anions measured are HCO_3^- and Cl^-. Unmeasured anions are plasma proteins (mainly albumin), phosphates, sulphates and other organic anions. The important unmeasured cations include Ca^{2+}, Mg^{2+} and K^+. Usually, the unmeasured anions exceed the unmeasured cations in the plasma. Difference between concentration of cations (other than Na^+) and the concentration of anions (other than Cl^- and HCO_3^-) in the plasma gives the **anion gap (Fig. 55.8)**. Normal value is 12 mEq/L. Plasma albumin accounts for most of the anion gap. The plasma anion gap is used mainly in diagnosing different causes of metabolic acidosis. In normochloremic metabolic acidosis anion gap will be increased whereas in hyperchloremic metabolic acidosis, the anion gap will be normal. Measurement of anion gap is of some value in the differential diagnosis of metabolic acidosis.

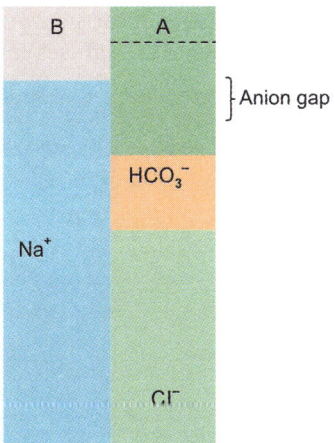

Fig. 55.8: Concept of anion gap: (A) Unmeasured anions like plasma protein (mainly albumin), inorganic phosphate, sulfates and ions of inorganic acids; (B) Minor cations like K^+, Ca^{2+} and Mg^{2+}. Difference between A and B gives anion gap (the portion below the dashed line in A).

Anion gap is increased in:
- Conditions of decreased plasma K^+, Ca^{2+} or Mg^{2+}.
- Increased concentration of plasma proteins.
- Metabolic acidosis due to accumulation of lactic acid, acetoacetic acid and other organic acids.
- In renal failure, the anion gap increases because sulfates, phosphates and organic acid anions are not excreted efficiently.

Anion gap is decreased in:
- Increase in cations.
- Decrease in plasma proteins.

Abnormalities of Renal Function

Proteinuria or Albuminuria

The amount of protein excreted through urine is very large in this condition and is typical of **nephrotic syndrome**. The liver is not able to synthesize all the protein that is lost through urine. This leads to hypoproteinemia and a reduction in blood oncotic pressure. The plasma volume falls and fluid accumulates in the tissues leading to edema.

In certain normal individuals, proteinuria is seen when they stand for a long time, which is referred to as **orthostatic albuminuria**. This is not a pathological condition and the exact cause is not known.

Polyuria and Nocturia

When the concentrating capacity of kidney is reduced in renal diseases, the urine becomes dilute and flow rate increases. The urine output becomes more than 3 L/day and urine osmolarity <250 mOsm/L. This condition is **polyuria**. Waking up at night frequently to void urine is **nocturia**.

Oliguria and Anuria

Decrease in urine volume to less than 500 mL/day is oliguria and is seen in advanced renal failure. When the kidneys stop functioning, it is called anuria. In anuria, urine volume will be less than 50 mL/day.

Uremia and Azotemia

Increase in plasma urea level above normal is **uremia**. Retention of nitrogenous waste products like urea, creatinine, etc., due to reduction in GFR is referred to as **azotemia**. It is usually seen in renal failure. The symptoms of azotemia include nausea, vomiting, loss of appetite, confusion, disorientation, convulsions and even coma. In chronic renal failure, where there is progressive and irreversible loss of nephron function, hemodialysis followed by renal transplantation is the treatment.

Acidosis

Causes of Acidosis

A plasma pH of 7.35 and less indicates acidosis.

In chronic renal failure, the acidic products of metabolism accumulate in the blood. NH_4^+ production and excretion are impaired leading to increased concentration of H^+ in blood leading to acidosis.

Hematuria

Presence of plenty of red blood cells in urine due to damage to the glomerular capillaries is called hematuria. Usually, it is a feature of **glomerulonephritis**. Other causes include renal stones, renal tuberculosis, trauma to the kidney, etc. Hematuria with **pyuria** (presence of pus cells in urine) and **bacteruria** is typical of infection of the urinary tract.

Dialysis

> **PY7.7:** Describe artificial kidney, dialysis and renal transplantation.

Removal of waste materials and toxic substances that accumulate in the blood in renal failure and restoration of normal volume and composition of body fluids is referred to as **dialysis**. It is a process of separating the soluble crystalloids from the colloid in a mixture, by means of a semipermeable membrane that is highly permeable to most solutes but impermeable to plasma proteins and blood cells.

Indications

Indications for dialysis are acute and chronic renal failure, snake bite, poisoning, drug overdose, etc. Early dialysis along with conservative medical management is the treatment of choice in **acute renal failure** because the damage to the kidney is reversible. Causes of acute renal failure are acute nephritis, poisoning with lead, mercury, etc., circulatory shock, severe transfusion reactions, ureteric obstruction, etc.

The causes of **chronic renal failure** are chronic nephritis, severe hypertension, carcinoma of kidney, etc. In chronic renal failure, the damage to the kidney is irreversible in nature, and so, **renal transplantation** is the treatment of choice. Body homeostasis is maintained by dialysis till transplantation is done. Chronic renal failure is diagnosed by ultrasound scan (USS) in which the kidney appears small and confirmed by renal biopsy.

Serum creatinine is the most sensitive index to measure the need for dialysis. Dialysis becomes a must when the serum creatinine level is **more than 6 mg%**.

Types of Dialysis

- Hemodialysis
- Peritoneal dialysis

Dialysis is indicated when signs and symptoms of azotemia develop due to renal shutdown.

Hemodialysis

Principle

Dialysis is based on the principle of diffusion equilibrium. Diffusion of substances across a semipermeable membrane with blood of the patient on one side and a cleansing solution called **dialysate** on the other side of the membrane is the principle. The waste materials from the blood diffuse into the dialysate while desirable components from the dialysate diffuse into the blood across the membrane. The dialysate or the dialysing fluid is a solution with the ionic composition similar or lower than that of normal plasma (Table 55.6). Thus, by dialysis, patients with renal failure can be maintained in a relatively healthy state.

Procedure

The apparatus used is called **artificial kidney or dialyzer**. The dialyzer usually used is the hollow fiber or capillary dialyzer in which the membrane material is spun into fine capillaries packed into bundles with blood flowing through the capillaries of the dialyzer while dialysate circulates outside the fibers. The flow of dialysate is counter current to blood flow (Fig. 55.9). The composition of dialysate is almost similar to normal plasma and its composition can be varied depending on the need. The capillaries are made of polyacryl nitrite, polymethylmethacrylate, etc., which are cellulose derivatives and are porous.

Normally, patients require 9–12 hours of dialysis/week, equally divided into several sessions. Before hemodialysis, an **arteriovenous (AV) fistula** is created in the arm by surgically anastomosing a superficial artery and a nearby vein. Usual site for AV fistula is the forearm 3–5 cm proximal to the wrist and the connection is made between the radial artery and the cephalic vein. This is because blood from a vein is not sufficient to maintain the pressure necessary for dialysis since a flow of 300–400 mL/min to the dialyzer is necessary. It is difficult to puncture a large artery repeatedly. Blood flows from the arterial side into the dialysis tubing and the purified blood flows back into the body through the vein of fistula. Blood is **heparinized** before entering the artificial kidney and is deheparinized using **protamine** before entering the body.

Complications of hemodialysis include septicemia with *Staphylococcus aureus*, embolization, and complications of heparinization like intracranial hemorrhage, hypotension and psychiatric problems like depression.

Peritoneal Dialysis

An indwelling catheter is introduced into the peritoneal cavity and 2 liters of dialysate is introduced into the peritoneal cavity. The dialysate remains in the peritoneal cavity and waste products and excess ECF diffuses into the dialysis

Table 55.6: Composition of extracellular fluid (ECF) and dialysate.

Substance	ECF (mmol/L)	Dialysate
Sodium	152	140–145
Potassium	4.5	1–3
Calcium	1.5	1.5
Magnesium	0.5	0.5
Chloride	109	100–110
Bicarbonate	32–38	32–38
Glucose	5	0–10

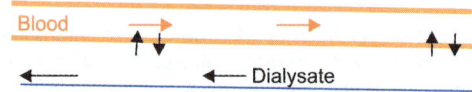

Fig. 55.9: Counter current flow of blood and dialysate through the artificial kidney.

solution. Every 4–6 hours empty the peritoneal cavity and replace the dialysate. Here the peritoneal membrane acts as the dialysis membrane.

Advantages of Peritoneal Dialysis
- Avoidance of heparinization and vascular surgery.
- Very useful in patients with severe cardiac insufficiency and diabetic retinopathy.
- The procedure can be performed at home.

Complication in peritoneal dialysis is peritonitis.
There are limitations in dialysis like:
- Dialysis cannot maintain normal homeostasis as kidney does
- Anemia is a rule in dialysis because of deficiency of erythropoietin which is produced by the kidney.

Renal Transplantation

In renal transplantation, a healthy kidney from a live or dead (deceased) donor is surgically placed in a person whose kidneys are not functioning properly due to irreversible renal damage (end stage renal disease where kidneys have lost 90% of their function). Renal transplantation is the most effective treatment in advanced chronic renal failure. The donor should be of the same blood group and should have compatibility for human leukocyte antigens (HLA).

Procedure
The existing kidneys of the patient are not removed. The donor kidney is usually placed in the iliac fossa. Renal artery of the donor kidney is connected to the external iliac artery and the renal vein connected to the external iliac vein of the recipient. The donor ureter is anastomosed to the urinary bladder of the recipient. Complications include hemorrhage, infection, thrombosis, myocardial infarction, rejection of the kidney received, etc. Success rate is more than 90%.

After transplantation, the patient should be given azathioprine, cyclosporine and glucocorticoids as immunosuppressive drugs to prevent rejection of the transplant. Erythropoietin is also administered to prevent anemia.

Rejection may be immediate (acute) or delayed (chronic) in which case rejection occurs after several years.

Hormones Acting on the Kidney
The main hormones acting on the kidney are ADH, angiotensin, aldosterone, ANP, prostaglandins, parathyroid hormone (PTH), calcitonin, calcitriol, dopamine, endothelins, leukotrienes and nitric oxide (NO).

ADH
In the kidney, ADH acts through V1 receptors and produce antidiuresis by:
- Increasing the permeability of the collecting duct to water (by inserting aquaporins into the luminal membrane) and urea
- Stimulating Na^+-K^+-$2Cl^-$ cotransport in the thick ascending limb.

Angiotensin II
Sources of Angiotensin II
- Angiotensin II in systemic circulation originating from the pulmonary circulation
- Renal arterioles locally
- Proximal tubular cells of kidney secrete angiotensin II into the tubular lumen.

The principal factor controlling blood angiotensin II levels is renin released from the granular cells of juxtaglomerular apparatus. **Renin** secreted by the juxtaglomerular cells of kidney enters circulation and acts on an a_2 globulin called **angiotensinogen** (renin substrate) synthesized in the liver and convert it into **angiotensin I** which is not physiologically active. Renin is a protease that cleaves a peptide bond near the C terminus of angiotensinogen, releasing the decapeptide angiotensin I. Angiotensin I is converted to the **angiotensin II** by **ACE** produced by the lungs. ACE removes the two C-terminal amino acids from angiotensin I to form the physiologically active octapeptide angiotensin II. ACE is present on the luminal surface of vascular endothelia throughout the body but it is abundantly present in the endothelium- rich lungs. ACE present in the endothelial cells of afferent and efferent arterioles of kidney can produce enough angiotensin II to exert local vascular effects. Proximal tubular cells also contain renin and ACE and are able to secrete angiotensin II into the tubular lumen. 20% of angiotensin I is converted to angiotensin II in the kidney by ACE in kidney. Angiotensin receptors are present in the afferent and efferent arterioles, proximal tubules and mesangial cells. Half-life of angiotensin II in circulation is 1–2 minutes.

Aminopeptidases present in the circulation further cleave angiotensin II to the heptapeptide **angiotensin III** by removing the aspartic acid residue from the amino terminal of angiotensin II. Angiotensin III has about 100% of the aldosterone stimulating activity of angiotensin II.

Renal Effects of Angiotensin II
- Angiotensin II constricts both afferent and efferent arterioles leading to a reduction in renal blood flow and GFR, however efferent arterioles are more sensitive to it. The reduction in GFR is less when compared to the reduction in RBF. So there is an increase in the filtration fraction which is given by the ratio of GFR and renal blood flow. Increase in the filtration fraction reduces the hydrostatic pressure and increases the colloid osmotic pressure (due to increase in the protein concentration) in the peritubular capillaries. This increases the uptake of solutes and fluid from the peritubular interstitium into the peritubular capillaries. This in turn enhances the reabsorption of Na^+ and fluid by the proximal tubule.
- Angiotensin II causes mesangial cell hypertrophy and an increase in the extracellular matrix production by mesangial cells. It also causes contraction of mesangial cells with a resultant decrease in GFR. Angiotensin II has been implicated in the cause for diabetic nephropathy.

- It increases reabsorption of Na$^+$ and HCO$_3^-$ by a direct action on proximal tubules.
- It directly stimulates aldosterone release from the glomerulosa cells in the adrenal cortex and aldosterone in turn increases the reabsorption of sodium and water from the distal nephron
- Angiotensin II act on the brain to increase ACTH release. ACTH acts on adrenal cortex to increase the release of aldosterone
- It acts on the hypothalamus and increases the sensation of thirst and stimulates the secretion of AVP. Both of these increase total-body free water.
- It enhances Na$^+$-H$^+$ exchange in the renal tubules and thus promotes Na$^+$ reabsorption.

> Angiotensin converting enzyme inactivates bradykinin to form its inactive metabolites. Many patients treated with ACE inhibitors like **captopril** and **enalapril** complain of cough which is an annoying side effect of ACE inhibitors. This is because when ACE is inhibited, the increased tissue bradykinin produced will stimulate the bradykinin (B$_2$) receptors in the respiratory tract to produce cough.

Aldosterone

Reduction in the dietary intake of salt increases aldosterone secretion from the adrenal cortex. The actions of aldosterone are localized to distal tubular and collecting duct cells.

Its actions in the kidney are:

- It stimulates the basolateral Na$^+$-K$^+$ ATPase and thus decreases the intracellular Na$^+$ concentration.
- It increases the permeability of apical membrane to Na$^+$ and water.
- It increases the number of active ENaCs in the collecting duct of the nephron.
- Increases K$^+$ secretion into the tubular lumen.

Atrial Natriuretic Peptide

Atrial natriuretic peptide is present as granules in the atrial muscle cells. ANP is released in response to small changes in the plasma Na$^+$ concentration. The effects of ANP are antagonistic to those of angiotensin II.
- It produces natriuresis due to increase in GFR
- It causes relaxation of mesangial cells of the glomerulus which causes increase in GFR
- It acts on the medullary collecting duct to decrease the reabsorption of Na$^+$
- ANP increases intracellular cGMP in the tubular cell and this inhibits Na$^+$ transport via ENaC
- It decreases the secretion of renin, aldosterone and ADH.

Prostaglandins

Renal vascular smooth muscle cells, endothelial cells, mesangial cells and interstitial cells of the renal medulla synthesise locally acting prostaglandins from arachidonic acid via the cyclooxygenase pathway. Local intrarenal effects of prostaglandins prevent excessive constriction especially during increased sympathetic discharge or activation of renin-angiotensin system. In conditions of high angiotensin II levels, increased prostaglandin release is responsible for maintaining fairly constant blood flow and GFR. PGE2 causes natriuresis possibly by inhibiting Na$^+$-K$^+$ ATPase and possibly by increasing intracellular Ca^{2+} which in turn inhibits transport of Na$^+$ via ENaCs. Endothelin and interleukin-1 causes natriuresis by increasing formation of PGE$_2$.

Calcitonin, Calcitriol and Parathormone (Calcitropic Hormones)

- **Calcitonin** increases the urinary excretion of calcium and phosphate ions.
- **Calcitriol** stimulates reabsorption of phosphate in the proximal tubule and reabsorption of calcium in the distal tubule.
- **PTH** increases calcitriol formation by stimulating 1α-hydroxylase activity in the proximal tubular cells of the kidney. It also increases calcium reabsorption in the distal nephron. PTH increases phosphate excretion (phosphaturic effect) by decreasing the proximal tubular reabsorption of phosphate.

Dopamine

Dopamine receptors (D$_1$ receptors) are present in the renal blood vessels. Proximal tubule cells synthesize dopamine locally and they express dopamine receptors. Sympathetic fibers also release dopamine at their endings in the kidney. In the kidney dopamine produces vasodilation and inhibition of sodium reabsorption by the tubules. Stimulation of dopamine receptors inhibits apical Na$^+$-H$^+$ exchanger and basolateral Na$^+$-K$^+$ pump in the proximal tubule leading to natriuresis. These effects are opposite to the effects of norepinephrine.

Endothelins

Endothelium of renal cortical vessels and mesangial cells release endothelins in response to shear stress, epinephrine, angiotensin II, etc. They act locally to constrict smooth muscles of the renal vessels. They are seen to constrict both afferent and efferent arterioles resulting in a sharp decline in renal blood flow and GFR. These actions of these locally produced endothelins are limited to the kidney.

Leukotrienes

In response to inflammation, the renal vascular smooth muscle cells and glomeruli synthesize several leukotrienes from arachidonic acid via lipooxygenase pathway. They act locally as strong vasoconstrictors and reduce renal blood flow and GFR.

Nitric Oxide

The endothelial cells of the kidney contain NO synthase and it generates NO from L-arginine. NO has a strong smooth muscle relaxing effect and it produces renal vasodilation.

NO opposes the vasoconstrictor effects of epinephrine and angiotensin II. NO increases renal blood flow and GFR.

MULTIPLE CHOICE QUESTIONS

1. Dehydration increases the plasma concentration of all the following hormones, *except*:
   a. Vasopressin
   b. Angiotensin-II
   c. Norepinephrine
   d. Atrial natriuretic peptide

2. Calculate the clearance of the substance from the following data: Plasma concentration: 5 mg/dL; concentration in urine: 50 mg/dL; urine flow rate: 2 mL/min.
   a. 2 mL/min
   b. 20 mL/min
   c. 100 mL/min
   d. 200 mL/min

3. Aldosterone increases the retention of sodium from the urine by its action on:
   a. Renal collecting duct
   b. Proximal convoluted tubule
   c. Ascending limb of loop of Henle
   d. Distal convoluted tubule

4. The most important determinant of ECF volume is:
   a. Amount of Na^+ in the ECF
   b. Amount of K^+ in the ECF
   c. Protein content in the ECF
   d. Antidiuretic hormone level

5. Normal plasma osmolality is:
   a. 250 mOsm/L
   b. 285 mOsm/L
   c. 300 mOsm/L
   d. 270 mOsm/L

6. Vasopressin secretion increases when plasma osmolality is changed by:
   a. 10%
   b. 5%
   c. 15%
   d. 1%

7. The principal buffer in the interstitial fluid is:
   a. Carbonic acid
   b. Phosphoric acid
   c. Proteins
   d. Compounds containing histidine

8. All the following are features of metabolic alkalosis, *except*:
   a. Rise in plasma HCO_3^- level
   b. Rise in pH
   c. HCO_3^- appears in urine when its plasma level exceeds 28 mEq/L
   d. Fall in PCO_2 level

9. Carbonic anhydrase is found in high concentration in the following areas, *except*:
   a. Red blood cells
   b. Parietal cells of stomach
   c. Renal tubular cells
   d. Intracellular fluid

10. The major buffers in blood include all the following, *except*:
    a. $H_2CO_3 \leftrightarrow H^+ + HCO_3^-$
    b. $HProt \leftrightarrow H^+ + Prot$
    c. $H_2PO_4^- \leftrightarrow H^+ + HPO_4^{2-}$
    d. $HHb \leftrightarrow H^+ + Hb^-$

11. The normal plasma clearance of PAH in adult is:
    a. 70 mL
    b. 120 mL
    c. 250 mL
    d. 630 mL

12. If an excessive amount of water is consumed:
    a. Only 50% of water is absorbed from the gut
    b. The osmolality of interstitial fluid increases
    c. Stretch receptors in the right atrium are stimulated
    d. There will be increase in GFR which is the main means of disposing water

13. All the following regarding renal tubules are correct, *except*:
    a. Urea is reabsorbed
    b. PAH is secreted
    c. Glucose clearance is 180 mg/min
    d. H^+ is secreted

14. Calcium reabsorption in the renal tubule is increased by:
    a. Hypercalcemia
    b. Calcitriol
    c. Calcitonin
    d. Increased sodium reabsorption

15. The indicator of the ability of the kidney to concentrate urine is:
    a. Blood urea
    b. Specific gravity of urine
    c. Inulin clearance
    d. Urinary sodium

16. During starvation, urine becomes more acidic due to:
    a. Mobilization of lipids
    b. Increased protein breakdown
    c. Increased glucose utilization
    d. Concentration of urine

17. Furosemide is a:
    a. Osmotic diuretic
    b. Loop diuretic
    c. Proton pump inhibitor
    d. Carbonic anhydrase inhibitor

18. The main buffer of H^+ in the proximal tubular fluid is:
    a. Phosphates
    b. Bicarbonates
    c. Ammonia
    d. Protein

19. Glomerular filtration rate is increased by:
    a. Afferent arteriolar constriction
    b. Fall in systemic arterial pressure
    c. Efferent arteriolar constriction
    d. Presence of glucose in tubular fluid

20. Filtration fraction in the kidney is:
    a. 0.18
    b. 0.8
    c. 1.2
    d. 1.8

21. The term anuria is used when the urine volume per day is less than:
    a. 2 mL
    b. 5 mL
    c. 50 mL
    d. 100 mL

22. **When there is increase in ADH secretion, the tonicity of tubular fluid in PCT will be:**
    a. Hypertonic with plasma
    b. Isotonic with plasma
    c. Hypotonic with plasma
    d. Maximally hypertonic

23. **Action of ANP include all the following, *except*:**
    a. Increased aldosterone secretion
    b. Decreased renin secretion
    c. Increase in GFR
    d. Decrease in blood pressure

24. **The substance used to measure GFR is:**
    a. PAH
    b. Inulin
    c. Urea
    d. Evans blue

25. **In a normal healthy adult, with regard to renal tubules which of the following statement is incorrect?**
    a. Urea is reabsorbed
    b. PAH is secreted
    c. Glucose clearance is 180 mg/min
    d. Tubular maximum for glucose is 375 mg/min

ANSWERS

1. d	2. b	3. a	4. a	5. b
6. d	7. a	8. d	9. d	10. c
11. b	12. c	13. c	14. b	15. b
16. a	17. b	18. b	19. c	20. a
21. d	22. b	23. a	24. b	25. c

Lower Urinary Tract

CHAPTER 56

LEARNING OBJECTIVES
- Describe the innervation of urinary bladder with the help of a diagram
- Explain the physiology of micturition and its abnormalities
- Describe cystometry and discuss the normal cystometrogram

INTRODUCTION

Renal pelvis continues as the **ureter** which is a muscular tube about 30 cm long. Ureters help in the passage of urine from renal pelvis into the urinary bladder. The ureter lumen is lined by transitional epithelium. The ureters, one from each kidney, enter the **urinary bladder** on its posterior aspect just above the posterior urethra or bladder neck. The upper part of urinary bladder is called **body or fundus**, and the lower part forms the **bladder neck**. The ureters pass obliquely through the wall of the urinary bladder for some distance, thus forming a **functional valve**. Ureters open into the bladder lumen 1 to 2 cm above and lateral to the urethral orifice. The two ureteral orifices connected by a ridge of tissue and the urethral orifice forms the corners of a triangle (**bladder trigone**). In this part of urinary bladder, the mucosa is firmly bound to the underlying muscular layer and hence has a smooth appearance.

A flap like valve of mucous membrane covers each ureteral orifice. This anatomical valve along with the functional valve-like effect created by the ureter's oblique pathway through the bladder wall prevents reflux of urine back into the ureters during contraction of bladder.

Peristaltic contractions of the muscular wall of ureters propel urine towards the urinary bladder in **spurts** at frequencies of 2 to 6 per minute. During the peristaltic waves, the intraureteral hydrostatic pressure increases to 20 to 80 cm H_2O from a baseline pressure of 0 to 5 cm H_2O. Gravity also contributes to filling of the bladder. As the urinary bladder gets distended, the pressure in the bladder compresses the part of the ureter passing obliquely through the bladder. This functional valve prevents **reflux** of urine into the ureters when the intravesical volume and pressure increase. If this mechanism is not functioning, urinary infection, especially cystitis (infection of the bladder) can spread to the kidneys due to reflux of urine. This leads to the development of **glomerulonephritis** (inflammation of glomeruli) which, if left untreated, can lead on to chronic renal failure.

In males, posterior urethra is continued as the anterior urethra which extends through the penis and opens to the outside as external urethral orifice. In males, the **urethra** is about 15–20 cm long and in females it is only 4 cm long. Ureters and urinary bladder are lined by **transitional epithelium** which has the ability to distend. The smooth muscle of the urinary bladder is called **detrusor muscle**. The muscle fibers of the detrusor muscle interspersed with elastic tissue in the bladder neck form the **internal urethral sphincter**. The lower part of the urethra is covered by a layer of skeletal muscle fibers called **external urethral sphincter**.

INNERVATION OF THE BLADDER

PY7.6: Describe the innervation of urinary bladder, physiology of micturition and its abnormalities.

Urinary bladder is innervated by sympathetic, parasympathetic and somatic divisions of nervous system (**Fig. 56.1**).

Sympathetic Innervation

Sympathetic fibers arise from the lateral horn cells of **L1,2,3** segments of spinal cord and relay in the sympathetic ganglion. Postganglionic fibers travel through the **hypogastric nerve** and supply the body, internal sphincter and urethra. β-**adrenergic receptors** are present on the body of the bladder, and when the sympathetic fibers are stimulated it causes **relaxation of detrusor muscle**. Due to discharge from the sympathetics, the detrusor muscle is tonically inhibited during filling of the bladder. The trigonal area and the internal urethral sphincter contain α-**adrenergic receptors** which on stimulation cause contraction of muscles in these areas.

Recent view is that the sympathetic nerves to the bladder play no part in micturition. Filling of the bladder occurs due to the property of distensibility and plasticity of the smooth muscle of the bladder. In males, sympathetic stimulation causes contraction of internal urethral sphincter which

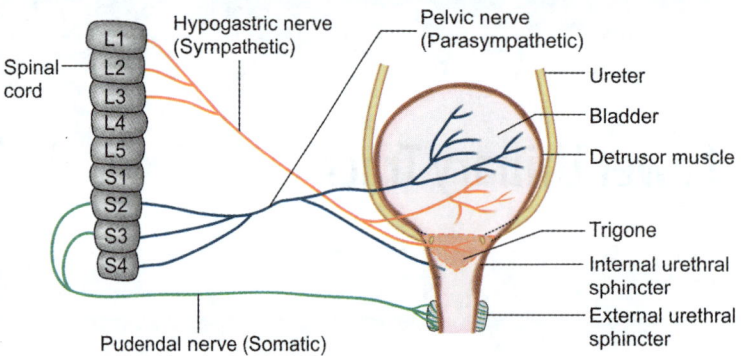

Fig. 56.1: Innervation of bladder.

prevents reflux of semen into the bladder during ejaculation. Sympathetic afferents carry pain sensation from the bladder.

Parasympathetic Innervation

Parasympathetic fibers originate from the intermediolateral horn cells in S2,3,4 segments of spinal cord, pass through **pelvic nerves** and relay in the parasympathetic ganglia present in the bladder wall. Postganglionic fibers innervate the fundus and neck of the urinary bladder. Pelvic nerves also carry sensory information of fullness, pain, etc., to the sacral segments forming the afferent limb of the spinal reflex of urination. These fibers also send input to higher centers. Parasympathetic stimulation causes **contraction** of the body of the bladder and relaxation of the internal urethral sphincter, resulting in urination.

Somatic Innervation

Somatic fibers to the bladder originates from the motor neurons coming from the sacral segments through the pudendal nerve (S2,3) and supply the **external urethral sphincter** which is a striated muscle and is under voluntary control.

■ MICTURITION

Micturition is the process of emptying the urinary bladder. Micturition reflex is an **automatic spinal reflex** which can be modified by higher centers in the brainstem and cerebral cortex.

Storage Phase

When the urinary bladder gets filled with urine, the stretch receptors on the bladder wall get stimulated. Sensory information from the stretch receptors reaches the spinal cord through the afferent fibers in the pelvic splanchnic nerve. There is a sense of urge to empty the bladder at a volume of approximately 150 mL. The sense of fullness occurs at 400 to 500 mL. Efferent impulses coming from the brain inhibit the parasympathetic neurons in the sacral spinal cord and thus inhibit contraction of detrusor muscle. Voluntary contraction of the external urinary sphincter also contributes to storage of urine.

Voiding Phase

Motor impulses from the spinal cord come through the parasympathetic efferent fibers in the pelvic nerve and cause contraction of the detrusor muscle and relaxation of the internal urethral sphincter. Urine flows into the posterior urethra. At the same time, sensory impulses also reach the cortex and the inhibition on the parasympathetic neurons innervating the detrusor muscle is removed and the bladder contracts. There will be a conscious desire to void urine. Voluntary relaxation of the external urethral sphincter causes flow of urine through the external urethral meatus to the outside. Voluntary urination also involves voluntary contraction of abdominal muscles, which further raises bladder pressure and thus contributes to complete bladder emptying. The complete emptying of bladder during micturition helps to keep the urinary system sterile.

Although micturition is basically an autonomic spinal cord reflex, it may be initiated voluntarily and can also be stopped voluntarily because of the cerebral cortical control to the external urethral sphincter.

Control of Micturition by Higher Centers

The spinal centers of micturition are influenced by higher centers of brainstem and cerebral cortex. Proprioceptive impulses like feeling of fullness and the desire to void urine pass through **fasciculus gracilis** into the cerebral cortex, and efferent fibers pass down to spinal cord through **pyramidal tract**. Cortical center can inhibit micturition once it has started and it can also initiate micturition even if there is no desire to void urine. This is mainly because of the voluntary control of external urethral sphincter and perineal muscles.

The first desire to void urine occurs when the intravesical volume is 150–250 mL. The impulses pass to the brainstem inhibitory center which causes inhibition of micturition. As the intravesical volume increases, the feeling of fullness increases, and there will be discomfort and pain. These impulses reach the cerebral cortex which in turn inhibits spinal centers. When conditions are favorable, cortical influences are lifted away and micturition is initiated.

The brainstem contains facilitatory centers and inhibitory centers for micturition. **Facilitatory center** is in the pons and it exerts a facilitatory effect on the spinal micturition center.

It causes contraction of detrusor and relaxation of external urethral sphincter. **Inhibitory center** is in the midbrain and it causes inhibition of spinal centers at the unconscious level.

The spinal micturition reflex starts by 5th month of intrauterine life and continues as a spinal reflex up to the age of three. Voluntary control is attained slowly by training the child.

Continence, Incontinence and Urinary Retention

In addition to collecting and voiding urine periodically, the urinary bladder can retain urine for some time. This is **continence**. This is due to the tone of the smooth muscle of internal urethral sphincter.

A lack of voluntary control over urination is called **incontinence**. It is normal in children less than 2 years of age. Incontinence in adults may be due to injury to spinal cord or to the spinal nerves innervating the bladder. Incontinence is also seen in states of unconsciousness.

Retention is the failure to void urine. It may be due to obstruction of urethra as in the case of enlarged prostate or due to lack of sensation to urinate. Urinary tract infection is a complication.

ABNORMALITIES OF BLADDER FUNCTION

Atonic Bladder or Tabetic Bladder (Afferent Limb Lesions)

De-afferentation due to tabes dorsalis (neurosyphilis) or due to injury to the afferent limb of the reflex arc of micturition reflex causes atonic bladder. Here only the sacral dorsal roots are interrupted. All reflex contractions of the bladder in response to stimulation of the stretch receptors are absent. Bladder becomes thin, hypotonic and **distended**. As a result, bladder cannot empty periodically. It gets filled to its maximum capacity so that urine overflows through urethra. This is called **overflow incontinence**. Some residual contractions of the bladder may be present because of the intrinsic contractile response of smooth muscle to stretch. Always residual volume of urine will be present.

Autonomous Bladder (Combined Afferent and Efferent Lesions)

Autonomous bladder also referred to as **decentralized bladder** is due to damage of both afferent and efferent nerves and is usually seen in tumors of cauda equina. Initially the bladder becomes flaccid and distended. Gradually detrusor muscles become active and small contraction waves appear so that urine is voided in drops. Later, bladder becomes **shrunken and hypertrophied**. Although small amounts of urine can be expelled, some amount of urine always remains in the bladder leading to infection.

Automatic Bladder (Spinal Cord Lesions)

Automatic bladder is seen in transection of spinal cord, e.g., paraplegia. Bladder becomes hypotonic, **distended** and there will be overflow incontinence during the initial stage of spinal shock. In this stage, if catheterization is done, with time, slowly the micturition reflex reappears, but there will be no voluntary control. These patients are trained to void urine by eliciting the mass reflex. Bladder capacity is often reduced and reflex hyperactivity may lead to the state of spastic neurogenic bladder.

Spastic Neurogenic Bladder

Lesion may be in the brainstem or spinal cord. All inhibitory signals are absent so that only facilitatory signals will be present. Urinary bladder becomes **hyperactive** and micturition becomes uncontrollable. Even then, residual urine volume will be there which leads to growth of bacteria. Catheterization of the bladder also predisposes to urinary tract infections.

Nocturnal Enuresis (Night Bedwetting)

Nocturnal enuresis may be due to poorly developed nervous control of the bladder. In children, it is normal but in adults it may be due to diseases of sacral spinal segments.

CYSTOMETRY

> **PY7.9:** Describe cystometry and discuss the normal cystometrogram.

Like other visceral smooth muscles, **detrusor muscle** has the property of **plasticity**. Because of this property, urine gets filled in the bladder without much increase in intravesical pressure up to a volume of 400 mL. Thus the urinary bladder can store urine without much discomfort.

The study of the relationship between intravesical pressure and volume is known as **cystometry**. A double lumen catheter is introduced into the bladder and the bladder is emptied completely. Then the urinary bladder is filled with 50 mL increments of water, simultaneously recording the intravesical pressure. A graph is plotted with volume on the X-axis and intravesical pressure on the Y-axis and the record obtained is called **cystometrogram (Fig. 56.2)**.

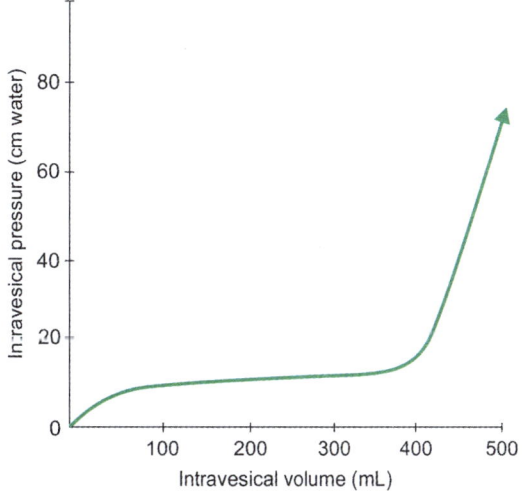

Fig. 56.2: Cystometrogram.

It is seen that initially there is a slight increase in pressure followed by a flat segment and a sharp rise in pressure when the intravesical volume exceeds 400 mL. The flat segment is a manifestation of **law of Laplace** which states that pressure is equal to twice the tension developed in the wall divided by radius in case of a hollow spherical organ ($P = 2T/R$). In the case of urinary bladder, there is simultaneous increase in radius as the tension increases.

The rise in tension is comparatively less because of the property of plasticity exhibited by the detrusor muscle. So, the pressure remains constant within the physiological limit.

DIURESIS AND DIURETICS

Diuresis

Increased excretion of water due to inhibition of water reabsorption by the kidney is called **diuresis**. There are two types of diuresis, water diuresis and solute or osmotic diuresis.

Water Diuresis

In **water diuresis**, there is an increase in water excretion but no increase in solute excretion. This may be due to excessive intake of water or inhibition of water reabsorption by the collecting tubules.

Osmotic Diuresis

The presence of large quantities of solutes that are not reabsorbed in the renal tubules causes an increase in urine volume called **osmotic diuresis**. In osmotic diuresis, solute and water excretion through the urine increases. This may be due to increased intake of solute or inhibition of solute reabsorption, both of which lead to an indirect inhibition of water reabsorption. Solutes that are not reabsorbed in the proximal tubules exert an appreciable osmotic effect and they hold water in the tubules decreasing reabsorption of Na^+ and water. The medullary hypertonicity is also decreased due to decreased reabsorption of Na^+ and Cl^-.

Commonly used osmotic diuretics are glycerine, mannitol, and related polysaccharides that are filtered but not reabsorbed. Since these substances are non-reabsorbable, they hold water in the tubule. The water retained in the tubule dilutes the tubular concentration of Na^+ and other electrolytes thereby reducing their reabsorption also. *Osmotic diuresis is seen in diabetes mellitus since the filtered load of glucose exceeds TmG and glucose remain in the tubules leading to polyuria.* Osmotic diuresis can also be produced by infusion of large amounts of NaCl and urea.

> In water diuresis, the amount of water reabsorbed in the proximal tubule is normal and the maximal urine flow that can be produced is 16 mL/min. In osmotic diuresis, increased urine flow is due to decreased water reabsorption in the proximal tubules and loop of Henle and very large urine flows can be produced.

Diuretics

Diuretics are substances that decrease reabsorption of water from the renal tubules and produce diuresis, thereby reducing

Table 56.1: Actions of the important diuretics.

Drug	Mechanism of action
Loop diuretics, e.g., Furosemide (Lasix), ethacrynic acid	Inhibit Na^+-K^+-$2Cl^-$ co-transporter of thick ascending limb of loop of Henle. May lead to hypokalemia
K^+ sparing diuretics, e.g., spironolactone (aldactone), triamterene, amiloride	Spironolactone inhibits the action of aldosterone and amiloride inhibits the action of ENaCs
Carbonic anhydrase inhibitors, e.g., acetazolamide (Diamox)	Inhibit H^+ secretion leading to increased excretion of Na^+ and K^+. Usually this drug is not advised
Osmotic diuretics, e.g., Mannitol, glycerin, etc.	Produce osmotic diuresis by increasing the concentration of osmotically active substances in urine
V_2 receptor antagonists	Inhibit the action of vasopressin on collecting duct. Used primarily for research purposes

blood volume. Diuretics are used to adjust the volume and composition of body fluids in the treatment of conditions like hypertension, congestive cardiac failure, edema, etc. The diuresis produced is almost always secondary to increased Na^+ loss in urine.

There are two groups of diuretics:
1. Naturally occurring diuretics:
   - Those which inhibit Na^+ reabsorption, e.g., caffeine in tea and coffee
   - Those which inhibit ADH secretion, e.g., alcohol, beer, wine, excess water, etc.
2. Drugs act on specific nephron segments and inhibit specific Na^+ transport mechanisms **(Table 56.1)**. Most diuretics have undesirable side effects like hypokalemia and pH disturbances.

MULTIPLE CHOICE QUESTIONS

1. **Stimulation of the parasympathetic nerve supplying the urinary bladder produces all the following effects, *except*:**
   a. Contraction of detrusor muscle
   b. Relaxation of trigone
   c. Relaxation of external urethral sphincter
   d. Relaxation of internal sphincter

2. **Stimulation of the following nerve supplying the urinary bladder causes retention of urine:**
   a. Parasympathetic efferent fibers
   b. Sympathetic efferent fibers
   c. Parasympathetic afferent fibers
   d. Pudendal nerve

3. **All the following features regarding automatic urinary bladder are correct, *except*:**
   a. It is due to damage of the afferent nerves of the reflex arc of micturition
   b. Bladder is distended
   c. Bladder is hypertonic
   d. Voluntary micturition is possible

4. **Pudendal nerve controls:**
   a. Detrusor muscle
   b. External urethral sphincter
   c. Internal urethral sphincter
   d. Trigone and detrusor muscle

5. **In infants micturition is:**
   a. Purely a spinal reflex
   b. Controlled by higher centers
   c. Voluntarily controlled
   d. Initiated when the urinary bladder volume is 200 mL

6. **All the following statements regarding micturition in a normal adult are correct, *except*:**
   a. Initiated when the bladder volume is about 150 mL
   b. Can be inhibited or facilitated by centers in the brain
   c. Sympathetic efferents to the bladder are reflexly inhibited during micturition
   d. Parasympathetic efferent nerve is not a component of micturition reflex

7. **Anatomical capacity of urinary bladder in adult is:**
   a. 200 mL
   b. 400 mL
   c. 600 mL
   d. 1000 mL

8. **Physiological capacity of the urinary bladder in adult is:**
   a. 200 mL
   b. 400 mL
   c. 600 mL
   d. 1000 mL

9. **Sensation of stretch of urinary bladder is transmitted through:**
   a. Sacral afferent parasympathetic nerves
   b. Afferent fibers in the sympathetic nerve
   c. Pudendal nerve
   d. Efferent sympathetic fibers

10. **Pain sensation from the urinary bladder is carried along:**
    a. Sacral afferent parasympathetic nerves
    b. Afferent fibers in the sympathetic nerve
    c. Pudendal nerve
    d. Efferent sympathetic fibers

11. **All the following statements regarding external urethral sphincter are correct, *except*:**
    a. It is a voluntary skeletal muscle
    b. Normally it remains tonically contracted
    c. It relaxes when the pudendal nerve is stimulated
    d. It prevents reflux of semen into the bladder during ejaculation

12. **A sudden sharp rise in pressure in the cystometrogram is obtained when the bladder volume is more than:**
    a. 400 mL
    b. 150 mL
    c. 600 mL
    d. 200 mL

ANSWERS

1. c   2. b   3. c   4. b   5. a
6. d   7. d   8. c   9. a   10. b
11. d 12. a

Renal Function Tests

CHAPTER 57

LEARNING OBJECTIVE
- Describe and discuss renal function tests

■ INTRODUCTION

PY7.8: Describe and discuss renal function tests.

Renal function tests (RFT) are mainly blood and urine tests done to evaluate renal function. It is also done in conditions like diabetes mellitus and hypertension which can cause damage to the kidneys. If there are problems like blood in urine, frequent urges to urinate, painful urination, generalized edema, etc. RFT is advised.

Renal function tests include the following:
- Urine analysis
- Blood examination
- Miscellaneous tests

■ URINE ANALYSIS

Volume
The normal volume of urine passed per day ranges from 500 to 2500 mL depending on fluid intake.
- Polyuria (output >2.5 L/day) occurs in diabetes insipidus and diabetes mellitus.
- Oliguria (output <400 mL/day) occurs in acute glomerulonephritis, hypotension and dehydration.
- Anuria (output <100 mL/day) occurs in lower urinary tract obstruction and in acute renal shut down.

Color
Normally urine is clear and straw colored.
- Cloudy urine is seen in urinary tract infection and in gout.
- Urine is yellow in bilirubinuria and red or brown in hematuria.

pH
Urine is normally slightly acidic except immediately after a meal due to post-prandial alkaline tide. The pH ranges from 4.6 to 8 normally.

Odor
On exposure to atmosphere, urea present in urine splits to form ammonia imparting the typical smell. Freshly voided urine has an aromatic smell.

Specific Gravity
Specific gravity of urine is 1.001–1.035. With maximum concentration, the specific gravity comes to 1.040. Specific gravity is inversely proportional to the quantity of urine. Specific gravity of urine depends on the concentration of electrolytes like Na^+, K^+, Cl^-, and urea.
- *Increase in specific gravity*
  - Decreased water intake
  - Diabetes mellitus (due to increased glucose in urine)
  - Albuminuria
  - Acute glomerulonephritis
- *Decrease in specific gravity*
  - Renal tubular damage
  - Deficiency of ADH

Composition
Urine is composed of 95% water and 5% solutes.
- *Solutes normally present in urine*:
  - Organic—urea, creatinine, uric acid, urobilinogen, mucin, enzymes and hormones; up to 150 mg of protein is excreted daily in urine. Of this, 15 mg is albumin.
  Inorganic—Na^+, K^+, Cl^-, Mg^{2+}, SO_4^{2-}, $H_2PO_4^-$, HPO_4^{2-}, PO_4^{3-}, NH_4^+, Ca^{2+}
- *Abnormal constituents of urine*: Albumin, glucose, red blood cells, white blood cells, ketone bodies, casts, microbes (bacteria, fungi, protozoa).

Microscopic Examination of Urine (Figs. 57.1A to C)
Freshly voided urine sample is centrifuged at a rate of 3000 revolutions/min for 15 minutes. The sediment obtained is examined under the high power of the microscope. Normal observation:

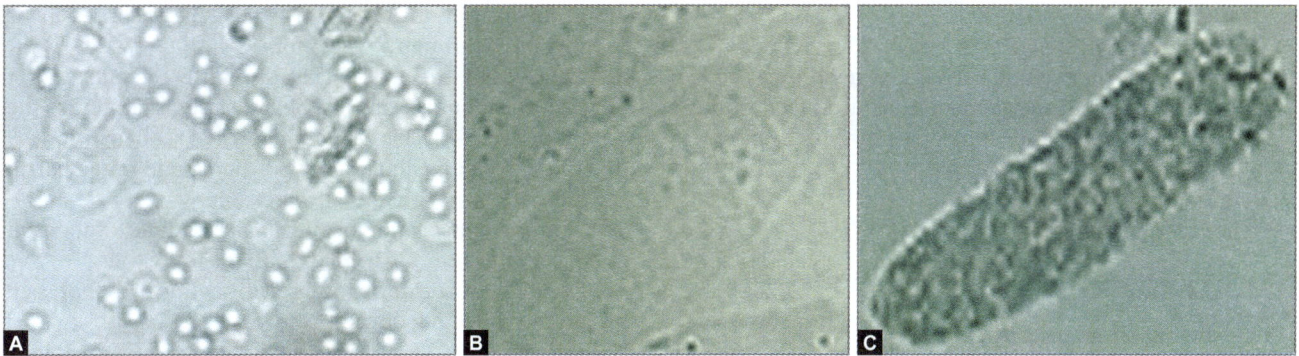

Figs. 57.1A to C: Microscopic examination of urine: (A) Red blood cells and epithelial cells; (B) Hyaline cast; (C) Granular cast.

- 1 to 2 pus cells/high power field (HPF)
- Hyaline cast which is formed of non-squamous epithelial cells shed from the epithelium of the DCT and collecting tubule. They are clear, colorless casts which are seen as small cylinders **(Fig. 57.1B).**

Abnormal Constituents

- Presence of granular casts which are hyaline casts embedded with red blood cells, leukocytes or degenerated glomerular cells in large numbers **(Fig. 57.1C).** Their presence indicates destruction of glomeruli or tubular cells.
- Presence of red blood cells, large number of pus cells (leukocytes), microbes, etc. is abnormal **(Fig. 57.1A).**

BLOOD EXAMINATION

- Blood urea—normal: 20–40 mg%. It is increased in azotemia.
- Serum creatinine—normal: 0.2–1.5 mg%. This is the most sensitive test to analyze renal function.
- Serum proteins—normal: 6–8 g/100 mL. In renal diseases with proteinuria, total proteins will be reduced. In nephrotic syndrome, serum albumin level decreases and globulin increases. There will be reversal of albumin/globulin ratio (normal ratio: 1.7:1).
- Serum uric acid level normally is 2–4 mg/dL
- Serum K$^+$ increases in oliguria and anuria.

MISCELLANEOUS TESTS

- *Concentration dilution tests:* Water is withheld for 24 hours, and the urine is collected and the specific gravity found out. Normally, it will be 1.020–1.025. Then, give 1 L of water to the subject. If specific gravity of the sample taken after some time is fixed at 1.010, it denotes impaired renal function. It indicates that the diluting and the concentrating functions of the kidney are lost.
- *Measurement of GFR and clearance tests:* Inulin clearance and creatinine clearance are used to measure glomerular filtration rate. Both will be reduced in impaired renal function and progressive reduction indicates chronic renal failure.
  Creatinine clearance
  Normal value: 90–130 mL/min.

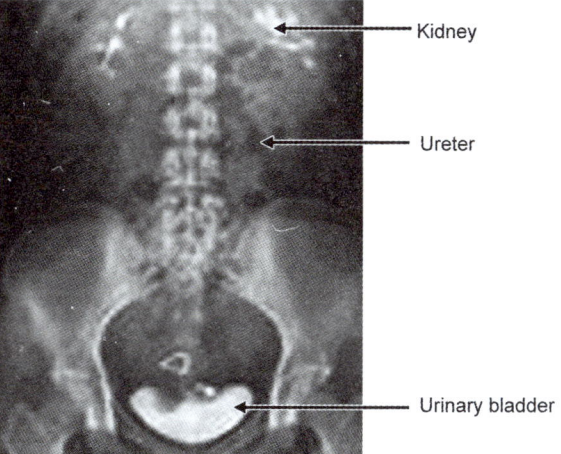

Fig. 57.2: Intravenous pyelography.

Creatinine clearance is decreased in old age and in impaired renal function.

- *Intravenous pyelography (IVP) (Fig. 57.2):* A radio-opaque dye **hypaque** 45% is given intravenously in a dose of 40–60 mL. X-ray pictures are taken at 5, 10, 15 and 25 min after administration of the dye. The dye appears in the calyx and pelvis normally 2 min after injection. In renal insufficiency, it may be delayed. Kidney, ureter and bladder can be visualized. Bladder emptying can also be visualized. IVP is also helpful in detecting stones, growth, etc. in the renal passage.
- *Ultrasound scan (USS):* The shape and size of kidney can be assessed. Small shrunken kidney is indicative of chronic renal failure. Hydronephrosis, polycystic kidney, stones, cysts, tumors of kidney, etc., can be detected by USS.
- *Cystoscopy:* By this technique, the interior of the bladder can be inspected. Dye **indocarmine** is given intravenously and see whether the dye appears at the ureteric orifice within 4–5 min, which is normal.
- *Retrograde pyelography*
- *Renal catheterization*
- *Cystography:*
  - Excretory cystography
  - Retrograde cystography
  - Micturating cystography

- *Urethroscopy*
- *Urethrography*
- *Renal biopsy:* The method used is **fine needle aspiration cytology** (FNAC). A special needle is introduced through the back of the body and biopsy specimen of the kidney is taken for histological examination.
- *Renal angiography*
- *Renal tomography*

MULTIPLE CHOICE QUESTIONS

1. **Normal blood urea level is:**
   a. 2–6 mg/dL
   b. 20–40 mg/dL
   c. 0.6–1.5 mg/dL
   d. 2–6 g/dL

2. **Normal serum creatinine level is about:**
   a. 2–5 mg/dL
   b. 20–40 mg/dL
   c. 0.6–1.5 mg/dL
   d. 2–5 g/dL

3. **Specific gravity of urine with maximum concentration is:**
   a. 1040
   b. 1001
   c. 1020
   d. 1060

ANSWERS

1. b   2. c   3. a

FILL IN THE BLANKS/GIVE THE NORMAL VALUE/NAME THE FOLLOWING

1. Percentage of erythropoietin produced by interstitial cells in the peritubular capillary beds of kidney: **85%**.
2. The stimulus for erythropoietin secretion is **hypoxia**.
3. Juxtaglomerular apparatus is formed by **macula densa of DCT, lacis cells** and **juxtaglomerular cells in the afferent arteriole**.
4. Three important hormones produced by the kidney - 1,25 dihydroxy cholecalciferol (calcitriol), renin and erythropoietin.
5. Renin is secreted by **juxtaglomerular cells** of juxtaglomerular apparatus.
6. Decreased delivery of Na^+ and Cl^- in the region of macula densa of DCT is associated with increased **renin** secretion.
7. Angiotensinogen is converted to angiotensin I by which hormone? Renin.
8. Aldosterone increases Na^+ and water reabsorption in the **DCT** and **cortical collecting duct**.
9. Aldosterone causes secretion of K^+ or H^+ in exchange for Na^+ in the distal nephron.
10. Aldosterone act by increasing the number of **epithelial sodium channels (ENaC)** primarily in the collecting duct.
11. Water reabsorption is mediated by **aquaporin-1** in the proximal convoluted tubule.
12. **ADH or arginine vasopressin** increases reabsorption of water in the collecting ducts by inserting more aquaporin-2 (water channels) on cell membrane.
13. Vasoconstriction effect of ADH or vasopressin is mediated through $\underline{V}_1$ receptor.
14. Antidiuretic effect of ADH is through $\underline{V}_2$ receptor.
15. Reabsorption of water in the collecting duct under the influence of ADH is called **facultative reabsorption**.
16. Thick ascending limb of loop of Henle and initial part of DCT are **impermeable** to water.
17. Sodium reabsorption occurs in all segments of nephron except **descending limb of loop of Henle**.
18. Osmolality of urine depends on the action of vasopressin on the collecting ducts.
19. Deficiency of vasopressin leads to diabetes insipidus characterized by **polyuria** and **polydipsia**.
20. 60% of filtered Na^+ is reabsorbed in the proximal tubule (by Na^+-H^+ exchange), 30% in the thick ascending limb (Na^+-$2Cl^-$-K^+ cotransport), 7% in the DCT (Na^+-Cl^- cotransport) and 3% in the collecting duct (via ENaC channels).
21. **Countercurrent flow** is one in which inflow runs parallel to, counter to and in close proximity to the outflow for some distance.
22. Loop of Henle establishes the medullary osmotic gradient and act as counter current multiplier.
23. Medullary osmotic gradient is maintained by vasa recta which act as countercurrent exchanger.
24. Acidification of renal tubular fluid occurs in the **collecting duct**.
25. **Macula densa** of juxtaglomerular apparatus senses the changes in NaCl concentration.
26. 80–90% of bicarbonate is reabsorbed in the proximal tubule.
27. 98% of total body potassium is present inside the cells and only 2% in the ECF.
28. The minimum volume of urine necessary to remove all waste products, with a normal diet, is 500 mL/day and is called **obligatory volume**.
29. When the urine output is <500 mL/day it is referred to as **oliguria**.
30. Normal GFR at rest: **125 mL/min or 180 L/day**.
31. Percentage of glomerular filtrate that is reabsorbed: **99%**.
32. The normal amount of protein in urine: **100 mg/day**.
33. Name two substances used to measure GFR: **Inulin and creatinine**.
34. If the renal clearance of a substance is same as that of GFR it means that the substance is **neither reabsorbed nor secreted**.
35. If the renal clearance is more than GFR the substance is **secreted**.
36. If the renal clearance of a substance is less than GFR then it means that it is **reabsorbed**.
37. Glucose is reabsorbed from the renal tubular fluid with the help of **sodium-dependant glucose transporter-2 (SGLT 2)**.
38. The tubular maximum for glucose (Tm_G): **375 mg/min in men and 300 mg/min in women**.

39. The plasma level at which glucose first appears in urine: **Renal threshold for glucose.**
40. Concentrating power of kidney can be assessed by measuring the **specific gravity** of urine.
41. The substance commonly used to measure renal plasma flow: **Paraaminohippuric acid (PAH).**
42. In humans effective renal plasma flow (ERPF) is about **625 mL/min**.
43. Actual renal plasma flow—**700 mL/min**.
44. The ratio of GFR to renal plasma flow: **Filtration fraction (0.16 to 0.20)**.
45. Net filtration pressure at afferent end of glomerular capillary: **15 mm Hg.**
46. Anion gap represents **unmeasured anions** in plasma and it is mostly due to **proteins**.
47. Normal anion gap: **10–12 mmol/L.**
48. Phosphate buffer is mainly present in the **intracellular fluid**.
49. The most important buffer in the interstitial fluid is **carbonic acid-bicarbonate buffer system**.
50. The maximal urine flow that can be produced during a water diuresis: **16 mL/min.**
51. A plot of intravesical pressure against the volume of fluid in the bladder: **Cystometrogram.**
52. Overflow incontinence is seen in the **stage of spinal shock** in spinal cord transection.

CLINICAL CASE SCENARIO

1. **A patient comes with complains of excessive thirst and passing large volumes of colorless urine frequently. Appetite is normal. On investigation his urine output is 15 L/day, urine specific gravity 1.002 to 1.004, no sugar, blood or albumin in urine. Answer the following questions.**
   a. Secretion of which hormone is affected in the patient and mention its site of secretion.
   b. What is the physiological basis of the above-mentioned symptoms?
   c. Explain the actions and mechanism of action of the affected hormone in the renal tubules.
   d. How is its secretion regulated?

   Ans:
   a. Decreased secretion of ADH. ADH is synthesized and secreted from the paraventricular nucleus of hypothalamus; stored and released from the posterior pituitary.

   OR (Same Q1; Sub questions are different).
   a. Identify the clinical condition in the above patient
   b. Explain the mechanism of reabsorption of water in different segments of nephron.
   b. Outline the mechanisms involved in the concentration of urine

   Ans:
   a. Diabetes insipidus

SECTION 7 SKIN AND TEMPERATURE REGULATION

Skin

CHAPTER 58

LEARNING OBJECTIVES
- Explain the structure and functions of skin
- Differentiate between eccrine and apocrine sweat glands

■ INTRODUCTION

Skin is a physiologically and morphologically specialized tissue which covers our body. It acts as the major interphase between our body and the environment. It is continuous with the mucous membrane lining the different openings of the body forming **mucocutaneous junction**. The external surface of skin shows numerous ridges visible to the naked eye, especially on sole and palm. Those ridges on the palmar aspect of fingers form the basis of fingerprints used for personal identification as they show marked individual variation and never change throughout life. Skin in other parts of the body has an average thickness of 0.5–4 mm.

■ STRUCTURE OF SKIN

Skin consists of two layers which are distinct in structure, function and embryological origin:
1. Epidermis
2. Dermis

Epidermis

Epidermis is the superficial layer of **ectodermal** origin, which is a **keratinized, stratified squamous epithelium** consisting of 5 layers. It is the primary barrier to mechanical, chemical and microbial invasions. The outer layer of epidermis (**stratum corneum**) is impermeable to water and is chemically inert. The innermost layer of epidermis called **stratum basale** or **Malpighian layer** consists of a single layer of columnar cells. Among these cells, there are occasional pigment cells of neural crest origin rich in **melanin**, called **melanocytes**. Epidermis has a very high capacity for regeneration after damage.

Dermis

Dermis is the layer deeper to epidermis which is a dense, vascular, connective tissue layer of **mesodermal origin**. It is a tough, flexible and highly elastic layer. It is very thick in palm and sole and very thin over the eyelids. Connective tissue of the dermis is arranged in two layers:
1. Superficial or papillary layer
2. Deep or reticular layer

The junction between epidermis and dermis shows a complex pattern: a peg and socket interdigitation. This prevents peeling off of epidermis from the dermis. Just beneath the dermis is a layer of loose connective tissue or the **superficial fascia**. The skin moves freely over the underlying tissues due to the presence of superficial fascia (**Fig. 58.1**).

■ APPENDAGES OF SKIN

Epidermis of skin gives rise to appendages of skin like hair, nails, sweat gland, sebaceous gland, etc.

Hair

Hair varies in length, thickness and color in different parts of the body. It consists of a **root**, implanted in the skin and a **shaft** which projects from the surface. The root has a proximal enlargement, the **hair bulb**, placed in an invagination of the epidermis and superficial portion of the dermis called the **hair follicle (Fig. 58.1)**.

Ducts of sebaceous gland open into the follicle near the skin surface. At the bottom of the hair follicle, there is a small conical vascular eminence called the **papilla**. The capillaries in the papilla provide nutrition to the hair.

Minute involuntary muscle fibers called *arrector pili or piloerector muscle* are connected to the hair follicle. They arise from the superficial layer of the dermis and are inserted to the hair follicle. Their contraction produces **piloerection**, i.e., hair standing on end, or goose skin. This is seen during exposure to cold or during emotional reaction.

Sebaceous Glands

Sebaceous glands are seen in the dermis in between the piloerector muscle and hair follicle. When the piloerector muscle contracts, it squeezes the gland expelling **sebum**.

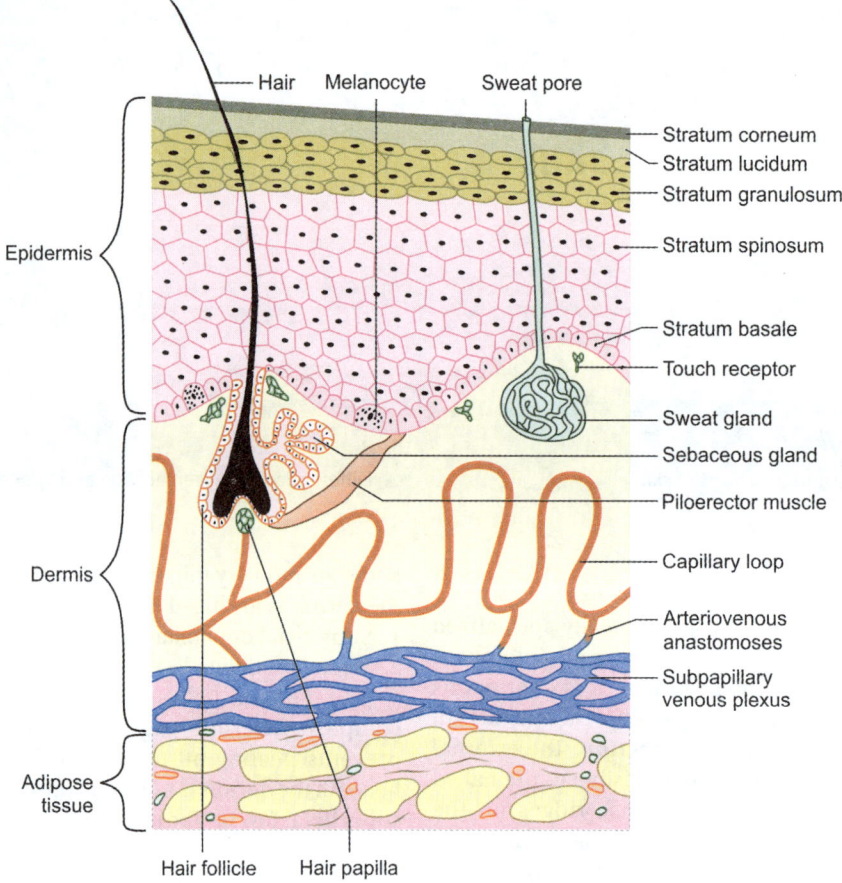

Fig. 58.1: Structure of skin.

Sweat Gland

Sweat glands are present all over the body in large numbers and they are of two types:
1. Eccrine gland
2. Apocrine gland

Eccrine Gland

Eccrine glands are the most numerous and seen all over the body. They are more in number over thick skin. It consists of a single tube which is coiled in its deeper part forming the body of the gland. The superficial part traverses the dermis and epidermis and opens on the surface of the skin by **sweat pore**. These glands are large in areas where perspiration is more as in axilla and more in number in the palm and sole. These glands are innervated by sympathetic cholinergic fibers. Eccrine gland produces merocrine secretion, which is a thin watery secretion. Secretion from eccrine gland is increased during increased temperature and emotional conditions. It plays an important role in regulating body temperature.

Apocrine Gland

Apocrine glands are larger than the eccrine glands and produce a thicker secretion **(Table 58.1)**. They are seen in axilla, areola, pubic area, eyelids, etc., and are supplied by sympathetic adrenergic fibers. These glands start functioning only from puberty onwards. *Pheromones are thought to be secreted by the apocrine glands*. Pheromones are chemical substances present in body secretions, such as sweat, vaginal

Table 58.1: Differences between eccrine and apocrine sweat glands.

Eccrine gland	Apocrine gland
Seen throughout the body, more on the palms and soles	Seen only in areas, such as axilla, mons pubis, areola, eye lids, etc.
Opens on the skin surface through sweat pore	Opens into the canal of the hair follicle
Supplied and stimulated by sympathetic cholinergic fibers, atropine blocks the secretion	Not innervated but stimulated by circulating epinephrine, atropine does not block the secretion
Start functioning from birth	Starts functioning only at puberty
Secrete profuse, watery, hypotonic sweat	Secretion is thick which is acted upon by bacteria to produce a characteristic odor
Function is to regulate body temperature	No role in temperature regulation
Secretion is increased during emotional states and in increased body temperature	Secretion is increased only during emotional states
Secretion is under nervous control	Secretion is under hormonal control. Adrenaline increases secretion

secretion, urine, etc., which can influence the behavior and reproductive cycle in individuals of the same species.

Ceruminous glands of external auditory canal and mammary glands are modified apocrine glands.

BLOOD SUPPLY OF THE SKIN

Blood vessels are distributed profusely in the subpapillary portion of the skin. Circulation to the skin serves two functions:
1. Nutrition
2. Conduction of heat from deeper tissues to the surface

Immediately beneath the skin is a continuous **venous plexus** supplied by blood from the skin capillaries. In areas, such as hands, feet, ears, etc., **arteriovenous anastomosis** is seen. Here, blood is supplied to the plexus directly from small arteries and arterioles. The venous plexus can accommodate as much as 30% of the total cardiac output. A high rate of blood flow causes heat to be conducted from the deeper structures to the skin, whereas reduction in the rate of blood flow leads to decrease in heat conduction from the core of the body.

Heat conduction to the skin by the blood is controlled by the degree of vasoconstriction of the arterioles and the arteriovenous anastomosis that supply blood to the venous plexus of skin.

SKIN COLOR

The three pigments that impart color to the skin are **hemoglobin, melanin and carotene**. Basic determinant of skin color is the quantity of **melanin** in the cells of epidermis. Of all body cells, only **melanocytes** present in the stratum basale of epidermis have the ability to convert the amino acid **tyrosine** into the dark brown melanin pigment with the help of the enzyme **tyrosinase** and the hormone, melanocyte stimulating hormone **(MSH)**. As age advances, tyrosinase activity is decreased leading to greying of hair.

If the enzyme tyrosinase is absent from birth, the condition called **albinism** results. Melanin is absent in the hair, skin and eyes of these individuals. **Vitiligo** is an autoimmune disease in which antibodies attack and destroy melanocytes in patches of skin, producing irregular white spots **(Fig. 58.2)**.

Prolonged exposure of the skin to sunlight causes melanocytes to increase melanin production and darken skin color. Excess secretion of adrenocorticotrophic hormone (ACTH) by the anterior pituitary also leads to hyperpigmentation of skin since ACTH has MSH like activity. Other pigments, such as **carotene** also contribute to skin color.

Skin color changes temporarily when there is change in the volume of blood flowing through the skin capillaries. The amount of blood in the venous plexus decides the color of the skin to some extent because the venous plexus lies parallel to the skin surface. Cold and pale skin denotes that the blood flow is very slow and venous plexus constricted. When the cutaneous blood vessels dilate, the skin appears pink, especially in fair individuals.

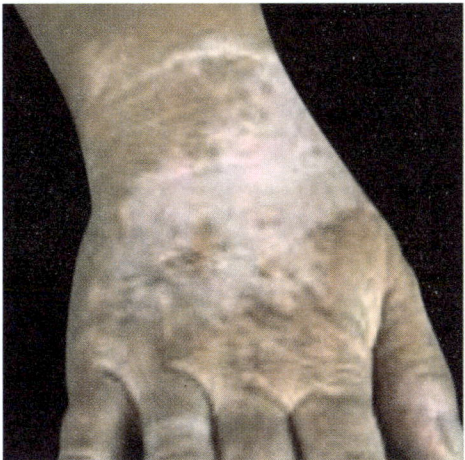

Fig. 58.2: Vitiligo.

In abnormal conditions, there will be bluish discoloration of skin called **cyanosis** where the amount of reduced hemoglobin in blood is more than 5 g% (*refer* **Fig. 39.17**). In **jaundice** where the serum bilirubin is more than 2 mg% there is yellowish discoloration of skin (*refer* **Fig. 48.3**). **Pallor** or paleness of the skin occurs in circulatory shock and anemia.

The vessels of the skin are supplied by **autonomic fibers**. Sympathetic stimulation causes vasoconstriction and parasympathetic stimulation produces vasodilatation.

FUNCTIONS OF SKIN

- Skin **protects** the body by preventing the entry of injurious agents into the tissues. It acts as a barrier between body and environment. As the superficial layers are keratinized, skin is resistant to the action of dilute acids and alkali.
- Skin acts as an **excretory organ**. For example, urea is excreted through sweat to some extent.
- Skin is the largest **sense organ**; receptors for touch, pain, temperature, pressure, etc., are situated in the skin.
- Skin does not allow **diffusion of water** from deeper tissues to outside as it is impermeable to water and thus prevents dehydration.
- Formation of **vitamin D**; sebum contains 7-dehydrocholesterol and when this is acted upon by ultraviolet rays, it is converted to vitamin D.
- Skin contains a pigment called **melanin** which protects the skin from solar radiation.
- Skin acts as a **blood reservoir**, i.e., when cutaneous vessels are dilated, it can accommodate 5–10% of blood volume. In times of emergency as in circulatory shock, these blood vessels constrict and blood is diverted to the vital organs.
- Skin is loosely attached to the subcutaneous tissue and can easily move over it. So it prevents transmission of the impact of a mechanical blow to deeper structures.
- The skin and the subcutaneous tissue act as a heat insulator for the body. This helps in maintaining normal internal core temperature.
- Skin also has absorptive function. Certain medications given as ointments and creams when applied on the skin

is absorbed and produces effects locally and systemically. Muscle relaxants when applied to the skin relieve muscle pain locally; hyoscine epidermal patch when applied prevents motion sickness. Vaccines, such as BCG vaccine (for tuberculosis) and antirabies vaccine are given intradermally.

- ❖ Skin helps in **temperature regulation** by the following mechanisms:
  - By producing sweat
  - By altering the blood flow through the skin.

Temperature Regulation

CHAPTER 59

LEARNING OBJECTIVES
- Describe the mechanism of temperature regulation
- Describe the adaptations to altered temperature (heat and cold)
- Explain the mechanism of production of fever, cold injuries and heat stroke
- Clinical application of hypothermia

INTRODUCTION

Based on body temperature, animals are divided into two groups:
1. Homeothermic animals
2. Poikilothermic animals

Homeothermic or warm-blooded animals maintain their body temperature within a narrow range in spite of wide fluctuation in environmental temperature, e.g., birds and mammals. **Poikilothermic** or cold-blooded animals have a body temperature which fluctuates with environmental temperature, e.g., reptiles, fishes and amphibians.

Hibernating mammals while active are homoeothermic, but during hibernation their body temperature falls.

Temperature of the deeper tissues of the body is known as **core temperature**. Core temperature is measured by taking the rectal temperature. Skin has a temperature lower than the core temperature and is called **shell** or **surface temperature**. Armpit temperature is measured to find out the shell temperature. The skin temperature in contrast to the core temperature varies with the temperature of the surroundings.

Maintenance of a constant body temperature is possible only if the net heat lost from the body exactly matches the amount of heat generated in the body. The skin, subcutaneous tissue and fat form an **insulator** system. Most of the body heat is produced in the deeper portions of the body and the insulation mentioned above is an effective means for preventing excessive heat loss from the body.

MEASUREMENT OF BODY TEMPERATURE

Body temperature is measured using a **clinical thermometer (mercury in glass thermometer)**. Oral, axillary or rectal temperature is usually taken. Rectal temperature more or less corresponds to core temperature. Axillary temperature varies with environmental temperature. Oral temperature also corresponds to core temperature, but hot or cold drinks should be avoided before taking oral temperature.

Other devices used to measure body temperature include:
- Electronic digital readout thermistors
- Infrared thermometer which measures temperature over the temporal artery

Normal body temperature in different parts of the body is as follows:
- Oral temperature – 37°C (36.3-37.1°C) or 98.6°F (97.3-98.8°F) [to convert °C to °F, multiply by 9/5 and add 32; and to convert °F to °C, (°F – 32) × 5/9].
- Axillary temperature – 0.5°C lower than oral temperature.
- Rectal temperature is 0.5°C more than oral temperature.
- Scrotal temperature is 32°C and this low temperature is essential for normal spermatogenesis.
- Body temperature shows a circadian rhythm normally, i.e., a diurnal fluctuation of 0.5–0.7°C. The core temperature is lowest at 6 am and highest in the evening. This is because basal metabolic rate (BMR) is low after a night's restful sleep and towards evening BMR is high due to the day's work.
- Extremities are generally cooler than the rest of the body due to counter current flow of blood in the arteries and veins.

Importance of Temperature Regulation

Maintenance of a constant body temperature is essential because, the rates of most physical and chemical reactions in the body depend on temperature. Many of the body functions depend on the activity of various enzymes. Most of the enzymes regulating metabolism are temperature dependent. The enzyme systems of the body have narrow temperature ranges in which their function is optimal. Therefore, marked alterations of body temperature adversely affects metabolism. The normal body temperature (core temperature) of an adult human is 37°C but individual variation is seen, it may be as low as 36°C or as high as 37.5°C in active, healthy people.

Maintenance of Body Temperature

The rate of heat production in the body can vary from 70 kcal/hour, at rest to 600 kcal/hour during exercise. Body temperature is maintained by a balance between heat production and heat loss from the body. When they are equal, person is said to be in **heat balance**. Lethal limits of temperature are not clearly defined, but the lower limit is around 24°C and upper limit is 43°C.

■ MECHANISMS OF HEAT GAIN AND HEAT LOSS FROM THE BODY

PY11.1: Describe and discus the mechanism of temperature regulation.

Thermogenesis or Heat Production in the Body

Heat production is the result of chemical reactions taking place in the body, i.e., heat is a by-product of metabolism. Therefore, heat production is otherwise called **chemical regulation of body temperature (Fig. 59.1)**.

Factors influencing heat production are:
- Basal metabolic rate (BMR)
- Specific dynamic action of food (SDA)
- Muscular activity
- Action of calorigenic hormones
- Environmental temperature
- Sympathetic discharge
- Brown fat (non-shivering thermogenesis)

Basal Metabolic Rate

Basal metabolic rate (BMR) is the metabolic rate under basal conditions, i.e., the person should be at rest, 12-14 hours after the last meal, in a room of comfortable temperature. It is the energy consumption necessary to maintain the basal functions of resting cell such as active transport across membranes as well as the activity of cardiac and respiratory muscles necessary for survival **(Table 59.1)**. Since by definition, at BMR, the body is performing no work on the environment, all the energy produced is ultimately dissipated as heat.

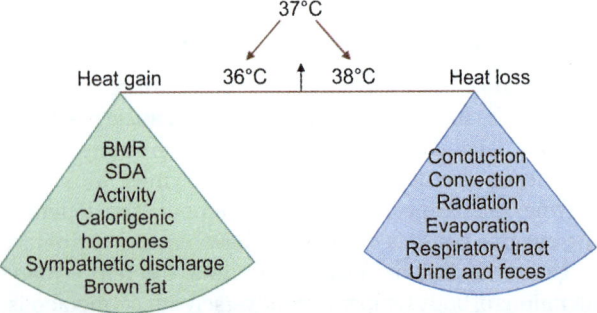

Fig. 59.1: Mechanisms of heat gain and heat loss in the body when there is variation in body temperature from normal.

Table 59.1: Percentage of BMR contributed by different body systems.

System	% of BMR
Respiratory and circulatory systems	15%
Nervous system	20%
Muscles (at rest)	20%
Abdominal viscera	45%
BMR	100% (70 kcal/hour)

BMR of a man of average size is about 1 kcal/kg body weight/hour or 2000 kcal/day or 70-80 kcal/hour or 40 kcal/m²/hr. BMR is usually expressed as a percentage of increase or decrease above or below a standard value. For example, a value of +65 means that the person's BMR is 65% above the standard for that age and sex.

The major portion of heat produced in the body is due to the metabolism of food stuffs. Most of the metabolic reactions occur in the liver. Heat production is more during metabolism of fat.

Since the body is composed chiefly of water, which has a specific heat of one, the body temperature should rise by 1°C if no heat is lost from the body. Exercise, fever, etc., increase metabolic rate and thereby increase heat production in the body. Fever increases metabolic rate by 13% for each degree rise in core temperature.

(0.8 kcal of heat is required to raise the temperature of one kilogram body weight by 1°C. So a person weighing 70 kg requires 56 kcal (70 × 0.8) of heat to raise the body temperature by 1°C.)

Food Intake or SDA

Main source of heat is from the metabolism of carbohydrates, fats and proteins. It is due to **specific dynamic action** (SDA) of food. SDA of a food is the extra heat produced over and above the caloric value of a given amount of food when this food is used by the body. For example, when 25 g of protein which contains 100 calories is metabolized, the heat produced in the body is not 100 calories but 130 calories. This extra 30 calories is due to SDA of protein. In the case of fat containing 100 calories, the heat generated is 113 calories, and carbohydrate it is 105 calories.

The origin of this extra heat may be:
- Due to the activity of the tissues which are metabolizing these food stuffs.
- Due to increased sympathetic discharge after food intake leading to increased release of adrenaline and noradrenaline which increases metabolic rate.

After food intake, there is also a second component in increased heat production other than SDA, i.e., heat production is increased in brown fat. Nerve discharge to brown fat is increased after food intake and there will be a somewhat slower increase in heat production.

Muscular Activity

Muscular activity increases the metabolic rate and thereby heat production. The heat produced during muscular activity is called **heat of activity.** About 80% of heat of activity is produced by skeletal muscles. Muscular activity can be voluntary or involuntary. Voluntary is muscular exercise and involuntary is shivering. During exercise, the heat produced by muscular contraction accumulates in the body and the rectal temperature normally rises to values as high as 40°C or 104°F.

Calorigenic Hormones

Thyroxin and catecholamines increase heat production by accelerating metabolic activities. **Thyroxine** produces a slowly developing prolonged increase in heat production, while **epinephrine and norepinephrine** produce a rapid but short-lived increase in heat production. It is seen that adrenal medullectomized rats die faster than normal rats when exposed to cold. Patients with cretinism and myxedema have subnormal body temperature and therefore, they prefer hot environment.

Climate or Environmental Temperature

If the environmental temperature is more than that of skin, body gains heat.

Sympathetic Discharge

Sympathetic stimulation increases heat production by the release of calorigenic hormones.

Brown Fat or Brown Adipose Tissue

Brown fat is a special type of fat (other being white fat which includes structural lipids and neutral fat in adipose tissues) seen abundantly in infants between and around the scapula, behind sternum, around kidney and adrenals. It is also present in adults in between scapula, at the nape of neck, along the great vessels in the thorax and abdomen and also in other parts of the body. This fat has a high rate of metabolism and is the source of considerable heat production in the body particularly in infants. Oxidative phosphorylation occurs in brown fat as usual, but it produces extra heat by uncoupled oxidative phosphorylation, i.e., all energy is converted to heat (uncoupled metabolism does not generate ATP). A special type of **uncoupling protein** (UPC) is present in brown fat called **UCP1 or thermogenin located on the inner mitochondrial membrane.** The cells contain numerous mitochondria, several small fat droplets and have extensive sympathetic innervation.

On exposure to cold, there will be increased sympathetic discharge and increased release of norepinephrine from the nerve endings supplying the fat cells of the brown fat. Via β_3-adrenergic receptors norepinephrine activates hormone sensitive lipase which in turn splits triglyceride to form free fatty acids. The increased fatty acid oxidation in the mitochondria increases heat production.

Brown fat also contributes to the regulation of body weight. **Leptin receptors** are present in brown adipose tissue, and leptin increases the activity of uncoupling proteins, thus producing a direct peripheral increase in energy expenditure. Mutation of leptin gene leads to obesity. Leptin is a hormone produced by adipose tissue, which acts on the hypothalamus to decrease food intake and increase energy consumption.

Non-shivering Thermogenesis

An increase in metabolic heat production in response to cold exposure that is not associated with muscular activity is called **non-shivering thermogenesis**. It occurs mainly through metabolism of **brown fat** or brown adipose tissue. Brown fat comprises 2 to 6% of the infant's total body weight. The brown color is due to the abundant content of mitochondria in the cytoplasm of the brown fat cells. These mitochondria are densely packed with cristae and have an increased content of respiratory-chain components. They have the ability to **uncouple oxidative phosphorylation**. Brown fat is highly vascularized and has a rich sympathetic innervation. Non-shivering thermogenesis of brown fat is mediated through the activation of β_3-receptors on mature brown fat cells. Exposure to cold increases sympathetic activity leading to release of norepinephrine. It causes increased lipase activity in the brown fat. The free fatty acids released act on **uncoupling protein-1** (**UCP-1**) and produce thermogenesis. **Glucocorticoids and thyroxine** have also a role in triggering non-shivering thermogenesis. The heat produced by non-shivering thermogenesis is mainly a by-product of fatty acid metabolism and to a minor degree from glucose metabolism. Clinically significant non-shivering thermogenesis persists from birth up to the age of two years. Infants are able to double their metabolic heat production during cold exposure by non-shivering thermogenesis. Non-shivering thermogenesis in adults does not appear to be functional or relevant. Non-shivering thermogenesis can be inhibited by β-receptor blockers and anesthetics.

Mechanisms of Heat Loss from the Body

Heat loss depends on physical factors and so, it is called **physical regulation of body temperature**. Most of the heat produced in the body is generated in the liver, brain, heart and in the skeletal muscles during exercise. The heat produced in the deeper tissues and organs is then transferred to the skin where it is lost to the outside. The rate at which heat is lost depends on two factors
1. Rapidity with which heat is conducted from the deeper tissues to the skin.
2. Rapidity with which heat is transferred from the skin to the surroundings.

Factors Influencing Heat Loss by Physical Methods

Physical methods include **conduction, convection, radiation, evaporation** of sweat and **insensible perspiration.**

The factors influencing heat loss by these methods include:
- Temperature gradient
- Degree of air movement
- Amount of subcutaneous fat
- Surface area of exposed part
- Extent of cutaneous blood flow

Methods by Which Heat is Lost from the Body (Fig. 59.1)
- Conduction (2%), convection (15%) and radiation (50%)
- Evaporation of sweat and insensible perspiration (30%)
- Through respiratory passage for warming and humidifying inspired air (1%)
- Through urine and feces (2%)
- Panting in animals.

Conduction
Transfer of heat from the body to another object with which it is in contact is conduction. The amount of heat transferred is proportionate to the temperature difference between the objects in contact (thermal gradient). When an individual is in a cold environment, heat is lost to the surrounding air in contact with the body by conduction. This can be aided by increasing the movement of air around the body as by a fan that blows air through a room.

Convection
Occurs by movement of air molecules away from the area of contact. Warm air rises and cold air falls because of changes in the specific gravity of air. Air molecules near the skin get heated up and move away from the body and this brings in cold air from the surrounding in contact with the body which in turn gets warmed and moves away. This reduces body temperature. Heat moves from the body core to the skin mainly by convection. Blood carries heat from the core of the body to the skin surface where the cutaneous capillaries are dilated.

If the body is immersed in water which has a temperature less than that of body temperature, the rate of heat loss from the body will be many times greater than the rate of heat loss to air. This is because water has a specific heat several thousand times as great as that of air and so the water adjacent to the skin can absorb far greater quantities of heat as can be absorbed by air.

Radiation
It is the transfer of heat by infrared electromagnetic radiation from one object to another at a different temperature with which it is not in contact. Heat is removed from the body by radiation to cool objects in the vicinity.

Heat loss by conduction, convection and radiation can occur only when the temperature of objects and air is less than that of the body. If the temperature of air and objects is higher than that of the body, then the body will only gain heat.

The amount of heat reaching the skin from the core varies with the change in blood flow through the skin. The rate of blood flow to the skin can vary from barely above zero to as great as 30% of the total cardiac output. When the rate of blood flow to the skin is increased, more heat will be conducted from the core of the body to the skin. The rate at which heat is transferred from deeper tissues to the skin is called **tissue conductance**.

In cutaneous vasodilation, more blood flows to the skin and more heat is lost. In vasoconstriction, less blood flows through the skin and heat loss is decreased. The degree of vasoconstriction is controlled by the sympathetic nervous system in response to changes in the environmental temperature.

Evaporation of Water from Skin
When the environmental temperature is same or higher than that of body temperature, heat cannot be lost by conduction, convection or radiation. Then, the chief method of heat loss from the body is by evaporation of water from the skin surface. Anything that prevents adequate evaporation from the skin when the surrounding temperature is higher than the skin temperature will cause the internal body temperature to rise.

Vaporization of 1 g of water removes 0.6 kcal of heat.
Evaporation from the skin occurs by two methods:
1. Insensible perspiration
2. Sweating

Insensible perspiration: Without our knowledge, some amount of water evaporates from the skin and lungs even if there is no sweating. It is called **insensible water loss** because it is *not seen or felt*. It diffuses from the deeper tissues through the epidermis to dry surface. The fluid is derived from the cutaneous capillaries. Amount of fluid lost by this method comes to about 600–800 mL/day or 50 mL/hr. It is always present unless the humidity is 100%. Insensible perspiration cannot be controlled for purposes of temperature regulation. But loss of heat by evaporation of sweat can be controlled by regulating the rate of sweating.

Sweating: Sweat is a weak solution of NaCl, urea and electrolytes in water.
- Specific gravity of sweat: 1.002–1.003
- pH: 4.2–7.5

Sweat is secreted from the deep sub-dermal coiled portion of the sweat gland. This secretion which is isotonic with plasma is called precursor secretion or **primary secretion**. As this flows up the tubular portion through the dermis and epidermis, NaCl and water are reabsorbed depending on the rate of secretion.

Normal amount of sweating in hot weather goes up to 700 mL/hour in an unacclimatized person. In an acclimatized person, the rate may go up to 1.5–2 L/hr. 25,00,000 sweat glands are seen in a person living in temperate climate.

The rate of evaporation of sweat is independent of the temperature gradient between skin and the environment. Instead, it is proportional to the water vapor pressure gradient between skin and the environment. The degree to which the sweat vaporizes depends on the humidity of the environment. If humidity is high, the rate of evaporation of sweat from the body decreases. This is the reason why one feels hotter on a humid day than on a dry day.

Innervation of sweat glands: Sweat glands that are involved in temperature regulation are innervated by postganglionic **cholinergic fibers of the sympathetic nervous system** which run in the sympathetic nerves along with the adrenergic fibers. These glands can also be stimulated by epinephrine or norepinephrine circulating in the blood. This is important during exercise when excessive amount of heat is produced by the active muscles.

Centers for sweating are:
- Preoptic area in the anterior part of hypothalamus
- Spinal center for sweating

Types of sweating:
- Thermal sweating
- Mental sweating
- Sweating in exercise
- Sweating due to sympathetic activity
- Gustatory sweating

- **Thermal sweating:** In hot weather, sweating occurs by:
  - Direct stimulation of the thermoreceptors in hypothalamus by the increased body temperature.
  - Reflexly by the receptors of skin.
- **Mental sweating:** In emotional conditions, sweating is confined to palm, sole and axilla. Some of the sweat glands in these areas are innervated by adrenergic fibers. Excessive sweating in these areas due to over activity of the centers controlling sweat secretion is called **hyperhidrosis**. This can be reduced by atropine and ganglion blocking agents. It can be abolished by sympathectomy. **Sweating in exercise** is due to mental and thermal factors.
- **Sweating in exercise:** During muscular exertion in a hot environment, sweat secretion reaches values as high as 1600 mL/hr. In a dry atmosphere, most of this sweat is vaporized. During exercise there is sympathetic stimulation as well as stimulation of adrenal medulla which leads to increased secretion of catecholamines. Sympathetic cholinergic fibers as well as circulating catecholamines stimulate the sweat glands.
- **Sweating due to sympathetic activity:** This type of sweating occurs during nausea, vomiting, fainting, hypoglycemia, etc. Sweating usually occurs with vasodilatation. But sometimes it occurs in vasoconstriction. This is called non-thermal sweating. This type of sweat is known as **cold sweat**; it occurs in forehead, palm, sole, etc. Some of the sweat glands in these areas are stimulated by circulating epinephrine and norepinephrine. So in emotional states like anxiety, there is increased sweating in palm and sole. Atropine does not inhibit this secretion.
- **Gustatory sweating:** Gustatory sweating is seen when spicy foods are taken in a hot climate. Pain nerve endings are stimulated to produce reflex sweating in head and neck.

Panting

Some mammals lose heat by panting which is rapid, shallow breathing. Panting increases the amount of water evaporated from the mouth and respiratory passages thus increasing the amount of heat lost from the body. Dogs have no sweat glands, so the important mechanism of heat loss from the body is by panting. Panting process is controlled by a panting center that is associated with the pneumotaxic respiratory center located in the pons.

Thermoregulation

The thermoregulatory system includes:
- Thermal sensors in the skin (warmth and cold receptors) and viscera
- Thermo-sensory afferent pathways within the CNS
- Integrating system in the central nervous system (preoptic anterior hypothalamus)
- Efferent pathways (autonomic and somatomotor)
- Thermal effectors capable of heat generation such as brown fat, skeletal muscle, sweat glands and cutaneous blood vessels.

Thermoregulatory receptors are receptors which detect any change in body temperature.
- Central thermoreceptors
- Peripheral or cutaneous thermoreceptors
- Deep body temperature receptors.

Central Thermoreceptors

Central thermoreceptors are specialized neurons sensitive to changes in the temperature of blood flowing through the area. It is seen mainly in the hypothalamus. There are heat-sensitive neurons and cold-sensitive neurons. Heat-sensitive neurons present in the preoptic area, increase their firing rate as the temperature rises.

Cutaneous Thermoreceptors

Thermoreceptors present in the skin provide the central nervous system (CNS) with information about the ambient temperature. They detect the temperature change in skin which in turn depends on the environmental temperature. They are of two types:
1. Cold receptors
2. Warmth receptors

Cold receptors are 3–10 times more in number than warm receptors. Pain receptors of skin are stimulated by extremes of heat and cold. Warmth receptors increase their firing rates as the local skin temperature increases from 32°C up to 45°C. Cold receptors increase their firing rate as local temperature decreases from 40°C down to 26°C. They inform the central thermoregulatory center on changes in the ambient temperature and are responsible for **reflex thermoregulation.** Information from the cutaneous thermoreceptors also travels through the thalamic pathways to the cerebral cortex. This is the basis for the conscious perception of the environmental temperature. This pathway is also responsible for the **behavioral thermoregulation** like moving from the sun to the shade when it is hot.

Some of the fibers carrying temperature sensation instead of going to the thalamus synapse in the parabrachial nucleus of pons which forms the third order neurons that provide sensory information to the preoptic hypothalamus. The neurons in the hypothalamus integrate cutaneous temperature information with the core temperature information. Increase in the activity of warmth sensory neurons in the thermal afferent pathway stimulates the preoptic warmth-sensitive neurons. Cutaneous cold sensory signals inhibit the discharge of the preoptic warmth-sensitive neurons. The efferent fibers from the preoptic warmth-sensitive neurons inhibit two types of spinal neurons: (1) Sympathetic preganglionic neurons that cause cutaneous vasoconstriction and brown adipose tissue thermogenesis, and (2) Alpha motor neurons that cause shivering in skeletal muscle.

Deep body temperature receptors are present in the spinal cord, abdominal viscera, and in or around the great veins in the upper abdomen and thorax. The cutaneous receptors and deep body temperature receptors are concerned with preventing hypothermia (low body temperature).

Thermoregulatory Centers and their Mechanism of Action

Hypothalamus is the chief center for temperature regulation. Heat production and heat loss are adjusted by thermoregulatory centers situated in the hypothalamus. Hypothalamus acts as a **thermostat**. There is a **set point** for the hypothalamic thermostat at 37°C.

There are two thermoregulatory centers, one **for heat loss** in the anterior part of hypothalamus (preoptic temperature sensitive neurons) which responds to increase in body temperature, and the other **for heat gain** in the posterior part of hypothalamus approximately at the level of the mammillary bodies which respond to decrease in body temperature. Stimulation of anterior hypothalamus causes cutaneous vasodilation and sweating. Lesions in this region cause hyperthermia with rectal temperature reaching about 43°C. Stimulation of posterior hypothalamus cause shivering and lesions of posterior hypothalamus causes fall in body temperature towards that of the environment. In the posterior hypothalamus, **serotonin** is the synaptic mediator and in the anterior hypothalamus, **norepinephrine** is the mediator for regulating body temperature.

Thermoregulatory Responses

Under physiological conditions, hypothalamic thermostat detects the temperature fluctuations and appropriate responses are brought into action to maintain the normal body temperature. The anterior hypothalamic-preoptic area contains large number of heat-sensitive neurons and about one-third as many cold-sensitive neurons which are stimulated by an increase or decrease in body temperature. For example, when body is exposed to hot environment, heat loss is increased and heat production is decreased. When exposed to cold, heat loss is decreased and heat production increased. *Thus the hypothalamic-preoptic area serves as a thermostatic body temperature control center.*

There are **threshold core temperatures** for each of the main temperature-regulating responses and when the threshold is reached, the response begins. The threshold is *37°C for sweating and vasodilatation, 36.8°C for vasoconstriction, 36°C for non-shivering thermogenesis and 35.5°C for shivering.*

Responses when Exposed to Cold (Flowchart 59.1)

❖ **Decrease in heat loss**
- Generalized cutaneous vasoconstriction by stimulation of sympathetic centers in the posterior hypothalamus
- Decreased sweating
- Behavioral responses like curling up to decrease the surface area exposed, moving into a heated room or wearing well-insulated clothing in cold weather. This is because the temperature controlling areas in the brain give the person a psychic sensation of cold.
- Piloerection or horripilation by contraction of piloerector muscles attached to the hair follicles caused by sympathetic stimulation. This mechanism is not important in human beings, but in animals upright position of hairs allows them to entrap a thick layer of air next to the skin which acts as an insulator. So transfer of heat to the surroundings is decreased significantly.

❖ **Increased heat production**
- Increased appetite which increases SDA
- Increased muscular activity (voluntary or involuntary as shivering)
- Increased secretion of calorigenic hormones (catecholamines and thyroxine)

Shivering

Shivering is rapid involuntary contractions of skeletal muscles. Shivering occurs when environmental temperature

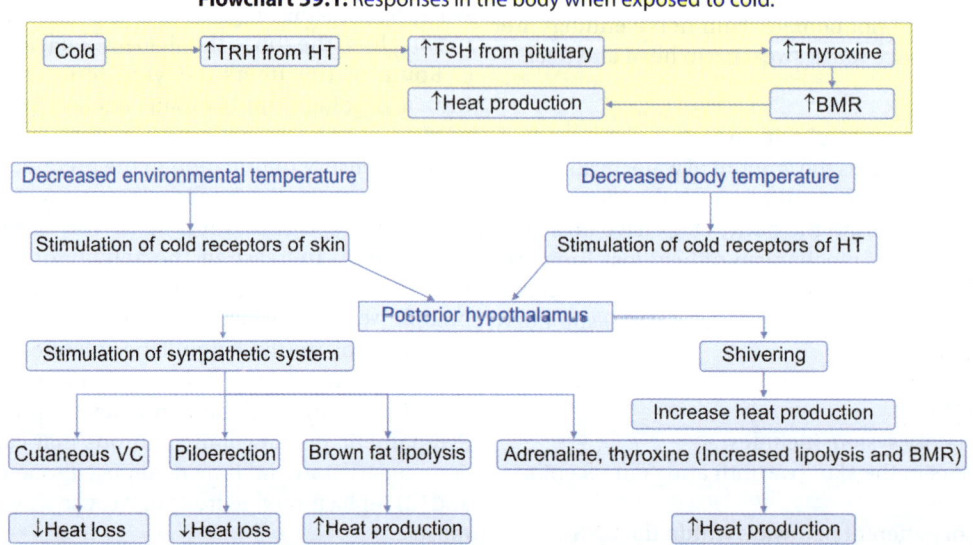

Flowchart 59.1: Responses in the body when exposed to cold.

falls below 23°C. Shivering increases body heat production. Dorsomedial portion of posterior hypothalamus near the wall of the third ventricle is called **primary motor center for shivering**. This area is normally inhibited by signals from the heat center in the preoptic area of anterior hypothalamus. But, it is excited by cold signals from the skin and spinal cord. When activated, this area sends impulses down the brain stem to the lateral column of spinal cord to end in the α-motor neurons supplying the skeletal muscles. This produces involuntary skeletal muscle contraction called shivering which increases heat production in the body. Shivering occurs when the core temperature falls below 35.5°C; shivering is also seen in fever. *During maximum shivering, heat production in the body can increase to four to five times normal.*

In muscular exercise, 25% of energy is converted to work and remaining 75% is liberated as heat.

Increased Secretion of Calorigenic Hormones

Increased catecholamine secretion is an important endocrine response to cold. Adrenaline increases lipolysis in adipose tissue, increases rate of cellular metabolism and increases brown fat lipolysis leading to increased heat production in the body. This is called *chemical thermogenesis or non-shivering thermogenesis*. This is due to the ability of epinephrine and norepinephrine to uncouple oxidative phosphorylation. This means that excess food stuffs are oxidized and release energy in the form of heat but do not cause ATP to be formed.

Exposure to cold increases the release of thyroxine which increases BMR and increase body temperature. It is seen that exposure of animals to extreme cold for several weeks can cause increase in the size of thyroid gland by 20–40%. This is the reason why incidence of toxic thyroid goiters is high in people who live in cold climates than in those who live in warm climates.

Responses when Exposed to Hot Climate (Table 59.2)

When exposed to hot climate, there should be increased heat loss and decreased heat production.
- ❖ **Increase in heat loss (Flowchart 59.2)**
  - The amount of heat reaching the skin from the deeper tissues can be varied by changing the blood flow to the skin. The rate at which heat is transferred from the deep tissues to the skin is called the **tissue conductance**. Vasodilation of skin blood vessels by inhibition of sympathetic center in the posterior hypothalamus brings large amount of warm blood to the skin. Due to conduction and radiation large amount of heat will be lost from the skin during vasodilation.
  - Increased sweating. There is a sharp increase in the rate of evaporation of sweat when the core temperature rises above 37°C.
  - Increase in cardiac output.
  - Increase in the rate of respiration increases evaporation of water from mouth and respiratory passages. For example, panting in dogs is a means of increasing heat loss through respiratory passages. Panting is rapid shallow breathing. Since, it is shallow, no change in the composition of alveolar air occurs. Dogs do not have sweat glands.
- ❖ **Decreased production of heat**
  - Decrease in appetite (anorexia) leads to decrease in SDA.
  - Apathy and inertia, i.e., decreased muscular activity.
  - Decreased liberation of calorigenic hormones.

Local Skin Temperature Reflexes

When a part of the body is heated or cooled, appropriate responses are seen locally to regulate the temperature locally. If the part is heated, local vasodilation and mild local sweating occurs. If the area is placed in cold water, there will be local vasoconstriction and local cessation of sweating. These reactions are caused by local effects of temperature directly on the blood vessels and also by local cord reflexes conducted from the skin receptors to the spinal cord and back to the same skin area and the sweat glands. These reflexes are very weak when compared to the hypothalamic control of body temperature.

Comfort Zone

Low environmental temperature is a stimulus for heat production. When the air temperature is below 28°C, the body loses heat rapidly. In the temperature range between **28°C and 31°C**, the body can easily maintain the balance between heat loss and heat production. There will be no sweating or

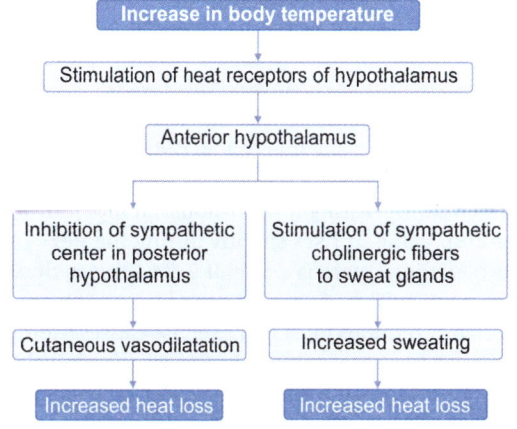

Flowchart 59.2: Main responses when there is increase in body temperature.

Table 59.2: Temperature regulating mechanisms.	
Activated by cold	**Activated by heat**
Cutaneous vasoconstriction	Vasodilatation
Decreased sweating	Increased sweating
Curling up	Increased respiration
Piloerection	Increased cardiac output
Increased appetite	Decreased appetite (anorexia)
Increased voluntary activity	Decreased muscular activity
Shivering	Apathy and inertia
Increased secretion of epinephrine, norepinephrine and thyroxine	Decreased release of catecholamines and thyroxine

shivering. This range of temperature is called **comfort zone**. It is broader for female, i.e., 27–33°C.

Critical Air Temperature

External temperature below which heat production should be increased to maintain the normal body temperature is **critical temperature**. Or, the ambient temperature at which there is no active heat loss or heat gain mechanism operating in the body. It is the lowest ambient temperature at which mammals can maintain its body temperature at the basal metabolic rate and is normally **23±2°C**. Any deviation from this temperature leads to heat production or heat loss mechanisms in the body. Both critical temperature and comfort zone depend on the nature and extent of clothing.

Lethal Temperature

When the core temperature goes below **26°C**, cardiac arrhythmia and death due to cardiac failure occur. When the core temperature is above **43°C**, death may result due to heat stroke. These are the lower and upper **lethal temperatures**.

VARIATIONS IN BODY TEMPERATURE

> **PY11.2:** Describe and discuss adaptation to altered temperature (heat and cold).
> **PY11.3:** Describe and discuss mechanism of fever, cold injuries and heat stroke.

- Physiological variations
- Pathological variations

Physiological Variations

- **Diurnal variation:** Diurnal variation is approximately 0.5–0.7°C normally. Minimum temperature is seen between 3 and 6'o clock in the morning. During day time, due to increased metabolism and muscular activity, heat production is increased and maximum temperature is recorded in the late afternoon (3 pm to 6 pm).
- **Age:** In infants, body temperature varies due to imperfect regulation of body temperature. Their body temperature is 0.5°C higher than that of adults mainly because of brown fat. They are more vulnerable to be affected by changes in external temperature than adults. Preterm infants are exceptionally vulnerable to hypothermia. In old people, temperature is subnormal because body is less active, circulation is feeble and sweat glands are atrophied. Their thermoregulatory mechanism is also weak.
- **Sex:** Females have a slightly low body temperature than males of the same age due to low BMR and thick layer of subcutaneous fat.
- **Menstruation:** During menstruation, temperature is at a minimum value. It rises slightly during the next 14 days. After ovulation, there is a rise of 0.5°C. This is due to the thermogenic effect of progesterone.
- **Exercise:** Strenuous muscular exercise causes a temporary rise in body temperature that is proportional to the severity of exercise. During muscular contraction, only 25% of energy liberated is used for work. Remaining 75% is liberated as heat.
- **Emotions:** Emotions like excitement, anger, fear, etc., can raise the body temperature. This may be due to unconscious tensing of the muscles.
- If the body temperature is chronically elevated in normal adults, it is called **constitutional hyperthermia**.

Pathological Variation

In hyperthyroidism, there is increase in body temperature due to increased secretion of thyroxine which increases the metabolic rate.

Fever or Pyrexia

Rise in body temperature above normal range is **fever**. Different types of fever are:
1. Infectious fever due to infections.
2. Surgical fever especially in operations in the region of hypothalamus.
3. Neurogenic fever is seen in injuries of brain and in compression of hypothalamus by brain tumors.
4. Fever of dehydration due to lack of sweating.
5. Fever produced by drugs and chemicals.

Mechanism of Production of Fever

Certain proteins, toxins of bacteria, etc., are capable of acting at the temperature regulating center and can raise the **set point** of the **hypothalamic thermostat**. Normal body temperature is 37°C. This means that the hypothalamus is set in a position to produce a temperature of 37°C. Under normal circumstances, all the temperature control mechanisms continually attempt to bring the body temperature back to this set-point level. But in fever, the toxins of bacteria raise the set point of the hypothalamic thermostat. So, the body temperature rises to this temperature. The body by heat conservation and heat production raises the body temperature to the new set point of hypothalamic temperature controller. Those substances that produce fever are called **pyrogens**.

Mechanism of Action of Pyrogens

Certain pyrogens can act directly on the hypothalamic temperature-regulating center to increase its set point. Certain others do not increase the body temperature soon and may require several hours of latency before causing their effects. The time interval is taken for the formation of **endogenous toxins**. Bacteria or breakdown products of bacteria are phagocytosed by leukocytes (monocytes and cytotoxic T cells) and tissue macrophages and the bacterial products are digested. Toxins of bacteria such as endotoxins thus formed stimulate monocytes, macrophages and Kupffer cells to produce **cytokines** (interleukins) that act as **endogenous pyrogens**. One of the important cytokines in producing fever is interleukin-1β (IL-1β), also called leukocyte pyrogen or endogenous pyrogen. This interleukin on reaching the hypothalamus produces fever in 8–10 minutes. Other cytokines producing fever include IL6, IFN-β, IFN-γ and TNF-α. These circulating cytokines are polypeptides and they cannot penetrate the blood-brain barrier (BBB). The cytokines act on organum vasculosum of the lamina terminalis (OVLT) which is a circumventricular organ. Circumventricular organs are outside the blood-brain barrier (BBB) and so substances can easily enter them. OVLT, in turn, activates the preoptic area of hypothalamus which contains the heat-sensitive neurons. In infections of brain, cytokines are produced by the cells in CNS and they can act directly on the thermoregulatory centers (**Flowchart 59.3**). The fever produced by cytokines is due to local release of **prostaglandin (PGE$_2$)** in the hypothalamus. This has been proved by intra-hypothalamic injection of prostaglandin which produced fever. Aspirin which is given for the treatment of fever, acts by inhibiting prostaglandin synthesis from arachidonic acid. Drugs such as aspirin that reduce fever are called **antipyretics.**

Characteristics of Fever

* Chills or shivering
* Flushing

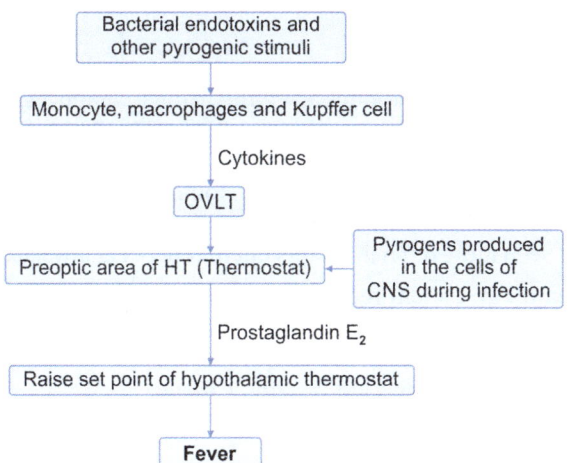

Flowchart 59.3: Mechanism of production of fever.

(OVLT: organum vasculosum of the lamina terminalis; HT: hypothalamus)

Chills: Once the **set point of hypothalamic thermostat** is raised to a higher level, the body tries to increase the temperature by heat production. This occurs mainly by shivering and this continues till the body temperature is equal to the set point of hypothalamic thermostat.

Along with shivering, the person feels cold because of vasoconstriction and thus conservation of heat is facilitated. There will be increased sympathetic activity and increased production of catecholamines. Along with chills, there will be piloerection also. Chills can continue until the body temperature reaches the new hypothalamic set point. Then the chills disappear and the person feels neither hot nor cold. As long as the causative factor for fever is present, the body temperature will be maintained at the high-temperature set-point level.

Crisis or flush: Once the cause for increased temperature is removed, the set-point of the hypothalamic temperature controller will be reduced to a lower value or even back to normal level. But the body temperature still remains high. The hypothalamus now attempts to regulate the temperature to 98.6°F. The body tries to lower the temperature by vasodilatation and sweating. This sudden change of events occurring in a febrile condition associated with profuse sweating and red hot skin is known as **crisis or flush** (**Fig. 59.2**).

Advantages of Fever

* A rise in temperature inhibits the growth of several microorganisms.
* Antibody production is increased when the body temperature is elevated.
* Hyperthermia is beneficial for individuals suffering from neurosyphilis, anthrax, pneumococcal pneumonia, leprosy and certain viral, fungal and rickettsial diseases.
* Hyperthermia slows down the growth of some tumors. But, very high temperature is harmful to the body.

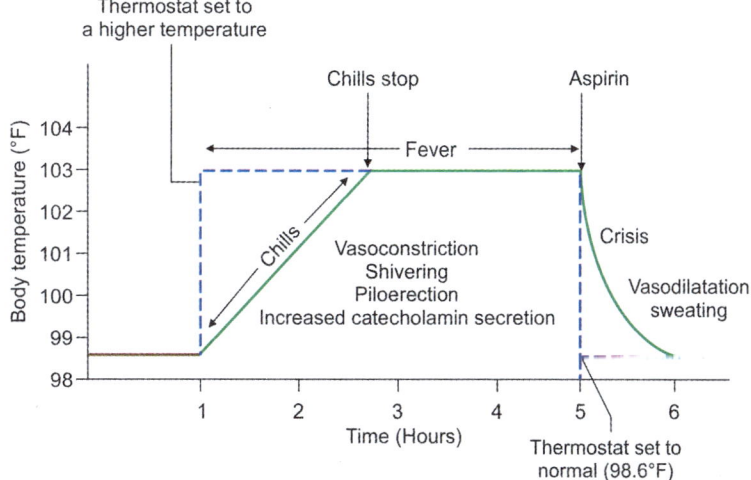

Fig. 59.2: Characteristics of fever. Note the changes occurring when the hypothalamic thermostat is set to a higher and lower temperature suddenly.

Body temperature greater than 41°C or 106°F sustained for prolonged periods will cause permanent damage to the brain tissue. When the over 43°C, heat stroke develops and death occurs.

Malignant Hyperthermia

Mutation of the gene coding for the ryanodine receptors in the sarcoplasmic reticulum leads to **malignant hyperthermia**. There will be excess release of calcium from the sarcoplasmic reticulum during muscle contraction. This in turn leads to contractures of muscles, increased muscle metabolism and a great increase in heat production in muscles. The increased heat production causes a marked rise in body temperature that is fatal if not treated.

EFFECTS OF EXPOSURE OF THE BODY TO EXTREMES OF TEMPERATURE

Exposure to Extreme Heat

- Heat exhaustion
- Dehydration exhaustion
- Heat cramps
- Heat stroke

Heat Exhaustion

Sudden exposure of the body to a high temperature causes peripheral vasodilatation. The blood pressure falls in spite of increase in heart rate and cardiac output. If physical work is also done, the BP still falls and the patient develops signs of cardiac insufficiency.

The person becomes confused, fatigued, and dyspneic and feels very hot. The skin will be moist and there will be profuse sweating. Pulse will be rapid and BP low. Finally, he may collapse and become unconscious. This condition responds to rest, cooling of the body and fluid replacement.

Dehydration Exhaustion

This occurs after exposure to heat for a longer period. If the fluid lost is not replaced, signs of cardiac insufficiency occur. Usually, dehydration exhaustion occurs when the body has lost 5% of its weight. This condition responds to cooling of the body and fluid replacement.

Heat Cramps

Large amounts of electrolytes and fluid are lost from the body by excessive sweating and low salt intake. When the person exerts, there will be severe painful muscle contractures. These painful cramps can be relieved by administration of NaCl orally or parenterally.

Heat Stroke

Heat stroke is a rare condition. This occurs when a person with dry skin is exposed to a very high temperature in a dry atmosphere. As the body core temperature rises, excessive cutaneous vasodilation can lead to a fall in arterial blood pressure. As the core temperature reaches 41°C, there is decrease in brain perfusion leading to confusion and ultimately loss of consciousness. The rectal temperature comes to 106–110°F. The core temperature >41°C leads to the clinical condition known as **heat stroke**. The extreme rise in temperature will damage the brain tissue. High temperature can cause fibrinolysis and consumption of clotting factors resulting in disseminated intravascular coagulation, uncontrolled vascular thrombosis and hemorrhage. Heat-induced damage to cell membranes of skeletal and cardiac muscle leads to **rhabdomyolysis** and **myocardial necrosis**. In rhabdomyolysis, disrupted muscle cells release their intracellular contents, including myoglobin, into the circulation. Cell damage also causes acute hepatic insufficiency and pancreatitis. Renal failure occurs due to high plasma levels of myoglobin and decreased renal perfusion. Metabolic disturbances also occur. When the temperature is over 43°C, death is common.

So, the temperature should be lowered suddenly. This is done by applying ice pieces or placing the patient in ice water bath.

Miliaria

Overheating may produce an erythematous, papulovesicular eruption due to closure of sweat ducts **(Fig. 59.3)**. It may be seen when there is excessive sweating due to high temperature, increased humidity, too much sun exposure, overprotective clothes in infants, steam baths, fever, coma, etc. Seen more often in infants but may occur at any age.

Treatment: Patient requires a cooler environment (fan, air conditioning, etc.). Cool starch baths, application of powder, calamine lotion or corticosteroid lotion are beneficial. If itching is severe, give antihistamine orally.

Exposure to Cold

Frost Bite

When the person is exposed to very low temperature, i.e., below 21°C, there will be impairment of circulation and the tissue shows local damage and gangrene. It is usually seen in earlobes, fingertips, etc.

Hypothermia

When the body temperature is between 28 and 31°C, it is known as hypothermia. When it is below 25°C, it is known as deep hypothermia. Hypothermia is seen in:
- Hypothyroidism
- Lesions of hypothalamus
- Pontine hemorrhage

Hypothermia may be accidental or induced. Accidental hypothermia occurs when the body is exposed to extreme cold.

Induced hypothermia: Hypothermia can be induced artificially by giving sedatives, anesthetic agents or by artificial cooling. When the skin or the blood is cooled enough to lower the body temperature in non-hibernating animals and in humans, metabolic and physiologic processes slow

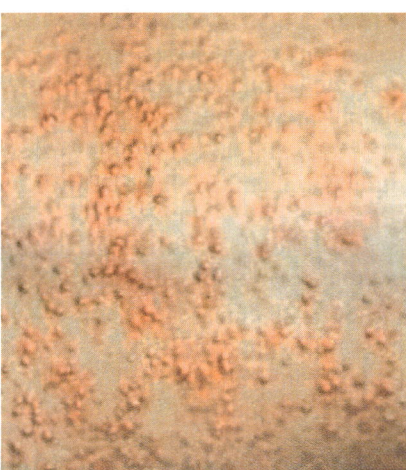

Fig. 59.3: Miliaria (note the papulovesicular eruptions in the skin).

down, respiration and heart rate fall to very low levels, blood pressure falls and consciousness is lost.

Tissue metabolism is also slowed down. At rectal temperature of about 28°C, the ability to spontaneously return the temperature to normal is lost, but the individual continues to survive and if rewarmed with external heat, returns to a normal state. Care should be taken to prevent the formation of ice crystals in the tissue.

Advantages of hypothermia: Humans tolerate body temperature of 21–24°C without permanent ill effects. So hypothermia is made use of in **cardiac and brain surgery**. The blood supply to these organs can be temporarily cut-off for relatively long periods because the oxygen need of the tissues is greatly reduced at low temperature. Blood pressure will be low and bleeding will be minimal during surgery. So it is possible under hypothermia to stop and open the heart and to perform brain operations.

MULTIPLE CHOICE QUESTIONS

1. **Heat is produced maximally in the body at rest in the:**
   a. Liver
   b. Skeletal muscle
   c. Heart
   d. Stomach

2. **Average oral body temperature is:**
   a. 36°C
   b. 98.6°F
   c. 96.8°F
   d. 95.6°F

3. **Comfort zone temperature normally is:**
   a. 29 ± 2°C
   b. 37 ± 2°C
   c. 40 ± 2°C
   d. 34 ± 2°C

4. **Normal scrotal temperature is:**
   a. 32°C
   b. 36°C
   c. 37°C
   d. 28°C

5. **Lower lethal core temperature:**
   a. 36°C
   b. 30°C
   c. 26°C
   d. 18°

6. **Upper lethal core temperature is:**
   a. 40°C
   b. 43°C
   c. 46°C
   d. 39°C

7. **In the menstrual cycle, temperature is minimal during:**
   a. Ovulation
   b. Proliferative phase
   c. Menstruation
   d. Secretory phase

8. **Average BMR in an adult male of average size is:**
   a. 1300 kcal/day
   b. 40 kcal/day
   c. 100 kcal/day
   d. 2000 kcal/day

9. **Maximum heat production occurs after ingestion of:**
   a. Carbohydrates
   b. Proteins
   c. Fats
   d. Water

10. **Rapid but short lived increase in heat production occurs after administration of:**
    a. Thyroxine
    b. Cortisol
    c. Epinephrine
    d. Progesterone

11. **Slowly developing but prolonged increase in heat production is produced by:**
    a. Thyroxine
    b. Cortisol
    c. Epinephrine
    d. Progesterone

12. **When the environmental temperature is more than body temperature, heat loss from the body is mainly accomplished by:**
    a. Radiation
    b. Conduction
    c. Convection
    d. Sweating

13. **The amount of heat removed from the body by vaporization of 1 mL of water is:**
    a. 0.2 kcal
    b. 0.6 kcal
    c. 1 kcal
    d. 20 kcal

14. **Apocrine glands are mainly responsible for:**
    a. Non-thermal sweating
    b. Thermal sweating
    c. Perspiration
    d. Increased sweating with rise in body temperature

15. **Apocrine sweat glands are innervated by:**
    a. Sympathetic cholinergic fibers
    b. Parasympathetic cholinergic fibers
    c. Sympathetic adrenergic fibers
    d. Fibers that release NO

16. **The following statements regarding temperature regulation are correct, *except*:**
    a. Eccrine sweat glands are supplied by sympathetic cholinergic fibers
    b. One feels hotter on a dry day than on a humid day
    c. Insensible water loss amounts to 50 mL/hour normally
    d. Atropine does not inhibit secretion from apocrine glands

17. **Sweating as a result of exertion is mediated through:**
    a. Adrenal hormones
    b. Sympathetic cholinergic discharge
    c. Sympathetic adrenergic discharge
    d. Parasympathetic cholinergic fibers

18. **Heat loss from the body depends mostly on:**
    a. Thermoregulatory center
    b. Warming of air during inspiration
    c. On the environmental temperature
    d. Radiation and evaporation

19. **The first physiological response to high environmental temperature is:**
    a. Sweating
    b. Vasodilatation
    c. Decreased heat production
    d. Non-shivering thermogenesis

20. **The physiological effect in unacclimatized person suddenly exposed to cold is:**
    a. Tachycardia
    b. Shift of blood from shell to core
    c. Non-shivering thermogenesis
    d. Hypertension

21. **Under physiological conditions, heat acclimatization is accompanied by all the following, except:**
    a. Decreased renal blood flow
    b. Increased urine sodium
    c. Increased aldosterone secretion
    d. Excessive sweating

22. **Non-shivering thermogenesis in adults is due to:**
    a. Thyroid hormone
    b. Brown fat between shoulders
    c. Noradrenaline
    d. Muscle metabolism

23. **Endogenous non-shivering thermogens are secreted by all, except:**
    a. Liver   b. Spleen
    c. Heart   d. Small intestine

24. **The hormone associated with cold adaptation is:**
    a. Growth hormone
    b. Thyroxine
    c. Insulin
    d. Melanocyte stimulating hormone

25. **Non-shivering thermogenesis is mediated by:**
    a. α_1-receptor   b. β_2-receptor
    c. β_3-receptor   d. UCP-2

26. **The center for heat loss is located in the:**
    a. Posterior hypothalamus
    b. Lateral hypothalamus
    c. Medulla oblongata
    d. Anterior hypothalamus

27. **The center for heat gain is present in:**
    a. Posterior hypothalamus
    b. Lateral hypothalamus
    c. Medulla oblongata
    d. Anterior hypothalamus

28. **All the following produces fever, except:**
    a. Bacterial endotoxins
    b. Cytokines and interleukin-I
    c. Prostaglandin E_2
    d. ACTH

29. **In the treatment of fever, aspirin acts by:**
    a. Inhibiting prostaglandin synthesis
    b. Inhibiting formation of endogenous toxins
    c. Inhibiting cytokine production
    d. Resetting hypothalamic thermostat

30. **Hypothermia occurs in all the following conditions, except:**
    a. Hypothyroidism   b. Hypothalamic lesions
    c. Pontine hemorrhage d. Cushing syndrome

31. **Hypothermia produces all the following, except:**
    a. Increase in blood pressure
    b. Decrease in heart rate
    c. Loss of consciousness
    d. Decreased O_2 needs of tissues

32. **A 10 degree decrease in body temperature causes a decrease in cerebral metabolic rate by:**
    a. 10%   b. 30%
    c. 50%   d. 70%

33. **In human being, the least useful physiological response to low environmental temperature is:**
    a. Shivering   b. Vasoconstriction
    c. Release of thyroxine d. Piloerection

34. **The hypothalamic thermostat is located in the:**
    a. Supraoptic nucleus
    b. Preoptic nucleus
    c. Paraventricular nucleus
    d. Median eminence

35. **All the following are controlled by the hypothalamus, except:**
    a. Increase in heart rate with exercise
    b. Food intake
    c. Pituitary hormone regulation
    d. Temperature regulation

36. **A major source of heat production in infants is:**
    a. Glycogen
    b. Stimulation of adrenal medulla
    c. Increased sympathetic activity
    d. Brown fat

37. **The maximum amount of cardiac output that can be accommodated in the venous plexus of skin is:**
    a. 30%   b. 5%
    c. 10%   d. 50%

38. **All the following are homeothermic animals, except:**
    a. Rat   b. Frog
    c. Man   d. Birds

39. **The synaptic mediator for regulating body temperature in the anterior hypothalamus is:**
    a. Serotonin   b. Acetylcholine
    c. Nor epinephrine d. Glutamate

40. **The mediator for regulating body temperature in the posterior hypothalamus is:**
    a. Serotonin   b. Acetylcholine
    c. Norepinephrine d. Glutamate

41. **Shivering starts when the core temperature falls to:**
    a. 36.5°C
    b. 35.5°C
    c. 31°C
    d. 32°C
42. **Mutations in the gene coding for ryanodine receptor in muscles lead to:**
    a. Frost bite
    b. Heat stroke
    c. Hypothermia
    d. Malignant hyperthermia
43. **Pyrogens raise body temperature by:**
    a. Setting the thermostat to higher level
    b. Releasing cytokines like interleukins
    c. Decreasing peripheral heat liberating mechanism
    d. Causing peripheral vasoconstriction
44. **Profound hypothermic signs include all, *except*:**
    a. Slow breathing
    b. Bradycardia
    c. Hypotension
    d. Hyperactivity
45. **Daily loss of water from the skin in the absence of visible sweating is:**
    a. 200–300 mL
    b. 500–700 mL
    c. 1 liter
    d. 1.5 liter
46. **At normal atmospheric temperature, most body heat loss is by:**
    a. Convection
    b. Direct conduction
    c. Radiation
    d. Sweating
47. **Which probably causes stimulation of thermal receptors?**
    a. Change in membrane structure caused by heat or cold
    b. Change in the metabolic rate of nerve ending
    c. Change in the concentration of Na⁺ outside the neuron caused by change in temperature
    d. Change in the velocity of fluid surrounding the neuron
48. **Cytokines that act as endogenous pyrogens are produced by:**
    a. Monocytes and macrophages
    b. Lymphocytes
    c. Hepatocytes
    d. Endothelium
49. **Major source of heat in the body is:**
    a. Cutaneous vasoconstriction
    b. Contraction of skeletal muscles
    c. Secretion of catecholamines
    d. Shivering
50. **All the following statements regarding hyperthermia are correct, *except*:**
    a. Hyperthermia inhibits growth of microorganisms
    b. Antibody production is decreased
    c. Slows the growth of some tumors
    d. Benefits individuals infected with leprosy, anthrax, etc.
51. **When the atmospheric temperature is 21°C and humidity 80%, maximum amount of heat is lost from the body through:**
    a. Respiratory tract
    b. Urination
    c. Evaporation of sweat
    d. Radiation and conduction
52. **Heat stroke and death occurs when the rectal temperature is over:**
    a. 43°C
    b. 45°C
    c. 41°C
    d. 40°C
53. **Normal set point of hypothalamic thermostat is:**
    a. 37°C
    b. 97.6°F
    c. 36°C
    d. 104°F
54. **There is mutation of the gene coding for ryanodine receptors in malignant hyperthermia. The explanation for the increased heat production in this condition is:**
    a. Increased muscle metabolism due to excess calcium ions
    b. Thermic effect of blood
    c. Increased sympathetic discharge
    d. Mitochondrial thermogenesis
55. **When environmental temperature is more than body temperature, heat loss from the body mainly occur by:**
    a. Radiation
    b. Evaporation
    c. Conduction
    d. Convection

ANSWERS

1. a	2. b	3. a	4. a	5. c
6. b	7. c	8. d	9. b	10. c
11. a	12. d	13. b	14. a	15. c
16. b	17. b	18. c	19. b	20. b
21. b	22. c	23. b	24. b	25. c
26. d	27. a	28. d	29. a	30. d
31. a	32. d	33. d	34. b	35. a
36. d	37. a	38. b	39. c	40. a
41. b	42. d	43. b	44. d	45. a
46. d	47. b	48. a	49. b	50. b
51. d	52. a	53. a	54. a	55. b

FILL IN THE BLANKS/GIVE THE NORMAL VALUE/NAME THE FOLLOWING

1. **Poikilothermic** animals are cold blooded animals because their body temperature fluctuates over a considerable range.
2. **Homeothermic** animals are warm blooded animals who maintain body temperature within a narrow range.
3. Average oral temperature: **37°C or 90.6°F.**
4. The average temperature of the scrotum: **32°C**.
5. The rectal temperature is **0.5°C** greater than oral temperature.
6. In females there is a rise in basal temperature by 0.5°C after ovulation due to the thermogenic action of **progesterone**.

7. **Constitutional hyperthermia** means, some normal adults chronically have a temperature above the normal range.
8. Ingestion of food increases heat production because of **specific dynamic action** of food.
9. The processes by which heat is lost from the body when the environmental temperature is below body temperature: **Conduction, convection and radiation.**
10. The rate at which heat is transferred from the deep tissues to the skin is called the **tissue conductance.**
11. When the environmental temperature is high, heat is lost from the body by evaporation of sweat.
12. Vaporization of 1 g of water removes about 0.6 kcal of heat.
13. Water vaporized from the body without our knowledge: **Insensible water loss.**
14. An individual in a humid climate feels **warmer** than an individual in a dry environment.
15. Secretion of which hormone is increased by cold and decreased by heat: **TSH.**
16. The reflex responses activated by cold are controlled by the **posterior hypothalamus**.
17. The reflex responses activated by warmth are controlled from **anterior hypothalamus**.
18. Lesions of anterior hypothalamus cause **hyperthermia**.
19. The threshold core temperature for sweating and vasodilatation: **37°C**.
20. The threshold core temperature for vasoconstriction: **36.8°C**.
21. The threshold core temperature for shivering: **35.5°C**.
22. The normal set point of hypothalamic thermostat: **37°C**.
23. Aspirin inhibits **prostaglandin** synthesis and the antipyretic effect is exerted directly on the **hypothalamus**.
24. Name one prostaglandin that produce fever: **PGE2**.
25. The rectal temperature over which heat stroke occurs: **43°C.**
26. Malignant hyperthermia is due to mutation of the gene coding for **ryanodine receptor** in the muscle.

SECTION 8: ENDOCRINE SYSTEM

Organization of the Endocrine System

CHAPTER 60

LEARNING OBJECTIVES
- Define the term hormone
- Describe the location of the major endocrine glands
- Explain the feedback regulation of hormone secretion with examples
- Describe the types of assay of hormones
- Explain the functions of growth factors

INTRODUCTION

Coordination of biological functions and homeostasis in humans is achieved by two main control systems, the nervous system and the endocrine system. Endocrinology is the branch of medicine that deals with endocrine glands and hormones. **Endocrine** means inwardly secreting (*endos*: inward, *krenein*: secreting). The main function of endocrine system is to maintain homeostasis throughout the body by means of hormone signaling pathways.

Endocrine glands are also known as **ductless glands** because they release their secretions directly into the circulatory system or into the interstitial fluid. They are scattered throughout the body and their secretion is known as **hormone**. Hormone is derived from the Greek word, **ormao**, which means to excite.

By **definition**, hormone is a **chemical messenger** secreted in small amounts from specific secretory cells into the blood stream and carried to distant target organs where they exert their action. Cells communicate with each other by means of these chemical signals. **Target cells** are cells that respond to the actions of hormones.

The distance through which the hormone travels to reach the target tissue varies. It may be long as in case of pituitary hormones, e.g., luteinizing hormone (LH), which has to travel to the ovary from the anterior pituitary, or it may be short as in the case of hypothalamic releasing hormones, which have to travel only a short distance, i.e., from the hypothalamus to the pituitary gland.

The hormone that was first isolated is **secretin**, which was discovered by **Bayliss and Starling** in 1902.

In addition to **endocrine secretion,** which occurs into the blood stream, cells also communicate with each other through **paracrine secretion**. Here, the chemical signals are released into the extracellular fluid (ECF) and reach the target cell by simple diffusion through the ECF. Sometimes, cells respond to their own secretion and this is called **autocrine secretion (Figs. 60.1A to C).** Autocrine response is defined as one in which the hormone secreting cell is also responsive to the hormone that it secretes. This may result in feedback inhibition of the hormone secreted by the cell or there may be increase in the hormone output from the same cell.

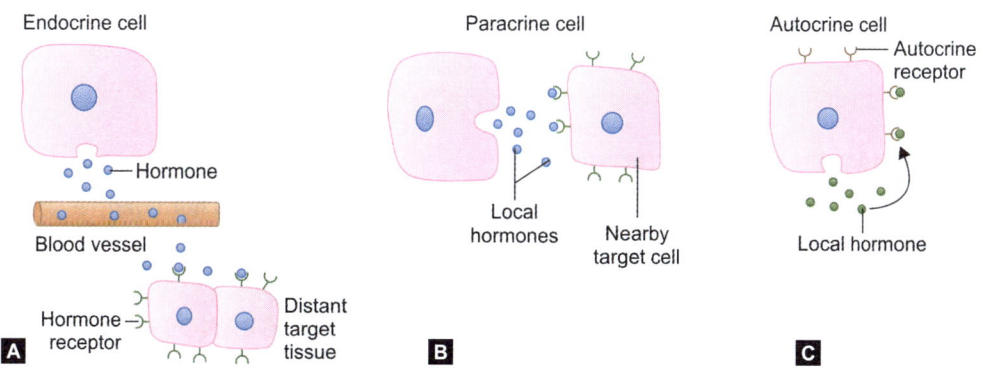

Figs. 60.1A to C: (A) Endocrine secretion; (B) Paracrine secretion; (C) Autocrine secretion.

Characteristics of Hormones

- Hormones are secretory products of ductless glands or of specialized cells which are released directly into the blood stream or to the extracellular fluid in response to a specific stimulus.
- Target cells are cells that respond to a particular hormone. These cells have receptors for the particular hormone. The hormone interact with the specific receptor to bring about the physiological effect.
- Hormones act as regulators of physiological processes occurring in the cell. As such they do not alter cellular reactions in the cell. They stimulate or inhibit specific enzymes which in turn bring about the biochemical reactions in the target tissue.
- Hormones are secreted in very low concentration.
- When compared to stimulation of nervous system, the latent period following stimulation of target cell by hormone is longer.
- Most hormones are metabolized rapidly after secretion in the liver or kidney.
- Different hormones exhibit synergistic effect. The combination of hormones produces a greater effect than when only one hormone is present. For example, epinephrine and glucagon increases blood glucose. When both are present together, the increase in blood sugar is far greater than the sum of the effects of the two hormones independently.
- Certain hormones show permissive effects. A particular hormone can exert its effect fully only if a second hormone is present.
- Some hormones have antagonistic effect on the same target tissue. For example, insulin decreases blood glucose while glucagon increases blood glucose by acting on the same tissue.
- Hormones can up regulate or down regulate their receptors. When the hormone concentration is increased in the extracellular fluid, the receptor number decreases and vice versa.

Functions of Hormones

The functions of hormones include regulation and integration of cellular function in general. There are five areas of hormonal action:

1. Regulation of constancy of internal environment by regulating its chemical composition and volume.
2. Smooth, sequential integration of growth and development.
3. Utilization, production and storage of energy; help the body cope with emergency situations such as infection, trauma, emotional stress, dehydration, starvation, hemorrhage and temperature extremes.
4. They contribute to the basic processes of reproduction including gamete production, fertilization, nourishment of the embryo and fetus, parturition and nourishment of newborn.
5. Role in behavior

RELATION BETWEEN ENDOCRINE SYSTEM AND NERVOUS SYSTEM

Nervous system and endocrine system are the two major systems that help to communicate and coordinate body functions. Endocrine system provides slow control over longer duration. Nervous system provides rapid control over shorter duration. These two systems are not independent of each other. They are interrelated and integrated. Nervous system integrates tissue functions through a network of neurons. The nerve endings release mediator molecules called **neurotransmitters**. The endocrine system integrates body functions via **hormones** secreted from endocrine glands into the extracellular fluid.

The **hypothalamus** is the highest center of control of endocrine system. It is also the highest center of autonomic nervous system (ANS). The hormones produced by the hypothalamus bridge the body's two major communication systems i.e., endocrine system and nervous system.

Nervous signals are converted to endocrine signals in some cases (e.g. neuroendocrine reflex like suckling reflex). A number of hormones act as mediators in the synapses. Several neurotransmitters are also hormones. For example, norepinephrine released at the postganglionic sympathetic ending acts as neurotransmitter. But the norepinephrine released by the cells of adrenal medulla acts as hormone.

Methods of Studying Endocrine Glands

- **Anatomical and histological methods:** The endocrine glands constitute ductless glands where, the organ has a glandular structure in histology. The gland is highly vascular because the hormone is secreted into the blood stream. Fenestrations are gaps in the capillary endothelium through which secretions escape into the blood stream.
- **Physiological methods**
  - *Ablation methods:* After ablation of the gland, look for deficiencies.
  - *Replacement:* Replacement of the gland will restore the original function.
  - *Transplantation studies:* Transplant a gland into a normal animal. Symptoms due to excess of hormones are seen.
- **Clinical methods:** Clinical syndromes due to deficiency or excess of hormones are seen (syndrome means group of symptoms).
- **Pathological methods:** Autopsy shows changes in a particular gland and we can confirm the diagnosis.
- **Biochemical methods**
  - Isolation
  - Purification
  - *Characterization* of hormone

Nowadays many hormones are being synthesized by biochemical methods, e.g., steroid hormones.

ENDOCRINE GLANDS (FIG. 60.2)

- Hypothalamus
- Anterior and posterior pituitary

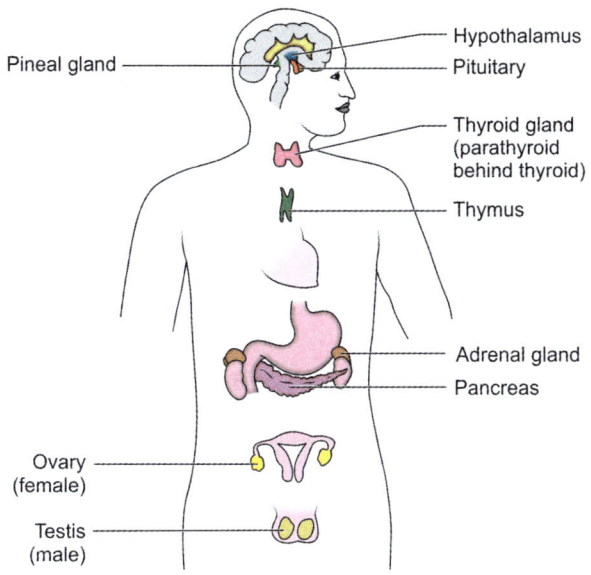

Fig. 60.2: Location of the major endocrine glands.

- Pineal gland
- Thyroid gland
- Parathyroid glands
- Adrenal cortex and medulla
- Islets of Langerhans of pancreas
- Thymus
- Ovary and testis
- Placenta.

The major endocrine glands and the hormones secreted by them are given in **Table 60.1**.

Tissues that Produce Hormones

Tissues that are not classically recognized as part of endocrine system produce hormones and play a vital role in endocrine regulation. These tissues include hypothalamus, gastrointestinal tract, adipose tissue, liver, heart, and kidney. Examples are:
- Juxtaglomerular cells of kidney: Erythropoietin
- Atrial cells of heart: Atrial natriuretic peptide (ANP)
- Gastrointestinal cells (APUD cells): Secretin, gastrin, cholecystokinin, etc.
- Salivary gland synthesizes nerve growth factor
- Endothelial cells: Endothelin, NO
- Lymphocytes, monocytes, macrophages: Interleukins, interferon, tumor necrosis factor
- Platelets and mesenchymal cells: Growth factor, integrins, annexin
- Adipose tissue: Leptin, resistin, interleukin-6, adiponectin etc.
- Liver cells: Insulin like growth factors (IGF-I and IGF-II).

With certain neoplasms, nonendocrine tissues can produce hormones, which are normally secreted only by endocrine tissues. For example, certain lung cancers secrete excessive amounts of arginine vasopressin (normally produced by hypothalamus) and some others like lung and gastrointestinal tumors produce ACTH (normally produced by the pituitary gland).

Table 60.1: Major endocrine glands and their hormones.

Endocrine gland	Hormones secreted
Anterior pituitary	Growth hormone (GH), thyroid stimulating hormone (TSH), adrenocorticotropic hormone (ACTH), follicle stimulating hormone (FSH), luteinizing hormone (LH) and prolactin
Posterior pituitary	Vasopressin and oxytocin
Thyroid gland	Thyroxine, tri-iodothyronine, calcitonin
Parathyroid gland	Parathyroid hormone (PTH)
Adrenal cortex	**Glucocorticoids:** Cortisol, corticosterone **Mineralocorticoids:** Aldosterone, 11-deoxycorticosterone **Sex steroids:** Androgen, estrogen, progesterone
Adrenal medulla	Epinephrine, norepinephrine, dopamine
Endocrine pancreas	Insulin, glucagon, somatostatin and pancreatic polypeptide
Pineal gland	Melatonin
Testis	Mullerian regression factor (MRF) in fetus, testosterone, dihydrotestosterone, and rostenedione, inhibin
Ovary	Estrogen, progesterone, inhibin, relaxin

Even though most of the endocrine glands produce 2 or more hormones, each hormone is secreted by individual cells within these glands. One exception is the gonadotropin producing cells of pituitary which secrete follicle stimulating hormone (FSH) and luteinizing hormone (LH).

Assessment of Endocrine Gland Function

- Assay of hormones
- Dynamic test for endocrine function

Assay of Hormones

Most of the hormones are present in very small concentrations in blood. So, very sensitive methods should be employed for hormonal assay.

Bioassay

One of the oldest methods is bioassay based on the effect of hormone on living animals. The hormone is injected into experimental animals and the effect studied. Bioassays are expensive, time consuming and sensitivity is less. Results are affected by several factors.

In Vitro Bioassays

Difficulties of bioassay to some extent have been overcome by in vitro bioassays. Incubation of the tissues, cells or cell membrane with the hormone is done and alteration in some function of the cell is studied.

Chemical Assay

Some hormones can be estimated by chemical methods. For example, steroids and catecholamines can be estimated by estimating their products of metabolism like vanillylmandelic acid (VMA).

Radioimmunoassay (RIA)

Radio-receptor assay: This method is related to RIA. Instead of antibody, the receptors on the tissues are made use of. This is used to assay the concentration of hormone in the plasma and also to study the receptor function.

Enzyme-linked immunosorbent assay: Enzyme linked immunosorbent assay (ELISA) is a colorimetric or flurometric assay. It is more sensitive and does not produce radioactive wastes.

Dynamic Test of Hormone Reserve and Regulation

This includes suppression test and stimulation tests, e.g., **metyrapone test** to assess adrenocortical status.

■ RADIOIMMUNOASSAY

Radioimmunoassay is the most important method of assay of hormones. **Berson and Talow** were awarded Nobel Prize for their work on this field in 1960. They first employed this method for the assay of insulin.

Principle

Radioimmunoassay depends on the competition between labeled hormone and unlabeled hormone for binding to specific antibody (Ab). The specific antibody to the hormone to be assayed is mixed with a small amount of labeled hormone (H*) and the plasma sample, which contains the hormone to be estimated.

$$H^* + H + Ab \rightarrow H^*Ab + HAb$$

The amount of labeled hormone getting bound to the antibody is inversely related to the amount of unlabeled hormone present in the mixture. In other words, when more unlabeled hormone is there in the mixture, only less of labelled hormone will bind to the antibody.

Reagents Required

- Specific antibody to the hormone to be assayed.
- Labeled hormone which is pure hormone labeled with 125I.
- Pure hormone in serial dilutions which is the standard.
- Plasma sample to be assayed.

Procedure

The standards and the plasma samples are taken in different small tubes. A small amount of the labeled hormone and small amount of antibody are added to this. It is important that the number of antibody molecules should not be enough to bind all the two types of hormone molecules so that there will be competition. The mixtures are incubated for 2–3 days at a low temperature to form the complex. The hormone antibody complex is separated and its radioactivity is determined. A standard curve is plotted with the concentration of the standard hormone on the X-axis and the % of binding of radioactivity on the Y-axis. It is plotted in a semi-log paper. The radioactivity of the hormone-antibody complexes is

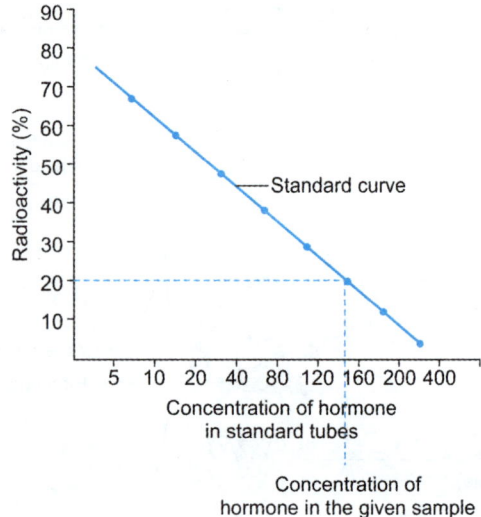

Fig. 60.3: Radioimmunoassay (RIA) of hormones.

calculated. Knowing the % binding of radioactivity in these labels we can read out the concentration of hormones in the given sample of plasma from a standard curve **(Fig. 60.3)**.

Advantages of RIA

- Highly sensitive
- Highly reproducible
- Large number of samples can be handled in less time
- Less expensive
- Less number of interfering factors.

■ CLINICAL SYNDROMES RELATED TO ENDOCRINE FUNCTIONS

Diseases of the endocrine system are numerous. Endocrine and metabolic disorders like diabetes mellitus, dyslipidemia, metabolic syndrome and thyroiditis are the most common diseases in developed countries. There are several syndromes due to deficiency or excess of hormones. Abnormality can be in the hypothalamus, pituitary or at any level. Sometimes, abnormal hormones are produced and at other times antibodies against receptors may be formed in the body. Excessive production of hormone may be due to some defect in the feedback regulation. There may be abnormal stimuli, which go on stimulating the gland. Tumors in other parts of the body may produce specific hormones.

Endocrine disorders can be due to:
- Hormone deficiency
- Hormone resistance
- Hormone excess.

Hormone Deficiency

- Deficiency of particular hormones is seen commonly when there is destruction of the gland producing the hormone mainly due to autoimmunity. For example, in type I diabetes mellitus there is destruction of the beta cells of pancreas leading to insulin deficiency, often from young age.

- Hormonal deficiency can also be due to inherited mutations in the genes responsible for their production.
- Defects in the enzymatic machinery needed for the hormone production or lack of the precursors for the hormone can lead to deficiency of the hormone. For example deficiency of iodine leads to decreased synthesis of thyroid hormones.

Hormone Resistance

- In certain endocrine disorders, adequate levels of the particular hormone are synthesized and released. But the target tissue will be resistant to the hormone's effects.
- Mutations in the hormone receptors may result in heritable syndromes of hormone resistance.
- Functional hormone resistance that develops over time is also seen. Target tissues gradually become more and more resistant to the action of the hormone secondary to reduced activation of intracellular signaling pathways. Type-II diabetes mellitus that occurs in adults is an example. Target tissues for insulin gradually become more and more resistant to the actions of insulin. This is secondary to reduced activation of phosphatidylinositol 3-kinase and other intracellular signaling pathways. Insulin sensitizers such as metformin help to prevent development of irreversible insulin resistance.
- An important feature of hormone resistance is that there will be overproduction of the hormone involved because the feedback loops that inhibit hormone synthesis and release are also desensitized. In case of type II diabetes mellitus this may lead to beta cell exhaustion and irreversible insulin resistance.

Hormone Excess

- A number of endocrine tumors may produce hormones in an excessive and uncontrolled manner. This type of hormone secretion is not regulated by normal feedback mechanisms of the hormone. For example, in tumor of the pituitary somatotropes, there is excessive secretion of growth hormone leading to gigantism.
- Certain tumors secrete hormones which are secreted at some other site from which they are not originally derived.
- Certain antibodies will mimic the action of certain hormones by binding to their specific receptors. Binding of the antibody to the receptor will stimulate the receptor. For example, in Grave's disease thyroid stimulating antibodies are produced which bind with the TSH receptors in the thyroid gland and stimulate it leading to hyperthyroidism. The excess hormone release is not subject to negative feedback in these conditions.
- Mutations in the receptors for hormonal action can also be associated with diseases due to hormone excess.

MULTIPLE CHOICE QUESTIONS

1. **An example of a single endocrine cell producing two different hormones:**
   a. Thyroid cell
   b. Delta cells of pancreas
   c. Gonadotrophs of pituitary
   d. Lactotrophs of pituitary

2. **Hormone produced by the APUD cells of gastrointestinal tract include all the following, *except*:**
   a. Calcitriol
   b. Somatostatin
   c. Gastrin
   d. Cholecystokinin

3. **In hormone resistance there will be:**
   a. Underproduction of the hormone concerned
   b. Overproduction of the hormone
   c. Normal production of the hormone
   d. The hormone will be absent

4. **False statement regarding antibodies produced against specific receptors:**
   a. Stimulate the receptors
   b. Inhibit the receptors
   c. Destroy the receptors
   d. Cause feedback regulation of the hormone secretion

5. **All the following hormones act as neurotransmitters, *except*:**
   a. Secretin
   b. Norepinephrine
   c. Nitric oxide
   d. Dopamine

6. **The hormone that was first isolated:**
   a. Insulin
   b. Secretin
   c. Growth hormone
   d. Gastrin

ANSWERS

1. c 2. a 3. b 4. d 5. a
6. b

Mechanism of Cellular Action of Hormones

CHAPTER 61

LEARNING OBJECTIVES
- Describe the mechanisms of hormone secretion, transport and degradation in the body
- Classify the various types of hormones
- Explain hormone receptors and their properties
- Describe and differentiate the mechanism of action of steroid, protein and amine hormones

INTRODUCTION

PY8.6: Describe and differentiate the mechanism of action of steroid, protein and amine hormones.

At the cellular level, hormones alter the functional level of the cell. Hormones bind to specific binding sites on the target cell called **receptors**. This binding results in a series of biochemical changes in the cell like increase in permeability of the cell, synthesis and degradation of substances, etc. Some hormones elicit responses within seconds (e.g. increase in heart rate by epinephrine) whereas, others may require hours or days (e.g. increase in protein synthesis by growth hormone). Receptors for hormones may be located in the cell membrane or in the cytoplasm or within the nucleus.
1. **Cell membrane receptors** for polypeptide hormones and catecholamines.
2. **Cytoplasmic receptors** in the case of steroid hormones.
3. **Intranuclear receptors** for thyroxine.

Hormones, which act by activation of genes, are steroid hormones and thyroid hormones.

HORMONE RECEPTORS

The hormones are recognized by specific high affinity receptors present in the target tissue. Receptors may be protein molecules or in the case of plasma membrane receptors, they are large glycoproteins composed of subunits. Each molecule extends completely through the plasma membrane. There are about 104–105 receptors in a target cell. The receptors are constantly being destroyed and synthesized and so, the receptor number is not static. Receptors are destroyed by lysosomes within the cell. Synthesis as well as recycling of receptors occurs in the cell.

The degree of hormone action depends not only on the concentration of hormones but also on the number and affinity of receptors. Receptors are always present in excess within the cell so that receptor availability will not be rate limiting for hormone action. A single target cell may have receptors for a number of hormones. Such multiple receptors allow interaction of a number of hormones. Once its target tissue recognizes a hormone, it can exert its biological action by a process known as **signal transduction**.

Receptors that directly gate ion channels are called **ionotropic receptors**. Those receptors that act through second messenger systems are called **metabotropic receptors**.

Up-regulation and Down-regulation of Receptors

The receptor's own hormone often regulates the receptor capacity. Usually, the regulation has an inverse relationship, i.e., a sustained excess of hormone decreases the number of its receptors per target cell. This limits its action. This process is called **down-regulation**. For example, increase in the concentration of insulin decreases the number of insulin receptors on the target cell. When the concentration of hormone decreases, the number of receptors will increase.

In certain cases, the hormone causes an increase in the number of its receptors in the target cell. For example, adrenocorticotropic hormone (ACTH) increases the number of ACTH receptors on the adrenal cortical cells. This type of regulation is called **up-regulation**.

Receptor Induction

Sometimes, heterologous hormones influence the receptor number. For example, follicle stimulating hormone (FSH) increases the number of luteinizing hormone (LH) receptors on the granulosa cells in the first half of the menstrual cycle. Thus, the follicle is capable of responding to the mid-cycle burst of LH secretion to cause ovulation.

Thyroxine increases the number of adrenergic receptors in heart. This is called **receptor induction**.

Receptor Specificity and Crossing over of Hormones

Most important feature of receptor is *receptor specificity*. A receptor will bind only its own specific hormone and a hormone will bind only with its own specific receptor, i.e., the match between the receptor and hormone is unique. But there are instances in which a hormone binds to receptors of other hormones, which have close resemblance with each other. For example, aldosterone receptor binds cortisol when cortisol is present in excess. This is called **crossing over of hormones**.

Complementary and Antagonistic Action of Hormones

For homeostasis, **complementary action** of several hormones may be necessary. For example, epinephrine, cortisol and glucagon have complementary action in maintaining blood glucose level to the body's response to severe short-term exercise like 100 meter dash. Lack of any of these hormones will adversely affect exercise performance. Growth hormone, IGF-1 and thyroid hormones are needed for normal growth. Deficiency of any of these hormones result in dwarfism.

Homeostasis also involves **antagonistic action** of certain hormones. The overall effect on the target tissue depends on the balance between the opposing effects. For example, glucagon and insulin have effects on the blood glucose levels. Insulin decreases blood glucose while glucagon increases blood glucose. A balance of actions of these hormones on blood glucose is responsible for maintaining normal blood glucose level. Deficiency of any one of these will lead to impaired blood glucose level.

Receptor Antibodies

- Antagonists or antibodies to receptors sometimes bind to receptors so that the hormonal effect is blocked. For example, the diuretic spironolactone acts by binding to aldosterone receptors and thereby **blocks** the action of aldosterone in the renal tubules, thus decreasing water and Na⁺ reabsorption.
- Alternatively, the antibody-receptor combination **mimics** the hormone-receptor interaction and enhances the function of the target cells, e.g., hyperthyroidism caused by Grave's disease, which is an autoimmune disorder. Here, the antibody combines with thyroid stimulating hormone (TSH) receptors in the thyroid gland and mediates the actions of TSH, which leads to hyperthyroidism.
- Sometimes, antibodies to receptors may **destroy** the receptors as in the case of myasthenia gravis where the acetyl choline receptors in the motor end plate are destroyed. This leads to muscle weakness.

Receptor Diseases

Receptor disease may be due to mutation of genes coding for the receptors or for the G protein subunits. Receptor mutation causing disease is seen for vasopressin receptor, thyroid hormone receptor, insulin receptor and 1, 25 dihydroxycholecalciferol receptor.

Chemical Nature of Hormones

Hormones may be peptides, amines, amino acid, steroid or glycoproteins.

1. **Peptide and protein hormones**—hypothalamic releasing hormones, pituitary hormones, insulin, parathormone, calcitonin, glucagon, cholecystokinin, secretin, vasoactive intestinal polypeptide. Peptide hormones are the most numerous among hormones.
2. **Monoamines**—catecholamines (adrenaline, noradrenaline and dopamine).
3. **Steroids and cholesterol derivatives**—estrogen, progesterone, testosterone, adrenal cortical hormones, calcitriol, etc.
4. **Amino acid derivatives**—thyroxine, triiodothyronine (tyrosine derivatives), melatonin (tryptophan derivative), serotonin.
5. **Arachidonic acid derivative**—prostaglandin family (PGF, PGE, PGA), prostacyclin and thromboxane.

Classification of Hormones Depending on Solubility

1. **Water-soluble hormones**: Pituitary hormones, parathormone, hormones of pancreas and adrenal medulla. The concerned glands are developed from ectoderm (adrenal medulla, pituitary) or endoderm (parathyroid, pancreas). Usually peptide hormones and catecholamines are water soluble.
2. **Lipid-soluble hormones**: Thyroid hormones, hormones of adrenal cortex, ovary and testis. The concerned glands develop from mesoderm.

Synthesis and Storage of Hormones

Hormones are synthesized in cell organelles, especially **rough endoplasmic reticulum** from precursors like amino acids, cholesterol, etc. The majority of peptide hormones are synthesized initially as much larger polypeptide chains. These are then processed intracellularly by specific proteases to form the final hormone molecule. The hormone precursors are by themselves inactive. Usually, the hormones are not stored in the endocrine gland in considerable amounts except thyroid gland in which large amount of thyroxine is stored. Protein hormones and catecholamines are stored in **secretory granules**. Thyroid hormones and steroid hormones are not stored in discrete granules but in cytoplasmic compartments.

Even though, most of the endocrine glands produce two or more hormones, individual cells within these glands secrete each hormone. One exception is the gonadotropin-producing cells (gonadotropes) of pituitary, which secrete both FSH and LH.

Release and Transport

Hormones are released into the blood stream by **exocytosis or by diffusion**. Hormones are transported through the blood stream with the help of specific transporting and binding proteins like thyroid binding globulin. In the blood, small amounts of hormone exist in the free form and this *free form is responsible for feedback regulatory mechanisms*. Peptide hormones and catecholamines get dissolved in plasma and is transported in the free form. Exception for peptide hormones that are transported in the bound form are IGF-I and IGF-II.

Normally, bound form is in equilibrium with the free form in plasma. When there is a fall in the plasma level of free form, more of hormone is released from the bound form. **Bound form** has the following functions

- Bound form provides a reservoir of the hormone in the blood so that minute-to-minute fluctuation in hormone concentration in blood is minimized
- Binding increases the half-life of the hormone in circulation. For example the half-life of bound T_4 is 7-8 days where as half-life of free T_4 is only several minutes. Most of the peptide hormones exist free in the circulation except for IGF-1 and IGF-2. Insulin like growth factors are tightly bound to plasma proteins in circulation.
- Hormones having long-term actions like induction of the synthesis of new proteins or enzymes in target tissues are usually in the bound form. Hormones like catecholamines, which have short-term role in the regulation of body homeostasis, circulate freely in blood without associated binding proteins.

Degradation of Hormones

The hormone in some cases is partially degraded in the target organ itself. After their function, most of the hormones are degraded in the liver and kidney and the degradation products are excreted through urine and bile.

INTERCELLULAR COMMUNICATION

PY1.3: Describe intercellular communication.

Intercellular communication is a fundamental biological process to coordinate the activities among neighboring and distant cells. This communication is mainly through chemical messengers. Most of the chemical messengers interact with specific receptors which may be cell surface receptors, cytosolic or nuclear receptors, and trigger a cascade of reactions within the cell. As discussed in chapter 60, the chemical messenger produced by one cell type can act on distant tissues by being transported through blood stream (endocrine), or on a neighboring cell in the same tissue (paracrine) or on the same cell that released the signaling molecule (autocrine).

Cells can also communicate by direct interactions. For example, neighboring cells can be electrically and metabolically coupled by means of gap junctions. These gap junctions play an important role in the flow of electrical current in cardiac and smooth muscle.

On the basis of signal transduction mechanisms, receptors are divided into 4 categories.

1. **Ligand gated ion channels or ionotropic receptors:** Ionotropic receptor is a part of an ion channel. Examples are ionotropic receptors for acetyl choline in muscle and nerve, serotonin, gamma amino butyric acid (GABA), glycine and ryanodine receptors (intracellular receptors in cell organelles like sarcoplasmic reticulum in muscle).
2. **Catalytic receptors:** When the catalytic receptors bind with a ligand, these membrane proteins themselves act as enzymes or part of an enzymatic complex. Atrial natriuretic peptide (ANP), insulin, growth hormone, erythropoietin, etc. act through catalytic receptors.
3. **Nuclear receptors:** These are proteins located in the cytosol or in the nucleus. They are ligand-activated transcription factors which produce specific gene transcription. Examples include receptors for steroid hormones, thyroid hormones, vitamin D, prostaglandin, etc.
4. **G-protein coupled receptors:** These receptors are coupled through intermediaries to activate or inactivate a separate membrane-associated enzyme or channel. The intermediary is a heterotrimeric (composed of α, β and γ subunits) guanosine triphosphate (GTP) binding complex called G-protein. Peptide hormones, norepinephrine, acetyl choline except in muscle and nerve and odorants act through these receptors.

■ G-PROTEINS

G-proteins are nucleotide regulatory proteins that are activated after binding guanosine triphosphate (GTP). They are members of the superfamily of GTP binding proteins. They play an important role in signal transduction in cells. When an activating signal reaches a G-protein, the protein exchanges guanosine diphosphate (GDP) for GTP. The GTP-protein complex brings about the effects of the G-protein. After action, the inherent GTPase activity of the protein then converts GTP to GDP restoring the G-protein to an inactive resting state.

Types of G-proteins

1. Small G-proteins
2. Large or heterotrimeric G-proteins.

Small G-proteins

There are 6 different subfamilies of small G-proteins. The important ones are **Rab, Rac** and **Ras** families. Some G-proteins which contain lipid modifications adhere to membranes, while others diffuse throughout the cytosol.

Functions of Small G-proteins

- **Rab family** regulates rate of vesicle movement between cell organelles and the cell membrane.
- **Rho/Rac** family mediates interaction between cytoskeleton and the cell membrane
- **Ras family** controls growth by regulating transmission of signals from the cell membrane to the nucleus.

Large G-proteins

Large G-proteins couple cell surface receptors to catalytic units that catalyze the intracellular formation of second messengers or couple the receptors directly to ion channels. Five families have been discovered: Gs, Gi, Gt, Gq and G_{13}. They are trimeric proteins consisting of 3 subunits; α, β and γ. Hence they are called **heterotrimeric G-proteins**. Both α and γ subunit have lipid modifications that anchor these proteins to the plasma membrane. The α-subunit is bound to GDP.

There are 16 different α subunits, 5 β subunits and 11 γ subunits in mammalian tissue. The multiple α, β and γ subunits demonstrate distinct tissue distributions and interact with different receptors and effectors. This provides the potential for several hundred combinations of the α, β and γ subunits. Hence, G proteins are ideally suited to link a diversity of effector molecules. For example, G protein Gs stimulates adenylyl cyclase whereas Gi inhibits adenylyl cyclase. The G protein αq subunit activates phospholipase C, which breaks phosphatidylinositol diphosphate into membrane associated diacylglycerol and cytosolic inosine triphosphate.

Alfred Gilman and Martin Rodbell received the 1994 Nobel Prize in physiology or medicine for their work in identifying G proteins and their functions.

Mechanism of Action

In the inactive state, G protein exists as a complex of α-GDP, β and γ subunits in which GDP occupies the guanosine nucleotide binding site of the α subunit **(Fig. 61.1A)**. When a hormone or ligand binds to a G-protein coupled receptor, a conformational change occurs in the receptor protein, which activates G-protein associated with it. This facilitates the release of bound GDP and simultaneous binding of GTP to the α-subunit. This GDP-GTP exchange stimulates dissociation of the complex from the receptor and the trimer splits into a free GTP bound α subunit and βγ complex.

The separated free GTP bound α-subunit interact with the effectors such as adenylyl cyclase and phospholipases and brings about many of the biological effects. The βγ-subunit complex is tightly bound to the cell and together form a signaling molecule that can also activate a variety of effectors like ion channels. The effectors of G-protein coupled receptors (GPCR) include ion channels (γβ subunit) and enzymes (GTP-α subunit).

The action via G protein is terminated by hydrolyzing GTP to GDP and inorganic phosphate. The intrinsic GTPase activity of the GTP-α subunit converts GTP to GDP and this leads to re-association of the α-GDP complex with the βγ complex and lead to termination of the effector activation **(Fig. 61.1A)**. Thus the cycle is completed.

MECHANISM BY WHICH COMBINATION OF HORMONE WITH RECEPTOR TRIGGERS CELLULAR FUNCTION

PY8.6: Describe and differentiate the mechanism of action of steroid, protein and amine hormones.

Conformational changes occur in the receptor when the hormone binds with it and the receptor gets activated. The

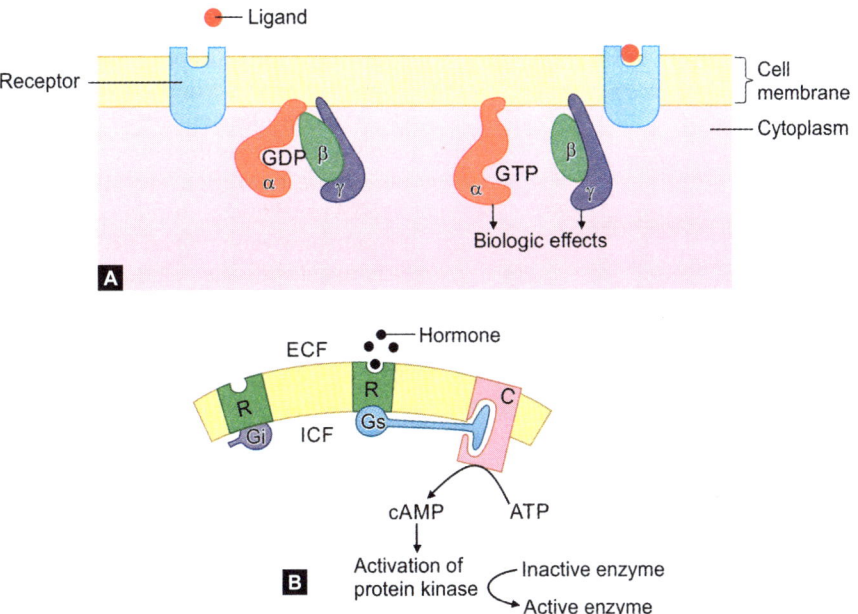

Figs. 61.1A and B: (A) Heterotrimeric G-protein. When the ligand binds to the G-protein coupled receptor, GTP replace GDP on the α-subunit. GTP-α separates from the βγ subunit. Both GTP-α and βγ subunit activates enzymes and produce physiological effects. GTP-α has intrinsic GTPase activity which converts GTP to GDP and the α, β and γ subunits reassociate; (B) Adenylyl cyclase - cAMP system.

(R: hormone sensitive receptor; Gs: stimulating G protein; C: catalytic unit (adenylyl cyclase); Gi: inhibiting G protein; GTP: guanosine triphosphate; GDP: guanosine diphosphate; ECF: extracellular fluid; ICF: intracellular fluid; ATP: adenosine triphosphate; cAMP: cyclic adenosine monophosphate)

activation of receptors in turn stimulates cellular functions by different mechanisms:
- By altering the permeability of cell membrane
- By generation of second messengers
- By activating genetic mechanisms
- By tyrosine kinase activation

Action through Change in Membrane Permeability

Certain hormones like adrenaline and noradrenaline bind to receptors present on the cell membrane. This binding leads to conformational change in the receptor causing either opening or closing of ion channels like Na$^+$ channel, K$^+$ channel, etc.

Action through Second Messengers

Most of the polypeptide hormones cannot enter the cells. They combine with specific receptors on the cell membrane and this combination of hormone and receptor leads to the formation of a second messenger within the cell (**Flowchart 61.1**).

The second messenger in turn triggers the actions in the cell. Enzyme activation by the second messenger is achieved largely by inducing the phosphorylation of specific proteins. Hence, the liberation of phosphate is an important feature of action via second messengers. The extracellular ligands (hormones) are called **first messengers** and the intracellular mediators are called **second messengers**. Not only do multiple hormones utilize the same second messenger system, but a single hormone can utilize more than one system (**Table 61.1**).

Flowchart 61.1: Mechanism of action of hormones through second messengers.

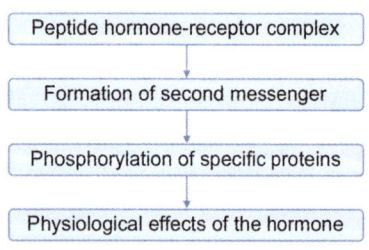

Peptide hormones that do not need second messengers for their action are growth hormone, insulin like growth factor (IGF), prolactin and insulin. These hormones act through a protein kinase cascade and the receptors for these hormones have intrinsic tyrosine kinase activity.

There are a number of second messengers like:
- Cyclic AMP (cAMP)
- Ca^{2+} and calcium binding proteins like calmodulin
- Cyclic GMP
- Prostaglandins
- Inositol triphosphate (IP$_3$) and diacylglycerol.

Adenylyl Cyclase-cAMP System

Cyclic adenosine mono phosphate (cAMP) is formed from ATP by the action of the enzyme adenylyl (adenylate) cyclase present on the cell membrane, with Mg^{2+} as cofactor. Three components are involved in the activation or inhibition of adenylyl cyclase:
1. Hormone-sensitive receptor (R)
2. Coupling units (Gs and Gi)
3. Catalytic cyclase or catalytic unit (C) which is the enzyme, adenylyl cyclase

The receptors acting through this system are **G-protein coupled receptors**. Coupling units may be stimulatory or inhibitory G proteins that link the receptor to the catalytic unit. *Gs is the stimulatory G protein and Gi is the inhibitory G protein.* When a hormone binds to the receptor which is coupled with Gs subunit it activates adenylyl cyclase to form cAMP. When a hormone binds to receptor coupled with Gi, it inhibits adenylyl cyclase (**Fig. 61.1B**) leading to an inhibitory action in the cell.

When the hormone binds to the receptor, it leads to coupling of the receptor to a G protein. If it is a stimulatory G protein (Gs), the receptor interacts with C through Gs so that coupling unit 'Gs' combines with GTP. Hormone-receptor-Gs-GTP complex activates the catalytic adenylyl cyclase (C) and this facilitates the conversion of ATP to cAMP liberating phosphate. cAMP activates cAMP-dependent protein kinase A (PKA) and this in turn leads to further enzyme activation by phosphorylation (**Fig. 61.2**). This produces biochemical reactions inside the cell that lead to the response of the cell to the hormone (**Flowchart 61.2**).

Table 61.1: Hormones and their second messengers.

Hormone	Second messenger	Membrane located enzyme	Kinase
CRH, ACTH, FSH, LH, MSH, TSH, hCG, ADH (V$_2$-receptors), parathormone, calcitonin, glucagon, somatostatin, secretin; and catecholamines acting through β-adrenergic receptors	cAMP	Adenylyl cyclase	cAMP dependent protein kinase
ANP and nitric oxide	cGMP	Guanylyl cyclase	cGMP dependent protein kinase
Angiotensin II (vascular smooth muscle), ADH (V$_1$A receptors in vascular smooth muscle), oxytocin, CCK, gastrin, gonadotropin-releasing hormone (GnRH) growth hormone–releasing hormone (GHRH) parathyroid hormone (PTH) oxytocin, thyrotropin-releasing hormone (TRH), substance P, ACh (muscarinic) and α$_1$ adrenergic catecholamines	Ca^{2+} Inositol triphosphate Diacylglycerol	Phospholipase-C	Protein kinase C, calmodulin dependent protein kinase

(CRH: corticotropin releasing hormone; ACTH: adenocorticotrophic hormone; FSH: follicle stimulating hormone; LH: luteinising hormone; MSH: melanocyte-stimulating hormones; TSH; thyroid stimulating hormone; hCG: human chorionic gonadotropin: ADH: antidiuretic hormone; CCK: Cholecystokinin; ACH: acetylcholine)

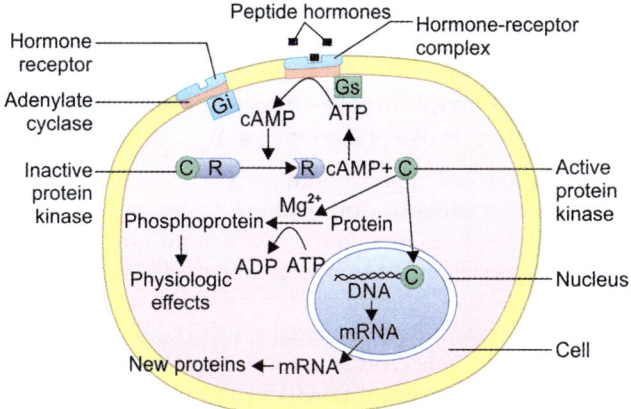

Fig. 61.2: Mechanism of action of peptide hormone.
(ADP: adenosine diphosphate; ATP: adenosine triphosphate; DNA: deoxyribonucleic acid; mRNA: messenger ribonucleic acid)

Flowchart 61.2: Role of cAMP as a second messenger.

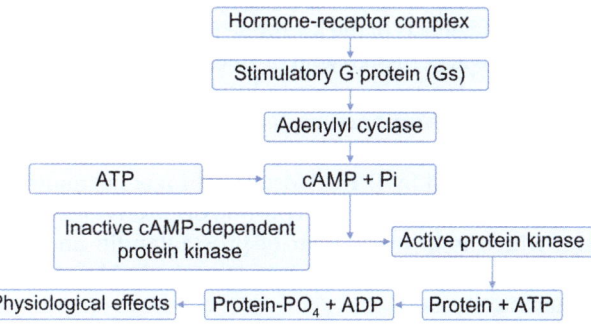

(Pi: inorganic phosphate)

Once cAMP is formed inside the cell, it activates a cascade of enzymes. The first enzyme that is activated activates a second enzyme which in turn activates a third enzyme and so on until a large amount of enzymes get activated. Thus a small amount of hormone can activate a large number of enzymes in the cell. Depending on the coupling of the hormone receptor to an inhibitory or stimulatory G protein, a hormone can either increase or decrease the concentration of cAMP and there by decrease the phosphorylation of proteins inside the cell. For his works on cAMP, **Earl Sutherland** was awarded Nobel Prize in 1970.

The activation of protein kinase is terminated in two ways:
1. The cytoplasmic enzyme **phosphodiesterase** in the cell degrade cAMP to 5'-AMP
2. **Phosphoprotein phosphatases** can dephosphorylate enzymes and proteins that had previously been phosphorylated by protein kinase A.

Summary of Adenylyl Cyclase-cAMP System

❖ The hormone binds to its receptor in the plasma membrane of target cells
❖ Coupling of hormone receptor to G protein
❖ If the G protein is a stimulatory G protein (Gs protein), it stimulates adenylyl cyclase, which is also an integral membrane protein **(Flowchart 61.2)**.
❖ Activated adenylyl cyclase converts ATP to cyclic AMP, resulting in an elevated intracellular concentration of cAMP.
❖ High levels of cAMP in the cytosol activate cAMP dependent protein kinase A
❖ Active protein kinase A add phosphates to other enzymes inside the cell, thereby changing their conformation and modulating their catalytic activity
❖ Levels of cAMP decrease due to the breakdown of cAMP by phosphodiesterase to physiologically inactive 5'AMP and due to the inactivation of adenylyl cyclase.
❖ If the hormone-receptor complex couples to an inhibitory G protein (Gi protein), it leads to inhibition of adenylyl cyclase. This decreases formation of cAMP leading to an inhibitory action in the cell.

> The hormones that act by inhibiting cAMP formation are norepinephrine acting via α_2 receptors and somatostatin.

Applied Aspect

Two bacterial toxins affect adenylyl cyclase system mediated by G protein. **Cholera toxin** causes prolonged stimulation of adenylyl cyclase system by inhibiting GTPase activity. In intestinal epithelial cells, cAMP decreases Na^+ absorption and increase Cl^- secretion. The increased NaCl content in the intestinal lumen increases the osmolarity of the contents. This retains water in the lumen leading to watery diarrhea and severe dehydration.

Pertussis toxin produced in whooping cough decreases adenylyl cyclase activity by activating inhibitory G-protein (Gi subunit). This impairs the defense mechanism of the patient.

The drug **forkolin** stimulates adenylyl cyclase activity by a direct action.

Hormones that Act through Adenylyl Cyclase–cAMP Second Messenger System

❖ Adrenocorticotropic hormone (ACTH)
❖ Angiotensin II (epithelial cells)
❖ Calcitonin
❖ Catecholamines (β receptors)
❖ Corticotropin-releasing hormone (CRH)
❖ Follicle-stimulating hormone (FSH)
❖ Glucagon
❖ Growth hormone–releasing hormone (GHRH)
❖ Human chorionic gonadotropin (hCG)
❖ Luteinizing hormone (LH)
❖ Parathyroid hormone (PTH)
❖ Secretin
❖ Somatostatin
❖ Thyroid-stimulating hormone (TSH)
❖ Vasopressin (V_2 receptor, epithelial cells).

Calcium-Calmodulin System

The combination of the hormone with the receptor increases the intracellular Ca^{2+} concentration. Hormones like angiotensin II, catecholamines acting through α1 receptors, oxytocin, etc., combine with specific receptors in the target cell membrane. This complex increases the intracellular Ca^{2+} concentration by the release of Ca^{2+} from intracellular stores or by increasing the entry of Ca^{2+} from extracellular fluid into the cell through ligand-gated Ca^{2+} channel. Ca^{2+} in the cytoplasm combines with specific Ca^{2+} binding protein called calmodulin. Ca^{2+}-calmodulin complex activates specific enzymes in the cell, thereby triggering biochemical changes within the cell (**Flowchart 61.3**). One of the actions of catecholamines through α-receptors is increasing glycogenolysis in liver. Ca^{2+}-calmodulin complex activates **phosphorylase kinase** enzyme which catalyzes the reaction. Another enzyme activated by Ca^{2+}-calmodulin complex is myosin light chain kinase, which causes contraction of smooth muscles. This complex in some cells brings about increased secretion.

> Calcineurin is a Ca^{2+}-calmodulin dependent protein phosphatase which causes dephosphorylation of Ca^{2+} channels and inactivates them. It activates T cells of the immune system. Calcineurin is inhibited by immunosuppressant drugs like cyclosporine.

Guanylyl Cyclase-cGMP System

Peptide hormones like atrial natriuretic peptide (ANP) bind to receptor which is itself guanylyl cyclase that converts cytoplasmic guanosine-tri-phosphate (GTP) to cGMP. The cGMP in turn can activate cGMP-dependent kinases, phosphatases, or ion channels. The action of nitric oxide on vascular smooth muscle and some actions of ANP are brought about by increasing cGMP. The effects of light on rods and cones of retina are by reducing cGMP.

Membrane Phospholipase-phospholipid System (Phosphatidyl Inositol Derivatives)

G protein coupled to phospholipase C

Phosphatidyl inositol diphosphate is derived from the phospholipid of cell membrane. The action is mediated by G protein, $G\alpha_q$ coupled to phospholipase C. When $G\alpha_q$ is activated by peptide hormones like arginine vasopressin, it activates the enzyme phospholipase C (PLC). Phosphatidyl inositol diphosphate cleaves to form **inositol triphosphate (IP_3)** and **diacylglycerol (DAG)** in the presence of PLC. IP_3 combines with receptors on the cytoplasmic surface of endoplasmic reticulum. This causes release of Ca^{2+} from endoplasmic reticulum and increase in intracellular Ca^{2+} several fold. Ca^{2+} activates calcium dependent kinases like protein kinase C (PKC), Ca^{2+}-calmodulin dependent kinases, etc. This leads to alteration in cell function and the physiological effects of the hormone (**Flowchart 61.4**).

DAG activates the enzyme protein kinase C (PKC). PKC is also activated by increase in intracellular Ca^{2+}. Protein kinase C then phosphorylates a number of proteins which are enzymes leading to the cell's response. The actions of TSH is mediated by DAG. Most of the local hormones act through this system. The lipid portion of DAG is arachidonic acid, which is the precursor of prostaglandin and other local hormones that causes a wide variety of local effects throughout the body.

G Protein Coupled to Membrane Bound Enzyme, Phospholipase A_2

Some G proteins are coupled to **phospholipase A_2**. Some peptide hormones like TRH combines with G protein coupled receptor $G\alpha_q$ or $G\alpha_{11}$. Stimulation of these receptors leads to the stimulation of membrane bound phospholipase A_2 (PLA_2). PLA_2 cleaves membrane phospholipids to produce **lysophospholipid** and **arachidonic acid**. Arachidonic acid is converted by enzymes into a variety of biologically active **eicosanoids** like prostaglandin, prostacyclin, thromboxane and leukotrienes.

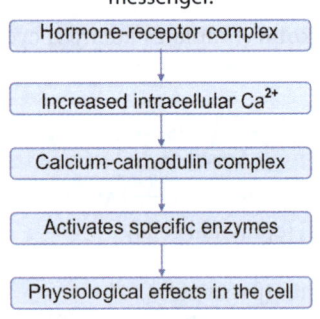

Flowchart 61.3: Mechanism by which Ca^{2+} act as a second messenger.

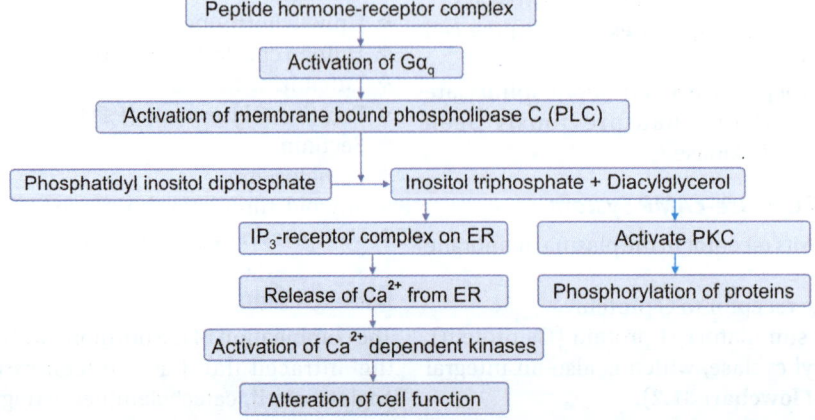

Flowchart 61.4: Mechanism of action of phospholipid-phospholipase system.

Specificity of hormonal action is due to the following reasons:

- Specificity of receptors
- Presence of specific enzymes. The effects of the same second messenger on different tissues vary because the enzyme systems in different tissues are different. For example, when cAMP acts on thyroid cells when these cells are activated by TSH, there is increased synthesis of thyroid hormones. Whereas, if cAMP acts on adrenocortical cells there will be increased secretion of adrenal cortical steroid hormones. In the collecting tubules of the kidney, cAMP increases its permeability to water.
- Specificity resulting from the activation of different second messengers. The activation of different receptors by the same hormone may result in a different response in the same cell. For example, adrenaline can act on α_2-receptors and produce an inhibitory response in the target cell while it can act on β-receptors in the same target cell and induce a stimulatory response. Binding of adrenaline to β-receptors activates $G\alpha_s$ protein which results in the activation of adenylyl cyclase and increase in cAMP. This leads to increase in the activity of PKA. Whereas binding of adrenaline to α_2 receptors activate $G\alpha_i$ protein which inhibit adenylyl cyclase and decrease cAMP. This decreases PKA activity. α_1-receptors which are linked to $G\alpha_q$ activates phospholipase C and increases IP_3 and DAG. This mechanism through the use of Ca^{2+} as second messenger exerts its effects. Dopamine D1 receptor is coupled to $G\alpha_s$ and D2 receptor is linked to $G\alpha_i$.

Activation of Genetic Mechanism

Activation of genetic mechanism is the most important mechanism of action of **steroid hormones** that enter the cells. The hormone binds with specific mobile receptors in the cytoplasm and the receptor-hormone complex stimulates genetic mechanism to increase the production of specific enzymes **(Fig. 61.3)**. The events are as follows:

- Steroid hormone being lipid soluble easily passes through the cell membrane.
- The hormone combines with mobile receptors in the cytoplasm.
- Receptor-hormone complex moves into the nucleus and binds to specific portion of DNA molecule.
- Specific genes are activated, transcription occurs and specific mRNA is formed.
- The mRNA move into the cytoplasm where they act at the ribosomal level and facilitate translation, and new enzymes are synthesized **(Flowchart 61.5)**.
- The enzymes activate specific biochemical reactions in the cell.

Thyroxine also acts by stimulating the genetic mechanism but the receptors are present within the nucleus.

Action through Tyrosine Kinase Activation

Activation of tyrosine kinase occurs by two mechanisms.
1. When the hormone binds with the receptor, the receptor itself becomes a tyrosine kinase
2. The receptor itself does not have kinase activity. But when the hormone binds with the extracellular portion of the receptor it can attract intra-cytoplasmic tyrosine kinases like Janus tyrosine kinases (JAKs).

In the **first mechanism**, the receptors have an intracellular tyrosine kinase domain. They themselves act as **protein kinases** when activated **(Fig. 61.4)**.

- These enzyme linked receptors have their hormone binding site on the outside of the cell membrane and their catalytic site on the inside.
- Binding of the hormone with the extracellular portion of the receptor causes dimerization of two similar receptors.
- The dimerization and cross phosphorylation of the receptors leads to its activation.
- These receptors when activated, functions directly as enzymes.
- The kinase activity associated with such receptors results in phosphorylation of tyrosine residues on other enzymes and they get activated **(Fig. 61.4)**.
- The activated tyrosine kinase receptor activates small G-protein Ras

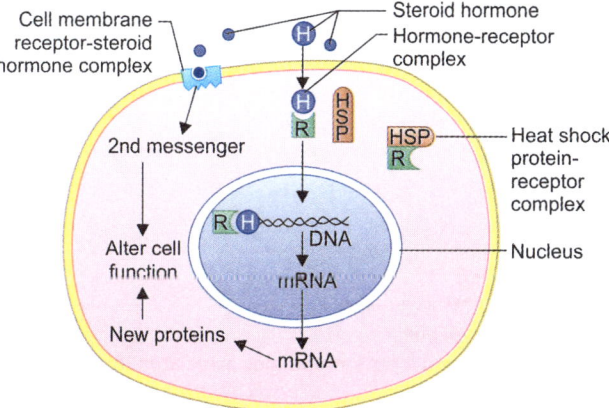

Fig. 61.3: Mechanism of action of steroid hormone. The figure shows both the genomic and the non-genomic actions.

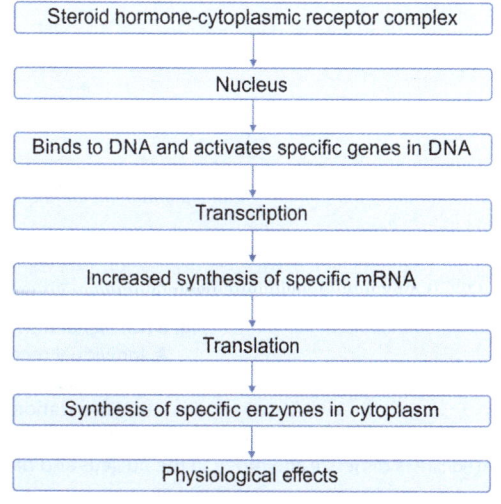

Flowchart 61.5: Action of steroid hormone by activation of genetic mechanism.

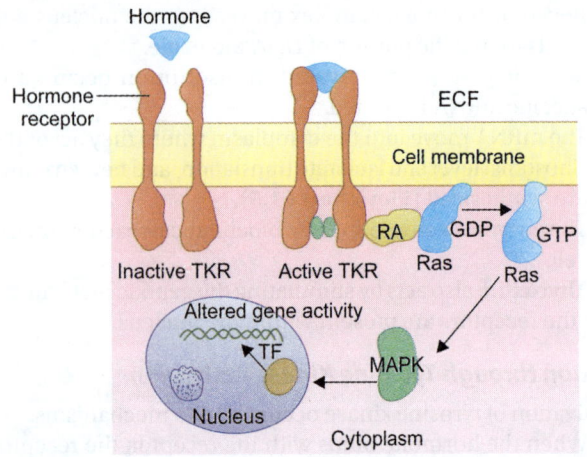

Fig. 61.4: Action of hormone through tyrosine kinase activation.

(TKR: tyrosine kinase domain of the receptor; RA: Ras activator; Ras: small G protein; MAPK: mitogen activated protein kinase; TF: transcription factor; GDP: guanosine diphosphate).

- Activated Ras activates mitogen activated protein kinases (MAP K)
- MAP kinases eventually lead to the production of transcription factors in the nucleus that alter gene expression.
- This mechanism of signal generation does not require G protein intermediates.

Insulin is an example of a hormone whose receptor is a tyrosine kinase. Other hormones acting through this system includes erythropoietin, and several growth factors like nerve growth factor, insulin-like growth factor, activin and epidermal growth factor.

In the **second mechanism** when the hormone binds to domains exposed on the cell surface it results in a conformational change in the receptor that activates kinase domains located in the cytoplasmic regions of the receptor. In many cases, the receptor phosphorylates itself as part of the kinase activation process. The activated receptor phosphorylates a variety of intracellular targets, many of which are enzymes that become activated or are inactivated upon phosphorylation. Hormones acting through this system include growth hormone, prolactin, oxytocin, leptin etc. One example of this system is the JAK- STAT pathway.

JAK-STAT Pathway (Fig. 61.5)

- Certain receptors are associated with inactive Janus tyrosine kinases.
- When the hormone binds to the extracellular portion of the receptor, it can phosphorylate the receptor and the associated **Janus tyrosine kinase (JAK).**
- Activated JAK in turn will attract STATs which then associates with the phosphorylated receptors **(Fig. 61.5).**

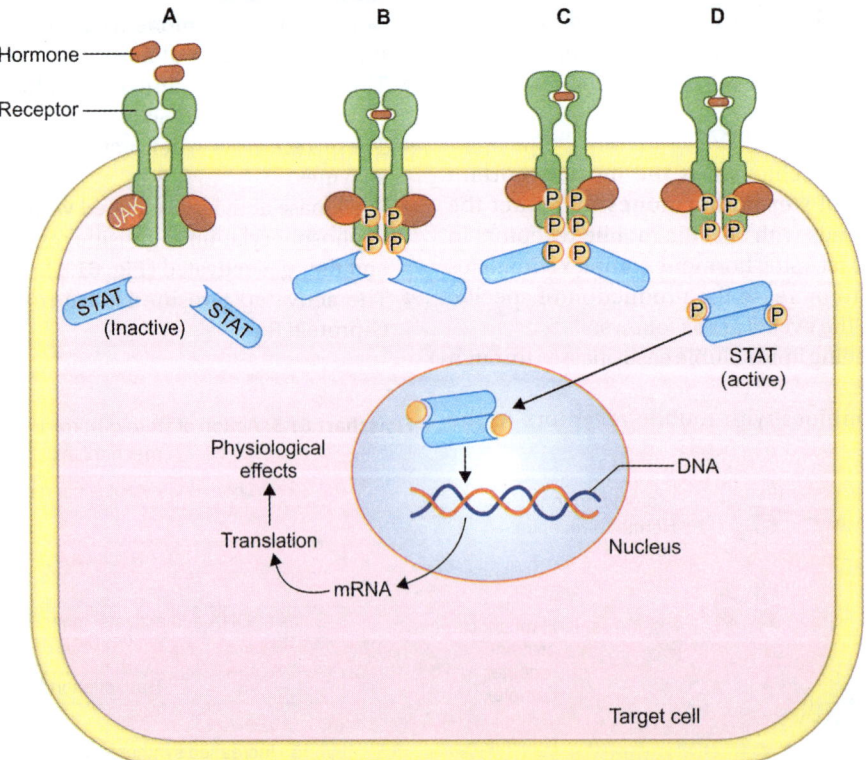

Fig. 61.5: Signal transduction through the JAK-STAT pathway.
A. Individual receptors associated with inactive JAKs,
B. Ligand binding to the receptor leads to phosphorylation of tyrosine residues on opposing receptors and their associated JAK. This leads to dimerization of receptor and activation of JAK,
C. STATs then associate with phosphorylated receptors and JAKs in turn phosphorylate these STATs,
D. Activated STATs dimerize and move to the nucleus and bind to target gene on the DNA. Specific mRNA is formed following transcription.
(JAK: Janus tyrosine kinase; STAT: signal transducer and activator of transcription)

- ❖ JAKs in turn will phosphorylate **signal transducers and activators of transcription (STAT)** proteins.
- ❖ Phosphorylated STATs will form dimers and move to the nucleus where they bind to specific sites in the DNA and act as transcription factors.
- ❖ Activation of target genes leads to the synthesis of proteins or enzymes which mediates the hormone action.

GENOMIC AND NONGENOMIC EFFECTS OF HORMONES

Some actions of steroid hormones are more rapid than those that are mediated via binding to DNA. This has led to the hypothesis of **non-genomic actions of steroid hormones**. These actions are mediated by membrane receptors and second messengers especially Ca^{2+} formed inside the cells (*see* **Fig. 61.3**). Steroid and thyroid hormones after binding to nuclear receptors, bind to DNA to either increase or decrease gene transcription in the target tissue.

Most of the hormones which act on receptors within the cell or nucleus causing gene transcription, target gene expression, and ultimately cellular responses are referred to as genomic effects of a hormone. Non-genomic effects of some hormones do not depend on gene transcription or protein synthesis. Signal transduction occurs through steroid hormone receptors that do not involve gene transcription. The hormones having both genomic and non-genomic effects include glucocorticoids, estrogen, progesterone, aldosterone and androgens. The characteristics of non-genomic effects are:
- ❖ Action is very rapid (seconds to minutes). For genomic actions there will be a time lag of hours or even days.
- ❖ Non-genomic effects can be elicited in steroid hormones even if they are prevented from crossing the cell membrane and entering the cell
- ❖ Non-genomic effects are not blocked by inhibitors of mRNA or protein synthesis
- ❖ Non-genomic effects are not blocked by antagonists of the genomic steroid receptors

REGULATION OF HORMONE SECRETION

Rate of secretion of hormones is regulated precisely to meet the needs of the body in different situations. The central nervous system ultimately regulates almost all the endocrine glands. The nerves directly control the pituitary and adrenal medulla. The anterior pituitary controls other important endocrine glands like thyroid, adrenal cortex and gonads. *Islets of Langerhans and parathyroid are not regulated by pituitary.* These are regulated by blood glucose and Ca^{2+} levels.

Fine adjustments of the secretion of hormones to meet the needs of the body are through feedback mechanisms acting either on the endocrine glands or on the nervous system. Feedback is normally negative and the net result of negative feedback is to restore homeostasis. There are examples of positive feedback as well. Feedback is usually provided by the secretion of the endocrine gland itself or by the blood concentration of a variable.

Feedback Mechanisms

1. Negative feedback
2. Positive feedback
3. Modifying feedback.

Negative Feedback

Negative feedback mechanism is the most common control mechanism or homeostatic mechanism and involves the inhibition of the initial hormone release mechanism or stimuli. Negative feedback mechanism helps the body to maintain a steady state. The synthesis and release of many hormones is subject to regulation by negative feedback loops. The hormone produced act back to inhibit its further release. The different types of negative feedback mechanisms are:

1. **Short-short loop feedback:** The hormone suppresses its own secretion by a local effect.
2. **Short loop feedback:** The hormone suppresses the factor which is responsible for its release. For example, estrogen produced by ovaries inhibits the secretion of FSH by the anterior pituitary. FSH is responsible for the secretion of estrogen by the ovary.
3. **Long loop feedback:** One hormone stimulates the secretion of another hormone from its target tissue. The second hormone secreted by the target gland (e.g., pituitary) stimulates the secretion of another hormone from an endocrine gland. The third hormone will inhibit the secretion of the first hormone by a long loop feedback mechanism. For example, cortisol inhibits the secretion of corticotrophin releasing hormone from the hypothalamus, estrogen and progesterone from ovaries inhibit the secretion of gonadotropin releasing hormone from hypothalamus (**Fig. 61.6**).

An example of negative feedback mechanism operating to maintain a steady state of the variable, blood osmolality is shown in **Flowchart 61.6**. Blood osmolality is maintained within a range of 275–299 mOsm/L to maintain homeostasis. Blood osmolality will increase in conditions like dehydration and decrease in conditions like over-hydration. When osmolality is increased by 10 mOsm, the osmoreceptors in the hypothalamus get stimulated leading to the release of ADH or vasopressin from the posterior pituitary. Vasopressin acts on the collecting duct of the renal tubule leading to increased reabsorption of water from the tubular fluid. The reabsorption of water into the blood brings back the osmolality to the physiological range. When homeostasis of blood osmolality is achieved, there will be a negative feedback on the cells of the hypothalamus and release of vasopressin is inhibited. This will prevent over-hydration of blood.

Positive Feedback

Positive feedback mechanism means that some consequence of hormonal secretion acts on the secretory cells to provide augmented drive for further secretion. The drive for secretion becomes progressively more intense and usually terminates in an explosive event. The action of the positive feedback system continues until it is interrupted by some mechanism outside the feedback system. If the action of the

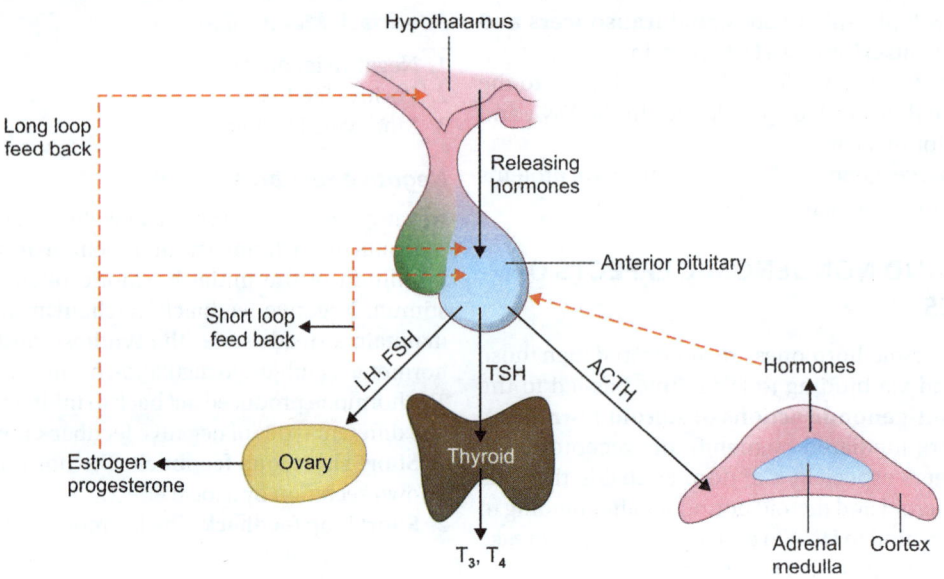

Fig. 61.6: Regulation of hormone secretion by negative feedback mechanisms. Dashed arrows indicate inhibition.
(FSH: follicle stimulating hormone; LH: luteinizing hormone; ACTH: adrenocorticotropic hormone; TSH: thyroid stimulating hormone)

Flowchart 61.6: Feedback mechanism operating to maintain blood osmolality within physiological range.

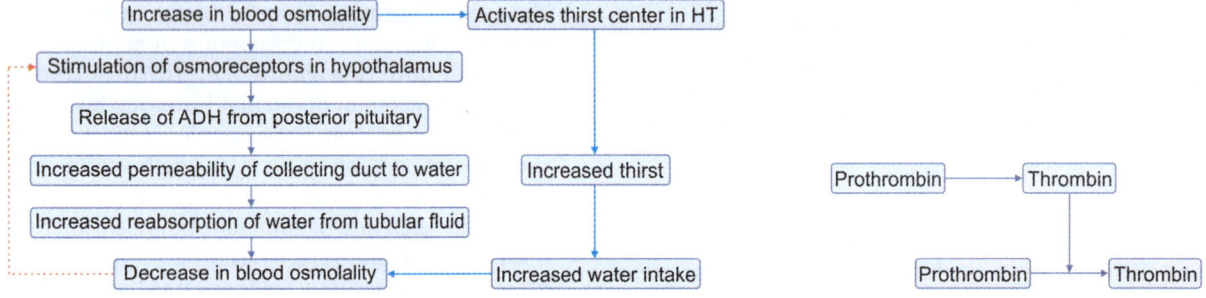

(HT: hypothalamus; ADH: antidiuretic hormone. Dashed line indicates negative feedback inhibition)

positive feedback system is not stopped, it may even produce life threatening conditions in the body as in the case of irreversible stage of circulatory shock. In contrast to negative feedback mechanism, positive feedback is not self-limiting. In negative feedback system, the action stops as the initial condition returns to normal state.

Positive feedback mechanisms rarely occur in the body. For example, during **childbirth**, the stimulus for oxytocin secretion is dilatation of uterine cervix by the descending part of the baby. Oxytocin causes uterine contraction, which pushes the baby further down, causing more dilatation of cervix. The impulses reach the hypothalamus and more and more oxytocin are being secreted which causes intense contraction of the uterus expelling the baby out **(Fig. 61.7)**. Another example is the **LH surge** occurring in the mid-luteal phase of ovarian cycle in female where, high circulating level of estrogen produces increased secretion of LH rather than inhibiting LH secretion. LH surge is followed by ovulation. Normally, moderate levels of estrogen have a negative feedback effect on LH secretion.

Other positive feedback mechanisms operating in the body include:

a. In **blood coagulation**, once a small amount of thrombin is formed it acts on prothrombin to form still more thrombin and it continues till interrupted. Blood coagulation is controlled by the fibrinolytic system operating in the body normally. But in disseminated intravascular coagulation (DIC) this control mechanism fails, leading to widespread coagulation in the body by positive feedback.

b. Irreversible stage of **circulatory shock** is also a positive feedback mechanism operating in the body.

c. When an excitable cell is stimulated, there is slight leakage of Na^+ through Na^+ channels into the interior of the cell. The change in membrane potential thus produced will make the membrane more and more permeable to Na^+ by opening up more Na^+ channels and an action potential is produced which spreads through the membrane by this positive feedback mechanism.

Modifying Feedback

In modifying feedback, it is the metabolite and not the hormone that is responsible for the feedback effect. For example, increase in blood sugar level stimulates insulin secretion and inhibits glucagon secretion. Increase in

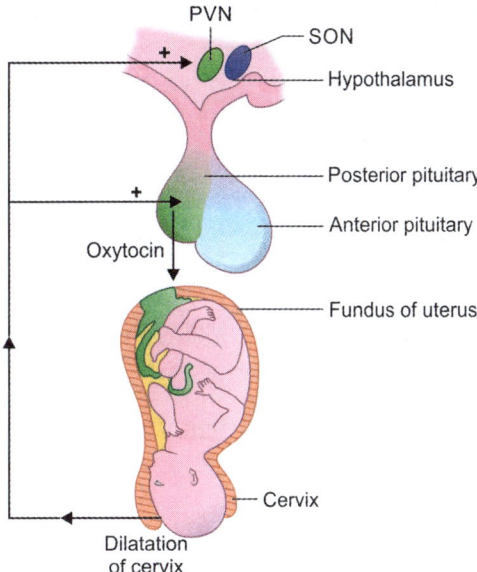

Fig. 61.7: Positive feedback mechanism by which intensely strong contractions of uterus occur during labor, expelling the baby.
(PVN: paraventricular nucleus; SON: supraoptic nucleus)

blood calcium inhibits parathyroid hormone secretion and stimulates calcitonin secretion. The secretion of renin by the kidney will be suppressed by retention of sodium and water produced by renin-angiotensin-aldosterone mechanism.

MULTIPLE CHOICE QUESTIONS

1. Which of the following is not mediated through negative feedback mechanism?
    a. Blood pressure
    b. GH secretion
    c. Thrombus formation
    d. ACTH release
2. About the homeostatic mechanism of the body, following are true, *except*:
    a. Values revolve around the mean
    b. Value of controlled variable is compared to the reference value
    c. Value of controlled variable oscillates near a set point
    d. System is stabilized by the positive feedback mechanism
3. Positive feedback is seen in all, *except*:
    a. LH surge
    b. Entry of calcium into sarcoplasmic reticulum
    c. Stimulation of gastric secretion by histamine and gastrin
    d. Thrombolytic activity in coagulation cascade
4. Which of the following is a membrane bound enzyme that catalyzes the formation of cyclic AMP from ATP?
    a. Tyrosine kinase   b. Polymerase
    c. ATP synthase   d. Adenylate cyclase
5. Cholera toxin:
    a. Increases the level of intracellular cyclic GMP
    b. Acts through the receptors for opiates
    c. Causes continued activation of adenylate cyclase
    d. Inhibits the enzyme phosphodiesterase
6. Which of the following acts as second messenger?
    a. Mg^{2+} b. Cl^-
    c. Ca^{2+} d. PO_4^{3-}
7. True about intracellular receptors
    a. Mainly on nuclear surface
    b. Steroids does act on them
    c. Estrogen does not act on them
    d. GH act on it
8. Receptors on cell membrane that activate ion channel after binding with agonists is:
    a. Nicotinic cholinergic
    b. Muscarinic cholinergic
    c. Opioid μ-receptors
    d. GABA-B
9. Following are true about G-protein, *except*:
    a. G-channels
    b. Phosphorylase formation
    c. Made up of 4 subunits
    d. Related to ras oncogene
10. Various cells respond differentially to a second messenger because they have different:
    a. Receptors   b. Enzymatic composition
    c. Nuclei   d. Membrane lipid
11. Second messengers respond differentially to a hormone because of:
    a. Receptors   b. Enzymatic composition
    c. Nuclei   d. Membrane lipid

SECTION 8 ⊃ Endocrine System

12. Which of the following acts through tyrosine kinase receptor?
    a. Insulin
    b. Glucagon
    c. GH
    d. FSH
13. Cyclic AMP action mediates the action of all, *except*:
    a. Glucagon
    b. FSH
    c. LH
    d. Estrogen
14. Cyclic AMP acts as the second messenger of:
    a. FSH
    b. Thyroxine
    c. Growth hormone
    d. Insulin
15. Cyclic GMP is the second messenger of:
    a. Growth hormone
    b. FSH
    c. Nitric oxide
    d. Thyroxine
16. All the following act as second messengers, *except*:
    a. Cyclic AMP
    b. DAG
    c. Ca^{2+}
    d. Mg^{2+}
17. Cyclic AMP activates which of the following?
    a. Phosphodiesterase
    b. Protein kinase
    c. Phosphoglucomutase
    d. Hexokinase
18. Adenylate cyclase is found in association with:
    a. Cyclic AMP
    b. Phosphodiesterase
    c. GTP regulating proteins
    d. Nuclear receptors
19. First messengers are the:
    a. Protein kinases
    b. Intracellular mediators
    c. Extracellular ligands
    d. Hormone receptors
20. A hormone that binds to nuclear receptor is:
    a. Glucocorticoid
    b. Thyroxine
    c. Progesterone
    d. Insulin
21. The following receptors are present in the presynaptic membrane, *except*:
    a. H_3 histamine receptors
    b. α_1 adrenergic receptors
    c. α_2 receptors
    d. NO receptors
22. The BMR is least affected by an increase in the plasma level of:
    a. TSH
    b. TRH
    c. Thyroxine binding globulin (TBG)
    d. Free T_3
23. Neuroendocrine secretion means:
    a. Chemical acting at the synapse
    b. Chemical act at peripheral nervous system
    c. Substances act on the cells that release it
    d. Substance is released into the blood from the nerve
24. To report that a person is obese, his body mass index (BMI) should be greater than:
    a. 25
    b. 20
    c. 30
    d. 40
25. The following are second messengers, *except*:
    a. Calmodulin
    b. Prostaglandin
    c. Cyclic GMP
    d. Calsequestrin
26. The following are water soluble hormones:
    a. Parathormone
    b. Thyroid hormone
    c. Glucocorticoids
    d. Testosterone
27. Hormones are synthesized mainly in the
    a. Smooth endoplasmic reticulum
    b. Rough endoplasmic reticulum
    c. Peroxisomes
    d. Golgi apparatus
28. The receptors for the following hormones are ionotropic receptors:
    a. Glycine
    b. Insulin
    c. Thyroxine
    d. Growth hormone
29. The following hormones act through second messengers:
    a. Adrenaline
    b. Insulin
    c. Prolactin
    d. Thyroid stimulating hormone
30. Catecholamines mediate their action by combining with
    a. Cell membrane receptors
    b. Intranuclear receptors
    c. Cytoplasmic receptors
    d. Both cytoplasmic and intranuclear receptors

ANSWERS

1. c	2. d	3. c	4. d	5. c
6. c	7. a	8. a	9. c	10. b
11. a	12. a	13. d	14. a	15. c
16. d	17. b	18. a	19. c	20. b
21. b	22. c	23. d	24. c	25. d
26. a	27. b	28. a	29. d	30. a

Anterior Pituitary Gland and Hypothalamus

CHAPTER 62

LEARNING OBJECTIVES
- Describe the functional anatomy of anterior pituitary gland
- Explain hypothalamo-hypophyseal portal system
- Enumerate the hormones secreted by the anterior pituitary
- Explain the actions of growth hormone
- Explain the mechanism of regulation of growth hormone secretion
- Describe the clinical features and their physiological basis in gigantism, dwarfism and acromegaly
- Explain the hypothalamic control of the anterior pituitary
- Describe the stages of growth and development
- Review the factors affecting growth and development

PITUITARY GLAND

PY8.2: Describe the synthesis, secretion, transport, physiological actions, regulation and effect of altered (hypo and hyper) secretion of anterior pituitary gland and hypothalamus.

Functional Anatomy

Pituitary gland or hypophysis is an ovoid, reddish gray gland situated in the pituitary fossa of sphenoid bone at the base of the brain.
Weight – 0.5 g Diameter – 1 cm
Larger in females than in males and becomes still larger in pregnancy.

Relation of Pituitary Gland to Hypothalamus

Pituitary is attached to the hypothalamus by **pituitary stalk or hypophyseal stalk**. There are neural connections between the hypothalamus and posterior lobe of pituitary forming the **hypothalamo-hypophyseal tract** and vascular connection between hypothalamus and anterior pituitary forming the **hypothalamo-hypophyseal portal system**.

The hypothalamo-hypophyseal portal vessels form a direct vascular link between hypothalamus and anterior pituitary. Pituitary and hypothalamus play important roles in the regulation of virtually all aspects of growth, development, metabolism and homeostasis.

Parts of Pituitary Gland

Pituitary gland has two anatomically and functionally separate portions:
1. Adenohypophysis or anterior pituitary
2. Neurohypophysis or posterior pituitary.

Between these two parts is a relatively avascular zone called **intermediate lobe or pars intermedia**. It is almost absent in human beings **(Fig. 62.1)**. The cells that secrete derivatives of proopiomelanocortin (POMC) are present in the anterior pituitary.

Development of the Pituitary Gland

Anterior and posterior pituitary develop from two different sources even though they are situated in close approximation and are entirely different in structure and functions.

Posterior pituitary arises from the floor of the hypothalamus as a downward diverticulum called **neurohypophyseal bud**. The **infundibulum** connects posterior pituitary to hypothalamus **(Fig. 62.2)**.

Anterior pituitary develops from **Rathke's pouch or hypophyseal pouch,** which is an embryonic invagination of the pharyngeal epithelium. The pouch grows towards the neurohypophyseal bud and eventually loses its connection with the roof of the mouth. The origin of anterior pituitary from the pharyngeal epithelium explains the epithelioid

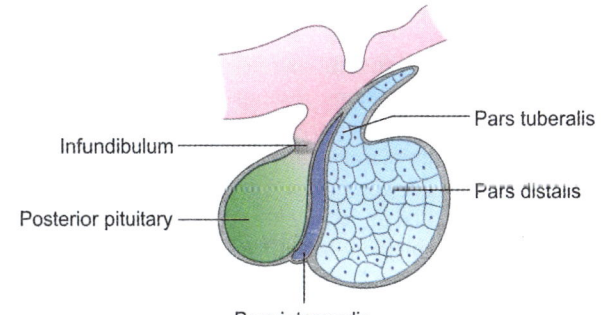

Fig. 62.1: Parts of pituitary gland. Anterior pituitary comprises pars tuberalis, pars distalis and pars intermedia.

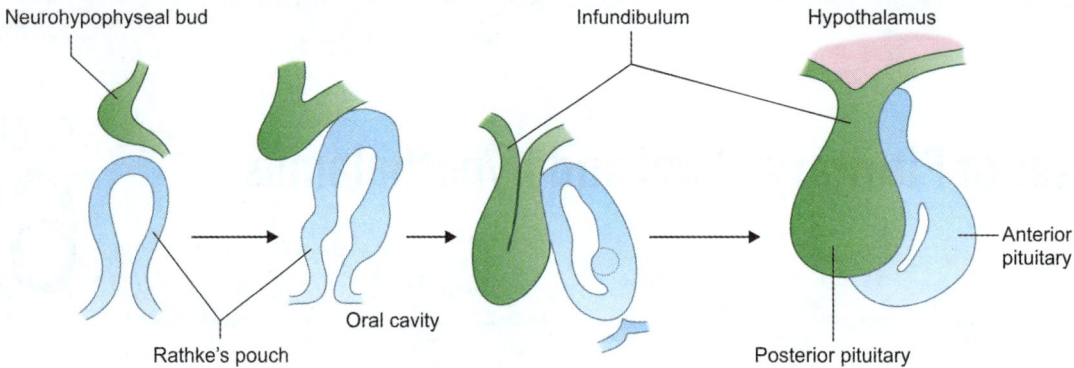

Fig. 62.2: Development of pituitary gland.

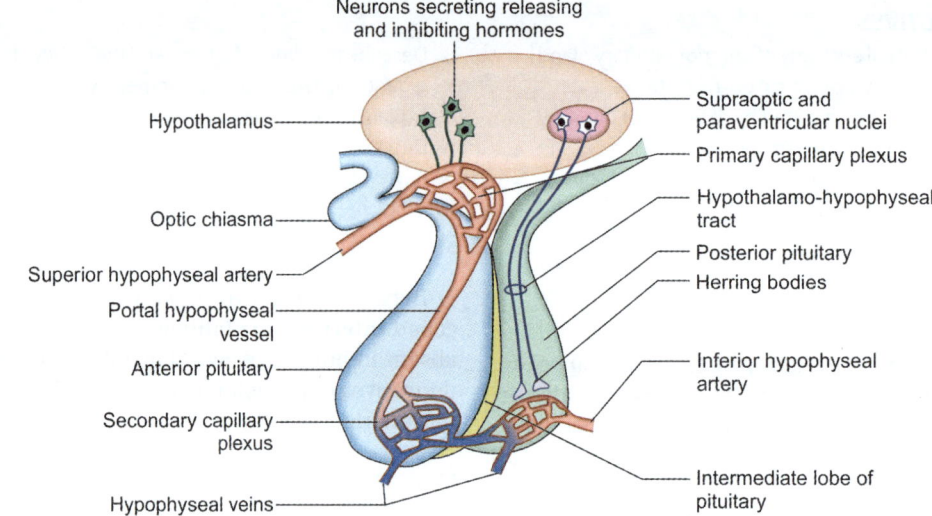

Fig. 62.3: Pituitary gland and hypothalamus showing the hypothalamo-hypophyseal tract and hypothalamo-hypophyseal portal system.

nature of the cells and the origin of posterior pituitary from neural tissue explains the presence of large number of glial cells in this part called **pituicytes**. *Pars intermedia* is formed from the posterior wall of **Rathke's pouch (Fig. 62.2)**.

Blood Supply

Pituitary is supplied by **superior and inferior hypophyseal arteries,** which are branches of internal carotid artery. The superior hypophyseal artery forms a capillary network called **primary plexus** on the ventral surface of hypothalamus referred to as **median eminence**. The primary plexus drains into the portal hypophyseal vessels that carry blood down the pituitary stalk to the capillary plexus of anterior pituitary called **secondary plexus**. This is referred to as **hypothalamo-hypophyseal portal system**. The hormones produced by the hypothalamus reach the anterior pituitary through this vascular connection. This direct route permits hypothalamic hormones to act quickly on the anterior pituitary gland cells before the hormones get diluted or destroyed in the systemic circulation.

Superior hypophyseal artery supplies 90% of anterior pituitary. The inferior hypophyseal artery forms a plexus around the lower part of pituitary stalk and supplies the rest 10% of adenohypophysis and whole of neurohypophysis **(Fig. 62.3)**.

Venous Drainage

Venous drainage occurs through anterior and posterior hypophyseal veins into the cavernous sinus, which in turn drains into the jugular vein.

■ HORMONES OF THE PITUITARY GLAND (FLOWCHART 62.1)

Anterior Pituitary

Anterior pituitary forms 75% of the weight of the pituitary. It is divided into three parts:
1. Pars distalis
2. Pars tuberalis
3. Pars intermedia.

Pars distalis forms the bulk of anterior pituitary **(Fig. 62.1)**.

Anterior pituitary synthesizes and secretes the following hormones:
- Thyroid stimulating hormone (TSH) or thyrotropin
- Adrenocorticotropic hormone (ACTH) or corticotropin
- Gonadotropins
  - FSH or follicle stimulating hormone
  - LH or ICSH (luteinizing hormone or interstitial cell stimulating hormone)

CHAPTER 62: Anterior Pituitary Gland and Hypothalamus

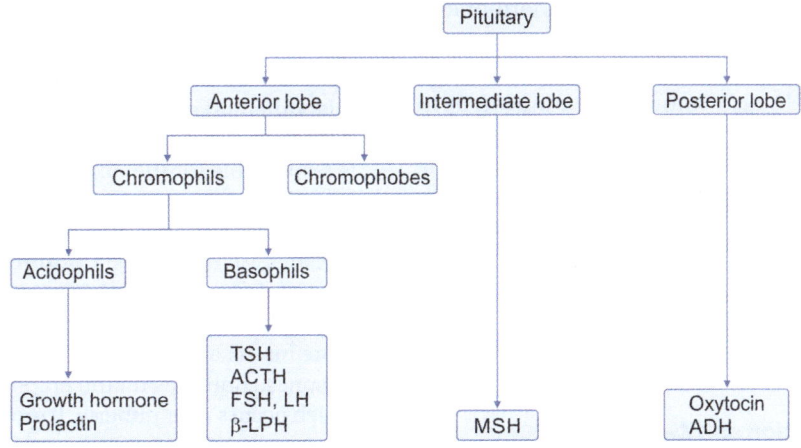

Flowchart 62.1: Hormones secreted by the different lobes of pituitary gland.

(ACTH: adrenocorticotropic hormone; ADH: antidiuretic hormone; β-LPH: β-lipotropin; FSH: follicle-stimulating hormone; LH: luteinizing hormone; MSH: melanocyte-stimulating hormone; TSH: thyroid-stimulating hormone)

- Growth hormone (GH) or somatotropin
- Prolactin or mammotropin
- β-LPH or β-lipotropin.

Pars intermedia of the anterior pituitary secrete the following hormones:
- α and β-MSH or melanocyte stimulating hormone
- γ-LPH or γ-lipotropin
- Pro-opiomelanocortin (POMC)
- Corticotropin like intermediate lobe peptide (CLIP)
- β-Endorphin.

Posterior Pituitary

Posterior pituitary *does not synthesize any hormone*, but it stores and releases two hormones, which are synthesized in the hypothalamus:
1. Antidiuretic hormone (ADH) or arginine vasopressin
2. Oxytocin.

ANTERIOR PITUITARY

The anterior pituitary is concerned with the regulation of reproduction, growth, energy metabolism and stress responses. The main targets for four of the anterior pituitary hormones i.e. TSH, ACTH, LH and FSH are other endocrine tissues. Action of growth hormone is mediated by somatomedins or insulin like growth factors. IGF-1 is produced in non-endocrine tissues like liver, kidney, muscle and cartilage.

Histology of Anterior Pituitary

Anterior pituitary is composed of interlacing cell cords and large number of sinusoids. Based on the staining character, cells are classified into two groups.
1. Agranular chromophobes
2. Granular chromophils.

Chromophobes are precursors of chromophil cells.

Depending on the staining nature, chromophils are classified into (Table 62.1):

Table 62.1: Cell types of anterior pituitary gland.

Cell type	Staining nature	Hormones secreted	% of total cells
Somatotrope	Acidophilic	Growth hormone	50
Lactotrope	Acidophilic	Prolactin	20
Corticotrope	Basophilic	ACTH	10
Thyrotrope	Basophilic	TSH	5
Gonadotrope	Basophilic	FSH, LH	15

1. Acidophils
2. Basophils.

The granules of chromophils contain stored hormones, which are released from the cells by exocytosis. The granules break down in the pericapillary space and the hormones enter the capillaries, which are fenestrated. The hormones of the anterior pituitary play major roles in the control of metabolic activities throughout the body.

Regulation of Secretion of Anterior Pituitary Hormones

All anterior pituitary hormones are secreted in a **pulsatile manner**. Secretion of anterior pituitary is regulated by hypothalamus. Some special nerve cells present in the hypothalamus synthesize and secrete the releasing and inhibiting hormones. These hormones are transported directly to the anterior pituitary by hypothalamo-hypophyseal portal system. Hypothalamus is part of central nervous system (CNS), whereas anterior pituitary is an endocrine gland. *Thus, the hypothalamic hormones finally act as a bridge between the CNS and endocrine system (for details refer Chapter 63).*

With the exception of prolactin, all the anterior pituitary hormones are under feedback regulation by the target tissue on which the pituitary hormones act. Prolactin acts on breast. Growth hormone acts on liver and other tissues. The rest of the anterior pituitary hormones are **tropic hormones**. Tropic hormones are hormones that have other endocrine glands as their target. There are short loop and long loop feedback mechanisms for controlling the secretion of the hormones.

Growth Hormone

Growth hormone (GH) also known as **somatotropin** is synthesized and secreted by somatotropes of adenohypophysis. It is a single chain polypeptide containing 191 amino acids with two intra-chain disulfide bridges with a molecular weight of 22,005. Structure of growth hormone is similar to prolactin and a placental hormone, human chorionic somatomammotropin. There are two forms of growth hormone depending on molecular weight:
1. 2 Kh growth hormone or normal growth hormone—75%
2. 20 KhGH—25%.

Secretion, Transportation and Metabolism of Growth Hormone

Secretion

Growth hormone is secreted by somatotropes in irregular spikes or **pulses**. Rate of secretion is more in late embryonic life and early childhood. The amount of growth hormone secreted is maximal during adolescence and decreases as age advances.

The amplitude of growth hormone secretory bursts is maximal during night, especially during sleep. Secretion is also increased after each meal.

Transport

Growth hormone is transported in blood bound to **growth hormone-binding protein (GHBP)** in plasma and one-half of growth hormone in circulation is in the bound form, which acts as a reservoir of the hormone. The GHBP is a large fragment of the extracellular domain of the growth hormone receptor. It is produced by cleavage of the receptors in humans.

Plasma growth hormone level: < 3 ng/mL
In children: 5 ng/mL

Metabolism

Growth hormone is metabolized rapidly in the liver. Half-life of growth hormone is 6–20 minutes.

Growth Hormone Receptor

Growth hormone receptor has a large extracellular portion, a transmembrane domain and a large cytoplasmic portion. It is a member of cytokine receptor superfamily. After binding with the receptor, growth hormone activates many different intracellular signaling cascades of which the important one is activation of **JAK2-STAT pathway.** Growth hormone has two domains that can bind to its receptor, and when it binds to one receptor, the second binding site attracts another receptor, producing a homodimer. Dimerization is essential for receptor activation. (*Refer* Chapter 61; Fig. 61.5).

Physiological Actions of Growth Hormone

a. Actions on somatic growth
b. Actions on metabolism.

Action on Somatic Growth

Growth hormone is responsible for the growth of almost all tissues of the body that are capable of growing. It increases the number as well as the size of the cells. It also causes cellular differentiation in the intrauterine life (IUL).

❖ *Action on skeletal growth*: During IUL, growth hormone is responsible for the differentiation and development of bone cells. After birth, growth hormone stimulates linear growth of long bones. It increases the length as well as the thickness of the bones. **Chondrogenesis** is accelerated. Rate of deposition of Ca^{2+} in the cartilage is increased. Epiphyseal plate gets widened. Growth hormone lays down more matrix at the ends of long bones. Increase in length of bones continues till the epiphysis fuses with the shaft, which occurs after puberty. If growth hormone is secreted in excess before puberty, it leads to **gigantism**.

❖ *Action on soft tissues*: Growth hormone stimulates mitosis, thereby increasing the number of cells. It also increases the size of the cells. Thus, it stimulates growth of the body as a whole. *Growth hormone can stimulate growth only in the presence of insulin and carbohydrates.*

Mechanism of Growth-promoting Action

Growth-promoting action of growth hormone is not a direct one, it is mediated by somatomedins. Growth hormone stimulates the release of small protein molecules from liver, fibroblast and other tissues known as **somatomedins**. Mechanism of action of somatomedin is by the formation of a second messenger called cAMP. In somatomedin deficiency, growth hormone cannot exert its growth promoting effects even if it is present in high concentrations. The effect of growth hormone on protein metabolism also depends on interaction between growth hormone and somatomedins.

In humans, the two important circulating somatomedins are **IGF-I (somatomedin C) and IGF-II (somatomedin A).** These factors are closely related to insulin and hence the name **insulin-like growth factor (IGF)**. They are synthesized mainly in the liver. IGF-I receptor is similar to insulin receptor. The growth-promoting action of somatomedins is helped by their insulin-like actions. Secretion of IGF-I is stimulated by growth hormone. IGF-II is independent of growth hormone and plays a role in the growth of the fetus before birth.

Growth hormone, through somatomedin, stimulates proliferation of chondrocytes and osteocytes resulting in increased deposition of cartilage and increased ossification of the newly formed cartilage. There will be widening of the cartilaginous epiphyseal plate and the bones grow longer, resulting in rapid increase in height. After epiphyseal closure, chondrogenesis does not occur and only sub-periosteal bone deposition occurs due to increased activity of osteocytes. Hence, there is no increase in bone length but bone thickening continues. GH promotes renal reabsorption of Ca^{2+} and phosphate that are important for bone growth.

In addition to GH, secretion of somatomedins is influenced by many factors like:

❖ Glucocorticoids and protein deficiency inhibit action of somatomedins.

- ❖ Increase in estrogen level inhibits somatomedin secretion.
- ❖ Hyperglycemia, as seen in untreated diabetes mellitus, inhibits somatomedins.

Recent view is that growth hormone also exerts a direct action on target tissues by activating the **JAK-STAT pathway**. It forms an important direct path from the cell surface to the nucleus. When the hormone binds to the cell membrane receptor, there is activation of **Janus tyrosine kinases (JAKs)** in the cytoplasm. These in turn phosphorylate **signal transducers and activators of transcription (STAT)** proteins. The phosphorylated STATs form dimers and move to the nucleus, where they act as transcription factors and activate various genes (**Fig. 61.5**).

Action of GH on Metabolism

Growth hormone is described as **anabolic, lipolytic and diabetogenic**.

- ❖ *Action on protein metabolism*

    Growth hormone is an **anabolic hormone**. It increases protein synthesis predominantly in skeletal and cardiac muscle. It produces a positive nitrogen and phosphorous balance. It promotes healing and tissue repair.

    Protein synthesis is increased by:
    - Increasing the transport of amino acid into the cell, thereby increasing the availability of amino acids for protein synthesis.
    - Increasing RNA translation leading to increased protein synthesis by ribosomes.
    - Stimulating transcription of DNA to RNA in nucleus leading to the formation of large quantities of RNA.
    - Decreasing the breakdown of cellular protein and thus helps in the building up of tissues.

- ❖ *Action on electrolyte metabolism*
    - Growth hormone increases intestinal absorption of calcium.
    - It causes retention of sodium, magnesium, calcium, chloride and phosphate ions. Growth hormone has lactogenic action (increase in yield of milk in lactating animals).

- ❖ *Action on fat metabolism*
    - Growth hormone is a **ketogenic hormone**. It mobilizes fat from adipose tissue and thus increases plasma free fatty acid level. In the tissues, growth hormone enhances the conversion of fatty acid to acetyl coenzyme A.
    - If growth hormone is present in excess, it leads to the formation of acetic acid in the liver leading to ketosis.
    - Under the influence of growth hormone, fat is utilized for energy rather than carbohydrate or protein. This protein-sparing action is responsible for growth.

- ❖ *Action on carbohydrate metabolism*

    Growth hormone is a **hyperglycemic** or **diabetogenic** hormone.

    It produces hyperglycemia by:
    - Decreasing the uptake of glucose by tissues, especially the liver. It also decreases the peripheral utilization of glucose.
    - Increasing glucose output from liver.
    - Stimulating gluconeogenesis.
    - Growth hormone utilizes fat for energy, thereby sparing carbohydrate. The above anti-insulin actions of growth hormone cause an increase in blood glucose level, which has been called **pituitary hyperglycemia** to differentiate it from diabetic hyperglycemia.
    - **Diabetogenic effect** of growth hormone — growth hormone does not directly stimulate β-cells of pancreas. But it increases the ability of pancreas to respond to insulinogenic stimuli like glucose.

Hyperglycemia produced by growth hormone stimulates the β cells of pancreas. More of insulin is secreted by pancreas and β cells get burnt out. This produces deficiency of insulin leading to frank diabetes mellitus. This effect of growth hormone is called **diabetogenic effect of GH.**

> While GH itself has anti-insulin effects, the somatomedins it produces have insulin-like effects. Somatomedins bind to insulin receptors and induce most of the metabolic effects of insulin, although to a lesser degree.

Regulation of Growth Hormone Secretion

The normal basal level of growth hormone in an adult is 300 ng/100 mL of blood. It is much more in growing children. Secretion of GH is stimulated in times of stress conditions like hypoglycemia, starvation, exercise and trauma. Glucose and free fatty acids inhibit secretion of GH. Pulsatile secretion of growth hormone from the anterior pituitary is regulated mainly by three hypothalamic regulatory hormones and somatomedins (**Fig. 62.4**). The hypothalamic hormones are:

- ❖ Growth hormone releasing hormone (GHRH).
- ❖ Growth hormone inhibiting hormone (GHIH) or somatotropin release inhibiting factor (SRIF) or somatostatin.
- ❖ Ghrelin, which is secreted by hypothalamus and stomach.

Growth hormone releasing hormone (GHRH): The GHRH, which contains 40–44 amino acids, directly stimulates somatotropes to secrete GH. It acts by stimulating adenylyl cyclase.

Growth hormone inhibiting hormone (GHIH) or somatostatin: Somatostatin is also secreted by other parts of the brain and also by the δ cells of pancreas. Somatostatin inhibits not only growth hormone but also thyrotropin releasing hormone (TRH). It acts by inhibiting adenylyl cyclase. The balance between the effects of GHRH and somatostatin on the pituitary will determine the level of growth hormone release.

Ghrelin: Ghrelin increases growth hormone secretion by stimulating somatotropes directly. It is also involved in the regulation of food intake.

Feedback Control

Whenever the blood level of growth hormone is decreased, there is increased secretion of GHRH from the hypothalamus. GHRH, in turn, increases the secretion of GH from the pituitary. Growth hormone secretion is also regulated by a

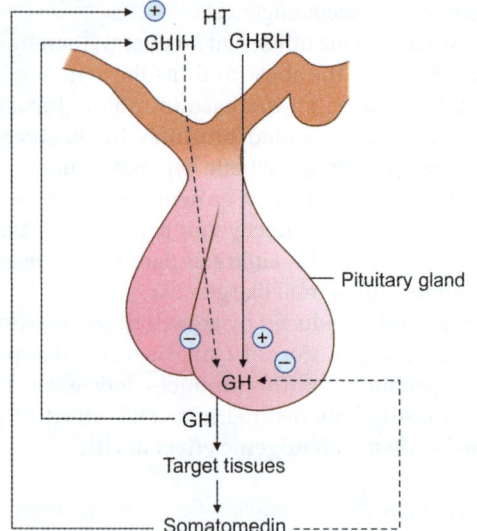

Fig. 62.4: Regulation of growth hormone (GH) secretion.
(GHIH: growth hormone inhibiting hormone; GHRH: growth hormone releasing hormone; HT: hypothalamus)

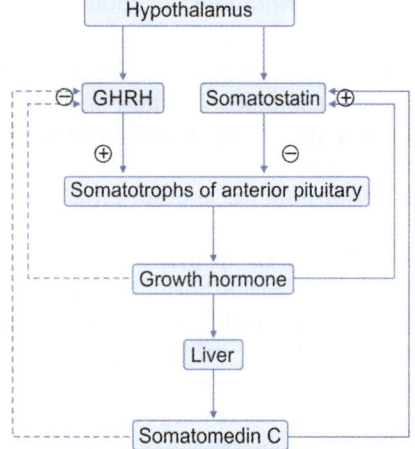

Fig. 62.5: Regulation of growth hormone secretion "+" sign denotes stimulation and "–" sign and dashed line denotes inhibition.
(GHRH: growth hormone releasing hormone)

direct negative feedback control mechanism. GH inhibits its own secretion by stimulating the release of GHIH from the hypothalamus. The inhibitory action of GH is also mediated through somatomedin-C (IGF-I) produced by the liver. GH increases secretion of somatomedin in the liver but somatomedin in turn inhibits GH secretion by a direct action on pituitary and also by stimulating the release of GHIH or somatostatin from the hypothalamus. Somatostatin inhibits release of GH from the pituitary. Similarly, GHRH inhibits its own secretion by an ultra-short feedback loop **(Fig. 62.5)**.

Factors Affecting Growth Hormone Secretion

Increase in Growth Hormone Secretion

- Deficiency of energy substrate as in:
  - Fasting
  - Hypoglycemia
  - Exercise
- Increase in circulating level of amino acid and decrease in level of fatty acids
- Stressful situations like fever and emotional trauma
- Deep sleep—stages 3 and 4 of non-rapid eye movement (NREM) sleep
- Hormones—estrogen, androgen, thyroid hormone
- Sympathetic stimulation.

Decrease in Growth Hormone Secretion

- Rapid eye movement (REM) sleep
- Hyperglycemia
- Increase in level of free fatty acids
- Increased glucocorticoids
- Progesterone (reason for decline in GH secretion in late pregnancy)
- GHIH
- Obesity
- Hypothyroidism
- Emotional deprivation
- Growth hormone by feedback regulation

Abnormalities in Growth Hormone Secretion

Hypersecretion of Growth Hormone

Causes

- Hypothalamic tumors lead to increased secretion of GHRH.
- Acidophilic adenoma of pituitary produces increased growth hormone and prolactin secretion.
- Tumors of somatotropes secrete large amounts of growth hormone.
- Ectopic GHRH and growth hormone secreting tumors.

Before Puberty

Gigantism

If hypersecretion of growth hormone occur before puberty there will be excessive growth of the body and the condition is called **gigantism**. The features are:

- Since hypersecretion of GH occur before the fusion of the epiphysis of long bone with the shaft, there will be abnormal increase in the length of long bones. As a result, the person becomes **very tall** (8–9 feet). The limbs will be disproportionately long **(Fig. 62.6)**.
- There will be hyperglycemia and glycosuria due to its anti-insulin effects. It is seen that 10% of giants develop **diabetes mellitus** usually referred to as **pituitary diabetes mellitus**. The hyperglycemia produced by GH causes excessive stimulation of β cells of islets of Langerhans. The over activity leads to degeneration of these cells and deficiency of insulin. Ultimately frank diabetes mellitus develops.
- Symptoms like **headache**, **visual disturbances,** etc., occur due to pressure exerted by the tumor. X-ray skull shows widened sella turcica. The tumor presses on optic chiasma leading to visual disturbances like **bitemporal hemianopia** (the temporal field of vision of both eyes will be absent).
- In most giants, **panhypopituitarism** eventually develops leading to death in early adulthood. This is because, the tumor producing gigantism will continue to grow until the

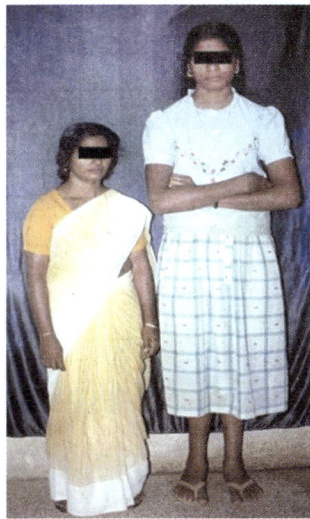

Fig. 62.6: Gigantism (right), the lady on the left side is of normal height.

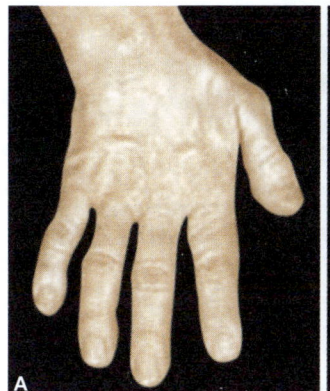 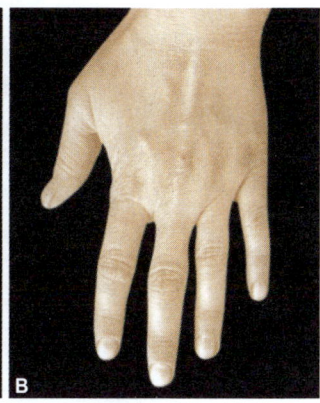

Figs. 62.7A and B: (A) Spade like hand in acromegaly; (B) Normal hand.

gland is destroyed, which leads to panhypopituitarism. This can be prevented by early diagnosis and destruction of the tumor.

Diagnosis: An elevated level of insulin-like growth factor-1 (IGF-1) establishes the diagnosis along with X-ray skull which shows widening of sella turcica.

Treatment: In medical management, dopamine agonists like cabergoline which is a D2 receptor agonist can be given that act on D2 receptors in somatotrophs and decrease GH secretion. GH receptor antagonists are also available. This antagonist binds to the first binding site and prevents dimerization and post receptor signaling. Selective surgical excision of the pituitary adenoma or irradiation of the pituitary gland is done if medical management fails. After surgery, treatment with somatostatin analogues is also helpful since it inhibits the secretion of GH from any ectopic sites. Hypopituitarism can occur as a result of surgery or irradiation of the gland. Annual assessment of pituitary hormones should be done and hormonal replacement should be done if needed.

After Puberty

Acromegaly

If hypersecretion of growth hormone occurs after puberty, i.e., after the fusion of epiphysis with the shaft of long bone, the condition is called **acromegaly**. The most common cause is pituitary acidophilic tumor. It is characterized by the enlargement, thickening and broadening of bones, particularly of hands and feet (acro means extremities). Membranous bones like cranium, nasal bones, lower jaw bone, portions of vertebrae, etc. are affected. The features of acromegaly are:

- The person cannot become taller because the epiphyseal plates are closed. So, the bone increases in thickness and this occurs mainly in the membranous bones, such as jaw bone, skull and bones of hands and feet. Extremities will be very large, e.g., spade like hand **(Fig. 62.7A)**.
- Enlarged and thickened jaws, protrusion of supraorbital ridge, thick and wrinkled forehead due to increase in skin thickness, enlarged tongue and lips due to soft tissue swelling. The nose increases to as much as twice the normal size. Protrusion of lower jaw is called **mandibular prognathism**. These features are collectively referred to as **acromegalic or gorilla facies (Fig. 62.8A)**.
- Visceral organs like lung, heart, kidney, liver, thyroid, spleen, thymus, etc. are enlarged due to soft tissue hypertrophy **(Fig. 62.8B)**. Cardiomyopathy is seen in most patients with acromegaly. Skin tags are present in 98% of cases due to epithelial cell hyperproliferation induced by GH.
- Deep voice and obstructive sleep apnea can occur due to soft tissue swelling of the upper airway and large tongue. Obstructive sleep apnea is seen in 70% of patients with acromegaly.
- Gonads atrophy and the reason for hypogonadism is hyperprolactinemia.
- Hyperglycemia and glycosuria are present (pituitary diabetes mellitus). About 25% of patients have abnormal glucose tolerance tests.
- Galactorrhea is present in 4% in the absence of pregnancy due to the lactogenic effect of growth hormone.
- Hypersecretion of growth hormone is accompanied by hypersecretion of prolactin in 20-40% of patients with acromegaly. This also causes galactorrhea.
- Bowing of spine called kyphosis is seen mainly due to osteoarthritis. In addition, portions of vertebrae continue to grow under the influence of growth hormone because their growth do not cease at adolescence.
- Increase in glomerular filtration rate because GH increases GFR and renal plasma flow in humans.
- Mild hypertension is seen in 45% of patients with acromegaly.

Diagnosis is confirmed by estimation of serum IGF-I. Pituitary magnetic resonance imaging helps in the diagnosis. Size of the tumor, its extent, optic chiasmal compression etc. can be assessed by MRI. Testing of visual field should be done if the tumor is in contact with optic chiasma.

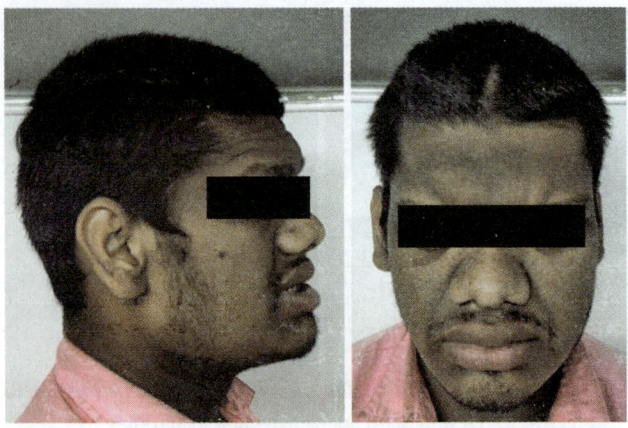

Fig. 62.8A: Acromegaly.
Courtesy: Dr Akhil Krishna.

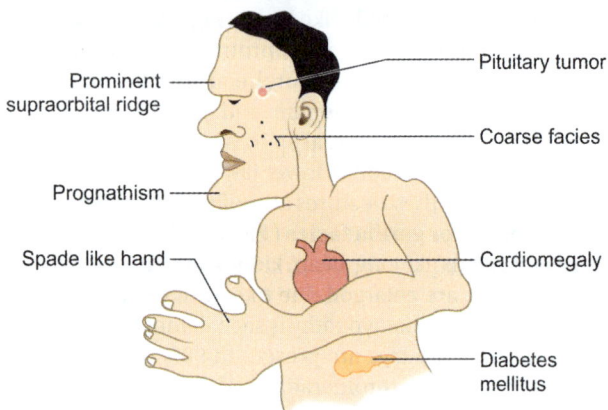

Fig. 62.8B: Features of acromegaly.

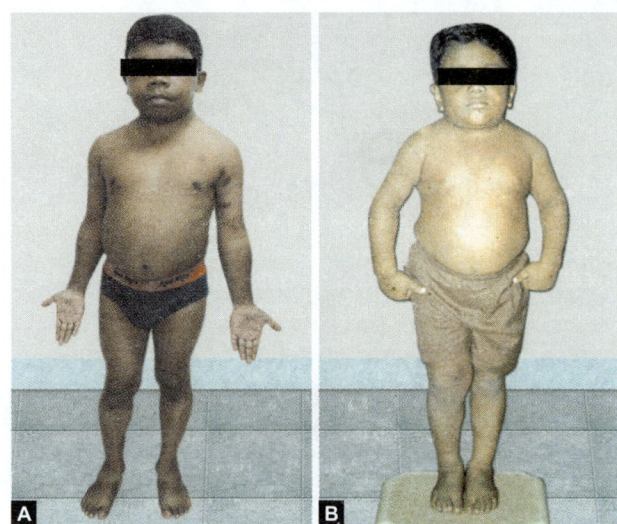

Figs. 62.9A and B: Dwarfism.
Courtesy: (A) Dr Abhilash Nair; (B) Dr RV Jayakumar.

Hyposecretion of Growth Hormone

Causes

- Hypothalamic and pituitary lesions lead to decreased GHRH and GH. Isolated GH deficiency is often due to GHRH deficiency, or due to abnormality in the growth hormone secreting cells or in some other cases, growth hormone receptors will be unresponsive as a result of loss-of-function mutations.
- Chromophobe tumor can compress and destroy the chromophils.
- Panhypopituitarism due to destruction of pituitary leads to lack of all anterior pituitary hormones.
- Deficient secretion of IGF-I.

Before Puberty

Dwarfism

- Bone growth is slow and epiphyseal plates close before normal height is reached. This condition is called **dwarfism**. Maximum height attained is 3 feet (**Figs. 62.9A and B**).
- Other organs of the body also fail to grow and the pituitary dwarf is childlike in appearance. If it is isolated growth hormone deficiency, there will be only growth retardation.
- Unlike cretins, the body proportions of the pituitary dwarf are not infantile but like those of an adult. Hypoglycemia may be a feature.
- There is no mental retardation.
- *Reproductive function is not affected if there is only isolated growth hormone deficiency.*

Treatment

- Dwarfism due to GH deficiency can be treated with **human growth hormone** (hGH). hGH is now being synthesized by Escherichia coli bacteria in sufficient quantities by recombinant DNA technology. If treated early in life, dwarfs having pure GH deficiency can be completely cured.
- Administration of growth hormone releasing hormone (GHRH) gives good response if it is due to GHRH deficiency.
- Dopamine agonists like bromocriptine stimulates GH secretion and have been used in the treatment of GH deficiency.

Laron Dwarfism or Growth Hormone Insensitivity

In Laron dwarfism, the secretion of growth hormone is either normal or elevated, but *there is impaired hepatic synthesis of somatomedin (IGF-1)*. Here, the GH receptors in the liver are resistant to the action of GH as a result of loss-of-function mutations of gene coding for the growth hormone receptor. It is autosomal recessive mutations of growth hormone receptor. This is one explanation for the short stature of African pygmies. Some patients with Laron dwarfism have absent or reduced levels of growth hormone binding protein (GHBP).

> Other causes of dwarfism include hypothyroidism and Cushing's syndrome in childhood, achondroplasia (most common cause of dwarfism in humans which is an autosomal dominant condition due to mutation in the gene that codes for fibroblast growth factor 3 present in cartilage), Turner's syndrome (XO chromosomal pattern), psychosocial dwarfism or Kasper Hauser syndrome (due to chronic abuse and neglect of children) and familial dwarfism.

Growth Hormone Deficiency in Adults

Acromicria

In adults, growth hormone deficiency leads to a condition called **acromicria,** which is characterized by:
- Atrophy and thinning of the extremities of the body.
- Hypoglycemia.
- Aging process is accelerated because of decreased protein deposition in the tissues and increased fat deposition.
- Mild anemia refractory to usual treatment may be a feature.
- There is loss of sexual function.

PHYSIOLOGY OF GROWTH AND DEVELOPMENT

Introduction

Growth is the process of physical maturation resulting in an increase in the size of the body and various organs. It is a characteristic feature of living organisms that includes increase in the size and number of cells leading to increase in the height and weight. In humans, growth involves accretion of proteins and increase in the weight and height of the individual measured in kilograms and centimeters. **Development** refers to the functional and physiological maturation of the individual i.e. it is the growth in psychomotor capacity. It occurs by progressive increase in the skill and capacity to function. Growth is related to quantitative changes of the body while development amounts to qualitative changes of the body. Both are interrelated. Growth and development together refers to the process of maturation, both in quality and in quantity. It begins in the embryonic life and continues till old age. In adulthood, growth is limited to repair and renewal process. Growth hormone is the most important hormone for post-natal growth although it is unimportant for fetal development. Both growth and development are dependent on genetic, nutritional and environmental factors.

Periods of Rapid Growth

In humans, two periods of rapid growth occurs. The first growth spurt occurs in **infancy** and the second in **late puberty** just before growth stops. The first period is a continuation of fetal growth period. The second growth spurt at the time of puberty is due to growth hormone, androgens and estrogens. In girls, the second growth spurt appears earlier. Growth stops due to closure of epiphysis in the long bones by estrogens. Further increase in height is not possible after this.

Stages in Growth and Development

1. Fetal stage
2. Postnatal stage
   - Infancy: Up to one year of age after birth
   - Toddler: One to five years of age
   - Childhood: Three to eleven years of age (early childhood is from three to eight years of age; middle childhood is from nine to eleven years of age)
   - Adolescence or teenage from twelve to eighteen years of age
   - Adulthood.

Factors Affecting Growth

Growth is a complex phenomenon that is affected not only by growth hormone and somatomedins, but also by other factors like:
- Hormones like thyroid hormones, androgen, estrogen, glucocorticoids and insulin
- Genetic factors
- Nutritional factors
- Environmental factors

Hormonal Factors (Fig. 62.10)

- Intrauterine growth is independent of growth hormone. Thyroid hormone plays an important role in growth and differentiation in late fetal and early postnatal life.
- Rapid growth during infancy is due to the action of thyroid hormone and GH.
- Growth spurt at puberty is due to androgens and GH. It is due to an interaction between sex steroids, growth hormone and IGF-1.
- In between, continuous growth occurs by the action of thyroid hormone and GH.
- After puberty, for the rest of the life growth occurs by thyroid hormone, growth hormone and androgens.

Growth Hormone

Growth hormone has very little role in the fetal and early postnatal period. During this period, thyroid hormone has the most important role in growth and development. During infancy, growth hormone and thyroid hormone have equal role in growth. During growth spurt, androgens and growth hormone play the important role. During rest of the life, thyroid hormones, growth hormone and androgens are responsible for growth and development.

Growth hormone does not function through a specific target gland but exerts its effects directly on all or almost all tissues of the body. Growth hormone is responsible for the growth of almost all tissues of the body, which are capable of growing. It increases the size and number of cells by increasing mitotic division. GH also causes specific differentiation of certain types of cells like bone cells and muscle cells. It increases body protein, decreases fat stores and conserves carbohydrate. It increases DNA transcription, which leads to increased formation of RNA, which in turn stimulates protein synthesis and growth provided, sufficient energy, amino acids, vitamins and other factors necessary for growth are available. It has a protein sparing action by decreasing the catabolism of proteins.

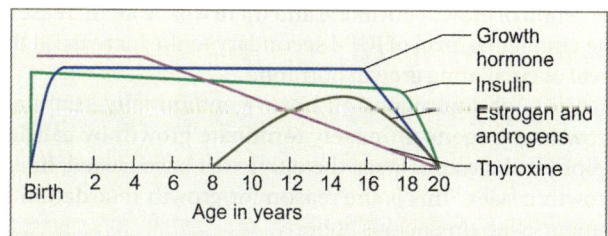

Fig. 62.10: Relative importance of hormones in human growth at various ages.

Plasma growth hormone level is elevated in newborns. The spikes of GH secretion are larger in children, especially during puberty. The growth promoting action of GH is mediated through IGF-1 (somatomedin C) and the plasma IGF-1 levels rise during childhood, reaching a peak at 13–17 years of age. In contrast, IGF-II levels are constant throughout postnatal growth. Deficiency of GH during childhood produces growth retardation known as pituitary dwarfism.

> GH is of little importance during fetal and early postnatal life. Infants with congenital deficiency of growth hormone have normal height and weight up to about 2 years of age provided, thyroid function is normal.

Thyroid Hormone

Thyroxine is essential for growth in the late fetal life and first few years of postnatal life. If the fetus does not secrete sufficient quantities of thyroid hormone, growth and maturation of the brain before birth and after birth are greatly retarded and the brain remains smaller than normal. Without specific thyroxine therapy, within days or weeks after birth, the child with thyroid hormone deficiency will remain mentally retarded throughout life.

Thyroid hormone is necessary for normal rate of GH secretion. GH and thyroid hormone show permissive action. Thyroid hormones alone have no effect on growth after birth. Their action is therefore permissive to that of GH, possibly via potentiation of the actions of somatomedins. When administered together, GH and thyroid hormones stimulate growth.

Thyroid hormone plays an important role in tissue differentiation and maturation, ossification of cartilage, growth of teeth, brain development, and the contours of the face and is responsible for normal body proportions. Cretins are dwarfed, mentally retarded and have infantile body proportion.

Androgen and Estrogen

Sex hormones are most essential around puberty and play an important role in the development of gonads as well as general growth. Androgen is a protein anabolic hormone and is responsible for the growth spurt at puberty. The secretion of adrenal androgen increases at the time of puberty in both sexes. It produces an increase in GH secretion that increases IGF-1 secretion. This, in turn, causes growth. The actions of sex hormones, GH and IGF-I, seem to potentiate each other at puberty. Increase in estrogens and androgens increases the secretion of growth hormone and there will be an increase in the circulating level of IGF-I secondary to the increase in the level of circulating growth hormone.

Although androgens and estrogens initially stimulate growth, estrogens ultimately terminate growth by causing epiphyseal closure. Once the epiphyses have closed, linear growth ceases. This is the reason for growth retardation in patients with precocious puberty.

Patients with panhypopituitarism in childhood have features consistent with their chronological age until puberty, but since they do not mature sexually, they possess juvenile features in adulthood.

Insulin

Insulin promotes growth due to its anabolic effect. The anabolic effect of insulin is aided by the protein sparing action of insulin by providing adequate intracellular glucose supplies. Failure to grow is a sign of diabetes in children. Insulin stimulates the growth of immature hypophysectomized rats to almost the same degree as growth hormone provided; large amounts of carbohydrate and protein are supplied with insulin. There is synergistic action of growth hormone and insulin on growth.

> The importance of insulin and GH in the growth of the body is demonstrated in **Houssay animal**. It is an animal in which both anterior pituitary and pancreas are removed. Administration of either insulin or GH alone does not induce growth in this animal. However, administration of both the hormones stimulates growth. This proves the synergistic action of these two hormones on growth.

Glucocorticoids

Glucocorticoids are potent inhibitors of growth because of their direct action on cells, and treatment of children with pharmacologic dose of steroids slows or stops growth for as long as the treatment is continued. It promotes protein catabolism and is potent inhibitor of growth hormone. Children with Cushing syndrome are of short stature.

Other hormones like **parathormone, calcitonin and vitamin D** are important for the growth of bone.

Genetic Factors

Genetic factors are very important in relation to growth and stature especially in the adolescence phase. It is mainly responsible for certain racial differences in height. *Dinkas of Sudan (6 feet average height) are the tallest and Pygmies of Congo are the shortest of the human beings.* Children will have almost the same stature of the parents. One of the best indicators of child's ultimate stature is **mid parental height**. **Achondroplasia,** which occurs due to failure of growth of long bones, is inherited as Mendelian dominant.

Nutritional Factors

Normal growth depends on adequate nutrition. Food supply is the most important extrinsic factor affecting growth. Requirements of proteins and various amino acids are increased during active periods of growth. These are essential for laying down new tissues, for wear and tear and for specific metabolic functions. Diet deficient in quantity, calories, proteins, minerals and vitamins inhibit growth markedly. Dietary deprivation has greater adverse effect on muscles and adipose tissue than on growth of bone. Deficiency of trace elements like zinc, selenium, iodine, manganese, and copper can affect growth and development. However, the age at which dietary deficiency occurs is a very important factor.

Under nutrition and malnutrition in childhood is responsible for short stature, poor muscular development and generalized apathy. Injury and diseases stunt growth because these factors increase protein catabolism.

Environmental Factors

* **Season:** Growth in height is faster in the spring season than in autumn; whereas gain in weight is faster in autumn than in spring. Cause is not known.
* **Diseases**: During acute **illness** or starvation, growth is temporarily slowed but during recovery, a period of **catch up growth** takes place during which the growth rate is greater than normal. The accelerated growth usually continues until the previous growth curve is reached, then slows to normal. The exact mechanism of this catch up growth is not known. Chronic long-standing illness in childhood can produce permanent growth retardation.
* **Emotional disturbances** like lack of love and security and a disturbed child-parent relationship can cause decrease in the rate of growth in children taking an adequate diet. Profound neglect during early childhood can impair development. Removal of the cause leads to restoration of normal growth rate. Emotional stress and psychological disorders can activate the pituitary-adrenal stress response and inhibit growth hormone secretion (**psychosocial dwarfism**).
* **Socioeconomic factors** also play important role in growth and development of child. Children of higher socio-economical groups are taller than children of the same age and sex in the lower socio-economic groups. Higher family educational levels have a positive impact on growth.
* Repeated **exercise** can lead to hypertrophy of skeletal muscles.
* **Aging** is characterized by cellular degeneration and impairment of various functions. A slight reduction in the height is seen in old age due to collapse of the vertebral discs. Elasticity of skin is reduced; there will be a reduction in memory, capacity to learn; osteoporosis, stiffness of joints, senile cataract, coronary and cerebral atherosclerosis in old age.

Growth Curves

Growth of different parts of the body does not follow a uniform pattern. The patterns of growth of different parts are described in the form of **growth curves** by **Richard E Scammon** in 1927 (**Fig. 62.11**). The different Scammon's growth curves are:
* General growth curve
* Neural growth curve
* Lymphoid growth curve
* Gonadal growth curve.

General Growth Curve

General growth curve includes growth of the skeleton as a whole, muscles and the thoracic and abdominal viscera. It shows two growth spurts, one in infancy and the other around puberty.

First growth spurt in infancy is characterized by increase in birth weight to two times by 6 months of age, three times

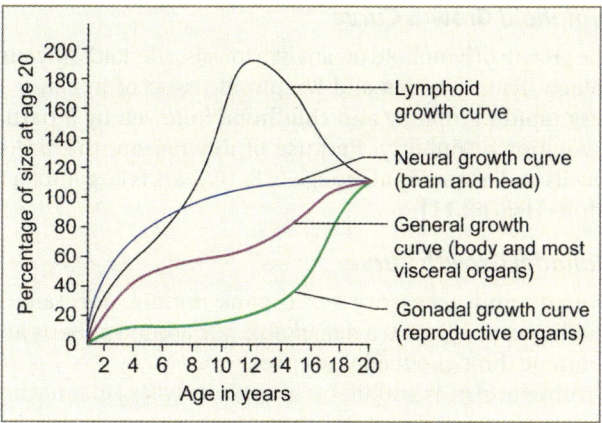

Fig. 62.11: Growth curves showing different tissues at various ages as a percentage of size at age 20.

at 1 year of age and four times at 2 years of age. After this, the weight increases by about 2 kg/year till about 12 years of age. Height increases in increments of 2–2.5 cm per month in the first year of life. Thereafter it slows down. This growth spurt is a continuation of fetal growth period.

Adolescent growth spurt is characterized by rapid increase in weight gain, about 3.5 kg/year between 12 and 18 years of age. Height increase during this period varies between 4 and 7 cm/year depending on genetic and endocrine factors. In girls, the rate of increase in height and weight is greatest at 12 to 13 years of age. In boys, it is at 14 to 15 years of age. Increase in weight in girls during adolescence is due to increased fat formation and in boys, it is due to increased muscular growth under the influence of testosterone. Adolescent growth spurt is due to (1) protein anabolic effects of androgen and (2) interaction between sex steroids, growth hormone and insulin like growth factor-I (IGF-I).

From 3 to 12 years of age, there is a slower progressive increase in growth. During this period, boys are slightly taller than girls. Even when the pubertal increase in growth is complete at 18 years in girls and 20 years in boys, a small slow growth occurs till the age of 30 years. After adolescence, boys are usually taller and heavier than females on an average.

Following illness or starvation there will be a period of catch up growth. During this period, the growth rate is greater than normal. Accelerated growth usually continues till the previous growth curve is reached, then comes to normal. The exact mechanism is unknown.

Neural Growth Curve

Brain, spinal cord and eyes grow very rapidly after birth. At the end of first year of postnatal life, the brain has already achieved 2/3rd and by the end of second year, 4/5th of adult size. By 5 years of age, brain is fully developed. Although the nerve cells do not increase in number after birth, some nerve cells increase enormously in mass up to 2 lakh times by elongation, ramification and myelination. Nerve cells become rich in RNA, which synthesizes cytoplasm, which migrates into the nerve fibers.

Lymphoid Growth Curve

The growth of lymphoid organs like tonsils, adenoids, thymus, spleen, lymph nodes and lymphoid tissue of intestine is very rapid in infancy and childhood followed by a partial involution at puberty. Because of this reason, the size of tonsils and adenoids at the age of 8–10 years is larger than in adults (**Fig. 62.11**).

Gonadal Growth Curve

Gonads and accessory sex organs remain dormant in childhood and grow at a remarkable rate around puberty and continue throughout adolescence.

Adrenal glands and uterus are relatively larger at birth. It loses weight rapidly after birth and regains birth weight just before puberty.

Growth Factors

Growth factors are biologically active polypeptides that perform hormone-like functions relating to control of proliferation and differentiation of cells. Like hormones, these are secreted by one cell type and regulate another cell or tissue. Most of the growth factors are produced in immediate proximity to the target cell so that the growth factor reaches the target cell by local diffusion. Some endocrinologists consider growth factors as a subclass of polypeptide hormones. But cells that have other functions besides growth factor secretion produce growth factors. For example, platelet derived growth factor (PDGF) is produced by platelets which causes proliferation of fibroblasts, endothelial cells of blood vessels, etc. On the other hand, platelets have many other important functions to perform like hemostasis and blood coagulation, clot retraction, etc. Contradictory to hormonal function, surgical removal of any single organ or part of the tissue that is believed to secrete the growth factor will not cause observable growth factor deficiency.

The important growth factors are:
- Neurotropic factors like nerve growth factor (NGF)
- Epidermal growth factor (EGF)
- Platelet derived growth factor (PDGF) and fibroblast growth factor (FGF)
- Insulin-like growth factor (IGF)
- Blood cell growth factors:
  - Erythropoietin
  - Colony stimulating factors (CSF)
  - Cytokines like interleukin 1, 2, 3

Growth factors are divided into three groups for convenience.
1. Factors that promote the multiplication and development of various types of cells; e.g., NGF, PDGF, IGF-I, activins, inhibins, EGF, etc.
2. Cytokines produced by macrophages and lymphocytes involved in the regulation of immune system form the second group, e.g., interleukins.
3. Colony-stimulating factors that regulate proliferation and maturation of red blood cells and white blood cells form the third group.

Nerve Growth Factor

Nerve growth factor is necessary for the embryonic development of sympathetic and sensory neurons and it enhances development of central nervous system. The chromaffin cells of adrenal medulla require NGF in small amounts for survival.

Epidermal Growth Factors

These factors stimulate cell mitosis and are referred to as **mitogens**. They stimulate proliferation of a wide variety of epithelial and fibroblastic cell types. They have a very important role in regulation of growth during embryonic development. It is present in plenty in the breast milk and may have a role in early postnatal development.

Platelet Derived Growth Factor

Platelet derived growth factor is produced from the α-granules of platelets. They are mitogens that cause proliferation of a number of mesodermal cell types including fibroblasts, glial cells, arterial smooth muscle cells and endothelial cells of blood vessels. During the period of rapid growth of the organism, the arterial cells must continually proliferate and in this stage, the endothelial cells produce their own growth factor. Later in development, these cells stop producing growth factor. Following injury to the vessel wall, endothelial cells resume production of PDGF.

> **APPLIED PHYSIOLOGY**
> - **Simian sarcoma**: A viral infection of fibroblasts causes production of PDGF. Since PDGF is a mitogen for fibroblasts, an autocrine stimulation of cell growth occurs, leading to the formation of a tumor. This is an example of autocrine hormonal response.
> - PDGF has been implicated in the development of **atherosclerosis**. Small arterial lesions may lead to local release of PDGF from endothelium and also from platelets that aggregate at the site of injury. This leads to excessive local proliferation of arterial smooth muscle cells causing the development of an atherosclerotic plaque.

Fibroblast Growth Factor

Fibroblast growth factor is structurally different from PDGF but the target cells are almost same for both growth factors. FGF stimulates proliferation and migration of vascular endothelial cells leading to **angiogenesis**, i.e., growth of the vasculature. Thus, it plays an important role in regulating tissue vascularization during development.

Insulin-like Growth Factors

Insulin-like growth factors are synthesized in the liver and its production is stimulated by growth hormone. Many biological effects of growth hormone are mediated by increased production of IGF. Thus, IGF is very important in regulating the growth and stature of children. The growth of many tissues should be regulated simultaneously in a coordinated manner during development and so, IGF stimulate the proliferation of different types of cells.

Insulin-like growth factors have close structural similarity to insulin and have mitogenic activity on a wide variety of cell types. These growth factors are also called **somatomedins or non-suppressible insulin-like activity (NSILA)**. IGF-1 is somatomedin C and IGF-2 is multiplication-stimulating activity (MSA). Because of the structural similarity of the receptors for insulin and IGF- 1, IGF-1 cross-reacts weakly with the insulin receptor and thus has weak insulin-like activity. On the other hand, insulin binds to IGF-1 receptor and has weak IGF-like activity.

Actions of IGF

- They stimulate proliferation of a very wide variety of cell types.
- Stimulates incorporation of chondroitin sulfate in chondrocytes of cartilage.
- They have a variety of insulin-like effects like alterations in the metabolism of adipocytes. These effects are due to cross-reaction with insulin receptors at high concentration of IGF.

Blood Cell Growth Factors

The differentiation of different types of blood cells from a common pluripotent stem cell is controlled by a number of specific growth factors. They include:
- **Erythropoietin:** Regulates production of erythrocytes by stimulating the proliferation of erythrocyte stem cells.
- **Granulocyte and macrophage colony stimulating factors (GM-CSF):** This causes a common stem cell to form either granulocyte or macrophage colonies. Low concentration of GM-CSF induces production of granulocytes and high concentration favors formation of macrophages.
- Interleukin-1, 2 and 3
  - **IL-3** is also known as **multi-colony stimulating factor** (CSF) because it stimulates the production of granulocytes, macrophages, erythroid cells, eosinophil, megakaryocyte and mast cell precursors. Splenic cells secrete IL-3.
  - **IL-2** is secreted by T lymphocytes and it stimulates proliferation of both T and B lymphocytes.
  - **IL-1** is produced by activated macrophages. Activities include stimulation of IL-2 release by T lymphocytes, stimulation of B lymphocyte proliferation and maturation, proliferation of fibroblasts, release of prostaglandin and collagenase by synovial cells.
- Antigens can act as growth factors for lymphocytes. T and B-lymphocytes have a specialized type of IgM antibodies on their surface. When antigen molecules corresponding to the antibody bind to the cell surface IgM, the lymphocyte becomes activated and proliferates producing a clone of cells with that antigenic specificity. Since these antigens stimulate the cell proliferation, they are grouped under growth factors.

Major Causes of Short Stature or Dwarfism

- **Familial**: There will be a family history of short stature. They have normal body proportion.
- **Endocrine** disorders:
  - Pituitary dwarf due to deficiency of growth hormone, IGF-I or growth hormone releasing hormone.
  - Laron dwarfism or growth hormone insensitivity syndrome which is due to deficiency of somatomedins. Here, GH level will be normal or elevated.
  - Cretinism or hypothyroid dwarf has infantile body proportion.
  - Cushing syndrome due to excess glucocorticoid secretion.
- **Nutritional** dwarfism due to inadequate nutrition:
  - Protein energy malnutrition (marasmus)
  - Vitamin D deficiency – rickets
- **Genetic cause**, e.g., achondroplasia – an autosomal dominant disease of the skeleton in which there is faulty endochondral ossification.
- **Chromosomal abnormalities** like Turner's syndrome.
- **Psychosocial dwarfism** or Kaspar Hauser syndrome due to emotional deprivation.

Other Hormones of Anterior Pituitary

Prolactin

Prolactin (PRL) is secreted by lactotrophs (pituitary acidophil cell) and it is also called *lactogenic or mammotrophic or galactopoietic hormone.* It is a polypeptide with 199 amino acids with three intra-chain disulfide bridges. It has considerable structural similarity to human growth hormone and human chorionic somatomammotropin (hCS). Plasma half-life of prolactin is 30–50 min.

Normal plasma level:
In male – 5 ng/mL
In female – 8 ng/mL

Late in the secretory phase of menstrual cycle, the endometrium produces prolactin, but the function of this endometrial prolactin is unknown. Placenta also secretes prolactin.

Actions of Prolactin

Prolactin receptors are present in the mammary gland of female and also on T lymphocytes. Action is mainly through JAK-STAT pathway.
- During pregnancy and in the postpartum period, prolactin-secreting cells constitute over 50% of pituitary acidophils. Prolactin along with estrogen and progesterone enhances the growth of lobulo-alveolar tissue of breast during pregnancy.
- Prolactin cannot initiate lactation during pregnancy because of the inhibitory effect of estrogen and progesterone in high levels. After delivery, estrogen and progesterone levels fall and prolactin initiates lactation.
- During lactation, high blood prolactin level (250 ng/ mL) suppresses LH secretion, which in turn inhibits ovulation. This is the reason for **lactational amenorrhea**.
- The function of prolactin in normal males is unsettled, but excess prolactin secreted by tumors cause erectile dysfunction.

Regulation of Secretion

Prolactin level is regulated by prolactin inhibiting hormone (PIH) or dopamine secreted by hypothalamus.

Stimuli which Affect Prolactin Secretion

Increased Secretion
- Stimulation of nipple
- Sleep
- Stress, exercise
- Hypoglycemia
- Drugs which inhibit dopamine receptors
- Pregnancy and lactation.

Decreased Secretion
- L- Dopa
- Bromocriptine and other dopamine agonists.

L-dopa decreases prolactin secretion by increasing the formation of dopamine. Bromocriptine and other dopamine agonists inhibit secretion by stimulating dopamine receptors.

Hypersecretion of Prolactin due to Tumor of Lactotrophs

Symptoms are:
- Galactorrhea
- Amenorrhea (refer reproductive system for details).

> **APPLIED PHYSIOLOGY**
>
> Hyperprolactinemia is a cause for infertility in females. High serum level of prolactin is associated with suppressed LH and FSH secretion from the anterior pituitary leading to its antigonadal effects. The condition is called **amenorrhea-galactorrhea syndrome**. The hypogonadism produced by hyperprolactinemia is associated with osteoporosis due to estrogen deficiency. In men, hyperprolactinemia leads to hypogonadism resulting in decreased spermatogenesis, loss of libido and erectile dysfunction. Dopamine agonists provide benefit in many cases.

Thyroid Stimulating Hormone

Thyroid stimulating hormone is necessary for the growth and secretory activity of thyroid gland (for details *refer* Chapter 65).

Adrenocorticotropic Hormone

Adrenocorticotropic hormone is a polypeptide hormone with 39 amino acids. The sequence of 4–11 amino acids of ACTH is identical with β-MSH and therefore it possesses some MSH activity. Its main action is on the adrenocortical cells to stimulate secretion of adrenocortical hormones. Mechanism of action is by activating adenylyl cyclase via Gs. ACTH secretion is very much increased during severe stress.

Follicle Stimulating Hormone

In males, FSH along with testosterone helps in spermatogenesis. In females, FSH is responsible for the development of Graafian follicle from primordial follicle. It also stimulates the theca cells of Graafian follicle to secrete estrogen.

Luteinizing Hormone

Action in Males

Luteinizing hormone stimulates the interstitial cells of Leydig to secrete testosterone. Hence, LH is also called interstitial cell stimulating hormone (ICTH).

Action in Females

- Along with FSH, LH helps in the formation of Graafian follicle.
- LH is the hormone responsible for ovulation.
- It is necessary for the formation of corpus luteum.
- It stimulates the secretory functions of corpus luteum.

β-Lipotropin

β-Lipotropin is a polypeptide hormone, which mobilizes fat from adipose tissue and promotes lipolysis. It acts through adenylyl cyclase. It forms the precursor of endorphins.

Intermediate Lobe of Pituitary

Intermediate lobe cells synthesize a pro-hormone called **pro-opiomelanocortin (POMC)**. POMC is hydrolyzed to corticotropin like intermediate-lobe peptide and β-endorphin. β-Endorphin is an opioid peptide like morphine. Intermediate cells also secrete **melanotropins, α and β-MSH**. The intermediate lobe in human is rudimentary. In humans, MSH is produced by corticotrophs. ACTH has MSH like activity.

Actions of Melanocyte Stimulating Hormone

In lower animals like reptiles and amphibia, MSH act on melanophores, which contain melanin pigment. Melanin pigment helps to change the color of their skin for thermoregulation, camouflage, etc.

Action of MSH is mediated via a **neuroendocrine reflex**. Receptors for this reflex are located in the retina. When the animal is exposed to dark, these receptors are stimulated and more of MSH is released, and this MSH causes dispersion of melanin granules and the skin darkens. On a white background, the MSH release is inhibited leading to aggregation of melanin granules and the skin becomes light.

In mammals, instead of melanophores, melanocytes are present which contain melanin granules. Administration of MSH in man causes increased melanin synthesis and leads to darkening of skin.

Since the amino acid sequence is similar for MSH and ACTH, ACTH has MSH-like activity. So, in conditions where ACTH level is high as in adrenal insufficiency there will be hyperpigmentation.

Abnormalities in Skin Pigmentation

- **Hyperpigmentation** of skin, e.g., adrenal insufficiency (due to adrenal disease).
- **Albinism** is due to congenital defect in the synthesis of melanin pigment.
- **Vitiligo** is a condition that develops after birth where there are patches of skin hypopigmentation (*refer* Chapter 58).

Pituitary Insufficiency or Panhypopituitarism (Flowchart 62.2)

In pituitary insufficiency, there will be deficiency of all the hormones controlled by the pituitary. The condition is also called **Simmonds disease** where there is complete destruction of the anterior pituitary.

Causes: Destruction of pituitary by infection, necrosis, tumors and surgical removal of the gland

Manifestations: Depend on the deficiency of the target organ hormone. First deficiency to be manifested is that of gonadotropins. This is followed by thyroid deficiency, which is followed by adrenals.
- Some of the secondary sex characteristics disappear.
- Cold intolerance due to decreased TSH.
- Hypoglycemia and decreased sensitivity to stress due to decrease in growth hormone and ACTH.
- Pallor due to decreased ACTH secretion, which has MSH like activity
- Senile decay, i.e., dry and wrinkled skin and accelerated aging due to decreased GH.
- Inhibition of growth in children.
- If posterior pituitary is also damaged, it leads to diabetes insipidus.
- Loss of hair over the body and loss of teeth.

Sheehan Syndrome

Following delivery, if there is excessive blood loss, it leads to hypotension. If hypotension is severe, it leads to **pituitary ischemia** and infarction leading to postpartum necrosis of the gland. This leads to pan-hypopituitarism referred to as **Sheehan syndrome**.

HYPOTHALAMUS

PY8.2: Describe the synthesis, secretion, transport, physiological actions, regulation and effect of altered (hypo and hyper) secretion of anterior pituitary gland and hypothalamus.

Anatomically, hypothalamus is situated at the center of the brain below the thalamus and above the pituitary gland. It is the primary link between nervous system and endocrine system. Hypothalamus is closely connected to the autonomic nervous system, limbic system and the pituitary gland. It plays a vital role in the regulation of visceral and endocrine functions. It controls all the secretions from the pituitary gland. Through its connections to the anterior pituitary, it controls thyroid gland, adrenal cortical secretions and gonadal functions. Via its influence on the sympathetic system, it controls the secretions of adrenal medulla. It directly controls the secretions of posterior pituitary (neurohormones). Since hypothalamus controls the major endocrine glands, it is considered as the **master of endocrine orchestra**. (Details of the connections and functions of hypothalamus are described in Chapter 92)

Hypothalamic Control of the Pituitary Gland

There are neural connections between the hypothalamus and the posterior pituitary and vascular connections between the hypothalamus and the anterior lobe of the pituitary gland. Releasing and inhibiting hormones produced by the hypothalamus control the secretory activity of the anterior lobe of pituitary gland. The hormones of the posterior pituitary, oxytocin and vasopressin are actually secreted by the supraoptic and paraventricular nuclei of the hypothalamus. In 1955, **Suffran and Schally** reported that extracts of median eminence of hypothalamus contain a substance that stimulates the release of ACTH from the anterior pituitary and they named this substance corticotropin-releasing factor. Later, many releasing and inhibiting hormones were isolated and their structures were determined. Before understanding the structure of the different hormones released from the hypothalamus, they were known as factors, but once their structure was determined they are referred to as hormones.

All the releasing and inhibiting hormones are small peptides synthesized in the ribosome of the neurosecretory cell. One exception is prolactin-inhibiting hormone, which is an amine, dopamine. In addition to acting as hormones, most of these hormones act as neurotransmitters.

The hormones secreted by the hypothalamus that regulate anterior pituitary are called **hypophysiotropic hormones.** They are:
- Corticotropin-releasing hormone (CRH)
- Gonadotropin-releasing hormone (GnRH)
- Thyrotropin-releasing hormone (TRH)

Flowchart 62.2: Disorders of pituitary gland.

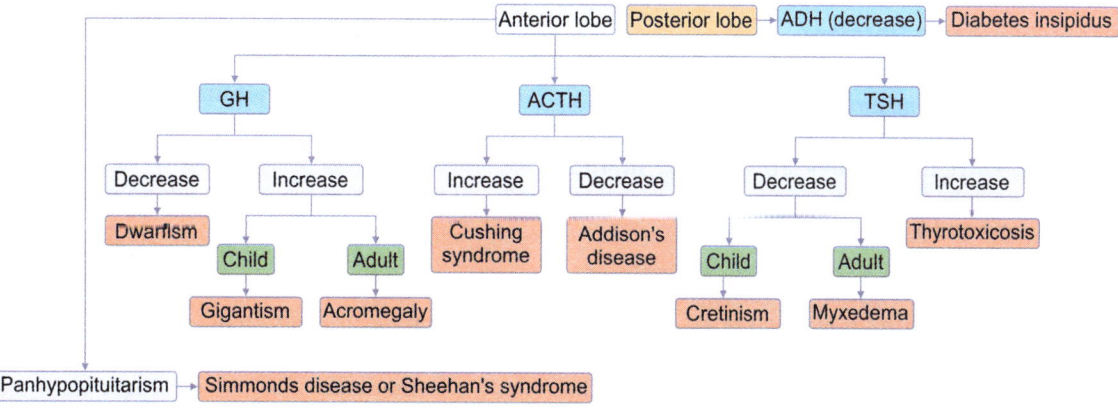

- Growth hormone-releasing hormone (GHRH)
- Growth hormone-inhibiting hormone (GHIH) or somatostatin
- Prolactin inhibiting hormone (PIH)
- Prolactin releasing hormone (PRH).

The releasing and inhibiting hormones reach the anterior pituitary through the hypothalamo-hypophyseal portal system. Under the influence of the hypothalamic releasing hormones, the anterior pituitary releases a set of hormones, which increase the secretory activity of the target glands like thyroid gland, adrenal cortex and gonads. These hormones act on target cells by acting through cAMP and IP_3 or DAG as second messengers.

The hormones produced by the target glands inhibit the hypothalamus and pituitary by feedback mechanisms leading to a decrease in the secretion of their tropic hormones. This is very essential for homeostasis. This hypothalamo-hypophyseal control of certain endocrine glands by feedback mechanisms is called **hypothalamo-hypophyseal axis**. Examples are hypothalamo-pituitary-thyroid axis, hypothalamo-pituitary-adrenocortical axis, hypothalamo-pituitary-gonadal axis, and hypothalamo-sympatho-adrenal axis.

Thyrotropin Releasing Hormone

Thyrotropin releasing hormone is the smallest of the releasing hormones and contains only three amino acids. Function is to *stimulate the release of thyroid stimulating hormone (TSH)* from anterior pituitary. It is also capable of *stimulating prolactin and growth hormone release*. It is secreted by neurosecretory neurons in the anterior paraventricular nucleus of hypothalamus. The axons of these neurosecretory cells end in the median eminence where they terminate on the capillary loops of the hypothalamo-hypophyseal portal system. TRH also acts as a neurotransmitter.

Gonadotropin Releasing Hormone or GnRH or LHRH

Gonadotropin releasing hormone regulates the *release of both LH and FSH*. It is a peptide containing 10 amino acids. The neurosecretory cells are found in the arcuate nucleus of hypothalamus mainly, but are also present in the pre-optic area. GnRH is also expressed in the placenta and it *stimulates secretion of growth hormone*.

Corticotropin Releasing Hormone

Corticotropin releasing hormone was the first releasing hormone to be detected in median eminence extracts. It is a 41 amino acid peptide that has potent ACTH stimulating properties. The CRH cell bodies are present in the paraventricular nucleus. CRH also stimulates the secretion of β- and γ-lipotropin and β-endorphins.

Prolactin Releasing Factor

A 31-amino acid polypeptide was isolated from human hypothalamus, which stimulated prolactin secretion from anterior pituitary. TRH, vasoactive intestinal polypeptide (VIP) and several other polypeptides found in hypothalamus also stimulate prolactin secretion. The actual physiologic prolactin releasing hormone (PRH) is yet to be isolated.

Prolactin Inhibiting Hormone

Prolactin-inhibiting hormone (PIH) is a simple monoamine, dopamine, which inhibits prolactin secretion from anterior pituitary. Prolactin is mostly under inhibitory control, since isolation of pituitary from hypothalamus leads to hypersecretion of prolactin. (The dopaminergic neurons are present mainly in the substantia nigra which project to the basal ganglia and act as neurotransmitter.) A group of dopaminergic neurons is present in the arcuate nucleus-medial eminence region of hypothalamus that secretes dopamine into portal circulation. Dopamine binds to prolactin secreting anterior pituitary cells and inhibits prolactin release.

Growth Hormone Releasing Hormone

Growth hormone releasing hormone consists of 44 amino acids and the cell bodies are present in the arcuate nucleus of hypothalamus. It increases the secretion of growth hormone from anterior pituitary.

Growth Hormone Inhibiting Hormone or Somatostatin

Somatostatin is a 14 amino acid peptide that inhibits secretion of growth hormone from anterior pituitary. The neurosecretory cells are present in the periventricular nucleus, supraoptic and paraventricular nuclei of hypothalamus. Only 30% of brain somatostatin is of hypothalamic origin. Rest is present in the cortex, thalamus and brainstem. These act as neurotransmitters and are not involved in the control of pituitary hormone release.

Ghrelin

Ghrelin is a hormone synthesized both in the hypothalamus and oxyntic cells of stomach. It acts on somatotrophs to increase growth hormone secretion. It also acts on hypothalamus to increase secretion of GHRH. Ghrelin stimulates the arcuate nucleus to release neuropeptide Y (NPY) which in turn enhance appetite.

■ MULTIPLE CHOICE QUESTIONS

1. **Basophilic cells of pituitary secretes all, *except*:**
   a. GH b. TSH
   c. ACTH d. LH
2. **Hormones secreted by adenohypophysis are all, *except*:**
   a. Oxytocin b. Gonadotropins
   c. ACTH d. Prolactin
3. **ACTH level is highest during:**
   a. Early morning b. Evening
   c. Afternoon d. Night

CHAPTER 62 — Anterior Pituitary Gland and Hypothalamus

4. The biological clock responsible for diurnal variation of ACTH is located in:
   a. Supraoptic nucleus
   b. Suprachiasmatic nucleus
   c. Cerebral cortex
   d. Amygdaloid nucleus

5. MSH is secreted by:
   a. Anterior lobe of pituitary
   b. Intermediate lobe of pituitary
   c. Posterior lobe of pituitary
   d. Pineal gland

6. Acromegaly is due to excess of:
   a. Somatomedin
   b. Somatostatin
   c. Thyroxine
   d. Growth hormone

7. Secretion of prolactin is affected by:
   a. GnRH
   b. Dopamine
   c. Serotonin
   d. FSH

8. Accidental transection of pituitary stalk causes all the following, *except*:
   a. Polyuria
   b. Galactorrhea
   c. Diabetes mellitus
   d. Diabetes insipidus

9. TRH stimulation testing is useful in the diagnosis of disorders of the following hormone:
   a. Insulin
   b. ACTH
   c. Growth hormone
   d. PTH

10. The transmitter which control the secretion of prolactin is:
    a. Serotonin
    b. GABA
    c. Somatostatin
    d. Dopamine

11. Transection of pituitary stalk leads to increase in:
    a. TSH
    b. ACTH
    c. GH
    d. Prolactin

12. The following are hormones secreted from the anterior pituitary, *except*:
    a. Growth hormone
    b. ACTH
    c. Somatostatin
    d. Prolactin

13. Which of the following are true of median eminence?
    a. Portion of ventral hypothalamus
    b. Hypothalamo-hypophyseal vessels arise here
    c. Outside the blood brain barrier
    d. All are correct

14. Panhypopituitarism causes all, *except*:
    a. Pigmentation
    b. Infertility
    c. Loss of secondary sexual characters
    d. Cold intolerance

15. The effect of hypophysectomy include all the following, *except*:
    a. Glucocorticoid deficiency
    b. Mineralocorticoid deficiency
    c. Menstrual failure
    d. Diabetes mellitus

16. The anterior lobe of hypophysis secretes the following, *except*:
    a. Somatotrophic hormones
    b. Prolactin
    c. Thyrotrophic hormone
    d. Antidiuretic hormone

17. Correct regarding beta endorphins:
    a. A lipoprotein
    b. Analogue of morphine
    c. Hormone of intermediate lobe of pituitary
    d. Morphine receptor in brain

18. The following parts of brain does not require insulin for the entry of glucose into cells, *except*:
    a. Cerebral cortex
    b. Cerebellum
    c. Posteroventral nucleus of thalamus
    d. Ventromedial nucleus of hypothalamus

19. Beta endorphin is:
    a. A lipoprotein
    b. Analog of morphine
    c. Hormone of intermediate lobe of pituitary
    d. Morphine receptor in brain

20. Anterior pituitary gland exerts very little control on the regulation of secretion of:
    a. Thyroxine
    b. Glucocorticoids
    c. Estrogen
    d. Adrenalin

21. Growth and development is promoted by all the following hormones, *except*:
    a. Thyroxine
    b. Insulin
    c. Somatostatin
    d. Somatotropic hormone

22. Sheehan's syndrome is due to:
    a. Adrenal hemorrhage
    b. Pituitary hemorrhage
    c. Hypothalamic hemorrhage
    d. Pancreatic hemorrhage

23. Pituitary diabetes mellitus is due to:
    a. Increase in ADH
    b. Decrease in ADH
    c. Decrease in insulin
    d. Increase in growth hormone

ANSWERS

1. a
2. a
3. a
4. b
5. b
6. d
7. b
8. c
9. c
10. d
11. d
12. c
13. d
14. a
15. d
16. c
17. d
18. c
19. c
20. d
21. c
22. b
23. d

Posterior Pituitary

CHAPTER 63

LEARNING OBJECTIVES
- Explain the actions of vasopressin
- Enumerate the functions of oxytocin
- Describe the disorders of posterior pituitary hormone secretion

INTRODUCTION

PY8.2: Describe the synthesis, secretion, transport, physiological actions, regulation and effect of altered (hypo and hyper) secretion of posterior pituitary gland.

Posterior pituitary consists of endings of unmyelinated axons of **hypothalamo-hypophyseal tract (Fig. 63.1)**. It also contains neuroglial cells called **pituicytes**. Pituicytes are stellate cells that are modified astrocytes. The posterior pituitary does not have secretory cells of its own but it stores and releases the neurohormones antidiuretic hormone (ADH) and oxytocin synthesized in the hypothalamus.

HORMONES OF POSTERIOR PITUITARY

- Arginine vasopressin (AVP) or antidiuretic hormone (ADH)
- Oxytocin.

The hormones vasopressin and oxytocin are synthesized in the cell bodies of the magnocellular neurons in the **supraoptic** and **paraventricular nuclei** of hypothalamus.

Oxytocin-containing and vasopressin-containing cells are found in both nuclei. But vasopressin is mainly synthesized in the supraoptic nucleus and oxytocin in the paraventricular nucleus. Both hormones are polypeptides with nine amino acids (nonapeptides) and one disulfide ring at one end. These hormones are transported bound to a carrier protein called **neurophysin** down the unmyelinated axons of these neurons to their endings in the posterior lobe. These axons form tracts that pass to the neurohypophysis through the pituitary stalk. Oxytocin is associated with neurophysin-I and vasopressin with neurophysin-II. They are stored in the axonal endings in the posterior pituitary in the free form in granules called **Herring bodies (Fig. 63.1)** and released in times of need along with the associated neurophysin. The nerve endings which are bulbous knobs containing the Herring bodies are in close proximity to the capillaries so that the hormones can be secreted directly into the blood stream.

Oxytocin and vasopressin are typical **neural hormones**, that is, they are hormones secreted into the circulation by nerve cells. Vasopressin-secreting neurons are also found in the suprachiasmatic nuclei, and vasopressin and oxytocin are also found in the neurons that project from the paraventricular nuclei to the brain stem and spinal cord. Oxytocin is also synthesized in the gonads.

Mechanism of Secretion of Hormones

When a stimulus for secretion of vasopressin or oxytocin acts on the appropriate magnocellular cell body, an action potential is generated. It is propagated down the long axon to the posterior pituitary. The action potential causes an influx of calcium ions, which induces neurosecretory granules to fuse with the cell membrane and exocytosis of the contents of the granules occur into the perivascular space. Subsequently the hormones enter the blood in the capillaries of the posterior pituitary.

Vasopressin or ADH

Actions of Vasopressin

There are three kinds of vasopressin receptors, namely, V_{1A}, V_{1B} and V_2. All are G-protein coupled receptors. V_{1A} and V_{1B}

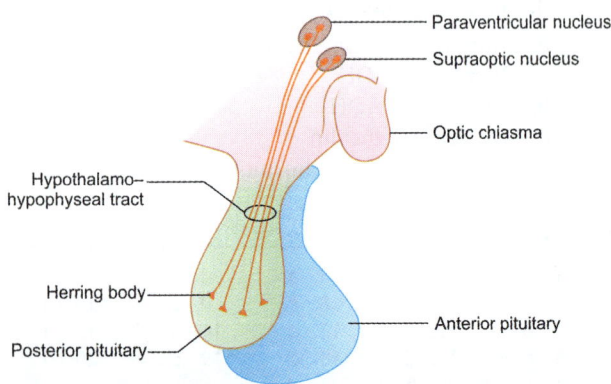

Fig. 63.1: Hypothalamo-hypophyseal tract.

receptors act through phosphatidylinositol hydrolysis to form inositol triphosphate and diacylglycerol to increase intracellular Ca^{2+} concentration. V_2 receptors act through Gs to increase cAMP levels. Actions depend on the type of receptors stimulated. V_1 receptors present on blood vessels mediate smooth muscle contraction and activated V_2 receptors promote antidiuresis. *Half-life of ADH in plasma is 15 minutes.*

The actions of vasopressin are:
- Vasoconstrictor and antidiuretic action
- Glycogenolysis in liver via V_{1A} receptors
- Stimulate release of ACTH from anterior pituitary via V_{1B} receptors
- Act as neurotransmitter in brain and spinal cord
- Vasopressin stimulates the production of clotting factor VIII and vWF via V_2 receptors

Vasopressor Effect of ADH

Vasopressin in large amount (pharmacological dose) is a potent stimulator of vascular smooth muscle producing peripheral vasoconstriction and increase in blood pressure. Because of this reason ADH is also called vasopressin. It causes constriction of arterioles in all parts of the body. This occurs mainly in times of hypotension, e.g., hemorrhage. **Vasoconstrictor effect** is mediated via V_{1A} receptors.

Antidiuretic Action

Since the principal physiologic effect of vasopressin is retention of water by the kidney, it is often called **antidiuretic hormone** (ADH). It promotes antidiuresis by the following mechanisms:
- When the osmotic pressure of blood is high, ADH is released and it increases the reabsorption of water in the distal convoluted tubules and collecting tubules of kidney. This is by increasing their permeability to water by increasing the number of aquaporins (protein water channels), especially **aquaporin-2** in the luminal cell membrane. Thus, the volume of urine decreases and urine becomes concentrated. The effective osmotic pressure of body fluids returns to normal. In the absence of vasopressin, the urine becomes hypotonic to plasma, urine volume is increased and there is net water loss. Consequently, the osmolality of body fluids rises. Antidiuretic action is mediated via **V_2 receptors**, which act by stimulating adenylyl cyclase to increase cAMP levels (for details, *refer* renal physiology, Chapter 55).
- ADH increases the permeability of collecting duct to urea by activating urea transporter proteins.
- It stimulates Na^+-K^+-$2Cl^-$ cotransport in the thick ascending limb of loop of Henle.

Action on Anterior Pituitary

Antidiuretic hormone (ADH) causes increased secretion of ACTH from anterior pituitary and this action is mediated via V_{1B} receptors, which act through phosphatidylinositol hydrolysis to increase intracellular Ca^{2+} concentration. Thus, it controls aldosterone secretion from adrenal cortex.

Regulation of ADH Secretion

- First mechanism is by changes in the osmolar concentration of body fluids
- Second mechanism is by changes in the extracellular fluid volume.

Mechanism of osmoregulation: There are receptors called **osmoreceptors** in the anterior hypothalamus near the supraoptic and paraventricular nuclei. They are stimulated by increase in osmotic pressure of body fluids above 285 mOsm/kg. When they lose water, these receptors are stimulated which in turn stimulate the neurons which secrete ADH, i.e., *hyperosmolality is the prime determinant of ADH secretion.* More of water is reabsorbed in the kidney and osmotic pressure of blood is brought back to normal. On the other hand, when plasma osmolality falls, ADH secretion falls and more water is excreted through urine. As little as 1% change in plasma osmolality cause significant changes in ADH secretion.

ECF volume effects: Vasopressin secretion is increased when ECF volume is low, and decreased when ECF volume is high. The receptors involved are **stretch receptors** in the blood vessels. There are low-pressure receptors and high-pressure receptors. Low-pressure receptors are present in the great veins and atria, and these receptors are the mediators of volume effects on vasopressin secretion. Stimulation of volume receptors inhibits ADH secretion. Increase in blood volume increases stretch of blood vessels and the low pressure volume receptors are stimulated. Via vagus nerve, inhibitory impulses reach the supraoptic nucleus and there will be inhibition of ADH secretion.

Hypovolemia and hypotension release large amounts of vasopressin. *Hypovolemia is a more potent stimulus to release ADH than hyperosmolality.*

Factors Affecting ADH Secretion

Increase in ADH Secretion

- Increase in the osmotic pressure of plasma as in dehydration.
- Decrease in extracellular fluid (ECF) volume.
- Pain, fear, anger, exercise, etc.
- Drugs such as nicotine, morphine, barbiturates
- Cirrhosis of liver and nephrosis increase ADH level in blood because it is mainly inactivated by liver and kidney.
- Surgical stress and nausea

Decrease in ADH secretion

- Decreased osmotic pressure of plasma.
- Increase in ECF volume.
- Alcohol, anticholinergic agents such as atropine; caffeine etc., decrease ADH release by their direct action on the supraoptic nucleus.
- Adrenaline or epinephrine

Abnormalities in ADH Secretion

Diabetes Insipidus (Tasteless Urine)

- **Central or neurogenic diabetes insipidus**
  Causes:
  - Hypothalamic lesion leads to ADH deficiency
  - Destruction of posterior pituitary

In central diabetes insipidus, there will be complete or partial failure of ADH secretion. Symptoms include **polyuria and polydipsia**, i.e., passage of large amounts of dilute urine and drinking large amounts of fluid. Urine volume may increase up to 3–20 L/day. Dehydration may occur in severe cases leading to hypotension.

❖ **Nephrogenic diabetes insipidus**
Nephrogenic diabetes insipidus is due to inability of kidney to respond to vasopressin or ADH. This may be due to defects in V_2 receptors or mutation of aquaporin-2.

Syndrome of Inappropriate Hypersecretion of ADH (SIADH) or Dilution Syndrome

In certain cerebral diseases and lung diseases such as lung tumors, the impulses from the volume receptors do not reach the hypothalamus to inhibit ADH secretion. The body osmolarity will be low, but ADH secretion will be high. ECF Na^+ level will be very much decreased and ECF volume will be high. There will be features of water intoxication, called **over-hydration or dilution syndrome**.

Prolonged exposure to elevated level of vasopressin eventually leads to down regulation of production of aquaporin-2. This decreases water reabsorption in the distal nephron; i.e., the individual escapes from the renal effects of vasopressin. This is called **vasopressin escape**.

OXYTOCIN

Oxytocin is a peptide hormone and a neuropeptide. In humans, oxytocin acts primarily on breasts and uterus. Its actions are mediated by specific oxytocin receptors. Oxytocin receptors present in the myometrium, mammary gland and ovary are **G-protein coupled receptors** and stimulation of these receptors increases intracellular Ca^{2+} levels. Oxytocin also has actions in the brain. The behavioral effects of oxytocin are mediated via oxytocin released from centrally projecting oxytocin neurons, which are different from those that project to the pituitary gland. Oxytocin receptors are expressed by neurons in many parts of brain and spinal cord, such as the amygdala, ventromedial hypothalamus, septum, and the brain stem.

Actions of Oxytocin

❖ Oxytocin stimulates contraction of smooth muscles of pregnant uterus and helps in the expulsion of the fetus. The sensitivity of the myometrium of uterus to oxytocin is enhanced by estrogen and inhibited by progesterone. Progesterone acts directly on the uterine oxytocin receptors and inhibit them. The number of oxytocin receptors in the uterus is increased in late pregnancy and oxytocin secretion is increased during parturition. There is a positive feedback effect on oxytocin secretion during labor till the baby is expelled.
❖ Oxytocin stimulates the release of prostaglandins in the placenta, which intensify uterine contractions induced by oxytocin.
❖ It also causes contraction of the myoepithelial cells that surround the alveoli of the mammary gland and help in milk ejection during lactation. Milk ejection is initiated by a neuroendocrine reflex.
❖ Oxytocin released during breastfeeding causes mild contractions of the uterus during the first few weeks of lactation. This helps in involution of uterus after delivery.
❖ Oxytocin plays a role in maternal behavior.
❖ It appears to be involved in luteolysis.
❖ Oxytocin act on non-pregnant uterus to facilitate sperm transport by producing uterine contractions towards the fallopian tube.
❖ At the time of ejaculation, there is increased oxytocin secretion in males, which causes increased contraction of the smooth muscles of vas deferens, propelling sperm towards the urethra.
❖ In high doses, oxytocin causes relaxation of blood vessels producing a fall in blood pressure. In high doses, oxytocin stimulates sodium excretion from the kidneys leading to hyponatremia.
❖ Secretion of oxytocin is increased by stressful stimuli and inhibited by alcohol
❖ Oxytocin has been implicated in the etiology of autism as a result of mutation on the oxytocin receptor gene.
❖ Oxytocin is found to have a role in social behavior and possibly plays a role in emotional bonding and it increases positive attitudes. Trust is increased by oxytocin.

Stimuli Increasing Oxytocin Secretion

❖ Stimulation of touch receptors of nipple during suckling
❖ Emotional stimulus, e.g., hearing the baby's cry
❖ Stimulation of cervix during parturition
❖ Genital stimulation during coitus
❖ Stimulation of cholinergic nerve fibers.

Stimuli Decreasing Oxytocin Secretion

❖ Emotional stress
❖ Stimulation of sympathetic neurons
❖ Drugs such as ethanol and enkephalins

Neuroendocrine Reflex

Neuroendocrine reflex is a reflex mechanism in which the nervous system and endocrine system interact in bringing about the reflex, e.g., milk ejection reflex or milk letdown reflex. Normally a reflex is a neural phenomenon where, the reflex arc consists of neurons in the afferent and efferent limbs. When the afferent limb is neural and a hormone forms part of the efferent limb, the reflex is referred to as **neuroendocrine reflex**. Thus this reflex involves both hormones and neurons in the reflex pathway.

Milk Ejection Reflex

In milk ejection reflex, receptors are the touch receptors around the nipple. Stimulus is **suckling of the breast** by the baby. Afferent impulses are relayed from the spinal

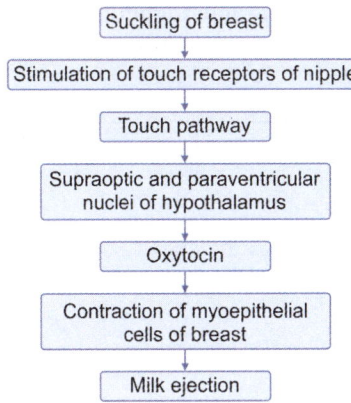

Flowchart 63.1: Pathway for milk ejection reflex.

nerves through the touch pathway to the **supraoptic and paraventricular nuclei** of hypothalamus (**Flowchart 63.1**). These neurons when stimulated fire action potentials in intermittent bursts. These bursts result in the secretion of pulses of oxytocin from the neurosecretory nerve terminals of the posterior pituitary gland. The oxytocin released from here reaches the breast and causes contraction of the myoepithelial cells (contractile cells that line the ducts of mammary gland) leading to milk ejection. This process by which milk is ejected from the alveoli of breast is called **milk ejection reflex or milk let down reflex**. As this reflex is initiated by nervous factors and completed by hormonal action, it is called neuroendocrine reflex.

Parturition: Another example of neuroendocrine reflex is increased uterine contraction **during labor or parturition**. Throughout the period of pregnancy, oxytocin secretion is inhibited by estrogen and progesterone. Towards term, secretion of estrogen and progesterone decreases and oxytocin secretion is increased. In late pregnancy, the uterus becomes very sensitive to oxytocin because there is a marked increase in the number of oxytocin receptors in the uterus. Descent of the baby during parturition causes dilation of the cervix. The receptors in the cervix are stimulated and afferent impulses from the cervix reach the supraoptic and paraventricular nuclei of hypothalamus through afferent nerve fibers. This causes further increase in the secretion of oxytocin, which increases the intensity of uterine contractions. This is a positive feedback mechanism (refer **Chapter 61, Fig. 61.7**) and it continues till the baby is born.

Other Examples of Neuroendocrine Reflexes

❖ During sexual intercourse, the receptors in the vagina are stimulated. They generate impulses in the afferent nerves, which are transmitted to the supraoptic and paraventricular nuclei of hypothalamus. There is increased release of oxytocin into the blood stream, which reaches the female genital tract. Oxytocin causes contraction of uterus towards the fallopian tube to facilitate sperm transport. This is also a neuroendocrine reflex.

❖ Reflex ovulation is another example. Female cats, rabbits, minks etc. have long period of estrus, during which they ovulate only after copulation. Such reflex ovulation is brought about by afferent impulses from the genitalia and the eye, ears and nose that converge on the ventral hypothalamus and provoke ovulation by inducing the release of LH from the pituitary.

❖ Melatonin secretion from the pineal gland is another example. Afferent is retinohypothalamic pathway. Efferent is secretion of melatonin (refer **Flowchart 64.2**).

Uses of Oxytocin

❖ Oxytocin is used as a therapeutic agent in the induction of labor.
❖ Along with estrogen, oxytocin is used therapeutically in arresting uterine bleeding.
❖ Oxytocin injections are given to dairy animals before milking them.

■ MULTIPLE CHOICE QUESTIONS

1. Posterior pituitary releases:
   a. Prolactin   b. MSH
   c. ADH   d. FSH
2. Milk ejection reflex is mediated by:
   a. Oxytocin   b. Vasopressin
   c. Growth hormone   d. Thyroxin
3. In the neurohypophysis, secretory granules accumulate in:
   a. Pituicytes
   b. Nerve endings
   c. Intercellular spaces
   d. Capillary endothelium
4. Oxytocin causes all, *except*:
   a. Lactogenesis
   b. Milk ejection
   c. Contraction of uterine muscle
   d. Myoepithelial cell contraction
5. Which of the following is true regarding oxytocin?
   a. Increased at the time of ovulation
   b. Secreted by paraventricular nucleus
   c. Effective in males
   d. Important for maintaining pregnancy
6. Hypertonic contraction of fluid volume is caused by:
   a. Addison's disease
   b. Cushing disease
   c. Salt losing nephropathy
   d. Diabetes insipidus
7. In which of the following form is ADH circulated in plasma?
   a. Bound to plasma albumin
   b. Bound to globulin
   c. Bound to neurophysin-I
   d. Free form

8. **In stress which of the following hormone is increased?**
   a. Insulin
   b. Vasopressin
   c. Parathormone
   d. Thyroxine

9. **All the following statements are true, *except*:**
   a. Vasopressin is the main hormone involved in the regulation of water homeostasis and osmolality
   b. Renin-angiotensin-aldosterone system is mainly responsible for regulation of blood pressure and blood volume
   c. V_2 vasopressin receptors stimulate ACTH secretion from the anterior pituitary
   d. V_{1a} receptors are mainly present in blood vessels

ANSWERS

| 1. c | 2. a | 3. b | 4. a | 5. b |
| 6. d | 7. d | 8. b | 9. c | |

Pineal Gland

CHAPTER 64

LEARNING OBJECTIVES
- Enumerate the functions of melatonin
- Explain the mechanism of circadian rhythm

INTRODUCTION

PY8.3: Describe the physiology of pineal gland.

Pineal gland is a small, conical structure having the size of a grain of rice about 6 mm long. It is a midline structure, located between the two cerebral hemispheres. It is attached by the pineal stalk to the posterior wall of the third ventricle. This gland is termed pineal gland because it resembles a pine cone. It has a role in circadian rhythm by producing melatonin. The pineal gland can alter its production of melatonin based on the amount of light perceived by the eyes. This gland is also known as the '**third eye**' of the body because of its ability to respond to the perception of light.

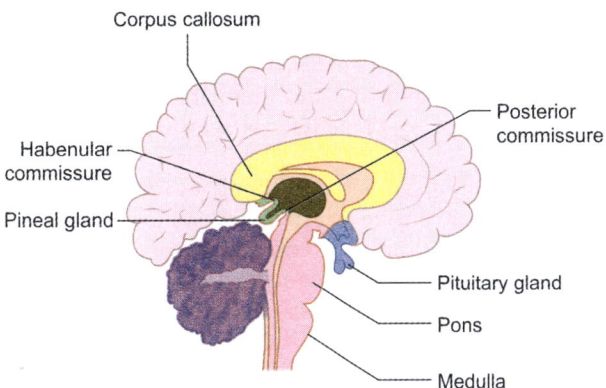

Fig. 64.1: Sagittal section of brain showing the location of pineal gland.

FUNCTIONAL ANATOMY

Pineal gland is located in the roof of the third ventricle posteriorly between the habenula and the posterior commissure. The gland is covered by pia mater and consists of masses of neuroglia and secretory cells called **pinealocytes**. The gland weighs about 0.1–0.2 g. *It is the smallest endocrine gland in the body.* Pineal gland is embryologically derived from an evagination of the ependymal cells of the roof of third ventricle and is **outside the blood-brain-barrier (Fig. 64.1).** It is a part of circumventricular organs (CVO).

Brain sand (pineal sand) is concretions of calcified material (carbonates and phosphates of calcium and magnesium) which progressively accumulate within the pineal gland with age. It is radiopaque and can be seen in X-ray pictures as pineal sand. Displacement of a calcified pineal gland from its normal position indicates the presence of a space-occupying lesion.

Innervation of the Gland

There is a circuitous innervation through postganglionic sympathetic nerve supply from the superior cervical ganglia. The sympathetic preganglionic fibers in the superior sympathetic chain arise in the lateral horn of spinal cord.

These nerve cells are regulated by descending fibers from the **suprachiasmatic nucleus** of hypothalamus, which receives a direct nerve input from the retina through the **retinohypothalamic tract (Fig. 64.2).** This tract conveys information about light and dark, independent of conscious perception. Suprachiasmatic nucleus is the primary pacemaker for the circadian rhythm. This pathway regulates pineal activity in response to external light. The sympathetic fibers end on the plasma membrane of pinealocytes. β-adrenergic blockers and damage to sympathetic innervation inhibit pineal metabolic activity.

> A small number of photoreceptors in the retina contain **melanopsin** rather than rhodopsin or cone pigments. The axons of these photoreceptors project to the suprachiasmatic nuclei (concerned with circadian rhythm) *and all the circadian entrainment responses to light-dark changes* are controlled by this system. In the absence of melanopsin, the circadian photo entrainment is found to be abolished.

Secretion of Pineal Gland

The pinealocytes secrete indoleamines like **melatonin** and some **peptide hormones**.

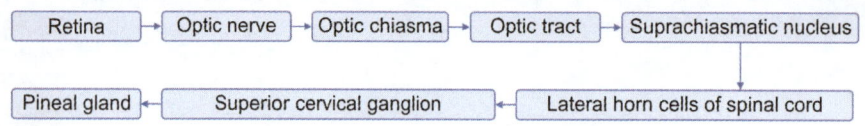

Fig. 64.2: Pathway from retina to pineal gland.

The peptides present in small amounts in the pineal gland are:
- Arginine vasopressin
- Oxytocin
- Adrenocorticotropic hormone (**ACTH**), α-melanocyte-stimulating hormone (**MSH**), β-endorphin

Synthesis of Melatonin (Flowchart 64.1)

Melatonin (N-acetyl-5-methoxytryptamine) is synthesized from the amino acid tryptophan.

Serotonin-N-acetyltransferase (SNAT) *is the rate limiting enzyme in the synthesis of melatonin* (**Flowchart 64.1**). SNAT is also known as **arylalkylamine-N-acetyltransferase (AANAT)**. The concentration of serotonin in the pineal gland is very high. The activity of SNAT and the concentration of melatonin in the pineal gland fluctuate with a circadian rhythm. Peak of SNAT activity is seen during hours of darkness.

Stimulation of sympathetic supply to the pineal gland releases norepinephrine, which in turn stimulate melatonin synthesis by binding to β-adrenergic receptors on the pinealocytes. This increases the synthesis of **cyclic adenosine monophosphate (cAMP)** from adenosine triphosphate by activating adenylyl cyclase. This is followed by increased RNA and protein synthesis. There is also stimulation of SNAT activity. Spontaneous activity in the sympathetic fibers innervating the pineal gland is highest in the darkness.

Regulation of Melatonin Secretion (Flowchart 64.2)

Pineal activity exhibits a **circadian rhythm** that is influenced by light. It is most active during darkness, i.e., melatonin level rises in darkness and falls during the day.

The pineal gland does not store appreciable quantities of melatonin. Melatonin acts through MT1 and MT2 receptors.

Maximum secretion of melatonin is seen in children of 1–3 years of age and it is approximately 250 pg/mL. In young adults, the blood level of melatonin is 70 pg/mL and in old age it is only 30 pg/mL. Melatonin secretion is controlled by sympathetic nerves originating from the superior cervical ganglion. The sympathetic fibers to the pineal gland are under the control of the suprachiasmatic nucleus of hypothalamus which is linked to the day-night cycle through the retinohypothalamic fibers (**Flowchart 64.2**). This can be considered as a **neuroendocrine reflex**.

Diurnal Variation

Melatonin secretion peaks between 2 am and 6 am, and probably serves to control the circadian rhythm of other physiological events. Melatonin synthesis and secretion are increased during darkness and maintained at a low level during day light hours (**Flowchart 64.3**).

Flowchart 64.1: Steps in the synthesis of melatonin.

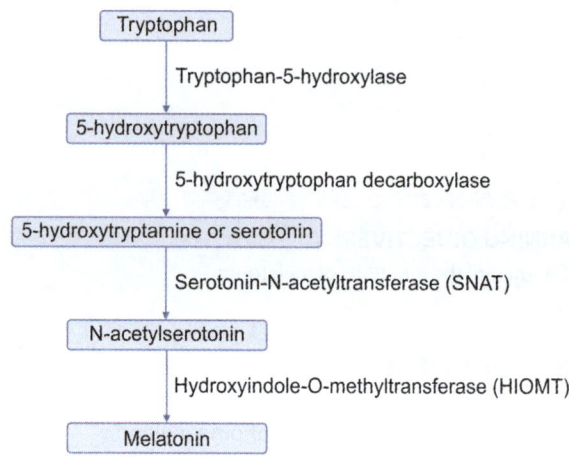

Flowchart 64.2: Regulation of melatonin secretion.

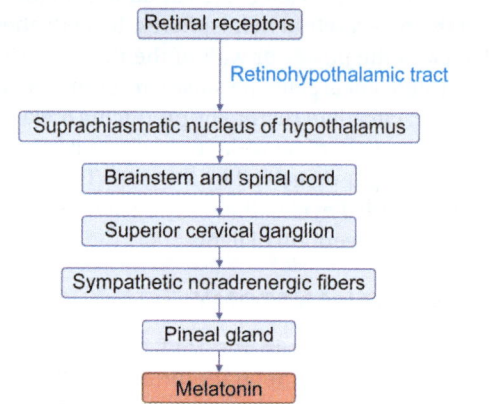

Flowchart 64.3: Circadian rhythm in melatonin secretion.

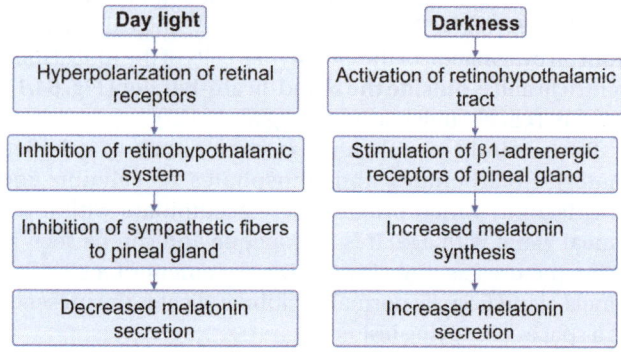

Functions and Uses of Melatonin

- Melatonin has an important role in the regulation of reproductive function. Melatonin is **antigonadotropic**. It is a regulator of seasonal reproductive cycles in most mammalian species by its effect on luteinizing hormone (LH) pulse frequency. Melatonin acts on the gonadotropin releasing hormone (GnRH) pulse generator. It inhibits GnRH secretion from hypothalamus. Main action is on anterior pituitary to inhibit the release of gonadotrophic hormones, follicle-stimulating hormone (FSH) and luteinizing hormone (LH).

- **Pineal gland and puberty**: It is seen that precocious puberty occurs in patients with pineal tumors that decrease melatonin secretion. In true pinealomas where there is increased secretion of melatonin, delayed puberty and hypogonadism are seen. *Puberty is also delayed in blind girls due to increased melatonin.*
- Role in **circadian rhythm**: Pineal gland functions as a timing device to keep internal events synchronized with the light-dark cycle in the environment.
- Melatonin influences the activity of adrenal gland, thyroid, parathyroid and endocrine pancreas. *The actions are mainly inhibitory.* It inhibits ACTH secretion. Pinealectomy leads to hypertrophy of adrenal cortex. The action of melatonin on corticosterone secretion and aldosterone secretion are primarily inhibitory.
- Melatonin inhibits thyroid function by directly acting on the gland and also by inhibiting TRH secretion.
- Melatonin inhibits insulin secretion by pancreas.
- It has a role in thermoregulation. It has a **hyperthermic** effect.
- Enhancement of immune function and inhibition of tumor growth. **Antitumor** activity is due to the antimitotic effect of melatonin.
- Melatonin is used to treat patients with depression.
- Melatonin **induces sleep** and also improves the quality and duration of sleep. REM sleep will be increased. In the darkness, norepinephrine released from the sympathetic fibers supplying the pineal gland stimulates synthesis and secretion of melatonin which produces sleepiness. It has a hypnotic effect in low doses.
- Melatonin is a very effective **antioxidant**. It is a potent scavenger of free radicals. As an antioxidant it is more effective than vitamin E. It protects neurons in the central nervous system from free radicals like nitric oxide and hydrogen peroxide. There is a high affinity binding site for melatonin (MT3) on the cytosolic enzyme **quinone reductase 2**, which is involved in cellular detoxification.
- Melatonin can slow down the progression of aging mainly due to its antioxidant effect.
- It can prevent ischemic damage after vascular reperfusion
- It is used for resetting circadian rhythms. Thus it is used to treat jet lag and certain sleep disorders.

CIRCADIAN RHYTHM

Circadian rhythm means a 24 hours (ranges from 20-28 hours) fluctuation in body functions. Circadian in Latin means 'about a day'. It refers to numerous physiological processes that are coupled to the timing of light and darkness.

It helps to adapt in the geographical locations. Normally all living organisms become entrained (entrain means gradually to fall into synchrony with the rhythm) to the day-night light cycle in the environment.

Factors Affecting Circadian Rhythm

- Variations of geophysical parameters caused by rotation of the earth round its axis is the main factor
- Genetic influences
- Information from suprachiasmatic nucleus of hypothalamus which is referred to as the biological clock.
- Light and darkness are exogenous factors that influence the internal environment greatly.

Mechanism

Hypothalamic nucleus maintaining the circadian rhythmicity is the suprachiasmatic nucleus (**Flowchart 64.2**). The suprachiasmatic nucleus (SCN) plays a major role in the entrainment process. The SCN receive information about the light-dark cycle via the retinohypothalamic fibers. Efferent fibers from the SCN initiate neural and humoral signals that entrain a wide variety of circadian rhythms like sleep-wake cycle, release of melatonin from the pineal gland, etc.

Two melatonin G-protein-coupled receptors referred to as melatonin receptor type 1 and 2 (MT_1 and MT_2) are found on the neurons in the SCN. Activation of MT_1 receptor inhibits adenylyl cyclase and results in sleepiness. Activation of MT_2 receptors stimulates phosphoinositide hydrolysis and helps to synchronize the light-dark cycle.

Melatonin inhibits the activity of the neurons in the suprachiasmatic nucleus of the hypothalamus which is considered as the **circadian pacemaker** in the brain. Melatonin can entrain several mammalian circadian rhythms, probably by inhibition of neurons in the SCN. Many effects of melatonin on circadian rhythm is mediated via MT_1 and MT_2 receptors present in the SCN, retina and pars tuberalis of adenohypophysis.

The diurnal change in melatonin secretion may function as a timing signal to coordinate events with the light-dark cycle in the environment (**Flowchart 64.3**). Melatonin secretion is increased during dark and decreased during daylight. This diurnal variation in secretion is due to norepinephrine released from the post-ganglionic sympathetic nerves that innervate the pineal gland. Norepinephrine via beta adrenergic receptors increases intracellular cAMP which in turn produces a marked increase in N-acetyltransferase activity. This results in increased melatonin synthesis and secretion.

Insomnia is difficulty in initiating or maintaining sleep several times a week. The two major types of sleep disorders are transient sleep disorders like jet lag, shift work and illness: and chronic sleep disorders like advanced sleep phase syndrome which is associated with old age and depression. Melatonin is used to treat jet lag and insomnia in elderly individuals.

MULTIPLE CHOICE QUESTIONS

1. **Melatonin is secreted by:**
   a. Hypothalamus
   b. Adrenal cortex
   c. Pineal gland
   d. Melanocytes

2. **Increased melatonin secretion in darkness is brought about by:**
   a. Decreasing the activity of suprachiasmatic nucleus
   b. Increasing serotonin N-acetyltransferase
   c. Decreasing hydroxyindole-O-methyltrans- ferase activity
   d. Blocking the release of norepinephrine from sympathetic nerve terminals

3. **Melatonin is:**
   a. Serotonergic
   b. Dopaminergic
   c. Adrenergic
   d. Estrogenic

4. **The rate limiting enzyme in the synthesis of melatonin is:**
   a. Serotonin-N-acetyl transferase
   b. Tryptophan-5-hydroxylase
   c. 5-hydroxytryptophan decarboxylase
   d. Hydroxyindole-O-methyltransferase

5. **Pineal gland is the chief source of:**
   a. Serotonin
   b. Bradykinin
   c. Melatonin
   d. Epinephrine

6. **The following are secreted by pineal gland, *except*:**
   a. Oxytocin
   b. Melatonin
   c. Vasopressin
   d. Thyroid stimulating hormone

7. **Circadian rhythm is controlled by:**
   a. Suprachiasmatic nucleus
   b. Posterior pituitary
   c. Thalamus
   d. Pineal gland

ANSWERS

1. c   2. b   3. a   4. a   5. c
6. d   7. a

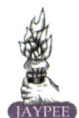

TOP DOC BANE WOHI | JISKA GUIDE HO SAHI

diginerve
A Jaypee Initiative

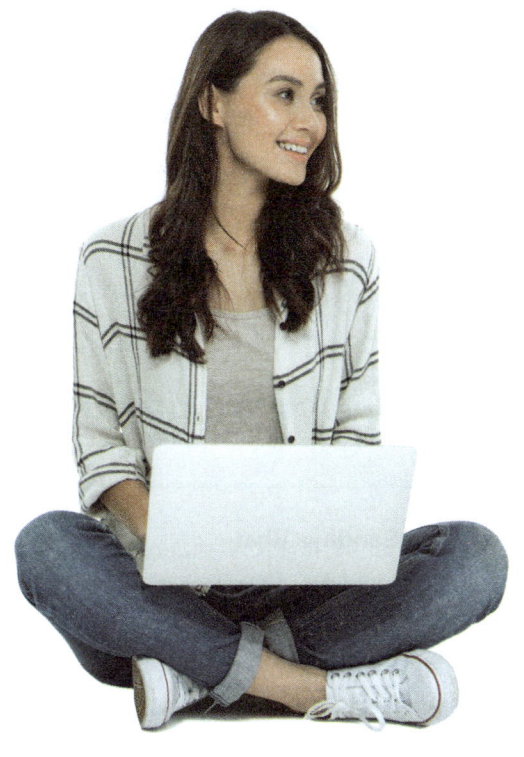

YOUR GUIDE AT EVERY STEP

Expert Knowledge Anytime, Anywhere

SCAN QR CODE FOR MORE DETAILS

WHY CHOOSE US

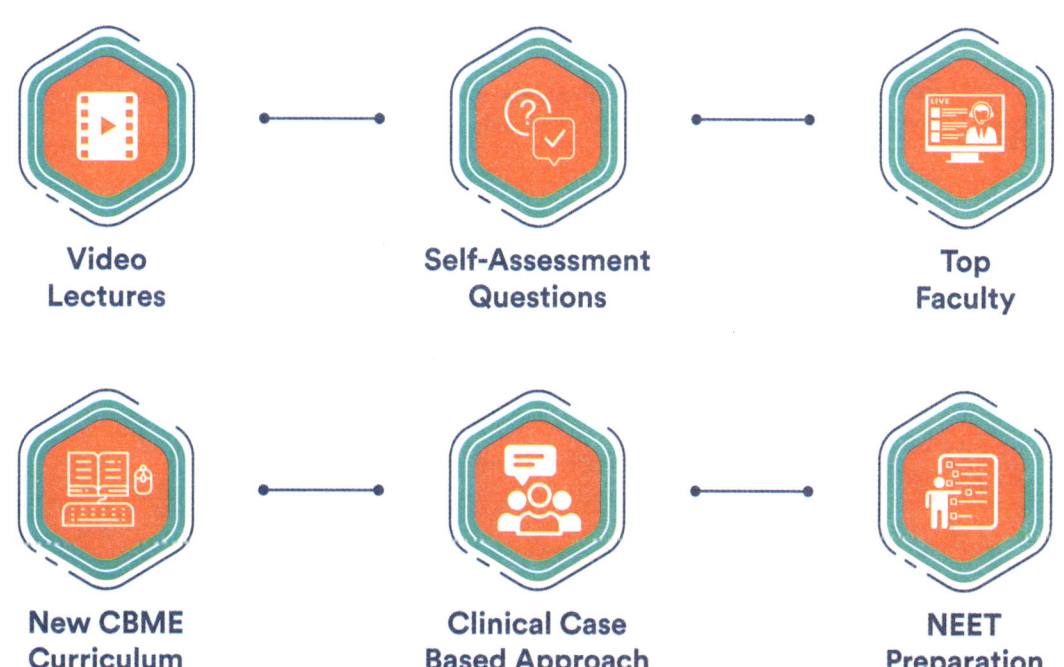

- Video Lectures
- Self-Assessment Questions
- Top Faculty
- New CBME Curriculum
- Clinical Case Based Approach
- NEET Preparation

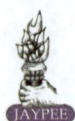 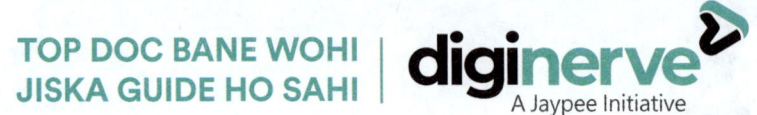

TOP DOC BANE WOHI | JISKA GUIDE HO SAHI

Video Lectures | Notes | Self-Assessment

UnderGrad Courses Available

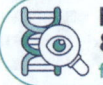 **Community Medicine** for UnderGrads — by Dr. Bratati Banerjee

Forensic Medicine & Toxicology for UnderGrads — by Dr. Gautam Biswas

 Medicine for UnderGrads — by Dr. Archith Boloor

 Microbiology for UnderGrads — by Dr. Apurba S Sastry, Dr. Sandhya Bhat & Dr. Deepashree R

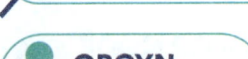 **OBGYN** for UnderGrads — by Dr. K. Srinivas

 Ophthalmology for UnderGrads — by Dr. Parul Ichhpujani & Dr. Talvir Sidhu

 Orthopaedics for UnderGrads — by Dr. Vivek Pandey

 Pathology for UnderGrads — by Prof. Harsh Mohan, Prof. Ramadas Nayak & Dr. Debasis Gochhait

 Pediatrics for UnderGrads — by Dr. Santosh Soans & Dr. Soundarya M

 Pharmacology for UnderGrads — by Dr. Sandeep Kaushal & Dr. Nirmal George

 Surgery for UnderGrads — by Dr. Sriram Bhat M (SRB)

 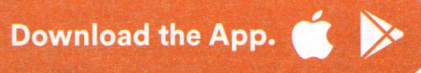

*T&C Apply

Contact:
+91 8800 418 418
marketing@diginerve.com

Thyroid Gland

CHAPTER 65

LEARNING OBJECTIVES
- Describe the steps in the synthesis of thyroid hormones.
- Describe the mechanism of secretion of thyroid hormones and their transport
- Explain the physiological actions of thyroid hormones
- Explain the effects of hyposecretion and hypersecretion of thyroid hormones
- Discuss the regulation of thyroid hormone secretion
- Describe thyroid function tests

INTRODUCTION

PY8.2: Describe the synthesis, secretion, transport, physiological actions, regulation and effect of altered (hypo and hyper) secretion of thyroid gland.

Peculiarities of Thyroid Gland

- Thyroid gland is the largest endocrine gland, which weighs about 15–25 g.
- It is the only visible endocrine gland. It is located in front of the trachea.
- Thyroid secretion is stored extracellularly in the colloid.
- Thyroid contains a large percent of the total I_2 content of the body. Total body iodine is about 15–20 µg of which 8 to 10 µg is present in the thyroid gland, i.e., 70–80% is contained in the thyroid.
- Thyroid gland is the only tissue that can oxidize iodide to iodine.
- The thyroid gland stores enough thyroid hormones to maintain a euthyroid state for about 3 months without hormone synthesis.
- It has a very high blood flow which comes to about 4–6 mL/g/minute

Thyroid gland is not essential for life, but its absence or hypo function during fetal and neonatal life results in severe mental retardation and dwarfism. Thyroid hormones act in almost all cells of the body and the net result is a generalized increase in the functional activity throughout the body.

Thyroid gland has two primary functions.
1. It secretes the thyroid hormones, T_4 and T_3 that maintain the level of metabolism in the tissues, which is optimal for their normal function.
2. The second function of thyroid gland is to secrete calcitonin, a hormone that regulates circulating levels of calcium (actions of calcitonin are discussed in detail in calcium homeostasis—Chapter 66).

Functional Anatomy of Thyroid Gland

Thyroid gland is a bilobed (butterfly-shaped) gland situated in front of the trachea. The two lobes are connected by a bridge of tissue called thyroid **isthmus (Fig. 65.1)**. The right lobe may be twice as large as the left. Rarely, a **pyramidal lobe** is seen which extends upwards from the isthmus.

Histology

Histologically, a number of lobes and lobules are present in the thyroid gland. Each lobule contains about 20–40 **acini** or follicles. *Acini form the structural and functional units of the thyroid gland,* and are spherical in shape.

Normal human thyroid contains about 3 million follicles each measuring about 100 to 300 µm in diameter depending on the activity of the gland. A rich capillary plexus surrounds the follicle. Each acinus is surrounded by a single layer of cuboidal **follicular cells or thyrocytes** and is filled with a pink-staining proteinaceous material called **colloid**. Main constituent of colloid is a big protein molecule called **thyroglobulin,** which contains thyroid hormones attached to it.

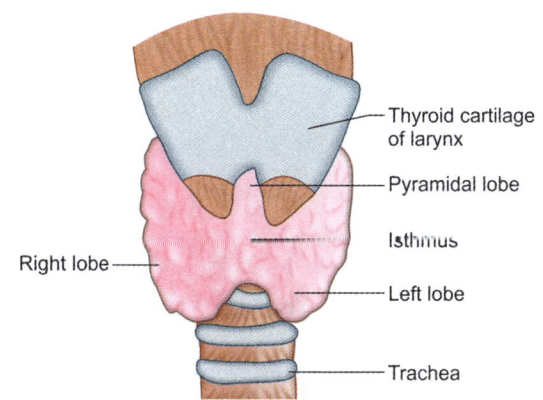

Fig. 65.1: Thyroid gland located anterior to trachea.

The free border of the epithelial cells lining the follicle has numerous microvilli projecting into the colloid.

Size of the follicle varies with the activity of the gland. When inactive, the amount of colloid is abundant and the follicle will be large with flat epithelial cells **(Fig. 65.2)**.

When the gland is active, the follicle is smaller in size, amount of colloid is less and cells lining are cuboidal or columnar. Active gland also shows scalloped edge of colloid showing small **reabsorption lacunae**. These are areas where the colloid is being actively reabsorbed into the thyrocytes when the gland is active.

By electron microscopy, numerous microvilli are seen projecting from the free surface of the thyroid cells into the colloid. Cells contain prominent rough endoplasmic reticulum involved in the synthesis of thyroglobulin. Secretory granules containing thyroglobulin are also seen in the cell. Each cell rests on a basal lamina, which separates the cells from the adjacent capillaries. The capillaries are fenestrated, such as those of other endocrine glands.

In between the thyroid follicles, groups of **parafollicular cells or 'C' cells** are seen which secrete **calcitonin**.

Functions of Follicular Cells

- Follicular cells collect and transport iodide from blood into the colloid for the synthesis of thyroid hormones.
- Synthesize thyroglobulin and secrete it into the colloid.
- They fix iodine to the thyroglobulin molecule to generate thyroid hormones.
- Remove the thyroid hormone from thyroglobulin and release it into the circulation.

Blood Supply

Thyroid gland has a rich blood supply from **superior thyroid artery** (arises from external carotid artery) **and inferior thyroid artery** (arises from the subclavian artery). Rate of blood flow is 4-6 mL/g/min. The whole of blood volume passes through the gland in 1 hr.

Lymphatic Supply

Thyroid gland has extensive lymphatic drainage into the inferior cervical lymph glands.

Nerve Supply

Sympathetic supply is from T_2-T_5 segments of spinal cord from the cervical ganglia. Parasympathetic supply is through superior and recurrent laryngeal nerve, branches of vagus.

Both are vasomotor in function, i.e., they regulate the rate of secretion of the gland by altering the blood supply.

Hormones of Thyroid Gland

- Thyroxine—T_4
- Triiodothyronine—T_3
- Reverse T_3—in small amounts
- Calcitonin secreted by the parafollicular C cells

Reverse T_3, diiodothyronine (DIT) and monoiodothyronine (MIT) are not physiologically important.

Biosynthesis of Thyroid Hormones

T_4 and T_3 are formed in the colloid by the iodination and condensation of **amino acid, tyrosine**. Raw materials are tyrosine and iodine. Both are obtained from food. Deficiency of thyroid hormone is mainly due to deficiency of iodine rather than tyrosine because iodine is not present in all foodstuffs.

Daily requirement of iodine is 150 µg normally in adults. Minimum iodine requirement is 75 µg/day. This ingested iodine is converted to iodide and absorbed into blood. This is carried to the thyroid gland where it is utilized for hormone synthesis.

Steps in Synthesis of Thyroid Hormones (Fig. 65.3)

The different steps are:
1. Synthesis of thyroglobulin
2. Iodide trapping
3. Oxidation of iodide and iodination of tyrosine (Organification)
4. Condensation or coupling.

Synthesis of Thyroglobulin

Thyroglobulin is a large glycoprotein that forms a stable dimer with a molecular weight of 660,000 Daltons. It is synthesized in the rough endoplasmic reticulum of thyrocytes.

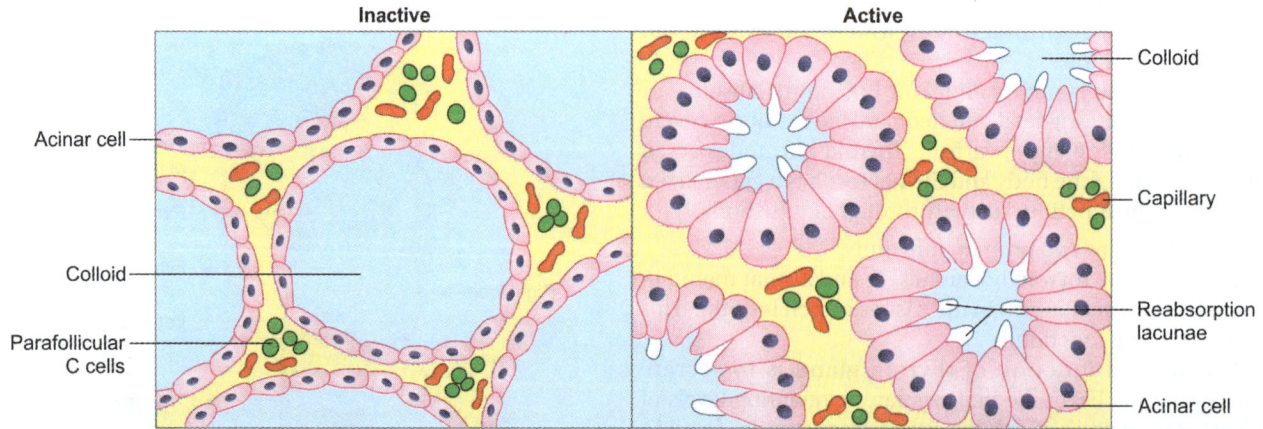

Fig. 65.2: Histology of thyroid gland showing variations in the follicular cell size with activity.

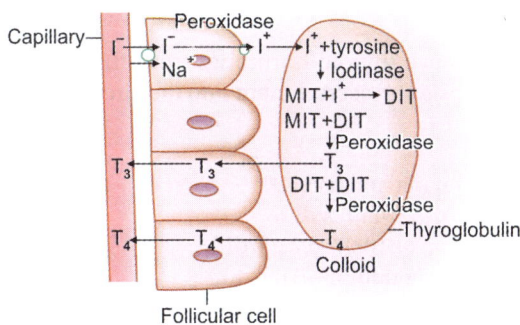

Fig. 65.3: Synthesis and release of thyroid hormones.
(MIT: monoiodotyrosine; DIT: diiodotyrosine)

TSH stimulates the synthesis and secretion of thyroglobulin. It is secreted by exocytosis into the cavity of the follicle forming the colloid. Each thyroglobulin molecule contains approximately 100–120 tyrosine residues. But only a few of these are subject to iodination by thyroperoxidase in the follicular colloid. Each thyroglobulin molecule forms approximately 10 thyroid hormone molecules.

Iodide Trapping

Iodide trapping is the first step in the biosynthesis of thyroid hormones. Iodide is transported from blood to thyroid cells and to colloid. This mechanism is called **iodide trapping or iodide pump**. The follicular cell is 50 mV negative (RMP −50 mV) when compared to interstitial area and colloid. Iodide is actively transported against the electrical gradient into the cell by **iodide pump or Na⁺-I⁻ symporter (NIS)**. The symporter present on the basolateral membrane of thyrocytes facing the capillaries transports two Na^+ and one I^- into the thyrocytes with each cycle. The NIS is capable of producing intracellular I^- concentrations that are 20–40 times as great as the concentration in plasma. TSH increases the number of NIS in the basolateral membrane.

The process involved is secondary active transport, with the energy provided by the active transport of Na^+ out of the thyroid cell by Na^+-K^+ ATPase. From the thyroid cell iodide is transported into the colloid by a **Cl^--I^- exchanger** known as **pendrin**. TSH stimulates iodide trapping.

Iodide pump is inhibited by perchlorate and thiocyanate which are drugs given in hyperthyroidism. Sodium-potassium pump also influences iodide pump.

> The salivary glands, gastric glands, placenta, ciliary body of the eye, the choroid plexus, mammary glands and certain cancers derived from these tissues also contain Na^+-I^- symporter (NIS) and can transport iodide against a concentration gradient. But TSH does not affect the transport of iodide in these tissues.

Oxidation of Iodide and Iodination of Tyrosine (Organification)

In the gland, at the interface between the thyrocyte and the colloid, iodide undergoes a process referred to as **organification**. First iodide is oxidized to iodine by **thyroid peroxidase**, a membrane bound enzyme present in the thyrocyte apical membrane. Iodine is then incorporated in the 3′ position of tyrosine molecule, which is a part of thyroglobulin molecule in the colloid to form **monoiodotyrosine (MIT)**. One more molecule of iodine is incorporated to the 5th position of MIT to form **diiodotyrosine (DIT)**. This reaction is also stimulated by thyroid peroxidase **(Fig. 65.3)**.

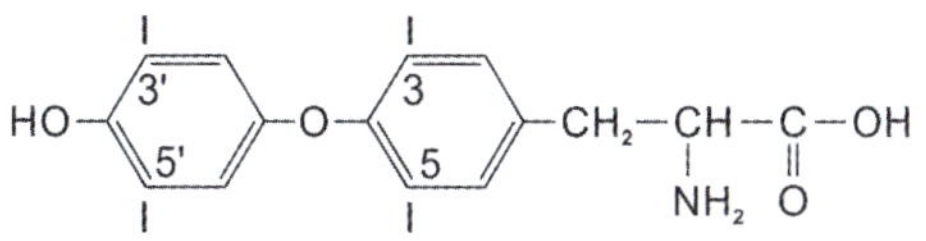

TSH promotes the reaction. *Thyroid gland is the only tissue that can oxidize iodide to iodine.* Conversion of I^- to I^+ prevents the back diffusion of iodide into circulation (iodide trapping).

Oxidation to iodine in the gland is inhibited by thiouracil and imidazole derivatives. Sulfonamide derivatives interfere with iodination of tyrosine.

Condensation or Coupling of Iodotyrosines

Condensation reaction is also stimulated by the enzyme thyroid peroxidase (TPO). Two molecules of DIT undergo oxidative condensation to form T_4 with the elimination of the alanine side chain from the molecule. One MIT and one DIT condense to form T_3 **(Fig. 65.4)**.

DIT + DIT = T_4 (Tetraiodothyronine)
MIT + DIT = T_3 (Triiodothyronine)
DIT + MIT = Reverse T_3.

The hormones are stored in combination with thyroglobulin in the lumen of the follicle as colloid for several months.

In the normal human thyroid, the average distribution of the different forms of iodinated compounds is:
MIT—3%
DIT—33%
T_4—35%
T_3—7%
Reverse T_3—2%.

Fig. 65.4: Structure of thyroid hormones - T_4, T_3 and reverse T_3.

3, 5, 3′, 5′ – Triiodothyronine (Thyroxine, T_4)

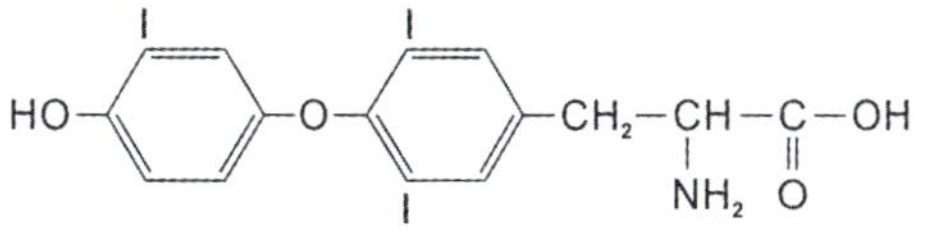

3, 5, 3′ – Triiodothyronine (T_3)

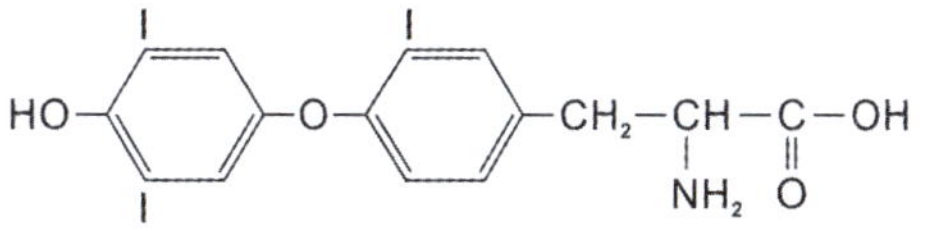

3, 3′, 5′ Triiodothyronine (reverse T_3)

> MIT and DIT that do not undergo oxidative condensation are deiodinated by the enzyme **iodotyrosine deiodinase**. The iodine liberated by deiodination of MIT and DIT provides twice the amount of iodine than obtained by iodide trapping. Deficiency of this enzyme leads to excretion of large amounts of iodine and leads to iodine deficiency goiter. In these patients, MIT and DIT appear in the urine.

Thyroglobulin

Thyroglobulin is a large glycoprotein molecule with two subunits.
1. Contains 10% CHO by weight.
2. Contains 123 tyrosine molecules.
3. Molecular weight—660,000.

Thyroglobulin is synthesized by the rough endoplasmic reticulum of thyroid follicular cells and enters the colloid by exocytosis. Thyroglobulin serves as the substrate for the formation of thyroid hormones since it contains large amounts of tyrosine molecules. The thyroid hormones produced remain part of thyroglobulin molecule until needed. When stimulated by thyroid stimulating hormone (TSH), the colloid is endocytosed from the follicular lumen into the surrounding thyroid follicular epithelial cells. The colloid is subsequently cleaved by proteases to release thyroglobulin from its T_3 and T_4 attachments. T_3 and T_4 are then released into circulation. The thyroglobulin is recycled back into the follicular lumen where it again serves as a substrate for thyroid hormone synthesis. Thus, the colloid represents a reservoir of thyroid hormones, and complete deficiency of iodine for up to 2 months can maintain a normal circulating level of thyroid hormones. Some amount of thyroglobulin also enters the bloodstream. The blood level is increased in hyperthyroidism and carcinoma thyroid. Thyroglobulin levels in the blood are mainly used as **tumor marker**.

Secretion of Hormone

Secretion of hormone is a complex process and is stimulated by thyroid stimulating hormone (TSH). Thyroid cells engulf the colloid by **endocytosis**. This chewing away of the edge of the colloid forms the **reabsorption lacunae** in the active state of the colloid. Once the colloid enters the cell, it fuses with the lysosomes present in the cell to form **phagolysosome**. This is rich in protease enzymes and these hydrolyze the peptide linkage and free the hormones, T3 and T4 from the thyroglobulin. This T3 and T4 traverse the basal membrane and enter circulation (**Fig. 65.3**). Only T3 and T4 diffuse out into the circulation. MIT and DIT are not secreted into the blood and they are acted upon by the intracellular enzyme, **iodotyrosine deiodinase**. The iodide thus released is utilized for new hormone synthesis. In patients with congenital absence of iodotyrosine deiodinase, MIT and DIT appear in urine leading to symptoms of iodine deficiency. Thyronines (T3 & T4) are resistant to the activity of iodotyrosine deiodinase.

The amount of thyroid hormones secreted per day is:
1. T_3—4 µg/day
2. T_4—80 µg/day
3. RT_3—2 µg/day.

Even though T_4 is the primary hormone secreted by the thyroid gland, T_3 has much greater biological activity than T_4. T_3 is specifically generated at its site of action in peripheral tissues by deiodination of T_4. Reverse T_3 is inert.

Functions of Thyrocytes

- They collect iodine from blood
- They synthesize thyroglobulin and secrete it into the colloid
- They fix iodine to the thyroglobulin to generate thyroid hormones
- They remove thyroid hormones from thyroglobulin by endocytosis and secrete them into the circulation.

Transport

Total normal plasma levels:
- T_4—8 µg/dL (4–11 µg/dL)
- T_3—0.15 µg/dL (0.07–0.2 µg/dL)
- Serum thyroglobulin—6 ng/mL
- Protein bound iodine—4–8 µg/dL (increased to 9–20 µg/dL in hyperthyroidism and reduced to 0.5 µg/dL–3.5 µg/dL in hypothyroidism)

In plasma, the hormones are bound to plasma proteins. Only minor quantity is in the free form. Both T_3 and T_4 are bound to plasma proteins such as:
1. Thyroxine-binding albumin (TBA)
2. Thyroxine-binding pre-albumin (TBPA) or transthyretin
3. Thyroxine-binding globulin (TBG).

T_4 is more bound to TBG and less to transthyretin and albumin. About 99.98% of T_4 is found in bound form and 0.02 in free form, i.e., 2 ng/dL. It is the free thyroid hormones that are physiologically active and that which feedback to inhibit pituitary secretion of TSH. When there is a sudden, sustained increase in the plasma concentration of thyroid-binding proteins, the concentration of free thyroid hormones falls. This decrease in the free form stimulates TSH secretion from the pituitary. This in turn causes an increase in the production of free thyroid hormones and the free hormone level come back to normal. A new equilibrium is reached at which the total quantity of thyroid hormones in blood is elevated but the concentration of free hormones is normal. Then the TSH secretion comes back to normal. Corresponding changes in the opposite direction occur when the concentration of thyroid-binding protein is reduced. Free form is released from the bound form according to need. Hormone-binding prevents excess uptake of the hormone by the first cells encountered and promotes uniform tissue distribution. TBG levels are increased in estrogen therapy and during pregnancy. It is decreased by glucocorticoids and androgens.

T_3 is bound largely to albumin. Thyroid hormone bound to TBG and TBPA is metabolically inactive. T_3 is less bound to plasma proteins. 99.8% is in the bound form and 0.2% in the free form. This less binding of T_3 accounts for the rapid action of T_3 and shorter half-life of T_3. Hence, T_3 is physiologically more active and T_4 is metabolically inert.

T_4 acts as a pro-hormone or stable precursor of T_3. It acts as a reservoir from which T_3 is continuously replenished. T_3 is specifically generated at its site of action in peripheral tissues by deiodination of T_4.

T_3 is more active than T_4 because of the following reasons:
- T_3 is seen more in the free form, i.e., it is less tightly bound to plasma proteins.
- It has greater affinity for nuclear thyroid hormone receptors.
- It has a shorter half-life of 1–3 days and action is rapid.
- T3 is easily absorbed than T_4.

❖ It penetrates into the cells and tissue fluids more rapidly than T_4.

Free T_3 and T_4 as well as bound form can be measured by radioimmunoassay (RIA). Measurement of **protein bound iodine (PBI)** is used as an index to assess thyroid function. *Normal plasma PBI level is 6 μg/dL.*

Metabolism of Thyroid Hormones

Thyroid hormones are metabolized in the **liver, kidney and many other tissues**. 80% of T_3 and T_4 are deiodinated to iodothyronines. 1/3 of the circulating T_4 is converted to T_3. Deiodination of T_4 in the tissues by the enzyme **deiodinase** provides a local supply of T_3 that is the physiologically active form. Only about 13% of T_3 is produced by thyroid gland as such, the rest is formed by deiodination of T_4. Three different deiodinases act on thyroid hormones: D_1, D_2 and D_3. D_1 (present in high concentration in liver, kidney, thyroid gland and pituitary) and D_2 (present in brain, pituitary and brown fat) are responsible for converting T_4 to T_3. D_3 converts T_3 and T_4 to reverse T_3 (RT_3) in the blood and tissues. *Two tissues that have very high T_3/T_4 ratio are the pituitary and the cerebral cortex, due to the expression of specific deiodinases.*

Rest of T_4 is converted to reverse T_3. 20% of T_3 and T_4 undergo conjugation in the liver to **glucuronides and sulfates**, respectively. These enter bile and in the intestine undergo hydrolysis. A portion of iodine released undergoes enterohepatic circulation and the rest is excreted through feces. The iodide lost by these routes amounts to about 4% of the total daily iodide loss. Unbound and unconjugated T_3 and T_4 undergo oxidation, decarboxylation, deamination and deiodination in liver and muscle. Deaminated product of T_4 is known as **tetraiodothyroacetic acid** (tetrae) and that of T_3 is **triiodothyroacetic acid** (triae). These can be measured to assess the level of T_3 and T_4.

Actions of Thyroid Hormones

❖ In general metabolism
  ▪ Calorigenic action
  ▪ Basal metabolism
❖ Special metabolism
❖ Role in growth and differentiation
❖ Systemic actions.

Calorigenic Actions

Thyroid hormone **increases the O_2 consumption** of all tissues *except testis, brain, anterior pituitary, uterus, spleen and lymph node*. Increase in metabolism and O_2 consumption is more marked in the heart and skeletal muscle.

The increase in metabolic reactions and the increase in the activity of Na^+-K^+ pump, result in increased demand for ATP. This is met by an increase in cellular respiration inside the mitochondria, which increases its oxygen consumption. Normally, 68% of the energy released in the mitochondria through oxidative phosphorylation is captured into ATP and 32% is wasted as heat. Hence, increase in oxidative phosphorylation not only increases ATP yield but also increases heat production (thermogenesis). This calorigenic action of thyroid hormones depends on the level of catecholamine secretion as well as on the initial metabolic rate. If the initial metabolic rate is high, then thyroxine does not have much calorigenic action.

Thyroid hormones also increase the activity of Na^+-K^+ ATPase in many tissues. T_4 has a latent period of few hours but the effect lasts for 6–7 days. T_3 has a short latent period for action, but the duration of action is also very short. In hyperthyroidism, the patient cannot tolerate high temperature and in hypothyroidism the patients are hypersensitive to cold.

Effect on Basal Metabolism

By increasing the metabolism in tissues at rest, thyroid hormones maintain the normal basal metabolic rate **(BMR)** which is about **40 kcal/m²/hour or 2000 kcal/day** in a man of average size. The metabolic rate determined at rest, in room temperature, 12–14 hours after the last meal is called the basal metabolic rate. In hyperthyroidism, BMR is increased to as much as 60–100% above the normal level. In hypothyroidism, BMR falls by 20–40% below the normal level.

Special Metabolism

Action on Protein Metabolism

In *physiological doses, thyroid hormone is mainly a protein **anabolic hormone***, i.e., it promotes protein synthesis. This is responsible for the growth-promoting action of thyroxine. Although the rate of protein synthesis is increased, at the same time the rate of protein catabolism is also increased. So, T_3 is very essential for normal growth. It increases protein synthesis by the following mechanisms:

❖ By increasing translation of RNA in the cells.
❖ By increasing the transcription of DNA to RNA by activating enzymes such as RNA polymerase and phosphoprotein kinases. A large number of mRNA is formed which activate the ribosomes to synthesize more proteins.

When the hormone is *present in excess, it promotes protein catabolism* by activating enzymes which accelerate the metabolism of proteins. Protein catabolism exceeds protein anabolism. There is increased breakdown of endogenous protein leading to wasting of muscles and muscle weakness. Urinary excretion of uric acid and creatinine increases. This leads to a negative nitrogen balance.

Action on Carbohydrate Metabolism

Thyroid hormone stimulates all aspects of carbohydrate metabolism and the balance maintains blood glucose normal. It has both hyperglycemic and hypoglycemic effects. Hypoglycemic effect is the increased glycolysis.

❖ Thyroid hormones *increase the absorption of glucose from GIT*. So, the blood glucose increases rapidly after a carbohydrate meal and it may exceed the renal threshold in hyperthyroidism. So, hyperthyroidism in a diabetic patient may worsen the hyperglycemic state. In severe hyperthyroidism, β-cells are destroyed due to excessive stimulation resulting in persistent glycosuria and the condition is called **metathyroid diabetes**.

- Increase **gluconeogenesis**.
- Increase the breakdown of glycogen into glucose (**glycogenolysis**).
- Increase glucose uptake by cells and also increase **glycolysis**.

Fat and Cholesterol Metabolism

- Thyroid hormone stimulates mobilization of lipids rapidly from fat tissue and degradation of lipids. This lead to a decrease in the fat stores in the body.
- Hormone-sensitive lipase mobilizes fat from adipose tissues, increasing the plasma concentrations of free fatty acid and glycerol.
- Free fatty acid level of blood increases after thyroxine administration due to **lipolysis**, but triglyceride level decreases. This is because triglycerides are broken down into FFA and glycerol by lipoprotein lipase. In hypothyroidism, triglyceride level increases and there is increased deposition of fat in tissues especially liver, leading to fatty liver.
- Thyroxine increases oxidation of free fatty acids in the cells
- Thyroxine decreases blood cholesterol, phospholipid and triglyceride level. Cholesterol is decreased due to increased synthesis of LDL receptors in the liver cells. This leads to rapid removal of low density lipoprotein from plasma by the liver and subsequent secretion of cholesterol in these lipoproteins through bile and it is excreted through feces. Thyroxine increases the synthesis, breakdown and excretion of cholesterol. So, the net effect is a **reduction in blood cholesterol**.

Fluid and Electrolyte Metabolism

Thyroid hormone helps in the distribution of fluid uniformly in the body. In hypothyroidism, there is accumulation of fluid, Na^+, K^+ and proteins in the extracellular space. Decrease in T3 and T4 increases ADH secretion which leads to increased water reabsorption. This leads to hypotonic hyponatremia. In hyperthyroidism, there is increased excretion of phosphate and Ca^{2+} from the body.

Mucopolysaccharide Metabolism

Normal level of thyroxine is necessary for the removal of certain proteins from the body, especially from skin. In hypothyroidism, glycosaminoglycans (GAGs) or mucopolysaccharides like chondroitin sulfate and hyaluronic acid form complexes and get accumulated in the subcutaneous area and cause water retention. There will be puffiness of skin and the skin becomes coarse and dry. This condition is called **myxedema** where, the edema is of the non-pitting type.

When thyroid hormones are administered, these proteins get metabolized, and diuresis continues until the myxedema is cleared.

Cellular Metabolism

- Thyroxine increases metabolism in almost all cells.
- It increases the permeability of cell membrane and mitochondrial membrane. It causes swelling of mitochondria and also increases the number of mitochondria.
- It stimulates sodium-potassium ATPase as well as adenylyl cyclase enzyme.
- It promotes transport of amino acids into the cell.

Vitamin Metabolism

- Thyroxine stimulates the hepatic conversion of β-**carotene to vitamin A** and also converts vitamin A to retinene. In hypothyroidism, there is accumulation of β-carotene leading to yellowish discoloration of skin called **carotenemia**. This is often mistaken for jaundice. In carotenemia, the sclera is not stained yellow but in jaundice, the sclera is stained yellow.
- Increases absorption of B-complex group of vitamins especially vitamin B_{12}.

Growth and Differentiation

- Normal level of thyroxine is needed for normal growth and development of all tissues especially for **skeletal maturation and brain development**.
- Thyroxine is more important to promote growth and development of the brain during fetal life and during the first few years of post-natal life. Development of the fetus is dependent on maternal T_4 that reaches it through the placenta and therefore, maternal hypothyroidism results in neonatal hypothyroidism. Thyroxine is necessary for myelination, arborization of neurons and normal synaptic development in the brain. If neonatal hypothyroidism is left untreated till 2 years of age, the changes in the brain are irreversible and result in mental retardation as seen in cretins.
- Thyroxine is essential for the normal ossification of cartilage and bone growth.
- Thyroxine also potentiates the action of growth hormone on tissues and promotes growth. Growth is retarded in cretins.
- Thyroxine has a role in the differentiation of tissues during development. It is seen that thyroidectomized tadpoles grow into large tadpoles, but will not get differentiated into frogs. This proves that thyroxine is necessary for amphibian **metamorphosis**.
- In fibroblasts, thyroxine maintain the production of glycosaminoglycan.

Systemic Effects (Table 65.1)

Effects on Cardiovascular System

- Thyroxine **increases heart rate, force of contraction and cardiac output**. This is by increasing the number and affinity of β-adrenergic receptors on heart and increasing their sensitivity to catecholamines. T3 and T4 also favor the synthesis of the α-isoform of myosin heavy chain in the heart which has greater ATPase activity than the β-isoform. This also increases the force of cardiac contraction. Increase in the metabolism of heart including nodal tissue and increased sensitivity to catecholamines increase the heart rate.

Tissue	Effects
Metabolically active tissues (except testes, uterus, lymph node, spleen, anterior pituitary)	Increase metabolic rate and O_2 consumption Thermogenesis, increase BMR
Heart	Positive chronotropic and inotropic effect Increased sensitivity to catecholamines by increasing the number of β-adrenergic receptors Increases synthesis of β-myosin heavy chain with higher ATPase activity
Muscle	Protein anabolism in physiological doses Increase protein breakdown in high doses
Bone	Necessary for normal ossification of cartilage and bone growth
Blood	Stimulate erythropoiesis
Adipose tissue	Stimulate lipolysis
Nervous system	Promote normal brain development
Intestine	Increases rate of carbohydrate absorption
Liver	Increased formation of LDL receptors and increased excretion of cholesterol

Table 65.1: Effects of thyroid hormones on different tissues.

- There is **widening of pulse pressure** because systolic pressure is increased due to increased cardiac output, and diastolic pressure is decreased due to reduction in peripheral resistance. Decrease in peripheral resistance is due to release of vasodilator metabolites from cells leading to peripheral vasodilatation. Increase in body temperature is also responsible for peripheral vasodilatation.

Action on Central Nervous System

Normal level of thyroid hormone is necessary for the normal functioning of CNS.

- Thyroxine regulates the activity of sympathetic nervous system by increasing the synthesis of β-adrenergic receptors. Major symptoms of hyperthyroidism are due to increased sympathetic activity. This can be blocked by β-adrenergic antagonists.
- Thyroxine does not increase the metabolism of brain, but it is essential for its normal functioning. It **increases the rapidity of cerebration**. In hyperthyroidism, there is increased irritability, sleeplessness and restlessness. This is due to increased responsiveness of the reticular activating system to catecholamines. In hypothyroidism, mentation is low and sleep is increased.
- Thyroxine shortens the reaction time of reflexes and reflex responses become brisk. In hypothyroidism, reflexes are sluggish.
- During fetal life and infancy, thyroxine enters the brain. It is essential for **myelination, axonal and dendritic development**. Mental retardation is a feature of hypothyroidism that sets in during fetal life and infancy. If the hormone is not replaced immediately after birth, synapses develop abnormally and the condition becomes irreversible.

Action on Skeletal System

Thyroxine is necessary for normal integrity of skeletal system and for normal skeletal maturation. In hypothyroid children, bone growth is slowed and epiphyseal closure is delayed. As a result, limbs are short compared to trunk as seen in cretins. Hypersecretion of thyroid hormones results in increased excretion of calcium and phosphate, which in turn, causes rarefaction of bone. The serum calcium will never increase because it is excreted through urine.

Action on Muscular System

Normal integrity of muscles needs thyroxine. It is necessary for the development, regeneration and contraction of muscles. In hyperthyroidism there is muscle weakness. This results in **thyrotoxic myopathy** due to increased breakdown of muscle protein and changes in myosin filament. Hyperthyroidism can also cause fine muscular tremor. This is due to increased excitability of the nerves that controls the muscles.

Action on Skin

Increases blood flow to skin, increases growth of hair and nails, increases sebum and sweat secretion.

Action on Blood

- Thyroxine **stimulates erythropoiesis** and stimulates maturation of RBC. So in hypothyroidism, anemia is a feature.
- It also increase the dissociation of oxygen from hemoglobin by increasing red cell 2,3-diphosphoglycerate (DPG).

Action on Alimentary System

- Thyroxine increases appetite, secretion of digestive juices and food intake.
- Thyroxine is necessary for **normal motility** of gastrointestinal tract (GIT). Hyperthyroidism results in diarrhea due to increased motility. In hypothyroidism, constipation and anorexia are seen.

Action on Reproductive System

- Thyroxine is necessary for normal sexual function.
- Irregularities of menstrual cycle (menorrhagia and polymenorrhea), sterility, etc., are seen in hypothyroidism in females and loss of libido is seen in males.
- Thyroxine increases milk secretion from mammary gland during lactation.

Mechanism of Action of Thyroxine

Genomic Action

Thyroid hormones enter nucleated cells and bind to thyroid hormone receptors in the nucleus which belong to superfamily of hormone sensitive nuclear transcription factors. The hormone-receptor complex then binds to the DNA molecule via zinc fingers. This increases the expression of a variety of different genes that code for proteins that regulate cell function. Before acting on the genes to increase gene transcription, T_4 is converted to triiodothyronine (T_3). Intracellular thyroid hormone receptors have a high affinity for T_3. More than 90% of thyroid hormones that bind with the receptors are T_3. After binding with the hormone, the thyroid hormone receptors become activated and initiate gene transcription. Large number of different types of specific mRNA is formed. The mRNA moves to the cytoplasm and RNA translation on the cytoplasmic ribosomes leads to the production of numerous new intracellular proteins which are mainly enzymes. The actions of thyroid hormones are mediated by the enzymatic and other functions of these proteins. The enzymes bring about increased activity in the cell. Thyroxine increases the synthesis of Na^+-K^+ ATPase and the cell utilizes more of ATP. T_3 acts more rapidly and is three to five times more potent than T_4.

Non-genomic Action

Thyroid hormones also have non-genomic cellular effects. Some actions of thyroid hormone that occur rapidly as that which occur in the heart are due to this action. The site of non-genomic action is on the plasma membrane, cytoplasm or in organelles such as mitochondria. Non-genomic actions include regulation of ion channels, oxidative phosphorylation etc. and this effect may be due to the activation of intracellular second messengers such as cAMP or protein kinase signaling cascades. There is a local effect on mitochondria. Thyroxine increases the number and size of mitochondria and leads to increased production of ATP. T_3 acts more rapidly.

Regulation of Secretion of Thyroid Hormones

Suprathyroid Mechanism

Hypothalamic-hypophyseal-thyroid Axis

Suprathyroid regulation is through the anterior pituitary hormone **TSH** secreted by thyrotrophs and by TRH secreted by the hypothalamus. The anterior pituitary regulates the synthesis and secretion of thyroid hormones through the release of TSH and the hypothalamus, in turn, stimulates the release of TSH through thyrotropin-releasing hormone (TRH). Finally, circulating thyroid hormones exert feedback control on both TRH and TSH secretion.

Role of Pituitary

Thyroid stimulating hormone (TSH) is a glycoprotein hormone secreted by the thyrotrophs of anterior pituitary. Action of TSH on thyroid gland is mediated through cAMP. TSH has multiple effects on the thyroid gland.

- All steps in the synthesis and release of thyroid hormones are facilitated by TSH.
- It increases proteolysis of thyroglobulin in the follicles releasing thyroid hormones into circulation.
- It also increases the size of thyroid cells and the acinar cells tend to become columnar and there is also increase in the number of infoldings of secretory epithelium.
- TSH also increases blood flow to the gland. It increases the size and the secretory activity of the follicular cells. The gland as a whole enlarges. When TSH stimulation is prolonged, the cells hypertrophy and the weight of the gland increases. The gland becomes detectably enlarged, a condition called **goiter**.

Role of Hypothalamus and Feedback Control by Thyroid Hormones

TSH secretion is in turn regulated by **TRH** secreted by hypothalamus and also by the feedback effect of the thyroid hormones, mainly, T_3. Both TRH and thyroid hormones interact at the level of thyrotrophs. TRH tries to increase the secretion of TSH, whereas thyroid hormones inhibit the secretion of TSH. Rate of secretion of TSH depends on the balance of these actions (**Fig. 65.5**). Although T_4 does not inhibit TSH secretion directly, it does so indirectly through its conversion to T_3 within the thyrotrophs. The negative feedback of T_4 and T_3 on TSH release occurs at the level of the pituitary thyrotrophs by both indirect and direct mechanisms. In the indirect feedback pathway, intracellular T_3 decreases the number of TRH receptors on the surface of the thyrotroph. Thus thyroid hormones indirectly inhibit TSH release by reducing the sensitivity of thyrotrophs to TRH. In the direct feedback pathway, intracellular T_3 inhibits the synthesis of both α and β chains of TSH.

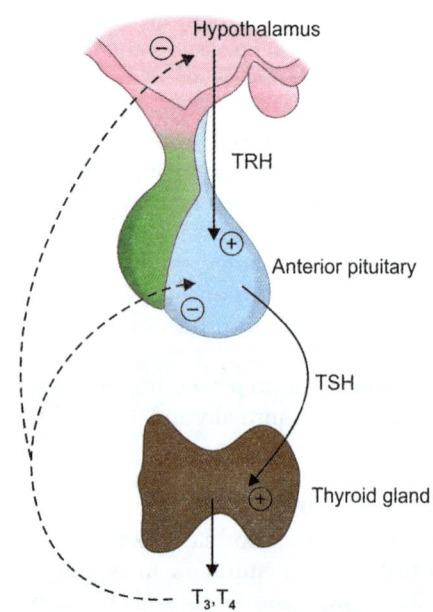

Fig. 65.5: Regulation of thyroid hormone secretion by negative feedback control mechanism. Dashed arrows indicate inhibition.

Intrathyroid Mechanism or Role of Iodide or Autoregulatory Mechanism

Iodide is an important factor regulating the synthesis of thyroid hormones. In spite of wide variation in iodine intake, a normal thyroxine level is maintained to a certain extent. Iodide is essential for normal thyroid function, but iodide deficiency and iodide excess both inhibit thyroid function. When iodine intake is increased (>2 μg), iodide concentration in the thyroid gland is increased. High intrathyroid iodide concentration inhibits organification of iodine and thus inhibits hormone synthesis. This effect of iodide is called **Wolff-Chaikoff effect** (for details *refer* Wolff-Chaikoff effect, page 606).

The rise in intrathyroid iodine autoregulates the iodine uptake, i.e., it reduces further iodine uptake by the gland. The intrathyroid iodide level therefore decreases and with it, the Wolff-Chaikoff effect subsides. If the autoregulation is absent due to thyroid dysfunction, the Wolff-Chaikoff effect will persist and keep the iodine organification suppressed. The effect is known as the **Jod-Basedow effect** and it explains the cause for **hypothyroid iodide goiter**.

Other Factors Regulating Thyroid Secretion

TRH secretion is increased on exposure to cold. Leptin from adipose tissue and α-MSH from pituitary increases TRH secretion and thus increase synthesis of thyroxine. Glucocorticoids, dopamine and somatostatin decrease TSH secretion. Secretion of TSH and TRH is also inhibited by stressful conditions such as burns, trauma, fever and starvation.

Thyroid Function Tests

> **PY8.4:** Describe thyroid function tests.

1. Thyroid radioactive iodine uptake test or radioisotope scans
2. Estimation of hormone (T_3 and T_4) level of blood
3. Determination of protein bound iodine
4. Metabolic tests—BMR, serum cholesterol and serum creatinine estimation
5. Thyroid suppression test
6. TRH and TSH stimulation test
7. Estimation of TSH by RIA
8. Measurement of antibodies against thyroid
9. Ultrasound scan
10. Achilles reflex time
11. Sleeping pulse rate
12. Fine needle aspiration cytology and thyroid biopsy.

Radioactive I_2 Uptake Test

This test is based on the capacity of the thyroid gland to accumulate iodine. A standard bolus of radioactive iodine (^{131}I) is administered to the subject. This is absorbed and taken up by the thyroid gland and the rest is excreted through urine. The amount of iodine taken up by the thyroid gland can be determined by thyroid scanning. In normal subjects, 10–30% of iodine is accumulated in the gland in 24 hrs. In hyperthyroidism, the uptake is increased to 50–70% of the administered dose by the gland. An underactive gland will take up subnormal amounts of iodine. This test is also done to distinguish between a 'hot' (functioning) and a 'cold' (nonfunctioning) solitary thyroid nodule. Cold nodules are more likely to be malignant.

Estimation of Hormone Level in Blood

The diagnosis of hypothyroidism or hyperthyroidism is confirmed by measuring the T_4 and TSH levels in blood. Hypothyroidism is characterized by a low T_4 and a high TSH level. The upper limit of normal TSH secretion is 5 IU/mL. When the TSH is high, but the T_4 level is normal, this condition is called subclinical hypothyroidism. Free hormone estimation (estimation of the concentration of hormones that are not bound to circulating proteins) is also useful as it measures the metabolically active component. Autoimmune thyroiditis is diagnosed by estimating the levels of anti-thyroid peroxidase (TPO) antibodies.

In significant thyrotoxicosis, TSH will be less than 0.1 IU/mL. The serum T_3 is proportionately more elevated than serum T_4 levels. Thyroglobulin antibodies and TPO antibodies are seen in 90% of patients with Graves' disease.

Determination of Protein Bound Iodine

Protein bound iodine (PBI) gives an idea of the amount of thyroid hormone in the bound form. The total amount of bound form depends on the amount of thyroid binding globulin. Normal range is 4–8 μg/dL of serum. It is increased in hyperthyroidism and decreased in hypothyroidism. By finding out PBI, the level of free hormones can be found out.

Thyroid Suppression Test

After administering thyroid hormone, the level of TSH in blood is estimated. If hypothalamic control is normal, TSH level will be decreased. Failure of feedback mechanism will not suppress TSH.

Thyroid Stimulation Test

TRH stimulation test is used to differentiate whether hypothyroidism is due to hypothalamic origin or pituitary origin. After giving TRH, if the level of T_3 and T_4 is increased, then it is of hypothalamic origin.

TSH stimulation test is used to differentiate hypothyroidism due to pituitary origin or thyroid origin. After giving TSH, if circulating T_3 and T_4 levels are increased then it is due to pituitary origin.

Achilles Reflex Time

Half relaxation time of ankle jerk is 230–350 msec. It is prolonged in hypothyroidism and shortened in hyperthyroidism.

Lipid Profile Estimation

Lipid profile estimation shows a raised LDL and triglyceride level in hypothyroidism. Total cholesterol will also be increased in hypothyroidism.

Diseases of Thyroid Gland

Normally, functioning thyroid gland is referred to as **euthyroid**.

Diseases result in hyper- or hypo-functioning of the gland. Most important clinical condition is **goiter (Flowchart 65.1)**.

Other Conditions

1. Thyroiditis
2. Carcinoma thyroid

Simple Goiter (Flowchart 65.2 and Fig. 65.6)

Most common cause is dietary iodine deficiency i.e. intake of iodine less than 10 µg/day.

In the beginning, follicles enlarge in size without any hypertrophy or hyperplasia of epithelium. This is the first stage of simple goiter. This is **colloid goiter**. Later there is hypertrophy and hyperplasia of the follicular epithelium. Because of decreased synthesis of hormone, the amount of colloid is decreased. This is **parenchymatous goiter**. Sometimes, the excessive enlargement of follicles results in tumor-like masses of thyroid tissue. This leads to asymmetrical enlargement of gland which is called **simple adenomatous goiter or Multinodular goiter**.

Hypothyroidism

Consequences of thyroid gland dysfunction depend on the life stage at which it occur. Its absence or hypo- functioning during fetal and neonatal life results in severe mental retardation and dwarfism. In adults, hypothyroidism is accompanied by mental and physical slowing and poor resistance to cold. Hypothyroidism may be **primary hypothyroidism** which is due to diseases of the thyroid gland such as Hashimoto's thyroiditis (autoimmune), iodine deficiency, after thyroidectomy and radiation therapy, radioactive iodine (^{131}I) therapy, viral thyroiditis, etc. **Secondary hypothyroidism** is due to defect in the pituitary where TSH production is impaired. **Tertiary hypothyroidism** is due to hypothalamic causes where there is TRH deficiency. Secondary and tertiary hypothyroidism are together called **central hypothyroidism**. The measurement of TSH and TRH level will help to differentiate between these two types. Secondary and tertiary hypothyroidism are due to hypothalamo-pituitary lesions like tumors, radiation, surgery, sarcoidosis and trauma.

Endemic Colloid Goiter

Endemic colloid goiter is caused by dietary iodine deficiency. Goiter means greatly enlarged thyroid gland. Adequate quantities of thyroxine and triiodothyronine are not produced. Due to feedback mechanism there is increased secretion of TSH from the pituitary. Increased TSH stimulates thyroid cells to secrete large amounts of thyroglobulin into the follicles and the amount of colloid in the follicles goes on increasing. The gland grows larger and larger and may increase to 10 to 20 times its normal size.

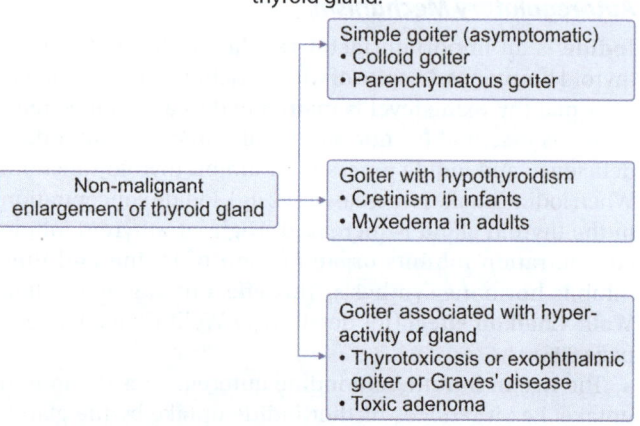

Flowchart 65.1: Classification of non-malignant enlargement of thyroid gland.

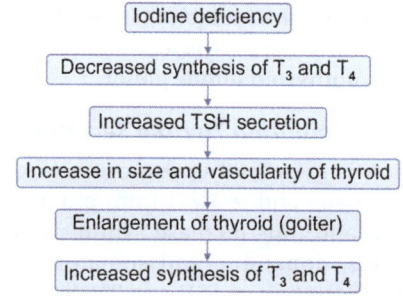

Flowchart 65.2: Steps in the development of simple goiter.

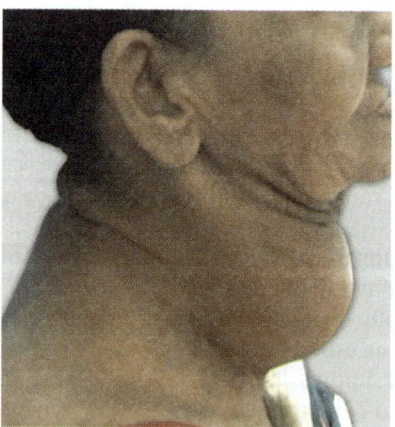

Fig. 65.6: Simple goiter.
Courtesy: Dr Devika.

Idiopathic Non-toxic Colloid Goiter or Multinodular Goiter

In idiopathic non-toxic colloid goiter, there is no iodine deficiency. The secretion of thyroid hormones is not severely affected. The exact cause of goiter is not clearly known. Most of the patients show signs of mild thyroiditis leading to mild hypothyroidism. This leads to increased TSH secretion and progressive growth of the non-inflamed portion of the gland leading to multinodular goiter. Here only the normal portions of the gland grow whereas the areas affected by thyroiditis fails to grow.

Hypothyroidism in Children

Cretinism or Congenital Hypothyroidism

When severe thyroid deficiency occurs during fetal life, infancy or childhood, the result is cretinism **(Fig. 65.7)**.

Causes of Cretinism

1. Maternal iodine deficiency and maternal hypothyroidism
2. Maternal antibody mediated destruction of baby's thyroid gland
3. Congenital absence of thyroid gland in the baby (thyroid agenesis) where there is no T3 and T4
4. Thyroid dysgenesis (improper formation of thyroid gland) where the amount of T3 and T4 secreted is less
5. TSH receptor mutation in the baby
6. Decreased expression of thyroid peroxidase gene (dyshormonogenetic goiter)
7. Use of medicines that inhibit thyroid hormone production such as antithyroid drugs, sulfonamides or lithium during pregnancy.
8. Lack of iodine in the diet (endemic cretinism)

Features of Cretinism

- **Prolonged neonatal jaundice**
- Cretins are mentally retarded dwarfs due to **poor brain development**. Mental retardation is due to defect in the growth, branching and myelination of the neurons of the central nervous system at the time of normal development of mental powers. The child's IQ drops. They show generalized cortical atrophy.
- Hypothyroid children usually present with delayed milestones, sluggish movements, delayed dentition, growth failure, declining academic performance, pubertal delay and menstrual irregularities.
- Different parts of the body are disproportionate. The upper part of the body is taller than the lower part (1.7:1).
- Skeletal growth in the cretin is characteristically more inhibited than the soft tissue growth. Due to this disproportionate rate of growth, soft tissues enlarge excessively, producing the characteristic appearance of cretins. (Differences between pituitary dwarf and cretin are given in **Table 65.2**).
- They are unpleasant in appearance; **puffy face**, broad nose with depressed bridge; large **protruded tongue**; **pot belly**, **protruded umbilicus**, etc. Tongue becomes so large that it obstructs swallowing and breathing. This produces a characteristic guttural breathing in a cretin. Chocking is also common in cretins.
- Croaking sound while crying due to thickening of vocal cords
- Skin is dry, cold, coarse, wrinkled, **pale**, edematous (non-pitting edema) and with scanty hair. Yellowish discoloration of skin due to hypercarotinemia
- Swelling in the neck due to thyroid enlargement (goiter)
- There will be hypogonadism. Decrease in thyroid hormones lead to decreased production of testosterone and estrogen.
- Severe constipation due to decreased gastrointestinal movements

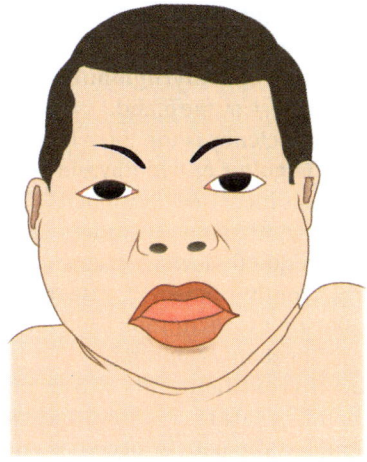

Fig. 65.7: Cretinism.
Courtesy: Dr Anil P.

Table 65.2: Differences between pituitary dwarf and thyroid dwarf.

Pituitary dwarf	Thyroid dwarf
Deficiency of growth hormone	Deficiency of thyroxine
No mental retardation	Mentally retarded
Milestones normal	Milestones delayed
BMR normal	BMR low
Parts of the body proportionate	Disproportionate body
Normal looking face	Face not pleasing
Normal skin	Dry, rough skin

- Lack of weight gain
- Excessive sleep
- Hypotonia
- Problems with memory and attention
- Vision and hearing problems

Diagnosis

About 24–48 hours after birth, estimate the TSH and free T4 levels. TSH will be increased very much and free T4 decreased.

Treatment

Thyroid hormone replacement therapy orally is the treatment of choice. Levothyroxine which is synthetic T4 is given. This is a reversible condition if treated on time. Newborn screening for hypothyroidism helps to totally avoid this condition. If hypothyroidism is recognized and corrected within 7–14 days after birth, development including mental development can proceed normally. Once the clinical signs of congenital hypothyroidism become apparent, the CNS abnormalities become irreversible.

Hypothyroidism in Adult

Causes

- Hypothyroidism can occur as an autoimmune disease where the antithyroid antibodies destroy the thyroid gland (**Hashimoto's thyroiditis**). The most common cause of primary hypothyroidism is Hashimoto's thyroiditis or chronic autoimmune thyroiditis. **Thyroid peroxidase (TPO) antibodies and thyroglobulin antibodies** are produced which destroy the gland.

- Severe iodine deficiency is the most common cause for **endemic colloid goiter** or hypothyroid goiter where the size of the gland is increased very much **(Fig. 65.6)**.
- Pituitary and hypothalamic disorders can also lead to hypothyroidism due to decreased secretion of TSH and TRH **(central hypothyroidism)**. Causes are brain trauma, tumor pressing on the thyrotrophs, infarction of anterior pituitary as in Sheehan's syndrome.
- **Postpartum thyroiditis** occurs within one year after giving birth. It is an acute condition and later there will be resolution and the patient becomes euthyroid. TPO antibodies and thyroglobulin antibodies are detected.
- Viral infections where the patient presents with flu like symptoms (**sub-acute granulomatous thyroiditis**). The thyroid gland is painful and tender. ESR will be very much increased.
- **Riedel's thyroiditis** where the thyroid gland is hard and painless. Pathology is fibrosis of the gland. IgG-4 antibodies are detected.
- Thyroidectomy not followed by adequate thyroid hormone intake.
- **Drugs** such as lithium, ^{131}I, and antithyroid drugs may lead to hypothyroidism.

Myxedema

Severe hypothyroidism in adults is called myxedema. This name has come from the skin changes associated with this condition. It is one of the most common of all endocrine diseases affecting 1–2% of adults. Women are much more commonly affected than males.

Features of Myxedema

- Face is puffy with swollen eyelids. Hyaluronic acid is hygroscopic, producing mucinous edema that is responsible for the thickened features and puffy appearance.
- Myxedematous tissue is responsible for the enlarged tongue and thickening of laryngeal and pharyngeal mucosa in severe hypothyroidism.
- Hoarseness of voice (voice is husky and in severe cases croaky) is a characteristic feature. It is said that *myxedema can be diagnosed over the telephone* because of the frog like husky voice. This is due to thickening of the vocal cords due to deposition of mucopolysaccharides.
- Coarse, dry, cold, edematous and yellowish skin **(Fig. 65.8)**. Skin is dry and coarse due to reduced secretions of the sweat gland and sebaceous gland. Cold skin is due to cutaneous vasoconstriction. Hypercarotinemia gives the yellow color to skin but sclera is not affected.
- Growth of hair is retarded and the hair becomes dry and brittle and easily fall off.
- Body swelling (edema) is due to a combination of fluid retention and glycosaminoglycan deposition and hence severe hypothyroidism is also referred to as myxedema.

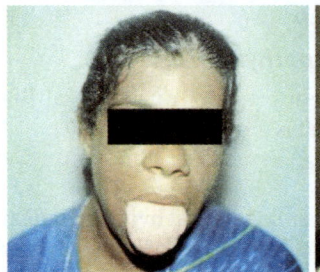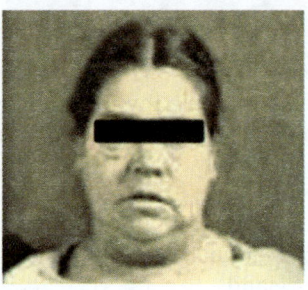

Fig. 65.8: Myxedema (note the facial puffiness, puffiness under the eyes, yellowish discoloration of skin and large tongue).

- Mental and physical lethargy, intolerance to cold, increased sleep, snoring, anemia, sterility, constipation, subnormal temperature of skin. Anemia which is normochromic, normocytic is due to decreased production of erythropoietin as a result of deficiency of T_3. Increased fatigability is due to decreased ATP production and muscle weakness as a result of decreased protein synthesis.
- The patient is slow in thought, speech and action
- There is weight gain despite a relative lack of appetite. This is due to fluid retention in the tissues by the hydrophilic glycoprotein deposits and decreased metabolic rate.
- In severe cases, mental symptoms are severe, leading to **myxedema madness**.
- There is decrease in heart rate, cardiac output, blood volume and blood pressure. Cardiac output is reduced due to decrease in stroke volume and heart rate. Stroke volume and heart rate are reduced due to loss of inotropic and chronotropic effects of thyroxine. The number of beta adrenergic receptors are decreased in the myocardium and there is decreased sensitivity to catecholamines. In severe cases, myocardial contractility is reduced very much leading to heart failure. Enlargement of heart in X-ray is seen in some patients due to accumulation of mucopolysaccharides in the heart. Low voltage ECG is a characteristic feature of hypothyroidism.
- More than 90% of subjects with primary hypothyroidism have increased levels of cholesterol and triglycerides. LDL cholesterol level will be high. Increase in cholesterol is due to altered fat and cholesterol metabolism due to reduced activity of **cholesterol-α-monooxygenase**, which breaks down cholesterol and increases the excretion of cholesterol by the liver through bile. A hypothyroid state results in decreased expression of hepatic LDL receptors resulting in decreased LDL clearance through bile. This leads to atherosclerosis, hypertension and coronary artery thrombosis.
- Reflexes are slow and relaxation time of reflexes is very much prolonged. This is caused by a decrease in the rate of muscle contraction and relaxation. The relaxation phase is much more affected. Reaction time of reflexes is increased. Classically the ankle jerks relax slowly after contraction in hypothyroidism.
- There will be features of carotinemia such as yellowish discoloration of skin.

- Hearing disturbances may be due to thickening of the ear drum and middle ear effusions. Fluid collects in the middle ear leading to conductive deafness.
- Fall in basal metabolic rate. BMR ranges between -30 and -50.
- Muscle weakness, cramps and muscle stiffness are seen. Muscle weakness and easy fatigability are due to decrease in the number and activity of mitochondria. The metabolic activities of almost all tissues of the body are reduced.
- In women, menorrhagia is the commonest menstrual irregularity. Menstrual cycles are anovulatory and the proliferative phase is prolonged leading to increased endometrial thickness.
- Non-pitting type of edema is due to accumulation of proteins like mucopolysaccharides, hyaluronic acid and chondroitin sulfate which form a tissue gel in the interstitial space under the skin with accumulation of water.
- Sometimes primary hypothyroidism may be associated with hyperprolactinemia which presents with galactorrhea (milk secretion in the absence of pregnancy). A high TRH level can stimulate prolactin secretion from anterior pituitary. Prolactin in turn causes amenorrhea and galactorrhea.

Myxedema Coma

A severe life threatening complication of hypothyroidism is **myxedema coma**. It is rare and coma occurs in elderly patients following severe untreated thyroid failure. Precipitating factors include stressful conditions like exposure to severe cold temperature, infections, heart failure, excessive alcohol intake, surgery, etc. Clinical features are hypoglycemia, hypothermia, hypotension, hyponatremia, bradycardia, hypoventilation and hypercapnia.

Sympathetic drive is decreased due to decreased T3 and T4. Heart rate will be decreased producing severe bradycardia. Myocardial contractility is decreased leading to decrease in cardiac output, decrease in blood pressure which finally leads to circulatory shock. Decreased sympathetic activity of CNS leads to altered mental status, confusion, lethargy and coma. Decreased metabolic activity drastically decrease heat production which leads to severe hypothermia. The findings are similar to adrenal insufficiency and so intravenous hydrocortisone is given until it is ruled out. Intravenous fluid therapy will increase blood pressure. T3 and T4 is also given intravenously.

Pathophysiology of Hypothyroidism

Goiter: In iodide deficiency, there is no iodination of thyroglobulin molecule and there is no phagocytosis of TG. This leads to increased formation and accumulation of TG in the follicle. When there is reduction in thyroid hormones no negative feedback occurs and there is increased secretion of TSH which stimulates the gland leading to goiter.

Nucleated cells: There is decreased metabolic activity. There is decrease in glycolysis, lipolysis, glycogenolysis and gluconeogenesis which lead to decreased blood glucose. Weight gain is due to decreased metabolism. There is decreased ATP production and heat production. There will be decrease in body temperature and cold intolerance.

Heart and blood vessels: There is decrease in the sensitivity of β-adrenergic receptors to catecholamines. This leads to decrease in heart rate (bradycardia) and decreased contractility of heart. Vasomotor tone is affected which leads to vasoconstriction, increase in peripheral resistance and increase in blood pressure. Thus there is hypertension and bradycardia.

Bone: There is decreased bone growth and decreased bone maturation which lead to short stature.

GIT: There is decrease in gastrointestinal secretions and motility which lead to constipation. There is decrease in appetite.

Nervous system: Decrease in sympathetic activity leads to depression, fatigue, lethargy and memory loss. Decrease in T3 and T4 delays relaxation phase of deep tendon reflexes referred to as **Woltman's sign**. This is a classic sign of hypothyroidism.

Muscle: There is decrease in muscle growth and regeneration. Muscle damage leads to myopathy and increased release of creatine kinase into blood. Muscle weakness is prominent in the proximal muscles. Muscle contraction is decreased due to decreased Ca^{2+}-ATPase activity.

Skin: Decreased blood flow to the skin due to vasoconstriction leads to hair loss and thin, brittle nails. Decreased sweating and decreased sebum production produces dry skin. Yellowish discoloration of skin is seen due to carotinemia.

Liver: LDL receptor expression is decreased which leads to increased blood LDL level and triglyceride level.

Reproductive system: There will be hyperprolactinemia due to increased secretion of TRH. TRH stimulates secretion of both TSH and prolactin. Prolactin inhibits FSH and LH secretion which in turn inhibit the secretion of estrogen and testosterone. In males, decrease in testosterone leads to decreased sperm production, decreased libido, erectile dysfunction and decreased masculinization which leads to gynecomastia. In females there will be no ovulation due to decrease in FSH and LH which leads to infertility. Menstrual cycle is affected. Increased prolactin secretion produce galactorrhea.

Fibroblast: Decrease in T3 and T4 lead to decreased degradation of glycosaminoglycans (GAGs) and accumulation of GAGs absorb more water leading to edema which is of the non-pitting type. GAGs usually accumulate in the dermis leading to myxedema. Accumulation of GAGs in the tissues around the eyes retain water leading to periorbital edema. GAGs also accumulate in the carpel tunnel of the wrist leading to edema of the muscles and tendon in that area which compress the median nerve leading to the symptoms of carpal tunnel syndrome.

Diagnosis

Primary hypothyroidism

- T3 and T4 will be decreased but TSH will be high.
- If it is due to iodide deficiency, serum iodide level and protein bound iodine (PBI) will be low.

- In Hashimotos thyroiditis, antibodies against thyroglobulin and thyroid peroxidase will be detected. Serum thyroglobulin will be increased due to leakage of thyroglobulin from the damaged gland. There will be no radioactive iodine uptake by the gland. Biopsy of the gland will confirm the diagnosis. Does not return to euthyroid state without treatment.
- In postpartum thyroiditis, there will be history of child birth within one year and the patient returns to euthyroid state after some time.
- In Riedel's thyroiditis IgG-4 antibodies are detected. Biopsy shows fibrosis of the gland.
- In subacute granulomatous thyroiditis, there will be flu like symptoms and ESR will be high.

Central hypothyroidism
- If the cause is in the hypothalamus T4, T3, TRH and TSH will be reduced.
- If the cause is in the pituitary, TRH will be increased but TSH, T3 and T4 will be decreased.

Treatment of Hypothyroidism

Administration of thyroid hormone orally.

Hyperthyroidism

Hyperthyroidism can be **primary** which is due to diseases of the thyroid gland or it can be **secondary** due to diseases of pituitary or hypothalamus.

Causes

1. Thyroid solitary **toxic adenoma and toxic multinodular goiter** where there are nodules in the gland which are hyperactive and produce large amounts of thyroxine **(Fig. 65.9)**.
2. TSH secreting **pituitary tumor** where there is increased secretion of TSH.
3. Graves' disease of **autoimmune etiology**.
4. **Iatrogenic** hyperthyroidism due to administration of thyroid hormones in excess of what is necessary.
5. **Hyperthyroidism associated with choriocarcinoma** where, beta-hCG and free T4 or T3 or both levels are increased. Glycosylated hCG can combine with TSH receptors and can induce thyroid over activity.

Graves' disease or Exophthalmic Goiter or Thyrotoxicosis

In thyrotoxicosis, there is diffused enlargement of thyroid gland, but *TSH level is normal*. This is an **autoimmune** disease in which antibodies are produced against the TSH receptors in the thyroid cells.

Most important of these antibodies is the **thyroid stimulating immunoglobulin (TSI)** whose structure is similar to TSH. These antibodies get attached to the TSH receptors on the thyroid cells and the cells are stimulated to secrete large quantities of thyroxine and triiodothyronine. These antibodies have a prolonged stimulatory effect on the gland lasting for about 12 hours. TSH acts only for about an hour. The TSI binds to the same TSH receptors and leads to continuous activation of the cAMP system in the thyroid cells leading to increased secretion of T_3 and T_4.

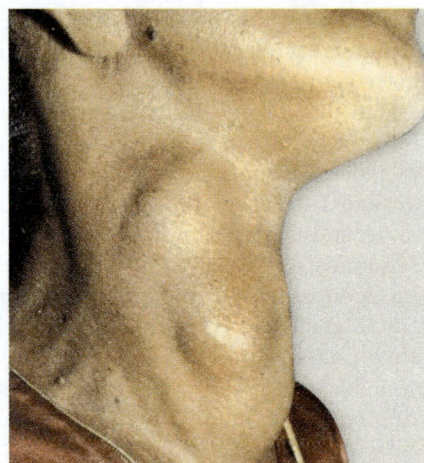

Fig. 65.9: Toxic multinodular goiter.
Courtesy: Dr Anil Sundaram, Surgeon.

Features

- Enlargement of the thyroid gland referred to as diffuse toxic goiter.
- Blood flow to the thyroid gland may exceed 1 L/minute and may be associated with a bruit (sound heard on auscultation) or even a thrill (palpable vibration)
- Warm, moist skin due to vasodilatation and increased sweating. Skin is oily due to increased sebum production.
- There is increase in the basal metabolic rate. The body temperature is increased due to increased metabolism and increased heat production. There will be intolerance to hot temperature.
- Increase in pulse rate and systolic blood pressure. Systolic blood pressure is increased due to increase in heart rate, stroke volume and cardiac output. Pulse rate is increased due to increased sympathetic discharge and increased body temperature.
- Diastolic pressure is reduced due to decrease in peripheral resistance. Peripheral resistance is reduced due to peripheral vasodilatation caused by metabolites released due to increased metabolism. There will be widening of pulse pressure because systolic pressure is increased and diastolic pressure is decreased.
- Fine tremor of hands and brisk reflexes due to increased neuronal excitability.
- Palpitation due to increased cardiac response to circulating catecholamines, and breathlessness on exertion
- Increase in appetite due to increased metabolism
- Loss of weight due to increased catabolism of endogenous protein, carbohydrate and fat stores. There will be muscle wasting.
- Diarrhea due to increased gastrointestinal motility. There is increased water loss leading to dehydration and hypovolemia.

- Decrease in serum cholesterol due to increased excretion of cholesterol by liver through bile. There is increased expression of LDL receptors in liver cells. There is increased uptake of LDL cholesterol which in turn decreases LDL in blood.
- Irritability, nervousness, insomnia (inability to sleep) due to increased sympathetic activity and increased activity of reticular activating system.
- In bone, there is increased osteoclastic activity leading to increased bone resorption. This leads to **osteoporosis** and increased risk of fractures.
- Increase in T4 and T3 causes increased synthesis and release of thyroxine binding globulin (TBG) from liver which binds with T4. At the same time, there is also increased release of sex hormone binding globulin from the liver which binds with estrogen and testosterone decreasing the circulating level of active estrogen and testosterone. In males, decrease in testosterone leads to decreased masculinization and **gynecomastia**. There will be decreased libido and decrease in sperm production.
- In females, decrease in free estrogen leads to anovulation and infertility. Menstrual abnormalities such as oligomenorrhea or amenorrhea occur since menstrual cycle is affected.
- Weakness of proximal muscles (**thyrotoxic myopathy**) due to increased breakdown of muscle protein. There will be increased release of creatine kinase (CK) into blood.
- **Pretibial edema** is a typical feature of Graves' disease which is due to deposition of glycosaminoglycan in the skin of pretibial area.
- **Exophthalmos** or **proptosis** is a condition where there is bulging of eyeball and the eyelids does not close completely when the person blinks or is asleep. It is seen only in Graves' disease among endocrine abnormalities. It is due to swelling of tissues in the eye, especially the extraocular muscles. There will be increased filling of the rigid orbital wall due to accumulation of fluid and cells in the retrobulbar tissues which causes pushing of eyeball forwards **(Fig. 65.10)**. The patient complaints of double vision, difficulty in moving eyes, blindness if there is involvement of optic nerve, pain in the eyes etc. It is more common in women and the condition affects 1 in every 3 people suffering from hyperthyroidism due to Graves' disease.

There are different views to explain exophthalmos in Graves' disease:
1. One view is that the swelling is due to deposition of immune complexes resulting in inflammatory reactions in the eyeball. There will be damage and inflammation of the extraocular muscles.
2. Current theory is that the preadipocyte fibroblasts in the orbit contain TSH receptors. TSH binds with these receptors and stimulates the fibroblasts to release cytokines that promote inflammation and edema in the retrobulbar tissue.
3. T cells present in the retro-orbital space contain TSH receptors. The antibodies combine with these receptors and the T cells produce interferon-gamma (IFγ) and tumor necrosis factor-alpha (TNFα). These substances stimulate the fibroblasts, which produce increased amounts of glycosaminoglycan. This in turn increases water retention leading to swelling of the retrobulbar tissues. There is also increase in the adipocytes. The immune system also attack the muscles and fatty tissues around and behind the eye, making them swollen.
4. Incomplete closure of eye lids in exophthalmos is also due to varying degree of spasm of the upper eyelid. In hyperthyroidism, there is increased sympathetic activity. The levator palpebrae superioris supplied by the sympathetic fibers remain contracted leading to lid retraction and lid lag.

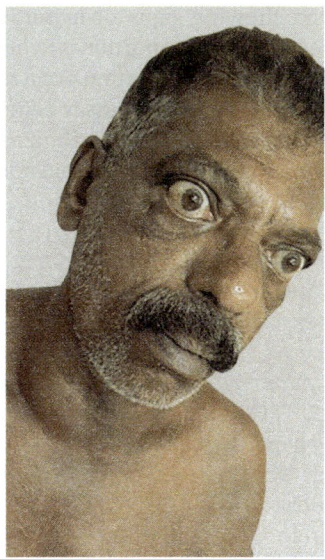

Fig. 65.10: Exophthalmos in thyrotoxicosis.
Courtesy: Dr Anil Sundaram, Surgeon.

If exophthalmos is severe, it leads to blindness. Pushing of the eyeball forwards by the swollen retrobulbar tissue will stretch the optic nerve and damage it. Another reason is that constant exposure of the cornea to the atmosphere leads to drying and ulceration of the cornea which result in blindness due to **exposure keratopathy.**

Thyroid Storm

Thyroid storm also known as **thyrotoxic crisis**, is an acute, life-threatening, hypermetabolic state induced by excessive release of thyroid hormones in individuals with thyrotoxicosis. It is precipitated by infections like pneumonia. It also occurs in patients poorly prepared for thyroid surgery. Normally the patient should be treated with antithyroid drug until euthyroidism is achieved, to prevent thyroid storm during surgery. Thyroid storm is characterized by high fever (the temperature may rise above 41°C), tachycardia, tremor, vomiting, dehydration, and coma. Death may be caused by cardiac arrhythmia, hyperthermia or cardiac failure.

Toxic Adenoma

A tumor which is localized in the thyroid gland may secrete large quantities of thyroid hormones. Toxic adenoma is simple adenoma showing signs of hyperactivity seen in elderly. Only the adenomatous portion is hyperactive and the rest of the gland atrophies. Estimation of thyroid stimulating immunoglobulin (TSI) by immunoassay helps to identify the condition. The concentration of the antibodies will be high in thyrotoxicosis but low or absent in thyroid adenoma.

There will be no exophthalmos in toxic adenoma.

Diagnosis of Hyperthyroidism

To differentiate between primary and secondary hyperthyroidism, estimate free T3, T4 and TSH levels in blood.
- In primary hyperthyroidism, free T3 and T4 will be increased and TSH is found to be decreased.
- In secondary hyperthyroidism, TSH, T3 and T4 levels will be increased. An MRI scan will confirm the presence of pituitary tumor.
- In choriocarcinoma (malignant growth arising in the body of uterus), β-hCG and free T4 will be increased. TSH level will be decreased. An ultrasound scan will rule out choriocarcinoma.

Treatment of Hyperthyroidism

1. Administration of antithyroid drugs.
2. Surgery, i.e., thyroidectomy (surgical removal of the gland).

Antithyroid drugs:

Antithyroid drugs act at various stages in the synthesis and release of thyroid hormones.
- **Thiocyanate and perchlorate** inhibit secretion of hormones by preventing iodide trapping by the gland.
- **Thiocarbamides or thionamides**, such as propylthiouracil and carbimazole inhibit iodination of tyrosine and coupling of iodotyrosines thus blocking the synthesis of thyroid hormones. Antithyroid drugs do not block the release of preformed thyroid hormones and so the action of antithyroid drugs may take about 1 to 6 weeks for euthyroidism to be obtained. Treatment is given for 12 to 24 months, after which treatment is discontinued.
- Administration of **iodine** inhibits synthesis of hormones (*refer* Wolff-Chaikoff effect).
- β-Adrenergic blocking agents like propranolol will relieve the symptoms of hyperthyroidism. Propranolol decreases the conversion of T4 to T3 within the cell. Many of the manifestations of thyrotoxicosis are due to hyperactivity of the sympathetic nervous system. Hence beta blockers are important in the early management of thyrotoxicosis.
- Large dose of ^{131}I is used in malignancy of thyroid gland. Radioiodine produces thyroid ablation without the complication of surgery. After oral administration, radioiodine is rapidly absorbed, concentrated and organified in the thyroid follicular cells. Thyroid cells are then destroyed by the ionizing effects of beta particles.

Wolff-Chaikoff Effect:

Even though iodide is needed for normal thyroid function, deficiency of iodide and excess of iodide cause abnormal thyroid function. In normal individuals, large doses of iodide act directly on the thyroid gland to produce a mild and transient inhibition of iodination of tyrosine and thereby hormone synthesis, irrespective of the serum levels of TSH. This effect is more pronounced and long lasting in patients with hyperthyroidism because iodide transport is increased in these patients. Lugols iodine or saturated solution of potassium iodide decreases its own transport into thyroid, inhibits iodine organification and blocks release of T_4 and T_3 from the gland.

This inhibition of thyroid hormone synthesis by excess iodide is known as **Wolff-Chaikoff effect**. This effect was first reported in 1948 by Jan Wolff and Israel Chaikoff. Other actions of increased iodides are, it reduces the effect of TSH on the gland by reducing cAMP response and it also inhibits proteolysis of thyroglobulin. This causes colloid to accumulate in the gland and the vascularity of the hyperplastic gland will be reduced. This reduces bleeding during thyroid surgery.

This effect lasts around 10 days after which it is followed by an escape phenomenon when there is resumption of normal organification of iodine and normal thyroid peroxidase function. So iodine therapy is useful only for short periods and is used in patients with thyrotoxic crisis, surgical emergencies, etc.

Goitrogens:

Goitrogens are substances that cause thyroid swelling and hypothyroidism. **Thiocyanate and thiouracil**-like substances are present in certain plants such as cabbage and turnips. The antithyroid agent present in plant is called **goitrin**. Goitrin inhibits synthesis of thyroid hormones and a reduction in the hormone level stimulates secretion of large amounts of TSH from pituitary by feedback mechanism. This TSH causes hyperplasia and enlargement of the thyroid gland. When the stored hormones in the gland are used up, features of hypothyroidism develop.

MULTIPLE CHOICE QUESTIONS

1. Thyroid hormones in blood is transported by the following, *except*:
   a. Albumin
   b. Globulin
   c. Prealbumin
   d. Transferrin
2. Regarding thyroid hormone, all are true, *except*:
   a. T3 is more avidly bound to nuclear receptors than T4
   b. T4 has the maximum plasma concentration
   c. T3 is more active than T4
   d. T4 has shorter half-life than T3
3. Plasma half-life of T4 is:
   a. 6–7 days
   b. 1–2 days
   c. 12–24 hours
   d. 10–12 days
4. Plasma half-life of T3 is:
   a. 6–7 days
   b. 1–2 days
   c. 12–24 hours
   d. 10–12 days
5. Iodine uptake is seen in the following organs, *except*:
   a. Thyroid
   b. Salivary gland
   c. Ovary
   d. Mammary gland

6. Thyroxine injected to rat produce all the following, *except*:
   a. Increased lipolysis
   b. Increased oxygen consumption
   c. Decreased BMR
   d. Increased myocardial contractility
7. BMR is decreased in:
   a. Hyperthyroidism
   b. Increased body temperature
   c. Cushing syndrome
   d. Addison's disease
8. BMR increase in all, *except*:
   a. Low environmental temperature
   b. Anxiety
   c. Thyrotoxicosis
   d. Sleep
9. BMR depends on:
   a. Body weight
   b. Surface area
   c. Amount of adipose tissue
   d. Amount of lean body mass
10. Which of the following statement is true regarding BMR?
    a. It is not affected by dietary changes
    b. It is not influenced by hormonal changes
    c. It is not affected by energy expenditure
    d. Decreased by 40% in starvation
11. TRH stimulates TSH and:
    a. FSH
    b. Oxytocin
    c. Prolactin
    d. Gonadotropin
12. A patient with hypothyroidism is likely to have all the following, *except*:
    a. Subnormal oral temperature
    b. Tendency to fall asleep frequently
    c. Decreased body hair
    d. Moist hands and feet
13. Full body stature is not attained by people who as children have experienced all the following, *except*:
    a. Thyroid deficiency
    b. Castration
    c. Chronic malnutrition
    d. Premature puberty
14. Regarding myxedema, the following are true, *except*:
    a. Swollen edematous look of face
    b. Impotency, amenorrhea
    c. BMR increased by 30-45%
    d. Dullness, loss of memory
15. In a person who has fasted for 5 days, all are seen, *except*:
    a. Growth hormone level decreased
    b. Glucose tolerance decreased
    c. Immunoreactive insulin decreased
    d. Plasma free fatty acids increased
16. Which of the following does not change in the old age?
    a. GFR
    b. Glucose tolerance
    c. Hematocrit
    d. Blood pressure
17. Thyroxine binding globulin is increased in:
    a. Pregnancy
    b. Nephrotic syndrome
    c. Glucocorticoid treatment
    d. Cancer chemotherapy
18. High levels of thyroxine can lead to all the following, *except*:
    a. Increased cardiac output
    b. Increased plasma triglyceride level
    c. Increased heart rate
    d. Increased metabolic rate
19. Features of hyperthyroidism include all, *except*:
    a. Weight loss
    b. Increased appetite
    c. Insomnia
    d. Constipation
20. Deficiency of thyroid hormone in children leads to:
    a. Cretinism
    b. Dwarfism
    c. Myxedema
    d. Cushing's syndrome
21. Hyperglycemia is seen in all the following conditions, *except*:
    a. Hypothyroidism
    b. Gigantism
    c. Diabetes mellitus
    d. Cushing's syndrome
22. Myxedema is due to:
    a. Cortisol excess
    b. Deficiency of insulin
    c. Deficiency of thyroxine
    d. Excess of calcitonin
23. A hypothyroid patient is likely to have a BMR of:
    a. +50
    b. –50
    c. 0
    d. +20
24. A patient with hyperthyroidism is likely to have all the following features, *except*:
    a. Increased BMR
    b. Tachycardia at rest
    c. Insomnia
    d. Increased total peripheral resistance
25. Autoimmunity against the thyroid gland leading to the destruction of the gland produces
    a. Hashimoto's disease
    b. Graves' disease
    c. Endemic colloid goiter
    d. Exophthalmos

ANSWERS

1. d	2. d	3. a	4. b	5. c
6. c	7. d	8. d	9. b	10. d
11. c	12. d	13. d	14. c	15. a
16. c	17. a	18. b	19. a	20. a
21. a	22. c	23. d	24. d	25. a

Calcium and Phosphate Homeostasis

CHAPTER 66

LEARNING OBJECTIVES
Must know
- Outline the hormonal regulation of calcium homeostasis
- Enumerate the functions of ionic calcium in the body
- Explain the physiological actions of parathormone (PTH)
- Describe the effects of deficiency and excess of parathormone
- Describe the actions of calcitonin
- Describe the steps in the synthesis of calcitriol
- Explain the actions of calcitriol and discuss the effects of its deficiency in children

Desirable to know
- Describe the functional anatomy of bone
- Role of phosphate in bone physiology
- Describe the pathophysiology of osteoporosis and osteopetrosis

PHYSIOLOGY OF BONE

PY8.1: Describe the physiology of bone and calcium metabolism.

Bone is a connective tissue composed of organic matrix in which mineral salts are impregnated. There is also a small population of cells. Bone consists of 20% organic matrix, 35% mineral salts and 45% water. 90% of organic substance is formed of collagen fibers and the rest forms the ground substance. Ground substance contains extracellular fluid and **proteoglycans**, namely, **chondroitin sulfate and hyaluronic acid**. Total blood flow to the bone is 200-400 mL/min in adults. The functions of bones are protection of the vital organs, enabling locomotion and supporting the body against gravity with the aid of muscles.

The mineral salts present in bones are mainly **hydroxyapatite crystals** ($Ca_{10}(PO_4)_6(OH)_2$). They are seen as long thin plates. Functions of hydroxyapatite are:
- It provides mechanical support to the bone.
- It serves as a reservoir of sparingly soluble minerals like Ca^{2+}, Mg^{2+} and PO_4^{3-}. Thus bone is involved in overall calcium and phosphate homeostasis.

The calcium and phosphate present in the bone are in dynamic equilibrium with these minerals in the extracellular fluid (ECF). Bone matrix also contains small amounts of $Mg(OH)_2$, fluoride and sulfate.

Insulin-like growth factors (IGF) are produced by bone tissue and liver. IGF promotes cell division at the epiphyseal plate and in the periosteum. It also increases the synthesis of proteins needed to build new bone.

Deposition and Resorption of Bone

Bone consists of two types of bone tissue: the **cortical (**also called **compact or lamellar)** bone and the **trabecular (cancellous or medullary or spongy)** bone. Cortical bone is the outer layer of all bones and represents about 80% of the total bone mass. Dense cortical bone provides much of the strength for weight bearing by the long bones. Trabecular bone constitutes 20% of the total bone mass and is found in the interior of bones. It is composed of thin spicules of bone that extend from the cortex into the medullary cavity.

The bone building cells are called osteoblasts. **Calcification** is the process by which mineral salts are deposited around collagen fibers of the matrix where they crystallize. This leads to hardening of the tissue. Bone consists of four types of cells:
1. Osteogenic cells
2. Osteoblasts
3. Osteocytes
4. Osteoclasts.

Osteogenic cells are stem cells derived from mesenchyme. They are the only bone cells that can divide. They divide many times and the daughter cells develop into osteoblasts.

Osteoblasts are the bone building cells. These are reticuloendothelial cells involved in laying down new bone. They synthesize collagen and other extracellular matrix proteins like **osteocalcin** and **osteonectin** and help in mineralizing bone. They are the principal target cells for the action of parathormone to stimulate bone growth. They secrete **alkaline phosphatase,** and PO_4 ions are released locally. Normally, the product of calcium and phosphate remains as a constant and these salts remain saturated. Product of calcium and phosphate goes above the solubility product during bone formation, and calcium and phosphate precipitate. The matrix around osteoblasts and osteocytes gets calcified.

Osteoblasts mature to form **osteocytes** and they are the main cells in the bone tissue **(Fig. 66.1)**. These cells maintain the bone tissue. They are found on the bone surface or within lacunae. The osteocytes send their cellular processes through the canaliculi of bone and make contact with other osteocytes and osteoblasts. They stimulate osteoblast by secreting growth factors. They also play a role in the transfer of Ca^{2+} from the interior of bone to the growth surface, a process called *osteocytic osteolysis*.

Osteoclasts are multinucleated giant cells formed by the fusion of many cells. These cells are concentrated in the endosteum. Their main function is **bone resorption**. Their activity is increased by cytokines. They secrete powerful lysosomal enzymes like **acid phosphatase** and acids. They phagocytose bone fragments and release calcium. Bone breakdown is essential for bone remodeling, and also helps to release calcium and phosphate in times of need.

The breakdown of bone matrix is called **bone resorption**. Resorption is a part of normal development, growth and repair of bone. Enzymes produced by osteoclasts digest collagen and other organic substances, while acids dissolve the bone minerals. To achieve homeostasis in bone, bone resorbing action of osteoclasts must balance the bone building actions of osteoblasts. Bone remodeling consists of a coordinated interplay of osteoblastic, osteocytic and osteoclastic activities.

Applied Aspect

Sex steroids slow down bone resorption and promote calcification of bone. Estrogen promotes apoptosis of osteoclasts, thus decreasing bone resorption. It increases osteoblast activity and also increases the synthesis of bone matrix. *After menopause, osteoporosis is seen due to deficiency of estrogen,* i.e., bone resorption outpaces bone deposition. The decreased rate of protein synthesis especially collagen, makes the bones brittle and there is *increased risk of fracture after menopause*.

In males, testosterone level starts declining only after the age of 60 years, that too, gradually. Only 3% of bone mass is lost every 10 years in males after this age, but in females, after menopause, the loss is about 8% every 10 years.

BODY CALCIUM

Calcium, magnesium and phosphate are very essential for life. As calcium and phosphate are major constituents of bone and all cells, there is a vast store of these substances in the body. These substances are usually ingested in excess and body homeostatic mechanisms are aimed primarily at maintaining their levels constant. This is achieved by three mechanisms:
1. Control of absorption from bowel.
2. Control of renal reabsorption of calcium that is filtered.
3. Increased release of calcium from bone when blood Ca^{2+} is reduced.

Total body calcium in a 70 kg adult man is 1100 g. 99% of this is present in the skeleton, 4–5 g in soft tissues and 1 g in the ECF. The ECF calcium is seen mainly in the plasma. Normal plasma calcium level is 9–11 mg/dL. This plasma calcium exists in two forms:
1. Diffusible form
2. Non-diffusible form or bound form.

Calcium is bound loosely to albumin mainly and to a lesser extent to globulin. Protein-bound calcium is physiologically inactive and acts as a reserve form of calcium. Diffusible calcium exists in two forms:
1. Ionized calcium which constitutes 50%.
2. Complex calcium, i.e., calcium bound to diffusible anions like citrate and HCO_3^-. This form is also physiologically inactive.

Ionized calcium is the physiologically active form. Plasma concentration of ionized calcium is maintained within a narrow range. It depends on the level of parathormone and calcitriol secretion, which increase the absorption of Ca^{2+} from the intestine and renal tubules. The hormones that affect blood calcium level are given in **Table 66.1**.

Factors Affecting Ionization of Calcium in the Plasma

- *Plasma pH:* In alkalosis, more of calcium gets bound to plasma proteins, causing a reduction in the ionic calcium level, whereas in acidosis binding is reduced and more of free Ca^{2+} will be available.
- Plasma protein concentration
- Concentration of plasma HCO_3^- and PO_4^{3-}
- Amount of parathormone and calcitriol

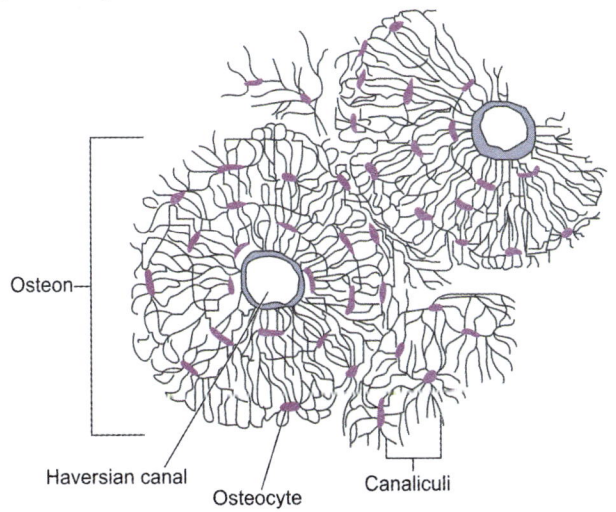

Fig. 66.1: Structure of bone.

Table 66.1: Hormones affecting blood calcium level.	
Increase in blood calcium	*Decrease in blood calcium*
• Parathormone • Calcitriol • Growth hormone • Thyroxine	• Calcitonin • Glucocorticoids

Functions of Ionic Calcium in the Body

- Helps in the formation of bone and teeth
- Necessary for blood coagulation
- Excitation-contraction coupling in muscles
- Necessary for secretion from glands by emeiocytosis (exceptions are **renin** secretion from the granular cells of juxtaglomerular apparatus of kidney and **parathyroid hormone** secretion by the chief cells of the parathyroid gland. Decrease in calcium concentration increases the secretion of both these hormones and increase in ionic calcium concentration decreases their secretion)
- Formation of milk
- Acts as intercellular cementing substance
- Acts as second messenger
- Activates amylase, lipase, thromboplastin, etc.
- Helps in the release of neurotransmitters and hormones
- Affects excitability of excitable tissue and helps in the stabilization of cell membrane.

PHOSPHORUS METABOLISM

Total body phosphorus is 500–800 g and 2/3rd of this is organic and 1/3rd inorganic phosphate (PO_4^{3-}, HPO_4^{2-} and $H_2PO_4^-$). 90% of phosphorus is incorporated in bone. It is also present in ATP, ADP, creatine phosphate, 1,2-diphosphoglycerate, etc. Since phosphate is part of ATP molecule, it plays a critical role in cellular energy metabolism. Plasma phosphate level is 12 mg/dL.

The sources of plasma phosphorus are from bone, reabsorption from kidney and absorption from intestine. Normally, 3 mg of phosphorus moves into and out of the bone daily. 90% of filtered phosphorus is reabsorbed from renal tubules. This reabsorption is inhibited by parathormone. In the intestine, phosphorus absorption is stimulated by parathormone. Unlike calcium, the plasma phosphate concentration is not strictly regulated, and its levels fluctuate throughout the day, particularly after meals.

Functions of Phosphorus in the Body

- Phosphorus is an essential component of cell membrane.
- Calcium phosphate is involved in the calcification process of bone [hydroxyapatite is $Ca_{10}(PO_4)_6(OH)_2$].
- Plays an important role in intracellular energy generation. PO_4^{3-} in blood, buffers Ca^{2+}, Mg^{2+} as well as other cations
- PO_4^{3-} is a major cytoplasmic buffer.
- Maintain pH of blood by buffering H^+ in blood and urine.
- Necessary for the formation of ATP, ADP, phospholipase, adenine and guanine nucleotides, etc.
- Necessary for enzymatic activities like glycolysis.

Concentration of phosphorus is inversely related to calcium concentration in plasma. The product of calcium (Ca^{2+}) and phosphate (PO_4^{3-}) concentration is called **solubility product**, and when it is normal these minerals remain saturated in solution. When this value exceeds normal limit of solubility product, these salts get precipitated and form calcium phosphate. This mechanism is involved in the calcification process of bone.

The three hormones that affect calcium and phosphorus metabolism are (**Flowchart 66.1**)
1. Parathormone
2. Calcitonin
3. 1, 25-dihydroxycholecalciferol or calcitriol.

PARATHYROID GLANDS

PY8.2: Describe the synthesis, secretion, transport, physiological actions, regulation and effect of altered (hypo and hyper) secretion of parathyroid gland.

There are four parathyroid glands in humans. They are found on the posterior surface of the upper and lower poles of each lobe of thyroid gland. Total weight is approximately 120 mg.

Histologically, there are two types of cells in the parathyroid: the **chief cells** that secrete **parathormone** (**PTH**) and the **oxyphil cells**. The oxyphil cells are found in clusters and are larger and lighter staining than the chief cells. They contain oxyphil granules and large number of mitochondria. The function of these cells is not known, but it is seen that these cells first appear at the time of puberty and their number increases throughout life.

PARATHORMONE

Parathormone (PTH) or parathyroid hormone is the hormone produced by the parathyroid gland which is a linear polypeptide with 84 amino acids. Half-life of PTH is <20 minutes. It is metabolized in the liver. The function of PTH is to increase the blood calcium level in times of hypocalcemia.

Synthesis and Release of Parathyroid Hormone

There are specific genes in the nucleus of the chief cells of the parathyroid gland which code for PTH. By transcription, it produces specific mRNA which enter the cytoplasm. In the

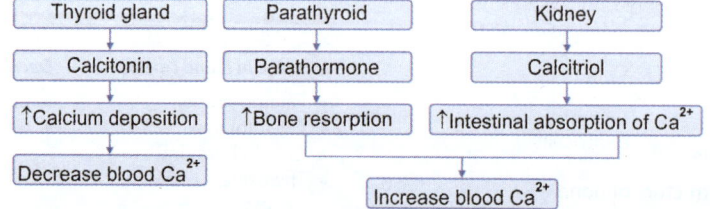

Flowchart 66.1: Important hormones regulating blood calcium level and their source.

ribosomes of the rough endoplasmic reticulum, by translation specific protein called **preproparathormone** with 115 amino acids is formed. This is cleaved in the endoplasmic reticulum to form **proparathormone (proPTH)** with 90 amino acids. It is further cleaved in the Golgi apparatus and six more amino acid residues are removed from the amino terminal of proPTH to form active PTH. From the Golgi apparatus secretory granules containing parathormone gets budded off. This will be released to the exterior by exocytosis in response to appropriate stimulus.

The chief cells of the parathyroid gland contain **calcium sensing receptors (CaSR)** which are G-protein-coupled receptors on their cell membrane. When there is increase in blood calcium level, Ca^{2+} binds with these receptors. This binding leads to activation of the CaSR, which in turn causes inhibition of release of parathormone from the secretory granules. In times of hypocalcemia, there is no stimulation of the calcium sensing receptors and there is no inhibition of exocytosis of granules containing PTH. This leads to release of PTH into the blood stream. There will be increased resorption of bone and blood Ca^{2+} level comes back to normal.

Actions of PTH (Flowchart 66.2)

*The overall effect of parathormone is to **increase the plasma calcium concentration and decrease the plasma phosphate concentration** by acting on three main target organs: bone, kidney and intestine.* PTH has direct action on bone and kidney. Action on intestine is mediated through 1,25-dihydroxycholecalciferol synthesized in the kidney. PTH is secreted in response to a fall in ionized calcium and acts mainly on bone and on the kidney tubule to increase blood calcium.

Action on Bone

In the bone, PTH promotes both bone resorption and bone synthesis.

❖ PTH acts directly on bone to increase **bone resorption** and thus mobilizes calcium and phosphate from hydroxyapatite crystals. Osteoblasts contain plenty of PTH receptors. PTH binds to PTH receptors which are G-protein coupled receptors (Gs). This leads to release of **receptor activator for nuclear factor kappa beta ligand (RANKL)** from the osteoblast. Action is mediated through cAMP. The osteoclasts contain receptors for the RANK-ligand. When this ligand combines with the receptors in the osteoclast, they become activated and release substances like H^+ which acidifies the area to a pH of 4 and acid phosphatases which causes bone resorption and release of Ca^{2+} and phosphate from hydroxyapatite into the blood stream. Thus, plasma Ca^{2+} level is increased. Acid proteases secreted by the osteoclast break down collagen and a shallow depression is formed in the bone where the osteoclast gets attached to the bone. The collagen breakdown products are **pyridinolines** and their measure in urine is used as an index of the rate of bone resorption.

❖ PTH receptors are present in both osteoblasts and osteoclasts. It increases permeability of osteoblasts and osteoclasts to calcium.

❖ PTH stimulates the precursor of osteoclasts in the bone marrow and increases the number of osteoclasts and **increases osteoclastic activity**. Vitamin D and PTH stimulate osteoblastic cells to secrete factors such as macrophage colony-stimulating factor (M-CSF) that cause osteoclast precursors to proliferate. These precursors differentiate into mononuclear osteoclasts which fuse to become multinucleated osteoclasts.

❖ PTH increases the release of lysosomal enzymes, which in turn increases breakdown of collagen. At the same time it stimulates osteoblastic activity and increases collagen synthesis. This simultaneous bone resorption and formation helps in the remodeling of bone. It is seen that low doses of PTH when given intermittently, stimulates bone formation in humans. But in high doses it increases bone resorption.

PTH promotes bone synthesis by three mechanisms:
1. PTH directly activates Ca^{2+} channels in the osteocytes, which leads to a net transfer of Ca^{2+} from bone fluid to the osteocyte. The osteocyte then transfers this Ca^{2+} to the osteoblast via gap junctions. This process is called **osteocytic-osteolysis**. The osteoblasts pump this Ca^{2+} into the extracellular matrix, which contributes to mineralization.
2. PTH promotes osteoblastic differentiation and also inhibits osteoblastic apoptosis. Thus osteoblastic activity is increased.
3. Third mechanism is an indirect one. Osteoclastic bone resorption due to the action of PTH, leads to the release of growth factors trapped within the matrix. These include insulin like growth factor (IGF-1 and IGF-2), fibroblast growth factor and transforming growth factor-β which stimulates bone synthesis.

Action on Kidney

❖ PTH **increases the reabsorption of Ca^{2+}** and H^+ from thick ascending limb of loop of Henle and distal convoluted tubule. The tubular cells contain PTH receptors which are G-protein coupled receptors. Binding of PTH with these receptors activates protein kinase. Specific mRNA is formed by transcription of specific genes. This mRNA in the cytoplasm after translation, produces specific proteins which are calcium channel proteins. The vesicles containing

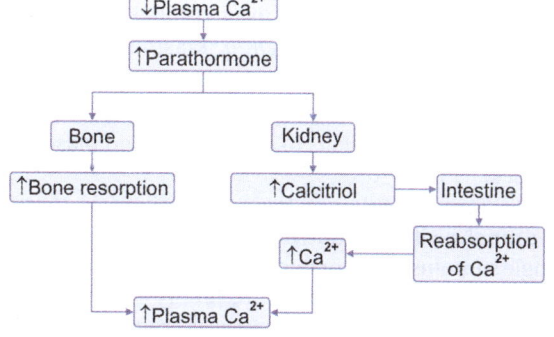

Flowchart 66.2: Mechanism of calcium homeostasis when blood calcium is decreased ('↑' denotes increase and '↓' denotes decrease).

these proteins move to the cell membrane on the luminal side and insert the proteins on the cell membrane. There will be increased reabsorption of Ca^{2+} from the tubular lumen through these calcium channels. This calcium will reach the peritubular space by secondary active transport in exchange for sodium which enter passively into the cell from the lateral interstitial space. Acute stimulation of PTH secretion by calcium deficiency helps to prevent hypocalcaemia by causing the kidney to reabsorb a greater fraction of the filtered calcium. But in hyperparathyroidism, Ca^{2+} excretion is increased due to increased filtered load of calcium.

- PTH increases PO_4^{3-} excretion and thus the plasma PO_4^{3-} level falls. This **phosphaturic action** is due to inhibition of reabsorption of PO_4^{3-} in the proximal convoluted tubule of nephron.
- It also increases excretion of Na^+, K^+ and HCO_3^- by decreasing their reabsorption in the proximal tubule.
- PTH stimulates the 1-hydroxylation of 25-hydroxycholecalciferol to 1,25-dihydroxycholecalciferol (calcitriol) in the mitochondria of the proximal tubule. Thus, by stimulating the **synthesis of calcitriol** PTH indirectly increases calcium absorption from the intestine.

Action on Intestine

The PTH has *indirect action* on intestine. It stimulates the formation of calcitriol in the kidney. Calcitriol, in turn, stimulates reabsorption of Ca^{2+} from intestine. PTH as such has no action on intestine.

Skin contains **7-dehydrocholesterol**. This is acted upon by ultraviolet light to form **cholecalciferol**. Cholecalciferol reaches the liver and is converted to **25-hydroxycholecalciferol** by the enzyme **25-hydroxylase**. Specific cells in the kidney contain the enzyme **1-α-hydroxylase** which is stimulated by parathormone. This enzyme converts 25-hydroxycholecalciferol to **1, 25-dihydroxycholecalciferol** which is the active form of vitamin D. It is also known as calcitriol. Calcitriol acts on its receptors in the duodenal cell cytoplasm and leads to the formation of calcium channel proteins which get inserted on the cell membrane. More calcium is absorbed from the duodenum through these channels.

Mechanism of Action of PTH

The PTH receptor is a G protein coupled receptor (GPCR). PTH is a polypeptide hormone which binds to $G\alpha_s$ and its action is mediated through cAMP with the help of **adenylyl cyclase**. cAMP stimulates protein kinase A. Kidney and bone has the greatest number of PTH receptors. In the kidney, they are abundant in the proximal and distal convoluted tubules. In the bone, osteoblasts appear to be the major target cells. Whenever blood Ca^{2+} level decreases, the receptors in the parathyroid gland detect the change and there is increase in cAMP production. cAMP acts on genes involved in PTH secretion and more PTH is synthesized and released into circulation. PTH increases the number and activity of osteoclasts which increase bone resorption. Ca^{2+} is released from bone to blood. PTH acts on kidney and increases Ca^{2+} reabsorption from renal tubules. It also stimulates formation of calcitriol in the kidney, which increases Ca^{2+} absorption from the GIT. Thus, the blood Ca^{2+} will be brought back to normal.

Binding of PTH to the receptor also stimulates $G\alpha_q$, which in turn stimulates **phospholipase C** to generate inositol triphosphate (IP_3) and diacylglycerol (DAG). The IP_3 release Ca^{2+} from endoplasmic reticulum, thus increasing intracellular Ca^{2+}. This Ca^{2+} activates Ca^{2+} dependent kinases. DAG activate protein kinase C (PKC).

Regulation of Secretion of PTH

- Most important regulatory factor for parathormone secretion is the level of Ca^{2+} in plasma. When plasma Ca^{2+} falls, the PTH secretion increases and more of Ca^{2+} is mobilized from bone to plasma. When Ca^{2+} level rises in plasma, PTH secretion decreases and more of Ca^{2+} gets deposited in bone.
- Plasma Mg^{2+} level has also a direct effect on PTH secretion. Magnesium is required to maintain normal parathyroid secretory responses. In magnesium deficiency, hypocalcemia occasionally occurs due to impaired PTH release along with diminished target organ responses to PTH.
- 1,25-dihydroxycholecalciferol or calcitriol acts directly on the parathyroid gland and decrease preproPTH mRNA.
- β-Adrenergic stimulation and cAMP can stimulate PTH secretion.
- Plasma PO_4^{3-} level has an indirect effect on PTH secretion. When PO_4^{3-} level increases, ionic calcium level decreases and this stimulates PTH secretion. It also inhibits the formation of 1,25-dihydroxycholecalciferol. When PO_4^{3-} level decreases, Ca^{2+} level increases and inhibits PTH secretion from parathyroid gland.

Abnormalities of PTH Secretion

- Hypoparathyroidism
- Hyperparathyroidism

Hypoparathyroidism

Causes

- Accidental removal of parathyroid along with thyroid gland during thyroidectomy
- Damage to the gland during radiation for carcinoma thyroid
- Autoimmune destruction of the gland
- Congenital absence of parathyroid gland is called **DiGeorge syndrome**.

Hypoparathyroidism is suspected when there is hypocalcemia and hyperphosphatemia. Plasma parathormone concentration will be low.

Symptoms: Symptoms are due to decreased level of plasma Ca^{2+}. Plasma Ca^{2+} level falls to half normal and plasma PO_4^{3-} level rises.

- When ionized calcium level falls, there is increased neuronal excitability and nerve fibers fire repetitively for a single stimulus. If motor nerve fibers are involved, muscular contraction called tetany is seen. **Tetany** is characterized by spontaneous tonic spasm of muscles limited to a particular group of muscles or to the entire body. Some nerve fibers are more sensitive than others. Accoucher's hand and laryngeal stridor are common.

- **Accoucher's hand** is flexion at wrist joint, flexion of metacarpophalangeal joint, extension of interphalangeal joint and adduction of thumb **(Fig. 66.2)**. Plantar flexion of feet with flexion of toes is also common. When both hands and feet are affected, it is called **carpopedal spasm**.
- **Laryngeal stridor** is due to rapid contraction of the laryngeal muscles resulting in closure of glottis. This leads to cyanosis due to hypoxia. After sometime, the muscles relax and air enters the respiratory tract with a crowing sound. If it is severe, it leads to asphyxia and death.

❖ Hypoparathyroidism is also associated with numbness, tingling and burning sensation of extremities due to increased sensitivity of sensory nerves to depolarization.
❖ Visceral manifestations like intestinal colic, biliary colic and bronchospasm are common.
❖ Profuse sweating will be present.
❖ ECG shows abnormalities like prolonged ST segment and abnormal T wave.
Sometimes, clinical manifestations do not develop with decreased Ca^{2+}. This is called **latent tetany** and can be diagnosed by the following tests.
- **Chvostek's sign:** Tapping the skin in front of the ear will stimulate the facial nerve and due to hyperexcitability or decreased threshold of the nerve, the facial muscles show spasm.
- **Trousseau's sign:** Obstruction of circulation of upper arm by inflating the BP cuff results in Accoucher's hand.
- **Erb's sign:** Stimulation of motor nerves using galvanic current will produce contraction of muscles supplied by the nerve.

Other conditions that produce tetany
❖ **Alkalosis** as in hyperventilation, excessive vomiting and excessive administration of alkaline salts especially HCO_3^-. When H^+ concentration falls, more of Ca^{2+} gets bound to plasma proteins and ionized calcium level falls. As a result tetany occurs. Here, the total plasma calcium level will be normal only the free calcium level falls.
❖ **Vitamin D deficiency** as in rickets and osteomalacia causes tetany. Vitamin D is necessary for the formation of calcitriol which is necessary for the absorption of calcium from the intestine and also from the renal tubules. It also mobilizes Ca^{2+} from bone. So, when the level of vitamin D falls, ionic calcium level also falls leading to tetany.
❖ **Malabsorption** of calcium from intestine as in tropical sprue
❖ Excessive administration of citrate and phosphate leads to a fall in the ionic calcium level because calcium citrate is formed.

Pseudohypoparathyroidism: Here, the plasma parathormone (PTH) level is increased and the defect is resistance at the tissue level for PTH. This may be due to defect in the receptors for PTH.

Treatment

Hypoparathyroidism is treated with oral calcium and calcitriol in order to return plasma calcium concentration to normal. PTH is not used therapeutically since it is antigenic. Synthetic PTH which has only 34 amino acids possesses all the biological effects of PTH. Marked increase in bone density occurs in response to injections of PTH once or twice daily.

Hyperparathyroidism

Causes

Primary hyperparathyroidism:
❖ Diffuse enlargement (hyperplasia) of the gland
❖ Adenoma of parathyroid
❖ Carcinoma of parathyroid is a rare cause.

Secondary hyperparathyroidism: Secondary hyperparathyroidism occurs in chronic renal disease where there is decreased formation of calcitriol in the kidney. This via feedback stimulation causes compensatory parathyroid hypertrophy referred to as secondary hyperparathyroidism.

Manifestations

Hypercalcemia, hypophosphatemia, hypercalciuria and renal calculi (stones) are typical manifestations. The blood Ca^{2+} level rises in hyperparathyroidism. Symptoms are due to hypercalcemia, formation of renal stones and deformities due to destruction of bone. **Pathological fracture and bone cysts** are common findings and it is referred to as **osteitis fibrosa**. Symptoms include bone pain, muscle weakness, lassitude, anorexia, nausea, vomiting, constipation, polyuria, increased thirst and mental symptoms. Polyuria is due to damage to the distal nephron and increased thirst is due to polyuria.

In hyperparathyroidism, the plasma calcium level can become high enough so that the hormone's primary renal tubular calcium reabsorbing action will be overwhelmed by the increased filtered load of calcium. This results in hypercalciuria and an increased frequency of renal calcium stone formation. Stones are mainly calcium oxalate and calcium citrate. Sometimes, renal stones may be the only

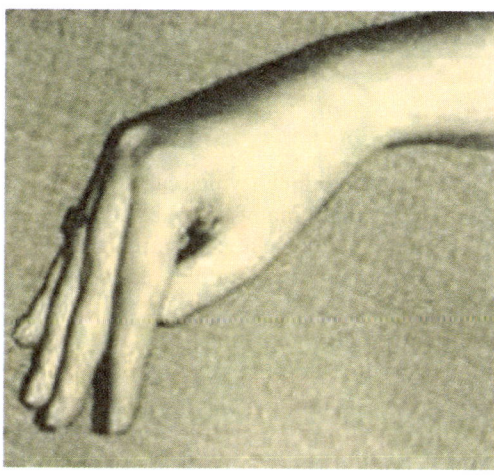

Fig. 66.2: Accoucher's hand in tetany.

manifestation of hyperparathyroidism and more than 50% of patients present with renal stone formation. There will be deposition of calcium in soft tissues.

Diagnosis
- Hypercalcemia (increase in serum calcium up to 22 mg/dL), low fasting serum phosphate level (<2.5 mg/dL) and increase in serum alkaline phosphatase are seen in hyperparathyroidism.
- Shortened ST segment in ECG.
- Radiological finding is subperiosteal erosions due to excessive bone resorption.

PTH-Related Protein

PTH-related peptide or protein (PTHrp) is a protein with PTH activity produced by tissues like skin keratinocytes, kidney, brain, lactating mammary epithelium, placenta and fetal parathyroid glands. It is also a product of human cancers that are of squamous cell origin. Because of the similarity between the N-terminal amino acids of PTHrp and PTH, PTHrp exhibits most of the actions of PTH on bone and kidney. But it has no action in kidney to stimulate calcitriol synthesis. So patients with hypercalcemia caused by PTHrp do not have elevated plasma levels of calcitriol. PTHrp appears to act locally as a growth factor for the development of skin, hair follicles, cartilage, teeth and breasts.

Hypersecretion of PTHrp is seen as a complication of cancer of breast, kidney, ovary, skin, etc. This results in hypercalcemia referred to as **humoral hypercalcemia of malignancy**. Clinically, it is associated with symptoms of hypercalcemia.

Physiological role of PTHrp
- In the intrauterine life and early infancy, PTHrp plays an important physiological role in the regulation of endochondral bone formation.
- PTHrp in the placenta and the fetus help in maintaining the 30–40% increased ionized calcium concentration gradient between the fetal and maternal plasma.
- PTHrp is also involved in breast development and lactation and it increases the calcium concentration in breast milk.
- Help in resorbing alveolar bone, so as to allow normal tooth development and eruption. In the absence of PTHrp teeth fail to erupt.
- Regulate the rate of differentiation of skin keratinocytes and growth of hair follicles.
- Protect central nervous system neurons from toxic overstimulation of glutamate receptors.

Calcitonin

Calcitonin is the calcium-lowering hormone secreted by parafollicular cells or C cells of the thyroid gland. Since it is produced by the C cells of thyroid gland it is also known as **thyrocalcitonin**. Calcitonin is also produced by thymus, brain, liver, gut, etc. Role of this extra thyroid calcitonin is not known.

Thyrocalcitonin is a polypeptide with 32 amino acids and molecular weight 3500. Half-life is less than 10 minutes.

Actions of Calcitonin

The release of calcitonin from the C cells is triggered by a rise in the extracellular Ca^{2+} concentration above normal. Calcitonin receptors are found in bone and kidney which are the main sites of action of the hormone and the actions are mediated through **cAMP**.

- Calcitonin inhibits bone resorption by inhibiting the osteoclasts. This is by a direct action on bone by decreasing the permeability of the membranes of osteoclasts to Ca^{2+}. Calcitonin receptors are present in plenty in the osteoclasts. Binding of calcitonin with the receptor inhibits osteoclastic activity. Normally there is a balance between osteoblastic activity and osteoclastic activity. When osteoclasts are inhibited, there will be increase in osteoblastic activity. Calcium and phosphate are taken from the blood into the osteoblast and this leads to increased bone deposition and the bone becomes thicker.
- It enhances excretion of Ca^{2+} by kidney and thus lowers blood Ca^{2+} level.
- It also lowers blood PO_4 level by increasing PO_4 excretion through kidney.
- It increases Na^+ excretion from renal tubules.
- It inhibits PTH effects on bone.
- Calcitonin plays a very important role in maintaining normal blood Ca^{2+} level when blood Ca^{2+} is increased.
- It plays an important role in bone remodeling. Clinically, calcitonin is given for the treatment of various diseases, for relieving bone pain and also for maintaining normal bone structure.
- In pregnancy and lactation, more Ca^{2+} is drained from the mother by the baby for its bone formation. Increased secretion of calcitonin will prevent bone resorption and bone loss in the mother during pregnancy.

Regulation of Secretion

Most important stimulus for calcitonin secretion is increase in the plasma ionic calcium level. Calcitonin is not secreted until the plasma Ca^{2+} is more than 9.5 mg%. Above this level, calcitonin secretion is directly proportional to rise in blood calcium. Other factors that stimulate calcitonin secretion are dopamine, estrogen, gastrin, cholecystokinin (CCK), secretin and glucagon. Gastrin is a potent stimulus for calcitonin secretion.

Abnormalities

There is no known condition in which calcitonin is decreased, but in medullary carcinoma of thyroid, there is increase in calcitonin secretion, but no clinical symptoms are seen.

After thyroidectomy, the parafollicular cells are absent, but bone density and plasma Ca^{2+} level are normal as long as the parathyroid glands are intact. This may be partly due to secretion of calcitonin from tissues other than thyroid. No syndrome due to calcitonin deficiency has been described. Patients with calcitonin-secreting tumor of the C cells who have calcitonin concentrations 50–100 times normal, maintain normal plasma levels of Ca^{2+}, vitamin D and PTH.

CALCITRIOL OR 1,25-HYDROXYCHOLECALCIFEROL

Calcitriol is an active metabolite of **vitamin D**. It is called a hormone because it is synthesized in one site and exerts its action at another site. It is synthesized from 7-dehydrocholesterol.

❖ Normal blood level is of calcitriol is 30 ng/mL.
❖ Vitamin D insufficiency means values between 21 ng/mL and 29 ng/mL
❖ Vitamin D deficiency means less than 20 ng/mL

Steps in the Formation of Calcitriol (Flowchart 66.3)

❖ *Formation of vitamin D_3 or cholecalciferol in the skin:* Vitamin D_3 is formed from 7-dehydrocholesterol present in the skin of mammals by the action of ultraviolet light non-enzymatically. Vitamin D_3 is also obtained from foods like fish, fish liver oil, egg yolk etc. Cholecalciferol enters circulation from the skin by facilitated diffusion with the help of D_3-binding proteins.

$$\text{7-dehydrocholesterol} \xrightarrow{\text{UV light}} \text{cholecalciferol or vitamin } D_3$$

❖ *Formation of 25-hydroxycholecalciferol:* Cholecalciferol is present in the blood bound to α-globulin and is transported to the liver. In the liver, it is converted to 25-hydroxycholecalciferol. This product has an inhibitory feedback control on this reaction. Excess cholecalciferol will be stored in the liver for long periods.

$$\text{Cholecalciferol} \xrightarrow{\text{25-hydroxylase}} \text{25-hydroxycholecalciferol}$$

❖ *Formation of 1,25 dihydroxycholecalciferol in the kidney:* 25-hydroxycholecalciferol reaches the kidney and in the PCT it is converted to 1,25-dihydroxycholecalciferol. Enzyme involved is mitochondrial **1α-hydroxylase**. *Proximal convoluted tubule is the only site of formation of this hormone in the human body.*

$$\text{25-hydroxycholecalciferol} \xrightarrow{\text{1α-hydroxylase}} \text{1,25-dihydroxycholecalciferol (calcitriol)}$$

Actions of Calcitriol

Receptors for calcitriol are present in the **intestine, bone and kidney**. Calcitriol exerts its action primarily by genomic effects that involve induction of the synthesis of epithelial Ca^{2+} channels and pumps and calcium binding proteins in the epithelial cells. The action of calcitriol is opposite to that of calcitonin.

Action on Intestine

❖ Calcitriol increases calcium absorption in the duodenum. It acts by entering the nuclei of the intestinal epithelial cells and stimulate the production of mRNA directly. There is increased synthesis of water-soluble calcium-binding proteins called **calbindin** which contains two binding sites for calcium. Calbindin helps in calcium absorption via the brush border cells of the gut.

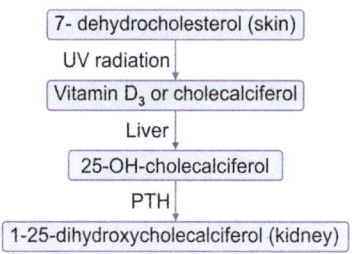

Flowchart 66.3: Summary of the steps in the synthesis of calcitriol.

Increased absorption of Ca^{2+} from the intestine occurs in three steps:

1. Ca^{2+} enters the intestinal cell via calcium channels in the apical membrane. Calcitriol increases the permeability of the brush border to Ca^{2+}
2. The calcium ions in the cell bind to binding proteins called calbindin. This maintains a favorable gradient for Ca^{2+} entry across the apical membrane of the enterocyte since the free cytosolic Ca^{2+} level is low.
3. The enterocyte extrudes Ca^{2+} across the basolateral membrane by means of a Ca^{2+} pump or Na^+-Ca^{2+} exchanger. Calcitriol increases production of calcium dependent ATPase which pumps calcium out of the enterocyte.

❖ Vitamin D stimulates PO_4 absorption by the small intestine by increasing the synthesis of the transporter protein, Na^+-PO_4^- co-transporter in the enterocyte.

Action on Bone

In bone, it mobilizes Ca^{2+} and PO_4. This is by increasing the permeability of the membrane of osteoblasts to Ca^{2+} and Ca^{2+} ion is pumped into the ECF. Increase in calcitriol causes bone resorption. Action of calcitriol on bone is the result of both indirect and direct actions.

❖ **Indirect action:** Vitamin D increases absorption of Ca^{2+} from the small intestine and kidney thereby increasing the plasma Ca^{2+} available to mineralize unmineralized osteoid.
❖ **Direct action:** Direct effect of calcitriol on bone is via both osteoblast and osteoclast precursor cells. Both these cells have vitamin D receptors. It increases both osteoblastic and osteoclastic differentiation, thereby increasing bone turn over. When calcitriol binds with its receptors on osteoblasts it produces some cytokines which activates osteoclasts. Activated osteoclasts produce phosphatase and collagenase that lyses bone matrix. Calcitriol in smaller quantities promotes bone calcification. Bone resorption and mineralization should occur in a controlled manner for proper bone remodeling.

But when calcitriol is present in excess, it favors bone resorption because it favors osteoclastogenesis and increase the number of mature osteoclasts. There will be increased osteoclast activity. Thus *indirectly calcitriol causes net bone mineralization since it increases the concentration of both Ca^{2+} and PO_4^- in the blood and ECF. On the other hand, if calcitriol is present in excess the direct effect predominates and there will be increased bone mobilization.* In the absence of calcitriol, bone resorption function of PTH is reduced.

Action on Kidney

In the kidney, calcitriol increases the reabsorption of Ca^{2+} by increasing the number of Ca^{2+} pump. It also increases the reabsorption of phosphate ions.

During Pregnancy

Calcitriol secretion is elevated during pregnancy to provide more Ca^{2+} for the developing fetus.

Regulation of Secretion of Calcitriol

Secretion of calcitriol is regulated by a feedback mechanism by plasma **Ca^{2+} and PO_4 level**. Decrease in calcium and phosphate level increases calcitriol synthesis.

- Most important stimulus for calcitriol secretion is parathormone (PTH). PTH stimulates conversion of 25-hydroxycholecalciferol to **1,25-dihydroxycholecalciferol** (1,25-DHCC) by activating 1α-hydroxylase enzyme. It is seen that the renal 1α-hydroxylase activity decreases to unstimulated levels within 24 hours of parathyroidectomy. PTH causes an increase in blood Ca^{2+} level and high blood calcium will inhibit PTH as well as calcitriol, thus bringing blood Ca^{2+} back to normal. Decrease in blood calcium will stimulate PTH secretion which in turn stimulates 1α-hydroxylase enzyme.
- Plasma PO_4 level also influences the secretion of calcitriol. Its formation is stimulated by low PO_4 level and inhibited by high PO_4 level. PO_4 mechanism acts directly through 1α-hydroxylase enzyme.
- By negative feedback mechanism calcitriol itself regulates its own production.
- Other stimuli are estrogen, progesterone, prolactin and insulin which facilitate the formation of calcitriol by activating the enzyme 1α-hydroxylase.
- Secretion of calcitriol is decreased in metabolic acidosis and insulin insufficiency.

Effects of Deficiency of Calcitriol

Deficiency of calcitriol leads to hypocalcemia and failure of mineralization of bones. In children the condition is called **rickets** and in adults it is called **osteomalacia**. Postmenopausal women are prone to develop fracture of bone due to demineralization.

Causes

- Inadequate exposure to sun
- Inadequate intake of calcium
- Mother's vitamin D deficiency during pregnancy
- Babies who are exclusively breast-fed should receive vitamin D drops. Breast milk does not contain enough vitamin D. all infants should receive 400 IU of vitamin D per day
- Chronic renal failure decreases calcitriol (1,25-DHCC) formation due to reduced activity of 1α- hydroxylase
- Liver dysfunction prevents 25-DHCC formation
- Defects in target cell receptors for calcitriol
- 1α-hydroxylase deficiency.

Rickets

In children prolonged deficiency of vitamin D is characterized by soft and weak bones due to deficient deposition of calcium salts. Vitamin D is necessary to absorb calcium and phosphorus from food. Therefore, bones get easily bent under the weight of the body. The condition is called rickets. Tetany may occur as a complication of rickets due to lowered serum calcium. Features of rickets are:

- Soft skull which yield under pressure
- Widening and thickening of wrist and ankle
- Beading of costochondral junction and breast bone projection
- Frontal bossing of skull
- Bowing of legs or knock knees **(Fig. 66.3)**
- Kyphosis and pelvic deformities
- Tetany and seizures
- Delayed growth and delayed motor skills
- Muscle weakness.

Osteomalacia

Vitamin D deficiency in adults is referred to as osteomalacia. It is characterized by skeletal pain, bone tenderness, muscle weakness, soft pelvis and ribs.

Osteoporosis

Osteoporosis is caused by a relative excess of osteoclastic activity which affects the trabecular bone more rapidly than the compact bone. There is marked loss of bone matrix leading to increased risk of fractures like Colles fracture, fracture of vertebral body and hip. These areas have a high content of trabecular bone. Humans lose bone as they become older which is referred to as **involutional osteoporosis**. When this loss is accelerated, as in females after menopause it leads to severe osteoporosis. The cause for the bone loss is estrogen deficiency. Estrogen replacement therapy soon after menopause can maintain bone density to some extent. But estrogen has several side effects. Drugs like **bisphosphonates,** which inhibit osteoclastic activity can be administered in a cyclical manner. They can inhibit bone

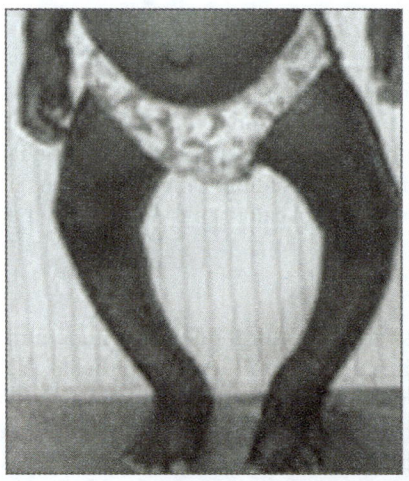
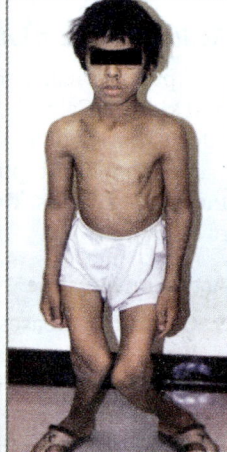

Fig. 66.3: Bone deformity in rickets.
Courtesy: Dr RV Jayakumar.

breakdown, increase mineral content of bone and increase bone density in hip and spine. Thus the risk of fractures can be reduced.

Inactivity is another cause for osteoporosis which is referred to as **disuse osteoporosis**. It is seen in immobilized patients where bone resorption exceeds bone formation.

Osteopetrosis

Osteopetrosis, a rare and often severe disease, is also referred to as **stone bone or marble bone disease**. It is an autosomal dominant inherited disease. Adult osteopetrosis is the most common type. Here about 40% of affected individuals are asymptomatic. The bones harden, and become denser. This condition is opposite to osteoporosis where the bones become less dense and more brittle and osteomalacia where the bones become soft. Osteopetrosis is due to malfunctioning of the osteoclasts. They fail to resorb bone since they fail to release the necessary lysosomal enzymes for bone resorption into the extracellular space. The osteoblastic activity becomes unopposed. As a consequence, bone modeling and remodeling are impaired. There is defective bone turn over and there is increased skeletal fragility. Symptoms include increased risk of fractures; there will be frequent infections of teeth and jaw bones, hemopoietic insufficiency and growth impairment in children. Radiographs reveal generalized osteosclerosis referred to as '**bone-within-bone appearance**'.

Other Hormones Regulating Calcium Metabolism

Other hormones regulating calcium metabolism are thyroxine, glucocorticoids, prolactin, growth hormone, prostaglandin, insulin and estrogen.

Estrogen

Most common cause for osteoporosis is the postmenopausal decline in estrogen levels. Estrogen **prevents osteoporosis** by inhibiting the secretion of cytokines such as interleukin-1 (IL-1), IL-6 and tumor necrosis factor (TNF-α). These cytokines foster the development of osteoclasts. Estrogen also stimulates the production of transforming growth factor (TGF-β) which increases apoptosis of osteoclasts. It is observed that at the time of **menopause**, there is an accelerated rate of bone loss in women. The same effect is seen after **ovariectomy**. When estrogen secretion is less, the actions of PTH in the bone are accelerated. Administration of small doses of estrogen to menopausal women leads to decrease in urinary excretion of calcium and total body calcium is maintained normal.

Glucocorticoid

Glucocorticoid excess leads to accelerated loss of bone since it interferes with intestinal calcium absorption. Glucocorticoid decreases the absorption of calcium and phosphate from the **gastrointestinal tract** (GIT) and increases their renal excretion by inhibiting the action of calcitriol on GIT and kidney. This leads to a decrease in blood calcium level. The response of bone to PTH is also increased by glucocorticoids. In glucocorticoid-induced **osteoporosis**, there is decreased bone formation and increased bone resorption. The decreased bone formation is due to inhibition of osteoblast differentiation and function. Glucocorticoids decrease blood Ca^{2+} levels by inhibiting osteoclast formation and activity. The decrease in calcium in turn increases secretion of parathyroid hormone. But prolonged administration of glucocorticoids causes osteoporosis by decreasing bone formation and increasing bone resorption. They decrease bone formation by inhibiting protein synthesis in osteoblasts.

Thyroid Hormones

In hyperthyroidism there is hypercalcemia, hypercalciuria and osteoporosis due to increased bone resorption. Intestinal absorption of calcium is also increased. In hypothyroidism, intestinal absorption of Ca^{2+} is decreased.

Growth Hormone

Growth hormone (GH) increases blood calcium by increasing the intestinal absorption of calcium resulting in positive calcium balance. IGF-I generated by the action of GH stimulates protein synthesis in bone.

Prostaglandins

The PGE_2 is a potent stimulator of bone resorption and increases blood calcium.

Insulin

Insulin increases bone formation. There is significant bone loss in untreated diabetes mellitus.

Interleukin-1

Interleukin-1 (IL-1) causes bone resorption. This effect of IL-1 is responsible for bone destruction in arthritis.

■ MULTIPLE CHOICE QUESTIONS

1. **Parathyroid hormone is responsible for all actions, *except*:**
   a. Increase in the absorption of phosphorus from renal tubules
   b. Increase in the absorption of vitamin D
   c. Mobilizes calcium from bone
   d. Increase intestinal absorption of calcium

2. **Calcium absorption occurs in:**
   a. Proximal small intestine
   b. Distal ileum
   c. Middle small intestine
   d. Ascending colon

3. **True of the following:**
   a. Calcium is mainly reabsorbed in the DCT
   b. 90% calcium is excreted by glomerulus
   c. Parathormone promotes absorption of calcium from intestine
   d. Parathormone promotes action of calcitonin

4. **Secondary hyperparathyroidism due to vitamin D deficiency shows:**
   a. Hypocalcemia   b. Hypercalcemia
   c. Hypophosphatemia d. Hyperphosphatemia

5. Which of these can cause hypocalcemia?
   a. Thyroxine
   b. Calcitonin
   c. Parathormone
   d. Cholecalciferol

6. Hypocalcemia due to calcitonin is by:
   a. Increased excretion in kidney
   b. Decreased bone resorption
   c. Decreased intestinal absorption
   d. Decreased renal reabsorption

7. Osteoclasts are inhibited by:
   a. Parathyroid hormone
   b. Calcitonin
   c. 1,25-dihydroxycholecalciferol
   d. Tumor necrosis factor

8. Osteoclasts have specific receptor for:
   a. Parathormone
   b. Calcitonin
   c. Thyroxin
   d. Vitamin D_3

9. Sudden decrease in serum calcium is associated with:
   a. Increased thyroxine and parathormone secretion
   b. Increased phosphate
   c. Increased excitability of muscle and nerve
   d. Cardiac conduction abnormalities

10. Hypocalcemia is characterized by all, *except*:
    a. Numbness and tingling of circumoral region
    b. Hyperactive tendon reflexes and positive Chvostek's sign
    c. Shortening of Q-T interval in ECG
    d. Carpopedal spasm

11. In tetany hyperexcitability is due to:
    a. Low Ca^{2+} causes increased permeability of Na^+
    b. Prevent K^+ release
    c. Prevent Na^+ and K^+ release
    d. Decreased Ca^{2+} produce generation of action potential

12. Which of the following organ is not involved in calcium metabolism?
    a. Skin
    b. Liver
    c. Spleen
    d. Kidney

13. Hypercalcemia associated with malignancy is most often mediated by:
    a. Parathormone
    b. Parathormone-related protein
    c. Interleukin-6
    d. Calcitonin

14. Which of the following organ is not involved in calcium homeostasis?
    a. Kidney
    b. Skin
    c. Intestine
    d. Lung

15. True statement about calcium:
    a. Absorbed in large intestine
    b. Absorbed in lower small intestine
    c. Absorption increased by alkaline pH
    d. Absorption increased by acidic pH

16. Calcitonin is produced by:
    a. Thyroid
    b. Parathyroid
    c. Thymus
    d. Kidney

17. Which of the following does not interfere with calcium metabolism?
    a. Calcitonin
    b. Cholecalciferol
    c. Vitamin D
    d. Thyroxine

18. Hyperparathyroidism is characterized by:
    a. Hypocalcemia
    b. Hyperphosphatemia
    c. Multiple bone cysts
    d. Increased bone formation

19. Osteoclasts are differentiated:
    a. Monocytes
    b. Osteoblasts
    c. Osteocytes
    d. Glial cells

20. Stimulus for parathyroid secretion is:
    a. Decreased ionized calcium
    b. Decreased total calcium
    c. Decreased serum phosphate
    d. Decreased non-ionized calcium

21. Hormones involved in calcium metabolism include all, *except*:
    a. Calcitonin
    b. Parathormone
    c. Thyroxine
    d. Calcitriol

22. In osteopetrosis, which of the following is defective?
    a. Osteoblasts
    b. Osteocytes
    c. Osteoclasts
    d. Bone collagen

23. The mechanism of action of calcitriol in the intestine is:
    a. Alteration in the activity of gene
    b. Activation of adenylyl cyclase
    c. Changes gastric acid secretion
    d. Decreases cell turn over

24. Ninety percent of protein in bone matrix is:
    a. Type I collagen
    b. Calbindin-D
    c. Osteoprotegerin
    d. Pyridinolines

25. Which hormone increases blood calcium level?
    a. Insulin
    b. Glucagon
    c. Parathormone
    d. Calcitonin

26. Fluoride ions act by inhibiting:
    a. Enolase
    b. Cytochrome oxidase
    c. Carbonic anhydrase
    d. Hexokinase

27. **Normal plasma ionic calcium level is:**
    a. 9–11 mg/dL
    b. 2–3 g/dL
    c. 14–16 mg/dL
    d. 2–3 mg/dL

28. **A high plasma Ca^{2+} level leads to:**
    a. Increased formation of calcitriol
    b. Increased secretion of calcitonin
    c. Decreased blood coagulability
    d. Increased secretion of parathormone

29. **Prolonged deficiency of calcium in the diet leads to:**
    a. Increased parathyroid hormone secretion
    b. High plasma calcitonin concentration
    c. Increased plasma phosphates
    d. Decrease in plasma parathyroid hormone level

30. **All the following can occur when calcium intake is reduced, *except*:**
    a. Acceleration in PTH synthesis
    b. Decreased calcitonin secretion
    c. Decreased renal absorption of calcium ions
    d. Increased mobilization of calcium ions from the bone

ANSWERS

1. a	2. a	3. c	4. c	5. b
6. b	7. b	8. b	9. c	10. c
11. a	12. c	13. b	14. d	15. d
16. a	17. d	18. c	19. a	20. a
21. c	22. c	23. a	24. a	25. c
26. a	27. a	28. b	29. a	30. c

Adrenal Gland

CHAPTER 67

LEARNING OBJECTIVES

- Describe the synthesis of adrenal cortical hormones
- Explain the physiological actions of cortisol
- Discuss the regulation of secretion of glucocorticoids
- Describe the effects of hypersecretion and hyposecretion of adrenal cortical hormones
- Explain the regulation of secretion of aldosterone
- Describe the steps in the synthesis of catecholamines
- Describe the actions of catecholamines in various systems
- Describe the tests to assess the functioning of adrenal cortex and medulla
- Comment on pheochromocytoma and Addisonian crisis

FUNCTIONAL ANATOMY OF ADRENAL GLAND

PY8.2: Describe the synthesis, secretion, transport, physiological actions, regulation and effect of altered (hypo and hyper) secretion of adrenal gland.
PY8.4: Describe function tests: Adrenal cortex, adrenal medulla.

Adrenal gland is a small, flattened, triangular, retro-peritoneal gland situated on the superior pole of the kidney **(Fig. 67.1A)**. Each gland weighs about 4–5 g. The gland is composed of two separate endocrine organs, **outer cortex and inner medulla**. Both differ in embryonic development, histology and functions. Embryologically, the cortex is derived from mesoderm, whereas the medulla is derived from neural crest cells that migrate into the developing cortex. The gland is larger in females and during intrauterine life. In the fetus, the gland is large because of the presence of large adrenal cortex which forms part of fetoplacental unit. After birth, adrenal cortex degenerates partially and the gland becomes normal in size. The adrenal gland produces four principal hormones, cortisol, aldosterone, epinephrine and norepinephrine. Cortisol and aldosterone are essential for survival.

Development of the Gland

Adrenal cortex develops from **coelomic epithelium** along the medial aspect of Wolffian ridge. The medulla develops from the ectodermal tissue from which the sympathetic ganglia are formed. This tissue migrates from **neural crest** and reaches the inner aspect of adrenal cortex to form adrenal medulla.

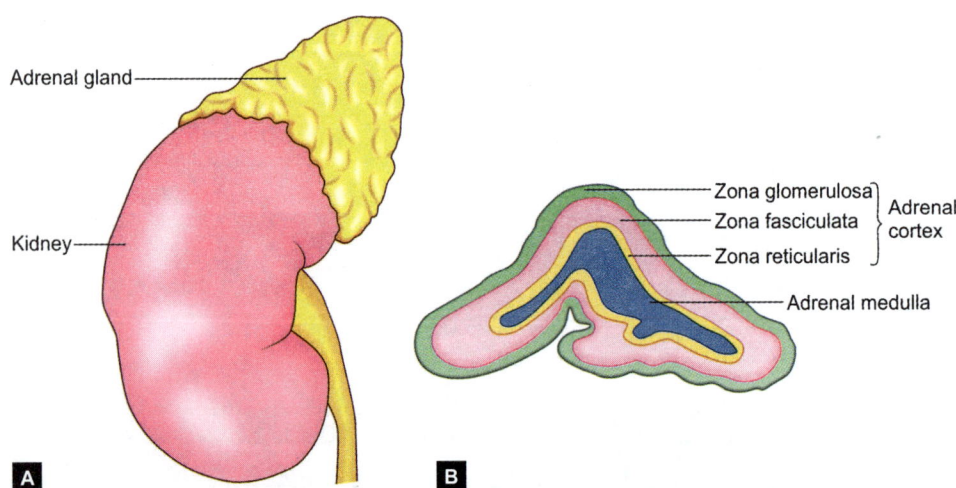

Figs. 67.1A and B: (A) Location of right adrenal gland; (B) Section through adrenal gland showing medulla and the three zones of cortex.

Blood supply to the adrenal gland is from aorta and small branches of inferior phrenic and renal artery. This forms a plexus in the capsule and from the plexus blood flows through the cortex to the sinusoids of the medulla. Blood from the medulla flows into the central adrenal vein.

Innervation of Adrenal Gland

Sympathetic fibers which supply the gland reach the gland via the **splanchnic nerves**. These fibers pierce the capsule of the gland, reach the cortex and pass through the cortex without supplying the cortical cells and finally end in the medullary cells. So, adrenal medullary cells are considered as postganglionic sympathetic cells which have lost their axons and became secretory cells **(Fig. 67.2)**.

Histology

Adrenal Cortex

Adrenal cortex consists of three layers **(Fig. 67.1B)**:
1. **Zona glomerulosa:** 15% of the total mass of gland constitutes this layer. It forms the outer zone and is made up of whorls of large cells with numerous rounded mitochondria.
2. **Zona fasciculata:** This is the widest zone and is seen in the midcortex and constitutes 50% of the total mass of the gland.
3. **Zona reticularis:** It is the innermost layer seen near the cortical-medullary junction and it constitutes 7% of the total weight of the adrenal.

Adrenal cortical cells are rich in lipid especially cholesterol, the precursor of steroid hormones. Middle layer is rich in ascorbic acid. Cortical cells contain numerous smooth endoplasmic reticulum, which are involved in steroid synthesis. Zona glomerulosa in addition to secreting mineralocorticoids is also capable of forming new cortical cells. After hypophysectomy the adrenal cortex atrophies. When adequate adrenocorticotropic hormone (ACTH) is replaced, the adrenal cortex is capable of regeneration from cells in the zona glomerulosa. The zona glomerulosa will not atrophy in the absence of ACTH since it is also maintained by angiotensin II. *Adrenal medulla does not regenerate.*

Adrenal Medulla

Adrenal medulla is composed of interlacing cords of densely innervated network of cells which contains granules.

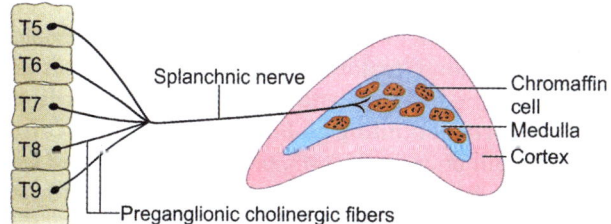

Figs. 67.2: Innervation of adrenal medulla. Preganglionic sympathetic fibers synapse directly on the chromaffin cells which contain adrenaline.

Two types of cells are distinguished:
1. Epinephrine-secreting cells which have large but less dense granules and constitute 90% of the total adrenal medullary cells.
2. Norepinephrine-secreting cells constitute 10% of cells which contain small but dense granules.

Even though dopamine is produced by adrenal medulla, the cells that produce dopamine have not been distinguished.

All adrenal medullary cells stain brown with chromium salts because of the oxidation of epinephrine, norepinephrine or dopamine. Since these cells have affinity for chromium, they are called **chromaffin cells**, and it is the granules that take up the stain.

Hormones of Adrenal Cortex (Table 67.1)

Three groups of steroid hormones are produced by adrenal cortex:
1. **Glucocorticoids** secreted by zona fasciculata (C_{21} steroids)
   - Cortisol
   - Corticosterone
   - Cortisone
2. **Mineralocorticoids** from zona glomerulosa
   - Aldosterone
   - 11-deoxycorticosterone
3. **Sex steroids** from zona reticularis
   - Androgens—dehydroepiandrosterone and androstenedione
   - Estrogen and progesterone in small amounts.

Biosynthesis of Cortical Hormones

The ACTH produced from anterior pituitary stimulates the adrenal cortical cells to synthesize the hormones. All steroid hormones have **cyclopentanoperhydrophenanthrene ring** structure. C_{19} steroids have androgenic activity and C_{21} steroids have mineralocorticoid or glucocorticoid activity. The main glucocorticoid in humans is **cortisol** and the main mineralocorticoid is **aldosterone**.

Steps in the Synthesis of Adrenal Cortical Hormones (Flowchart 67.1)

- Precursor of adrenal cortical hormones is cholesterol. Cholesterol is synthesized from acetate present inside the cortical cell or it is obtained from blood. From blood, low-density lipoprotein (LDL)-cholesterol enters the cortical cells by means of **LDL receptor-mediated endocytosis**. There are numerous low-density lipoprotein cholesterol receptors in the cortical cell membrane.

Table 67.1: Hormones secreted by adrenal cortex and adrenal medulla.

Hormones of adrenal cortex	Hormones of adrenal medulla
• Glucocorticoids—cortisol, corticosterone	• Norepinephrine
• Mineralocorticoid—aldosterone	• Epinephrine
• Sex steroids—mainly androgens (dehydroepiandrosterone); estrogen and progesterone in very small amounts	• Dopamine

Flowchart 67.1: Steps in the synthesis of adrenal cortical hormones. The major hormones of the gland are underlined.

- The cholesterol is transported into the mitochondria by means of a carrier protein. In the mitochondria it is converted to pregnenolone by the enzyme **cholesterol desmolase or side-chain cleavage enzyme.** This is the rate limiting step in the formation of adrenal steroids.
- Pregnenolone moves into the smooth endoplasmic reticulum where some of it is dehydrogenated to form progesterone by **3β-hydroxysteroid dehydrogenase enzyme.**
- By the action of **17α-hydroxylase** enzyme pregnenolone is converted to 17α-hydroxypregnenolone and progesterone to 17α-hydroxyprogesterone.
- These are then converted to C_{19} steroids dehydroepiandrosterone and androstenedione by **17,20- desmolase**.
- Hydroxylation of progesterone to 11-deoxycorticosterone and 17α-hydroxyprogesterone to 11-deoxycortisol occurs in the smooth endoplasmic reticulum catalyzed by the enzyme **21β-hydroxylase**.
- 11-deoxycorticosterone and 11-deoxycortisol move back to the mitochondria where they are 11-hydroxylated to form corticosterone and cortisol catalyzed by the enzyme **11β-hydroxylase**. These reactions occur both in zona fasciculate and zona reticularis.
- In the zona glomerulosa, there is no 11β-hydroxylase enzyme but another enzyme called **aldosterone synthase** is present which converts corticosterone to aldosterone. This occurs in the mitochondria. The zona glomerulosa also lacks 17α-hydroxylase and this is *the reason why zona glomerulosa fails to produce cortisol or sex steroids.*

Plasma concentration of the hormones:
- Cortisol—13.9 µg/dL
- Corticosterone—0.4 µg/dL
- Aldosterone—0.006 µg/dL
- Deoxycorticosterone—0.006 µg/dL.

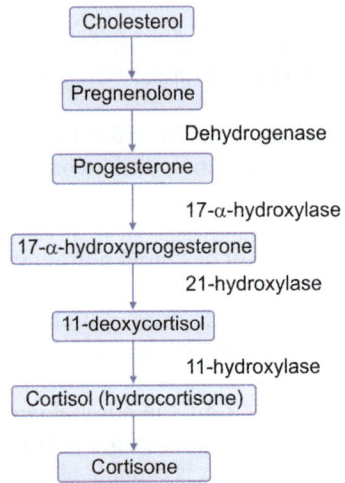

Flowchart 67.2: Steps in the synthesis of glucocorticoids.

GLUCOCORTICOIDS

The main glucocorticoids are **cortisol and corticosterone** which are secreted by zona fasciculata of adrenal cortex. **Cortisone** is formed in very small amounts. Steps in the synthesis of glucocorticoids are given in **Flowchart 67.2**.

Transport of Glucocorticoids

Steroids are relatively insoluble in water and are approximately 95% protein bound, mainly to **albumin**. In blood, cortisol is present in the free form and bound form. 90% cortisol is bound to **cortisol binding globulin (CBG)** or transcortin, 7% is albumin bound and 3–4% of circulating cortisol is in the free form. Free form is the physiologically active form and bound form is the reservoir form. Since 95% of cortisol is in the bound form, its half-life is about 60–90 minutes.

Transcortin is synthesized in the liver and its synthesis is stimulated by estrogen. So, during pregnancy, bound form is more than free form. Since free form is responsible for feedback regulation of cortisol secretion, there is stimulation of secretion of ACTH, which in turn increases the production of cortisol in pregnancy. Thus, free cortisol level comes back to normal. *This is the reason for increased level of glucocorticoids in pregnancy without symptoms of hypersecretion of glucocorticoids.* In liver disease, nephritis, etc. bound form is less and free form is more because there is decrease in transcortin level. So, less ACTH is secreted.

Metabolism

Cortisol is metabolized in the liver and kidney. Most of the cortisol is converted to **dihydrocortisol and then to tetrahydrocortisol** in the liver. A small portion is converted to **cortisone** which is an inactive steroid. Both the above metabolites are conjugated with **glucuronic acid** in the liver. The conjugated product is water-soluble and excreted through bile and urine. 10% of cortisol is converted to **17-ketosteroid** which is conjugated with **sulfate** and excreted through urine. Estimation of 17-ketosteroids in urine is used as an index to assess the function of adrenal cortex. A small fraction of cortisol enters enterohepatic circulation and a small amount is excreted through feces. Fate of corticosterone is same as that of cortisol but it is not converted to 17-ketosteroids. The half-life of cortisol in circulation is 60–90 minutes and that of corticosterone is 50 minutes.

Rate of Excretion of 17-Ketosteroids

❖ In males—15 mg/day
❖ In females—10 mg/day.

Mechanism of Action of Glucocorticoids

Glucocorticoids act by binding to specific receptors in the cytosol of target cells. Hormone-receptor complexes accumulate in the target cell nucleus and bind with high affinity to chromosomal DNA. This induces DNA transcription and synthesis of new mRNA which codes for the synthesis of specific enzyme.

Physiological Actions of Glucocorticoids

Cortisol is the most important glucocorticoid and 95% of glucocorticoid activity is contributed by cortisol.

Almost all body tissues like liver, fat, muscle, bone, skin, other viscera, hemopoietic and lymphoid tissue and the central nervous system are the target sites for glucocorticoid action.

Actions include the following:
❖ Metabolic actions
❖ Systemic actions
❖ Permissive actions
❖ Role of cortisol in stress
❖ Anti-inflammatory actions
❖ Antiallergic actions
❖ Action on other endocrine glands.

Metabolic Effects of Cortisol

Effect on Carbohydrate Metabolism

❖ Cortisol exhibits an **anti-insulin** action, i.e., it decreases peripheral utilization of glucose *except in brain and heart*. It decreases the sensitivity of peripheral tissues to insulin and blocks glucose transport into muscle and adipose tissue leading to hyperglycemia. *Cortisol excess produces **adrenal diabetes** which is moderately insulin resistant.* So, cortisol is contraindicated in diabetes mellitus.
❖ **Glycogen synthesis** and deposition in the liver is also increased by cortisol.
❖ Cortisol stimulates **gluconeogenesis** in liver and muscle thereby increasing blood glucose level. Gluconeogenesis is production of glucose from substances like amino acids, lactic acid, glycerol, free fatty acid, etc. Increase in gluconeogenesis occurs mainly due to two reasons: (i) Cortisol increases protein breakdown in muscles and bones and (ii) stimulates lipolysis in adipose tissue. This leads to increased availability of amino acids, free fatty acids and glycerol for gluconeogenesis **(Flowchart 67.3)**.

Effect on Protein Metabolism

❖ Glucocorticoid is both **anabolic and catabolic** in action in physiological levels. If glucocorticoid is present in excess, **catabolic** action predominates.
❖ Cortisol enhances the release of amino acids from proteins in skeletal muscle and bone matrix. It also decreases amino acid uptake by extrahepatic cells and when present in excess, **inhibits protein synthesis**. So, glucocorticoid excess leads to growth retardation, muscle wasting, thinning of skin and osteoporosis.
❖ The amino acids released, especially alanine are transported to the liver and are deaminated for gluconeogenesis,

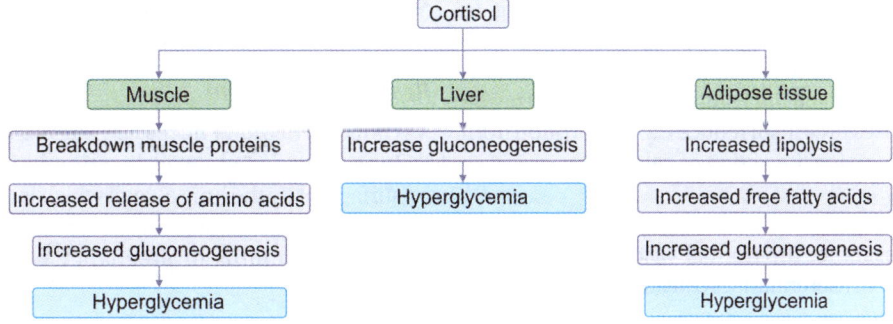

Flowchart 67.3: Mechanisms by which cortisol increases blood glucose.

i.e., they are utilized for the synthesis of glucose. Due to deamination, there is increased nitrogen excretion which leads to **negative nitrogen balance**.
- Cortisol increases the synthesis of plasma proteins by enhancing amino acid transport into liver cells.

Effect on Fat Metabolism
- Glucocorticoids stimulate absorption of fat from intestine.
- It causes lipolysis in adipose tissue by stimulating hormone-sensitive lipase. The concentration of fatty acids is increased in blood.
- Cortisol potentiates the lipolytic effects of catecholamines and glucagon (permissive action) which causes **selective lipolysis** (loss of body fat in the limbs). This leads to increased availability of fatty acids for **gluconeogenesis**.
- Despite the lipolysis, cortisol produces **lipogenesis**, i.e., synthesis of new fat probably due to the hyperinsulinemia produced by cortisol.
- In excess, cortisol causes **redistribution of fat** with more fat deposition in the trunk at the expense of extremities (characteristic centripetal distribution that is seen in Cushing's syndrome). Deposition of more fat in the face and neck leads to moon face. Deposition of excess fat in the shoulder leads to buffalo hump.
- Serum cholesterol is increased.
- More fat is converted into ketone bodies when cortisol is present in excess.

Effect on Water and Electrolyte Metabolism
- Glucocorticoids are necessary for the normal distribution of water and electrolytes between extracellular fluid (ECF) and intracellular fluid (ICF).
- Excess cortisol leads to retention of sodium and water, leading to edema and hypertension.
- Excess glucocorticoid also causes K^+ depletion, leading to muscular weakness and ECG changes.

Action on Various Systems (Table 67.2)
Musculoskeletal System
- Glucocorticoid is necessary for normal functioning of muscles. Excess cortisol leads to muscle wasting and thinning of skin due to endogenous breakdown of protein. Because of thinning of skin and due to subcutaneous deposition of fat in the trunk, the skin may break, leading to **purplish striae in the skin**.
- Excess cortisol decreases glucose utilization and decreases the sensitivity of muscle cells to insulin leading to hyperglycemia.
- Excess glucocorticoids also results in osteoporosis. Cortisol increases osteoclastic activity leading to demineralization of bone. Large doses of cortisol reduce Ca^{2+} absorption from the gut by antagonizing the action of calcitriol.

Cardiovascular System
- Cortisol is necessary for the normal vascular response of catecholamines. Cortisol enhances catecholamine synthesis by activating phenylethanolamine N-methyltransferase (PNMT). It also increases the responsiveness of vascular smooth muscle to epinephrine and norepinephrine by an inhibitory effect on prostaglandin synthesis, especially prostacyclin. Prostacyclin in excess produces vasodilatation and hypotension. Adrenocortical insufficiency or absence of cortisol is characterized by vasodilatation and hypotension which can be reversed by glucocorticoid therapy. Thus, cortisol helps to maintain normal tone of blood vessels of microcirculation.
- It increases formation of angiotensin, which in turn increases the secretion of aldosterone. Aldosterone increases reabsorption of sodium and water from the renal tubules which leads to hypertension if cortisol is present in excess.
- It increases the force of myocardial contraction.
- It increases plasma volume by increasing the movement of fluid into the vascular system.

Respiratory System
- Glucocorticoid is necessary for the **maturation of fetal lung**. This is achieved by stimulating the secretion of surfactant by the lung alveoli which is an essential factor for lung maturation. Glucocorticoid level is increased towards the later months of pregnancy when lung maturation occurs.

Table 67.2: Sites of actions of glucocorticoids and consequences of glucocorticoid excess.

Site of action	Actions
Brain	Depression and psychosis
Pituitary gland	Decrease secretion of luteinizing hormone (LH), follicle stimulating hormone (FSH), thyroid stimulating hormone (TSH), and growth hormone (GH)
Eyes	Glaucoma
Renal and cardiovascular system	• Salt and water retention • Hypertension
Immune system	• Anti-inflammatory action • Immunosuppression
Gastrointestinal system	Peptic ulceration
Skin, muscle, connective tissue	• Protein catabolism, collagen breakdown • Thinning of skin • Muscular atrophy
Bone and calcium metabolism	• Decrease bone formation • Decrease bone mass • Leads to osteoporosis
Adipose tissue	Produces visceral obesity
Growth and development	Decrease linear growth
Carbohydrate and lipid metabolism	• Increased hepatic glycogen deposition • Peripheral insulin resistance and hyperglycemia • Gluconeogenesis • Increased fatty acid production • Overall diabetogenic effect

- Cortisol exerts a permissive effect on the bronchodilator effect of catecholamines

Central Nervous System
- Normal levels of glucocorticoids are necessary for normal functioning of nervous system.
- It influences brain growth and development especially in the neonatal period. Treatment with glucocorticoids in neonates inhibits CNS cell proliferation and there will be a decrease in the brain weight. It also interferes with synapse formation and influences the differentiation of glial cells in the brain.
- Excess or deficiency will produce symptoms. Excess cortisol lowers the threshold of excitation and thus precipitates fits in epileptic patients. Excess is also associated with psychosis (depression), insomnia, amnesia, etc.
- Deficiency of glucocorticoids results in personality changes as seen in adrenal insufficiency. There will be irritability, apprehension and inability to concentrate.

Gastrointestinal System
- Cortisol increases absorption of water and soluble fats from intestine.
- It stimulates gastric acid and pepsin secretion.
- It decreases gastric mucosal cell proliferation and so prolonged cortisol treatment predisposes to acid peptic disease.
- Stress which is invariably associated with excessive glucocorticoid secretion, often results in gastric ulcers usually referred to as **stress ulcers.**

Blood and Immune System
- Glucocorticoids decrease the number of eosinophils in circulation by increasing the sequestration and destruction of eosinophils in spleen.
- It also decreases the number of basophils, monocytes and lymphocytes in circulation by promoting their migration from blood into tissues.
- It stimulates hemopoiesis and increases the number of platelets, neutrophils and red blood cells in circulation. Neutrophilia occurs due to excess release from bone marrow, reduced margination and reduced diapedesis into tissues.
- In therapeutic doses, cortisol is anti-inflammatory, antiallergic and immunosuppressive. In high doses, corticosteroids suppress both humoral (by reducing B-cell proliferation) and cell-mediated immunity (by inhibiting T-cell proliferation and cytokine release). The size of lymph node, spleen and thymus are decreased on glucocorticoid administration.

Permissive Action of Glucocorticoids
Normal level of glucocorticoid secretion is necessary for a number of metabolic actions exerted by other hormones. This action is known as **permissive action**. This includes:
- Gluconeogenetic action of glucagon
- Vasoconstrictor action of catecholamines

- Calorigenic action of catecholamines
- Bronchodilator effect of catecholamines
- Fatty acid mobilizing action of catecholamines.

Role of Glucocorticoids in Reactions to Stress Situation
Any condition that disrupts or threatens to disrupt homeostasis is called a **stress**.
- During stress, ACTH secretion is increased, and this in turn increases glucocorticoid secretion. This is necessary for the survival of the animal.
- During stress, sympathoadrenal system is also stimulated and there is increased secretion of catecholamines. Glucocorticoids exert permissive action on catecholamines.
- Cortisol enhances catecholamine synthesis by activating PNMT. Catecholamines produce vascular effects and helps in maintaining normal blood pressure and volume.
- It also mobilizes free fatty acids which form the most important source of energy during stress.
- It is seen that stress produces pharmacological levels of glucocorticoid secretion necessary for survival in short duration, but harmful to life in long duration.

Stressful situations that increase ACTH secretion include severe pain, surgery, circulatory shock, fever, hypothermia, hypoglycemia, infections, emotional trauma and severe exercise. **Selye** named the noxious stimuli as **stress or "stressors."**

Anti-inflammatory Action
- Glucocorticoids inhibit inflammatory reactions and promote healing. This is achieved by the following mechanisms:
- Glucocorticoids stabilize the lysosomal membrane and inhibit the release of proteolytic enzymes.
- It inhibits the release of inflammatory mediators like serotonin, histamine and hydrolases from granulocytes, mast cells and macrophages.
- It decreases the permeability of capillaries there by inhibiting leukocytic diapedesis and reducing inflammatory exudations.
- It suppresses immune system, especially T lymphocytes.
- Inhibits fever by inhibiting prostaglandin synthesis and thus arrest vasodilatation.

Antiallergic Action
- Glucocorticoids act as an antiallergic agent and thus relieve the symptoms of conditions like asthma, hypersensitivity reactions, etc.
- When certain antibodies react with antigen, histamine is released from mast cells, which is responsible for the symptoms of allergy. Glucocorticoid prevents antigen-antibody reaction and thus prevents release of histamine by mast cells.

Action on Other Endocrine Organs

- Glucocorticoids inhibit secretion of ACTH, thyroid-stimulating hormone (TSH) and growth hormone from pituitary. Thus, it inhibits somatic growth.
- Inhibit conversion of T_4 to T_3.
- In the pancreas, it inhibits insulin secretion and stimulates secretion of glucagon.
- Facilitates β-adrenergic effects of epinephrine.
- Inhibits ADH secretion and increases glomerular filtration rate (GFR). Cortisol has a negative feedback effect on ADH secretion.

Antigrowth Effects of Cortisol

- Large doses of cortisol reduce Ca^{2+} absorption from the gut by antagonizing the actions of calcitriol.
- It inhibits proliferation of fibroblasts and cause degradation of collagen leading to osteoporosis.
- Connective tissue is reduced in quantity and strength when cortisol is present in excess.
- Cortisol inhibits the anabolic actions of growth hormone and IGF-I, particularly in the bone.
- Excess cortisol suppresses growth hormone secretion and inhibits somatic growth.
- In large doses, cortisol cause muscle atrophy and weakness referred to as **steroid myopathy**.

Regulation of Secretion of Glucocorticoids

Both basal secretion and increased secretion of glucocorticoid is regulated by adrenocorticotropic hormone (ACTH) from anterior pituitary. ACTH is a polypeptide hormone having a half-life of 10 minutes. It is produced in **episodic bursts** and these bursts are more frequent towards morning and least frequent towards evening. Plasma cortisol level varies according to these bursts of ACTH secretion. Episodic bursts of ACTH secretion is known as **circadian rhythm**. In a healthy adult individual, ACTH secretion towards morning is 25 pg/mL. ACTH secretion is controlled by two factors:
1. Hypothalamic factors
2. Circulating level of cortisol.

Hypothalamic Control

This control is through the secretion of **corticotropin releasing hormone (CRH)**. CRH is a peptide released from the median eminence of hypothalamus and reaches the pituitary through the hypothalamohypophysial portal system. This CRH stimulate secretion of ACTH from pituitary. ACTH in turn increases secretion of glucocorticoids from adrenal cortex. This is referred to as **hypothalamus-pituitary-adrenal axis.**

Many afferent pathways from different parts of the body converge on the median eminence and regulate secretion of CRH. These include emotions, stress, fear, anxiety, etc.

Control by the Circulating Cortisol Level (Feedback Control)

If circulating level of cortisol is high, it acts both at the pituitary and at the hypothalamic level by feedback loops to inhibit secretion of ACTH and CRH (**Flowchart 67.4**). If circulating cortisol level is less, it stimulates the release of CRH and ACTH by the feedback mechanism.

Mechanism of Action of ACTH in Adrenal Cortical Cells

The ACTH binds to specific receptors on the plasma membrane of adrenocortical cells. The receptors are G-protein coupled receptors. Binding of the hormone activates adenylyl cyclase via stimulatory G-protein (Gs). The cAMP produced stimulates protein kinase. **Protein kinase A** phosphorylates **cholesteryl ester hydrolase (CEH)** and increases its activity. More free cholesterol is formed from cholesteryl esters which enters the mitochondria. Cholesterol is converted to pregnenolone. It is transferred to the smooth endoplasmic reticulum where it forms 17-OH pregnenolone. It is converted to 11-deoxycortisol. 11-deoxycortisol enters the mitochondria and is converted to cortisol. Cortisol is secreted out of the cell and it enters the circulation (**Fig. 67.3**).

Flowchart 67.4: Regulation of secretion of glucocorticoids (Dashed line denotes inhibition).

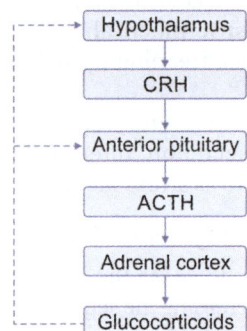

(CRH: corticotropin releasing hormone; ACTH: adrenocorticotropic hormone)

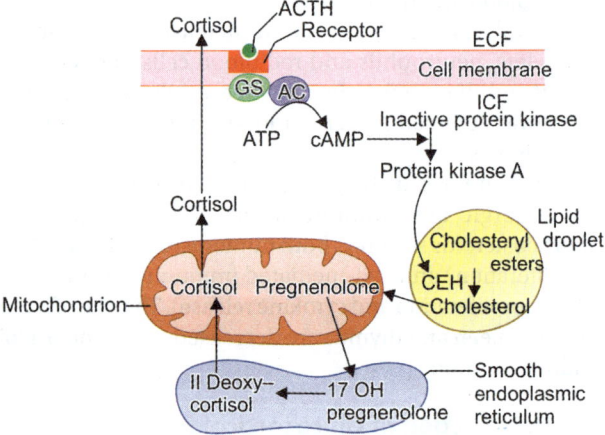

Fig. 67.3: Mechanism of action of ACTH on adrenal cortical cells in the production of glucocorticoids.

(ACTH: adrenocorticotropic hormone; GS: stimulatory G-protein; AC: adenylyl cyclase; cAMP: cyclic adenosine monophosphate; ATP: adenosine triphosphate; CEH: cholesteryl ester hydrolase; ECF: extracellular fluid; ICF: intracellular fluid)

Abnormalities in Glucocorticoid Secretion

- Hypersecretion of Glucocorticoids leads to **Cushing syndrome**
- Hyposecretion leads to **Addison's disease.**

Cushing Syndrome

Causes

- Prolonged administration of glucocorticoids
- Tumor of adrenal cortex
- Tumor of pituitary leading to hypersecretion of ACTH
- Hypothalamic diseases causing increased CRH secretion
- **Ectopic Cushing syndrome**—in this condition, a tumor of extrarenal or nonendocrine origin often in the lungs, produces substances having CRH or ACTH activity.
- When anterior pituitary tumors are responsible for the glucocorticoid excess, the disorder is referred to as **Cushing disease**. In this condition, there is excess secretion of ACTH.

Features of Cushing Syndrome (Figs. 67.4A and B)

- Loss of muscle tone is the most common presenting symptom of Cushing's syndrome.
- Since patients are protein depleted as a result of excess protein catabolism, there will be muscle wasting and thinning of skin. Wasting of muscle tissue leads to generalized weakness that is most prominent in the proximal muscles of lower extremities. Wounds heal poorly, and minor injuries cause bruises and ecchymosis as the skin is thin.
- Scalp hair becomes scanty, but facial hair appears in females (hirsutism). There will be increased acne formation due to increased secretion of adrenal androgens that often accompanies the increase in glucocorticoid secretion.
- There is redistribution of fat called **truncal adiposity**; more fat is deposited on face, neck, abdomen and upper back leading to mooning of face, pendulous abdomen and appearance of buffalo hump.
- Extremities become thin because of redistribution of subcutaneous adipose tissue to the trunk, loss of connective tissue and due to protein breakdown.
- Subcutaneous tissue especially collagen fibers will rupture due to thinning of skin and stretching of the skin by fat. Deposition of fat in the abdomen stretches the thin skin and makes the blood vessels prominent producing the **purplish striae** seen in the abdomen.
- Hyperglycemia leads to **adrenal diabetes mellitus** resistant to insulin.
- Cholesterol and lipid content in blood is increased and there will be ketosis.
- K^+ depletion leads to hypokalemia characterized by arrhythmia, lethargy, muscle weakness, etc. This is due to mineralocorticoid activity of cortisol.
- Excess glucocorticoids lead to bone dissolution by decreasing bone formation and increasing bone resorption. This leads to **osteoporosis**, a loss of bone mass that lead eventually to increased risk of fractures.
- Frank psychosis, insomnia, euphoria, etc., are commonly encountered.
- Skin pigmentation due to increased circulating level of ACTH or MSH is seen and may be severe in cases of ectopic ACTH secretion, pituitary tumors, etc. *The hyperpigmentation is not seen if hypersecretion of glucocorticoid is due to adrenal tumor.*
- Due to increased red cell count the cheeks appear red referred to as 'tomato cheeks.'
- 85% of patients are hypertensive due to salt and water retention and also due to the effect of glucocorticoid on blood vessels. Salt and water retention is due to the weak mineralocorticoid action of cortisol. Exogenous synthetic glucocorticoid therapy rarely produces hypertension

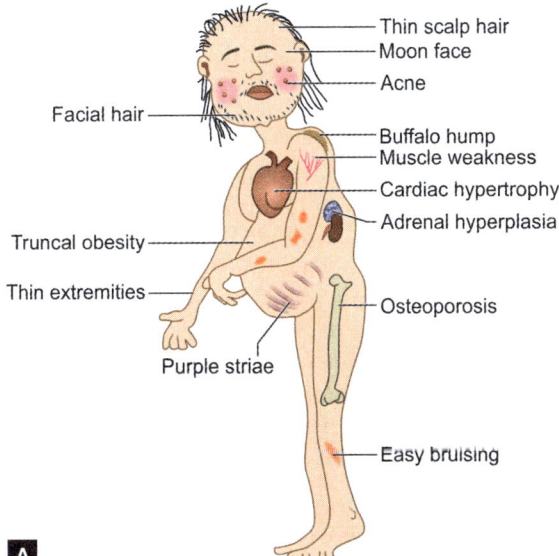
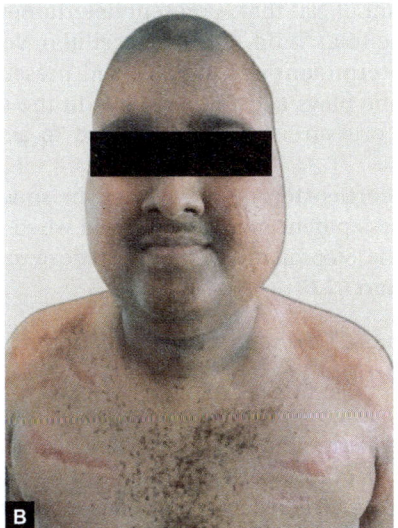

Figs. 67.4A and B: Features of Cushing syndrome.
Courtesy: Dr Anil P and Dr Abhilash Nair.

because these drugs lack the mineralocorticoid activity of the endogenous hormone.

Diagnosis is confirmed by estimating urinary 17-hydroxycorticosteroids and 17-ketosteroids which are very much elevated in Cushing's syndrome.

Therapeutic Uses of Glucocorticoids

- Used for substitution therapy in adrenal insufficiency.
- Because of its anti-inflammatory and immunosuppressive effects, corticosteroids are used in the treatment of chronic inflammatory disorders like rheumatoid arthritis and systemic lupus erythematosus (SLE).
- Used to prevent graft rejection in organ transplantation.
- Due to antiallergic effects, used to treat bronchial asthma and skin diseases.
- Used in malignancies like lymphomas and lymphocytic leukemia because of its antilymphocytic effect.
- Used to treat cerebral edema.
- Used in circulatory shock to increase blood pressure.

■ MINERALOCORTICOIDS

Mineralocorticoids are secreted by zona glomerulosa of adrenal cortex. *Since glomerulosa cells are the only cells that contain aldosterone synthase, these cells are the exclusive site of aldosterone synthesis.* The important mineralocorticoids are:
- Aldosterone
- Deoxycorticosterone

Mineralocorticoid activity is also shown by corticosterone and cortisol. Aldosterone is the potent mineralocorticoid which exerts 95% of mineralocorticoid activity. It is the primary regulator of salt balance and extracellular fluid volume. It acts by controlling the extent to which the kidney excretes or reabsorbs the Na^+ filtered at the renal glomerulus. Na^+ which is the primary osmotically active particle in the extracellular space retains water and thus the amount of Na^+ that is present determines the volume of extracellular fluid. The extracellular volume is the prime determinant of arterial blood pressure and thus aldosterone plays an important role in the maintenance of blood pressure. It is also referred to as a *lifesaving hormone*.

Deoxycorticosterone is secreted in small quantities and is a less potent mineralocorticoid when compared to aldosterone. Steps in the synthesis of aldosterone are shown in **Flowchart 67.5**.

Actions of ACTH and Angiotensin II in the Formation of Aldosterone

Adrenocortical secretion is controlled primarily by ACTH from the anterior pituitary, but mineralocorticoid secretion is also subject to independent control by angiotensin II. **ACTH** binds to its receptors on the plasma membrane of adrenocortical cells. This activates adenylyl cyclase via Gs. This leads to increase in the formation of pregnenolone and its derivatives.

Flowchart 67.5: Steps in the synthesis of aldosterone in the zona glomerulosa of adrenal cortex.

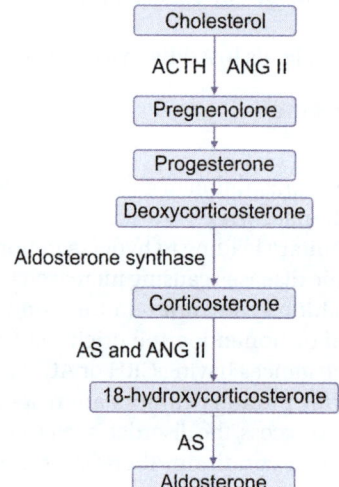

(AS: aldosterone synthase; ANG II: angiotensin II; ACTH: adrenocorticotropic hormone)

Angiotensin II binds to AT_1 receptors in the zona glomerulosa that act via a G-protein to activate phospholipase C. The resulting increase in protein kinase C stimulates the conversion of cholesterol to pregnenolone. It also facilitates the action of aldosterone synthase resulting in increased secretion of aldosterone.

Actions of Aldosterone

Action on Kidney

The important site of action of aldosterone is **kidney**. It promotes transport of Na^+, K^+ and H^+ across the tubular epithelium of distal convoluted tubule, collecting tubule and collecting duct. It enhances reabsorption of Na^+ from the tubular fluid and increases excretion of K^+ and H^+ through urine. Na^+ is retained in the extracellular fluid (ECF) with the help of aldosterone and an excess of aldosterone increases plasma sodium ion and decreases plasma potassium ion concentration.

Aldosterone Escape

When there is excess of aldosterone, Na^+ is reabsorbed from the renal tubule and at the same time, an equivalent amount of H_2O is also reabsorbed by **obligatory mechanism**. When Na^+ is reabsorbed into renal tubule, an osmotic gradient is created from the tubule to the peritubular fluid. So, water also follows the reabsorbed Na^+. So, there is increase in ECF volume. But there will be no edema. This is because, when aldosterone is administered there is increase in Na^+ and H_2O reabsorption in the first 2–3 days. After that there is Na^+ and H_2O excretion. This secondary effect is known as **aldosterone escape**.

Causes of aldosterone escape:
- Aldosterone escape is due to an increased production of **atrial natriuretic peptide (ANP)** from the heart which causes natriuresis and diuresis. When there is increase in

the blood volume the atria get stretched and ANP will be released from the atria. Aldosterone also facilitates active transport of Na⁺ from the renal tubular cell into the ECF. This is by activating sodium-potassium pump which pumps Na⁺ actively into the peritubular space. Thus, the concentration of Na⁺ inside the cell decreases and this facilitates entry of more sodium into the cells. When Na⁺ is reabsorbed along with water there is increase in ECF volume. This, in turn, stimulates production of ANP. Most important action of ANP is natriuresis and diuresis. As a result, more of water and sodium escapes and no edema develops.

- Another reason is that prolonged elevation of mineralocorticoid levels causes unresponsiveness of the Na⁺ channels and Na⁺ will be excreted despite the high mineralocorticoid level.
- Aldosterone escape is also due to **pressure natriuresis and diuresis** that occurs when the arterial pressure rises. Increase in renal arterial pressure increases glomerular filtration and causes large increases in urine and sodium output. Renal perfusion pressure can directly regulate sodium reabsorption in the proximal tubule.

Aldosterone escape is clinically very significant. *This is the explanation for the absence of edema in patients with hyperaldosteronism.*

But such patients will develop metabolic alkalosis and hypokalemia due to increased K⁺ and H⁺ excretion due to the action of aldosterone.

When aldosterone is present in excess, more of K⁺ is excreted through urine and this leads to muscle weakness. In aldosterone deficiency, plasma K⁺ level rises and if it doubles the normal value, cardiac toxicity results, e.g., arrhythmia.

In the renal tubule, aldosterone also enhances excretion of H⁺. But, excretion of H⁺ in exchange for Na⁺ is very minimal when compared to K⁺.

Action on Salivary Gland, Sweat Gland and Intestine

Primary secretion of saliva and sweat is rich in Na⁺ and Cl⁻. As this secretion passes through the duct system of the gland, Na⁺ and Cl⁻ are reabsorbed in the presence of aldosterone. Because of this action of aldosterone, excess salt is not lost in hot environment or during excessive salivation.

In the intestine, aldosterone facilitates absorption of Na⁺. If aldosterone is deficient, more of Na⁺ and water will be lost in stools resulting in diarrhea and dehydration.

Action on Circulatory System

Due to increased reabsorption of Na⁺ and H₂O from the renal tubules there is increase in ECF volume. If there is a deficiency of the hormone, ECF volume falls, and if severe, it leads to circulatory shock.

Mechanism of Action of Aldosterone

Mechanism of action is same as that for any steroid hormone. There are two types of receptors for adrenal steroids:
1. Mineralocorticoid or type I receptors
2. Glucocorticoid or type II receptors.

Type I receptors have high affinity for aldosterone and deoxycorticosterone. These receptors are found in distal nephron, salivary gland and gut mucosa.

Type II receptors have affinity for glucocorticoid, especially synthetic glucocorticoid like dexamethasone.

Regulation of Secretion of Aldosterone (Flowchart 67.6)

Approximately, 37% of circulating aldosterone remains free in plasma. The rest is weakly bound to albumin or cortisol binding globulin (CBG). The factors which regulate the secretion of aldosterone are:
- Renin-angiotensin-aldosterone mechanism
- Plasma K⁺ concentration
- Plasma Na⁺ concentration
- Extracellular fluid volume
- ACTH.

The factors that stimulate aldosterone secretion are increase in plasma K⁺ concentration, decrease in plasma Na⁺ concentration, decrease in ECF volume and ACTH (**Flowchart 67.5**).

Renin-Angiotensin-Aldosterone Mechanism (Flowchart 67.7)

Renin is a hormone produced by the juxtaglomerular apparatus of kidney. The important stimuli for renin secretion

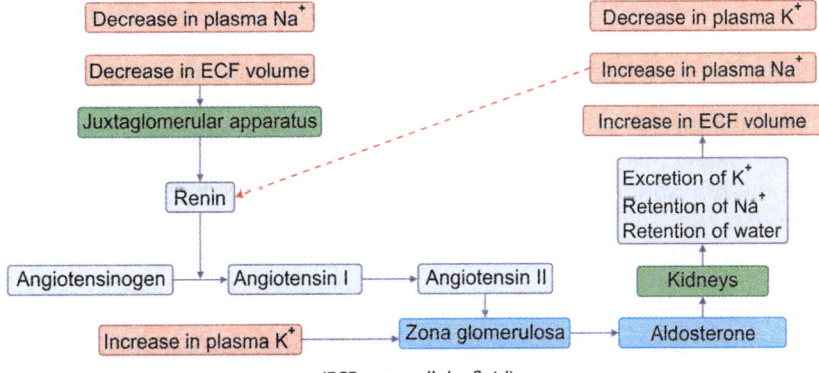

Flowchart 67.6: Regulation of secretion of aldosterone (dashed line indicates inhibition).

(ECF: extracellular fluid)

Flowchart 67.7: Renin-angiotensin-aldosterone system.

```
Decreased ECF volume and plasma Na⁺
               ↓
             Renin                    ACE
               ↓                       ↓
Angiotensinogen → Angiotensin I → Angiotensin II → Angiotensin III
                                        ↓                ↓
ECF volume increases ← Increased Na⁺ and water reabsorption ← Aldosterone
```

(ACE: angiotensin converting enzyme; ECF: extracellular fluid)

are a fall in ECF volume, fall in plasma Na⁺ and decrease in renal arterial pressure. Renin acts on angiotensinogen which is an α_2-globulin present in plasma and it is converted to angiotensin I. This is converted to angiotensin II by **angiotensin converting enzyme** in lungs. Angiotensin II acts on the proximal tubule of kidney to increase Na⁺ and water reabsorption. It also stimulates zona glomerulosa of adrenal cortex to increase aldosterone secretion. Aldosterone acts on distal nephron to increase Na⁺ and water reabsorption. Thus, ECF volume, Na⁺ concentration and blood pressure are brought back to normal. Action of angiotensin II is mediated by diacylglycerol and protein kinase C.

Plasma K⁺ Concentration

An increase in plasma K⁺ concentration is the most effective stimulant for secretion of aldosterone. K⁺ acts directly on zona glomerulosa and increases the secretion of aldosterone **(Flowchart 67.5).** This aldosterone, in turn, acts on the renal tubule and enhances the excretion of K⁺. Thus plasma K⁺ level is brought back to normal.

Plasma Na⁺ Concentration and ECF Volume

A decrease in plasma Na⁺ increases aldosterone secretion. This is brought about by the following mechanisms:
* A decrease in Na⁺ decreases the extracellular fluid (ECF) volume and decreases blood pressure. Both these factors stimulate renin secretion. Renin through renin-angiotensin-aldosterone mechanism brings back Na⁺ concentration and ECF volume back to normal.
* A decrease in Na⁺ increases the plasma K⁺ level which acts on zona glomerulosa and increases aldosterone secretion.
* A decrease in Na⁺ directly stimulates zona glomerulosa.
* A decrease in plasma Na⁺ increases the number of angiotensin II receptors and also increases the affinity of the receptors to angiotensin II in the zona glomerulosa cells.
* Aldosterone acts in the renal tubules and increases the retention of sodium and water. This increases plasma sodium concentration and ECF volume is also brought back to normal. Increased plasma sodium inhibits renin secretion by feedback mechanism.

Role of ACTH

The ACTH plays a minor role in the regulation of aldosterone secretion under normal conditions.

During stressful conditions, aldosterone secretion is stimulated by ACTH. The amount of ACTH required to stimulate secretion of aldosterone is very high. In the absence of ACTH, aldosterone secretion is reduced very much.

After hypophysectomy, basal secretion of mineralocorticoid never falls, but glucocorticoid concentration immediately falls. Long time after hypophysectomy, the zona glomerulosa also start to atrophy. This shows that ACTH is necessary for the functioning of zona glomerulosa.

Abnormalities in Aldosterone Secretion

* Primary hyperaldosteronism or Conn's syndrome
* Secondary hyperaldosteronism

Primary Hyperaldosteronism or Conn Syndrome

Causes are aldosterone-secreting adenoma of the zona glomerulosa, adrenal hyperplasia, adrenal carcinoma etc. In patients with primary hyperaldosteronism, renin secretion is depressed.

Features

* **Hypokalemia, hypernatremia** and increase in plasma volume. There will be no edema or marked hypertension because of aldosterone escape phenomenon. But, severe hypokalemia leads to renal damage and defect in the concentrating mechanism which leads to **polyuria**. This is called **hypokalemic nephropathy**. *Due to aldosterone escape and also due to the polyuria associated with hypokalemic nephropathy, edema almost never occurs in Conn's syndrome.*
* Hypokalemia also leads to **muscle weakness**.
* Increase in aldosterone also produces, **metabolic alkalosis,** and this lowers plasma ionic calcium level which leads to latent or frank **tetany**. Alkalosis is due to increased secretion of H⁺ in exchange for Na⁺ that is being reabsorbed in the distal nephron. There is increased loss of H⁺ from the body.
* **Glucose intolerance** due to impaired insulin secretion caused by hypokalemia.

Secondary Hyperaldosteronism

Causes

* All factors that cause increased secretion of renin
* Congestive cardiac failure (CCF)
* Nephrosis and liver diseases like cirrhosis

Secondary hyperaldosteronism is *characterized by edema* because aldosterone escape phenomenon does not occur in secondary hyperaldosteronism. If it is due to increased renin secretion it stimulates renin-angiotensin-aldosterone mechanism leading to hyperaldosteronism. Since aldosterone is metabolized in the liver, liver diseases lead to decreased metabolic clearance of aldosterone. CCF also leads to decreased clearance of aldosterone.

Effect of Deficiency of Aldosterone

Isolated aldosterone deficiency is seen in patients with renal disease and a low circulating renin level. This is referred to as **hyporeninemic hypoaldosteronism**. **Pseudohypoaldosteronism** is produced when there is resistance to the action of aldosterone. Primary effect in hypoaldosteronism will be loss of Na$^+$ through urine. Water is lost along with Na$^+$ leading to a reduction in the ECF volume leading to severe circulatory shock. If medical treatment is not given immediately, fatal hypotension and death follow. Since there is retention of K$^+$ and H$^+$ there will be hyperkalemia and metabolic acidosis which may lead to cardiac arrhythmias. Normal plasma potassium level is 4.5 mEq/L.

Adrenal Androgens and Estrogens

Androgens and small amounts of estrogens are secreted by the zona reticularis layer of adrenal cortex. Androgenic steroids are to a large extent byproducts of cortisol production. Adrenal androgens exert only 20% of the masculinizing effect in the body. The important adrenal androgen is dehydroepiandrosterone and it is less potent than testosterone and dihydrotestosterone. However, peripheral tissues can convert androstenedione to testosterone with the help of 17-ketosteroid reductase. In this manner, the adrenal gland can contribute significant amounts of circulating androgen. Testosterone can be converted to estrogen in fat and other peripheral tissues by the enzyme aromatase. This is an important source of estrogen in men and postmenopausal women.

The plasma level of **dehydroepiandrosterone (DHEA)** is about 300 µg/dL in both sexes. After menopause, the level of DHEA is decreased to 90 µg/dL in female. Adrenal androgen secretion is low in childhood and maximum secretion is seen by about 13 years. Increase in adrenal androgen production is seen 1–2 years before the increase in gonadal steroid production that occurs with puberty. This is responsible for the growth of axillary and pubic hair at the time of puberty in both sexes. **Adrenarche** is the time of development of pubic and axillary hair.

Actions of Adrenal Androgens

- Adrenal androgens are responsible for adrenarche at the time of puberty
- Enhances protein synthesis and promote growth
- Contributes to the growth of sex organs and development of secondary sex characteristics
- The adrenal androgen, androstenedione is converted to testosterone and aromatized to estrogens in fat and other peripheral tissues. This is an important source of estrogens in men and postmenopausal women.

- Excess androgen secretion leads to masculinization (adrenogenital syndrome) and precocious pseudopuberty or female pseudohermaphroditism.

Variation in Secretion of Adrenal Androgens

Adrenogenital Syndrome

Cause of adrenogenital syndrome is tumor of adrenal cortex limited to zona reticularis layer in females. Excessive secretion of adrenal androgens in female leads to **virilism or masculinization**, i.e., appearance of beard, development of muscles like that of males, baldness, conversion of female genital organs to that of male like enlargement of clitoris, peculiar distribution of body hair, deep low-pitched voice, stoppage of menstruation etc. If excessive secretion occurs in the prepubertal or adult female the condition is called adrenogenital syndrome.

If excessive secretion of adrenal androgens occurs in the first 12 weeks of intrauterine life, **pseudohermaphroditism** of genetic females occurs.

If the above condition occurs in prepubertal male child, all the above-said features will be present along with early development of genital organs and development of sexual desire. This is **precocious puberty**. If it occurs in adult male, the symptoms are not prominent because it is masked by the masculinizing effect of testosterone from the testis.

Virilizing Congenital Adrenal Hyperplasia

Congenital virilizing adrenal hyperplasia is due to deficiency of some of the enzymes involved in steroidogenesis like cholesterol desmolase, 21α-hydroxylase, etc. The result is greater than normal activity of 17α-hydroxylase and 11β-hydroxylase. The net effect is all the precursors of steroid hormone synthesis in the adrenal cortex will be diverted to the sex steroid pathway. If the defect is severe, it results in masculinization of female fetus during sexual differentiation which alerts the pediatrician to the potential diagnosis.

There is no cortisol secretion and hence ACTH secretion will be high. ACTH causes enhanced growth of the adrenal gland. There will be accumulation of pregnenolone. The combination of inadequate production of glucocorticoids and mineralocorticoids leading to hypoglycemia, dehydration, hypotension, and hyperkalemia; excessive production of androgens, and enhanced growth of the adrenal gland is the classical clinical syndrome of salt losing, virilizing congenital adrenal hyperplasia.

Hypofunctioning of Adrenal Cortex

- Primary adrenal insufficiency or Addison's disease
- Secondary adrenal insufficiency

Primary Adrenal Insufficiency or Addison's Disease or Hypoadrenalism

Primary adrenal insufficiency may occur rapidly as a life-threatening collapse or it may develop gradually. If not treated with glucocorticoids and mineralocorticoids, the condition is fatal. Causes are:

- Autoimmune adrenal disease that destroy the adrenal cortex
- Infections like tuberculosis affecting the adrenal gland, meningococcal infection (which can cause bilateral adrenal hemorrhage), etc.
- Cancer of adrenal gland
- Adrenalectomy
- Congenital unresponsiveness of adrenal gland to ACTH

In the initial stages, steroid production may be adequate to meet normal demands, but stress like fasting may provoke a sudden total failure and precipitate severe symptoms due to fatal hypoglycemia and hypotension. This is called **adrenal crisis or Addisonian crisis** due to mineralocorticoid and glucocorticoid deficiency.

Features of Addison's Disease

- Electrolyte loss due to mineralocorticoid deficiency. There will be increased excretion of NaCl and decreased excretion of potassium through urine. This leads to hyponatremia and hyperkalemia.
- Acidosis develops because of failure of H^+ to be secreted in exchange for sodium reabsorption due to aldosterone deficiency.
- Decrease in blood pressure due to hyponatremia, dehydration, decrease in blood volume, decreased vascular tone and decreased cardiac output.
- Hyperkalemia leads to cardiac arrhythmias.
- Hypoglycemia in between meals can cause coma if severe. It is due to deficiency of glucocorticoids.
- Lethargy because fat and protein is not utilized by the body. There will be muscle weakness, weight loss and easy fatigability.
- Gastrointestinal disturbances like vomiting, anorexia, etc.
- Increased susceptibility to infections.
- Since adrenal androgens are absent, it leads to loss of axillary and pubic hair in females.
- Since there is reduction in the level of adrenal steroids, there is reduction in the feedback suppression of ACTH. High ACTH level will cause hyperpigmentation of skin and mucosa because high levels of ACTH has MSH-like activity. ACTH acts on melanocytes and stimulates the secretion of melanin in the same way that MSH does. There is also increase in other products, such as pro-opiomelanocortin (POMC), such as α-MSH and γ-MSH which cause skin pigmentation.

Treatment: Addison's disease is treated with synthetic steroids. A number of synthetic steroids have been prepared for therapeutic uses. They slightly differ from cortisol in their structure. Examples are **prednisolone, dexamethasone, betamethasone,** etc. Mineralocorticoids are also administered to correct electrolyte imbalance.

Secondary and Tertiary Adrenal Insufficiency

Secondary adrenal insufficiency is due to deficiency of ACTH secretion from anterior pituitary and **tertiary adrenal insufficiency** is caused by hypothalamic disorders disrupting corticotropin-releasing hormone (CRH) secretion. Since aldosterone is secreted in response to renin-angiotensin system, defects in electrolyte balance are not seen. *Pigmentation of skin is not seen as in Addison's disease because in both these conditions, plasma ACTH is low.* Since ACTH is deficient, glucocorticoid secretion is severely affected. Hypoglycemia, hypotension, weight loss and gastrointestinal problems are seen. In women, there will be loss of pubic and axillary hair.

ADRENAL MEDULLA

Introduction

Adrenal medulla derived from the **neural crest** is essentially a sympathetic ganglion in which the postganglionic cells have lost their axons and have become specialized for secretion of their products directly into the bloodstream. Thus it forms a bridge between sympathetic nervous system and endocrine system. It is composed of **chromaffin cells** or **pheochromocytes** which correspond to the sympathetic postganglionic neurons. Normally, stimuli that activate adrenal medulla also activate sympathetic nervous system. Hence, the two systems are considered as a functional unit termed **sympathomedullary system**. The secretions are stored in granules inside the cell (*refer* **Fig. 67.2**).

The vascular supply of adrenal medulla is typical. Normal adrenal medullary function is dependent on the normal adrenal cortical function. The blood vessels beginning in the subcapsular plexus of adrenal cortex form a capillary network in the cortex and then merge to form small venous vessels. They again branch into a second capillary network within the medulla thus forming a **portal system**. The venous blood from the adrenal cortex thus passes through the adrenal medulla and is drained out from the medulla. Thus, the medulla is exposed to high levels of adrenal cortical hormones, which is of great significance especially in stressful situations. This allows the corticosteroids to increase epinephrine secretion from adrenal medulla through a permissive action which is very essential to combat stress. Deficiency of cortisol inhibits formation of epinephrine.

Hormones of Adrenal Medulla

The hormones of adrenal medulla are collectively called **catecholamines**. They are:
- Epinephrine or adrenaline
- Norepinephrine or noradrenaline
- Dopamine

Epinephrine is the predominant catecholamine synthesized, stored and secreted by the adrenal medulla.

Norepinephrine is mainly synthesized and stored in the sympathetic nerve endings.

Small amounts of opioid peptides like **enkephalin** (met-enkephalin and leu-enkephalin) are also present in the adrenal medulla. Stress-induced analgesia is also due to the action of these opioid peptides released from adrenal medulla.

Epinephrine-secreting neurons are also present in the medulla oblongata that project to the thalamus, periaqueductal gray matter, hypothalamus and spinal cord.

Biosynthesis of Catecholamines

Catecholamines are synthesized from the amino acid **tyrosine or phenylalanine** by the following steps **(Fig. 67.5)**.
- Phenylalanine is converted to tyrosine by *phenylalanine hydroxylase* in the liver.
- Tyrosine from blood is taken up by chromaffin cells of adrenal medulla by active transport.
- *Tyrosine hydroxylase* catalyzes the conversion of tyrosine to 3,4-dihydroxyphenylalanine (DOPA). **Tetrahydrobiopterin** is a cofactor for tyrosine hydroxylase as well as phenyl alanine hydroxylase. *The rate-limiting enzyme of the pathway is tyrosine hydroxylase.* It is inhibited by norepinephrine and dopamine by negative feedback.
- DOPA is decarboxylated to dopamine by *DOPA decarboxylase or aromatic L-amino acid decarboxylase.*
- Dopamine is transported into the chromaffin granule where *dopamine-b-hydroxylase* catalyzes the conversion of dopamine to norepinephrine. This reaction requires O and H⁺ donor such as ascorbic acid.
- Norepinephrine moves out of the granule and is methylated to epinephrine by cytoplasmic enzyme **phenylethanolamine-N-methyltransferase (PNMT)**. Cortisol is necessary for the activation of PNMT. After hypophysectomy, glucocorticoid concentration in the blood reaching the adrenal medulla falls and there will be a decrease in the synthesis of epinephrine.
- Epinephrine is then transported back into the chromaffin granule before release.

The enzyme PNMT is absent in postganglionic sympathetic nerve endings and hence epinephrine is not produced in postganglionic sympathetic nerve endings. Chromaffin cells of adrenal medulla and certain neurons in the central nervous system are the only cells that have the enzyme to synthesize epinephrine.

> **APPLIED PHYSIOLOGY**
>
> *Phenylketonuria* or phenylpyruvic oligophrenia is a disorder where there is accumulation of phenylalanine and its ketoacid derivatives in blood, tissues and urine. The condition is mainly due to deficiency of phenylalanine hydroxylase which may bedue to mutation of the gene coding for it. Here, catecholamines can be synthesized from tyrosine.
>
> In tetrahydrobiopterin deficiency, catecholamine synthesis is also defective. This is because tetrahydro-biopterin is a cofactor for tyrosine hydroxylase as well as phenylalanine hydroxylase.

Storage of Hormones

Catecholamines are stored in the **chromaffin granules** with ATP. Epinephrine comprises 80% of the catecholamine content of chromaffin granule. Rest is formed by norepinephrine and dopamine. Small amounts of binding protein called **chromogranin A and enkephalins** are also present in the granule. Contents of the chromaffin granules are expelled by exocytosis when the cholinergic preganglionic fibers coming through splanchnic nerve to adrenal medulla are stimulated. Acetylcholine activates cation channels and Ca^{2+} enters the secretory cells from the ECF and triggers the exocytosis of the granules. Catecholamines, ATP and proteins from the granules are released into the blood.

Transport

50% of circulating catecholamines is bound to plasma proteins. Conjugates of catecholamines with sulfate are the inactive forms. Free epinephrine level in plasma is normally about 30 pg/mL. Circulating level of norepinephrine is 5–10 times higher than circulating epinephrine. Plasma dopamine levels are normally very low, about 0.13 nmol/L.

Metabolism (Flowchart 67.8)

Catecholamines are inactivated by two enzymes by oxidation and methylation. The enzymes are **monoamine oxidase (MAO) and catecholamine-O-methyltransferase (COMT)**, which are present in liver and kidney. MAO is present in the mitochondria and COMT in the cytoplasm. Half-life of catecholamines is 2 minutes. The catecholamines are methylated to metanephrine and normetanephrine by

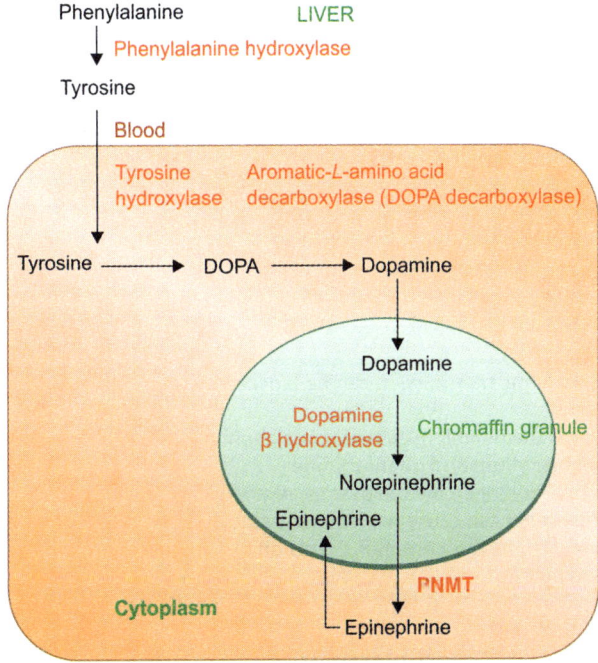

Fig. 67.5: Synthesis of catecholamines in the chromaffin cell of adrenal medulla.
(PNMT: phenylethanolamine-N-methyltransferase; DOPA: 3, 4-dihydroxyphenylalanine)

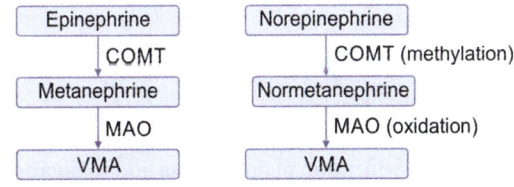

Flowchart 67.8: Metabolism of catecholamines.

(VMA: vanillylmandelic acid; COMT: catecholamine-O-methyltransferase; MAO: monoamine oxidase)

COMT. They are then oxidized by MAO to **3-methoxy-4-hydroxy mandelic acid or vanillylmandelic acid (VMA)** which is excreted through urine **(Fig. 67.5)**. About 700 µg of VMA is excreted per day. *Estimation of VMA in urine is used as an index for assessing the function of adrenal medulla.* Very small quantities of free forms of catecholamines are excreted through urine.

Mechanism of Action of Catecholamines

Catecholamines exert their action through five types of receptors—α_1, α_2, β_1, β_2 and β_3. The receptors are classified depending on the basis of sensitivity of receptors to certain drugs and blocking agents. Stimulation of each type of receptor gives rise to specific effect different from those caused by others **(Table 67.3)**.

- α_1**-receptors** are present mainly in the postjunctional membrane on the effector organ and are mainly excitatory. They are found in the smooth muscle of all blood vessels except skeletal muscle blood vessels. They are also present in glands, gut wall, liver and heart. They exert their effect through phospholipase C.
- α_2**-receptors** are present in the presynaptic membrane of both cholinergic and adrenergic neurons. They are inhibitory in action. They exert their action by inhibiting adenylate cyclase enzyme, thereby inhibiting cAMP. In noradrenergic neurons, stimulation of these receptors by norepinephrine inhibits further release of norepinephrine, thus providing a feedback control. α_2-receptors are present in the postjunctional membrane in brain, pituitary and pancreatic B-cells.
- β_1**-receptors** are mainly found in the heart and juxtaglomerular cells in kidney.
- β_2**-receptors** are present in skeletal muscle blood vessels, smooth muscles of intestine, urinary bladder, bronchioles, uterus, etc. Both the β-receptors exert their effects by activating adenylate cyclase, thereby increasing cAMP production.
- β_3**-receptors** present in adipose tissue cause lipolysis and thermogenesis.

Norepinephrine stimulates mainly α-receptors and epinephrine stimulates both α- and β-receptors equally. β-receptors respond more to epinephrine. Norepinephrine has no β effect.

Drugs Acting on Different Adrenergic Receptors

Adrenergic Agonists

- α-*Agonists*: Phenylephrine (α_1), clonidine (α_2)
- β-*Agonists*: Dobutamine (β_1), salbutamol, terbutaline (β_2), BRL 37344 (β_3).

Uses of Adrenergic Agonists

- Adrenalin is the drug of choice in anaphylactic shock.
- 1 in 1,00,000 adrenalin is given along with local anesthetics to increase the duration of anesthesia and to decrease the systemic toxicity of the local anesthetic.
- Used as a nasal decongestant.

Table 67.3: Effects of stimulation of different adrenergic receptors.

α_1-effect	β_1-effect	β_2-effect
• Vasoconstriction • Pupillary dilatation • Piloerection • Contraction of intestinal sphincters • Bladder sphincter contraction	• Increases heart rate • Increases force of contraction of myocardium • Glycogenolysis • Lipolysis	• Vasodilatation • Calorigenesis • Uterine relaxation • Relaxation of bladder • Bronchiolar dilatation • Intestinal relaxation

- Cardiac arrest (given intravenously).
- Bronchial asthma.
- Uterine relaxant.
- Clonidine is used to treat hypertension.

α- Receptor Blocking Drugs

Ergot alkaloids like ergotamine, phentolamine, piperoxan, phenoxybenzamine, etc.

Uses of α-receptor Blockers

α-receptor blockers are used to treat:
- Pheochromocytoma
- Hypertension
- Benign prostatic hypertrophy (BPH)

β-receptor Blockers

- Propranolol which blocks both β_1 and β_2 receptors.
- Practalol blocks only β_2 receptors.
- Cardioselective β_1-blockers are atenolol and metaprolol.

Uses of β-blockers

β-blockers are used in the treatment of:
- Hypertension
- Angina pectoris
- Cardiac arrhythmias
- Thyrotoxicosis
- Pheochromocytoma
- Anxiety.

Adrenergic transmission can be blocked by drugs like α-methyl dopa.
Drugs that inhibit release of norepinephrine from nerve endings are **bretylium and guanethidine**.
6-hydroxydopamine can destroy adrenergic neurons.
Reserpine can cause depletion of catecholamines at tissue level and also in the chromaffin cells and in the adrenergic nerve endings.

Actions of Catecholamines

- Metabolic effect
- Calorigenic effect
- Systemic effect

Metabolic Effect

On Carbohydrate Metabolism

- Catecholamines are **diabetogenic** hormones. They increase blood glucose level through adenylate cyclase mechanism.
- It causes glycogenolysis in muscle. Muscle glycogen is converted to lactic acid. This lactic acid is taken up by the liver where resynthesis of glycogen occurs. This glycogen is converted to blood glucose.
- Stimulation of α_2-receptors in the beta cells of pancreas inhibits insulin secretion, and β-receptor stimulation stimulates insulin secretion. But the net effect is inhibition of insulin secretion.
- Stimulation of β_2-receptors of the alpha cells of pancreatic islets increases glucagon secretion and produce glycogenolysis and lipolysis.

On Lipid Metabolism

Catecholamines are **lipolytic** hormones. They increase free fatty acid level by stimulating hormone sensitive lipase.

On Mineral Metabolism

Catecholamines play an important role in the distribution of intracellular and extracellular potassium.

Calorigenic Action

Adrenaline increases tissue metabolism leading to increased O_2 consumption and increased CO_2 production. This causes **increase in basal metabolic rate (BMR)** and temperature. But this calorigenic action is not seen in the absence of thyroid and adrenal cortical hormones.

Thyroxine increases the formation of β-adrenergic receptors in the presence of glucocorticoids. This action of glucocorticoid and thyroxine is called **permissive action**.

Systemic Actions (Table 67.4)

- Action of catecholamines on cardiovascular system (**Fig. 67.6**)
- *Action of adrenaline on skeletal muscle:* Adrenalin increases contractility and excitability of skeletal muscles.

Table 67.4: Systemic actions of adrenaline and noradrenaline.

Adrenaline	Noradrenaline
On blood vessels	
Contraction of all blood vessels (via α_1-receptors) except skeletal muscle blood vessels (via β_2-receptors), cerebral, hepatic and coronary vessels. Since skeletal muscle blood vessels constitute 80% of blood vessels in the body and adrenaline being a vasodilator of these vessels, adrenaline is considered as a net vasodilator	Contraction of all blood vessels via α_1- receptors except cerebral and coronary vessels. Hence it is considered as a net vasoconstrictor
Contraction of systemic veins	Contraction of systemic veins
On heart	
In isolated heart, there is increase in heart rate and force of contraction via β_1-receptors	Increase force and rate in isolated heart via β_1-receptors
In intact heart and blood pressure	
It increases systolic pressure and decreases diastolic pressure and widens pulse pressure Increase in heart rate and cardiac output Decrease total peripheral resistance and is a net vasodilator If adrenaline is infused to an intact animal, there is a rapid increase in blood pressure which lasts for a few seconds. This is due to stimulation of both α- and β-receptors. After some time BP falls and again comes back to normal. As adrenaline is metabolized in the body the concentration is lowered and β-receptor stimulation predominates. This called **biphasic action of adrenalin**	Both systolic and diastolic pressure increases. It is a **net vasoconstrictor** and increases peripheral resistance. The rise in blood pressure operates the reflex baroreceptor mechanism or sinoaortic reflex. This in turn lowers heart rate, i.e., **reflex bradycardia** is seen. There is decrease in cardiac output Biphasic action is not seen with nor-adrenaline
On coronary blood vessels	
Increases coronary blood flow partly by increasing metabolism and partly by vasodilatation.	Increases coronary blood flow
Effect on respiration	
By its vasoconstrictor effect on pulmonary vessels, it decreases the secretion of mucus. Administration of adrenaline causes **adrenaline apnea** due to irradiation of impulses from the vasomotor center to respiratory center.	Less effective than adrenaline
Actions on gastrointestinal tract (GIT)	
Relaxation of intestinal smooth muscles, decreased movements and contraction of sphincters.	
On urinary bladder	
Relaxation of the detrusor muscle, contraction of trigone of bladder and contraction of the sphincter of bladder.	Less effective than adrenaline
On uterus	
Adrenaline produces contraction of uterus irrespective of the stage of gestation, but at full term it inhibits uterine contractions.	
On eyes	
Pupillary dilatation and retraction of upper eye lid.	Less effective
On skin	
Cutaneous vasoconstriction and piloerection.	Less effective

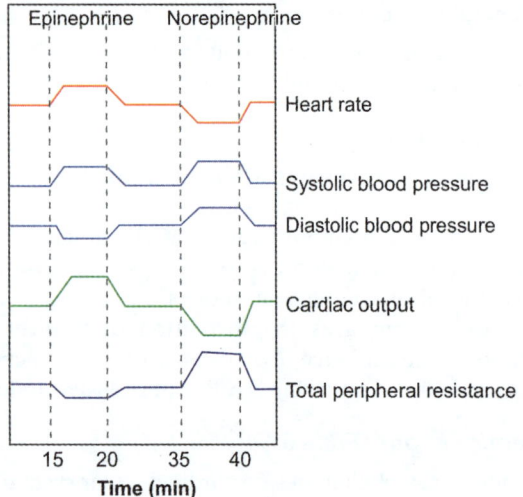

Fig. 67.6: Circulatory changes produced by slow intravenous infusion of epinephrine and norepinephrine.

It postpones fatigue, lowers chronaxie value and prevents loss of intracellular potassium.
- **On adipose tissue:** Causes release of free fatty acid from adipose tissue by acting via β-receptors.
- **On blood:**
  - Adrenaline increases blood glucose and blood lactic acid level.
  - It increases RBC count, hemoglobin concentration and plasma protein content. Thus, it produces hemoconcentration.
  - Decreases eosinophil and lymphocyte count.
  - Coagulation time is shortened.
- **On spleen:** Adrenaline causes contraction of splenic capsule, but produces relaxation of plain muscles of spleen.
- **Action on CNS:** Adrenaline lowers the threshold of ARAS and stimulates it by producing alert and arousal phenomenon. Large doses of adrenaline inhibit spinal reflexes.

Action on Other Endocrine Glands

- Adrenaline stimulates anterior pituitary via hypothalamus, which in turn stimulates adrenal cortex to increase secretion of glucocorticoids.
- It inhibits ADH secretion.
- It also inhibits insulin secretion from pancreas and stimulates glucagon secretion.

Dopamine

Physiological role of dopamine in adrenal medulla is unknown, but when injected, dopamine produces the following effects:
- Renal vasodilatation, vasodilatation of mesenteric vessels
- In some regions, it produces vasoconstriction probably by releasing noradrenaline
- Dopamine produces cardioacceration via $β_1$-receptors.
- It increases systolic blood pressure, but diastolic pressure remains unchanged. So, dopamine is used for the treatment of traumatic and cardiogenic shock to increase blood pressure. All other functions are similar to adrenaline and noradrenaline.

There are 5 dopamine receptors D1 to D5. D1 and D5 increase cAMP levels. D2, D3 and D4 decrease cAMP levels. Prolactin-inhibiting factor released by hypothalamus is dopamine.

Dopamine acts as a neurotransmitter in dopaminergic pathways like nigrostriatal pathway in basal ganglia. It is also the principal transmitter in carotid and aortic bodies.

Regulation of Secretion of Adrenal Medulla

Basal resting secretion of adrenal medulla is very little. It becomes very low during sleep. Usually, adrenal medulla is stimulated only during stress. Increase in the secretion of adrenal medulla is a part of stimulation of sympathetic system. Preganglionic fibers coming through the splanchnic nerves of the sympathetic nervous system stimulate the chromaffin cells of medulla. So, together they are known as **sympathoadrenal system**.

According to Cannon, emergency-induced secretion from sympathoadrenal system is considered as the preparation for flight, fright or fight. During stress, due to stimulation of sympathoadrenal system, eye is relaxed, pupils dilate, heart rate and blood pressure are increased, cutaneous vessels constrict, there will be increase in the level of blood sugar, free fatty acids, etc., to provide more energy. All these changes are preparations for facing a stress situation. Medullary center situated in the floor of the fourth ventricle controls this situation.

Hypoglycemia is a potent stimulus for adrenal medullary secretion. Catecholamines increase blood sugar level by inducing glycogenolysis in muscle. Other stimuli include rage, anxiety, anesthesia, pain, hemorrhage, fasting, exposure to cold, etc. On exposure to cold, catecholamines significantly increase muscular activity and sometimes produce shivering so that, the body temperature is increased.

Glucocorticoids increase the synthesis of phenylethanolamine-N-methyltransferase (PNMT) in adrenal medulla and promote the conversion of norepinephrine to epinephrine. The functional integrity of adrenal medulla indirectly depends on the secretion of ACTH from pituitary and CRH from hypothalamus since catecholamine synthesis depends on glucocorticoids. Blood flowing from adrenal cortex to medulla maintain high concentration of glucocorticoids in the medulla necessary for catecholamine synthesis.

Importance of Adrenal Medulla in the Body

- Adrenal medulla is stimulated by sympathetic nervous system and the catecholamines released from the adrenal medulla make the sympathetic stimulation prolonged.
- Adrenal medulla is involved in day-to-day regulatory mechanisms of the body such as regulation of blood pressure, blood glucose, etc.
- Catecholamines allow the sympathetic nervous system to cope up with adverse conditions and emergency

situations. For example, when the body is exposed to cold, there is increase in heat production due to increased secretion of calorigenic hormones. There is also peripheral vasoconstriction to decrease heat loss from the surface of the body. Adrenalectomized animals may die when exposed to cold.
- In times of starvation, catecholamines maintain blood glucose level.
- Adrenal medulla is involved in the reactions associated with fight, fright and flight.

Abnormalities in Catecholamine Secretion

Pheochromocytoma

Pheochromocytoma is a rare, benign tumor arising from the chromaffin cells of adrenal medulla or paravertebral sympathetic ganglia. This tumor produces large quantities of catecholamines. Most of the tumors produce norepinephrine. In such cases, **paroxysmal hypertension** is the main feature. If the secretion is adrenaline, the hypertension is not severe, but hyperglycemia, glycosuria and other metabolic effects may be severe.

The cardinal features of pheochromocytoma are:
- Paroxysmal hypertension (endocrine or secondary hypertension)
- Hyperglycemia
- Glycosuria, polyuria
- Dyspnea, chest pain, shortness of breath
- Palpitation, headache, sweating, tremor, nervousness, symptoms of panic attack, etc.
- Loss of weight, nausea, vomiting, etc.

On examination, patient is pale, cold and moist, with increased heart rate, increased blood-pressure and extrasystole. Sweating is due to stimulation of hypothalamus by the rising temperature and also due to direct stimulation of sweat glands by the increased catecholamines. Pheochromocytoma is detected by measuring metanephrine, nor-metanephrine and vanillylmandelic acid (VMA) in urine and catecholamine level in plasma. These are found to be increased in pheochromocytoma. Surgery to remove pheochromocytoma usually returns blood pressure to normal.

MULTIPLE CHOICE QUESTIONS

1. When NaCl is injected into the internal carotid artery, it causes release of ADH by acting on?
   a. Paramedian nucleus
   b. Anterior pituitary
   c. Paraoptic nucleus
   d. Supraoptic nucleus

2. An increase in ECF osmolality stimulates osmoreceptors in:
   a. Anterior hypothalamus
   b. Posterior hypothalamus
   c. Lateral hypothalamus
   d. Ventromedial hypothalamus

3. All the following statements regarding adrenals are correct, *except*:
   a. Chromaffin granules are seen in pheochromocytoma
   b. Adrenal medulla normally secretes norepinephrine in excess of epinephrine
   c. Tumors of adrenal medulla secrete norepinephrine in excess of epinephrine
   d. Adrenal medulla is not essential for life

4. Hormones secreted by adrenal medulla are:
   a. Glucagon
   b. Cortisol
   c. Aldosterone
   d. Norepinephrine

5. Aldosterone synthesis is inhibited by:
   a. Renin
   b. Endothelin
   c. Dopamine
   d. Hypernatremia

6. Action of epinephrine in liver:
   a. Glycogenolysis
   b. Gluconeogenesis
   c. Glycolysis
   d. Lipolysis

7. Increase in the reabsorption of Na^+ from urine, sweat, saliva and colon occurs under the influence of:
   a. Cortisol
   b. Calcitonin
   c. Aldosterone
   d. Parathormone

8. Stress induced hyperglycemia is mediated through the following hormones, *except*:
   a. Glucagon
   b. Epinephrine
   c. Cortisol
   d. Thyroxine

9. During stress, increased secretion of cortisol cause all the following, *except*:
   a. Gluconeogenesis
   b. Lipolysis
   c. Protein breakdown
   d. Glycolysis

10. The following is seen in Addison's disease:
    a. Hyperkalemia
    b. Hypernatremia
    c. Hyperglycemia
    d. Hypertension

11. Hyperaldosteronism causes:
    a. Hyperkalemia
    b. Hyponatremia
    c. Decreased water reabsorption
    d. Hypokalemia

12. Which of the following has natriuretic actions?
    a. Aldosterone
    b. ANP
    c. Angiotensin
    d. Prednisolone

13. Excess aldosterone is associated with all, *except*:
    a. Water retention
    b. Hypokalemia
    c. Hyperkalemia
    d. Hypertension

14. Adrenal insufficiency causes:
    a. A rise in plasma sodium/potassium ratio
    b. High blood pressure
    c. Increased breakdown of protein
    d. A fall in extracellular fluid volume

15. **What is not true of aldosterone?**
    a. Secreted in increased amounts when blood volume falls
    b. Is a polypeptide
    c. Secretion tends to increase renal arterial pressure
    d. Secretion results in a reduction in urinary volume

16. **Postural hypotension develop in all the following conditions, *except*:**
    a. Hypovolemia
    b. Autonomic neuropathy
    c. Primary hyperaldosteronism
    d. Addison's disease

17. **All the following statements regarding ACTH are correct, *except*:**
    a. Secreted by basophil cells
    b. Controls secretion of adrenal cortex
    c. It is not protein in nature
    d. It can withstand heating up to 100oC

18. **In Cushing syndrome the following features are found, *except*:**
    a. Rapidly increasing adiposity
    b. Polycythemia
    c. Hypotension
    d. Impotence with atrophy of testis

19. **Cushing syndrome is characterized by:**
    a. Eosinophilia
    b. Hyperkalemia
    c. Nitrogen retention
    d. Poor wound healing

20. **In the adrenal gland, androgens are produced by the cells in the:**
    a. Zona glomerulosa
    b. Zona reticularis
    c. Zona fasciculate
    d. Adrenal medulla

21. **Drugs used in the treatment of congenital adrenal hyperplasia inhibits:**
    a. 17-alpha hydroxylase
    b. 21-alpha hydroxylase
    c. 11-beta hydroxylase
    d. Desmolase

22. **Correct statement regarding cortisol is:**
    a. Secretion increases following injury
    b. Favors protein synthesis
    c. Enhances effects of antigen-antibody reactions
    d. Tends to lower blood pressure

23. **The excretion of estrogens and progesterone are through:**
    a. Bile
    b. Sweat
    c. Urine
    d. Feces

24. **Angiotensinogen is produced by:**
    a. Kidney
    b. Liver
    c. Atrium
    d. Hypothalamus

25. **Most potent vasopressor is:**
    a. Angiotensin II
    b. Renin
    c. Aldosterone
    d. Cortisol

26. **BMR is decreased in:**
    a. Hyperthyroidism
    b. Increased body temperature
    c. Cushing syndrome
    d. Addison's disease

27. **Which of the following is released during "flight, fright and fight" reaction?**
    a. Adrenaline
    b. Noradrenaline
    c. Acetylcholine
    d. Glutamate

28. **Dopamine α-hydroxylase catalyze the step:**
    a. Dopamine to norepinephrine
    b. Dopa to dopamine
    c. Norepinephrine to epinephrine
    d. Tyrosine to DOPA

29. **Secondary hypertension is not seen in:**
    a. Hyperthyroidism
    b. Cushing's syndrome
    c. Addison's disease
    d. Conn syndrome

30. **The chemical nature of hormones of adrenal cortex is:**
    a. Amino acid
    b. Steroid
    c. Protein
    d. Glycoprotein

31. **Defective water excretion in adrenal insufficiency may be due to all the following, *except*:**
    a. Rise in plasma ADH
    b. Fall in GFR
    c. Fall in plasma cortisol
    d. Rise in blood glucose

32. **Pheochromocytoma is a tumor of:**
    a. Adenohypophysis
    b. Adrenal cortex
    c. Parathyroid
    d. Adrenal medulla

33. **Marked skin pigmentation is seen in:**
    a. Cushing's syndrome
    b. Addison's disease
    c. Down's syndrome
    d. Conn's syndrome

34. **Sodium retention is brought about by:**
    a. Androgen
    b. Glucagon
    c. Thyroxine
    d. Aldosterone

35. **In Addison's disease the following is raised:**
    a. Blood glucose
    b. Blood pressure
    c. Serum K$^+$
    d. Serum Na$^+$

36. **Action of norepinephrine is terminated by:**
    a. Reuptake into the presynaptic vesicle
    b. Reuptake into postsynaptic membrane
    c. Extraneuronal uptake
    d. Destroyed immediately in the synaptic cleft

37. All the following are involved in the degradation of catecholamines, *except*:
    a. MAO-A
    b. MAO-B
    c. COMT
    d. Dopamine hydroxylase

38. All are involved in the synthesis of norepinephrine, *except*:
    a. DOPA decarboxylase
    b. Dopamine hydroxylase
    c. Catecholamine-O-methyltransferase
    d. Tyrosine hydroxylase

39. The cofactor or coenzyme for tyrosine hydroxylase is:
    a. Vitamin B_{12}
    b. Tetrahydrobiopterin
    c. Calcium
    d. NAD

40. Tetrahydrobiopterin is a cofactor for all the following enzymes, *except*:
    a. Tyrosine hydroxylase
    b. Phenylalanine hydroxylase
    c. 17α-hydroxylase
    d. Tryptophan hydroxylase

ANSWERS

1. d	2. a	3. b	4. d	5. d
6. a	7. c	8. d	9. d	10. a
11. d	12. b	13. c	14. d	15. b
16. c	17. c	18. c	19. d	20. b
21. c	22. a	23. c	24. b	25. a
26. d	27. b	28. a	29. c	30. b
31. d	32. d	33. b	34. d	35. c
36. a	37. d	38. c	39. b	40. c

Endocrine Pancreas

CHAPTER 68

LEARNING OBJECTIVES

- Describe the structure of islets of Langerhans and name the hormones secreted by each cell
- Describe the structure of insulin receptors and the mechanism by which they mediate insulin action
- Name the types of glucose transporters in the body and explain their mechanism of action
- Explain the actions of insulin
- List the types of diabetes mellitus and outline the major differences between them
- State the regulation of secretion of insulin
- Describe the actions of glucagon and the factors that regulate its secretion
- Describe the tests to assess endocrine pancreas
- Describe the metabolic and endocrine consequences of obesity and metabolic syndrome
- Outline the psychiatry component pertaining to metabolic syndrome

■ INTRODUCTION

PY8.2: Describe the synthesis, secretion, transport, physiological actions, regulation and effect of altered (hypo and hyper) secretion of pancreas.
PY8.4: Describe function tests: Thyroid gland, adrenal cortex, adrenal medulla and pancreas.

Pancreas is a **dual gland or heterocrine gland** having an exocrine and an endocrine portion. Exocrine portion which constitute 99% of the gland consists of acini, which produce pancreatic juice. Endocrine portion (1%) consists of cell groups called **islets of Langerhans**. Function of endocrine pancreas is to maintain the plasma level of glucose within a narrow range. It accomplishes this function by changing the rate of secretion of hormones insulin and glucagon. Blood levels of nutrients such as glucose, amino acids and fatty acids are the major signals controlling the release of insulin and glucagon from the endocrine pancreas.

The circulating level of glucose is the primary controller. For example, when a carbohydrate-rich meal is taken, the plasma glucose level increases and this stimulates insulin secretion and suppresses glucagon secretion from the endocrine pancreas. The high level of insulin promotes storage of glucose as glycogen in liver and muscle, thereby preventing hyperglycemia. In contrast, during fasting, the blood glucose level falls and there will be inhibition of insulin secretion and stimulation of glucagon secretion from pancreas. Glucagon increases hepatic glucose production by increasing glycogenolysis and gluconeogenesis. Thus, the plasma level of glucose is maintained. This is very important because brain function is absolutely dependent on an adequate level of glucose in blood. *In hypoglycemia, there will be severe impairment of brain function.*

■ FUNCTIONAL ANATOMY

The islets of Langerhans constitute 1–2% of the total weight of the gland. There are about 1–2 million islets in the human pancreas. Each islet consists of 50–200 cells which are of different types. The islets are ovoid in shape, 76 × 175 μm in size and scattered throughout the gland, but more towards the tail than in the body and head. Depending on the staining properties and morphology, the cells are classified into A, B, D and F cells.

There is a specific arrangement for the different cells of the islets. In the central portion of the islets are the β-cells that form 70% of the total cells. Surrounding these cells are the other types of cells. Cells show all the features of secretory cells and they contain secretory granules. Granules of β-cells are large but less in number **(Fig. 68.1)**. Hormones secreted by the different cells of the islets are given in **Table 68.1**. Glucagon, somatostatin and pancreatic polypeptide are also secreted by the mucosal cells of the gastrointestinal tract.

Blood Supply

Pancreas lies between spleen and duodenum and shares the blood supply of these two organs. Unlike any other endocrine organ the venous blood from the islets of the pancreas drains into the hepatic portal vein so that the liver is exposed to high concentration of insulin and glucagon.

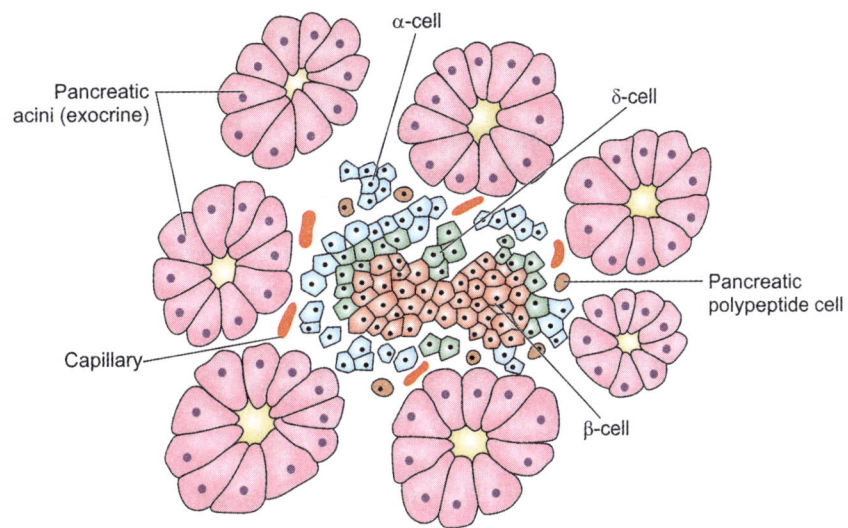

Fig. 68.1: Histological structure of pancreas; the islets of Langerhans are seen in the center surrounded by exocrine pancreatic acini.

Table 68.1: Types of cells and the hormones secreted by endocrine pancreas.

Cell type	% of total cells	Hormone
A or α-cell	20	Glucagon
B or β-cell	60–70	Insulin
D or δ-cell	10	Somatostatin
F cell or PP cell	<10%	Pancreatic-polypeptide

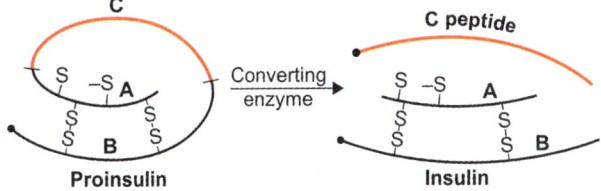

Fig. 68.2: Structure of proinsulin and insulin.
(A: A chain; B: B chain; C: connecting peptide)

Innervation of Endocrine Pancreas

The endocrine pancreas is supplied by unmyelinated fibers of sympathetic and parasympathetic nervous system. The sympathetic adrenergic fibers are postganglionic and originate from **celiac ganglion**. They innervate blood vessels and islets and influence the islet cells in times of stress. Stimulation of sympathetic fibers to endocrine pancreas inhibits insulin secretion. The norepinephrine released acts on $α_2$-adrenergic receptors and causes inhibition.

Parasympathetic cholinergic fibers are preganglionic branches of **right vagus**. They terminate in the intrapancreatic ganglia. The cholinergic postganglionic fibers innervate islets and are responsible for food-related release of pancreatic hormones. Stimulation of parasympathetic fibers causes increased insulin secretion via M_3 receptors. Atropine blocks this response and acetyl choline stimulates insulin secretion.

Some autonomic nerves innervating the islets, release the polypeptide **galanin** which inhibits insulin secretion by activating K^+ channels.

INSULIN

Insulin is the only hypoglycemic hormone in the body whose deficiency leads to diabetes mellitus. **Banting and Best** in 1922 first extracted insulin from pancreas. Insulin is synthesized in the rough endoplasmic reticulum of β-cells of the islets and then transported into Golgi apparatus where it is stored in membrane-bound vesicles from where hormone is released by the process of exocytosis. The vesicles contain granules filled with insulin.

Insulin is synthesized from **preproinsulin**, a large polypeptide which has a leader sequence of 23 amino acids. This leader sequence is split off while the hormone is in the endoplasmic reticulum. After removal of the above segment, it becomes **proinsulin (Fig. 68.2)**. It has a folded structure with disulfide bridges. Proinsulin contains A-chain, B-chain and a connecting peptide or **C peptide** with 31 amino acids. From proinsulin, C peptide is split off to form active insulin. In active insulin, there are two polypeptide chains that contain 21 and 30 amino acids respectively, and are joined by two disulfide bridges. Both insulin and C-peptide are stored in the secretory granules of β-cell. Equimolar amounts of C peptide are also released along with insulin from the beta cells into the blood stream. Only negligible amount of C-peptide is metabolized in the liver. *Level of C peptide in blood can be measured by radioimmunoassay and it is a better index of β-cell function especially in patients receiving insulin.* Otherwise, C peptide is not significant and has no physiological action. In type 2 diabetes mellitus, the level of C-peptide is found to be increased.

Normal daily secretion of insulin is 40 units/day (1 unit = 40 μg).

The main target organs for insulin are liver, adipose tissue and muscle **(Table 68.2)**.

Table 68.2: Effect of insulin in different tissues.

Tissue	Liver	Muscle	Adipose tissue
Glucose receptor present	GLUT 2	GLUT 4	GLUT 4
Insulin dependence	Insulin independent	Insulin dependent	Insulin dependent
Actions	• Glycogenesis • Glycolysis	• Stimulate GLUT4 and increase glucose uptake • Glycolysis • Glycogen synthesis • Increased amino acid uptake and increased protein synthesis	• Increased glucose uptake • Lipogenesis and increase triglyceride level

Secretion of Insulin

Biosynthesis of insulin in the β-cells increases with increase in blood glucose level.

Insulin secretion in response to rise in plasma glucose occurs in **two phases**.

1. Immediately following a rise in plasma glucose level, there is a rapid increase in the secretion of insulin within 1–2 minutes which comes back to the basal level in 3 minutes. This rise is due to the release of already stored insulin in the β-cell granules.
2. Then after some time the level of insulin increases slowly and reaches a peak in about 1 hour and comes to the resting level by about 5 hours. This response is due to increase in insulin synthesis and secretion from the β–cell.

When there is hyperglycemia, glucose enter the beta cells through **GLUT-2** receptors. *This entry of glucose does not require insulin.* Glucose is converted to glucose-6-phosphate which is converted to pyruvate and then to acetyl coenzyme A. This enters the citric acid cycle and forms FADH2 and NADH. These enter the mitochondria and release ATP. This ATP binds with K^+ channels in the beta cell membrane and closes it. So K^+ accumulate in the cell leading to depolarization of the membrane. This stimulates Ca^{2+} channel in the cell membrane and there is influx of Ca^{2+} into the beta cell. Synapto-proteins in the vesicular membrane and the cell membrane link together in the presence of Ca^{2+} leading to exocytosis of the insulin vesicles. Along with insulin, C-peptide is also released into the extracellular fluid. They enter the blood stream and reaches the different tissues where insulin exerts its action (**Table 68.2**).

Glucose-stimulated insulin secretion is abolished by somatostatin, but insulin synthesis remains unaffected. So, even if synthesis occurs normally, if release is affected it leads to insulin deficiency.

Insulin-like Substances in the Body

Non-suppressible Insulin-like Activity (NSILA)

There are a variety of substances in plasma with insulin-like activity in addition to insulin. When anti-insulin antibody is administered, only 7% of insulin activity is suppressed. This means that only 7% of insulin-like activity is due to insulin secreted by islet cells. The rest 93% is due to the presence of **non-suppressible insulin-like activity (NSILA)** whose activity is not suppressed by anti-insulin antibodies. This is contributed mainly by somatomedins or insulin-like growth factors (**IGF-I and IGF-II**). These are polypeptides. In spite of the presence of large amounts of NSILA, diabetes mellitus results from insulin deficiency. This is because their insulin-like activity is very poor when compared to that of insulin. All the actions of insulin are necessary for maintaining normal blood glucose level.

Insulin Metabolism

Half-life of insulin is 5 min. About 80% of insulin is destroyed in **liver and kidney**. There are three systems which inactivate insulin. Of these, two systems destroy disulfide bridges and the third one breaks the polypeptide chain. All enzymes that are required for destruction of insulin are grouped under the general term **insulinases**.

Actions of Insulin

1. Action on cell membrane
2. Action on metabolism
3. Action on growth.

Action on Cell Membrane

Glucose enters the cells by facilitated diffusion or in the intestine and kidneys by secondary active transport. Insulin promotes entry of glucose into the cells of the body *except liver cells, brain cells and red blood cells*. In the brain, hypothalamus requires insulin for the entry of glucose into it. In muscle, fat and some other tissues insulin increases the number of glucose transporters in the cell membrane like sodium dependent glucose transporter (SGLT-1, SGLT-2) and glucose transporters (GLUT). There are 7 types of glucose transporters, GLUT-1 to GLUT-7. GLUT-4 is the transporter that is stimulated by insulin. The GLUT-4 receptors are concentrated in vesicles in the cytoplasm of insulin-sensitive cells. When insulin combines with insulin receptors, the receptors get activated and the vesicles move rapidly to the cell membrane and fuse with it inserting the glucose transporters into the cell membrane. This increases the entry of glucose into the cell. Activation of the insulin receptor causes activation of **phosphatidyl inositol 3-kinase** (PI3K), which speeds up the translocation of GLUT-4 containing vesicles into the cell membrane. When insulin action stops the transporter containing patches of the cell membrane are endocytosed which again form vesicles in the cytoplasm.

Muscle cells also contain a population of GLUT-4 vesicles that move into the cell membrane in response to exercise and insert more glucose transporters on the cell membrane. Thus, more of glucose enters the muscle cells during exercise. This mechanism of glucose entry in exercise is independent of the action of insulin. A 5'-AMP activated kinase may trigger insertion of these vesicles into the cell membrane. *This is the reason why diabetic patients are advised to do exercise regularly to lower the blood sugar level even though there is deficiency of insulin.*

The increase in the entry of glucose into liver cells is not by increasing the number of glucose transporters. Instead, it induces glucokinase which increases phosphorylation of glucose so that intracellular free glucose concentration stays low, facilitating the entry of more glucose into the cell along the concentration gradient. *Absorption of glucose from the intestine and from the proximal tubules of kidney is not influenced by insulin.* It occurs by secondary active transport with Na^+.

- Insulin enhances entry of amino acids into the cell. It acts directly on the cell membrane of muscle cells and stimulates transport of amino acids by activating amino acid channels.
- Insulin promotes entry of fatty acids into the cell by acting on the cell membrane of adipose tissue.
- It stimulates entry of K^+ into the cell. It activates Na^+-K^+ ATPase in cell membrane and stimulates the transport of K^+ into the cell.

Action of Insulin on Carbohydrate Metabolism

After a carbohydrate meal, glucose is absorbed into circulation and this glucose stimulates insulin secretion. Insulin in turn lowers blood glucose level by the following mechanisms:

- Insulin stimulates glycogen synthesis in the liver by activating enzymes phosphofructokinase and glycogen synthetase. Liver glycogen can be converted to glucose in between meals.
- It also enhances glycogen synthesis in the muscle. Insulin acts directly on muscle membrane and enhances the transport of glucose into the cell and this glucose is converted to glycogen in muscle cell. This glycogen cannot be converted to glucose in between meals because muscle lacks the enzyme glucose-6-phosphatase. But muscle glycogen is utilized in the muscle to supply energy.
- Insulin stimulates glycogen synthesis in adipose tissue.
- Insulin is a glycogenetic hormone. It inhibits glycogenolysis in liver by inhibiting the enzyme phosphorylase.
- It converts excess glucose in liver to fatty acids and these fatty acids are transported to adipose tissue where fat is synthesized and stored.
- It prevents gluconeogenesis.
- It increases peripheral utilization of glucose, i.e., oxidation of glucose to CO_2 and water, releasing energy in the peripheral tissues (glycolysis).
- With a large dose of insulin, blood glucose falls tremendously, resulting in hypoglycemia. If hypoglycemia is severe it leads to convulsions and coma.

On Protein Metabolism

Insulin is a protein anabolic hormone. The growth promoting, protein anabolic effects of insulin are mediated by phosphatidyl inositol-3 kinase.

- It acts directly on the cell membrane of muscle cells and promotes the entry of amino acids into the cell necessary for protein synthesis.
- It acts directly on ribosome and stimulate translation of mRNA.
- Inhibits protein catabolism.
- Inhibits gluconeogenesis so that more amino acids are available for protein synthesis.

On Fat Metabolism

- In the tissues, glucose is mainly utilized for energy so that fat is spared. This **fat-sparing action** of insulin makes fatty acids available for fat synthesis.
- In the liver, excess glucose is converted to fatty acids and insulin stimulates formation of triglycerides from fatty acid.
- Some of the fatty acids are transported to adipose tissue where fat is synthesized and stored. Fatty acids directly enter into the adipose tissue by the action of insulin and facilitate fat synthesis.
- Fat breakdown or lipolysis is inhibited by insulin by inhibiting the enzyme lipase. In the absence of insulin, more of fat is broken down and increases free fatty acid level in plasma.
- Absence of insulin also promotes formation of ketone bodies leading to ketoacidosis. One of the main complications of diabetes mellitus is ketoacidosis.

On Mineral Metabolism

Insulin stimulates entry of K^+ into the cell leading to hypokalemia.

Action on Nucleic Acid Metabolism

Insulin stimulates both DNA and RNA synthesis in the cells.

Action on Growth

- Growth hormone and insulin act synergistically to stimulate growth of the individual. This is because of its **anabolic action** on proteins.
- Increase in protein synthesis from amino acids and inhibition of protein degradation stimulates growth.
- Protein-sparing action of insulin by increasing adequate intracellular glucose supplies for energy needs also favors growth. Failure to grow is a symptom of diabetes mellitus in children.
- The net effect of insulin is storage of carbohydrate, protein and fat and therefore insulin is called "**the hormone of abundance**."

Insulin Receptors

Insulin binds to specific receptors in the cell membrane. The insulin receptor with molecular weight 340,000 is a tetramer which has 2 α and 2 β glycoprotein subunits. The alpha subunit is extracellular and binds insulin whereas beta subunit is intracellular (**Fig. 68.3**). The gene that codes for insulin receptor is located on chromosome 19. When insulin combines with receptors, the complex is engulfed into the cytoplasm, which is called **internalization**. These are then

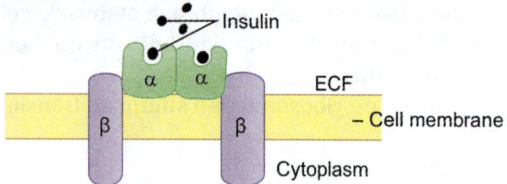

Fig. 68.3: Structure of insulin receptor.

broken down by lysosomal enzyme and some of the receptors are recycled. When insulin concentration is low, the number of receptors and their affinity to insulin increases and vice versa. This is known as **up-regulation and down-regulation of receptors**.

Mechanism of Action of Insulin

Even though insulin is a peptide hormone; its action is not mediated by second messengers. Insulin combines with the alpha subunit of insulin receptor which is extracellular. The beta subunit spans the cell membrane and the intracellular portion of the beta subunit has tyrosine kinase activity. This result in auto phosphorylation of the beta subunit and phosphorylation of tyrosine residues present on the cytoplasmic portion called **insulin receptor substrate (IRS)**. This initiates a series of events that culminate into a cascade of phosphorylation and dephosphorylation reactions.

- Insulin also binds to the insulin-like growth factor-1 (IGF-I) receptor since insulin receptor is very similar to IGF-I receptor.
- Insulin also stimulates the synthesis and insertion of more glucose transporters (GLUT-4) in insulin sensitive cells by ATP-dependent translocation of GLUT-4 to the cell membrane.
- Inhibits cAMP mechanism.
- Facilitates Na^+-K^+ pump and increases the transport of more K^+ into the cell.

Regulation of Insulin Secretion (Table 68.3)

Regulation by Blood Glucose Level

Most important factor that regulates insulin secretion is blood glucose. When blood glucose is at the fasting level, insulin secretion is minimal. But when there is increase in blood glucose, insulin secretion increases in two stages. There is a sharp rise in insulin secretion within 3–5 min. After 15 min, again there is a rise which lasts for few hours. The first peak is due to release of stored insulin and the second rise is due to increased synthesis and secretion. Response depends on the route of administration of glucose. The initial rapid rise that occurs within one minute is usually seen during intravenous glucose administration. But the slow rise in insulin secretion after orally administered glucose is more than that seen after intravenous administration. This is because orally administered glucose also stimulates the secretion of gastrointestinal insulinogenic hormones such as incretins (GLP1 and GIP), gastrin, secretin etc.

Table 68.3: Factors affecting insulin secretion.

Increased secretion	Decreased secretion
• Hyperglycemia • Increased plasma amino acids and free fatty acids • Hormones such as glucagon, growth hormone, cortisol, gastrin, cholecystokinin • Parasympathetic stimulation • Incretins • β-adrenergic stimulation • Insulin resistance • Sulfonyl urea drugs	• Hypoglycemia • Somatostatin • α_2 adrenergic stimulation • Leptin

Mechanism

Glucose enters the cell via GLUT-2 transporters. Increased glycolysis in the β-cell increases intracellular ATP. This ATP inhibits ATP-sensitive K^+ channels and there is a decrease in K^+ efflux. This depolarizes the cell which in turn opens Ca^{2+} channels. Influx of Ca^{2+} stimulates Ca^{2+}-mediated exocytosis of insulin granules. Glucose regulates insulin synthesis at both the transcriptional and translational level. The increased level of insulin enhances the transport of glucose into adipose tissue, muscle and other tissues and thus blood glucose is brought back to normal.

Amino Acids

Many amino acids stimulate insulin secretion, of which the most important are **arginine and lysine**. Amino acids can stimulate insulin secretion in the absence of glucose. But presence of glucose potentiates the stimulating effect of amino acids. Insulin in turn stimulates the entry of amino acids into the cell and promotes protein synthesis.

Fatty Acids

Fatty acids have no role in insulin secretion.

Hormonal Regulation

- Gastrointestinal hormones such as *gastrin, secretin, CCK, GIP, glucagon and glucagon-like polypeptide (GLP-1) stimulate insulin secretion.* Secretion of these hormones is stimulated by food intake. Orally administered glucose and amino acids exerts a greater insulin stimulating effect than intravenously administered glucose and amino acids because of the simultaneous release of these gastrointestinal hormones.
- Paracrine hormones: Hormones that enter the β-cells to modify their secretion are paracrine hormones. Glucagon and somatostatin act as paracrine hormones. Glucagon stimulates insulin secretion, while somatostatin inhibits insulin secretion.
- Other endocrine hormones such as cortisol, ACTH, thyroxine, growth hormone, human placental lactogen, estrogen and progesterone stimulate insulin secretion indirectly. These hormones increase blood glucose level, which in turn stimulates insulin secretion.

Neural Regulation

β-Cells of islets receive both sympathetic and parasympathetic fibers. Parasympathetic stimulation increases insulin secretion and the parasympathetic supply is through right vagus. In the case of sympathetic system, stimulation of adrenergic β-receptors increases insulin secretion while α_2-receptor stimulation inhibits insulin secretion. The net effect of epinephrine and norepinephrine on islet cell is inhibition of insulin secretion.

Abnormalities of Insulin Secretion

Diabetes Mellitus

Diabetes mellitus is a collection of abnormalities caused by deficiency of insulin. It can also be due to insulin resistance where the abnormality is at the receptor level.

There will be alterations in carbohydrate, lipid and protein metabolism. Diabetes mellitus is characterized by **polyuria, polydipsia, polyphagia, weight loss, hyperglycemia, glycosuria, ketosis, acidosis and coma** (in severe cases). Hyperglycemia can also be due to glucagon excess and somatostatin excess.

It is clinically diagnosed when the fasting blood sugar is more than 140 mg/100 mL. Diabetes mellitus should be differentiated from diabetes insipidus which is caused by deficiency of ADH. In diabetes insipidus, there is polyuria and polydipsia but there is no hyperglycemia or glycosuria as in diabetes mellitus. Specific gravity of urine is less in diabetes insipidus but it is high in diabetes mellitus. The term diabetes alone refers to diabetes mellitus.

Types of Diabetes (Table 68.4)

I. Type I diabetes or Insulin dependent diabetes mellitus (IDDM) or juvenile diabetes mellitus.
II. Type II diabetes or non-insulin dependent diabetes mellitus (NIDDM) or maturity-onset diabetes mellitus.

Type I diabetes or IDDM

IDDM is seen in young individuals and is of rapid onset. If it occurs at infancy or in childhood, it is called juvenile diabetes. Causes are autoimmune etiology where antibodies are developed against B-cells of islets, degeneration of B-cell due to some viral infections or idiopathic degeneration, i.e., without any specific cause. The symptoms of type I diabetes appear when more than 80% of the islets are destroyed.

Type II or NIDDM or adult-onset diabetes

NIDDM is seen in adults especially in obese people due to progressive degeneration of β-cells with aging. Insulin resistance is a common feature of NIDDM. Precise molecular mechanism of insulin resistance in type II diabetes mellitus has not been explained.

- Post receptor defects are believed to play a prominent role in insulin resistance. Polymorphism in insulin receptor substrate (IRS-I) may be associated with glucose intolerance, raising the possibility that polymorphism in various post receptor molecules combine to create an insulin resistant state.
- Pathogenesis of insulin resistance is currently focused on a phosphatidyl inositol-3 kinase signaling defect, which reduces translocation of GLUT-4 to the plasma membrane.
- Obesity is the most important environmental factor causing insulin resistance. Elevated levels of free fatty acids may contribute to the pathogenesis of insulin resistance and type II diabetes mellitus.
- Rare insulin-resistance syndromes occur in patients who develop antibodies that block the interaction of insulin with its receptor. This may be associated with other autoimmune disorders such as systemic lupus erythematosus (SLE), Sjogren's syndrome, etc.

Effects of Lack of Insulin in Diabetes Mellitus

- Decrease in the peripheral utilization of glucose.
- Increased glycogenolysis and gluconeogenesis in liver and liberation of more glucose into circulation.
- Decreased entry of amino acids into the cells and decreased protein synthesis.
- Increased lipolysis and increase in ketone bodies.
- Increased secretion of glucagon which is a hyperglycemic hormone.
- Even though there is plenty of glucose in the ECF, there is intracellular glucose deficiency because glucose is not entering the cells. This situation has been called *"starvation in the midst of plenty."* A similar metabolic picture is seen in starvation except that there is no hyperglycemia.
- There is increased filtration of glucose in the glomerulus and when it exceeds tubular maximum, excess glucose is excreted through urine, resulting in glycosuria.
- Increased urinary loss of Na^+ and K^+.

Signs and Symptoms of Diabetes Mellitus

- Cardinal symptoms of diabetes mellitus are polyuria, polydipsia and polyphagia
- Hyperglycemia and glycosuria
- Protein depletion and muscle weakness
- Weight loss
- Acidosis and coma
- Hyperlipidemia and atherosclerosis.

Table 68.4: Comparison of type I and type II diabetes mellitus.		
	Type I diabetes (IDDM)	**Type II (NIDDM)**
Genetic predisposition	Moderate	Very strong
Cause	Destruction of B-cells of islets	Insulin resistance
Insulin level in blood	Decreased or absent	Normal or increased
Age of onset	Less than 30 years	More than 40 years
Mode of onset	Rapid	Gradual
Prevalence	10% of all diabetics have type I diabetes	90% of all diabetics have type II diabetes
Body weight	Normal	Obese
Metabolic disturbance	Ketoacidosis	Hyperosmolar coma
Treatment	Insulin injection	Oral hypoglycemic drugs

Polyuria, polydipsia and polyphagia: *The classic triad of manifestation of diabetes mellitus include polyuria (excessive passage of urine), polydipsia (excessive thirst), and polyphagia (excessive eating).*

- When the blood glucose increases due to insulin lack, more of glucose is filtered through urine and there is increased osmotic tension in the renal tubules. As a result, more water is lost through urine leading to frequent urination referred to as **polyuria**. This is an example of **osmotic diuresis**.
- When excess water is lost through urine, there will be dehydration, hypovolemia and hyperosmolality of plasma. Thirst center of hypothalamus will be stimulated by the hyperosmolality of plasma and by the hypovolemia and the patient drinks more water. This is **polydipsia**.
- In the satiety center of hypothalamus, there are certain cells known as **glucoreceptors**. These cells require insulin for the entry of glucose into them. In the absence of insulin, glucose does not enter these cells and they do not get stimulated. They inhibit the feeding center in hypothalamus only when glucose enters them. Since feeding center is not inhibited in diabetes, there will be increased appetite resulting in increased food intake. This is the explanation for **polyphagia**.

Hyperglycemia and glycosuria: Hyperglycemia in diabetes mellitus is due to a reduction in glucose uptake by liver cells and stimulation of gluconeogenesis. Since insulin deficiency reduces protein synthesis, large quantities of amino acids are available for gluconeogenesis **(Flowchart 68.1)**. When the blood glucose exceeds the renal threshold for glucose, glucose appears in urine which is referred to as **glycosuria**.

In untreated cases of diabetes mellitus, glucose is converted to other sugars such as sorbitol. This leads to osmotic fluid shifts leading to swelling of the lens of the eye resulting in blurred vision and formation of **cataract**. Numerous proteins such as hemoglobin, albumin and collagen are non-enzymatically glycosylated in long standing hyperglycemia. End products of protein glycosylation contribute to **damage in the retina, kidneys, nerves and cardiovascular system**.

Protein depletion and muscle wasting: In diabetes, protein catabolism is stimulated and at the same time protein synthesis is inhibited. Both these factors lead to **muscle wasting and weight loss** even if there is increased food intake.

Due to this effect there is growth retardation in children with diabetes. Due to increased catabolism of protein, there will be protein depletion in the body and negative nitrogen balance. This protein depletion makes the individual more susceptible to infection. Glucose-rich ECF acts as a culture medium for pathogenic organisms and the patients are prone to infections.

Ketoacidosis and coma: Because of increased lipolysis, free fatty acid level in blood increases. Glucagon, which is increased in diabetes, causes mobilization of free fatty acids from fat depots. Because of insulin lack, fatty acid is not converted to fat. All these lead to increase in free fatty acid level in plasma. In the liver and other tissues this fatty acid is metabolized to acetyl coenzyme-A. If it is present in excess, it is converted to acetoacetyl CoA and then to acetoacetate. Thus acetoacetic acid and β-hydroxybutyric acid which are called **ketone bodies** accumulate in the blood stream leading to **diabetic ketoacidosis**. Acidosis stimulates the respiratory center producing rapid deep respiration called **Kussmaul breathing (Flowchart 68.2)**. Urine becomes highly acidic. Along with H^+, large quantities of Na^+ and K^+ are also lost through urine. Polyuria leads to hypovolemia, dehydration and hypotension.

Because of acidosis and hypotension, unconsciousness may occur which finally leads to coma. Coma can also occur if the blood sugar is very high, then it is called **hyperosmolar coma**.

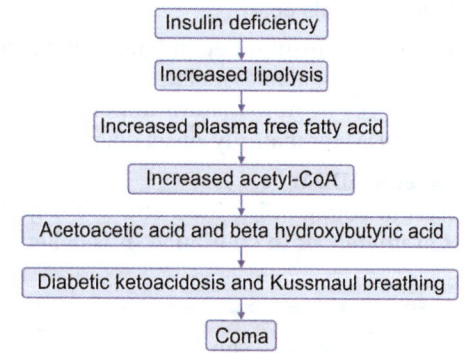

Flowchart 68.2: Mechanism of production of ketoacidosis and coma in diabetes mellitus.

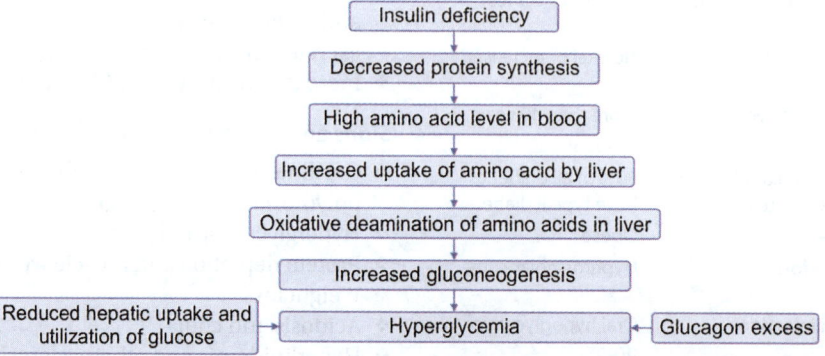

Flowchart 68.1: Causes of hyperglycemia in diabetes mellitus.

Hyperlipidemia, atherosclerosis and coronary artery disease: In diabetes, plasma cholesterol level is elevated and this plays an important role in the development of atherosclerotic vascular disease which is a major complication of diabetes. This is due to increased plasma level of VLDL and LDL which is due to increased hepatic production of VLDL and decreased removal of VLDL and LDL from circulation. The hyperlipidemia and related hypercholesterolemia results in hypertension and coronary artery disease (CAD) in uncontrolled diabetes mellitus **(Flowchart 68.3)**.

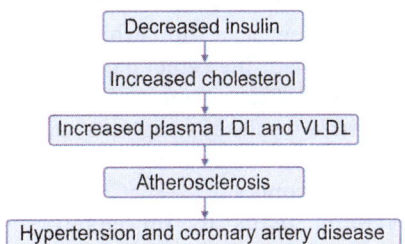

Flowchart 68.3: Mechanism of production of hypertension and CAD in diabetes mellitus.

Diagnosis of Diabetes Mellitus

- Clinically, diabetes mellitus is diagnosed when the fasting blood sugar is more than 130 mg/100 mL and random blood glucose more than 200 mg/dL. Normal fasting blood glucose level is 70–110 mg/100 mL.
- Oral glucose tolerance test (GTT): If a glucose load is given to a diabetic, the plasma glucose rises higher in the graph and returns to the baseline more slowly than it does in normal individuals **(Fig. 68.4)**.
- Measurement of the concentration of plasma glycated hemoglobin (**GHb** or **HbA1c**). When plasma glucose is elevated, small amounts of hemoglobin-A are non-enzymatically glycated to form HbA1c. Periodic measurement of this parameter during treatment for diabetes is very important to assess the control of diabetes with treatment.

The level of HbA1c in individuals without diabetes is 4 to 5.6%. Levels between 5.7 and 6.4% indicate increased risk of diabetes mellitus. Levels of 6.5% and higher indicate diabetes. The goal for people with diabetes mellitus is an HbA1c less than 7%.

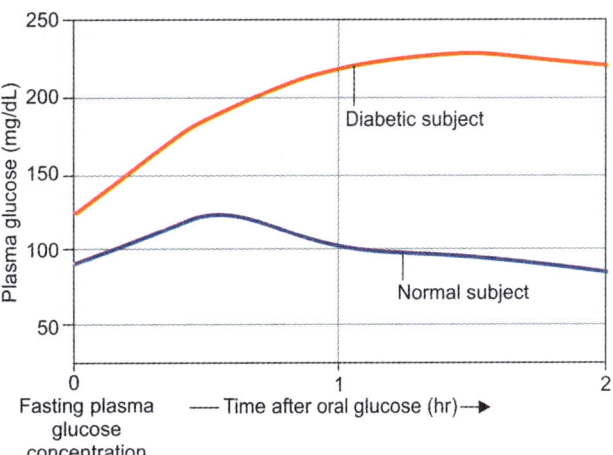

Fig. 68.4: Glucose tolerance test in a normal subject and in a diabetic subject.

Treatment of Diabetes Mellitus

a. Insulin administration is the treatment of choice in IDDM. Fast acting insulin that is injected subcutaneously is crystalline zinc insulin (CZI).
b. Oral hypoglycemic drugs are advised in NIDDM:
  - **Sulfonylurea** derivatives such as tolbutamide, glipizide, etc., act by increasing the secretion of insulin from islets. It is ineffective after pancreatectomy and in type I diabetes.
    - **Biguanides** such as metformin decrease gluconeogenesis and decrease hepatic glucose output.
    - Thiazolidinediones reduce insulin resistance.
c. Healthy eating habits [low fat (<30%), high-fiber carbohydrates (>55%) and 10–15% proteins in diet], regular exercise and stopping smoking is beneficial. About 20% of type II diabetes mellitus can be controlled by diet and exercise alone.
d. Weight reduction is important in type II diabetes since these people are obese.

Hyperinsulinemia or Insulin Excess

Hypersecretion of insulin is usually caused by a tumor of the β-cells. The cardinal manifestation is a low plasma glucose level; the fasting blood glucose will be less than 50 mg/dL. Insulin excess causes hypoglycemia which affects mainly the nervous system. Hypoglycemia is a more serious condition than hyperglycemia. Symptoms include palpitation, sweating, nervousness, etc., due to increased sympathetic discharge. If severe, it leads to lethargy, coma, convulsions and even death. The condition is diagnosed by estimating fasting plasma insulin and C-peptide levels, both will be elevated in β-cell tumor. Insulin excess is treated by the drug **diazoxide** which inhibits insulin release from β-cells. Subtotal pancreatectomy is done in severe cases.

Hypoglycemia

Normal fasting blood glucose level is 70–110 mg/dL. Decrease in blood glucose level below the normal range is called **hypoglycemia**. In normal individuals, symptoms of hypoglycemia occur when the blood glucose is less than 60 mg/dL. In patients with diabetes mellitus, signs and symptoms of hypoglycemia are produced when the blood glucose level falls below 100 mg/dL.

Causes

- Overdose of insulin or oral hypoglycemic agents.
- Insulinomas (insulin secreting tumors) such as β-islet cell adenoma.
- Severe exercise in diabetic patients on insulin.

Signs and Symptoms

- Normal functioning of brain depends on a continuous glucose supply because the carbohydrate reserve of brain is very limited. The cerebral cortex also has a high metabolic rate. Deficient supply of glucose to the brain in hypoglycemia results in symptoms such as giddiness, mental confusion, irritability, fatigue and in extreme cases convulsions and coma.
- Hypoglycemia leads to increased secretion of catecholamines from the adrenal medulla due to over activity of the sympathetic system. This produces nervousness, anxiety, headache, tremor, tachycardia and increased sweating. These symptoms warn the patient about imminent hypoglycemic coma (referred to as hypoglycemia awareness).
- If the vital centers of medulla oblongata are involved the condition may be fatal due to cardiorespiratory center involvement.

Compensatory Mechanisms in Hypoglycemia

The blood glucose level can be increased by stimulating the secretion of hormones which increases blood glucose level. The important hyperglycemic hormones are glucagon, catecholamines, ACTH, GH and TSH. These hormones increase blood glucose by promoting glycogenolysis and gluconeogenesis thus increasing glucose output from liver. There is also decreased peripheral utilization of glucose. Thyroxine also increases glucose absorption from the GIT.

OBESITY AND METABOLIC SYNDROME OR SYNDROME-X

> **PY8.5:** Describe the metabolic and endocrine consequences of obesity and metabolic syndrome. Outline the psychiatry component pertaining to metabolic syndrome.

Metabolic syndrome is a cluster of multiple risk factors including elevated insulin level, insulin resistance, hyperglycemia, visceral obesity, hyperlipidemia and hypertension. Elevated intracellular glucocorticoid tone is thought to be an etiology of metabolic syndrome. The release of cortisol by the adrenal gland is dependent on hypothalamo-pituitary-adrenal axis regulated by an integrated feedback of three separate control systems. These include:
1. Circadian rhythm regulated by suprachiasmatic nucleus
2. Stress responsive circuit (inputs to hypothalamus from brain stem, limbic system and cerebral cortex)
3. Feedback control

Obesity leads to disordered carbohydrate metabolism and diabetes mellitus. In obesity, there is increased **insulin resistance** and the ability of insulin to move glucose into adipose tissue and muscle is inhibited leading to **hyperglycemia**. As a compensatory mechanism, there will be **hyperinsulinemia** induced by high blood glucose level. There is also **dyslipidemia** characterized by high circulating triglycerides and low HDL. This combination of findings is commonly called metabolic syndrome or **syndrome-X**.

It is now clear that white fat is an endocrine tissue that secretes hormones such as leptin and other adipokines like resistin, adiponectin, etc. **Leptin and adiponectin** decrease insulin resistance. Leptin acts on hypothalamus to decrease food intake and thus prevents obesity. Leptin secretion is decreased in fasting. Mutation in the leptin gene leads to obesity.

Psychiatry Component Pertaining to Metabolic Syndrome

Psychological support and patient education is an essential part in treating metabolic syndrome. The patient must be made aware of the disease especially its complications. Reassurance is the key for the patient's well being.

The role of stress in the functioning of hypothalamo-pituitary-adrenal (HPA) axis has been extensively studied, first by Hans Selye in his earliest conceptualization of stress response. Psychoneuroendocrinology involves the structural and functional relationships between hormonal systems and the central nervous system and the behavioral pattern derived from both.

Corticotropin releasing hormone (CRH), adrenocorticotropic hormone (ACTH) and cortisol are elevated in response to a variety of physical and psychological stresses and serve as prime factors in the maintenance of homeostasis and the development of adaptive responses to any challenging stimuli. A normal glucocorticoid stress response helps the body to recover after the challenge. The hormonal response is dependent not only on the characteristics of the stressor but also on how the individual is able to cope with it.

Exposure to chronic stress produces increased concentration of CRH in the paraventricular nucleus of hypothalamus. Over time, continued stress (chronic stress) produces increasing allostatic load. Allostasis is the process of achieving stability, or homeostasis, through physiological or behavioral change. This can be carried out by means of alteration in HPA axis hormones, the autonomic nervous system, cytokines, or a number of other systems. The higher the allostatic load, the more damage stress is doing to the body. The sustained effects of hypercortisolemia in chronic stress lead to hyperglycemia, increased visceral fat, elevated blood pressure, hyperlipidemia and changes in immune response. If allostatic load is reduced by proper eating, proper sleeping and proper knowledge of allostasis, the ill effects of chronic stress can be reduced.

Psychiatric patients have a greater risk of premature mortality due to cardiovascular diseases. Evidences show that psychiatric conditions are characterized by an increased risk of metabolic syndrome. This increased risk is present for a range of psychiatric conditions, including major depressive disorder, schizophrenia, anxiety disorder, bipolar disorder and post-traumatic stress disorder. Contributing factors are an unhealthy life style and poor adherence to medical regimen.

HOUSSAY ANIMAL

Houssay animal is an animal in which both the pancreas and the pituitary are removed. Houssay demonstrated that features of hyperglycemia, glycosuria and ketosis seen in a pancreatectomized animal disappeared when it was further subjected to hypophysectomy.

ACTH, TSH and growth hormone secreted by the anterior pituitary, produces hyperglycemia in the pancreatectomized animal due to lack of insulin. Hypophysectomy relieves the diabetogenic symptoms in the Houssay animal. This experiment proves the antagonistic effects of insulin and hormones of the anterior pituitary.

GLUCAGON

Glucagon is a polypeptide hormone containing 29 amino acid residues secreted by A-cells of islets of pancreas. It is synthesized from **preproglucagon** in the islet cells. Preproglucagon contains **glycentin-related polypeptide (GRPP)**, glucagon and two glucagon-like peptides (GLP-1 and GLP-2) **(Flowchart 68.4)**. GRPP is also stored in the A-granules along with glucagon, and is also secreted along with glucagon and has glucagon-like activity. Glycentin is produced as such from gastrointestinal mucosa along with glucagon by the APUD cells of gastrointestinal tract. Glycentin is a polypeptide that has some glucagon activity, and consists of glucagon and GRPP. The physiological role of GLP-1 is to stimulate insulin secretion after a meal. It is a potent incretin hormone produced by L-cells of the distal ileum and colon. The role of GLP-2 is not yet known.

Metabolism

Glucagon is metabolized in the liver. Half-life is 5–10 min.

Actions of Glucagon

Glucagon is a hormone of energy release, whereas insulin is a hormone of energy storage. Glucagon is an **anti-insulin hormone** or hyperglycemic hormone which is **glycogenolytic, gluconeogenic, lipolytic and ketogenic**.

- Stimulates glycogenolysis by stimulating the enzyme adenylate cyclase and thus increasing intracellular cAMP in liver. This via protein kinase-A activates phosphorylase enzyme and causes breakdown of glycogen to glucose which is released into circulation causing hyperglycemia. *Glucagon does not cause glycogenolysis in muscle.*
- Stimulates gluconeogenesis by increasing hepatic uptake of amino acids, thus making it available for conversion into glucose.
- Decreases metabolism of glucose 6-phosphate in the liver cells and the consequent buildup of glucose 6-phosphate leads to increased release of glucose into circulation.
- Stimulates lipolysis and increases the free fatty acid level in plasma.
- Glucagon stimulates the secretion of growth hormone, insulin and pancreatic somatostatin.
- Calorigenic action is due to hepatic deamination and not due to hyperglycemia.
- Large doses of glucagon increases force of contraction of heart by increasing myocardial cAMP.

> Insulin and glucagon have opposing effects. Insulin is anabolic and it increases the storage of glucose, amino acids and fatty acids. Glucagon is catabolic and it mobilizes glucose, amino acids and fatty acids and increases their blood level.

Regulation of Secretion of Glucagon

See **Table 68.5**.

Differences between insulin and glucagon are given in **Table 68.6**.

SOMATOSTATIN

Somatostatin is a hormone secreted by the D-cells of pancreatic islets. Types of somatostatin are:
1. Somatostatin-14 (SS-14)
2. Somatostatin-28 (SS-28)

Actions of Somatostatin

- Somatostatin inhibits secretion of insulin, glucagon and pancreatic polypeptide by its **paracrine action**. SS-28 is more potent than SS-14 in inhibiting insulin secretion. Excess pancreatic production of somatostatin causes hyperglycemia and other manifestations of diabetes.
- It decreases the motility of stomach, duodenum and gallbladder. As a result, gastric emptying is delayed and results in dyspepsia. Due to decreased motility of

Table 68.5: Factors affecting glucagon secretion.

Stimulants of glucagon secretion	Inhibitors
• Amino acids such as alanine, serine, glycine, cysteine	• Hyperglycemia
• Hormones such as gastrin, CCK, cortisol	• Insulin, somatostatin
	• Secretin
• Hypoglycemia, exercise	• Ketone bodies
• Vagal stimulation	• Free fatty acids
• Adrenergic β-receptor stimulation	• α-adrenergic stimulation
	• GABA

Table 68.6: Differences between insulin and glucagon.

Insulin	Glucagon
Secreted by B cells or beta cells of islets of Langerhans	Secreted by A cells or alpha cells of islets
Anabolic hormone I.e., it increases storage of glucose, fatty acids and amino acids	Catabolic in action. It increases mobilization of glucose, amino acids and fatty acids from the storage depots into the blood
Deficiency leads to hyperglycemia and excess leads to hypoglycemia	Deficiency leads to hypoglycemia and excess leads to hyperglycemia

Flowchart 68.4: Structure of preproglucagon.

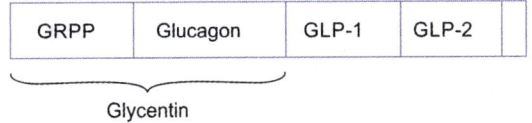

gallbladder, gallstones are formed if somatostatin is present in excess.

Somatostatin is also released from the GIT into the peripheral blood.

Stimuli that Increase Somatostatin Secretion

- Hyperglycemia
- Amino acids such as arginine and leucine
- Hormones such as CCK
- Free fatty acids.

PANCREATIC POLYPEPTIDE

Pancreatic polypeptide (PP) is secreted by F cells of pancreatic islets. It is a polypeptide with 36 amino acid residues. It is closely related to polypeptide YY and neuropeptide Y. Only known function of pancreatic polypeptide is that it slows down the absorption of food from GIT.

Regulation of Secretion of PP

Secretion of pancreatic polypeptide is increased by a meal containing proteins, during fasting, in exercise and in acute hypoglycemia. It is decreased by somatostatin and intravenous glucose administration.

Pancreatic hormones and their main actions are summarised in **Table 68.9**.

CONTROL OF BLOOD GLUCOSE

Normally, blood glucose level is kept within a narrow range (fasting blood glucose: 70–110 mg/dL) by stimulating or depressing processes such as glycogenolysis, glycogenesis, gluconeogenesis, glycolysis, etc. This occurs by the activity of different hormones and organs that control blood glucose level.

Hormones Affecting Blood Glucose (Tables 68.7 and 68.8)

1. **Insulin** lowers blood glucose level by stimulating glycogenesis and increasing peripheral utilization of glucose. It also inhibits glycogenolysis and gluconeogenesis.
2. **Glucagon** increases blood glucose level by promoting glycogenolysis and gluconeogenesis. It inhibits glycogenesis (glycogen synthesis).
3. **Epinephrine and norepinephrine** increase blood glucose by stimulating glycogenolysis and gluconeogenesis. It also inhibits peripheral utilization of glucose.
4. **Cortisol** increases blood glucose by exerting anti-insulin action on peripheral tissues.
5. **Thyroxine and growth hormone** (GH) also increase blood glucose. Thyroxine increases glucose absorption from the intestine. It increases glycogenolysis in the liver, heart and skeletal muscle and increases gluconeogenesis in the liver. GH produces hyperglycemia by increasing hepatic glucose output and by decreasing glucose uptake by skeletal muscle and adipose tissue. In excess, thyroxine and GH precipitate diabetes mellitus.

Table 68.7: Hormones affecting blood glucose levels.

Increase in blood glucose	Decrease
Cortisol, ACTH, glucagon, thyroxine, catecholamines, growth hormone, estrogen and progesterone	Insulin, incretins

Table 68.8: Actions of hormones on blood glucose level.

Hormone	Effects
Insulin	• Decreases blood glucose • Increases glycogen synthesis • Promotes glycolysis • Inhibits gluconeogenesis
Glucagon	• Increases blood glucose • Stimulates glycogenolysis • Increases gluconeogenesis • Decreases glycogen synthesis • Inhibits glycolysis
ACTH and cortisol	• Increase blood glucose • Increase gluconeogenesis • Release amino acids from muscle
Catecholamines	• Increase blood glucose level • Stimulate glycogenolysis • Increase gluconeogenesis
Growth hormone	• Increases blood glucose level • Decreases glycolysis • Mobilizes fatty acids from adipose tissue
Thyroxine	• Increases blood glucose level • Increases absorption of glucose from the intestine
Incretins	• Decreases blood glucose level indirectly • Stimulates insulin secretion from pancreas

6. **Incretins** such as gastric inhibitory polypeptide (GIP) decrease blood glucose level by increasing release of insulin from the β-cells of pancreas.

Organs that Control Blood Glucose

- **Liver** plays a major role in maintaining blood glucose level constant. In hypoglycemia, glycogenolysis and gluconeogenesis are stimulated in the liver and hepatic glucose output increases bringing back blood glucose to normal. When blood glucose level is high, glycogen synthesis (glycogenesis) is stimulated in the liver. At the same time, glycogenolysis and gluconeogenesis are inhibited. This results in lowering of blood glucose level.
- **Skeletal muscle** also plays a role in maintaining blood glucose. Excess of glucose is stored in the skeletal muscle as glycogen. Peripheral utilization of glucose is increased in the skeletal muscle during exercise. Exercise is advised in diabetic patients to decrease blood glucose level.

Paracrine Function of the Hormones of the Islets of Langerhans

The islet cell hormones released into the extracellular fluid diffuse to other islet cells and influence their function in a paracrine fashion and help in the regulation of nutrient

CHAPTER 68 — Endocrine Pancreas

Table 68.9: Pancreatic islet hormones and their main actions.

Hormone	Source	Main actions	Control of secretion
Glucagon	Alpha (α) cells	Increases blood glucose by: • Glycogenolysis in liver • Gluconeogenesis • Lipolysis	• Stimulated by hypoglycemia, exercise and high protein diet • Inhibited by somatostatin and insulin
Insulin	Beta (β) cells	Decrease blood glucose by: • Transport of glucose into cells • Increased glycogenesis • Increased lipogenesis • Increased protein synthesis • Inhibiting glycogenolysis and gluconeogenesis	• Stimulated by hyperglycemia, vagal stimulation, glucagon, ACTH; arginine and leucine • Inhibited by somatostatin
Somatostatin	Delta (δ) cells	• Inhibit glucagon and insulin secretion • Inhibit gastrointestinal motility	Inhibited by pancreatic polypeptide
Pancreatic polypeptide	F cells	• Inhibit somatostatin secretion • Inhibit absorption of food in GIT • Causes gallbladder contraction	• Stimulated by high protein diet, fasting exercise and hypoglycemia • Inhibited by hyperglycemia and somatostatin

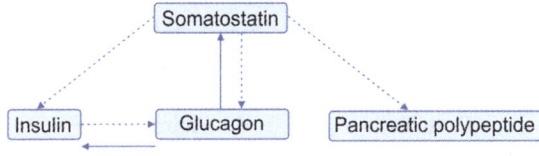

Flowchart 68.5: Paracrine control of pancreatic hormones.

homeostasis. Somatostatin inhibits the secretion of insulin, glucagon and pancreatic polypeptide. Insulin inhibits the secretion of glucagon and glucagon stimulates the secretion of insulin and somatostatin (**Flowchart 68.5**).

■ MULTIPLE CHOICE QUESTIONS

1. **Delta cells or D cells of pancreas secrete:**
   a. Glucagon
   b. Insulin
   c. Somatostatin
   d. Pancreatic polypeptide

2. **The substances secreted by the endocrine part of pancreas are all, except:**
   a. Somatostatin
   b. Pancreatic polypeptide
   c. Chymotrypsin
   d. Glucagon

3. **The mechanism that protects the normal pancreatic tissue from auto digestion is:**
   a. Secretion of bicarbonate
   b. Protease inhibitors present in plasma
   c. Proteolytic enzymes secreted in the inactive form
   d. The resistance of pancreatic cells

4. **All the following changes are seen on the 5th day of fasting, except:**
   a. Increase in free fatty acid level
   b. Decreased glucose tolerance
   c. Decreased growth hormone
   d. Decreased level of insulin

5. **Glycogen reserve get exhausted in the first how many hours of fasting?**
   a. 12 hours
   b. 24 hours
   c. 36 hours
   d. 48 hours

6. **All the following are seen in hypoglycemia, except:**
   a. Increase in gluconeogenesis
   b. Decrease in glucagon
   c. Decrease in insulin
   d. Increase in growth hormone

7. **All the following cause hyperglycemia, except:**
   a. Insulin
   b. Growth hormone
   c. Catecholamines
   d. Cortisol

8. **True about the action of insulin is:**
   a. Causes gluconeogenesis
   b. Not useful for growth and development
   c. Required for the transport of glucose, amino acid, Na^+ and K^+
   d. Catabolic hormone

9. **In the fetus, insulin and thyroxin secretion begins by:**
   a. 3rd month
   b. 5th month
   c. 7th month
   d. 9th month

10. **Glucose-mediated insulin release is mediated through:**
    a. ATP dependent K^+ channels
    b. cAMP
    c. Carrier modulators
    d. Receptor phosphorylation

11. **Insulin secretion is decreased by:**
    a. Glucagon
    b. Glucose
    c. Adrenaline
    d. Vagal stimulation

12. **Increased ratio of insulin to glucagon causes:**
    a. Decreased levels of cAMP
    b. Decreased levels of lipoprotein lipase
    c. Decreased amino acid synthesis
    d. Enhanced lipolysis in adipose tissue

13. All the following are actions of insulin on adipose tissue, *except*:
    a. Decreased glucose entry into adipose tissue
    b. Increased fatty acid synthesis
    c. Activation of lipoprotein lipase
    d. Inhibition of lipolysis
14. Human insulin differs from bovine insulin by how many amino acid residues?
    a. 1
    b. 2
    c. 3
    d. 4
15. Diet devoid of carbohydrate causes:
    a. Ketosis
    b. Diabetes mellitus
    c. No effect
    d. Obesity
16. Energy of brain during prolonged starvation is mainly from:
    a. Glucose
    b. Ketones
    c. Fatty acids
    d. Amino acids
17. How many parts are there in insulin receptor?
    a. 1
    b. 2
    c. 3
    d. 4
18. Ketoacidosis is seen in all the following conditions, *except*:
    a. Starvation
    b. Diabetes mellitus
    c. High fat, low carbohydrate diet
    d. High carbohydrate diet
19. Insulin secretion is increased with the following, *except*:
    a. Glucose
    b. Vagal stimulation
    c. Adrenaline
    d. Acetyl choline
20. Stress induced hyperglycemia is due to all, *except*:
    a. Glucocorticoids
    b. Growth hormone
    c. Catecholamines
    d. Thyroxine
21. Endogenous triglycerides are maximum in:
    a. VLDL
    b. LDL
    c. HDL
    d. Chylomicrons
22. The normal non-fasting blood ketone level is:
    a. 0.1–9.5 mg%
    b. 0.5–2 mg%
    c. 2–10 mg%
    d. 100–500 mg%
23. Anabolic action on protein is mediated by:
    a. ACTH
    b. TSH
    c. Insulin
    d. Adrenaline
24. Experimental diabetes is caused by:
    a. Alloxan
    b. PgE1
    c. Radioactive sodium
    d. Gold chloride
25. Somyogi phenomenon is:
    a. Hypoglycemia followed by hyperglycemia
    b. Hyperglycemia followed by hypoglycemia
    c. Glycosuria with normal blood sugar
    d. Reactive hyperglycemia
26. Insulin stress test assay estimates:
    a. Diabetes mellitus
    b. Growth hormone
    c. Glucagon assay
    d. Catecholamines
27. Insulin facilitates glucose uptake in:
    a. Kidney tubules
    b. Red blood cells
    c. Brain
    d. Skeletal muscle
28. Glucagon stimulates:
    a. Glycogenolysis
    b. Bile secretion
    c. Hydrochloric acid secretion
    d. Intestinal secretion
29. Increase in insulin receptor is seen in:
    a. Starvation
    b. Obesity
    c. Acromegaly
    d. Diabetes mellitus
30. An adult human pancreas has about:
    a. 100–2000 islets
    b. 1 lakh–2 lakhs islets
    c. 2.5 lakhs–7.5 lakhs islets
    d. Above 10 lakhs islets
31. Somatostatin is produced by which cells of pancreas?
    a. Alpha cells
    b. Beta cells
    c. Delta cells
    d. Acinar cells
32. Beta cells of pancreas produce:
    a. Glucagon
    b. Gastrin
    c. Insulin
    d. Pancreatic polypeptide
33. Which is false regarding insulin?
    a. Secreted by beta cells
    b. Glycopeptides
    c. Causes lipogenesis
    d. Promotes glycogenesis
34. Insulin helps entry of glucose into the following cells, *except*:
    a. Liver
    b. Muscle
    c. Adipose tissue
    d. Brain tissue
35. Glucose transport across the following cells does not require insulin, *except*:
    a. Gastrointestinal tract
    b. Kidney tubules
    c. Red blood cells
    d. Adipose tissue cell
36. Insulin secretion is stimulated by all, *except*:
    a. Amino acid
    b. Fat
    c. Gastrointestinal peptide
    d. Hyperglycemia
37. Most abundant islet cell type is:
    a. D cell
    b. A cell
    c. F cell
    d. B cell
38. Somatostatin is produced by:
    a. A cell
    b. B cell
    c. D cell
    d. F cell

39. **Which is the hormone that contain sulfur:**
    a. Insulin
    b. Thyroxine
    c. LH
    d. FSH

40. **Insulin release occurs by:**
    a. Endocytosis
    b. Exocytosis
    c. Active transport
    d. Facilitated diffusion

41. **Glycogenolysis is mediated by:**
    a. Alpha 1 receptor
    b. Alpha 1 + Beta 2 receptor
    c. Beta 2 receptor
    d. Alpha 2 + Beta 1 receptor

42. **Most important side effect of insulin is:**
    a. Hypoglycemia
    b. Lipodystrophy
    c. Insulin resistance
    d. Production of antibodies to insulin

43. **All are true of insulin, *except*:**
    a. It is secreted by the beta cells of pancreas
    b. It promotes lipogenesis
    c. It is a steroid hormone
    d. It promotes glycogenesis

44. **Insulin is required for the transport of glucose into:**
    a. Intestinal epithelial cells
    b. Renal tubular cells
    c. Liver cells
    d. Adipose tissue cells

45. **Which of the following is related to type-2 diabetes mellitus?**
    a. Obesity
    b. Insulin resistance
    c. Target defect
    d. Beta cell destruction

46. **Somatostatin is produced in the:**
    a. Hypothalamus
    b. Anterior pituitary
    c. Delta cells of pancreas
    d. Alpha cells of pancreas

47. **The satiety center is located in the:**
    a. Dorsomedian nucleus of hypothalamus
    b. Ventromedian nucleus of hypothalamus
    c. Perifornical region
    d. Lateral hypothalamic area

ANSWERS

1. c	2. c	3. c	4. c	5. d
6. b	7. a	8. c	9. a	10. a
11. c	12. a	13. a	14. a	15. a
16. b	17. d	18. d	19. c	20. d
21. a	22. b	23. c	24. a	25. a
26. b	27. d	28. a	29. a	30. d
31. c	32. c	33. b	34. d	35. d
36. b	37. d	38. c	39. a	40. b
41. b	42. a	43. c	44. d	45. b
46. c	47. b			

Other Endocrine Organs and Local Hormones

CHAPTER 69

LEARNING OBJECTIVES
- Explain the physiological role of thymus
- Describe the functions of prostaglandins
- Discuss the functions of atrial natriuretic hormone
- Explain the role of local hormones in the body

INTRODUCTION

Other organs that secrete hormones include thymus, heart, kidney, placenta and intestine. The hormones produced by the gastrointestinal system are discussed in detail in Chapter 53. The hormones produced by other organs and tissues are given in **Table 69.1**.

THYMUS

PY8.3: Describe the physiology of thymus and pineal gland.

Introduction

Primary lymphoid organs are thymus and bone marrow. Thymus is a bilobed gland derived from the 3rd and 4th pharyngeal pouches. It is located in the mediastinum between the sternum and aorta. Each lobe consists of **outer cortex and inner medulla**. During childhood, thymus has a well-defined cortex and medulla. As age advances, it is replaced by connective tissue. Cortex is composed of T cells, dendritic cells, epithelial cells and macrophages. The endocrine epithelium of thymus is derived from the **neural crest**.

At birth, it weighs about 10 g and the weight progressively increases and reaches a maximum of 20–30 g during adolescence. Later it degenerates and weighs only 3–6 g in old age. Sex hormones have a role in thymic involution. After castration in children it is seen that the thymus fails to involute.

Functions

- Thymus plays a very important role in processing T lymphocytes. Thymus is the site of initial T lymphocyte differentiation. Immature T cells migrate from the red bone marrow to the cortex of thymus where they proliferate and mature. Most of the preprocessing of T lymphocytes in the thymus occurs shortly before birth of a baby and for a few months after birth. Beyond this period, removal of the thymus gland diminishes (but does not eliminate) the T-lymphocytic immune system. However, removal of the thymus several months before birth can prevent development of cell-mediated immunity.

- The epithelial cells of the thymus secrete **thymosin**, a hormone that controls the proliferation and maturation of primitive lymphocytes into immunologically competent T cells. It also secretes **thymopoietin**, another hormone which is a polypeptide that induces the differentiation of prolymphocytes into immunologically competent T cells. Medulla contains more mature T cells. T cells that leave the thymus are carried to lymph node, spleen, etc.

- Auto reactive clones (clones of cells that react with self-antigens) are eliminated in the thymus. The thymus makes certain that any T lymphocytes leaving the thymus will not react against proteins or other antigens that are present in the body's own tissues; otherwise, the T lymphocytes would be lethal to the person's own body.

Table 69.1: Hormones produced by other organs and tissues.

Organ/Tissue	Hormones
Thymus	• Thymosin • Thymopoietin
Heart	Atrial natriuretic peptide
Kidney	• Erythropoietin • Renin • Calcitriol • Prostaglandin E_2
Placenta	• HCG, HCS estrogen, progesterone • Relaxin
Intestine	Gastrin, secretin, CCK, VIP, GIP, GRP, somatostatin, glucagon, glicentin, motilin, bombesin, ghrelin, peptide YY, neurotensin and guanylin
Endothelium	Endothelin, nitric oxide (NO)
Adipose tissue	Leptin, resistin

Clinical Importance

- In children with genetic immunodeficiency disease and in patients with lymphocytopenia secondary to radiation or chemotherapy for cancer, significant clinical improvement has been reported after injections of thymosin.
- In myasthenia gravis, there is enlargement of the thymus. It is seen that thymectomy relieves the symptoms of myasthenia gravis.
- In endocrine disorders like acromegaly, grave's disease, etc. the thymus enlarges.

KIDNEY

Kidney produces many important hormones like renin, erythropoietin, 1,25-dihydroxycholecalciferol, prostaglandin, etc.

Renin

Renin is an acid protease with 340 amino acid residues secreted by the juxtaglomerular cells of juxtaglomerular apparatus. Half-life of renin in circulation is 80 min or less.

Stimuli for renin secretion are:
- Na^+ depletion and dehydration
- Hemorrhage and hypotension
- Decrease in renal perfusion pressure, e.g., constriction of renal artery
- Cardiac failure
- Cirrhosis liver
- Drugs like diuretics
- Prostaglandins.

Stimuli that inhibit renin secretion:
- Increased Na^+ and Cl^- reabsorption across macula densa
- Increased afferent arteriolar pressure
- Angiotensin II
- Vasopressin.

Action of Renin

Renin acts on α_2-globulin called angiotensinogen secreted by liver. The only known function of renin is to convert angiotensinogen to angiotensin-I which is a decapeptide. Angiotensin-I is acted upon by angiotensin converting enzyme **(ACE)** to form angiotensin-II which is an octapeptide. Enzyme **angiotensinase** converts angiotensin-II to angiotensin-III.

Regulation of Renin Secretion

- Intrarenal baroreceptor mechanism - When the arteriolar pressure at the level of juxtaglomerular cells decreases as in hypotension, there will be an increase in renin secretion and vice versa. Renal artery constriction and constriction of the aorta proximal to the renal arteries also decreases renal arteriolar pressure.
- Renin secretion is inversely proportional to the amount of Na^+ and Cl^- entering the distal tubules from the loop of Henle. These electrolytes enter the macula densa via the Na^+-K^+-$2Cl^-$ transporters present in their apical membranes. This increase triggers a signal that decreases renin secretion from the juxtaglomerular cells in the adjacent afferent arteriole. The signal is assumed to be NO.
- Renin secretion also varies inversely with the plasma K^+ level.
- Angiotensin II feedback to inhibit renin secretion by a direct action on the juxtaglomerular cell
- Vasopressin also inhibits renin secretion
- Sympathetic stimulation increases renin secretion. A decrease in central venous pressure increases sympathetic activity. The increased renin secretion is mediated by increased circulating catecholamines and by the norepinephrine secreted by the postganglionic renal sympathetic nerves. It acts on β_1-adrenergic receptors on the juxtaglomerular cells and renin release is mediated by an increase in intracellular cAMP.

> **Plasma renin activity (PRA)** or random plasma renin is a measure of the activity of the enzyme renin in plasma. It is determined by incubating the sample to be assayed and measuring by immunoassay the amount of angiotensin I generated. Deficiency of angiotensinogen as well as renin can lead to low PRA value. To avoid this, exogenous angiotensinogen is often added, so that plasma renin concentration (PRC) is measured. The normal PRA is approximately 1 ng of angiotensin-I generated per milliliter per hour for normal sodium diet. The plasma angiotensin-II concentration in such subjects is about 25 pg/mL. PRA is measured in certain diseases which present with hypertension or hypotension. It is also measured in some tumors. Patients with secondary hyperaldosteronism will have increased plasma levels of renin. Plasma renin activity is reduced in patients with hypertension due to primary hyperaldosteronism. PRA is increased in 50-80% of patients with renal hypertension.

Actions of Angiotensin-II

- It is a powerful vasoconstrictor and produces a rise in systolic and diastolic pressure. It is 4–8 times more potent than noradrenaline in increasing blood pressure.
- It acts on zona glomerulosa of adrenal cortex and stimulates aldosterone secretion. Renin-angiotensin-aldosterone mechanism is an important regulatory mechanism in maintaining blood pressure.
- It stimulates release of norepinephrine from the sympathetic nerve endings by direct action.
- It causes contraction of mesangial cells of renal glomerulus and decreases GFR, and exerts a direct effect on the renal tubules to increase Na^+ reabsorption
- It acts directly on brain to increase blood pressure by increasing water intake due to its direct action on hypothalamus.
- It stimulates release of ADH and ACTH
- Renin-angiotensin systems are found in the walls of blood vessels, eyes, exocrine pancreas, heart, adrenal cortex, gonads, brain, etc. Tissue renin contributes very little to the circulating renin pool. Tissue angiotensin II is a significant growth factor in the heart and blood vessels. ACE inhibitors or angiotensin II receptor blockers are used in the treatment of heart failure due to the inhibition of the growth effects of angiotensin II.

Actions of Angiotensin-III

Angiotensin III has 40% pressor activity and 100% aldosterone secreting activity.

Erythropoietin

Erythropoietin is a glycoprotein with 166 amino acid residues. In adults, 85% of erythropoietin is secreted by kidney and 15% by liver. Fetal liver also produces large amounts of erythropoietin. Half-life is 5 hrs.

Main function of erythropoietin is to stimulate erythropoiesis. It acts on stem cells in the bone marrow and converts them into proerythroblasts. Most important stimulus for erythropoietin secretion is hypoxia. Other stimulants include cobalt salts, androgens, catecholamines, etc.

HEART

Atrial Natriuretic Peptide

The most important hormone produced by the heart is **atrial natriuretic peptide** (ANP). It is produced by the atrial cells. ANP is a polypeptide with 28 amino acid residues and is synthesized from a precursor molecule called preprohormone which is a large polypeptide. A second natriuretic peptide known as brain natriuretic peptide (**BNP**) or **B-type natriuretic peptide** is present in brain and heart including ventricles. Some of the amino acid residues in this type are different from atrial natriuretic peptide. A third member of this family has been isolated from brain, kidneys and vascular endothelial cells named **C-type natriuretic peptide (CNP)**. But the actions of all these three peptides are similar.

Actions of ANP

- ANP produces **natriuresis and diuresis**. The receptors for ANP are situated in the mesangial cells of glomeruli.
  - ANP causes relaxation of the mesangial cells and dilation of afferent arteriole thereby increases the surface area for filtration. Thus, glomerular filtration rate (GFR) is increased. As a result, Na^+ and water excretion are increased.
  - ANP also acts directly on renal tubule and inhibit Na^+ reabsorption thus enhancing Na^+ excretion.
- ANP lowers blood pressure by the following mechanisms:
  - Decrease the responsiveness of vascular smooth muscle to circulating catecholamines, angiotensin-II, vasopressin, serotonin, etc.
  - Increases capillary permeability leading to extravasation of fluid into the tissue spaces producing a decrease in blood volume and a decline in blood pressure.
  - Inhibit renin secretion and thus counteract the pressor effect of catecholamines and angiotensin II. Effect of ANP is opposite to angiotensin II.
  - Relax vascular smooth muscles of arterioles and venules.
- It also decreases responsiveness of zona glomerulosa to stimuli that increase aldosterone secretion.
- ANP is responsible for aldosterone escape in primary hyperaldosteronism (refer aldosterone escape). This is the reason for absence of edema in these patients.

Regulation of Secretion

Secretion of ANP is proportionate to the degree to which atria is stretched by increase in central venous pressure. ANP is increased by an increase in Na^+ intake and by an increase in extracellular fluid volume. BNP secretion from heart is increased when the ventricles are stretched. ANP is decreased when there is decrease in central venous pressure. Normal plasma level is 5 fmol/mL. Plasma level of ANP and BNP is increased in heart failure.

LOCAL HORMONES (TABLE 69.2)

Local hormones are produced by different tissues of the body and exert their action locally. Examples are **histamine, serotonin, prostaglandin, bradykinin, acetylcholine, noradrenaline, gastrointestinal hormones; and neurotransmitters like ACh, substance P, etc.**

Histamine

Histamine is formed from amino acid **histidine** by the action of **histidine decarboxylase**. In our body, histamine is found in mast cells, basophils, gastric mucosal cells and brain cells (hypothalamus, limbic cortex, etc.).

It is also present in some bee venom and in the stings of certain insects. The highest concentration of histamine occurs in skin, intestine and lungs i.e. at surfaces in contact with the outside world.

Fate of Histamine

Histamine is excreted as free form or conjugated form in urine. Conjugated form is *N*-acetyl histamine. It is oxidized to 4-imidazole acetic acid and is excreted in urine.

Actions of Histamine

- It causes relaxation of arterioles and pre-capillary sphincter. Intravenous injection of histamine produces vasodilatation of skin vessels, a rise in body temperature, a fall in systolic and diastolic pressure and increase in heart rate.
- Increases the tone of smooth muscle of intestine, bladder and bronchioles. In GIT, histamine increases motility.
- It is a potent stimulus for HCl secretion in stomach and a moderate stimulant for pepsin secretion.
- Stimulates secretion from pancreas, salivary glands and intestine.

Table 69.2: Sites of synthesis of local hormones.	
Local hormones synthesized in tissues	*Local hormones synthesized in blood*
• Prostaglandins, thromboxanes, prostacyclin, leukotrienes, and lipoxins • Acetylcholine, norepinephrine, serotonin, histamine, substance P, and gastrointestinal hormones	• Serotonin • Angiotensinogen • Bradykinin

- Plays a role in the production of pain and itching.
- Release of histamine occurs in response to physical stimuli like firm pressure, application of heat or cold.
- In allergy to foreign proteins, it is responsible for anaphylaxis. Antigen reacts with tissue antibody and cause release of histamine and slow reacting substance (SRS). It causes severe bronchoconstriction and profound fall in arterial BP.

Mechanism of Action

There are two receptors for histamine, H_1 and H_2 receptors. Action on smooth muscle is mediated through H_1 receptors and increase in HCl secretion is mediated through H_2 receptors. H_2 receptor antagonists, cimetidine, ranitidine, famotidine, etc., are used in the treatment of peptic ulcer.

Serotonin or 5-Hydroxytryptamine

Serotonin is formed from amino acid **tryptophan**. In our body, serotonin is produced by enterochromaffin cells, platelets, lungs and brain cells (hypothalamus, limbic system, and cerebellum). Serotonin containing neurons are present in the midline raphe nucleus of brain stem. The hallucinogen, LSD is a serotonin agonist.

Serotonin is metabolized in the liver to 5-hydroxy indole acetic acid and is excreted through urine.

Actions of Serotonin

- It is a cardiac stimulant.
- It is a powerful vasoconstrictor.
- It increases systolic and diastolic pressure.
- Produces bronchospasm and hyperpnoea.
- Increases tone of smooth muscle of eye, intestine, urinary bladder, bronchioles and uterus.
- In the kidney, it has antidiuretic effect due to afferent arteriolar constriction and decrease in GFR.
- Stimulates pain nerve endings in the skin.
- Acts as a neurotransmitter.
- Serotonergic neurons in the brain have important physiological effects on mood, behavior, sleep induction, analgesic action and regulation of body temperature.

Prostaglandins

Prostaglandins (PG) are membrane-associated, biologically active lipids synthesized by every mammalian cell and tissue. It was first isolated from prostatic secretion and hence the name. It is synthesized from **arachidonic acid (Flowchart 69.1).**

Prostaglandins are composed of 20-carbon unsaturated fatty acids containing 5 carbon atoms joined to form a cyclopentane ring. They are modulators of cAMP-induced responses. Different types of prostaglandins are:
- PGA_1, PGA_2
- PGE_1, PGE_2
- PGF_1, PGF_2.

Functions of Prostaglandins

- On cardiovascular system, PGA produces vasodilatation and is used in the treatment of hypertension. PGA_2 increases renal blood flow and increases urinary excretion of sodium, potassium and water.

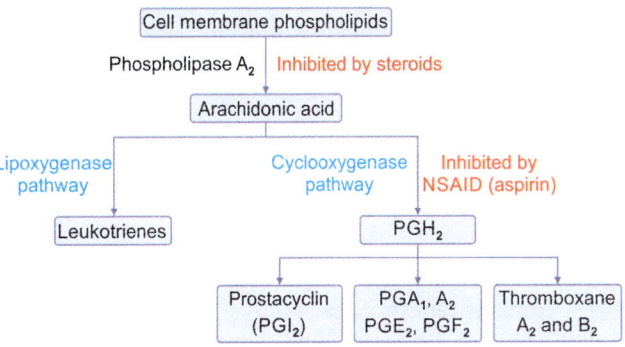

Flowchart 69.1: Synthesis of prostaglandins.

- On reproductive system, actions of PGE and PGF are:
  - Stimulate contraction of gravid uterus and induce labor.
  - Luteolysis
  - Decrease progesterone secretion.
  - Stimulates release of GnRH from hypothalamus.
  - Used in the treatment of infertility in males.
  - Used for medical termination of pregnancy (MTP)
  - $PGF_{2\alpha}$ found in menstrual blood causes painful uterine contractions (dysmenorrhea). Its concentration in the amniotic fluid is increased during labor.
- On respiratory system, PGE_2 produces bronchial relaxation, so, used in the treatment of asthma.
- Inhibit secretion of glucagon, epinephrine and steroids. Decreases cAMP by inhibiting adenylate cyclase, thus inhibiting the actions of glucagon and epinephrine.
- Inhibit the release of naturally induced norepinephrine.
- Acts as a neurotransmitter.
- PGE_2 and $PGF_{2\alpha}$ produce miosis (pupillary constriction) and increase in intraocular pressure.
- PGE_2 inhibits HCl secretion and help in the healing of peptic ulcer.
- PGE and PGF stimulate intestinal motility.
- Produce natriuresis.
- PGI_2 inhibits blood coagulation by preventing platelet aggregation, whereas PGE_2 and PGF_2 favor clotting.
- PGE_2 & F_2 act as natural mediators of inflammation and cause pain and increase in temperature. Systemic administration of PG produces headache and fever.
- Prostaglandins maintain the patency of ductus arteriosus prior to birth. So, in patients with patent ductus arteriosus (PDA), prostaglandin inhibitors are used for treatment.

> Synthetic prostaglandins are used to induce labor, as a vasodilator in pulmonary hypertension, to reduce gastric acid secretion and treat peptic ulcers.

Prostaglandin Inhibitors

- Nonsteroidal anti-inflammatory drugs like aspirin, indomethacin, phenybutazone, etc. act by inhibiting cyclooxygenase enzyme by acetylation.

- Steroidal anti-inflammatory drugs like hydrocortisone, prednisolone, etc. act by inhibiting phospholipase A_2, which is the rate limiting enzyme in prostaglandin synthesis (*see* **Flowchart 69.1**).

Bradykinin

Bradykinin is a member of the kinin family having 9 amino acids (non a peptide).

Actions

- It is considered as the third factor for the reabsorption of Na^+ from the renal tubules.
- It is a potent vasodilator and is responsible for cutaneous vasodilatation during sweating. This is because bradykinin-forming enzyme is released from the sweat gland along with sweat.
- It is involved in producing pain and inflammation by inducing changes in vascular permeability and by eliciting vasodilatation.
- Stimulates the release of arachidonic acid from phospholipid stores.

Acetylcholine

Acetylcholine is found in:
- All ganglia where transmission occurs from preganglionic neuron to postganglionic neuron.
- Parasympathetic postganglionic endings.
- Neuromuscular junction.
- Sympathetic cholinergic endings supplying sweat glands and sympathetic vasodilator system seen in muscle blood vessels.
- Certain synapses in CNS.

Synthesis and Degradation of Acetylcholine

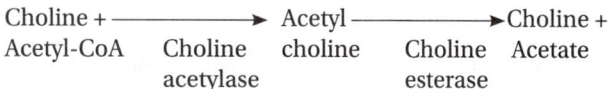

Cholinergic Receptors

There are two types of receptors:
- **Muscarinic receptors** are present in heart, smooth muscles and glands.
- **Nicotinic receptors** are present in the autonomic ganglia and in the motor endplate of neuromuscular junction.

Action of muscarinic receptors is similar to the alkaloid muscarine. The effects are blocked by the drug *atropine*. Nicotinic receptor action is similar to the actions of nicotine. Small doses of acetylcholine in the ganglia facilitate transmission and large doses inhibit. The effects are blocked by ganglion blocking drugs. The effect of acetylcholine at the neuromuscular junction is blocked by curare.

Brain contains both muscarinic and nicotinic receptors. *Presynaptic nicotinic cholinergic receptors* are present in the brain. They are located on glutamate-secreting axon terminals. Stimulation of these receptors facilitates the release of glutamate into the synaptic cleft. *Glutamate is responsible for 75% of excitatory transmission in the brain.*

ENDOTHELIUM

Endothelium constitutes a large and important tissue. They secrete many growth factors and vasoactive substances. The vasoactive substances include prostacyclin and thromboxane, nitric oxide, carbon monoxide and endothelins.

Prostacyclin and Thromboxane

Prostacyclin is produced by endothelial cells and **thromboxane A_2** by the platelets from a common precursor, arachidonic acid via cyclo-oxygenase pathway. Prostacyclin inhibits platelet aggregation and produce vasodilatation. On the other hand, thromboxane A_2 promotes platelet aggregation and produce vasoconstriction. The balance between prostacyclin and thromboxane A_2 prevent extension of a clot and maintain blood flow.

Nitric Oxide

Endothelium-derived relaxing factor (EDRF), a substance now known to be **nitric oxide (NO)** is produced by the endothelial cells. NO is synthesized from L-arginine in a reaction catalysed by nitric oxide synthase (NOS). NOS-3 is found in endothelial cells. NO acts through cGMP as the second messenger. NO is inactivated by hemoglobin.

Actions of Nitric Oxide

- NO diffuses to the smooth muscle of blood vessel and causes *relaxation of vascular smooth muscle* via cGMP. NO checks the excessive action of various vasoconstrictors that act directly on vascular smooth muscle. If NO is absent, the degree of constriction of vessels will be much greater.
- When blood flow to a tissue is to be increased, there will be arteriolar dilatation. Along with arteriolar dilatation there will be *dilatation of large arteries*. This flow induced dilatation is due to the local release of NO.
- Tonic release of NO is necessary to maintain normal *blood pressure*. When drugs that inhibit nitric oxide synthase are administered, there is a prompt rise in blood pressure due to deficiency of NO.
- NO is also involved in *vascular remodeling and angiogenesis*.
- *Penile erection* is produced by release of NO in the blood vessels of penis which lead to vasodilatation and engorgement of corpora cavernosa. The drug Viagra (sildenafil), promotes penile erection by inhibiting the inactivation of NO. This drug is a selective inhibitor of cGMP-specific phosphodiesterase which inactivates NO.
- NO inhibits superoxide anion (O^-) production by inhibiting NADPH reductase activity and decreases LDL oxidation. Thus NO has strong anti-atherosclerotic effect.
- NO is necessary for the cytotoxic activity of macrophages including its ability to kill cancer cells.
- NO inhibits platelet adhesion and aggregation. This effect along with its vasodilatory effect makes NO important for the maintenance of normal flow of blood.
- In the GIT, NO produces smooth muscle relaxation.

The drug nitroglycerin, used in the treatment of angina, exerts its vasodilator action by being converted to NO.

Table 69.3: Stimulators and inhibitors of secretion of endothelin-1.

Stimulators	Inhibitors
• Angiotensin-II • Catecholamines • Growth factors • Hypoxia • Insulin • HDL • Thrombin • Shear stress	• Nitric oxide • ANP • Prostaglandin E_2 • Prostacyclin

Carbon Monoxide

Carbon monoxide (CO) acts as a blood vessel relaxant, as signaling molecule and also acts as neurotransmitter in the brain. Carbon monoxide is produced as a byproduct during hemoglobin degradation.

ENDOTHELINS

Endothelins are a family of three highly potent vasoconstrictor peptides. They are:
1. Endothelin-1 produced by vascular endothelial cells, brain and kidney.
2. Endothelin-2 produced by kidney and intestine.
3. Endothelin-3 present in blood, brain, kidney and GIT.
    - **Endothelin-1** is a 21 amino acid polypeptide produced by endothelial cells. It is one of the most potent vasoconstrictor agents. It is secreted into the tunica media of blood vessels and act in a paracrine manner. Endothelin-1 plays a role in the pathophysiology of heart failure and myocardial infarction. In both these conditions, the circulating level of endothelin-1 is elevated.
    - Endothelin-1 is a potent growth factor for smooth muscle and a chemo-attractant for monocytes.
    - Endothelin is secreted when blood flows over the endothelium at high velocity (increased shear stress).
    - Endothelin is responsible for mesangial cell mediated decrease in glomerular filtration rate. Endothelin receptors are present in the mesangial cells of kidney.
    - Endothelin also play a role in closing the ductus arteriosus at birth.
    - Abnormality in endothelin-1 gene is seen to be associated with Hirschsprung's disease. This is because the cells that normally form the myenteric plexus fail to migrate to the distal colon. It is also associated with severe craniofacial abnormalities and die of respiratory failure at birth.
    - Regulation of secretion of endothelin-1 is given in **Table 69.3**.

MULTIPLE CHOICE QUESTIONS

1. **Prostaglandin secretion is maximum in:**
   a. Urine
   b. Semen
   c. Amniotic fluid
   d. Saliva

2. **Which of the following is true about prostaglandins?**
   a. It is a precursor to arachidonic acid
   b. It causes uterine contraction and cervical dilatation
   c. It produces vasoconstriction and increases blood pressure
   d. It increases acid secretion and decreases mucus secretion in stomach

3. **Following are local hormones, *except*:**
   a. Insulin   b. Bradykinin
   c. Heparin   d. Acetyl choline

4. **Action of ANF is mediated by:**
   a. Inositol phosphate   b. DAG
   c. Cyclic AMP   d. Cyclic GMP

ANSWERS

1. b   2. b   3. a   4. d

FILL IN THE BLANKS/ GIVE THE NORMAL VALUE/NAME THE FOLLOWING (ENDOCRINOLOGY)

1. Cell membrane receptors are specific for **protein, peptide** and **catecholamine** hormones.
2. The primary receptors for steroid hormones are found in the **cytoplasm**.
3. The receptors for thyroid hormones are found in the **nucleus**.
4. Hormones which are amino acid derivatives: **Catecholamines and thyroid hormones**.
5. Name three peptide hormones: **Calcitonin, insulin, glucagon.**
6. Name three second messengers: **cAMP, cGMP, and Ca^{2+}**.
7. Name three peptide hormones that do not require second messengers for their action: **Insulin, growth hormone and prolactin**
8. Adenylate cyclase is the enzyme present on the surface of cell membranes that catalyzes the formation of **cAMP** from **ATP**.
9. Name three hormones for which cAMP is the second messenger: **CRH, ACTH, calcitonin.**
10. cGMP is the second messenger for **ANP** and **NO**.
11. Insulin, epidermal growth factor and IGF-I receptors have intrinsic **tyrosine kinase** activities located in their cytoplasmic domains.
12. Name three receptors with intrinsic ion channels: **Nicotinic cholinergic receptor, glutamate receptor, glycine receptor.**
13. Cholera toxin increases intracellular cAMP by the persistent activation of **adenylate cyclase**.
14. Name two hormones that inhibit growth hormone secretion: **Cortisol, and medroxyprogesterone.**
15. Injury and diseases stunt growth because they increase **protein catabolism**.

16. Cessation of growth is due in large part to closure of epiphysis in the long bones by **estrogens**.
17. The hyperglycemia seen in growth hormone excess is referred to as **pituitary diabetes mellitus**.
18. In women who have an episode of shock due to postpartum hemorrhage, with the subsequent development of postpartum necrosis and pituitary insufficiency the condition is referred to as **Sheehan syndrome**.
19. Gastrointestinal motility is **increased** in hyperthyroidism and **decreased** in hypothyroidism.
20. Diabetes mellitus is characterized by **polyuria, polydipsia, polyphagia**.
21. Name three intestinal hormones that stimulate insulin secretion: **GIP, gastrin, secretin**.
22. **Pheochromocytoma** is adrenal medullary tumor which secretes norepinephrine or epinephrine or both and produce sustained hypertension.
23. Normally in the adrenal medulla, **epinephrine** is secreted more than that of **norepinephrine**.
24. In adrenal insufficiency, Na⁺ loss and circulatory shock occurs due to lack of **mineralocorticoid** and lack of **glucocorticoids**.
25. Parathyroid hormone (PTH) **increases** phosphate excretion in the urine.
26. PTH **increase** calcium reabsorption in distal tubule.
27. In hypocalcemia, the excitability of nerve and muscle cells increases markedly and can in extreme cases result in **tetany**.
28. Ca²⁺ is actively absorbed into the blood from which part of GIT: **Duodenum**.
29. Calcium absorption from the intestine is inhibited by **phosphates** and **oxalates**.
30. PTH increases formation of **1,25-dihydroxy cholecalciferol** in kidney and this in turn increases Ca²⁺ absorption from the intestine.
31. Tendon reflexes are **hyperactive** in hypocalcemia.
32. Calcitonin secreted by the parafollicular cells (C cells) of thyroid gland lowers serum **calcium level**.
33. Calcitonin inhibits the activity of **osteoclasts** and prevents bone resorption.
34. Osteoblasts contain receptors for **PTH** and **calcitriol**.
35. Alkalosis **decreases** the ionized calcium levels in blood
36. During fasting, insulin secretion is **decreased**.
37. The only hormone in the body that decreases blood glucose level: **insulin**.
38. Name three hyperglycemic hormones: **Catecholamines, glucagon, growth hormone**.
39. Two conditions that produce ketoacidosis: **Starvation, diabetes mellitus.**
40. Acetyl choline and beta adrenergic stimulation **increases** insulin secretion.
41. Alpha adrenergic stimulation **decreases** insulin secretion.
42. Name three hormones increased by stress: **Glucagon, cortisol, catecholamines**.
43. Exogenous triglycerides are maximal in **chylomicrons** and endogenous triglycerides are maximal in **VLDL**.
44. ADH is synthesized in **supraoptic nucleus** and oxytocin is synthesized in the **paraventricular nuclei** of hypothalamus.
45. Name two neurohormones: **Oxytocin and vasopressin**
46. Secretory granules associated with oxytocin and vasopressin is called **Herring bodies**.
47. Hormones secreted by anterior pituitary: **TSH, ACTH, FSH, LH, prolactin and growth hormone**.
48. The effect of growth hormone on growth, cartilage and in protein metabolism depends on the interaction between GH and **somatomedins**.
49. Hypersecretion of growth hormone leads to **gigantism** in children and **acromegaly** in adult
50. **Dopamine** is the hypothalamic prolactin inhibiting hormone.
51. Increase in the effective osmotic pressure of plasma **increases** ADH secretion.
52. Circadian rhythm is mediated by **suprachiasmatic nucleus** of hypothalamus.
53. T_3 is **5** times more potent than T_4.
54. In physiological levels thyroxine produces protein **anabolism** but at higher levels it promotes protein **catabolism**.
55. TRH stimulates release of **TSH, prolactin and growth hormone.**
56. Marked skin pigmentation is seen in **Addison's disease**
57. Catecholamines stimulate **glucagon** secretion and inhibit **insulin** secretion.
58. Catecholamines produce hyperglycemia by increasing **glycogenolysis** in liver.
59. **Neuroendocrine glands** are those glands in which substance is released directly from nerve to blood.
60. Osteoclasts are differentiated **monocytes.**
61. 90% of protein in bone matrix is **type-I collagen.**
62. Name two hormones that act by inhibiting cAMP formation: **Somatostatin and norepinephrine (acting through α_2 receptors)**

CLINICAL CASE SCENARIO

1. **A 40-year-old woman complains of palpitation, heat intolerance, increased sweating, diarrhea and loss of weight in spite of increased appetite. On examination swelling of neck and exophthalmos were noted. Heart rate was 100/min and blood pressure 150/70 mm Hg.**
    a. What endocrine abnormality is responsible for the problems in the patient?
    b. Explain the physiological basis of the signs and symptoms in the patient?

CHAPTER 69 → Other Endocrine Organs and Local Hormones

c. Write two tests to confirm the diagnosis.
d. What are the actions of the hormone in protein and carbohydrate metabolism.

Ans:
Exophthalmic goitre or Graves disease (hyperthyroidism)

2. **A patient with autoimmune disease on steroids for the past 6 months presents with truncal obesity, mooning of face and purplish striae in the abdomen. On examination, fasting blood sugar was 220 mg%, BP 160/100 mm Hg and PCV 60%. Answer the following:**
   a. What is the probable diagnosis?
   b. Explain the physiological basis of mooning, purplish striae, hyperglycemia, hypertension and increased PCV in the patient.
   c. What is the reason for increased risk of fracture in this patient?
   d. What are the actions of glucocorticoid in inflammatory and immune response?

   Ans:
   Cushing syndrome due to excess glucocorticoids

3. **A 40-year-old lady complains of weight gain, recent onset of hoarseness of voice, lethargy, menstrual irregularities and cold intolerance. On examination she was anemic, pulse rate 66/min and serum cholesterol level was 350 mg%.**
   a. Identify the probable condition.
   b. Explain the physiological basis of the above symptoms and findings.
   c. What is the effect of the affected hormone on nervous system?
   d. How is the secretion of the hormone regulated?

   Ans:
   a. Myxedema or hypothyroidism

4. **A 50-year-old man complains of increased frequency of urination, increased thirst and appetite. In spite of increased food intake, there was weight loss. On examination:**
   BP – 140/84 mm Hg
   Fasting blood sugar – 270 mg/100mL
   HbA1c – 9%
   a. What is the probable diagnosis.
   b. Explain the physiological basis of weight loss, polyuria, polydipsia and polyphagia.
   c. Describe the actions of the affected hormone on carbohydrate metabolism.
   d. What is the significance of glycated hemoglobin. Give its normal value.

   Ans:
   a. Diabetes mellitus

5. **A 40-year-old female complains of weight loss, increased tiredness, hyperpigmentation; excessive sweating and fainting on fasting for the past few months. On investigation:**
   Blood pressure – 90/50 mm Hg
   Fasting blood glucose – 40 mg/100 mL
   Serum sodium – 127 mEq/L
   Blood cortisol and aldosterone levels were very low
   a. What is the probable diagnosis?
   b. What is the physiological basis of the above signs and symptoms?
   c. Explain the regulation of aldosterone secretion.
   d. Give the normal fasting blood glucose and serum sodium levels.

   Ans:
   Addison disease

SECTION 9 REPRODUCTIVE SYSTEM

Introduction to Reproductive Physiology

CHAPTER 70

LEARNING OBJECTIVES
- Enumerate the secondary sex characters in male and female
- Differentiate between genetic sex and sex phenotype

INTRODUCTION

The process by which an organism produces offspring of its own kind to continue its very existence and to transfer genetic material from generation to generation is called **reproduction**. Reproduction also includes the formation of new cells for tissue growth, repair or replacement in the individual. Reproduction is mainly of two types:

1. **Asexual reproduction** is the production of offspring from parts of a single organism without the formation of gametes, e.g., ameba, hydra, etc.
2. **Sexual reproduction** is the formation of offspring by the fusion of gametes, e.g., mammals, birds, etc.

With evolution, males and females were involved in sexual reproduction. The organs involved in the production of gametes are called **gonads**. Union of gametes occurs outside the body in frogs. Union of gametes occurs within the body of female in birds, but development occurs outside the body.

In humans, who occupy the highest position in evolution, the ovum is fertilized within the body of female which later develops to form the zygote, and development of zygote occurs for a definite period of time within the uterus. At the end of this period the child is born.

CHARACTERISTICS WHICH DIFFERENTIATE AN ADULT HUMAN MALE FROM AN ADULT FEMALE

- Primary sex organs **(Table 70.1)**
- Secondary or accessory sex organs **(Table 70.2)**
- Secondary sex characters **(Table 70.3)**

Various differences in characteristics between male and female depend on a single chromosome, the Y chromosome, and a pair of endocrine organs, testis in male and ovary in female.

Table 70.1: Primary sex organs and their secretions.

Primary sex organ	Secretions
Testis	Sperm, testosterone, androgen binding protein, inhibin, small amounts of estrogen
Ovary	Ovum, estrogen, progesterone, relaxin, inhibin, small amounts of androgen

Table 70.2: Accessory sex organs.

Male	Female
Epididymis, vas deferens, seminal vesicle, urethra, prostate, Cowper's gland or bulbourethral gland and external genitalia	Fallopian tube, uterus, vagina, external genitalia and accessory glands

Table 70.3: Secondary sex characters in male and female.

Male	Female
• Moustache and beard	• Scanty body hair
• Abundant body hair	• Apex of pubic hair downwards (female escutcheon)
• Tendency to baldness	
• Apex of pubic hair towards umbilicus (male escutcheon)	• Well-developed mammary gland
• Narrow male type pelvis	• High pitched voice
• Highly developed muscles	• Broad pelvis
• Low pitched voice	• Muscles less developed than males
• High BMR	
• Low ESR when compared to females	• BMR less than males
	• ESR more than that of males
• Initiative and idealistic	• Emotional and affectionate

Primary Sex Organs

Functions of primary sex organs are gametogenesis and production of hormones.

Accessory Sex Organs

These include ducts which transport gametes to the outside and the glands which empty their secretions into the ducts.

Secondary Sex Characters

Secondary sex characters is shown in **Table 70.3.**

Sex

- *Genetic sex or chromosomal sex or nuclear sex* depends on the chromosomal pattern of the individual.
- *Gonadal sex* depends on the presence of ovary or testis. If ovary is present, it is female, and if testis is present then the individual is considered as male.
- *Genital sex or gender sex or sex phenotype* depends on the genitalia or accessory sex organs.
- *Psychological sex* depends on the psychosexual behavior of the individual. It is the sex which the individual believes that he or she belongs to.

Sexual Development in the Embryo

CHAPTER 71

LEARNING OBJECTIVES
- Describe the mechanism of sex determination and sex differentiation in the embryo
- Discuss the physiological significance of Barr body
- Explain the abnormalities in sex differentiation

■ INTRODUCTION

Sexual development in embryo involves two processes:
1. Sex determination
2. Sex differentiation

■ SEX DETERMINATION

PY9.1: Describe and discuss sex determination; sex differentiation and their abnormalities and outline psychiatry and practical implication of sex determination.

Sex determination is a **genetic phenomenon**. It depends on the genetic sex, i.e., the constitution of sex chromosomes. It is determined at the time of fertilization by two chromosomes, called the sex chromosomes, to distinguish them from the somatic chromosomes. The sex chromosomes are called X and Y chromosomes. All cells, including oogonia and spermatogonia, contain 23 pairs of chromosomes, out of which 22 pairs are **somatic chromosomes or autosomes** responsible for somatic functions. The remaining one pair is **sex chromosomes**. In females, sex chromosomes are 2 X chromosomes, i.e., 44+XX pattern; and in male, sex chromosomes are one X and another Y chromosome, i.e., 44+XY pattern.

Chromosomal studies are done to determine genetic sex. Human cells can be grown in tissue cultures. They are treated with a drug called **colchicine** which arrests mitosis at the metaphase stage of cell division. It is then exposed to hypotonic solution. The chromosomes swell up and get dispersed. Spread it on a slide, squash and stain it using fluorescent or other staining techniques. The morphology of individual chromosomes can be studied under the microscope.

During gametogenesis, reduction division occurs and each gamete contains only 23 chromosomes, i.e., 22 autosomes and one sex chromosome. Each ovum has 22+X chromosomal pattern, and sperm has either 22+X or 22+Y chromosomal patterns. When an ovum is fertilized by a sperm containing X chromosome, the zygote will be a genetic female with 44XX chromosomal pattern. When the ovum is fertilized by a sperm containing Y chromosome, the zygote will be a genetic male with chromosomal pattern 44XY **(Fig. 71.1)**.

It is clear from **Figure 71.1**, that the genetic sex is exclusively determined by sperms and is independent of ovum. Y chromosomes are smaller and lighter than X chromosome and so the sperms containing Y chromosome swim faster in the female genital tract and can fertilize the ovum earlier. This is the cause for slight increase in male population than females.

Functions of Sex Chromosomes

❖ Y chromosome contains strong **testis-determining gene called SRY gene** (sex determining region of the Y chromosome) which is essential for the development of testes in genetic male. **SRY protein** produced by SRY gene is

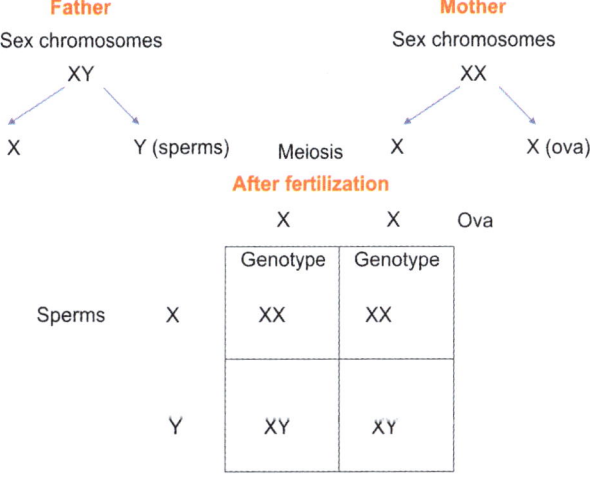

Fig. 71.1: Zygote genotypes after fertilization.

a DNA-binding regulatory protein. It acts as a transcription factor that initiates transcription of a cascade of genes necessary for testicular differentiation, including the gene for mullerian inhibiting substance (MIS). Y chromosome also affects the stature of the individual.
- ❖ X chromosome carries X determining genes necessary for ovarian differentiation. Extra-gonadal characteristic differentiation is also determined by X chromosome.
- ❖ Another importance of sex chromosome is that it contains genes which transmit diseases like hemophilia, color blindness, etc.

Sex Chromatin or Barr Body

Nucleus of the somatic cell of male and female can be differentiated by the presence of a special mass of chromatin known as sex chromatin or Barr body. Soon after cell division has started during embryonic development in normal female zygote, one of the two X-chromosomes of the somatic cells becomes functionally inactive. *Barr body is the condensation of the functionally inactive X chromosome.* In normal females, there will be only one Barr body in each cell which means that the cell contains two X chromosomes. In abnormal individuals with more than two X chromosomes, only one X chromosome remains active. The others become Barr bodies, e.g., super females with XXX chromosomal pattern have two Barr bodies in their somatic cells.

Number of Barr body + 1 = Number of X chromosomes in the cell.

Sex chromatin is seen as a plano-convex dark staining body present just beneath the nuclear membrane, 1 μm in diameter. It is a condensation of DNA. 50% of buccal smears in females show the presence of sex chromatin. It is also seen in vaginal smears and in the epidermal spinous layer. It is also seen as a drumstick-like projection from the nucleus of neutrophils of females **(Figs. 71.2A and B)**. It can be demonstrated in 1–15% of neutrophils.

The process that is responsible for inactivation of X chromosome appears to be initiated in an X-inactivation center in the chromosome. Inactivation is probably due to methylation of DNA. The choice of which X chromosome remains active is random, so normally one X chromosome remains active in approximately one-half of the somatic cells and the other X chromosome is active in the other half.

Thus, some of the somatic cells in adult female contain an active X chromosome of paternal origin and some contain active X chromosome of maternal origin.

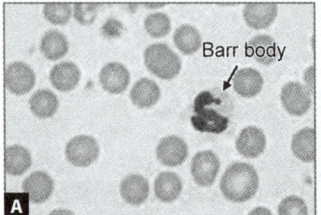 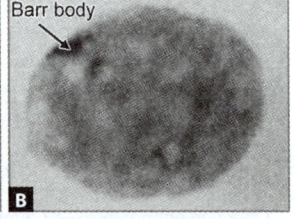

Figs. 71.2A and B: Barr body in the nucleus of: (A) Neutrophil; (B) Cheek cell.

Sex chromatin can be stained by **Pap stain or Orcin stain**, fixed in ether-alcohol mixture. The chromatin mass also stains deeply with **cresyl violet**.

■ SEX DIFFERENTIATION

Sex differentiation includes development of gonads and accessory sex organs. Sex determination occurs soon after fertilization but sex differentiation begins only after a few weeks of development but continues to early adult life.

Both male and female embryos develop identically until about 7 weeks after fertilization. At this point, the male determining gene called **sex determining region of Y chromosome (SRY gene)** is activated in male embryo. Only if the SRY gene is present and functional in a fertilized ovum, will the fetus develop testes and differentiate into a male. *In the absence of SRY gene, the fetus will develop ovaries and differentiate into a female.* SRY gene encodes a protein called **testes determining factor (TDF) or SRY protein**. This protein initiates a cascade of gene activation that causes the genital ridge cells to differentiate into testes which secretes testosterone.

> A histocompatibility antigen known as **H-Y antigen** is present on the surface of all male cells. It is a male tissue specific antigen. This antigen is thought to help in the development of male gonads, and masculinization. If H-Y antigen is not expressed, individuals with XY chromosomal pattern develop as females. H-Y antigen is the first cell surface protein to which a specific organogenesis function has been assigned. H-Y antigen causes rejection of male skin grafts by female recipients. H-Y antigen secreted by testes is found to be identical to mullerian inhibiting substance.

Sex Differentiation Occurs in Different Stages

- ❖ Gonadogenesis or development of gonads
- ❖ Formation of genital ducts
- ❖ Development of external genitalia
- ❖ Differentiation of brain

Gonadogenesis

On either side of the embryo, a primitive gonad arises from the **genital ridge**, which is a condensation of tissue near suprarenal gland. This primitive gonad develops into an **outer cortex and inner medulla**. Until the 6th week of development, the primitive gonads are identical in both sexes.

In genetic males (XY pattern) by about 7th week, medulla of the primitive gonad develop into testis and cortex degenerates. The SRY gene or the testes determining factor (TDF) is responsible for this development. By 8th week of intrauterine development, Leydig cells and sertoli cells appear in the fetal testis; and the Leydig cells secrete **testosterone** and sertoli cells secrete **Mullerian duct regression factor (MRF) or Mullerian inhibiting substance (MIS) or antimullerian hormone (AMH).** Testosterone secretion in the 8th week is stimulated by **human chorionic gonadotropin (hCG).**

In genetic females with XX pattern, by about 11th week of development, the cortex differentiates into the ovary and medulla degenerates due to the absence of Y chromosome and testes determining factor (TDF). Both X chromosomes are necessary for the development of ovary. *Fetal ovary does not secrete any hormone.* Hormonal treatment to the mother does not produce any change in gonadal differentiation in fetus as opposed to ductal and genital differentiation. Thus, *it is the absence of hormones that leads to the development of the ovary in the female fetus.*

Gonadal sex is determined to a large extent by genetic sex. In most cases, gonadal and genetic sex is the same.

Formation of Genital Ducts

Up to 7th week of intrauterine life (IUL), the embryo contains both male and female primordial germinal ducts. An early embryo has the potential to follow either the male or the female pattern of development since it contains both the germinal ducts. In the male embryo, germinal duct is **Wolffian duct** and in female, it is **mullerian duct**, which are paired duct systems **(Fig. 71.3)**. Further development depends on the gonads.

In the female fetus, due to the absence of antimullerian hormone, the mullerian duct differentiates into uterus, fallopian tubes and upper part of vagina. The Wolffian duct regresses. In a male fetus, under the influence of testosterone, Wolffian duct differentiates into epididymis, vas deferens and seminal vesicles. Mullerian duct degenerates by the action of mullerian regression factor (MRF) secreted by the fetal testis. *Mullerian inhibiting substance and testosterone act unilaterally in their effects on the internal genitalia.*

The natural tendency of the fetus is to develop female phenotype. *Only when the embryo has functional testes, the male internal and external genitalia develop.* In a fetus with genotype XY if testis is removed around 7th week of IUL, it will develop female type of genital ducts. When born, the child will have fallopian tube, uterus, vagina and vulva.

Development of External Genitalia

Up to 8th week of IUL, external genitalia are identical in both sexes. In the presence of testosterone, the urogenital slit disappears and male external genitalia develop. If testosterone is absent, the urogenital slit remains open and develops into female external genitalia. **Dihydrotestosterone (DHT)** formed from testosterone by the action of **5α-reductase** is responsible for the development of urethra, scrotum, penis and prostate. 5α-reductase deficiency leads to male pseudohermaphroditism, i.e., the external genitalia will be that of female. As opposed to the effects on internal genitalia, *testosterone acts bilaterally on their effects on the external genitalia.*

Hormonal Control of Development of Genitalia

If the embryo contains a functional testis, male type of internal and external genitalia develops. The Leydig cells of fetal testis produce **testosterone** and sertoli cells produce **MIS**. Both these are important for the development of internal genitalia. MIS alone is necessary for the regression of mullerian duct.

Actions of MRF and Testosterone in Fetus

- **Mullerian regression factor (MRF)** or mullerian inhibiting substance (MIS) or antimullerian hormone (AMH) stimulates the growth of the mesenchymal cells surrounding the mullerian duct which causes active regression of mullerian duct in the fetus. MIS is a polypeptide hormone related to inhibin. Leydig cells secrete testosterone from 8th week of intrauterine life. In their effects on internal genitalia, MIS and testosterone act unilaterally. MIS causes regression of mullerian duct by apoptosis on the side from which it is secreted and **testosterone** stimulates the development of vas deferens and related structures of male internal genitalia from Wolffian duct. Testosterone alone is necessary for the formation of male external genitalia. Testosterone is converted to dihydrotestosterone by the enzyme **5-α reductase.**
- **Dihydrotestosterone** (DHT) is responsible for the development of prostate and penis. Thus, testosterone acts directly or indirectly (through DHT) in the formation of male genitalia.

MIS is also produced by granulosa cells of ovarian follicles. MIS requires a high androgen to estrogen ratio to exert its effects on mullerian duct and this ratio is present in the male but not in the female fetus. So, the mullerian duct persists in the female despite the MIS in the ovaries. MIS is secreted in both sexes even after puberty and the plasma level of MIS is about the same in adult male and female, that is, about 2 ng/mL. It is seen that MIS is involved in germ cell maturation in both sexes and in the control of testicular descent in boys.

Functions of MIS or antimullerian hormone (AMH):

- Regression of mullerian duct in male by apoptosis
- Helps in germ cell maturation in both sexes
- Controls testicular descent in boys
- Plasma MIS level is an indicator of ovarian reserve of follicles in female. Its plasma level is assessed during treatment for infertility.

Differentiation of Brain

Presence of androgen is necessary for the development of male pattern of sexual behavior and also for the development of constant gonadotropin secretion after puberty in males. Evidence indicates that male sexual behavior and male pattern of gonadotropin secretion are due to the action of

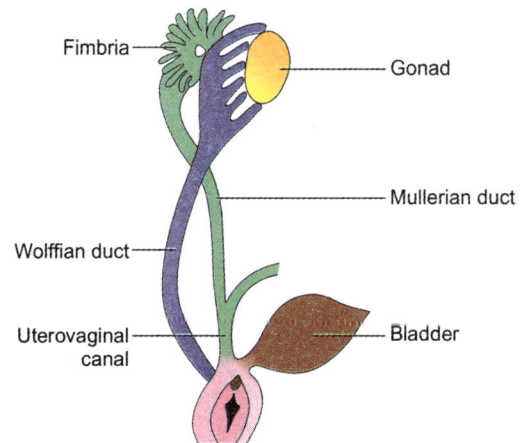

Fig. 71.3: Embryonic undifferentiated internal and external genitalia.

androgens on the brain in early development. In the absence of androgen, a cyclic gonadotropin secretion occurs after puberty and a female pattern of sexual behavior is seen. A cyclic center for gonadotropin secretion develops in the hypothalamus in the absence of androgen. When fetal hypothalamus is exposed to androgens, some histological changes occur in the cells of hypothalamus.

Psychological sex refers to the behavioral pattern and psychosexual identification of the individual with others in the society. Usually, psychological sex is same as genetic sex. A child cannot be identified as male or female before the age of 2 years by psychological sex. Thereafter, psychosexual differentiation occurs by dress, hairstyle, behavior, etc.

Sexual Identity and Gender Identity

Sexual identity is the pattern of a biological sexual characteristic. It depends on chromosomal pattern, external and internal genitalia, hormonal composition, gonads and secondary sexual characteristics.

Gender identity is an individual's sense of maleness or femaleness. It is fixed by 3 years and results from the experiences with family members, peers and cultural phenomena. The physiological basis of gender identity is said to be masculinization or feminization of the fetal brain. It signifies one's persistent inner sense of belonging to either the male or female gender category. Gender identity may be described as masculine, feminine or somewhere in between. **Transgenderism** (concept of third gender) involves identifying oneself as a member of the other gender or desiring to be the other gender.

ABNORMALITIES IN SEXUAL DIFFERENTIATION

Classification of Abnormalities Chromosomal Disorders

- Nondisjunction of sex chromosomes
- Nondisjunction of autosomes
- Transposition of parts of chromosomes to other sex chromosomes

Developmental Disorders

- Hormonal disorders
- Non-hormonal disorders having nonspecific causes

Chromosomal disorders: Main cause of chromosomal disorder is **non-disjunction** of homologous chromosomes. This is a phenomenon where a homologous pair of chromosomes fails to separate so that both chromosomes enter one of the daughter cells during cell division, either mitosis or meiosis.

Aneuploid cell means a cell that has one or more chromosomes of a set added or deleted. **A monosomic cell** is missing one chromosome (2n−1) and a **trisomic cell** has an added chromosome (2n+1). Non-disjunction of chromosomes is of three types:
1. Non-disjunction of sex chromosome during oogenesis
2. Non-disjunction of sex chromosomes during spermatogenesis
3. Non-disjunction of autosomes

1. *Non-disjunction of sex chromosomes during oogenesis* (Fig. 71.4): Four types of zygotes can be formed when there is meiotic non-disjunction of X chromosomes during oogenesis (Fig. 71.4):
    a. 44XO: Turner's syndrome
    b. 44XXX: Super female
    c. 44OY: The fetus does not survive
    d. 44XXY: Klinefelter's syndrome

   a. **Turner's syndrome or gonadal dysgenesis or ovarian agenesis**
      - Number of chromosomes—45
      - Chromosomal pattern—XO
      - Phenotype—female
      - Genetic sex—sexless
      - Gonadal sex—nil (no testis or ovary)
      - Sex chromatin test—negative
      - Genitalia—female type of internal and external genitalia due to absence of testosterone.

      At the time of puberty, menstruation does not occur and this is referred to as **primary amenorrhea**. Amenorrhea means absence of menstruation. Breast development does not occur due to absence of estrogen. Gonadal dysgenesis may lead to **dwarfism**. Other congenital abnormalities like webbing of neck, renal dysgenesis, abnormalities of heart, etc., are seen.

   b. **Super female**
      - Chromosomal pattern—XXX
      - Number of chromosomes—47
      - Phenotype—female
      - Genetic sex—female
      - Gonadal sex—female
      - Sex chromatin test—2 Barr bodies seen
      - Genitalia—female type

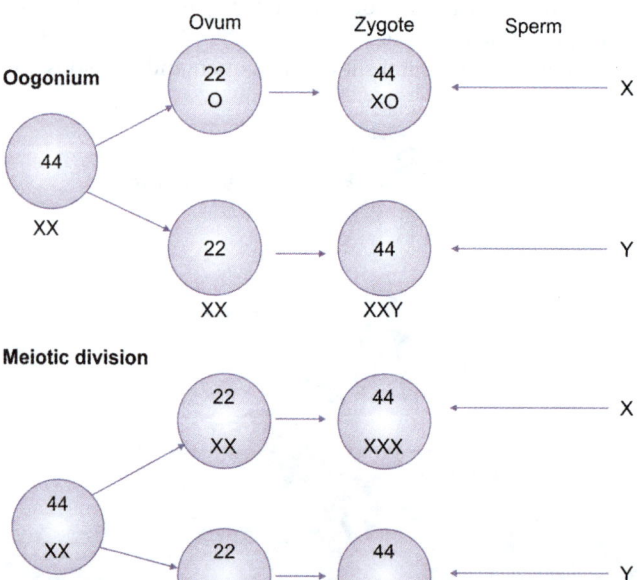

Fig. 71.4: Nondisjunction of sex chromosomes during oogenesis.

This abnormality is *second in frequency* among chromosomal disjunctions. It does not seem to be associated with any characteristic abnormalities. They have less feminine characters.

c. YO chromosomal pattern

This is a lethal condition and the child does not survive.

d. Klinefelter's syndrome or seminiferous tubule dysgenesis
- Chromosomal pattern—XXY
- Number of chromosomes—47
- Phenotype—male
- Genetic sex—female due to XX chromosomes
- Gonadal sex—male due to the presence of Y chromosome
- Sex chromatin test—positive, one barr body (an extra X chromosome is present)
- Genitalia—male type

Both MRF and androgens are produced, so male type of internal and external genitalia are present. Testicular differentiation is seen due to Y chromosome but testis is small and seminiferous tubules are abnormal. So spermatogenesis does not occur and this results in **sterility**. The patients show mental retardation, gynecomastia, abnormal hair distribution, etc. They are **tall** and this abnormality is the *most common sex chromosomal abnormality*.

2. ***Non-disjunction of sex chromosomes during spermatogenesis:***

   XYY pattern: They are tall males with severe acne. Incidence is high in **prison population**. This condition may be due to non- disjunction of Y chromosomes in the second meiotic division of spermatogenesis.

❖ ***Chromosomal mosaicism/true hermaphroditism:*** In true hermaphroditism, the same individual will be having cells with different chromosomal pattern. Some cells contain XX and others contain XY pattern. They have **both ovary and testis**. Hence, this condition is called true hermaphroditism. **Hermaphroditism** is the presence of both male and female sex organs in the same individual. This condition is due to non-disjunction of sex chromosome during the early mitotic division after fertilization. The person is called a **mosaic** because the individual contains two or more populations of cells with different chromosome complements.

3. ***Nonisjunction of autosomes:*** Non-disjunction of chromosome 21 produces trisomy 21. This chromosomal abnormality is associated with **Down's syndrome or mongolism**. The excess genes are responsible for the abnormalities seen in Down's syndrome. *This is the most common chromosomal disorder.*

Chromosomal abnormalities also include defects in single genes which lead to several abnormalities.

- **Transposition of parts of chromosomes**

  Another abnormality can occur due to transposition of parts of chromosomes to other chromosomes. Genetic males having XX chromosomal pattern are detected. This is because the short arm of their father's Y chromosome was transposed to the X chromosome during meiosis and the sperm carrying this X chromosome fertilized the ovum to form the zygote which developed into such individuals.

  Since the short arm of Y chromosome contains the SRY gene, these individuals develop testis and male genitalia even though they have XX karyotype. Similarly, deletion of the small portion of Y chromosome containing SRY produces females with the XY karyotype.

- **Detection of chromosomal abnormalities in the intrauterine life (IUL)**

  Genetic screening of mutations and genetic human diseases can be done prenatally (before birth) by ultrasound scan, amniocentesis and chorionic villus sampling.

  An **ultrasound scan** done at 12 to 13 weeks of pregnancy, measures the thickness of fluid behind the baby's neck, called **nuchal translucency**. This is lager in babies with Down syndrome. A **non-invasive prenatal test or NIPT** involves a blood test that analyzes DNA from baby that has passed into the mother's blood. This test is more than 99% accurate for Down syndrome.

  Chromosomal abnormalities, such as Down syndrome, Turner's syndrome as well as numerous diseases due to defects in single genes (mutant genes), such as sickle cell anemia can be diagnosed during intrauterine life by the analysis of fetal cells present in the amniotic fluid. Amniotic fluid is collected by introducing a needle into the amniotic sac through the anterior abdominal wall, and the process is called **amniocentesis**. It is done during 15 to 18 weeks of gestation.

  The defects can also be detected very early in pregnancy by studying fetal cells obtained by chorionic villi biopsy. This technique is called **chorionic villus sampling**. It is done by 10 to 12 weeks of gestation. But these tests increases the risk of miscarriage.

Developmental disorders

I. Hormonal abnormalities

- *Pseudohermaphrodite:* In pseudohermaphroditism genetic pattern and gonads are of one sex and genitalia that of opposite sex.
- *Female pseudohermaphrodite:* In female pseudohermaphrodite, genetic pattern is that of female and genitalia that of male. This is due to exposure of genetic female fetus to androgens between 8th and 13th week of IUL. After 13 weeks, if there is exposure to androgen then hypertrophy of clitoris occurs.

  Causes of female pseudohermaphroditism are congenital virilizing adrenal hyperplasia, administration of an-drogens to pregnant females, etc.
- *Male pseudohermaphrodite:* In male pseudohermaphrodite, genetic pattern is that of male but genitalia is that of female.

Causes of male pseudohermaphroditism:
- Due to defective embryonic testes. Both internal and external genitalia will be that of female since there is no secretion of testosterone and MIS.
- Due to androgen resistance, i.e., the tissues are not responding to androgen.

Androgen resistance can be due to:
- Deficiency of 5α-reductase enzyme necessary for the conversion of testosterone to its active form dihydrotestosterone. DHT is the most potent natural androgen and is necessary for virilization.
- Mutation in the androgen receptor gene
- Reduction in the number of androgen receptors.
- Presence of abnormal receptors.
- Receptor may be normal but there is something wrong in the molecular events after the combination of hormone and receptor. This is called **receptor-positive androgen resistance**.
- When there is complete loss of receptor function, it is called **testicular feminizing syndrome** now known as **complete androgen resistance syndrome**. In this condition, MIS is present and testosterone is secreted at normal or even elevated rates. The internal genitalia is that of male and external genitalia that of female because the androgen receptors are not functioning. Vagina ends blindly because there are no female internal genitalia.

These individuals have breast enlargement at puberty and are considered as females. But there will be no menstruation.

Causes of testicular feminizing syndrome are:
- Congenital deficiency of 17α-hydroxylase enzyme necessary for the synthesis of androgens from pregnenolone.
- Genetic male with congenital blockage of formation of pregnenolone is pseudohermaphrodite because testicular as well as adrenal androgens are formed from pregnenolone.
- LH receptor mutation leads to impaired testosterone production in Leydig cells. Severe defects in LH receptors leads to male pseudohermaphroditism.

II. **Non-hormonal disorders**

These defects are due to teratogenic effects. A **teratogen** is any agent or environmental factor that causes developmental defects in the embryo. Fetal teratogens include alcohol, pesticides, some hormones, antibiotics, etc.

PUBERTY

> **PY9.2:** Describe and discuss puberty: onset, progression, stages; early and delayed puberty and outline adolescent clinical and psychological association.

Puberty is defined as the stage of development in which gametogenic and endocrine functions of gonads have first developed to the point where reproduction is possible. This period of growth and sexual maturation is also called **adolescence**. Age at the time of puberty is variable; usually, it is between 8–13 in girls and 9–14 in boys. Spermatogenesis in boys and folliculogenesis in girls begin at puberty.

A burst of testosterone secretion occurs in the male fetus before birth which is necessary for the development of male genitalia. After birth, the gonads of both sexes remain quiescent because there is no gonadotropin secretion. During adolescence, the gonads are activated in both sexes by gonadotropins secreted by the pituitary to bring about the final maturation of the reproductive system. This period of final maturation is called adolescence. After puberty, in males gonadotropin secretion is noncyclic. But in post-pubertal females an orderly, sequential secretion of gonadotropins is necessary for the occurrence of menstruation and pregnancy.

Puberty coincides with a surge of sex hormone secretion resulting in the development of secondary sexual characters. *It is the pulsatile secretion of GnRH that brings on puberty.* There is accelerated growth spurt. In girls, first event is development of breasts. This is known as **thelarche**. This is followed by development of axillary and pubic hair known as **pubarche**. **Menarche** is first menstrual bleeding. At this time, adrenals produce large quantities of androgens with no change in cortisone secretion. This change in adrenals is called **adrenarche** which occurs at the age of 8–10 years in girls and at age 10–12 years in boys. This occurs probably due to an adrenal androgen-stimulating hormone secreted from the pituitary gland. The initial menstrual periods are generally anovulatory and regular ovulation occurs about a year later.

Even though hypothalamus and pituitary contain secretions, they do not secrete gonadotropin releasing hormone (GnRH) and gonadotropins in childhood. There are different views to explain this:

- Some neural mechanism is operating during childhood which prevents normal pulsatile secretion of GnRH. This is due to lack of signals from some part of brain or due to inhibition of some genes that stimulate GnRH release from hypothalamus. At the time of puberty, signals arise from limbic system to stimulate hypothalamus for pulsatile secretion of GnRH.
- During childhood, hypothalamus is very sensitive to the inhibitory effect of sex hormones. At the time of puberty, as the brain matures, the sensitivity of brain decreases and puberty occurs.
- Some product of pineal gland inhibits gonadotropin secretion. At puberty, this inhibitory effect is removed.
- **Leptin**, a satiety-producing hormone secreted by the fat cells facilitates the release of GnRH, thereby helping in pubertal onset. Onset of puberty occurs at an earlier age in well-nourished girls because of the action of leptin. A critical body weight is required for leptin release and pubertal onset. It has been seen that leptin treatment induces precocious puberty in immature female mice.

Abnormalities of Pubertal Onset

Precocious Puberty (Fig. 71.5)

Precocious puberty is generally caused by a premature activation of the hypothalamic-pituitary-gonadal axis due

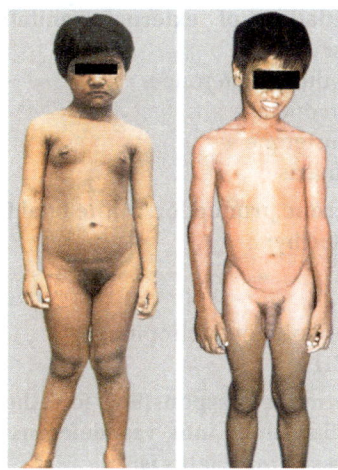

Fig. 71.5: Precocious puberty in a four-year-old girl and five-year-old boy.
Courtesy: Dr RV Jayakumar

to brain tumors; or it may be due to excess sex hormone production. Precocious puberty may be:
1. True precocious puberty (gametogenesis present)
2. Precocious pseudo puberty (gametogenesis absent)

True Precocious Puberty

In this condition, there is early but normal pattern of gonadotropin secretion from pituitary, and precocious sexual development is seen. *Gametogenesis is present.* Causes are:
❖ Constitutional (without definite cause)
❖ Hypothalamic disorders especially lesions of ventral hypothalamus near the infundibulum interrupt a pathway that normally holds pulsatile GnRH secretion in check.
❖ Pineal tumors, especially when hypothalamus is also involved

Precocious gametogenesis can occur without the pubertal pattern of gonadotropin secretion. This condition is called **gonadotropin-independent precocity**. In some of these cases, the sensitivity of LH receptors to gonadotropins is increased because of an activating mutation in the G-protein that couples the receptors to adenylyl cyclase.

Precocious Pseudopuberty

The syndrome in which there is early development of secondary sexual characters *without gametogenic function* is called precocious pseudopuberty. This is due to early exposure of immature boys to androgen and girls to estrogen. Usually seen in:
❖ Congenital virilizing adrenal hyperplasia
❖ Hormone producing tumor of ovary and testes
❖ Androgen and estrogen secreting tumors of adrenal

Delayed or Absent Puberty

Puberty is said to be delayed if menarche has failed to occur by 17 years in females and testicular development and sexual characters fail to develop by 20 years of age in males. In females, this condition is called **primary amenorrhea** and in males, it is called **eunuchoidism**. Usual causes are:
❖ Panhypopituitarism where dwarfism and other endocrine abnormalities are present.
❖ Gonadal dysgenesis or Turner's syndrome (XO chromosomal pattern).
❖ Primary amenorrhea in females is seen where there is no menstruation but other endocrine functions are normal.

MULTIPLE CHOICE QUESTIONS

1. **The primitive gonad remains undifferentiated up to:**
   a. 5th week of intrauterine life
   b. 7th week of IUL
   c. 9th week of IUL
   d. 3rd month of IUL

2. **The following are due to non-disjunction of sex chromosomes, *except*:**
   a. Klinefelter's syndrome
   b. Down syndrome
   c. Turner's syndrome
   d. Super female

3. **The gene coding for androgen receptors is located in:**
   a. Short arm of X chromosome
   b. Short arm of Y chromosome
   c. Long arm of X chromosome
   d. Long arm of Y chromosome

4. **Female pseudohermaphroditism is present in:**
   a. 21-β hydroxylase deficiency
   b. 17-hydroxylase deficiency
   c. 3-beta-hydroxylase deficiency
   d. Aromatase deficiency

5. **Barr body is found in the following phase of the cell cycle:**
   a. Interphase   b. Metaphase
   c. G1 phase   d. Telophase

6. **Barr body is seen in:**
   a. Turner syndrome
   b. Klinefelter's syndrome
   c. Testicular feminization
   d. 46 XY pattern

7. **Father to son inheritance is never seen in case of:**
   a. Autosomal dominant inheritance
   b. Autosomal recessive inheritance
   c. X-linked recessive inheritance
   d. Multifactorial inheritance

8. **Chromosomal pattern in Klinefelter's syndrome is:**
   a. XO   b. XXY
   c. YO   d. XXX

9. **Chromosomal pattern in Turner's syndrome is:**
   a. XO   b. XXY
   c. YO   d. XXX

10. Period of gestation up to which gonads of males and females are indistinguishable:
    a. 5 weeks   b. 8 weeks
    c. 2 weeks   d. 12 weeks

11. Sex chromatin (Barr body) is:
    a. Inactive Y chromosome
    b. Found in all males
    c. Attached to nuclear membrane
    d. Found only in males with chromosomal abnormalities

12. Testis determining gene or sex determining region is located on:
    a. X chromosome   b. Y chromosome
    c. Chromosome 21   d. Chromosome 18

13. Most common chromosomal defect is:
    a. Down syndrome   b. Turner
    c. Edward   d. Superfemale

14. Nondisjunction of autosomes leads to:
    a. Mosaicism
    b. Klinefelter's syndrome
    c. Down's syndrome
    d. Pseudohermaphroditism

15. Hormonal abnormalities during sex differentiation in the fetus lead to:
    a. True hermaphroditism
    b. Down's syndrome
    c. Turner's syndrome
    d. Pseudohermaphroditism

16. All the following statements are true, *except*:
    a. In female fetus, due to lack of testosterone Wolffian duct regress
    b. In the absence of MIF, the mullerian duct differentiate into female internal genitalia
    c. In the absence of the enzyme 5-α-reductase, male pseudohermaphroditism results
    d. Active hormonal participation of testosterone and mullerian inhibiting factor results in the development of normal male internal and external genitalia.

17. Growth and differentiation of Wolffian ducts in male is by the action of:
    a. Dihydrotestosterone
    b. 5-α reductase
    c. Testosterone
    d. Aromatase

18. The gestational age at which external genitalia of both sexes begin to differentiate:
    a. 12–14 weeks   b. 15–18 weeks
    c. 7–0 weeks   d. 9–10 weeks

19. Differentiation of external genitalia in males requires:
    a. Dihydrotestosterone
    b. 5-α reductase
    c. Testosterone
    d. Aromatase

20. Testosterone production by the fetal Leydig cells is stimulated by:
    a. FSH
    b. LH
    c. Chorionic gonadotropin
    d. GnRH

21. The hormone responsible for the conversion of Wolffian duct into vas deferens and related structures in male fetus is:
    a. Estrogen   b. Progesterone
    c. Testosterone   d. Cortisone

22. The hormone that is responsible for the formation of male external genitalia and male external sex characteristics:
    a. Dihydrotestosterone
    b. FSH
    c. Testosterone
    d. Mullerian inhibiting substance

23. Nondisjunction of sex chromosomes during mitotic division after fertilization gives rise to:
    a. Male pseudohermaphroditism
    b. Female pseudohermaphroditism
    c. True hermaphroditism
    d. Down's syndrome

24. Female pseudohermaphroditism is seen in all the following conditions, *except*:
    a. Congenital virilizing adrenal hyperplasia
    b. Virilizing ovarian tumor
    c. Androgen resistance
    d. Maternal androgen excess

25. Nondisjunction of chromosome 21 produces:
    a. Down syndrome
    b. Turner syndrome
    c. True hermaphroditism
    d. Klinefelter's syndrome

ANSWERS

1. a	2. b	3. c	4. a	5. a
6. b	7. c	8. b	9. a	10. a
11. c	12. b	13. a	14. c	15. d
16. d	17. c	18. d	19. a	20. c
21. c	22. a	23. c	24. c	25. a

Male Reproductive System

CHAPTER 72

LEARNING OBJECTIVES
- Describe the functional anatomy of male reproductive system
- Discuss the functions of testis
- Explain the steps in spermatogenesis and the factors affecting it
- Describe the physiological effects of testosterone
- Discuss the effects of removal of testes on physiological functions
- Interpret a normal semen analysis report as per WHO guidelines

FUNCTIONAL ANATOMY OF MALE REPRODUCTIVE SYSTEM

PY9.3: Describe male reproductive system: Functions of testis and control of spermatogenesis and factors modifying it and outline its association with psychiatric illness.

Primary sex organ is **testis** which has a dual function, i.e., **spermatogenesis and endocrine function**. Testis is developed within the abdomen in the embryo. By the end of 7th month of intrauterine life (IUL), the testis descends into the scrotum through the inguinal canal. When the testes do not descend into the scrotum, the condition is called **cryptorchidism**. It is seen in 3% of full-term infants and 30% of premature babies. If it persists at puberty, it results in sterility. Chance of testicular cancer is also more.

Weight of each testis—10–15 g.

Structure of Testis

There are **200–300 lobules** in each testis and 1–3 **seminiferous tubules** in each lobule. There are about 500 seminiferous tubules per testis. Each seminiferous tubule is about 70 cm in length.

Lining cells of seminiferous tubule contain **germinal epithelium** from which spermatozoa or sperms are formed. In adult testis, sperms are seen towards the lumen of the seminiferous tubule. In between spermatogenic cells, there are large pyramidal-shaped supporting cells or sustentacular cells called **Sertoli cells.** They rest on the basal lamina of the seminiferous tubule and extend from basement membrane to the lumen of the tubule. The spermatogenic cells are seen in the clefts between Sertoli cells.

The spermatogenic cells are attached to the cytoplasm of Sertoli cells. In between seminiferous tubules, there are clusters or nests of lipid-containing cells called **Leydig cells or interstitial cells of Leydig**. These cells produce **testosterone**, the male sex hormone (**Fig. 72.1**).

The seminiferous tubules open into **rete testis**. From this arise a number of efferent ducts and they join and form **epididymis**. Epididymis is a highly convoluted tube about 4–6 m long when uncoiled and it opens into the **vas deferens** where sperms are stored. Spermatozoa released from the seminiferous tubule are non-motile, but when they reach epididymis they become motile and mature. The vas deferens enlarges to form **ampulla** before it enters the prostate.

Seminal vesicles are situated on either side just above the prostate; they secrete spermatozoa activating substances, such as fructose, citrate, inositol, prostaglandins and several proteins. The ducts of the seminal vesicles join the ampulla to form a common duct called **ejaculatory duct**. Ejaculatory duct opens into the prostatic part of urethra. The prostatic duct also empties into the ejaculatory duct. **Urethra** is the last portion which connects testes to the exterior (**Fig. 72.2**).

Testicular Vessels

The spermatic arteries are tortuous blood vessels that lie parallel and counter to the **pampiniform plexus** of spermatic veins. The direction of blood flow in the artery and vein is opposite to that of each other. Heat and testosterone can be exchanged between the artery and the vein. This is known as **countercurrent exchange system**. Because of this mechanism, the temperature of testis is maintained 2°C lower than body temperature and the local concentration of testosterone is maintained at high levels. Both these factors are very essential for normal spermatogenesis.

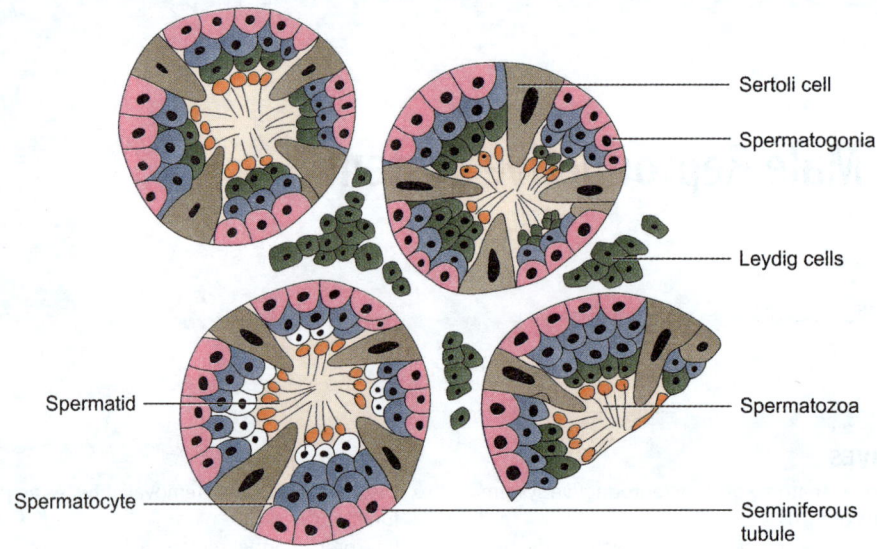

Fig. 72.1: Histology of testis.

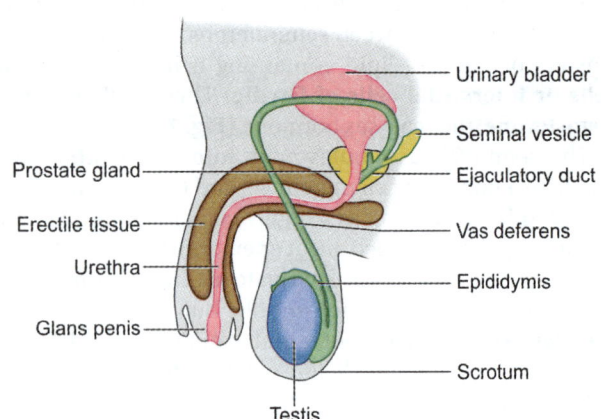

Fig. 72.2: Male reproductive system.

SPERMATOGENESIS

The process by which primitive germ cells (2n) in the seminiferous tubules of the testis are converted into mature haploid (n) spermatozoa is called **spermatogenesis**. This process begins during adolescence, i.e., by about 13 years (the primordial germ cells do not undergo meiosis until puberty). The process continues throughout life, but there is a sharp decline at old age. Spermatogenesis depends upon both LH and FSH.

Spermatogonia develop from primordial germ cells that arise from yolk sac endoderm and enter the testis early in development. The primordial germ cell differentiates into spermatogonia.

Stages of Spermatogenesis

- Spermatocytogenesis
- Meiosis
- Spermiogenesis

Spermatocytogenesis

In spermatocytogenesis, the spermatogonia divide and produce successive generations of cells that give rise to **spermatocytes**. Spermatogonia are small cells, 12 μm in diameter. At puberty, these cells divide by mitosis several times to produce large number of spermatogonia. They are of three types:

1. **Type A spermatogonia** (dark cells) which serve as reserve stem cells, have large, round nucleus containing 46 chromosomes and swollen cytoplasm. They do not undergo mitosis.
2. **Type A spermatogonia (pale cells)** are stem cells that undergo mitosis to form type B cells.
3. **Type B spermatogonia,** which are progenitor cells or precursors of sperms. These cells undergo differentiation to form **primary spermatocytes** with 46 chromosomes. These are the most conspicuous cells on cross-section of seminiferous tubule.

Meiosis

In the next stage, primary spermatocytes undergo first meiotic division. The homologous pairs of chromosomes line up in the center of the cell. In this stage, **crossing over** occurs, which permits exchange of genes among maternal and paternal chromosomes. Such an exchange of genes is termed **recombination**. When the first meiotic division is completed, the daughter cells are called **secondary spermatocytes,** which have **haploid** number (n) of chromosomes **(Fig. 72.3)**. The second meiotic division follows and the daughter cells are called **spermatids** with 23 chromosomes. *Each primary spermatocyte thus produces 4 spermatids.* Spermatids lie close to the lumen of the seminiferous tubule. *The number of spermatids formed from a single spermatogonium is 512.* Summary of the steps in spermatogenesis is shown in **Flowchart 72.1**.

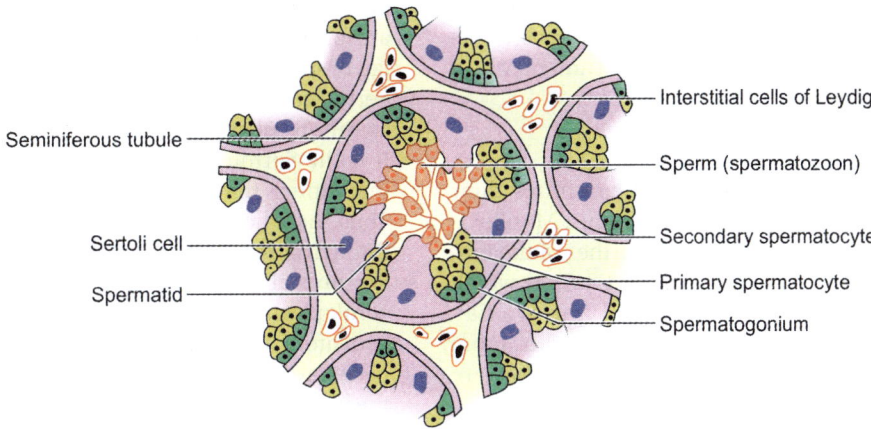

Fig. 72.3: Cross section of seminiferous tubule showing different stages in the development of sperm from spermatogonia.

Flowchart 72.1: Steps in spermatogenesis. Note that from one primary spermatocyte, 4 spermatozoa or mature sperms are formed.

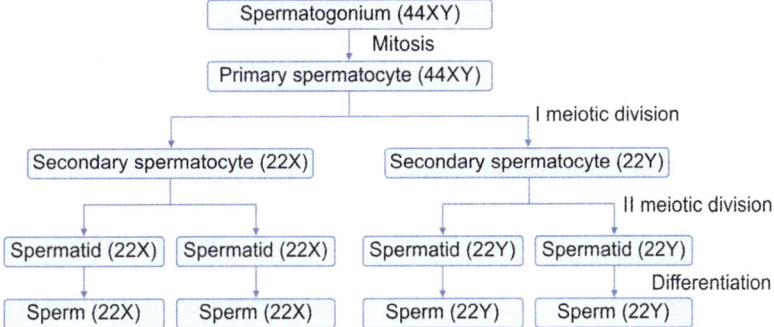

Spermiogenesis

Conversion of spermatids to spermatozoa is called **spermiogenesis**. During spermiogenesis, changes occur in the nucleus and cytoplasm. Nucleus becomes smaller and ovoid and chromatin gets condensed. This forms the **head** of the sperm. Some amount of cytoplasm is lost from the spermatid and nucleus is surrounded by a thin film of cytoplasm and cell membrane. There is a thick cap-like structure in the head called **acrosomal cap or acrosome**, derived from the Golgi apparatus. Acrosome contains many types of enzymes, such as **hyaluronidase** and proteolytic enzymes. These enzymes are important for fertilization, i.e., they help the sperm to penetrate the ovum. The rest of the cytoplasm and cell membrane form the **tail** portion. It consists of a central axoneme which contains microtubules. This axoneme is surrounded by cell membrane. In the proximal part of the tail, the axoneme is surrounded by a number of mitochondria called **body piece or mid-piece** of tail. There is also a **chief piece and a tail piece**. There is a neck at the junction of head and tail. From head to tail a human sperm cell measures about 50 μm in length. The energy for flagellar movement of tail is obtained from ATP provided by mitochondria **(Fig. 72.4)**. The membrane of late spermatids and spermatozoa contains a special small form of angiotensin converting enzyme called **germinal angiotensin converting enzyme (gACE)**. Its exact function is not yet established but its deficiency leads to sterility.

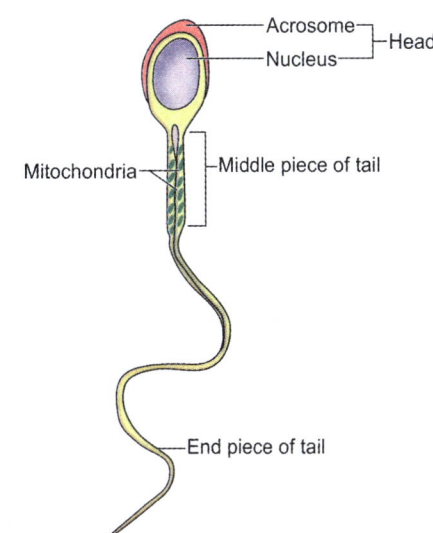

Fig. 72.4: Structure of spermatozoon (Sperm).

Developing sperm cells are connected to the Sertoli cells. The release of a sperm cell from its connection to the Sertoli cell is known as **spermiation**. Sperm then enters the lumen of the seminiferous tubule and flows towards the epididymis where it is stored.

- ❖ Velocity of movement of sperm is 1–4 mm/min.
- ❖ Normal duration of spermatogenesis: 65–70 days.

In the region of rete testis, fluid is reabsorbed and the spermatozoa are concentrated. Otherwise, the sperms entering the epididymis become much diluted and may lead to sterility.

Maturation of Spermatozoa

The spermatozoa leaving the rete testis continues their maturation as they pass through the epididymis. Motility is also acquired as the spermatozoa are stored in the epididymis. This involves activation of a protein called **CatSper** which is present in the principal piece of sperm tail. This is a Ca^{2+} ion channel and when activated it helps in Ca^{2+} influx. From epididymis, the sperms enter vas deferens where they are stored.

Functions of Sertoli Cells

- Contribute to blood-testis barrier
- Role in spermatogenesis
- Endocrine function

Blood-testis Barrier

There are tight junctions between the adjacent Sertoli cells near the basement membrane which forms the **blood-testis barrier**. This barrier is important because spermatogenic cells have surface antigens that are recognized as foreign by the immune system. Thus, immune response is prevented by isolating the spermatogenic cells from blood.

Functions of Blood-testis Barrier

- Prevents the passage of proteins and large molecules from the interstitial spaces and basal parts of seminiferous tubules into the lumen; but steroids can easily pass through this barrier, e.g., androgens.
- This barrier maintains the composition of the seminiferous tubular fluid constant for proper spermatogenesis. Glucose and protein are very less in the tubule. It is rich in androgens, estrogen, K^+, inositol, glutamic acid and aspartic acid.
- Protects the germ cells from blood-borne noxious agents.
- Prevents the occurrence of autoimmune response by preventing the entry of antigenic substances released during cell division and maturation of spermatozoa into the blood stream.
- Helps to establish an osmotic gradient which facilitates fluid movement through the tubular lumen.

Role of Sertoli Cells in Spermatogenesis

- Sertoli cells provide the specific environment for spermatogenesis and provide support to maturing germ cells. With the help of cytoplasmic bridges germ cells stay in contact with the Sertoli cells. This is essential for the survival of germ cells.
- Sertoli cells secrete a large amount of fluid which provides nutrition to the sperms and also assists in moving the immotile spermatozoa into the epididymis.
- They have a role in **spermiogenesis**. Spermatids mature in the cytoplasmic folds of Sertoli cells. This is by liberating certain nutritious factors, enzymes and hormones. The digestive enzymes produced by Sertoli cells remove most of the cytoplasm from the spermatids before spermatozoa are formed. Sertoli cells also help in shaping the head and tail of sperms.
- Sertoli cells can engulf damaged germ cells and injured sperms by phagocytosis.
- It is the Sertoli cell and not the developing sperm cell that express the androgen receptor and the FSH receptor. Thus, these hormones support spermatogenesis indirectly through stimulation of Sertoli cell function.
- Sertoli cells produce proteins, such as transferrin, ceruloplasmin and plasminogen activators. Plasminogen activators are responsible for the proteolytic reactions necessary for migration of maturing germ cells towards the lumen.
- **Androgen binding protein** (ABP) produced by Sertoli cells can bind androgen as well as estrogen and maintain the level of androgens in the seminiferous tubule at a high level.

Endocrine Function of Sertoli Cells

- In the fetal testis, Sertoli cells produce hormones, such as **mullerian regression factor (MRF)** or **antimullerian hormone (AMH)** which inhibits the development of mullerian duct.
- Some amount of **estrogen** is secreted by Sertoli cell which is necessary for spermiogenesis. Sertoli cells ex- press the enzyme aromatase which convert testosterone produced by the Leydig cell to the potent estrogen, 17-beta estradiol. This estrogen enhances spermatogenesis in humans.
- **Inhibin-B** produced by Sertoli cells inhibits FSH secretion from anterior pituitary by feedback mechanism. FSH stimulates androgen, estrogen and inhibin production. Inhibin in turn inhibits FSH secretion. Thus inhibin keeps FSH levels within a set point.

Factors Influencing Spermatogenesis

- Hormonal factors
- Sertoli cells
- General factors

Hormonal Factors

Hormones affecting spermatogenesis in **Table 72.1**

- **Testosterone** is necessary for the conversion of primary spermatocyte to secondary spermatocyte.
- **LH** or interstitial cell stimulating hormone (ICSH) stimulates the Leydig cells to secrete testosterone.
- **FSH** stimulates spermatogenesis and it also stimulates Sertoli cells to produce estrogen that is necessary for spermiogenesis.

Table 72.1: Hormones affecting spermatogenesis.	
Hormones stimulating spermatogenesis	**Inhibiting spermatogenesis**
• Testosterone • LH, FSH • Estrogen • Growth hormone	Inhibin

Flowchart 72.2: Hormonal regulation of FSH secretion in males; antimullerian hormone (AMH) (dashed line indicates negative feedback inhibition).

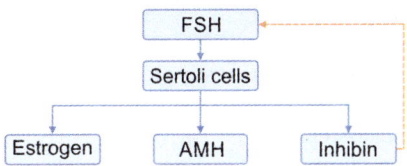

- **Growth hormone** helps in the metabolic effects of testis and helps in the first few stages in the development of sperms. In growth hormone deficiency, spermatogenesis may be defective as seen in pituitary dwarfs.
- **Inhibin** inhibits FSH secretion from anterior pituitary (Flowchart 72.2).

Role of Sertoli Cells
Refer functions of Sertoli cells.

General Factors
- *Temperature*: Temperature is the most important factor that affects spermatogenesis. It requires a temperature lower than the body temperature, i.e., **34°C**. This low temperature is maintained in the testis by the following factors:
  - Constant circulation of air around the scrotum.
  - By the contraction of dartos and cremaster muscles, the distance between the scrotum and the body can be adjusted.
  - Heat exchange between spermatic artery and pampiniform plexus of veins by countercurrent exchange mechanism.

  In cases of undescended testis, the temperature of testis is 37°C. The seminiferous tubules gradually degenerate and this leads to sterility. Hot baths daily, use of insulated athletic supports, etc., lead to decreased sperm count.
- **Diseases**: Diseases, such as mumps may cause **orchitis** (infection and inflammation of testis) which damages the seminiferous tubules. The blood-testis barrier will be disrupted leading to autoimmune destruction of gametogenic cells leading to sterility.
- Irradiation: Irradiation damages seminiferous tubules but interstitial cells are unaffected.
- *Vasectomy*: Ligation of vas deferens leads to degeneration of seminiferous tubules because the sperms formed accumulate in the tubules increasing the pressure and damaging the tubules in 50% of cases.
- *Age*: Spermatogenesis decreases with advancing age.
- Germinal angiotensin-converting enzyme (gACE): The membrane of spermatozoa contains a special form of angiotensin converting enzyme called gACE. Although its full function is not known absence of gACE leads to sterility.

Secretion of Seminal Vesicle
Seminal vesicle secretes a mucoid material, **yellow** in color due to the presence of **flavin pigments**. It also contains large amount of fructose (2–6 mg/mL), amino acids, ascorbic acid, inositol, fibrinogen, prostaglandin, phosphoryl choline, etc., *60% of semen is contributed by the secretion of seminal vesicle*. Fructose and other nutrients provide nutrition to the sperm. The functions of prostaglandin are:
- It acts on cervical mucus and makes it more receptive to sperms.
- It causes a reverse peristalsis in the female genital tract and thus helps the sperm to move towards the ovum in the fallopian tube.

Secretion of Prostate
Prostatic secretion is a thin, milky, **alkaline fluid** which contains spermine, citric acid, acid phosphatase, profibrinolysin, fibrinogenase, cholesterol, phospholipids, hyaluronidase, Ca^{2+}, Zn^{2+}, PO_4^{3-}, HCO_3^-, etc., *20% of semen is contributed by prostatic secretion*.

Spermine is a polyamine which has an important role in cell growth and differentiation. Deficiency of spermine leads to arrest of cell growth, differentiation and division. It is so called because it was first isolated from semen by Leeuwenhock in 1678. Now, it is known that it is present in all eukaryotic cells. Function of spermine is to stabilize the double helical structure of DNA by binding the two strands together.

Prostate is very small in children, grows at puberty and maximum growth is attained by 20 years, and is maintained up to 50 years. Testosterone is very essential for maintaining prostate. After 50 years, testosterone secretion falls and the prostate degenerates.

Bulbourethral gland secretes an alkaline fluid rich in mucus, HCO_3^- and PO_4^{3-}.

Prostate Specific Antigen (PSA)
PSA is a 30 kD a serine protease produced by prostate and secreted into the semen. PSA hydrolyzes the sperm motility inhibitor 4 called **semenogelin** in semen. Plasma PSA is found to be elevated in benign prostatic hyperplasia, prostatitis and in prostate cancer. Estimation of plasma PSA is widely used as a screening test for prostate cancer.

ERECTION AND EJACULATION

Erection is initiated by dilatation of the arterioles of penis. The erectile tissues of the penis, **two corpora cavernosa and one corpus spongiosum**, get filled with blood. The veins get compressed blocking outflow and this adds to the turgor of the organ. The afferent impulses reach the lumbar segments from the genitalia and efferent impulses from the descending tracts mediate erection in response to psychological stimuli. The efferent parasympathetic fibers are in the pelvic splanchnic nerves, (nervi erigentes) and the neurotransmitters are acetylcholine and VIP. Fibers that help to synthesize NO are also present in nervi erigentes. NO activates guanylyl cyclase and leads to increased production of cGMP which is a potent vasodilator. NO synthase inhibitors prevent erection. **Viagra**, a drug used for the treatment of erectile dysfunction (previously referred to as impotence), inhibits the breakdown of cGMP by **phosphodiesterases**. *Since the phosphodiesterases of retina are also inhibited by Viagra, this drug produces transient blue-green color blindness.*

Erection is terminated by sympathetic vasoconstrictor fibers to the arterioles of penis.

Ejaculation helps in expelling the sperms out of the urethra. It is a spinal reflex which includes **emission and ejaculation**. Emission involves movement of semen into the urethra and ejaculation is the propulsion of semen out of the urethra during **orgasm**. *Emission is a sympathetic reflex.* Afferent fibers for emission arise from the touch receptors of glans penis which travel through internal pudendal nerve, the center is the upper lumbar segments of spinal cord and efferents comes through hypogastric nerve. Effect is contraction of smooth muscle of vas deferens and seminal vesicles and the semen reaches the urethra. *Ejaculation is a parasympathetic reflex* and the center is in the lower lumbar and upper sacral segments of spinal cord. The semen is propelled out of the urethra by the contraction of bulbocavernosus muscle of penis. It has been proved that **carbon monoxide** is involved in the control of ejaculation.

Semen

The fluid that is ejaculated at the time of orgasm is called semen, which contains **sperms, secretions of seminal vesicle, prostate, Cowper's gland and urethral glands**. It is a milky, opalescent fluid. The milky appearance is due to prostatic secretion. Secretion of seminal vesicle and Cowper's gland give a mucoid nature. The secretion of seminal vesicle contains fibrinogen and so the semen clots soon after ejaculation. The sperms get entangled in this coagulum. After 15–20 min, dissolution of the coagulum occurs and sperms are freed. Buffers like HCO_3, PO_4, etc., present in the semen help to neutralize the acid present in the vagina. Vaginal pH is 3.5–4.5.

Semen Analysis

PY 9.9: Interpret a normal semen analysis report including (a) sperm count (b) sperm morphology and (c) sperm motility, as per WHO guidelines and discuss the results.

- Normal volume of semen—2.5–3.5 mL
- pH—7.35–7.5
- Specific gravity—1.028
- Sperm count—100 million/mL
- Motility—70%
- Speed of movement of sperms in female genital tract—3-5 mm/min
- Life span of sperms in the female reproductive tract—48 hours

When the sperm count is less than 20 million/mL, the condition is called **sterility**. Motility is also a very important factor. Activity and motility depend on the pH of the medium. The activity is reduced in acidic medium. Activity is increased in neutral and alkaline medium.

ENDOCRINE FUNCTION OF TESTIS

PY9.5: Describe and discuss the physiological effects of male sex hormones.

Hormones secreted by the testis are:
- Testosterone
- Dihydrotestosterone
- Androstenedione
- Estrogen
- Inhibin

Sources of the Hormones (Table 72.2)

Leydig cells form 20% of the total mass of testis and are the source of **androgen**. Leydig cells are seen in newborn male and after puberty. In childhood, Leydig cells are not seen. Tumors of Leydig cells secrete large quantities of testosterone. In females, **arrhenoblastoma**, which is an ovarian tumor, secrete androgen.

Androgens are secreted by the adrenal cortex in both sexes. Some of the androgens are converted to estrogens in fat and other extra-gonadal and extra-adrenal tissues.

Sertoli cells secrete estrogen and inhibin. About 90% of estrogens in the plasma of adult male are formed by aromatization of circulating testosterone and androstenedione. The rest comes from testes. Leydig secrete some amount of estrogen. In the Sertoli cells, aromatization of androgens occurs, producing estrogens.

Testosterone

Chemistry of Testosterone

Testosterone is a C19-17-hydroxy steroid. It is synthesized from cholesterol in the Leydig cell. It is also formed from androstenedione secreted by adrenal cortex. In Leydig cell 17α-hydroxylase is present and it hydroxylate pregnenolone in the 17th position to form **dehydroepiandrosterone**. **Androstenedione** is also formed from progesterone. Androstenedione and dehydroepiandrosterone are then converted to testosterone **(Flowchart 72.3)**. LH secreted by the anterior pituitary stimulates the Leydig cells to secrete testosterone. cAMP is the second messenger involved in

Table 72.2: Testicular hormones.	
Hormone and source	**Main actions**
Androgens (Leydig cells)	Sex differentiation and descent of testis in fetus
Testosterone	Development of secondary sex characters at puberty
Dihydrotestosterone (DHT)	Regulates spermatogenesis
Androstenedione	Maintains male secondary sexual characters in adults
Inhibin (Sertoli cells)	Inhibits FSH secretion from anterior pituitary
MRF (Sertoli cells)	Degeneration of mullerian duct in fetus
Estrogen (Sertoli cells)	Helps in spermiogenesis

Flowchart 72.3: Steps in the synthesis of androgens.

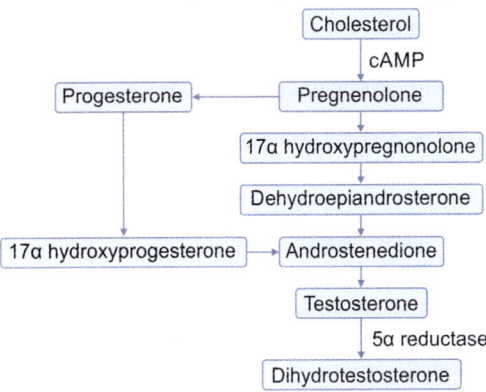

stimulating Leydig cell. cAMP increases the formation of cholesterol and stimulates the conversion of cholesterol to pregnenolone via activation of protein kinase A.

Transport and Metabolism of Testosterone

About 98% of testosterone in plasma is transported in the bound form. About 65% is bound to **gonadal steroid binding globulin (GBG)** and 33% to **albumin**. 2% is present in the **free form**.

Total plasma testosterone level—300–1000 ng/dL in adult males and 30–70 ng/dL in adult females.

There are two metabolic pathways for testosterone;
1. Reduction
   5α-reductase
   Testosterone→Dihydrotestosterone
2. Oxidation
   Testosterone reaches liver and is converted to **17-ketosteroids, androsterone and etiocholanolone**. These are excreted through urine. 2/3rd of urinary 17-ketosteroids are of adrenocortical origin and 1/3rd is of testicular origin. 17-ketosteroids are conjugated with glucuronides and sulfates, and are excreted through bile and feces as well.

Actions of Testosterone

Androgenic Effects

❖ **In fetus**: Testosterone is responsible for sex differentiation and descent of testis (during the last two months of pregnancy). Cryptorchidism is mainly caused by abnormally formed testis that is unable to produce enough testosterone. Testosterone causes the formation of prostate gland, seminal vesicles and male genital ducts. Dihydrotestosterone is necessary for the development of male external genitalia. Exposure of fetal brain to testosterone is necessary for normal male sexual behavior.
❖ **At puberty**: For the growth of both internal and external genitalia and for the appearance of secondary sex characters. Dihydrotestosterone (DHT) is responsible for the enlargement of prostate and penis at the time of puberty. Testosterone increases protein synthesis and muscle development. It increases calcium deposition in bone and increase bone strength. It also increases RBC count.
❖ **In adults**: Testosterone is necessary for the further growth and maintenance of sex organs, male secondary sex characteristics and for proper spermatogenesis.
  ▪ Change in voice is due to enlargement of larynx, hypertrophy of laryngeal mucosa, increase in length and thickness of vocal cords. The voice becomes deeper in adult males.
  ▪ Hair distribution: Beard and moustache appear, male pattern of pubic hair, hair appear in the axilla and chest wall. Baldness in male is mainly due to dihydrotestosterone, but genetic factor also has a role.
  ▪ Changes occur in the skeletal system and muscles. Shoulders become broad and muscles become well-built and strong. Pelvis becomes long and funnel shaped with extreme strength for load bearing.
  ▪ Changes in the skin include excessive stimulation of sebaceous glands producing thick abundant secretion leading to acne formation.
  ▪ Behavioral changes, such as aggressiveness, interest in opposite sex, etc., are seen.

Anabolic Actions

Testosterone stimulates protein synthesis and inhibits protein breakdown, thus producing a **positive nitrogen balance**. It stimulates growth; especially **muscle growth**, the muscle mass gets doubled. It also causes fusion of epiphysis. BMR is increased by 5–10% of normal. The kidney size will be increased.

Secondary to anabolic effect there will be retention of Na, K, H_2O, SO_4, PO_4, etc.

Other Actions

❖ Testosterone stimulates **erythropoiesis** leading to increase in RBC count in males.
❖ It has negative feedback action on LH secretion.
❖ Testosterone along with FSH helps in spermatogenesis and maintenance of germinal cells.

Mechanism of Action of Testosterone

In the cytoplasm of the target cell, testosterone or dihydrotestosterone (DHT) combines with cytoplasmic receptors and the complex migrates to the nucleus. In the nucleus, it binds to DNA and stimulates nuclear proteins. This causes transcription of various genes in DNA leading to protein synthesis through mRNA. In some target cells, testosterone is converted to DHT by **5α-reductase**. DHT also binds to the same intracellular receptor as testosterone. This complex is more stable than testosterone-receptor complex.

Congenital 5α-reductase deficiency produces male pseudo hermaphroditism. These individuals have testis and male internal genitalia, but the external genitalia are that of female. So these children are brought up as girls. At puberty, due to the action of testosterone they develop male characteristics and due to very high levels of LH and testosterone their clitoris enlarges. This condition is known as **penis-at-12 syndrome**.

5α-reductase inhibiting drugs are used to treat benign prostatic hyperplasia.

Regulation of Secretion of Testosterone (Flowchart 72.4)

In the fetus, human chorionic gonadotropin (hCG) has got LH-like activity and hCG stimulates Leydig cells to secrete fetal testosterone.

During childhood there is no gonadotropin secretion from anterior pituitary.

At the time of puberty, hypothalamus produces GnRH in a pulsatile manner, which stimulates pituitary to secrete LH and FSH. In males, gonadotropin secretion is noncyclic.

FSH stimulates Sertoli cells, and FSH and androgens together maintain gametogenesis. FSH also stimulates secretion of inhibin from Sertoli cells. Inhibin inhibits further FSH secretion by a feedback regulation on pituitary.

LH is tropic to Leydig cells and stimulates testosterone secretion. Testosterone in turn inhibits LH and gonadotropin releasing hormone (GnRH) secretion by negative feedback mechanism. GnRH released from hypothalamus is necessary for secretion of LH and FSH from anterior pituitary. So, decrease in GnRH leads to decreased secretion of LH and FSH. Thus when secretion of testosterone is too great, this negative feedback effect on hypothalamus and anterior pituitary reduces testosterone level back to normal. The opposite effect occurs when secretion of testosterone is reduced. Hypothalamic lesions lead to testicular atrophy due to lack of GnRH.

Abnormalities

Cryptorchidism

Cryptorchidism means **undescended testis**. In 10% of male newborns, the testis will be undescended on one side or both sides. By 1 year of life after birth, 2% becomes the incidence. At puberty, only 0.3% will have undescended testis. The undescended testis may be in the abdominal cavity or in the inguinal canal. **Malignant tumors** are more prone to occur in undescended testis. High temperature causes irreversible damage to seminiferous tubules leading to **sterility**.

Treatment: Gonadotropic treatment or surgery before puberty.

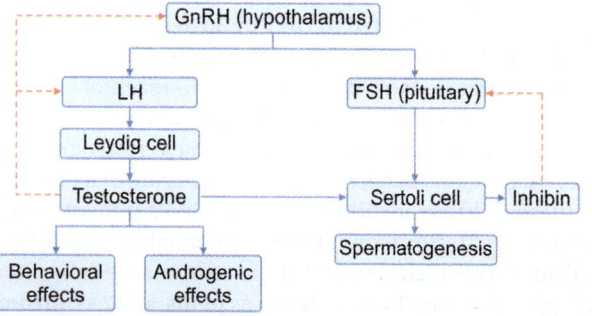

Flowchart 72.4: Regulation of secretion of testosterone (dashed line indicates negative feedback inhibition).

Infertility

Infertility is seen in the following conditions:
- Sperm count <20 million/mL of semen
- Sperms with abnormal morphology
- Decreased motility of sperms

Male Hypogonadism

Causes

- Primary hypogonadism or hypergonadotropic hypogonadism.
- Secondary hypogonadism or hypogonadotropic hypogonadism. e.g., Kallmann syndrome.
- Hormonal disorders

In **primary hypogonadism**, defect is in the testis. The circulating gonadotropin levels are elevated. In **secondary hypogonadism**, defect is in the hypothalamus or pituitary. The circulating gonadotropin levels are depressed.

Clinical features depend on whether hypogonadism occurs before puberty or after puberty.

Hypogonadism during fetal life: When the testes of a male fetus are nonfunctional during fetal life, none of the male sexual characteristics develop in the fetus. Instead, female organs are formed. The reason for this is that the basic genetic characteristic of the fetus, whether male or female, is to form female sexual organs if there are no sex hormones. However, in the presence of testosterone, formation of female sexual organs is suppressed and male organs are induced.

> **PY9.7:** Describe and discuss the effects of removal of gonads on physiological functions.

Hypogonadism before puberty: When the testes are removed from a boy before puberty, accessory sex organs and secondary sex characters do not develop. Eunuch will have childlike voice, narrow shoulders, soft muscles, female type of body configuration, etc. He continues to have infantile sex organs and other infantile sexual characteristics throughout life. They are tall because of late fusion of epiphysis. Pubic hair and axillary hair develop due to adrenal androgens, but the pubic hair will be of female type. This condition is called **eunuchoidism or eunuchism**.

Hypogonadism may be caused by a genetic inability of the hypothalamus to secrete GnRH. This condition is often associated with abnormality of the feeding center of the hypothalamus. Due to overeating, obesity is also present in these individuals along with eunuchoidism. The condition is called **adiposogenital syndrome or Frohlich's syndrome or hypothalamic eunuchism.**

Hypogonadism after puberty: If gametogenic function is affected, it leads to sterility. If endocrine function is affected, it leads to regression of accessory sex organs. There will be no change in the voice since the growth of larynx is permanent. There will be loss of libido and frequently experiences hot flushes. Psychologically, they will be irritable, passive and depressed.

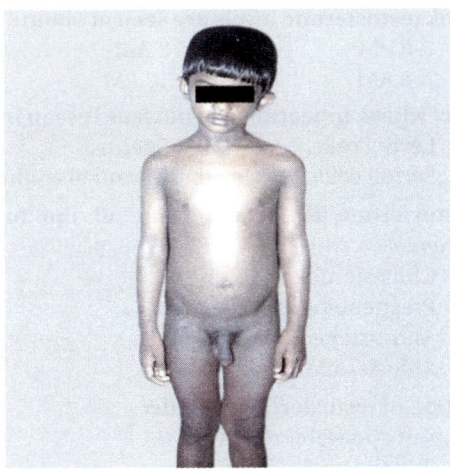

Fig. 72.5: Precocious puberty in a five-year-old boy.

Male Precocious Pseudopuberty

Androgen-secreting Leydig cell tumors in pre-pubertal boys lead to this condition **(Fig. 72.5)**. Spermatogenesis is absent and it is a very rare condition.

MULTIPLE CHOICE QUESTIONS

1. **FSH receptors in males are present in:**
   a. Sertoli cells
   b. Leydig cells
   c. Germinal epithelium
   d. Primary spermatocyte

2. **LH receptors in males are present on:**
   a. Leydig cells
   b. Sertoli cells
   c. Primary spermatocyte
   d. Spermatozoa

3. **Sertoli cells have receptors for:**
   a. FSH only
   b. Testosterone only
   c. Both FSH and testosterone
   d. Progesterone

4. **Spermatozoa get nourishment from:**
   a. Glucose
   b. Fructose
   c. Galactose
   d. Lactose

5. **Testosterone:**
   a. Causes salt and water retention
   b. Has protein catabolic effect
   c. Inhibits erythropoiesis
   d. Has positive feedback effect on LH secretion

6. **Sertoli cells are present in:**
   a. Epididymis
   b. Seminiferous tubule
   c. Rete testis
   d. Vas deferens

7. **Sertoli cells secrete:**
   a. Testosterone
   b. Progesterone
   c. Androstenedione
   d. Inhibin

8. **Testosterone production is mainly contributed by:**
   a. Leydig cells
   b. Sertoli cells
   c. Seminiferous tubules
   d. Epididymis

9. **Which of the following statements can be regarded as primary action of inhibin?**
   a. It inhibits secretion of prolactin
   b. It stimulates synthesis of estradiol
   c. It stimulates secretion of TSH
   d. It inhibits secretion of FSH

10. **Sperms are stored in the:**
    a. Seminal vesicle
    b. Seminiferous tubules
    c. Vas deferens
    d. Epididymis

11. **Sperms are produced in the:**
    a. Seminal vesicle
    b. Seminiferous tubules
    c. Vas deferens
    d. Epididymis

12. **Sperm acquire motility in:**
    a. Seminal vesicle
    b. Epididymis
    c. Rete testes
    d. Vas deferens

13. **Capacitation of sperm occur in:**
    a. Seminiferous tubule
    b. Sertoli cell
    c. Female genital tract
    d. Epididymis

14. **Which of the following hormone is mainly responsible for skeletal maturation?**
    a. Testosterone
    b. Estrogen
    c. Growth hormone
    d. Testosterone/estrogen ratio

15. **Antibodies against sperms may develop after all of the following, *except*:**
    a. Trauma
    b. Infection
    c. Vasectomy
    d. Orchidectomy

16. **Which of the following organs secretes zinc in large amount in man?**
    a. Seminal vesicle
    b. Prostate
    c. Epididymis
    d. Vas deferens

17. **Prostaglandin is mainly secreted from:**
    a. Seminal vesicle
    b. Prostate
    c. Epididymis
    d. Vas deferens

18. **60% of total volume of semen is contributed by:**
    a. Prostate
    b. Seminiferous tubules
    c. Seminal vesicle
    d. Cowper's gland

19. **Total duration of spermatogenesis from primitive germ cell to mature sperm is:**
    a. 74 days
    b. 48 hours
    c. 120 hours
    d. 72 hours

20. **Concentration of fructose in semen is:**
    a. 1.5–6.5 mg/mL
    b. 0.5–1 mg/mL
    c. 0.05–0.5 mg/mL
    d. 10–15 mg/mL

21. **The approximate speed at which human sperm move through the female genital tract:**
    a. 0–1 mm/min
    b. 2–3 mm/min
    c. 5–6 mm/min
    d. 7–10 mm/min

22. **Semen contain all the following, *except*:**
    a. Citric acid
    b. Ascorbic acid
    c. Alkaline phosphatase
    d. Fibrinolysin
23. **Failure of descent of testis is called:**
    a. Cryptorchidism
    b. Eunuchoidism
    c. Sterility
    d. Pseudohermaphroditism
24. **Sperm motility inhibitor in semen is:**
    a. Spermine
    b. Semenogelin
    c. Prostaglandin
    d. Hyaluronidase
25. **The following are involved in penile erection *except*:**
    a. Acetylcholine
    b. Vasoactive intestinal polypeptide
    c. Nitric oxide
    d. Prostaglandins
26. **Average sperm count in semen is normally:**
    a. 100 million/mL
    b. 80 million/mL
    c. 100 lakhs/mL
    d. 80 lakhs/mL
27. **Normal temperature of testis is:**
    a. 37°C
    b. 32°C
    c. 34°C
    d. 30°C
28. **Capacitation of spermatozoa occurs in the:**
    a. Vagina
    b. Isthmus of the uterine tubes
    c. Epididymis
    d. Vas deferens
29. **Following are the effects of testosterone, *except*:**
    a. Hemopoiesis
    b. Calcium retention
    c. Increase in the total quantity of bone matrix
    d. Decrease in BMR
30. **Testis does not produce:**
    a. Estradiol
    b. Testosterone
    c. Fructose
    d. Inhibin
31. **Baldness in male is due to the effect of:**
    a. Estrogen
    b. Dihydrotestosterone
    c. Testosterone
    d. Androstenedione
32. **Prostaglandin secretion is maximum in:**
    a. Urine
    b. Semen
    c. Amniotic fluid
    d. Saliva
33. **FSH is secreted by:**
    a. Chromophobes
    b. Basophils
    c. Acidophils
    d. Theca interna cells
34. **Spermatozoa mature in which of the following organs?**
    a. Epididymis
    b. Vas deferens
    c. Rete testes
    d. Prostate
35. **Precursor of testosterone is:**
    a. Methyl testosterone
    b. Pregnenolone
    c. Aldosterone
    d. Cortisone
36. **Peak testosterone levels are seen at about:**
    a. 7–8 PM
    b. 2 AM
    c. 7–8 AM
    d. 12 PM
37. **Cart wheel appearance of nucleus is seen in:**
    a. Leydig cell
    b. Sperms
    c. Sertoli cells
    d. Germinal epithelium
38. **Testosterone is formed from all the following, *except*:**
    a. Cholesterol
    b. Pregnenolone
    c. Androstenedione
    d. Aldosterone
39. **Action of testosterone include:**
    a. Salt and water retention
    b. Protein catabolic effect
    c. Inhibits erythropoiesis
    d. Development of male external genitalia
40. **Blood-testis barrier is formed by:**
    a. Sertoli cells
    b. Leydig cells
    c. Epididymis
    d. Vas deferens
41. **Mumps virus affects all, *except*:**
    a. Pancreas
    b. Parotid
    c. Testis
    d. Adrenals
42. **Blood-testis barrier is mainly formed by the presence of:**
    a. Tight junctions between germ cells
    b. Tight junctions between sertoli cells
    c. Presence of basal lamina
    d. Tight junction between stromal cells
43. **Sertoli cells produce all the following, *except*:**
    a. Androgen
    b. Androgen binding protein
    c. Inhibin
    d. Estradiol
44. **The cells in the ovary that is homologous to the sertoli cells of testis:**
    a. Theca interna
    b. Granulosa cells
    c. Theca externa
    d. Cumulus oophorus
45. **All the following statements regarding human spermatozoa are correct, *except*:**
    a. Contains 23 chromosomes
    b. Contain X or Y sex chromosome
    c. Get capacitated in the epididymis
    d. Are activated by secretions of accessory sex organs
46. **All the following statements are true regarding semen, *except*:**
    a. Average volume is 2–5 mL/ejaculate
    b. Sperm count is 80–200 million/mL
    c. Coagulate once it is ejaculated
    d. Does not contain prostaglandin
47. **Testosterone secretion by Leydig cell is inhibited by:**
    a. LH
    b. Inhibin
    c. Activin
    d. TNF-a

CHAPTER 72 — Male Reproductive System

48. Testosterone secretion by fetal Leydig cell is stimulated by:
    a. FSH
    b. LH
    c. GnRH
    d. Chorionic gonadotropin

49. The life span of spermatozoa in the female genital tract is approximately:
    a. 72 hours
    b. 48 hours
    c. 12 hours
    d. 3 days

50. Mullerian inhibiting substance is produced by:
    a. Sertoli cells
    b. Leydig cells
    c. Germ cells
    d. Granulosa cells

51. Full development and function of seminiferous tubule requires:
    a. Somatostatin and LH
    b. LH and oxytocin
    c. Androgens and FSH
    d. Oxytocin and FSH

52. Capacitation of sperm occurs in the:
    a. Epididymis
    b. Female genital tract
    c. Seminiferous tubules
    d. Vas deferens

53. Blackheads and acne are due to the action of the following hormone on sebaceous glands:
    a. Testosterone
    b. Estradiol
    c. Progesterone
    d. Estriol

54. Normal duration of spermatogenesis is:
    a. 120 days
    b. 30 days
    c. 74 days
    d. 92 days

55. The enzyme that converts androgen to estrogen in the testis is:
    a. Aromatase
    b. 5α-reductase
    c. 17α-hydroxylase
    d. 17-hydroxyprogesterone

56. Testosterone causes:
    a. Increase in sperm motility
    b. Increase in scalp hair
    c. Negative nitrogen balance
    d. Fusion of epiphysis of long bones

57. Normal length of sperm cell:
    a. 3 mm
    b. 50 μm
    c. 500 μm
    d. 3 μm

ANSWERS

1. a	2. a	3. c	4. b	5. a
6. b	7. d	8. a	9. d	10. d
11. b	12. b	13. c	14. b	15. d
16. b	17. a	18. c	19. a	20. a
21. b	22. c	23. a	24. b	25. d
26. a	27. b	28. b	29. d	30. c
31. b	32. b	33. b	34. a	35. b
36. d	37. c	38. d	39. a	40. a
41. d	42. b	43. a	44. b	45. c
46. d	47. c	48. d	49. b	50. a
51. c	52. b	53. a	54. c	55. a
56. d	57. b			

Female Reproductive System

CHAPTER 73

LEARNING OBJECTIVES
- Describe the functional anatomy of female reproductive system
- Describe the functions of ovary and control of its secretions
- Describe the menstrual cycle (hormonal, uterine and ovarian changes)
- Draw and label Graafian follicle
- Explain the actions of estrogen and progesterone

FUNCTIONAL ANATOMY

PY9.4: Describe female reproductive system: (a) functions of ovary and its control (b) menstrual cycle – hormonal, uterine and ovarian changes.

Female reproductive system consists of a pair of **ovaries** which produce ova, two **fallopian tubes** where fertilization of ovum by sperm occurs, **uterus** in which growth of the fetus and nourishment occur, the **vagina and cervix** which help in the transport of sperms **(Fig. 73.1)**, and a pair of **mammary glands** to nourish the baby after birth.

The branch of medicine that deals with the diagnosis and treatment of diseases of female reproductive system is called **gynecology**. The branch that deals with the management of pregnancy, labor and the neonatal period is **obstetrics and neonatology**.

Ovaries

Ovaries, two in number, are the primary sex organs in female. They are situated in the pelvic cavity on each side of the uterus, behind and below the fallopian tube held in position by ligaments. Ovary is held suspended in a fold of peritoneum called **mesovarium**. Each ovary measures about 4 × 3 × 2 cm in size and weighs about 10–20 g. Weight decreases with increasing age.

Each ovary consists of an **outer cortex and inner medulla**. A dense connective tissue layer, the **tunica albuginea**, covers the cortex and this layer imparts the whitish color to the ovary. Outside the tunica albuginea is located the **germinal epithelium** of Waldeyer formed of cuboidal cells. Ovarian follicles in different stages of maturation are embedded in the stroma of cortex **(Fig. 73.2)**. The medulla is composed of loose connective tissue and blood vessels.

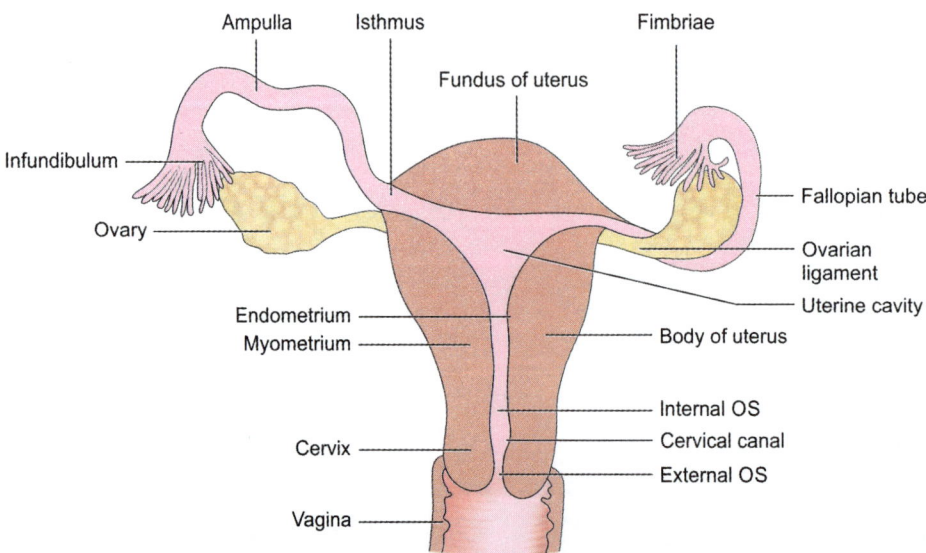

Fig. 73.1: Female reproductive organs.

In the ovary, some of the theca interna cells of atretic (degenerated) follicles present in the stroma are called **interstitial cells**. They secrete small amounts of **androgen** which is converted to estradiol.

Functions of Ovaries

- Production of gametes.
- Production of female sex hormones, estrogen and progesterone. It also produces inhibin and small amounts of activin, androgen and relaxin.

■ SECONDARY SEXUAL ORGANS IN FEMALE

The fallopian tubes, uterus, vagina, accessory glands, clitoris and mammary glands constitute the secondary sexual organs in the female.

The fallopian tube or oviduct is a muscular tube about 12 cm in length, lined by **ciliated** secretory epithelium. It is situated above and behind the urinary bladder. The secretory cells of the epithelium secrete a viscous fluid that provides nutrition and protection to the ovum. The oviduct opens into the uterus. The fimbriated end of the fallopian tube is in close relation to the ovary so that it can receive the ovum as soon as it is liberated. The ovum moves along the fallopian tube by the ciliary movement and by the peristaltic contraction of the wall of the oviduct. Usually, *fertilization occurs in the fallopian tube*.

Uterus is a thick pear-shaped organ consisting of a **body** and a lower cylindrical part, the **cervix**. The wall of the uterus is three layered. Inner layer, the **endometrium**, is made up of columnar ciliated secretory epithelium and **lamina propria**. Lamina propria is made up of simple tubular glands and connective tissue formed of fibroblasts, blood vessels and nerves. Middle layer of uterus is the thick **myometrium** made up of bundles of smooth muscles. The outermost layer is the **serosa or perimetrium**. Weight of a non-pregnant uterus is 50 g. But during pregnancy it weighs about 1000 g due to hypertrophy and hyperplasia of the smooth muscle of uterus.

The **cervix** projects into the vagina and is about 2.5 cm in length (*refer* **Fig. 73.1**). The opening of the vagina to the outside is partially covered by a thin ring of tissue called **hymen**.

The female external genitalia consist of clitoris, labia minora and labia majora. The clitoris is homologous to the male glans penis.

■ OOGENESIS

Oogenesis is the formation of ovum in the ovary. During fetal life, ovary is covered by a layer of germinal epithelium. They differentiate into **oogonia** and migrate into the substance of the ovarian cortex. Oogonia multiply rapidly and differentiate to form **primary oocyte**. Primary oocyte is covered by a single layer of cuboidal epithelium. This forms the **primordial follicle**.

There are 6–7 million oogonia at 5th month of intrauterine life (IUL). By 7th month of IUL, proliferation of oogonia stops. After 7th month, atresia or regression of oogonia occurs, and *at birth, the number of oogonia is only 2 million.* In humans, no new ova are formed after birth.

The primary oocyte undergoes *first meiotic division and stops at prophase* at the time of birth. Period of arrest in the prophase continues up to puberty or up to first ovulation. This is due to the secretion of **oocyte maturation inhibitor (OMI)** by the follicular cells. At puberty, number of oocytes is 3-4 lakhs. *Just before ovulation first meiotic division is completed.* LH surge stimulates the completion of the first meiotic division and formation of **secondary oocyte and the first polar body**.

Most of the cytoplasm of the primary oocyte goes to one of the daughter cells, and this cell forms the secondary oocyte with 23 chromosomes; and the other cell with very little cytoplasm and 23 chromosomes forms the first polar body. In humans, first polar body fragments and degenerates normally. If it persists, it undergoes second meiotic division to form 2 polar bodies which fragment and degenerate.

Secondary oocyte undergoes **second meiotic division** and stops at the stage of **metaphase**. The arrest in metaphase is due to the formation of the protein **pp39mos** a product of the **c-mos proto-oncogene**. Mos protein was previously known as endogenous meiotic inhibitor in vertebrate eggs. When fertilization occurs, this protein is destroyed by **calpain**, a calcium dependent cysteine protease (proteolytic enzyme). If fertilization does not occur the secondary oocyte

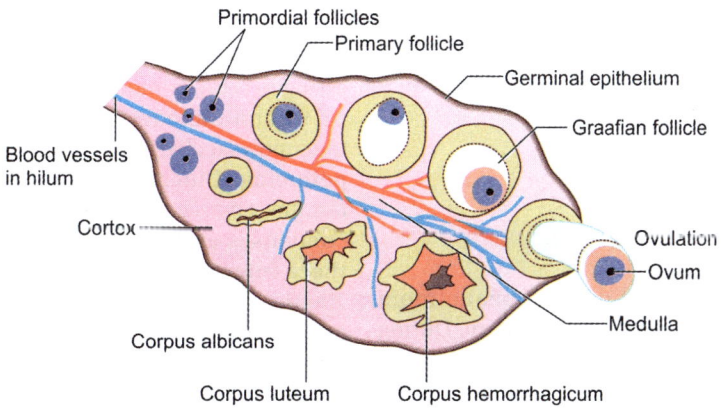

Fig. 73.2: Structure of ovary.

Flowchart 73.1: Steps in oogenesis. Note that only one haploid ovum is formed from a primary oocyte whereas from a primary spermatocyte 4 haploid sperms are formed.

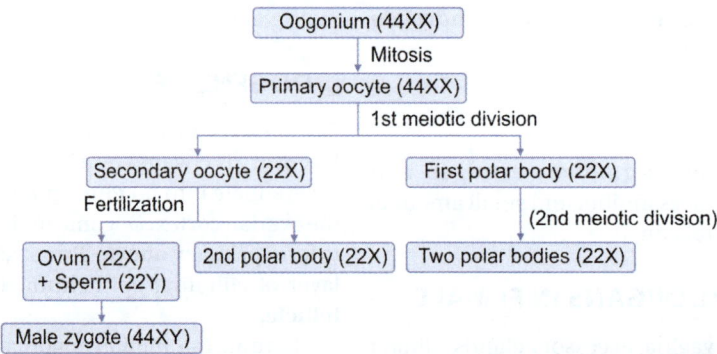

degenerates. *Second meiotic division is completed only when the sperm fertilizes the ovum.* If fertilization occurs, second meiotic division is completed leading to the formation of mature ovum and second polar body. Thus, *one primary oocyte finally gives rise to 1 haploid ovum and 3 haploid polar bodies* **(Flowchart 73.1)**. The polar bodies degenerate (one primary spermatocyte produces 4 mature sperms).

About 450 ova are produced during the reproductive period of a female, and during ovulation only one ovum is liberated.

Both spermatozoa and ova originate from primordial germ cells which are extra-gonadal in origin. During the early embryonic development the primordial germ cells originate from the extra embryonic mesoderm. Later, they migrate to the yolk sac and then to the gonads where they undergo further development.

■ FEMALE REPRODUCTIVE CYCLE OR MENSTRUAL CYCLE

In mammals other than primates, the reproductive cycle in female is called **estrous cycle**. The number of cycles/year varies in different animals. In animals, period of heat is the period of ovulation. Sexual interest is aroused only during this period and the females become more receptive to males.

In primates, reproductive cycle is known as **menstrual cycle** where, regular, rhythmic changes are seen in the reproductive system. Main characteristic is periodic vaginal bleeding associated with shedding of endometrium. The duration of each cycle varies between 20 days and 45 days and the average duration is considered as 28 days. Cyclical changes occur in the sex organs like ovary, uterus and vagina, and the menstrual cycle is divided into three phases:
1. Ovarian cycle
2. Uterine cycle
3. Vaginal cycle

Ovarian Cycle

The changes in the ovary depend on the gonadotropin (FSH and LH) secretion from the anterior pituitary. During childhood there is no gonadotropin secretion and hence primordial follicles remain inactive. The primary oocyte surrounded by a basal lamina containing flat spindle-shaped cells is called **primordial follicle**. Between the ages of 11 and 15 years, there is cyclical secretion of FSH and LH producing cyclical changes in the ovaries. The phases are:
* Follicular phase
* Ovulation phase
* Luteal phase

Follicular Phase

At the time of puberty, ovaries contain about 3–4 lakhs primordial follicles. FSH and LH from the anterior pituitary cause growth of the entire ovary along with the follicles. Follicular growth has two stages:
1. Conversion of primordial follicle to primary follicle.
2. Conversion of primary follicle to Graafian follicle.

About 1 year is required for a primordial follicle to mature into a Graafian follicle.

Follicle stimulating hormone (FSH) acts on primordial follicle and it enlarges 2–3 times. The spindle cells of primordial follicle get converted into a single layer of cuboidal epithelium surrounded by a basal lamina. Now the follicle is called **primary follicle (Figs. 73.2 and 73.6A)**.

Conversion of primary follicle to Graafian follicle includes two phases:
1. Proliferative phase
2. Antral phase

Proliferative Phase

By the action of FSH, 6–12 primary follicles begin to enlarge each month. The cuboidal cells surrounding the oocyte multiply and form several layers of cells and these cells are called **granulosa cells**. The primary source of circulating estrogen is the granulosa cells of the ovaries.

Around the oocyte of the dominant follicle, a layer of mucopolysaccharide is formed and this layer is called **zona pellucida**. Outermost layer of granulosa cell is the basal lamina. Ovarian stroma containing spindle-shaped cells condenses around the follicle. The inner layer is called **theca interna** and the outer layer is called **theca externa**. The theca interna has an epithelioid character. It secretes **androgens** that are taken up by the granulosa cells and aromatized to estrogen. Theca externa is highly vascular with thick connective tissue and it forms the capsule of the follicle.

Antral Phase

After the proliferative phase, the granulosa cells secrete a fluid which contains high concentration of estradiol. A cavity appears in the mass of granulosa cells, called **antrum**. The antrum gets filled with a fluid called **liquor folliculi**.

Granulosa and theca cells proliferate rapidly. The resulting follicle is called **vesicular follicle or Graafian follicle or antral follicle**. The Graafian follicle measures about 10–12 mm in diameter (**Fig. 73.3**). Of the several primary follicles developing in the ovary, only one becomes Graafian follicle each month. By day 7 of the menstrual cycle, the dominant follicle is selected and the rest of the developing follicles begin to undergo atresia.

Ovum occupies an eccentric position in the Graafian follicle and it is surrounded by 2–3 layers of granulosa cells called **cumulus oophorus**. FSH is responsible for early growth of the follicle. Both FSH and LH are necessary for the final maturation of the follicle to form Graafian follicle (**Fig. 73.3**).

The dominant follicle in the pre-antral phase contains FSH receptors only on the granulosa cells and LH receptors only on the theca cells. The theca cells produce androgen in response to LH and granulosa cells produce estrogen in response to FSH. This androgen will be taken up by the granulosa cells and are aromatized to estrogens. This is called the **two-cell theory of steroidogenesis**. Estrogen in the follicle increases the number of FSH receptors in the granulosa cells and thus increases the sensitivity of these cells to FSH.

Estrogen level peaks towards the end of the follicular phase of the menstrual cycle. This increasing estradiol exerts a negative feedback effect on FSH secretion from the pituitary. The granulosa cells also produce inhibin-B which also exerts a negative feedback on FSH secretion. This decrease in FSH has a negative effect on the non-dominant follicles leading to their destruction.

Because of the higher density of FSH receptors in the dominant follicle, it continues to produce estrogen and aromatize androgen to estrogen. Activin is also produced by the granulosa cells in response to FSH stimulation. It increases the number of FSH receptors on the granulosa cells. The net effect is a high concentration of estradiol in the dominant follicle. In the late stages of follicular development, FSH also induces LH receptors on the granulosa cells. LH acts synergistically with FSH. This is essential for the granulosa cells to be able to respond to LH surge in mid-cycle. Increase in FSH precedes increase in LH.

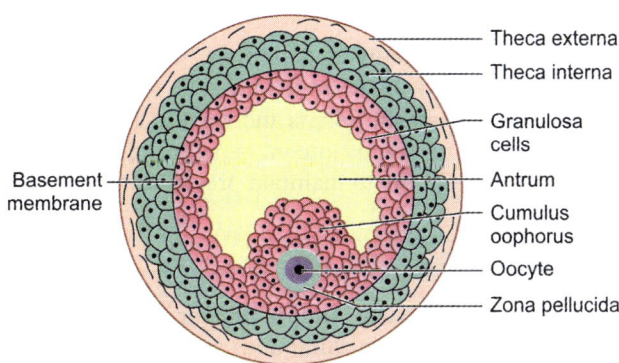

Fig. 73.3: Structure of a Graafian follicle.

Ovulation

Rupture of the mature Graafian follicle and release of ovum (secondary oocyte) surrounded by cumulus oophorus into the abdominal cavity is called ovulation. It occurs on the 14th day of a 28-day cycle.

Mechanism of Ovulation

Graafian follicle secretes large quantities of estrogen mainly estradiol. When the plasma estradiol level reaches 200 pg/mL, it exerts a positive feedback effect on LH secretion. Two days before ovulation, LH secretion from anterior pituitary is increased 6–10 times due to positive feedback effect of estrogen. This is called **LH surge**. *Increase in circulating estradiol to a critical level and of sufficient duration (for a minimum of 2 days) is necessary to initiate LH surge.* The dominant follicle reaches a size of 20–26 mm before the LH surge. LH surge lasts for 48 hours and is necessary for the complete maturation of the oocyte. Ovulation normally occurs about 9 hours after the peak of LH surge. Immediately before LH surge, a sudden depression of estrogen secretion by the ovarian follicles is seen. There is also a 2-fold increase in FSH secretion. Increase in FSH secretion is due to the strong stimulation of gonadotropes by GnRH (*refer* Fig. 73.5). The significance of the midcycle burst of FSH secretion is uncertain.

Increase in estrogen level in the midcycle has two effects:
1. Increasing estradiol levels in the preovulatory phase sensitizes the gonadotropes in the anterior pituitary to GnRH pulses.
2. Increasing estrogen levels modulate hypothalamic neuronal activity and induce GnRH surge.

Exact mechanism of LH surge is not clearly understood. Recent studies show that the negative and positive feedback effects of estrogen are exerted in the hypothalamus. There are neurons in the hypothalamus that express a peptide called **kisspeptin**. Estrogen and progesterone modulate kisspeptin activity through receptors expressed on kisspeptin neurons in the infundibular nucleus of hypothalamus. In the positive feedback effect of estrogen, there is increase in the frequency of GnRH bursts from the hypothalamus which in turn strongly stimulate the gonadotropes of anterior pituitary to produce the LH surge. Episodic bursts of GnRH secretion are essential for the normal secretion of gonadotropins (LH and FSH). Just before LH surge the sensitivity of gonadotropes to GnRH is greatly increased because of their exposure to GnRH pulses at a specific frequency.

The mature Graafian follicle moves towards the surface of the ovary. At the time of ovulation, progesterone levels in the mature follicle rise. Progesterone is produced by the granulosa cells and theca cells which are stimulated by LH. The midcycle LH and FSH surge also result in plasminogen activator production in the mature follicle. It converts plasminogen to plasmin. Plasmin causes detachment of the cumulus oophorus from the surrounding granulosa cells. The oocyte now floats in the follicular fluid. Plasmin, FSH, LH and progesterone stimulates the theca externa to release proteolytic enzymes like collagenase which cause digestion of the collagen in the follicular wall and dissolution of the capsule. FSH and LH also stimulate production of prostaglandins (PGF2α, PGE2) and histamine in the follicle which also aids in the rupture of the follicular wall and extrusion of the oocyte.

A small area on the central part of the capsule protrudes like a nipple called **stigma**, towards the outer part of the ovary. The follicular fluid escapes into the stigma because it is thin and avascular and finally the stigma ruptures, releasing the secondary oocyte into the abdominal cavity. The oocyte or ovum is arrested in the second stage of metaphase of second meiotic division, and is covered by granulosa cells. The exact reason for the arrest in metaphase is not clear. It may be due to formation in the ovum of the protein **pp39mos**, which is encoded by the **cmos protooncogene**. If fertilization occurs, the pp39mos is destroyed within 30 minutes by **calpain**, a calcium-dependent cysteine protease. The ovum in the abdominal cavity is carried or sucked into the fimbrial end of the fallopian tube. If the ovum is not fertilized it degenerates and is expelled out.

The released ovum is haploid (22X) and is one of the largest cells in the body, measures about 120-130 micrometer in diameter. It has an eccentric round nucleus with prominent nucleolus.

Role of LH in Ovulation

- LH is the hormone of ovulation.
- Along with FSH helps in rapid growth of Graafian follicle.
- It stimulates secretion of follicular steroids.
- Along with FSH and progesterone stimulates theca externa to produce proteolytic enzymes which cause dissolution of the capsule.
- It is responsible for the rapid growth of new blood vessels into the follicular wall.
- It causes secretion of prostaglandin which is a vasodilator.
- It increases plasma transudation into the follicle which causes further swelling of the follicle.

> The rapidly growing follicle contains excess amount of estradiol and this causes positive feedback in the granulosa cells leading to increased proliferation of granulosa cells. Estrogen also increases the FSH receptors in the granulosa cells and this increases the action of FSH on granulosa cells leading to increase in the number of granulosa cells. The net effect is rapid increase in the size of that follicle. When estrogen level in the blood increases, it exerts a negative feedback effect on FSH and LH secretion by acting on hypothalamus and pituitary. As the FSH level decreases, the follicles other than the dominant follicle which contains less number of FSH receptors cannot produce the requisite amount of estradiol. This decreases the development of these less developed follicles resulting in their regression by apoptosis. The dominant follicle, with its high concentration of FSH receptors, continues to synthesize estradiol. Estradiol in turn increases the number of FSH receptors in the granulosa cells leading to the complete maturation of the dominant follicle. *This is the reason why only one Graafian follicle is formed in one cycle normally.* It has also been observed that the dominant follicle always expresses an abundance of FSH receptors. If pituitary gonadotropins are given by injection, many follicles develop simultaneously.

Luteal Phase

Once ovulation has occurred, the wall of the follicle collapses and blood accumulates in the cavity of the follicle. This is called **corpus hemorrhagicum**. During ovulation, minor bleeding occurs into the peritoneal cavity producing a fleeting lower abdominal pain called **mittelschmerz**. This is an indication of ovulation.

Under the influence of luteinizing hormone (LH), the granulosa cells and theca interna cells proliferate in the corpus hemorrhagicum and the cavity gets filled with lipid-rich luteal cells. The luteal cells form a yellow pigment called lutein similar to carotene and hence these cells are called luteal cells. This process is called **luteinization**. The structure formed is **corpus luteum** which is about 15 to 20 mm in size **(Fig. 73.2)**. Formation and maintenance of corpus luteum is by LH.

The granulosa cell layer becomes vascularized after ovulation. When blood flow increases, more cholesterol is delivered to the luteinized granulosa cells by low density lipoprotein (LDL). This is necessary for the production of progesterone and estradiol. LH increases LDL receptors in the granulosa cells. The corpus luteum secretes **estrogen, progesterone, inhibin and relaxin**. After LH surge the granulosa cells express new LH receptors and its affinity for LH increases and that for FSH decreases. As a result there is increased progesterone synthesis in the granulosa cells than estrogen. Hence progesterone becomes the dominant steroid in the luteal phase. Progesterone levels continue to rise as long as LH is present.

High progesterone levels exert a negative feedback effect on GnRH and subsequently GnRH pulse frequency decreases. As a result LH and FSH secretion also decreases. Reduction of FSH and LH also occurs in this phase due to negative feedback effect of estrogen and progesterone on the pituitary. The stimulation of corpus luteum by LH and FSH decreases. Both lead to a gradual decrease in estrogen and progesterone in the late luteal phase. If the ovum is not fertilized, there is no human chorionic gonadotropin (hCG) secreted by the trophoblastic cells of the blastocyst to maintain the corpus luteum. By about the 24th day of the 28-day cycle, corpus luteum degenerates and forms **corpus albicans** which is a mass of fibrous scar tissue. This is called **luteolysis**. Prostaglandin has a role in luteolysis.

When corpus luteum degenerates, no estrogen and progesterone are formed and the negative feedback effect is removed, FSH secretion starts and the next cycle begin. If fertilization occurs corpus luteum persists and is the main source of progesterone to maintain pregnancy in the early stages.

Uterine Cycle or Endometrial Cycle

Endometrium consists of simple tubular glands lined by epithelial cells which are continuous with the lining of the rest of the endometrium. In between the tubular glands, the

endometrium contains stromal cells. Endometrium consists of two layers:
1. **Stratum basale** which forms the basal 1/3rd.
2. **Stratum functionale** which forms the superficial 2/3rd of endometrium (Fig. 73.6B).

Blood Supply of Endometrium
Endometrium is supplied by two types of arteries:
1. **Basilar artery or straight artery** which supplies the stratum basale. This part is not shed during menstruation.
2. **Spiral artery** supplies stratum functionale. This layer is shed during menstruation. In human beings, the menstrual cycle is counted from the day menstrual bleeding occurs.

Phases of Uterine Cycle (Fig. 73.4)
❖ Menstrual phase: 1–4 days
❖ Proliferative phase: 5–14 days
❖ Secretory phase: 15–28 days of 28-day cycle

Menstrual Phase
In human beings, the menstrual cycle is counted from the day menstrual bleeding occurs. Menstruation will occur exactly 14 days after ovulation. During this period, the superficial part of endometrium or stratum functionale is desquamated or shed and it lasts for 4–5 days. At the end of menstruation, all the layers of endometrium will be sloughed except the deep layers.

Proliferative Phase or Preovulatory Phase
Shedding of the stratum functionale leaves only the basal portions of the tubular glands. The endometrium will be only 2 mm thick. The endometrium increases rapidly in thickness from the 5th to the 14th days of the 28 day menstrual cycle. Changes occurring in the proliferative phase are mainly due to estrogen from the developing ovarian follicle and hence this phase is also known as **estrogenic phase**. It corresponds to the follicular phase of ovarian cycle.

The main changes are stromal cells and epithelial cells of the tubular glands proliferate and the endometrium gets covered by epithelial cells derived from the tubular glands, i.e., **epithelization** occurs within 7 days of menstrual cycle. Blood vessels grow into the endometrium and the glands increase in length. At the end of this phase, the endometrium becomes 4–7 mm thick. As the thickness increases, the uterine glands increase in length but they do not secrete. This part of the menstrual cycle is called proliferative phase.

Changes in the Cervical Secretion
Mucous membrane of cervix shows no change, but the cervical secretion becomes **thin, elastic and alkaline** in response to estrogen. It helps in the survival, motility and transport of spermatozoa. When a thin layer of cervical mucus is spread on a slide, it dries up forming a **fern pattern** due to the presence of NaCl in it. Cervical mucus is thinnest at the time of ovulation. The elasticity of cervical mucus or **spinnbarkeit** is maximal in the mid-cycle so that a drop of mucus can be stretched into a long thin thread about 8–12 cm in length. The mucosa of the uterine cervix does not undergo cyclical desquamation although it is continuous with the body of the uterus.

Secretory Phase
During the second half of menstrual cycle, large quantities of **estrogen and progesterone** are secreted by corpus luteum and these hormones are responsible for the secretory phase of uterine cycle. Estrogen produces slight additional cellular proliferation and progesterone is responsible for the swelling and secretory activity of the endometrium. Progesterone is the main hormone responsible for this phase. The endometrium becomes highly vascularized and the glands secrete a clear fluid. This phase corresponds to the luteal phase of ovarian cycle and is called the secretory phase. The secretory phase represents the preparation of endometrium for implantation. *The duration of secretory phase is relatively constant and menstruation occurs exactly 14 days after ovulation.*

Main Changes in the Endometrium
❖ Endometrial glands increase in length and diameter, and they become coiled more tortuous. Towards the late secretory phase the endometrial glands become increasingly tortuous and the stroma becomes edematous and highly vascular.
❖ Epithelial cells lining the glands show secretory products, and the lumen of the gland gets filled with clear secretion. Progesterone is responsible for the secretory activity. Progesterone induces secretory changes only if the endometrium is primed by estrogen which increases progesterone receptors in the endometrial cells.
❖ There is increased deposition of glycogen and lipid in the stromal cells.
❖ Spiral artery becomes more tortuous and the vascularity of the endometrium increases. Arteriovenous and venovenous anastomosis occurs and they open into sinusoids or venous lakes.
❖ The thickness of the endometrium increases to 8–12 mm.

Changes in the Cervical Secretion
Cervical mucus becomes **thick**, tenacious, and cellular and fails to form the fern pattern due to the influence of progesterone.

Menstrual Phase
If the ovum is not fertilized, the corpus luteum regresses and fails to produce estrogen and progesterone. This reduction in the hormone level is responsible for menstruation.

Main changes are:
❖ Due to lack of estrogen and progesterone, endometrium becomes thinner due to **involution**. This leads to more coiling of spiral arteries. The coiled arteries undergo vasoconstriction a few hours before the onset of menstrual bleeding.

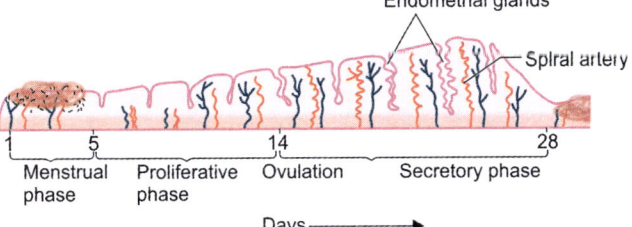

Fig. 73.4: Uterine changes during a 28-day menstrual cycle.

- Areas of **necrosis** appear in the endometrium due to lack of blood supply.
- The necrotic endometrium releases **prostaglandin F_2 alpha** which causes spasm of spiral arteries and uterine muscle contractions. Release of prostaglandin is the reason for dysmenorrhea.
- Spots of hemorrhages occur into the superficial layers of endometrium and gradually the superficial parts of the endometrium gets sloughed off leading to menstrual flow. Complete shedding occurs within 4–5 days.

Blood in the menstrual flow is mainly arterial. Only 25% is venous. Menstrual blood consists of tissue debris, blood, serous fluid, secretions from glands, prostaglandin, fibrinolysin from the endometrial tissue, etc. The fibrinolysin lyses the clot formed during menstruation, and so menstrual blood does not clot unless the flow is excessive. During menstruation large number of leukocytes is released along with blood. As a result, the uterus is highly resistant to infection during menstruation. During each menstrual flow about 30 mL of blood and 35 mL of serous fluid is lost. Loss of more than 80 mL of blood is abnormal. Bleeding is stopped by local vasoconstriction of the spiral arteries, clotting and re-epithelialization of the sloughed endometrium. Vasoconstriction is mediated by endothelins and $PGF_2\alpha$. After menstruation, a new endometrium regenerates from the stratum basale. Regeneration begins 36 hours after menstruation. Menstruation is referred to as crying of the uterus for lack of baby.

The length of the secretory phase is constant, i.e., about 14 days. Variations seen in the length of the menstrual cycle is due to variations in the length of the proliferative phase.
- **Menarche**—First menstrual period
- **Menopause**—Stoppage of menstruation for more than one year

Vaginal Cycle

During proliferative phase, estrogen from ovary causes **cornification** of vaginal epithelial cells. Cornified epithelial cells can be identified in the vaginal smear.

During secretory phase, due to the action of progesterone, there will be proliferation of vaginal epithelium and it gets infiltrated with leukocytes. Thick mucus is also secreted.

CHANGES IN THE BREAST

Estrogen stimulates growth of mammary ducts. Progesterone is responsible for growth of alveoli and lobules, distention of ducts, hyperemia and edema of interstitial tissue of breast causing pain and tenderness during the 10 days preceding menstruation. All these changes regress along with the symptoms, during menstruation.

ENDOCRINE FUNCTION OF OVARY

> **PY9.5:** Describe and discuss the physiological effects of female sex hormones.

Ovary produces female sex hormones *estrogen and progesterone* (**Table 73.1**). It also secretes *inhibin, activin, follistatin* and *relaxin*. Inhibin is secreted by granulosa cells and it inhibits FSH production by the gonadotrophs. Activin activates FSH production. Both inhibin and activin are glycoproteins. Follistatin is a polypeptide that inhibits FSH production by binding to activin and thereby inhibiting it.

Estrogen

Sources of Estrogen

- Ovary: Theca interna, granulosa cells and corpus luteum
- Placenta in pregnancy
- Adrenal cortex
- Testis in male: Sertoli cells

Forms of Estrogen

Estrone, 17β-estradiol and estriol are the biologically important natural estrogens. Estrone is produced in the ovary by the aromatization of androstenedione. It is also produced in the adipose tissue and muscle by the peripheral conversion of circulating androstenedione. It is less active than estradiol. *Estradiol is the most potent estrogen* and is mainly produced by the ovary. Androstenedione can be converted to testosterone which is then aromatized to estradiol. Estrone can also be converted to estradiol peripherally. Estriol is the weakest of the natural estrogens. It is a metabolic by-product of estrone and estradiol during their inactivation.

Synthesis of Estrogen (Flowchart 73.2)

Steps in the synthesis of estrogens is described in **Flowchart 73.2.**

Table 73.1: Ovarian hormones and their main actions.

Hormone	Main actions
Estrogens and progesterone	• Maintain female secondary sex characters • Regulate reproductive cycles oogenesis • Maintenance of pregnancy lactation
Relaxin	• Relaxes pubic symphysis • Dilates uterine cervix during parturition
Inhibin	Inhibits FSH secretion from anterior pituitary

Flowchart 73.2: Steps in the synthesis of estrogens.

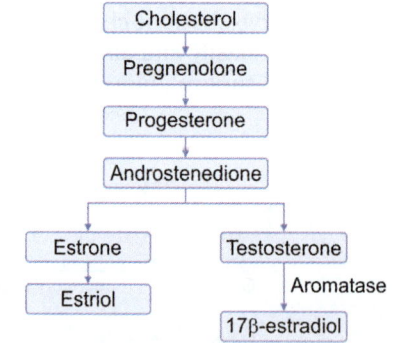

Transport of Estrogen
- 3% transported in blood in the free form
- 60% bound to albumin
- 37% to gonadal steroid binding globulin (GBG)

Rate of Secretion
In adult females:
- Just before ovulation: 0.5 mg/day
- In the mid-luteal phase: 0.25 mg/day
- Early follicular phase: 0.07 mg/day

After menopause, estrogen secretion declines to low levels.

Metabolism and Excretion
Estradiol, estrone and estriol are degraded in the liver. They are conjugated with **glucuronides and sulfates**, and excreted through urine and bile. Appreciable amounts undergo enterohepatic circulation.

Actions of Estrogen
- **Ovary**: Causes growth of ovarian follicles.
- **Uterus**:
  - *Myometrium*: Increases the size and vascularity of uterus, increases excitability and increases the sensitivity of uterus to oxytocin. It increases the content of contractile proteins in the uterine muscle.
  - *Endometrium*: Responsible for the proliferative changes during menstrual cycle. Prolonged exposure of the endometrium to estrogen is a risk factor in the development of endometrial cancer.
  - *Cervix*: Secretion becomes thin, alkaline and elastic. Fern pattern is observed.
- **Fallopian tube**: Estrogen causes proliferation of epithelial cells and increased activity of cilia in the fallopian tube. The motility of the uterine tubes is also increased.
- **Vagina**: Cornification of vaginal epithelium. Vaginal epithelium changes from cuboidal to stratified type. pH of vagina becomes more acidic and this prevents vaginal infections.
- **Breast**: Estrogen stimulates duct growth in breasts and causes enlargement of breasts at the time of puberty. There is also increased fat deposition and causes pigmentation of areola.
- **Secondary sexual characters**: Estrogen is responsible for the development of secondary sexual characters in females. Estrogen is referred to as the **feminizing hormone**.
- **Bone**: Estrogen increases osteoblastic activity so that at puberty growth rate increases. But, it also causes early fusion of epiphysis with the shaft of the bone. Absence of estrogen leads to osteoporosis as in old age. Estrogens inhibit osteoclastic activity due to stimulation of **osteoprotegerin**, also called **osteoclastogenesis-inhibitory factor**, a cytokine that inhibits bone resorption.
- **Skin**: Estrogen makes sebaceous gland secrete more fluid and inhibits formation of black heads (comedones) and acne. Estrogen rapidly produces vasodilatation by increasing the local production of NO.
- **Effects on endocrine glands**: Estrogen decreases FSH secretion from anterior pituitary. It has a negative feedback effect on LH secretion, but high concentration of estrogen has a positive feedback effect on LH secretion as at the time of ovulation. Estrogen increases secretion of angiotensinogen and thyroid binding globulin.
- **Central nervous system and behavior:** Estrogens increase libido in humans due to its direct effect on certain neurons in the hypothalamus probably in the suprachiasmatic area. Estrogens also increase the proliferation of dendrites on neurons.

Metabolism
- *Protein metabolism*: Estrogen has anabolic action and produce positive nitrogen balance. Due to its anabolic effect, estrogen treatment has been used commercially to increase the weight in chickens and cattle.
- *Fat metabolism*: Estrogen causes deposition of fat in subcutaneous tissue, breasts, buttocks and thighs. It decreases total blood cholesterol and LDL level, and so these values are less in female up to menopause. HDL increases under estrogen influence.
- *Electrolyte and water*: Causes sodium and water retention. This is responsible for **premenstrual syndrome or premenstrual tension**. There is weight gain before the onset of menstruation due to water retention.

Mechanism of Action
There are two principal types of nuclear estrogen receptors—estrogen receptor-α (ER-α) and estrogen receptor-β (ER-β). Most of the tissues contain one type of receptor or the other but certain tissues contain both types of receptors. ER-alpha is found in the uterus, kidney, liver and heart. ER-beta is found in the ovaries, prostate, lungs, GIT, hemopoietic system and CNS.

Most of the effects of estrogen are due to actions on the nucleus. But, rapid actions of estrogen like effects on neuronal discharge in brain and feedback effects on gonadotropin secretion are mediated by cell membrane receptors acting via protein kinase pathways. The cell membrane receptors are structurally related to the nuclear receptors.

Regulation of Secretion
Estrogen secretion is regulated by **FSH** from pituitary and **GnRH** from hypothalamus.

Synthetic Estrogens
Estrogens are used clinically in situations like postmenopausal hormone replacement therapy, dysfunctional uterine bleeding (DUB), and in carcinoma prostate in males. Naturally occurring estrogens cannot be given orally because they will be metabolized in the liver. So, synthetic estrogens are used because they are resistant to hepatic metabolism. Usually used synthetic estrogen is **stilbesterol (ethinyl estradiol)**. It is used as an oral contraceptive and also advised after menopause to prevent osteoporosis. Others include mestranol and quinestrol. An undesirable effect of estrogen

therapy is that it produces uterine and breast cancer. Two compounds **tamoxifen and raloxifene**, have the bone-preserving effects of estradiol. These compounds are referred to as selective estrogen receptor modulators (**SERMs**) and they do not stimulate the breast or the uterus.

Progesterone

Sources

Progesterone is a C_{21} steroid secreted by **corpus luteum, placenta, adrenal cortex and** small amounts by **ovarian follicle and testes**.

Biosynthesis

Progesterone is an intermediate product in steroid biosynthesis.

Cholesterol →Pregnenolone →Progesterone

Transport

- 2% transported in free form
- 80% bound to albumin
- 18% bound to corticosteroid binding globulin

Secretion

- Adult male: 0.3 ng/mL of blood
- Adult female:
  - Follicular phase – 0.9 ng/mL of blood
  - Secretory phase (luteal phase) – 18 ng/mL of blood

Metabolism

Progesterone is metabolized in the liver to pregnanediol, and is conjugated with glucuronic acid and excreted through urine.

Actions of Progesterone

Uterus

- *In myometrium*: In myometrium, progesterone has **anti-estrogenic** action. Uterus becomes less active, less sensitive to oxytocin and less excitable because there is a rise in membrane potential, i.e., the membrane becomes hyperpolarized. This prevents expulsion of implanted zygote.
- *Endometrium*: Progesterone is responsible for the secretory changes in the endometrium which is previously primed with estrogen. It decreases the number of estrogen receptors in the endometrium and increases the conversion of 17β-estradiol to less active estrogens.
- *Cervix:* Cervical mucus becomes thick, tenacious and cellular. Fern pattern disappears.

Vagina

Progesterone causes proliferation of vaginal epithelium and infiltration with leukocytes.

Fallopian Tube

Secretory changes occur in the epithelium and the secretions are necessary for the nutrition and protection of fertilized ovum.

- **Breast**: Progesterone stimulates growth of lobules and alveoli of breast. It supports the secretory function of the breast during lactation which is previously estrogen primed.
- **Endocrine glands**: Progesterone has a negative feedback effect on LH secretion from pituitary and GnRH secretion from hypothalamus. It potentiates the inhibitory effects of estrogen in preventing ovulation.
- **Electrolyte metabolism**: In large doses, progesterone causes excretion of sodium by competing with aldosterone for the same receptor in the kidney.
- **Pregnancy**: Progesterone is essential for the continuation of pregnancy. It prevents abortion.

Thermogenic action: Due to the action of progesterone, basal body temperature increases by 0.5°C after ovulation and this temperature is maintained throughout the luteal phase. The metabolites of progesterone like **etiocholanolone and pregnanediol** are responsible for the thermogenic action.

Respiratory system: Progesterone stimulates respiration and alveolar PCO_2 is decreased during luteal phase and in pregnancy.

Mechanism of Action

Action of progesterone is on the DNA to initiate synthesis of new mRNA. The progesterone receptor in the nucleus is bound to a **heat shock protein** and binding of progesterone to the receptor releases the heat shock protein, exposing the DNA binding domain of the receptor.

Mifepristone, a synthetic steroid, binds to the receptor but does not release the heat shock protein and competitively inhibits the binding of progesterone to the receptor. When given in the early stages of pregnancy, mifepristone **causes abortion**. This is by inhibiting the actions of progesterone on pregnant uterus. Progesterone is very essential for the maintenance of early pregnancy. Mifepristone combined with prostaglandin is used to induce abortion.

Synthetic Progesterone

Gestagens or progestin or progestational agents mimic the actions of progesterone. They are used with synthetic estrogens as oral contraceptive agents. Synthetic progesterone includes norethindrone, norethynodrel, ethynodiol and norgestrel.

Uses of Synthetic Progesterone

- Used as a contraceptive agent in females.
- Prevent abortion especially in the first trimester.
- It is also used to prevent preterm labor.
- Facilitate placenta formation.
- Decrease uterine contractility.
- Stimulate endometrial growth.
- Used in in vitro fertilization cycles along with GnRH.
- Used along with estrogen in hormone replacement therapy (HRT) to counter the unopposed effects of estrogen.

Relaxin

Relaxin is a polypeptide hormone.

Sources

Corpus luteum, secretory endometrium, placenta, mammary glands in female and prostate in men.

Actions

- Relaxation of pubic symphysis and other pelvic joints during pregnancy.
- Dilatation and softening of cervix, thus facilitating delivery.
- Decrease uterine contractility during pregnancy.
- Helps in the development of mammary glands.
- In men it is present in semen and is necessary for sperm motility.

CONTROL OF OVARIAN FUNCTION

Cyclic changes in the ovaries are controlled by pituitary gonadotropic hormones, which in turn are controlled by hypothalamus and also by feedback effects of the ovarian hormones. After puberty, GnRH is secreted throughout the day in a pulsatile fashion. The frequency and amplitude of GnRH pulses differ in different phases of the reproductive cycle. Follicular phase is characterized by continuous small amplitude pulses once in 60 minutes. In the late follicular phase, there is increase in both frequency and amplitude of the pulses. In the luteal phase, the frequency of pulses decreases but the amplitude increases. This variation in the GnRH pulses is responsible for the variation in secretion of gonadotropins throughout the menstrual cycle. Gonadotropic hormones are FSH and LH.

FSH and LH

FSH is responsible for early follicular growth. LH regulates the theca interna cells whereas the granulosa cells are regulated by both LH and FSH. Both FSH and LH are responsible for maturation of follicle. LH surge is responsible for ovulation and formation of corpus luteum. There is also increase in FSH secretion at the time of ovulation.

During luteal phase, LH and FSH are at basal levels due to increase in progesterone and estrogen secreted by corpus luteum. Peak of progesterone secretion occurs in the mid-luteal phase. Estrogen and progesterone exert negative feedback effect on FSH and LH secretion. *Progesterone inhibits positive feedback effect of estrogen on LH secretion.* In the late luteal phase, if fertilization does not occur, estrogen and progesterone level fall due to luteolysis. So, there is no feedback inhibition on hypothalamus and pituitary. Gonadotropic hormone secretion increases. Rise in FSH precedes rise in LH. Rise in FSH occurs just before menstruation.

In the early follicular phase, FSH is responsible for the initial growth of follicle. Small amount of estrogen is secreted by follicles. Moderate and constant level of estrogen inhibits LH secretion. The progesterone level is at its lowest throughout follicular phase.

In the late follicular phase, the follicles further grow by FSH and final maturation requires both FSH and LH. The mature follicle begins to secrete large amounts of estrogen 2–3 days before ovulation and so FSH level falls. Inhibin secreted by the mature follicle also inhibits FSH secretion.

The peak of estrogen secretion occurs 24 hours before ovulation. This high level of estrogen is responsible for LH surge in midcycle. This is by a **positive feedback** mechanism on hypothalamus and pituitary. During LH surge, LH secretion increases 6–10 times normal. An FSH surge is also seen at the time of LH surge **(Fig. 73.5)**.

LH surge is responsible for ovulation and initiation of corpus luteum formation. Estrogen level begins to decline just before ovulation but increases in the luteal phase. *The high circulating level of progesterone inhibits the positive feedback effect of estrogen on LH secretion in the luteal phase.*

Summary of the changes occurring in the female reproductive system during the different phases of a 28-day menstrual cycle is shown in **Figures 73.6A to C**.

Role of Hypothalamus in Controlling Gonadotropin Secretion

Luteinizing hormone releasing hormone (LHRH) or gonadotropin releasing hormone (**GnRH**) is released from medial basal portion of hypothalamus (especially arcuate and infundibular nuclei) to hypothalamo-hypophyseal portal vessels. LHRH stimulates LH and FSH secretion from anterior pituitary. LHRH is liberated in **episodic bursts** and this type of secretion is necessary for normal gonadotropin secretion **(Table 73.2)**. Continuous secretion of GnRH down-regulate GnRH receptors in the anterior pituitary and LH secretion declines to zero. Long acting GnRH analogs inhibit LH secretion and are used to treat precocious puberty and cancer prostate.

Fluctuations in the frequency and amplitude of these bursts are responsible for various changes that take place in the hormonal secretion that occur during menstrual cycle. Estrogen increases the frequency of bursts and progesterone decreases the frequency of bursts.

Various inputs coming from hypothalamus can cause change in the frequency of bursts, e.g., emotional states

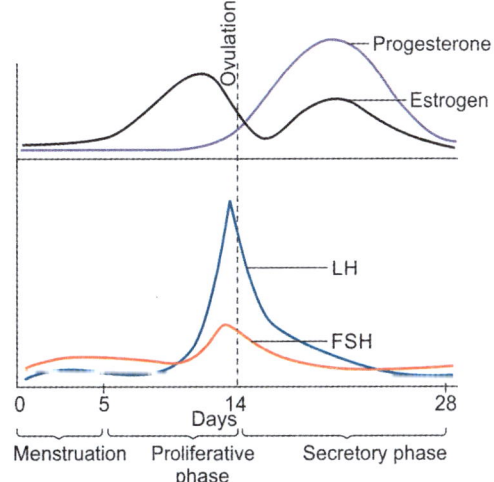

Fig. 73.5: Variation in the levels of LH, FSH, estrogen and progesterone in different phases of a 28-day menstrual cycle.

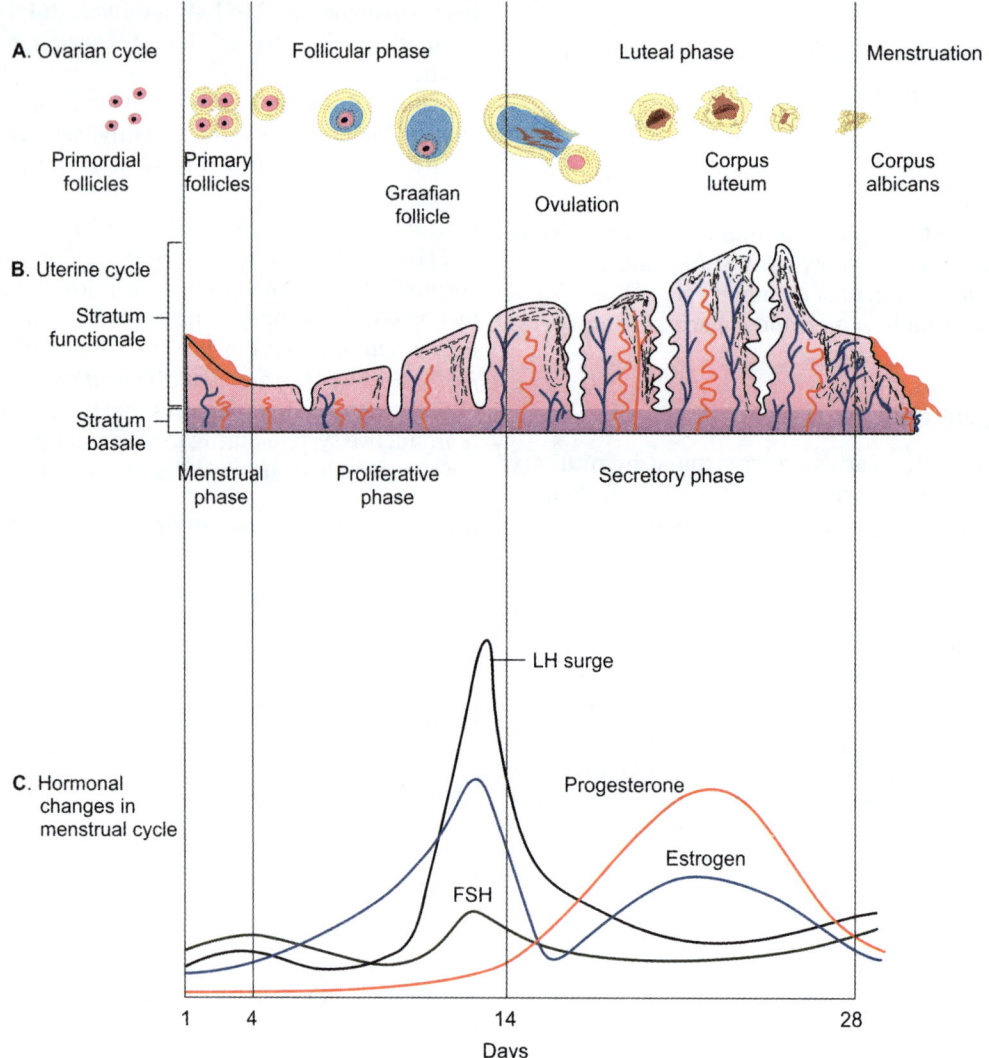

Figs. 73.6A to C: Changes occurring in the different phases of a 28-day menstrual cycle.

Table 73.2: Factors influencing LHRH bursts from hypothalamus.	
Increase in the frequency of bursts	*Decrease in the frequency of bursts*
• Estrogen • Norepinephrine in HT • Epinephrine	• Progesterone • β-endorphin • Encephalin

cause changes in the limbic system which influence the hypothalamus and cause change in the pattern of menstrual cycle. High concentration of estrogen increases the frequency of LHRH bursts, and this is responsible for LH surge. In the luteal phase, high levels of progesterone decrease the frequency of LHRH bursts. This decrease both FSH and LH secretion. On pituitary, estrogen increases the responsiveness of pituitary to LHRH. In the late luteal phase, frequency of LHRH bursts increases.

ABNORMALITIES OF MENSTRUATION

Anovulatory Cycles

In **anovulatory cycle**, LH surge is absent and hence no ovulation occurs. Corpus luteum is not formed and there will be deficiency of progesterone. So, secretory changes will be absent in the endometrium. Estrogen secretion from the follicle continues and hence endometrium becomes thick and at a stage the endometrium gets shed. When an endometrial biopsy is taken, only proliferative changes are seen throughout the cycle. Usually, the cycles occur in less than 28 days and the flow is variable. Anovulatory cycles are seen normally in a few cycles following menarche and before menopause. In adult females it is the main cause of infertility.

❖ **Amenorrhea**: Absence of menstruation
❖ **Polymenorrhea**: Increased frequency of menstruation
❖ **Dysmenorrhea**: Painful menstruation

Amenorrhea

Amenorrhea means absence of menstruation. It is classified into:
- Primary amenorrhea
- Secondary amenorrhea

If menstrual bleeding has never occurred at the pubertal age, the condition is called **primary amenorrhea**. Causes may be hypothalamic or pituitary disorders, primary ovarian disorders, etc.

Absence of menstruation in a female with previous normal periods is **secondary amenorrhea**. Most common cause is pregnancy. Other causes are lactation, emotional disturbances, environmental changes, systemic diseases, Sheehan's syndrome, etc.

- **Hypomenorrhea** means scanty flow during menstruation.
- **Menorrhagia** means profuse bleeding during regular periods and increased duration of bleeding.
- **Oligomenorrhea** is infrequent menstrual periods.
- **Metrorrhagia** means uterine bleeding in between menstrual periods.
- **Dysmenorrhea** means painful menstruation. Severe uterine cramps or spasms are common in young females and this is mainly due to accumulation of prostaglandin in the uterus. Usually, this disappears after the first delivery. Prostaglandin inhibitors give relief to this condition.

Premenstrual Syndrome

7–10 days before menstruation, some females experience certain symptoms like irritability, reduced ability to concentrate, puffiness, constipation, headache, etc. This is referred to as premenstrual syndrome. Main cause is retention of salt and water. Usually, the peak of estrogen secretion is seen before the onset of these symptoms.

Polycystic Ovary Syndrome or Stein-Leventhal Syndrome

Polycystic ovary syndrome (PCOS) is the most common endocrine condition which affects females in the reproductive age group. About 10% of women in the child-bearing age suffer from this disease. It is characterized by chronic anovulation, androgen excess, hirsutism, amenorrhea or oligomenorrhea, insulin resistance, acanthosis nigricans and polycystic ovaries. The ovary contains multiple follicular cysts on both sides and the ovarian capsule is thickened. There is compensatory hyperinsulinemia, risk of type 2 diabetes mellitus, dyslipidemia and increased risk of coronary artery disease. In females, PCOS is considered equivalent to metabolic syndrome or syndrome X. The subject shows hirsutism (excess body and facial hair), increased acne and masculinization due to excess production of androgens by the ovaries. The cause of PCOS is not well understood. But, it is known to involve a combination of genetic and environmental factors.

Insulin resistance is due to a defect in the post-receptor mechanisms in insulin receptor signaling. An abnormality in insulin receptor phosphorylation inhibits the intrinsic tyrosine kinase activity of the insulin receptor. Hyperinsulinemia secondary to insulin resistance causes several metabolic dysfunctions. Excess of insulin inhibits sex steroid binding globulin synthesis in the liver thus increasing the levels of free bioactive androgens. Hyperinsulinemia also decreases the production of IGF-1 binding proteins in liver, thereby increasing the levels of free IGF-1 in circulation. IGF-1 and excess insulin act as growth factors and stimulate excess androgen production in the ovaries and stimulate the development of more preanteral follicles which grow relatively bigger.

Excess insulin and free IGF-1 stimulate IGF-1 receptors present on the keratocytes in skin leading to their proliferation. This results in hyperpigmentation of skin particularly in the areas of skin folds. This condition is called acanthosis nigricans.

Ovary is the primary source of androgens in PCOS. About 25% of testosterone in the blood of female comes from the adrenals, 25% from the ovaries and 50% from the peripheral conversion of precursors to testosterone by enzymes such as 5α-reductase in the skin and fat cells. Most of the women having elevated serum androgen levels have mainly testosterone, androstenedione, dehydroepiandrosterone and dehydroepiandrosterone sulphate. Excess androgen is secondary to hyperinsulinemia as explained previously. Due to androgen excess an androgenic microenvironment is created in the preanteral follicles. A conversion of microenvironment to estrogenic is essential for the selection of the dominant follicle. But androgen in excess inhibit aromatase enzyme function of converting androgens to estrone. So the dominant follicle selection fails. Thus oocyte production and ovulation does not occur. Excess androgens also increase the size and number of potentially recruitable follicles by about 2 to 3 times than in normal ovary. Thus multiple follicles larger than normal are seen. These are the polycysts characteristic of PCOS.

In women with PCOS there is enhanced activity of 5α-reductase enzyme. This enzyme is responsible for the 5-α-reduction of testosterone to 5α-dihydrotestosterone in the skin. Thus increased activity of 5α-reductase mediates hirsutism in females with PCOS. Hirsutism refers to the presence of course hairs in the androgen dependent areas on the face and body of women and is due to excess levels of dehydroepiandrosterone (DHEA) and 5α-dihydrotestosterone.

In PCOS, there is increased secretion of inhibin which leads to low FSH secretion from the anterior pituitary and is responsible for anovulation. High androgen levels also inhibit secretion of FSH and LH. They have irregular prolonged menstrual cycles with menorrhagia (heavy bleeding). Infertility is a common finding. These people are prone to develop type II diabetes mellitus, fatty liver, depression, obstructive sleep apnea, and metabolic syndrome. Obesity associated with PCOS can worsen the complications of the disorder. They are more prone for endometrial cancer. The condition is treated with weight loss, exercise, birth control pills, metformin and anti-androgens.

Ovarian Tumors

If the ovarian tumors secrete hormones it leads to endocrine abnormalities. If estrogen is produced in excess in small girls it leads to **precocious puberty**. If the tumor produces large amounts of androgen, then masculinization occurs.

Genetic Defects

A number of single gene mutations produce menstrual abnormalities in female. For example, **Kallmann's syndrome** causes hypogonadotropic hypogonadism. GnRH resistance, FSH and LH resistance, etc., occur due to defects in the respective receptors. Aromatase deficiency prevents formation of estrogen.

TESTS OF OVULATION

- Basal body temperature is recorded every morning before getting up from bed. There will be a rise in body temperature by 0.5°C above normal 1–2 days after ovulation and this temperature is maintained throughout the luteal phase. This rise in temperature is due to the thermogenic action of progesterone.
- *Endometrial biopsy*: Secretory changes in the endometrium indicate the presence of a functioning corpus luteum.
- *Vaginal smear*: Absence of cornification of vaginal epithelium indicates ovulation.
- *Cervical mucus*: The cervical mucus will be thick; cellular and fern pattern will be absent if ovulation has occurred.
- *Pregnanediol in urine*: Pregnanediol appears in urine a day after ovulation and disappears a day before menstruation.
- *Estrogen level*: Maximum level of estrogen in blood is seen just before ovulation.
- FSH and LH levels are high at the time of ovulation
- *Mittelschmerz*: This is a fleeting lower abdominal pain in midcycle due to irritation of peritoneum at the time of ovulation. This is a clear indication of ovulation.

Reflex Ovulation

In cats, rabbits, etc., ovulation is induced by copulation. This is called reflex ovulation. Here, afferent impulses from the genitalia converge on ventral hypothalamus and induce ovulation by increasing LH secretion from pituitary.

PERIMENOPAUSE

PY9.11: Discuss the hormonal changes and their effects during perimenopause and menopause.

Perimenopause means around menopause. It is the period that occurs in females before menopause usually between ages of 45 and 55 years. It lasts for about 10 years. It marks the end of the reproductive years. It is also known as menopausal transition.

- The level of estrogen and progesterone in the body rises and falls unevenly during perimenopause. Changes experienced during perimenopause are as a result of declining estrogen levels.
- Menstrual cycles may lengthen or shorten. The cycles are usually anovulatory.
- There will be symptoms such as hot flashes, night sweats, insomnia and vaginal dryness due to low estrogen level. Urinary and vaginal infections are common. Some complain of urinary incontinence.
- Mood swings, irritability and increased risk of depression occur during perimenopause.
- Due to decrease in estrogen, there is increased risk of osteoporosis as a result of increased bone loss.
- Cholesterol level increases. There is increase in LDL cholesterol and decrease in HDL cholesterol. Both these contribute to increased risk of coronary artery disease.

Perimenopausal period is over when there is no menstruation for 12 consecutive months. Then menopause is said to be attained.

MENOPAUSE

The period in which human ovaries fail to respond to gonadotropins with advancing age and the sexual cycles disappear continuously for 12 consecutive months is known as **menopause**. Secretion of sex hormones (estrogen and progesterone) slowly declines and stops. This is because of the decrease in the number of primordial follicles. Menstrual cycles become irregular at first and finally stop. Average age of menopause is 52 years (45–55 years).

Since estrogen and progesterone level falls, there is no negative feedback effect on gonadotropin secretion, and LH and FSH levels increase. Uterus and vagina atrophy. Some physiological changes occur in the body. Spreading of warmth from chest to face occurs which is referred to as **hot flushes or hot flashes,** occur in 75% of menopausal women. These vasomotor symptoms are due to dysfunction of the central thermoregulatory center in the hypothalamus. It is due to estrogen withdrawal which leads to increased secretion of norepinephrine and serotonin which lower the set point of the hypothalamic thermostat. (Previously it was thought that hot flush was due to large LH surge since there is no feedback inhibition on LH secretion. But hot flushes continue even after removal of pituitary.) Psychological symptoms like dyspnea, irritability, anxiety, insomnia, fatigue, depression, increased sweating, etc., are seen in some individuals. 15% of postmenopausal females require treatment with small doses of estrogen.

There is no menopause in males (**andropause**) but the function of testes declines slowly with advancing age.

PHYSIOLOGY OF HUMAN SEXUAL RESPONSES

Sexual intercourse is called **coitus**. During coitus, spermatozoa are ejaculated from male urethra into the vagina. The sequence of physiological and emotional changes experienced by the individuals before, during and after intercourse is called human sexual response.

Changes in the Male

The arterioles of the penis are supplied by parasympathetic nerves originating from the second, third and fourth sacral segments of the spinal cord along the **nervi erigentes.** The first sign of sexual excitement is **erection** which is enlargement and stiffening of the penis. Parasympathetic stimulation causes release of neurotransmitters like **nitric oxide** which relaxes the vascular smooth muscle of penis. The arteries of penis dilate and blood gets filled in the blood sinuses of the three corpora of penis. In addition to this, there is obstruction to the venous drainage. This is because the expansion of the erectile tissues compresses the superficial veins draining the penis. The penis becomes hard and enlarged in size which is called erection. Parasympathetic stimulation also causes increased secretion of mucus from the bulbourethral gland which serves as a lubricant during intercourse. If there is damage or degeneration of the parasympathetic nerve as in advanced diabetes mellitus, there will be no erection and the condition is called **erectile dysfunction** also called impotence. During erection there is increased sympathetic discharge through the hypogastric nerve to the internal urethral sphincter causing the sphincter to contract. This prevents regurgitation of semen into the bladder during ejaculation.

At the time of **orgasm**, rhythmic sympathetic impulses cause peristaltic contraction of the smooth muscles of epididymis and vas deferens. There is also increased secretion from seminal vesicle and prostate along with contraction of the walls of these glands. These rhythmic contractions propel sperm and other secretions into the urethra which is called **emission**. Emission is followed by ejaculation. During ejaculation there is rhythmic contraction of skeletal muscles of perineum which help to propel the semen to the exterior.

Other changes in both sexes include increase in heart rate and blood pressure, increased tone of skeletal muscles of the body, and hyperventilation.

Changes in the Female

Parasympathetic impulses to the female genital tract stimulate release of fluids that lubricate the vaginal walls. Vagina is devoid of glands and the fluid is mainly derived from the engorged blood vessels of the vagina by **transudation**. A small quantity of lubricating fluid is derived from the cervical mucosa and Bartholin's glands. During sexual excitement, there is engorgement of labia and relaxation of vaginal smooth muscle. The breasts also swell due to vasodilatation. Rhythmic contraction of the vagina, uterus and perineal muscles are also observed in females during orgasm.

The semen is deposited in the upper part of vagina. The spermatozoa are sucked into the uterus by rhythmic uterine contractions. These contractions are mainly due to release of **oxytocin** (released due to stimulation of the genital tract and also due to emotional stimuli to hypothalamus) and **noradrenaline** (by increased sympathetic activity during intercourse) from the body and it is also contributed by the **prostaglandins** present in the semen.

The peristaltic contraction and action of cilia help in the transport of sperm through the fallopian tube. The acrosome of the sperm produces an enzyme called **acrosin** which stimulates sperm motility. In addition, spermatozoa express olfactory receptors, and ovaries produce odorant- like molecules. These molecules and their receptors in the sperm interact, promoting movement of spermatozoa towards the ovum. This is an example of chemotaxis.

MULTIPLE CHOICE QUESTIONS

1. **Ovulation is associated with sudden rise in:**
   a. Prolactin
   b. Testosterone
   c. LH
   d. Oxytocin

2. **Ovulation corresponds with:**
   a. FSH surge
   b. LH surge
   c. Progesterone surge
   d. Estradiol surge

3. **Positive feedback action of estrogen for inducing LH surge is associated with which of the following steroid hormone ratios in peripheral circulation?**
   a. High estrogen : low progesterone
   b. Low estrogen : high progesterone
   c. Low estrogen : low progesterone
   d. High estrogen : high progesterone

4. **Corpus luteum is maintained by:**
   a. Progesterone
   b. LH
   c. FSH
   d. Estrogen

5. **The phase of uterine cycle occurring after ovulation is called:**
   a. Bleeding phase
   b. Proliferative phase
   c. Secretory phase
   d. Mid-luteal phase

6. **Follicular stimulating hormone receptors are present on:**
   a. Theca cells
   b. Granulosa cells
   c. Leydig cells
   d. Basement membrane of ovarian follicle

7. **LH receptors in females are present in the pre-ovulatory follicle on:**
   a. Theca interna cells only
   b. Granulosa cells only
   c. Both theca interna and granulosa cells
   d. Ovum

8. **The important hormone that is responsible for the early growth of ovarian follicle is:**
   a. FSH
   b. LH
   c. Estrogen
   d. Progesterone

9. **Whether menstrual cycle is ovulatory or not can be assessed by estimating the serum level of which hormone on the 20th day of menstrual cycle in a young woman?**
   a. FSH
   b. LH
   c. Estradiol
   d. Progesterone

10. In a 28-day menstrual cycle, ovulation occurs on which day?
    a. 7th day
    b. 10th day
    c. 14th day
    d. 21st day
11. Corpus luteum salvage hormone is:
    a. hCG
    b. FSH
    c. LH
    d. Progesterone
12. The second meiotic division is completed in the ovum at:
    a. Fertilization
    b. Puberty
    c. Birth
    d. Seventh month of intrauterine life
13. Mitosis occurs in the developing ovum till:
    a. Birth
    b. Puberty
    c. Menopause
    d. Fifth month of intrauterine life
14. The enzyme associated with the conversion of androgen to estrogen in the growing ovarian follicle is:
    a. Desmolase
    b. Isomerase
    c. Aromatase
    d. Hydroxylase
15. Elasticity of cervical mucus is seen in:
    a. Proliferative phase
    b. Midcycle
    c. Luteal phase
    d. Menstruation
16. Oogonia are derived from:
    a. Amnion
    b. Yolk sac
    c. Stroma of ovary
    d. Germinal epithelium
17. Ovum released from the ovary is viable for:
    a. 12 hours
    b. 24 hours
    c. 36 hours
    d. 72 hours
18. If a lady presents with a very regular 29 days menstrual cycle, ovulation should occur on day:
    a. 14
    b. 15
    c. 17
    d. 19
19. Levels of which of the following hormones are increased in post-menopausal women:
    a. Estrogen
    b. FSH
    c. Progesterone
    d. Cortisone
20. Function of luteinizing hormone is:
    a. Follicle maturation and ovulation
    b. Milk secretion
    c. Causes progesterone secretion during ovulation
    d. Maintains placenta
21. Menopause is defined as cessation of menstruation for:
    a. 3 consecutive month
    b. 6 consecutive months
    c. 9 consecutive months
    d. 12 consecutive months
22. Which of the following is increased in blood after hepatectomy?
    a. Fibrinogen
    b. Lipoprotein
    c. Angiotensin
    d. Estrogen
23. Menstrual blood does not clot because:
    a. It is arterial in origin
    b. It is venous in origin
    c. It contains fibrinolysin
    d. It does not contain calcium ions
24. Fern pattern of cervical mucus is due to:
    a. The action of estrogen
    b. The action of progesterone
    c. Action of both estrogen and progesterone
    d. Secretory changes in the endometrium
25. Spinnbarkeit phenomenon refers to:
    a. Property of elasticity of cervical mucus
    b. Ferning pattern of cervical mucus
    c. Lower abdominal pain at the time of ovulation
    d. Cornification of vaginal epithelium
26. Ovulation corresponds to:
    a. 14 days before menstruation
    b. 14 days after menstruation
    c. The day of menstruation
    d. Increase in basal body temperature
27. During the fertile period of a female:
    a. Estrogen decreases
    b. Estrogen increases
    c. Progesterone increases
    d. Progesterone decreases
28. Menopause is defined as cessation of menstruation for:
    a. Three consecutive months
    b. 6 consecutive months
    c. 9 consecutive months
    d. 12 consecutive months
29. The hormone that increases basal body temperature is:
    a. Progesterone
    b. Estrogen
    c. LH
    d. FSH
30. The hormone required for the development of corpus luteum is:
    a. Estrogen
    b. FSH
    c. Luteinizing hormone
    d. Progesterone
31. Ovulation is associated with sudden rise in:
    a. Prolactin
    b. Cortisol
    c. LH
    d. Progesterone
32. The mid-cycle rise in the basal body temperature after ovulation is caused by:
    a. FSH peak
    b. LH peak
    c. Estradiol
    d. Progesterone

33. In a 28-day cycle, which hormone assay gives a clear indication of ovulation if blood sample is taken on the 20th day of the cycle?
    a. FSH
    b. LH
    c. Estradiol
    d. Progesterone
34. FSH acts on which of the following?
    a. Granulosa cell
    b. Theca cell
    c. Endometrium
    d. Myometrium
35. Estrogen therapy in menopausal females is associated with increased risk of:
    a. Breast cancer
    b. Endometrial cancer
    c. Cancer ovary
    d. Lung cancer
36. Intrafollicular pressure of Graafian follicle is:
    a. 2–4 mm Hg
    b. 5–10 mm Hg
    c. 30–40 mm Hg
    d. 16–20 mm Hg
37. The average diameter of Graafian follicle just before ovulation is about:
    a. 5 mm
    b. 20 mm
    c. 10 mm
    d. 8 mm
38. The main estrogen secreted by the ovary and the most biologically active estrogen is:
    a. Estradiol
    b. Estrone
    c. Estriol
    d. 16-α hydroxyestrone
39. The estrogen that is not secreted by the ovary but secreted by the placenta in large amounts is:
    a. Estriol
    b. Estrone
    c. Estradiol
    d. 16-α hydroxyestrone
40. On the 21st day of anovulatory cycle in a non-pregnant woman, all the following are true, *except*:
    a. Basal body temperature does not increase
    b. Endometrial biopsy shows secretory pattern
    c. Cervical mucus smear shows a fern like pattern
    d. Plasma progesterone level is very low
41. Regarding human female reproduction the correct statement is:
    a. Each ovary releases one ovum every month
    b. Fertilized ovum contains 46 autosomes
    c. Fertilization of the ovum occurs in the fallopian tube
    d. Twin pregnancy occurs due to entry of two sperms into an ovum
42. Mittelschmerz refers to:
    a. Property of elasticity of cervical mucus
    b. Ferning pattern of cervical mucus
    c. Fleeting lower abdominal pain at the time of ovulation
    d. Cornification of vaginal epithelium
43. All the following statements are true, *except*:
    a. In humans, no new ova are formed after birth
    b. At the time of birth, there are 7 million ova
    c. At the time of puberty, the number of ova in both ovaries is less than 3 lakhs
    d. Just before ovulation, the first meiotic division is completed
44. Secretory phase of endometrium is due to the action of:
    a. Estradiol
    b. LH
    c. FSH
    d. Progesterone
45. The dominant hormones in the follicular stage of menstrual cycle are:
    a. Estrogen and progesterone
    b. FSH and LH
    c. FSH and estrogen
    d. LH and estrogen
46. The first meiotic division in the ova of primordial follicle get arrested in which stage?
    a. Prophase
    b. Metaphase
    c. Anaphase
    d. Telophase
47. In which stage is second meiotic division of the secondary oocyte arrested until fertilization?
    a. Prophase
    b. Metaphase
    c. Anaphase
    d. Telophase
48. The vasospasm occurring in the endometrium at the onset of menstruation is mainly due to:
    a. Prostaglandin
    b. Estrogen
    c. Progesterone
    d. Serotonin
49. Ovulation occurs how many hours after LH surge?
    a. 24 hours
    b. 48 hours
    c. 9 hours
    d. 2 hours
50. Both estrogen and progesterone peak occur on which day of a 28-day menstrual cycle?
    a. 21st day
    b. 16th day
    c. 24th day
    d. 18th day
51. Which hormone shows two peaks during a menstrual cycle?
    a. Progesterone
    b. LH
    c. GnRH
    d. Estrogen
52. Maximum estrogen secretion occurs in:
    a. Middle luteal phase
    b. Just prior to ovulation
    c. Early part of follicular phase
    d. Late luteal phase
53. Weight gain in the premenstrual phase is due to:
    a. Salt and water retention caused by estrogen
    b. Salt and water retention due to progesterone
    c. Increased fat deposition
    d. Protein anabolic effect of estrogen
54. Osteoporosis seen after menopause is due to deficiency of:
    a. Progesterone
    b. FSH
    c. GnRH
    d. Estrogen
55. Fertile period in a woman can be determined by detecting urinary concentration of:
    a. LH
    b. FSH
    c. hCG
    d. Estrogen
56. Sheehan's syndrome is due to:
    a. Adrenal hemorrhage
    b. Pituitary hemorrhage

c. Hypothalamic hemorrhage
d. Pancreatic hemorrhage

57. The most important corpus luteum maintaining hormone is:
    a. FSH
    b. LH
    c. hCG
    d. Estrogen

58. On the 21st day of an anovulatory cycle, in an otherwise normal non-pregnant woman, all the following are true, *except*:
    a. Basal body temperature does not increase
    b. Endometrial biopsy shows secretory pattern
    c. The cervical mucus smear shows a fern like pattern
    d. Plasma progesterone level is very low

59. **Regarding human female reproduction:**
    a. Each ovary releases one ovum every month
    b. Fertilized ovum contains 46 autosomes
    c. Fertilization of the ovum occurs in the fallopian tube
    d. Twin pregnancy occurs due to entry of two sperms into an ovum

60. **Ovulation occurs as a result of:**
    a. Excessive estrogen level
    b. Surge of luteinizing hormone
    c. Excessive progesterone
    d. Low estrogen level

ANSWERS

1. c	2. b	3. a	4. b	5. c
6. b	7. c	8. a	9. d	10. c
11. a	12. a	13. d	14. c	15. b
16. b	17. b	18. b	19. b	20. a
21. d	22. d	23. c	24. a	25. a
26. a	27. c	28. b	29. a	30. d
31. c	32. d	33. d	34. a	35. b
36. d	37. b	38. a	39. a	40. b
41. c	42. c	43. b	44. d	45. c
46. a	47. b	48. a	49. c	50. a
51. d	52. b	53. a	54. d	55. a
56. b	57. c	58. b	59. c	60. b

Fertilization and Pregnancy

CHAPTER 74

LEARNING OBJECTIVES
- Describe the physiology of pregnancy and parturition
- Discuss the physiological basis of various pregnancy tests
- Explain the functions of placenta
- Discuss the importance of fetoplacental unit in pregnancy

INTRODUCTION

PY9.8: Describe and discuss the physiology of pregnancy, parturition and outline the psychology and psychiatry disorders associated with it.

Once ovum is released after ovulation, it can survive for 72 hours, but is fertilizable only for less than 36 hours. Once the ovum is released into the peritoneal cavity, it is sucked into the fallopian tube by the fimbriated end of fallopian tube. The cilia and the peristaltic movement of the fallopian tube aid in the transport of ovum through the oviduct.

Sperms can survive in the female genital tract for 48 hours. Only one sperm can fertilize the ovum. Of the millions of sperms deposited in the vagina during intercourse, only 50-100 sperms reach the ovum and some of them make contact with zona pellucida of ovum through sperm receptors in the zona.

CHANGES IN THE SPERM BEFORE FERTILIZATION

Capacitation

Ejaculated sperms can fertilize the ovum only after **capacitation** (gain the ability to fertilize egg). For capacitation to occur, the decapacitation factors acquired in the epididymis have to be removed. Capacitation usually occurs in the fallopian tube and it takes about 6–7 hrs. Once a sperm is capacitated, its tail shows increased activity and its head acquires the capability to undergo the acrosome reaction. Only capacitated sperm can pass through the corona radiata and zona pellucida of the ovum. Capacitation of spermatozoa occurs by the following mechanisms:

- ❖ The uterine and fallopian tube fluids wash away the various inhibitory factors or decapacitation factors that suppress sperm activity in the male genital ducts.
- ❖ While the spermatozoa remain in the fluid of the male genital ducts, they are continually exposed to vesicles containing large amounts of cholesterol. This cholesterol is continually added to the cellular membrane covering the sperm acrosome, toughening this membrane and preventing release of its enzymes. After ejaculation, the sperm deposited in the vagina swim away from the cholesterol vesicles upward into the uterine cavity, and they gradually lose much of their excess cholesterol during the next few hours. In so doing, the acrosome becomes much weaker.
- ❖ The membrane of the sperm also becomes much more permeable to calcium ions, so calcium now enters the sperm in abundance and changes the activity of the flagellum, giving it a powerful whiplash motion in contrast to its previously weak undulating motion. In addition, the calcium ions cause changes in the cellular membrane that cover the leading edge of the acrosome, making it possible for the acrosome to release its enzymes rapidly so that the sperm can easily penetrate the granulosa layer and zona pellucida.

Recent evidence indicates that spermatozoa move towards the ovary by **chemotaxis**. Ovaries produce odorant molecules and spermatozoa express olfactory receptors so that sperms will be attracted towards the ovary.

Acrosomal Reaction

Capacitation is followed by **acrosomal reaction**. This occurs after the sperm binds to zona pellucida. Contact of **zona pellucida protein, ZP3**, to its sperm receptor triggers the acrosomal reaction. The acrosome of the sperm breaks down and enzymes, such as acrosin, trypsinases and hyaluronidase are released, of which the most important one is the protease, **acrosin**. Acrosin facilitates the penetration of sperm through the zona pellucida. As soon as the nucleus of the sperm enters the ovum, the membrane of the ovum fuses, which is aided by **fertilin**, a protein on the surface of sperm head.

A barrier is formed around the ovum which prevents further entry of sperms into the ovum, i.e., **polyspermy** is prevented.

Prevention of polyspermy: Normally only one sperm cell penetrates and enters a secondary oocyte. This event is called **syngamy**. When one sperm penetrates the zona pellucida, there is a reduction in the membrane potential of the ovum. This depolarization triggers the release of calcium ions inside the ovum. Calcium ions stimulate the release of certain cortical granules that are superficially situated in the oocyte. This is followed by a structural alteration in vitelline membrane and zona pellucida to block entry of other sperms into the egg. Thus, block occurs at two levels which constitute the *vitelline block to polyspermy and the zona block to polyspermy*. This prevents **polyspermy** (the fertilization of ovum by more than one sperm) permanently.

FERTILIZATION

Fertilization occurs in the **ampulla** of fallopian tube. *During nuclear fusion, second meiotic division of ovum is completed and second polar body is extruded.* Fertilized ovum is called **zygote** which contains 46 chromosomes. *The genetic sex of the individual is determined at the time of fertilization.*

Zygote immediately undergoes mitotic division to form a cell mass called **morula** (morum = mulberry). It gets its nutrition from the secretions of oviduct. The morula is transported to the uterine cavity by 3–4 days after fertilization. A cavity is formed inside the morula and forms the **blastocyst**. It floats in the fluid in the uterine cavity for another 3–4 days and gets nutrition from the secretions of oviduct and uterine cavity and reaches 8 or 16 cell stage. The inner cells form the **embryo proper** while the outer cells form the **trophoblast** which develops into the placenta.

Implantation

Blastocyst comes in contact with endometrium and implantation occurs 5–7 days after fertilization. During this time, endometrium is prepared to receive the fertilized ovum. Normal site of implantation is the upper posterior wall of the uterus. When the blastocyst comes in contact with endometrium the blastocyst is covered with **trophoblast cells** in two layers:
1. **Syncytiotrophoblast**, a multinucleate mass with no cell boundaries.
2. **Cytotrophoblast**, made up of individual cells.

Syncytiotrophoblast produces certain proteolytic enzymes which digest and liquefy the endometrial cells and burrows into the endometrium. This process is called **implantation**. Trophoblast cells proliferate and form the placenta and fetal membranes. *Pregnancy is said to be established at the time of implantation of the fertilized ovum* (Fig. 74.1).

Under normal conditions, the fetus is not rejected even though it is a transplant of foreign tissue in the mother. This is because the placental trophoblasts that separate maternal and fetal tissues do not express class I and class II MHC genes that are responsible for rejection. So, antibodies against fetal proteins do not develop in the mother. Also, certain substances in the placenta like **Fas ligand** on its surface binds to T cells and produce apoptosis of T lymphocytes that mediate cellular immunity.

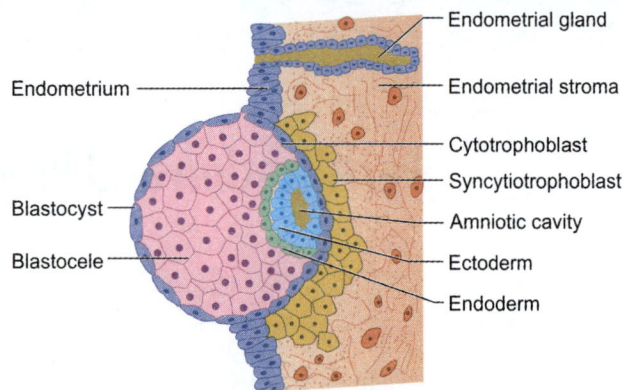

Fig. 74.1: Implantation of blastocyst to endometrium.

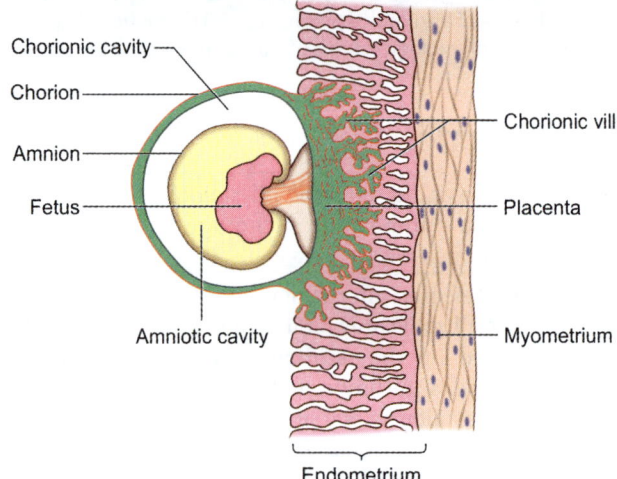

Fig. 74.2: Fetal membranes and placenta of implanted embryo.

One week after implantation, the placenta begins to provide nutrition for the developing ovum. The placenta attains full size by 12 weeks. Fetal portion of placenta contains numerous villi with capillaries and these villi project into the maternal sinusoids and is called **fetal membrane (Fig. 74.2)**. After 12 weeks, fetus and placenta function as a single unit, especially for the synthesis of steroid hormones.

Placental Barrier

The fetal and maternal blood is never in direct contact **(Fig. 74.3)**. They are separated by the **placental barrier**. The layers of the barrier are:
❖ Syncytiotrophoblast
❖ Cytotrophoblast
❖ Basement membrane
❖ Mesoderm
❖ Endothelium of fetal capillaries

Hormonal Changes in Pregnancy

Syncytiotrophoblast of placenta produces a hormone called **human chorionic gonadotropin (hCG)** which prevents involution of corpus luteum. The corpus luteum produces more progesterone, estrogen and relaxin. Relaxin and progesterone helps to maintain pregnancy by inhibiting

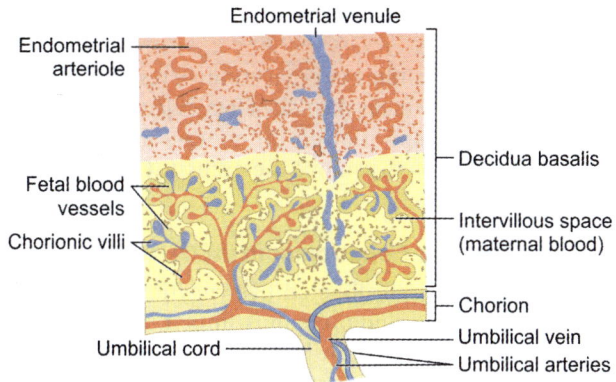

Fig. 74.3: Structure of placenta and umbilical cord. Decidua basalis is the maternal portion of placenta and chorion is the fetal portion.

uterine contractions. Prostaglandin production by the uterus is inhibited by progesterone.

Progesterone acts on the endometrium and causes swelling of the stromal cells and accumulation of abundant nutrient materials in the cells. These cells are called **decidual cells**. The embryo initially depends on the decidual cells for nutrition. The function of corpus luteum begins to decline after 8 weeks of pregnancy, but it persists throughout pregnancy.

FUNCTIONS OF PLACENTA

- Respiratory function
- Nutritive and storage function
- Excretory function
- Immunological function
- Endocrine function

Respiratory Function

- *Diffusion of O_2*: Usually dissolved O_2 from the maternal blood diffuses into fetal blood. In the mother, mean PO_2 is 50 mm Hg in the later months of pregnancy. The PO_2 of fetal blood in placenta is only 30 mm Hg.
  Due to the pressure gradient of 20 mm Hg, the fetus gets enough O_2.
    There is increased extraction of O_2 from the maternal blood due to the following reasons:
    - Affinity of fetal hemoglobin for O_2 is very high.
    - The hemoglobin content is more in the fetus than in the mother.
    - Bohr effect on the maternal side and opposite of Bohr Effect on the fetal side **(double Bohr effect)** leads to increased extraction of O_2 from maternal blood. When the fetal blood passes through the placenta, CO_2 diffuses from fetal side to maternal blood. The fetal blood becomes alkaline and the maternal blood becomes more acidic. Due to Bohr Effect more O_2 is liberated from maternal blood and more O_2 is taken up by fetal blood because it is alkaline. There is a shift to right of ODC on the maternal side and a shift to left on the fetal side.

- *Diffusion of CO_2*: The PCO_2 of fetal blood is 2–3 mm Hg higher than that of maternal blood. Even though pressure gradient is less, CO_2 diffuses with ease because:
    - The diffusion capacity of CO_2 is 20 times more than that of O_2 through the placental membrane.
    - The PCO_2 of maternal sinuses is lower than 40 mm Hg and this also helps in easy diffusion of CO_2 from fetus to mother.

Nutritive and Storage Function

Substances diffuse across the placental membrane depending on their molecular weight. If molecular weight is less than 1000, the substance can pass very easily through the placental membrane. Glucose is transported by carrier-mediated facilitated diffusion. Fatty acids are soluble in the membrane, but are transported at a slower rate than glucose. Amino acids and ascorbic acid are actively transported across the membrane. Ketoacids and ions are also transported across the membrane. Various drugs can also cross the placenta, such as anesthetics; pethidine and morphine, antibiotics, etc., and some of them may even damage the fetus.

During early stages of pregnancy, substances like glucose, Na^+, Ca^{2+}, iron, etc., are stored in the placenta and are utilized by the fetus in later pregnancy.

Excretory Function

Excretory products of the fetus, such as urea, uric acid, creatinine, etc., diffuse across the placenta into the maternal blood. Urea content is slightly higher in the fetal blood than in the mother's blood.

Immunological Function

The fetus contains paternally derived antigens which are foreign to the mother's body. Placenta protects the fetus from incompatibility produced between mother and fetus. It restricts entry of antigens and toxic materials from maternal blood to the fetus. Placenta prevents immunological maternal attacks by destroying T lymphocytes. Thus, placenta is partially responsible for the prevention of rejection of the fetal tissue.

Placental membrane allows passage of some antibodies from the mother to the fetus and this provides passive immunity to the fetus against various infections until the baby is capable of producing its own antibodies after birth. *IgG antibodies can cross the placenta from 14 weeks onwards.*

Endocrine Function

The hormones synthesized and secreted by the placenta are:
1. Estrogen and progesterone
2. Human chorionic gonadotropin (hCG)
3. Human chorionic somatomammotropin (hCS)
4. Human chorionic thyrotropin (hCT)
5. Relaxin
6. Inhibin and GnRH
7. CRH, β-endorphin, α MSH and dynorphin A.

Estrogen and Progesterone

Fetoplacental Unit (Flowchart 74.1)

By 12th week of development, fetus and placenta function as a single unit called **fetoplacental unit**. This unit has a very important role in **steroidogenesis** especially in the synthesis of **estrogen and progesterone**. From the mother cholesterol enters the placenta, and in the placenta, pregnenolone and progesterone are formed. A part of progesterone reaches the fetal adrenals and is converted to cortisol and corticosterone. The rest escapes into the maternal circulation. Pregnenolone reaches the fetal adrenal and liver and is converted to dehydroepiandrosterone sulfate (DHEAS) and 16-hydroxy dehydroepiandrosterone sulfate (16-OH-DHEAS). The principal estrogen formed by the fetoplacental unit is estriol, and fetal 16-OH-DHEA is the principal source of estriol. Urinary estimation of estriol in the mother is used as an index to monitor the state of the fetus.

Functions of Estrogen

- Helps in the growth of uterus.
- Development of duct system of breast.
- Relaxation of pelvic ligaments and pubic symphysis in conjunction with relaxin.
- Helps in the growth of the fetus by stimulating cell multiplication.

Functions of Progesterone in Pregnancy

- Progesterone helps in the development of decidual cells and it is the *most important hormone necessary for the maintenance of pregnancy*.
- Reduces uterine contractility and thus prevents abortion.
- Increases the secretions of fallopian tube and endometrium in the early stages of pregnancy for the nourishment of the zygote.
- Growth of the lobulo-alveolar system of breast requires progesterone.
- Progesterone inhibits maternal immune responses to fetal antigens. This reduces the risk of fetal rejection.
- It stimulates respiration in the mother and the hyperventilation helps to remove the excess CO_2 produced in pregnancy.

Human Chorionic Gonadotropin (hCG)

hCG is a glycoprotein formed by syncytiotrophoblast. It has α and β chains, and α chain is similar to LH, FSH and TSH. β-chain is specific for hCG. hCG can be detected in blood by about 6th day of pregnancy by radioimmunoassay and by about 14th day it can be estimated in the urine of pregnant woman. Peak level of hCG is attained by 6–9 weeks and then the level declines by about 16–20 weeks.

Throughout the rest of pregnancy, the level will be low. Detection of hCG in urine is the basis of immunological test of pregnancy. TSH-like activity of placental extracts is due to hCG.

The level of hCG is found to be increased in multiple pregnancy, Down's syndrome and in hydatidiform mole.

Functions of hCG

- Maintenance of corpus luteum of pregnancy. The size of corpus luteum doubles due to the action of hCG.
- Increases estrogen and progesterone secretion from the ovary. Progesterone in turn stimulates formation of decidual cells.
- In the male fetus, hCG stimulates the Leydig cells of fetal testis to secrete testosterone so that male genitalia are formed. It also helps in the descent of testes.
- Because of its structural similarity to TSH, hCG stimulates maternal thyroid gland function.

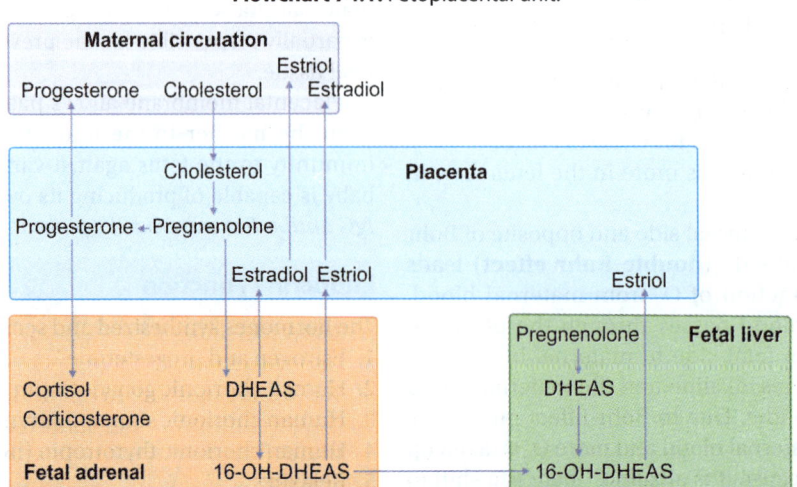

Flowchart 74.1: Fetoplacental unit.

(DHEAS: dehydroepiandrosterone sulfate).

* Immunosuppressive action of hCG helps in the maintenance of pregnancy.

Human Chorionic Somatomammotropin (hCS) or Human Placental Lactogen (hPL) or Chorionic Growth Hormone Prolactin (CGP) or Placental Growth Hormone

This hormone is also formed in syncytiotrophoblast and is secreted by 5th week of pregnancy onwards. hPL is mainly responsible for the diabetogenic state of the mother in pregnancy by producing insulin resistance. The rate of secretion progressively increases to term and its plasma level in maternal blood depends on the weight of placenta. If hCS level is low, it indicates some dysfunction of placenta like placental insufficiency.

Functions of hCS

* Lactogenic function, i.e., hCS has milk producing effect and it also causes slight enlargement of breasts.
* It has a mild growth-promoting activity. It is known as **maternal growth hormone of pregnancy**. The structure of hCS is similar to human growth hormone and prolactin. Prolactin and hCS help in linear growth of fetus before birth since growth hormone receptors are deficient in fetus. IGF-II produced in the placenta under the influence of hCS, probably helps in fetal growth.
* Metabolic actions—large quantity of hCS is present in maternal blood during pregnancy, but very little reaches the fetus. Since the structure of hCS is similar to growth hormone, it inhibits the secretion of GH in the mother in a feedback manner. But, hCS has GH like activity. It reduces glucose utilization in the mother by its anti-insulin action and the excess glucose is made available for the growing fetus. It also produces lipolysis in the mother and the fatty acids released form a source of energy for the fetus.
* It causes retention of Na^+, K^+, Ca^{2+} and N_2 in the mother.

Human Chorionic Thyrotropin (hCT)

hCT is a glycoprotein similar to pituitary TSH. Its physiological function in pregnancy is not known. The plasma level of hCT follows a curve similar to that of hCG.

Relaxin

Relaxin is produced by corpus luteum and placenta. In late pregnancy, large amount of relaxin is produced by placenta.

Functions

* Relaxes pelvic ligaments.
* Causes dilatation and softening of cervix.
* Reduces uterine contractility and helps to maintain pregnancy.
* Causes slight enlargement of lobules and alveoli of breasts.

Inhibin and GnRH

GnRH stimulates while inhibin inhibits hCG secretion. Thus, locally produced GnRH and inhibin may act in a paracrine fashion to regulate hCG secretion.

PREGNANCY TESTS

PY9.10: Discuss the physiological basis of various pregnancy tests.

Detection of hCG quantitatively or qualitatively in urine or blood is the basis of pregnancy tests and all pregnancy tests done today are immunological.
1. Biological tests
2. Immunological tests

Note: Ultrasonography in the first trimester helps to confirm pregnancy.

Biological Tests

Biological tests are usually done in animals. Urine containing hCG is injected into animals and ovulation is watched for. This is more time consuming and is only of historical importance at present.

Immunological Test of Pregnancy or Gravindex Test

Principle

Gravindex test is based on the latex agglutination inhibition technique. Absence of agglutination indicates a positive test. hCG is injected into rabbit's body and antibodies against hCG can be isolated from rabbit's plasma and this antiserum is used to detect the presence of hCG in the urine or serum of pregnant women.

Requirements

* Suspected urine sample of the lady
* Antiserum containing antibodies against hCG
* Latex particles coated with hCG

Procedure

Mix urine sample with antiserum. If hCG is present in the sample it will react with the antibodies and antigen-antibody complex will be formed. No free antibodies will be present. Now add hCG-coated latex particles. If there is no agglutination of latex particles, the test is positive, i.e., the woman is pregnant. This is because antibodies are not available to react with hCG-coated latex particles because it has been used up by the hCG present in the urine sample. If there is agglutination of latex particles it shows that the lady is not pregnant. Kits are available and it takes only few minutes to get the result. This test becomes positive 2 days after a missed period or 16 days after conception. Serum hCG assays can be positive 8–10 days after conception by radioimmunoassay. Two methods are there:
1. Rapid slide method
2. Tube method
* **Rapid slide method**: In a slide, take a drop of urine and a drop of antiserum. After some time, add hCG-coated latex particles and observe under a microscope. If there is no agglutination, pregnancy test is positive. Result is obtained within minutes; it is reliable and cheap. Instead of latex particles, sheep's RBC can be used.

- **Tube method**: It is more accurate but is time consuming.

  False-positive tests are obtained in the following conditions:
- Vesicular mole or hydatidiform mole
- Choriocarcinoma
- Chorioepithelioma
- Certain other tumors like tumors of GIT which produce hCG.

AMNIOCENTESIS

The volume of amniotic fluid surrounding the fetus at 36 weeks is about 800–1000 mL. A wide-bored long needle is introduced into the amniotic cavity through the abdominal wall after giving local anesthesia. The fetal parts and the location of placenta should be detected by ultrasound scan before doing the procedure to prevent harm to the fetus and placenta. This procedure is usually done at 14–18 weeks of gestation.

The cells seen in the amniotic fluid are fetal epithelial cells, amniotic cells and dermal fibroblasts. These fibroblasts are used for karyotyping.

Advantages of Amniocentesis

- Early detection of genetic disorders, such as Down's syndrome, Tay-Sachs disease, sickle cell disease, muscular dystrophies, etc., is possible.
- All gross chromosomal abnormalities and more than 50 biochemical defects can be detected by this method. The baby's sex can also be determined so that sex-linked disorders that affect the male child only can be detected.
- Prenatal estimation of lecithin: Sphingomyelin (L:S) ratio in amniotic fluid is useful to predict the chances of developing respiratory distress syndrome (RDS). If L:S ratio is less than 1.5 the risk is high. If L:S ratio is more than 2, the risk of RDS is minimal.

PARTURITION OR LABOR

> **PY9.8:** Describe and discuss the physiology of pregnancy, parturition and outline the psychology and psychiatry disorders associated with it.

Introduction

Duration of pregnancy is 270 days from the date of fertilization or 284 days (40 weeks) from the first day of last menstrual period (LMP). **Parturition** is the process by which baby is born. Throughout pregnancy there are episodes of mild rhythmic contractions of the uterus called **Braxton-Hicks contractions**. These are contractions of the uterus that are perceived by the mother towards the end of gestation. Initially, these contractions are uncoordinated and ineffective. As pregnancy advances, these contractions become stronger and stronger, and finally, they will be exceptionally strong and cause stretching and dilatation of the cervix and the baby is forced through the birth canal to the outside. This is parturition. Strong contractions of the uterus that cause parturition are called **labor contractions**. Many factors come into play during the onset of labor. They are:
1. Hormonal factors
2. Mechanical factors

Hormonal Factors

Estrogen and Progesterone

Ratio between **estrogen and progesterone** is very important. During early pregnancy, high levels of progesterone and low level of estrogen inhibit uterine contractility. Progesterone reduces muscle excitability by increasing calcium binding, thereby reducing free intracellular calcium. After 7 months of pregnancy, estrogen level increases rapidly and progesterone level decreases. Estrogen increases the contractility of uterus. It also stimulates prostaglandin synthesis and increases oxytocin receptors. Estrogen to progesterone ratio is increased at term which leads to labor contractions.

Oxytocin

Oxytocin increases uterine contractility. During the later months of pregnancy, the responsiveness of uterus to oxytocin is increased. The number of oxytocin receptors in the myometrium increases 100 times than that of non-pregnant uterus in the later stages of pregnancy. Distention of uterus and estrogen increases the number of oxytocin receptors. Dilatation of cervix produces a positive feedback effect on oxytocin secretion by the hypothalamus, and more of oxytocin is released; this causes increase in the force of contraction of uterus which in turn causes the cervix to dilate more and thus a **positive feedback loop** is formed. This leads to expulsion of the baby. Oxytocin also increases prostaglandin secretion from the uterus, which in turn increases uterine contractility.

Prostaglandin

Prostaglandin has a major role for the onset of labor. Prostaglandin concentration increases during labor. It is present in the decidua, placenta, fetal membranes and amniotic fluid. It infuses into the myometrium and initiate labor. Prostaglandin and oxytocin act synergistically in stimulating uterine contraction. Both causes increase in the intracellular free Ca^{2+} level in the myometrial cells by inhibiting calcium binding. Increase in free calcium level stimulates uterine contraction. Prostaglandin also induces the formation of gap junctions between the myometrial cells so that the myometrium can perform as a functional syncytium. Estrogen also stimulates prostaglandin synthesis at term.

CRH and Role of Fetus

Placental corticotropin releasing hormone (CRH) increase and maternal free CRH levels also increase at the time of onset of labor. CRH potentiate the contractile response of uterus to prostaglandin and oxytocin. CRH also stimulates fetal pituitary to secrete ACTH which in turn stimulates the fetal adrenal to increase fetal cortisol and DHEA production. DHEA increases estradiol production in the placenta.

Fetus produces hormones, such as cortisol, oxytocin, prostaglandin, etc., which increases uterine contractility. Increased cortisol in the fetus inhibits progesterone synthesis in the mother. This leads to increase in the estrogen-progesterone ratio which induces prostaglandin synthesis leading to initiation of labor. Fetal cortisol also exerts a positive feedback effect on placental CRH synthesis.

Role of Cortisol on Fetus and Mother towards Term
- Stimulates fetal lung maturation
- Increases glycogen content in liver
- Stimulates closure of ductus arteriosus
- Stimulates uterine contraction since fetal cortisol secretion is increased at the time of parturition. It also helps the fetus to overcome the stress during delivery.
- At term there is increased secretion of cortisol by the fetal adrenals and this inhibits progesterone synthesis in the mother.

Mechanical Factors
- Intermittent fetal movements cause stretching of uterus and these initiate uterine contractions. Distension of uterus and overstretching of muscle fibers at term increases the excitability of uterus and initiate labor.
- Stretching of the cervix or irritation of the cervix causes uterine contractions by a reflex mechanism. Artificial rupture of membrane (ARM) causes irritation and stretching of the cervix, and this induces uterine contractions.
- Contraction of abdominal muscle also aids in labor. Reflex contraction of abdominal muscles occurs by pain signals reaching the spinal cord from uterus. In the later stages of labor, voluntary contraction of the abdominal muscles occurs usually referred to as **bearing down**. After delivery of the baby, expulsion of placenta follows. The uterus involutes and reaches the normal size after some time. In lactating females, the uterus comes back to the normal size within 4 weeks of delivery.

Summary of Factors Leading to Parturition
- Increase in fetal cortisol.
- Increase in placental and maternal CRH level.
- Decrease in progesterone leads to softening and dilatation of cervix which is aided by estradiol and relaxin.
- Increase in the local concentration of prostaglandin which increases myometrial contractility by increasing intracellular calcium.
- Number of oxytocin receptors increases in the uterus towards term and there is also increased local synthesis of oxytocin by decidua and fetal membranes.
- Estradiol and prostaglandin increase α-adrenergic receptors in myometrium, which on stimulation causes uterine contraction. Catecholamine release is increased due to maternal stress during delivery.
- There is increase in the concentration of actin and myosin in myometrium which help in coordinated contraction of the uterus.

PUERPERIUM

The 6-week period after delivery during which, the mother's reproductive system returns to the pre-pregnancy state is called **puerperium**. By tissue catabolism and by the action of oxytocin released during lactation, decrease in the size of the uterus occurs, which is referred to as **involution**. For 2–4 weeks after delivery, women have uterine discharge called **lochia** which consists of secretions and sloughed tissue from the site of detachment of placenta.

MULTIPLE CHOICE QUESTIONS

1. Maximum production of hCG occurs during:
   a. First trimester
   b. Second trimester
   c. Third trimester
   d. Implantation
2. The viability of the spermatozoa within the female genital tract is up to:
   a. 6 hours
   b. 120 hours
   c. 24 hours
   d. 48 hours
3. Once deposited in the female genital tract, spermatozoa is capable of fertilizing the ovum up to:
   a. 6 hours
   b. 12 hours
   c. 24 hours
   d. 48 hours
4. Fertilization occurs in the:
   a. Fallopian tube
   b. Uterus
   c. Cervix
   d. Vagina
5. Increased fetal cortisol just before birth results in:
   a. Uterine contraction
   b. Release of oxytocin
   c. Placental steroid biogenesis
   d. Fetal lung maturation
6. Braxton—Hicks contractions:
   a. Is a positive feedback system
   b. Is another term for labor contraction
   c. Occur during most of the months of pregnancy
   d. Result in hypoxia of the fetus
7. Uterine contractions can be enhanced during parturition by giving synthetic:
   a. Estrogen
   b. Progesterone
   c. Oxytocin
   d. LH
8. The role of human placental lactogen is:
   a. Stimulate milk production
   b. Fetal breast development
   c. Growth of fetus
   d. Endocrine regulation
9. Hormone which does not cross the placenta is:
   a. Insulin
   b. Estrogen
   c. Cortisol
   d. Progesterone

10. **A premature infant is more likely to:**
    a. Suffer from jaundice of hepatic origin
    b. Maintain normal body temperature in cold environment
    c. Excrete urine with a uniform specific gravity
    d. Suffer from anemia

11. **Prenatal diagnosis at 16 weeks of pregnancy can be performed using all of the following, *except*:**
    a. Amniotic fluid
    b. Maternal blood
    c. Fetal blood
    d. Chorionic villi

12. **Corpus luteum saving hormone is:**
    a. hCG
    b. FSH
    c. LH
    d. Progesterone

13. **Weight of placenta at term is:**
    a. 300 g
    b. 500 g
    c. 700 g
    d. 900 g

14. **Which of the following probably triggers the onset of labor?**
    a. ACTH in fetus
    b. ACTH in mother
    c. Oxytocin
    d. Prostaglandin

15. **Regarding human chorionic gonadotropic hormone, the correct statement is:**
    a. It maintains corpus luteum
    b. It stimulates growth
    c. It inhibits LH and FSH
    d. It relaxes pelvic ligaments

16. **Zygote reaches the uterine cavity as:**
    a. 2 celled
    b. 8 celled
    c. 16 celled
    d. 32 celled

17. **Life span of sperms in the female reproductive tract is:**
    a. 48 hours
    b. 24 hours
    c. 72 hours
    d. 12 hours

18. **The hormone that is not secreted by placenta is:**
    a. hCG
    b. HPL
    c. Progesterone
    d. Prolactin

19. **Uterine contractility is increased by:**
    a. Vasopressin
    b. Oxytocin
    c. Luteinizing hormone
    d. Progesterone

20. **Immunological test of pregnancy is based on the urinary detection of:**
    a. hCG
    b. Estrogen
    c. Progesterone
    d. Estrogen and progesterone

21. **Somatomammotropin hormone is produced by:**
    a. Testis
    b. Ovary
    c. Pituitary
    d. Placenta

22. **All the following are hormones produced by placenta, *except*:**
    a. hCG
    b. Estrogen
    c. Oxytocin
    d. Progesterone

23. **The hormone which increases the availability of glucose and fatty acids to the developing fetus is:**
    a. hCG
    b. hCS
    c. Estrogen
    d. Progesterone

24. **Principal estrogen secreted by the placenta is:**
    a. Estriol
    b. β-estradiol
    c. Estrone
    d. 16-α hydroxyestrone

25. **Peak level of hCG is in urine is attained by .... weeks of pregnancy.**
    a. 2–3 weeks
    b. 9–12 weeks
    c. 16–20 weeks
    d. 20–24 weeks

26. **The placental hormone which reduces the possibilities of fetal rejection is:**
    a. hCG
    b. Estrogen
    c. Progesterone
    d. Relaxin

27. **The hormone whose concentration gives a good index of placental function is:**
    a. hCG
    b. hCS
    c. Progesterone
    d. Estrogen

28. **A good index of fetal well-being is measurement of:**
    a. Urinary estriol of mother
    b. Urinary hCG level
    c. Plasma progesterone
    d. Plasma hCS level

29. **All the following statements regarding hCG is correct, *except*:**
    a. hCG is produced by cytotrophoblast
    b. It can be detected in blood as early as 6 days after conception
    c. Fetal liver and kidney normally produce small amounts of hCG
    d. hCG is not absolutely specific for pregnancy

30. **The hormone referred to as the maternal growth hormone of pregnancy is:**
    a. hCS
    b. hCG
    c. Progesterone
    d. Prolactin

31. **The most common cause for secondary amenorrhea is:**
    a. Stein-Levinthal syndrome
    b. Pregnancy
    c. Sheehan's syndrome
    d. Lactation

32. **In humans, fertilization usually occurs in the:**
    a. Abdominal cavity
    b. Cervix
    c. Uterine tube
    d. Uterine cavity

33. **The most dominant endocrine factor during parturition is:**
    a. Decrease in the sensitivity of myometrium to estrogen
    b. Increased release of prostaglandins
    c. Decrease in progesterone effect and increase in sensitivity to relaxin
    d. Decrease in progesterone effect and increase in estrogen effect

34. The hormone that is produced in the mother's kidney exclusively during pregnancy is:
    a. Aldosterone
    b. Deoxycorticosterone
    c. Calcitriol
    d. Cortisol

35. Relaxin suppresses myocardial contractility by:
    a. Inhibiting prostaglandin synthesis
    b. Increasing the sensitivity of myometrium to progesterone
    c. Inhibiting myosin light chain phosphorylation
    d. Increasing the sensitivity of myometrium to estrogen

36. Growth of myometrium during pregnancy is stimulated mainly by:
    a. Estrogen
    b. Progesterone
    c. hCG
    d. hCS

37. The actions of progesterone during pregnancy includes all the following, *except*:
    a. Inhibits uterine contractions
    b. Maintain the decidual lining of uterus
    c. Modulate the secretion of hCG and hCS
    d. Stimulates production of prostaglandin

38. The hormone that is directly responsible for the establishment and sustenance of the fetus in the uterine cavity is:
    a. Estrogen
    b. Progesterone
    c. FSH
    d. hCG

39. Corpus luteum of pregnancy is maintained by:
    a. hCG
    b. hCS
    c. Progesterone
    d. Estrogen

40. Peak hCG plasma level is reached at:
    a. 20–24 weeks
    b. 9–12 weeks
    c. 4–6 weeks
    d. 30–32 weeks

41. hCG of pregnancy is secreted by:
    a. Corpus luteum of pregnancy
    b. Fetal liver
    c. Syncytiotrophoblast cells
    d. Fetal adrenal gland

ANSWERS

1. a	2. b	3. d	4. a	5. a
6. c	7. c	8. c	9. a	10. a
11. c	12. a	13. b	14. a	15. a
16. c	17. a	18. d	19. b	20. a
21. d	22. c	23. b	24. a	25. b
26. c	27. b	28. a	29. a	30. a
31. b	32. c	33. d	34. b	35. c
36. a	37. d	38. b	39. a	40. b
41. c				

Cardiorespiratory Adjustments of the Baby after Birth

CHAPTER 75

■ INTRODUCTION

In the intrauterine life (IUL), the fetus is totally dependent on the mother for O_2, nutrients, protection, etc., and also for the elimination of waste products, such as CO_2, other waste products, excess heat, etc.

■ RESPIRATORY ADJUSTMENTS AFTER BIRTH

Fetal lungs do not function till birth. Exchange of gases occur through the placenta, i.e., placenta perform the function of lungs. Once umbilical cord is cut, the baby takes the first breath and independent life starts. Life also ends with stoppage of respiration.

In the IUL, the fetal lungs are collapsed and filled with amniotic fluid. Surfactant production begins by 7th month of IUL and the lung becomes mature by 36 weeks of pregnancy. When the umbilical cord is cut after delivery, the baby's supply of O_2 from the mother stops and the baby suffers from **hypoxia**. Metabolism is continuing and so the CO_2 content of blood also increases and this **hypercapnia** stimulates the respiratory center causing the respiratory muscles to contract, and the baby draws its first breath. When the child exhales deeply naturally, it cries during the first few breaths. Violent respiratory efforts are seen during the first few breaths because the work of breathing is more. Rate of respiration is about 45/min for the first 2 weeks after delivery. Slowly it declines to normal rate.

■ CARDIOVASCULAR ADJUSTMENTS

After the first breath, the foramen ovale, the opening between right and left atria closes so that, deoxygenated blood passes to the right ventricle and is diverted to the lungs. The remnant of foramen ovale is called **fossa ovalis**. The ductus arteriosus also shuts off due to contraction of smooth muscle of its wall and it becomes **ligamentum arteriosum**. The smooth muscle contraction is mediated by bradykinin. Complete closure occurs by 3 months after birth. If it persists, the condition is called **patent ductus arteriosus (PDA)**. When the umbilical cord is cut, no blood flows through the umbilical arteries, and it gets filled with connective tissue and the distal portion becomes **medial umbilical ligament**. The umbilical vein becomes **ligamentum teres** of the liver.

In fetus, ductus venosus connects umbilical vein to inferior vena cava so that placental blood bypasses fetal liver. After birth, ductus venosus collapses and venous blood from fetal viscera flows into hepatic portal vein of the baby into the liver and via hepatic vein to inferior vena cava. Remnants of ductus venosus becomes **ligamentum venosum**.

Lactation

CHAPTER 76

LEARNING OBJECTIVE
- Describe the physiology of lactation

INTRODUCTION

PY9.8: Describe and discuss the physiology of lactation.

At the time of puberty, breasts enlarge due to the action of **estrogen and progesterone**. Estrogen causes proliferation of duct system whereas progesterone is responsible for the development of lobules. In subsequent menstrual cycles, further growth occurs and adult size is attained by the age of 19 years. Other hormones responsible for the development of breasts are **growth hormone, cortisone, insulin, thyroxine and prolactin**.

Final growth of breasts occurs during pregnancy in response to high circulating levels of estrogen, progesterone, prolactin, hCG and hCS. Placenta produces large amounts of these hormones. Prolactin and hCS have lactogenic (milk producing effect) action also **(Fig. 76.1)**.

Prolactin secretion starts by 5th month of pregnancy, gradually increases and peak secretion occurs at term. At term, estrogen level and prolactin levels are high.

Lactogenic action of prolactin is inhibited by estrogen. So, there is no milk secretion during pregnancy. *Prolactin and estrogen synergize in their action in producing breast growth, but estrogen antagonizes the lactogenic effect of prolactin.* Prolactin acts only on estrogen and progesterone primed breasts. Just before delivery, few mL of fluid is secreted by breasts called **colostrum**. It contains no fat, but is rich in lactose, protein, lactoferrin, oligosaccharides, antibodies, cells, such as polymorphonuclear leukocytes, monocytes, etc. After birth, baby is protected by colostrum due to the presence of **IgA** which is absorbed by the intestinal mucosa of the baby by endocytosis. It provides passive immunity to the baby against infection till the baby's immune system starts functioning. Lactation involves two processes:
1. Milk secretion
2. Milk ejection

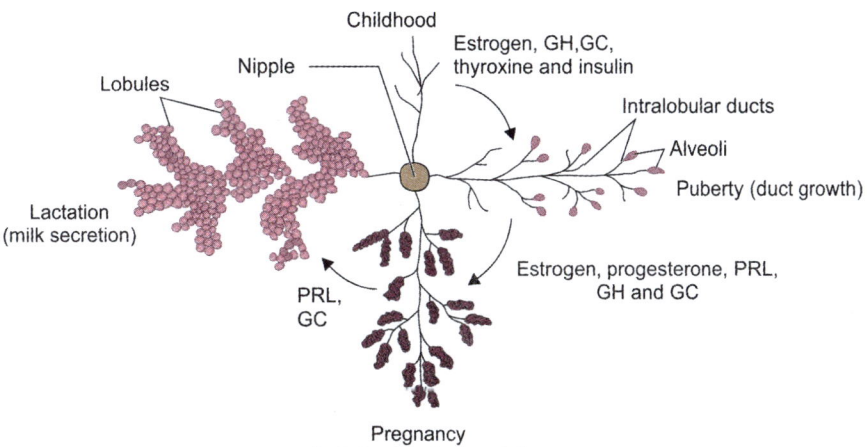

Fig. 76.1: Development of mammary gland and the hormones involved in different stages.
(GH: growth hormone; GC: glucocorticoid; PRL: prolactin)

MILK SECRETION

Synthesis and passage of milk into the lumen of the gland includes:
1. Initiation of lactation or lactogenesis
2. Maintenance of lactation or galactopoiesis

Initiation of Lactation

From 5th month of pregnancy, some amount of fluid is secreted by the breasts. After delivery, when placenta is expelled out, estrogen and progesterone levels fall and the inhibitory effect on the lactogenic action of prolactin is removed. This is one mechanism of initiation of lactation. Rate of prolactin secretion is increased so much after delivery that it increases milk production. Due to the stress of delivery, glucocorticoid secretion is also increased which can initiate lactation. Lactation is established only after 2-3 days after delivery in humans.

Maintenance of Lactation

When baby suckles the breast, the nerve signals are transmitted to the hypothalamus and this stimulates anterior pituitary to liberate **prolactin** and this increase persists for 1 hour. This helps in the synthesis of milk for the next nursing period **(Fig. 76.2A)**. Even though the basal prolactin level falls after 2 months of delivery, there is acute rise in prolactin level during each period of suckling. This repeated acute rise in prolactin is very essential to maintain milk secretion. Other hormones, such as **growth hormone, glucocorticoid, parathormone,** etc., help to maintain lactation by providing glucose, fatty acid, protein, Ca^{2+}, etc., for the synthesis of milk. TRH also stimulates release of **prolactin**. As long as the baby suckles, there will be milk production. The rate of milk production decreases by 7-9 months. Composition of human milk is given in **Table 76.1**.

MILK EJECTION

Milk is continuously secreted from the alveolar epithelium to the lumen. Milk has to flow to the duct before the baby gets milk. The process by which milk is ejected from lumen to duct is called **milk ejection or milk let down**.

This is a reflex phenomenon usually referred to as a **neuroendocrine reflex**. Oxytocin is responsible for milk ejection.

Table 76.1: Composition of human milk.	
Constituent	Percentage
Water	88.5
Fat	3.3
Lactose	6.8
Casein	0.9
Lactalbumin and other proteins	0.4
Ash	0.2

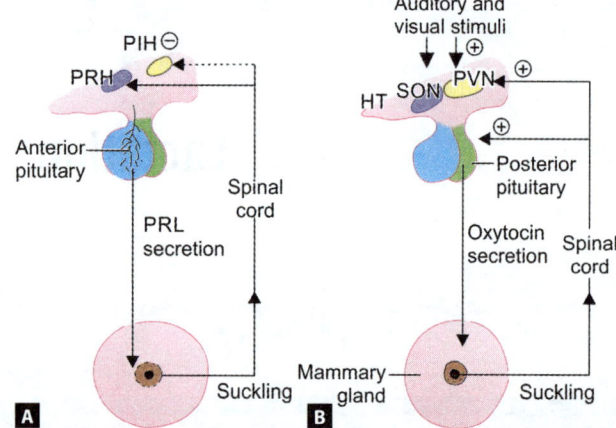

Figs. 76.2A and B: Pathways for: (A) Milk secretion; (B) Milk ejection.
(HT: hypothalamus; PIH: prolactin inhibiting hormone)

- *Receptors:* Touch receptors of breast especially of nipple.
- *Center:* Supraoptic and paraventricular nuclei of hypothalamus.
- *Effect:* Release of oxytocin which causes contraction of myoepithelial cells leading to milk ejection **(Fig. 76.2B)**.

Myoepithelial cells are smooth muscle cells that line the ducts of the breast. When the baby sucks one breast, signals go to the hypothalamus and milk ejection occurs from both breasts. Fondling of the baby, hearing the cry of the baby, etc., causes release of oxytocin. Temporary inhibition of milk ejection is seen at times of fear, anxiety, sympathetic stimulation, etc.

Actions of Prolactin

- Initiation of lactation.
- Maintenance of lactation.
- Prevents ovulation by inhibiting LH secretion in mother.
- Reduces the responsiveness of ovaries to FSH.
- Acts in different areas of the brain of mother to stimulate maternal behavior.
- Increases appetite in mother so that the calories and nutrients needed for breast feeding is met with.
- Helps in the concentration of lactose, protein, calcium, phosphorus, etc., in the vesicles of mammary gland.
- Prolactin along with placental growth hormone (hCS) helps in the linear growth of fetus.

LACTATION AND MENSTRUATION

If the mother does not nurse the baby, within 6 weeks of delivery the menstrual cycle starts. If the mother continues to nurse the baby, there will be increased prolactin secretion which has the following effects:

- Acts on hypothalamus and inhibits GnRH secretion.
- Acts on pituitary and inhibits the action of GnRH on pituitary and thus inhibits FSH and LH secretion.
- In the ovaries, prolactin antagonizes the action of gonadotropins on ovary.

Net effect is inhibition of ovulation. Ovary becomes inactive and progesterone and estrogen levels fall. So, *there* will be no ovulation and menstruation during lactation, and this is called **lactational amenorrhea**. About 50% of mothers do not ovulate till the baby is weaned. Nursing the baby has long been known as an effective method of contraception.

Milk that is secreted is a balanced diet for the baby. It contains fat, surplus proteins, lactose, Ca^{2+}, Mg^{2+}, phosphorus, vitamins, etc. At the peak of lactation, about 1.5 L of milk is secreted per day.

Chiari-Frommel Syndrome

In some females, there is persistence of lactation even if the baby is not nursed. Here, galactorrhea, amenorrhea and gonadal atrophy are seen with persistent prolactin secretion. There is no secretion of LH and FSH and so there is no stimulation of gonads and hence no ovulation. This condition is **Chiari-Frommel syndrome**. In pituitary chromophobe tumor, this condition is seen without delivery, i.e., in non-pregnant females.

Gynecomastia

Enlargement of breasts in male is called **gynecomastia**. It is common at the time of puberty. It is also seen in 75% of newborns due to the effect of maternal estrogens.

Pathological conditions are:
- Androgen resistance
- Estrogen therapy
- Estrogen-secreting tumors in males
- Hyperthyroidism
- Cirrhosis of liver
- Eunuchoidism
- Digitalis therapy (because cardiac glycosides have weak estrogenic action).

MULTIPLE CHOICE QUESTIONS

1. Milk ejection reflex is mediated by:
   a. Oxytocin
   b. Vasopressin
   c. Growth hormone
   d. Thyroxin

2. Milk is deficient in:
   a. Calcium   b. Vitamin A
   c. Vitamin D   d. Iron

3. The correct statement regarding prolactin is:
   a. It is not produced in male
   b. It is present in high concentration in later months of pregnancy
   c. Causes secretion of milk in later months of pregnancy
   d. Causes ejection of milk during lactation

4. Prolactin inhibiting hormone is:
   a. Somatostatin   b. TRH
   c. Dopamine   d. Growth hormone

5. Hormone responsible for milk secretion is:
   a. Oxytocin   b. Prolactin
   c. Estrogen   d. FSH

6. The following hormones are necessary for maintaining lactation, *except*:
   a. Growth hormone   b. Glucocorticoid
   c. Parathormone   d. Estrogen

7. One of the prolactin releasing hormones is thought to be:
   a. TRH   b. TSH
   c. ACTH   d. Dopamine

8. Prolactin inhibiting factor is secreted by:
   a. Anterior pituitary   b. Posterior pituitary
   c. Hypothalamus   d. Thalamus

9. The hormone that is responsible for pigmentation of areola is:
   a. Estrogen   b. Progesterone
   c. Melatonin   d. LH

10. The hormone that promotes growth of ductules of breast:
    a. Progesterone   b. FSH
    c. Estrogen   d. Prolactin

ANSWERS

| 1. a | 2. d | 3. b | 4. c | 5. b |
| 6. d | 7. a | 8. c | 9. a | 10. c |

Contraception and Infertility

CHAPTER 77

LEARNING OBJECTIVES
- Enumerate the contraceptive methods for male and female. Discuss their advantages and disadvantages
- Discuss the causes of infertility and the role of IVF in its management

CONTRACEPTION

PY9.6: Enumerate the contraceptive methods for male and female. Discuss their advantages and disadvantages.

Contraception means prevention of conception or unwanted pregnancies. It includes:
- Temporary methods or spacing methods
- Permanent or terminal methods

Temporary Methods

Natural Methods
- *Coitus interruptus*: This method involves withdrawal of the penis before ejaculation. Failure rate is 4 per 100 women.
- *Lactational amenorrhea*: Since prolactin inhibits gonadotropin secretion and blocks the action of gonadotropins on the ovaries, ovulation is suppressed in lactating women. On an average, ovulation suppression is seen for 6 months in completely breastfeeding mothers.
- *Periodic abstinence or safe period*: Intercourse is avoided during the fertile period. In a woman with 28-day cycle or with regular periods, this method is effective. In a 28-day cycle, ovulation occurs on the 14th day of the cycle. Fertilization is possible 3 days before and 3 days after ovulation. This is taken as the fertile period which is usually between. This method is also called **rhythm method**. Before 9th day and after 19th day is usually said to be the safe period. First find out the duration of the menstrual cycle. Ovulation occurs 14 days before the onset of bleeding. Avoidance of intercourse for 4 days before the calculated day of ovulation and 3 days afterward prevents conception. This method does not offer much protection because even in normal women ovulation can occur between 6th and 21st days and sperms may survive in the female genital tract for 5–7 days. Failure rate is 6%.

Barrier Method
Barrier methods prevent sperms from reaching the ovum. They are:
- *Physical methods*: **Condom** in males and diaphragm or **cervical cap** in females. Female condoms are also available but it is expensive. This method prevents sperms from meeting the ovum. The advantages of condom are: (a) it prevents sexually transmitted diseases (b) it is free from side effects. They also provide protection from cervical cancer since they protect against human papilloma virus infection.
- *Chemical methods:* Jelly, suppositories, pastes or creams which are spermicidal are used alone or along with physical methods. These chemicals contain sperm-killing agents called **spermicides**. Most widely used spermicide is **nonoxynol-9** which is a non-ionic surface- active detergent that immobilizes sperms.

Intrauterine Contraceptive Devices (IUCD or IUDs)
Intrauterine devices (IUD) are metal or plastic appliances introduced into the uterine cavity to prevent pregnancy.

They are effective, safe and convenient. They are inserted soon after menstruation. These include:
- Non-medicated intrauterine devices
- Copper-releasing IUDs
- Medicated (hormone releasing) intrauterine devices.

Non-medicated IUDs
These include **Lippes loop, Ota ring,** etc., which are inert IUDs. Lippes loop is a plastic double S-shaped device which is non-toxic and non-tissue reactive (**Fig. 77.1 C**). Even though the exact mechanism is not known they prevent sperms from fertilizing the ovum. The inert IUDs are not used nowadays.

Copper Releasing IUDs

The medicated or copper releasing IUDs are widely used. They consist of a T-shaped plastic frame with copper wire wound around the stem and arms. These include CuT200, multiload Cu250, CuT380A, etc. **(Figs. 77.1A and B)**. The number denotes the surface area of copper in square mm. The surface area of copper determines the efficacy and lifespan of the device. Copper appears to have a spermatocidal effect and it also alters the composition of cervical mucus. Multiload Cu250 has flexible serrated arms that hold the device in place **(Fig. 77.1A)**.

Hormone Releasing IUDs

In **medicated IUDs**, hormones, such as progesterone will be incorporated in the device which slowly releases progesterone. Mechanisms of action are:

- IUDs causes a sterile local inflammatory reaction in the endometrium that is not suitable for implantation.
- Certain phagocytes are formed in the uterus during the inflammatory response, which phagocytose the sperms.
- Progesterone thickens the cervical mucus and decreases sperm motility. It also makes the endometrium unfavorable for implantation of fertilized ovum.

Disadvantage of IUDs is that, it causes intrauterine infections. IUDs have to be replaced periodically at intervals of 2–4 years. IUDs are contraindicated in those with pelvic inflammatory disease, sexually transmitted disease, uterine fibroids, cancer of genital tract, AIDS.

Oral Contraceptives

Estrogen or progesterone alone can be used as a contraceptive. Estrogen inhibits ovulation and progesterone induces change in cervical mucus and endometrium. Combination of estrogen and progesterone (combined pill) can also be used to prevent pregnancy. Naturally occurring hormones, if given orally, will be metabolized in the liver. So, synthetic forms are used. Estrogen secreted by the ovary is estradiol. Addition of an ethinyl group to estradiol makes it orally active. Ethinyl estradiol is a very potent oral estrogen and is the commonly used oral contraceptive. The other estrogen used is mestranol. Oral contraceptives include:

- Combined pill or classical pill
- Mini pill or micro-pill
- Morning-after pill or post-coital contraceptive pill
- Long acting pill
- Male pill.

Combined Pill

Almost all pills used for the control of fertility consist of some combination of synthetic estrogens and synthetic progestins. The main reason for using synthetic estrogens and progestins is that the natural hormones are almost entirely destroyed by the liver within a short time after they are absorbed from the gastrointestinal tract into the portal circulation. However, many of the synthetic hormones can resist this destructive propensity of the liver, thus allowing oral administration. Commonly used synthetic estrogens are ethinyl estradiol and mestranol. Commonly used synthetic progestins are norethindrone, norethynodrel, ethynodiol, and norgestrel. Combination of synthetic estrogen and progesterone is given daily for 21 days starting from the 5th day of the menstrual cycle. A break of 7 days is given during which withdrawal bleeding occurs and a new cycle begins. During these days vitamin tablets are given **(Fig. 77.2)**. Estrogen and progesterone lead to hypertrophy of the endometrium.

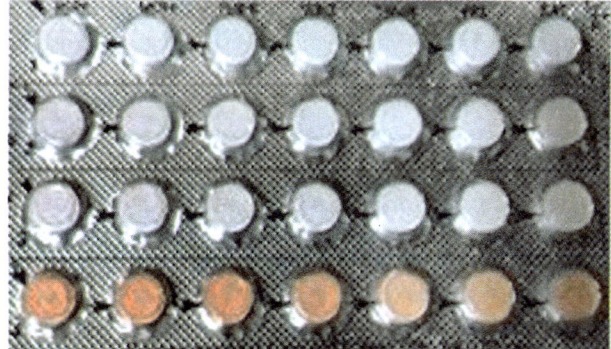

Fig. 77.2: Oral contraceptive pills.

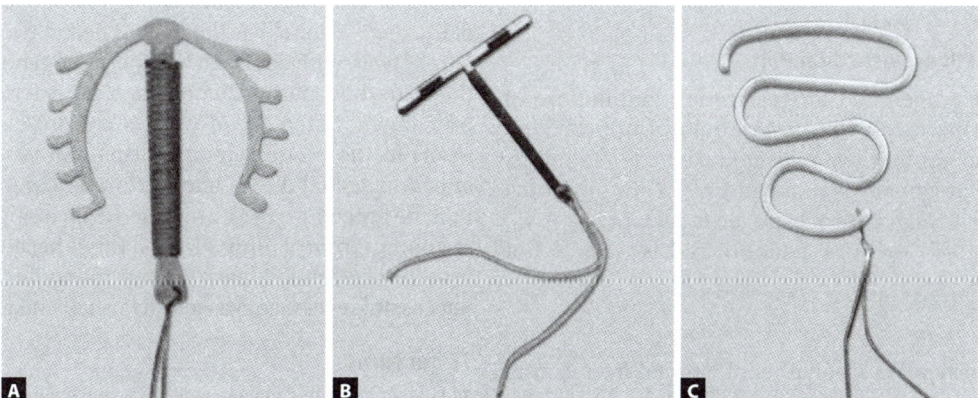

Figs. 77.1A to C: Intrauterine contraceptive devices: (A and B) Copper T; (C) Lippes loop.

Bleeding is due to sudden withdrawal of hormones, known as **withdrawal bleeding**. If taken properly, combined pill is 100% effective in preventing fertilization. This is the most popular and widely accepted contraceptive pill.

Mechanism of Action of Combined Pill
- When estrogen and progesterone are given there is inhibition of LH surge by progesterone and FSH secretion by estrogen from the anterior pituitary by negative feedback. The low levels of FSH and LH usually inhibit the development of ovarian follicle. As a result, estrogen level does not rise to produce the mid-cycle LH surge. Since there is no LH surge, ovulation does not occur.
- By feedback inhibition, gonadotropin releasing hormone (GnRH) secretion from the hypothalamus is also inhibited.
- In the ovary, follicular growth is inhibited.
- In the cervix, the secretion becomes thick due to the action of progesterone and this prevents entry of sperms.
- Estrogen makes the endometrium hyper-proliferative thereby preventing implantation.

Side effects of combined pill include weight gain, venous thromboembolism, arterial thrombosis, stroke, hypertension, diabetes mellitus and liver disorders, cancerous conditions especially of breast and endometrium, and rarely myocardial infarction. Women who take pill and smoke have a higher risk of heart attack and stroke than nonsmoking pill users. Most common complication is venous thromboembolism. Estrogen increases the production of clotting factors, such as factor V, VIII, X and fibrinogen resulting in hypercoagulability of blood and increased risk of venous thrombosis. Progesterone in the pill increases the risk of arterial thrombosis which may lead to myocardial infarction and stroke.

Contraindications for oral contraceptives are arterial or venous thrombosis, ischemic heart disease, carcinoma breast, hypertension, migraine, epilepsy, liver diseases, breast feeding, etc.

Minipill or Micropill

Minipill contains very small amounts of progesterone and is given throughout the cycle. This prevents fertility without inhibiting ovulation. This is due to change in cervical mucus and endometrium, and decreased motility of fallopian tubes.

Morning-after Pill or Post-coital Pill

High dose of estrogen and progesterone (double dose of combined pill) is taken within 48 hours of unprotected intercourse and another two pills are taken after 12 hours. The chance of pregnancy is reduced by 75%. In postcoital contraceptive pill, high dose of estrogen is present.

Long-acting pill or once-a-month pill is usually not recommended.

Male Pill

Male pill or **gossypol** is a polyphenol derived from cotton seed. It produces reduction in sperm count. Due to its toxicity, it is not recommended as a male contraceptive pill.

Testosterone and Inhibin as Contraceptives in Men

Administration of **testosterone** in high doses decreases sperm count by its inhibitory feedback effect on LH (ICSH) secretion by the anterior pituitary. Testosterone in high doses also inhibits the release of GnRH from the hypothalamus, but it is not safe as a contraceptive because high doses of testosterone cause sodium and water retention.

Inhibin inhibits FSH secretion by a feedback effect on the pituitary. Use of inhibin as a potential contraceptive measure is under trial.

Vas-occlusive Plugs in Males

Polyurethane or silicone rubber is injected in the liquid form into the vas deferens where it hardens within 20 min forming a plug in the vas deferens. This forms a barrier against sperms. This type of contraception is reversible and fertility is restored after the plugs are removed.

Depot Forms in Females

Depot forms include Norplant, Depo-Provera and vaginal ring.
- **Norplant**: Hormone-containing capsules are implanted subcutaneously in the arm. These slowly release progestin which inhibits ovulation. The effect lasts for 5 years.
- **Depo-provera**: Intramuscular injection of medroxy-progesterone acetate (synthetic progesterone) is given once in 3 months. It acts by inhibiting ovulation and by thickening cervical secretions.
- **Vaginal ring**: A ring that fits in the vagina is introduced which releases estrogen and progestin slowly. This ring is worn for 3 weeks and removed for 1 week to allow menstruation to occur.

Permanent Methods

Sterilization is the procedure that renders an individual incapable of reproduction.

Vasectomy

Vasectomy is the principal method for sterilization of males where, bilateral ligation of vas deferens after cutting a portion of the duct is done. Vas deferens is tied at two places and the part between the ties is cut off. Spermatogenesis continues in the testes but sperms do not reach the exterior and produce pregnancy. Since blood vessels are not cut, testosterone levels in the blood remain normal. So vasectomy has no effect on sexual desire and performance. Another merit is that the procedure can be reversed even though the chance of regaining fertility is only 30–40%. This is because about 50% of vasectomized individuals develop antibodies against sperms. Successful reversal of vasectomy usually takes about 2 years.

Tubectomy

Tubectomy is done in females. It can be done by **laparoscopy** or by **minilaparotomy**. The fallopian tubes are cut and the

cut ends are ligated. It is also a reversible process. Advantages of tubectomy are:
- It avoids pregnancy.
- Reduces the risk of pelvic inflammatory disease in females with sexually transmitted diseases.
- Reduces the risk of ovarian cancer.
- It is a reversible process

Summary
Female Contraception
- Barriers, such as diaphragm and cervical cap
- Intrauterine contraceptive devices, such as copper T and Lippes loop
- Oral contraceptives containing estrogen, progesterone or both
- Long-acting injectable and implants
- Tubectomy

Male Contraception
- Coitus interruptus
- Condoms
- Drugs causing azoospermia, such as testosterone, gossypol, nifedipine (antihypertensive drug), etc. are not usually recommended for male contraception
- Vas-occlusive plugs
- Vasectomy

INFERTILITY

> **PY9.12:** Discuss the common causes of infertility in a couple and role of IVF in managing a case of infertility.

Female infertility occurs in 10% of women of the reproductive age group. Causes may be ovarian diseases, obstruction of fallopian tube, abnormalities of uterus or autoimmunity. Lack of ovulation due to hyposecretion of pituitary gonadotropic hormones can be treated by administration of human chorionic gonadotropin (hCG) extracted from human placenta. hCG has almost the same effects of LH and can stimulate ovulation.

Male infertility is different from erectile dysfunction previously referred to as impotence. Causes of infertility may be decreased sperm count, obstruction to ducts, destruction of germinal epithelium by X-rays, infections, such as mumps in adults, high scrotal temperature as in undescended testes.

In 30% of infertility cases, the problem is in the man; in 45% problem is in the woman; in 20% both have a problem and in 5% no cause can be found.

Treatment (Assisted Reproduction)
In Vitro Fertilization (IVF)

In vitro fertilization is a type of **assisted reproductive technology (ART)** for the treatment of infertility or genetic problems. It is the most effective form of assisted reproductive technology. It is the process of fertilization where an ovum is combined with sperm outside the body. First of all, ovulation is induced in the woman (**ovulation induction**). The woman is given FSH soon after menstruation, which leads to the development of several follicles in the ovary. After maturation of the follicles, the secondary oocytes are aspirated by laparoscopy (**egg retrieval**) and transferred to a solution containing sperms where the secondary oocyte is fertilized to form the zygote. If the sperms have lower motility, they may be injected directly into the eggs to promote fertilization. Embryo culture takes about 2–6 days. When the zygote reaches 8 cell or 16 cell stage, it is introduced into the uterus for implantation and development (**embryo transfer**). Progesterone is administered orally or by injection daily for the first 8–10 weeks after the embryo transfer. The hormone makes it easier for the embryo to survive in the uterus.

The sperms are obtained from the epididymis or from the testis. IVF has a 5–10% chance of producing a live birth. IVF is time-consuming, highly expensive and invasive. It can also result in multiple pregnancy. Anxiety and depression are usually observed in the couple undergoing treatment throughout the process.

In 1978, Louise Brown was the first child born by this method for which **Robert G Edwards** was awarded the **Nobel Prize** in Physiology or Medicine in 2010.

Intracytoplasmic Sperm Injection (ICSI)

This is done when infertility is due to impaired sperm motility. The oocyte is fertilized in vitro by suctioning a sperm into a tiny pipette and then injecting it into the oocyte's cytoplasm. When the zygote reaches 8–16 cell stage it is introduced into the uterus.

Embryo Transfer

Artificial insemination of semen is done into a fertile female who is a donor. After fertilization in the donor's fallopian tube, the blastocyst is transferred from the donor to the infertile woman. This is usually done in infertile woman who does not ovulate and also in those who are carriers of serious genetic disorders, such as hemophilia, sickle cell disease, thalassemia major, etc.

Intrauterine Insemination (IUI)

In IUI, sperms are placed directly in the uterus and are therefore not exposed to the acidic environment of the vagina.

Gamete Intrafallopian Transfer (GIFT)

Here, the normal process of conception is mimicked by uniting sperm and ovum in the woman's fallopian tube. This is usually done when the sperm count is very low. The woman is given FSH and LH to stimulate production of several ova which are aspirated from mature follicles, mixed outside with sperms and then immediately introduced into the fallopian tubes.

Post-conceptional Fertility Control
Menstrual Regulation

In menstrual regulation 6–14 days after the missed period, uterine contents are aspirated.

Menstrual Induction

Here, uterine contractions are produced by injecting PGF into the uterine cavity. Strong uterine contractions produce bleeding and evacuation of the uterine contents.

Abortion or Medical Termination of Pregnancy

Medical termination of pregnancy (MTP) is done before the fetus becomes viable. Premature expulsion of the products of conception from the uterus before 20th week of pregnancy is called **abortion**. It is induced by vacuum aspiration (suction), infusion of saline into the uterine cavity or by scraping the endometrium.

Nonsurgical abortion can be induced by **mifepristone** which is a progesterone antagonist. It binds to progesterone receptors and blocks them. When the action of progesterone is blocked, menstruation occurs and the embryo sloughs off. **Misoprostol**, a form of PGE, stimulates uterine contraction and helps in abortion.

MULTIPLE CHOICE QUESTIONS

1. Male contraceptive pill contains:
   a. Bromocryptine b. Cyproheptadine
   c. Cyproterone acetate d. Gossypol

2. Which of the following is a rare complication of the use of hormonal contraceptives?
   a. Contraceptive failure
   b. Cardiovascular effects
   c. Carcinogenesis
   d. Liver disorders

3. Post-coital contraception is recommended within...... hours of unprotected intercourse:
   a. 24 hours b. 48 hours
   c. 72 hours d. 12 hours

4. Which of the following is barrier contraception?
   a. Male sterilization b. Tubectomy
   c. Spermicidal jelly d. Minipill

5. Which can be used as an emergency postcoital contraceptive?
   a. Spermicidal jelly b. Copper-T
   c. Vaginal sponge d. Progesterone

6. Combined oral contraceptive pill act mainly by:
   a. Inhibition of ovulation
   b. Increasing motility of fallopian tube
   c. Preventing ovum from reaching the uterus
   d. Making cervical secretion watery

7. Which of the following is the constituent of minipill?
   a. Only progesterone
   b. Only estrogen
   c. Estrogen + progesterone
   d. Norethisterone + estradiol

8. Which of the following is the constituent of mini pill?
   a. Progesterone only
   b. Estrogen only
   c. Estrogen and progesterone
   d. Norethisterone and estradiol

ANSWERS

| 1. d | 2. a | 3. c | 4. c | 5. d |
| 6. a. | 7. a | 8. a | | |

NAME THE FOLLOWING/GIVE THE NORMAL VALUE/FILL IN THE BLANKS

1. The neurotransmitter that exerts an inhibitory action on GnRH secretion before the onset of puberty: **GABA**.
2. Increase in GnRH secretion at the onset of puberty is due to the excitatory effect of **glutamate**.
3. Episodic bursts of **GnRH** from the hypothalamus are essential for the normal secretion of FSH and LH.
4. Primordial follicle is converted to **primary follicle** at the time of puberty.
5. Size of Graafian follicle: **1–1.5 cm**.
6. The **second meiotic** division is completed in the ovum at the time of fertilization.
7. The hormone responsible for ovulation: **LH**.
8. Absence of ferning of cervical mucus is an indicator of **ovulation**.
9. Estrogens cause **cornification** of vaginal epithelium.
10. Leukocytic infiltration in the vaginal epithelium is due to the action of **progesterone** after ovulation.
11. If fertilization fails to occur, corpus luteum becomes corpus albicans on the **24th** day of 28 day cycle.
12. The receptors present on the granulosa cells in female and on the sertoli cells in male: **FSH receptors**.
13. FSH stimulates first half of spermatogenesis while testosterone stimulates **last half** of spermatogenesis.
14. At the time of ovulation (mid-cycle) in the cervical mucus, **fern pattern** can be demonstrated.
15. After ovulation LH level falls due to **negative feedback** effect of progesterone secreted by the corpus luteum.
16. The ovum which is released at the time of ovulation is known as **secondary oocyte**.
17. Fertilization occurs normally in the **ampulla** of the fallopian tube.
18. Fertilized ovum is called **zygote**.
19. Name the hormone which is responsible for the rise in basal body temperature by 0.5°C after ovulation: **Progesterone**.
20. Down syndrome is due to non-disjunction in **chromosome 21**.
21. The enzyme that catalyzes conversion of testosterone to estradiol and androstenedione to estrone: **Aromatase**.
22. Name the naturally occurring estrogens: **17-β. estradiol, estrone and estriol**.
23. Sertoli cells have receptors for **FSH** and **testosterone**.
24. Tight junctions between sertoli cells contribute to **blood-testis-barrier**.
25. Name the substances secreted by the Sertoli cells: **Androgen binding protein (ABP), inhibin, activin and mullerian inhibiting substance (MIS)**.

26. Inhibin is secreted by Sertoli cells in males and **granulosa cells** in females.
27. Inhibin inhibits **FSH** secretion.
28. Activin secreted by Sertoli cells in males and granulosa cells in females stimulate **FSH** secretion.
29. Name the cells that secrete testosterone: **Leydig cells**.
30. Capacitation of sperm occur in the **female genital tract**.
31. Name the hormone responsible for skeletal maturation, epiphyseal fusion and cessation of growth: **Estrogen**.
32. 21-hydroxylase deficiency and 11-hydroxylase deficiency leads to **female** pseudohermaphroditism.
33. 17-hydroxylase deficiency and 3-hydroxylase deficiency leads to **male** pseudohermaphroditism.
34. Average volume of semen per ejaculation: **2.5–3.5 mL**.
35. Normal sperm count: **100 million/mL of semen**.
36. Sperm count less than 20 million/mL leads to sterility.
37. pH of semen: **7.35–7.5**.
38. Sperms are stored in the **epididymis**.
39. Normal menstrual flow: **50 mL**.
40. Onset of menstruation is called **menarche**.
41. Normal duration of pregnancy in humans: **280 days**.
42. Name the hormones produced by the placenta: **hCG, hCS, progesterone, estrogen, relaxin, inhibin**.
43. Before 7th week of pregnancy, estrogen and progesterone are produced by **corpus luteum**.
44. The hormone that is necessary for the maintenance of corpus luteum after fertilization: **hCG**.
45. The conditions where very high level of hCG is seen: **Multiple pregnancy, Down's syndrome, choriocarinoma**.
46. The principal estrogen secreted by the placenta is **estriol** whereas β-**estradiol** is the principal estrogen secreted by the ovaries.
47. Deficiency of **progesterone** in pregnancy leads to abortion.
48. The basis of immunological test of pregnancy is detection of **hCG** in blood or urine.
49. Blastocyst is surrounded by an outer layer of **syncytiotrophoblast** and inner layer of **cytotrophoblast**.
50. The endometrial cells at the site of implantation become **decidual** cells containing glycogen, protein and lipids.
51. Double Bohr Effect is seen in the **placenta**.
52. Name the hormone that increases excitability of the uterine myometrium: **Estrogen**.
53. Name the prostaglandins which increase uterine contractility: **Prostaglandins E_1 and $F_2\alpha$**.
54. Milk ejection reflex is mediated by oxytocin.
55. Prolactin inhibiting substance is **dopamine**.
56. Estrogen and progesterone are transported in blood in combination with **albumin**.
57. Testosterone is transported in blood in combination with **globulin**.
58. Precursor of progesterone is **cholesterol**.
59. Name the hormones influencing spermatogenesis: **LH, FSH, testosterone, inhibin, activin**.
60. Failure of descent of testis is called **cryptorchidism**.
61. Permanent methods of sterilization are **tubectomy** in female and **vasectomy** in male.
62. During pregnancy ovulation is inhibited by progesterone from **corpus luteum** and placenta.
63. Systemic administration of testosterone inhibits **LH** secretion and decrease sperm count.
64. Estrogen lower plasma cholesterol and is responsible for the low incidence of myocardial infarction in **premenopausal** women.
65. **Dihydrotestosterone** leads to the development of male external genitalia and male secondary sexual characters.
66. Penis-at-12 syndrome is seen in congenital **5α-reductase** deficiency.
67. Chromosomal pattern in **Turner's syndrome** is XO, in **Klinefelter's syndrome** it is XXY and in super-females it is XXX.

CLINICAL CASE SCENARIO

1. **An endometrial biopsy was taken after 22 days of last menstruation from a 35-year-old female complaining of not conceiving after 5 years of married life. Her menstrual cycles were regular (30-day cycle). The biopsy report was non-secretory endometrium. Answer the following questions:**
   1. Comment on the biopsy report.
   2. What will be the pattern of cervical mucus and vaginal smear taken on the same day in this lady?
   3. Explain the hormonal and uterine changes in the different phases of menstrual cycle.

SECTION 10: NERVOUS SYSTEM

CHAPTER 78: Organization of Nervous System

LEARNING OBJECTIVES
- Describe the organization of nervous system
- Explain the functions of neuroglial cells
- Draw and label the nuclei and laminas in spinal cord at the thoracic level

INTRODUCTION

PY10.1: Describe and discuss the organization of nervous system.

The two major controlling and coordinating systems of the body are endocrine system and nervous system. Any change in the internal or external environment produces changes in the nervous system. *Nervous system and endocrine system function together in maintaining homeostasis.* Most of the endocrine secretions are directly or indirectly influenced by the nervous system and most of the hormones influence different parts of the nervous system. The central nervous system correlates, coordinates and integrates the functioning of the different organ systems of the body. Differences between nervous system and endocrine system are shown in **Table 78.1**.

The branch of medicine that deals with the functioning and disorders of nervous system is called **neurology**.

FUNCTIONS OF NERVOUS SYSTEM

- ❖ **Sensory function:** Sensory receptors respond to different stimuli from within and outside the body, and the information is carried through the sensory neurons to the higher level. This information reaches the spinal cord, reticular formation, cerebellum, thalamus and sensory areas of the cerebral cortex.

Table 78.1: Differences between nervous system and endocrine system.

Nervous system	Endocrine system
Quick acting system but short lived	Has a latent period but action is prolonged
Action is mediated through action potentials	Action is mediated through hormones
Localized effect	Generalized effect
Controls rapid activities of the body like muscle contraction	Controls metabolic activities, growth, reproduction, etc.

- ❖ **Integrative function:** Nervous system integrates sensory information by analyzing it and making appropriate responses in the effector organ. Nervous system can inhibit or modify sensory signals so that unimportant sensory impulses can be ignored without responding to it. When important information excites the nervous system, it is channeled to the appropriate areas of the nervous system where it is processed to cause the desired responses. This processing of important and significant information is called integrative function of the nervous system. The correlation and integration of nervous information occur in the brain and spinal cord. *Interneurons have a very important role in the integration of sensory information.*
- ❖ **Motor function:** It involves responses to the sensory information. Efferent neurons are involved in this function. They carry motor information from the motor cortex, reticular formation, basal ganglia, cerebellum and spinal cord directly or indirectly through spinal nerves and cranial nerves. Motor functions of the nervous system include:
  - Contraction of skeletal muscles.
  - Contraction of smooth muscles in the internal organs.
  - Secretion of substances by exocrine and endocrine glands in different parts of the body.
- ❖ **Storage of information (memory):** Only a fraction of the sensory information that reaches the nervous system causes immediate response. Much of the information is stored for future control of motor activities and for use in the thinking process. Storage of information is also called memory and it is a function of the synapses. **Synapse** is the junctional point between neurons. Nervous system can store sensory information received during past experiences for minutes, weeks or years in the memory and appropriate modifications can be made in the future responses. The thinking process of the brain compares new sensory information with the stored memories and the memories help to select the important new information. Thus, memories become part of the brain processing mechanism. This process helps to (a) select the important

new sensory information and direct it to the motor areas to cause immediate responses or (b) to channel the new information to appropriate memory storage areas for future use.
- **Homeostasis:** Nervous system along with endocrine system controls the overall functions of the body, i.e., helps in homeostasis.
- Sympathetic division of autonomic nervous system (ANS) prepares the body to overcome emergency situations.
- Parasympathetic division of the ANS is concerned with conservation and restoration of energy.

ORGANIZATION OF NERVOUS SYSTEM

Structurally, nervous system is divided into:
- **Central nervous system (CNS)**, which includes brain and spinal cord
- **Peripheral nervous system (PNS)** consists of those parts of the nervous system that lie outside the dura mater. It includes 12 pairs of cranial nerves and 31 pairs of spinal nerves, and their ganglia. Sensory ganglia are present along the course of the cranial nerves V, VII, VIII, IX and X. Structurally, PNS also includes the paravertebral sympathetic chains and the preganglionic and post-ganglionic autonomic nerves even though functionally ANS is a distinct entity **(Flowchart 78.1)**

Functionally, nervous system is classified into:
- **Somatic nervous system**, which is divided into central nervous system (CNS) and peripheral nervous system (functionally, PNS consists of 12 pairs of cranial nerves and 31 pairs of spinal nerves).
- **Autonomic nervous system** (ANS), which controls viscera, such as heart, lungs, and gastrointestinal tract that are concerned with involuntary activities. It is divided into sympathetic nervous system and parasympathetic nervous system **(Flowchart 78.2)**. ANS is mainly responsible for maintaining a constant internal environment (For details, *refer* **Chapter 94**).

Both somatic and autonomic nervous systems consist of sensory and motor divisions. Differences between somatic nervous system and autonomic nervous system are given in **Table 78.2**.

Table 78.2: Differences between somatic and autonomic efferent pathways.

Somatic nervous system	Autonomic nervous system
The somatic efferent pathway consists of only one neuron which passes directly to the effector organ, i.e., the skeletal muscle	Autonomic efferent pathway consists of two neurons, i.e., preganglionic and postganglionic neurons. The postganglionic fiber supplies the effector organs, such as glands, visceral smooth muscles, blood vessels, heart, etc.
The neurotransmitter released at the efferent nerve ending is ACh	The transmitter released by the postganglionic fiber depends on the division of ANS (acetylcholine or norepinephrine)
Stimulation of the motor neuron to skeletal muscle leads to muscle contraction, i.e., excitation	Stimulation of postganglionic autonomic fiber can lead to either excitation or inhibition of the effector organ

BASIS OF NEURAL ACTIVITY

Basic unit of integrated neural activity is a **reflex arc**. It is the neural pathway involved in a reflex action where both the peripheral and central nervous systems are involved. Reflex

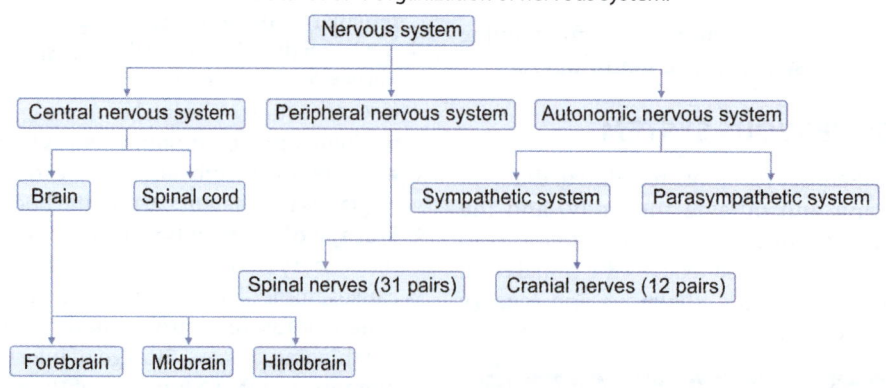

Flowchart 78.1: Organization of nervous system.

Flowchart 78.2: Divisions of autonomic nervous system.

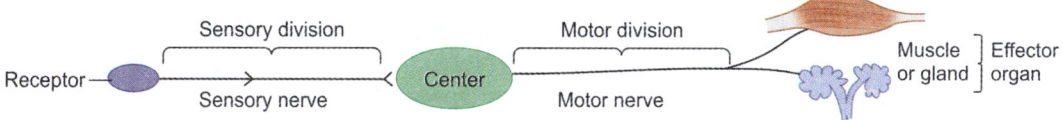

Fig. 78.1: Reflex arc.

arc consists of a sense organ or receptor, afferent neuron, one or more synapses in the central integrating station, efferent neuron and effector organ. Afferent neuron is present in the dorsal root ganglion or ganglion of cranial nerve **(Fig. 78.1)**.

The primary function of nervous system is to receive millions of sensory information from either the external or internal environment by special structures called **sensory receptors**. Receptors are present in the skin, mucous membrane, muscles, tendons, joints, viscera and special sense organs (*refer* **Chapter 81**).

Receptor may be part of a neuron or a specialized cell which can generate action potentials. It can act as **transducer** and convert various forms of energy into action potentials. Action potentials are transmitted through afferent nerve fibers or sensory fibers to the center.

Nervous system has a sensory part and a motor part. Sensory receptor with the sensory nerve is called the **sensory portion of the nervous system (Fig. 78.1)**. **Motor part of the nervous system** controls the various motor functions, such as contraction of skeletal muscles, smooth muscles, secretion of substances by exocrine and endocrine glands in many parts of the body. Motor part includes the motor nerve and the effector organ. The muscles and the glands are called **effectors** since they perform the functions directed by the nerve signals.

■ CENTERS OF NERVOUS SYSTEM

Major levels of central nervous system function include:
- Spinal cord level
- Lower brain level
- Higher brain level.

Spinal Cord Level

The afferent fibers pass through the dorsal root and reach the concerned segment of spinal cord and produce a localized motor response. Spinal reflexes include simple spinal reflexes, such as stretch reflex, withdrawal reflex, micturition reflex, defecation reflex, etc. The upper levels of the nervous system often operate by sending signals to the control centers of the spinal cord and the effect is performed by the spinal cord centers and not directly by the higher centers.

Lower Brain or Subcortical Level

The subconscious activities of the body are controlled by lower areas of the brain. These centers include reticular substance of medulla, pons and midbrain; thalamus, hypothalamus, cerebellum and basal ganglia. Centers in medulla and pons control the subconscious activities of the body like maintenance of normal arterial blood pressure, respiration, etc. Posture and equilibrium are controlled by cerebellum, reticular formation, midbrain and basal ganglia. Feeding reflexes are controlled by areas in the medulla, pons, midbrain, amygdala and hypothalamus. Emotional states, such as anger, excitement, sexual response, reaction to pain or pleasure, etc., can still occur after destruction of much of the cerebral cortex. This proves that they can be integrated at the subcortical level. But precise functioning of the lower center does not occur without the cerebral cortex.

Higher Brain or Cortical Level

Highest center for the control of body functions is the cerebral cortex. It controls voluntary activities. It is essential for thought processes and is the storehouse of memory. Cerebral cortex always functions in association with the lower centers of the nervous system. The lower centers can execute their functions precisely only by the control from cerebral cortex. Cerebral cortex is the source of intelligence, thinking process, emotions and memories. Even though, the cortex is essential for most of our thought processes, it cannot function by itself.

Thus, each portion of the nervous system performs specific functions. The lower regions are concerned primarily with automatic, instantaneous muscle responses to sensory stimuli, and the higher regions are concerned with complex muscle movements controlled by the thought processes of the brain. The autonomic nervous system controls the smooth muscles, glands and other internal body systems.

■ PROCESSING OF SENSORY INFORMATION

The neurons in the different centers process the incoming sensory information so that appropriate responses can occur. *More than 99% of sensory information is discarded by brain as unimportant.* After the selection of important information, it is directed to the motor regions of brain for appropriate motor events. This function of the nervous system is called **integrative function of nervous system**.

Instruction from the center is carried by efferent fibers or motor fibers to the effector organ which may be a muscle or a gland. Efferent fibers and effector organ together form **motor part of nervous system (Fig. 78.1)**.

Information from the receptor enters the spinal cord through the dorsal root and reaches the brain through the spinal cord. The cell body of afferent nerve is located in the **dorsal root ganglion** of spinal cord in the case of spinal nerves and **cranial nerve ganglia** in the case of cranial nerves. The efferent fibers leave through the ventral root of spinal cord or through the motor cranial nerves from brainstem.

The nervous system can be compared to an **electronic computer** which receives millions of information. Sensory portion can be compared to **input circuit** and motor system can be compared to **output circuit** of the computer. The output signals depend both on the input signals and also on the information stored in the **memory** of the computer. This can be compared to complex motor activities executed by higher centers of nervous system, such as cerebral cortex which is the seat of memory. In computers, there is a **central processing unit** which performs sequence of operations. A similar mechanism in our brain allows us to direct our information to one thought process or to a motor response and then to the next one until the complex action is completed.

FUNCTIONAL ANATOMY OF THE BRAIN

Functionally and structurally, brain has the highest position in the body. It lies within the cranial cavity and is continued as the spinal cord at the level of **foramen magnum** which is an opening at the base of the skull. The brain and spinal cord are covered by 3 coverings called pia mater, arachnoid mater and dura mater. Subdural space between dura and arachnoid mater is a potential space containing tissue fluid. Subarachnoid space contains cerebrospinal fluid (CSF) which circulates throughout the space and is continuous in the brain and spinal cord. Brain constitutes 3% of total body weight, i.e., it weighs about 1.5 kg in an adult. Brain is divided into three parts **(Fig. 78.2)**:

- **Forebrain** or prosencephalon, which consists of two parts:
  1. *Telencephalon* or cerebrum
  2. *Diencephalon* which includes thalamus, subthalamus, epithalamus and hypothalamus. Subthalamus includes cranial ends of red nuclei and subthalamic nucleus. Epithalamus includes habenular nuclei and pineal gland.
- **Midbrain** or mesencephalon (divided into ventral and dorsal part by aqueduct of Sylvius)
  - Ventral part called cerebral peduncle comprises the tegmentum and the substantia nigra
  - Dorsal part called tectum constitutes superior and inferior colliculi
- **Hindbrain** or rhombencephalon, which includes:
  - Cerebellum
  - Pons
  - Medulla.

Ventricles of Brain

Cavities in the brain are called **ventricles** of brain. Each cerebral hemisphere contains one **lateral ventricle**. The lateral ventricles of both sides are connected by interventricular foramen. Lateral ventricles open into **third ventricle** in the midline. Third ventricle passes down through the midbrain as **aqueduct of Sylvius** or **cerebral aqueduct** and opens into the **fourth ventricle** in the medulla. The fourth ventricle continues as the **central canal** of spinal cord **(Fig. 78.2)**. The roof of fourth ventricle contains certain openings and through these openings it is connected to the subarachnoid space. Ventricles are filled with cerebrospinal fluid (CSF) which is in constant motion (*refer* **Chapter 97**).

CRANIAL NERVES

There are 12 pairs of cranial nerves (**Table 78.3**).

STRUCTURE OF CENTRAL NERVOUS SYSTEM

Nervous system consists of two main types of cells:
1. Neurons
2. Neuroglial cells.

Neurons

A neuron is an excitable cell that receives processes and transmits information in the form of action potentials. It is the fundamental unit of the nervous system. The area where cell bodies of neurons are accumulated in the central nervous system is called **gray matter**. Gray matter appears grayish because of the presence of Nissl granules in the cell bodies and due to the absence of myelin. Area where axons or nerve fibers are accumulated is called **white matter**. White matter appears whitish because of the presence of myelin sheath. Collections of nerve cell bodies that serve similar functions seen inside the white matter are called nuclear masses or **nuclei**. Collections of nerve cell bodies seen outside the central nervous system are called **ganglia**. Exception is basal ganglia located in the brain; actually the term is a misnomer. *In cerebrum, gray matter is seen outside and white matter inside, whereas in the spinal cord gray matter is seen inside and white matter outside.* Beneath and between cerebral hemispheres, there are two nerve cell masses called thalamus and hypothalamus. Midbrain, pons and medulla contain nuclear masses and nerve tracts.

Neuroglia

Neuroglia (glia means glue) or supporting cells of CNS are smaller than neurons but more in number. They make up ¾ the volume of CNS. They are not excitable and so cannot transmit impulses like neurons. Unlike neurons, they can divide by mitosis throughout life.

The glial cells seen in the peripheral nervous system are **Schwann cells and satellite cells**. Schwann cells are responsible for the myelination of nerve fibers of peripheral nervous system. Satellite cells encapsulate dorsal root ganglion cells and cranial nerve ganglion cells, and regulate their microenvironment in the same way as that of astrocytes. They are also present in the autonomic ganglia. In the CNS, there are four types of neuroglia **(Fig. 78.3)**:
1. Astrocytes
2. Oligodendrocytes

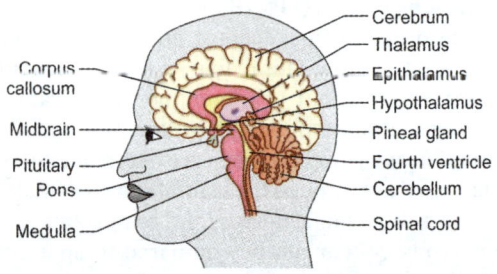

Fig. 78.2: Parts of the brain.

CHAPTER 78 — Organization of Nervous System

Table 78.3: Cranial nerves and their important functions.

Cranial nerve	Fiber type	Function
Olfactory nerve	Sensory	Olfaction
Optic nerve	Sensory	Vision
Oculomotor nerve	Mixed (contain both sensory and motor fibers)	• Sensory part brings proprioceptive information from eye muscles • Motor part innervate extrinsic muscles of eye ball (except superior oblique and lateral rectus); intrinsic muscles, constrictor pupillae and ciliary muscle
Trochlear nerve	Mixed	• Sensory part brings proprioceptive information from superior oblique muscle • Motor part innervates superior oblique muscle of eye
Trigeminal nerve	Mixed	• Sensory fibers bring information from receptors in skin and skeletal muscles of face; mucosa of oral and nasal cavity; and from teeth sockets • Efferent fibers innervate muscles of mastication
Abducens nerve	Mixed	• Afferents bring proprioception from eye muscles • Efferents supply lateral rectus muscle
Facial nerve	Mixed	• Afferents bring taste sensation from anterior 2/3rd of tongue and touch sensation from external auditory meatus • Efferents supply muscles of facial expression; lacrimal and salivary glands (sublingual and submaxillary glands)
Vestibulo-cochlear nerve	Sensory	Hearing; maintenance of balance and equilibrium
Glossopharyngeal nerve	Mixed	• Afferents bring taste sensation from posterior 1/3rd of tongue • Motor supply to muscles of swallowing; parotid gland
Vagus nerve	Mixed	• Bring sensory information from thoracic and abdominal viscera • Innervate muscles of heart, pharynx, larynx, and GIT; glands of thorax and abdomen
Spinal accessory nerve	Primarily motor	• Innervate sternocleidomastoid and trapezius muscles • Sensory fibers carry proprioceptive information from these muscles
Hypoglossal nerve	• Primarily motor • Contain some proprioceptive fibers from the tongue	Innervate muscles of tongue

3. Microglia
4. Ependymal cells.

Astrocytes

Astrocytes are star-shaped or stellate cells which are ectodermal in origin. They are of two types:
1. Fibrous astrocytes
2. Protoplasmic astrocytes.

Fibrous astrocyte contains numerous filaments in the cytoplasm and their processes are long, slender, smooth and less branched. They are seen between nerve fibers, i.e., in the white matter (**Fig. 78.3**).

Protoplasmic astrocytes contain few filaments in cytoplasm. Their processes are shorter, thicker and more branched. These are seen in between the nerve cell bodies, i.e., in the gray matter. The processes are called **end feet**. End feet come in contact with pia mater outside and ependymal cells inside the brain. They are also seen around blood vessels (perivascular).

Functions of Astrocytes

❖ Protoplasmic astrocytes support neurons in gray matter and fibrous astrocytes support nerve fibers of white matter of CNS. The glial filaments of astrocytes are responsible for this mechanical support to CNS. It also produces extracellular matrix molecules, such as laminin.
❖ Act as an insulator in the CNS. Processes of astrocytes surround groups of synaptic endings and isolate them from adjacent synapses. This prevents impulses from spreading in unwanted directions.
❖ Help in repair by scar formation. The glial filaments are responsible for the formation of glial scar after injury to nervous system. Astrocytes respond to injury by multiplying rapidly and closing the gaps of injured area.
❖ The end feet of protoplasmic astrocytes encircle the blood vessels of brain contributing to blood-brain barrier (BBB).
❖ Astrocytes take part in metabolic activities of neurons. They form a route for the transfer of nutrients from blood to brain

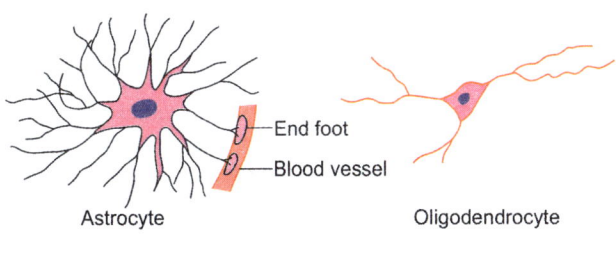
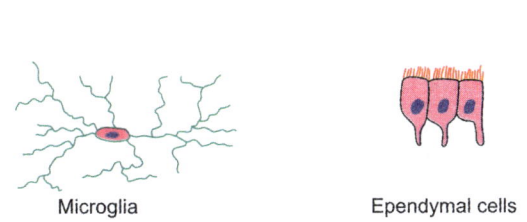

Fig. 78.3: Neuroglial cells.

tissue. They produce certain trophic substances (trophic means nourishing or providing nutrition) necessary for the nourishment of neurons like growth factors such as nerve growth factor, fibroblast growth factors and brain derived neurotrophic factor.

- Maintain the composition of the interstitial fluid of brain by actively taking up excess K^+ and neurotransmitter substances which they can metabolize. Astrocytes play an important role in terminating neuronal responses to glutamate, the most abundant excitatory transmitter in the brain. If glutamate is present in excess it leads to neuronal death. Glutamate transporters on the astrocyte cell membrane take up glutamate and the glutamine synthase present convert glutamate to glutamine.
- Astrocytes have a role in neurovascular communication. The processes of protoplasmic astrocytes make contact with neurons and the surrounding blood vessels, providing a sort of neurovascular communication. The processes of astrocytes cover most synapses and large foot processes are closely opposed to the vascular wall. When the excitatory glutaminergic neurons are highly active, it leads to increase in the intracellular calcium ion concentration in the astrocyte foot processes and cause vasodilatation of nearby arterioles. Local vasodilatation in response to stimulation of adjacent excitatory neurons is mediated by vasoactive metabolites released from the astrocytes, such as nitric oxide, potassium ions, adenosine, etc.
- Astrocytes store almost all the glycogen present in the brain. It contains the enzymes necessary for metabolizing glycogen. Normally, brain's metabolic needs are met by the glucose transferred from blood. Very little glycogen is stored in the brain. In the absence of glucose from blood, astrocytic glycogen can sustain the brain activity for only less than 10 minutes. Astrocytes break down glycogen to glucose and then to lactate by glycolysis. This lactic acid is transferred to nearby neurons, where it can be aerobically metabolized. In times of excess neuronal activity when the demand for glucose exceeds the supply from blood, astrocytes can provide lactate derived directly from glucose, independent of glycogen. Even though glucose can enter the brain cells, the usual route is to deliver it through the astrocytic end feet that too after conversion into lactic acid by astrocytic glycolysis.

Oligodendrocytes

Oligodendrocytes are small cells of *ectodermal* origin containing dense cytoplasm and large nucleus with few short processes. They are seen in the white matter and contain rough endoplasmic reticulum. Their main function is **myelination** in the CNS. A single oligodendrocyte myelinate part of many axons and therefore a neurilemmal sheath is not seen around CNS axons. This is because the oligodendrocyte cell body and nucleus do not envelop the axon to form the neurilemma. As a result, axons in the CNS do not regenerate after injury.

Oligodendrocytes are involved in iron metabolism in the brain. They contain iron storage protein ferritin and iron transport protein transferrin. Iron acts as a cofactor for certain enzymes in the brain.

Microglia

Microglial cells are *mesodermal* in origin. They are the *smallest of the glial cells* and have dense cytoplasm and large nucleus. They have got wavy branches which give off short spine-like processes. These cells are probably derived from circulating monocytes which migrate into the CNS during late fetal life. They resemble tissue macrophages and their main function is **phagocytosis** and hence known as **scavenger cells** of the nervous system. They are part of the immune system and belong to reticuloendothelial system. They are activated by brain injury, infection, and neuronal degeneration, such as multiple sclerosis, dementia, Parkinson disease, and Alzheimer disease. They remove debris resulting from these conditions. Phagocytic action of microglia is assisted by other phagocytes that invade the damaged area from the circulation.

Ependymal Cells

Ependymal cells are elongated cells with processes that go deep into the brain substance. They appear like columnar cells and have numerous cilia. They are *ectodermal* in origin and line the epithelium that separates brain tissue from cerebrospinal fluid (CSF) in the ventricles. It also lines the central canal of spinal cord. The cilia help in the circulation of CSF. They are seen in the choroid plexus and help in the secretion of CSF. They also have absorptive function (**Fig. 78.3**).

Applied Physiology

Unlike neurons, glial cells have the ability to divide and multiply throughout life and so, most of the brain tumors arise from neuroglial cells (**glioma**). When there is brain injury, neuroglia multiply to fill the space and excessive multiplication leads to glioma. Examples are *astrocytoma, oligodendroglioma, ependymoma,* etc. *Acoustic neuroma* is a tumor formed from the Schwann cells of the VIII cranial nerve. **Exceptions** of brain tumors not arising from glial cells are *meningioma,* which arise from meninges, and *retinoblastoma,* which arises from nervous tissue of the eye in infants.

Microglia on activation expresses surface receptors, such as CD45, MHC class I and II and immunoglobulin Fc receptors; secretes several cytokines, reactive oxygen intermediates, and proteinases. Even though this response helps to remove dead tissue and destroy invading organisms, it may contribute to central nervous system (CNS) damage, particularly in certain CNS inflammatory and degenerative diseases.

STRUCTURE OF SPINAL CORD

Spinal cord is roughly a cylindrical structure which begins superiorly at the **foramen magnum** in the skull and is the continuation of the medulla oblongata into the vertebral canal. Spinal cord terminates in the lumbar region and the lower part of spinal cord is conical in shape and hence known as **conus medullaris**. Pia mater closely envelops the spinal cord and it extends up to the upper border of second lumbar vertebra. Conus medullaris is attached to the back of coccyx by a prolongation of pia mater called **filum terminale** meaning terminal filament.

Spinal cord consists of 31 segments and 31 pairs of spinal nerves are attached to these segments. Area of the skin supplied by a single spinal segment is called a **dermatome**. A group of anatomically and functionally related skeletal muscles supplied by a single spinal segment is called a **myotome**.

Each spinal nerve is connected with the spinal cord by two roots, a ventral root which is motor in function and a dorsal root which is sensory in function. The two roots unite in the intervertebral foramen to form a **mixed spinal nerve**.

The spinal nerves are named according to the names of the segments from which they arise. They are:
- Cervical—8
- Thoracic—12
- Lumbar—5
- Sacral—5
- Coccygeal—1.

Since the spinal cord is shorter than the vertebral column, the spinal cord segments do not correspond numerically with the vertebrae that lie at the same level. Each spinal segment is higher than the corresponding vertebra and this should be kept in mind when dealing with spinal cord injuries.

Because of the disproportionate growth in length of the vertebral column and the spinal cord during development, the length of the spinal nerve roots increases progressively from above downward. In the cervical region, the spinal nerve roots take a horizontal course, in the thoracic region horizontal or oblique course, and in the lumbar and sacral region the spinal nerve roots run vertically downward. The bundle of spinal nerve roots of the lumbar and sacral segments running vertically downward surrounding the filum terminale is called **cauda equina**, meaning "horse tail."

There are two fusiform enlargements in the upper and lower parts of spinal cord, the **cervical enlargement** from C_4 to T_2 segments, and **lumbosacral enlargement** from L_2 to S_3 segments. These enlargements are due to presence of large number of motor neurons to supply the muscles of upper and lower limbs respectively. Here, the anterior horn is larger than the rest of the spinal segments. From these enlargements, nerve plexuses to the limbs arise.

In adults, the spinal cord terminates at the lower border of **first lumbar vertebra**. In young children, the spinal cord is longer and extends up to the upper border of **third lumbar vertebra**. This fact should be remembered while performing lumbar puncture in children.

Like brain, spinal cord is also covered by dura mater, arachnoid mater and pia mater. Pia mater extends only up to the level of spinal cord.

Arachnoid and dura mater extend up to the lower border of second sacral vertebra (**Fig. 78.4**). CSF can be collected without injuring the spinal cord if a needle is introduced into

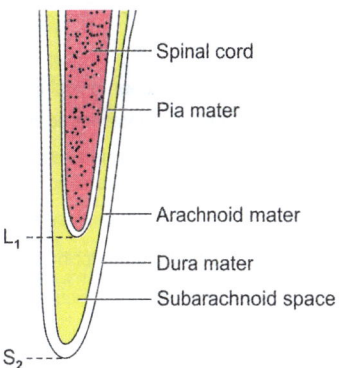

Fig. 78.4: Lower extent of spinal cord and meninges.

the subarachnoid space below the level of second lumbar vertebra in adults. The procedure is called **lumbar puncture**.

The spinal cord is incompletely divided into two lateral halves by a **posterior or dorsal median septum and anterior or ventral median fissure**. On the lateral surface is a *dorsolateral sulcus* through which the dorsal root or posterior root (sensory) enters the spinal cord. Dorsal root ganglion contains pseudounipolar neurons with central and peripheral processes. The peripheral process ends in the sensory receptor and the central process enters the spinal cord. The neurons in the dorsal root ganglion are called *first order neurons* in the sensory pathway. There is also an anterior or ventral root which carries motor impulses from spinal cord to the effector organ. The ventral root in the thoracolumbar segments also contains axons of the preganglionic sympathetic neurons. The ventral root is attached to the *ventrolateral sulcus* of spinal cord. Spinal cord contains a central core of gray matter surrounded by white matter (**Fig. 78.5**).

Bell-Magendie Law

The general principle in the spinal cord that the dorsal (posterior) nerve root contains only sensory fibers and the ventral (anterior) nerve root contain only motor fibers and the impulses travel only in one direction in each root is called **Bell**-**Magendie law**. This principle is named after Charles Bell (surgeon) and Francois Magendie (physiologist).

Cross-section of Spinal Cord

On cross-section, gray matter of spinal cord is seen in the shape of an H. It has got a broad **anterior horn** and a narrow **posterior horn**. Anterior and posterior horns on either side are connected by a thin **gray commissure**. The **central canal** is situated in the center of the gray commissure. The part of gray matter in front of central canal is the **anterior gray commissure** and the part situated posterior to central canal is called **posterior gray commissure**. The central canal is lined by ependymal cells and it contains CSF. **Terminal ventricle** is the fusiform expanded part of central canal of spinal cord in the region of conus medullaris. In the thoracic and upper lumbar segments, in addition to anterior and posterior horn, there is a lateral projection of gray matter called **lateral horn**

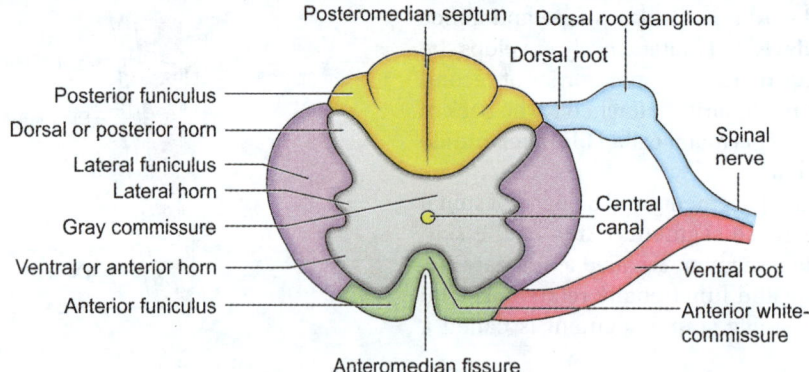

Fig. 78.5: Cross-section of spinal cord at the thoracic level.

or **intermediolateral horn (Fig. 78.5)**. *The amount of gray matter present in any level of the spinal cord is related to the amount of muscles innervated at that level.* For example, the anterior horn is larger in the cervical and lumbosacral enlargements of spinal cord because of the large number of motor neurons present in these segments innervating the large number of muscles of the upper and lower limbs.

The white matter consists of various ascending and descending tracts. Each tract is made up of bundles of axons extending up or down the spinal cord. **Sensory tracts** or ascending tracts consists of axons that conduct impulses towards brain. **Motor** or **descending tracts** consist of axons that carry nerve impulses from brain to spinal cord. White matter is divided into three broad areas on each side called **columns or funiculi**. They are:

1. Anterior funiculus or ventral white column
2. Posterior funiculus or dorsal white column
3. Lateral funiculus or lateral white column

There is an **anterior white commissure** and a **posterior white commissure** in the middle of the spinal cord through which the nerve fibers cross from one side to the opposite side **(Fig. 78.5)**.

Cell Groups in the Gray Matter of Spinal Cord (Fig. 78.6)

Cells of spinal cord are seen in groups in the posterior horn, lateral horn and anterior horn. Actually, the spinal nuclei are columns of cells extending vertically through several spinal segments as seen in a longitudinal section.

Cell Groups in the Posterior Horn

There are four cell groups in the posterior horn, of which, two extend throughout the length of the spinal cord and two are restricted to thoracic and lumbar segments. Substantia gelatinosa and nucleus proprius extend throughout the length of spinal cord.

1. **Substantia gelatinosa of Rolando** is a group of small Golgi type II neurons with many dendrites. It is present at the apex of the posterior horn and receives afferent fibers of pain and temperature sensations. They have a role in the gate control of pain sensation.
2. **Clarke's column or nucleus dorsalis** is composed of large neurons at the base of the posterior horn. It extends from C_8 to L_4 segments of spinal cord and receives afferents from muscle spindle and Golgi tendon organ. Axons of these cells ascend as the uncrossed posterior spinocerebellar tract.
3. **Chief sensory nucleus or nucleus proprius** is composed of large cells and is present in between the above two groups. It receives afferent fibers associated with proprioception, two-point discrimination and vibration sense.
4. **Visceral afferent nucleus** is situated lateral to Clarke's column and extends from T_1 to L_3 segments of spinal cord. It is concerned with receiving visceral afferent fibers.

Cells in the Anterior Horn

- Gamma motor neurons are small multipolar neurons supplying the muscle spindle.
- Alpha motor neurons are large multipolar neurons that supply skeletal muscles.

Lateral Horn Cells

Lateral horn present from T_1 to L_3 segments of spinal cord contains certain neurons (intermediolateral group of cells) which give rise to **preganglionic sympathetic efferent fibers (Fig. 78.6)**. The fibers are carried along with the ventral root. These fibers constitute visceral motor nerves. Similar group of neurons are present in S_2 to S_4 segments of spinal cord which give rise to **preganglionic parasympathetic fibers**. These fibers leave the spinal nerve as the pelvic splanchnic nerves.

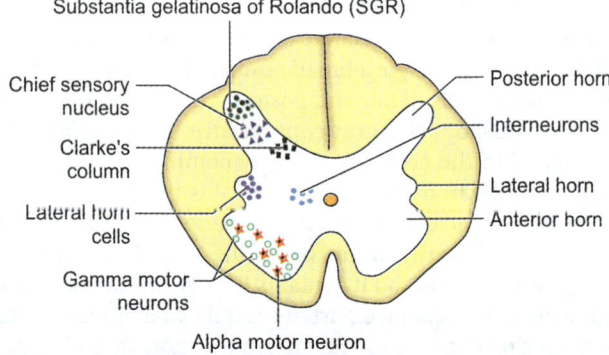

Fig. 78.6: Nuclei in the gray matter of spinal cord at the thoracic level.

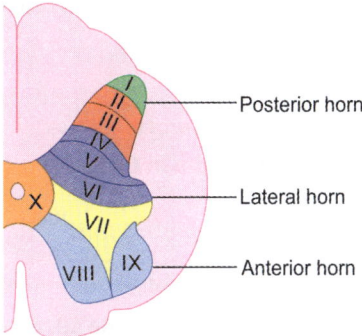

Fig. 78.7: Laminae in the gray matter of spinal cord at the thoracic level.

In addition to the above groups of neurons, certain **interneurons** which receive sensory information from the periphery and motor signals from the higher centers are also present in the spinal cord gray matter. Some of these interneurons may be excitatory in function, while some others are inhibitory in function. They also have interneuronal connections.

Rexed's Laminae of Spinal Gray Matter

In 1952, Rexed classified the gray matter into laminations called Rexed laminae I to X. The laminae in the dorsal horn are called **sensory laminae**. The nerve fibers with different diameters terminate in the different sensory laminas. There are 7 laminas in the dorsal horn (I to VI), with I being the most superficial and VI the deepest. Lamina I receive small nociceptive Aδ and C fibers. Lamina II and part of lamina III constitutes substantia gelatinosa of Rolando **(Fig. 78.7)**. Lamina III to VI receives myelinated Aα and Aβ fibers which mediates proprioception, vibration and fine touch. Lamina VII in the lateral horn is composed of preganglionic autonomic neurons.

The laminae in the ventral horn are called **motor laminae**. Lamina IX is composed of alpha and gamma motor neurons and several interneurons. Lamina VIII contains mainly interneurons even though some motor neurons are also present. Lamina X forms the gray matter around the central canal and is called inter-commissural lamina. It consists mainly of neuroglial cells. The descending tracts primarily terminate directly or indirectly on the motor neurons in the anterior horn. But a significant number of descending fibers also terminate in the sensory laminae. This helps to bring about **sensory-motor coordination** so that the sensory information reaching the CNS can be modified according to the motor needs of the body. For example, the corticospinal tract has terminations in laminae III to VI of the dorsal roots.

■ MULTIPLE CHOICE QUESTIONS

1. **The following are parts of diencephalon, *except*:**
   a. Thalamus
   b. Hypothalamus
   c. Epithalamus
   d. Basal ganglia

2. **Largest cranial nerve is:**
   a. Trigeminal nerve
   b. Facial nerve
   c. Vestibulo-cochlear nerve
   d. Glossopharyngeal nerve

3. **Longest cranial nerve is:**
   a. Trigeminal nerve
   b. Facial nerve
   c. Vagus
   d. Glossopharyngeal nerve

4. **Regarding brain all the following statements are true, *except*:**
   a. Sensitive to hypoxia
   b. Dependent on glucose
   c. Use fatty acids in starvation
   d. Does not store energy

5. **White color of the white matter of nervous system is due to the presence of:**
   a. Myelin sheath
   b. Nerve cell bodies
   c. Astrocytes
   d. Pia mater

6. **Hind brain include all the following, *except*:**
   a. Midbrain
   b. Pons
   c. Medulla oblongata
   d. Cerebellum

7. **Brain stem consists of all the following, *except*:**
   a. Midbrain
   b. Pons
   c. Medulla oblongata
   d. Cerebellum

8. **The number of coccygeal spinal nerve is:**
   a. 4 pairs
   b. 1 pair
   c. 3 pairs
   d. 5 pairs

9. **Total number of cervical spinal nerve is:**
   a. 7
   b. 18
   c. 16
   d. 8

10. **Sensory ganglia are present along the course of the following cranial nerves, *except*:**
    a. II
    b. VII
    c. VIII
    d. V

11. **The dendrites and axons are referred to as:**
    a. Nerve fibers
    b. Neuron
    c. Gray matter
    d. Nerve

12. **The non-excitable cells in the central nervous system is called:**
    a. Neuroglia
    b. Interneuron
    c. Ganglia
    d. White matter

13. **The glial cell that contribute to blood brain barrier is:**
    a. Oligodendrocyte
    b. Microglia
    c. Ependyma
    d. Astrocyte

14. **The glial cell in the brain that secrete cytokines which regulate the activity of immune cells entering brain is:**
    a. Astrocyte
    b. Microglia
    c. Oligodendrocyte
    d. Ependyma

15. **Tanycyte is a type of:**
    a. Antigen presenting cell
    b. Ependyma
    c. Motor neuron
    d. Interneuron
16. **In the CNS, the dead neurons and parts of injured neurons are removed by:**
    a. Microglia
    b. Schwann cell
    c. Oligodendrocyte
    d. Ependyma
17. **The neuroglia that possesses microvilli and cilia is:**
    a. Schwann cell
    b. Ependyma
    c. Astrocyte
    d. Microglia
18. **All of the following are of neural crest origin, *except*:**
    a. Oligodendrocytes
    b. Astrocyte
    c. Microglia
    d. Schwann cells
19. **Most common CNS disease is:**
    a. Glioma
    b. Multiple sclerosis
    c. Paraplegia
    d. Tabes dorsalis
20. **The neuroglia that can absorb GABA, glutamic acid and excess K⁺ ions from extracellular fluid is:**
    a. Ependyma
    b. Oligodendrocyte
    c. Astrocyte
    d. Microglia
21. **The cell that is responsible for myelination in the CNS is:**
    a. Astrocyte
    b. Oligodendrocyte
    c. Microglia
    d. Schwann cell
22. **The neuroglial cell that is derived from macrophages outside nervous system is:**
    a. Astrocyte
    b. Ependyma
    c. Microglia
    d. Oligodendrocyte
23. **Myelin in spinal cord is synthesized by:**
    a. Schwann cells
    b. Oligodendrocytes
    c. Microglia
    d. Protoplasmic astrocyte
24. **Function of microglia in CNS is:**
    a. Phagocytosis
    b. Myelination
    c. Fibrosis
    d. Conduction of impulse
25. **Features of neuroglia include all, *except*:**
    a. Protoplasmic astrocytes are found in gray matter
    b. Oligodendrocytes are derived from ectoderm
    c. Microglia is mesodermal in origin
    d. Central neuroglial cells are derived from Schwann cells
26. **The cranial nerve which contains both afferent and efferent fibers is:**
    a. Olfactory
    b. Glossopharyngeal
    c. Optic
    d. Vestibulo-cochlear
27. **Satellite cells or capsular cells are present in the:**
    a. Sensory ganglia
    b. Thalamus
    c. Basal ganglia
    d. Cerebellum

ANSWERS

1. d	2. a	3. c	4. c	5. a
6. a	7. d	8. a	9. c	10. a
11. a	12. a	13. d	14. a	15. b
16. a	17. b	18. c	19. b	20. c
21. b	22. c	23. a	24. a	25. d
26. b	27. a			

Physiology of Nervous System

CHAPTER 79

LEARNING OBJECTIVES

Must know
- Describe the functions and properties of synapse
- Classify synapses
- Explain synaptic inhibition
- Differentiate between EPSP and IPSP
- Explain the transmission of impulse across a chemical synapse

Desirable to know
- Describe the physiological role of neurotransmitters and neuromodulators

INTRODUCTION

The main function of nervous system is to receive millions of information each minute coming through the sensory nerves and to integrate all these information (discarding unwanted signals) in order to determine the appropriate responses to be made by the body. Information is carried through the nervous system in the form of action potentials. The action potentials or impulses are carried by a series of neurons in the conducting pathway. Even though there is no anatomical continuity between the neurons, there is functional union between the neurons. Synapse is a structure specialized for the transfer of information from the axon terminal to muscle, to glands or to another neuron. For example, neuromuscular junction is a synapse. But action potential is generated in the postsynaptic cell only if it is an excitable cell.

SYNAPSE

PY10.2: Describe and discuss the functions and properties of synapse, reflex, receptors.

In the nervous system, synapse is the junction between two neurons. Impulses are transmitted from one neuron to another neuron at the synapse. The term 'synapse' was coined by **Sherrington**, and is derived from the Greek word meaning to clasp. Synapse is considered to be the most important single determinant of central nervous system (CNS) function. Functions of synapse are:
- Transmission or conduction of impulses
- Certain synapses can block or inhibit impulse transmission
- Synapse can change an impulse to repetitive impulses
- Modification of impulses
- Integration of impulses.
- Learning and memory (storage of information) is also a function of synapse.

The neuron which makes contact with another neuron is called **presynaptic neuron**. The neuron with which contact is made is called **postsynaptic neuron**. Presynaptic neuron conducts impulses towards the postsynaptic membrane and postsynaptic neuron conducts impulses away from a neuron. *Even though the number of neurons is constant, the number of synapses in the nervous system can increase or decrease with use and experience.*

Types of Synapse

Structural Classification of Synapse

Usually, axon of presynaptic neuron makes contact with either dendrite or soma or axon of the postsynaptic neuron. There are 4 types of synapses **structurally (Fig. 79.1)**:

1. **Axo-dendritic** synapse is the most common type (80–90%). For example, the climbing fibers form axo-dendritic connection with the dendrite of Purkinje cell in cerebellum.
2. **Axo-somatic** synapse is less common and is seen in the motor neuron of spinal cord, basket cells in the cerebellum and in autonomic ganglia. Synaptic connection between basket cell and Purkinje cell in the cerebellum is axo-somatic. Axons of basket cell make synapse with the soma of Purkinje cell.
3. **Axo-axonal** is the least common type and is seen in spinal cord in areas of presynaptic inhibition and presynaptic facilitation.
4. **Dendrodendritic** synapse is present in the olfactory bulb between mitral cells and granule cells.

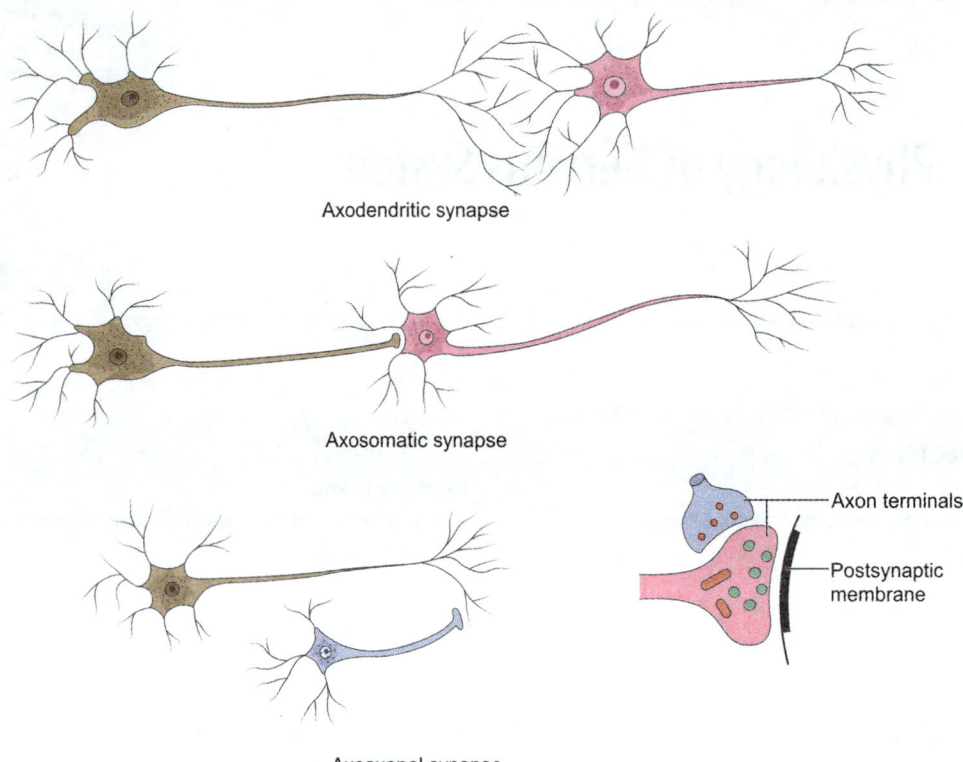

Fig. 79.1: Structural classification of synapse.

Functional Classification of Synapse

According to the type of **transmission** across the synapse, synapses are classified into the following:

- **Chemical synapse**, where the presynaptic neuron liberates certain chemical transmitters which alter the permeability of the postsynaptic membrane. Conduction of impulse is *unidirectional*, i.e., from presynaptic to postsynaptic membrane. This is the most common type of synapse functionally **(Fig. 79.2)**.

- **Electrical synapse** is one in which the presynaptic and the postsynaptic neurons come close together so that the cytoplasm of the adjacent cells are directly connected by clusters of ion channels called gap junctions **(Fig. 79.2)**. They form low-resistance bridges through which ions can easily pass from the interior of one cell to the interior of the next cell. This type is seen in the lateral vestibular nuclei, hippocampus and cerebral cortex. There is no synaptic delay in electrical synapse and conduction is *bidirectional*.

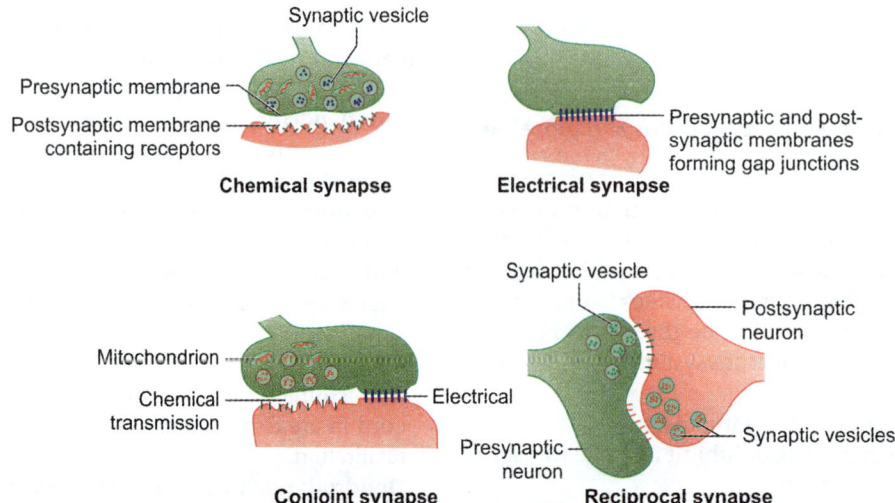

Fig. 79.2: Types of synapse depending on the nature of transmission. In conjoint synapse, there is electrical and chemical transmission. In reciprocal synapse, secretory vesicles as well as receptors for neurotransmitters are present in the presynaptic and postsynaptic membranes.

Table 79.1: Differences between chemical synapse and electrical synapse.	
Chemical synapse	**Electrical synapse**
Impulse transmission is by the release of neurotransmitter from the presynaptic ending	Ions pass directly from presynaptic to postsynaptic cell through gap junctions, no neurotransmitters involved
Impulse pass only in one direction, i.e., from presynaptic to postsynaptic neuron	Impulse transmission is bidirectional
Definite synaptic cleft 20-40 nm wide is present	No synaptic cleft, the presynaptic and the postsynaptic membranes are connected by gap junctions
Synaptic delay present	No synaptic delay since the gap junctions act as low resistance bridges
Seen in almost all areas of the nervous system	Seen only in certain areas of CNS, such as hippocampus, lateral vestibular nucleus and cerebral cortex
Sensitive to hypoxia	Insensitive to hypoxia

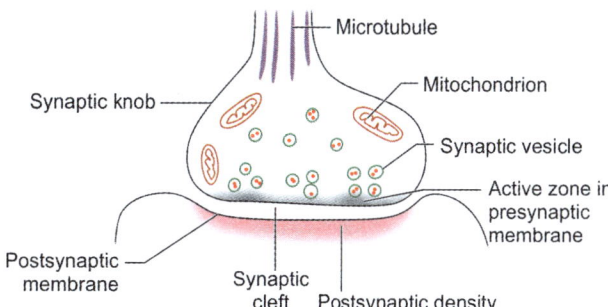

Fig. 79.3: Structure of chemical synapse.

This bidirectional transmission permits them to help in coordinating the activities of large groups of interconnected neurons. This enables increased neuronal sensitivity and promotes synchronous firing of a group of interconnected neurons. Differences between chemical synapse and electrical synapse are given in **Table 79.1**.

❖ **Conjoint synapse** where there are both types of transmission, i.e., chemical and electrical transmission in the same synapse **(Fig. 79.2)**.

❖ **Reciprocal synapse**: In reciprocal synapse, both the pre- and the postsynaptic membranes contain receptors for the neurotransmitter and vesicles that release neurotransmitters **(Fig. 79.2)**. So, this synapse does not obey the property of one-way conduction of impulses at the synapse. It is usually seen in association with anaxonic neurons which make *dendrodendritic synapse*. For example, in the olfactory bulb, **mitral cell** stimulates **granule cells**, while granule cells inhibit mitral cells through the dendrodendritic reciprocal synapse **(Chapter 101, Fig. 101.2)**. Gamma-amino butyric acid (GABA) is the inhibitory neurotransmitter in the granule cell.

Functional Anatomy of Chemical Synapse

The axon of the presynaptic neuron divides into a number of branches. On an average, each axon divides to form over 2000 synaptic endings. The end of each branch is enlarged to form **terminal bouton or end foot or synaptic knob**. There are two important structures in the synaptic knob, vesicles or granules and numerous mitochondria **(Fig. 79.3)**. Mitochondria are necessary for the synthesis of neurotransmitters. A few lysosomes are also seen. But there are no neurofibrils. Instead of synaptic knob, **basket-like axon terminal** is seen in cerebellum and autonomic ganglia.

Vesicles

Vesicles contain small packets of chemical transmitters. The vesicles and the neurotransmitters are synthesized in the neuronal cell body and transported along the axon to the nerve endings by fast axoplasmic transport. Small clear vesicles and small dense core vesicles can also recycle in the nerve ending. The synaptic vesicle discharges its content through a small hole in the presynaptic membrane, then the membrane reseals rapidly and the main vesicle stays inside the cell (**kiss-and-run discharge**). The large dense core vesicles release their neuropeptide contents by exocytosis from all parts of the nerve terminal. As the small synaptic vesicles are located near the synaptic cleft, they discharge their contents only at the active zones on the presynaptic membrane. Morphology of the vesicles varies according to the type of transmitter:

❖ Round or spherical, small clear vesicles contain excitatory transmitter, e.g., acetylcholine and glutamate.
❖ Flat clear vesicles contain inhibitory transmitters, such as GABA, glycine, etc.
❖ Small dense core vesicles contain catecholamines, e.g., epinephrine, norepinephrine and dopamine.
❖ Large dense core vesicles contain peptide transmitters like endorphin, enkephalin, substance P, etc.

Membrane thickening in the presynaptic membrane of the axon is called **active zone**, which contains many proteins and rows of Ca^{2+} channels. The presynaptic membrane and postsynaptic membrane are separated by a gap called **synaptic cleft**, which is about 20–40 nm wide. This cleft contains extracellular fluid (ECF) and some polysaccharides. The postsynaptic membrane is thickened and is known as **synaptic web or postsynaptic density (Fig. 79.3)**. It contains a complex of specific receptors, binding proteins and enzymes induced by the postsynaptic effects. **Receptor proteins** consist of two parts:

1. A **binding component** which projects outwards from the membrane into the synaptic cleft. It binds with the transmitter coming from the presynaptic terminal.
2. An **intracellular component** which passes through the membrane and project into the cytoplasmic part of postsynaptic membrane. There are two types of intracellular components:
   a. One type contains ligand-gated ion channels which allow passage of specific type of ions through the membrane. The receptors that directly gate ion channels are called **ionotropic receptors**.
   b. The second type can activate one or more substances inside the postsynaptic neuron. They can mediate a

number of activities in the postsynaptic neuron via second messengers. The receptors that act through second messenger systems are called **metabotropic receptors**.

Ion channels in the ionophore component are of four types:
1. Na$^+$ channel
2. K$^+$ channel
3. Cl$^-$ channel
4. Ca^{2+} channel

Upon activation, some postsynaptic receptors cause excitation of the postsynaptic neuron and others cause inhibition. Excitatory transmitters open Na$^+$ channels. Inhibitory transmitters open either K$^+$ or Cl$^-$ channels. They can also close Na$^+$ or Ca^{2+} channels. The summation of all the excitatory and inhibitory effects determines whether an action potential is generated or not in the postsynaptic neuron. This permits the grading and adjustment of neural activity necessary for normal function. Thus, the neurotransmitter can alter the reactivity of the synapse and this property is known as **synaptic modulation**.

Action potentials are not produced at the postsynaptic membrane. The change in the postsynaptic membrane potential (depolarization or hyperpolarization) is conducted electrotonically through the membrane of the postsynaptic neuron and eventually reaches the axon hillock. The action potential is generated in the initial segment if the potential reaches the firing level (**Chapter 6, Fig. 6.2**). This part of the cell has a lower threshold than the rest of the plasma membrane of the postsynaptic neuron. *This is because initial segment contains the maximum number of Na$^+$ channels per unit area.*

Neurexins

Neurexins are proteins that hold the presynaptic and the postsynaptic membranes together at the synapse thus providing structural stability to the synapse. Close proximity of presynaptic and postsynaptic membranes is very essential for the transmitter to be effective. Neurexins are present in the presynaptic membrane and they bind to the specific neurexin receptor present in the postsynaptic membrane. In humans, neurexins are encoded by three genes and both α and β isoforms are produced. More than 1000 different neurexins are present. Thus, neurexins are also responsible for the production of **synaptic specificity** in addition to holding synapses together.

MECHANISM OF TRANSMISSION AT THE EXCITATORY CHEMICAL SYNAPSE

Transmission at the synapse is very similar to that in the neuromuscular junction. When an action potential reaches the synaptic knob the voltage-gated calcium channels in the presynaptic membrane opens. Ca^{2+} from extracellular fluid (ECF) enters the synaptic knob. Ca^{2+} binds with certain special protein molecules on the cytoplasmic surface of presynaptic membrane called **active zone** or **release sites** of presynaptic membrane. Small vesicles discharge their contents by exocytosis only at the release sites but, large dense core vesicles release their neuropeptide contents by exocytosis from all parts of the presynaptic terminal. The quantity of neurotransmitter that is released from the nerve terminal into the synaptic cleft is directly related to the number of calcium ions that enter the synaptic terminal.

Normally, the synaptic vesicles do not release their contents into the synaptic cleft unnecessarily. The vesicles remain anchored to the cytoskeleton of the nerve terminal by a group of proteins called **synapsins**. When an action potential reaches the presynaptic membrane, Ca^{2+} enters the presynaptic terminal and the synapsins become phosphorylated by activated kinases. Activation of kinases is triggered by a rise in intracellular Ca^{2+}. The vesicles are freed from the cytoskeleton and move towards the active zone. **Rab protein (rab3)**, a small guanosine tri phosphatase (GTPase) guides the vesicles to the releasing site. These vesicles concentrated at the active zone undergo docking and priming. **Docking** is the process by which vesicles attach with the membrane and **priming** is the process by which vesicles become ready to discharge their content in response to a stimulus. Both docking and priming requires the interaction between syntaxin and synaptobrevin.

The binding of the synaptic vesicle to the presynaptic membrane requires integral membrane proteins called **SNARE proteins**. The snare protein present in the vesicular membrane is **synaptobrevin (v-snare protein)** and that present in the presynaptic membrane is called **syntaxin (t-snare protein)**. *During exocytosis, synaptobrevin in the vesicle membrane locks with syntaxin in the postsynaptic membrane* (**Fig. 79.4**). Vesicles come in contact with the presynaptic membrane and the site of contact breaks and the neurotransmitter is released into the synaptic cleft. The transmitter is released in a quantized manner and this quantal release of neurotransmitter is referred to as **Dale's phenomenon**. It takes about 200 microseconds from calcium influx to the release of neurotransmitter. Most of the neurotoxins inhibit release of neurotransmitters by preventing the attachment of synaptobrevin and syntaxin.

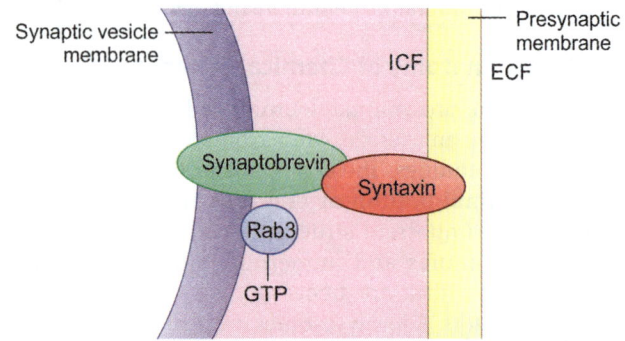

Fig. 79.4: Main snare proteins synaptobrevin (v-snare protein) in the vesicle membrane locking with the t-snare protein syntaxin in the presynaptic membrane regulated by small GTPases like Rab3. This process leads to the fusion of vesicles with the nerve ending and exocytosis.

Flowchart 79.1: Summary of transmission at a chemical synapse.

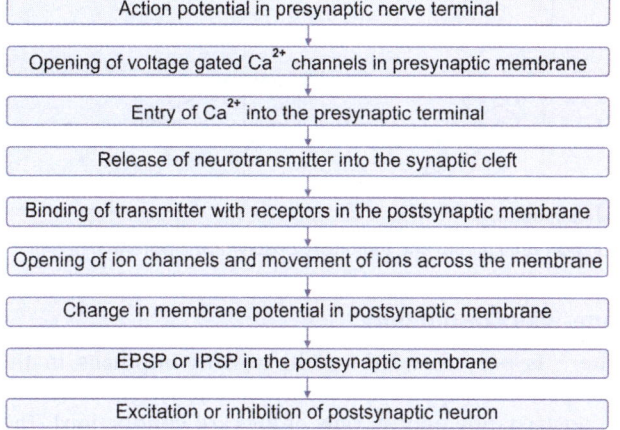

Action of the Neurotransmitter on the Postsynaptic Neuron

The postsynaptic membrane contains large number of receptor proteins. If the transmitter is an *excitatory neurotransmitter and if the receptor is an ionotropic receptor,* the transmitter binds to the binding component of the receptor specific to that transmitter and chemically gated Na⁺ channels open. Na⁺ enters the postsynaptic membrane from the synaptic cleft. This causes depolarization of the postsynaptic membrane, and when the summated potentials in the postsynaptic neuron reach the threshold value, an action potential is produced in the initial segment, which is propagated through the nerve fiber. The action potential produced in the initial segment spreads anterogradely along the axon and also retrogradely to the soma and dendrites. This retrograde conduction of action potential brings the soma and dendrites to the resting potential so that fresh summation of subsequently generated excitatory postsynaptic potentials (EPSPs) and inhibitory postsynaptic potentials (IPSPs) is possible.

If the transmitter released at the synapse is an *inhibitory transmitter,* summation of IPSPs will inhibit impulse transmission in the postsynaptic neuron or it decreases the excitability of the postsynaptic neuron. *Synaptic transmission can thus produce either excitation or inhibition of the postsynaptic neuron. Excitatory synapses evoke EPSP in the postsynaptic membrane and inhibitory synapses produce IPSP in the postsynaptic membrane* (**Flowchart 79.1**).

> Toxins which block neurotransmitter release are zinc endopeptidases that cleave and inactivate snare proteins. Tetanus toxin and botulinum toxins B, D, F and G inactivate synaptobrevin and botulinum toxin C inactivates syntaxin and prevents its attachment with synaptobrevin. This prevents the release of neurotransmitters.

ELECTRICAL EVENTS AT SYNAPSES

Excitatory Postsynaptic Potential (EPSP) and Inhibitory Postsynaptic Potential (IPSP)

A single stimulus reaching a synaptic knob may not lead to the formation of a propagated action potential in the postsynaptic neuron. Instead, it produces a transient partial depolarization (EPSP) or a transient hyperpolarization (IPSP) depending on the neurotransmitter released. The axons of neurons have only voltage gated Na⁺ and K⁺ channels whereas the cell body, dendrites and axonal endings have both voltage gated and ligand gated channels. So, the response produced by the transmitter depends on the type of channel associated with the synapse. The algebraic sum of all EPSPs and IPSPs on the postsynaptic neuron determines the membrane potential. If the summated potential reaches the firing level, a propagated action potential will be generated in the initial segment of the postsynaptic neuron.

Excitatory Postsynaptic Potential (EPSP)

If the response in the postsynaptic membrane is depolarizing, it has a latency of 0.5 milliseconds (ms) and reaches a peak at 5 ms and then declines exponentially. During this potential, the excitability of the postsynaptic neuron to other stimuli is increased since the potential moves towards the firing level. So, this potential is called **excitatory postsynaptic potential (EPSP) (Fig. 79.5A).**

Causes of EPSP

- Opening of sodium channels when the transmitter binds with the specific receptor. Large number of sodium ions move into the interior of the postsynaptic cell. This raises the membrane potential in the positive direction leading to depolarization.
- Closure of chloride or potassium channels. This decreases the influx of chloride ions into the interior or decreases the exit of potassium ions to the outside of the postsynaptic neuron. In both cases, the internal membrane potential become more positive than normal, which is excitatory.
- Some changes in the internal metabolism of the postsynaptic neuron may increase the number of excitatory membrane receptors or decrease the number of inhibitory membrane receptors.

The EPSPs produced by several active synaptic knobs in the same postsynaptic neuron can summate and if the summated potential reaches the firing level, a propagated impulse can be produced in the postsynaptic neuron.

Types of Summation of EPSPs

- *Spatial summation*: When the strength of the stimulus is increased, several synaptic knobs are stimulated at the same time and spatial summation of EPSPs occurs in the postsynaptic neuron. The postsynaptic potential reaches the firing level producing an action potential which is propagated.
- *Temporal summation*: If the stimuli of same strength are repeated at very short intervals so that new EPSPs are produced before previous EPSPs have decayed, it leads to temporal summation of EPSPs. The summated potential may reach the firing level and produce an action potential.

Inhibitory Postsynaptic Potential (IPSP)

If the neurotransmitter released at the synapse is an inhibitory transmitter, then a hyperpolarizing response is produced

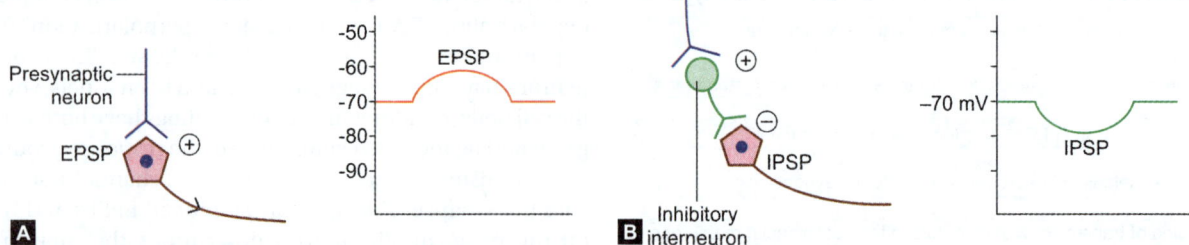

Figs. 79.5A and B: Mechanism of production of excitatory postsynaptic potential (EPSP) and inhibitory postsynaptic potential (IPSP).

Table 79.2: Differences between EPSP and IPSP.	
EPSP	**IPSP**
Produced by excitatory neurotransmitters like glutamate	Produced by inhibitory transmitters like GABA and glycine
Produced by opening of ligand-gated Na⁺ channel	Produced by opening of Cl⁻ or K⁺ channels or closing of Na⁺ or Ca²⁺ channel
Depolarizing potential magnitude of EPSP is about +8 mV	Hyperpolarizing potential Magnitude of IPSP is about -2 mV
When EPSPs are summated, an action potential can be produced	Cannot produce action potential in the postsynaptic neuron

in the postsynaptic membrane. During this potential, the excitability of the postsynaptic neuron is decreased because the membrane potential moves away from the firing level (**Fig. 79.5B**). So, this potential is called **inhibitory postsynaptic potential** (*refer* Synaptic Inhibition). Both spatial and temporal summation is seen in the case of IPSPs as well. However, the change in permeability is short lived and resting conditions are rapidly restored. Differences between EPSP and IPSP are given in **Table 79.2**.

Slow Postsynaptic Potentials

Slow EPSPs and IPSPs are seen in autonomic ganglia, cardiac and smooth muscles, and cortical neurons. These postsynaptic potentials have a latency of 100-500 ms and last several seconds. Slow EPSPs are due to decrease in K⁺ conductance and slow IPSPs are due to increase in K⁺ conductance.

PROPERTIES OF SYNAPSE

- One-way conduction
- Synaptic delay
- Synaptic inhibition
- Presynaptic facilitation
- Integration (convergence and divergence)
- After-discharge
- Summation
- Occlusion
- Post-tetanic potentiation
- Synaptic fatigue
- Synaptic plasticity.

One-Way Conduction

There is only forward conduction of impulses in the synapse, i.e., impulses pass only from presynaptic neuron to postsynaptic neuron (law of forward conduction). This is because the receptors for the neurotransmitter released are present only on the postsynaptic membrane. Another reason is that the neurotransmitters are present only in the presynaptic membrane and not in the postsynaptic membrane. So, impulse is not transmitted from post- to presynaptic membrane. *This is the reason why antidromic impulses transmitted through the axon stop in the soma of the neurons.* This is necessary for orderly neuronal function. **Exceptions** are reciprocal synapse and electrical synapse where transmission is bidirectional.

Synaptic Delay

When an impulse reaches the presynaptic terminal of a chemical synapse, there is an interval of at least **0.5 ms** before a response is obtained in the postsynaptic neuron. This delay is called **synaptic delay**. Because of this delay, conduction in a pathway that contains many synapses is slower than if there are only a few synapses. Since the synaptic delay is 0.5 ms, the number of synapses in a reflex pathway can be assessed. *Synaptic delay is negligible in electrical synapse.*

Causes of Synaptic Delay

- Time taken for the release of the transmitter from the presynaptic membrane
- Diffusion of the transmitter to the postsynaptic membrane
- Action of the transmitter on the postsynaptic receptor
- Changes in the receptor to increase membrane permeability
- Inward diffusion of Na⁺ to raise the EPSP to the firing level and produce an action potential.

Synaptic Inhibition

In some synapses in the CNS, the impulses are blocked or inhibited instead of being transmitted. This is synaptic inhibition. Here, the transmitter released is an **inhibitory transmitter** like GABA, glycine, etc. They act on the postsynaptic membrane and produce hyperpolarization. The excitability of the postsynaptic neuron to other stimuli is decreased. So, this hyper-polarizing response is called **inhibitory postsynaptic potential or IPSP**. The interior of the cell becomes more negative and the potential moves away from the firing level. For example, if the RMP was initially

−70 mV and after stimulation if the new potential is −75 mV, then IPSP is −5 mV (**Fig. 79.5B**). IPSPs can be summated, i.e., spatial and temporal summation of IPSP occurs. IPSP is responsible for synaptic inhibition. Synaptic inhibition plays a very important role in preventing widespread activation of many neurons by an ordinary or insignificant stimulus and thus preventing unnecessary spread of impulses.

Causes of IPSP

- Binding of the inhibitory transmitter to the receptor in the postsynaptic membrane opens Cl^- channels. Cl^- moves into the postsynaptic membrane along the concentration gradient. This increases the negativity inside producing hyperpolarization in the postsynaptic membrane. The membrane potential moves away from the firing level and so the excitability of the cell is decreased.
- IPSP can also be produced by opening K^+ channels and K^+ moves out of the postsynaptic cell along the concentration gradient, increasing the negativity inside.
- Closure of Na^+ or Ca^{2+} channel is also responsible for IPSP.
- Binding of the inhibitory transmitter to the receptor, may cause activation of receptor enzymes that alter cellular functions leading to increase in the number of inhibitory synaptic receptors or decrease in the number of excitatory receptors.

There are two types of synaptic inhibition:
1. Postsynaptic inhibition
2. Presynaptic inhibition.

Postsynaptic Inhibition

Inhibition of the postsynaptic neuron by producing IPSP in that neuron is called postsynaptic inhibition.

Types of postsynaptic inhibition (Figs. 79.6A to D):
- Direct inhibition
- Feedback inhibition or Renshaw cell inhibition
- Feed-forward inhibition.

A. *Direct inhibition*: When the postsynaptic neuron is directly inhibited by the formation of IPSP on the postsynaptic neuron, it is called direct inhibition. This is seen in the spinal cord. Stimulation of a sensory nerve fiber produces two types of effects in the spinal motor neurons. Stimulation of this neuron produces EPSP in one motor neuron and at the same time, it produces IPSP in some other neuron. Thus, there are two pathways, an excitatory and an inhibitory pathway. In the inhibitory pathway, the sensory fiber does not directly end in the spinal motor neuron; instead, an inhibitory interneuron is interposed between afferent nerve and spinal motor neuron. This inhibitory interneuron is called **Golgi bottle neuron**. This interneuron is short, plump and has a thick axon. The inhibitory transmitter is **glycine**. This type of inhibition is responsible for *reciprocal innervation*. For example, when biceps are contracting, triceps will be relaxing; otherwise, flexion at the elbow will not be possible (**Fig. 79.6A**). Golgi tendon organ inhibition (when a skeletal muscle is excessively stretched it relaxes) is another example for direct inhibition.

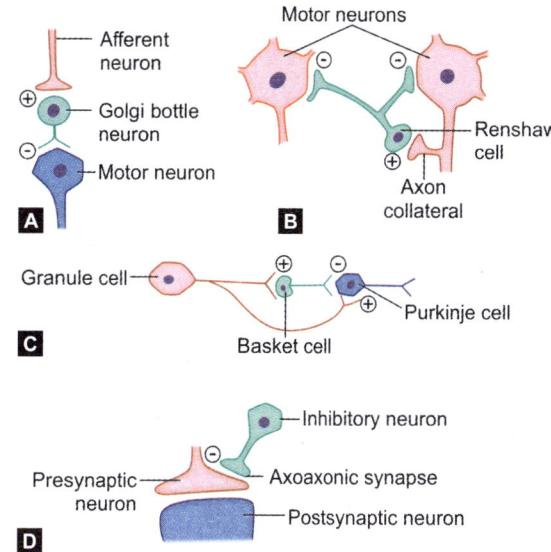

Figs. 79.6A to D: Types of inhibition at synapses: (A) Direct inhibition; (B) Feedback inhibition; (C) Feed-forward inhibition; (D) Presynaptic inhibition.

B. *Feedback inhibition or Renshaw cell inhibition or recurrent collateral inhibition*: Certain neurons may inhibit themselves in a feedback manner. Spinal motor neuron which supplies the skeletal muscle, gives off a recurrent collateral branch which terminates on an inhibitory interneuron called **Renshaw cell**. Renshaw cell in turn synapses with the same motor neuron and other neighboring motor neurons. Collateral from the Renshaw cell inhibiting neighboring motor neurons is an example of **lateral inhibition (Fig. 79.6B).**

When the motor neuron is stimulated, impulse that is transmitted also passes through the collateral (refer the diagram) and stimulates the Renshaw cell. Renshaw cell releases inhibitory transmitter **glycine** which produces IPSP in the same motor neuron, thus slowing or stopping impulse discharge from that motor neuron. Thus, the same motor neuron can control its rate of discharge. This type of inhibition is seen in different parts of nervous system like cerebral cortex and limbic system.

Applied aspect: Strychnine is an alkaloid obtained from the seeds of *Strychnos nuxvomica*. When ingested, it produces convulsions. In **strychnine poisoning**, the poison binds to glycine receptor in the motor neuron and blocks it. So, there is no feedback inhibition and excitation predominate. All skeletal muscles including diaphragm remain contracted in strychnine poisoning.

C. *Feed forward inhibition*: Feed forward inhibition is seen in cerebellum. There are flask-shaped cells called **Purkinje cells** and small cells called **basket cells** in the cerebellum. The basket cells act as inhibitory interneurons. When impulse passes through the parallel fibers of granule cells, both basket cells and Purkinje cells are stimulated. But basket cell in turn inhibits Purkinje cell. Thus, duration of discharge by Purkinje cell is reduced and output discharge from Purkinje cell is controlled. This type of inhibition is feed forward inhibition (**Fig. 79.6C**).

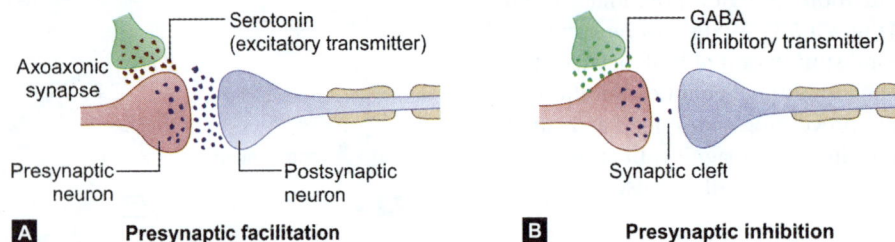

Figs. 79.7A and B: Mechanism of presynaptic facilitation and presynaptic inhibition. In presynaptic facilitation, the amount of transmitter released from the presynaptic membrane is increased due to the release of excitatory transmitter at the axo-axonic synapse. In presynaptic inhibition, the inhibitory transmitter (GABA) released at the axo-axonic synapse decrease the amount of transmitter released from presynaptic neuron.

Presynaptic Inhibition

Inhibition at the level of presynaptic terminal is known as **presynaptic inhibition or indirect inhibition**. The process is mediated by inhibitory interneurons whose terminals end on the presynaptic excitatory endings, forming **axo-axonal synapses (Fig. 79.6D)**. The amount of Ca^{2+} entering the presynaptic terminal is reduced, thereby reducing the amount of neurotransmitter released from the presynaptic terminal. This reduces the magnitude of action potential in the postsynaptic neuron (the 'all or none law' for action potential is applicable only under a given set of experimental conditions). For example, the descending pathway that terminates on afferent pathway in the dorsal horn is involved in the gating of pain transmission by presynaptic inhibition (refer 'pain control at the supraspinal level').

Mechanism of pesynaptic inhibition

an interneuron makes *axo-axonal synapse* with the presynaptic terminal. This synapse is called presynaptic synapse **(Fig. 79.7B)**. The first transmitter shown to produce presynaptic inhibition was GABA. Other transmitters also mediate presynaptic inhibition by G-protein-mediated effect on Ca^{2+} channels and K^+ channels. Three mechanisms have been described by which GABA produces presynaptic inhibition.

- GABA released at the axo-axonal synapse, increases Cl^- conductance in the presynaptic membrane through $GABA_A$ receptors. This decreases the magnitude of the action potential reaching the excitatory nerve ending. The amount of Ca^{2+} entering the presynaptic membrane is reduced and this decreases the amount of transmitter released from the excitatory ending **(Figs. 79.7A and B)**.
- $GABA_B$ receptors act via a G-protein that increase K^+ conductance in the presynaptic membrane by opening voltage-gated K^+ channels. The resulting K^+ efflux from the presynaptic membrane decreases the amount of Ca^{2+} entering the presynaptic membrane and this decreases the amount of excitatory transmitter released.
- Direct inhibition of transmitter release from the presynaptic membrane independent of Ca^{2+} influx into the excitatory ending.

Significance of presynaptic inhibition

- Presynaptic inhibition is responsible for inhibition of pain transmission in the dorsal horn of spinal cord (*refer* 'gate control hypothesis').
- It is responsible for lateral inhibition occurring in the CNS necessary for accurate localization of stimulus. For example, fine touch pathway from finger tips has significant lateral inhibition whereas pathway for temperature lacks lateral inhibition. So, fine touch can be localized clearly.
- Responsible for the relaxation of antagonist muscle during contraction of agonist in movements (reciprocal innervation).
- Certain drugs that produce convulsions act by antagonizing presynaptic inhibition.
- Barbiturates facilitate presynaptic inhibition.
- Baclofen, a $GABA_B$ receptor agonist is used in the treatment of spasticity of spinal cord injury. It acts by presynaptic inhibition.

Presynaptic Facilitation

In presynaptic facilitation, the action potential in the presynaptic membrane is prolonged and the L-type Ca^{2+} channels are open for a longer period. The transmitter responsible for the production of presynaptic facilitation is **serotonin (Fig. 79.7A)**. Serotonin released at the *axo-axonal* ending increases cAMP levels in the presynaptic neuron. This results in the phosphorylation of one group of K^+ channels which closes the channels, slowing repolarization and causing prolongation of depolarization. This keeps Ca^{2+} channels in the presynaptic membrane open for longer periods. This leads to increase in the transmitter release from the presynaptic terminal. Thus, transmission through the synapse is facilitated. *Presynaptic inhibition and facilitation may last for several minutes or hours. These properties are important in learning and memory.*

Presynaptic inhibition is mediated mainly by **GABA** whereas, presynaptic facilitation is mediated by **serotonin**.

Integration

The soma and dendrites act as an **integrator** that summates all the EPSPs and IPSPs produced at the postsynaptic endings. Depending on the summated potential, synaptic transmission may or may not occur.

Divergence

One axon may terminate on one postsynaptic neuron. Sometimes, a single axon divides into a number of branches, and each of these branches can terminate on

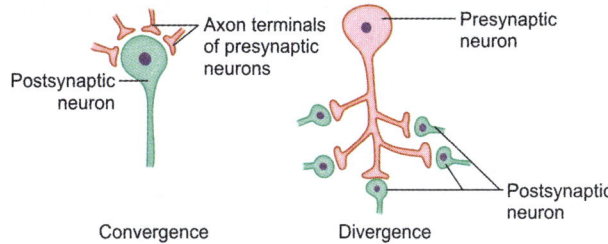

Fig. 79.8: Convergence and divergence at synapses.

different postsynaptic neurons. Thus, information from one presynaptic neuron passes to many postsynaptic neurons. This is known as **divergence (Fig. 79.8)**.

Convergence

A number of presynaptic neurons can converge on a single postsynaptic neuron. This is **convergence (Fig. 79.8)**.

A single neuron can diverge on to 1000 other neurons or a single neuron can have thousands of inputs. Convergence and divergence play important role in the phenomena of occlusion and facilitation. The number of synaptic knobs in a postsynaptic neuron may vary. In midbrain, one synaptic knob for one postsynaptic neuron is seen. Numerous synaptic knobs in one postsynaptic neuron are seen in spinal motor neurons. About 10,000 synaptic knobs are seen in spinal motor neuron, 8000 in dendrites and about 2000 in the soma. According to the transmitter released, either excitation or inhibition occurs at the synapse.

Some of the synaptic knobs may be excitatory producing EPSP and some may be inhibitory producing IPSP (*refer* Fig. 79.5). Thus, the motor neuron shows a fluctuating membrane potential. The membrane potential at a particular time is the algebraic sum of all the EPSPs and IPSPs. This potential is called **summated potential**.

Depending on the summated potential, synaptic transmission may or may not occur. When the summated potential is towards excitation, the neuron is said to be in the **central excitatory state** and the neuron is facilitated. When the summated potential reaches the threshold level, a propagated action potential is produced. If the summated potential is towards inhibition, it is called **central inhibitory state**. As the postsynaptic neuron integrates all the above mechanisms it is called an **integrator**.

Reciprocal Inhibition Circuit

This type of circuit involves both excitatory and inhibitory output signals. The neuronal pool causes one output signal to go in one direction and at the same time, causes an inhibitory signal to go in another direction. An inhibitory interneuron is involved in the inhibitory pathway. For example, when the arm is flexed, the biceps contracts and at the same time, triceps relaxes. Biceps contracts as a result of the excitatory pathway in the circuit and the triceps relaxes due to the inhibitory pathway involved in the circuit. This type of circuit is involved in controlling all antagonistic pairs of muscles and is called **reciprocal inhibition circuit**.

The input fibers directly excite the excitatory output pathway, but it stimulates an inhibitory interneuron which releases an inhibitory neurotransmitter to inhibit the second output pathway in the neuronal pool **(Fig. 79.6A)**. This type of circuit also helps to prevent over activity in many parts of the central nervous system.

After-discharge or Synaptic Modification

After-discharge is due to the presence of multiple connections between sensory afferent fibers and motor efferent fibers. This function is seen in synapses of neuronal pools in brain and spinal cord. A single input signal is converted to repetitive discharges as it passes through the synapse and there will be prolonged output discharge from the circuit. This is called **after-discharge**. This after-discharge lasts even after the input signal is over. Duration may be few milliseconds to minutes. There are three basic mechanisms for after-discharge:

1. Synaptic after-discharge.
2. Parallel circuit type of after-discharge.
3. Reverberating circuit or oscillatory type of after-discharge.

Synaptic After-discharge

The postsynaptic potential produced by the stimulation of the excitatory synapse will last for many milliseconds. In spinal motor neuron, this will last for 15 milliseconds. Certain other synapses have longer duration especially when a **long-acting transmitter** is released. As long as the central excitatory state is above the threshold level, the neurons can spontaneously discharge impulses repeatedly until the potential is maintained above the threshold level. Frequency of impulses produced depends on the degree of excitation, or in other words it depends on the level of central excitatory state above the threshold level. As long as central excitatory state or postsynaptic potential is above threshold value, it can discharge continuously. Thus, an instantaneous signal can be converted to a continuous sustained output discharge of long duration. This is synaptic after-discharge.

Parallel Circuit Type of After-discharge

As the input signal goes to the output neuron, this inputs signal stretches to a series of neurons that form parallel pathways that finally converge on the postsynaptic neuron or the output neuron. The number of synapses in the parallel pathways varies. This is called **parallel circuit**. The impulses reach the output neuron one after the other since there is a synaptic delay of 0.5 ms at each synapse in each parallel pathway. As a result, the output discharge neuron discharges repeatedly and for long duration. The duration depends on the number of synapses in the different parallel circuits. This is known as parallel circuit type of after-discharge **(Fig. 79.9)**.

Reverberatory (Oscillatory) Circuit Type of After-discharge

Reverberatory circuit type of after-discharge is the *most common type* of circuit seen in the nervous system. This is

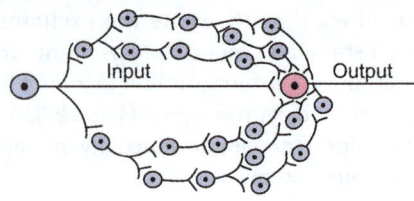

Fig. 79.9: Parallel circuit type of after-discharge.

produced by a positive feedback from the output discharge within the neuronal pool. Here, the impulse passes from the output neuron back to the same neuron through collaterals. In other words, the output discharge feeds back to the same circuit to re-stimulate it or re-excite the input of the same circuit. As a result, once stimulated, the input discharge is converted to prolonged, continuous output discharge **(Fig. 79.10)**. This can be checked by the phenomenon of synaptic fatigue. Different types of reverberating circuits are:

- **Simple type:** A single neuron is involved. Here, output neuron sends collateral to the dendrite or soma of same neuron, and there is continuous output neuronal discharge due to repeated signals.
- **Complex type:** Additional neurons are included in the feedback circuit.
- **Highly complex type** of reverberatory circuit consists of parallel fibers and cell stations containing several neurons. Terminals of nerve fibers diffuse widely. This complex reverberatory circuit is seen in respiratory neural pool. In ascending reticular activating system (ARAS), this type of circuit is responsible for wakeful state **(Fig. 79.10)**.

The reverberatory circuit is a complex system in which both facilitatory and inhibitory fibers are involved in the circuit. A facilitatory signal enhances the intensity and frequency of reverberation, whereas the inhibitory signal depresses or stops the reverberation.

The reverberation will not continue for long. There will be a sudden cessation of reverberation due to fatigue of the synaptic junctions in the circuit. The duration of reverberation is also controlled by signals coming from other parts of the brain that inhibit or facilitate the circuit.

Many neuronal circuits produce rhythmical output signals. For example, a rhythmical respiratory signal originates in the respiratory centers of the medulla and pons. This signal continues throughout life.

Summation

Since the synaptic potentials are graded, individual potentials (EPSP or IPSP) can be summated. This occurs when many presynaptic endings converge on a single postsynaptic membrane. There are two types of summation; spatial and temporal summation.

1. In **spatial summation**, a number of synaptic knobs converging on one postsynaptic membrane are simultaneously stimulated. The postsynaptic response evoked by all inputs becomes larger than the response to their individual stimulation. If the inputs are all excitatory, the postsynaptic response evoked by all inputs becomes larger than the response that would have occurred in response to their individual application.
2. In **temporal summation**, a single presynaptic knob is repeatedly stimulated in such a way that the second synaptic potential arrives before the membrane recovers from the previous synaptic potential **(Fig. 79.11)**. The potentials get summated.

Occlusion (Fig. 79.11)

When two excitatory afferent nerve fibers to a skeletal muscle are stimulated simultaneously, sometimes it is seen that the tension developed in the muscle is less than the sum of the tension developed when the two afferent fibers are stimulated separately. In this case, when a presynaptic neuron fires, a particular number of neurons fire and when another presynaptic neuron fires separately a fixed number of neurons fire. Simultaneous firing of these two presynaptic neurons results in activation of less number of postsynaptic neurons than when they are stimulated separately. This is because the two presynaptic neurons share same postsynaptic neurons on their discharge zone.

As shown in **Figure 79.11**:
- Stimulation of neuron A: EPSP is produced in neuron X.
- Stimulation of neuron B: EPSP is produced in neurons X and Y.
- Simultaneous stimulation of A and B: The two EPSPs in X neuron are summated, i.e., spatial summation. Neuron X can discharge impulse and hence it is said to be in the

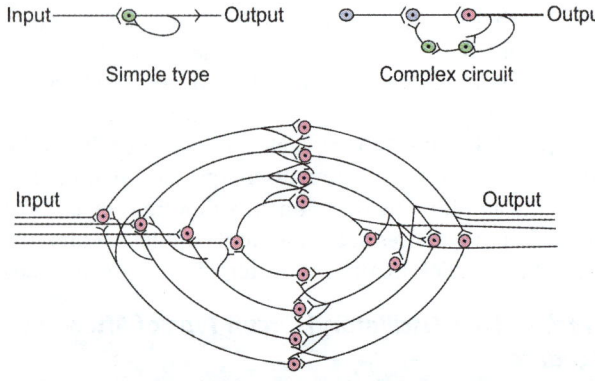

Fig. 79.10: Reverberatory circuit types of synaptic after-discharge.

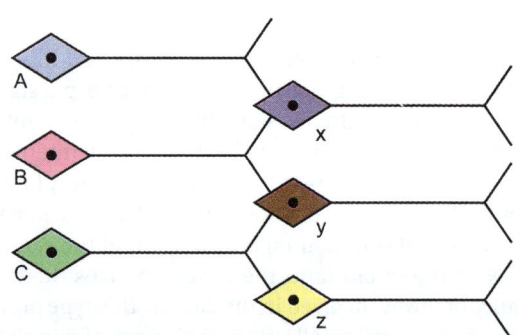

Fig. 79.11: Occlusion and summation (For details refer text).

discharge zone. In the case of Y neuron, excitability is increased but not to that extent to discharge impulse. So, Y neuron is said to be in the **subliminal fringe** *(occurs when a neuron receiving an excitatory input can affect synapses in its adjacent (fringe) area whose excitability is increased but not to the firing level)*

- Repeated stimulation of neuron B: Temporal summation in X and Y neurons and both can discharge impulses.
- Stimulation of neuron C repeatedly: Temporal summation in Y and Z neurons and both discharge impulses.
- Simultaneous stimulation of B and C repeatedly: X, Y and Z neurons discharge impulses. Sum of the response is less when B and C are simultaneously stimulated than when they are repeatedly stimulated separately. This property is known as **occlusion (Fig. 79.11)**. This is because, different presynaptic neurons share the same postsynaptic neuron and hence the sum of the responses or potentials obtained is less when the two presynaptic neurons are stimulated simultaneously (*refer* **Chapter 80, Fig. 80.12**).

Post-tetanic Potentiation or Facilitation

When excitatory synapses are stimulated repeatedly and rapidly for a short period and a period of rest is allowed, the postsynaptic neuron becomes more responsive to subsequent stimulation and they show an enhanced postsynaptic potential. This is *post-tetanic potentiation or post-tetanic facilitation*. Because of this property, some neurons can store information from few seconds to hours. This is one of the explanations for *short-term memory*.

Causes of Post-tetanic Potentiation

- Post-tetanic potentiation is due to accumulation of Ca^{2+} in the previous action potentials in the presynaptic neuron. Vesicles become more mobile towards presynaptic membrane and hence, the release of transmitter occurs with ease. There is also increase in the amount of transmitter released.
- The postsynaptic neuron becomes more responsive to the transmitter.

Synaptic Fatigue

If synapses are stimulated repeatedly and rapidly for some time, the number of discharges produced by postsynaptic neuron is at first great, but progressively becomes less and finally stops. This phenomenon is called *synaptic fatigue*. Electrical synapse is much less susceptible to fatigue on repeated stimulation. Causes of fatigue are:

1. Depletion of neurotransmitter.
2. Gradual inactivation of Ca^{2+} channels in the presynaptic membrane due to repeated stimulation which leads to decreased release of neurotransmitter.
3. Inactivation of postsynaptic receptors due to repeated stimulation.

> **CLINICAL IMPORTANCE OF SYNAPTIC FATIGUE**
>
> Synaptic fatigue is a protective phenomenon against excess neuronal activity. *This is the cause for the cessation of fits during an epileptic attack without treatment.*

Synaptic Plasticity

Synaptic transmission can be increased or decreased for short or long periods on the basis of past experience to suit the need of the body. These changes can occur due to changes in the presynaptic or postsynaptic areas at the synapses in the brain. This is called **synaptic plasticity**. This helps to react against a particular stimulus in an appropriate manner. Plastic change often results from alteration of the number of neurotransmitter receptors located on a synapse or changes in the quantity of neurotransmitters released into the synaptic cleft. Synaptic plasticity includes:

- Post-tetanic potentiation
- Long-term potentiation (LTP)
- Long-term depression (LTD)
- Habituation
- Sensitization.

- **Post-tetanic potentiation** is due to increase in the intracellular Ca^{2+} in the presynaptic neuron due to tetanizing stimuli. Each action potential is associated with increased release of neurotransmitter.
- **Long-term potentiation** is due to increase in the intracellular Ca^{2+} in the postsynaptic neuron and also due to structural changes in the postsynaptic neuron. This occurs when the post-tetanic potentiation is much more prolonged. LTP occurs due to the growth of new presynaptic release sites as well as synthesis of new postsynaptic receptors. There is also increase in the number of dendritic spines in the postsynaptic neuron. Thus, the number of synapses in the postsynaptic neuron is also increased. LTP is involved in **learning and memory**.
- **Long-term depression** is opposite to that of LTP. Here, stimulation of presynaptic neuron is associated with a smaller rise in intracellular calcium. There is also decrease in the number of receptors synthesized by the endoplasmic reticular–Golgi apparatus system in the postsynaptic neuron. LTD is also involved in learning.
- **Habituation:** When a neutral or benign stimulus is repeated over and over, the response to the stimulus gradually decreases and finally disappears. This phenomenon is called **habituation**. Habituation is due to decreased release of neurotransmitter from presynaptic membrane as a result of decrease in Ca^{2+} influx. When the synapse is repeatedly stimulated, there will be gradual inactivation of Ca^{2+} channels in the presynaptic terminal. It can be short-term or long-term depending on the duration of repeated exposure to the benign stimulus. For example, we ignore the continuous touch sensation produced by the clothes we are wearing; we are not bothered about the sound of the fan while we are sleeping, etc. This is because we become habituated to these repeated stimuli since we learn that the stimulus is not important.
- **Sensitization:** Sensitization is the facilitation of a stimulus. It is due to *presynaptic facilitation* and the transmitter involved is **serotonin**. Sensitization occur when a benign or neutral stimulus to which the animal has become habituated is paired once or several times with a noxious stimulus (pain). The noxious stimulus causes discharge of

serotonergic neurons that end on the presynaptic endings of sensory neurons. Serotonin at the axo-axonic synapse leads to presynaptic facilitation due to increased Ca^{2+} entry into the presynaptic terminal. The postsynaptic response will be more and prolonged. Due to reinforcement, sensitization is very important in establishing short-term and long-term memory. The short-term prolongation of sensitization is due to increased production of cAMP, and long-term prolongation is due to increased protein synthesis in postsynaptic neuron. It is also due to growth of presynaptic and postsynaptic neurons and their connections.

❖ Sensitization can also occur by pairing the stimulus with a non-noxious stimulus. For example, mothers wake up on hearing the baby's cry even though they are sleeping through many kinds of noises.

Neuroplasticity

> **Neuroplasticity** or brain plasticity refers to the ability of brain to change with learning throughout life. Brain has the ability to reorganize itself by forming new connections between neurons. Neuroplasticity occurs in the brain in the following situations:
> - In the fetal life when the immature brain organizes itself.
> - In case of brain injury, the brain compensates for the damage by reorganizing and forming new connections between intact neurons. But to achieve this, the neurons need to be stimulated through activity.
> - Throughout life whenever something new is learned and memorized.

EFFECT OF ENVIRONMENTAL FACTORS ON SYNAPTIC TRANSMISSION

Effect of pH

Alkalosis increases neuronal excitability. When the pH is increased to 7.8, convulsions are seen due to increased neuronal activity. In **acidosis**, neuronal activity is depressed. When pH is reduced to 7 from 7.4, as seen in diabetic acidosis, metabolic and respiratory acidosis coma occurs due to depression of neuronal activity.

Effect of Hypoxia

O_2 is necessary for normal functioning of neuron. Neuronal activity is depressed in hypoxia and person becomes unconscious when cerebral circulation is interrupted even for 5 sec.

Effect of Drugs on Neuronal Activity

❖ Certain drugs like caffeine, theophylline, etc., increase neuronal activity. Mechanism is by lowering the threshold of excitation.
❖ Strychnine blocks the action of inhibitory transmitters especially glycine in the spinal cord so that the action of excitatory transmitter becomes predominant leading to convulsions (severe tonic muscle spasms).
❖ Anesthetics depress neuronal activity by increasing the threshold of excitation.

NEUROTRANSMITTERS AND NEUROMODULATORS

Neurotransmitters

Definition

Neurotransmitters are chemical substances stored in the axon terminal, which are responsible for the transmission of impulse across a chemical synapse. Neurotransmitters are also released from neurons supplying a muscle or gland. A substance can be designated as a neurotransmitter only if it satisfies the following *criteria*:
❖ The presynaptic neuron must contain the substance.
❖ The presynaptic cell must contain the enzymes involved in the biosynthesis of the substance or the transporters for the reuptake of the substance into the presynaptic terminal.
❖ The substance should be released from the presynaptic terminal on appropriate stimulation.
❖ The postsynaptic membrane should contain the receptors specific for the substance.
❖ Application of the substance experimentally to the postsynaptic membrane must mimic the effects of stimulation of the presynaptic neuron.
❖ The effects of presynaptic stimulation and microapplication of the substance to the postsynaptic membrane should be altered in the same way by drugs.

Neurotransmitters are released when an action potential reaches the nerve terminal. They are synthesized by the presynaptic neuron which contains the enzymes responsible for the synthesis. There are specific receptors for the neurotransmitters in the presynaptic or postsynaptic membranes. Some neurotransmitters can stimulate both presynaptic and postsynaptic receptors, e.g., norepinephrine. Some neurons release more than one transmitter at their endings, e.g., ACh and VIP are stored in the same nerve ending in the GIT. *Usually, the coexistence of transmitters in the same neuron includes a transmitter and a neuropeptide*, e.g., ACh and GRP in the vagus nerve, glutamate and dynorphin in the hippocampus, ACh and substance P in the nociceptors, serotonin and substance P in the nociceptive fibers. About 50 neurotransmitters have been identified so far. There are excitatory neurotransmitters and inhibitory neurotransmitters. **Excitatory transmitters** produce *depolarizing* excitatory postsynaptic potential **(EPSP)** in the postsynaptic membrane, e.g., glutamate, acetylcholine, aspartic acid, serotonin, norepinephrine, histamine, etc. **Inhibitory neurotransmitters** produce *hyperpolarizing* inhibitory postsynaptic potential (**IPSP**) in the postsynaptic membrane.

Inhibitory neurotransmitters in the CNS are glycine, gamma-aminobutyric acid (GABA), dopamine, etc.

Classification of Neurotransmitters

❖ **Small molecule transmitters**: Monoamines, biogenic amines and amino acids.
❖ **Large molecule transmitters**: Neuropeptides or neuroactive peptides – VIP, substance P, neurotensin, endorphin, dynorphin, etc.
❖ **Gases**: Nitric oxide and carbon monoxide.

Small Molecule Transmitters

Small molecule neurotransmitters are synthesized in all parts of the neurons especially nerve terminal. For example, glutamate, GABA, glycine, catecholamines, ACh, serotonin, etc., are small-molecule neurotransmitters.
1. Acetylcholine
2. Biogenic amine transmitters: Norepinephrine, epinephrine, dopamine, serotonin and histamine.
3. Amino acid transmitters: Glycine, γ-aminobutyric acid (GABA), glutamate and aspartate.

Acetylcholine
1. ACh is the transmitter released by all motor neurons that arise from the spinal cord.
2. It is the transmitter for all preganglionic autonomic neurons and for all postganglionic parasympathetic fibers.
3. Sympathetic cholinergic fibers innervating skeletal muscle blood vessels and sweat glands release ACh as the neurotransmitter.
4. The Betz cells of the motor cortex use ACh as their transmitter.
5. ACh is an important transmitter in basal ganglia.
6. It is the transmitter in many other central neural pathways.

(For details, *refer* autonomic nervous system, Chapter 94).

Catecholamines: Dopamine, norepinephrine and epinephrine are the catecholamines. They are all synthesized from the amino acid *tyrosine*. Tyrosine is converted to L-Dopa by tyrosine hydroxylase. L-Dopa is converted to dopamine by Dopa decarboxylase. In dopaminergic neurons, the pathway stops here. Dopaminergic neurons are concentrated in the substantia nigra, ventral tegmentum of midbrain and posterior hypothalamus.

Dopamine
- Dopamine is the transmitter in the neurons of substantia nigra which terminate in corpus striatum. Degeneration of dopaminergic synapses in the corpus striatum leads to *Parkinson's disease*.
- Dopaminergic neurons of posterior hypothalamus give rise to the descending autonomic fibers to sympathetic preganglionic neurons of spinal cord.
- The small intensely fluorescent (SIF) cells in the autonomic ganglia are dopaminergic interneurons.
- *Prolactin inhibiting hormone* is dopamine, produced by tubuloinfundibular tract extending from arcuate nucleus to infundibulum of hypothalamus.
- The periglomerular cells of olfactory bulb, amacrine cells of retina and cells in the medullary chemoreceptor trigger zone are dopaminergic.

Norepinephrine: In noradrenergic neurons, dopamine β-hydroxylase converts dopamine to norepinephrine. Norepinephrine is the primary transmitter in postganglionic sympathetic fibers. Norepinephrine is the transmitter in locus coeruleus and lateral tegmentum. Lateral tegmentum includes nucleus ambiguus, nucleus of tractus solitarius and dorsal motor nucleus of vagus. Catecholaminergic receptors are present in almost all tissues of the body. Norepinephrine acts through α_1 and α_2 receptors. α_1 receptor is present in the postsynaptic membrane. α_2 receptors are present in the presynaptic membrane and are *inhibitory auto-receptors*. When stimulated, these receptors reduce the amount of neurotransmitter released from the presynaptic membrane.

Epinephrine: Chromaffin cells in the adrenal medulla convert norepinephrine to epinephrine by catecholamine- O-methyl transferase which is present only in adrenal medulla.

Serotonin: **Serotonin** is synthesized from the amino acid *tryptophan*. It is inactivated by monoamine oxidase (MAO) after an active reuptake mechanism to 5-hydroxy- indole acetic acid (5-HIAA) and this is excreted through urine. In the pineal gland, serotonin is converted to *melatonin* by the enzymes, N-acetyl transferase and hydroxyl-indole-o-methyltransferase (HIOMT).

Serotonin is present in the brain as a neurotransmitter. It is also present in non-neural cells. In the brain, serotonergic neurons have their cell bodies in the raphe magnus nucleus of the brainstem. They project to hypothalamus, limbic system, neocortex and spinal cord. Serotonergic neurons may be involved in sensory perception, onset of sleep, control of mood, etc. Serotonin has excitatory effect on motor pathways and inhibitory effect on sensory pathways. Its activity is high in alert wakeful conditions when it increases motor responsiveness to stimuli. Serotonin along with norepinephrine is involved in food intake and regulation of body temperature. It potentiates the analgesic action of morphine in the central analgesia system. Decreased activity of serotonergic neurons leads to depression. Serotonin receptors have a high affinity for antidepressant drugs. The antidepressant drug escitalopram is a **selective serotonin reuptake inhibitor** (SSRI). It increases the availability of serotonin.

Among non-neuronal cells, serotonin is present in the highest concentration in blood platelets. It is also present in mast cells, basophils, and retina and enterochromaffin cells. It is also present in the myenteric plexus of GIT.

Histamine: Histamine is formed by decarboxylation of amino acid **histidine**. Histaminergic neurons have their cell bodies in the tuberomammillary nucleus of posterior hypothalamus and limbic system. The axons project to all parts of the brain and spinal cord. Non-neural cells that contain histamine include mast cells and cells of gastric mucosa. Histaminergic receptors are H_1, H_2 and H_3 receptors. H_3 receptors are seen in the presynaptic membrane. They inhibit the release of histamine and other transmitters via a G-protein.

Role of histamine in brain includes arousal and sexual behavior and it is an *excitatory* transmitter in CNS. It is involved in the sensation of itch.

Amino Acid Transmitters
Glycine and GABA: **Glycine** is an *inhibitory* neurotransmitter released by certain spinal interneurons that inhibit antagonistic muscles. **Gamma-amino butyric acid (GABA)** is synthesized from glutamic acid by a specific glutamate decarboxylase enzyme present only in certain neurons of CNS. GABA-containing neurons are present in basal ganglia

(striatum), cerebellar Purkinje fibers, reticular nuclei of thalamus and certain spinal interneurons. It functions as an *inhibitory* transmitter and is the most common transmitter in brain. It is the neurotransmitter in as many as 1/3 of synapses in brain.

The postganglionic receptors for GABA and glycine contain Cl⁻ channels that cause Cl⁻ influx into the postsynaptic neuron leading to hyperpolarization and inhibition. GABA acts through two types of receptors, $GABA_A$ and $GABA_B$ receptors. Stimulation of $GABA_A$ receptor increases Cl⁻ influx. GABA receptors are present in the pre- and postsynaptic membranes and their stimulation increases K⁺ efflux in postsynaptic membrane and closes Ca^{2+} channels in the presynaptic membrane, both producing hyperpolarization of synaptic membranes.

APPLIED PHYSIOLOGY

General anesthetics act mainly by stimulating GABA receptors. $GABA_A$ agonists include antianxiety, muscle relaxant, anticonvulsant and sedative drugs. Drugs like diazepam and barbiturates (phenobarbitone) bind to $GABA_A$ receptors and enhance the opening of Cl⁻ channels in the ionophore part of the receptor. Diazepam is an antianxiety and muscle relaxant drug while phenobarbitone is used as sedative and anticonvulsant.

Glutamate: Glutamate is synthesized by glial cells from **glutamine**. It is an *excitatory transmitter in the CNS and is responsible for about 75% of excitatory transmission in brain*. Reuptake of released glutamate occurs into the nerve terminal or glial cells.

APPLIED PHYSIOLOGY

Normally, reuptake of glutamate in the CNS occurs into the glial cells especially astrocytes through secondary active transport with Na⁺ ions. If glutamate is present in high concentration in the brain, it is toxic to neurons and is called **glutamate excitotoxicity**. This occurs in cerebral ischemia following cerebral stroke, head injury, epilepsy, etc.

Large Molecule Transmitter

Neuropeptides: Neuropeptides like **opioid peptides** (enkephalin, β-endorphin and methionine), **neurohormones**, etc., are synthesized in the soma and transported to the axon terminal. Peptides that bind to opioid receptors are called opioid peptides. The large dense core vesicles that contain the neuropeptides lack the SNARE proteins required for the localized release of the transmitter at the active sites in the presynaptic membrane. So, exocytosis can occur anywhere along the membrane of the presynaptic terminal. Ca^{2+} alone is responsible for the movement of vesicles to the presynaptic membrane.

Enkephalins (met-enkephalin and leu-enkephalin) are found in the region of substantia gelatinosa and have analgesic activity. Pro-opiomelanocortin present in the pituitary contains β-endorphin. *The opioid peptides inhibit adenylyl cyclase and produce analgesia.* It also acts by increasing K⁺ conductance, and closing Ca^{2+} channels thereby producing hyperpolarization and decreased excitability of central neurons and primary afferents.

The physiologic effects produced by stimulation of opioid receptors include analgesia, euphoria, sedation, miosis and rarely respiratory depression.

Other neuropeptides include **calcitonin gene-related peptide (CGRP) and neuropeptide-Y**. CGRP is present along with substance P in the primary afferent neurons that end near blood vessels and the effect is vasodilatation (refer axon reflex).

Neuropeptide-Y is found throughout the brain and the autonomic nervous system. It is a potent orexigenic neurotransmitter that has a stimulatory effect on food intake. Neuropeptide-Y antagonists are used to decrease food intake.

Differences between small molecule neurotransmitters and neuropeptides are given in **Table 79.3**.

Neurohormones like substance P, somatostatin, vasopressin, oxytocin, angiotensin II, endothelin, VIP, GRP, etc., are peptides that act as hormones in some areas like gastrointestinal tract, kidney, etc., and as neurotransmitters in the central nervous system.

Gases acting as neurotransmitters: Nitric oxide (NO) and CO are gases that act as neurotransmitters. Being lipid soluble, these gases can easily diffuse into the neurons. NO also acts as a retrograde transmitter at some synapses where it carries information from postsynaptic neuron to presynaptic neuron, e.g., in long-term potentiation and long-term depression.

NO is synthesized in the brain from **arginine** catalyzed by the enzyme **NO synthase**. It is also released by the endothelium of blood vessels as endothelium-derived relaxing factor (EDRF). On entering the cell NO binds directly to guanylyl cyclase and activates it. CO is formed in the course of metabolism of heme by heme-oxygenase, and like NO, it also *activates guanylyl cyclase*.

Classification of neurotransmitters based on their chemical structure:
- acetylcholine
- Amines: Norepinephrine, epinephrine, dopamine, serotonin, histamine

Table 79.3: Differences between small molecule neurotransmitters and neuropeptides.

Small molecule neurotransmitter	Neuropeptide
Synthesized in all parts of neuron	Synthesized in the soma of the neuron
Packaged in small clear or small dense core vesicles	Packaged in large dense core vesicles
Released only at the active zone	Released all along the presynaptic membrane
For exocytosis, v-SNARE proteins must bind to t-SNARE proteins in the presynaptic membrane	Exocytosis depends only on Ca^{2+} influx since vesicles lack SNARE proteins
Neurotransmitter is immediately removed from the synaptic cleft by reuptake or by degradation	Removed from synaptic cleft slowly by diffusion and proteolysis by peptidases
Duration of action is less	Duration of action is long
Recycling present	No recycling is present. Fresh supply of neurotransmitter must arrive from the cell body for next release

- Amino acids: Glutamate and aspartate (excitatory transmitters); GABA and glycine (inhibitory)
- Polypeptides: Oxytocin, ADH, substance P, CGRP, neuropeptide-Y, somatostatin, endorphins, encephalins
- Gases: Nitric oxide, carbon monoxide.

Neuromodulators

Neuromodulators are substances that modulate synaptic transmission in the nervous system. They are chemicals released by neurons that have little or no direct effects on their own but can modify the effects of neurotransmitters. They enhance the excitatory or inhibitory responses of the receptors. Neuromodulation has a very important role in cortical plasticity. Major neuromodulators in the central nervous system include **dopamine, serotonin, acetylcholine, histamine, noradrenaline and several neuropeptides**. Many forms of synaptic modulation influence the nervous system. For example axons from the locus coeruleus synapse on the pyramidal cells in the cerebral cortex and the transmitter involved is norepinephrine. Norepinephrine acts on the beta-adrenergic receptors in the pyramidal cell membrane. But it produces no response on the resting cell. When this pyramidal cell is stimulated by a strong excitatory input e.g., by glutamate, the cell will react more powerfully. In this situation norepinephrine modulates the pyramidal cell's response to other inputs and norepinephrine acts as a neuromodulator. Other examples include:

- Acetylcholine, catecholamines, and neuropeptides act as vasoactive neuromodulators in the region of synaptic activity in controlling blood vessels.
- Enteric nervous system involves many different neurotransmitters and neuromodulators.
- Noradrenergic neurons in the locus coeruleus innervate spinal cord, cerebellum, thalamus and neocortex and modulate the action of the neurons in response to the neurotransmitters.
- Serotonergic neurons in the raphe nuclei project to the hypothalamus, limbic system, neocortex, cerebellum and spinal cord and modulate their functions.
- Dopaminergic neurons in the substantia nigra project to striatum and influence neuronal activity in striatum.
- Cholinergic neurons in the basal forebrain complex projecting to the hippocampus and the neocortex act as neuromodulators.
- Cholecystokinin act as a neuromodulator in potentiating the stimulatory effects of secretin in pancreatic juice secretion.
- Serotonin and norepinephrine act as neuromodulators in the determination of taste thresholds. When the levels of these substances are altered, taste disturbances occur as in anxiety and depression.
- There are drugs that act as neuromodulators. GABA is an inhibitory transmitter. The increase in Cl⁻ conductance produced by $GABA_A$ receptors is potentiated by benzodiazepines like diazepam. Thus this drug acts as a neuromodulator. This drug has antianxiety and muscle relaxant action. They bind to alpha subunits of $GABA_A$ receptor and modulate the action of GABA.

The mechanism of action of neuromodulators is complex. Neuromodulators typically bind to metabotropic, G-protein coupled receptors (GPCRS) to initiate a second messenger signaling cascade that induces long lasting effects. This modulation can last for hundreds of milliseconds to several minutes. Adenylyl cyclase is stimulated which increase intracellular cAMP level. The cAMP acts as second messenger which in turn stimulates other enzymes by phosphorylation. Phosphorylation of some types of K^+ channel prevents them from opening. This leads to decreased efflux of K^+ and greater excitability of the neuron.

■ MULTIPLE CHOICE QUESTIONS

1. All are features of neurotransmitters, *except*:
   a. Released from presynaptic membrane
   b. Degraded in the synaptic cleft
   c. Exogenous administration will not have any effect
   d. Produced in neurons only

2. Glycine is a neurotransmitter that is found principally in the synapses of:
   a. Spinal cord   b. Cerebral cortex
   c. Cerebellum   d. Substantia nigra

3. The transmitter that produces inhibitory postsynaptic potential is:
   a. Acetylcholine   b. L-glutamate
   c. GABA   d. Serotonin

4. The neurotransmitter that is taken back into the presynaptic membrane after its release into the synaptic cleft is:
   a. Catecholamine   b. Acetylcholine
   c. Endorphin   d. Serotonin

5. Inhibitory postsynaptic potential is mainly due to increase in the permeability of postsynaptic membrane to:
   a. Chloride ions   b. Potassium ions
   c. Sodium ions   d. Calcium ions

6. Neuropeptides in CNS includes all the following, except:
   a. Substance P   b. Somatostatin
   c. Norepinephrine   d. Cholecystokinin

7. The toxin that inhibit the release of acetyl choline at the neuromuscular junction is:
   a. δ-Tubocurarine   b. Botulinum toxin
   c. Tetanus toxin   d. Endotoxin

8. Drugs that compete with acetyl choline receptor include all the following, *except*:
   a. Atropine   b. Scopolamine
   c. δ-Tubocurarine   d. Succinyl choline

9. The neuromuscular blocking action of curare is brought about by:
   a. Blocking ACh synthesis
   b. Preventing release of ACh
   c. Causing depolarization block
   d. Competitive inhibition

10. The inhibitory transmitter in CNS neurons is:
    a. Glutamate
    b. Aspartate
    c. GABA
    d. Taurine

11. False statement about excitatory postsynaptic potential is:
    a. It is localized
    b. Show summation
    c. Weans in exponential rate
    d. Produce hyper polarization

12. Strychnine acts as an anticonvulsant by:
    a. Exciting all excitatory synapses in spinal cord
    b. Lowering intracellular Ca^{2+} level
    c. Blocking inhibitory synapses
    d. Directly stimulating skeletal muscles

13. Neurotransmitter in the retino-hypothalamic tract is:
    a. Glycine
    b. Aspartate
    c. Glutamate
    d. Serotonin

14. The main excitatory neurotransmitter in the CNS is:
    a. Glutamate
    b. Aspartate
    c. Acetyl choline
    d. Glycine

15. The neurotransmitter substance released from the major output unit of basal ganglia is mainly:
    a. GABA
    b. Glutamate
    c. Dopamine
    d. Acetyl choline

16. Which of the following synaptic transmitters is not a peptide or protein?
    a. Serotonin
    b. Substance P
    c. β endorphin
    d. Metencephalin

17. The correct statement regarding EPSP is:
    a. It cannot be summated
    b. It cannot be decreased by curare
    c. It is propagated
    d. It is initiated by acetyl choline always
    e. It is not associated with increase in sodium permeability

18. IPSP is due to:
    a. Cl^- influx
    b. Na^+ influx
    c. K^+ influx
    d. Ca^{2+} influx

19. Beta-endorphins are present in high concentration in the:
    a. Substantia gelatinosa
    b. Posterior pituitary
    c. Spinal cord
    d. Medulla

20. Most common type of synapse is:
    a. Electrical synapse
    b. Conjoint synapse
    c. Axodendritic synapse
    d. Axoaxonic synapse

21. True about Renshaw cell inhibition is:
    a. Add on collateral sensation
    b. Increases by local anesthetics
    c. Has memory for spinal cord
    d. Inhibition of feedback propagation

ANSWERS

1. c	2. a	3. c	4. a	5. a
6. c	7. b	8. d	9. d	10. c
11. d	12. c	13. c	14. a	15. a
16. a	17. d	18. a	19. c	20. c
21. d				

Reflex Action

CHAPTER 80

LEARNING OBJECTIVES
- Describe the basic elements of a reflex pathway
- Describe the functions and properties of reflexes
- Explain stretch reflex and its clinical importance
- Explain the components, function and innervation of muscle spindle
- Describe the role of Golgi tendon organ in the control of skeletal muscle tension
- Describe the physiological basis of tremor, clonus and muscle tone
- Explain the role of gamma motor neuron in the control of muscle tone
- Identify the components and function of withdrawal reflex

INTRODUCTION

PY10.2: Describe and discuss the functions and properties of synapse, reflex, receptors.

The involuntary response produced as a result of the application of an adequate stimulus is called **reflex action** or, a *reflex* is a rapid, fixed motor response to a particular sensory stimulus. Examples are withdrawal of hand when we touch a hot object, constriction of pupil when light is thrown into the eye, etc. These are inborn reflexes or unconditioned reflexes. Acquired reflexes are called conditioned reflexes. Reflex activity is specific, i.e., a particular stimulus elicits a particular response. Basis for all integrated neuronal activity is reflex action and the basic unit of integrated reflex activity is the **reflex arc**.

REFLEX ARC

Structural basis of reflex action is reflex arc. It has three components (**Fig. 80.1**):
1. Afferent limb, which consists of sense organ or receptor and afferent neuron
2. Center
3. Efferent limb.

Receptor

Receptor may be located:
- Superficially in the skin or mucous membrane
- Deeply in the muscle or tendon
- In the viscera
- In sense organs concerned with special senses like vision, olfaction, taste, etc.

In a reflex arc, activity starts with the stimulation of the sensory receptor. When the receptors are stimulated and if the **receptor potential** reaches firing level, they generate impulses or action potentials in the afferent neuron. The magnitude of receptor potential is proportional to the strength of the stimulus. The number of action potentials produced in the afferent nerve is proportional to the size of the receptor potential. The impulses in the form of action potentials are conveyed to the spinal cord or brain through the afferent nerve.

Afferent Neuron

The afferent neuron enters the spinal cord through the dorsal root, and other afferents from the head and neck region enter the brain through the cranial nerves. Cell body of afferent neuron is located in the dorsal root ganglion (DRG) in spinal reflexes and in the ganglia of cranial nerves in cranial reflexes.

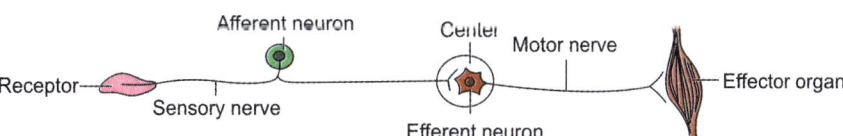

Fig. 80.1: Reflex arc.

Center

The center is situated in the brain or spinal cord and is constituted by the synapse between the afferent and efferent neuron. Center is also known as *central integrating station*, and it contains one to many hundred synapses.

Several interneurons may be present between the afferent and the efferent neuron in the central nervous system (CNS). Thus the activity in the reflex arc is modified by the multiple inputs converging on the efferent neurons within the reflex arc. In the center, the response in the postsynaptic neuron depends on the sum of the excitatory postsynaptic potentials (EPSP) and inhibitory postsynaptic potentials (IPSPs). If the summated potential is excitatory, action potential is generated in the efferent motor nerve.

Efferent Limb

Efferent limb consists of efferent neuron and effector organ. Efferent neuron conveys impulses from CNS to the periphery (effector organ). The action potential generated in the efferent motor nerve reaches the effector where a graded response is produced. Cell bodies are situated in the ventral horn of spinal cord and impulses are carried through the anterior nerve root. From brain, impulses are carried through cranial nerves from nuclei of brain, especially brainstem nuclei.

Effector Organ

Effector organ is either a muscle or gland and the effect is contraction of muscle or secretion from gland. If the sum of the graded potentials generated in the effector is adequate to produce action potentials in the muscle, it leads to muscle contraction. If the effector is a gland it leads to secretion from the gland.

Simple reflex consists of only one synapse and is called *monosynaptic reflex*. If the reflex pathway consists of more than two synapses it is called a *polysynaptic reflex*. The number of synapses in the reflex arc varies from two to many hundreds. Many interneurons are interposed between the afferent and efferent neurons in polysynaptic reflexes. In the reflex arcs, summation, occlusion, subliminal fringe effects and other effects modify the activity. This is because the center for the reflex is in the CNS and multiple inputs converge on the efferent neurons (*refer* final common pathway).

Central nervous system is not a part in some reflex pathways, e.g., local gut reflexes, axon reflex, etc. In **axon reflex,** which is a **pseudoreflex,** when skin is stimulated, the impulse is transmitted antidromically through collaterals arising from the afferent nerves innervating a nearby cutaneous blood vessel **(Fig. 80.2)**. The effect is dilation of the cutaneous blood vessel. Here, there is no center. Hence, it is called a pseudoreflex.

Spinal cord is the center of all the reflex activities in the limbs. The responses produced by the spinal cord are modified by the influences from other parts of the nervous system. The anterior horn of spinal cord contains two types of motor neurons: (i) α-**motor neurons** innervate the main force

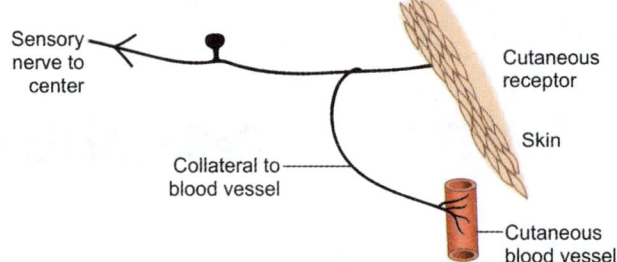

Fig. 80.2: Axon reflex or pseudoreflex.

generating muscle fibers (the extrafusal fibers), whereas (ii) **gamma motor neurons** innervate only the fibers of the muscle spindles (intrafusal fibers). The group of all motor neurons innervating a single muscle is called a **motor neuron pool.**

CLASSIFICATION OF REFLEXES

I. **Whether present from birth onwards:**
   - Unconditioned reflex or inborn reflex
   - Acquired or conditioned reflex (*refer* Chapter 96)

II. **Depending on the effector organ:**
   - *Somatic reflexes* include the responses from skeletal muscles mediated through CNS.
     - Flexor reflexes
     - Extensor reflexes.
   - Somatic reflex (another classification)
     - Superficial reflex
     - Deep reflex.
   - *Visceral or autonomic reflexes*
     Autonomic reflexes include responses from smooth muscles of viscera. These reflexes are mediated through autonomic nervous system (ANS).

III. **According to the response produced:**
   - Motor reflexes in which skeletal muscle is the effector organ.
   - Secretory reflexes in which glands are the effector organs.
   - Vasomotor reflexes in which smooth muscle of blood vessel is the effector organ.

IV. **Clinical classification:**
   - Superficial reflexes which are elicited from the surface of the body like abdominal reflex, plantar reflex, corneal reflex, etc.
   - Deep reflexes or tendon reflexes like knee jerk, biceps jerk, etc.
   - Visceral reflexes are reflexes originating from internal organs; e.g., deglutition, defecation, carotid sinus reflex, etc.
   - Pathological reflexes like extensor plantar reflex.

V. **According to the number of synapses in the pathway:**
   - Monosynaptic reflex if there is only one synapse, e.g., deep tendon reflexes (stretch reflexes).
   - Bisynaptic reflex where there are two synapses in the center, e.g., inverse stretch reflex and reciprocal innervation.

- Polysynaptic reflex where there are more than two synapses in the central integrating station, e.g., withdrawal reflex, superficial reflexes, etc. Here many interneurons are interposed between the afferent and efferent neurons.

Monosynaptic Reflex or Stretch Reflex or Myotatic Reflex

Passive abrupt stretching of a skeletal muscle with intact nerve supply causes a reflexive contraction of that same muscle. It is sometimes called the **myotatic reflex** because it is specific for the same muscle that is stretched. This response is called **stretch reflex (Fig. 80.3)**. *Stretch reflex is the only monosynaptic reflex in the human body. The physiological basis of tendon jerks is the monosynaptic stretch reflex.*
- **Stimulus**: Sudden stretch of the skeletal muscle.
- **Receptor**: Muscle spindle.
- **Afferent neuron**: Dorsal root ganglion (DRG) cell of spinal cord, the central process enters the spinal cord through the posterior root.
- **Center**: Spinal cord α-motor neuron or brainstem nucleus with which afferent nerve fiber synapse. The neurotransmitter involved is **glutamate**.
- **Efferent:** The axon of α-motor neuron, which leaves the spinal cord through the ventral nerve root and supplies the same muscle.
- **Effector organ**: The same muscle that has been stretched
- **Effect**: Contraction of the same muscle.

Reaction time is the time interval between the application of the stimulus and the response. For a stretch reflex, reaction time is only 19–24 msec. **Central delay** for stretch reflex is only 0.6–0.9 msec since there is only one synapse in the pathway. *Stretch reflex is the quickest of all reflexes.*

Muscle Spindle

Muscle spindles are the receptors of stretch reflex present in all skeletal muscles. Function of muscle spindle is to signal changes in the length and rate of change of length of the muscle in which it is located. Changes in muscle length are associated with changes in joint angle; thus muscle spindles provide information on position of joints, i.e., proprioception.

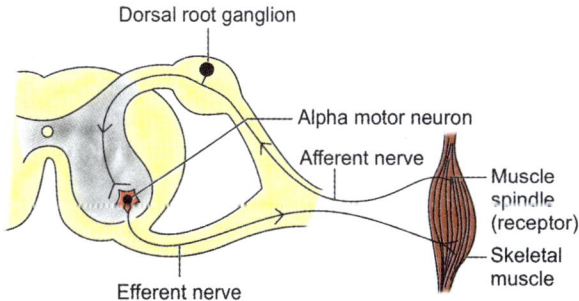

Fig. 80.3: Monosynaptic reflex (stretch reflex).

Muscle spindles are small spindle shaped structures, 5–10 mm long, 100 μm in diameter and embryonic in nature. They are constituted by 3–10 small muscle fibers enclosed in a connective tissue capsule, distributed throughout the belly of the skeletal muscle. These fibers are called **intrafusal fibers** and the regular contractile units of the muscle form **extrafusal fibers or skeletal muscle fibers (Fig. 80.4)**. The muscle spindle is spindle shaped and the ends of the spindle capsule are attached to the tendon or to the glycocalyx of the adjacent extrafusal skeletal muscle fibers. *They are arranged parallel to the extrafusal fibers.* The number of muscle spindles in a muscle is proportionate to the degree of precision required for the contraction of the muscle. For example, the gastrocnemius muscle contains few spindles while the interossei muscles of hand contain numerous spindles. They are also present in plenty in muscles involved in the control of posture.
- Intrafusal fibers: Fibers in the muscle spindle
- Extrafusal fibers: Skeletal muscle fibers.

In the muscle spindle, contractile elements are seen only in the peripheral portion of the intrafusal fibers. Central portion is devoid of contractile elements (actin and myosin). *It is the non-contractile central part of the muscle spindle, which is sensitive to stretch.* The receptor portion of the muscle spindle is its central portion. There are two types of intrafusal fibers:
1. Nuclear bag fibers
2. Nuclear chain fibers

Nuclear bag has a central bulging containing many nuclei in the central portion. The two subtypes of nuclear bag fibers are **dynamic and static nuclear bag fibers**. Static nuclear bag fiber has the same function as nuclear chain fiber. Nuclear chain fibers are smaller and their ends are attached to nuclear bag fibers. Nuclei are arranged in a chain in the nuclear chain fibers at the center, with no central bulging. Each muscle spindle contains two nuclear bag fibers and four or five nuclear chain fibers.

Innervation of Muscle Spindle

Sensory Supply

Two types of sensory nerve fibers innervate each muscle spindle:
1. A single rapidly conducting type Ia (Aα) afferent fiber, 12–20 μm in diameter with a conduction velocity of 70–120 m/sec. It winds round the central portion of the nuclear bag and nuclear chain fibers. It is also called **annulospiral nerve endings or primary endings**. These endings are stimulated by both the nuclear bag and the nuclear chain intrafusal fibers.
2. **Flower spray nerve endings or secondary endings** (8 μm in diameter) usually eight in number are seen in the nuclear chain fibers and static nuclear bag fibers on either side of annulospiral nerve ending. These are type II (Aβ) sensory nerve endings **(Fig. 80.4)**. *These fibers do not innervate the dynamic nuclear bag fibers.* The secondary ending is usually excited only by nuclear chain fibers.

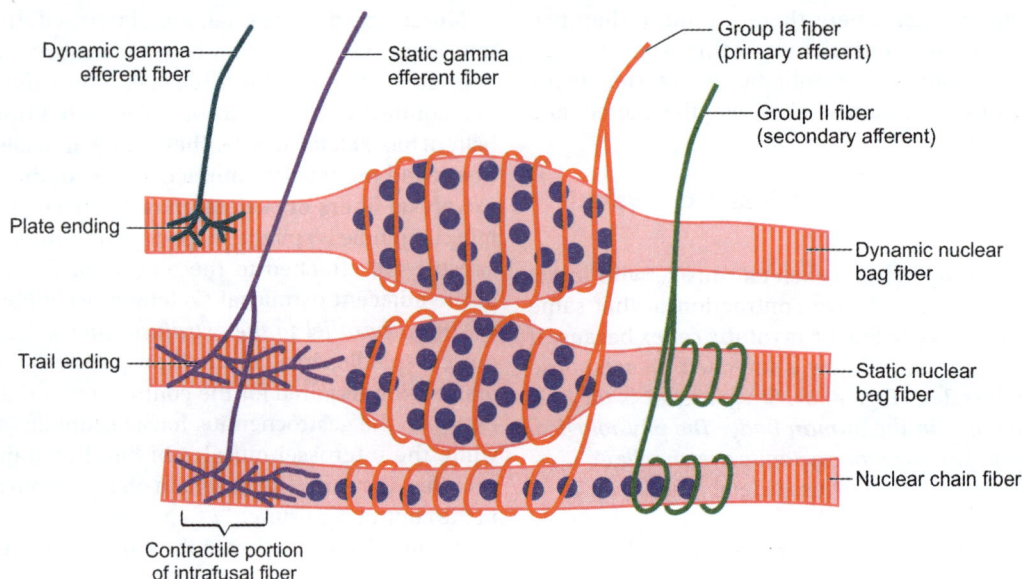

Fig. 80.4: Structure and innervation of muscle spindle. A single Ia afferent fiber innervates all three types of intrafusal fibers (dynamic and static nuclear bag and nuclear chain fibers). Group II sensory fibers innervates only nuclear chain and static nuclear bag fibers.

Motor Supply to Muscle Spindle

Unlike any other receptor, muscle spindle has a motor nerve supply, a unique situation in which a receptor is having a motor supply of its own. Motor supply comes from special neurons in the anterior horn of spinal cord called γ **motor neurons**. They are small motor neurons, the axons of which supply only the muscle spindle. Axons belong to Aγ fiber type and leave the spinal cord through the anterior root and supply only the peripheral portions of the muscle spindle and thus cause contraction of the peripheral portion of muscle spindle **(Fig. 80.5)**. There will be stretching of the central portion of the muscle spindle when the peripheral portions of the intrafusal fiber contract. This in turn stimulates the sensory nerve endings which can lead to reflex contraction of the muscle (refer spindle loading). The γ-motor neurons constitute 30% of the fibers in the ventral root of spinal cord.

The γ-efferent endings in the muscle spindle are of two histological types. They are **plate endings** which end on the motor endplates of nuclear bag fiber and **trail endings** that form extensive networks on the nuclear chain fibers. The gamma efferents are further subdivided into two groups: γ_1 and γ_2 fibers. Gamma-1 or gamma-dynamic (γ- d) fibers supply the ends of dynamic nuclear bag fibers and γ_2-fibers or gamma-static (γ-s) fibers supply static nuclear bag and nuclear chain fibers. Gamma-d fibers excite the dynamic nuclear bag fibers and gamma-s fibers excite the nuclear chain fibers and static nuclear bag fibers. When the gamma-d fibers excite the dynamic nuclear bag fibers, the dynamic response of the muscle spindle becomes tremendously enhanced, whereas the static response is hardly affected. On the other hand, stimulation of the gamma-s fibers enhances the static response while having little influence on the dynamic response.

Factors Affecting Gamma Efferent Discharge

- Anxiety increases gamma efferent discharge
- **Alpha-gamma coactivation**: When alpha motor neurons are stimulated, the gamma motor neurons are also stimulated at the same time. This helps in sustained contraction
- Noxious stimuli increase γ-efferent discharge in the ipsilateral flexor muscles and decrease γ discharge in ipsilateral extensors.
- Other motor activities like Jendrassik's maneuver increases γ-discharge and causes augmentation of reflexes.
- Increased activity of bulboreticular facilitatory area increase γ-efferent discharge and lead to hypertonia.

Spindle Loading and Unloading

Stretching of the equatorial region of the intrafusal fiber is called **spindle loading**. The muscle spindle becomes loaded when the muscle is stretched or when descending motor influences from the brain stimulates the γ-motor neurons.

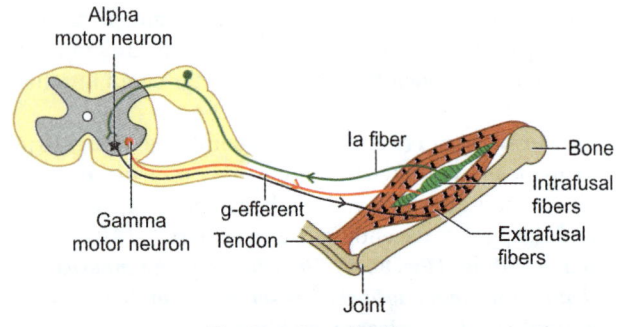

Fig. 80.5: Stretch reflex.

When a muscle is stretched, the spindle is also stretched. Stretching of the equatorial region of the intrafusal fiber stimulates the sensory afferents originating there. When the γ-motor neurons are stimulated, the peripheral parts of the intrafusal fiber contract. Contraction of the peripheral part of the spindle results in stretching of its central part and stimulates the spindle afferents.

Stimulation of α-motor neurons produces contraction of the extrafusal fiber. Since the ends of the spindle are attached to the extrafusal fibers, the spindle folds up when the extrafusal fibers contract and the spindle afferent discharge decreases. This is called **spindle unloading (Figs. 80.6A to D)**. Thus α-motor neuron discharge decreases the spindle afferent discharge.

Functions of Muscle Spindle

❖ Muscle spindle send information to the nervous system about muscle length or rate of change in length.
❖ The muscle spindle and its reflex connections operate as a feedback device to maintain muscle length. When a muscle is stretched, spindle discharge increases and reflex shortening of the muscle occurs. When a muscle is shortened without a change in gamma efferent discharge, spindle afferent activity decreases and the muscle relaxes.
❖ Dynamic and static responses of the muscle spindle afferents help to minimize physiological tremor. This is because of the sensitivity of the muscle spindle to the velocity of stretch. **Physiological tremor** manifests as a mild high frequency (10–12 Hz), postural or action tremor which is not visible. It is a normal phenomenon which affect everyone while maintaining posture or during movements. Physiological tremor is the result of a small oscillation in the feedback loop regulating muscle length. The oscillations caused by conduction delays in this feedback loop is dampened by the prompt, marked phasic response of Ia sensory fiber endings in the muscle spindle to dynamic (phasic) events in the muscle.
Enhanced physiological tremor which is clearly visible is seen in 10% of the population in association with anxiety, fatigue, etc. It is also seen in hyperthyroidism, electrolyte abnormalities and alcoholism.

❖ For determining joint angulations in midranges of motion, the muscle spindles are among the most important receptors. When the angle of a joint is changing, some muscles are being stretched while others become lax, and the net information from the spindle is transmitted into the integrating centers of spinal cord and higher regions of the dorsal column system for interpreting joint angulations. Thus muscle spindles provide information on position, i.e., proprioception.

(At the extremes of joint angulation, stretch of the ligaments and deep tissues around the joints is an additional important factor in determining position. Types of sensory endings used for this are the Pacinian corpuscles, Ruffini's endings, and receptors similar to the Golgi tendon receptors found in muscle tendons).

Static and Dynamic Spindle Responses

Muscle spindle is stimulated whenever the skeletal muscle is stretched and action potentials are set up in the sensory nerve, proportionate to the degree of stretching. So, stretch is the stimulus for muscle spindle and the effect is reflex contraction of the skeletal muscle. Whenever a small stretch is applied, immediate contraction is seen for a short duration (phasic response). If the stretch is sustained, contraction of muscle is also prolonged due to reflex firing of impulses. This is **static contraction** or sustained contraction of muscle.

Muscle spindle shows static and dynamic responses, i.e., muscle spindle can respond to change in the length of muscle fiber (degree of stretch) and also to the rate of change in length of muscle fiber.

Nuclear bag fibers show **dynamic response**, whereas nuclear chain fibers show **static response**. Afferents originating in the nuclear bag fibers discharge impulses at a frequency proportional to the rate at which the muscle is being stretched (dynamic response). The afferents originating in the nuclear chain fibers discharge with a frequency proportional to the degree of stretch (static response), i.e., afferents from nuclear chain fibers are stimulated only by a sustained stretch.

The primary and secondary nerve endings in the muscle spindle respond differently to stretch. Since group-Ia afferents

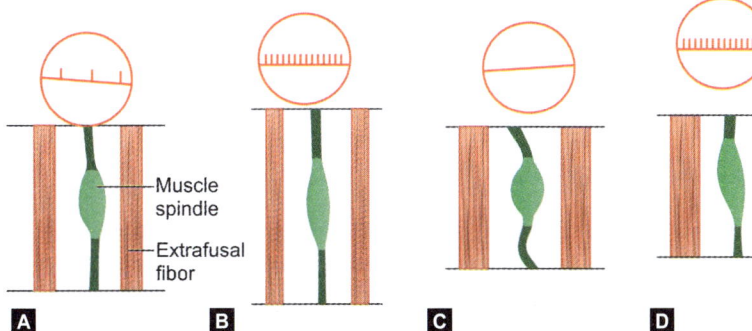

Figs. 80.6A to D: Loading and unloading the muscle spindle: (A) Muscle at rest; (B) Muscle stretched (the spindle is also stretched and the sensory endings are activated). This is loading the spindle; (C) Muscle contracted. Spindle sensory endings stop firing. This is unloading the spindle; (D) Muscle contracted but gamma efferent discharge to spindle increased. This causes contractile ends of spindle to shorten and the nuclear bag region stretches and sensory endings fire rapidly.

originate from both nuclear bag and chain fibers, they show both static as well as dynamic responses. The primary nerve ending in the nuclear bag region discharge most rapidly while the muscle is being stretched suddenly and less rapidly during sustained stretch. Ia afferents are very sensitive to the velocity of the change in muscle length during a stretch. This is called a *dynamic response*. A branch of the primary ending (type Ia fiber) from the muscle spindle terminate directly on the alpha motor neurons supplying the extrafusal fibers of the same muscle from which the type Ia fiber originated. Thus they provide information about the speed of movement and helps in quick corrective movements.

The primary nerve endings in the nuclear chain fibers discharge at an increased rate throughout the period of sustained stretch. This is called *static response*.

Group II secondary afferents originate only from the nuclear chain fibers and therefore show only static response, i.e., they are stimulated when the muscle spindle is stretched slowly. Most of the type II fibers from the muscle spindle terminate on multiple interneurons in the gray matter of spinal cord and transmit delayed signals to the alpha motor neurons in contrast to type Ia fibers. These endings continue to transmit impulses for some time if the spindle remains stretched. The primary ending or annulospiral nerve ending (group Ia) is sensitive both to the amount of stretch and to its rate, whereas secondary ending in nuclear chain fibers responds chiefly to the amount of stretch. In other words, the primary endings signal both the length of the muscle and the rate of change in length, whereas secondary endings signal only the length of the muscle, i.e., sustained stretch.

Clinically stretch reflexes are elicited by applying small sudden stretch to the muscle using a knee hammer (reflex hammer). Examples of clinically tested stretch reflexes are knee jerk, ankle jerk, biceps and triceps jerk, jaw jerk and supinator jerk.

Knee Jerk

Knee jerk is elicited by a light tap on the patellar tendon with a reflex hammer. The tap deflects the tendon, which then pulls on and briefly stretches the quadriceps femoris muscle. A reflexive contraction of the quadriceps quickly follows observed as a forward movement of leg. Thus, stretching of a skeletal muscle causes rapid feedback excitation of the same muscle through the shortest circuit involving one sensory neuron, one synapse, and one alpha motor neuron.

- **Receptors**: Muscle spindles in the quadriceps.
- **Afferent limb**: Ia fiber
- **Center**: α-motor neurons in the L3, L4 segments of spinal cord.
- **Efferent limb**: Axon of α-motor neuron supplying the quadriceps muscle
- **Effect**: Contraction of quadriceps femoris and forward movement of leg.

Absence of knee jerk may indicate some abnormality or lesion anywhere in the reflex arc. It may be in the muscle spindle, the afferent Ia fibers or in the motor neurons to the quadriceps femoris muscle, e.g., peripheral neuropathy.

A *hyperactive knee jerk* may be due to interruption of the descending pathways that suppress the activity of the reflex arc, e.g., UMN lesion.

Ankle Jerk

In ankle jerk, the gastrocnemius muscle is stretched by tapping the Achilles tendon at the ankle joint and the effect is contraction of gastrocnemius and plantar flexion of foot. Center is motor neuron in S_1 segment of spinal cord.

Other deep tendon reflexes (DTR) elicited during neurological examination are triceps jerk (C7), biceps jerk (C5, C6), supinator jerk and jaw jerk.

Sustained Stretch

In sustained stretch, impulses pass through group Ia and group II fibers, resulting in static or sustained contraction of muscle. This is necessary for maintaining posture of the body. The gravitational pull is stretching the muscles of the back of leg, body and neck leading to sustained contraction of these muscles for maintaining the standing posture. These muscles are also called *antigravity muscles*.

Stretch is not the only stimulus for muscle spindle. When the γ-motor neurons are stimulated experimentally, it causes contraction of muscle spindle which in turn causes reflex contraction of muscle in which the muscle spindle is present.

If a stretch is applied to a muscle when the γ-motor neuron activity is more in the body, the force of contraction of the muscle will be greater than normal. γ-motor neuron activity increases the sensitivity of muscle spindle to stretch and thus γ-*motor neurons play a very important role in maintaining normal muscle tone.*

Exaggerated stretch reflex will be seen if there is increased γ-motor neuron firing as in upper motor neuron lesion.

Alpha-gamma Coactivation

Continuous contraction of a muscle is made possible by activation of gamma motor neurons along with α-motor neurons. When γ-motor neurons are stimulated, there is contraction of the peripheral portions of the intrafusal fiber. When the two ends of the spindle contract, it stretches the central part of the spindle stimulating the primary nerve endings. Thus when a muscle contracts, due to alpha-gamma coactivation, its spindle remains active and this leads to contraction of the extrafusal fibers and intrafusal fibers at the same time **(Fig. 80.6D)**. If the muscle is shortened without a change in gamma efferent discharge, the muscle spindle discharge decreases and the muscle relaxes.

Continuous contraction of the antigravity muscles helps in maintaining a standing posture. When γ-motor neurons are stimulated along with α-motor neurons, the stretch on the central part of the spindle becomes continuous and the contraction of the extrafusal fibers continues. This is α-γ **coactivation**. This coactivation can produce sustained contraction of a muscle because the spindle discharge continues throughout the muscle contraction.

Table 80.1: Differences between alpha motor neuron and gamma motor neuron.

Alpha motor neuron	Gamma motor neuron
Large, multipolar neuron having a soma diameter of 70 μm	Small neuron with a soma diameter of 35 μm
Supplies ordinary skeletal muscle fibers (extrafusal fibers)	Supplies intrafusal fibers of muscle spindle (receptor)
Form final common pathway since all impulses for skeletal muscle contraction pass through α-motor neuron	Not responsible for muscle contraction directly
Controlled mainly by pyramidal tract	Controlled by extrapyramidal tracts
Does not affect the sensitivity of muscle spindle	Increases muscle spindle sensitivity
Only one type is seen in the anterior horn of spinal cord	Static and dynamic γ-motor neurons are present in the anterior horn

Differences between alpha motor neuron and gamma motor neuron are summarized in **Table 80.1**.

Higher Control of Stretch Reflex

Since there are connections between afferent and efferent neurons in the CNS, the reflex activity can be modified by higher centers. For a normal reflex action, there will be a balance between the excitatory and inhibitory influence of higher centers on the reflex. The gamma motor neuron activity is regulated mainly by the descending tracts from different brain areas.

❖ Facilitatory area of reticular formation in the brain stem increases the sensitivity of muscle spindle and the stretch reflex becomes hyperactive.
❖ Inhibitory area of reticular formation inhibits gamma efferent discharge and decrease spindle sensitivity.
  Fibers from the cerebral cortex and cerebellum stimulate the inhibitory reticular formation and reflexly inhibit the stretch reflex. Basal ganglia inhibit stretch reflex by stimulating the inhibitory area or by inhibiting the facilitatory reticular formation.
❖ Anxiety produces hyperactive tendon reflexes because it increases gamma efferent discharge.

Physiological Importance of Stretch Reflex

Stretch reflex is responsible for maintaining muscle tone and thus maintains posture and equilibrium of the body. Excitatory impulses from the alpha motor neurons alone cannot control muscle function. It also needs a continuous feedback of sensory information from each muscle to the spinal cord, indicating the functional status of the muscle at each instant. The muscle spindle as well as the Golgi tendon organ provides this information and muscle contraction will be adjusted unconsciously without oscillations.

Clinical Importance of Stretch Reflex

In clinical examination, tendon jerks like knee jerk, biceps jerk, triceps jerk, supinator jerk, ankle jerk and jaw jerk are elicited. In certain diseases of the nervous system where reflex arc is affected as in lower motor neuron lesion, these jerks are abolished. In certain other neurological conditions like hemiplegia or upper motor neuron lesion these tendon jerks are exaggerated.

Spinal cord is the center of all the reflex activities in the limbs. The responses produced by the spinal cord are modified by the influences from other parts of the nervous system. The modification may suppress a normal spinal reflex or may facilitate the appearance of such new reflexes, which would not have been offered by the cord alone. Those lesions which do not damage the spinal reflex arc directly but which affect these modifying influences are therefore capable of altering the reflex function. Thus in diseases, a reflex seen in health might change its pattern or even may get abolished; otherwise reflexes not seen during health might now appear. Such apparently new reflexes, which appear because of a disease are described as **pathological reflexes,** e.g., extensor plantar response.

Hypoactive stretch reflexes are seen in destruction of afferent or efferent nerve to muscle, hypothyroidism and lesion in the excitatory reticular formation. Hyperactive stretch reflexes are seen in hyperthyroidism, anxiety, stimulation of facilitatory reticular formation, inhibition of inhibitory area, etc.

During neurological examination, the deep tendon reflexes are graded on the following scale:
❖ Grade 0: No response (absent)
❖ Grade 1+: Hypoactive
❖ Grade 2+: Brisk (normal)
❖ Grade 3+: Hyperactive without clonus
❖ Grade 4+: Hyperactive with mild clonus
❖ Grade 5+: Hyperactive with sustained clonus.

Bisynaptic Reflex

There are two synapses in the bisynaptic reflex pathway. Examples are **reciprocal innervation** to antagonistic muscle and **inverse stretch reflex**.

Passive stretching of a skeletal muscle with intact nerve supply causes a reflexive contraction of that same muscle which is referred to as stretch reflex. At the same time as the stretched muscle is being stimulated to contract, parallel circuits are inhibiting the alpha motor neurons of its *antagonist* muscles (i.e., those muscles that move a joint in the opposite direction). Thus, as the knee jerk reflex causes contraction of the quadriceps muscle, it simultaneously causes relaxation of its antagonists, including the semitendinosus muscle. To achieve inhibition, branches of the group Ia sensory axons excite specific interneurons that *inhibit* the alpha motor neurons of the antagonists. This **reciprocal innervation** increases the effectiveness of the stretch reflex by minimizing the antagonistic forces of the antagonist muscles.

Reciprocal Innervation

During movement the muscle that contracts and brings about the movement, is the **agonist**. The muscle that opposes the agonist is the **antagonist**. For example, during flexion at the elbow, the biceps contracts and is the agonist. At the same time, the triceps relaxes, which is the antagonist. Due to reciprocal innervation, the movement of agonist muscle is not opposed by the contraction of the antagonist.

The afferent nerve fiber from the agonist muscle entering the spinal cord gives collateral to an inhibitory interneuron which makes synapse with the α-motor neuron that supplies the antagonistic muscle. This is **reciprocal innervation** and the interneuron is **Golgi bottle neuron**. When the muscle is stretched, the motor neuron supplying the stretched muscle is stimulated and the muscle contracts. At the same time, the collateral from the afferent fiber inhibits the motor neuron supplying the antagonistic muscle through the inhibitory interneuron. This is **reciprocal inhibition** through reciprocal innervation **(Fig. 80.7)**.

Inverse Stretch Reflex

Another example for bisynaptic reflex is **inverse stretch reflex**. As seen in the stretch reflex, the harder a muscle is stretched, the stronger is its reflex contraction. But there is a limit to this stretch. If a very strong stretch is applied, instead of muscle contraction there is reflex relaxation of that muscle and this is referred to as *inverse stretch reflex* or Golgi tendon reflex or autogenic inhibition **(Fig. 80.8)**. It is a protective reflex that prevents excessive rise in muscle tension and tearing of the muscle when a muscle is strongly stretched or when it undergoes severe contraction.

Receptor is Golgi tendon organ (GTO) or **neurotendinous spindle** which is located in the muscle tendon. Like muscle spindle, Golgi tendon organs are also stretch receptors. However, unlike the muscle spindle which acts as a muscle length-detector, the Golgi tendon organ acts as a muscle tension-detector. They transmit information regarding tendon tension and rate of change in tension.

Golgi afferent fibers belong to group Ib fiber. The sensory endings of the group Ib fiber in the Golgi tendon organ is arranged in series with the extrafusal fibers **(Fig. 80.9B)**, in contrast to the parallel arrangement of muscle spindle with the extrafusal fibers **(Fig. 80.9A)**. Because of their arrangement in series with the extrafusal fibers, GTO can be activated either by muscle stretch or by strong contraction of the muscle. Muscle contraction is a more effective stimulus for GTO than muscle stretch.

When the muscle contracts isometrically, or when a muscle is stretched excessively, the tendon is stretched and the tension in the tendon rises markedly. This rise in tension stimulates the Golgi tendon organ. Afferent Ib fibers from the GTO terminate on inhibitory interneurons in the spinal cord. These interneurons which release inhibitory neurotransmitter terminate on the α-motor neuron in the anterior horn and inhibit them so that the firing from α-motor neurons is suppressed and the muscle relaxes. This reflex relaxation of the extrafusal fibers in response to a rise in muscle tension is called inverse stretch reflex. *Golgi tendon organ thus acts as a transducer regulating the tension of the*

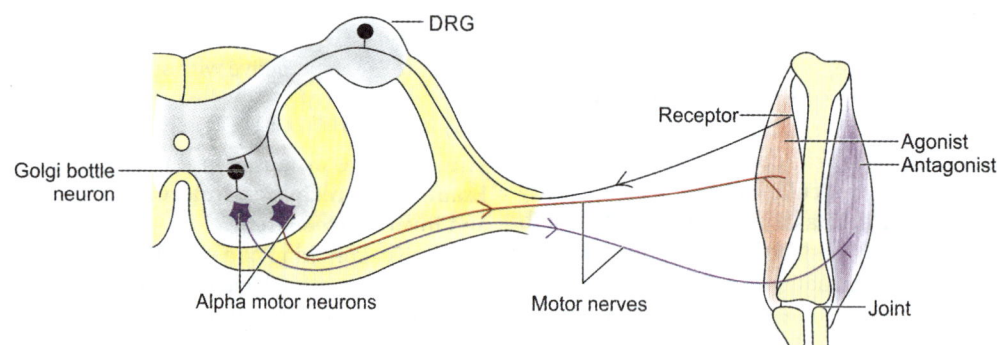

Fig. 80.7: Bisynaptic reflex (reciprocal innervation and inhibition).
(DRG: dorsal root ganglion)

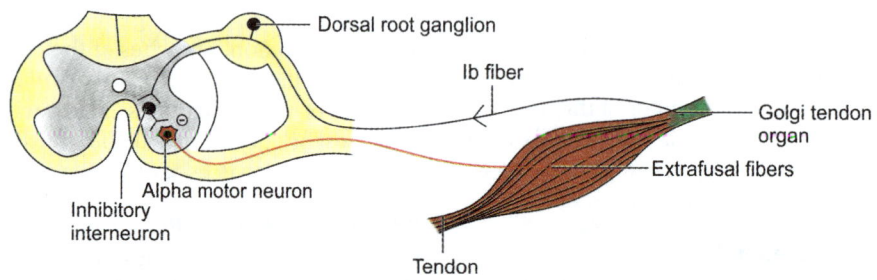

Fig. 80.8: Inverse stretch reflex.

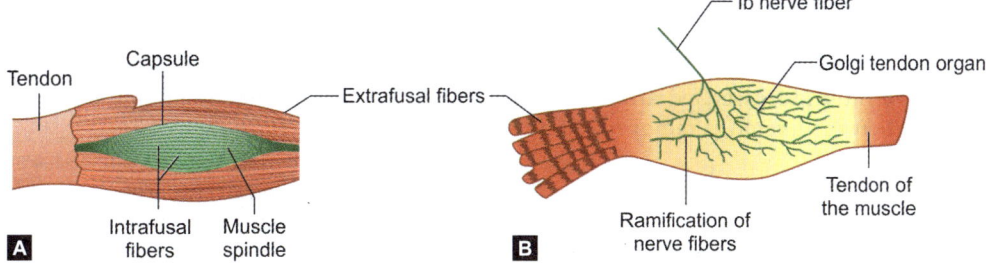

Figs. 80.9A and B: Difference between muscle spindle and Golgi tendon organ. The muscle spindle is arranged in parallel with the extrafusal fibers whereas Golgi tendon organ is arranged in series with the extrafusal fibers (muscle fibers): (A) Muscle spindle; (B) Golgi tendon organ.

muscle. *Muscle spindles are excitatory to muscle tone, whereas Golgi tendon organs are inhibitory to muscle tone.*

Golgi tendon organ decides the tension in the muscle, and muscle spindle regulates the length of muscle. Thus impulses from the muscle spindle and Golgi tendon organ help the nervous system to know the status of muscle contraction and the tension in the muscle tendon at each instant. The signals from these two receptors operate at a subconscious level in intrinsic muscle control at the level of spinal cord. In addition to the spinal cord, they also transmit information to the cerebellum and cerebral cortex helping these areas of the nervous system to control muscle contraction. For the differences between muscle spindle and Golgi tendon organ (**Table 80.2**).

The sequence of moderate stretch producing contraction and stronger stretch causing relaxation can be better studied in cases of hypertonia where clasp-knife phenomenon and clonus are seen.

Clasp Knife Effect or Lengthening Reaction

Clasp-knife effect is a phenomenon seen in upper motor neuron lesion where there is hypertonia. It is the response of a spastic muscle to stretching and is due to the operation of stretch reflex and inverse stretch reflex. If the hypertonic limb is flexed forcefully there is an initial resistance and then suddenly the limb flexes. This is clasp-knife effect (because of its resemblance to the closing of a pocket knife) or **lengthening reaction** (because it is the response of a spastic muscle to lengthening). When the hypertonic muscle is flexed forcefully, it relaxes due to excessive stretch and gives way, leading to sudden flexion compared to a pocketknife or clasp knife. This is due to the operation of inverse stretch reflex.

Clonus

Regular, rhythmic contraction of a skeletal muscle when it is subjected to sudden, maintained stretch is called **clonus**. It is a feature of hypertonia and is due to increased gamma efferent discharge to the muscle spindles of the hypertonic muscle. Here, stretch reflex and inverse stretch reflex alternate.

Ankle clonus is a neurological sign elicited in the gastrocnemius muscle in **hypertonia**. When the foot is extended forcefully there will be repeated contraction and relaxation of the gastrocnemius muscle as long as the stretch is maintained. This is ankle clonus. Similarly, **patellar clonus** can be elicited in these patients, where the patella is pushed

Table 80.2: Comparison between muscle spindle and Golgi tendon organ (GTO).	
Muscle spindle	*Golgi tendon organ*
Receptor for stretch reflex	Receptor for inverse stretch reflex
Located in between extrafusal fibers	Located in the muscle tendon
Arranged in parallel to the extrafusal fibers	Arranged in series with the extrafusal fibers
Innervated by type Ia and type II afferent fibers	Innervated by type Ib afferent fibers
Afferent fiber synapses with alpha motor neuron in the anterior horn of spinal cord	Afferent fiber synapses with inhibitory interneurons in the dorsal gray horn of spinal cord
Has a motor supply of its own through gamma motor neuron	Has no motor innervation
It is a stretch receptor that acts as a muscle length-detector. Sends information to the nervous system about muscle length or rate of change in length	Stretch receptor which acts as muscle tension-detector. GTO transmit information about tendon tension or rate of change of tension
Stimulated when the skeletal muscle is stretched within a limit	Stimulated during excessive stretch as well as during excessive contraction of skeletal muscle
Stimulation of the muscle spindle causes contraction of the stretched muscle	Stimulation of GTO causes relaxation of the skeletal muscle
Excitatory to muscle tone	Inhibitory to muscle tone
Function is to maintain muscle tone and posture	Function is to prevent excessive rise in muscle tension

downwards, which stretches the quadriceps muscle leading to repeated contraction and relaxation of quadriceps. Here, inverse stretch reflex is being repeated and since there is clonic contraction of muscle it is called ankle clonus and patellar clonus. When the stretch is removed, clonus stops.

Polysynaptic Reflex

In polysynaptic reflex, there are more than two synapses in the reflex pathway. Interneurons are interposed between the afferent and the efferent neurons in polysynaptic reflexes. The superficial reflexes like abdominal and cremasteric reflexes are polysynaptic reflexes. Typical example for polysynaptic reflex is **flexor reflex or withdrawal reflex** in response to a noxious stimulus (painful stimulus). Effect is flexion of the limb and hence called flexor reflex. Since the body tries to move away from the stimulus it is called withdrawal reflex **(Fig. 80.10)**.

Withdrawal reflex

- **Receptor**: Pain receptor or free nerve ending
- **Afferent neuron:** DRG cell
- **Center**: Spinal cord.

The afferent limb divides into a number of branches in a complex pattern. The reflex pathway branches in a complex fashion and the number of synapses in each of their branches vary from two to many hundreds. Thus impulse has to pass through a series of neurons before it reaches the α-motor neuron that supplies the flexor muscle. Output discharge will be prolonged since there are after-discharges and reverberatory circuits in the pathway. Reciprocal innervation is also seen in the circuit that supplies the antagonistic muscle.

- **Efferent**: Axon of α-motor neuron is the final common pathway.
- **Effector organ**: Flexor muscle.
- **Effect:** Contraction of flexor muscle and relaxation of extensor muscle of the same limb. Limb that is stimulated is flexed and withdrawn from the stimulus. Withdrawal reflex is more evident in the limbs, but is present in all parts of the body. With a stronger stimulus, in addition to flexor reflex there will be extension of the opposite limb

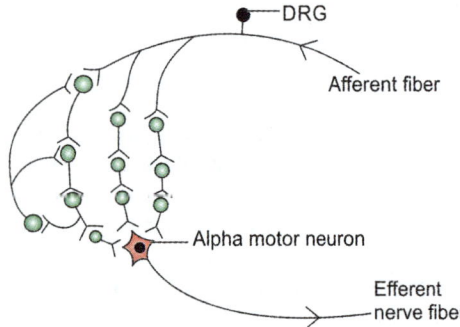

Fig. 80.10: Polysynaptic reflex (withdrawal reflex; DRG—dorsal root ganglion).

also. This is called **crossed extensor reflex**. This is because a strong stimulus causes spread of excitatory impulses up and down the spinal cord to more and more motor units. This is called irradiation of impulses and recruitment of motor units.

The superficial reflexes are elicited by stimulation of skin or mucous membrane. They are either withdrawal reflexes or their modifications. When an adequate sensory stimulus is applied, the motor response occurs in the form of contraction of an appropriate group of muscles. The severity of contraction depends on the number of the receptors (sensory units) stimulated.

The superficial reflexes result from the activity of the spinal cord neurons that are modified by the influence of higher neurons. Impulses ascend to the parietal areas of the brain and have connections with the motor centers in the pyramidal and the extrapyramidal cortical areas. Efferent impulses then descend in the pyramidal or extrapyramidal pathways. As a consequence, not only a sensory interruption but also an interruption in the descending pathways from the upper motor neurons can cause diminution, abolition or modification of the superficial reflexes. Superficial reflexes will be brisk in anxiety; psychosis, etc. There is a center in the midbrain, which normally inhibits the superficial reflexes. In Parkinson's disease and other extrapyramidal diseases, this center is involved leading to brisk superficial reflexes.

Local Sign

The exact pattern of flexor reflex response depends on the location of stimulus. If the stimulus is applied on the medial side of the limb, in addition to flexion there will be abduction of limb. If the stimulus is applied on the lateral aspect of limb, the limb is flexed and adducted. This dependence of reflex response on the location of stimulus is called **local sign**.

Crossed Extensor Reflex

When a reflex on one side of the body is elicited, it causes opposite effects on the contralateral limb (the limb of the other side of the body). For example, when a strong stimulus is applied to one limb, in addition to flexion and withdrawal of that limb there will be extension of the contralateral limb to support the body. This is crossed extensor reflex which is also a withdrawal reflex. Withdrawal reflex has a very important role in the regulation of posture of the body.

Once the sensory fibers enter the spinal cord from the posterior root, they bifurcate and branch and go both up and down the spinal cord and transmit signals to many segments. These ascending and descending fibers in the spinal cord are mainly responsible for the multisegmental reflexes like reflexes that coordinate simultaneous movements in the forelimbs and hind limbs. There is also irradiation of impulses from one side of the spinal cord to the opposite side through the commissures. This can be better demonstrated in a spinal animal.

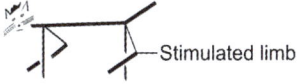

Fig. 80.11: Spinal cat.

Spinal Animal

The above responses, i.e., local sign and crossed extensor reflex can be studied in a spinal animal. A **spinal animal** is one whose spinal cord is interrupted from the influence of higher centers by sectioning the spinal cord. In a spinal cat, if a stronger stimulus is applied on one of the hind limb the following effects are seen:
- Flexion of stimulated hind limb
- Extension of opposite hind limb
- Extension of ipsilateral fore limb
- Flexion of contralateral fore limb.

This response is called **shifting reaction** or four limb reflex response. Here, impulses spread to all the four limbs by irradiation in order to keep the body erect. These effects can be elicited only in a spinal animal **(Fig. 80.11)**.

■ GENERAL PROPERTIES OF REFLEXES

All the properties of synapses are included in the properties of reflexes because synapse is a part of reflex pathway (*refer* **properties of synapse**).
- One-way conduction
- Reaction time and central delay
- Summation
- After-discharge or reflex momentum
- Reciprocal inhibition
- Irradiation and recruitment
- Grading of reflex
- Fractionation and occlusion
- Summation of subliminal fringe
- Post-tetanic potentiation
- Fatigue
- Habituation and sensitization
- Adequate stimulus
- Principle of final common pathway
- Central excitatory and inhibitory states
- Adaptation and modification of reflexes.

Reaction Time

The duration from the time of application of stimulus to the time when response is obtained is called reaction time. For knee jerk, reaction time is 19–24 msec.

Central Delay

The time taken by the impulse to traverse the spinal cord is called central delay. It includes synaptic delay. For knee jerk, it is 0.6–0.9 msec.

Irradiation of Impulses

The impulses can move up and down the spinal cord, and can spread to more and more motor neurons. This property is called irradiation of impulses. It is responsible for crossed extensor reflex.

Recruitment

When more and more neurons are involved, more and more motor units are included. This is called recruitment.

Grading of Reflex

Stronger stimulus can produce a greater response by irradiation and recruitment. This is called grading of reflex.

Fractionation and Occlusion (Fig. 80.12)

When a muscle is stimulated directly or through the motor nerve, the magnitude of contraction is greater than when it is stimulated by stimulating the sensory nerve to the muscle. When sensory nerve is stimulated, only a fraction or portion of motor units is activated and hence contraction will be less. This is due to **occlusion**.
- Simulation of A = 9
- Stimulation of B = 9
- A + B = 12.

When nerve A is stimulated, 9 neurons are activated. Stimulation of nerve B stimulates 9 neurons. Stimulation of these of A and B together causes stimulation of only 12 neurons. If two afferent nerves are stimulated simultaneously, the response obtained is smaller than the sum of maximum response expected by summation of these two nerves separately.

This is due to central overlapping by afferent nerves, i.e., different afferent nerves share the same motor neurons. This property is called **occlusion**.

Summation of Subliminal Fringe (Fig. 80.13)

- A = 3
- B = 3
- A + B = 12

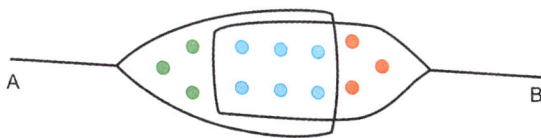

Fig. 80.12: Occlusion: When nerve A is stimulated 9 neurons are activated and when nerve B stimulated 9 neurons are stimulated. But stimulation of A and B together activate only 12 neurons.
A = 9; B = 9; A + B = 12.

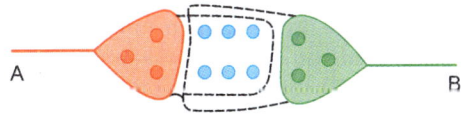

Fig. 80.13: Summation of subliminal fringe. When A and B are stimulated separately, each can activate only 3 neurons. But stimulation of A and B together produce action potentials in 12 neurons. This is because excitability of 6 neurons were high, i.e., they are in the subliminal fringe, only A or B is stimulated.
A = 3, B = 3, A + B = 12.

Stimulation of A stimulates 3 neurons and B stimulates 3 neurons. Simultaneous stimulation of A and B together stimulates 12 neurons instead of 6. Here, when the two afferent nerves are simultaneously stimulated, the response obtained is greater than the sum of the responses obtained when these nerves are stimulated separately. When one afferent fiber alone is stimulated, 3 neurons reach the discharge zone and can produce impulses. But, 6 neurons are in the subliminal fringe (excitability is increased but has not reached the threshold level or firing level), so, cannot produce impulses. Simultaneous stimulation of A and B together causes **summation of subliminal fringe** and all the twelve neurons start discharging impulses.

Habituation and Sensitization of Reflex Responses

Reflex responses can be modified by experience. If the stimulus is benign and repeated at intervals, the response declines and disappears. This phenomenon is called **habituation**.

Prolonged facilitation of synaptic conduction in a reflex can be produced by a noxious stimulus and can last from hours to days. This is called **sensitization** of reflex response.

Adequate Stimulus

The reflex activity is specific in terms of both the stimulus and the response. The receptors respond only when an appropriate specific stimulus is applied. A particular stimulus produces a particular response. The stimulus that produces a reflex is very precise and is called the **adequate stimulus** for the particular reflex.

Final Common Path

Lower motor neurons are the neurons that directly innervate the skeletal muscle fibers. The cell body of these neurons is located in the ventral horn of the spinal cord or in the corresponding cranial nerve nuclei. They are called α-motor neurons because they are of the Aα type of nerve fiber. They receive and integrate inputs from various parts of the brain as well as from sensory receptors.

All neuronal influences affecting muscular contraction ultimately come through these motor neurons to the muscles even though there are multiple inputs both excitatory and inhibitory (through inhibitory interneurons) into the alpha motor neurons. So, they are called the **final common paths**. The dendrites of an α-motor neuron accommodates about 10,000 synaptic knobs, some coming from the same spinal segment, some from other segments of spinal cord, and some others are multiple long descending tracts from the brain.

All these converge on the same α-motor neuron. All the inputs are analyzed and the summated effect is discharged through the single fiber arising from the α-motor neuron. The two types of inputs funneled through the final common pathway are:
1. Segmental inputs originating from receptors in the muscle (muscle spindle), the tendon (Golgi tendon organ) the skin (nociceptors). The alpha motor neurons supplying the skeletal muscle fibers are the efferent limbs of many reflex arcs.
2. Supraspinal inputs descending from various parts of the brain like the cerebral cortex, reticular formation, etc.

The inputs converging on the motor neurons have three main functions:
1. To produce voluntary activity
2. To adjust body posture
3. To make movements smooth and precise.

Central Excitatory and Inhibitory States

The spinal cord neurons show prolonged changes in excitability due to reverberating circuits or prolonged effects of neurotransmitters. This state of the neurons where the excitatory influences exceed inhibitory influences is called **central excitatory state.** When the summated potential is towards inhibition inhibitory state predominates and this is called **central inhibitory state**. For example, after complete transection of spinal cord, in the stage of reflex activity the neurons below the level of lesion will be in the central excitatory state where the excitability is very much increased. So a mild noxious stimulus in the thigh may cause withdrawal reflex and autonomic reflexes like urination, defecation, sweating, etc., which is referred to as mass reflex.

Adaptation and Modification of Reflexes

Reflex activity is specific in that a particular stimulus elicits a particular response. But the reflex responses can be modified by experience. Reflexes are adaptable and can be modified to perform motor tasks and maintain balance. Spinal reflexes undergo modification and adaptation with the help of descending inputs from higher brain regions into the central integrating station of the reflex arc.

Effects of Injury to the Motor Neuron

If the motor nerve to a muscle is damaged, that muscle may develop **paresis** (weakness) or complete **paralysis** (loss of motor function). When motor axons cannot trigger contractions, there will be no reflexes (**areflexia**). Normal muscles are slightly contracted even at rest that is, they have some *tone*. If their motor nerves are transected, muscles become flaccid (**atonia**) and eventually develop profound **atrophy** (loss of muscle mass) because of the absence of trophic influences from the nerves.

■ MULTIPLE CHOICE QUESTIONS

1. The only monosynaptic reflex in the human body is:
   a. Stretch reflex
   b. Withdrawal reflex
   c. Crossed extensor reflex
   d. Inverse stretch reflex

2. **Correct statement regarding muscle spindle is:**
   a. Intrafusal fibers are positioned in series to the extrafusal fibers
   b. Primary (group Ia) endings discharge most rapidly while the muscle is being stretched
   c. Increased γ-motor neuron activity decreases spindle sensitivity during stretch
   d. When the muscle shortens, spindle afferent activity increases

3. **The transmitter released at the central integrating station in the case of stretch reflex is:**
   a. GABA
   b. Glycine
   c. Glutamate
   d. Acetylcholine

4. **The muscle stretch receptors are:**
   a. Muscle spindle
   b. Merkel's disc
   c. Golgi tendon organ
   d. Muscle spindle and Golgi tendon organ

5. **The sensitivity of muscle spindle to stretch is determined by:**
   a. Gamma efferent discharge
   b. Type I-a afferent discharge
   c. Type II afferent discharge
   d. Alpha efferent discharge

6. **Stretch reflex and inverse stretch reflex can be studied most effectively in:**
   a. Spinal animal
   b. Decorticate preparation
   c. Decerebrate preparation
   d. Thalamic preparation

7. **The percentage of fibers in the ventral root of spinal cord constituted by γ-motor neuron is:**
   a. 30%
   b. 3%
   c. 5%
   d. 50%

8. **The inhibitory interneuron involved in reciprocal innervation is:**
   a. Stellate cell
   b. Renshaw cell
   c. Golgi bottle neuron
   d. Basket cell

9. **The receptor involved in inverse stretch reflex is:**
   a. Muscle spindle
   b. Golgi tendon organ
   c. Crista ampullaris
   d. Free nerve endings

10. **Final common path refers to:**
    a. Alpha motor neuron
    b. Gamma motor neuron
    c. Interneuron
    d. Substantia Gelatinosa of Rolando

11. **The sense organ that has a motor supply of its own is:**
    a. Organ of Corti
    b. Taste bud
    c. Muscle spindle
    d. Crista ampullaris

12. **Stretch reflex alternating with inverse stretch reflex is called:**
    a. Clonus
    b. Tetanus
    c. Chorea
    d. Athetosis

13. **The type of motor neuron that supplies the intrafusal fibers of skeletal muscles is:**
    a. Alpha motor neuron
    b. Beta motor neuron
    c. Gamma motor neuron
    d. Delta motor neuron

14. **The termination of gamma motor nerve fibers is:**
    a. Extrafusal fibers
    b. Equatorial region of nuclear bag fiber
    c. Equatorial region of nuclear chain fiber
    d. Both ends of intrafusal fibers

15. **The receptor that provide the central nervous system with sensory information regarding the tension of muscles:**
    a. Golgi tendon organ
    b. Pacinian corpuscle
    c. Muscle spindle
    d. Ruffini's corpuscle

16. **The primary sensory nerve ending of a muscle spindle in a voluntary muscle is stimulated by:**
    a. Shortening of extrafusal fibers
    b. Shortening of intrafusal fibers
    c. Stimulation of alpha motor neuron
    d. Inhibition of gamma motor neuron

17. **Receptor for inverse stretch reflex is:**
    a. Pacinian corpuscle
    b. Golgi tendon organ
    c. Muscle spindle
    d. Free nerve ending

18. **Golgi tendon organ receptor is:**
    a. Stimulated by simple stretching of the muscle
    b. Innervated by Ia nerve fibers
    c. The receptor for inverse stretch reflex
    d. The receptor for myotatic reflex

19. **While eliciting knee jerk, the receptor stimulated is:**
    a. Free nerve ending
    b. Annulospiral nerve ending
    c. Flower spray nerve ending
    d. Golgi tendon organ

20. **Muscle spindle is:**
    a. Receptor for a variety of polysynaptic reflexes
    b. Receptor for myotatic or stretch reflex
    c. Seen only in antigravity extensor muscles
    d. Excited by both stretch and contraction of the muscles in which it is situated

21. **Gag reflex is mediated by which cranial nerve?**
    a. VII
    b. IX
    c. X
    d. XII

22. **Increased gamma efferent discharge is seen in all the following, *except*:**
    a. Jendrassik's maneuver
    b. Anxiety
    c. Rapid shallow breathing
    d. Stimulation of skin

23. **Lower most level of integration of stretch reflex is:**
    a. Cerebral cortex
    b. Upper medulla
    c. Lower medulla
    d. Spinal cord

24. **Crossed extensor reflex is a:**
    a. Withdrawal reflex
    b. Postural reflex
    c. Monosynaptic reflex
    d. Sympathetic reflex

ANSWERS

1. a	2. b	3. c	4. d	5. a
6. c	7. a	8. c	9. b	10. a
11. c	12. a	13. c	14. d	15. a
16. b	17. b	18. c	19. b	20. b
21. b	22. c	23. d	24. a	

Sensory Division of Nervous System

CHAPTER 81

LEARNING OBJECTIVES
- Classify receptors
- Describe the functions and properties of receptors
- Explain the physiology of generator potential
- Explain how stimuli are converted to signals that are carried to the central nervous system
- Differentiate between EPSP and IPSP
- Describe cortical sensations

INTRODUCTION

PY10.2: Describe and discuss the functions and properties of synapse, reflex, receptors.

Those portions of the nervous system concerned with **receiving** information (reception) from the external and internal environment (sensory receptors), **transmission** of information (ascending neural pathways), **integration** of information in the brainstem and **analysis** of information in the cortical areas (somatosensory cortex) are included in the sensory division of nervous system. In short, the sensory nervous system makes us aware of our external and internal environments. It consists of receptors and sensory pathway.

SENSATION

PY10.3: Describe and discuss somatic sensations and sensory tracts.

Sensation or **aesthesia** is the sensory information that reaches consciousness, e.g., touch sensation, pain sensation, etc. Absence of sensation is called anesthesia. *Each of the principal sensations, we experience is called **sensory modality***. For example, modality of tactile sensation is touch. The major sensory modalities are classified as conscious senses and unconscious senses. We can experience almost **11 conscious senses**. **Conscious senses** are senses that reach consciousness while **unconscious senses** are those that do not reach consciousness.

Sensations are also classified into **somatic, visceral and special sensations**. Somatic sensations arise from receptors present on the body surface, muscles, tendons, joints, connective tissue and bones. These include touch, pain, temperature, vibration sense and proprioception. Visceral sensations arise from receptors located in the visceral organs (wall or connective tissue) present in skull, thorax, abdomen and pelvis and the sensation is mainly pain. Special sensations originate from the receptors of the special sense organs (eye, ear, nose and tongue) and include vision, audition, olfaction and taste. Equilibrium is also considered as a special sensation. The attributes of sensation are quality, intensity, duration and localization.

Perception is the appreciation and interpretation of a sensation, i.e., the understanding and awareness of the sensation's meaning. For example, pain is a sensation but awareness of pain is perception. Perception occurs not at the level of sensory receptor, but at the brain level.

Intensity, Affect and Acuity of Sensation

Intensity is the degree of perception of a stimulus. It depends on the rate of action potentials produced by the sensory receptor. Thus an intense stimulus will produce a more rapid train of action potentials. A weak stimulus will slow the rate of production of action potentials. Another mechanism to discriminate intensity depends on the number of receptors stimulated. An intense stimulus may produce action potentials in a large number of adjacent receptors. A less intense stimulus might stimulate fewer receptors. Integration of information occurs in the central nervous system.

The emotional component of a sensation is called **affect**. A sensation may have **positive, negative or neutral affect.** The sensation that do not have emotional component is said to be neutral. Positive affect means, the sensation evokes pleasant emotional response and negative affect is one which evokes unpleasant emotional response. For example, pain sensation has negative affect.

Acuity of a sensation is the precision of stimulus localization. Acuity depends on the number of receptors per unit area and the size of the cortical area of representation. For example, maximum acuity of vision occurs when the image falls on the macula where the number of cones per unit area is very high and macula has a large area of representation in the visual cortex.

SENSORY RECEPTORS

Sensory receptors are specialized **dendritic** endings of sensory neurons or **specialized cells** that can convert various forms of energy in the environment into action potentials in the sensory neurons connected to them. They monitor changes in the external or internal environment and they may be neural or non-neural cells. In the olfactory epithelium, the cell body of the neuron is modified into olfactory receptor. The photoreceptors, rods and cones are modified epithelial cells. Pain receptors are free nerve endings.

Receptors can respond to a particular type of stimulus by undergoing depolarization and in turn can generate action potentials in the sensory nerve. Thus, they act as **transducers** that convert various forms of energy in the environment into action potentials (electrical energy) in the sensory neuron. These electrical impulses are carried by the sensory nerve to the CNS.

> The term receptor alone is used to refer to proteins that bind neurotransmitters, hormones, etc., and are present in different parts of the cell like cell membrane, cytoplasm, etc. These receptors should not be confused with sensory receptors.

Sense Organ

The sensory receptor may be part of a neuron as in the case of free nerve endings that mediate pain sensation. Sometimes sensory receptor may be a specialized cell, such as taste receptor that receives an afferent nerve fiber and can generate action potential in the sensory neuron. When the sensory receptor is associated with non-neuronal cells or supporting cells it forms a **sense organ**, e.g., taste bud in the tongue, organ of Corti in the inner ear, etc. Each sense organ or receptor is specialized to respond to one type of sensation. Though the stimuli and receptors are different, information is carried along the nerve tracts in the form of action potentials.

Functions of Sensory Receptors

- Sensory receptors receive information from the internal as well as the external environment.
- Receptors act as transducers, i.e., they convert various forms of energy in the environment into action potentials in neurons. The stimulus generates receptor potential or generator potential in the receptor, which is converted into action potentials in the sensory nerve and transmitted to the center.

Types of Stimuli that Stimulate the Sensory Receptors

- Mechanical—Touch, pressure, etc.
- Thermal—Heat, cold
- Electromagnetic—Light
- Chemical—Taste, smell, chemical composition of blood, such as arterial PO_2, PCO_2, pH, etc.
- Sound energy (stimulate the hair cells of organ of Corti).

Classification of Sensory Receptors

Traditional or Anatomical Classification

- Receptors for special senses (vision, hearing, smell, taste, rotational and linear acceleration). Receptors are located at one area in the head and they are specialized for detecting only one type of sensation. Information from them is carried by cranial nerves.
- Receptors for cutaneous or superficial senses (mediate touch, pressure, pain, and temperature). Receptors are located in the skin and information is carried by cutaneous branches of spinal nerves.
- Receptors for deep senses (those mediating sensation of joints, muscles and tendons where information is carried by spinal or cranial nerves).
- Receptors for visceral senses (stretch and pain receptors of viscera where information is carried by the autonomic nervous system).

Classification Depending on the Adequate Stimulus

- **Mechanoreceptors, which respond to application of a mechanical stimulus:**
  - Skin (epidermis and dermis)
    - Rapidly adapting receptors, such as hair follicle receptor, Meissner's corpuscle and Pacinian corpuscle.
    - Slowly adapting receptors, such as Merkel's disc, Ruffini endings, and unmyelinated C-mechano-receptors.
  - Deep tissue: Free nerve endings, Pacinian corpuscle, Ruffini endings, muscle spindle, Golgi tendon receptors
  - Hearing—hair cells in the cochlea
  - Equilibrium—vestibular receptors
  - Arterial pressure—baroreceptors in carotid sinus and aortic arch
- **Thermoreceptors:** They are moderate heat and cold receptors in the skin, which are free nerve endings. Aδ fibers mediate cold sensation, while C fibers mediate warmth.
- **Nociceptors or pain receptors:** Harmful stimuli, such as pain, extreme heat and cold stimulate them. They detect physical or chemical damage occurring in the tissues.
  - Aδ nociceptors, the fibers of which are thinly myelinated. They respond to fast pain.
  - C-nociceptors, whose nerve fibers are unmyelinated and these nociceptors contain **vanilloid receptors** (VR_1 receptors) in their membrane activated by heat, low pH and capsaicin.
- **Electromagnetic receptors or photoreceptors:** Rods and cones of retina
- **Chemoreceptors:** They respond to chemical stimuli, e.g., Taste and smell receptors; receptors responding to blood chemistry (PO_2, PCO_2, H^+, osmolality, glucose, etc.)

Sherrington's Classification (According to the Type of Receptors)

- **Telereceptors** are receptors that receive stimuli which are far away from the body, e.g., receptors for vision, hearing and smell
- **Exteroceptors** are present in the skin and subcutaneous tissue and include receptors for touch, pressure, pain, external temperature and smell. These receptors are concerned with perception of the external environment.
- **Interoceptors:** These are receptors that detect changes in the internal environment of the body e.g., baroreceptors, chemoreceptors, stretch receptors, osmoreceptors and glucoreceptors
- **Proprioceptors:** Provide information about the position of the body in space, muscle length and tension, movement of joints and sense of equilibrium. Proprioceptors include muscle spindle, Golgi tendon organ, hair cells of utricle, saccule and semicircular canal.

Encapsulated and Non-encapsulated Receptors

- **Encapsulated receptors** are Meissner's corpuscle, Pacinian corpuscle, Ruffini's corpuscle, Krause's end-bulbs, muscle spindle and Golgi tendon organ (neuro-tendinous spindle). They form the expanded tips and encapsulated endings respectively on the sensory nerve terminals of Aβ and Aδ fibers.
- **Non-encapsulated receptors** are free nerve endings, Merkel's disc and hair follicle receptors.

Phasic Receptors and Tonic Receptors

The receptors that adapt rapidly are called phasic receptors, e.g., touch and pressure receptors. For example, we do not feel the clothes we are wearing. The receptors that adapt slowly or do not adapt at all are tonic receptors. Examples are pain receptors, baroreceptors, chemoreceptors, etc.

PACINIAN CORPUSCLE

Pacinian corpuscles or lamellar corpuscles are rapidly adapting large mechanoreceptors (1 mm in length) located in the skin and deep tissues. They mediate the sensation of vibration and deep pressure. It was described by Pacini in 1835. Pacinian corpuscle is formed of straight, non-myelinated sensory nerve ending surrounded by concentric lamellae of connective tissue giving it the appearance of an onion (*refer* **Chapter 82; Fig. 82.4**). There are about 20 to 60 lamellae separated by gelatinous material. The actual receptor is the unmyelinated nerve ending within the corpuscle. Myelination of sensory nerve begins inside the corpuscle and the first node of Ranvier is seen inside the corpuscle and the second node is seen at the point where the sensory nerve leaves the corpuscle. These receptors are seen in the skin, subcutaneous tissue and mesentery and in the neighborhood of tendons and joints. They respond to deep pressure and vibration sensation. Optimal sensitivity is 250 Hz. Touch, pressure and vibration are different forms of the same sensation. When the force applied on the skin is more, the Pacinian corpuscle will be stimulated and pressure sensation is felt. When the force is insufficient to reach deep receptors, fine touch is felt. Rhythmic variation in pressure is vibration sense.

The function of various cutaneous sensory receptors has been studied in humans using a technique called **microneurography**. Here, recording can be made from a single sensory axon and the receptive field of the sensory nerve fiber can be mapped. Most of the studies of sensory receptor function are carried out in Pacinian corpuscle because of its large size, accessibility and the ease with which microelectrodes can be introduced.

GENERATOR POTENTIAL OR RECEPTOR POTENTIAL

When a stimulus is applied, a potential change is produced in the concerned receptor. This is similar to excitatory post synaptic potential (EPSP) and since this potential can generate an action potential in the sensory nerve, it is referred to as **receptor potential or generator potential**.

Receptor potential is studied in detail in the Pacinian corpuscle because of its relatively large size. It can be easily isolated from the mesentery of experimental animals and can be subjected to microdissection for introducing microelectrodes. Recording electrodes are placed on the sensory nerve as it leaves the Pacinian corpuscle and graded pressure is applied to the corpuscle by a rod. Certain potential changes occur in the receptor when a small amount of pressure is applied, resulting in localized depolarizing potentials called receptor potential or generator potential. This is similar to excitatory postsynaptic potential (EPSP). As the pressure is increased, the magnitude of receptor potential also increases. When it reaches a threshold level, which is about 10–15 mV, an action potential is generated in the sensory nerve at the first node of Ranvier, which is located in the lamellae of the corpuscle. The receptor thus converts the mechanical energy into electrical energy, the magnitude of which is proportional to the intensity of the stimulus. *Since the receptor potential can generate action potentials in the sensory nerve, it is called **generator potential***. The generator potential originates from the unmyelinated nerve ending and it electrotonically depolarizes the first node of Ranvier. The generator potential alone can be recorded by placing the recording electrodes on the unmyelinated nerve ending within the lamellae and applying pressure on the naked ending. Differences between receptor potential and action potential are given in **Table 81.1**.

Ionic Basis of Receptor Potential

The **generator potential or receptor potential** is produced in the unmyelinated nerve terminal inside the Pacinian corpuscle. Thus the nerve terminal is the actual receptor. When pressure is applied on the Pacinian corpuscle, displacement of the different layers of the corpuscle occur leading to distortion of the unmyelinated nerve terminal. This opens **stretch sensitive sodium channels** in the

Table 81.1: Differences between generator potential and action potential.	
Receptor potential	**Action potential**
• Recorded from sensory receptors • Non-propagated • Does not obey all or none law • Can be summated, they are graded potentials • Can generate action potentials in the sensory nerve, i.e., can act as transducer	• Recorded from excitable tissues like nerve and muscle • Propagated • Obey all or none law • Cannot be summated • No transducer function

unmyelinated nerve terminal. The permeability of the nerve membrane to Na⁺ is increased, leading to depolarization of the nerve ending. Thus, the receptor converts mechanical energy into an electrical response, the magnitude of which is proportionate to the intensity of the stimulus. Thus, the receptor acts as a **transducer** i.e., the sensory receptor translates a sensory signal to an electrical signal in the nervous system. The receptor potentials are graded potentials and they can be summated to produce an action potential in the sensory nerve. The generator potential thus produced in turn depolarizes the sensory nerve at the first node of Ranvier. Once the firing level is reached, an action potential is produced at the first node of Ranvier which is propagated. Thus, the node of Ranvier converts graded response of the receptor into action potentials. Graded potentials are similar to EPSPs and can be summated to produce an action potential in the sensory nerve. The frequency of action potentials depends on the intensity of the stimulus. If the intensity is high, the nerve continues to fire as long as it is applied.

■ PROPERTIES OF RECEPTORS

Specificity

Receptors are specialized according to the type of stimulus they sense. Thus they have receptor specificity. This specificity arises from the sensory endings that are used by each sensory pathway. The receptors respond maximally only when an appropriate specific stimulus is applied. That is, receptors are specific to a particular type of stimulus; for example, touch receptors are stimulated by tactile stimuli, rods and cones by light and sound receptors by sound. Touch receptors are not sensitive to light or sound. They are sensitive only to touch or pressure.

Adequate Stimulus

The particular form of energy to which a receptor is most sensitive is called its **adequate stimulus**. Receptors can respond to other forms of energy other than their adequate stimuli, but the threshold for these nonspecific stimuli is very high. For example, the adequate stimulus for rods and cones is light energy. Pressure on the eyeball can also stimulate rods and cones but the threshold of these receptors to pressure is very high when compared to the pressure receptors in the skin.

Adaptation or Desensitization

If a maintained stimulus of constant strength is applied to a receptor, the frequency of action potentials in its sensory nerve declines over time. This phenomenon is known as **adaptation or desensitization**. Adaptation depends on the type of receptors. The degree to which adaptation occurs varies from one sense to another. Depending on the degree of adaptation, receptors are of three types:

1. Rapidly adapting receptors or **phasic** receptors, e.g., Meissner's corpuscle, Pacinian corpuscle and olfactory receptors.
2. Slowly adapting receptors or **tonic** receptors, e.g., Merkel's disc, Ruffini ending, muscle spindle, baroreceptors, etc. They continue to transmit information for many hours even if the intensity of stimulus remains constant over a long period. This is important because if these receptors get adapted, it will damage the body. For example, the muscle spindle discharge continues as long as the muscle is stretched. This is important in maintaining posture. Baroreceptors and chemoreceptors also adapt very slowly for precise operation of the regulatory systems.
3. Non-adapting receptors, e.g., nociceptors. If the nociceptors adapt, they will lose their warning values.

Mechanism of Adaptation

Mechanism of adaptation is different for each type of receptor.
❖ Rods and cones adapt by changing the concentration of their photosensitive pigments.
❖ Some receptors adapt by **accommodation**. This occurs by progressive inactivation of the Na⁺ channel in the receptor membrane.
❖ Pacinian corpuscles adapt by readjustment in the structure of the corpuscle itself.

Sensitization of Receptors

Sensitization is opposite to desensitization. In sensitization, repeated application of an unpleasant stimulus produces greater and greater response. Nociceptors are receptors that do not adapt since pain is a protective phenomenon. Nociceptors can be sensitized by injury or inflammation. The damaged cells at the site of injury release K⁺, bradykinin, serotonin, histamine, prostaglandin, etc. These substances contribute to the sensitization of the receptors by opening up ion channels or by activating second messenger system. After sensitization, the nociceptors respond to stimuli like stretch, weak pressure, etc., which normally do not activate the nociceptors **(allodynia)**. They were neutral stimuli or benign stimuli before injury. Also, sensitized nociceptors respond more vigorously to a noxious stimulus because the threshold of activation is lowered. *Pain and tenderness at the site of tissue injury is due to sensitization of nociceptors.*

■ SENSORY UNIT

A single sensory axon with all its peripheral branches terminating in sensory receptors constitutes a **sensory unit**

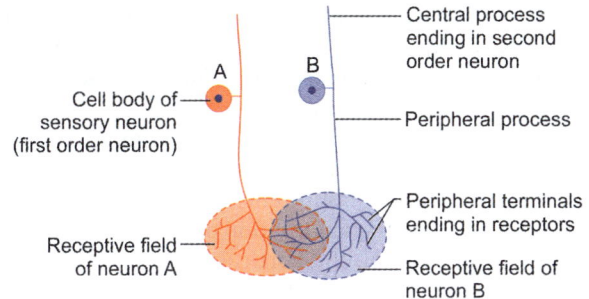

Fig. 81.1: Sensory units showing overlapping of receptive fields of two sensory neurons.

(Fig. 81.1). The number of branches varies. The **receptive field** of a sensory unit is the sensory area from which a stimulus can produce a response in that unit or in other words, the particular sensory area from which each sensory neuron receives information is its receptive field. This area of the body surface, when stimulated, produce activity in that particular sensory neuron. There is overlapping of areas supplied by different sensory units. Precise localization of the stimulus is possible only if the receptive field is small. For example, the receptive fields are much smaller and overlap considerably in the fingertips and lips than on the back of the body where the sensory units are large and widely spaced. So, tactile localization is precise in the lips and fingertips.

> All the receptors of a particular sensory unit are sensitive to the same type of stimulus. If the afferent neuron of a particular sensory unit carries fine touch sensation, then all the receptors of that sensory unit will be that of fine touch. In the internal organs, the afferent neurons are few in number and each has large receptive fields. So localization of sensation from the internal organs is less precise.

Recruitment of Sensory Units

A high intensity stimulus can increase the number of receptors stimulated because the stimulus spreads over a large area. Thus, more and more sensory units are recruited. Weak stimulus activates only the receptors with the lowest threshold, but stronger stimulus can activate receptors with lower as well as higher thresholds. Because of the overlapping of sensory units, more sensory units are stimulated with strong stimuli and this is known as **recruitment of sensory units**. Thus, more afferent pathways are activated and brain interprets it as an increase in the intensity of the sensation.

INTENSITY DISCRIMINATION BY CEREBRAL CORTEX

Intensity discrimination of different stimuli occurs in the cortex by the following mechanisms:
- by variation in the frequency of action potentials generated in a receptor
- by variation in the number of receptors activated
  When the frequency of action potentials reaching the cerebral cortex is increased, the cortex distinguishes it as high-intensity stimulus.

WEBER-FECHNER LAW

Weber-Fechner law states that the magnitude of sensation felt is proportionate to the logarithm of the intensity of the stimulus. If intensity is 10 units, then the magnitude of sensation is 1. Similarly if it is 100, magnitude of sensation will be 2, if it is 1000 magnitude will be 3 and so on. This law is usually applicable in audition. The ability of discrimination is more for low intensity than for high intensity stimuli.

CODING OF SENSORY INFORMATION (SENSORY CODING)

Sensory coding means converting a receptor stimulus to a recognizable sensation. All sensory systems code for four attributes of a stimulus: modality, location, intensity and duration.

Modality

Modality is the type of energy transmitted by the stimulus. Depending on the modality, there are four classes of receptors: mechanical, thermal, electromagnetic and chemical. The particular form of energy to which the receptor is most sensitive is called its adequate stimulus.

Location

Location is the site on the body where the stimulus originated. Representation of the senses in the skin is punctate. A particular sensation can be produced by stimulation of the skin only over the spots where the receptors for that particular modality are located. The area supplied by one sensory unit usually overlaps with the areas supplied by others **(Fig. 81.1)**. One of the most important mechanisms that enable localization of a stimulus site is lateral inhibition.

Intensity

Intensity is determined by the strength of the stimulus applied to the receptor and the frequency of action potential generation in the nerve fiber transmitting information to the CNS. Weak stimulus activates receptors with the lowest thresholds, and stronger stimuli also activate those with higher thresholds. If more number of receptors in the same sensory unit is activated, impulse frequency in that sensory fiber increases. As the strength of the stimulus is increased, it spreads over a large area and recruits more and more sensory units in the surrounding area because of overlap and interdigitation of one sensory unit with another. Thus more sensory units fire and more afferent pathways are activated, which is interpreted in the brain as an increase in the intensity of sensation.

Duration

Duration refers to the time from the start to the end of a response in the sensory receptor. If a stimulus of constant strength is maintained on some sensory receptors, the frequency of action potentials in its sensory nerve declines over time (*Refer* receptor adaptation).

MULLER'S DOCTRINE OF SPECIFIC NERVE ENERGIES

Action potentials in all the nerve fibers reaching the brain are identical. But stimulation of different receptors evokes different sensations even though the action potentials are same. For example, stimulation of touch receptor produces only touch sensation and not any other sensation, and we can also distinguish whether it is light touch or heavy touch. This is because the *sensory pathways are discrete from the sense organ to cerebral cortex*. Each sensory pathway terminates on specific areas of sensory cortex.

When the sensory nerve pathway from a particular sensory receptor or sense organ is stimulated anywhere in its course, the sensation evoked depends on the area of the cortex, where the sensory pathway terminates. This specificity of nerve fiber to transmit only one modality of sensation to the brain is called *labeled line principle*. Johannes Muller in 1835 described this as *law of specific nerve energies*. For example, if the sensory nerve fiber from a Pacinian corpuscle in the hand is stimulated at the region of elbow, the sensation evoked is pressure in the hand. When the sensory nerve for touch is stimulated by any type of stimuli anywhere along its course to the cerebral cortex, the sensation evoked is touch. This is because the pathways are specific and discrete from the sense organ to the cortex.

LAW OF PROJECTION

When a sensory pathway is stimulated anywhere along its course from the receptor to the sensory cortex, the conscious sensation is felt at the location of the receptors from which the pathway originated. This principle is called the **law of projection**. For example, if the cortical area for pain sensation from the left hand is stimulated, pain sensation is felt on the left hand and not in the head. If pain fibers from the receptors in the little finger are stimulated at the elbow, the subject experiences pain in the little finger and not in the elbow. Another example is seen in amputees. When the nerve fibers at the amputated end are irritated due to pressure, the patient complains of pain and proprioceptive sensations in the absent limb, i.e., the sensations evoked are projected to where the receptors used to be present. This is called **phantom limb** because the sensation is felt in a part of the body which is removed from the body. Phantom means ghost. Phantom sensations also occur after the removal of body parts other than limb like **phantom tooth pain** (after tooth extraction), **phantom eye syndrome** (after removal of an eye), etc. Another explanation for this phenomenon is **cortical plasticity**. The ventral posterior thalamic nucleus can reorganize if sensory input is cut off. In leg amputees, studies have shown that the thalamic region that once received input from the leg and foot now respond to stimulation of the stump in the thigh. Similarly changes occur in the cerebral cortex.

CORTICAL PLASTICITY

Cortical plasticity refers to brain's ability to change and adapt as a result of experience. Rapid reorganization of cortical neural pathways occurs by experience. Long lasting functional changes in the brain occur when we learn new things or memorize new information. Plasticity also occur as a result of damage to the brain.

Use, disuse and lesions are the strong stimuli for plasticity and reorganization in the adult cortex. Cortical reorganization plays an important role in the phantom limb phenomenon following amputation of hands, arm, leg, etc. If a digit is amputated, the cortical representation of the neighboring digits spreads into the cortical area that was formerly occupied by the representation of the amputated digit. Conversely, if the cortical area representing a digit is removed, the somatosensory map of the digit moves to the surrounding cortex. **Functional plasticity** refers to the ability of brain to shift functions from damaged area of brain to other undamaged areas. The cells that are close in the sensory periphery are also close in the cortical representation.

This reorganization is because cortical connections of sensory units to the cortex have extensive convergence and divergence, with connections that can become weak with disuse and strong with use. Plastic changes can also occur from one sensory modality to another. It is seen that tactile and auditory stimuli increase metabolic activity in the visual cortex in blind individuals. Conversely, deaf individuals respond faster and more accurately than normal individuals to moving stimuli in the visual periphery. This shows that brain has the ability to be easily molded and to adapt. Plasticity also occurs in the motor cortex (for details, *refer* **Chapter 96**).

SUPERFICIAL SENSES

There are four superficial or cutaneous senses; touch-pressure, cold, warmth and pain. Pressure is sustained deep touch **(Table 81.2)**. Receptors present in the skin are called cutaneous receptors. Combination of the superficial senses can produce different sensations called synthetic senses e.g., vibration sense, stereognosis, etc.

Head's Classification of Superficial Senses

- Epicritic sensation
- Protopathic sensation.

Epicritic sensation includes finer aspects of sensation like fine touch, light pressure, tactile localization, tactile discrimination, stereognosis and vibration sense. Epicritic sensations are mediated by encapsulated receptors. These sensations are transmitted in type Aβ nerve fibers having conduction velocities ranging from 30–70 m/sec.

Protopathic sensations include cruder aspects of sensations, such as crude touch, deep pressure, pain, temperature, itching, tickling, etc. These sensations are mediated by receptors with bare nerve endings. These sensations are transmitted by Aδ nerve fibers with conduction velocity of 5–30 m/sec and unmyelinated C fibers with conduction velocity less than 2 m/sec. Protopathic sensations have a protective function of warning of injury.

Table 81.2: Different sensory modalities and the receptors concerned.

Conscious sensations	Receptor and sense organ
• Vision	• Rods and cones of eye
• Audition (hearing)	• Hair cells of organ of Corti
• Olfaction (smell)	• Olfactory neurons of olfactory epithelium
• Gustation (taste)	• Taste receptor cells of taste bud
• Linear acceleration	• Hair cells of utricle and saccule in inner ear
• Rotational acceleration	• Hair cells of semicircular canals in ear
• Touch and pressure	• Nerve endings in Merkel's disc, Meissner's corpuscle, Pacinian corpuscle
• Warmth	• Nerve endings sensitive to warmth
• Cold	• Nerve endings sensitive to cold
• Pain	• Free nerve endings
• Joint position and movement	• Receptors in and around joint
Unconscious sensations	
• Muscle	• Nerve endings in muscle spindle
• Muscle tension	• Nerve endings in Golgi tendon orga
• Arterial blood pressure	• Stretch receptors in carotid sinus and aortic arch
• Central venous pressure	• Stretch receptors in the wall of great veins and atria
• Inflation of lung	• Stretch receptors in lung parenchyma
• Body temperature	• Neurons in hypothalamus
• Arterial PO_2	• Glomus cells in carotid and aortic bodies
• Arterial PCO_2 or pH of CSF	• Central chemoreceptors in medulla
• Osmotic pressure of plasma	• Osmoreceptors in the circumventricular organs of anterior hypothalamus
• Blood glucose level	• Glucostats of hypothalamus

CORTICAL SENSATIONS

Tactile localization, two point discrimination and stereognosis are called cortical sensations since these finer aspects of sensations are integrated in the cerebral cortex. These sensations are severely impaired in cortical lesions.

Tactile Localization

Tactile localization is the ability to localize the exact position of a light touch to the skin as when tested with a wisp of cotton or the finger.

Two-point Discrimination

Two-point discrimination is the ability to discriminate two touch spots as two separate points. Receptors are touch receptors and discrimination is the function of sensory cortex. The minimal distance by which two touch stimuli must be separated to be perceived as separate is called **two-point discrimination threshold**. It is a measure of **tactile acuity**. The distance varies from place to place in the body and it depends on the number of receptors per unit area. For example, in the fingertips 3 mm distance between the two fine touch points can be distinguished as two separate touch points. In the back of the body, this is possible only if the distance between the two-points is more than 65 mm. The sensation is carried through dorsal column pathway. **Lateral inhibition** occurring at different levels in the sensory pathway is also responsible for two-point discrimination. Two-point discrimination is used to test the integrity of the dorsal column pathway.

Stereognosis

Stereognosis is the ability to identify familiar objects by handling them with eyes closed. Receptors are touch and pressure receptors (*refer* synthetic senses).

LATERAL INHIBITION OR SURROUND INHIBITION

Lateral inhibition or afferent inhibition or surround inhibition is that form of inhibition in which activation of a particular neural unit is associated with inhibition of the activity of nearby units. Every sensory pathway, when excited, gives rise simultaneously to lateral *inhibitory* signals; these inhibitory signals spread to the sides of the excitatory signal and inhibit adjacent neurons. This phenomenon helps to sharpen the edges of a stimulus and improve discrimination. Lateral inhibition helps to increase the degree of contrast in the perceived spacial pattern.

In pathways providing the most accurate localization, it is seen that stronger inputs are enhanced and the weaker inputs of adjacent sensory units are simultaneously inhibited. For example, fine touch due to movement of hair can be localized accurately because it has greater degree of lateral inhibition. Whereas, temperature sensation can be localized only poorly as it activates pathways that lack lateral inhibition.

In any receptive field, its central portion stimulation results in accurate localization. As one goes away from the center, lateral inhibition goes on increasing resulting in poor localization even with same intensity of stimulus.

Information from sensory neurons whose receptors are at the peripheral edge of the stimulus is inhibited in the CNS when compared to information from the sensory neurons which innervate receptors at the center of the stimulus. This is called lateral inhibition which is very important in the pathways providing the most accurate localization like fine touch. This enhances the contrast between the center and periphery of a stimulated area and increases the ability of the brain to localize a sensory input. Thus, lateral inhibition contributes much to tactile localization and two-point discrimination. It also increases the contrast between relevant and irrelevant information.

In the case of dorsal column pathway, lateral inhibition occurs at the synaptic levels of second order neurons in medulla, third order neurons in the thalamus as well as neurons in the cortex itself. When a sensory pathway is stimulated, as it sends excitatory signal to the next neuron in the pathway, it simultaneously sends short inhibitory lateral pathways to the surrounding neurons through inhibitory interneurons. These in turn inhibit the surrounding neurons by releasing inhibitory neurotransmitters. The importance of lateral inhibition is that it blocks lateral spread of excitatory signals and thus increases the degree of contrast in the sensory pattern perceived in the cerebral cortex. Exact localization of the stimulus thus becomes possible.

Fine touch pathway in dorsal column has significant lateral inhibition. Pathways in the spinothalamic tract, such as slow pain and temperature sensations, which are poorly localized activates sensory pathways that lack lateral inhibition. Lateral inhibition is also seen in the visual pathway; auditory pathway; cerebellum, etc. Examples of lateral inhibition seen in different areas are:

- Basket cells and stellate cells located in the molecular layer of cerebellar cortex are stimulated by the parallel fibers which are axons of granule cells. These cells in turn cause lateral inhibition of the adjacent Purkinje cells, thus sharpening the signal (for details, *refer* **Chapter 87**).
- During itching, if the scratch is strong enough to elicit pain, the pain signals are believed to suppress the itch signals in the spinal cord by lateral inhibition.
- In two point discrimination, the capability of the sensorium to distinguish the presence of two points of stimulation on the skin is due to the mechanism of *lateral inhibition.*
- Stimulation of large Aβ sensory fibers from the peripheral tactile receptors can depress transmission of pain signals from the same area of the body. This effect results from local lateral inhibition in the spinal cord. It explains why simple maneuvers, such as rubbing the skin near painful areas is often effective in relieving pain, and it probably also explains why liniments are often useful for pain relief.
- The horizontal cells in the retina connect laterally between the synaptic bodies of the rods and cones and also connect with the dendrites of the bipolar cells. The outputs of the horizontal cells *are always inhibitory.* Therefore, this lateral connection provides the same phenomenon of lateral inhibition that is operating in other sensory systems. It helps to ensure transmission of visual patterns with proper visual contrast. This process is essential to allow high visual accuracy in transmitting contrast borders in the visual image. Some of the amacrine cells probably provide additional lateral inhibition and further enhancement of visual contrast in the inner plexiform layer of the retina (for details, *refer* **Chapter 98**).
- The frequency range to which each individual neuron in the auditory cortex responds is much narrower than that in the cochlear and brain stem relay nuclei. The basilar membrane near the base of the cochlea is stimulated by sounds of all frequencies, and in the cochlear nuclei, this same breadth of sound representation is found. Yet, by the time the excitation reaches the cerebral cortex, most sound responsive neurons respond only to a narrow range of frequencies rather than to a broad range. Therefore somewhere along the pathway, processing mechanisms sharpen the frequency response. It is believed that this sharpening effect is caused mainly by the phenomenon of lateral inhibition. That is, stimulation of the cochlea at one frequency inhibits sound frequencies on both sides of this primary frequency; this inhibition is caused by collateral fibers arising from the primary signal pathway and exerting inhibitory influences on adjacent pathways.
- Renshaw cell inhibition in the spinal cord is another example of lateral inhibition. Located in the anterior horns of the spinal cord, in close association with the motor neurons are a large number of small inhibitory neurons called *Renshaw cells.* Almost immediately after the anterior motor neuron axon leaves the body of the neuron, collateral branches from the axon pass to adjacent Renshaw cells. Renshaw cells are *inhibitory cells* that transmit inhibitory signals to the surrounding motor neurons. Thus, stimulation of each motor neuron tends to inhibit adjacent motor neurons, an effect called *lateral inhibition.* The motor system uses this lateral inhibition to focus, or sharpen, its signals.

SYNTHETIC CUTANEOUS SENSES

Synthetic senses are combination of touch, pressure, temperature and pain sensations. They are:

- **Vibration sense:** Vibratory sensation is due to rapidly repetitive vibratory signals and can be detected as vibration sense up to 700 cycles per second. It is a combination of touch and pressure senses. This sensation is transmitted through the dorsal column pathway. There is no specific receptor for detecting vibration sense. Different tactile receptors are differentially stimulated depending on the frequency of stimuli. This sensation is most marked over bones. A pattern of rhythmic pressure stimuli is interpreted as vibration and is demonstrated using the foot of a vibrating tuning fork placed over a bony prominence. The normal response is a buzzing sensation. Different receptors respond to different frequencies. For example, Pacinian corpuscle responds to high-frequency stimuli (600/sec) and Meissner's corpuscle respond to low-frequency stimuli (<80/sec). Vibratory sensation is diminished in conditions where there is degeneration of dorsal columns, such as uncontrolled diabetes mellitus associated with peripheral neuropathy, pernicious anemia (vitamin B_{12} deficiency) and tabes dorsalis. *Testing for vibration sense is a specific test to detect the integrity of dorsal column pathway.*
- **Stereognosis**: The ability to identify familiar objects by handling them (perception of the form and nature of the object) without looking at them is called stereognosis. This ability depends on intact touch and pressure sensations, and it is lost when the dorsal columns are damaged. Stereognosis also depends on intact somatic sensory area-I (**SSA-I) and sensory association areas 5 and** 7 in the parietal lobe. Sensory association area is necessary for the detailed analysis of sensory information since sensory processing occurs in this area. If there is a lesion in the sensory association area, it will result in **astereognosis** (loss of stereognosis) or **tactile agnosia**, but touch and pressure sensations will be normal.

❖ **Itching (pruritus) and tickling**: Mild stimulation of the skin by something that moves across the skin produces itch and tickle. Itching or pruritus is also due to stimulation of skin produced by chemical agents, such as histamine and kinins (e.g. bradykinin) that are released in the skin in response to tissue damage. Kinins cause severe itching. Itch sensation originates from stimulation of free nerve endings in the skin and is mainly carried by the **lateral spinothalamic tract** in the spinal cord. There is evidence that there is an itch-specific path in the sensory pathway. Itch specific unmyelinated C fibers have been demonstrated in the ventrolateral spinothalamic tracts. Uncontrolled itching occurs in obstructive jaundice, chronic renal failure and atopic dermatitis.

Very sensitive free nerve endings that elicit only itch and tickle sensations are found almost exclusively in the superficial layers of the skin from where itch and tickle sensations can be elicited. Tickling originates from stimulation of free nerve endings and touch receptors in the skin. Tickling sensation is regarded as pleasurable, whereas itching is annoying. Itch sensation activates the **scratch reflex** which helps the animal to get rid of the irritant from the body surface.

MULTIPLE CHOICE QUESTIONS

1. **The intensity of sensory stimuli is determined by:**
   a. Duration of latent period
   b. Amplitude of action potential
   c. Frequency of action potential
   d. Amplitude of generator potential

2. **Weber Fechner law deals with:**
   a. Frequency discrimination
   b. Receptive field organization
   c. Intensity discrimination
   d. Two point discrimination

3. **All the following modalities of sensations are detected by free nerve endings, *except*:**
   a. Crude touch   b. Pain
   c. Tickle sensation   d. Muscle stretch

4. **Intensity and amplitude are proportional to:**
   a. Weber-Fechner law
   b. Starling law
   c. Mary's law
   d. Hardy's law

5. **Perception of objects without stimulus is called:**
   a. Hallucination
   b. Illusion
   c. Delusion
   d. Delirium

6. **The inability to perceive the texture and shape of an object occurs in lesion of:**
   a. Nucleus gracilis
   b. Nucleus cuneatus
   c. Lateral spinothalamic tract
   d. Spinoreticular tract

7. **The law which states that in the spinal cord, dorsal roots are sensory and ventral roots are motor is called:**
   a. Bell-Magendie law
   b. Doctrine of specific nerve energies
   c. Law of projection
   d. Marey's law

8. **Weber-Fechner law is related with:**
   a. Amplitude
   b. Surface area
   c. Number of sensory fiber involvement
   d. Stimulus discrimination

9. **Phantom limb sensations are best described by:**
   a. Weber-Fechner law
   b. Power law
   c. Bell-Magendie law
   d. Law of projection

10. **Intensity of sensory stimulation is directly related to:**
    a. Duration of action potential
    b. Frequency of action potential
    c. Amplitude of action potential
    d. All of the above

11. **Phantom limb is an example of:**
    a. Law of projection
    b. Bell-Magendie law
    c. Marey's law
    d. Doctrine of specific nerve energies

12. **A person cannot identify a familiar object when placed in the palm when he is blindfolded, the condition is called:**
    a. Aphonia   b. Astereognosis
    c. Aphasia   d. Adiadokokinesia

ANSWERS

1. c   2. c   3. d   4. a   5. a
6. b   7. a   8. d   9. d   10. b
11. a   12. b

Ascending Sensory Pathways

CHAPTER 82

LEARNING OBJECTIVES
- Differentiate between dorsal column pathway and spinothalamic pathway
- Describe and discuss the functions of somatic sensory area I and II
- Explain fine and crude touch pathway from the right side of the body
- Explain slow and fast pain pathway
- Explain the physiological basis of referred pain giving examples
- Explain the gate control theory of pain perception
- Describe the mechanism of pain modulation

INTRODUCTION

PY10.3: Describe and discuss somatic sensations and sensory tracts.

The sensory pathways or the ascending pathways contain group of sensory fibers which carry sensations from the peripheral parts of the body to the sensory cortex. These pathways include neurons connected in series. Almost all sensory pathways are three neuronal pathways (there are exceptions, e.g., auditory pathway). The **first order** neuron is the primary afferent neuron which starts from the receptor and travel along the spinal nerve to reach the spinal cord. It is called so because it is the first neuron that enters the central nervous system (CNS) in the synaptically linked chain of neurons in the afferent pathway. Its cell body is located in the dorsal root ganglion.

After entering the spinal cord, the first order neuron may terminate on the second order neuron in the posterior horn or may ascend up in the dorsal column to end on the second order neuron in the medulla. The **second order** neuron may be in the spinal cord or in the brainstem and the function of this neuron is to transmit impulse from the first order neuron to the thalamus. The axon of the second order neuron crosses to the opposite side in the spinal cord or in the medulla. Thus, the second order neurons transmit impulses originating in one side of the body to the thalamus on the opposite side. Exception is taste pathway where the second order neuron does not cross to the opposite side.

The **third order** neuron is in the thalamus. The thalamus forms the main sensory relay center in the brain. From the specific nuclei of the thalamus the third order neuron projects to specific areas in the sensory cortex (refer sensory homunculus).

The main sensory pathways are:
- **Dorsal column pathway** or posterior column pathway (medial lemniscal system)
- **Spinothalamic pathway** or anterolateral system

> The ascending pathways that do not reach the cerebral cortex include spinocerebellar tract (which carries unconscious proprioception); spinoreticular tract (slow pain), etc.

Dermatome

The entire body from neck downwards is divided into 31 segments, and each segment is supplied by one pair of spinal nerves. The cutaneous area supplied by a dorsal root ganglion is called a **dermatome**. Thus the cutaneous area is divided into different dermatomes each being supplied by a specific sensory nerve arising from a dorsal root ganglion. This is called **somatosensory map**. A lesion of a particular sensory nerve or a dorsal root results in loss of sensation in the corresponding skin area supplied by that nerve. This helps in localizing the nerve or the spinal cord segment involved in the disease condition. For example, compression of the dorsal root occurs in herniation of intervertebral disc. This may lead to pain, paresthesia or hyperesthesia of the affected dermatome. If there is damage to a dorsal root it may lead to segmental anesthesia (loss of sensations).

Information reaching the spinal cord:
- **Exteroceptive information**, which originates from the body surface like pain, temperature and touch.
- **Proprioceptive information**, which originates from inside the body like muscles and joints.
- Information from the viscera also reaches the spinal cord.
  All the sensory fibers enter the spinal cord through the posterior nerve root. These fibers are axons of the neurons in

the dorsal root ganglion (DRG). The diameter and conduction velocity of the sensory nerve fibers depends on the receptors they innervate and the sensation carried by them. Large myelinated Aα and Aβ fibers transmit impulses generated in mechanoreceptors. Small myelinated Aδ fibers transmit impulses from nociceptors (fast pain) and cold receptors. Small unmyelinated C fibers transmit slow pain, itching and tickling sensation.

In the posterior nerve root, sensory fibers are grouped into two portions, a *larger medial portion* containing Aα and Aβ fibers and a *smaller lateral portion* which contains Aδ as well as C fibers. After entering the spinal cord, the sensory nerve ascends up the spinal cord to brainstem and sub-cortical areas. At the same time, it gives collaterals to anterior horn cells of spinal cord for reflex actions. The sensory nerve ends in the spinal cord if the second order neuron is in the spinal cord.

DORSAL COLUMN PATHWAY OR MEDIAL LEMNISCAL SYSTEM

The major part of the medial portion of the posterior nerve root containing thickly medullated fibers after entering the spinal cord move to the posterior white matter and ascend up as the dorsal column pathway or the posterior column tract. The lower sacral and lumbar fibers are pushed more and more medially by the fibers entering from the upper thoracic and cervical parts **(Fig. 82.1A)**. Dorsal column is seen as two bundles:
1. Tractus gracilis or fasciculus gracilis or tract of Goll.
2. Tractus cuneatus or fasciculus cuneatus or tract of Burdach.

Fasciculus gracilis is present throughout the length of the spinal cord and contain ascending fibers from sacral, lumbar and lower 6 thoracic spinal nerves. It carries sensations from the lower limbs and lower part of the trunk. Fasciculus cuneatus is situated laterally in the upper thoracic and cervical segments of spinal cord. It transmits impulses from the upper limb and upper part of the trunk. Thus in the dorsal column tract, the fibers are represented as sacral to cervical segments from medial to lateral aspect.

The two tracts end in medulla in the **nucleus gracilis and nucleus cuneatus**.

The sensations carried through the dorsal column are:
❖ Fine touch having high degree of localization of stimulus
❖ Tactile localization and tactile discrimination
❖ Proprioception (sense of position and joint movement)
❖ Vibration sense
❖ Stereognosis
❖ Pressure sensations related to fine degrees of judgment of pressure intensity
❖ From afferents for some superficial reflexes.

First order neuron of dorsal column pathway is in the dorsal root ganglion. The *second order neurons* are in the **nucleus gracilis and nucleus cuneatus** in medulla. The axons of these neurons cross to the opposite side and the arching fibers are known as **internal arcuate fibers**. They ascend up as the **medial lemniscus** and end in the ventral posterolateral nucleus (VPLN) of thalamus. Each medial lemniscus is joined by fibers from the sensory nucleus of the trigeminal nerve which carries similar sensations from the head. The *third order neurons* are situated in the VPLN. The axons of the third order neurons enter the posterior limb of internal capsule and then radiate as **corona radiata** and end in the **somatic sensory area I and area II** in the post-central gyrus of the cerebral cortex.

The ventral posterior nucleus (VPN) or posteroventral nucleus of thalamus is subdivided into two parts (*refer* **Fig. 83.2**):
1. **Ventral posteromedial nucleus (VPMN)**
2. **Ventral posterolateral nucleus (VPLN)**.

VPMN receives the ascending trigeminal and gustatory (taste) pathways while VPLN receives important ascending sensory tracts, the medial and lateral lemnisci.

The dorsal column nuclei have two parts, **cluster region and non-cluster region.** Cluster region is the main part in which cells are arranged in clusters. This region receives fibers in the dorsal column pathway. The second order neurons cross to the opposite side and transmit sensory information to the cerebral cortex. The non-cluster region receives inputs from the dorsal column pathway and also from the descending fibers from the cerebral cortex. The fibers arising from this area project to cerebellum, tectum, inferior olivary nucleus, red nucleus and also to other areas involved in motor control. Thus this part provides sensory input to the different motor areas of the brain to bring about regulation of movement by appropriate sensory feedback.

SPINOTHALAMIC PATHWAY OR ANTEROLATERAL SYSTEM

The *first order neurons* are the primary afferent fibers originating from nociceptors, thermoreceptors and mechanoreceptors. These fibers form the smaller lateral portion of the posterior nerve root which after entering the spinal cord ends in the posterior horn cells. They synapse

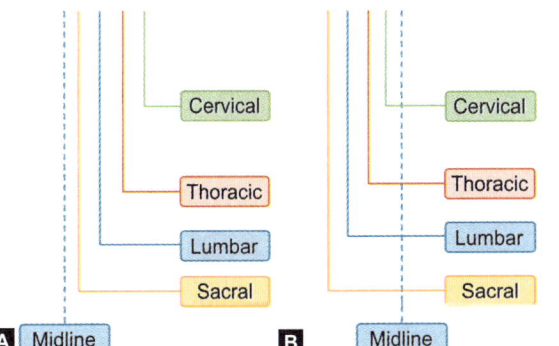

Figs. 82.1A and B: Pattern of lamination of sensory fibers in the spinal cord; in the dorsal column pathway, the cervical fibers are placed laterally and the sacral fibers medially. Whereas, in the spinothalamic pathway, the sacral fibers are pushed laterally by the crossing fibers as they ascend: (A) Dorsal column pathway; (B) Spinothalamic pathway.

with the *second order neurons present in laminas I, II and V in the posterior horn*. Pain and temperature fibers relay in the **substantia gelatinosa of Rolando (SGR)** and crude aspects of touch relay in the **chief sensory nuclei (CSN)**. Some of the fibers carrying pain and temperature may go up or down two or three segments of the spinal cord before ending in the posterior horn cells. These fibers form the **tractusdorsolateralis or Lissauer's tract**. The axons of the second order neurons cross to the opposite side in the anterior white commissure to form the spinothalamic pathway (anterolateral system) in the spinal cord. The sensations carried are:

- Crude touch
- Deep pressure sensation having crude localizing ability on the surface of the body
- Pain and temperature
- Itch and tickle sensation
- Sexual sensations
- Visceral sensations.

Fibers from substantia gelatinosa of Rolando (SGR) cross to the opposite side and ascend up as the **lateral spinothalamic tract,** which carries pain and temperature sensations. The axons from the chief sensory nuclei go to the anterior funiculus and ascend up as the **anterior spinothalamic tract**. It carries crude touch. In the spinothalamic tract, the lower fibers are pushed more and more laterally by the crossing upper fibers **(Fig. 82.1B)**.

In the medulla, the spinothalamic tract is called **spinal lemniscus**, which ends mainly in the ventral-posterolateral nucleus (VPLN) of thalamus. Some fibers end in the intralaminar and midline nuclei of thalamus. From the thalamus, **thalamocortical** projection fibers pass through the posterior limb of internal capsule and corona radiata to end in the primary somatic sensory area I and II **(SSAI & II)** in the post-central gyrus. In the brain stem, the spinothalamic tract sends several collaterals to the reticular formation before reaching the thalamus.

Differences between dorsal column and spinothalamic pathways is discussed in **Table 82.1**.

ASCENDING TRACTS OF SPINAL CORD (FIG. 82.2)

There are different types of classification:
1. **Long projection tracts** connect spinal cord and other higher centers.
   - **Intersegmental or association tracts** connect various segments of spinal cord.
2. **Sensory tracts** convey impulses to consciousness, i.e., they reach cerebral cortex.
   - **Nonsensory tracts** carry information from muscles, tendons, joints, etc., to other parts of brain other than cerebral cortex.
3. Ascending tracts connecting spinal cord and cerebral cortex.
   - Ascending tracts ending in brainstem (spinoreticular tract, spino-olivary tract and spinotectal tract).
   - Spinocerebellar pathways.

Table 82.1: Differences between dorsal column and spinothalamic pathways.

Dorsal column pathway	Spinothalamic pathway
• Composed of thickly medullated fibers which are axons of DRG cells	• Thinly medullated or non-medullated fibers which are axons of posterior horn cells
• Velocity of conduction is fast	• Velocity of conduction slow
• Second order neuron in nucleus Gracilis and nucleus cuneatus of medulla	• Second order neuron in posterior horn substantia gelatinosa of Rolando and chief sensory nucleus
• Carry sensations from the same side of the body, i.e. uncrossed tract	• Crossed tract, i.e. carries sensations from opposite side
• Lamination-lower segment fibers seen medially and cervical fibers laterally **(Fig. 82.1A)**	• Lower fibers are seen laterally and cervical fibers medially
• Carries finer aspects of sensations, i.e. epicritic sensations	• Carries cruder aspects of sensations, i.e. protopathic sensations
• Tract end at the medullary level in nucleus Gracilis and nucleus cuneatus	• The tract end in the posteroventral nucleus of thalamus
• Form medial lemniscus in medulla	• Form spinal lemniscus in medulla
• Damage to dorsal column leads to ipsilateral inability to detect light touch, vibration, and proprioception below the level of damage	• Damage to the spinothalamic pathway leads to contralateral loss of pain and temperature sensation below the level of lesion

Sensory Tracts
- Lissauer's tract
- Lateral spinothalamic tract
- Anterior or ventral spinothalamic tract
- Spinoreticular tract
- Fasciculus gracilis or tract of Goll
- Fasciculus cuneatus or tract of Burdach

Non-sensory Tracts
- Dorsal or posterior or direct spinocerebellar tract
- Ventral or anterior or indirect spinocerebellar tract
- Spino-tectal tract

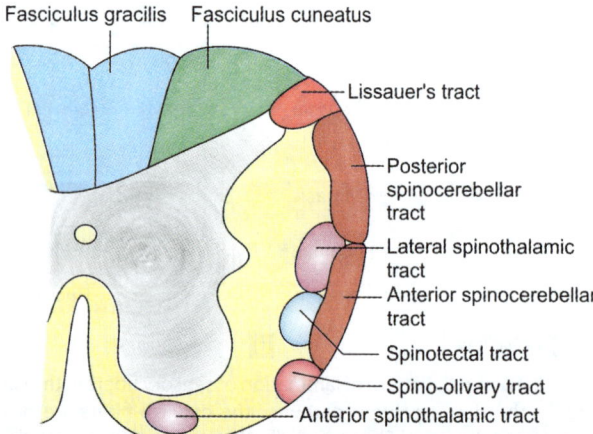

Fig. 82.2: Cross-section of spinal cord at the level of T_5 vertebra showing the ascending tracts.

- ❖ Spino-olivary tract
- ❖ Fasciculus proprius or propriospinal tract.

SENSORY TRACTS

Lissauer's Tract or Tractus Dorsolateralis

Posterior root fibers in the lateral portion, after entering the spinal cord ascend or descend 2 or 3 segments and then synapse with the cells of SGR. This forms the Lissauer's tract. They contain fibers that carry **pain and temperature** sensations.

Lateral Spinothalamic Tract

Lateral spinothalamic tract originates from substantia gelatinosa of Rolando **(SGR)** of opposite side and the axons of the second order neurons *cross* through the anterior commissure and ascend along the lateral funiculus as lateral spinothalamic tract. In the lateral spinothalamic tract, the fibers show laminations, the fibers from the lower segments are pushed more laterally by fibers that enter from the segments above, i.e., sacral fibers are seen laterally and cervical fibers medially. They ascend to the medulla and here the tract moves medially towards the anterior spinothalamic tract and the two together form the **spinal fillet or spinal lemniscus**. This ascends through pons and in the midbrain lies close to medial lemniscus and end in the ventral posterior nucleus of thalamus. The axons of the third order neurons pass through the internal capsule and corona radiata to reach the cerebral cortex where the sensations are appreciated. This tract carries **pain, temperature, deep pressure, itching, tickling, and sexual and bladder sensations**.

> Unilateral destruction of the lateral spinothalamic tract leads to complete loss of pain and temperature sensations on the opposite side of the body to a level one segment below the level of lesion. In anterolateral cordotomy, the lateral spinothalamic tract is cut using a special knife so that the person will not feel the severe intractable pain below the level of sectioning. This was usually done in patients suffering from advanced metastatic carcinomas.

Anterior Spinothalamic Tract

Fibers carrying sensation of **crude touch** and **deep pressure** in the posterior root terminate in the **chief sensory nucleus** of posterior horn. The axons of these second order neurons cross to the opposite side and reach the anterior funiculus and ascend as anterior spinothalamic tract. As the tract ascends, more and more fibers join at various levels and it reaches the medulla. In the medulla, the tract is known as **spinal fillet** which ascends through pons and midbrain close to medial lemniscus. The fibers relay in the **ventral posterolateral nucleus (VPLN)** of thalamus. The third order neurons end in the sensory cortex in the postcentral gyrus in the concerned area, which appreciates crude touch.

Spinoreticular Tract

Some of the fibers in the lateral spinothalamic tract separate out in the region of medulla and end in the reticular formation of medulla, pons and midbrain. A few other fibers terminate in the nonspecific nuclei of thalamus (midline and intralaminar nuclei). From there, the fibers go to all parts of the cerebral cortex. These fibers form the **ascending reticular activating system (ARAS)**. ARAS maintains the cerebral cortex in an alert state. This tract carries mainly **pain sensations** (*refer* **Chapter 88; Fig. 88.1**).

Tractus Gracilis and Tractus Cuneatus or Dorsal Column Pathway

The fibers forming the dorsal column pathway enter the spinal cord through the medial division of the posterior root and contain thickly medullated Aα **and** Aβ fibers. There is no relay and no crossing in the spinal cord, and the fibers ascend in the posterior funiculus as the dorsal column pathway. Fasciculus gracilis arises from lower segments of spinal cord up to the mid-thoracic level. Fasciculus cuneatus originates from mid-thoracic region. Laminations are seen in the dorsal column also, the sacral fibers are seen medially and the cervical fibers laterally. This tract ends in **nucleus gracilis and nucleus cuneatus** of medulla, and synapse with the second order neurons. Axons of the second order neurons cross to the opposite side in the medulla as **internal arcuate fibers or sensory decussation**. They ascend as **medial lemniscus** through pons and midbrain and end in the ventral posterior nucleus of thalamus. The axons of the third order neurons pass through internal capsule and corona radiata to reach the sensory cortex. The sensations carried are **fine touch-pressure, tactile localization and tactile discrimination, sense of position and sense of movement**.

NONSENSORY TRACTS

Spinocerebellar Tract

Thickly medullated fibers in the posterior root whose *second order neurons are in the posterior horn of spinal cord* form the spinocerebellar tract. The central process of the first order neurons of this tract located in the dorsal root ganglion enter the spinal cord through the medial division of posterior root. Spinocerebellar tract carries unconscious proprioceptive information from skeletal muscles, joints, tendons, etc. and is relayed to the paleocerebellum or spinocerebellum which includes the vermis and the adjoining medial portions of the cerebellar hemispheres via the dorsal and ventral spinocerebellar tract. Functions of this tract are:
- ❖ Sensory control of motor activity
- ❖ Maintain muscle tone especially of the extensor group of muscles
- ❖ Coordinate movements.

Dorsal or Direct or Posterior Spinocerebellar Tract

Some fibers in the medial part of the posterior root synapse with the cells of **Clarke's column** in the posterior horn of spinal cord. Axons of these second order neurons ascend through the posterior part of lateral funiculus more peripherally. There is **no crossing** of these fibers in the spinal cord. The fibers enter the medulla and from there through *inferior cerebellar peduncle* reach the vermis of the cerebellum from where third order neurons arise. Its axons pass to the cerebellar cortex (anterior and posterior lobe of cerebellum). The dorsal spinocerebellar tracts carry instantaneous information from both the muscle spindles and the Golgi tendon organs directly to the cerebellum at a conduction velocity of about 120 m/sec, the most rapid conduction anywhere in the brain or spinal cord.

Ventral or Indirect or Anterior Spinocerebellar Tract

Some of the fibers from the medial division of posterior root enter the spinal cord and synapse with the **chief sensory nucleus** and the axons of these cells ascend on the same side or some may cross to the opposite side. So, this tract contains fibers of both sides of the body, i.e., it contains *both crossed and uncrossed fibers*.

The fibers ascend through lateral funiculus anterior to dorsal or posterior spinocerebellar tract and reach medulla, pons and midbrain up to the level of red nucleus. Then, it descends backwards and downwards and enters the cerebellum through the *superior cerebellar peduncle*.

Spinotectal Tract

Spinotectal tract is formed of axons from the **chief sensory nucleus** of opposite side. It ascends in the lateral funiculus in front of the lateral spinothalamic tract, reaches medulla, pons and midbrain, and ends in the **superior colliculus** of the midbrain. This tract plays an important role in spino-visual reflexes, i.e., coordination of movements of muscles of head and neck in response to visual impulses.

Spino-olivary Tract

Spino-olivary tract is not of much importance in humans. It is formed of axons of **chief sensory nucleus** and is seen anterior to ventral spinocerebellar tract. They pass along with olivospinal tract. The tract terminates in inferior olivary nucleus of medulla and the fibers pass to cerebellum. It has a minor role in motor function.

Propriofascicular Tract

There are interconnecting fibers coming from an upper segment to a lower segment or from lower segment to upper segment. This is seen as a tract all around the gray matter of spinal cord called fasciculus proprius or propriofascicular tract.

■ SENSORY CORTICAL AREA

Introduction

Sensory cortex is called **somesthetic cortex**, located in the postcentral gyrus of parietal lobe (Brodmann's area 3,1,2). Body is represented in the upside down manner in this area. Certain regions of the body are represented over a larger area. Lips, tongue, hands, etc., have a larger area of representation.

Cortical area of appreciation of sensations is called **somesthetic cortex or sensory cortex** located in the parietal lobe. There are two areas:
1. Somatic sensory area-I (SSA-I)
2. Somatic sensory area-II (SSA-II)

Somatic Sensory Area-I (SSA-I)

SSA-I and SSA-II are the two specific areas in the cortex where sensory fibers project. Of these two areas, **SSA-I** is the important one for appreciation of sensation. This is situated in the postcentral gyrus. According to *Brodmann's classification*, SSA-I is divided into area 3, 1 and 2 (*refer* **Chapter 91; Fig. 91.1**). The entire body is represented in this area. Face area is represented down, body up and leg at the top, i.e., **an inverted representation of the body** is seen here. The map of the surface of the body and face of a human on the postcentral gyrus is called **sensory homunculus**. The representation is unilateral, i.e., only one-half of the body is represented on one side of the cortex. *Face has bilateral representation, i.e., upper half of the face is represented on both halves of the sensory cortex and another peculiarity is that face is represented in the erect position* (**Fig. 82.3**).

The area of representation in the sensory cortex is proportionate to the number of receptors in the periphery. Hand and tongue have a greater area of representation because of large number of receptors per unit area. If there is any damage to the area of representation, the particular sensation will be lost.

Functions of SSA-I

❖ Appreciation of almost all sensations (Crude sensations like pain can also be appreciated at the thalamic level).
❖ Localization of sensation as in tactile localization.
❖ Recognition of spatial relationship of body, i.e., sense of position and movement.
❖ Discriminative and synthesizing ability. For example, intensity discrimination of different stimuli, two-point discrimination, stereognosis, texture discrimination, etc.

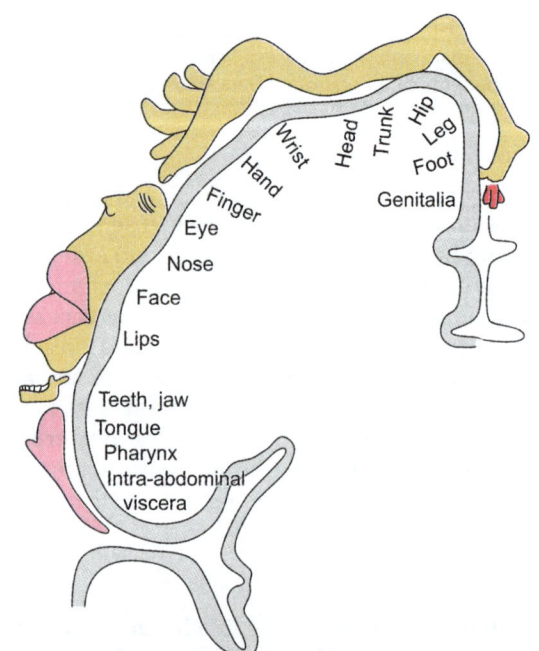

Fig. 82.3: Sensory homunculus (Representation of the body in the post-central gyrus).

Somatic Sensory Area-II (SSA-II)

SSA-II is not seen on the surface of the brain. It is seen inferior and posterior to SSA-I and extends up to sylvian fissure. It forms the roof of the posterior end of the lateral fissure where a second representation of the entire body is seen. The sensory fibers also go to this area but appreciation of sensation is very minimal except for some amount of pain sensation. Here, body is represented in upright position and the representation is not complete and detailed as in the case of SSA-I. Damage to this area does not produce loss of sensation. This area has a role in the sensory control of motor activity. Evidence suggests that electrical stimulation of this area produces some complex movements. Another function is its role in pain perception. Neurons in the posterior part of this area can also be excited by auditory and visual stimuli.

■ SENSORY ASSOCIATION AREA

Posterior to SSA-I is the **sensory association area**, Brodmann's area 5 and 7. This area is very essential for correlation and proper understanding of the sensation, i.e., correlation with previous experiences. This area receives information from SSA-I, thalamus, auditory cortex and visual cortex. All the sensory areas are closely interconnected.

Functions of Sensory Association Area

- Helps in the detailed analysis of sensory information.
- Helps in meaningful interpretation of various sensory experiences.
- The formation of thoughts and even most of the choices of the words to be used are the function of sensory association areas of the brain. It is closely associated with the Wernicke's area.

Amorphosynthesis

In lesions of sensory association area, there is loss of analysis and interpretation of the sense of form of the body. If the lesion is on one side, when feeling objects, the person tends to recognize only one side of the object and forgets that the other side even exists. The person also often forgets to use the other side for motor functions as well. The person is mainly ignorant to the opposite side of the body that is, he forgets that it is there. This complex sensory deficit is called **amorphosynthesis**. For example, if the left sensory association area is removed, the person loses the ability to recognize complex objects felt on the right side of the body. He is also not bothered about the right side of the body and he does not use the right side for motor functions also. He also recognizes only the left side of an object.

■ SENSE OF TOUCH

Introduction

Touch is a cutaneous sensation and it is very important in blind people where it substitutes the sense of vision. Different types of touch receptors are there on the skin and mucous membrane. So, the sensitivity of touch varies in different parts of the body. Most of the touch receptors are rapidly adapting receptors. Touch sensation is divided into fine touch and crude touch. In fine touch, very accurate localization and discrimination is possible. In crude touch, exact localization is not possible. Fine touch includes:

- Tactile localization
- Tactile discrimination
- Deep touch or light pressure
- Gradations of pressure.

Deep touch is felt as light pressure, fine touch and light pressure sensations are carried through dorsal column pathway. Crude touch sensation is carried through anterior spinothalamic tract.

Fine Touch Pathway

Stimulus: Non-uniform pressure or light pressure on the skin and movement of hair.

Receptors (Fig. 82.4)

- Free nerve endings
- Meissner's corpuscles present in abundance in the skin of palm and sole, nipple, lips, and tip of tongue
- Merkel's disc found in fingertips, lips and mouth
- Hair follicle receptors, which are stimulated just by bending the hair without touching the skin
- Basket-like nerve endings surrounding hair follicles
- Pacinian corpuscle.

Touch receptors are present in plenty in the finger tips and lips and very less on the back of the trunk. The receptors are present in more numbers around the hair follicle. Therefore movement of the hair without touching the skin can elicit touch sensation.

First order neuron is in the dorsal root ganglion (DRG) or the corresponding cranial nerve ganglion. Afferent fibers are Aβ fibers which are axons of **DRG cells**. The fibers enter the spinal cord through the posterior root. The fibers in the spinal cord are of two types, small fibers and long fibers. **Long fibers** ascend up through the dorsal column and small fibers go to the interneurons or anterior horn cells. These **short branches** give collaterals which modify cutaneous sensations carried through spinothalamic tract especially pain sensation (*refer* gate control theory). Some collateral terminate in the motor neurons directly or through interneurons for reflex activities.

The dorsal column fibers (tract of Goll and tract of Burdach) ascend up the spinal cord as the **dorsal column pathway** and end in the **nucleus gracilis** and **nucleus cuneatus** of medulla and synapse with the second order neurons. The axons of these neurons cross to the opposite side as internal arcuate fibers (sensory decussation) and ascend up as **medial lemniscus** through pons and midbrain and synapse with the third order neurons in the **ventral posterolateral nucleus (VPLN)** of thalamus. The axons of these neurons pass through the posterior limb of internal capsule and corona radiata to end in the SSA-I and SSA-II in the postcentral gyrus. Fibers also reach the sensory association areas **(Fig. 82.5)**. When there is a lesion to the dorsal columns, touch threshold is elevated and localization of touch sensation is impaired.

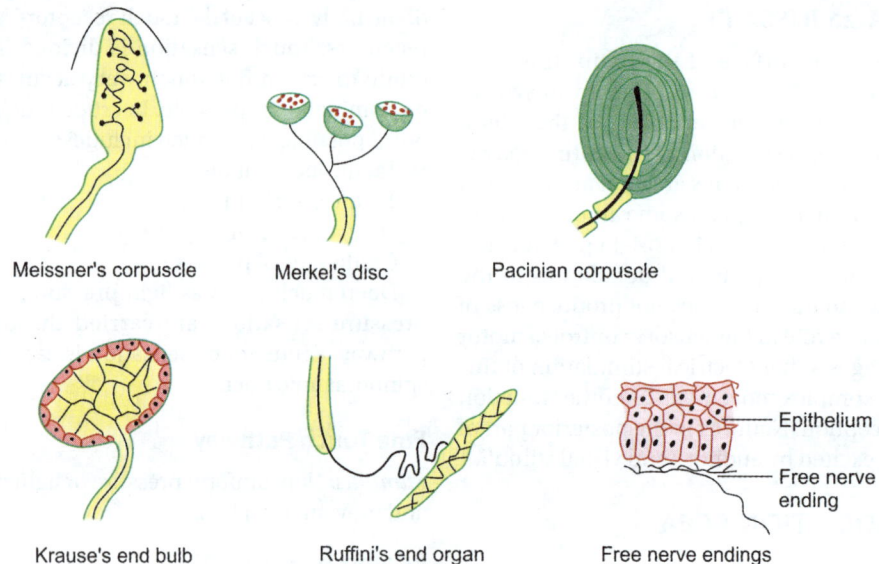

Fig. 82.4: Cutaneous receptors.

Touch Sensation from Face

Pathway for fine touch and crude touch is same from face. Trigeminal nerve supplies face, oral cavity, and head. Sensory fibers from the receptors in these areas go through the trigeminal nerve and the first order neurons are located in the **trigeminal ganglion** or gasserian ganglion or semilunar ganglion. The axons of these neurons form the trigeminal root of trigeminal nerve and end in the **chief/main sensory nucleus of trigeminal nerve** in brainstem where second order neurons are located (The spinal nucleus

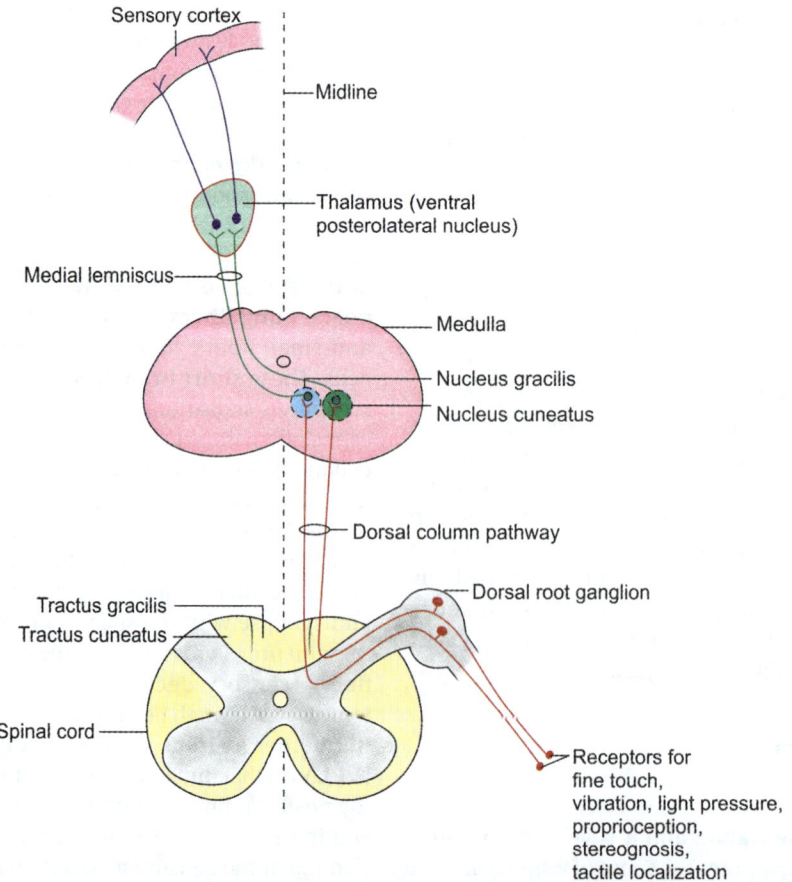

Fig. 82.5: Ascending (Sensory pathway) for fine touch, vibration sense, light pressure, conscious proprioception, stereognosis, tactile localization, and two point discrimination (Dorsal column pathway).

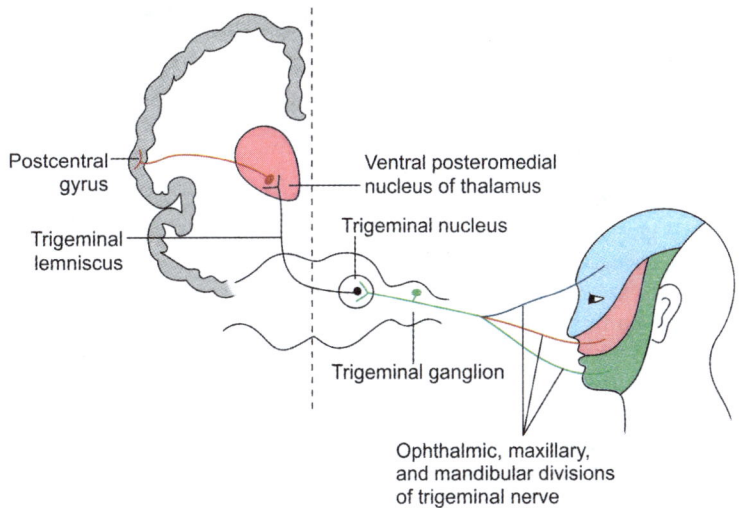

Fig. 82.6: Touch sensation from face.

of the trigeminal nerve receives nociceptive afferent fibers from face and head). Chief sensory nucleus is considered as the trigeminal homologue of dorsal column nuclei. Axons of these neurons cross to the opposite side and ascend as the **trigeminal lemniscus** which lies medial to the medial lemniscus to reach the **ventral posteromedial nucleus of thalamus (VPMN)**. The fibers from trigeminal nucleus to thalamus is also called **trigeminothalamic tract**. The axons of the third order neurons go as thalamocortical fibers to the somatic sensory area for face **(Fig. 82.6)**. The cortical representation of the face is very large due to its high innervation density.

Pathway for Crude Touch

Anterior (Ventral) Spinothalamic Tract

Crude touch is a sensory modality where the person senses touch sensation without having the ability to exactly localize where the stimulus was applied. It has a high threshold of excitation. The receptors for crude touch are Ruffini endings and free nerve endings which are not encapsulated. The afferent fibers from the touch receptors reaching the DRG are dendrites of **DRG** cells which form the *first order neurons*. The fibers carrying crude touch sensation enter the spinal cord through the posterior root and relay in the **chief sensory nucleus** in the posterior horn. These cells form the *second order neurons* and the axons of these cells cross to the opposite side through the anterior gray commissure and ascend up on the opposite side as the **anterior (ventral) spinothalamic tract**. They relay in the *third order neurons* in the **ventral posterolateral nucleus** of thalamus and the axons go to the somatic sensory area (SSA) in the postcentral gyrus and the sensation is appreciated as crude touch **(Fig. 82.7)**. When there is a lesion to the anterior spinothalamic tract, touch deficit is slight and touch localization remains normal.

Crude touch sensation from the face is carried through the trigeminal nerve and the pathway is same as that for fine touch.

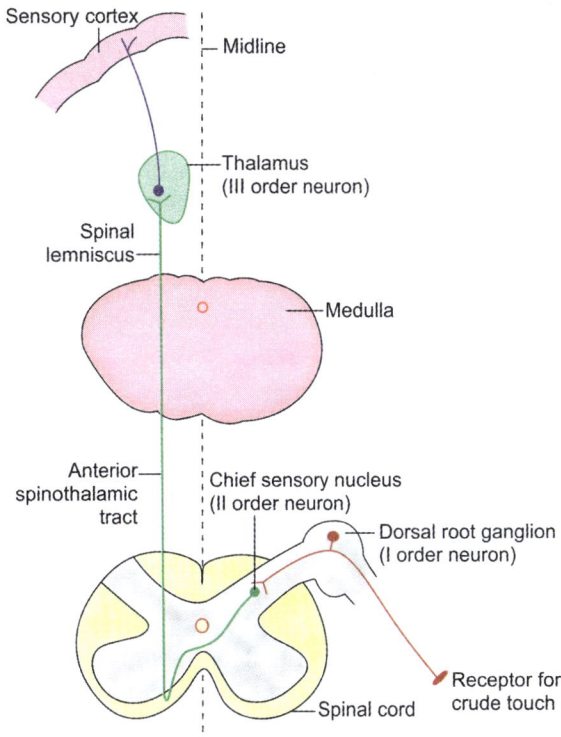

Fig. 82.7: Pathway for crude touch.

A number of afferent fibers for crude touch converge on one chief sensory nucleus and many fibers from chief sensory nucleus converge on one-third order neuron in the ventral posterolateral nucleus of thalamus. So, exact localization is not possible in the case of crude touch. But in the case of fine touch, the ratio is 1:1 and so, precise localization is possible for fine touch sensation.

Abnormalities of Touch Sensation

Anesthesia

Complete loss of all sensations is called anesthesia. It usually occurs in peripheral nerve lesions like leprosy which leads to anesthesia corresponding to the distribution of the sensory fibers. It is also seen in complete transection of spinal cord where there is complete loss of sensations below the level of lesion. Anesthetics are drugs used to control pain during a surgery and it is a temporarily induced loss of sensations.

In **dissociated anesthesia**, the sensation of pain and temperature is lost with the preservation of touch. It occurs in diseases where the spinal cord gray matter surrounding the central canal is damaged like syringomyelia. The fibers of the dorsal column pathway are spared because they are placed at the periphery of the spinal cord. The fibers of the spinothalamic tract (carrying pain and temperature sensation) cross to the opposite side very close to the central canal. So they will be affected by the disease.

Hemianesthesia is loss of sensations of one half of the body. It is seen in lesions of thalamus, internal capsule or cerebral cortex of the opposite side.

Hypoesthesia or Hypesthesia

Partial loss of sensation is called hypoesthesia. It is seen in **beri-beri** caused by thiamine deficiency. It affects feet, fingers, lips, etc. It also occurs in decompression sickness.

Paresthesia

Abnormal sensations like numbness, tingling, tickling, pricking or burning is referred to as paresthesia. Patient complains of pins and needle sensation. It is seen in cases of nerve compression as seen in Saturday night paralysis which is temporary. It is also seen in stroke, multiple sclerosis, transverse myelitis, thalamic lesions and encephalitis.

Dissociated Anesthesia

Dissociated sensory loss is a condition where there is loss of fine touch and proprioception without loss of pain and temperature or vice versa. It is seen in Brown-Sequard syndrome, tabes dorsalis, intramedullary spinal cord tumors, syringomyelia, etc. It usually occurs in isolated tract lesion of spinal cord.

Hyperesthesia

Increased receptor sensitivity to various stimuli is called hyperesthesia. It is seen in thalamic syndrome, herpes, peripheral neuropathy, etc. For example, a non-noxious stimulus like touch causes the sensation of pain in this case.

Agraphesthesia

Loss of the sense of writing figures on the body is called agraphesthesia, i.e., loss of graphesthesia. It is seen in lesions of the sensory cortex.

Astereognosis

Inability to identify a familiar object by feeling it with eyes closed even though the primary tactile sensibility is intact. It is seen in cortical lesions.

■ PATHWAY FOR TEMPERATURE SENSATION

Temperature receptors are free nerve endings. There are warmth receptors which respond to temperatures above

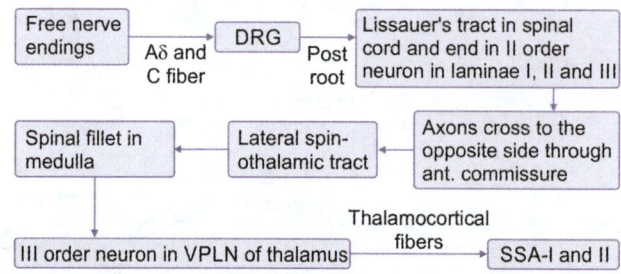

Flowchart 82.1: Schematic representation of the pathway for temperature.

(VPLN: ventral posterolateral nucleus; DRG: dorsal root ganglion; SSA: somatic sensory area).

the body temperature and cold receptors that respond to temperature below body temperature. Cold receptors respond to temperatures ranging from 10 to 40°C and warm receptors respond to temperatures ranging from 30 to 50°C (Previously it was thought that Ruffini's end organ is the receptor for warmth and Krause's end bulb for cold (**Fig. 82.4**). There are three sets of temperature receptors which are ion channels which belong to transient receptor potential (TRP) subfamily:

- **Cold and menthol sensitive receptors 1** (CMR-1) which respond to moderate cold
- **Vanilloid receptor 1** (VR-1) respond to very high temperature
- **Vanilloid receptor-like protein 1** (VRL-1) receptors respond to moderate to high temperature.

The temperature receptors show adaptation between 20°C and 40°C. Above and below these temperatures there is no adaptation. Freezing cold and burning hot stimulate pain receptors. Temperatures above 45°C lead to tissue damage and pain sensation is also felt at extremes of temperatures. Cold sensation is carried by Aδ fibers with velocity 20 m/sec **(Flowchart 82.1 and Fig. 82.8)** and the afferents for heat are C fibers.

Temperature sensations are transmitted in pathways similar to those for pain signals **(Fig. 82.8)**. Upon entering the spinal cord, the signals travel for a few segments upward or downward in the *tract of Lissauer* and then terminate mainly in laminae I, II, and III of the dorsal horn. From here axons of the second order neurons cross to the opposite side and ascend as lateral spinothalamic tract along with pain fibers. Some of the fibers terminate in the reticular formation of the brain stem and rest of the fibers end in the ventral posterolateral nucleus of the thalamus. From the thalamus, thermal signals are relayed to the cerebral somatic sensory cortex. Some amount of appreciation of temperature sensation occurs at the subcortical level because removal of the entire cortical postcentral gyrus in the human being reduces but does not abolish the ability to distinguish gradations of temperature.

Mechanism of Stimulation of Temperature Receptors

The cold and warmth receptors are stimulated by changes in their metabolic rates because temperature alters the rate of intracellular chemical reactions more than two fold for each 10°C change in external temperature. That is thermal

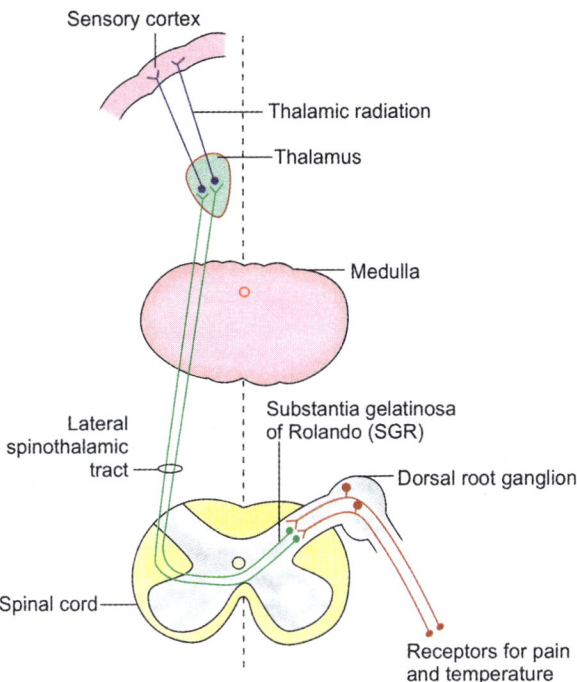

Fig. 82.8: Pathway for fast pain and temperature from the body except head.

the body and also to recognize the rate of movement of different parts of the body. Impulses from sensory receptors in and around joints, touch receptors and muscle spindle are synthesized in the cortex into a conscious picture of the position of the body in space.

Unconscious proprioception gives information from muscle, tendon and ligament about which we are not aware of, i.e., regarding length and tension of muscle. It is carried by the anterior and posterior spinocerebellar tracts and is necessary for the control of muscle tone, motor activity, etc. This information may not reach the cortex.

Another classification of position sense or proprioceptive sense

- *Static position sense,* which means conscious perception of the orientation of the different parts of the body with respect to one another
- *Rate of movement sense,* also called *kinesthesia* or *dynamic proprioception.*

Knowledge of position, both static and dynamic, depends on knowing the degrees of angulation of all joints in all planes and their rates of change. So, different types of receptors are involved in determining joint angulation. Some define proprioception as sense of joint position, i.e., position sense and kinesthesia as awareness of motion of the human body, i.e., motion sense.

Pathway for Conscious Proprioception

Receptors are present in and around joints, i.e., in ligaments, joint capsule, synovial membrane, or in the deep tissues around joint and muscles. Cutaneous tactile receptors are also involved in determining position sense. The important receptors are:

- Ruffini endings which are slowly adapting spray endings
- Golgi tendon organ like receptors
- Pacinian corpuscles in the synovia and ligaments

Afferent fibers are large sensory Aβ fibers whose cell bodies are present in the dorsal root ganglion. The central process of this first order neuron enters the spinal cord through the posterior root and ascends on the same side as the dorsal column pathway. They also give collaterals in the spinal cord to a motor neuron for reflex activity. The ascending fibers reaches the medulla, and fibers in fasciculus gracilis (from lower segments) synapse with the second order neurons in **nucleus gracilis**, and fibers in fasciculus cuneatus (those fibers entering the upper segments of the spinal cord) synapse with neurons in **nucleus cuneatus**. Axons of these second order neurons cross to the opposite side as internal arcuate fibers and ascend as **medial lemniscus** through pons and midbrain. The fibers end in the third order neurons in the ventral posterolateral nucleus (**VPLN**) of **thalamus** and axons of these neurons reach the somatic sensory area I and II through internal capsule and corona radiata (*refer* **Fig. 82.5**).

Pathway for Unconscious Proprioception

Receptors are:
- Muscle spindle
- Golgi tendon organ.

detection results not from direct physical effects of heat or cold on the nerve endings but from chemical stimulation of the endings which is induced by variations in temperature.

Trigeminothalamic Tract (Temperature and Pain Sensation from Face)

Sensory afferent fibers carrying pain and temperature sensations from the *face, teeth, oral and nasal cavities* relay in the **spinal nucleus of trigeminal nerve**. The axons of the second order neurons in this nucleus cross to the opposite side and constitute the **trigeminothalamic tract** which relays pain and temperature information to the contralateral ventral posteromedial nucleus (VPMN) of thalamus.

■ KINESTHETIC SENSATION (KINESTHESIA) OR PROPRIOCEPTION

Information from joints, muscles, tendons and ligaments that inform about the movement of joints and body parts in space and in relation to one another is called proprioceptive information. It is sometimes described as the *sixth sense.* (*Proprioception does not include the sense of position and orientation of the body occurring due to stimulation of visual and vestibular receptors.*) Proprioception or position sense is of two subtypes:
1. Conscious proprioception
2. Unconscious proprioception

Conscious proprioception includes sense of position and movement, i.e., conscious aspect of information which proceeds to cortex through the dorsal column pathway. We are aware of conscious proprioception. It helps to analyze movements of parts of body with respect to other parts of

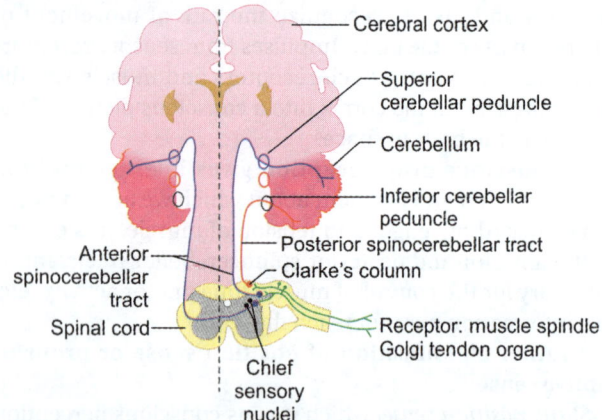

Fig. 82.9: Pathway for unconscious proprioception (unconscious proprioceptive information from head and face passes through trigeminal nerve to the cerebellum of same side after relaying in the mesencephalic nucleus of trigeminal nerve).

Afferent fibers: Large sensory Ia and Ib fibers whose cell bodies are in the dorsal root ganglion (DRG). The central processes enter the spinal cord through the posterior nerve root and end in the **Clarke's column and chief sensory nucleus** which form the second order neurons. The axons of the second order neurons in Clarke's column ascend in the spinal cord on the same side as the **posterior or direct spinocerebellar tract**. From the medulla, the fibers pass through the **inferior cerebellar peduncle** and reach cerebellar cortex.

The axons of the second order neurons in chief sensory nucleus either cross to the opposite side or ascend through the same side as the **anterior or indirect spinocerebellar tract**. This tract contains fibers from both sides of the body, i.e., both crossed and uncrossed fibers. The anterior spinocerebellar tract ascends through medulla, pons and midbrain, then descends and enters the cerebellar cortex through the **superior cerebellar peduncle (Fig. 82.9)**.

> For determining joint angulation in midranges of motion, the *muscle spindles* are among the most important receptors. They are also very important in helping to control muscle movement. When the angle of a joint is changing, some muscles are being stretched while others are loosened, and the net stretch information from the spindles is transmitted into the integrating areas of the spinal cord and higher regions of the dorsal column system for interpreting joint angulations.
> At the extremes of joint angulation, stretch of the ligaments and deep tissues around the joints is an additional important factor in determining position. Types of sensory endings used for this are the Pacinian corpuscles, Ruffini's endings, and Golgi tendon organ like receptors found in muscle tendons. The Pacinian corpuscles and muscle spindles are especially adapted for detecting rapid rates of change. It is likely that these are the receptors most responsible for detecting rate of movement.

Functions of Spinocerebellar Pathway

❖ Maintenance of muscle tone, posture and coordination of various motor activities. Proprioception helps with the planning of movements, sport performance, playing a musical instrument, etc.
❖ Posterior spinocerebellar pathway is concerned with movements of individual muscles whereas anterior spinocerebellar pathway is concerned with movement of whole limb.
❖ An intact sense of proprioception is essential to learn a new skill as sport performance, artistic activity, driving a car, etc. Appropriate integration of proprioceptive input specific to that activity should become familiar to perform the task with ease.

Proprioception from Head and Face

Fibers which carry the **conscious proprioceptive** information from head and face pass through the trigeminal nerve. The fibers go to the **mesencephalic nucleus** of trigeminal nerve which contains pseudounipolar neurons which form the first order neurons. *This is the only first order neuron present in the brain.* Mesencephalic nucleus of trigeminal nerve contains the cell bodies of primary afferent proprioceptive neurons innervating the stretch receptors in the muscles of mastication and in the other muscles of head.

The axons of the first order neurons end in the **main sensory nucleus** of trigeminal nerve which forms the second order neuron. The axons of these neurons cross to the opposite side and ascend as the trigeminal lemniscus to reach the thalamus and from there third order neurons project to the somatic sensory area.

Unconscious proprioception from head and face is carried through inferior cerebellar peduncle to cerebellum of same side.

Abnormalities of Proprioception

Sense of position and passive movement can be lost in lesions of posterior column. Poor proprioception at a joint may lead to increased risk of injury. Impaired proprioception is seen in tabes dorsalis, subacute combined degeneration of spinal cord, multiple sclerosis, Parkinson's disease and in lesions of the sensory cortex and cerebellum. Temporary impairment is seen following alcohol consumption.

Impaired proprioception can be detected by doing Romberg's test. Inability to maintain the standing posture with bare feet together and eyes closed without support is referred to as **Romberg's sign**. This is called **sensory ataxia** which occurs in posterior column lesion due to lack of sense of position in both legs. It is because, from the non-cluster region of the dorsal column nuclei, significant proprioceptive information goes to the cerebellum. This should not be confused with ataxia occurring in cerebellar lesion and vestibular dysfunction.

■ ITCHING AND TICKLING

Low-frequency mechanoreceptors when stimulated produce **itching and tickling**. Mild stimulation by something which moves through skin, chemicals like histamine, etc., produce tickling and itching. Specific free nerve endings present only in the superficial layers of skin are the receptors for itching and tickling. These receptors are rapidly adapting mechanoreceptors. Itching produces the **scratch reflex**.

Itching and tickling sensations are carried through unmyelinated type C fibers. First order neurons are in the dorsal root ganglion (DRG) which enter the spinal cord and form the Lissauer's tract and end in the **substantia gelatinosa of Rolando**. The axons of these neurons cross to the opposite side and ascend as **lateral spinothalamic tract** and reach the medulla. From medulla, it ascends as **spinal lemniscus** and reaches posteroventral nucleus (PVN) of thalamus and synapse with the third order neurons. From there, axons project to Brodmann's area 3,1,2.

VISCERAL SENSATIONS

Information about visceral distension arises from stretch receptors in the wall of the hollow viscus. The visceral sensation travels along the same spinothalamic tracts as somatic sensation. The cortical receiving areas for visceral sensation are intermixed with the somatic receiving areas.

PAIN SENSATION

Introduction

Pain is an **unpleasant sensation** which **protects** the organism against injurious agents. It draws the attention of the individual as a whole. For an individual, pain sensation gives a warning about tissue damage and helps to take immediate measures against those factors which produce the damage. For example, in angina, during exertion the patient feels pain over the chest and the pain disappears on taking rest. In occlusive vascular disorders, while walking, the patient complains of intense pain in the leg and pain disappears on taking rest and is known as **intermittent claudication**.

Pain sensation differs from other sensations in that it has an emotional or affective component. It is also associated with reflex withdrawal response and autonomic changes mediated via the autonomic nervous system such as sweating, changes in blood pressure, heart rate and respiration.

Regarding a physician, the location, quality, intensity and duration of pain gives a clue to come at a correct conclusion. Depending on the quality, pain is classified into:
- **Pricking pain:** Sharp, localized pain as in needle prick.
- **Burning pain:** Diffuse, intense pain as in burns.
- **Aching pain** due to deep muscle spasm.
- **Throbbing pain** in which the intensity increases and decreases with pulsations.
- **Colicky pain:** Pain is felt intermittently in hollow organs as in intestinal colic, ureteric colic, etc.
- **Ischemic pain:** Intense pain due to loss of blood supply.
- **Nauseating pain**
- **Electric pain**.

Pain Receptors or Nociceptors

Pain sensations arise from receptors located on unmyelinated dendrites of sensory neurons located throughout the skin as well as deep tissue. Pain receptors are also called **nociceptors**.

- **Mechanical nociceptors** respond to strong pressure applied by a sharp object.
- **Thermal nociceptors** are stimulated by skin temperatures above 45°C or below 20°C.
- **Chemically sensitive nociceptors** respond to chemicals such as bradykinin, histamine, acids and irritants.
- **Polymodal nociceptors** respond to combinations of these stimuli.

Many of the receptors on the endings of nociceptive sensory nerves are part of a superfamily of non-selective cation channels gated by noxious heat, vanilloids and extracellular protons called **transient receptor potential (TRP) channels**. Among the TRP channel superfamily, TRPV1, TRPV2, TRPV3, TRPV4, TRPM8 and TRPA1 are thermoreceptors which responds to extremes of temperature that cause pain sensation. These channels are also activated by chemical agents such as capsaicin (TRPV1), menthol (TRPM8), camphor (TRPV3) and mustard (TRPA1).

TRPV1 receptors also called **capsaicin receptors** (V refers to a group of chemicals called **vanilloids**) are activated by intense heat, acids, and chemicals such as **capsaicin.** Capsaicin is the active ingredient in hot peppers and an example of vanilloid. TRPV1 receptors can also be activated indirectly by initial activation of TRPV3 receptors in the keratinocytes in the skin. **TRPV3** and **TRPV4** receptors on sensory nerve endings are activated when the skin temperature reach 33–39°C and 25–34°C, respectively. Noxious mechanical, cold and chemical stimuli may activate **TRPA1-receptors** (A, for **ankyrin**) on sensory nerve terminals. Sensory nerve endings also have **acid-sensing ion channel (ASIC) receptors** that are activated by acid and are responsible for mediating acid induced pain.

Instead of directly activating nociceptors, some nociceptive stimuli release intermediate molecules that then activate receptors on the nerve endings. For example, nociceptive mechanical stimuli can cause the release of adenosine tri-phosphate (ATP) that acts on **purinergic receptors** like **P2X**, an ionotropic receptor, and **P2Y**, a G-protein coupled receptor. **Tyrosine receptor kinase A (TrkA)** is activated by **nerve growth factor (NGF)** that is released due to tissue damage.

Nociceptive sensory nerve endings also have a variety of receptors that respond to immune mediators that are released in response to tissue injury and mediate inflammatory pain. These include **B1 and B2 receptors** (bradykinin), **prostanoid receptors** (prostaglandins), and **cytokine receptors** (interleukins).

Causes of Pain

Tissue damage is the causes of pain which may be due to different stimuli.
- Physical factors:
  - Mechanical – wounds
  - Thermal – extremes of temperature (above 45°C or below 0°C) produce tissue damage
  - Electrical stimulus
- Chemical factors:
  - Strong acids and alkali
  - Chemical agents produced in the body as bradykinin, histamine, etc.

- Ischemia produce factor P of Lewis which is identified as K⁺
- Bacterial infection releases many pain-producing substances in the body like:
  - Bradykinin
  - Histamine
  - Substance P
  - Factor P of Lewis, acetylcholine, serotonin, prostaglandin, lactic acid, proteolytic enzymes, K⁺, etc. Prostaglandin and substance P cannot stimulate pain nerve ending directly but can lower the threshold for pain endings.

Components of Pain Sensation

Pain has two components:
1. Sensory discriminative component
2. Motivational-affective component

Sensory discriminative component includes processing of sensory inputs in the primary somatosensory cortex and helps in perception of the quality of pain, location of the stimulus, assess the intensity of pain and its duration. The pain pathway to the primary somatosensory cortex is responsible for the discriminative aspect of pain (pain localization).

Motivational-affective component includes attention and arousal; somatic and autonomic reflexes; endocrine reflexes and emotional changes associated with pain. These are responsible for the unpleasant nature of pain and are mainly due to the connection of pain pathway to the cingulate gyrus of limbic system. Some dorsal horn neurons that receive nociceptive input synapse in the reticular formation of the brainstem (**spinoreticular pathway**) and then project to the centrolateral nucleus of the thalamus. The pathway that includes synapses in the brainstem reticular formation and centrolateral thalamic nucleus projects to the frontal lobe, limbic system, and insular cortex. This pathway mediates the motivational-affective component of pain.

Areas in the brain concerned with reception and interpretation of pain sensation are:
- **Postcentral gyrus** interprets pain with past experiences.
- **Cingulate gyrus** of limbic system is concerned with the emotional aspect of pain.
- **Insular gyrus** brings about autonomic responses associated with pain.

Types of Pain

- Superficial pain (cutaneous pain)
- Deep pain.

Receptors for **superficial pain** are free nerve endings in skin and mucous membrane. For **deep pain**, receptors which are also free nerve endings are in the deep structures like tendon, joint surfaces, ligaments, synovial membrane, muscles, periosteum, parietal pericardium and pleura, arterial wall, dentine and pulp of teeth, etc. The difference between superficial pain and deep pain is shown in **Table 82.2**.

Organs like liver and lungs are devoid of pain receptors. Pain receptors show no adaptation. This is a protective mechanism which helps to warn the subject of the injurious process in the body.

Table 82.2: Differences between superficial pain and deep pain.

Superficial pain	Deep pain
Involves skin, mucous membrane of oral and nasal cavity and subcutaneous tissue	Involves muscle, tendon, bone, hollow viscera, parietal pleura, pericardium, etc.
Fast pain can be well localized and is sharp in character	Poorly localized and dull in character
Fast pain conducted along Aδ fibers with conduction velocity 12–30 m/sec which release glutamate as the neurotransmitter. Slow pain via C fibers	Conducted along unmyelinated C fibers with velocity 0.5–2 m/sec which release substance P as the neurotransmitter
Associated with reflex withdrawal movements, increase in heart rate and blood pressure	Associated with autonomic symptoms like sweating, hypotension, vomiting, etc.
Not referred to other areas	Pain is felt locally and may radiate/refer to a distant site

Peripheral Sensitization of Nociceptors

By continuous stimulation of pain receptors, the threshold for excitation becomes lower and lower, i.e., the receptor becomes **more sensitive**. When exposed to strong noxious stimulus, the nociceptor becomes sensitized and it responds more vigorously to another noxious stimulus since its threshold for activation is lowered. This may lead to **hyperalgesia** or increased sensitivity to pain. Substances like K⁺, prostaglandins, histamine, serotonin, eicosanoids, etc., contribute to sensitization by opening ion channels or by activating second messenger systems in the receptor. Activation of nociceptor releases various peptides like **substance P, calcitonin gene-related peptide (CGRP)**, etc. These are released from the terminal of the afferent pain fiber that is stimulated and also from other collateral terminals of the same nociceptor through an **axon reflex** (*refer* 'axon reflex'). This leads to *neurogenic edema* of the area stimulated, which is characterized by reddening, warming, swelling and pain.

Pain Pathway

The primary pain afferents are Aδ and 'C' group of nerve fibers. Information about pain sensation is transmitted to the higher centers through **specific and non-specific ascending pathways**. The specific pathways convey information regarding location and intensity of pain. It also helps to identify sharp pain, i.e., the nature of pain. Whereas, non-specific pathways convey information regarding the duration of pain, e.g., long lasting pain. It helps to identify dull pain which is poorly localized.

Neurons in the reticular formation and thalamus are activated by pain pathways. Pain pathway is also connected to hypothalamus and limbic system that integrate autonomic and endocrine responses associated with pain (**Fig. 82.10**). Discrimination and meaningful interpretation of pain requires cerebral cortex. But perception of pain alone does not require the cerebral cortex and it can occur at the subcortical level like thalamus.

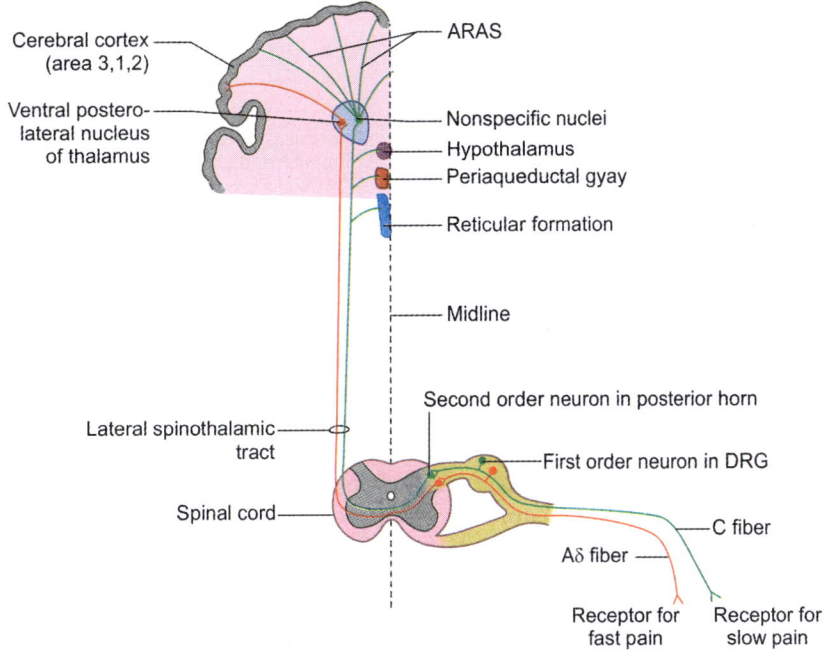

Fig. 82.10: Pathway for fast pain and slow pain from the body. Fast pain is transmitted via Aδ fibers and slow pain via C fibers. Pathway for pain sensation from face is shown in **Figure 82.6**.
(ARAS: ascending reticular activating system)

Pathway for Superficial Pain Sensation

Types of Superficial Pain Sensations

Superficial pain sensation is of two types whose pathways are different:
1. **Sharp pricking pain** or first pain or fast pain
2. **Dull aching pain** or second pain or slow pain.

Introduction

If the skin is pricked by a sharp pin, immediately the person can localize the area of prick. This helps to react immediately and move away from the source of stimulus (avoidance or withdrawal reflex). A little later, a diffuse intense burning sensation is felt in that area without clear localization. Thus, a *double sensation* is felt. The first sensation is first pain or sharp pain which is due to stimulation of fast conducting Aδ fibers. The second sensation is second pain or prolonged burning and aching pain due to stimulation of slow conducting "C" fibers.

The neurotransmitter released at the Aδ fiber ending is **glutamate** and that released from C fibers is **substance P**. The glutamate transmitter acts instantaneously and lasts for only a few milliseconds. Substance P is released much more slowly, and lasts over a period of seconds or even minutes. The "double" pain sensation one feels after a pinprick might result partly from the fact that the glutamate transmitter gives a faster pain sensation of short duration, whereas the substance P transmitter gives a more lasting pain sensation.

Fast pain is almost confined to the skin and is experienced within 0.1 sec after the pain stimulus is applied. Slow pain is produced due to tissue destruction and can occur in any tissue of the body. Fast pain activates the primary somatosensory cortex and is responsible for the discriminative aspect of pain. Slow pain activates cingulate gyrus, amygdala, frontal lobe and the insular cortex. This pathway mediates the motivational-affective component of pain.

Table 82.3 shows differences between fast pain and slow pain.

Table 82.3: Differences between fast pain and slow pain.	
Fast pain	**Slow pain**
Precisely localized	Poorly localized
Experienced 0.1 sec after the application of pain stimulus	Experienced 1 sec or later after the application of stimulus
Sharp, acute pricking type of pain confined to the skin	Burning, aching or throbbing type of pain which can occur in any tissue
Elicited by mechanical and thermal stimuli	Elicited by mechanical, thermal and chemical stimuli
Carried by **Aδ fibers** with velocity of conduction 30 m/sec	Carried by **'C' fiber** with velocity of conduction 2 m/sec
Aδ fibers release **glutamate** which is a fast acting localized neurotransmitter	C fibers release **substance P** which has a slow release and can diffuse widely and thus can influence many neurons of posterior horn
Produce reflex withdrawal movements, increase in heart rate and blood pressure	Produces sweating, bradycardia and fall in blood pressure
Afferent Aδ pain fibers end in lamina I of posterior horn	C fibers mediating slow pain end in laminas II and III of posterior horn
Responsible for the discriminative aspect of pain	Responsible for the motivational affective component of pain

Pathway for Fast Pain

Fast pain is also referred to as *sharp pain, pricking pain, acute pain, or electric pain*. This type of pain is felt when a needle is stuck into the skin, when the skin is cut with a knife, or when the skin is acutely burned. It is also felt when the skin is subjected to electric shock. Fast pain is usually not felt in the deep tissues of the body.

The pathway for fast pain is also known as **neospinothalamic pathway**. The fast type Aδ pain fibers terminate mainly in **lamina I** of the dorsal horn where they synapse with the second order neurons. The neurotransmitter released by the Aδ fibers is **glutamate**. The second-order neurons give rise to long fibers that cross immediately to the opposite side of the cord through the anterior commissure and then turn upward, ascending up to the brain as the **lateral spinothalamic tract** (**Figs. 82.10 and Flowchart 82.2**). In the brain stem a few fibers of the neospinothalamic tract terminate in the reticular formation of the brain stem, but majority of fibers pass all the way to the thalamus terminating in the *ventral posterolateral nucleus of thalamus*. From the thalamus, the third order neurons reach the somatosensory cortex.

Fibers entering the SSA-I and SSA-II help in localization and appreciation of pain sensation and also for the detailed analysis of the sensation, i.e., pain discrimination and its meaningful interpretation. In addition to SSA-I and SSA-II, pain fibers also activate cingulate gyrus, mediofrontal cortex, insular cortex and cerebellum. If there is a lesion in the insular cortex there will be analgesia to some extent.

Even if cortex is removed, pain perception is possible but exact localization is not possible. This is because crude pain perception occurs at the thalamic level, i.e., in the **ventral posterolateral nucleus** of thalamus. Emotional reactions in response to crude pain are initiated at this level.

Pathway for Slow Pain

Slow pain is also referred to as *slow burning pain, aching pain, throbbing pain, nauseating pain* and *chronic pain*. This type of pain is usually associated with *tissue destruction*. It can be sometimes unbearable. Slow pain can occur both in the skin and in the deep tissues or organs. The slow pain tends to become greater over time and may eventually produce intolerable pain. Exact localization of slow pain is not possible. This is mainly due to the multisynaptic, diffuse connectivity of this pathway.

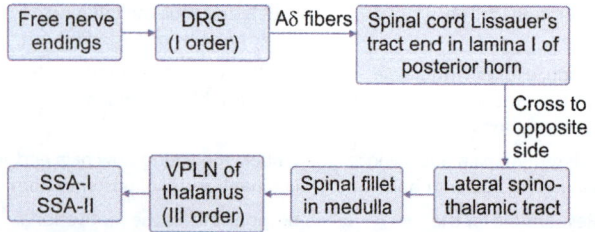

Flowchart 82.2: Pathway for pricking pain.

(DRG: dorsal root ganglion; VPLN: ventral posterolateral nucleus)

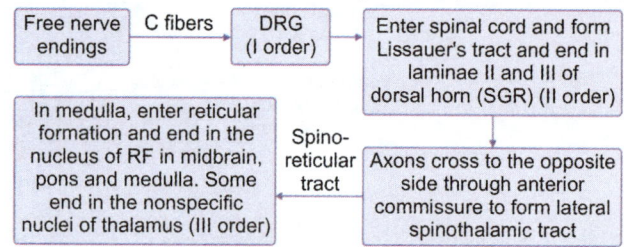

Flowchart 82.3: Pathway for slow pain.

(SGR: substantia gelatinosa of Rolando)

Following tissue injury, the chemicals that excite the chemical type of pain receptors are *bradykinin, serotonin, histamine, potassium ions, acids, acetylcholine,* and *proteolytic enzymes*. In addition, *prostaglandins* and *substance P* enhance the sensitivity of pain endings but do not directly excite them. The chemical that seems to be more painful than others is *bradykinin*. The chemical substances released during tissue injury are especially important in producing the slow, suffering type of pain that occurs after tissue injury.

The slow pain pathway is also referred to as **paleospinothalamic pathway** for transmitting slow chronic pain. This slow-pain pathway transmits pain mainly from the peripheral type C pain fibers which release **substance P** as the neurotransmitter. The afferent fibers terminate in the spinal cord in **laminae II and III** of the dorsal horn, which together form the *substantia gelatinosa of Rolando (SGR)*. The second order neurons in the SGR, give rise to long axons that mostly join the fibers of the fast pain pathway, passing first through the anterior commissure to the opposite side of the cord, then upward to the brain in the **lateral spinothalamic pathway** (**Flowchart 82.3**).

Majority of type C pain fibers in the lateral spinothalamic tract separate from the main pain pathway and instead of going to the thalamus, end in the nuclei of reticular formation which form the third order neurons. This forms the **spino-reticular pathway**. Axons of third order neurons diffusely go to the entire cerebral cortex. This system of fibers forms **ascending reticular activating system (ARAS)**. It increases the excitability of the entire cortex and can even wake up a person from sleep. It makes the person aware of some injurious process occurring in the body (**Fig. 82.11**). This explains why it is almost impossible for a person to sleep when he is in severe pain. From the brain stem pain areas multiple interneurons relay the pain signals upward into the intralaminar and ventrolateral nuclei of the thalamus (nonspecific nuclei of thalamus) and into certain portions of the hypothalamus and other basal regions of the brain.

In the brain stem, instead of going to the thalamus, most of the slow pain fibers terminate in one of the following three areas:

1. The *reticular nuclei* of the medulla, pons, and midbrain
2. The *tectal area* of the mesencephalon deep to the superior and inferior colliculi
3. The *periaqueductal gray region* surrounding the aqueduct of Sylvius.

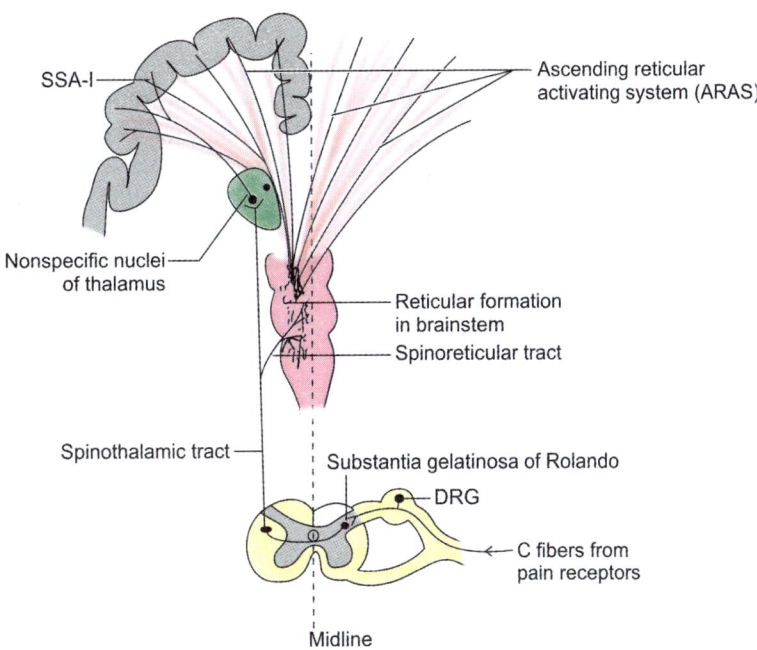

Fig. 82.11: Pathway for slow pain.

These lower regions of the brain appear to be important for feeling the suffering types of pain, because animals whose brains have been sectioned above the midbrain to block pain signals from reaching the cerebrum still have definite evidence of suffering from pain when any part of the body is traumatized. Therefore, it is likely that pain impulses entering the brain stem reticular formation, the thalamus, and other lower brain centers cause conscious perception of pain. However, the cortex plays an especially important role in interpreting pain quality, even though pain perception might be principally the function of lower centers.

Reaction to Pain

Reaction to pain varies from individual to individual and in the same person it varies from time to time.
- Reflex motor reactions and autonomic response
- Psychic reaction.

Reflex Motor Reaction and Autonomic Response

Reflex motor reaction includes withdrawal reflex which is very much modified in humans by influence from higher centers. Voluntary and planned motor activity occurs in man to avoid the injurious stimulus. There is also reflex increase in heart rate, blood pressure, etc.

Psychic Reaction

Worrying, crying, depression, anxiety, etc., are the psychic responses to pain. Pain always has an unpleasant emotional component due to certain connections from the thalamic level to the prefrontal areas. The spinoreticular tract that carries slow pain after synapsing in the reticular formation and centrolateral thalamic nucleus projects to the frontal lobe, limbic system and insular cortex on the side opposite the stimulus. This pathway mediates the motivational-affective component of pain.

If a prefrontal lobotomy is done it is seen that the person feels pain sensation but he is not bothered about it. Here, there is no emotional component of pain. This method was previously done in terminal stages of cancer where the excruciating pain can be abolished. Nowadays strong analgesics like morphine are given to relieve pain.

Deep Pain

Slow pain pathway is predominant in deeper structures. This is because, Aδ fibers are relatively deficient in deeper structures and so there is little fast, localized pain. Deep pain is poorly localized, unpleasant, nauseating and associated with autonomic symptoms like fall in blood pressure, bradycardia, vomiting, sweating, etc. There is reflex contraction of nearby skeletal muscles. This leads to ischemia which in turn stimulates pain receptors leading to more spasm and a vicious cycle develops. Deep pain is of two types:
1. Deep somatic pain
2. Visceral pain.

Deep Somatic Pain

Deep somatic pain arises from muscles, periosteum, tendons, ligaments, fascia, joints, etc. The pathway is same as that of superficial pain through C fibers. Its features are similar to that of **slow pain pathway**. Deep somatic pain initiates reflex contraction of nearby skeletal muscles. This protects the underlying inflamed structures from further trauma. This reflex spasm is referred to as muscle **guarding**. For example, in fracture, the nearby skeletal muscles contract so that the injured part is immobilized.

Ischemic Muscular Pain

When muscle contracts in the presence of inadequate blood supply it causes pain, e.g., intermittent claudication in occlusive vascular disorders, angina pectoris, severe exercise, etc. The ischemic muscle releases a chemical called **P factor of Lewis** during contraction. *Factor P is now identified to be K^+. When present in excess, it stimulates pain nerve endings leading to pain. The pain seen in angina pectoris is also due to release of P factor by the ischemic myocardium. Other substances producing ischemic pain are adenine nucleotides and accumulation of large amounts of lactic acid in the tissues formed as a result of anaerobic metabolism.* Other chemical agents, such as bradykinin and proteolytic enzymes, are formed in the tissues because of cell damage and these agents, in addition to lactic acid, stimulate the pain nerve endings.

Pain due to muscle spasm probably results partially from the direct effect of muscle spasm in stimulating mechanosensitive pain receptors, but it might also result from the indirect effect of muscle spasm to compress the blood vessels and cause ischemia. The spasm also increases the rate of metabolism in the muscle tissue thus making the relative ischemia even greater, leading to the release of pain inducing chemical substances.

Visceral Pain

There are no proprioceptors in the viscera. Temperature and touch receptors are few but pain receptors are present in the viscera. **Visceral pain** arises from the viscera like heart, stomach, intestine, etc. It is poorly localized, nauseating pain associated with other autonomic symptoms. Visceral pain is referred to other somatic structures or it radiates to other sites.

A few visceral areas are almost completely insensitive to pain of any type. These areas include the parenchyma of the liver and the alveoli of the lungs. Yet the liver *capsule* is extremely sensitive to both direct trauma and stretch, and the *bile ducts* are also sensitive to pain. In the lungs, even though the alveoli are insensitive, both the *bronchi* and the *parietal pleura* are very sensitive to pain.

Causes of Visceral Pain

Any stimulus that excites pain nerve endings in diffuse areas of the viscera can cause visceral pain. Essentially all visceral pain that originates in the thoracic and abdominal cavities is transmitted through type C pain fibers and, therefore, can transmit only the chronic-aching-suffering type of pain. The following conditions can lead to visceral pain:

- ❖ Ischemia of viscera produce substances such as bradykinin, proteolytic enzymes, etc., which produce pain.
- ❖ Spasm of smooth muscle of hollow viscous, e.g., intestinal colic, ureteric colic, etc.
- ❖ Chemical damage to surface of viscera as in ruptured gastric ulcer.
- ❖ Over distension of hollow viscera produces colicky pain as in stones in ureter, biliary duct, etc.
- ❖ Cramping pain occurs in structures like uterus as in dysmenorrhea, labor pain, etc.
- ❖ Traction on mesentery, stretching of the connective tissue surrounding the hollow viscus or within the viscus
- ❖ Inflammation of viscera as in appendicitis, pancreatitis, etc. Mild stimulation of inflamed viscera produces hyperalgesia.
  - Ischemia causes visceral pain in the same way that it does in other tissues, presumably because of the formation of acidic metabolic end products or tissue degenerative products such as bradykinin, proteolytic enzymes, or others that stimulate pain nerve endings.
  - Chemical stimuli can cause visceral pain. In certain conditions, damaging chemical substances leak from the gastrointestinal tract into the peritoneal cavity. For example, proteolytic acidic gastric juice may leak through a ruptured gastric or duodenal ulcer into the peritoneal cavity. This juice causes widespread digestion of the visceral peritoneum, thus stimulating large number of pain fibers. The pain is usually excruciating in this condition.
  - Spasm of a portion of the gut, the gallbladder, bile duct, ureter, or any other hollow viscus (singular form of viscera) can cause pain, possibly by mechanical stimulation of the pain nerve endings. Another possibility is that the spasm may cause diminished blood flow to the muscle, combined with the muscle's increased metabolic need for nutrients, thus causing severe pain. Often pain from a spastic viscus occurs in the form of *cramps,* with the pain increasing to a high degree of severity and then subsiding. This process continues intermittently, once in every few minutes. The intermittent cycles result from periods of contraction of the smooth muscle. For example, each time a peristaltic wave travels along an excessively excitable spastic gut, a cramp occurs. The cramping type of pain frequently occurs in persons with appendicitis, gastroenteritis, constipation, menstruation, parturition, gallbladder disease, or ureteral obstruction.
  - Extreme overfilling of a hollow viscus also can result in pain; presumably because of overstretch of the tissues themselves. Over distention can also cause compression of the blood vessels that encircle the viscus or that pass into its wall, thus leading to ischemic pain.

Pathway for Visceral Pain

The receptors which are **unmyelinated C fiber** endings are present in the walls of the hollow viscera and the stimulus is distension or chemical irritation of these organs. Visceral pain sensation is carried from the visceral receptors through sympathetic and parasympathetic divisions of autonomic nervous system (ANS) to the center. From trachea, pharynx and esophagus pain sensation is carried through **vagus and glossopharyngeal** nerve. From thorax, pain fibers are carried along with sympathetic fibers to reach the sympathetic ganglia and from there enter the spinal cord through the posterior root from T_1 to L_2 level. From pelvic organs afferent pain fibers pass through sacral parasympathetic nerves. The afferent fibers are carried to the posterior root of spinal cord. Their cell bodies are located in the dorsal root ganglia or in the homologous cranial nerve ganglia. Once within the

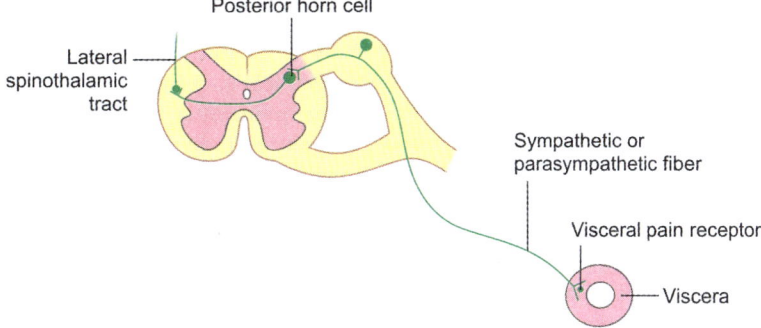

Fig. 82.12: Pathway for visceral pain.

central nervous system, the visceral pain impulses travel in the same ascending tracts as does the somatic slow pain, i.e., through the lateral spinothalamic tract **(Fig. 82.12)**. The fibers project either to the thalamus to reach the postcentral gyrus or enter the reticular formation.

Some substance P containing afferent pain fibers send collaterals to postganglionic sympathetic neurons in the sympathetic ganglia. These connections play a part in the *reflex control of viscera* independent of CNS.

Characteristic Features of Deep Pain or Visceral Pain
- Less localized and more diffuse because pain receptors in viscera are comparatively few.
- Very unpleasant and very severe. When severe, the pain is associated with autonomic manifestations like nausea, vomiting, sweating, alteration in heart rate and blood pressure. For example, in myocardial infarction there is sudden fall in BP, sweating, etc.
- Visceral pain causes reflex contraction of nearby skeletal muscle. It is more marked when inflammation of the viscera involves the peritoneum. For example, in appendicitis the abdominal muscles contract, referred to as **guarding,** in order to make the part immobile.
- The visceral pain sometimes may not be felt at the local site from which it arises. But, the pain may be felt in some somatic structure that may be a considerable distance away from the local site and this is called **referred pain**. Sometimes it spreads from the local site to the referred area and this is called **radiating pain**, i.e., it will be felt at the site where pain is originating as well as at the referred site. For example, in myocardial infarction, pain is felt retrosternally and from there it radiates to medial side of left arm. Another example is, in appendicitis, pain starts in the right iliac fossa and radiates towards the umbilicus.

Referred Pain

Sometimes pain arising from a deeper structure (especially viscera) is not felt in the same organ but is felt in a superficial somatic area at a considerable distance belonging to the same dermatome. The pain is said to be referred to the somatic structure **(Fig. 82.13)**. For example, pain arising from the heart is referred to the inner aspect of left arm. This is **referred pain**. Other examples include:
- Pain from diaphragm referred to the tip of the shoulder.

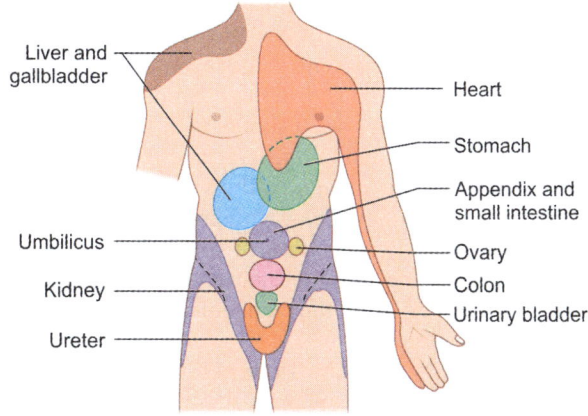

Fig. 82.13: Sites of referred pain from different visceral organs.

- Ureteric pain referred to testicular area in male and labia in female.
- Pain in appendicitis first felt around the skin of umbilicus.
- Maxillary sinus pain referred to nearby tooth.

Unusual reference sites are also seen as in the case of cardiac pain which may be referred to epigastrium or neck or right arm. Knowledge of the different types of referred pain is important in clinical diagnosis because in much visceral pathology, the only clinical sign is referred pain.

Mechanism of Referred Pain

Dermatomal Rule

Pain is referred to a superficial structure that has developed from the same embryonic structure from which the organ has developed. In other words, the organ from which pain is arising and the dermatome to which pain is referred belong to the same embryonic segment. This is called **dermatomal rule of pain reference**. The dermatome and the organ from which pain is arising belong to the same spinal segment. Pain fibers from the internal organ and the superficial somatic structure to which pain is referred enter the spinal cord through the same posterior root and ends in the same spinal segment. Motor innervation is also from the same spinal segment. The medial side of left arm and heart develop from the same embryonic segment. Diaphragm and tip of shoulder are supplied by $C_{3,4,5}$ segments of spinal cord.

Two mechanisms have been postulated to explain pain reference:
1. Convergence theory of pain reference
2. Facilitation theory.

Convergence-projection theory: Pain fibers from viscera and fibers from skin to which pain is referred enter through the same dorsal root and converge on the **same second order neuron** in substantia gelatinosa of Rolando (SGR). Here, **law of projection** comes into play. Since pain from somatic structures is more common than visceral pain, even though pain originates from viscera, brain interprets it as coming from somatic structure due to law of projection **(Fig. 82.14A)**.

Facilitation theory: Pain fibers from viscera as it enters the dorsal horn, gives collateral to the second order neuron in the somatic pain pathway. The collateral is given before the pain afferents from viscera end in the second order neuron of its pathway. As the visceral pain fiber stimulates the second order neuron of its pathway, it simultaneously increases the excitability of the second order neuron in the somatic pain pathway through the collateral. The second order neuron of the somatic pain pathway comes to the **subliminal fringe**. Now a mild stimulation of somatic pain pathway can stimulate the second order neuron of somatic pain and intense pain will be felt in the cutaneous area to which pain is referred **(Fig. 82.14B)**.

Previous experience plays a role in referred pain. In pain due to abdominal diseases, pain is usually referred to midline of abdomen. If the patient had a previous abdominal surgery, the pain is referred to the region of the scar.

Parietal Pain Caused by Visceral Disease

When there is a disease of the viscera, the inflammatory process often spreads to the parietal peritoneum, pleura, or pericardium. These parietal surfaces, like the skin, are supplied with extensive pain fibers from the peripheral spinal nerves. So the pathway is different for parietal pain than for visceral pain.

Control of Pain Sensation

It is well known that wounded soldiers are not aware of pain until the battle is over **(stress-induced analgesia)**; touching or rubbing the injured area relieves pain and acupuncture relieves pain. All these examples show that pain transmission undergoes certain inhibition and modification. There are certain intrinsic pain-controlling mechanisms occurring at two levels:
1. Spinal level or segmental level
2. Supraspinal level.

Pain Control at the Spinal Level (Gate-control Theory of Pain Perception)

Mechanical stimulation of the injured area may sometimes relieve pain. After a hit if we rub or massage that area the intensity of pain decreases. This is due to stimulation of mechanoreceptors in the area, which exerts a suppressor effect on pain sensation.

The first order neuron of the pain pathway ends in the substantia gelatinosa of Rolando (SGR) in the dorsal horn. The neurotransmitter released at the primary pain ending in SGR is substance P. The mechanoreceptor fibers pass through the dorsal column pathway. As the large sensory fibers (Aβ) carrying touch sensation ascends through the dorsal column, they give off collaterals to the dorsal horn cells. These collaterals end in certain interneurons in the dorsal horn which release enkephalin at their endings. These interneurons make **axo-axonic synapse** with the primary endings of pain pathway and inhibit the release of transmitter at the pain nerve endings (refer presynaptic inhibition). The primary afferent ending in the dorsal horn contains receptors for encephalin.

As the touch receptors are stimulated by rubbing the affected area, impulses passing through the Aβ touch fibers are carried through the collaterals to activate the interneuron which releases enkephalin **[substantia gelatinosa (SG) inhibitory enkephalinergic interneurons]**. This enkephalin binds with the receptors in the membrane of primary nerve endings in the pain pathway. The amplitude of action potential is reduced when it reaches the pain nerve ending due to presynaptic inhibition by the collateral of the touch fiber through the inhibitory interneuron. The amount of substance P and glutamate released at the pain nerve ending (type C and Aδ fibers) is reduced and the transmission of pain signals to the second order neurons in SGR is inhibited. The conduction of pain through the spinothalamic tract is inhibited. Thus, the substantia gelatinosa cells serve as a gate in the pain pathway. The gate remains open only when Aδ and C fibers are stimulated but tends to close down when Aβ fibers are stimulated simultaneously. This is referred to as **gate-control theory of pain perception or dorsal horn gating (Fig. 82.15)**.

The gate-control theory provides the basis for using vibratory stimulation for reducing pain. A medical therapy designed to activate the gate control mechanism is

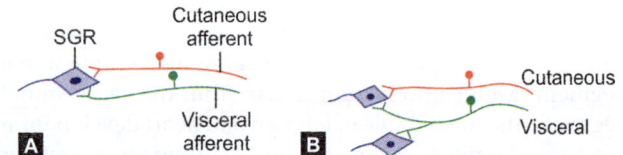

Figs. 82.14A and B: Pain reference: (A) Convergence; (B) Facilitation.

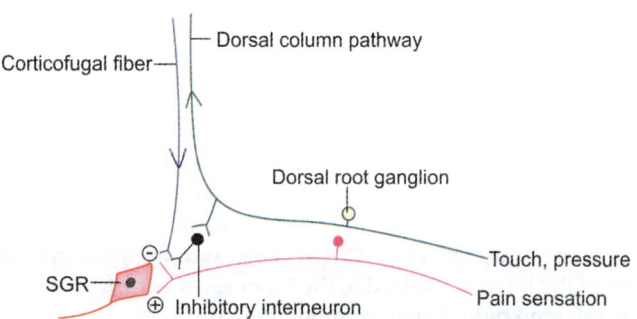

Fig. 82.15: Gate control theory of pain perception.

transcutaneous electrical nerve stimulation (TENS), where the large-diameter afferent sensory fibers are stimulated at the site of pain. In this procedure, application of electric shocks to the skin with surface electrodes in the painful area stimulates Aβ fibers that overlap the area of injury and reduces pain. Acupuncture resembles TENS. During acupuncture analgesia, needles are introduced into specific parts of the body to stimulate large afferent fibers, which cause analgesia. Even simple massage over the area of pain relieves pain due to the gate control of pain sensation in the dorsal horn.

In severe cases of pernicious anemia, there will be degeneration of dorsal column pathway. In this case, pain becomes unbearable because of the absence of pain inhibition in the dorsal horn. Thus impulses passing through dorsal column pathway can modulate pain sensation (**Fig. 82.15**).

> **Morphine** is a substance which relieves pain sensation, i.e., it is an **analgesic**. The receptors that bind morphine can also bind opioid peptides produced in the body. About a dozen such opiate-like substances have now been found at different points of the nervous system. All are breakdown products of three large protein molecules *pro-opiomelanocortin, proenkephalin,* and *prodynorphin*. The important opiate-like substances are **dynorphin, β-endorphin and met-enkephalin and leu-enkephalin**. The two encephalins are released mainly from brain and spinal cord from portions of the analgesia system, and their receptors are also located in the brain and spinal cord. They inhibit the release of substance P in the posterior gray column. β-endorphin is present in both the hypothalamus and the pituitary gland. Opiate analgesia can be prevented by the narcotic antagonist **naloxone**.

Pain Control at the Supraspinal Level

Endogenous Analgesia System

Transmission in the pain pathway to the brain is regulated by descending control system arising from the brain. This system suppresses excessive pain under special circumstances. This is the reason why wounded soldiers in the battle field and accident victims often feel no pain at the time of accident. But later pain becomes severe. This system of pain control is called **endogenous analgesia system**.

- **Corticofugal fibers** arising from the sensory cortex pass down up to the dorsal horn of spinal cord. The **corticofugal fibers** suppress pain sensation at the first synapse of the afferent pain pathway, i.e., at the substantia gelatinosa of Rolando (SGR) by presynaptic inhibition (*refer* 'Presynaptic inhibition'). Thus, SGR is the gate through which the pain information enters the central nervous system (CNS) and modulation of pain occurs at this level. Thus, the gate, i.e., **SGR**, controls pain sensation to a large extent and this is called **gate control theory of pain perception (Fig. 82.15)**.
- **Central analgesic system or mesencephalic pain inhibiting system:** Central analgesic system includes:
  - Periventricular gray matter of diencephalon around third ventricle
  - Periaqueductal gray matter of midbrain around aqueduct of Sylvius
  - Locus coeruleus
  - Medullary raphe nuclei

From these areas, fibers descend down and suppress pain transmission by presynaptic inhibition at the SGR and in the brainstem through inhibitory interneurons. Central analgesia system acts by inhibiting the release of substance P in the posterior gray column. Other pain inhibitory pathways originate in the sensory-motor cortex, hypothalamus and reticular formation.

Neurons in the **raphe nuclei** in the medulla release **serotonin** as the neurotransmitter. Serotonin can inhibit nociceptive neurons and thus has an important role in endogenous analgesia system. The descending serotonergic neurons act by stimulating substantia gelatinosa inhibitory enkephalinergic interneurons leading to presynaptic inhibition of pain transmission (**Fig. 82.16**).

Enkephalinergic and dynorphinergic neurons descending from the **periaqueductal gray matter** in the midbrain inhibit pain by stimulating the raphe nuclei. Neurons containing β-endorphin descend from the hypothalamus to terminate on the periaqueductal gray matter. It is surprising that although opioids like enkephalin are inhibitory neurotransmitters, they can stimulate descending pain inhibiting pathways. The exact mechanism by which they stimulate the analgesia system is not exactly known. The reason may be the descending pain-inhibiting pathways are normally inhibited by neurons in the brain stem. Opioids by antagonizing this inhibition stimulate the analgesia system.

Other components of the endogenous analgesia system release **epinephrine and norepinephrine** in the spinal cord which also inhibit nociceptive neurons. Central analgesia system can suppress both sharp pricking pain and burning pain sensations. Thus, *activation of the analgesia system* by nervous signals entering the periaqueductal gray and periventricular

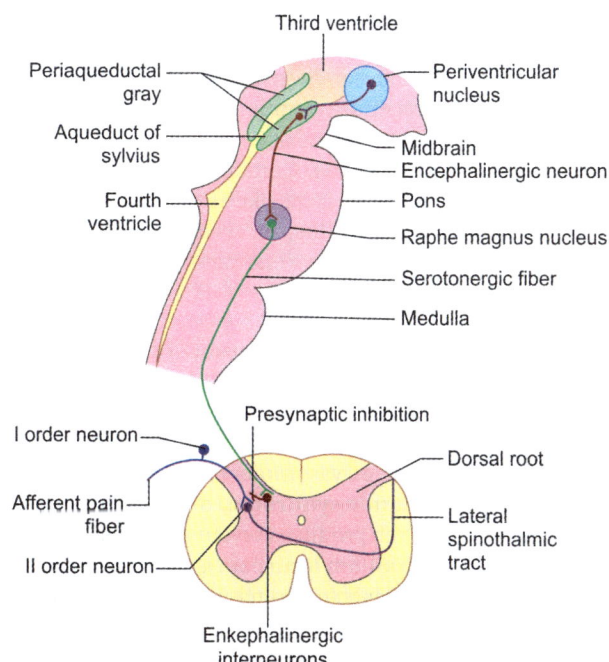

Fig. 82.16: Central analgesia system.

Flowchart 82.4: Pathway for endogenous pain inhibition (red arrow indicates stimulation and blue arrow indicates inhibition).

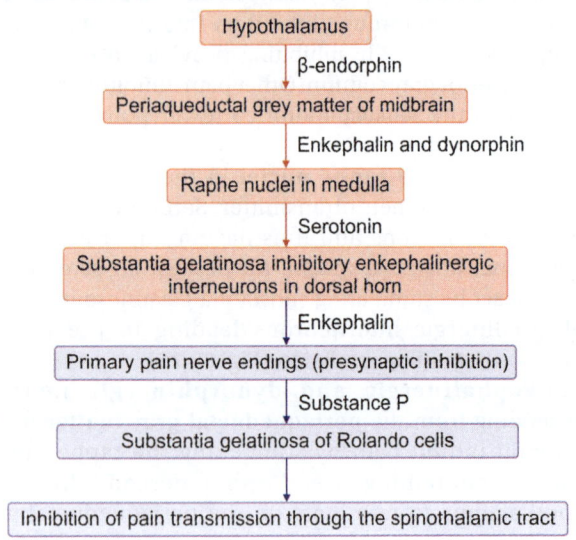

areas, or *inactivation of pain pathways* by morphine-like drugs, can almost totally suppress many pain signals entering through the peripheral nerves **(Flowchart 82.4)**.

Abnormalities in Pain Sensation

Hyperalgesia

Increased sensitivity to pain is called **hyperalgesia**. In this condition, pain threshold is decreased and so a painful stimulus becomes even more painful because the nociceptive afferents discharge at higher rates in response to a given stimulus. Even non-noxious stimulus produces pain. It is divided into primary and secondary hyperalgesia.

Primary Hyperalgesia

The pain is felt in the area of tissue damage due to infection, inflammation, burns, etc. It may be due to increased sensitivity of pain receptors or due to decrease in the pain threshold. Even non-noxious stimuli like touch produce pain. This is called **allodynia**. Certain chemical substances released during tissue damage like serotonin, histamine, prostaglandin, plasma kinins, etc., which sensitizes the unmyelinated 'C' afferent nerve endings may be the cause.

Secondary Hyperalgesia

Here, pain is felt in an intact area adjacent to or away from the site of injury. This is due to facilitation of pain transmission and spread of excitation in the CNS. There is no lowering of pain threshold in this condition. It is usually associated with spasm of skeletal muscles, vasomotor changes and secretion from glands. In **thalamic syndrome**, overreaction to pain occurs. Even light touch produces severe pain even if there is no tissue damage. **Phantom limb** pain is due to damage to a peripheral nerve. If the nerve endings in the amputated area are gently touched, excruciating pain is felt at the receptor level. This is an example of **neuropathic pain** which occurs when nerve fibers are injured.

Herpes Zoster (Shingles)

Occasionally *herpesvirus* infects a dorsal root ganglion. This infection causes severe pain in the dermatomal segment innervated by the ganglion, thus eliciting a segmental type of pain that circles halfway around the body. The disease is called *herpes zoster,* or "shingles," because of a skin eruption that often follows. The cause of the pain is presumably infection of the pain neurons in the dorsal root ganglion by the virus. In addition to causing pain, the virus is carried by neuronal cytoplasmic flow through the peripheral axons to their cutaneous origins. Here the virus causes a rash that become vesicles within a few days and then crusts over within another few days, all of this occurring within the dermatomal area supplied by the infected dorsal root.

Trigeminal Neuralgia

Stabbing type of pain occasionally occurs in some people over one side of the face in the sensory distribution area of the fifth cranial nerve called *trigeminal neuralgia*. The pain feels like sudden electrical shocks, and it may appear for only a few seconds at a time or may be almost continuous. Often it is set off by highly sensitive trigger areas on the surface of the face, in the mouth, or inside the throat almost always by a stimulus from a mechanoreceptor rather than a pain stimulus. For instance, when the patient swallows a bolus of food, as the food touches a tonsil, it might set off a severe lancinating pain in the mandibular portion of the fifth nerve. The pain of trigeminal neuralgia can usually be blocked by surgically cutting the peripheral nerve from the hypersensitive area. Trigeminal neuralgia and glossopharyngeal neuralgia together is referred to as **tic douloureux.**

Causalgia

Causalgia is a condition where there is spontaneous burning pain in the skin long after minor injuries like crush injury where there is incomplete peripheral nerve injury. It is associated with hyperalgesia and allodynia. This pain is not relieved by local anesthetics but sympathectomy relieves pain of causalgia.

Sympathetic discharge reflexly causes pain in the injured area due to **reflex sympathetic dystrophy**. In the injured area, damage of the sympathetic nerves leads to sprouting and overgrowth of sympathetic noradrenergic endings. Discharge through these noradrenergic endings is responsible for causalgia in that area of skin. The descending impulses in the sympathetic postganglionic fibers evoke ascending impulses in the afferent pain fibers at the site of injury. This is because at the site of damage to peripheral nerve, efferent sympathetic fibers may make connection with afferent somatic pain fibers producing a short circuit. Sympathetic discharge then brings on pain.

Analgesia

Substances that relieve pain are called **analgesics** and relief of pain is **analgesia**. Drugs like **aspirin and ibuprofen** inhibit prostaglandin synthesis, which is an important mediator of pain. Prostaglandin sensitizes free nerve endings to painful stimuli. Thus these drugs block pain receptors and inhibit pain transmission. Local anesthetics like **lignocaine** temporarily block conduction of nerve impulses along the axon of first order pain neuron. Drugs like **morphine** (narcotic analgesics) modulate pain perception in the CNS and produce analgesia. Morphine and related drugs act on opiate receptor sites and inhibit the release of glutamate and substance-P from sensory pain nerve endings. Hence, intrathecal or epidural injection of morphine into the spinal subarachnoid space is effective in abolishing postoperative pain and cancer pain. Receptor sites for endogenous opiates like endorphin and enkephalin are found in the posterior horn and thalamus. Electrical stimulation of **periaqueductal gray** matter can inhibit pain perception.

Stressful conditions may cause temporary analgesia. When the stress is over, the subject feels severe pain. This type of painless condition is called **stress analgesia**.

MULTIPLE CHOICE QUESTIONS

1. A person with intractable pain in the right leg is benefited by:
   a. Right spinothalamic tract cordotomy
   b. Left spinothalamic tract cordotomy
   c. Right hemicordotomy
   d. Left hemicordotomy

2. The visceral organ that has the broadest area for referred pain is:
   a. Kidney
   b. Liver
   c. Stomach
   d. Testis

3. The sensory deficit produced due to damage to the right spinothalamic tract is:
   a. Loss of pain and temperature sensations on the right side
   b. Loss of pain and temperature sensations on the left side
   c. Loss of kinesthetic sensations on the right side
   d. Loss of kinesthetic sensations on the left side

4. Kinesthetic sensation is:
   a. Transmitted by β-type of sensory nerve
   b. Located in Merkel's disc
   c. Transmitted by Meissner's corpuscle
   d. Means abnormal perception of sensation

5. Conscious proprioception is carried by:
   a. Dorsal column fibers
   b. Anterior spinothalamic tract
   c. Lateral spinothalamic tract
   d. Vestibular tract

6. An anterolateral cordotomy for relieving pain in right leg is effective because it interrupts the:
   a. Left dorsal column
   b. Left ventral spinothalamic tract
   c. Left lateral spinothalamic tract
   d. Right lateral spinothalamic tract

7. In the spinal cord, which of the following tracts contain first order neurons?
   a. Fasciculus gracilis
   b. Lateral spinothalamic tract
   c. Ventral spinothalamic tract
   d. Spinocerebellar tract

8. Ablation of the somatosensory area-I (SSA-I) of the cerebral cortex leads to:
   a. Total loss of pain sensation
   b. Total loss of touch sensation
   c. Loss of tactile localization but no loss of two point discrimination
   d. Loss of tactile localization and two point discrimination

9. Ability to appreciate the shape and size of an object placed in the hand is lost in lesion of:
   a. Tractus gracilis
   b. Tractus cuneatus
   c. Lateral spinothalamic tract
   d. Spinoreticular tract

10. Mechanism of analgesia is by all the following, *except*:
    a. Nociceptin stimulation
    b. Nocistatin stimulation
    c. Anadamide receptors
    d. Nicotinic and cholinergic receptors

11. All the following are thermal modalities, *except*:
    a. Cold receptor   b. Warm receptor
    c. Pain receptor   d. Pressure receptor

12. Vanilloid receptors are activated by:
    a. Pain   b. Vibration
    c. Touch   d. Pressure

13. Pacinian corpuscle transmits which sensation?
    a. Light touch   b. Vibration
    c. Cold   d. Heat

14. Which of the following phrase adequately describes Pacinian corpuscles?
    a. A type of pain receptor
    b. Slowly adapting touch receptor
    c. Rapidly adapting touch receptor
    d. Located in the joints

15. Massage and application of liniments to painful areas in the body relieves pain due to:
    a. Stimulation of endogenous analgesic system
    b. Release of endorphins by the first order neurons in the brain stem
    c. Release of glutamate and substance P in the spinal cord
    d. Inhibition of pain pathway by large myelinated afferent fibers

16. Repetitive stimulation increases pain sensation. The probable cause is:
    a. Hyper sensitization
    b. Decreased reflex time
    c. Increase in pain threshold
    d. Decreased receptor area

17. All the following are tonic receptors, *except*:
    a. Baroreceptor
    b. Muscle spindle
    c. Pain receptors
    d. Pacinian corpuscle
18. The following are grouped under encapsulated receptors, *except*:
    a. Ruffini's corpuscle
    b. Meissner's corpuscle
    c. Pacinian corpuscle
    d. Merkel's disc
19. The receptor that is responsible for two point tactile discrimination is:
    a. Pacinian corpuscle
    b. Meissner's corpuscle
    c. Merkel's disc
    d. Free nerve endings
20. The receptor that is most sensitive to vibration sense is:
    a. Pacinian corpuscle
    b. Meissner's corpuscle
    c. Merkel's disc
    d. Golgi tendon organ
21. Normally pain from viscera arises due to:
    a. Distension
    b. Irritation
    c. Compression
    d. Chemical stimulation
22. Decussation of lemnisci takes place:
    a. Posterior to the pyramids of medulla oblongata
    b. In the anterior white commissure of spinal cord
    c. Pons
    d. Posterior white commissure of spinal cord
23. Medial lemniscus is formed of second order neurons of the:
    a. Dorsal column pathway
    b. Spinothalamic pathway
    c. Spinocerebellar tract
    d. Spinotectal tract
24. All the following relay in the sensory cortex, *except*:
    a. Pain
    b. Touch
    c. Temperature
    d. Olfaction
25. The area in the body where a neuron is closest to the external environment is:
    a. Taste bud
    b. Skin
    c. Cornea
    d. Olfactory mucous membrane
26. Wernicke's encephalopathy is due to deficiency of:
    a. Niacin
    b. Cyanocobalamin
    c. Pantothenic acid
    d. Thiamine
27. Most rapidly adapting receptors are:
    a. Pain receptors
    b. Thermoreceptors
    c. Photoreceptors
    d. Pacinian corpuscles
28. Itching is produced by the stimulation of:
    a. B fibers
    b. Touch receptors
    c. Dorsal root C fibers
    d. Motor fibers
29. Which of the following is a phasic receptor?
    a. Carotid sinus receptor
    b. Muscle spindle
    c. Pain
    d. Touch
30. The analgesia induced by acupuncture is due to:
    a. Excitation of central analgesic system
    b. Blocking of local pain fibers
    c. Stimulation of sympathetic afferents
    d. Stimulation of release of substance P
31. The peripheral receptor for pressure sensation is:
    a. Free nerve ending
    b. Pacinian corpuscle
    c. Meissner's corpuscle
    d. Carotid sinus receptors
32. Pacinian corpuscles are the major receptors for:
    a. Pressure
    b. Pain
    c. Touch
    d. Temperature
33. The average number of muscle fibers attached to one Golgi tendon organ is:
    a. 1–3
    b. 5–10
    c. 10–15
    d. 15–75
34. Spinothalamic tract transmits all the following sensations, *except*:
    a. Proprioception
    b. Pain
    c. Temperature
    d. Touch
35. Which of the following stimulus does not induce visceral pain?
    a. Distension
    b. Pressure
    c. Cauterization
    d. Traction
36. Interneurons are:
    a. Essential part of stretch reflex
    b. Always excitatory
    c. Always inhibitory
    d. Most numerous neurons in CNS
37. Warmth sensation is sensed by:
    a. Pacinian corpuscle
    b. Meissner's corpuscle
    c. Ruffini's end organ
    d. Free nerve endings
38. Inhibition of the spinal cord may be brought about by:
    a. Glutamic acid
    b. Aspartic acid
    c. Glycine
    d. Strychnine
39. True visceral pain arise from:
    a. Distension
    b. Mechanical irritation
    c. Excessive heat
    d. Chemical stimulation
40. Nucleus gracilis and nucleus cuneatus are the first synapse for:
    a. Dorsal columns
    b. Ventral spinothalamic tract
    c. Lateral spinothalamic tract
    d. Dorsolateral tact

CHAPTER 82 — Ascending Sensory Pathways

41. **Crude touch sensations are carried by:**
    a. Lateral spinothalamic tract
    b. Ventral spinothalamic tract
    c. Posterior column
    d. Pyramidal tract
42. **The fiber which is thickest in human nerve is:**
    a. Touch
    b. Pain
    c. Temperature
    d. Proprioception
43. **Headache can be produced by all, *except*:**
    a. Mechanical damage to parietal cortex
    b. Dilatation of intracranial blood vessels
    c. Presence of blood in CSF
    d. Loss of CSF following lumbar puncture

ANSWERS

1. b	2. a	3. b	4. a	5. a
6. c	7. a	8. d	9. b	10. a
11. d	12. a	13. b	14. c	15. d
16. a	17. d	18. d	19. b	20. a
21. a	22. a	23. a	24. d	25. d
26. d	27. d	28. c	29. d	30. b
31. b	32. a	33. c	34. a	35. c
36. d	37. d	38. c	39. a	40. a
41. b	42. d	43. a		

Thalamus

CHAPTER 83

LEARNING OBJECTIVES
- Describe the connections and functions of thalamus
- Classify thalamic nuclei
- Explain the effects of lesion to one-half of the thalamus

FUNCTIONAL ANATOMY OF THALAMUS

PY10.7: Describe and discuss functions of cerebral cortex, basal ganglia, thalamus, hypothalamus, cerebellum and limbic system and their abnormalities.

Thalamus is a large subcortical mass of gray matter situated obliquely in the dorsal part of the diencephalon one on either side of third ventricle. **Isthmus** or **intermediate mass** is a bridge of gray matter that crosses the third ventricle to join the right and left halves of the thalamus. It is situated between the cerebral cortex and the midbrain **(Fig. 83.1)**. *Thalamus, subthalamus, epithalamus and hypothalamus together constitute the diencephalon.*

Thalamus measures about 3 cm in length and makes up 80% of diencephalon. The anterior end of the thalamus is narrow and the posterior expanded end forms the pulvinar. Reticular nuclei of thalamus separate it from the internal capsule.

The thalamus derives its blood supply from branches of the posterior cerebral artery like the posterior communicating artery, paramedian thalamic-subthalamic arteries, thalamogeniculate arteries and posterior choroidal arteries.

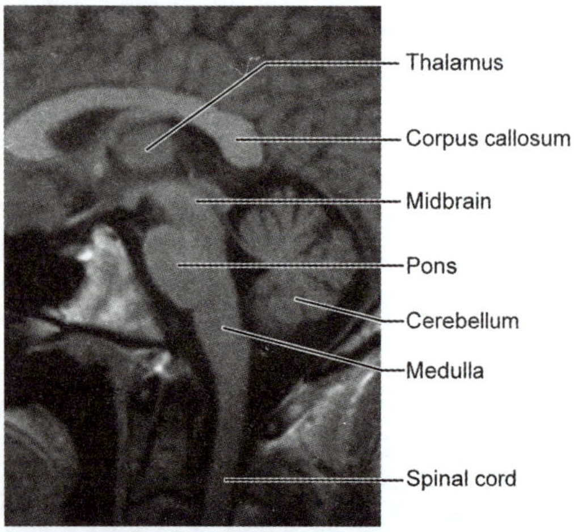

Thalamus consists of mainly gray matter. There is an external medullary lamina and an internal medullary lamina in the thalamus which contain white matter. **External medullary lamina** situated on the lateral aspect of thalamus consists of thalamocortical and cortico-thalamic fibers. **Internal medullary lamina** is a Y-shaped sheet of white matter seen inside the thalamus. It consists of nerve fibers that pass from one thalamic nucleus to another. Interconnecting nuclei are present here. Internal medullary lamina divides thalamus into an anterior, medial and lateral group **(Fig. 83.2)**.

The cerebral cortex operates in close association with the thalamus so that both are considered anatomically and functionally as a unit referred to as the **thalamocortical system**. All information that reaches the cortex is processed in the thalamus. So it is also called gateway to the cerebral cortex.

Subthalamus is located between the substantia nigra and the thalamus. It contains subthalamic nucleus (body of Luys), fibers from cerebellum and globus pallidus. The subthalamic nucleus has reciprocal connection with the globus pallidus. Lesion of the subthalamic nucleus leads to hemiballismus.

Epithalamus includes pineal gland, habenular nuclei and the stria medullaris. These are structures that form the roof of the third ventricle.

ANATOMICAL CLASSIFICATION OF THALAMIC NUCLEI

- ❖ Medial group
  - Anterior nucleus
  - Dorsomedial nucleus
- ❖ Lateral group
  - Ventral group
    - ♦ Ventral posterolateral nucleus
    - ♦ Ventral posteromedial nucleus
    - ♦ Lateroventral nucleus
    - ♦ Anteroventral nucleus

Fig. 83.1: Location of thalamus in the brain.

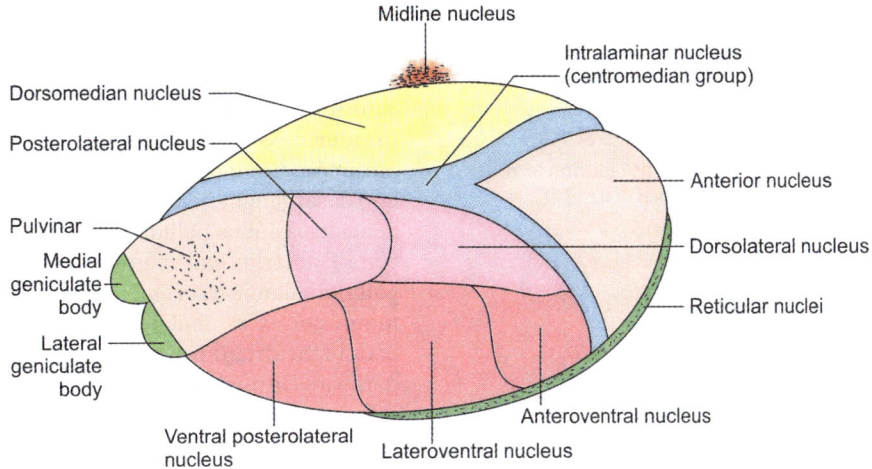

Fig. 83.2: Thalamic nuclei.

- Dorsal group
  - Posterolateral
  - Dorsolateral
- Midline nucleus or massa intermedia.
- Centromedian group or nuclei in internal medullary lamina.
- Pulvinar group, medial geniculate body, lateral geniculate body and reticular nuclei.

FUNCTIONAL CLASSIFICATION OF THALAMIC NUCLEI

- Specific relay nuclei
- Nonspecific projection nuclei
- Association nuclei.

Specific Relay Nuclei

- Medial geniculate body (MGB)
- Lateral geniculate body (LGB)
- Ventralis posterior or posteroventral nucleus (PVN) which consists of two parts, ventral posterolateral nucleus and ventral posteromedial nucleus (**Fig. 83.3**)
- Ventralis lateralis or lateroventral nucleus (LVN)
- Ventralis anterior or anteroventral nucleus (AVN)
- Anterior nucleus.

Nonspecific Projection Nuclei

- Midline nuclei
- Intralaminar nuclei
- Reticular nuclei.

Association Nuclei

- Pulvinar
- Lateralis posterior [posterolateral nucleus (PLN)]
- Lateralis dorsalis [dorsolateral nucleus (DLN)]
- Dorsalis medialis or dorsomedial nucleus.

CONNECTIONS OF THALAMUS

Connection of thalamus in **Tables 83.1 to 83.3**.

FUNCTIONS OF THALAMUS

- **Relay station for somatic and special sensations:** Thalamus is the most important **subcortical relay center** for all main sensory pathways. Modification of impulses also occurs in the thalamus.
- **Subcortical perception of sensations:** Thalamus plays a role in appreciation of protopathic sensations like pain, crude touch, crude temperature, etc. Although crude perception of these sensations occurs at the level of

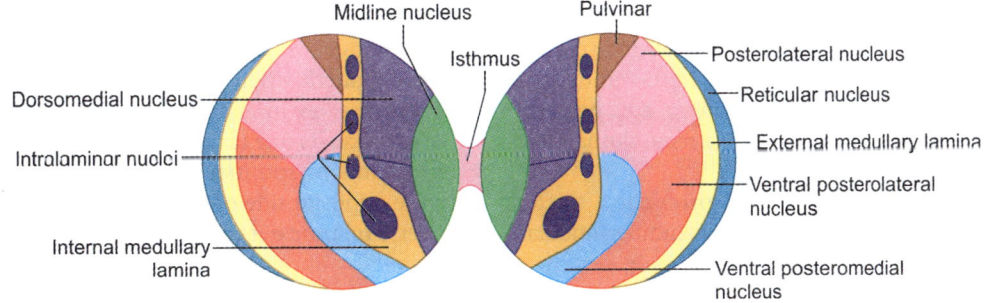

Fig. 83.3: Transverse section of thalamus through the isthmus showing thalamic nuclei.

Table 83.1: Afferent and efferent connections of specific relay nuclei of thalamus.

Nucleus	Afferent fibers	Efferent fibers
MGB	Auditory fibers through lateral lemniscus	Fibers to auditory cortex (area 41)
LGB	Visual fibers through optic tract	Optic radiation to visual cortex (area 17)
Ventral posteromedial nucleus	Trigeminothalamic tract, solitariothalamic tract (taste)	Face area of SSA I
Ventral posterolateral nucleus	Spinal lemniscus, medial lemniscus	SSA I
LVN	Dentato-thalamic and dentatorubrothalamic tract (cerebellum)	Primary motor area (area 4) Premotor area (area 6)
AVN	Globus pallidus of basal ganglia, reticular formation	Area 6 Area 4
Anterior nucleus	Mamillothalamic tract of Vicq de Azyr from hypothalamus	Cingulated gyrus of limbic cortex – papez circuit

(MGB: medial geniculate body; LGB: lateral geniculate body; LVN: lateroventral nucleus; AVN: anteroventral nucleus)

Table 83.2: Connections of nonspecific projection nuclei of thalamus.

Nuclei	Afferent fibers	Efferent fibers
Midline	Reticular formation	Neocortex
Intralaminar	Corpus striatum, hypothalamus, cerebellum	Project to all parts of neocortex
Reticular	Fibers from different parts of cerebral cortex	To reticular formation

Table 83.3: Connections of association nuclei of thalamus.

Nucleus	Afferent fibers	Efferent fibers
Pulvinar	• Amygdaloid complex • Other thalamic nuclei	Association areas of cerebral cortex
PLN	Other thalamic nuclei	Superior parietal lobe
DLN	Other thalamic nuclei	Cingulate gyrus
Dorsomedial nucleus	• Other thalamic nuclei • Amygdaloid nucleus • Hypothalamus	Prefrontal cortex

(PLN: posterolateral nucleus; DLN: dorsolateral nucleus)

thalamus, precise localization of these sensations depends on the nerve impulses reaching the primary sensory areas of the cerebral cortex.

* Thalamus plays a role in the **affective nature of pain** sensation because of its connection with prefrontal cortex.
* **Emotion and memory:** It plays a role in the emotional behavior of the individual, recent memory, etc., because of its connection with limbic cortex via mamillothalamic tract (*refer* 'Papez circuit').
* **Arousal mechanism:** Nonspecific projection nuclei of thalamus form important part of ascending reticular activating system (ARAS). This system is responsible for regulation and maintenance of consciousness, alertness and attention of the individual. Almost all sensations can activate ARAS. The level of activity in the ARAS determines the **alertness** of the individual.
* **Motor function:** Because of its connection with cerebellum and basal ganglia, it acts as an integrating center for motor activities. Globus pallidus of basal ganglia projects to the ventral anterior and ventral lateral nuclei of thalamus via pallidothalamic tract and thalamus in turn projects to the motor cortex via thalamocortical fibers. Cortex projects back to the striatum of basal ganglia through corticostriate pathway. Through this circuitous connection, thalamus influences postural movements. Thalamus also connects cerebellum and motor cortex via dentato-rubro-thalamo-cortical tract. Through this connection, thalamus influences the planning and programming of movements.
* **Association or modulation function:** Association nuclei connect thalamus to different parts of cerebral cortex, and thalamus and cortex function as a single unit. This helps to integrate sensory and motor function (**sensory-motor coordination**) and also somatic and visceral function.
* **Language and speech:** Thalamus has a role in language development. Dorsolateral nucleus of thalamus is connected to the parietal lobe and is concerned with language and speech.

LESIONS OF THALAMUS

Neoplasm or diseases affecting blood supply to the thalamus lead to degeneration of thalamic nuclei especially posteroventral nucleus. **Thalamo-geniculate branch of posterior cerebral artery** is usually blocked due to thrombosis. Bleeding or hemorrhage following very high blood pressure is another cause.

Depending on the degree and site of block other areas are also affected. When the thalamus is damaged, in addition to loss of thalamic functions, many cortical functions are also affected, as cortex is intimately connected with thalamus. Collectively the manifestations are called **thalamic syndrome**.

Thalamic Syndrome

Thalamic syndrome was described by Dejerine and Roussy. The features of lesion of lesion of one side are:

* **Hemianesthesia** or loss of sensations in the opposite half of the body.
* **Sensory ataxia** where there is loss of kinesthetic sensation. Movements are in-coordinated and clumsy.
* **Astereognosis** due to defect in touch-pressure system.
* Paroxysms of spontaneous excruciating burning pain in the opposite side of the body are present. This pain is called **thalamic overreaction or thalamic pain**. The pain

is aroused by light touch or cold, and does not respond to powerful analgesic drugs. Even minor stimulus leads to prolonged, severe and very unpleasant pain. Such sudden attacks of pain may occur spontaneously.

- ❖ The person is unable to localize the position of limb, and is called **thalamic phantom limb** or **amelognosia or position agnosia**.
- ❖ Involuntary movements like **choreoathetosis** and **intention tremor** are seen. This is due to involvement of ventral anterior nucleus or ventral lateral nucleus of thalamus, and the manifestations will be similar to basal ganglia or cerebellar lesions.
- ❖ If LGB or MGB is involved, vision or hearing will be affected.
- ❖ A particular position of the hand called **thalamic hand** is observed. This is due to flexion at wrist and metacarpophalangeal joints and extension of interphalangeal joints due to alterations in muscle tone in different groups of muscles.
- ❖ Emotional disturbances are usually present.
- ❖ Hemiparesis and defects in the visual field are seen if internal capsule is also affected.

MULTIPLE CHOICE QUESTIONS

1. **Primary function of thalamus is:**
   a. Long-term memory
   b. Planning voluntary movements
   c. Sensory relay station
   d. Error control

2. **Thalamic lesion will not produce:**
   a. Sensory loss
   b. Cogwheel rigidity
   c. Sensory disturbance of one-half of the body
   d. Tingling sensation

3. **The nucleus that separate thalamus from internal capsule is:**
   a. Reticular nucleus   b. Anterior nucleus
   c. Midline nucleus   d. Dorsomedial nucleus

ANSWERS

1. c   2. b   3. a

Motor Division of Nervous System

CHAPTER 84

LEARNING OBJECTIVES
- Define muscle tone
- Describe the mechanism of maintenance of muscle tone
- Explain the origin, course and termination of the pyramidal tract with the help of a diagram
- Differentiate between upper motor neuron lesion and lower motor neuron lesion
- Explain the effects of lesion of the pyramidal tract at different levels
- Discuss the physiological basis of crossed hemiplegia
- Briefly discuss LMN facial palsy

INTRODUCTION

PY10.4: Describe and discuss motor tracts, mechanism of maintenance of tone, control of body movements, posture and equilibrium and vestibular apparatus.

Motor means movement by contraction of effector organ. Motor functions of the nervous system include control of various bodily activities. Motor effects are seen in the somatic nervous system and autonomic nervous system (ANS). Muscles and glands are called effectors because they are the structures that perform the motor function. The effector organ in somatic nervous system is skeletal muscle and the effector organs in ANS are smooth muscles, cardiac muscle and glands (both endocrine and exocrine).

Two types of motor fibers in ANS are:
1. Sympathetic fibers
2. Parasympathetic fibers

Autonomic descending fibers are not seen as a separate tract; instead, these fibers are seen scattered among other nerve fibers. They carry information from hypothalamus, respiratory centers and cardiovascular centers in the brainstem to preganglionic autonomic neurons in the lateral horn of spinal cord.

SOMATIC NERVOUS SYSTEM

Effector organ of somatic nervous system is skeletal muscle. Muscle fibers are innervated by axons of α-motor neurons in spinal cord. The cranial nerve nuclei in the brainstem also innervate skeletal muscles of the head and neck. The alpha motor neurons are controlled by many levels of the central nervous system like the reticular formation in the brainstem, basal ganglia, cerebellum and the motor cortex. The higher centers are concerned with complex muscle movements controlled by the thought processes of the brain.

The neurons in the motor system can be divided into lower motor neurons and upper motor neurons. **Lower motor neurons (LMN)** refer to the spinal and cranial alpha motor neurons that directly innervate skeletal muscles. **Upper motor neurons (UMN)** are the neurons (**pyramidal**) in the pre-central gyrus and neighboring cortical regions that terminate on the lower motor neurons directly or through interneurons. Axons of the upper motor neurons comprise the corticospinal and corticobulbar tracts. Lowest level of motor neuron is the α-**motor neuron** or **lower motor neuron** which comprises the output of the motor system. **Final common pathway** for motor information to the muscle is α-motor neuron and its axon. **Gamma-motor neurons** also come under motor neurons, but they innervate only the skeletal muscle receptor called muscle spindle.

The motor cortex and spinal cord are connected with other deep cerebral and brainstem motor nuclei like the caudate nucleus, putamen, globus pallidus, red nuclei, sub-thalamic nuclei, substantia nigra, reticular nuclei and neurons of cerebellum. Neurons in these structures are referred to as **extrapyramidal neurons**.

Motor activity can arise in the body at the spinal cord level, which is called spinal reflex action, or at the brainstem level, called cranial reflex action. Highest level of motor activity is the cerebral cortex. Thus, motor activity can occur at three levels:
1. Spinal cord level as a spinal reflex action (*refer* **Chapter 00**)
2. Brainstem level as cranial reflex action
3. Cortical level as voluntary action

MUSCLE TONE

Slight (minimal) degree of contraction of muscle in the resting state is called **muscle tone**. It is a state of partial tetanus. Skeletal muscle tone results entirely from a slow rate of nerve impulses coming from the spinal cord.

These nerve impulses, in turn, are controlled partly by signals transmitted from the brain to the appropriate spinal cord anterior motor neurons and partly by signals that originate in *muscle spindles* located in the muscle itself.

Tone is defined as the resistance against stretch and is clinically examined by doing passive movement. Normal tone is reflexly maintained and the reflex concerned is **stretch reflex**. A muscle attached to a tendon is slightly stretched in the resting state. This stretch has slight stretching effect on the muscle spindle and this leads to slight contraction of muscle reflexly. This occurs only if the spindle sensitivity is normal or slightly increased due to continuous slow stream of impulses coming from the brain through γ-motor neurons **(Fig. 84.1)**. Some gamma motor neurons are active at rest, making the spindle fibers taut and sensitive to stretch.

Tendon reflexes and muscle tone depend on the activity of alpha motor neurons, muscle spindles, and gamma motor neurons whose axons innervate the spindle. Damage to lower motor neurons or their axons causes flaccid weakness of the innervated muscles. In addition muscle tone and deep tendon reflexes are impaired or lost. If the posterior nerve root is cut, hypotonia results because the reflex arc is not complete since the afferent limb of the reflex arc is cut.

γ-efferent discharge and α-efferent discharge are controlled by various descending tracts coming from higher centers. This is referred to as supra-spinal control of γ-motor neurons, especially fibers of the reticulospinal tract **(Fig. 84.1)**.

The descending tract directly exerting its effect on γ-motor neuron is **reticulospinal tract**. Descending fibers may be *excitatory to γ-motor neurons or inhibitory to γ-motor neurons*. Normally, inhibitory influences counteract excitatory influences so that only a minimal degree of firing is seen in the resting stage in γ-motor neuron. If there is a lesion in the descending tract, excitatory effect will be more and muscles go into a state of **hypertonia** where the resistance of the spastic muscle to stretch is high. But, if γ-motor neuron is damaged, then there will be **hypotonia** where the flaccid muscle offers little or no resistance to stretching. Muscle tone is assessed clinically by moving the muscle passively at various joints.

Rigidity and Spasticity

Rigidity is increase in muscle tone associated with muscle stiffness as seen in extrapyramidal lesion, e.g., Parkinson disease. *In rigidity, tendon reflexes are not affected and hypertonia is seen in both flexors and extensors equally.*

Spasticity is muscle stiffness or increased muscle tone associated with exaggerated tendon reflexes as seen in upper motor neuron lesion or lesion of internal capsule. *In spasticity, hypertonia is confined to only one group of muscles either flexors or extensors.*

Alpha-Gamma Linkage

For every muscle contraction, when the α-motor neuron is stimulated, γ-motor neuron is also stimulated simultaneously. This α-γ **co-activation** increases the sensitivity of muscle spindle to stretch and can produce sustained contraction of the muscle. This is very important in the maintenance of posture. It is seen that any cortical or brainstem system that influence α-motor neuron also influences γ-motor neurons and the effect, either excitation or inhibition, will be the same in the two motor neurons. Thus, the tone of the body is adjusted according to body needs.

Anxiety increases γ-efferent discharge. A noxious stimulus can stimulate the γ-motor neurons of the flexors, simultaneously inhibiting the γ-motor neurons of extensors.

Jendrassik's Maneuver or Reinforcement

Reinforcement is carried out if it is difficult to elicit the deep tendon reflex. This technique should be done before concluding that the reflex is absent. The act of reinforcement brings the muscle tone to the optimum level. If the subject is anxious there will be hypertonicity of the muscles. Jendrassik's maneuver carried out by the subject is of great help. It consists of hooking the flexed fingers of the two hands of the subject and pulling them apart while the reflex in the lower limbs is being elicited. This effort diverts the subject's attention and thus causes relaxation of the hypertonic muscles. Clenching the fists, grasping firmly the arm of the chair or side of the bed, etc., has also been used to obtain the same results. To reinforce the reflexes in the upper limbs, the subject is asked to clench his jaws tightly while eliciting the reflex. Even after reinforcement if a reflex cannot be elicited, it has pathological significance.

■ UPPER MOTOR NEURON PATHWAYS

Upper motor neurons (UMN) are the neurons in the cerebral cortex and brainstem that terminate on the lower motor neurons (LMN) in the brainstem or in the spinal cord directly or through interneurons, which in turn directly influences the skeletal muscle activity. Most of the upper motor neurons synapse with interneurons, which, in turn, synapse with the lower motor neurons. Some upper motor neurons synapse directly with LMN especially the neurons coming from the primary motor area.

Clinically, the term UMN is used to describe descending motor neurons forming the corticospinal and corticobulbar tracts which control voluntary activity. These upper motor neurons originate from cerebral cortex which includes primary motor area (Brodmann's area 4), premotor cortex (area 6), supplementary motor cortex and primary sensory

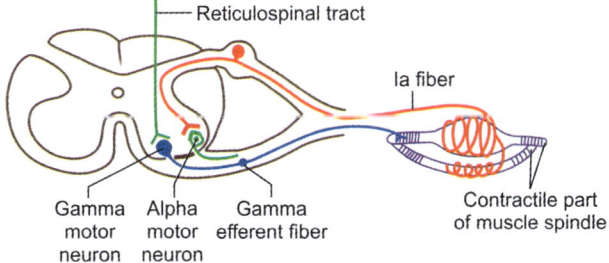

Fig. 84.1: Role of muscle spindle and gamma efferent discharge in maintaining normal muscle tone.

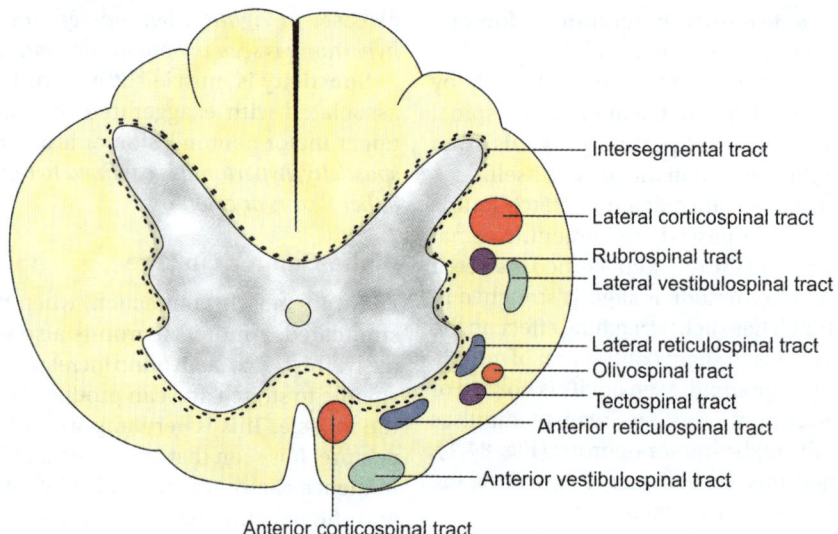

Fig. 84.2: Descending tracts of spinal cord.

cortex (area 3, 1 and 2). Extrapyramidal neurons originate from motor centers of brainstem like red nucleus, vestibular nucleus, superior colliculus and reticular formation. *The upper motor neurons from cerebral cortex regulate voluntary motor activity, whereas the extrapyramidal neurons from the brainstem regulate muscle tone, posture and equilibrium.*

Classification of Somatic Motor Pathways or Descending Pathways

- **Clinical classification (Fig. 84.2)**
  - Direct motor pathway or pyramidal pathway
    - Corticobulbar tract
    - Anterior corticospinal tract
    - Lateral corticospinal tract
  - Indirect motor pathway or extrapyramidal pathways
    - Reticulospinal tract (lateral and medial or anterior)
    - Tectospinal tract
    - Vestibulospinal tract (lateral and medial or anterior)
    - Rubrospinal tract
    - Olivospinal tract

Pyramidal system or direct motor pathway includes all the motor fibers travelling in the pyramids of medulla oblongata. Direct motor pathway input to lower motor neuron is through axons that extend directly from cerebral cortex.

Indirect motor pathway provides input to lower motor neurons from motor centers in the brainstem. These centers in turn receive signals from neurons in basal ganglia, cerebellum and cerebral cortex. Impulses from both the direct and indirect pathways are necessary for normal movements.

- **Functional classification of descending motor fibers**
  - **Lateral descending pathways or lateral system** terminate either directly on motor neurons or on interneurons in the lateral cell groups of the anterior horn of spinal cord. These fibers control the movements of the distal limb muscles and these muscles are innervated unilaterally. It includes the *lateral corticospinal tract and the rubrospinal tract* (Flowchart 84.1). The

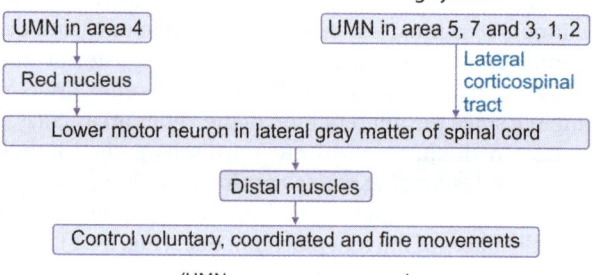

Flowchart 84.1: Lateral descending system.

rubrospinal tract contains less than 200 fibers in man and is less important in humans. Lateral pathways also include *corticobulbar fibers supplying the lower part of facial nerve nucleus and the hypoglossal nucleus.* Lateral system controls finely coordinated movements of the extremities.

- **Medial descending pathways or medial system** end in the anterior horn on the medial group of interneurons. These interneurons synapse with lower motor neurons that control the axial and girdle musculature bilaterally. Medial system controls coarse trunk and whole limb movements. They are also concerned with maintenance of muscle tone, balance and posture. Medial pathways include the *anterior corticospinal tract, most of the corticobulbar tracts, the vestibulospinal tract, reticulospinal tract and tectospinal tract* (Flowchart 84.2).

VOLUNTARY MOTOR ACTIVITY

Information for voluntary motor activity always arises from **cerebral cortex**. Whether the action is voluntary or reflex, the information should pass through the motor neurons in spinal cord or cranial motor nuclei in brainstem to reach the muscles. All excitatory and inhibitory signals that control movement converge on the α-motor neuron which is called the **final common pathway**. The information can reach muscles from central nervous system (CNS), only through the

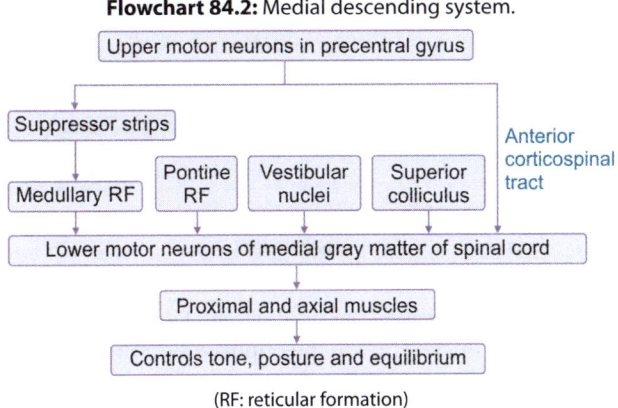

Flowchart 84.2: Medial descending system.

(RF: reticular formation)

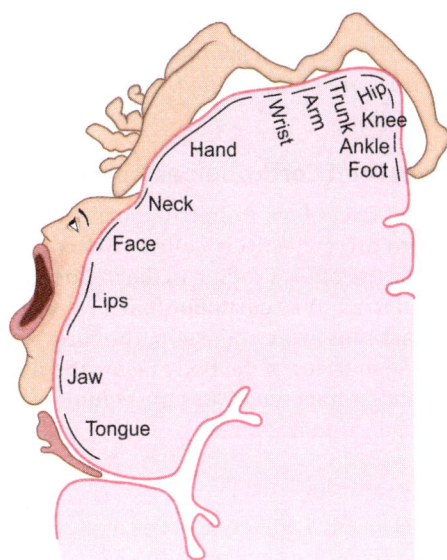

Fig. 84.3: Motor homunculus in the precentral gyrus of the right cerebral hemisphere.

final common pathway, i.e., through the α-motor neurons. The axons of the α-motor neurons innervate the skeletal muscles of the head and body and these neurons are called **lower motor neurons (LMN)**, and they have their cell bodies in the brainstem and spinal cord.

MOTOR AREAS OF CEREBRAL CORTEX

The motor cortex is divided into three subareas: (1) the *primary motor cortex*, (2) the *premotor cortex*, and (3) the *supplementary motor area*. 31% of fibers in the pyramidal tract arise from the **primary motor cortex** (Brodmann's area 4). The main area from which information for motor activity comes is called the **primary motor area**, located in the precentral gyrus of cerebral cortex. Primary motor area is called **Brodmann's area 4**. Large pyramidal cells called **Betz cells** are the characteristic feature of primary motor area. About 35,000 Betz cells are present in the primary motor area.

Topographical representation **(motor homunculus)** of the entire body is seen in the primary motor area. The body representation in this area is **inverted** and unilateral with the head represented down and foot up **(Fig. 84.3)**. The face and mouth region are represented near the Sylvian fissure; the arm and hand area, in the midportion of the primary motor cortex; the trunk near the apex of the brain; and the leg and foot areas, in the part of the primary motor cortex that dips into the longitudinal fissure. This topographical organization of the different muscle areas was mapped by **Penfield and Rasmussen.** If different areas in this part are electrically stimulated, muscle contractions are seen in different parts of the body depending on the area stimulated.

Bilateral representation is seen to lower motor neurons innervating the upper half of face, muscles of eyes, jaws, pharynx, larynx, neck, thorax and abdomen. Area of representation depends on the skill of the activity. Greater area of representation is seen in the motor cortex for muscles involved in speech, muscles of hand, etc., since the movements in these areas are fine and complex.

Apart from primary motor area an additional or **supplementary motor area** is seen on the medial part of the frontal lobe to the upper part of cingulate sulcus where the entire body representation is seen. Here, the strength of the stimulus needed is more and groups of muscles contract when the supplementary motor area is stimulated rather than single muscles.

Anterior to area 4 is area 6, which is called the **premotor area or motor association area**. Nerve signals generated in the premotor area cause much more complex patterns of movement than the discrete patterns generated in the primary motor cortex. If this area is stimulated, gross rotatory movements of eyes, head and body to the opposite side are seen. All the motor areas are intimately interconnected. The motor areas also have connection with the sensory areas. So they are together known as **sensory- motor area**. The major descending tracts which arise from these areas which control voluntary motor activity are collectively called **pyramidal tract**.

MIRROR NEURONS

A special class of neurons called *mirror neurons* becomes active when a person performs a specific motor task or when he or she observes the same task performed by others. Thus, the activity of these neurons mirrors the behavior of another person as though the observer was performing the specific motor task. Brain imaging studies indicate that these neurons transform sensory representation of acts that are heard or seen into motor representation of these acts. These mirror neurons are important for understanding the actions of other people and for learning new skills by imitation. For example, if a person yawns, another person seeing him yawn, also yawns due to the activity of mirror neurons. The premotor cortex, primary motor cortex, basal ganglia and thalamus constitute an overall system for the control of complex patterns of coordinated muscle activity.

PYRAMIDAL TRACT

Pyramidal tract or direct motor pathway is the major motor tract of the body which carries information from cerebral cortex for **voluntary motor activity**. There are about *1 million nerve fibers in each pyramidal tract. 50% of fibers in pyramidal tract are unmyelinated.* Therefore, it is a slowly conducting tract.

Corticospinal and Corticobulbar Tracts

The pyramidal tract fibers ending in the anterior horn cells of spinal cord are collectively called **corticospinal tract**. The pyramidal tract fibers ending in the motor cranial nerve nuclei are referred to as **corticobulbar or corticonuclear tract**. This tract ends in the brainstem. The corticospinal tract innervates the muscles of the body below the neck region. The corticobulbar tract innervates the voluntary muscles of eye, face, tongue, throat and neck.

Origin of Pyramidal Tract

Pyramidal cells which are the neurons of corticospinal and corticobulbar tracts are situated in the 5th layer of cerebral cortex. Betz cell (giant pyramidal cells 60 μm in diameter) fibers constitute about 2–3% of pyramidal tract fibers, i.e., it comes to about 35,000. 29% of the fibers arise from **supplementary or secondary motor area** and from **premotor cortex** (area 6). 60% of pyramidal tract fibers arise from motor areas and 40% from sensory areas of cerebral cortex.

Course of the Pyramidal Tract

The pyramidal tract fibers converge to **corona radiata,** to reach the internal capsule. **Internal capsule** is a mass of white matter containing nerve fibers lying between the lenticular nucleus of basal ganglia laterally and caudate nucleus of basal ganglia and thalamus medially. All motor and sensory nerve fibers connecting the cerebral cortex and spinal cord pass through the internal capsule. In the internal capsule, the pyramidal tract forms a bundle which occupies the genu (the bend in the internal capsule) and anterior 2/3rd of the **posterior limb of internal capsule**. Fibers from the head area are seen anteriorly and fibers from foot area posteriorly. The fibers of the pyramidal tract pass down through the brainstem, i.e., **midbrain, pons and medulla**.

Course in the Midbrain

In the midbrain pyramidal tract occupies the **crus cerebra**. It lies ventral to the substantia nigra and occupies the middle 3/5th of the crus. There is well marked localization of the fibers subserving different parts of the body. Fibers to the motor cranial nerve nuclei cross to the opposite side and end in the IV and V nuclei.

In the Pons

In the pons, the pyramidal tract occupies the most ventral aspect and splits into discrete bundles due to the presence of pontine nuclei. Fibers to the motor cranial nerve nuclei cross to the opposite side and end in the VI and VII nuclei.

In the Medulla

After passing pons, it again forms a bundle and occupies the pyramids of the medulla (ventral bulges of medulla) and

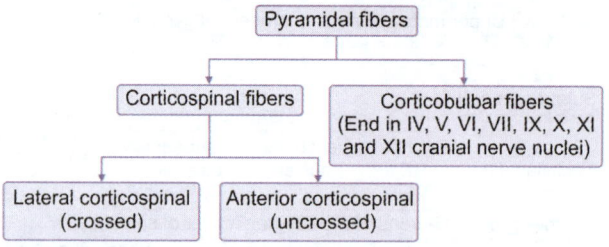

Flowchart 84.3: Divisions of the pyramidal tract.

hence this tract is called pyramidal tract. Fibers to the motor cranial nerve nuclei cross to the opposite side and end in the IX, X, XI and XII nuclei.

In the medulla, 80% of fibers cross to the opposite side (**contralateral** side) as **pyramidal decussation** and 20% pass uncrossed (**ipsilateral** fibers).

Course in the Spinal Cord and Termination of the Pyramidal Tract

The crossed fibers occupy the lateral funiculus of the spinal cord and descend as the **lateral corticospinal tract or indirect tract (Flowchart 84.3)**. A somatotopic organization is seen in the lateral corticospinal tract of the cervical cord. Here, fibers to the motor neurons that control leg muscles lie laterally and fibers to cervical motor neurons lie medially. The lateral corticospinal tract finally terminate principally on the interneurons in the intermediate regions of the spinal cord gray matter; a few terminate on sensory relay neurons in the dorsal horn, and a very few terminate directly on the anterior motor neurons that cause muscle contraction.

20% of uncrossed fibers in the spinal cord form the **anterior corticospinal tract or direct corticospinal tract**. These fibers also cross to the opposite side at different levels in spinal cord via the anterior white commissure before they end in the spinal motor neurons. Before crossing, the anterior corticospinal fibers give collaterals to the motor neurons of that side and thus it innervates the axial muscles bilaterally. These fibers are concerned with the control of bilateral postural movements controlled by the supplementary motor area. *55% of pyramidal tract fibers end in the cervical region, 20% ends in the thoracic region and 25% ends in the lumbosacral region of the spinal cord.*

The cortex has almost a direct pathway to the anterior motor neurons of the cord, bypassing some motor centers on the way. This is especially involved in the control of the fine expert movements of the fingers and hands. Only the largest corticospinal fibers end directly in the α-motor neurons. These are mainly the axons of Betz cells. The rest synapse with interneurons which in turn synapse with α-motor neuron or γ-motor neuron. Leg fibers come down up to the lumbar segments.

Corticobulbar Tract

As the pyramidal fibers descend through the diencephalon and brainstem, fibers separate to innervate extrapyramidal and cranial motor nuclei. Fibers to the muscles of head and neck region cross to the opposite side to end in the corresponding

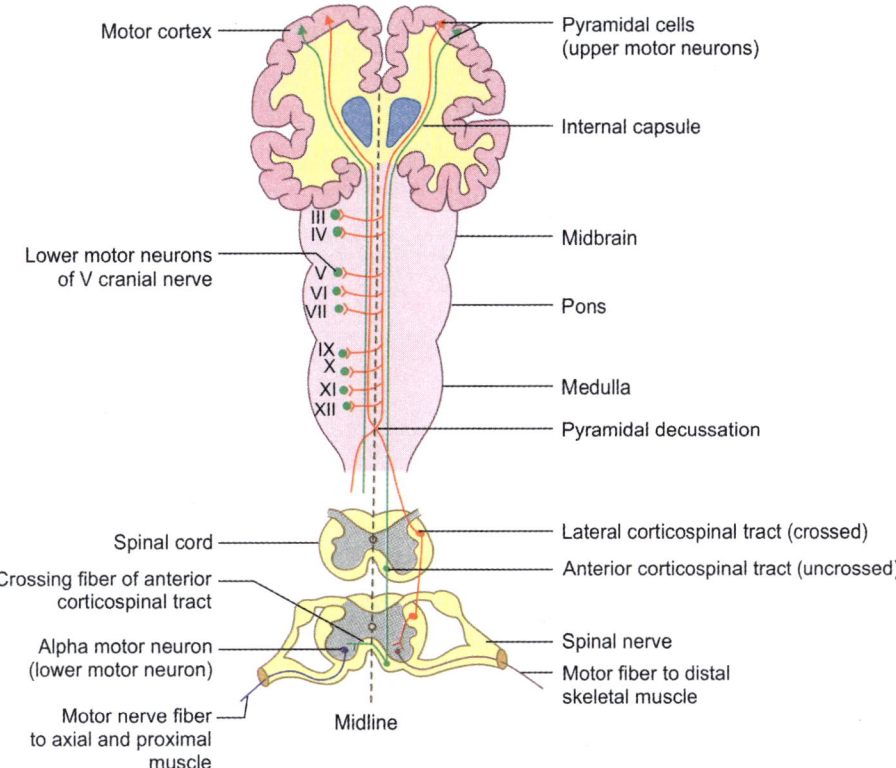

Fig. 84.4: Pyramidal pathways (corticobulbar and corticospinal tracts). The fibers to the cranial nerve nuclei cross to the opposite side in the midbrain, pons and medulla to end in the lower motor neuron of the corresponding cranial nerve nucleus. This forms the corticobulbar or corticonuclear tract. The other form corticospinal tract.

cranial nerve nuclei in the brainstem. Motor nuclei of the cranial nerves in which these axons terminate are that of III, IV, V, VI, VII, IX, X, XI and XII cranial nerves (I, II and VIII cranial nerves are purely sensory in function). These fibers of the pyramidal tract are called **corticonuclear or corticobulbar** fibers. The rest form **corticospinal** fibers **(Fig. 84.4)**. The lower motor neurons of cranial nerves convey impulses that control precise, voluntary movements of eyes, tongue and neck, and coordinate the activities of the muscles of mastication, facial expression and speech. The lower brainstem motor neurons receive input from crossed and uncrossed corticobulbar fibers, although neurons that innervate lower facial muscles receive primarily crossed fibers.

Bilateral connections are present for all the cranial nerve motor nuclei except for part of the facial nerve nucleus that supplies the muscles of the lower half of the face and a part of the hypoglossal nucleus that supplies the genioglossus muscle of the tongue.

The right cerebral cortex controls mainly the muscles of the left side of the body and the left cerebral cortex controls mainly the muscles on the right side of the body.

As the corticospinal tract descends, in addition to sending fibers to the brainstem motor cranial nerve nuclei, it also sends collaterals to the basal ganglia, thalamus, cerebellum and other centers of the brainstem either directly or indirectly. It includes the following:

❖ The axons from the Betz cells send short collaterals back to the motor cortex. These collaterals are believed to inhibit adjacent regions of the cortex when the Betz cells discharge, thereby sharpening the boundaries of the excitatory signal (lateral inhibition).

❖ A large number of fibers pass from the motor cortex into the *caudate nucleus* and *putamen (striatum)* of the basal ganglia. From there, additional pathways extend into the brainstem and spinal cord, mainly to control postural muscle contractions.

❖ A moderate number of motor fibers pass to *red nuclei* of the midbrain. From these nuclei, fibers pass down the spinal cord through the *rubrospinal tract.*

❖ A number of motor fibers send collaterals into the *reticular formation* and *vestibular nuclei* of the brainstem. From there, signals go to the spinal cord through the *reticulospinal* and *vestibulospinal tracts.* Fibers also go to the cerebellum by way of *reticulocerebellar* and *vestibulocerebellar tracts.*

❖ A large number of motor fibers synapse in the pontine nuclei, which give rise to the *pontocerebellar fibers,* carrying signals into the cerebellar hemispheres.

❖ Collaterals from the descending motor fibers also terminate in the *inferior olivary nuclei,* and from there, *olivocerebellar fibers* transmit signals to the cerebellum.

Thus, the basal ganglia, brainstem, and cerebellum all receive strong motor signals from the corticospinal system every time a signal is transmitted down the spinal cord to cause a motor activity.

Functions of the Corticospinal Tract

❖ Lateral corticospinal tract controls the voluntary activities of the distal limb muscles and are concerned with precise,

fine and quick movements of the fingers and hand to perform skilled motor activities like writing, typing, etc.
- Anterior corticospinal tract controls the muscles of the trunk and proximal muscles of the limbs. It is involved in postural adjustments and gross movements.
- Some of the fibers in the corticospinal tract make connections with the ascending sensory tracts and this helps in the sensory control of motor activities.
- Corticospinal tracts arising from the sensory cortex are concerned with sensory-motor coordination. Lesion to these areas leads to inability to perform learned sequences of movements like eating, driving, etc.
- The basal ganglia, brainstem, and cerebellum all receive strong motor signals from the corticospinal system every time a signal is transmitted down the spinal cord to cause a perfect motor activity after proper planning and programming.

EXTRAPYRAMIDAL TRACTS

All the descending tracts other than the pyramidal tract are called extrapyramidal tracts. It is important to note that the descending motor tract in brainstem contains not only corticospinal fibers or corticobulbar fibers, but also fibers that terminate on brainstem neurons like that of reticular formation, inferior olivary nucleus, etc., which are extrapyramidal fibers.

The pyramidal and the extrapyramidal tracts should function together for smooth activity. Planning and programming of each movement occurs in the basal ganglia or cerebellum or both. The information from these areas goes to the primary motor area from where information for activity comes down to the spinal cord. Background tone, posture, equilibrium, etc., are maintained by extrapyramidal system. Voluntary activity is controlled by pyramidal system.

Extrapyramidal fibers arise from cerebral cortex and from subcortical structures like basal ganglia, brainstem reticular formation, red nucleus, tectal nucleus, vestibular nucleus and olivary nucleus.

CORTICALLY ORIGINATING EXTRAPYRAMIDAL FIBERS

- Facilitatory fibers which stimulate muscle tone and stretch reflexes.
- Inhibitory fibers which inhibit or suppress motor activity or reflexes.

Facilitatory fibers arise from area 6, supplementary motor area and area 4. **Inhibitory fibers** arise from suppressor strips of different areas of cortex like 4S, 2S, 8S, 19S, 24S, etc. The cortically originating extrapyramidal fibers descend intermingled with pyramidal tract fibers. So, any lesion of the pyramidal tract in the brain will be associated with extrapyramidal manifestations.

Cortically originating extrapyramidal fibers do not go directly to the α-motor neurons; instead, relay in the reticular formation directly or indirectly through the basal ganglia. Thus, reticular formation forms the most important relay and integrating center for extrapyramidal influences.

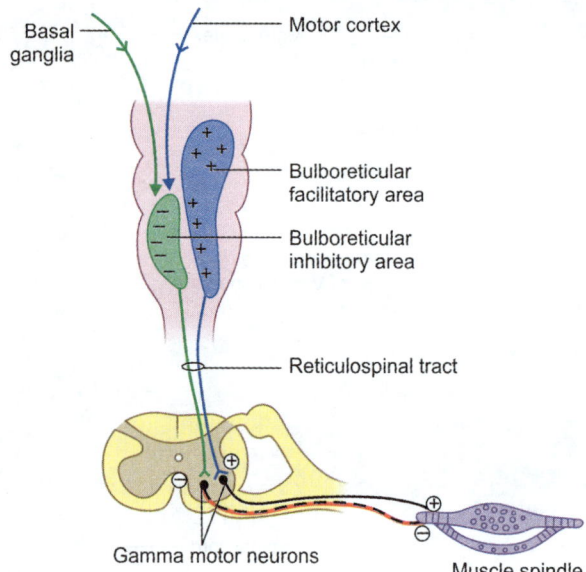

Fig. 84.5: Higher control of muscle tone and stretch reflex by modulation of gamma-motor neuronal activity.
(+: stimulation; –: inhibition)

Reticulospinal Tract

Fibers arising from the reticular formation descend as anterior and lateral reticulospinal tract. These fibers end on different segments of the spinal cord mainly in the γ-**motor neurons** which supply the muscle spindle. Some fibers also end in α-motor neurons and interneurons. The reticular formation consists of two parts:
1. A larger upper facilitatory area
2. A small caudal inhibitory area

The **bulboreticular facilitatory area** is capable of spontaneous firing of impulses. But, **caudal inhibitory area** is driven by fibers arising from inhibitory suppressor strips of cerebral cortex or fibers from basal ganglia. Normally, there is a balance between the facilitatory and inhibitory areas (**Fig. 84.5**). The slow stream of facilitatory impulses maintains normal **muscle tone**. Reticular formation in turn is controlled by cerebral cortex and basal ganglia. If there is damage to the extrapyramidal fibers from cortex or basal ganglia, the inhibitory influence to the reticular formation is lost. Since the facilitatory area can spontaneously generate impulses, there will be **hypertonia**.

Anterior reticulospinal tract arise from neurons in pons and is an uncrossed tract. **Lateral reticulospinal tract** arise from medulla which consists of crossed and uncrossed fibers. Pontine reticulospinal neurons are primarily excitatory and medullary reticulospinal neurons are primarily inhibitory.

Vestibulospinal Tract

The vestibulospinal tract arises from the neurons of vestibular nucleus. Vestibular nucleus receives connections from inner ear, cerebellum, basal ganglia, cerebral cortex, reticular formation, etc. This tract is seen in the anterior and lateral funiculus as anterior and lateral vestibulospinal tract. The

anterior vestibulospinal tract originates in the medial and inferior vestibular nuclei and projects *bilaterally* to cervical spinal motor neurons that control neck musculature. The **lateral vestibulospinal tract** originates in the lateral vestibular nucleus and projects *ipsilaterally* to end in the α-motor neurons of each segment of spinal cord directly or through interneurons. These motor neurons facilitate the activity of the **extensor group** of muscles, especially those that maintain posture. They inhibit the activity of flexor muscles.

Rubrospinal Tract

Fibers descending from red nucleus of midbrain form the rubrospinal tract. Red nucleus is connected to the cerebral cortex, cerebellum and reticular formation. Red nucleus has two parts:
1. **Magnocellular** portion, which contains large neurons
2. **Parvocellular** portion, which contains small neurons

The descending fibers cross to the opposite side and the decussation is called **Forrel's decussation**. The rubrospinal tract ends in α-motor neuron or in gamma motor neuron or in interneurons. But, mainly they end in α-motor neurons supplying **flexor group** of muscles, and is the functional antagonist to vestibulospinal tract which supplies extensor group of muscles. In other words, rubrospinal tract facilitates the activity of flexor muscles, and inhibit the activity of extensor or antigravity muscles.

Olivospinal Tract

Olivospinal tract arises from the **inferior olivary nucleus** in the medulla, and is seen in the lateral funiculus of spinal cord anteriorly. Inferior olivary nucleus is connected to cerebellum, thalamus, cortex, red nucleus and to reticular formation. They end in the spinal cord motor neurons. Function is not clearly understood.

Tectospinal Tract

Tectospinal tract arises from neurons in the **superior colliculus** of midbrain and is seen anterior to the olivospinal tract. The fibers cross and descend down to end in the spinal cord motor neurons. They terminate in the upper segments of spinal cord. It is concerned with spino-visual reflex (reflex neck movements in response to visual stimuli) which is better developed in lower animals than in humans **(Flowchart 84.4)**.

Medial Longitudinal Bundle

This is a well-developed tract seen in the brainstem area, but extensions are seen to upper segments of spinal cord. III, IV and VI cranial nerve nuclei are interconnected and are connected to the tectal region and upper segments of spinal cord. The medial longitudinal bundle plays a role in the coordination of neck movements with eye movements, both voluntary and reflex movements.

Intersegmental Tract

Intersegmental tract arises from interneurons of one segment of spinal cord, ascend or descend a few segments and end in

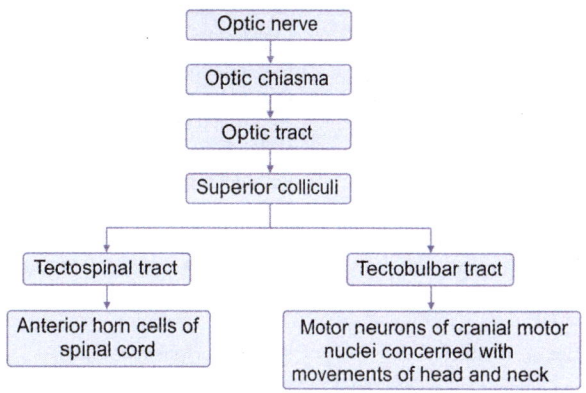

Flowchart 84.4: Pathway for spino-visual reflex (tectospinal tract).

the interneurons of another segment. This helps to coordinate functions of different segments of the spinal cord.

APPLIED PHYSIOLOGY

Amyotrophic Lateral Sclerosis

Amyotrophic lateral sclerosis is a progressive degenerative disease which affects the lower motor neuron cell bodies. It causes progressing muscle weakness and atrophy. Symptoms such as flaccid paralysis, muscular atrophy, fasciculation, hypotonia and hyporeflexia or areflexia are due to lower motor neuron damage. Cause of this disease is unclear, but possibilities include viruses, neurotoxins, heavy metals, DNA defects, immune system abnormalities and enzyme abnormalities. Intellect and sensations are unaffected in this disease.

Paralysis

If damage occurs to upper motor neuron or lower motor neuron, voluntary motor activity does not occur. Upper motor neuron (UMN) and lower motor neuron (LMN) should be intact for performing voluntary motor activity. Inability to do a motor activity voluntarily or to contract a muscle voluntarily is called **paralysis**. It can be due to **UMN lesion or LMN lesion**.

Damage or disease of the LMN produces **flaccid paralysis** of muscles of same side of lesion. Voluntary as well as reflex action of the innervated muscle is lost, muscle tone is lost and the muscle remains flaccid. Injury or disease of UMN causes **spastic paralysis** of muscles, where the muscle tone is increased, deep reflexes exaggerated and pathological reflexes such as Babinski sign appear.

UMN and LMN Lesions

In UMN lesion, reflex action is present, but voluntary activity is lost. In LMN lesion, both voluntary as well as reflex activities are lost. Muscle tone cannot be maintained in LMN lesion because reflex arc is interrupted, and this leads to **flaccid paralysis**.

In UMN lesion, the muscle tone can be maintained because the reflex arc is intact. But, if extrapyramidal inhibitory fibers

Table 84.1: Differences between UMN and LMN lesion.	
UMN lesion	**LMN lesion**
Due to lesion of UMN that influence the activity of LMN	Due to lesion of LMN in the motor cranial nerve nuclei or in spinal cord that directly innervate skeletal muscles
Voluntary activity lost, reflex activity present	Both voluntary and reflex activity lost
Spastic paralysis due to hypertonia, clasp-knife phenomenon and clonus can be elicited	Flaccid paralysis due to hypotonia and loss of innervation of muscle
Reflex arc is intact	Integrity of reflex arc is lost
Deep reflexes are exaggerated due to increase in muscle tone. Superficial reflexes are lost and some altered, e.g., extensor plantar reflex	Both superficial and deep reflexes are absent at the level of lesion since reflex arc is disrupted
Since nerve supply to the muscle is intact, muscle atrophy occurs slowly	Rapid muscular atrophy and muscle wasting occurs within 2–3 days
Reaction of degeneration is absent	Reaction of degeneration is present
Positive Babinski sign elicited	Babinski sign not elicited since plantar reflex is absent
EMG normal	EMG shows fibrillations

are also damaged, there will be hypertonia due to over activity of facilitatory area. If it is a pure pyramidal tract lesion, then there will not be hypertonia. All paralyzed muscles become spastic in UMN lesion, and is called **spastic paralysis**. The reason is due to associated damage of the extrapyramidal inhibitory fibers. Pyramidal fibers closely intermingle with extrapyramidal fibers which inhibit muscle tone. Since these fibers are damaged along with pyramidal fibers, there is increase in the facilitatory impulses from the facilitatory area of reticular formation leading to spasticity. Reflexes are exaggerated especially deep tendon reflexes **(Table 84.1)**. Clasp-knife phenomenon is present, and ankle clonus and patellar clonus can be elicited (*refer* 'inverse stretch reflex'). Some of the superficial reflexes are absent like abdominal reflex, cremasteric reflex, etc. because the reflex pathway involves the cerebral cortex unlike the deep tendon reflexes which occurs at the spinal cord level. Superficial reflexes are polysynaptic reflexes. Some superficial reflexes are altered as in the case of plantar reflex. Scratch the lateral aspect of sole of the foot, there will be dorsiflexion of toes and fanning out of toes which is called **extensor plantar reflex or positive Babinski sign**. This is a specific test for pyramidal tract lesion.

Causes for Positive Babinski Sign

- Corticospinal tract normally produces plantar flexion and adduction of toes when the lateral aspect of sole is stroked. When there is a lesion of the corticospinal tract, the influence of the extrapyramidal tracts on the toes become apparent. The effect will be dorsiflexion of great toe and fanning out of other toes.
- Most of the extrapyramidal fibers are uncrossed fibers which terminate in the α-motor neurons or γ-motor neurons of spinal cord through interneurons. So, even if some of the extrapyramidal fibers are affected on the side of lesion along with corticospinal fibers, Babinski sign will be positive on the affected limb. For example, the lateral vestibulospinal tract, which is an uncrossed tract, facilitates activity of extensor muscles and inhibits the activity of flexor muscles of the toes.
- *Normally, Babinski sign is positive in infants,* i.e., before the child starts walking. Pyramidal tract becomes fully developed and myelination is completed only after the child starts walking.

In LMN lesion, all reflexes are absent because the reflex arc is not complete. Here, since there is denervation of muscle, the muscle atrophies at an earlier date. In UMN lesion it is slow disuse atrophy. Reaction of degeneration will be present in LMN lesion because of denervation.

Reaction of Degeneration

When normally innervated muscles are stimulated with faradic current, the muscle contraction continues as long as the current is passing. Galvanic current or direct current causes contraction only when the current is turned on or turned off. When the lower motor nerve is cut, i.e., in LMN lesion, the affected muscle will no longer respond to faradic current after 7 days of nerve injury, and after 10 days the response to direct current also stops. This change in muscle response to electrical stimulation is known as reaction of degeneration.

Pyramidal Tract Lesion

Lesion can occur anywhere from cortex to the termination of pyramidal tract. If all the pyramidal tract fibers of one side are damaged, i.e., if the lesion is above the level of pyramidal decussation, there will be paralysis of opposite side of the body. This is called **contralateral hemiplegia**. If the lesion is in the cervical region of spinal cord then it produces **quadriplegia**, where all the four limbs are paralyzed. If it is in the lumbar region, then it produce **paraplegia**, where the lower two limbs are paralyzed. If the pyramidal fibers supplying only one limb are affected, it leads to **monoplegia**. Monoplegia occurs when there is a lesion in the cortical motor area 4 where the motor neurons remain scattered.

If the lesion is in the cortex or in the corona radiata, it should be very extensive to produce hemiplegia. In the case of lesion in the internal capsule, a very small lesion can produce hemiplegia because the fibers are thickly packed in this part. If the lesion is extensive in the internal capsule, then the sensory fibers will also be affected and sensations will also be lost. If the face fibers are affected, there will be paralysis of only the lower half of face because there is bilateral innervation for the upper half of face. So, in UMN facial palsy, only the contralateral lower half of face is affected. But, if the facial nerve nucleus is affected, then the whole half of face innervated by that facial nerve will be affected on the ipsilateral side. This finding helps to distinguish between UMN and LMN facial palsy.

Bell's Palsy

- Bell's palsy occurs when the seventh cranial nerve become inflamed or compressed. Sometimes it may follow a viral infection like chicken pox, mononucleosis, human immunodeficiency virus (HIV) infection, etc.
- This is an LMN type of facial palsy.
- It usually affects one side.
- There will be sudden weakness of the facial muscles of one side.
- The affected half of the face seems to droop.
- There will be deviation of the angle of the mouth to the opposite side while smiling. This is because of weakness of the facial muscles on the affected side. This will cause pulling of the angle of the mouth to the opposite side by the normal muscles on the opposite side.
- It will be difficult to close the eye on the affected side (**Fig. 84.6**).
- There will be drooling of saliva from the affected side.
- When asked to wrinkle the forehead, there will be no wrinkles on the affected side.
- There will be difficulty in eating also.

> The part of the motor nucleus of facial nerve that supplies the muscles of the upper half of the face receives corticonuclear fibers from both cerebral hemispheres. The part of the facial motor nucleus that supplies the muscles of the lower part of the face receives only corticonuclear fibers from the opposite cerebral hemisphere.

Crossed Hemiplegia

If there is a lesion in the **midbrain** on one side, the cranial nerve nuclei of that side are also affected. Since the third cranial nerve nucleus is present in the midbrain, this lesion produces **ipsilateral ophthalmoplegia** and **contralateral hemiplegia**. Cranial nerve paralysis will be of the LMN type since the cranial nerve nucleus contains the LMN neurons. This type of hemiplegia in which there is same-sided cranial nerve palsy and opposite side hemiplegia is called **crossed hemiplegia**. This is seen when the lesion to the pyramidal tract is in the brainstem where the cranial nerve nuclei are present.

If the lesion is on one side of **pons**, it produces ipsilateral facial palsy and contralateral hemiplegia. If the lesion is in the **medulla**, since all the vital centers are located in the medulla, the condition is fatal. The important centers located in the medulla are:

- *Respiratory centers,* which include pre-Botzinger complex, dorsal respiratory group and ventral respiratory group of neurons involved in the normal rhythmic control of respiration.
- *Vasomotor center and cardioinhibitory center,* involved in the regulation of cardiac function and maintenance of normal blood pressure.
- *Deglutition center,* controlling the muscles of deglutition.
- *Vomiting center,* in the chemoreceptor trigger zone of medulla, induces vomiting in gastrointestinal disorders and is also associated with central vomiting.
- *Superior and inferior salivatory nuclei,* in medulla, control salivary secretion.

The nuclei present in the medulla are 8th, 9th, 10th, 11th and 12th cranial nerve nuclei.

Stages of Hemiplegia

Initial Stage

Immediately after the damage to the pyramidal tract of one side, there will be a stage of flaccid paralysis on the opposite side of the body due to **hypotonia** similar to the stage of spinal shock. Usually, the muscles of face, leg and arm are affected. *Respiratory movements, movements of head and trunk and abdominal movements are not affected because these muscles have bilateral innervation of pyramidal tract.* If the lesion is above the brainstem level, eyeball movements also persist. All reflexes will be absent in the initial stage. This stage lasts for about two to three weeks.

Stage of Recovery

Reflex activity slowly returns by about 2–3 weeks. There will be **hypertonia** and the muscles become spastic referred to as spastic paralysis. *Hypertonia is due to loss of inhibitory control of lower centers by the higher centers and due to denervation hypersensitivity of centers below the level of lesion.* The deep tendon reflexes will be exaggerated due to increased muscle tone. Patellar and ankle clonus can be elicited in the affected limb. The superficial reflexes are lost because they are mediated by the pyramidal tract. Abnormal extensor plantar reflex is obtained (positive Babinski sign) instead of the normal flexor plantar response. If all the pyramidal fibers of the affected side are not damaged, some degree of power returns to the muscles. The patient can walk on a narrow base but has difficulty in bending his knee joint

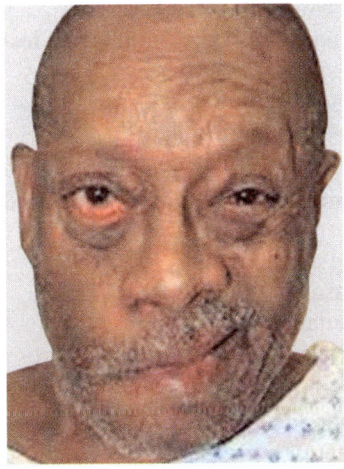

Fig. 84.6: LMN facial palsy. (Note the deviation of angle of the mouth to the left and absence of wrinkling of forehead, loss of nasolabial fold and difficulty to close the eye on the right side. The right side is affected.

and so drags his feet along. The gait is referred to as **spastic hemiplegic gait**.

MULTIPLE CHOICE QUESTIONS

1. All the following statements regarding corticospinal tract are true, *except*:
   a. 50% of fibers are unmyelinated
   b. 80% of fibers arise from area 4 of precentral gyrus
   c. Cranial motor neurons in the brainstem is not a part of pyramidal tract
   d. Lie in the genu and anterior 2/3rd of the posterior limb of the internal capsule

2. All are seen in third nerve palsy, *except*:
   a. Mydriasis
   b. Ptosis
   c. Outward deviation of eye
   d. Miosis

3. Which of the following is true about pyramidal system?
   a. Substantia nigra + basal ganglia
   b. Mainly concerned with sensory system
   c. Fine motor coordination
   d. Initiating voluntary control of large muscle groups

4. All the following tracts are involved in precise voluntary movements, *except*:
   a. Corticospinal tract
   b. Corticobulbar tract
   c. Reticulospinal tract
   d. Rubrospinal tract

5. Transection of medullary pyramid result in:
   a. Hypotonia
   b. Atrophy of muscles
   c. Forced grasping
   d. Negative Babinski sign

6. Skilled voluntary movement is initiated at:
   a. Motor cortex
   b. Basal ganglia
   c. Cortical association area
   d. Cerebellum

7. A unilateral upper motor neuron lesion in the internal capsule is best characterized by:
   a. Diminished use of contralateral appendages below the lesion
   b. Muscle fasciculation
   c. Ipsilateral hypotonia
   d. Flexion of the leg

8. Motor area of Brodmann's area is:
   a. Area 1
   b. Area 4
   c. Area 5
   d. Area 7

9. All the following are true about upper motor neuron lesion, *except*:
   a. Spasticity is a characteristic feature
   b. Babinski sign is positive
   c. Muscle atrophy is a marked feature
   d. Deep tendon reflexes are exaggerated

10. The extrapyramidal tract that increases the extensor tone of skeletal muscle is:
    a. Rubrospinal tract
    b. Vestibulospinal tract
    c. Reticulospinal tract
    d. Tectospinal tract

11. The extrapyramidal tract that completely crosses to the opposite side is:
    a. Rubrospinal tract
    b. Vestibulospinal tract
    c. Reticulospinal tract
    d. Olivospinal tract

12. Left hemiparesis and right hypoglossal nerve palsy with no signs of facial paralysis suggest that the site of lesion is in the:
    a. Midbrain
    b. Pons
    c. Medulla oblongata
    d. Internal capsule

13. Cranial nerve nuclei that are not present in the brainstem include:
    a. I and II
    b. I and VIII
    c. VIII and IX
    d. IX and X

14. Olives are present in the following part:
    a. Midbrain
    b. Pons
    c. Medulla oblongata
    d. Cerebellum

15. Features of pyramidal tract lesion are all, *except*:
    a. Clasp knife rigidity
    b. Involuntary movements
    c. Positive Babinski sign
    d. Exaggerated reflexes

16. All are features of pyramidal tract lesion, *except*:
    a. Clasp knife rigidity
    b. Increased tone
    c. Positive Babinski sign
    d. Involuntary movement

17. Following are features of corticospinal involvement, *except*:
    a. Cog-wheel rigidity
    b. Spasticity
    c. Plantar extensor response
    d. Exaggerated deep tendon reflexes

18. UMN includes:
    a. Pyramidal cells
    b. Anterior horn cells
    c. Peripheral nerves
    d. Schwann cells

19. Which part of the motor neuron has the lowest threshold of excitation?
    a. Soma
    b. Dendrite
    c. Axon hillock
    d. Initial segment

20. Following are features of upper motor neuron lesion, *except*:
    a. Spasticity
    b. Exaggerated deep tendon reflexes
    c. Intention tremor
    d. Positive Babinski sign

21. The percentage of pyramidal fibers that is unmyelinated:
    a. 20
    b. 35
    c. 50
    d. 75

22. The most common cause for hemiplegia in a patient with hypertension is due to rupture of:
    a. Lenticulostriate artery
    b. Middle meningeal artery
    c. Posterior cerebral artery
    d. Anterior cerebral artery

23. Spasticity seen in pyramidal tract lesion is due to:
    a. Destruction of pyramidal fibers
    b. Destruction of extrapyramidal fibers
    c. Damage to alpha motor neuron
    d. Inhibition of gamma motor neuron

24. Increased activity of supplementary motor area may lead to:
    a. Stuttering
    b. Tremor
    c. Rigidity
    d. Dysmetria

ANSWERS

1. b	2. d	3. d	4. c	5. a
6. a	7. a	8. b	9. c	10. b
11. a	12. c	13. a	14. b	15. b
16. d	17. a	18. a	19. d	20. c
21. c	22. a	23. b	24. a	

Lesions of Spinal Cord

CHAPTER 85

LEARNING OBJECTIVES
- Describe the effects of complete section of spinal cord
- Explain the pathophysiology of Brown-Sequard syndrome
- Discuss the effects of cutting the posterior nerve root of spinal cord
- Define sensory ataxia
- Explain the physiological basis of mass reflex

■ INTRODUCTION

PY10.6: Describe and discuss spinal cord, its functions, lesions and sensory disturbances.

The defects seen after spinal cord injury depend on the level of injury. The effects seen after spinal cord injury illustrate the degree of integration of reflexes at the spinal cord level. The main causes of spinal cord injury are road traffic accidents, fall from a height and sports injuries. Approximately 52% of cases of spinal cord injury results in quadriplegia and about 42% leads to paraplegia.

Motor neurons normally receive strong excitatory influences from the upper parts of the motor system, including regions of the spinal cord, the brainstem, and the cerebral cortex. When upper regions of the motor system are injured by stroke, trauma, or demyelinating disease, the signs and symptoms are distinctly different from those caused by damage to the lower regions. Complete transection of the spinal cord leads to profound paralysis below the level of the lesion. This is called **paraplegia** when only both legs are selectively affected, **hemiplegia** when one side of the body is affected, and **quadriplegia** when the legs, trunk, and arms are involved. For a few days after an acute injury, there is also **areflexia** (reflexes absent) and reduced muscle tone (**hypotonia**), a condition called **spinal shock**. The muscles are limp and cannot be controlled by the brain or by the remaining circuits of the spinal cord. Spinal shock is temporary; after days to months, it is replaced by both an exaggerated muscle tone (**hypertonia**) and heightened stretch reflexes (**hyperreflexia**). This combination of hypertonia and hyperreflexia is called **spasticity**. The mechanisms of spasticity are largely unknown, although the hypertonia is the consequence of tonically overactive stretch reflex circuitry, driven by spinal neurons that have become chronically hyper excitable.

■ TYPES OF LESIONS OF SPINAL CORD

- Complete section of spinal cord
- Incomplete section of spinal cord
- Hemisection of spinal cord.

Complete Section of Spinal Cord

Causes
- Gunshot injuries
- Road accidents
- Infections like transverse myelitis
- Sports injuries
- Expanding tumors.

Here, all ascending and descending tracts are cut and α-motor neurons of that segment are also damaged. So, there will be complete sensory and motor paralysis below the level of lesion, i.e., UMN type of paralysis. At the level of lesion, the paralysis is of the LMN type because the reflex arc is disrupted due to damage to the α-motor neurons. If the section occurs at the cervical level, there will be complete loss of motor function below the level of lesion, including all 4 limbs. The condition is called **quadriplegia**. If the section is at the lumbar region, lower 2 limbs will be paralyzed and the condition is **paraplegia**. The patient feels himself cut into two. Higher functions are normal and mind is clear.

The patient passes through three stages after the section of spinal cord:
1. Stage of spinal shock
2. Stage of reflex activity
3. Stage of degeneration.

Stage of Spinal Shock

Stage of spinal shock is seen immediately after the injury. The effects below the level of lesion are:
- Complete **flaccid paralysis** of muscles below the level of lesion and loss of muscle tone.
- All somatic, visceral and vascular reflexes are abolished below the level of section. Vascular smooth muscle loses its tone and fluctuations in blood pressure are seen. Micturition and defecation reflexes are absent and there will be severe constipation and overflow incontinence of bladder.
- Skin becomes cold and blue.

Duration of spinal shock is proportionate to the degree of encephalization of motor functions in various species. *Duration of spinal shock in humans is about 2–3 weeks in the absence of any complications*, whereas in rats it is only a few minutes. It is much longer in humans if complications such as infection, malnutrition, etc. are present. In spinal shock, if the lesion is at a higher level there will be severe hypotension due to loss of sympathetic vasomotor tone.

Causes of spinal shock

the spinal cord neurons are under the influence of higher centers. About 10,000 synapses are seen in each anterior horn cell. When a section is made in the spinal cord, there is sudden cessation of excitatory impulses reaching the spinal neurons through the descending pathways. The neuronal excitability is suddenly lowered and the peripheral nerve stimulation is incapable of producing a reflex activity. It takes time for the neuron to regain its excitability and produce a reflex action.

At this stage, the patient needs more care. Bed sores should be prevented, they should be given adequate nutrition and there should be continuous bladder drainage with an indwelling catheter to prevent urinary infection. Large doses of glucocorticoids if given soon after injury is of great benefit to foster recovery and minimize loss of function after spinal cord injury. Glucocorticoids reduce the inflammatory response in the damaged tissue.

Stage of Reflex Activity

If the management is proper during the stage of spinal shock, the reflexes will return slowly, but there will be *no voluntary control*. Muscle tone gradually returns, first, in the flexor group of muscles. The patient assumes an attitude of flexion. This is called **"paraplegia in flexion."** In about 6 months, extensor tone also returns. This is called **"paraplegia in extension."** Smooth muscle regains its activity and blood pressure becomes normal at rest. Bouts of sweating and blanching of the skin occur. Visceral reflexes also appear. Bladder becomes automatic; there will be reflex urination, but no voluntary control.

The spinal cord neurons become hyper-excitable with no higher control. Muscle tone will be increased and reflexes become exaggerated. Of the tendon reflexes, knee jerk comes back first. All classical features of UMN lesion set in, like spastic paralysis, clonus, positive Babinski sign, etc. **Mass reflex** is present.

Recovery may be satisfactory if the patient is properly treated. Give antibiotics, care for skin and bladder, and give sufficient nutrients and fluids. Proper nursing care is very important to prevent bed sores, urinary tract infection, etc.

Causes for the stage of reflex activity are:
- Denervation hypersensitivity to the mediators released by the remaining spinal excitatory endings (*refer* 'denervation hypersensitivity').
- Sprouting of collaterals from existing neurons, with the formation of additional excitatory endings on interneurons and motor neurons.

Mass reflex

in chronic spinal animals, afferent stimuli irradiate from one reflex center to another, producing a mass reflex. When a minor noxious stimulus is applied to skin, the afferent stimuli may irradiate to autonomic neurons and produce micturition, defecation, sweating, pallor, swinging of blood pressure in addition to the withdrawal response. This mass reflex is used to give paraplegic patients some degree of bladder and bowel control. They are trained to stroke the medial aspect of thigh which causes evacuation of bladder and rectum. In quadriplegic humans, there will be prolonged withdrawal of the stimulated limb and marked flexion-extension patterns in the other three limbs (*refer* 'spinal animal').

Stage of Degeneration

If the management is poor, the patient goes to the stage of degeneration. **Bed sores** appear on the skin over bony prominences as a result of compression of blood vessels due to the weight of the body. Normally, when the skin becomes painful as a result of the ischemia, the person shifts weight subconsciously. However, a person who has lost the pain sensation after spinal cord injury fails to feel the pain and, therefore, fails to shift the body. This results in total breakdown and desquamation of the skin at the areas of pressure. These ulcers get infected mainly due to malnutrition. This lesion is called bed sore.

Tissues including bone breakdown and Ca^{2+} ions are released in large amounts leading to hypercalcemia and hypercalciuria, leading to formation of renal stones. Septicemia and uremia finally lead to death.

Incomplete Section of Spinal Cord

Manifestations below the level of lesion depend on which all tracts are damaged and which tracts are spared.

Hemisection of Spinal Cord (Brown-Sequard Syndrome)

Causes of hemisection of spinal cord include tumors, disc prolapse, blood clots, accidents with fracture-dislocation of vertebral column, etc.

Exactly one-half of spinal cord is damaged. Effects and symptoms are collectively called **Brown-Sequard syndrome**.

Effects can be classified under three headings:
1. Below the level of lesion
2. At the level of lesion
3. Above the level of lesion.

Effects Below the Level of Lesion

Below the level of section initially there will be a stage of **spinal shock** on the same side of lesion. In hemisection, there will be sensory as well as motor loss. All motor functions are blocked on the side of the transection in all segments below the level of the transection. But only some of the modalities of sensation are lost on the transected side, and others are lost on the opposite side.

Sensory Loss

In the same side of lesion

sensations carried through dorsal column like fine touch, tactile localization, tactile discrimination, vibration sense, stereognosis and sense of position and movement are lost on the side of the transection in all dermatomes below the level of the transection. Discrete light touch is impaired on the side of the transection because the principal pathway for the transmission of light touch, i.e., the dorsal column, is transected. This is because the fibers in this column do not cross to the opposite side until they reach the medulla of the brain. Crude touch, which is poorly localized, still persists because of its transmission in the opposite spinothalamic tract.

In the opposite side of lesion

the sensations carried through the lateral and anterior spinothalamic tract, like pain, temperature and crude touch are lost in all dermatomes two to six segments below the level of the transection. Touch is impaired on both sides, but there is no complete loss of touch sensation. There is **dissociated sensory loss**, i.e., some sensations are affected on one side and some others on the opposite side and hence called **dissociated anesthesia (Fig. 85.1)**.

Motor Loss

Lateral and anterior corticospinal tract are damaged and **upper motor neuron (UMN) type** of paralysis is seen. 80% of motor loss is on the same side because 80% of pyramidal fibers cross at the medullary level. 20% of motor loss will be on the opposite side. Muscles become hypertonic, tendon reflexes will be exaggerated and there will be rigidity on the affected side. Vasomotor reflexes are lost on the same side.

Effects at the Level of Lesion

Anterior horn cells and posterior horn cells are damaged in that half of spinal cord at the level of lesion. There will be segmental motor loss of **lower motor neuron (LMN) type** (hypotonia and loss of reflexes) and loss of all sensations at the level of lesion. Vasomotor paralysis of same side is seen.

Effects Just Above the Level of Lesion

There will be a layer of cutaneous **hyperesthesia** (intensified sensations) due to hyperirritability of neurons just above the sectioned spinal cord segment.

COMPLICATIONS OF SPINAL CORD TRANSECTION

- All immobilized patients develop a **negative nitrogen balance** and catabolize large amounts of body protein.
- The weight of the body compresses on the circulation to the skin over bony prominences, so that unless the

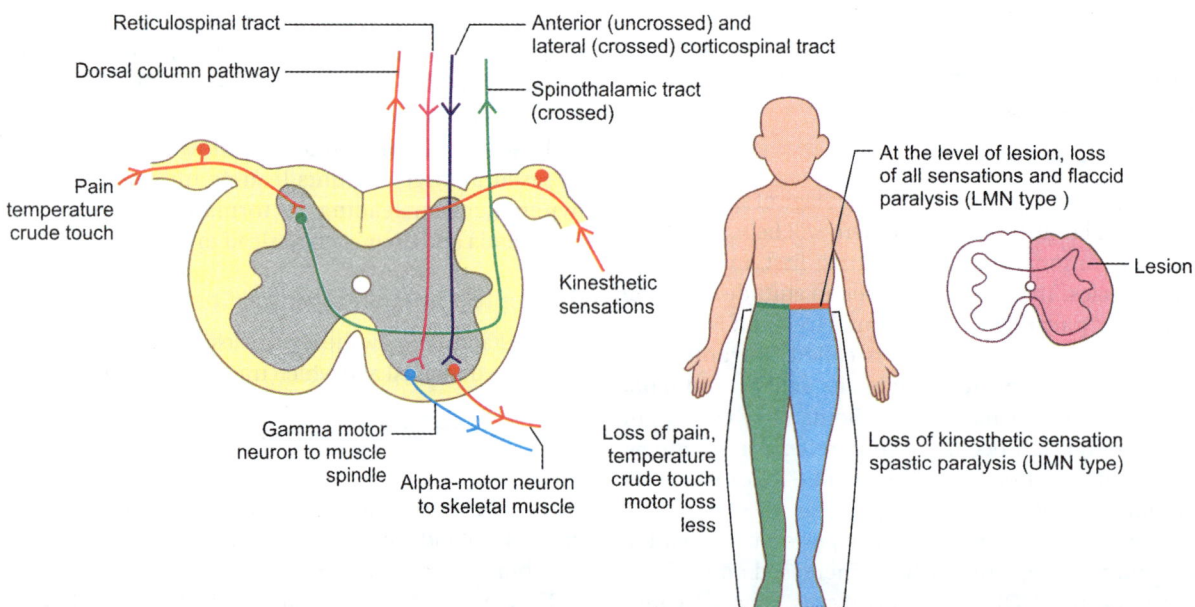

Fig. 85.1: Effects of hemisection of spinal cord (Brown-Sequard syndrome).

patient is moved frequently the skin breaks down at these points and **decubitus ulcers** form. These ulcers heal poorly and are prone to infection because of body protein depletion.
- The tissues that are broken down include the protein matrix of bone leading to hypercalcemia and hypercalciuria, and formation of calcium stones in the urinary tract.
- The stones and stasis of urine due to bladder paralysis predisposes to urinary tract infection which is the most common complication of spinal cord injury.

Management
- Two recent treatments that foster recovery and minimize loss of function after spinal cord injury are administration of large doses of glucocorticoids soon after injury (to minimize loss of function) and ganglioside GM-1. Glucocorticoids reduce the inflammatory response in the damaged tissue.
- If the spinal cord section is incomplete, the flexor spasms initiated by noxious stimuli can be associated with bursts of pain that are particularly bothersome. They can be treated with baclofen, a $GABA_B$ receptor agonist that crosses the blood-brain barrier and facilitates inhibition of pain.
- Administration of neurotrophins is of some benefit.
- Implantation of embryonic stem cells at the site of injury is under trial.
- The most important aspect of treatment is giving the patient proper nursing care.

SECTION OF POSTERIOR NERVE ROOT IN SPINAL CORD
- Segmental loss of all sensations
- Segmental loss of reflexes
- Hypotonia
- Incoordinated voluntary activity. There will be sensory ataxia but no paralysis.

SECTION OF ANTERIOR NERVE ROOT
Features are same as that in poliomyelitis where anterior horn cell is affected.
- Segmental loss of motor activity
- Loss of reflexes
- Hypotonia
- No sensory loss.

SECTION OF PERIPHERAL NERVE
If damage occurs to a peripheral nerve which contains both sensory and motor fibers, there will be motor and sensory loss.
- Complete segmental loss of all sensations
- Loss of reflexes
- Loss of muscle tone in areas supplied by the nerve
- Loss of voluntary activity, motor paralysis is of the LMN type.

DISEASES AFFECTING SPINAL CORD

Syringomyelia
Syringomyelia (syrinx means cavity) is a disease that affects the gray matter of spinal cord. It is due to proliferation of neuroglial cells and the proliferated tissue undergoes degeneration and cavities are formed around the central canal filled with gelatinous material. The crossing fibers are mainly affected. There will be unilateral or bilateral segmental loss of pain and temperature. Only crude touch is affected. This is known as **dissociated sensory loss**. If cavity formation extends to the anterior horn then there will be segmental motor loss of LMN type.

Tabes Dorsalis or Neurosyphilis
Neurosyphilis is a late stage of syphilis. Tabes means atrophy and dorsalis means dorsal column. It specifically affects the posterior nerve root. The lesion may extend to the spinal cord, and the dorsal column and spinocerebellar tract will be affected.
- In the early stages, there will be irritability and hyper-excitability of the neurons of the affected segments and the patient complains of shooting or lightning pain in the limbs. It is due to stimulation of pain fibers which are hyper-excitable. Later, when degeneration is complete all sensations carried through posterior root will be lost.
- All reflexes in the affected segment are lost.
- Muscle tone is lost.
- Movements are clumsy and incoordinated, i.e., there will be ataxia which is referred to as **sensory ataxia.** Sense of position and passive movement are lost and **Romberg's test** will be positive. There will be loss of vibration sense. Gait is referred to as **stamping gait**.
- Since the patient does not feel pain, trophic perforating ulcers occur.
- Painless degeneration of joints due to repeated trauma is referred to as **Charcot joints**.
- Atonic bladder or tabetic bladder is seen
- In neurosyphilis, the pretectal region in the brain is affected and a peculiar pupillary reaction is seen called **Argyll Robertson pupil (ARP)**. Here, pupillary reflex is absent but accommodation reflex is present.

Sensory Ataxia
Sensory ataxia is a form of ataxia (loss of coordination of movement) caused by loss of sensory input for controlling movements. It is not caused by cerebellar lesion. It is seen in patients with significant proprioceptive loss. The gait is referred to as **stamping gait**. The foot strikes the ground hard with each step. Romberg's sign will be positive, i.e., there will be normal coordination when the movement occurs with eyes open but there will be marked incoordination when the eyes are closed. The patients usually complain of loss of balance in the dark or after closing their eyes. In tabes

dorsalis, there is syphilitic damage to the dorsal columns of spinal cord which carries the conscious proprioceptive sense. When a patient with tabes dorsalis stands and closes his eyes, he immediately begins to move from side to side and finally falls to the ground if not supported. This is **positive Romberg's sign.** Sensory ataxia is also seen in vitamin B_{12} deficiency, peripheral neuropathy, multiple sclerosis, etc.

Sub-acute Combined Degeneration of Spinal Cord

This condition is seen in **pernicious anemia** due to deficiency of vitamin B_{12}. White matter of spinal cord is affected, especially the posterior column and spinocerebellar pathway.

Initially, there is atonia but at a later stage there will be hypertonia. All posterior column sensations are affected. Usually, the condition is associated with peripheral neuropathy. Burning, pricking and tickling sensations are present referred to as **paresthesia**. Treatment is parenteral administration of vitamin B_{12}.

Poliomyelitis

Poliomyelitis is an acute viral infection affecting anterior gray column of spinal cord and motor nuclei of cranial nerves. There will be paralysis and wasting of muscles supplied by the affected segments.

■ MULTIPLE CHOICE QUESTIONS

1. **Lesion in the following area leads to sensory ataxia:**
    a. Posterior column
    b. Vermis
    c. Flocculonodular lobe
    d. Vestibular apparatus

2. **A patient with tabes dorsalis will exhibit:**
    a. Some loss of pain sensation from face
    b. Diminished vibration sensibility
    c. Hypertonia of limb muscles
    d. Positive Babinski sign

3. **Brown-Sequard syndrome is seen in:**
    a. Complete section of spinal cord
    b. Lesion of thalamus
    c. Mid-collicular section
    d. Hemisection of spinal cord

4. **In hemisection of spinal cord the findings on the opposite side of the body below the level of lesion include all the following, *except*:**
    a. Analgesia
    b. Thermoanesthesia
    c. Loss of crude touch sensation
    d. Astereognosis

5. **If a single spinal nerve is cut, the area of tactile loss is always greater than the area of loss of pain sensation because:**
    a. Tactile information is carried by myelinated fast conducting fibers
    b. Tactile receptors adapt quickly
    c. Degree of overlap of fibers carrying tactile sensation is much less
    d. In the primary sensory cortex tactile sensation is represented on a larger area

6. **Modality that is lost in the ipsilateral side in Brown-Sequard syndrome is:**
    a. Pain
    b. Temperature
    c. Crude touch
    d. Proprioception

7. **Unlikely to be involved in lesion of anterior spinal artery is:**
    a. Pain and temperature
    b. Vibration and proprioception
    c. Pyramidal tract
    d. Sphincters

8. **Amyotrophic lateral sclerosis involves:**
    a. Both upper motor neurons and lower motor neurons
    b. Posterior column only
    c. Lower motor neuron only
    d. Raphe nucleus

9. **The first reflex response to appear as spinal shock wears off in humans is:**
    a. Tympanic reflex
    b. Withdrawal reflex
    c. Neck righting reflex
    d. Labyrinthine reflex

10. **A lesion of ventrolateral part of spinal cord will lead to loss (below the level of lesion) of:**
    a. Pain sensation on the ipsilateral side
    b. Proprioception on the contralateral side
    c. Pain sensation on the contralateral side
    d. Proprioception on the ipsilateral side

11. **Horner's syndrome may be present in the following condition:**
    a. Syringomyelia
    b. Complete cord transection
    c. Anterior cord syndrome
    d. Brown-Sequard syndrome

12. **Which of the following reflexes disappear in the absence of functional connections between the spinal cord and the brain?**
    a. Swallowing reflex
    b. Withdrawal reflex
    c. Erection of penis
    d. Micturition reflex

ANSWERS

1. a	2. b	3. d	4. d	5. c
6. d	7. b	8. a	9. b	10. c
11. a	12. a			

Basal Ganglia or Basal Nuclei

CHAPTER 86

LEARNING OBJECTIVES
- Describe the connections and functions of basal ganglia
- Explain the pathophysiology of Parkinson's disease
- Discuss the physiological basis of the treatment of Parkinson's disease

INTRODUCTION

PY10.7: Describe and discuss functions of cerebral cortex, basal ganglia, thalamus, hypothalamus, cerebellum and limbic system and their abnormalities.

Basal ganglia or basal nuclei are a group of five large nuclear masses on each side of the brain situated sub-cortically **(Fig. 86.1)** which functions in close association with the cerebral cortex and the corticospinal motor control system.

It is an important organ for extrapyramidal control. It is called so because of its position at the base of the fore brain. The important nuclear masses are:
- Caudate nucleus (tailed nucleus)
- Putamen
- Globus pallidus or pallidium which consists of an **external segment and an internal segment**
- Subthalamic nucleus (Body of Luys) of diencephalon
- Substantia nigra in the midbrain which consists of **pars compacta and pars reticulata**.

The thalamic nuclei associated with basal ganglia are:
- Ventral anterior group
- Ventral lateral group
- Intralaminar nuclei.

FUNCTIONAL ANATOMY

Globus pallidus and putamen are seen in the concavity of the internal capsule on the lateral side. Thalamus and caudate nucleus are situated on the medial side of internal capsule (the space between the caudate nucleus and the putamen through which all motor and sensory nerve fibers connecting the cerebral cortex and the spinal cord pass through is called internal capsule). Globus pallidus and putamen together show the similarity to lens and hence they are referred to as **lenticular or lentiform nucleus**. The internal capsule separates the caudate nucleus from lenticular nucleus. Putamen is the darker lateral portion of the lentiform nucleus and globus pallidus is the inner lighter portion (pallid means pale). Globus pallidus is lighter due to the presence of high concentration of myelinated nerve fibers **(Fig. 86.1)**.

Caudate nucleus is a highly curved comma-shaped band of gray matter seen medial to internal capsule. It is separated from lentiform nucleus by the fibers of internal capsule. It consists of head, body and tail and the head of caudate nucleus is connected to putamen of the lentiform nucleus. Amygdaloid nucleus is connected to the tail of caudate nucleus anteriorly.

The anterior limb of internal capsule lies between the head of caudate nucleus and the putamen. Numerous grey strands extend between the caudate nucleus and putamen passing across the internal capsule. This gives a striated appearance to caudate nucleus and putamen and so, together they are referred to as **striatum**.
- Caudate nucleus and putamen—**striatum** or corpus striatum or neostriatum (phylogenetically newer)
- Putamen and globus pallidus—**lenticular nucleus** or lentiform nucleus

Globus pallidus is the efferent portion and caudate nucleus and putamen (striatum) form the afferent portion of basal ganglia.

Substantia nigra—substantia nigra is a large motor nucleus situated between the tegmentum and the crus cerebri in the midbrain. The nucleus contains multipolar neurons which contain melanin pigment. Substantia nigra (black substance) derives its name from its content of **melanin** pigment, a by-product of dopamine synthesis. It also has a high copper content. Substantia nigra is connected to the cerebral cortex, spinal cord, hypothalamus and basal ganglia. It is connected to reticular formation and is concerned with muscle tone.

The substantia nigra consists of **pars reticularis** in front and **pars compacta** behind. The pars compacta (SNpc) contains mostly dopaminergic neurons. About a quarter of

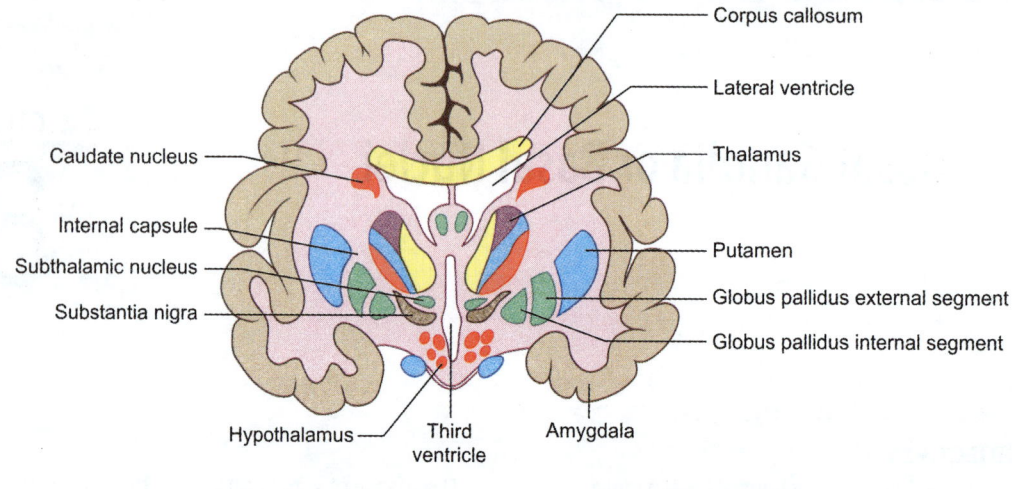

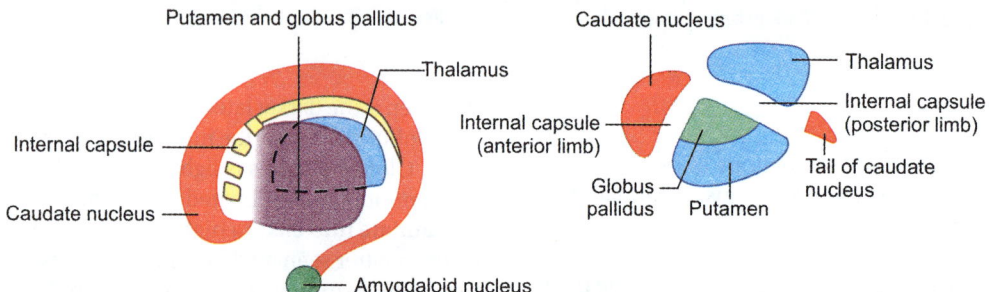

Fig. 86.1: Basal ganglia and surroundings structures.

pars compacta neurons are cholinergic. The pars reticularis (SNpr) contains large multipolar GABAergic neurons.

Subthalamic nucleus is a biconvex mass of gray matter situated lateral to red nucleus and dorsal to substantia nigra in the diencephalon. The neurons of the subthalamic nucleus are glutaminergic and excitatory. They are connected to globus pallidus internal segment (GPi) and substantia nigra pars reticularis (SNpr).

■ CONNECTIONS OF BASAL GANGLIA

The basal ganglia receive most of their input signals from the cerebral cortex and almost all their output signals go to the cerebral cortex itself.

Afferent Connections to Striatum

- From motor and sensory cortex
  - Primary motor area
  - Motor association area
  - Supplementary motor area
  - Suppressor strips of motor cortex
  - Sensory areas of cerebral cortex
- Pars compacta part of substantia nigra (dopaminergic fibers, inhibitory in function)
- Raphe nucleus in reticular formation (serotonergic fibers)
- Locus coeruleus (noradrenergic fibers)
- Intralaminar nuclei of thalamus (thalamostriatal pathway)
- Limbic areas, such as hippocampus and amygdala.

Of these the three major input systems are:
1. Corticostriatal system
2. Nigrostriatal system
3. Thalamostriatal system.

Efferent Connections from Globus Pallidus

All the efferents of basal ganglia are from globus pallidus mainly, and they emerge as a bundle called **ansa lenticularis**. *The neurons of globus pallidus release the inhibitory transmitter, GABA at their endings.* Efferent connections are mainly to:

- Thalamus (ventral anterior, ventrolateral and intralaminar nuclei)
- Reticular formation (caudal inhibitory area)
- Hypothalamus
- Red nucleus
- Subthalamic nucleus and substantia nigra

  The basal ganglia receive no direct input from or output to the spinal cord.

> All efferent projections of basal ganglia are inhibitory in nature except one, i.e., from subthalamic nucleus to internal segment of globus pallidus and pars reticulata.

Basal ganglia function in close association with the cerebral cortex and the corticospinal motor control system. Neurons of putamen and caudate nucleus (striatum) begin to discharge before movements occur. These neurons help to select the movement that is to be made. Most important input to striatum is from motor cortex, layer V, and glutamate is the

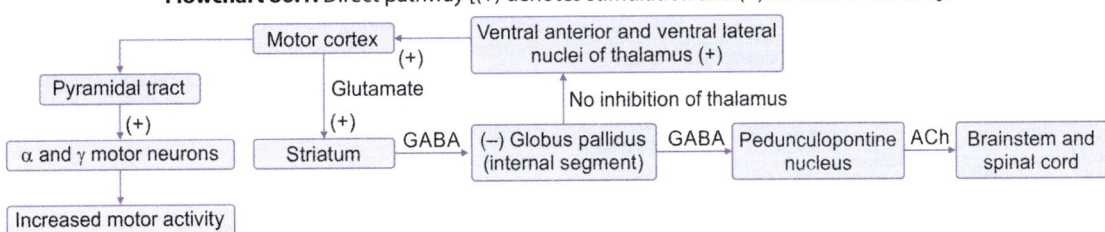

Flowchart 86.1: Direct pathway [(+) denotes stimulation and (−) denotes inhibition].

(ACh: acetylcholine; GABA: gamma-aminobutyric acid; VA: ventral anterior; VL: ventral lateral)

excitatory transmitter. The striatum in turn sends impulses to ventral anterior (VA) and ventrolateral (VL) group of nuclei in the thalamus. The thalamic neurons in turn excite neurons of the motor areas of the cerebral cortex and appropriate motor activity occurs. The striatum influences neurons in the VA and VL nuclei of thalamus by two pathways:
1. Direct pathway
2. Indirect pathway.

Direct Pathway

The direct pathway through basal ganglia to motor areas of cortex is to *enhance motor activity*.

Inhibitory pathways in the direct pathway in which GABA is the neurotransmitter are:
- Striatum → Globus pallidus internal segment (GPIS)
- Striatum → Pars reticulata of substantia nigra (SNpr)
- GPIS and SNpr → Ventral-anterior and ventrolateral nuclei of thalamus

Ventral-anterior and ventrolateral nuclei send excitatory connections to prefrontal, premotor and supplementary motor cortex. This influences motor planning and also influences discharges through corticospinal and corticobulbar pathways.

Neurons in the striatum have little background activity. At the onset of movements or during movements, they are activated by inputs from cortex. Neurons in the globus pallidus internal segment (GPIS) have a high level of background activity at rest. When striatum is stimulated during movement, its inhibitory projections to globus pallidus inhibit the background activity in globus pallidus. Globus pallidus internal segment normally at rest is inhibitory to ventral-anterior and ventrolateral nuclei of thalamus and provides a tonic inhibition of neurons of these nuclei. When GPIS is inhibited, this inhibition on ventral-anterior and ventrolateral nuclei are lost and they become excited, which in turn excites the motor neurons in the prefrontal and premotor areas of cerebral cortex (**Flowchart 86.1**). The excitatory thalamic projections to the motor cortex are mainly cholinergic. *The circuitous connection is known as* **cortico-striato-pallido-thalamo-cortical pathway** (**Fig. 86.2**). Through this pathway, basal ganglia can influence motor activity in the lateral descending system, i.e., fine skillful movements in the distal joints. Disturbances in the lateral control system result in involuntary automatic, purposeless movements at the distal joints, such as pill rolling tremor of fingers.

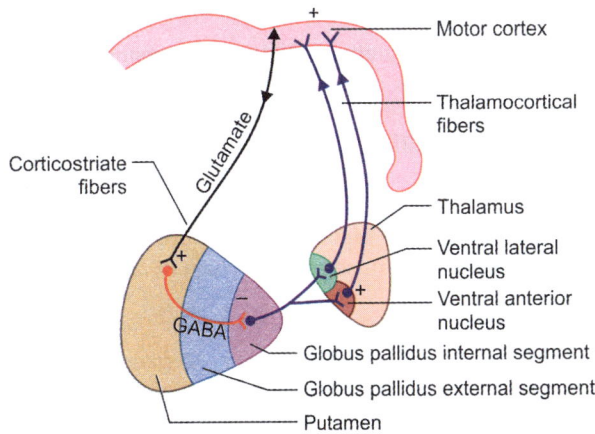

Fig. 86.2: Cortico-striato-pallido-thalamo-cortical circuitous connection of basal ganglia in the direct pathway during activity.

The internal segment of globus pallidus also relays to the pedunculopontine nucleus located in the upper pons where the neurotransmitter released is GABA. Pedunculopontine nucleus projects to the motor neurons in the brain stem and spinal cord. Through these connections, basal ganglia can influence the activity of the medial descending motor system which is concerned with maintenance of tone and posture in the proximal group of muscles. Disturbances in the medial system result in changes in muscle tone like rigidity, changes in posture (flexed posture) and balance.

Motor cortex in turn stimulates α- and γ-motor neurons in the anterior horn of spinal cord and brainstem through the pyramidal tract and evokes appropriate movements. Thus, the basal ganglia can regulate movements by enhancing the activity of neurons in the motor cortex through the direct pathway.

Indirect Pathway

The effect of indirect pathway is reduction in the activity of neurons in the motor areas of cerebral cortex. Inhibitory connections extend from striatum to external segment of globus pallidus (GPES). GPES in turn sends inhibitory projections to the subthalamic nucleus. The subthalamic nucleus in turn sends excitatory projection back to the internal segment of globus pallidus and substantia nigra pars reticulata.

Normally, the subthalamic neurons are active and their activity is increased when the inhibition from GPES is removed. The subthalamic nucleus in turn stimulates the

Flowchart 86.2: Indirect pathway [(+) denotes stimulation and (–) denotes inhibition].

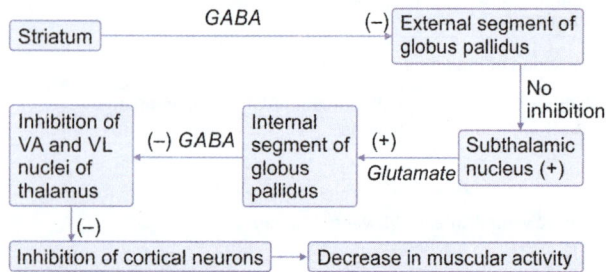

internal segment of globus pallidus by releasing glutamate. This excites neurons of internal segment of globus pallidus and this in turn inhibits ventral-anterior and ventrolateral nuclei of thalamus. The activity of thalamic neurons decreases and their action on cortical neurons is inhibited. This leads to reduction in the stimulatory impulses from cortex to the motor neurons in the brainstem and spinal cord leading to decreased activity of muscles **(Flowchart 86.2)**.

Conclusion

The direct and indirect pathways of basal ganglia thus have opposing actions. Direct pathway has a positive feedback effect and indirect pathway exerts a negative feedback effect on motor activity. Indirect pathway helps to prevent unwanted muscle contractions. Normally, there will be a balance between the two pathways. When there is increase in activity in any one of these pathways, it leads to an imbalance in motor control. This is due to alteration in the motor output from the cortex.

Thus the basal ganglia modify the timing and amount of activity from the cortex through the pyramidal pathway to the muscles involved in that activity. It amplify the activity that leads to a positive outcome and simultaneously suppress activity that leads to a deleterious outcome in a particular situation through the direct and the indirect pathway.

Effect of Substantia Nigra on Corpus Striatum

Dopamine is the neurotransmitter in the neurons of the pars compacta of substantia nigra (SNpc). In the nigrostriatal pathway, dopamine has an excitatory action on direct pathway and inhibitory action on indirect pathway **(Flowchart 86.3)**. Striatum contains interneurons that release acetylcholine at their endings. ACh stimulates neurons in the striatum that project to globus pallidus and substantia nigra. Striatum also contains two populations of medium sized spiny projection neurons which release GABA as the neurotransmitter. 50% of these neurons express neuropeptides substance P and dynorphin and express D_1 receptor subtype. These neurons project to globus pallidus internal segment and substantia nigra pars reticulata. They are responsible for direct striatal output pathway.

Other 50% spiny neurons express neuropeptide encephalin and have D_2 receptor subtype. They project to globus pallidus external segment. Dopamine receptors in these interneurons of the striatum are of two types, D_1 receptors

Flowchart 86.3: Mechanism by which dopamine stimulates direct pathway and inhibits indirect pathway in basal ganglia. (Red arrow indicates direct pathway and blue arrows indicate indirect pathway. Note that dopamine acting through D_2 receptor inhibits the striatum thereby inhibiting the indirect pathway. Glutamate is the excitatory transmitter and GABA is the inhibitory transmitter. Dashed arrows denote inhibition).

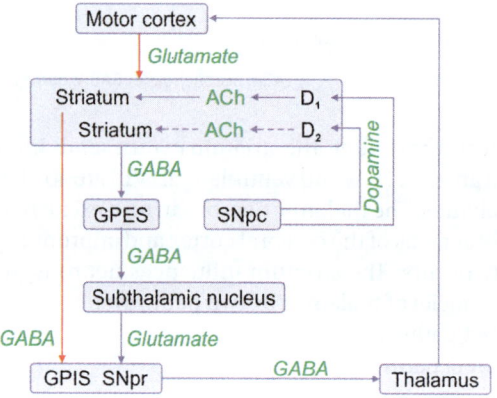

(GPES: globus pallidus external segment; GPIS: globus pallidus internal segment; SNpc: substantia nigra pars compacta; SNpr: substantia nigra pars reticulata; ACh: acetylcholine; GABA: gamma-aminobutyric acid; D: dopamine receptor)

which are excitatory and D_2 receptors which are inhibitory. The striatal neurons projecting to the direct pathway contain D_1 receptors and striatal neurons projecting to the indirect pathway contain D_2 receptors. The overall effect of dopamine is reduction in thalamocortical inhibition and facilitation of activity in the motor cortex, i.e., facilitation of movements. So, a loss of dopaminergic neurons leads to bradykinesia or decreased movements as that found in Parkinson's disease.

When D_1 receptors are stimulated, there is increased release of ACh in the striatum which in turn stimulate the direct pathway. In the direct pathway, striatal neurons (GABAergic) project to GPIS and SNpr and inhibit them. Since these areas are inhibited, there is no inhibition of thalamic neurons and there will be increased motor activity. More over there should be a balance in the ratio of acetylcholine and dopamine in the striatum. Alteration in this ratio results in abnormalities in motor activities.

Stimulation of D_2 receptors inhibits the indirect pathway by inhibiting the striatal neurons projecting to globus pallidus external segment. So there is no inhibition of GPES which releases GABA at its ending on subthalamic nucleus. There is inhibition of subthalamic nucleus which when active stimulates GPIS and SNpr. Since there is no stimulation of GPIS and SNpr, there is no inhibition of thalamic neurons and there will be increased motor activity.

Connections between Parts of Basal Ganglia

The connections between parts of basal ganglia include:
* Dopaminergic nigrostriatal projection from pars compacta of substantia nigra to the striatum and GABAergic projection from striatum to pars reticulata of substantia nigra.

Pars compacta →(Dopamine)→ Striatum →(GABA)→ Pars reticulata

Flowchart 86.4: Connections of basal ganglia showing the neurotransmitters involved. (Dashed lines indicate inhibitory pathways).

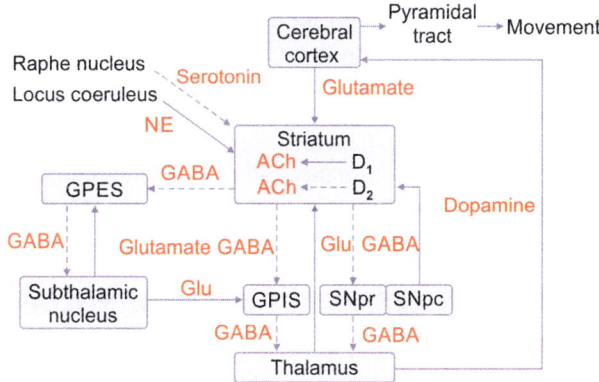

(Glu: glutamate; GPES : globus pallidus external segment; GPIS: globus pallidus internal segment; SNpc: substantia nigra pars compacta; SNpr: substantia nigra pars reticulata; ACh: acetylcholine; NE: norepinephrine; D: dopamine receptor)

❖ The striatum projects to both segments of globus pallidus. The external segment of globus pallidus projects to subthalamic nucleus, which in turn projects to both segments of globus pallidus and substantia nigra.

Neurotransmitters Involved in the Connections of Basal Ganglia (Flowchart 86.4)

❖ The neurons of substantia nigra pars compacta are **dopaminergic**.
❖ The neurons of the subthalamic nuclei are **glutaminergic** and excitatory in function.
❖ **Glutamate** is the neurotransmitter of the corticostriate fibers.
❖ Ascending fibers from the brainstem which end in the corpus striatum liberate **serotonin** at their endings. They are inhibitory in function.
❖ Striatopallidal fibers release **GABA** at their endings as neurotransmitter.
❖ Fibers from corpus striatum to substantia nigra (striatonigral fibers) release **GABA or acetylcholine or substance P** at their endings.
❖ **Acetylcholine** is the neurotransmitter in the intrastriatal interneurons which contain dopamine receptors.

■ PUTAMEN CIRCUIT AND THE CAUDATE CIRCUIT

Based on motor control and cognitive functions of basal ganglia, the connections are divided into two major circuits, i.e., the putamen circuit and the caudate circuit.

The Putamen Circuit

One important function of basal ganglia is to control complex patterns of motor activity like writing, throwing a basketball, other skilled movements which are performed subconsciously. This circuit is important for executing learned patterns of movement. This circuit does not involve the caudate nucleus. Fibers from the premotor, supplementary motor area and from the somatosensory areas of the sensory cortex reach the putamen. From the putamen fibers reach the internal segment of globus pallidus and from there to the ventroanterior and ventrolateral nuclei of the thalamus. From the thalamus fibers return to the primary motor cortex and the supplementary and premotor areas which are closely associated with the primary motor cortex **(Flowchart 86.5)**.

Flowchart 86.5: Putamen circuit for subconscious execution of learned patterns of movement.

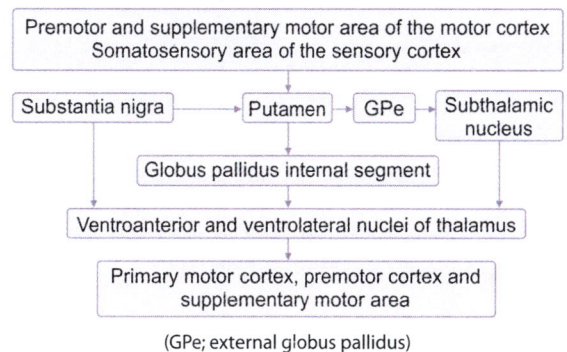

(GPe; external globus pallidus)

Fibers also pass from the putamen to the external segment of globus pallidus and from there to the subthalamic nucleus. Fibers from the subthalamic nucleus pass through the substantia nigra and finally return to the motor cortex via the thalamus.

Abnormal function of putamen circuit leads to athetosis, hemiballism and chorea. Lesions in the substantia nigra lead to Parkinson disease.

The Caudate Circuit

The caudate circuit is involved in the cognitive control of motor activity. Cognition means thinking processes of the brain using sensory information reaching the brain and information already stored in memory. One can respond quickly and appropriately without thinking for too long only by the cognitive control of motor activity which occurs subconsciously.

The caudate nucleus is connected to all lobes of the cerebrum, i.e., the frontal lobes, parietal lobes, occipital lobes and the temporal lobes. Caudate nucleus also receives large amounts of inputs from the association areas of the cerebral cortex which are concerned with the integration of different types of sensory and motor information into thought patterns.

In the caudate circuit, information from the cerebral cortex reaches the caudate nucleus and from there it is transmitted to the globus pallidus internal segment. From there to the ventroanterior and ventrolateral nuclei of thalamus and back to the prefrontal, premotor and supplementary motor areas of the cerebral cortex **(Flowchart 86.6)**. In contrary to the putamen circuit, in the caudate circuit none of the signals pass directly to the primary motor cortex. Here instead of exciting individual muscle movements, sequential patterns of movement are put together to achieve a complex specific conscious goal.

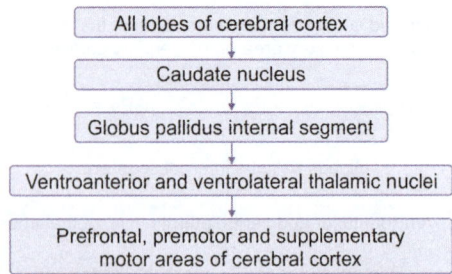

Flowchart 86.6: Caudate circuit for the cognitive planning of complex motor goals.

FUNCTIONS OF BASAL GANGLIA

Studies have proved that neurons in the basal ganglia discharge even before movements begin. It functions in close association with the corticospinal system in controlling subconsciously performed complex, skilled motor activities, such as writing, vocalization, cutting paper with scissors, etc.

- **Maintenance of muscle tone:** Basal ganglia is **inhibitory** to muscle tone. It causes suppression of stretch reflex. Inhibitory influence on muscle tone is by stimulating the caudal inhibitory area of reticular formation or by suppressing the bulboreticular facilitatory area. In lesions of basal ganglia, muscle rigidity due to increased muscle tone is a feature.
- **Role in voluntary and associated involuntary muscular activity:** During activity, basal ganglia influence posture and background tone. Apart from voluntary activity, basal ganglia also control all other associated unconscious activities, such as swinging of hands while walking, emotional facial expressions, etc. In lesions of basal ganglia, movements will be statue-like and face will be expressionless, i.e., mask-like face.
- **Planning, programming and initiation of voluntary activity:** It is seen experimentally that there is firing of impulses even before starting activity and also throughout slow activity from the basal ganglia. In basal ganglia, "abstract thought is converted to voluntary activity," i.e., an idea of voluntary movement is converted into the precise action. Thus, it plays an important role in planning actions that are required to achieve a particular goal e.g., using hands to catch a ball. It is also important in executing well-practiced actions and in learning new actions in novel situations.
- Oscillations and after discharges in the motor system are prevented by basal ganglia so that, movements occur in a smooth and appropriate manner. This is mainly coordinated by the to and fro connections between globus pallidus and subthalamic nucleus. Subthalamic nucleus stimulates globus pallidus and globus pallidus in turn inhibits subthalamic nucleus. This circuit plays an important role in maintaining movements appropriately.
- **Role of basal ganglia in cognitive process:** Cognition is a psychological term which involves the processes of thinking and perceiving, such as memory, attention, planning, etc. This is due to the connections of caudate nucleus with the prefrontal portions of neocortex. A lesion of the left caudate nucleus (dominant side) is associated with a dysarthric form of aphasia, which is different from Wernicke's aphasia. There is difficulty in articulating words and the patient cannot communicate in words what he wishes to say.
- All prefrontal cortical areas are under the influence of basal ganglia and so it is concerned with motor, cognitive, executive and emotional-motivational functions. Basal ganglia functions in close association with the limbic system in regulating emotional behavior.

EFFECTS OF LESIONS OF BASAL GANGLIA

Lesions of basal ganglia are most commonly associated with hyperkinetic and hypokinetic movement disorders. The movements in basal ganglia lesions are of two kinds, **hyperkinetic and hypokinetic**. *Hypokinetic movements are akinesia and bradykinesia. Others are hyperkinetic movements.*

1. **Abnormal hyperkinetic movements or dyskinesia**
   Abnormal movements are characterized by:
   - **Resting tremor** as in the case of pill-rolling tremor in the limbs.
   - **Athetosis**, which is continuous, slow, writhing (turning and twisting as if in pain, but here there is no pain) movements of distal parts of limbs. Groups of muscles are affected. This is due to a lesion affecting lenticular nucleus. The slow movement may sometimes be associated with jerky movement in between and is known as **choreoathetosis**.
   - **Chorea:** Rapid, involuntary, dancing or jerky type of movements of extremities and facial muscles (facial grimacing). This is usually associated with degenerative changes of caudate nucleus. (**Sydenham's chorea** is associated with rheumatic fever.)
   - **Ballism** is violent, flailing (ballistic), involuntary movements of limbs involving large groups of muscles. The whole limb may be affected and may be thrown into extension or sometimes the whole body may go into extension. This condition is due to damage to the subthalamic nucleus. If only one side is affected it is called **hemiballism.**
   - **Dystonia** is slow truncal movement that distorts body positions.
2. **Akinesia** is difficulty in initiating movement and inhibition of spontaneous movement.
3. Increased muscle tone or cogwheel **rigidity**.
4. **Bradykinesia** is slowness of voluntary movements.
5. Disorders of mood, cognition and non-motor behavior

PARKINSON'S DISEASE OR PARALYSIS AGITANS

Parkinson's disease or paralysis agitans (shaking palsy) was described by James Parkinson in 1817. It is due to degenerative change affecting the corpus striatum or substantia nigra or it

may be due to a reduction in the dopamine content. Other causes include:
a. Arteriosclerosis (in elderly hypertensive patients)
b. Post-encephalitic Parkinsonism
c. Wilson's disease
d. Idiopathic—without any known cause
e. Drug-induced (iatrogenic)—reserpine, chlorpromazine, and drugs that block the D_2 receptors, such as metoclopramide, droperidol etc.

The main cause is loss of neurons in the pars compacta of substantia nigra and the nigrostriatal pathway is affected. With aging there is loss of dopaminergic neurons and dopamine receptors. Symptoms appear when 60–80% of these neurons are lost. The striatum especially putamen suffers from severe loss of dopamine. Neurons of locus coeruleus, raphe nuclei and other mono-aminergic nuclei are also destroyed. Decrease in dopamine decreases the activity in direct pathway and increases the activity in indirect pathway. Net effect is increase in the activity of neurons in the subthalamic nucleus and globus pallidus. This leads to inhibition of ventral-anterior and ventrolateral nuclei of thalamus and decreased activation of motor cortical areas leading to bradykinesia.

In Parkinson's disease, there is no loss of muscle power and no loss of sensibility. Superficial reflexes and deep tendon reflexes are normal. But in advanced cases, tendon jerks become progressively more difficult to elicit as the rigidity increases.

Manifestations

Manifestations may be due to decrease in dopamine content or due to acetylcholine excess. Two types of manifestations are:
1. Hyperkinetic manifestations, such as rigidity and tremor.
2. Hypokinetic manifestations as evidenced by poverty of movement.

Hyperkinetic Manifestations

Rigidity
Rigidity is increase in muscle tone, which may be localized or generalized. Muscle tone is increased both in extensors and flexors (protagonists and antagonists), and rigidity is felt throughout passive movement and is referred to as **leadpipe rigidity or plastic rigidity** (since resistance is uniform). If rigidity is intermittent then it is called **cogwheel rigidity**. Tremor is absent in lead-pipe rigidity, whereas in cogwheel rigidity tremor is present.

Usually large proximal group of muscles of the limbs are affected. Rigidity is due to increased discharge of gamma efferents supplying the muscle spindle. There is also an imbalance between the activity of the inhibitory dopaminergic neurons and excitatory cholinergic neurons in the striatum. Lack of dopamine shifts the balance towards the excitatory cholinergic fibers. This leads to the hyperkinetic features of the disease. If anticholinergic agents like atropine are given to the patient, there will be a reduction in the hyperkinetic movements like tremor.

Tremor
Tremors are regular, rhythmic involuntary movements that result from the alternate contraction of opposing muscle groups, i.e., agonist and antagonist. Tremor may be **slow** in Parkinson's disease. Tremor may affect head or limbs. To start with, it occurs in the fingers and then spreads to the entire limb. A characteristic feature of Parkinson's disease is that the tremor is seen only when the patient is at rest, i.e., *resting tremor or static tremor*. It is due to regular, alternating 8-Hz contractions of antagonistic muscles. The tremor disappears when the patient is sleeping, during activity, etc. But it is increased in emotional states, excitement and anxiety. In well-established cases, thumb is seen moving over the first two fingers and is called **pillrolling tremor**. Alternate flexion and extension or alternate supination and pronation are also seen.

Hypokinetic Manifestations (Akinesia and Bradykinesia)

Hypokinetic manifestation seen in Parkinson's disease is poverty of movement or **bradykinesia**. There will be difficulty in initiating any movement and there is also slowness of movement. The patient cannot stand up from the sitting posture with ease. If the initial difficulty is overcome, then the patient moves in short, quick steps, bending forwards as if trying to catch up his center of gravity or preventing himself from falling. This gait is referred to as **shuffling gait or festinant type gait**. When a walking patient is suddenly pulled backwards, he begins to walk backwards and is unable to stop which is referred to as **retropulsion**. Associated involuntary movements during walking, such as swinging of the hands are not seen and it is referred to as **statuelike posture**. Facial expression is emotionless which is referred to as **masklike facies (Fig. 86.3)**.

In later stages, muscles of speech, swallowing, etc., will be affected leading to dysarthria and dysphagia. Other manifestations include depression, sleep disorders, loss of smell, autonomic dysfunctions, etc.

Treatment of Parkinson's Disease

L-Dopa is the drug of choice in Parkinson's disease. If dopamine is given to treat Parkinson's disease, it does not cross the blood-brain barrier. **LDopa** can cross the blood-brain barrier and it is converted to dopamine in the brain. Along with L-dopa, **carbidopa** is used to treat Parkinson's disease. Carbidopa prevents conversion of L-dopa into dopamine in the liver and thus prevents the side effects that can occur due to excessive dopamine content in the liver. Carbidopa cannot cross the blood-brain-barrier and so in the brain, L-dopa is readily converted into dopamine.

Normally, there is a delicate balance between the dopaminergic system and the cholinergic system in the striatum. When the dopaminergic system becomes weaker the excitatory effect of the cholinergic system takes the upper hand and produce hyperkinetic features like tremor.

So, **anticholinergic** drugs, such as atropine can be given to reduce tremor.

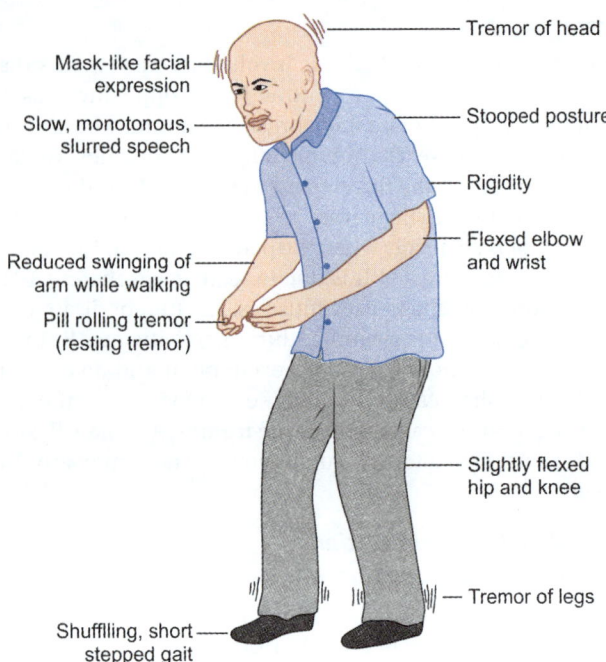

Fig. 86.3: Parkinson's disease.
Courtesy: Dr Rageeth.

Selegiline is a drug that inhibits monoamine oxidase (MAO), which destroys dopamine. It also slows the process of degeneration of the DOPA-secreting neurons of substantia nigra.

Works are going on for the transplantation of dopamine-synthesizing neurons into striatum. **Transplantation** of human embryonic dopamine-secreting neurons or stem cells into the caudate nucleus and putamen improve motor functions in the patient. Auto-transplantation of the suprarenal medullary cells is also done.

Surgical lesions of globus pallidus alleviate parkinsonian signs. The procedure is called **pallidotomy**. **Deep brain stimulation** is also of benefit in alleviating symptoms. It improves the quality of life, improves gait, and reduces tremor, stiffness, bradykinesia and dyskinesia. The procedure also helps to reduce medications.

Deep Brain Stimulation (DBS)

Deep brain stimulation is a neurosurgical procedure involving the placement of a medical device called neurostimulator which sends electrical impulses through implanted electrodes to specific targets in the brain. In 1987, French neurosurgeon Alim Benabid introduced DBS for Parkinson's disease. DBS is currently indicated in movement disorders, such as idiopathic Parkinson's disease, essential tremor, primary dystonia, obsessive-compulsive disorder, etc.

Mechanism

Several theories have been proposed
1. **Inhibition theory:**
   - Electrical stimulation of the target neuron inhibits its activity thereby decreasing neural output.
   - Depolarization block through K$^+$ mediated inactivation of Na$^+$ channels.
   - Pre-synaptic inhibition of excitatory afferents
   - Hyperpolarization of neuronal bodies and dendrites
   - Glutamate reduction with coincident increase of inhibitory neurotransmitter, such as GABA
2. **Activation theory:**
   Some studies observed
   - Increase in excitatory neurotransmitter and dopamine
   - Increase in blood flow
   - Stimulation of neurogenesis
   - Increase in reactive astrocytes
3. **Simultaneous excitatory and inhibitory theory of DBS mechanism:**
   - Inhibition of cell body and excitation in the axon
   - Decoupling causes change in the network activity and overall positive benefits.

Procedure

A detailed brain imaging is done with computed tomography (CT) or magnetic resonance imaging (MRI). General anesthesia is not preferred. A small burr hole is created in the skull for the insertion of microelectrodes and DBS lead is inserted. Burr hole is fitted with a capping device. Fluoroscopy can be used to monitor DBS lead migration, once it has been placed. Therapeutic stimulation can be done to assess response in tremor, rigidity, etc. and also to assess the minimal thresholds that evoke side effects. An extension cable is attached to the lead and it is tunneled under the skin of scalp and neck and placed in the anterior chest wall where subcutaneous pocket is created for insertion of impulse generator or neurostimulator that delivers the current. Neurostimulator is a titanium unit containing the electronics and power supply of the DBS system. Appropriate stimulation parameters like voltage, pulse width, frequency, polarity, etc., should be selected to provide the patient with maximum therapeutic benefit and minimum side effects.

HUNTINGTON'S DISEASE

Destruction of neurons in caudate nucleus and putamen (striatum) leads to Huntington's disease. It is an **autosomal dominant** inherited disease and is due to a single gene defect on **chromosome 4**. The protein encoded by the gene is **huntingtin** whose function is unknown. Movements become disorganized. Hyperkinetic choreiform movements are seen. Speech becomes slurred and progressive dementia is followed by death after 10–15 years of onset of symptoms. In basal ganglia, three pathways operate in a balanced manner, which are:
1. Nigrostriatal dopaminergic system
2. Intrastriatal cholinergic system
3. GABAergic system from striatum to globus pallidus and substantia nigra

In Huntington's disease, there is degeneration of GABA-ergic neurons of striatum that project to the external segment of globus pallidus. The loss of inhibitory impulses to external segment of globus pallidus releases inhibition on thalamus leading to the hyperkinetic features in the disease (Degeneration of dopaminergic system causes Parkinson's disease).

HEMIBALLISM OR HEMIBALLISMUS

Smooth movements of different parts of the body are integrated mainly in the subthalamic nucleus. Lesion of the subthalamic nucleus of one side leads to hemiballism on the opposite limb. Damage to the subthalamic nucleus reduces inhibitory output from globus pallidus internal segment (GPIS) and substantia nigra pars reticulata (SNpr) to thalamus. This leads to increased thalamic output to cortex resulting in hyperkinetic movements like involuntary violent movements of the proximal limbs. Pallidotomy relieves the symptoms mediated by the corticospinal tract.

WILSON'S DISEASE OR PROGRESSIVE HEPATOLENTICULAR DEGENERATION

Wilson's disease is a disorder of **copper metabolism** where there is reduction in copper-binding protein **ceruloplasmin**. This leads to accumulation of copper in the basal ganglia leading to manifestations similar to Parkinson's disease. It is also associated with degeneration of liver, greenish pigmentation of cornea, etc. It is treated with chelating agents, such as **penicillamine**, which remove copper.

KERNICTERUS

Kernicterus is a condition seen in hemolytic disease of newborn due to Rh incompatibility between mother and fetus. There is increase in unconjugated bilirubin in blood, which crosses the blood-brain barrier of the fetus. *Kernicterus occurs when serum bilirubin level is more than 18 mg%.* Bilirubin destroys the globus pallidus. Usually, the baby does not survive. If the child survives, there may be rigidity, chorea, athetosis and mental retardation.

MULTIPLE CHOICE QUESTIONS

1. Hyperkinetic syndromes, such as chorea and athetosis are usually associated with pathological change in:
   a. Motor areas of cerebral cortex
   b. Anterior hypothalamus
   c. Pathways for recurrent collateral inhibition in the spinal cord
   d. Basal ganglia complex

2. Neurotransmitter in nigrostriatal pathway is:
   a. Dopamine   b. GABA
   c. Acetyl choline d. Norepinephrine

3. In Parkinsonism, tremor is:
   a. 6-8/sec   b. 2/sec
   c. 2-4/sec   d. Uncountable

4. Parkinson's disease is characterized by:
   a. Paralysis of one-half of the body
   b. Tremor which becomes worse when a skilled movement is being carried out than at rest
   c. An increase in muscle tone which is maintained throughout
   d. Motor aphasia

5. Nucleus of basal ganglia include:
   a. Dentate nucleus   b. Caudate nucleus
   c. Red nucleus   d. Nucleus globosus

6. The efferent fibers from substantia nigra transmits dopamine to the following areas:
   a. Thalamus
   b. Corpus striatum
   c. Tegmentum of pons
   d. Tectum of midbrain

7. Functions of basal ganglia include:
   a. Skilled movements
   b. Emotions
   c. Maintenance of equilibrium
   d. Gross motor

8. Which of the following act as the major neurotransmitter in substantia nigra?
   a. Dopamine   b. Adrenaline
   c. Acetylcholine d. Serotonin

9. Which of the following clearly states the role of basal ganglia in motor function?
   a. Planning   b. Skilled function
   c. Coordinate function d. Coarse movements

10. Abnormal slowness of movement is called:
    a. Akinesia   b. Bradykinesia
    c. Ballism   d. Athetosis

11. The nigrostriatal system is:
    a. Adrenergic   b. Dopaminergic
    c. Cholinergic d. Serotonergic

12. The following are hyperkinetic conditions, *except*:
    a. Chorea   b. Athetosis
    c. Akinesia   d. Ballism

13. Kernicterus in newborn damages the:
    a. Globus pallidus
    b. Substantia nigra
    c. Subthalamic nucleus
    d. Caudate nucleus

14. In Huntington's disease, extensive degeneration is seen in:
    a. Caudate nucleus and putamen
    b. Globus pallidus
    c. Substantia nigra
    d. Thalamus

15. Lesion of the caudate nucleus produces:
    a. Athetosis   b. Chorea
    c. Hemiballism   d. All of the above

16. **Gait in Parkinsonism is referred to as:**
    a. Ataxic gait
    b. Festinant gait
    c. High stepping gait
    d. Dancing gait

17. **Static tremor or resting tremor is seen in lesion of:**
    a. Medulla
    b. Thalamus
    c. Cerebellum
    d. Basal ganglia

18. **The hyperkinetic features of Huntington's disease are due to the loss of:**
    a. Nigrostriatal dopaminergic system
    b. Intrastriatal cholinergic system
    c. GABAergic and cholinergic system
    d. Intrastriatal GABAergic system

19. **The primary function of basal ganglia is:**
    a. Neuroendocrine control
    b. Planning movements
    c. Short-term memory
    d. Sensory integration

20. **Hypotonia is seen in all the following conditions, *except*:**
    a. Cerebellar lesion
    b. Spinal shock
    c. Myopathies
    d. Parkinson's disease

21. **Melanin granules are present in the brain in the cytoplasm of the cells of:**
    a. Substantia nigra
    b. Subthalamic nucleus
    c. Dentate nucleus
    d. Caudate nucleus

ANSWERS

1. d	2. a	3. a	4. c	5. b
6. b	7. a	8. a	9. a	10. b
11. b	12. c	13. a	14. a	15. b
16. b	17. d	18. c	19. b	20. d
21. a				

Cerebellum

CHAPTER 87

LEARNING OBJECTIVES
- Describe the connections and functions of cerebellum
- Describe the pathophysiology of cerebellar lesion

INTRODUCTION

PY10.7: Describe and discuss functions of cerebral cortex, basal ganglia, thalamus, hypothalamus, cerebellum and limbic system and their abnormalities.

Cerebellum is situated in the posterior cranial fossa. It is connected to brainstem on each side through three peduncles that are located above and around the fourth ventricle. They are:
1. Superior cerebellar peduncle (brachium conjunctivum)
2. Middle cerebellar peduncle (brachium pontis)
3. Inferior cerebellar peduncle (restiform body).

The superior cerebellar peduncle connects the cerebellum to the midbrain, the middle cerebellar peduncle connects the cerebellum to the pons and the inferior cerebellar peduncle connects the cerebellum to the medulla oblongata.

Experimental stimulation of cerebellar region did not produce any movements. But ablation studies of cerebellum showed that control and coordination of motor activities, as well as control of equilibrium and posture, was lost. But there were no sensory disturbances. The studies proved that sense of position, muscle length and muscle tension are integrated in the cerebellar cortex.

FUNCTIONAL ANATOMY

Cerebellum is extremely folded and fissured to increase the surface area very much. Surface area of cerebellum is equal to 75% of surface area of cerebral cortex but weighs only 10% as much as cerebral cortex. The entire body representation is there in the cerebellum.

PARTS OF CEREBELLUM

Cerebellum has a central portion called vermis and lateral expansion called cerebellar hemisphere. Vermis is divided into 10 primary lobules numbered I to X from superior aspect to inferior aspect. They are **lingula, lobulus centralis, culmen, lobulus simplex, declive, folium, tuber, pyramid, uvula and nodulus.**

Anatomically, cerebellum is divided into three lobes by two deep fissures (**Fig. 87.1**):
1. **Anterior lobe**, constituted by lingula, lobulus centralis and culmen of vermis.
2. **Posterior lobe**, constituted by lobulus simplex, declive, folium, tuber, pyramid, uvula, paraflocculus and cerebellar hemispheres
3. **Flocculonodular lobe**, constituted by nodulus and flocculus.

Anterior lobe is separated from posterior lobe by **primary fissure**. The cerebellar hemisphere is divided into exterior cerebellar cortex containing gray matter and interior of cerebellum contains white matter. The intracerebellar nuclei are 4 masses of gray matter embedded in the white matter of cerebellum on each side of the midline.

The deep cerebellar nuclei are (**Fig. 87.2**):
a. **Fastigial nucleus** connected to archicerebellum.
b. **Nucleus emboliformis and nucleus globosus** together known as interpositus nucleus is connected to paleocerebellum.
c. **Dentate nucleus** connected to neocerebellum.

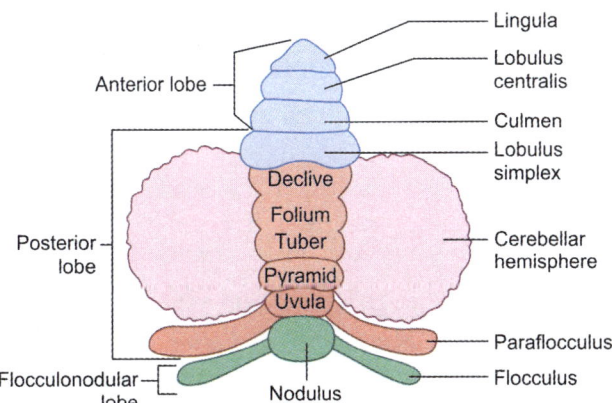

Fig. 87.1: Parts of cerebellum showing the ten primary lobules of vermis. Anatomical division is also shown.

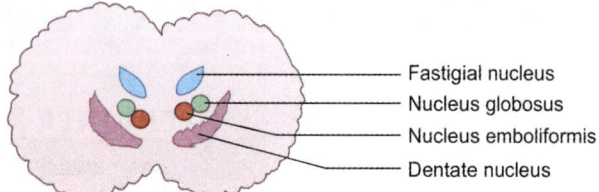

Fig. 87.2: Deep cerebellar nuclei.

PHYLOGENETIC CLASSIFICATION

Older classification of cerebellum is based on the development of the lobes of cerebellum at different times during evolution. The divisions are:
1. Archicerebellum is the oldest portion of cerebellum phylogenetically
2. Paleocerebellum
3. Neocerebellum is the newest portion from phylogenetic point of view.

Archicerebellum is constituted by flocculonodular lobe and has vestibular connections. It is concerned with control of equilibrium.

Paleocerebellum is constituted by anterior lobe and vermis portion of posterior lobe along with paraflocculus. This part is concerned with control of posture and postural activities.

Neocerebellum is constituted by the cerebellar hemispheres on both sides, and control and coordinate voluntary motor activity. They interact with the motor cortex in planning and programming movements.

FUNCTIONAL CLASSIFICATION

Functionally, cerebellum is divided into three parts **(Fig. 87.3)**:
1. Vestibulocerebellum
2. Spinocerebellum
3. Neocerebellum or cerebrocerebellum.

Vestibulocerebellum

Vestibulocerebellum or flocculonodular lobe is composed of nodulus of vermis and flocculus of the cerebellar hemisphere

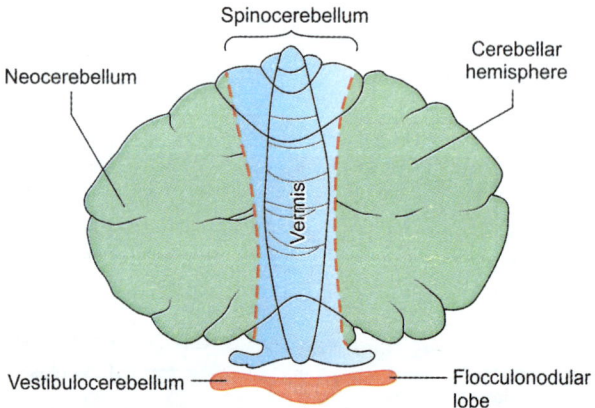

Fig. 87.3: Functional divisions of cerebellum and parts of cerebellum.

on each side. It receives afferents from vestibular apparatus and sends efferents to the vestibular nuclei. Functions are:
- Maintains posture and equilibrium.
- Coordinates eye movements with movements of head (learning-induced changes in the vestibulo-ocular reflex).

Spinocerebellum

The rest of the vermis and the adjacent medial portions of the cerebellar hemispheres form the spinocerebellum.

Afferents to spinocerebellum are from:
- Spinal cord which provides information about the position of limbs and degree of contraction of muscles.
- Visual, auditory and vestibular system which provide information about the environment.
- Sensory cortex.
- Primary motor cortex.

Efferents go to:
- Reticular formation
- Red nucleus
- Vestibular nuclei
- Motor cortex

Functions of Spinocerebellum

- Spinocerebellum receives proprioceptive inputs from the body as well as a copy of the motor plan from motor cortex. By comparing plan with performance, spinocerebellum smoothens and coordinates movements.
- Spinocerebellum is concerned with control of axial (trunk) and limb muscles and postural reflexes.
- Through its projection to the reticular formation and red nucleus it also regulates muscle tone.

Neocerebellum or Cerebrocerebellum

The lateral portions of the cerebellar hemispheres form the neocerebellum or cerebrocerebellum. It is essentially an extension of the cerebral cortex. Afferents are from sensory cortex, primary motor cortex and premotor cortex. Efferents go to thalamus, premotor cortex and primary motor cortex. Functions are:
- Neocerebellum interacts with the motor cortex in planning and coordination of body's sequential muscular activities that occur one after another within fraction of a second.
- It is concerned with learning of skilled voluntary movements.

CEREBELLAR CORTEX

Gray matter of cerebellar cortex is divided into three layers and contains five types of neurons; **Purkinje cells, granule cells, basket cells, stellate cells and Golgi cells**.

The cells are arranged in three layers **(Fig. 87.4)**:
1. External molecular layer
2. Middle Purkinje cell layer
3. Internal granular layer.

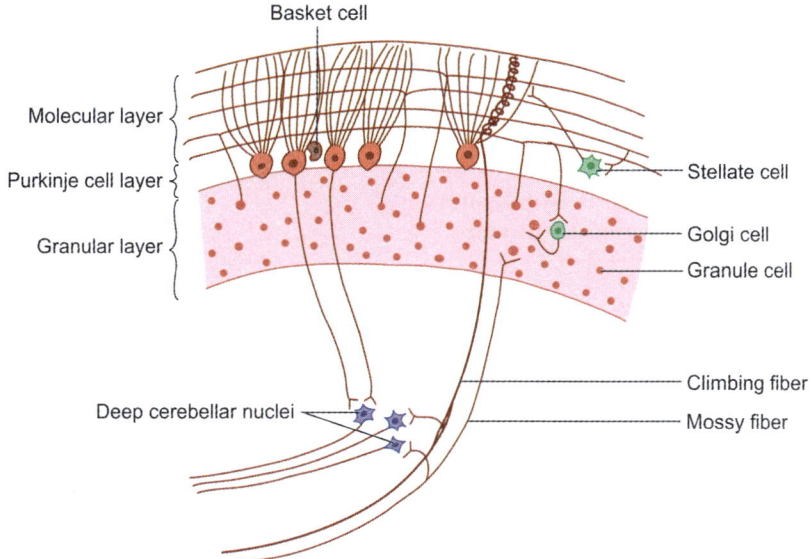

Fig. 87.4: Histology of cerebellar cortex.

Molecular Layer

Molecular layer contains unmyelinated nerve endings and nerve cells.

The nerve endings are:
- Dendrites of Purkinje cells forming dendritic tree
- Axons of granule cells forming parallel fibers
- Climbing fibers from inferior olivary nucleus which synapses with the dendrites of Purkinje cells.

The nerve cells are:
- Star-shaped stellate cells located superficially
- Basket cells located deeply in the molecular layer.

Purkinje Cell Layer

Purkinje cell layer consists of a single layer of large flask-shaped cells. There are about 30 million cells and form one of the largest neurons in the body. The dendrites form a large extensive dendritic tree projecting into the molecular layer and the terminal branches show dendritic spines.

Dendritic spines make synaptic contacts with the parallel fibers derived from the granule cell axons. The Purkinje cell axons come down through the granular layer and end on the deep cerebellar nuclei in the white matter of cerebellum.

Few Purkinje cell axons in the flocculonodular lobe and from parts of vermis bypass the cerebellar nuclei without synapsing and pass directly to end in the vestibular nuclei of the brainstem.

The only output from the cerebellar cortex is the axons of the Purkinje cells. Axons of the deep cerebellar nuclei go out as efferent fibers. Efferent fibers that leave the dentate nucleus form a large part of the superior cerebellar peduncle. Efferent fibers from the other cerebellar nuclei pass through the inferior cerebellar peduncle. *Purkinje cells are inhibitory cells and inhibit the deep cerebellar nuclei.*

Granular Layer

Granular layer is full of **granule cells**. Axons of the granule cells project into the molecular layer and on reaching the molecular layer divide into two branches arranged in the form of "T" constituting the parallel fibers of the molecular layer. They receive input from the mossy fibers and innervate the Purkinje cells. They have multiple synaptic connections with the dendritic spines of the Purkinje cells and stimulate Purkinje cells. *Granule cells are the only excitatory neurons in cerebellar cortex.*

The granule cells can either stimulate the Purkinje cell or can inhibit Purkinje cell through inhibitory interneurons. The Purkinje cells are inhibitory to deep cerebellar nuclei.

Deep cerebellar nuclei receive excitatory inputs via collaterals from the incoming **mossy and climbing fibers**. Total effect depends on the balance between inhibitory and excitatory effects. The output of the deep cerebellar nuclei to the brainstem and thalamus is always excitatory. Thus, almost all the cerebellar circuitry seems to be concerned with modulating or timing the excitatory output of the deep cerebellar nuclei to the brain stem and thalamus.

Inhibitory Interneurons in Cerebellar Cortex

The three inhibitory interneurons in the cerebellar cortex are **basket cells, Golgi cells and stellate cells**. Instead of stimulating the Purkinje cells directly, the granular cells synapse with inhibitory interneurons, such as basket cells located in the molecular layer, which in turn inhibit Purkinje cells. Basket cell axon forms a basket around the cell body and axon hillock of each Purkinje cell it innervates. The granular cells can directly stimulate the Purkinje cells, and through inhibitory interneurons can inhibit them. This is an example of **feed-forward inhibition**. Another inhibitory neuron in the molecular layer of cerebellar cortex is **stellate cell**.

Golgi cells are inhibitory cells in the granular layer. Their dendrites project into the molecular layer and receive excitatory input from parallel fibers of granule cells. Axons of Golgi cells synapse with the dendrites of granule cells. Axons of granule cells stimulate Golgi cells, which in turn inhibit granule cells. Cell bodies of Golgi cells receive excitatory input via collaterals from incoming mossy fibers.

The neurotransmitter released by the stellate, basket, Golgi and Purkinje cells is **GABA**, which is an inhibitory transmitter, whereas the granule cells release **glutamate**, which is excitatory.

Lateral Inhibition in the Cerebellum

Basket cells and *stellate cells* are inhibitory cells in the cerebellar cortex with short axons. Both the basket cells and the stellate cells are located in the molecular layer of the cerebellar cortex, and stimulated by the parallel fibers which are axons of granule cells. These inhibitory cells in turn send their axons to Purkinje cells and cause *lateral inhibition* of adjacent Purkinje cells, thus sharpening the signal.

Input Fibers to the Cerebellum

Two types of afferent fibers come through the inferior and middle cerebellar peduncles:
1. Climbing fibers
2. Mossy fibers

Climbing fibers and mossy fibers are excitatory fibers to the Purkinje cells. Climbing fibers come from a single source, the **inferior olivary nuclei**. Proprioceptive input to the inferior olivary nuclei comes from all parts of the body. All the other fibers are mossy fibers, which form the majority. All the fibers going to the cerebellar cortex give collaterals to deep cerebellar nuclei and are excitatory to the cerebellar nuclei. Thus, the intra-cerebellar nuclei are stimulated by afferent climbing and mossy fibers and inhibited by the Purkinje cell axon. After giving collateral, the climbing fiber goes up to the cerebellar cortex and in the molecular layer twines round the dendrites of a single Purkinje cell like a climbing plant and hence the name climbing fiber.

The mossy fibers also give collateral to the deep cerebellar nuclei and ends on the dendrites of granule cells in complex synaptic groups called **glomeruli**.

The glomerulus also contains inhibitory endings of Golgi cells. The mossy fibers provide direct proprioceptive input from all parts of the body plus input from the cerebral cortex via the pontine nuclei to the cerebellar cortex. One climbing fiber makes contact with a single Purkinje cell whereas; one mossy fiber may stimulate thousands of Purkinje cells through granule cells **(Fig. 87.5)**. Even though one Purkinje cell receives input from a single climbing fiber, it makes 2000–3000 synapses on it. So climbing fiber input exerts a strong excitatory effect on a single Purkinje cell. Mossy fiber inputs through granule cells exert a weak excitatory effect on many Purkinje cells.

Hypothalamo-cerebellar Fibers

There are to and fro connections between cerebellum and hypothalamus. There are direct connections between cerebellar nuclei and the hypothalamus and between several regions of hypothalamus and cerebellar cortex. Direct

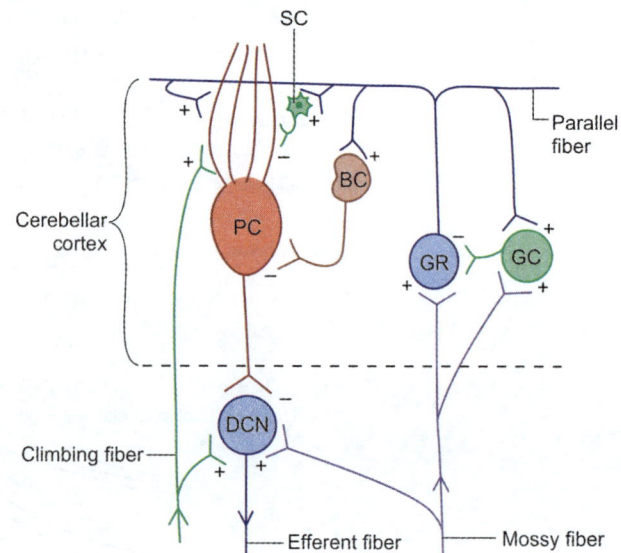

Fig. 87.5: Neural connections in the cerebellum. Plus (+) signs indicate that the endings are excitatory and minus (–) signs indicate that the endings are inhibitory.

(BC: basket cell; DCN: deep cerebellar nuclei; GC: Golgi cell; GR: granule cell; PC: Purkinje cell; SC: stellate cell)

Note that PC, BC, SC and GC are inhibitory.

hypothalamo-cerebellar fibers are uncrossed and reach all parts of cerebellar cortex and the cerebellar nuclei. They are neither mossy nor climbing fibers. Some of these fibers are histaminergic and some contain gamma amino butyric acid (GABA) as the neurotransmitter.

The direct cerebellohypothalamic fibers originate from all cerebellar nuclei, pass through the superior cerebellar peduncle and terminate in the posterior hypothalamic nuclei and in the posterior parts of the dorsomedian hypothalamic nucleus.

CONNECTIONS OF CEREBELLUM

Cerebellar Afferent Fibers

- From cerebral cortex
  - Cortico-pontocerebellar pathway (crossed)
  - Cerebro-olivocerebellar pathway (crossed)
  - Cerebro-reticulocerebellar pathway (uncrossed).
- From spinal cord
  - Anterior or ventral spinocerebellar tract
  - Posterior or dorsal spinocerebellar tract
  - Cuneocerebellar tract
- From vestibular apparatus (vestibulocerebellar fibers)
- From red nucleus and tectum (rubrocerebellar and tectocerebellar tracts)
- From inferior olivary nuclei (olivocerebellar tract)
- From hypothalamus (hypothalamo-cerebellar fibers)
- *All the afferent fibers except olivocerebellar tract and hypothalamo-cerebellar fibers constitute mossy fibers.*

Cerebellar Efferent Fibers

- Globose emboliform rubral pathway
- Dentatothalamic pathway

- Fastigial vestibular pathway
- Fastigial reticular pathway
- Cerebellohypothalamic pathway

Functions of the Dorsal Spinocerebellar and Ventral Spinocerebellar Tracts

The signals transmitted in the **dorsal spinocerebellar tracts** come mainly from the muscle spindles and to a lesser extent from other somatic receptors, such as Golgi tendon organs, large tactile receptors of the skin like Pacinian corpuscles, and joint receptors. All these signals inform the cerebellum of the momentary status of the following events:
- Degree of muscle contraction
- Degree of tension on the muscle tendons
- Position and rate of movement of the different parts of the body
- Forces acting on the surfaces of the body.

The **ventral spinocerebellar tracts** receive much less information from the peripheral receptors. Instead, they are excited mainly by motor signals arriving in the anterior horns of the spinal cord from:
- The brain through the corticospinal and rubrospinal tracts
- The internal motor pattern generators in the spinal cord itself.

Thus, this ventral spinocerebellar pathway informs the cerebellum of all motor signals that have arrived at the anterior horns.

The spinocerebellar pathways can transmit impulses at velocities up to 120 m/sec, which is the most rapid conduction in any pathway in the central nervous system. This speed is important for instantaneous judgment of the cerebellum of changes in peripheral muscle actions.

In addition to signals from the spinocerebellar tracts, signals are transmitted into the cerebellum from the body periphery through the following:
a. Collaterals from the spinal dorsal column tracts to the dorsal column nuclei of the medulla are relayed to the cerebellum.
b. Signals are transmitted up the spinal cord through the *spinoreticular pathway* to the reticular formation of the brain stem and from there to the inferior olivary nucleus.
c. Through the *spino-olivary pathway* to the inferior olivary nucleus. Signals are then relayed from both of these areas to the cerebellum. Thus, the cerebellum continually collects information about the movements and positions of all parts of the body even though it is operating at a subconscious level.

PEDUNCLES OF CEREBELLUM

The fibers coming to or going out of cerebellum go through the three peduncles. The different tracts passing through the peduncles are:
- All sensory and proprioceptive information reaches the cerebellum through the **anterior and posterior spinocerebellar tract or through spinoolivary or spinotectal tract**.
- From head and neck region, the fibers pass through **cuneocerebellar tract**.
- Visual and auditory fibers come through **tectocerebellar tract**.
- From vestibular apparatus fibers reach the vestibular nucleus, and from there the fibers reach the cerebellum through the **vestibulocerebellar tract** to terminate as mossy fibers in the flocculonodular lobe of cerebellum.
- Another important tract coming to cerebellum is from the cerebral cortex. From the motor cortical areas, fibers come along with the pyramidal tract and extrapyramidal tract and end in the pontine nuclei and from there fibers go to the cerebellum and the tract is called **cortico-ponto-cerebellar tract**.
- Fibers go back to the cortex from cerebellum as **dentato-rubro-thalamo-cortical** fibers.
- Fibers also go to other parts, such as reticular formation, thalamus, etc.

There are no direct fibers from cerebellum to spinal cord.

Fibers Going Through the Different Peduncles of Cerebellum

Inferior Cerebellar Peduncle
See **Table 87.1**.

Middle Cerebellar Peduncle

Afferent Fibers
1. Cortico-ponto-cerebellar fibers from cerebral hemispheres.
2. Commissural fibers coming from one side of cerebellar cortex to the opposite side so that the two sides function as a unit.

Efferent Fibers
Commissural fibers

Superior Cerebellar Peduncle
See **Table. 87.2**.

Table 87.1: Fibers passing through inferior cerebellar peduncle.

Afferent fibers	Efferent fibers
- Posterior spinocerebellar tract - Cuneocerebellar - Olivocerebellar - Vestibulocerebellar - Reticulocerebellar - Fibers from cranial nerve nuclei	- Fastigiovestibular tract - Fastigio-olivary fibers - Fastigioreticular

Table 87.2: Fibers passing through superior cerebellar peduncle.

Afferent fibers	Efferent fibers
- Anterior spinocerebellar tract - Tectocerebellar tract - Rubrocerebellar fibers - Cortico-ponto-cerebellar tract - Hypothalamo-cerebellar tract	- Dentatorubral tract - Dentato-rubro-thalamic tract - Dentato-rubro-thalamo-cortical tract - Dentato-thalamic tract - Cerebellotectal tract - Cerebellohypothalamic tract - Cerebelloreticular tract

FUNCTIONS OF CEREBELLUM

a. Role in muscle tone
b. Role in control of voluntary activity
c. Control of involuntary activity
d. Control of equilibrium
e. Role in learning motor skills
f. Influence on autonomic centers and affective behavior.

Role of Cerebellum in Muscle Tone

Cerebellum has afferent and efferent connections to reticular formation that controls muscle tone through gamma motor neurons.

In experimental animals, cerebellum has an inhibitory effect on muscle tone and lesions of cerebellum in animals lead to spasticity. In humans, cerebellum exerts a facilitatory influence on muscle tone and in lesions of cerebellum there will be hypotonia. *Cerebellum has no effect on the activity of smooth muscles.*

Control of Voluntary Motor Activity

Control of voluntary activity is through the circuitous connections between cerebral cortex and cerebellum. Cerebral hemisphere controls muscles of opposite side through the pyramidal tract. Cerebral hemisphere is connected to cerebellum of opposite side that controls muscles of same side. Thus cerebral hemisphere controls muscles of opposite side, whereas *cerebellar hemispheres control muscles of the same side of the body because of the double crossing* (Fig. 87.6).

Error Detection and Correction

Cerebellum compares the intentions of cerebral cortex with the actual performance at the periphery. If movement is more or fast, error is detected and corrective signals are sent to the cerebral cortex from cerebellum, and the firing from the cerebrum is corrected. Since the position of the moving limb changes from moment to moment, the cerebellar correction also changes continuously. Thus, movements are made smooth, precise and well-coordinated. This particular property of cerebellum is known as **error detection and correction** function.

Predictive Functions of Cerebellum

Normally, the rate of firing from cerebral cortex is much more than what is needed. Cerebellum is capable of predicting or determining the future position of a moving limb. Without cerebellum, all movements become jerky, pendular and rapid, e.g., overshooting, past-pointing, etc. Due to the functioning of cerebellum, damping of firing levels occurs and correct and precise movements occur. These are the predictive functions of cerebellum.

Damping and Braking Action

Due to the **damping effect** and due to the **braking action** through error detection, cerebellum is capable of producing a suppressor effect on cerebral firing level. Cerebellum is capable of completely stopping the range of movement by the braking action. **Rate, range, force and direction of movement** can be controlled by cerebellum, and movements become smooth, controlled, coordinated and precise to the point. For rapid, repeated, progressive, sequential activities, such as running, walking, talking, writing, etc., cerebellum is required. Cerebellum also plays a role in establishing new motor skills by conditioning.

Role in Involuntary Motor Activity

Cerebellum has afferent and efferent connections to structures, such as red nucleus, reticular formation, tectal nucleus, vestibular nucleus, olivary nucleus, etc., which control muscle tone, posture, etc. Cerebellum controls the rate of firing through the extrapyramidal tract. Reflex

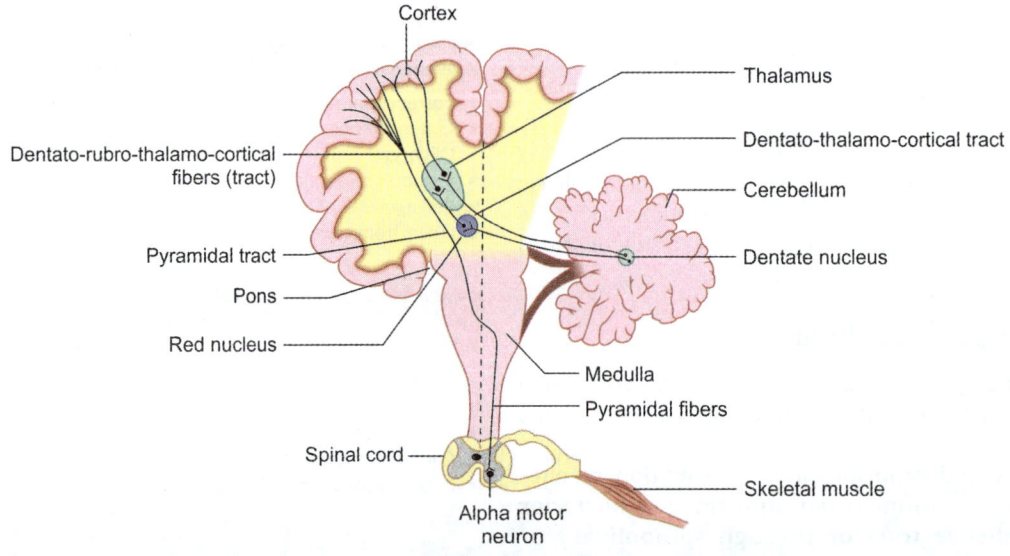

Fig. 87.6: Double crossing of fibers concerned with cerebellar functions.

contractions are controlled, coordinated and made precise by cerebellum. In cerebellar lesions, **knee jerk is pendular**. Hypotonia, absence of coordination and absence of braking action are responsible for the pendular movement of leg.

Control of Equilibrium

Most important organ in controlling equilibrium is vestibular apparatus. Static equilibrating signals arising from utricle, saccule and semicircular canals during movement (linear and angular acceleration) will be reaching vestibular nucleus and from there, the impulses reach the flocculonodular lobe of cerebellum. Cerebellum is able to predict whether mal-equilibrium is occurring. All reflex actions will be coordinated, made accurate and smooth to control equilibrium. Cerebellum inhibits the contraction of the antagonistic muscles.

Role of Cerebellum in Learning

Cerebellum is concerned with learned adjustments, which make coordination easier when a task is performed over and over. The basis of this learning is probably the input via the olivary nuclei. Climbing fiber activity is increased when a new movement is being learned and selective lesions of the olivary complex abolish the ability to produce long-term adjustments in certain motor responses.

Non-somatic Functions of Cerebellum (Influence on Autonomic Centers and Affective Behavior)

Cerebellum has been previously considered only as a subcortical center for motor control. Now, it has been proved that there are interconnections between hypothalamus and cerebellum. Hypothalamo-cerebellar circuits act as an essential modulator and coordinator for integrating motor, visceral and behavioral responses. Because of the cerebello-hypothalamic projections and the resultant descending hypothalamic projections to the visceral centers, the cerebellum can influence autonomic centers. The interconnections between hypothalamus and the cerebellum are also responsible for the affective responses seen in cerebellar diseases.

Cerebellum has a role in feeding. The decrease in body weight following lesion of the cerebellar cortex is due to alteration in food intake behavior. Thus the direct bidirectional cerebello-hypothalamic circuits are responsible for the non-somatic functions of cerebellum.

■ LESIONS OF CEREBELLUM

Cerebellar disease may be due to abscess, hemorrhage, trauma or tumor in the cerebellum. Manifestations of cerebellar lesion may be generalized or localized depending on the extent of lesion. If only a small area of cerebellar cortex is involved it may not manifest prominently. If a lesion occurs to a major extent in the cerebellar cortex or to the deep cerebellar nuclei, manifestations will be classical. Main defects in cerebellar lesion are **hypotonia** and loss of influence of cerebellum on the activities of cerebral cortex.

Muscle atrophy, sensory changes and paralysis are not present in cerebellar lesions. The classical manifestations are:
1. **Hypotonia** (decreased muscle tone)
2. **Asthenia** (weakness of muscle, slowness of movement and easy fatigability)
3. **Ataxia** or incoordination
4. **Disequilibrium and Vertigo**.

Hypotonia

Hypotonia refers to a decrease in the resistance to passive movements of the limbs. Through its projection to the reticular formation and red nucleus spinocerebellum regulates muscle tone. Hypotonia is usually a feature in acute cerebellar damage. In unilateral cerebellar disease, there is deviation of the body to the side of the lesion, probably due to hypotonia. Patients with chronic cerebellar lesion usually have normal muscle tone. The exact reason for the hypotonia is not clear.

It may be due to disruption of afferent input from the muscle spindle or it may be due to the lack of the facilitatory effect of cerebellum on spindle sensitivity. Cerebellum influences the activity of the gamma motor neurons which innervate the intrafusal fibers. When the activity of these neurons is decreased, the tonic stretch response of the muscle spindle afferents is lowered. Hypotonia is the reason for pendular knee jerk in cerebellar disease.

Asthenia

Most abnormalities associated with cerebellar lesion become apparent during movement. There is delay in the initiation of movements especially when there is lesion to the cerebrocerebellum. If the patient is asked to clench both hands simultaneously, it is seen that the normal hand clenches earlier than the affected hand.

Ataxia

Ataxia is loss of control over voluntary movements (muscular incoordination). Incoordination is due to errors in rate, range, force and direction of movement. During rest, ataxia is not seen. Muscular incoordination due to lesions of the cerebellum is called **cerebellar ataxia.** (Muscular incoordination due to defective sensory information as a result of lesions in the dorsal column pathway is called **sensory ataxia**.)

- *Past-pointing or dysmetria*: Dysmetria, i.e., overshooting to one side is seen when finger-nose test is performed. When correction is done, correction overshoots to the other side. The finger oscillates back and forth. This tremulous movement is called **intention tremor**. It is absent at rest, appears whenever the patient attempts to perform some voluntary action.

    This is due to failure of the cerebellum to inhibit the cerebral cortex after movement has begun. This leads to incoordination, lack of predictive function and lack of braking action of cerebellum. In the complex movement, different components are called into play at wrong times and an attempt at compensation results in irregular and jerky movements.

- *Nystagmus:* Intention tremor is seen for eye movement, i.e., oscillatory movement of eyeball called **cerebellar nystagmus**. Nystagmus in cerebellar lesion is due to lack of muscle coordination in eye. The quick component is to the side of lesion.
- *Rebound phenomenon*: Another characteristic feature of cerebellar disease is inability to put on the brakes, i.e., to stop movements promptly. Ask the patient to flex the forearm against resistance and withdraw the resistance suddenly. It is seen that the forearm strikes against the body due to absence of braking action. This is **rebound phenomenon**.

3. *Pendular knee jerk*: This is another finding in cerebellar lesion, which is due to hypotonia and lack of braking action. When knee jerk is elicited, normally the leg moves forwards and comes back to the original position. In cerebellar lesion, the leg swings like a pendulum when knee jerk is elicited.
4. *Adiadochokinesis:* In cerebellar disease, there is inability to perform rapidly alternating opposite movements such as repeated pronation and supination of forearm, due to lack of coordination of motor activity. This is called **dysdiadochokinesis or adiadochokinesis**.
5. *Decomposition of movement*: Patients with cerebellar disease have difficulty in performing actions that involve simultaneous motion at more than one joint. They dissect such movements and carry them out with one joint at a time, a phenomenon known as **decomposition of movement**.

    Each voluntary act is usually complex and can be analyzed into simple components. All the component movements of each activity are always carried out coordinately. When lack of coordination occurs because of errors in rate, range, direction and force, decomposition of the components of the movement occurs.
6. *Gait:* Gait in cerebellar disease is wide based, unsteady, **staggering gait called drunken gait,** which is due to ataxia of limbs. Degeneration of vermis and fastigial nucleus can result from thiamine deficiency in alcoholics and malnourished individuals.
7. *Disturbance of speech*: Speech is referred to as **slurring or scanning speech** (cerebellar dysarthria), which is due to ataxia. Scanning speech is usually seen when there is damage to the vermis and the fastigial nucleus.

Disequilibrium of the Body and Vertigo

Damage to the vestibulocerebellum leads to ataxia, disequilibrium and nystagmus. **Vertigo** will also be an important feature. When there is extensive damage; the person may not be able to stand up properly. Vertigo means dizziness where the subject feels like he is spinning or the world around him is spinning.

MULTIPLE CHOICE QUESTIONS

1. **The cerebellum:**
    a. Has a totally inhibitory output from its cortex
    b. Has only excitatory signal output from its deep nuclear layers
    c. Has a conscious interpretation of motor activity
    d. Has inhibitory influence on muscle tone in humans
2. **Purkinje cell is:**
    a. Output cell   b. Input cell
    c. Interneuron   d. Connector neuron
3. **Vestibular fibers relay in the:**
    a. Vermis
    b. Lateral geniculate body
    c. Flocculonodular lobe of cerebellum
    d. Auditory cortex
4. **In cerebellar disease all the following statements are correct,** *except*:
    a. Romberg's sign is positive
    b. There is adiadokokinesia
    c. Pendular knee jerk present
    d. There will be involuntary tremor
5. **Mossy fibers in cerebellum relay in:**
    a. Basket cell   b. Granule cell
    c. Purkinje cell   d. Stellate cell
6. **In cerebellum all are inhibitory cells,** *except*:
    a. Basket cell   b. Golgi cell
    c. Stellate cell   d. Granule cell
7. **Climbing fibers arise from:**
    a. Inferior olivary nucleus
    b. Superior olivary nucleus
    c. Inferior colliculus
    d. Red nucleus
8. **The most important site of linkage of α-γ systems in the maintenance of muscle tone is:**
    a. Basal ganglia   b. Cerebellum
    c. Cerebral cortex   d. Spinal cord
9. **Planning and programming of movement is the function of:**
    a. Cerebral cortex   b. Basal ganglia
    c. Cerebellum   d. Thalamus
10. **Flocculonodular lobe of cerebellum is concerned with:**
    a. Past-pointing
    b. Posture and equilibrium
    c. Coordination
    d. Reflex action
11. **In cerebellar lesion, tremor is seen:**
    a. At rest   b. With action
    c. With emotions   d. In sleep
12. **Which one of the following symptoms is not seen in cerebellar lesion?**
    a. Resting tremor
    b. Dysdiadochokinesia
    c. Ataxia
    d. Hypotonia
13. **All the following occur in lesion of cerebellum,** *except*:
    a. Scanning speech   b. Ataxia
    c. Intension tremor   d. Loss of memory

14. **Vestibular fibers relay in:**
    a. Vermis
    b. Lateral geniculate body
    c. Flocculonodular lobe of cerebellum
    d. Auditory cortex
15. **Coordination of movement is the function of:**
    a. Cerebellum
    b. Basal ganglia
    c. Cerebral cortex
    d. Limbic system
16. **Incoordination in movements is known as:**
    a. Ataxia
    b. Athetosis
    c. Atonia
    d. Akinesia
17. **Signs and symptoms of cerebellar disease includes all the following, *except*:**
    a. Hypotonia
    b. Ataxia
    c. Paralysis
    d. Nystagmus
18. **Dysdiadochokinesia is a feature of the lesion of:**
    a. Dorsal column tract
    b. Cerebellum
    c. Basal ganglia
    d. Internal capsule
19. **The transverse fibers connecting the two cerebellar hemispheres are mainly present in the:**
    a. Corona radiata
    b. Pons
    c. Medulla oblongata
    d. Corpus callosum
20. **Vermis is a part of:**
    a. Cerebellum
    b. Medulla oblongata
    c. Spinal cord
    d. Basal ganglia
21. **The largest nucleus in cerebellum is:**
    a. Nucleus globosus
    b. Dentate nucleus
    c. Nucleus emboliformis
    d. Caudate nucleus
22. **Neocerebellar syndrome is characterized by all the following, *except*:**
    a. Intention tremor
    b. Absence of knee jerk
    c. Hypotonia of skeletal muscle
    d. Nystagmus
23. **Flocculonodular lobe has direct connection with:**
    a. Red nucleus
    b. Inferior olivary nucleus
    c. Vestibular nucleus
    d. Dentate nucleus
24. **Cerebellar connection to other parts of the brain is projected through which cell?**
    a. Golgi cell
    b. Basket cell
    c. Purkinje cell
    d. Oligodendrocytes
25. **Output from cerebellum is solely from:**
    a. Basket cell
    b. Granular cell
    c. Treitz cell
    d. Purkinje cell
26. **True about cerebellum is:**
    a. Cerebral cortex has mostly inhibitory effects on cerebellum
    b. Coordination
    c. Planning of motor movements
    d. Decrease muscle tone
27. **All are true about cerebellum, *except*:**
    a. It has 3 layers, 4 nuclei and 5 cells
    b. Climbing fibers are afferent inputs
    c. Mossy fibers inhibit Purkinje cells
    d. Climbing fibers excite Purkinje cells
28. **Which one of the following clearly states the role of cerebellum in motor performance?**
    a. Planning and programming of movement
    b. Converts abstract thought into voluntary action
    c. Initiation of skilled voluntary action
    d. Smoothens and coordinates ongoing movements
29. **The following neurons in the cerebellar cortex are inhibitory, *except*:**
    a. Granule cell
    b. Golgi cell
    c. Purkinje cell
    d. Stellate cell
30. **Vestibulocerebellum is associated to which cerebellar nucleus?**
    a. Dentate
    b. Emboliform
    c. Globose
    d. Fastigial
31. **The only output fibers from cerebellar cortex are axons of:**
    a. Granule cell
    b. Golgi cell
    c. Purkinje cell
    d. Stellate cell
32. **The only output from spinocerebellum and neocerebellum is from:**
    a. Deep cerebellar nuclei
    b. Granule cell
    c. Mossy fibers
    d. Purkinje cell
33. **The axons of deep cerebellar nuclei project to all the following parts, *except*:**
    a. Nuclei of III, IV and VI cranial nerves
    b. Red nucleus
    c. Spinal cord motor neurons
    d. Vestibular nuclei
34. **Pendular knee jerk is seen in:**
    a. Basal ganglia lesion
    b. Cerebellar lesion
    c. Complete section of spinal cord
    d. Thalamic syndrome
35. **The following are features of cerebellar lesion, *except*:**
    a. Dysmetria
    b. Hypotonia
    c. Intension tremor
    d. Motor weakness
36. **Mossy fibers relay and transmit in:**
    a. Basket cells
    b. Granule cells
    c. Purkinje cells
    d. Stellate cells
37. **Correct statement regarding connections of cerebellar neurons**
    a. Basket cells release glutamate to activate Purkinje cells
    b. Mossy fiber collateral inputs exert a strong inhibitory effect on Golgi cells

c. Granule cells release glutamate to excite basket cells and stellate cells
d. Purkinje cells release glutamate to stimulate deep cerebellar nuclei

38. Interpositus nucleus is formed of:
a. Dentate and globose nuclei
b. Dentate and fastigial nuclei
c. Globose and emboliform nuclei
d. Globose and fastigial nuclei

ANSWERS

1. a	2. a	3. c	4. d	5. b
6. d	7. a	8. b	9. b	10. b
11. b	12. a	13. d	14. c	15. a
16. a	17. c	18. b	19. b	20. a
21. b	22. b	23. c	24. c	25. d
26. b	27. c	28. d	29. a	30. d
31. c	32. a	33. c	34. b	35. d
36. a	37. c	38. c		

Reticular Formation

CHAPTER 88

LEARNING OBJECTIVES
- Explain the functional anatomy of reticular formation
- Describe the components and functions of ascending reticular activating system

INTRODUCTION

PY10.5: Describe and discuss structure and functions of reticular activating system, autonomic nervous system (ANS).

Reticular formation consists of a diffuse network of neurons scattered throughout the brainstem, i.e., midbrain, pons and medulla extending into the cortex and to the thalamus. Billions of cells are seen in the reticular formation. Very long axons and dendrites is a characteristic feature of the neurons of reticular formation. All the vital centers like vasomotor center, cardioinhibitory center, deglutition center, respiratory center, etc., are situated in the reticular formation.

Red nucleus, olivary nucleus, vestibular nucleus, etc., are seen in close relation to reticular formation with afferent and efferent connections. Reticular formation is constituted by dispersed neurons mainly, but some are aggregated at places to form the nuclei of reticular formation.

In the **medulla**, the nuclei are:
- Median raphe nucleus
- Nucleus magnus
- Medial and lateral reticular nuclei

In the **pons**, pontine reticular nuclei form part of reticular formation.

In the **midbrain**, the nuclei are:
- Periaqueductal gray matter
- Deep tegmental nucleus
- Deep tectal nuclei

In the **thalamus**:
- Intralaminar nucleus
- Midline nucleus
- Reticular nucleus

CONNECTIONS OF RETICULAR FORMATION

Afferent Connections

- All the ascending tracts carrying general somatic sensation on reaching the brainstem give collateral fibers to reticular formation. Trigeminal pathway from face, visual, auditory, gustatory and vestibular pathways also give information to reticular formation. Pain sensations carried by type C fibers separate out as **spinoreticular pathway** and end in reticular formation.
- From the entire cortical area, afferent information reaches the reticular formation. Afferent information also comes from subcortical structures like basal ganglia, hypothalamus, thalamus, cerebellum, red nucleus, olivary nucleus, vestibular nucleus, etc. Nearby motor nuclei are also connected to the reticular formation.
- Apart from neural factors, chemical factors and hormonal factors like epinephrine, norepinephrine; CO_2; drugs like barbiturates, general anesthetics, etc., also influence reticular formation.

Efferent Connections

The axons of the neurons of reticular formation have numerous collaterals which make wide spread synaptic connections. Some of the collaterals ascend to the fore brain whereas some descend to the spinal cord. Efferent connections are seen to:
- All nearby structures from which afferent fibers are coming to reticular formation
- Major long efferent fibers are fibers which go up to the cerebral cortex
- Fibers go to spinal cord as reticulospinal tract.

The efferent fibers are classified under two headings:
I. Ascending reticular activating system (ARAS).
II. Descending reticular system of fibers (reticulospinal tract).

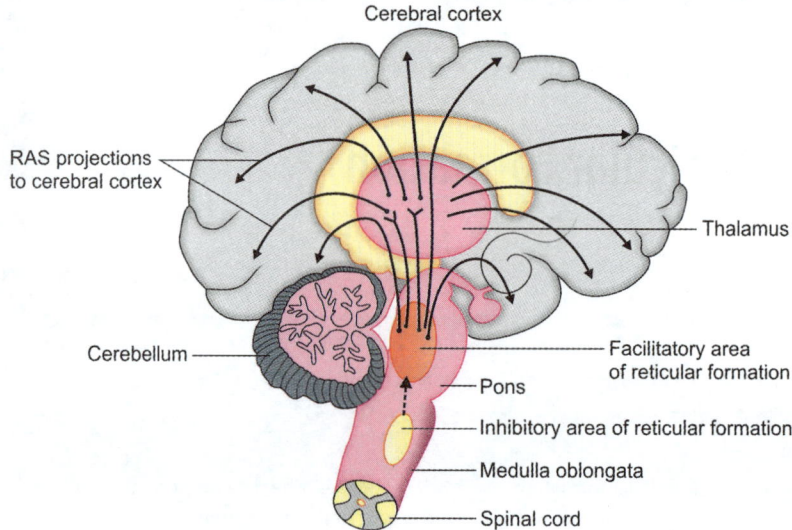

Fig. 88.1: Sagittal section of brain showing ascending reticular activating system (ARAS).

- Larger bulboreticular facilitatory fibers
- Smaller caudal inhibitory fibers.

Ascending Reticular Activating System (ARAS)

ARAS consists of:
- Fibers from reticular formation (bulboreticular facilitatory area) directly projecting to the entire cerebral cortex. They are mainly **cholinergic**.
- Fibers from reticular formation going through the thalamus and projecting to the entire cortex as the nonspecific thalamic projection **(Fig. 88.1)**. They are mainly **adrenergic**.
- Reticular formation also contains **serotonergic** fibers.

Reticulospinal Tract

The neurons of reticular formation are organized into two columns: medial column and lateral column. Lateral column contains small neurons and is referred to as the **parvocellular part.** Medial group contains large cells and is referred to as **gigantocellular part**. The descending fibers from the medial part of the reticular formation form the reticulospinal tract whose action is on γ-**motor neurons** or α-motor neurons or interneurons of spinal cord. The fibers arising from the **bulboreticular facilitatory area** have a facilitatory action on the motor neurons on which they end, and the neurons of this area of reticular formation exhibit spontaneous activity (*refer* Chapter 84, **Fig. 84.5**).

Fibers from the **caudal inhibitory area** of reticular formation descend to the spinal cord and end in interneurons which in turn inhibit the motor neurons. So, these fibers are inhibitory in action. This caudal inhibitory area is influenced by cerebral cortex and basal ganglia. When there is lesion in the cortex or basal ganglia, there will be unopposed action of bulboreticular facilitatory area.

FUNCTIONS OF RETICULAR FORMATION

Functions of Reticulospinal Tract

- Control of muscle tone – γ-motor neuron has connection from bulboreticular facilitatory area of reticular formation directly and from caudal inhibitory area indirectly through interneurons. Facilitatory impulses are counterbalanced by inhibitory impulses. Normally, there is a balance between these two effects and the muscle tone is maintained normally.
- Reticular formation is the most important integrating and relay center for extrapyramidal fibers. Impulses coming down through these fibers influence the γ-motor neuron to maintain muscle tone in the resting state. This also helps in the reflex control of muscle tone in various postures, in various reflex actions and in voluntary activity.
- Reticulospinal tract has an important role in deciding the background tone and posture of the body. It helps to maintain the tone of the antigravity muscles. The pontine part or the bulboreticular facilitatory area facilitates spinal stretch reflexes by exciting the antigravity muscles and is important for maintaining posture.
- Medullary part of caudal inhibitory area of reticular formation inhibits spinal motor neurons that innervate extensor group of muscles.

Functions of Ascending Reticular Activating System

Ascending reticular activating system (ARAS) is a complex polysynaptic pathway arising from the facilitatory area of reticular formation which may go directly to the cortex or via the thalamus. This is a **nonspecific projection** to the cortical area. *No specific sensation is carried by the ARAS.*
- It maintains **cortical neuronal excitability**. These fibers synapse with the dendrites of cortical neurons and maintain partial depolarization or the excitability of

cortical neurons is increased. EEG pattern at rest gives an idea about the rate of firing through ARAS. Experimental stimulation of ARAS causes diffuse stimulation of cortical neurons, even capable of arousing a person from sleep. Reticular formation influences the state of consciousness, and damage to the reticular formation [due to hemorrhage, tumor, sleeping sickness (encephalitis lethargica), etc.] may lead to persistent unconsciousness and even coma. The person cannot be aroused even with the most painful stimulus. Loss of consciousness in epilepsy is due to inhibition of the activity of the reticular formation in the upper part of diencephalon.

- ARAS is responsible for maintaining the **state of wakefulness, alertness and consciousness** of an individual. ARAS can be stimulated by sensory stimulation and by muscular activity. Fibers from limbic system and cerebral cortex (emotional upset, anxiety, intense thinking, anger, worries, etc.) can cause an increase in the activity of ARAS. A **reverberating circuit** sets in due to afferent and efferent connections between reticular formation and cortex. The information thus goes on and activity is maintained for prolonged periods. Once ARAS is stimulated, the wakefulness can be maintained as long as the reverberating circuit is continuing, i.e., for about 12 hours. This decides the wakefulness of an individual. When rate of firing in ARAS decreases, there will be neuronal fatigue and the person goes to sleep. The degree of wakefulness and alertness depends on the rate of firing of impulses through ARAS. If firing level is high, an extremely high degree of alertness is seen. If firing level is low, the person will be just awake.

- ARAS has an important role in the **appreciation of sensation**. Many of the ascending sensory pathways send collaterals to the reticular formation. So, when a stimulus is applied, it not only evokes conscious perception of the sensation, but also activates ARAS to make the individual aware of the different aspects of the sensation like its nature. A person can perceive sensation only if ARAS is active. The most important stimulus for stimulating ARAS is pain and this is a protective phenomenon. During sleep all sensations are dull.

- Ability to **concentrate** or to focus attention also depends on the activity of certain areas of ARAS especially the thalamic nuclei of reticular formation.

The field of awareness is narrowed and this is done by facilitating certain cortical areas and simultaneously suppressing certain other areas. For example, soldiers do not feel pain in the battlefield unless the fight is over. This is due to the suppression of pain fibers by corticofugal fibers and fibers from reticular formation (periaqueductal gray matter) that suppress pain pathway at the first synapse, i.e., substantia gelatinosa of Rolando.

This was experimentally proved by implanting recording electrodes into the cochlear nucleus of a cat. When a click sound is produced at regular intervals, an action potential is produced each time and this is called **click response**. If a rat is put in the cage, the cat watches the rat and even if the click sound is produced there will be no action potential in the recording.

- Pain sensation coming through type C fibers, i.e., spinoreticular fibers directly project into ARAS.

MULTIPLE CHOICE QUESTIONS

1. The most important part of nervous system responsible for maintaining wakeful, alert, active state of an individual is:
    a. Pyramidal system
    b. Reticular activating system
    c. Spinothalamic system
    d. Vestibular system

2. The reticular formation is a diffuse collection of:
    a. Sensory neurons
    b. Motor neurons
    c. Autonomic centers
    d. All of the above

3. The true statement regarding gamma efferent neuron is:
    a. An A group motor neuron with a smaller diameter than that of alpha efferent neuron
    b. Innervates intrafusal fibers
    c. Innervates muscle fibers that stretch annulo-spiral endings
    d. All of the above

ANSWERS

1. b   2. d   3. d

Vestibular Apparatus

CHAPTER 89

LEARNING OBJECTIVES
- Describe the functions of vestibular apparatus
- Explain the mechanism of stimulation of crista ampullaris and macula
- Discuss the vestibular function tests

INTRODUCTION

PY10.4: Describe and discuss motor tracts, mechanism of maintenance of tone, control of body movements, posture and equilibrium and vestibular apparatus.

Vestibular apparatus is a very complex sensitive sense organ, which can detect position and motion of the head and body. The concerned receptors can be stimulated by acceleration, i.e., linear acceleration and angular acceleration or rotational movement; and gravitational force. When stimulated, the vestibular apparatus initiates postural and ocular reflexes. Postural reflexes lead to reflex contraction of groups of muscles, can change muscle tone and bring about reflex postural movement. This helps to maintain posture and equilibrium. Ocular reflexes help in achieving stability of visual images despite movement of the body.

Impulses from the vestibular apparatus can go to the cortical area where the sensation can be appreciated. This does not have conscious awareness like other sensations. But, we become aware of these sensations when malfunction occurs in their function. The person feels dizziness, vertigo, nausea, etc. in vestibular dysfunction.

Two sensory modalities are present in the inner ear or labyrinth, **cochlea** for hearing and **vestibular apparatus** for maintaining equilibrium. Labyrinth is located in the petrous part of temporal bone. It consists of a bony labyrinth and inside the bony labyrinth is the membranous labyrinth. The membranous labyrinth contains endolymph whose composition is similar to intracellular fluid (ICF) and contains more K^+. Between the bony labyrinth and membranous labyrinth is the perilymph whose concentration is similar to ECF and has a high Na^+ content.

FUNCTIONAL ANATOMY OF VESTIBULAR APPARATUS

Vestibular apparatus is two in number, one on each side. Each vestibular apparatus consists of two sac-like structures, **utricle and saccule**, and **three semicircular canals**. The semicircular canals open into the utricle, and utricle in turn communicates with the saccule (*refer* Chapter 99, Fig. 99.1 in Section XI). The saccule communicates with the cochlea via the ductus reuniens.

Semicircular Canals

- Anterior or superior semicircular canal
- Posterior or inferior semicircular canal
- Lateral or horizontal or external semicircular canal

The three semicircular canals are located at right angles to each other representing three planes in space, i.e., two horizontal and one vertical plane. When semicircular canals of both sides are compared, it is seen that one pair of semicircular canals will be in the same plane. These pairs are called **synergistic pairs**. They are:
1. Right anterior canal and left posterior canal
2. Left anterior and right posterior
3. Two horizontal canals function together in one plane

When the head is held erect and slightly tilted forwards to about 30°, then the horizontal canals are exactly horizontal. In this position, the anterior canal is directed forwards and 45° outwards from the mid-vertical plane. The posterior canal is directed backwards and 45° outwards from the midline.

The three semicircular canals open into the utricle through 5 openings. One opening is common for superior and posterior canals. The part where each canal opens into the utricle is enlarged and this part is called **ampulla**. The

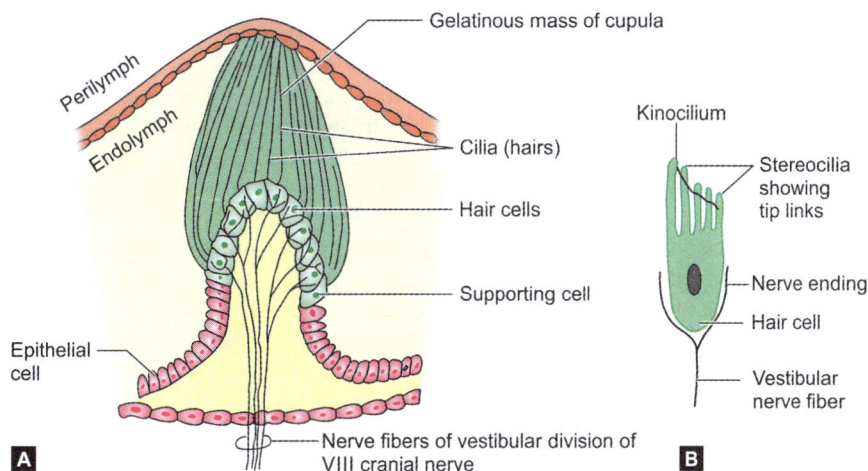

Figs. 89.1A and B: (A) Structure of crista ampullaris; (B) Structure of a hair cell.

ampulla contains the sense organ of semicircular canal, the **crista ampullaris**. The semicircular canals respond to **angular acceleration** or rotational movement.

Crista Ampullaris

The sense organ in the semicircular canal is crista ampullaris **(Figs. 89.1A and B)**. Both sensory cells and supporting cells are seen in the sense organ. The sensory cells are ciliated columnar cells and the hairs or the cilia project into a gelatinous material called **cupula**. The cupula divides the ampulla into two compartments by forming a movable partition. The cavity of ampulla contains endolymph.

Each sensory cell or hair cell has 60-100 hairs or cilia, of which, one hair is long and is called **kinocilium**. The other cilia are known as **stereocilia**. The kinocilium is present on one side of the ampulla. Stimulus for the sensory cell in angular movement, which in turn moves the hair of the sensory cell. Bending of the stereocilia towards kinocilium produces a depolarizing receptor potential and the frequency of discharge in the afferent nerve fiber increases. Bending of stereocilia away from the kinocilium produces a hyperpolarizing effect or inhibition. In the horizontal canals, the kinocilia are located towards the utricular side. So bending of cupula towards utricle stimulates the hair cells. In the anterior and posterior canals, the kinocilia are located away from the utricle. Therefore, in these canals, bending of cupula away from the utricle leads to stimulation of the hair cells. The bases of the hair cells or sensory cells are in close contact with the afferent fibers of the vestibular division of the VIII cranial nerve.

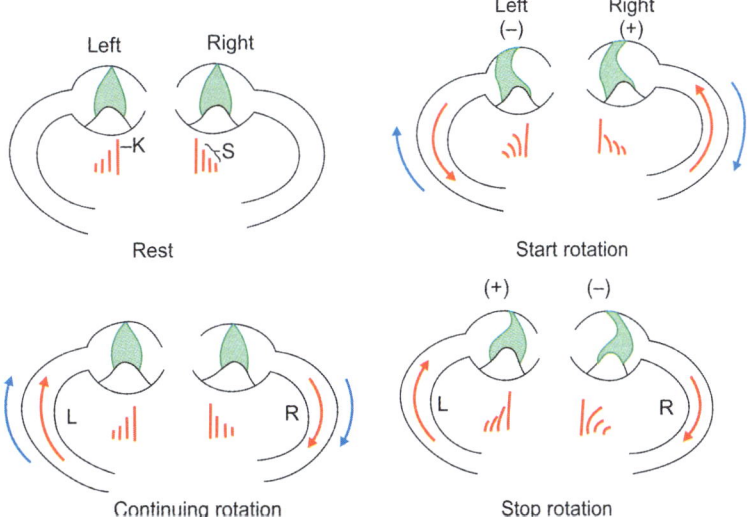

Fig. 89.2: Mechanism of stimulation of horizontal semicircular canals when the head rotates to the right in the horizontal plane. Blue arrows indicate the direction of movement of head and red arrows indicate the direction of movement of endolymph. In horizontal canals, kinocilia are towards the utricle and bending of stereocilia towards the kinocilium produces depolarization denoted by (+) sign and bending of stereocilia away from kinocilium produces hyperpolarization as denoted by (–) sign.
(K: kinocilium; S: stereocilia).

Mechanism of Stimulation of Crista Ampullaris

Only angular acceleration or rotatory movement can cause movement in semicircular canal and can stimulate the crista ampullaris. In an angular acceleration, one **synergistic pair** of canals will be functioning maximally. Depending on the plane on which rotation is occurring, one pair is maximally stimulated. In any rotatory movement, stimulation occurs at the beginning and end of rotation. In any pair of canal functioning, there will be increased firing on one side and decreased firing on the opposite side. *This forms the basis for the interpretation of direction of movement and the rate of firing determines the rate of acceleration.*

There is bending of hair and stimulation of the receptor cells only at the beginning and at the end of rotation. At the start of rotational acceleration, the endolymph, because of its inertia is displaced in a direction opposite to the direction of rotation. The fluid pushes on the cupula, thereby bending the cilia of the hair cells. When a constant speed of rotation is reached, the fluid in the semicircular canals moves at the same rate as the body is moving and the cupula swings back to the original upright position. When rotation is stopped, deceleration produces displacement of endolymph in the direction of rotation since the fluid continues to move and cupula bends in the opposite direction, i.e., in the direction of rotation. Thus, bending of cupula in one direction produces depolarization of hair cells and increased impulse transmission through the afferent nerve, whereas movement in the opposite direction produces hyperpolarization and inhibits afferent neuronal activity. Thus, stimulation of afferent nerve occurs only at the beginning or at the end of rotation depending on whether the hair cell is depolarized or hyperpolarized and not during rotation (**Fig. 89.2**).

Utricle and Saccule

The sense organ in utricle and saccule is called **macula or otolith organ**. The receptors are stimulated by linear acceleration and gravitational pull. Macula is about 2 mm in diameter and is lined by sensory cells and supporting cells. A gelatinous material covers the macula which contains small dust-like particles made up of calcium carbonate crystals combined with a matrix protein called **otoconia or ear dust** (**Figs. 89.3A and B**). Average size of otoconia is 10 micrometers. Hence, macula is also known as otolith organ.

Mechanism of Stimulation of Macula

Gravitational pull causes the otoconia to settle down and press on the hair cells leading to bending of the hair. Bending of the hair in one direction is excitatory and in the opposite direction is inhibitory. In the utricle, macula is placed horizontally with the hair projecting vertically up; and in the saccule, macula is placed vertically with the hair projecting horizontally when the head is held erect. Macular receptors are **static receptors** and are continuously stimulated by gravitational forces. When the head is held erect, in the normal resting position there is a particular pattern of firing from both macula, i.e., in the saccule, as well as in the utricle. A tilt of even half a degree in the vertical direction can cause change in the normal pattern of firing from the macula, i.e., the receptor is very sensitive. Normally, utricular hair cells signal horizontal acceleration and saccule signals vertical acceleration.

Since the macula of utricle is oriented horizontally, its hair cells respond to horizontally directed linear acceleration, e.g., travelling in a car.

The macula of the saccule is oriented vertically. So its hair cells are stimulated by vertically directed linear acceleration, e.g., travelling in a lift.

Electrical Responses in the Hair Cells

A hair bundle projects from the apical end of each hair cell in the inner ear. The hairs are called stereocilia and along an axis towards the kinocilium the stereocilia increase progressively in height (The kinocilium is not present in the cochlear hair cells in adults). Stereocilia about 30 to 150 in number are found in all hair cells in the inner ear. The mechanism of stimulation is also the same. The processes of the hair cells project into the endolymph.

Very fine processes called tip links (*refer* **Fig. 89.1A**) tie the tip of each stereocilium to the side of its higher neighbor. Mechanically sensitive cation channels are present at the junction of each tip link with its taller neighbor (**Fig. 89.4A**). When the shorter stereocilia are pushed towards the taller ones, the cation channel opens. K^+ and Ca^{2+} from the endolymph enter the stereocilium via the cation channel and induce depolarization (**Fig. 89.4B**). Depolarization of the hair cells causes them to release an excitatory neurotransmitter, glutamate, which generates depolarization of the associated afferent neuron. When the hairs move back to the resting state the cation channel closes.

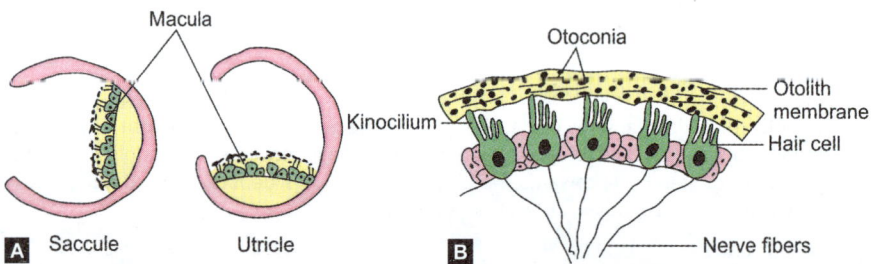

Figs. 89.3A and B: (A) Position of macula in saccule (vertically placed) and utricle (horizontally placed); (B) Structure of macula.

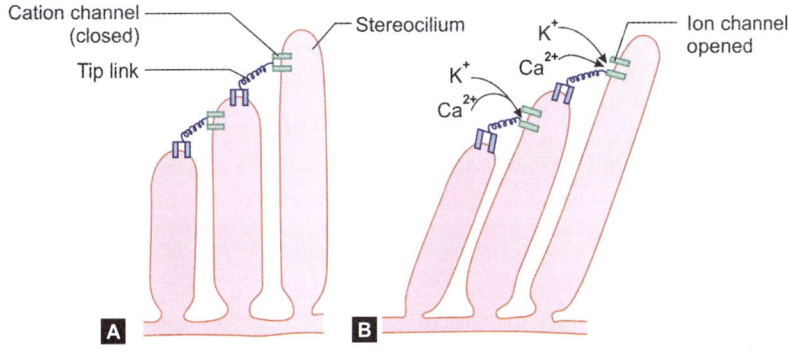

Figs. 89.4A and B: Mechanism of depolarization of hair cells: (A) Resting state where the cation channels in the stereocilia are closed; (B) When a stereocilium is pushed towards a taller one, the tip link is stretched and opens a cation channel in its taller neighbor. Ca^{2+} and K^+ enters the cells and depolarizes the hair cell. When the hairs return to the resting position the tip links closes the channel.

VESTIBULAR PATHWAY

First order neuron in vestibular pathway is situated in the **vestibular ganglion or Scarpa's ganglion**. The central process of the neuron enters the brainstem and majority of fibers end in the **vestibular nuclear complex** where these fibers synapse with the second order neurons here. A few fibers just pass through the vestibular nucleus without relay and end in the **flocculonodular lobe** of cerebellum.

The vestibular nuclei receive afferent fibers from inner ear and deep cerebellar nuclei.

Vestibular nuclear complex is composed of the following nuclei:
- Medial vestibular nucleus
- Inferior vestibular nucleus
- Lateral vestibular nucleus or Deiters' nucleus
- Superior vestibular nucleus

All the vestibular nuclei (superior, inferior, medial and lateral) function as a single unit **(Fig. 89.5)**.
- Majority of fibers from the vestibular nuclei pass through the inferior cerebellar peduncle as the **vestibulo-fastigial tract** to the flocculonodular lobe of cerebellum.
- **Vestibulo-reticular fibers** from the vestibular nuclei go to the reticular formation.
- Some of the fibers arising from the superior and medial divisions of the vestibular nucleus ascend up as the **medial longitudinal bundle** and end in the motor nuclei that control eye movements, i.e., 3rd, 4th and 6th cranial nerve nuclei. The afferent fibers to superior and medial vestibular nuclei come from the semicircular canals.
- The **vestibulo-thalamo-cortical fibers** go up along with medial lemniscal fibers to end in the posteroventral nucleus of thalamus. From here, fibers go to the equilibrium appreciation area in parietal lobe deep to Sylvian fissure and also extend into the temporal area **(Fig. 89.5)**. The vestibular apparatus thus provides us with conscious senses of head tilt and head rotation.
- **Vestibulospinal tract** descends down in the spinal cord and ends in anterior horn cells of different segments of spinal cord. This pathway is responsible for tonic labyrinthine reflexes. *The neurons of the lateral vestibular nucleus give rise to the axons that form the vestibulospinal tract* which is mainly an **uncrossed** tract.

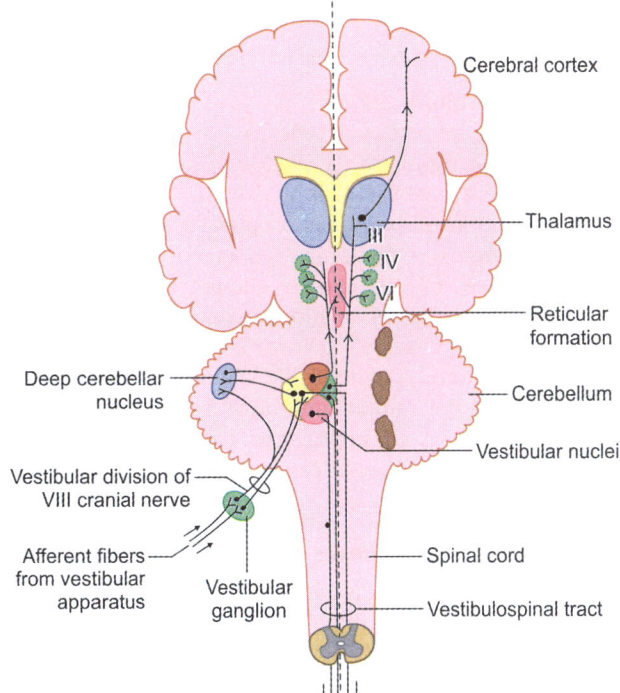

Fig. 89.5: Connections of vestibular apparatus in the central nervous system.

The afferents to the lateral vestibular nucleus are mainly from utricle and saccule.

Majority of the efferent fibers end in interneurons of the anterior horn of spinal cord, some end in the α-motor neurons supplying essentially extensor group of muscles. Some of the fibers end in the γ-motor neurons. The inner ear and cerebellum through this tract facilitate the activity of extensor group of muscles and inhibit the activity of flexor muscles in order to maintain the balance of the body.

MECHANISM OF CONTROL OF EQUILIBRIUM

The utricle and saccule play an important role to maintain static equilibrium and equilibrium during linear acceleration, whereas semicircular canals play a role in the maintenance of equilibrium in angular acceleration and rotational movement. A particular pattern of firing is seen from the utricle and saccule continuously depending on the pattern of posture. Gravitational pull on otoconia in different postures is different and hence firing of impulses is of different patterns. This plays an important role in maintaining the reflex tonic contraction of different groups of muscles for maintaining different postures. So, for static equilibrium, saccule and utricle are very important and also to maintain the posture during linear acceleration.

In rotational movement or angular acceleration, i.e., in changes in the direction of movement the semicircular canals are stimulated. We do not fall during rotational movement or angular acceleration because of reflex muscle contractions occurring immediately. Vestibular apparatus is concerned mainly with the reflex adjustments in posture and eye movements. These reflexes are collectively called **vestibular reflexes**.

Vestibular Reflexes

- Tonic labyrinthine reflexes
- Phasic postural vestibular reflexes
- Labyrinthine righting reflexes
- Labyrinthine placing reactions
- Visual fixation reflex and reflex optical movements

Even though the vestibular reflexes operate in intact animals, these reflexes can be elicited more clearly in experimental animals by ablation studies. This is because in the intact animal, these reflexes are masked and complicated by voluntary motor activity. Tonic labyrinthine reflexes are best studied in decerebrate animal where a mid-collicular section is made in the brain stem. Labyrinthine righting reflexes are studied in decorticate animal where the cerebral cortex alone is removed.

Tonic Labyrinthine Reflexes

Tonic labyrinthine reflex is usually elicited in a decerebrate animal placed in the supine position. Maximum tone is seen in the antigravity (extensor) muscles of its limbs. If the head of the animal is dorsiflexed, it shows extension of all the four limbs. Afferents for tonic labyrinthine reflexes originate in the otolith organs. Information reaches the vestibular and reticular nuclei in brain stem. Efferents travel in the vestibulospinal and reticulospinal tracts to the motor neurons in the spinal cord.

Phasic Postural Vestibular Reflexes

Afferents for phasic postural vestibular reflexes originate in the semicircular canals.

Labyrinthine Righting Reflex

Labyrinthine righting reflex is elicited in a decorticate animal. If the head is turned to one side, the animal tends to assume the upright posture. The stimulus for the reflex is tilting of the head, which stimulates the otolith organs. The response is compensatory contraction of the neck muscles to keep the head erect. Stretch of the muscles of neck causes reflex contraction of muscles which brings the animal to the upright posture. These reflexes are mainly integrated in the nuclei of midbrain. In the intact animal, the pressure receptors which are stimulated on the side which is in contact with the floor and visual information also contribute to righting reflex.

Visual Reflex (Vestibulo-ocular Reflex)

The **vestibulo-ocular reflex (VOR)** occurs when the eye is fixed on a target and the head moves suddenly. The direction of head movement is sensed by the semicircular canals. Afferent impulses from semicircular canals relay in the vestibular nuclei. Second order neurons project from vestibular nuclei to the oculomotor nuclei through medial longitudinal bundle. The third order neuron projects from the oculomotor nuclei to the extraocular muscles and activate corrective movements of the eye in the opposite direction. This prevents blurring of vision during head movement. Thus, vestibulo-ocular reflex helps in the stabilization of the foveal image.

The characteristic jerky movement of the eye observed at the start and end of a period of rotation is called **nystagmus**. It is actually a reflex that maintains visual fixation on stationary points while the body rotates. If the head rotates to the left, eyes move at the same rate to the right so that the retinal image remains constant. This slow movement of the eye forms the **slow vestibular component** of nystagmus seen during head movement. However, if the rotation exceeds 60°, rapid movement of the eyes occurs in the same direction in which rotation of head is occurring. This rapid movement of the eye is called saccadic movement and it forms the **fast saccadic component** of vestibular nystagmus. This movement leads to fixation of eyes on a new object. *Thus, in vestibulo-ocular reflex, the nystagmus consists of slow movement of eyeballs alternating with a rapid movement in the opposite direction.* Only the slow component is attributable to information originating from the vestibular apparatus. The rapid component depends on visual information and is integrated in visual centers like superior colliculi. Studying the pattern of nystagmus can be used as a diagnostic indicator of the integrity of the vestibular system. Nystagmus is seen at rest in patients with lesions of brain stem, damage to semicircular canals or after damage to the flocculonodular lobe of cerebellum.

> **Vestibular nystagmus** is jerky movement of eyeball to fix a point (gaze fixation). This is due to reflex movement of eyeball due to stimulation of vestibular apparatus. Nystagmus in cerebellar lesion is due to incoordination. Vestibular nystagmus can be elicited clinically, and this test is used as a clinical test to assess vestibular function.

FUNCTIONS OF VESTIBULAR APPARATUS

- Vestibular apparatus plays an important role in the maintenance of muscle tone, posture and equilibrium. The medial vestibulospinal tract controls the antigravity muscles of neck and upper limbs while the lateral vestibulospinal tract controls the muscles of trunk and lower limbs.
- It sends information to the higher centers about the position and rotation of the head so that corrective measures can be taken to maintain equilibrium.

- Macula in the utricle and saccule detect linear acceleration; the utricle is responsible for detecting horizontal acceleration while the saccule detects vertical acceleration. Thus maculae help in detecting orientation of head with respect to gravity and helps in the maintenance of static equilibrium.
- The crista ampullaris of the semicircular canals detect angular acceleration (head rotation). This enables the body to take corrective measures before a particular movement can throw the body off balance. In other words, the semicircular canals predict that disequilibrium is going to occur when a person is rapidly turning to one side and thereby causes the equilibrium centers to make appropriate anticipatory preventive adjustments. This is mainly due to the connection of vestibular apparatus with the flocculonodular lobe of cerebellum.

❖ Through the vestibular righting reflex it maintains the erect position of head. Tilting of the head stimulates the otolith organs which lead to compensatory contraction of the neck muscles to keep the head erect.

❖ It also adjusts the relative position of head to that of the trunk and limbs. When the head moves, the vestibular apparatus readjusts the posture to stabilize it against gravity through the tonic labyrinthine reflexes.

❖ The vestibulo-ocular reflex helps to keep visual fixation unchanged. This is a function of semicircular canal. As the head rotates in a particular direction, the eye slowly moves in the opposite direction to keep visual fixation unchanged (refer vestibular nystagmus). This reflex is transmitted through the vestibular nuclei and the medial longitudinal fasciculus to the oculomotor nuclei.

❖ The vestibular apparatus also provides us with conscious senses of head tilt and head rotation. This information is necessary for orientation in space. This is enabled by the vestibulo-thalamo-cortical fibers which reach the cerebral cortex after relaying in the ventrolateral and ventroposterior thalamic nuclei.

■ VESTIBULAR FUNCTION TESTS

Tests for Semicircular Canals

The functional integrity of the semicircular canals is tested clinically by eliciting the vestibulo-ocular reflex. It is elicited by two ways:
1. Post-rotatory nystagmus test
2. Caloric test

Post-rotatory Nystagmus Test or Barany Test

The subject is seated in the Barany chair and the chair can be rotated **(Fig. 89.6)**. Each pair of semicircular canals can be stimulated separately by tilting the head at different positions. For example, if the head is tilted at 30°, the horizontal canals are stimulated maximally. The chair is rotated 10 times in 20 seconds and then abruptly stopped. Vestibulo-ocular reflex forms the basis of vestibular function tests.

Nystagmus is seen at the beginning and at the end of rotation. It is the post-rotational nystagmus that is usually

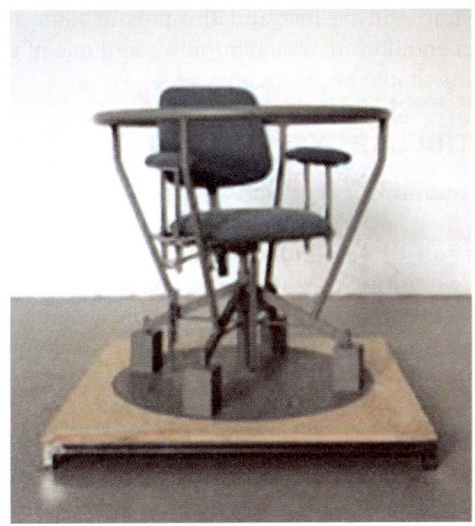

Fig. 89.6: Barany chair.

studied. Rate, duration and direction of nystagmus is studied and compared with the standard nystagmus pattern recorded from a normal individual. This is called **Barany test** or post-rotatory nystagmus test. Post-rotatory nystagmus occurs as the endolymph in the semicircular canals continues to flow due to inertia even after rotation has stopped.

Caloric Test or Ice Water Test

Warm (40°C) or cold (30°C) saline is instilled into the external auditory canal to stimulate the semicircular canals (SCC).

The temperature difference sets up convection currents in the endolymph with consequent motion of the cupula of the semicircular canals resulting in nystagmus. The integrity of the SCC can be studied by observing the pattern of nystagmus. Irrigation of auditory canal with warm saline results in nystagmus to the same side and irrigation with cold saline results in caloric nystagmus to the opposite side. This test is usually associated with giddiness, nausea, vomiting, hypotension, etc. When the ear canal is irrigated for the treatment of ear infections, it is important that the fluid used should be at the body temperature. Otherwise, the above symptoms are likely to occur.

Test for Utricle and Saccule

Balancing Test

Orientation in space depends on four inputs:
1. Vestibular input from vestibular apparatus through vestibular pathway.
2. Proprioceptive or kinesthetic sensation through dorsal column pathway.
3. Non-uniformity of pressure-touch system through dorsal column.
4. Visual impulses through visual pathway.

All these inputs are synthesized in the cortex into one's orientation in space. Out of the above four pathways, if two are disrupted, orientation becomes defective. If vestibular pathway alone is lost, the moment he closes the eyes, equilibrium will be lost and the person falls down. To maintain equilibrium, visual impulses and one of the other two inputs should be present.

VESTIBULAR DYSFUNCTION

Inflammation, local infection, fluid imbalance in the canal system and all other conditions that cause excessive stimulation of vestibular apparatus leads to vertigo, nausea, vomiting, dizziness and sometimes nystagmus. **Vertigo** is the sensation of rotation, in the absence of actual rotation and is the prominent symptom in labyrinthine inflammation.

Meniere's Disease

Vestibular dysfunction with progressive hearing loss is **Meniere's disease**. Here, there is abnormal distension of the membranous labyrinth due to increase in endolymph volume.

The disease is associated with attacks of dizziness, vertigo and vestibular nystagmus which are frequently accompanied by nausea and vomiting. There is also loss of sensitivity to low frequency sounds. Similar condition is seen following long-term streptomycin therapy.

Motion Sickness or Sea Sickness

Motion sickness or sea sickness is due to excessive stimulation of vestibular apparatus during travelling, especially in ship. There will be vertigo, headache, disorientation, and variation in blood pressure, sweating, nausea and vomiting. Motion sickness is actually due to abnormal side-to-side movement and forward movement, i.e., simultaneous movement in two accelerations, leading to sea sickness. In some people (who are extremely sensitive) even travelling in bus or swimming produces nausea, vertigo, vomiting and dizziness. Motion sickness is due to reflexes mediated via the vestibular connections in the brainstem and flocculonodular lobe of cerebellum. It is seen that surgical removal of flocculonodular lobe eliminates motion sickness. There is also a conflict in visual and vestibular signals. Closing the eyes while travelling might help in reducing the symptoms of motion sickness.

Treatment: Suppression of nausea with antiemetic drugs.

EFFECTS OF REMOVAL OF VESTIBULAR APPARATUS

Effects of Unilateral Labyrinthectomy

Effects are due to firing of impulses from one side alone. Complex postural changes with skew deviation of eye occur in this condition. There may be ataxia, nausea, vomiting and dizziness, which become more during movement. In unilateral labyrinthectomy, human beings learn to adapt slowly to one-side information.

Bilateral Labyrinthectomy

The person can lead an almost normal life if his visual pathway and dorsal column pathway are normal. But if he is under water while swimming, vision is impaired and since the pressure is equal all over the body, there will be no orientation of whether he is ascending or descending in water, i.e., he has no idea about his position in space.

MULTIPLE CHOICE QUESTIONS

1. **Semicircular canals are stimulated by:**
   a. Rotational acceleration
   b. Vertical acceleration
   c. Horizontal acceleration
   d. Gravity

2. **The rotational movement of head (angular acceleration) causes effective stimulation of the receptors in:**
   a. Utricle and saccule
   b. Organ of Corti
   c. Semicircular canals
   d. Middle ear cavity

3. **Utricle and saccule is stimulated by:**
   a. Gravity
   b. Rotational movement
   c. Angular acceleration
   d. Sound

4. **Sense organ of balance or equilibrium is:**
   a. Vestibular apparatus
   b. Organ of Corti
   c. Cerebellum
   d. Middle ear

5. **Information about linear acceleration is provided by:**
   a. Utricle and saccule
   b. Organ of Corti
   c. Semicircular canals
   d. Middle ear cavity

6. **Information regarding vertical acceleration is provided by:**
   a. Utricle
   b. Saccule
   c. Organ of Corti
   d. Semicircular canal

7. **Information: regarding horizontal acceleration is provided by:**
   a. Utricle
   b. Saccule
   c. Organ of Corti
   d. Semicircular canal

ANSWERS

1. a   2. c   3. a   4. a   5. a
6. b   7. a

Posture and Equilibrium

CHAPTER 90

LEARNING OBJECTIVES
- Explain the mechanism of maintenance of muscle tone, posture and equilibrium
- Describe the righting reflexes
- Differentiate between decerebrate and decorticate preparations

INTRODUCTION

PY10.4: Describe and discuss motor tracts, mechanism of maintenance of tone, control of body movements, posture and equilibrium and vestibular apparatus.

Posture is the attitude taken by the body in any particular situation like standing, sitting, walking, running, etc. Even during movement, there is a continuously changing posture. Every movement starts in one posture and ends in another posture. The basis of posture is the ability to keep certain groups of muscles in sustained contraction. Variation in the degree of contraction and tone in different groups of muscles decides the posture of the individual. The muscles which maintain posture should have the ability to remain contracted for long periods. There should not be fatigue and the energy expenditure should be minimal for maintaining a particular posture. This is achieved by two factors:
1. Posture-maintaining muscles contain more of **red muscle** fibers, which are slowly contracting and not easily fatigued. All muscles in the body are a mixture of red and pale (white) muscles. Muscles of hand, eye, etc., have a preponderance of white muscle fibers which are easily fatigued.
2. Only a fraction of the muscle fibers are active at any given time due to **asynchronous contraction**.

The basic reflex operating in maintaining posture is stretch reflex and the receptor involved is the muscle spindle. Any posture can be voluntarily assumed, but maintenance of posture is reflexly done. The degree of contraction of any muscle depends on the degree of firing from α-motor neuron. Motor neuron activity is influenced by pyramidal and extrapyramidal tracts ending directly on α-motor neuron or through γ-motor neurons or interneurons.

Maintenance of Posture

Decision for a particular posture occur in the cerebral cortex, planning and programming occur in the basal ganglia and cerebellum, and the information comes down through the pyramidal tract to the motor neurons supplying the muscles involved. In the standing posture, the center of gravity is acting in such a way that the body tends to fall forwards. So, the antigravity muscles like extensors of neck, back, hip, legs, etc., should be in a continuously contracted state. In the normal standing posture of humans, the upper limbs are slightly flexed, and the *flexor group of muscles are the antigravity muscles in upper limb*. The vestibular receptors, proprioceptors, visual receptors, cutaneous receptors, etc., play important role in maintaining posture. In the standing posture, impulses coming through vestibulospinal tract and reticulospinal tract also play an important role. If there is a change in the position of head while standing, the receptors in the utricle and saccule are stimulated and some group of muscles contract and the head is held erect or in the desired posture. If an animal is pushed to one side, the limbs of that side extend or there will be a hopping movement in order to maintain the posture.

POSTURAL REFLEXES

A number of reflexes take part in maintaining posture and equilibrium and these reflexes are called **postural reflexes**. In the **reflex arc** for postural reflexes, the afferents come from eyes, vestibular apparatus and proprioceptors. Center is in the cerebral cortex, brainstem or spinal cord **(Table 90.1)**. Efferents pass through α-motor neurons to skeletal muscles. Postural reflexes are classified into two groups:
1. Tonic or static postural reflexes
2. Dynamic or phasic postural reflexes

Static or Tonic Reflexes

Static reflexes are continuously acting and are called **attitudinal reflexes**. It involves sustained contraction of muscles due to the effect of gravity. They are:
- Antigravity muscle tone
- Positive supporting reaction

Table 90.1: Postural reflexes and their centers.

Postural reflex	Center
Muscle tone (stretch reflex)	Spinal cord
Positive supporting reaction	Spinal cord
Crossed extensor reflex	Spinal cord
Tonic labyrinthine reflexes	Medulla
Tonic neck reflexes	Medulla
Righting reflexes	Midbrain (red nucleus)
Hopping and placing reaction	Cerebral cortex
Visual righting reflex	Calcarine (visual) cortex

- Tonic labyrinthine or tonic vestibular reflexes
- Tonic neck reflexes

Dynamic Reflexes or Phasic Reflexes

Dynamic reflexes or phasic reflexes which involve transient movements are of two types:
1. Phasic postural reflexes:
   - Phasic postural stretch reflexes
   - Phasic postural labyrinthine reflexes
2. Righting reflexes:
   - Labyrinthine righting reflex
   - Neck righting reflex
   - Body on head righting reflex
   - Body on body righting reflex
   - Visual righting reflex

Except for visual righting reflex, the center for the other four righting reflexes is the **red nucleus** in the midbrain.

Other righting reflexes are:
- Placing reaction
- Hopping reaction

In placing and hopping reaction, cerebral cortex is also involved.

Experimental Study of Postural Reflexes

Even though, postural reflexes operate in intact animals and human beings, these reflexes can be studied more clearly by making sections in the brain at various levels in experimental animals. This is because in the intact animal these reflexes are masked and complicated by voluntary motor activity. Different types of experimental preparations are:
1. Section just below medulla oblongata—spinal animal
2. Mid-collicular section—decerebrate animal
3. Section just above the midbrain—midbrain animal
4. Section above the level of thalamus—thalamic animal
5. Above basal ganglia or after removal of cortex—decorticate preparation.

Spinal Animal

The entire spinal cord is intact in spinal animal. Immediately following section the animal goes into a stage of **spinal shock** where complete flaccid paralysis occurs. Slowly the spinal cord neurons regain excitability and may become hyperirritable.

The muscle tone can be maintained, but due to hyperirritability may be slightly more as in UMN lesion. The animal cannot maintain the standing posture even though the muscle tone has returned.

Segmental stretch reflexes can be elicited in the stage of **reflex activity**. Spinal cord is able to maintain muscle tone, but there will be no voluntary activity. Stretch reflex, withdrawal reflex, crossed extensor reflex, positive supporting reaction and mass reflex will be present. Superficial reflexes will be absent since the pathway involves cerebral cortex.

Positive Supporting Reaction

Application of pressure on the foot of spinal animal using a finger leads to extension of limbs as solid pillars by reflex contraction of muscles to resist gravity and to support the body. This is because of simultaneous reflex contraction of both extensors and flexors of a limb. This is **positive supporting reaction**. The foot follows the fingers as it is withdrawn and hence this is also called **magnet reaction**. If pressure is applied on all the four limbs, the animal can assume standing posture for a minute or two on the basis of positive supporting reaction. All righting reflexes will be absent in the spinal animal.

Decerebrate Animal

When a **mid-collicular section** (section between superior and inferior colliculi) is made the animal is referred to as decerebrate animal. Extensive **rigidity** is seen in all the muscles especially in the **extensor group** of muscles. The animal assumes a characteristic posture. Maximum rigidity is seen in the antigravity muscles. The rigidity is called **decerebrate rigidity**. Decerebrate rigidity is a **release phenomenon**. The impulses from basal ganglia and cortex to the caudal inhibitory area of reticular formation are removed in decerebrate animal. As a result, there will be over activity of the facilitatory area leading to increased stimulation of γ-motor neurons and increase in the muscle tone. This leads to the rigidity.

All reflexes elicited in the spinal animal can be elicited in the decerebrate preparation also. In addition, tonic labyrinthine and tonic neck reflexes are present, but *all the righting reflexes will be absent*. The animal can maintain the standing posture. But if it is pushed to one side it falls down, which denotes that righting reflexes are absent. The animal cannot stand up voluntarily.

Tonic Labyrinthine Reflexes

Variation in the degree of tone with change in position seen in decerebrate animal is due to **tonic labyrinthine reflexes**. It includes reflexes produced in response to changes in the position of head in the horizontal plane.
- *Stimulus*: Gravity
- *Receptors*: Hair cells in the otolith organ
- *Afferents*: Vestibular division of VIII cranial nerve
- *Center*: Vestibular nucleus
- *Efferents*: Vestibulospinal and reticulospinal tracts
- *Response*: Contraction of extensors of limbs.

Tonic Neck Reflexes or Attitudinal Reflexes

Tonic neck reflexes can be elicited in a decerebrate animal. If the otolith organ is removed from the animal and if the head is bent, tonic neck reflexes can be observed. If the head is turned to one side, the jaw limbs extend and the vertex limb flex. If the head is bent forwards, there is flexion of upper limbs and extension of lower limbs putting the animal into a position of **looking under the shelf**. If the head is pushed backwards, there is extension of upper limbs and flexion of lower limbs. This gives the animal an attitude of **looking over a shelf**. If the lower cervical vertebra is pressed anteriorly, all the limbs flex putting the animal into an attitude of **crawling into a hole**. All the above reflexes together form **attitudinal reflexes**. It is because moving the neck in different directions causes stretch of the neck muscles which causes the change in the attitude of the animal.

Midbrain Animal

Section is made above the level of midbrain. The important nuclei are intact. Integration of righting reflexes occurs in the upper part of midbrain and so in the midbrain animal righting reflexes will be present except visual righting reflex. If the animal is pushed to one side, it does not fall down because some *righting reflexes are present*. Soon after the section, there will be increased rigidity which will be manifested only when the animal is at rest. The rigidity is not that marked as in decerebrate animal. It can assume standing posture and can walk reflexly. But voluntary or purposeful walking is not possible. Temperature regulation is not possible in midbrain animal because hypothalamus is above the level of section.

Righting Reflexes

Labyrinthine Righting Reflex

In whatever position the animal is kept it tries to keep its head erect. It is due to information arising from vestibular apparatus which causes contraction of muscles which keep the head erect. This is labyrinthine righting reflex.

Body-on-Head Righting Reflex

If labyrinthectomy is done, then also if the animal is laid on one side it keeps its head erect. This is due to stimulation of cutaneous receptors which corrects the position of the head. This is body-on-head righting reflex.

Neck Righting Reflex

When the head is held erect, there is stretch of muscles on one side of the neck. The neck righting reflexes operate to correct the body and the body comes to the erect posture. This is neck righting reflex.

Body-on-Body Righting Reflex

If the above animal is prevented from correcting its head, then also the body tries to come to the erect posture. This is body-on-body righting reflex.

Visual Righting Reflex

In animals, visual information can correct the posture. These reflexes are called visual righting reflexes. This reflex is absent in midbrain animal because calcarine cortex is not intact in midbrain animal.

Table 90.2: Differences between decerebrate and decorticate preparations.

Decerebrate preparation	Decorticate preparation
Transection is made in between the superior and inferior colliculi	Cerebral cortex is removed from the rest of the brain
Extensive extensor rigidity and decerebrate posture	Moderate rigidity of antigravity muscles as in hemiplegia
Righting reflexes absent	Righting reflexes present
Temperature regulation absent	Temperature regulation normal
Only a standing posture can be maintained	Can stand and walk reflexly but, placing and hopping reactions are absent

Hopping Reaction

If an animal is pushed to one side, the limbs of that side extend. This may be due to stretch reflex. In an intact animal, not only extension of limb occurs but the animal goes into a series of jumping reactions so that posture is maintained. The cerebral cortex should be intact for hopping reaction. In a midbrain animal, the extension of limb is seen, but there is no hopping reaction.

Placing Reaction

If an intact animal is made to fall, the limbs spread out as if to place the body on the floor. Visual reflexes should be intact and the cortex is very essential for this reaction. If the cortex is intact, even a blindfolded cat can show this reaction.

Thalamic Preparation

Postural pattern and reflexes are almost same as that of midbrain animal. Here, temperature regulation and autonomic functions are normal because thalamus and hypothalamus are intact. So it is difficult to maintain a midbrain animal, but easy to maintain a thalamic preparation.

Decorticate Preparation

Only cortex is removed, basal ganglia are intact and so rigidity is less than that of decerebrate animal. Postural reactions which are absent in decorticate animal are visual righting reflex, placing and hopping reactions **(Table 90.2)**.

■ MULTIPLE CHOICE QUESTIONS

1. The maintenance of posture in a normal human being depends on:
    a. Integrity of reflex arc
    b. Muscle power
    c. Type of muscle fibers
    d. Joint movements in physiological range
2. The pathway that connects the vestibulo-cochlear nuclei with the III, IV and VI cranial nerve nuclei is:
    a. Medial lemniscus
    b. Spinal lemniscus
    c. Medial longitudinal fasciculus
    d. Lateral lemniscus

3. The basic postural reflex is:
   a. Crossed extensor reflex
   b. Golgi tendon reflex
   c. Stretch reflex
   d. Positive supporting reflex

4. All the following statements are true, *except*:
   a. Decorticate rigidity is greater than decerebrate rigidity
   b. Righting reflexes are absent in decerebrate animal
   c. Visual righting reflex is present in a thalamic preparation
   d. Decorticate rigidity is seen only when the animal is at rest

5. Decerebrate animal results from the following experimental procedure:
   a. Removal of the cerebrum
   b. Transection at the upper border of midbrain
   c. Intercollicular transection
   d. Section above the thalamus

6. Mid-collicular transection leads to:
   a. Decerebrate animal
   b. Decorticate animal
   c. Spinal animal
   d. Midbrain animal

ANSWERS

1. a   2. c   3. c   4. a   5. c
6. a

Cerebral Cortex

CHAPTER 91

LEARNING OBJECTIVES
- Describe the functional areas of cerebral cortex
- Explain the functions of prefrontal lobe and parietal lobe
- Discuss the lesions of prefrontal area

FUNCTIONAL ANATOMY OF CEREBRAL CORTEX

PY10.7: Describe and discuss functions of cerebral cortex, basal ganglia, thalamus, hypothalamus, cerebellum and limbic system and their abnormalities.

The cerebral hemispheres form the largest part of the brain and its functions include thinking, learning, memory and consciousness. The two hemispheres are separated by a deep midline **sagittal fissure** or the median longitudinal fissure. In the depths of the fissure, is the great white commissure, the **corpus callosum**, which connects the two cerebral hemispheres across the midline.

The surface of cerebral hemisphere is covered by a thin layer (2–4 mm thick) of gray matter called the **cerebral cortex (cerebral gray matter)** which is the most conspicuous part of the cerebral hemispheres. In order to increase the surface area of the cerebral cortex, the surface of each hemisphere is thrown into folds called **gyri (singular: gyrus)**. The gyri are separated from each other by grooves called **sulci** or fissures. The surface area of the cerebral cortex is approximately 2,200 cm² and contains about 2×10^{10} neurons. Each cerebral hemisphere is divided into lobes and each lobe is named according to the cranial bones under which they lie. The lobes are **frontal lobe, parietal lobe, temporal lobe and occipital lobe**. These lobes are separated by **central sulcus, parieto-occipital sulcus, lateral sulcus and calcarine sulcus**. Calcarine sulcus is seen on the medial aspect of the posterior part of cerebral hemisphere and it is Y-shaped. The **central sulcus** is of great importance because of the following reasons.
- The gyrus that lies anterior to the central sulcus contains the motor cells that initiate the movements of the opposite side of the body.
- Posterior to the central sulcus is the general sensory cortex that receives sensory information from the opposite side of the body.

Frontal lobe occupies the area anterior to the central sulcus and superior to the lateral sulcus. It is mainly concerned with motor functions. **Parietal lobe** (sensory in function) occupies the area posterior to the central sulcus and superior to the lateral sulcus. It extends posteriorly as far as the parieto-occipital sulcus. **Temporal lobe** concerned mainly with hearing occupies the area inferior to the lateral sulcus. The **occipital lobe** occupies a small area behind the parieto-occipital sulcus (**Fig. 91.1**) and it is concerned with vision. In addition, there is a **limbic lobe** that lies on the medial side of the cerebral cortex adjacent to the corpus callosum. Limbic lobe includes cingulate gyrus, isthmus, hippocampal gyrus and uncus.

Phylogenetically, cerebral cortex is divided into **allocortex, mesocortex and neocortex. Allocortex** or limbic cortex forms 10% of entire cortex and it includes hippocampus, dentate gyrus, uncus; and part of parahippocampal gyrus, which is concerned with olfaction. **Mesocortex** is the transitional zone between allocortex and neocortex and comprises the cingulate gyrus and the rest of the parahippocampal gyrus. The rest 90% of cerebral cortex in human brain is formed of **neocortex**. In lower animals, neocortex is not well developed. Intelligence, memory, ability to learn, speak, etc. are controlled by the neocortex.

Beneath the cerebral cortex lies the **subcortical white matter** in which is embedded masses of gray matter called subcortical nuclear masses, e.g., basal ganglia.

Cerebral Dominance

Previously, in right-handed individuals, the left cerebral hemisphere was considered as the **dominant hemisphere** as it controls the motor activities of the right hand. But the term dominant is misleading because the **non-dominant hemisphere** (right hemisphere) has equally important visuo-spatial functions. So the terms dominant and non-dominant hemispheres have been replaced by categorical and representational hemispheres, respectively. Since visual

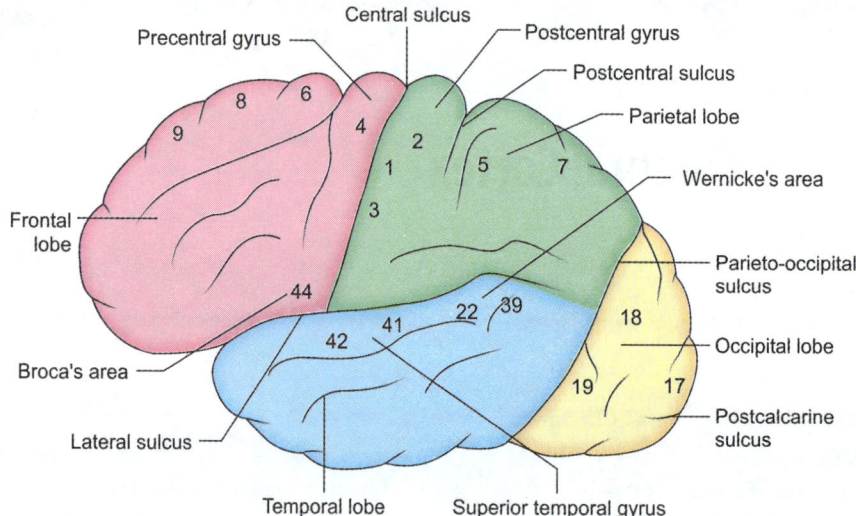

Fig. 91.1: Superolateral surface of left cerebral hemisphere showing lobes, important sulci and gyri and Brodmann's areas.

processing of written language, auditory processing of spoken language and language related motor functions like speech, reading and writing are performed by the left hemisphere in great majority of people, it is called the **categorical hemisphere**. The right hemisphere is responsible for the ability to appreciate music, stereognosis, artistic skills, etc. and it is called the **representational hemisphere (Table 91.1)**.

Histology of Cerebral Cortex

Histologically, allocortex is composed of three layers while neocortex has six layers numbered I–VI from outside to inside. Neocortex is 2–4 mm thick and the six layers are:
1. Molecular or plexiform layer
2. External granule cell layer
3. Outer pyramidal cell layer
4. Internal granule cell layer
5. Inner pyramidal cell layer
6. Multiform or polymorphic or fusiform layer.

Table 91.1: Differences between categorical and representational hemisphere.

Categorical hemisphere	Representational hemisphere
Specialized for sequential-analytic processes	Specialized for visuo-spatial relations
Concerned with language functions	Concerned with recognition of musical themes and in facial recognition
Left hemisphere in 96% of right handed individuals	Right hemisphere in 4% individuals
Left hemisphere in 70% of left handed individuals	Right hemisphere in 15% of left handed people
Lesion leads to language disorders	Lesion leads to agnosias like astereognosis
Patients are disturbed about their disability and are depressed	Patients with lesions are often unconcerned and sometimes euphoric

In the motor cortex, there is predominance of pyramidal layer when compared to granular layer and in the sensory cortex there is predominance of granule cell layer. The classical six layered structure is not found everywhere in the cerebral cortex. The areas of the cortex where the number of layers is less than six is called **allocortex**. Allocortex includes uncus, hippocampus and dentate gyrus. **Neocortex** contains all the six layers.

Cell Types in Cerebral Cortex

Four types of cells are identified in the cerebral cortex.
1. Pyramidal cells
2. Stellate or granule cells
3. Fusiform cells
4. Horizontal cells of Cajal.

Pyramidal cell has triangular cell body and these cells constitute 2/3rd of cortical neurons. They are present in layer II, III and V of neocortex. Layer V or inner pyramidal layer of primary motor area (Brodmann's area 4) contains giant pyramidal cells called **Betz cells**. Pyramidal cells with short axons are called **Martinotti cells**.

Stellate or granule cells have small cell bodies and they constitute 1/3rd of cortical neurons. Layer II and IV of neocortex contain these cells in large numbers.

Fusiform cells are few in number and have spindle-shaped cell body. Their dendrites form network in the outer layer and the axons project to sub-cortical nuclear groups. They are present in layer VI of cerebral cortex. **Horizontal cells of Cajal** are seen in the plexiform layer or molecular layer and are very few in number.

Pyramidal cells are projection cells (Golgi type I) that leave the cerebral cortex while granule cells are interneurons (Golgi type II cells) that are confined to the cortical laminae. Pyramidal cells and granule cells are excitatory in function and the neurotransmitters released are glutamate and aspartate. The rest of the cells of cortex contain inhibitory neurotransmitter GABA.

Layer I of cerebral cortex contains dense network of dendrites of pyramidal cells and axons of granule cells. Lamina II contains mainly granule cells and some small pyramidal cells. Lamina III contains predominantly medium sized pyramidal cells. Lamina IV contains predominantly granule cells. Lamina V contains predominantly large sized pyramidal cells. Layer VI contains all types of cells.

Connections of Cerebral Cortex

Beneath the gray matter of cerebral cortex lies the white matter, which is made up of fibers that originate or terminate in the cortex. The fibers are broadly classified into:
- **Projection fibers** that descend from the cerebral cortex that originates in the pyramidal cells of lamina V. This includes cortico-striate, corticobulbar and corticospinal fibers. Cortical fibers to the thalamus arise in layer VI.

    The ascending thalamocortical projection fibers are of two types: (i) Those from the specific thalamic nuclei terminate in lamina IV, while (ii) the sensory afferents from nonspecific thalamic nuclei terminate mostly in lamina I.
- Pyramidal cells of lamina II and III give rise to **association fibers and commissural fibers**. Association fibers are axons interconnecting different cortical areas of the same hemisphere. For example, those fibers connecting Wernicke's area and Broca's area; those fibers connecting the visual cortex with the frontal eye field are association fibers. Commissural fibers interconnect the two hemispheres. The major commissural pathway is the corpus callosum.

Afferent Connections of Cerebral Cortex

Afferent connections to the cerebral cortex are from the thalamus, reticular formation, basal ganglia, hypothalamus and cerebellum.

Thalamus and Reticular Formation
- Specific thalamic projection fibers
- Nonspecific thalamic projection fibers.

    Specific thalamic projection fibers carry sensory information. It includes fibers from specific nuclei and association nuclei of thalamus and they project to specific areas of cerebral cortex. The specific fibers end mainly in layers III and IV of cerebral cortex. Conduction through specific fibers is faster than in nonspecific fibers and the action dies out fast in specific projection areas.

    Nonspecific thalamocortical projection fibers go diffusely to the entire cortex and these fibers along with the nonspecific fibers from the reticular formation form the **ascending reticular activating system**. Nonspecific fibers end mainly in layers I and II of cerebral cortex. The action in the nonspecific projection areas of cortex lasts for a longer time than in specific projection areas.

Efferent Connections of Cerebral Cortex
- Pyramidal fibers
- Extrapyramidal fibers.

Pyramidal Fibers
- Corticonuclear fibers
- Corticospinal fibers:
    - Anterior corticospinal fibers
    - Lateral corticospinal fibers.

Extrapyramidal Fibers
From cortex descend down to basal ganglia, thalamus, reticular formation, red nucleus, tectal, olivary, vestibular nuclei, etc. Cortically originating extrapyramidal fibers end above the level of spinal cord. Cortically originating extrapyramidal fibers are:
- Corticostriate fibers to basal ganglia
- Corticothalamic fibers
- Corticoreticular fibers
- **Corticopontine fibers:**
    - Frontopontine fibers
    - Temperopontine fibers
    - Occipitopontine fibers
    - Parietopontine fibers

Interconnections
- Commissural fibers
- Association fibers:

Commissural fibers connect one hemisphere to the other hemisphere. Largest commissural fibers collectively form the **corpus callosum**. Association fibers connect different parts of the same hemisphere.

METHODS OF STUDY OF CEREBROCORTICAL FUNCTION
- Anatomical methods
- Physiological methods
- Pharmacological methods
- Clinical methods
- Pathological methods.

Anatomical Methods
- Macroscopic method
- Microscopic method.

    In macroscopic method, gross appearance, sulci, gyri, etc., are studied.

    In microscopic method, histology, staining characteristics of cells, correlation of structure with function, etc., are studied.

Physiological Methods
- Ablation studies
- Stimulation studies.

    In **ablation studies**, a particular area is removed or destroyed and the effect is studied.

    Stimulation study is done by electrophysiological methods. By stereotaxic surgery, an electrode can be introduced into any particular area of brain. The area is stimulated using stimulating electrodes and the potential changes are recorded using recording electrodes. A sensory nerve can be stimulated and the effect produced in the cerebral cortex can be studied and this study is called **evoked cortical potential study**.

Evoked potential study shows two responses, a primary response and a secondary response. The **primary response** is due to impulses going through specific sensory pathway to specific areas in brain. Specific areas of brain produce the primary response and have a short latent period (10 ms). First, there appears a surface positive wave, which is followed by a small negative wave. Evoked potential study is done in mapping the sensory areas.

Secondary response: This is a more diffuse wave seen after 30–50 ms after the primary response. It consists of a large and prolonged positive wave. Spread of impulses through the ascending reticular activating system (ARAS) to the cerebral cortex is responsible for this response. This is due to complex polysynaptic connections. Secondary response is obtained from specific areas of cortex and also from areas far away, i.e., it is not highly localized.

The association areas can be studied by keeping the recording electrode in one area and the stimulating electrode in another area of cerebral cortex.

Pharmacological Methods

Substances that stimulate, inhibit or block neuronal activity are used in this method.

Clinical Methods

- Infection, inflammation, hemorrhage, nutritional deficiency, injury, vascular anomalies, poisoning, etc., will help to elicit some **neurological signs** that give an idea about the functions of different areas of the cortex.
- **Plain X-ray** of skull helps to localize tumors, calcification, etc.
- **Pneumoencephalography** is a procedure in which air is introduced into the ventricles after removing cerebrospinal fluid, and plain X-rays are taken.
- **Angiography** is a technique in which a radiopaque dye is introduced into the carotid artery and then X-ray pictures are taken. Vascular anomalies like hemangioma can be detected by this method.
- **Radio uptake studies** using radioactive counters after giving radioactive substances are useful in locating tumors since the uptake is more in the tumor areas.
- **Computed axial tomography** (CAT scan) help to locate lesions. Here, the body can be studied layer-by-layer using a narrow beam of X-ray. Any abnormality in the density, structure, etc., can be detected.
- **Electroencephalography (EEG)** is done using surface electrodes. Here, total electrical activity of brain can be studied.
- **Echoencephalography** where an ultrasound generator is used. Structural anomaly can be studied.

Pathological Studies

Postmortem findings give information regarding the exact location of lesion.

FUNCTIONALLY IMPORTANT AREAS OF CEREBRAL CORTEX

Campbell in 1905 studied 20 areas in cerebral cortex. **Brodmann** described 47 areas (**see Fig. 91.1**). **Vogt** and others increased it into 200 areas. They represented the areas in alphabets. **Brodmann**, a histologist represented the cortical areas in numbers and his classification is the most accepted one. He did experiments on monkey brain and classified areas depending on the cell type, i.e., on their histological characteristics.

Sensorimotor cortex includes all those parts of the cerebral cortex that act together in the control of movement. It includes primary motor cortex, premotor cortex, somatosensory cortex and sensory association area.

Frontal Lobe Areas

- Precentral gyrus is Brodmann **area 4 or primary motor area**. Here, the body is represented upside down. The area of representation is proportional to the skill with which the part is used for fine voluntary movements. Thus, hands, fingers, face, lips, tongue, pharynx and vocal cords have large areas of representation. Area 4 is concerned with initiation of voluntary movements of the contralateral half of the body and initiation of speech. However, pharynx, vocal cords and the jaw muscles have bilateral representation. **Giant pyramidal cells** called Betz cells (in layer V of cerebral cortex) predominate in this area.
- **Supplementary motor area** is the medial extension of area 4 where a second representation of the body is seen. This area functions in association with premotor area. It is involved in programming complex motor movements. Lesions of this area produce difficulty in performing complex activities.
- A narrow strip of cortex anteriorly in area 4, inhibits motor activity and has a suppressor effect on muscle tone and this area is called area **4s** (suppressor strip).
- Anterior to area 4 is **area 6 or premotor area**. Stimulation of this area produces gross rotatory movement of body with head to the opposite side. This area helps to maintain background posture during voluntary activity. Area 6 coordinates the actions of area 4 and extrapyramidal system. Thus, skilled movements are made accurate and smooth. Lesions of area 6 lead to loss of skilled movements. Lesions involving area 6 along with area 4 produce severe symptoms of hemiplegia with spastic paralysis.
- Anterior to area 6 is **area 8**, which is also called **frontal eye field**. Stimulation of this area produces conjugate deviation of eyeballs to the opposite side and hence called frontal eye field. This area receives afferents from the occipital lobe. Efferents from area 8 go to nuclei of third, fourth and sixth cranial nerves. It is concerned with control of eye movements.
- Anterior to face area of area 4 or primary motor area is **area 44** or **motor speech area** or **Broca's area**. This area controls motor activities of speech and is present only on one side of the cerebral cortex, which is called the dominant hemisphere or categorical hemisphere. In right-handed

individuals, area 44 is in the left hemisphere. This area is closely related to the muscles involved in speech. Lesion to this area produces motor aphasia (inability to speak out words).

Anterior to areas 8 and 44, there are areas such as **9 to 14, 23, 24, 29, 32, 45, 46, and 47** on the frontal lobe. These areas together form **prefrontal area or prefrontal cortex or orbitofrontal cortex**. On the medial aspect, also there are extensions of these areas. **Area 13** is seen only on the medial aspect. Prefrontal areas control thought, memory, autonomic functions, etc.

Connections and Functions of Prefrontal Area

Afferent Connections

Prefrontal area receives afferent fibers from thalamus (dorsomedial and anterior nuclei), hypothalamus, amygdala, medial septal nucleus, etc. There is direct connection from hypothalamus and also indirect connection through mammillo-thalamic tract of Vicq-d' Azyr, which reaches areas 23 and 24 of cingulate gyrus. Nonspecific thalamic nuclei projects to prefrontal area as well.

Efferent Connections

Efferent connections from prefrontal area are to thalamus, hypothalamus, reticular formation, to cerebellum via the basal ganglia, etc.

Functions of Prefrontal Area

- Prefrontal area plays an important role in controlling the **autonomic functions** of the body due to its intimate connection with hypothalamus.
- Plays a role in the **emotional** and sexual behavior of the individual since it is intimately associated with the limbic system. Circuitous connection between thalamus and prefrontal cortex (**Papez circuit**) plays an important role in emotions.
- Plays an important role in higher **intellectual functions** like thought, memory, ability to concentrate, elaboration of thought, ability to consider the consequences of one's own motor activity, control one's behavior, i.e., self-control or a restraining effect on one's activities (cultured or polished behavior), etc.
- It is considered as the seat of intelligence since short-term memories are registered in the prefrontal cortex. It also has the ability to recall this information.

Effects of Lesion to the Prefrontal Area

Bilateral extensive damage to the prefrontal area is called **prefrontal syndrome or frontal lobe syndrome**. The effects are:
- Lack of restrain; the person starts boasting and goes on doing whatever he feels.
- Inability to plan for future, inability to concentrate and has no ideas.
- Rapidly changing moods.
- Becomes aggressive and hostile with no moral sense.
- Some people show complete indifference to every sensation, even to pain (even though they feel the pain they are not bothered about it).
- Euphoria is another feature, i.e., a false sense of well-being.
- Loss of recent memory. Memory of remote events is not lost.

Prefrontal Lobotomy or Prefrontal Leucotomy

Cutting the connection between the thalamus and the prefrontal lobe is called **prefrontal leucotomy**. This procedure was carried out in severe troublesome psychological disorders. Due to the availability of very effective drugs (tranquilizers), this procedure is not carried out nowadays to control mental illness. Connections to the prefrontal cortex are cut in terminal stages of cancer to relieve intolerable pain. Personality changes are seen and the manifestations will be that of prefrontal syndrome.

Parietal Lobe Areas

The postcentral gyrus contains **Brodmann areas 3, 1 and 2 or somatic sensory area I,** which lies immediately behind the central sulcus. All sensations are appreciated in this area and the whole body is represented in an inverted manner. Accurate localization of sensations is possible only in this area (*refer* SSA-I).

The sensory area that extends deep into the Sylvian fissure is called **somatic sensory area II**. A second representation of the body is seen here. The sensory fibers project both to SSA-I and SSA-II.

Posterior to SSA-I are the areas **5 and 7 known as sensory association area**. Critical analysis of sensations and actual understanding of sensations occur in this area.

Occipital Lobe Areas

Area 17 seen on either side of the calcarine fissure is the **primary visual area** necessary for the appreciation of visual information. **Visual association areas** are the areas 18 and 19 seen around area 17. Understanding and critical analysis of visual information occur in the visual association area. It is involved in the recognition and identification of objects in the light of past experience.

Afferents to visual cortex come from lateral geniculate body in the form of optic radiations. *Efferents* from visual cortex go to frontal eye field (area 8), superior colliculus, pretectal region, nuclei of third, fourth and sixth cranial nerves and thalamus (pulvinar).

Temporal Lobe Areas

On the superior temporal gyrus on the inferior wall of lateral fissure or Hesche's gyrus is the **primary auditory area or area 41**. Around area 41 is the **auditory association area or area 42**. Areas 20 and 21 are seen inferiorly.

At the posterior end of the lateral fissure, in the posterior part of superior temporal gyrus behind areas 41 and 42, is a very important area concerned with higher function called the **knowing area or gnostic area or sensory speech area**

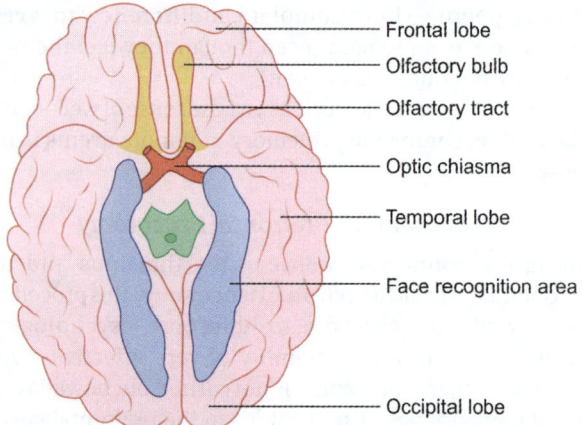

Fig. 91.2: Inferior view of the brain after removing medulla oblongata, pons and cerebellum to show the face recognition area.

or Wernicke's area (area 22). This area is well developed for language function, i.e., understanding of written and spoken speech occurs here. This area is well developed in the dominant or categorical hemisphere, which is the left one in right-handed individuals. Same area on the opposite side is well developed for understanding music, artistic talents, somatic senses, etc.

Lesion to Wernicke's area leads to **sensory aphasia**. They are not able to understand the meaning of spoken or written words. They can talk fluently but the speech does not make much sense.

Face Recognition Area

On the undersurface of brain in the inferior temporal gyrus (**area 20**), is a large area extending on to the occipital lobe responsible for face recognition. This is the face recognition area (**Fig. 91.2**). If lesion occurs in this area, the patient can recognize a person from his voice but not by seeing his face. This condition is called **prosopagnosia**, the inability to recognize faces.

Area 20 is also important for facial expressions. It is connected to the amygdala, which has an important role in emotions. Facial expression is very important in emotions.

MULTIPLE CHOICE QUESTIONS

1. Stereo anesthesia is due to lesion of:
   a. Nucleus gracilis
   b. Nucleus cuneatus
   c. Cerebral cortex
   d. Spinothalamic tract

2. Which of the following cortical layers is stimulated by the diffuse thalamocortical system?
   a. Layer II
   b. Layer III
   c. Layer IV
   d. Layer VI

3. Right and the left temporal lobes are connected by:
   a. Posterior commissure
   b. Anterior commissure
   c. Corpus callosum
   d. Habenular commissure

4. Extensive damage to the left cerebral cortex is likely to produce:
   a. Left sided hemiplegia
   b. Crossed hemiplegia
   c. Right sided hemiplegia
   d. Quadriplegia

ANSWERS

1. c   2. c   3. b   4. c

Hypothalamus

CHAPTER 92

LEARNING OBJECTIVES
- Explain the functions of hypothalamus
- Discuss the effects of lesion of hypothalamus

FUNCTIONAL ANATOMY

PY10.7: Describe and discuss functions of cerebral cortex, basal ganglia, thalamus, hypothalamus, cerebellum and limbic system and their abnormalities.

Hypothalamus is the part of diencephalon concerned with **visceral, autonomic and endocrine** functions. These functions are related to the affective and emotional behavior of the individual. Hypothalamus plays a very important role in the maintenance of homeostasis.

Hypothalamus consists of a diffuse nuclear mass situated below the thalamus. It extends from optic chiasma anteriorly to the caudal border of mammillary bodies posteriorly and lies in the wall of the third ventricle. It weighs about 10 g. The zone forming the floor of the third ventricle is called the **median eminence** and it represents the final point of convergence of pathways from CNS upon the peripheral endocrine system. The ventral protrusion of hypothalamus and the third ventricular recess forms the **infundibulum**. The thalamus lies dorsal to the hypothalamus and the subthalamic region lies lateral and caudal to it. The median eminence, the infundibulum and the posterior lobe of hypophysis cerebri together form the **neurohypophysis** (*refer* Chapter 63, Fig. 63.1).

Hypothalamic Nuclei (Fig. 92.1)

1. Anterior group
   a. Paraventricular nucleus
   b. Preoptic nucleus
   c. Supraoptic nucleus
   d. Suprachiasmatic nucleus
2. Middle group
   a. Median eminence
   b. Ventromedial nucleus
   c. Dorsomedial nucleus
   d. Anterior nucleus
   e. Lateral nucleus
   f. Nucleus tuberalis
   g. Infundibular nucleus or arcuate nucleus
3. Posterior group
   a. Posterior hypothalamic nucleus
   b. Mammillary body

Connections of Hypothalamus

Afferent Connections

1. Midbrain —— Medial forebrain bundle ——→ Hypothalamus
2. Hippocampus —— Fornix ——→ Hypothalamus
3. Midbrain —— Bundle of Schutz ——→ Hypothalamus
4. Amygdala —— Stria terminalis ——→ Hypothalamus
5. Thalamus —— Thalamohypothalamic fibers ——→ Hypothalamus
6. Basal ganglia —— Pallidohypothalamic fibers ——→ Hypothalamus
7. Midbrain —— Mammillary peduncle ——→ Mammillary body
8. Reticular formation ——→ Hypothalamus
9. Eyes —— Retinohypothalamic fibers ——→ Suprachiasmatic nucleus
10. Cerebral cortex ——→ Hypothalamus

Afferents According to the Transmitter Released

The neurotransmitters involved in afferent impulses to the hypothalamus are largely **norepinephrine, acetylcholine and serotonin**.

1. Raphe nucleus of midbrain —— Serotonergic fibers ——→ Hypothalamus
2. Locus coeruleus —— Noradrenergic fibers ——→ Hypothalamus
3. Medulla —— Adrenergic bundle ——→ Hypothalamus

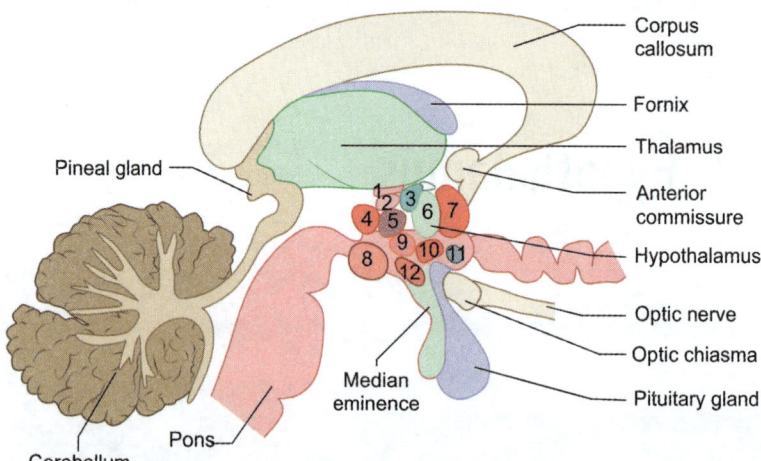

Fig. 92.1: Sagittal section of brain showing hypothalamic nuclei and the surrounding structures: (1) Lateral hypothalamic nucleus; (2) Dorsal hypothalamic nucleus; (3) Paraventricular nucleus; (4) Posterior hypothalamic nucleus; (5) Dorsomedial nucleus; (6) Anterior hypothalamic nucleus; (7) Medial preoptic nucleus; (8) Mammillary body; (9) Ventromedial nucleus; (10) Supraoptic nucleus; (11) Suprachiasmatic nucleus; (12) Arcuate nucleus.

Efferent Connections

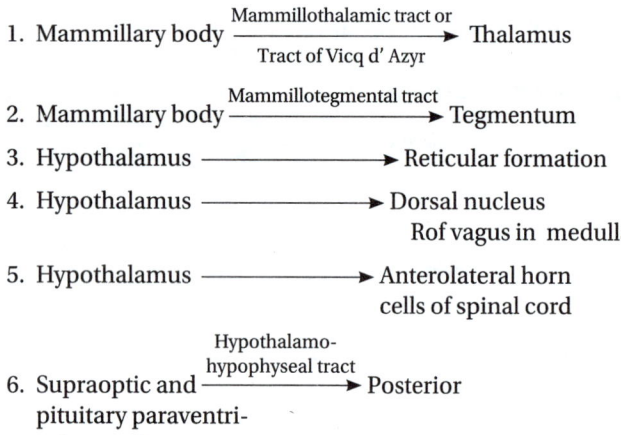

The neurotransmitters for efferent impulse to the median eminence include dopamine, GABA and β-endorphin.

Functions of Hypothalamus

- Regulation of autonomic activities
- Regulation of food intake
- Regulation of water intake and maintenance of water balance
- Temperature regulation
- Role in circadian rhythm
- Endocrine function
- Role in sexual behavior
- Role in emotional behavior
- Regulation of fat and carbohydrate metabolism.

Regulation of Autonomic Activities

Hypothalamus acts as the head ganglion of the autonomic nervous system. It is the chief subcortical center for the regulation of both sympathetic and parasympathetic activities.

Parasympathetic activities are controlled by **anterior and medial hypothalamic regions**. Stimulation of these regions results in increased vagal and sacral autonomic responses characterized by decrease in the heart rate, cardiac output and blood pressure, increased activity of GIT and bladder.

Sympathetic activities are controlled by the **lateral and posterior hypothalamic regions**. Stimulation of these regions activates thoracolumbar outflow characterized by increase in metabolic and somatic activities characteristic of emotional stress or flight reactions. These include dilatation of pupil, piloerection, increase in heart rate and blood pressure, increase in the rate and depth of respiration, and inhibition of gut and bladder.

A lesion in the posterior hypothalamus produces emotional lethargy, abnormal sleepiness and decrease in body temperature.

Hypothalamus also regulates adrenal medulla. Stimulation of dorsomedial nucleus and posterior hypothalamic area causes increased secretion of catecholamines from adrenal medulla. Stimulation of mid-dorsal area of the hypothalamus causes cholinergic sympathetic vasodilatation.

Regulation of Food Intake

There is a **feeding center** situated in the lateral hypothalamic nucleus and a **satiety center** in the ventromedial nucleus of hypothalamus. *The conscious sensation that causes cessation of eating is called satiety.* Feeding center is composed of adrenergic neurons. Stimulation of feeding center evokes eating behavior in animals and lesion of it causes anorexia (lack of appetite) and weight loss.

Feeding center is tonically active and is transiently inhibited by the satiety center after food intake. Stimulation of satiety center causes stoppage of eating. Lesions of satiety center cause hyperphagia (excessive eating) and if the food supply is abundant it leads to **hypothalamic obesity**. Normally, satiety center is not tonically active.

There are receptors in the satiety center which can respond to glucose levels in the satiety center called **glucostats**. These cells become active only when glucose enters these cells which require the presence of insulin. This is known as **glucostatic hypothesis** of food intake.

Other Brain Areas Affecting Feeding Behavior

Other than hypothalamus, food intake is affected by brain stem centers, limbic system and neocortex. The **mechanical features** of feeding like salivation, chewing of food and swallowing are controlled by brainstem centers.

The **discriminative aspect** of food intake is controlled by the limbic system (amygdala) and the prefrontal cortex. In bilateral lesions of the amygdala, this aspect is lost and a vegetarian monkey starts eating all sorts of food, i.e., psychic blindness in the choice of foods.

The **psychological aspect** of food intake as to the site and time of eating, likes and dislikes for certain food, etc. is controlled by the neocortex. The neocortex modifies feeding behavior through learning.

Other Factors Determining Food Intake

- **Lipostatic hypothesis** – The fat depots of body send signals to brain, and appetite is controlled accordingly. **Leptin** (leptin: thin) is a 167 amino acid protein hormone produced by adipocytes in the subcutaneous fat. Leptin acts on hypothalamus to reduce food intake, decreases lipogenesis, and increases lipolysis thereby reducing the body fat stores.
  Plasma leptin level is proportional to the amount of body fat and is therefore higher in women and obese individuals.
  Leptin receptors are present in the hypothalamus. Neuropeptide Y produced by the hypothalamus is a potent stimulator of food intake. Stimulation of leptin receptors inhibits neuropeptide Y secretion leading to decreased food intake and thus prevents obesity. Lack of leptin or lack of leptin receptors in the hypothalamus produces higher neuropeptide Y levels leading to decreased satiety signals in the hypothalamus. This leads to increased food intake and obesity. Insulin is a potent stimulator of leptin production. Leptin secretion is decreased in the adipocytes by insulin resistance. This is one reason for the hyperphagia seen in diabetes mellitus.
- Environmental factors – Food intake is increased in cold weather and decreased in hot environment.
- Hypoglycemia increases appetite.
- Hormones like CCK, GRP, α-MSH, glucagon, somatostatin and calcitonin decrease appetite. Incretins and insulin suppress appetite (*refer* gastrointestinal hormones).
- Drugs like amphetamine decrease appetite.
- **Ghrelin**, a hormone released mainly by the oxyntic cells of stomach, increases appetite and decreases insulin secretion. It has receptors in pituitary (to stimulate growth hormone secretion) and hypothalamus (to regulate appetite). Ghrelin stimulates the arcuate nucleus to release neuropeptide Y which in turn increases appetite. Blood levels of ghrelin rise during fasting and hypoglycemia. It falls rapidly after a meal, in hyperglycemia and obesity.
- Distension of stomach stimulates the stretch receptors of stomach and the impulses reach the brain through the vagus and inhibit appetite. Vagotomy abolishes this effect leading to hyperphagia.

Regulation of Water Intake and Maintenance of Water Balance

Thirst

Intake of water is regulated by plasma osmolality and extracellular fluid volume. Water intake is increased when there is increase in plasma osmolality or when there is decrease in **extracellular fluid** (ECF) volume or both. **Thirst center** is located in the hypothalamus. Stimulation of this area causes the animal to drink water. Lesion causes decrease in thirst. Thirst center is composed of **cholinergic neurons**. Osmolality of body fluids is sensed by **osmoreceptors** located in the anterior hypothalamus and these are stimulated by an increase in osmotic pressure of body fluids and initiate thirst. Lesions in the diencephalon lead to dehydration and hypernatremia. Anterior communicating artery supplies the hypothalamic areas concerned with thirst and so lesion of the anterior communicating artery prevents thirst sensation.

Decrease in ECF volume stimulates thirst by another mechanism different from that mediating thirst in response to increased plasma osmolality. Even though there is no change in blood osmolality, decrease in ECF volume stimulates thirst as in hemorrhage. This response to decrease in ECF volume is mediated through renin-angiotensin mechanism. Renin secretion from the kidney is stimulated by hypovolemia. Renin converts angiotensinogen to angiotensin I and angiotensin converting enzyme converts angiotensin I to angiotensin II Angiotensin II acts on the **subfornical organ** in the diencephalon and on the **organum vasculosum of the lamina terminalis (OVLT)** to stimulate areas concerned with thirst. These are circumventricular organs which are located outside the blood brain barrier.

Role of ADH in Water Balance

Supraoptic nucleus of hypothalamus secretes antidiuretic hormone (ADH) or vasopressin which causes increased reabsorption of water by the collecting ducts of the kidney. This decreases the effective osmotic pressure of body fluids. Stimuli are increase in osmotic pressure of plasma and decrease in ECF volume. ADH secretion is found to be maximal when the osmolality of body fluid reaches 290 mOsm/L. Thirst response is most important when body fluid osmolality rises above 290 mOsm/L.

Temperature Regulation

There is a center for heat loss in the anterior part of hypothalamus and a center for heat gain in the posterior part of hypothalamus. The reflex responses activated by cold are controlled from the posterior hypothalamus and those activated by warmth are controlled from the anterior hypothalamus. Stimulation of the anterior hypothalamus causes cutaneous vasodilation and sweating and lesions of this region leads to hyperthermia. Posterior hypothalamic stimulation leads to shivering, vasoconstriction, increased appetite, etc. Lesion of posterior hypothalamus brings the body temperature towards that of the environment. (For details, *refer* Chapter 59—'Temperature regulation').

Role of Hypothalamus in Maintaining Circadian Rhythm

Hypothalamus functions as a **biological clock**. Many tissues, organs and systems of the body show a cyclical variation in some of their functional activities, usually a 24-hr periodicity. This is called **circadian rhythm**. An intact hypothalamus is essential for maintaining this rhythm. Examples are:
1. Sleep wakefulness cycle
2. Adrenocortical activity
3. Melatonin secretion
4. Fluctuations in body temperature.

Lesions of suprachiasmatic nucleus of hypothalamus can result in variations in adrenocortical activity, melatonin secretion, etc. Retinohypothalamic tract is mainly responsible for this rhythm.

Sleep-wakefulness cycle: Hypothalamus forms part of ARAS. No definite center is there in the hypothalamus for sleep-wakefulness cycle. Lesion of posterior hypothalamus can induce prolonged sleep, whereas stimulation of posterior hypothalamus can lead to alertness. Stimulation of dorsal hypothalamus causes sleep. Hypothalamic lesion is a cause for narcolepsy.

Role of Hypothalamus in Endocrine Functions

Hypothalamus regulates the activity of anterior pituitary. Releasing hormones and inhibiting hormones released from the median eminence of hypothalamus through the hypothalamo-hypophyseal portal system controls the secretion of anterior pituitary hormones. Hormones synthesized in the supraoptic and paraventricular nuclei of hypothalamus (ADH and oxytocin) reach the posterior pituitary through the hypothalamo-hypophyseal tract.

Role of Hypothalamus in Sexual Behavior

Sexual behavior depends on the level of sex hormones in circulation. These hormones are under the influence of gonadotropic hormones secreted by anterior pituitary. Anterior pituitary in turn is controlled by the hypothalamus. Thus, hypothalamus plays an important role in maturation and maintenance of sexual behavior, gametogenesis and cyclic variation in the reproductive tract.

Stimulation of median forebrain bundle induces male receptivity in females and copulatory movement in male.

Mating is a basic complex phenomenon involving many parts of brain including hypothalamus. It consists of a series of reflexes initiated in spinal cord and brain. In humans, sexual functions have become extensively encephalized and conditioned by psychic and social factors.

Role in Emotional Behavior

Hypothalamus is regarded as one of the principal centers concerned with emotional expression. The physiological expression of emotion is controlled partly by sympathetic and parasympathetic nervous system, which in turn is controlled by hypothalamus. Stimulation of different hypothalamic areas produces different responses. For example, stimulation of anterior and lateral hypothalamic area causes flight reactions. Stimulation of ventromedian nucleus produces rage. This includes hissing, growling, piloerection, pupillary dilatation, etc. This experiment was conducted in a decorticate cat and is called reaction of **sham rage**.

In humans, emotion has an objective (emotional expression) and a subjective part (feeling). For the integration of these two aspects, limbic system and hypothalamus should function together. Hypothalamus is part of limbic system and it has afferent and efferent connections with parts of limbic system. There are areas called **positive and negative reward areas** in the hypothalamus. Stimulation of positive reward center causes pleasurable sensations and stimulation of negative reward center causes painful sensation.

Regulation of Fat and Carbohydrate Metabolism

Hypothalamus controls peripheral lipid metabolism through the sympathetic nervous system. The ventromedial hypothalamus and arcuate nucleus of the hypothalamus play an important role in the regulation of glucose and fat metabolism in the skeletal muscle and liver. Leptin secreted by white adipose tissue and ghrelin secreted by stomach and present in the hypothalamus alter both central and peripheral lipid metabolism and thus control feeding behavior and energy expenditure. Leptin is a satiety hormone which informs the hypothalamus of the status of energy stores. Leptin receptors are present in the hypothalamus. Leptin stimulate glucose uptake and fatty acid oxidation in skeletal muscle by stimulating ventromedial hypothalamus. Leptin suppress **AMP-activated protein kinase (AMPK)** activity in the ventromedial hypothalamus and this is responsible for the anorexic and weight loss effects of leptin. The key hormones in fat metabolism are **insulin, leptin** and **adiponectin**. In **dystrophia adiposogenitalis** and **Laurence-Beidel-Moon syndrome**, which are due to lesion of hypothalamus or anterior pituitary, there is abnormal deposition of fat in the body, sugar intolerance, etc.

Features of Hypothalamic Disorders

- Autonomic disturbances
- Lethargy and somnolence which are sleep disorders
- Hyperthermia in lesion of anterior hypothalamus
- Disorders of sexual function
- Diabetes insipidus due to decreased ADH secretion from supraoptic nucleus
- Obesity due to disturbance in fat and carbohydrate metabolism
- Emotional disturbances
- Narcolepsy and cataplexy. **Narcolepsy** is irresistible desire to sleep during daytime. **Cataplexy** occurs in anger, amusement, fear, etc., where there will be sudden helplessness of the body and the patient falls. Consciousness is not lost, but muscles are weak and deep tendon reflexes

will be absent. The attack is brief and last for few seconds to a few minutes.

MULTIPLE CHOICE QUESTIONS

1. **Destruction of lateral nucleus of hypothalamus leads to:**
   a. Aphagia (inability to swallow)
   b. Hyperphagia
   c. Satiety
   d. Somnolence

2. **The cell bodies of orexinergic neurons are present in:**
   a. Locus coeruleus
   b. Dorsal raphe
   c. Lateral hypothalamic area
   d. Hippocampus

3. **Stria terminalis emerges from the posterior aspect of:**
   a. Mammillary body
   b. Amygdaloid nucleus
   c. Hippocampus
   d. Olfactory bulb

4. **Amygdaloid nuclei is situated in the following area:**
   a. Temporal lobe
   b. Parietal lobe
   c. Occipital lobe
   d. Midbrain

5. **Location of osmoreceptors is in the:**
   a. Wall of atria
   b. Anterior hypothalamus
   c. Juxtaglomerular apparatus
   d. Walls of veins

6. **Injection of hypertonic saline in which region of hypothalamus produces intense thirst:**
   a. Posterior region
   b. Paraventricular area
   c. Preoptic area
   d. Supraoptic area

7. **Drinking can be induced by:**
   a. Electrical stimulation of posterior hypothalamus
   b. Osmotic stimulation of supraoptic nucleus
   c. Lesions in the paraventricular nucleus
   d. Neuronal lesion in the preoptic nucleus

8. **Thirst center is situated in:**
   a. Preoptic nucleus
   b. Supraoptic nucleus
   c. Posterior hypothalamus
   d. Paraventricular nucleus

9. **Lesion in which of the following structure leads to Kluver-Bucy syndrome:**
   a. Amygdala
   b. Hippocampus
   c. Hypothalamus
   d. Thalamus

10. **The following is not a function of hypothalamus:**
    a. Regulation of autonomic functions
    b. Production of certain hormones
    c. Temperature regulation
    d. Co-ordination of motor activities

11. **Sham rage is produced when?**
    a. Section is made at L_2 vertebra
    b. Pons is removed
    c. Medulla is removed
    d. All the cortex is removed from brain

ANSWERS

1. c 2. c 3. b 4. a 5. b
6. c 7. b 8. a 9. a 10. d
11. d

Limbic System

CHAPTER 93

LEARNING OBJECTIVES
- Describe the functions of limbic system
- Discuss the effects of lesion of limbic system

INTRODUCTION

PY10.7: Describe and discuss functions of cerebral cortex, basal ganglia, thalamus, hypothalamus, cerebellum and limbic system and their abnormalities.

The term limbic system is given to a group of **cortical and subcortical** structures that lie beneath the neocortex forming a limbus (Limbus = border) around the hilum of cerebral hemispheres. The cortical structures are arranged in the form of an inner ring and an outer ring. Inside these rings are the subcortical limbic structures. Limbic system is the site of origin of instinctive behavior, motivation and emotion.

The most important function of limbic system is to control emotional behavior in part, by its influence on hypothalamus through the **Papez circuit**. This is a circuit that connects the limbic lobe with the hypothalamus which regulates emotional behavior.

PARTS OF LIMBIC SYSTEM (FIG. 93.1)

- **Limbic lobe** formed by two gyri of cerebral hemisphere, cingulate gyrus and hippocampal gyrus. *The limbic lobe is phylogenetically the oldest part of the cerebral cortex (allocortex) having primitive histological structure, i.e., three layers.*
- Parts of olfactory cortex and parahippocampal gyrus
- Hippocampus is an extension of the hippocampal gyrus that extends into the floor of the lateral ventricle.
- Amygdaloid nucleus located at the tail end of the caudate nucleus
- Mammillary bodies of hypothalamus
- Anterior nucleus of thalamus located in the floor of the lateral ventricle

Although behavior is a function of the entire nervous system, the limbic system controls most of its involuntary aspects. Experiments on the limbic system of monkeys and other animals indicate that the **amygdaloid nucleus** assumes

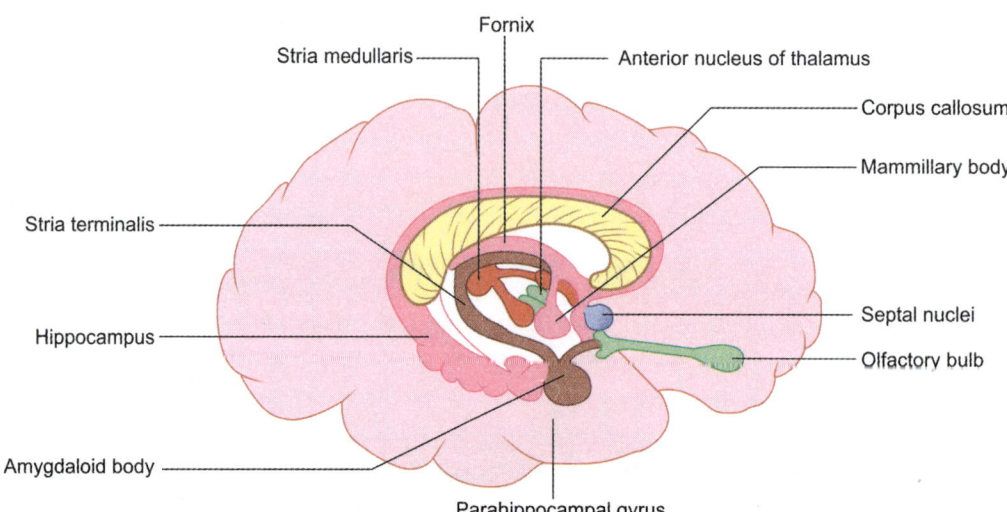

Fig. 93.1: Sagittal section of brain showing the components of limbic system.

a major role in controlling the overall pattern of **behavior**. Other experiments show that limbic system is associated with **pleasure and pain**. Still other studies show that stimulation of the perifornical nuclei of hypothalamus results in a behavioral pattern called **rage**. Stimulating other areas of limbic system, results in an opposite behavioral pattern which includes docility, tameness and affection. **Docile** means quiet and willing to obey.

Since the limbic system assumes a primary function in emotions such as pain, pleasure, anger, rage, fear, sorrow, sexual feelings, docility and affection, it is sometimes referred to as the **visceral or emotional brain**.

Connections of Limbic System

The connecting pathways of limbic system are the fornix, mammillo-thalamic tract and stria terminalis.

- **Fornix** connect hippocampus and the mammillary body and it forms part of the Papez circuit.
- **Mammillothalamic tract (of Vicq d' Azyr)** connects mammillary body to anterior nucleus of thalamus.
- **Stria terminalis** connects amygdaloid body to the preoptic and anterior nucleus of hypothalamus.
- Medial forebrain bundle connects anterior olfactory area to hypothalamic nuclei and raphe nuclei of reticular formation.
- **Papez circuit** which regulates emotional behavior connects limbic cortex to hypothalamus.

FUNCTIONS OF LIMBIC SYSTEM

- Role in olfaction (*refer* olfaction)
- Control of autonomic function
- Regulation of feeding
- Somatic responses
- Regulation of circadian rhythm due to its connection with the hypothalamus
- Role in sexual behavior
- Maternal behavior
- Role in consciousness, memory and emotion.

Control of Autonomic Function

Amygdala has an important role in the control of autonomic functions. Stimulation of limbic system produces changes in heart rate, blood pressure, pupillary reactions and gastrointestinal movements.

Role in Food Intake

Deprivation of food produces the sensation of hunger and thirst and this is due to impulses originating from the hypothalamus. When food and water are taken, the ultimate **satisfaction** is due to the activity of limbic cortex. Lesion of amygdala produces moderate hyperphagia. The amygdala and the prefrontal cortex are important for discriminative appetite.

Role of Limbic System in Somatic Responses

Stimulation of limbic system produces somatic responses in the facial muscles of ipsilateral side, especially orbital and oral muscles. These responses form part of emotional expression. If the neocortex is separated from limbic control, the voluntary aspect of this response is lost. This is called **dissociation of function of limbic system and cortex**.

Role of Limbic System in Sexual Behavior

Endocrine system and limbic system together control sexual function. There are two circuits in limbic system that control sexual function. They are a **positive feedback** mechanism and **negative feedback** mechanism. The positive feedback mechanism is:

Hippocampus → Hypothalamus → Pituitary → Gonads

The negative feedback mechanism is:

Amygdala → Hypothalamus → Pituitary → Gonads

For normal sexual behavior, integration of function of all these areas is essential. Damage of these areas results in abnormal sexual behavior.

Role in Maternal Behavior

Maternal behavior is the function of cingulate gyrus and retrosplenial portion of limbic cortex. It is concerned with breastfeeding and protection of offspring by the mother. Hormones such as prolactin and oxytocin also play an important role in maternal behavior. Lesions of the cingulate gyrus and retrosplenial gyrus abolish maternal behavior.

Role of Limbic System in Consciousness, Memory and Emotion

Consciousness is the simultaneous awareness of self and environment. Limbic system is concerned with the emotional aspect of consciousness, i.e., the feeling part.

Memory is the ability to recall a thought at least once or again and again. Lesion of hippocampus and amygdala produces loss of recent memory (anterograde amnesia). Hippocampus is concerned with converting recent memory to long-term memory.

Role in Emotions

Limbic system and hypothalamus are intimately concerned with the **genesis and expression of emotions**. **Papez circuit** connects limbic lobe with hypothalamus and regulates emotional behavior **(Flowchart 93.1)**. Information passes from the cingulate gyrus to the entorhinal cortex and hippocampus and from there to the mammillary bodies in the hypothalamus. The **mammillo-thalamic tract** then connects the mammillary body with the anterior thalamic nuclei, which project back to the cingulate gyrus.

Emotion has a physical aspect and a mental aspect.

Flowchart 93.1: Papez circuit.

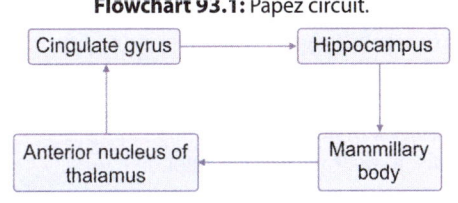

Physical part includes changes in activity of internal organs and skeletal muscles such as tachycardia, sweating, restlessness, etc.

Mental part has three components; cognition, affect and conation.

Cognition

Cognition involves an awareness of sensation and its cause through thought, experience and the senses.

Affect

Affect is the reflection of the mental state. It involves the feeling itself.

Conation or Motivation of Behavior

Conation involves the urge to take action. The desire arising in the mind or that is produced by any external stimulus to do something physical or mental is called **motivation**.

Behavior is motivated by promise of reward and avoidance of punishment. This is explained by self-stimulation technique. 35% of limbic system includes **reward area** and 5% includes **punishment area**. Dopamine acts as the main transmitter in the reward system. Other neurotransmitters involved in the reward area are norepinephrine, morphine and encephalins. Emotion is prolonged even after the stimulus is stopped. This is due to after-discharge of limbic system. It cannot be stopped at will.

> Tobacco, alcohol, opiates, cocaine, etc., act by increasing dopamine content in the reward center. Use of these substances lead to **addiction**, i.e., a strong motive to use them again and again despite its negative health consequences.

Manifestations of Emotional Expression

Fear or Fleeing Reaction or Avoidance Reaction

Manifestations of fear are due to stimulation of sympathetic nervous system and release of hormones from adrenal medulla such as adrenaline and noradrenaline. Fear reaction is associated with autonomic responses such as tachycardia, tachypnea, sweating, pupillary dilatation, piloerection, dryness of mouth, muscular tremor and turning the head from side to side to look for escape. This response is also called **fleeing or avoidance reaction**. This reaction can be produced experimentally by stimulation of the hypothalamic and amygdaloid nuclei. Lesion of amygdala produces loss of fear.

Rage or Fighting or Attack Reactions

Rage and fear are protective responses to threats in environment and are closely related emotions. Rage reaction in animals is associated with hissing, spitting, growling, piloerection, biting and clawing. Normally, minor irritating stimuli are usually ignored but major stimuli make an individual lose his temper. Rage responses to minor stimuli are seen in the following conditions:
- ❖ After removal of neocortex
- ❖ Stimulation of amygdaloid nuclei
- ❖ Destruction of ventromedial nuclei of hypothalamus
- ❖ Androgen excess.

Cerebral cortex especially prefrontal cortex has a control over hypothalamus. *Rage reaction is due to release of hypothalamus from the cortex.* Cerebral cortex inhibits the hypothalamus. Normally, hypothalamus tonically stimulates amygdala, and excessive stimulation is checked by the inhibitory impulses coming from cortex to the hypothalamus.

Cerebral cortex → Hypothalamus → Amygdala

*Bilateral lesion of amygdala leads to **placidity** (calmness).*

Grief is manifested as pallor of skin, lacrimation, muscular hypotonia, etc.

Delight is manifested as increase in heart rate, smiling, etc.

Kluver-Bucy Syndrome

Bilateral lesion of anterior part of temporal lobe along with amygdala leads to this condition. Manifestations of Kluver-Bucy syndrome are:
- ❖ **Psychic blindness** or **visual agnosia**, i.e., loss of ability to recognize and relate significance or meaning of objects on the basis of visual cues (criteria) alone.
- ❖ **Loss of memory**; usually there will be lack of retention of ongoing memories, but past memories may be retained.
- ❖ **Hypersexuality**
- ❖ **Hyperorality**, i.e., takes everything into the mouth, i.e., animal eats both edible and inedible things. The discriminative aspect is lost.
- ❖ Decreased aggressiveness.
- ❖ **Docility**, i.e., reduction of affectional and fear responses.
- ❖ Decreased emotionality.

MULTIPLE CHOICE QUESTIONS

1. Sham rage is seen in lesion of:
    a. Limbic system   b. Cerebellum
    c. Hypothalamus   d. Basal ganglia
2. The function of limbic system is:
    a. Control of motor activities
    b. Control of hearing
    c. Control of autonomic functions
    d. Control of emotions such as rage and fear
3. The area of the brain that is not concerned with emotional expression:
    a. Limbic system   b. Hypothalamus
    c. Cerebellum   d. Thalamus
4. True regarding limbic cortex:
    a. Formed of neocortex
    b. Phylogenetically the oldest part of cerebral cortex
    c. Lesion leads to muscular tremor
    d. Very much evolved in humans

ANSWERS

1. a   2. d   3. c   4. b

Autonomic Nervous System

CHAPTER 94

LEARNING OBJECTIVES
- Describe the organization of the autonomic nervous system
- Explain the functions of sympathetic and parasympathetic nervous systems
- Explain the physiology of stress

INTRODUCTION

PY10.5: Describe and discuss structure and functions of reticular activating system, autonomic nervous system (ANS).

Autonomic nervous system (ANS) is that portion of nervous system, which is concerned with the **visceral functions** of the body i.e., the functions that occur without our conscious knowledge. Sympathetic and parasympathetic divisions of the ANS are the two major efferent pathways controlling target tissues other than skeletal muscle. It controls the functions of the involuntary organs of the body such as heart and blood vessels, secretory epithelia, glands and all visceral organs. So it is also known as **involuntary nervous system or vegetative nervous system or visceral nervous system**. Vegetative functions are those bodily processes directly concerned with maintenance of life. This includes nutritional, metabolic and endocrine functions including eating, sleeping, bowel and bladder activity, etc. **John Newport Langley** in 1898 divided ANS into two divisions, sympathetic and parasympathetic nervous system.

Skeletal muscles receive only excitatory inputs through alpha motor neuron whereas; most of the visceral organs receive both inhibitory and excitatory synaptic inputs through the sympathetic and parasympathetic divisions of the ANS. Although as a general rule, the two divisions of ANS have antagonistic effects, there are exceptions. For example, salivary gland is excited by both divisions even though the nature of secretion differs. In addition, some organs receive innervation from only one of these two divisions of ANS. For example, sweat glands, piloerector muscle of skin and most peripheral blood vessels receive input only from the sympathetic division.

GENERAL ORGANIZATION OF ANS

The ANS has three divisions:
1. **Sympathetic nervous system**, or **thoracolumbar outflow**, it is called so because it takes origin from first thoracic to second or third lumbar segments of spinal cord (T_1–L_2).
2. **Parasympathetic nervous system**, also known as **craniosacral outflow** since it originates from 3rd, 7th, 9th and 10th cranial nerves and from the 2nd, 3rd and 4th sacral segments of spinal cord.
3. **Enteric nervous system** (details given in Chapter 44).

The sympathetic and the parasympathetic systems can act independently of each other but generally they work synergistically to control visceral activity. Increased sympathetic discharge occurs in conditions of stress, anxiety, physical activity, fear or excitement while increased parasympathetic discharge occurs during sedentary activity such as eating or at rest. The enteric nervous system present in the gastrointestinal tract can function independently, but it is normally controlled by the CNS through sympathetic and parasympathetic fibers.

Autonomic nervous system functions are mainly based on autonomic or visceral reflexes, which consist of receptor, afferent limb, center, efferent limb and effector organ. For example, cardiovascular reflex such as baroreceptor reflex, gastrointestinal reflex (defecation, sexual reflexes, etc.) are autonomic reflexes.

In somatic nervous system, the efferent neuron, which is the alpha motor neuron in the anterior horn of spinal cord, directly innervates the effector organ, which is the skeletal muscle. Here there is only one efferent neuron. In contrast to this, the ANS innervates target tissue by a two synapse pathway. The first neuron in the efferent pathway, which is called the preganglionic neuron, has its cell body in the brain stem or spinal cord. Axons of these neurons come out of the CNS to make synapse with the postganglionic neurons in the peripheral ganglia interposed between the CNS and the target cell. Axons of the postganglionic neurons supply their target cells.

I. **Receptors** in the ANS are situated in the internal visceral organs called **visceroceptors**. They are baroreceptors, chemoreceptors, thermoreceptors, osmoreceptors and nociceptors which are sensitive to stretch of heart, blood vessels and hollow viscera; PCO_2, PO_2 and pH, blood glucose; temperature of skin and internal organs; osmolarity of body fluids; and painful stimuli.

II. **Afferents:** All internal organs are densely innervated by visceral afferents. Afferents from receptors mainly travel with parasympathetic fibers to the center (spinal cord or brain). The cell bodies of the visceral afferent fibers are located in the dorsal root ganglia or cranial nerve ganglia. About 90% of the visceral afferents are unmyelinated. Vagus nerve carries non-nociceptive afferents to the CNS (medulla) from all viscera of the thorax and abdomen. Most of the visceral nociceptive afferents travel with the sympathetic fibers and enter the spinal cord at segmental levels along with the spinal nerve.

III. **Center:** Organization of ANS occurs at five different levels:
   1. Spinal cord
   2. Brain stem
   3. Hypothalamus
   4. Limbic system (amygdaloid complex)
   5. Prefrontal cortex.

Spinal cord is the lowest level for the control of autonomic function. Here, simple reflexes such as micturition and defecation are integrated. Sympathetic fibers originate from T_1 to $L_{2\ or\ 3}$ segments of spinal cord. The spinal component of parasympathetic nervous system originates from S_2 to S_4 segments of spinal cord. The afferent neurons of ANS enter the spinal cord through the dorsal root and terminate on the autonomic efferent neurons in the intermediolateral horn cell of spinal cord. In contrast to the somatic nervous system, there is another efferent neuron in the ganglion outside the spinal cord with which the first efferent neuron synapses.

Brain stem contains the major nuclei of ANS.
- *The cranial outflow of parasympathetic nervous system* originates from the cranial nerve nuclei (III, VII, IX and X) located in the brain stem.
- *Reticular formation* in the brain stem is one of the highest centers of autonomic function where respiratory center, vasomotor center and cardiac centers are integrated. Sympathetic fibers originate from the vasomotor center in the medulla.
- Pupillary reflexes such as light reflex and accommodation reflex are integrated in the *Edinger-Westphal nucleus* of midbrain.
- *Nucleus tractus solitarius* (NTS) in the medulla mediate respiratory and cardiovascular responses to autonomic activation. Special visceral sensations in VII, IX and X cranial nerves reach NTS. Salivary nucleus is located in pons and the dorsal motor nucleus of vagus is in the medulla.

Hypothalamus controls most of the endocrine glands and is also responsible for temperature regulation. The posterior and lateral portions of the hypothalamus control the sympathetic division of ANS. Stimulation of posterior hypothalamus can activate the vasomotor center of medulla strongly enough to increase arterial blood pressure to more than twice normal. Sherrington described hypothalamus as the **head-ganglion** of the sympathetic nervous system. Anterior and medial portions of hypothalamus control the parasympathetic division. The axons of these neurons relay in the reticular formation, and descend along with reticulospinal tract and reticulobulbar tract to the sympathetic and parasympathetic preganglionic neurons in the brainstem nuclei and spinal cord. The autonomic centers in the brain stem to some extent act as relay stations for the control of activities initiated at higher levels of the brain, especially in the hypothalamus.

Limbic system along with hypothalamus controls the emotional behavior of the individual such as fear, rage, sexual behavior, etc.

Prefrontal lobe is highly developed in man and is concerned with the intellectual behavior of man. Control of ANS by cerebral cortex occurs primarily during emotional stress. In extreme anxiety, cerebral cortex can stimulate hypothalamus, which in turn stimulates the vasomotor center in the medulla oblongata. This increases rate and force of heart beat and blood pressure.

IV. **Efferents:** The autonomic fibers from higher centers located in the brain stem, hypothalamus, limbic system, and the prefrontal lobe of cerebral cortex cross the midline in the brainstem and form part of **reticulospinal tract** and end in the lateral horn cells of spinal cord or the parasympathetic cranial nerve nuclei.

Autonomic efferents (**motor neurons**) are pre-ganglionic and postganglionic neurons. Preganglionic neuron conveys nerve impulses from brain or spinal cord to the autonomic ganglion. The postganglionic neuron conducts impulses from the autonomic ganglion to the visceral effector organ.

V. **Autonomic effector organs** are smooth muscles, cardiac muscle and glands.

FUNCTIONAL ANATOMY OF SYMPATHETIC NERVOUS SYSTEM

Sympathetic fibers take origin from T_1 to $L_{2\ or\ 3}$ segments of spinal cord. Afferent fibers synapse with the lateral horn cells in the intermediolateral horn of spinal cord. Axons of preganglionic neurons arise from their cell body, which are *myelinated* slow-conducting *type B fibers*. They pass out of the spinal cord through the ventral root along with the axons of alpha motor neurons of somatic nervous system. The sympathetic efferents separate from the somatic motor axons and enter the **white rami** communicantes and enter the ganglia of paravertebral sympathetic chain [sympathetic trunk] **(Fig. 94.1)**. Although the preganglionic sympathetic fibers emerge only from T_1 to L_2 segments, the paravertebral sympathetic chain of ganglia extends from the base of the skull to the tip of coccyx on either side. There are approximately 22 ganglia in a chain. In general, one ganglion is positioned at the level of each spinal root, but adjacent ganglia are fused in some cases. The most rostral ganglion, the **superior cervical ganglion** is formed by the

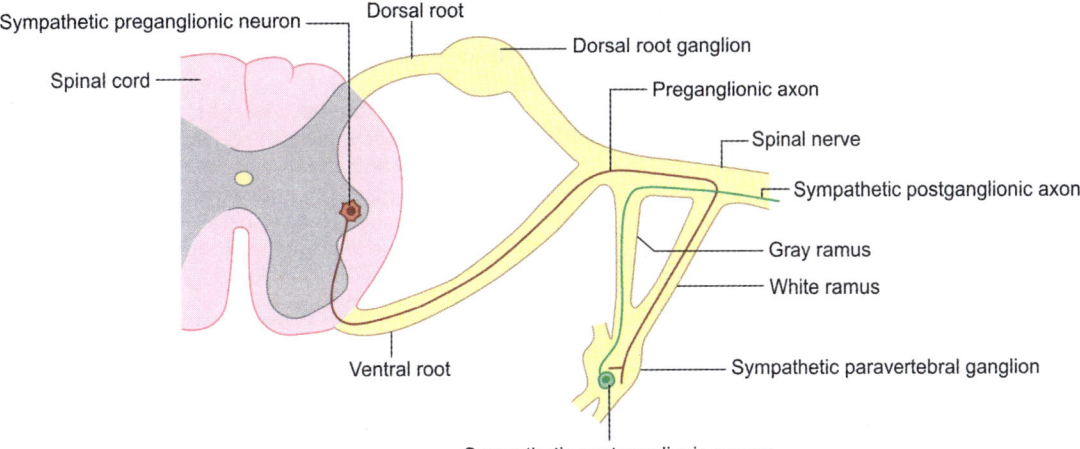

Fig. 94.1: Peripheral organization of the sympathetic division of autonomic nervous system.

fusion of C1 to C4 and supplies the head and neck. The **middle cervical ganglion** is formed by the fusion of C5 and C6 and the **inferior cervical ganglion** by the fusion of C7 and C8. The inferior cervical ganglion is usually fused with the first thoracic ganglion to form the **stellate ganglion.** The middle cervical ganglion, the stellate ganglion and the upper thoracic ganglia innervate the heart, lungs and bronchi. The remaining paravertebral ganglia supply organs and portions of body wall in a segmental manner. After entering the paravertebral ganglion, the preganglionic sympathetic axons have the following fates:

- The preganglionic fibers can either ascend or descend to make a synapse with the postganglionic neurons in the neighboring ganglia. From the cell bodies of postganglionic neurons, axons arise which are *unmyelinated C type* fibers. They pass out through the **gray rami communicantes** and rejoin the spinal nerve **(Fig. 94.1)** and supply the effector organs such as blood vessels, sweat glands and piloerector muscle of hairs. About 8% of the fibers in the spinal nerve are sympathetic fibers. These fibers primarily innervate organs above the diaphragm.
- Another group of preganglionic fibers synapse in the paravertebral sympathetic chain ganglion and the postganglionic fibers directly supply the viscera without passing through the spinal nerve.
- Some of the axons of preganglionic fibers arising from the cell body in the lateral horn of spinal cord pass through the paravertebral ganglia without synapsing there and enter the greater or lesser splanchnic nerve and reach prevertebral ganglia. The prevertebral plexus of ganglia lies in front of the aorta and along its major arterial branches. The major prevertebral ganglia are named according to the arteries that they are adjacent to and include the **celiac, superior and inferior mesenteric ganglia.** The preganglionic fibers synapse in the prevertebral ganglia, from where, postganglionic fibers arise and supply the viscera. The post ganglionic sympathetic axons from paravertebral and prevertebral ganglia travel to their target organs within other nerves or by travelling along with blood vessels.

Since the preganglionic sympathetic neurons are present only in the thoracic and upper lumbar spinal segments, white rami are found only at these levels. But, since each sympathetic ganglion sends out postganglionic fibers, gray rami are present at all spinal levels from C_2 to the coccyx.

Segmental Distribution of Sympathetic Fibers

- T_1 and T_2: Head and Neck (through superior, middle and inferior cervical ganglia)
- T_3 to T_6: Thorax (paravertebral ganglia)
- T_7 to T_{11}: Abdomen and pelvis [paravertebral ganglia, celiac plexus along the abdominal aorta and hypogastric plexus along the internal iliac artery]
- T_{12} to L_2: Leg.

FUNCTIONAL ANATOMY OF PARASYMPATHETIC NERVOUS SYSTEM

Parasympathetic efferents arise from 3rd, 7th, 9th and 10th cranial nerve nuclei and from 2nd, 3rd and 4th sacral segments of spinal cord. Thus, it has got two divisions, cranial and sacral divisions.

The preganglionic parasympathetic neurons distributed along with the II, VII, IX and X cranial nerves originate in four groups of nuclei: (a) the Edinger-Westphal nucleus in the midbrain, (b) the superior salivatory nucleus in upper medulla, (c) the inferior salivatory nucleus and upper part of nucleus ambiguus in the medulla, (d) the nucleus ambiguus and dorsal motor nucleus of vagus in the medulla. Cranial division supplies visceral structures of head and upper half of the body through oculomotor, facial, vagus and glossopharyngeal nerves.

- Parasympathetic preganglionic fibers travel in the oculomotor nerve (III) and synapse in the postganglionic neurons in the **ciliary ganglion**. The postganglionic fibers supply the circular muscle of iris and the ciliary muscles of eye.
- The preganglionic fibers from the superior salivatory nucleus pass through the facial nerve (VII) and synapse

with the postganglionic neurons in the **pterygopalatine ganglion**. The postganglionic fibers supplies lacrimal and nasal glands. Another branch of facial nerve carries preganglionic fibers to the **submandibular ganglion** and the postganglionic fibers supply the submandibular and sublingual salivary glands.

- The preganglionic fibers from the inferior salivatory nucleus pass through the glossopharyngeal nerve (IX) and synapse in the postganglionic neurons in the **otic ganglion**. The postsynaptic neurons supply the parotid gland.
- Preganglionic parasympathetic fibers of vagus (X) join the esophageal, pulmonary and cardiac plexus and travel to terminal ganglia located within their target organs. Postganglionic vagal fibers supply the viscera of thorax and upper abdomen. About 75% of all parasympathetic nerve fibers are in the vagus nerves, passing to the entire thoracic and abdominal regions of the body. It supplies the heart, lungs, esophagus, stomach, small intestine, proximal part of colon, liver, gallbladder, pancreas, kidneys, and upper portions of the uterus.

The sacral parasympathetic preganglionic neurons are located in S_2 to S_4 segments of spinal cord in a part similar to that of preganglionic sympathetic neurons although they do not form a distinct intermediolateral column. Sacral preganglionic parasympathetic axons leave through the ventral roots and travel with the **pelvic** splanchnic **nerves** to their terminal ganglia in the visceral structures of lower abdomen and pelvis (descending colon, rectum, urinary bladder, and lower portions of uterus). It also supplies nerve signals to the external genitalia to cause erection.

The parasympathetic preganglionic fibers are long and end in ganglia which are located near the organ or within the organ. The postganglionic fibers supply the concerned organ. So, the postganglionic fibers are short in contrast to the sympathetic fibers which have long postganglionic fibers (Fig. 94.2).

The postganglionic sympathetic as well as parasympathetic fibers pass over the cells to be stimulated and they have bulbous enlargements called varicosities as they reach each effector cells (*refer* synapse en passant). It is in these varicosities that the transmitter vesicles of acetylcholine or norepinephrine are synthesized and stored and many varicosities form synapses with their targets. This arrangement results in an increase in the number of targets that a single axonal branch can influence, with wider distribution of autonomic output.

Sympathetic and Parasympathetic Tone

Normally, the sympathetic and the parasympathetic systems are continually active, and the basal rates of activity are called **sympathetic and parasympathetic tone** respectively. The normal sympathetic tone to the systemic arterioles keeps them constricted to about one half their maximum diameters. The parasympathetic tone to the blood vessels is negligible. In times of need, the degree of sympathetic stimulation can be increased above normal, so that the vessels can be constricted more. Conversely, by decreasing the sympathetic stimulation below normal, the arterioles can be dilated. If the background sympathetic tone was not there, the sympathetic system could cause only vasoconstriction, never vasodilation.

Parasympathetic tone is prominent in the heart and the gastrointestinal tract (exception is sphincters of GIT which has a resting sympathetic tone). When the vagal supply to the heart is cut, the heart rate may increase to about 160/minute. When the parasympathetic discharge to the gut is cut, there will be decreased gastrointestinal motility (atony) and when there is increased parasympathetic stimulation the gastrointestinal activity increases.

■ TYPES OF TRANSMISSION IN THE AUTONOMIC NERVOUS SYSTEM

Sympathetic and parasympathetic nerve endings release neurotransmitters, such as **acetylcholine** and

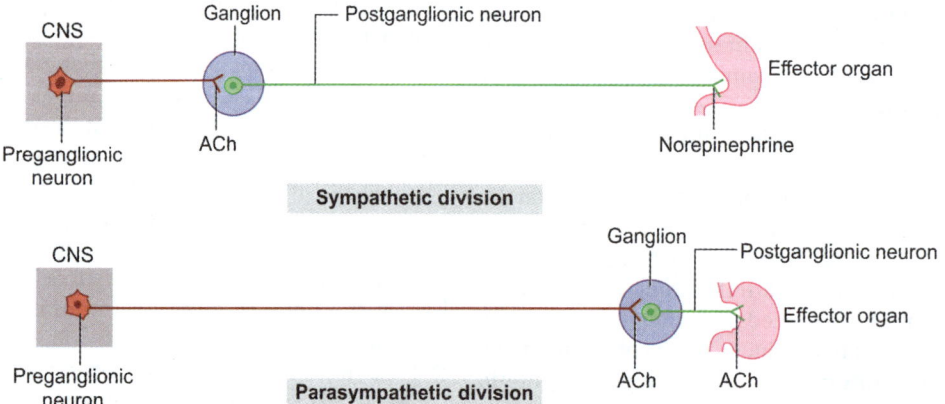

Fig. 94.2: Comparison of the organization and transmitters released by the sympathetic and parasympathetic divisions of autonomic nervous system.
Note that the sympathetic division has short preganglionic and long postganglionic fibers. Whereas, parasympathetic division has long preganglionic and short postganglionic fibers.

(ACh: acetylcholine; CNS: central nervous system)

norepinephrine (noradrenaline). Depending on the type of neurotransmitter, the fibers are classified into cholinergic and adrenergic fibers. In some areas, **nitric oxide** is the neurotransmitter where the fibers are termed non-adrenergic non-cholinergic fibers. The enteric nervous system, which is now considered as a third division of ANS release many amines, amino acids and active peptides as **co-neurotransmitters** along with acetyl choline or adrenaline, e.g. VIP with acetyl choline and neuropeptide Y with noradrenaline (*refer* enteric nervous system).

Cholinergic transmission is seen in:
* Preganglionic sympathetic nerve endings
* Preganglionic parasympathetic nerve endings
* Postganglionic parasympathetic nerve endings
* Postganglionic sympathetic nerve endings supplying skeletal muscle blood vessels and sweat gland (Cholinergic transmission also occurs in the neuromuscular junction in the somatic nervous system)

Adrenergic transmission is seen in:
* Rest of the postganglionic neurons of sympathetic nervous system.
* Adrenal medulla is considered as a specialized sympathetic ganglion (the chromaffin cells of adrenal medulla are considered as postganglionic sympathetic neurons that do not have axon. Adrenaline and noradrenaline released from these cells due to sympathetic stimulation enter the bloodstream and act as hormones)

Cholinergic Transmission

Cholinergic transmission is similar to transmission at the neuromuscular junction. The nerve endings end in the effector cells as varicosities which contain vesicles of acetylcholine. Acetyl choline is synthesized in the nerve endings and varicosities. When an action potential reaches the nerve ending the presynaptic membrane becomes permeable to Ca^{2+} and Ca^{2+} enter the nerve ending. This leads to the release of **acetylcholine** to the synaptic cleft by exocytosis. When the effect is over, acetylcholine is destroyed by acetylcholine esterase into choline and acetate. Choline is taken back into the nerve terminal.

Actions of Acetylcholine in the Postsynaptic Membrane (Table 94.1)

There are two types of receptors in the postsynaptic membrane for acetyl choline, **muscarinic and nicotinic receptors**. Muscarine activates only muscarinic receptors and will not activate nicotinic receptors. Nicotine activates only nicotinic receptors; acetyl choline activates both the receptors. Specific drugs are frequently used as medicine to stimulate or block one or the other of the two types of receptors.

Muscarinic Receptors

All postganglionic parasympathetic neurons act through muscarinic Ach receptors on the postsynaptic target cell. When stimulated, the action of these receptors resembles the action of muscarine which is a mushroom poison. Muscarinic receptor is a G protein-coupled receptor which is blocked by *atropine*. Because the actions are mediated by second messengers such as Ca^{2+}, inositol 1,4,5-triphosphate (IP_3) and diacylglycerol, muscarinic responses unlike the rapid responses evoked by nicotinic receptors are slow and prolonged. There are five subtypes of muscarinic receptors, M_1 to M_5 that are coded by five different genes. M_1, M_3 and M_5 activate phospholipase C while M_2 and M_4 inhibit adenylyl cyclase and thus decrease cAMP.

Sites of Muscarinic Receptors
a. Postsynaptic membrane of effector organs supplied by postganglionic parasympathetic nerve endings
b. Postganglionic cholinergic sympathetic nerve endings

Nicotinic Receptors

Nicotinic receptors on stimulation produce effects similar to that of **nicotine**. Nicotine in small doses stimulates the autonomic ganglia. Nicotinic receptors (subtype N_2) are present on the membrane of autonomic ganglia, i.e., at the synapses between preganglionic and postganglionic neurons of both sympathetic and parasympathetic system. [Nicotinic receptors (subtype N_1) are also present at many non-autonomic nerve endings like that on the membrane of skeletal muscle fibers at the neuromuscular junction.] Nicotinic receptors are ligand-gated ion channels activated by Ach or nicotine. Binding of the ligand with the receptor opens up the ion channel.

The nicotinic receptor can be blocked by *hexamethonium* in the autonomic ganglia and by d-tubo*curarine* at the neuromuscular junction.

Adrenergic Transmission

The neurotransmitter involved in adrenergic transmission is norepinephrine (NE). It is synthesized in the axoplasm of the terminal nerve endings of adrenergic fibers and transported into the vesicle.

$$\text{Tyrosine} \xrightarrow{\text{Hydroxylase}} \text{DOPA} \xrightarrow{\text{Decarboxylase}} \text{Dopamine} \xrightarrow{\beta\text{-hydroxylase}} \text{NE}$$

In the adrenal medulla, 80% of norepinephrine is converted to epinephrine by the enzyme **methyl transferase** which is present only in the adrenal medulla.

Once norepinephrine is released into the synaptic cleft, after its action there are three fates for norepinephrine:
1. Reuptake into the adrenergic nerve ending by active transport.
2. Diffusion into the surrounding body fluid and blood.
3. Destruction by enzymes such as monoamine oxidase (MAO) and catecholamine-O-methyl transferase (COMT).

$$\text{Norepinephrine} \xrightarrow{\text{COMT}} \text{Normetanephrine} \xrightarrow{\text{MAO}} \text{3 methoxy 4-hydroxy mandelic acid or vanillylmandelic acid (VMA)}$$

$$\text{Norepinephrine} \xrightarrow{\text{MAO}} \text{3,4 dihydroxy mandelic acid} \xrightarrow{\text{COMT}} \text{3 methoxy 4-hydroxy mandelic acid (VMA)}$$

Adrenergic Receptors (Table 94.1)

The adrenergic receptors are a class of G protein-coupled receptors. There are two major types of adrenergic receptors, **alpha receptors and beta receptors.** Their distribution in different organs differs. They are again subdivided as shown below, because certain chemicals affect only certain receptors. Norepinephrine excites mainly alpha receptors but excites beta receptors to a lesser extent. Epinephrine excites both types of receptors approximately equally. Therefore, the relative effects of norepinephrine and epinephrine on different effector tissues are determined by the types of receptors in the tissues.

Table 94.1: Characteristics of adrenergic and cholinergic receptors in the ANS.

Receptor type	Location	G protein	Mechanism	Second messenger	Effect	Agonist	Antagonist
Nicotinic ACh N_1 (Ligand gated channels)	Neuromuscular junction (motor end plate)	–	Increases permeability of Na^+ and K^+	–	Rapid depolarization	Nicotine, decamethonium	d-tubocurarine, α-bungarotoxin
Nicotinic ACh N_2 (Ligand gated channels)	Postsynaptic membrane of postganglionic autonomic neurons in the ganglia, chromaffin cells of adrenal medulla	–	Increases permeability of Na^+ and K^+	–	Depolarization	Nicotine	Hexamethonium
Muscarinic ACh M_1, M_3, M_5	M_1-Autonomic ganglia, exocrine gland, CNS M_3-endocrine and exocrine gland, eye, lungs, vascular smooth muscle and sweat glands innervated by cholinergic sympathetic fibers M_5-CNS	$G\alpha_q$	Activate phospholipase-C	IP_3, DAG	Excitation of parasympathetic neuroeffector organs and increased secretion Increased sweating and increased blood flow to skeletal muscles	Muscarine	Atropine, pirenzepine (M_1)
Muscarinic ACh M_2, M_4	M_2 - SA node, atria M_4 - CNS	$G\alpha_i$	Inhibit adenylyl cyclase	Decrease cAMP, Open K^+ channel	Decreases heart rate, decreases velocity of conduction in AV node	Muscarine	Atropine, gallamine, chlorpromazine
Adrenergic α_1	Vascular smooth muscle, GI and urinary sphincters, dilator pupillae, arrector pili, CNS	$G\alpha_q$	Activate phospholipase-C	IP_3, DAG	Vasoconstriction, increased tone of urinary and gastrointestinal sphincters, pupillary dilation, piloerection	Phenylephrine	Phentolamine
Adrenergic α_2	Presynaptic adrenergic terminals	$G\alpha_i$	Inhibit adenylyl cyclase	Decrease cAMP	Decreases the release of norepinephrine from presynaptic membrane	Clonidine	Yohimbine
Adrenergic β_1	Heart, salivary gland duct, eccrine and apocrine sweat glands, juxtaglomerular cells	$G\alpha_s$	Activates adenylyl cyclase	Increase cAMP	Increase heart rate, and myocardial contraction, increase water reabsorption from salivary duct, increase sweating	Isoproterenol, dobutamine	Metoprolol
Adrenergic β_2	Smooth muscle of bronchioles, GIT, urinary bladder, skeletal muscle blood vessels, some coronary vessels	$G\alpha_s$	Activates adenylyl cyclase	Increase cAMP	Decreases muscle tone and motility of GIT, relaxation of urinary bladder, bronchodilation, increase skeletal muscle blood flow	Terbutaline, isoproterenol	Butoxamine
Adrenergic β_3	Brown adipose tissue	$G\alpha_s$	Activates adenylyl cyclase	Increase cAMP	Lipolysis and thermogenesis	Isoproterenol	SR59230A

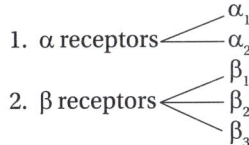

1. α receptors — α₁, α₂
2. β receptors — β₁, β₂, β₃

- Combination of norepinephrine with α_1 receptors produces increase in intracellular Ca^{2+}, which in turn activates protein kinase and produce metabolic effects in the cells.
- NE + α_2 receptors inhibit the enzyme adenylyl cyclase and decrease cAMP.
- NE + β_1 or β_2 receptors stimulate adenylyl cyclase and increase cAMP.

All the four types of receptors are present in the postsynaptic membrane. α_2 receptors are also present in the presynaptic membrane (autoreceptors). Norepinephrine once released into the synaptic cleft, combines with the α_2 receptors in the presynaptic membrane and prevents excessive release of norepinephrine. Norepinephrine has more affinity for α receptors than for β receptors. When NE combines with alpha-2 receptors, it decreases cAMP by inhibiting adenylyl cyclase.

β_3 **adrenergic receptors** are located in the adipose tissue and causes lipolysis and release of free fatty acids. Mechanism of action is by increasing cAMP.

The tissue-specific distribution of adrenergic receptor subtypes has permitted the development of drugs that are selective for different subtypes and tissues.

FUNCTIONS OF AUTONOMIC NERVOUS SYSTEM

1. Autonomic nervous system (ANS) controls the motor functions of smooth muscles, cardiac muscle and glands.
2. It maintains homeostasis.

Almost all the organs are supplied by both sympathetic and parasympathetic nerves. Sympathetic and parasympathetic divisions of ANS have opposite actions on different tissues. When the activity of one division is increased, the activity in the other division will be decreased i.e., they act reciprocally to each other. Parasympathetic system usually checks the over-activity of the sympathetic system and controls the autonomic responses. For example, the normal heart rate is 70–80/min. If the vagal supply to the heart is interrupted, the heart rate will become very high. This means that the over activity of sympathetic system is held in check by the simultaneous action of parasympathetic system. Normally, the two systems act synergistically to meet the specific demands of any given situation.

- Parasympathetic nervous system is effective in peaceful day-to-day life. It is also known as **anabolic nervous system** since it is concerned with conservative, restorative and vegetative aspects of day-to-day activities.
- Sympathetic system becomes more active during emergency conditions and stressful situations.
- Sympathetic stimulation increases blood glucose and free fatty acid levels for supplying more energy
- Sympathetic nervous system is also known as **catabolic nervous system**. The difference between the divisions of sympathetic and parasympathetic nervous system and their effects on various tissues is described in **Tables 94.2 and 94.3** respectively.

Alarm or Stress Response of the Sympathetic Nervous System

In times of stress as in fright, flight, fight, etc., large portions of sympathetic system become stimulated, producing **mass sympathetic discharge.** This result in widespread reaction throughout the body called the sympathetic **alarm or stress response.** This helps the animal to cope up with stress and situations of emergency. The ability of the body to perform vigorous muscle activity is increased in many ways. The following reactions occur in times of stress:

- Dilatation of pupil letting more light to enter the eye.
- Increase in heart rate and arterial blood pressure helps in better perfusion of vital organs and muscles.
- Constriction of cutaneous blood vessels and decreased blood flow to gastrointestinal tract and kidneys help to increase the blood flow to active muscles.
- Decreased threshold in the neurons of reticular formation and thus increasing mental alertness by activating ascending reticular activating system (ARAS).

Table 94.2: Differences between sympathetic and parasympathetic divisions of ANS.

Sympathetic nervous system	Parasympathetic nervous system
Cell bodies of preganglionic neurons are present in the lateral horn of T_1 to L_2 segments of spinal cord (thoracolumbar division of ANS)	Present in the III, VII, IX and X cranial nerve nuclei and $S_{2,3,4}$ segments of spinal cord (craniosacral division of ANS)
Preganglionic fibers are short and myelinated	Preganglionic fibers are long and myelinated
Postganglionic neurons are in the sympathetic trunk or prevertebral ganglia and postganglionic fibers are long and unmyelinated	Postganglionic neurons are present in the terminal ganglia in or near the effector organ and postganglionic fibers are short and unmyelinated
Effects of stimulation are long lasting and more widespread	Less than that of sympathetic stimulation and effect is localized to a single organ or system
Postganglionic fibers release acetylcholine or norepinephrine	Postganglionic fibers release acetylcholine
Adrenergic receptors are α and β receptors	Cholinergic receptors are nicotinic and muscarinic receptors
Prepares the body for emergency situations such as flight or fight reactions (catabolic nervous system)	Regulates activities that conserve and restore body energy (anabolic nervous system)
Excitatory to organs stimulated during physical activity and inhibitory to organs active during rest (heart rate increases during physical activity)	Inhibitory to organs that are stimulated during physical activity and stimulatory to organs active during rest (e.g., peristalsis in gut is increased and heart rate decreased during rest)

Table 94.3: Differences between sympathetic and parasympathetic effects.

Tissue	Sympathetic stimulation	Parasympathetic stimulation
Eye	Dilatation of pupil and relaxation of ciliary muscle (flattens lens)	Constriction of pupil and contraction of ciliary muscle (lens become more convex)
Heart	Increases heart rate Increases conduction velocity	Decreases heart rate Decreases conduction velocity
Respiratory tract	Bronchodilatation via β_2 receptors. Decreased secretion of mucus via α_1 and increased secretion via β_2 receptors	Bronchoconstriction and increased secretion of mucus
GIT	Decrease motility of GIT, contraction of sphincters	Increases gastrointestinal motility, relaxation of sphincters
Exocrine glands	Decreases secretions, except from salivary gland	Increases secretions of all glands, except mammary gland
Sweat glands	Localized sweating (adrenergic, via α_1)	Generalized cholinergic sweating
Salivary gland	Thick, viscous secretion via α_1	Profuse watery secretion
Blood vessels	Vasoconstriction mainly, but sympathetic cholinergic fibers produce vasodilatation	Vasodilatation
Urinary bladder	Relaxes detrusor muscle and constricts sphincters	Contracts detrusor and relaxes sphincters
Gallbladder	Relaxation	Contraction

- Increase in blood glucose and free fatty acid level, supplying more energy. There is also increased rate of cellular metabolism throughout the body.
- Increased glycolysis in liver and muscle

All the above reactions called the **sympathetic stress response** make the animal to decide whether to stand and fight or to run. This is also called **fight or flight reaction**.

DISORDERS OF AUTONOMIC NERVOUS SYSTEM

- Following sympathectomy, the person will not be able to overcome stressful situations.
- **Horner's syndrome** is due to lesion of the cervical sympathetics. There will be **ptosis** (drooping of eyelids due to paralysis of elevator palpebrae superioris), pupillary constriction (**miosis**) due to paralysis of dilator pupillae muscle, flushing of face on the affected side and reduced sweating on the ipsilateral face and neck (**hypohidrosis**).
- **Hirschsprung's disease** is a condition where there is congenital absence of myenteric plexus in a part of large intestine.
- **Raynaud's disease** is due to defective peripheral vascular innervation. It is especially seen in young women. Tips of fingers, toes, earlobes, tip of nose, etc., become pale and cyanosed and, if severe, lead to death of tissues and gangrene.
- **Multiple system atrophy (MSA)** is an adult onset, sporadic, rapidly progressive, multisystem neurodegenerative fatal disease characterized by features of Parkinsonism (bradykinesia); cerebellar gait, ataxia, nystagmus; autonomic and urogenital dysfunction and corticospinal disorders (extensor plantar response with hyper-reflexia). When autonomic failure predominates, MSA was previously termed *Shy-Drager syndrome*. The patient suffers from severe orthostatic hypotension and erectile dysfunctions (in male).
- **Haddad syndrome** is a combination of **congenital central hypoventilation syndrome (CCHS)** and **Hirschsprung's disease.** This condition is due to mutations in the **PHOX2B gene** which lead to loss of development of the neurons of the visceral control system. PHOX2B is considered as the **master gene** of the visceral control system. PHOX2B is a transcription factor required for the development of almost all neurons of the visceral control system, neurons of locus coeruleus in the pons and certain cranial nerve nuclei controlling respiration and feeding. CCHS is a congenital form of Ondine curse due to heterozygous mutations in the PHOX2B gene. Infants with this condition have problems in breathing while they sleep.

GENERAL ADAPTATION SYNDROME (GAS)

Stress

Stress is primarily a physical response, the body's way of responding to any kind of demand or threat. It is a change in the environment that is perceived as a challenge or difficult situation, threat or danger which has negative or positive effects. Factors in the environment that trigger stress response are called **stressors**. During stress, there is increased secretion of ACTH from the pituitary gland and blood cortisol level will be elevated normally. There is also increased secretion of adrenaline and noradrenaline to prepare the body for physical action, **fight or flight reaction** or stress response. When stressed, the body thinks it is under attack and switches to fight or flight mode. Stress is essential for survival. The reactions occurring in the body by the action of these hormones enables us to focus our attention so that we can quickly respond to the situation. But too much stress can lead to health problems. When there are too many stressors at one time, it can adversely affect a person's mental and physical health. The reaction following stress can be negative or positive. If we become agitated in times of stress, it can have negative effect on interpersonal relationships. But it is a natural reaction to stress.

Symptoms of stress include palpitation, fatigue, irritability, difficulty in concentrating, lack of sleep, hair loss (alopecia areata), abdominal pain typical of acid peptic disease, etc.

Hans Selye in 1936 proposed an integrative model for the stress response known as **general adaptation syndrome (GAS).** GAS is a term used to describe the body's short-term and long-term reactions to stress. Stressors include physical and mental stressors which have positive or negative effects. Examples of stressors having negative effects are starvation, injuries, infections and other disease conditions, fear, anxiety, assault, abuse, loss of loved ones, inability to solve a problem, having a difficult day at work, academic examinations, etc. Intense pleasure or joy such as travel, job promotion, marriage, etc. can also cause stress which is referred to as **eustress**. Opposite of eustress is **distress** which has negative effects. GAS represents a three-stage reaction to stress. This syndrome is called general adaptation syndrome because it is produced by agents, which have a general effect upon large portions of the body. Selye noted a triad in subjects with chronic stress (1) enlargement of adrenal cortex, (2) atrophy of thymus and other lymphoid tissues, and (3) development of bleeding ulcers in the stomach and duodenum.

The three stages of GAS are:
1. Alarm reaction
2. Stage of resistance
3. Stage of exhaustion.

Alarm Reaction

Alarm reaction is the immediate reaction to a stressor. In this initial phase, humans exhibit fight or flight response, which prepares the body for physical activity. There will be a decrease in the functioning of the immune system, making the subject susceptible to illness. There is increase in muscle tone; increase in blood pressure due to vasoconstriction and tachycardia; hyperglycemia, increased secretion of ACTH and catecholamines, loss of appetite, weight loss, etc.

Stage of Resistance or Stage of Adaptation

If the stress continues, the body adapts to the stressors. Changes occur in the body to reduce the effect of the stressor. There is increased secretion of glucocorticoids. There is increase in the level of glucose, fatty acids and amino acids in blood due to the lipolytic, catabolic and anti-anabolic actions of glucocorticoids. There will be neutrophilia, polycythemia, lymphocytopenia and eosinopenia. In high doses cortisol has mineralocorticoid-like activity and there may be features of hyperaldosteronism. Recovery follows when the compensatory mechanisms have successfully overcome the stressor effect.

Stage of Exhaustion

This stage occurs when the stress has continued for some. Although the body (in the second stage) tries to adapt to the demands of the environment initially, the body cannot maintain it indefinitely and so its resources get gradually depleted. The body's resistance to the stress gradually decreases or may collapse quickly. There will be a drastic reduction in immunity. Long-term stress may lead to severe infection; or hypertension due to prolonged vasoconstriction and an eventual heart attack. Mucosal ischemia is the main reason for stress ulcers.

Treatment and Prevention

Treatment includes avoiding stressors, changing one's reaction to the stressors or relieving stress after the reaction to stress. Listening to music, aromatherapy, exercising, relaxation techniques, acceptance of a stressful situation etc., may relieve stress after it has occurred. A healthy life style is very important such as a balanced diet, enough rest and sleep, regular exercise, improvement of social skills, avoiding smoking and drinking, strengthening relationships, etc.

Applied Aspects

The concept of general adaptation syndrome (GAS) has important application in sports training. The purpose of training is to make the body adapt to the sport-specific stressors. Training should strengthen the physiological system.

MULTIPLE CHOICE QUESTIONS

1. True regarding ANS is:
    a. Higher center of integration in the medulla oblongata
    b. Conduction in autonomic fibers is same as in somatic motor fibers
    c. Preganglionic parasympathetic fibers are more lengthy
    d. Ratio of preganglionic and postganglionic fiber is 20:1

2. All are effects of sympathetic stimulation, *except*:
    a. Increased conduction velocity
    b. Increased heart rate
    c. Increased refractory period
    d. Increased contractility of heart

3. During flight and fight reaction, which of the following is responsible for increase in local blood flow?
    a. Sympathetic system mediated cholinergic release
    b. Local hormones
    c. Parasympathetic cholinergic discharge
    d. Endocrine factors only

4. Alpha adrenergic receptor stimulation effects are:
    a. Vasoconstriction   b. Vasodilatation
    c. Bronchodilation   d. Bronchoconstriction

5. Parasympathetic stimulation causes:
    a. Decreased gastrointestinal secretion
    b. Bronchodilation
    c. Increased sweating
    d. Pupillary constriction

6. All the following are controlled by ANS, *except*:
    a. Aldosterone   b. Insulin
    c. Growth hormone   d. Somatostatin

7. Which of the following statement is true about ANS?
    a. The sympathetic outflow from the CNS is through both the cranial nerves and sympathetic chain
    b. The parasympathetic outflow from the CNS is through cranial nerves only
    c. The superior hypogastric plexus is located at the anterior aspect of the aortic bifurcation and fifth lumbar vertebra
    d. The superior hypogastric plexus contain sympathetic fibers only

8. Vagal stimulation causes all the following, *except*:
   a. Increase in intestinal secretion
   b. Constriction of intestinal musculature
   c. Relaxation of bronchial musculature
   d. Fall in blood pressure

9. Vessels not under sympathetic control are:
   a. Cerebral
   b. Splanchnic
   c. Cardiac
   d. Cutaneous

10. Which of the following is caused by acetylcholine through nicotinic receptors?
    a. Contraction of skeletal muscle
    b. Decrease in heart rate
    c. Secretion of saliva
    d. Contraction of pupils

11. Stimulation of postganglionic sympathetic neurons leads to:
    a. Fast EPSP
    b. Slow EPSP
    c. Fast IPSP
    d. Slow IPSP

12. Slow IPSP in autonomic fibers is generated by:
    a. Nicotinic cholinergic
    b. Muscarinic cholinergic
    c. Dopamine
    d. Adrenaline

13. Enzyme acetylcholine esterase is synthesized in:
    a. Liver
    b. Plasma
    c. Bone marrow
    d. Spleen

14. The parasympathetic outflow in the spinal cord occurs at the following levels:
    a. S3, 4, 5
    b. S2, 3, 4
    c. S1, 2, 3
    d. S1, 2

15. Parasympathetic stimulation will decrease the following, *except*:
    a. Heart rate
    b. AV conduction time
    c. SA node rhythmicity
    d. Atrial contractility

16. The neurotransmitter in the small intensely fluorescent cells in the autonomic ganglia is:
    a. Acetyl choline
    b. Serotonin
    c. Dopamine
    d. Nor epinephrine

17. The single ganglion that is formed by joining together of the two sympathetic trunks is called:
    a. Ganglion impar or Walther ganglion
    b. Celiac ganglion
    c. Inferior mesenteric ganglion
    d. Superior mesenteric ganglion

18. The neurons of autonomic ganglia are:
    a. Unipolar
    b. Bipolar
    c. Multipolar
    d. Anaxonic

19. Highest concentration of norepinephrine in the brain is found in the:
    a. Hypothalamus
    b. Basal ganglia
    c. Cerebellum
    d. Substantia nigra

ANSWERS

1. c	2. c	3. a	4. a	5. d
6. a	7. c	8. c	9. a	10. a
11. d	12. c	13. a	14. b	15. b
16. c	17. a	18. c	19. a	

Electroencephalography, Sleep, Yoga and Meditation

CHAPTER 95

LEARNING OBJECTIVES

Must know
- Describe the different waves of EEG
- Explain the EEG characteristics during sleep
- Differentiate between REM and NREM sleep
- Discuss the various theories of sleep

Desirable to know
- Describe the electrophysiological basis of EEG

ELECTROENCEPHALOGRAPHY (EEG)

PY10.8: Describe and discuss behavioral and EEG characteristics during sleep and mechanism responsible for its production.

Introduction

Electroencephalogram is a record of the electrical activity of the cortical neural units. The instrument used to record electrical activity of brain is called **electroencephalograph**. It includes electrodes, amplifier and recording device. Very small silver chloride electrodes, 0.5 cm in diameter are applied on the scalp with the help of a jelly. Background electrical activity is recorded by the electrode. The record obtained is called **electroencephalogram (EEG)** coined by **Hans Berger**, a German psychiatrist in 1929.

Amplifier is a **differential amplifier**. The potential should be amplified a million times. Recording device is a pen writing device or cathode-ray oscilloscope.

Procedure

Recording is done in a special room so that, interference signals can be avoided. The subject should relax physically and mentally. The electrode positions are selected. In EEG, a complicated wave pattern is obtained unlike that obtained in ECG. It is irregular and not systematic **(Figs. 95.1 and 95.2A to D)**.

EEG Pattern (Table 95.1)

EEG waves are described in terms of their **frequency** in hertz and **amplitude** in μV. There are four types of EEG wave patterns: α, β, θ and δ according to their frequency.

β-**Rhythm** is described as fast and irregular waves. They are high frequency, low amplitude waves.

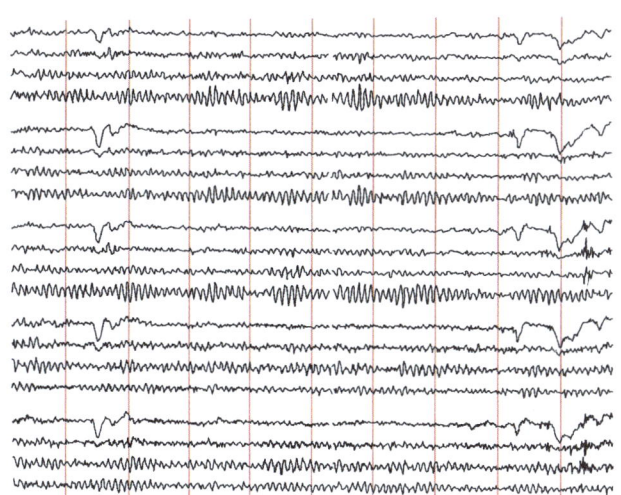

Fig. 95.1: Normal EEG pattern.

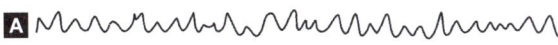
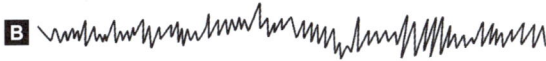
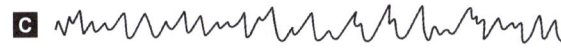
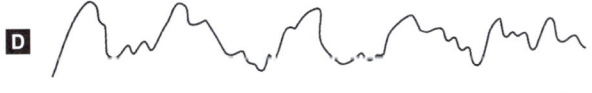

Time (s)

Figs. 95.2A to D: Waves recorded in an electroencephalogram: (A) Alpha waves; (B) Beta waves; (C) Theta waves; (D) Delta waves.

Table 95.1: Description of waves of EEG.

Wave of EEG	Frequency/second	Amplitude (µV)	Area of brain from where recorded	Condition of the subject
Alpha waves	8–12	30–50	Occipital lobe	Awake, relaxed, inattentive state with eyes closed
Beta waves	15–30	5–10	Parietal lobe	Awake, active state of brain
Delta waves	1–5	20–200	Frontal lobe	Deep sleep, newborn, deep anesthesia
Theta waves	4–7	5–100	Temporal lobe	Awake, but has emotional stress or frustration. Obtained normally during falling asleep

α-**Rhythm** is due to synchronized activity in the thalamocortical projection system. This pattern is seen in a normal adult, fully relaxed with eyes closed. It is mainly recorded from the parieto-occipital regions.

Alpha block

α-rhythm can be removed by asking the person to open the eyes. Then, α-rhythm will be converted to fast irregular β-like rhythm. When eyes are closed, again alpha rhythm is obtained. Disappearance of α rhythm when the person opens his eyes is known as α-**block or desynchronization or arousal or alerting response** (Fig. 95.3).

For α-wave to occur, the connection between reticular activating system and cortex is a must. Transection between reticular activating system and cortex produces δ waves. Decrease in the frequency of alpha rhythm is obtained in low blood glucose level, low body temperature, low glucocorticoid level, high arterial PCO_2, etc.

δ–**Rhythm** occurs normally during deep sleep. If it is recorded in the wakeful state in adult, it indicates some abnormality in the brain like serious brain damage.

Theta waves are low frequency, high amplitude waves. Theta rhythm is seen in children and while falling asleep. In adults, it appears in severe depression.

Basis of EEG

EEG waves are thought to be due to current flow in the fluctuating dipoles formed on the dendrites and the cell body of the layers of cerebral cortex.

Clinical Application of EEG

The following conditions can be detected using EEG:
- **Subdural hematoma** can be diagnosed and localized by EEG. The EEG activity recorded from the area overlying the clot may be damped.
- Detection and localization of **brain tumors**—the brain tumor may compress the neurons in the surrounding area and increase their excitability. It may be manifested as an epileptic attack. High-amplitude, high-frequency waves are obtained in this condition. Normally, if it is high frequency, the amplitude will be less.
- EEG can be used as a **biofeedback**.

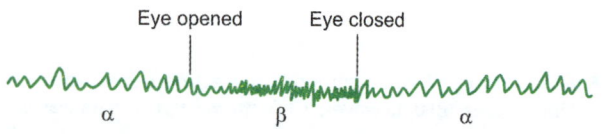

Fig. 95.3: EEG recording showing alpha block.

- **Brain death** is defined as a maintained flat EEG for more than 24 hours.
- Epileptogenic foci sometimes generate high-voltage waves that can be localized by EEG.
- Different types of **epilepsies** can be distinguished with the help of EEG **(Figs. 95.4A to C)**. For example:
  - In **grand mal epilepsy**, high-frequency, high-amplitude waves (100 mV) are obtained. A large region of brain or spinal cord will be involved. There will be severe tonic, clonic convulsions lasting for 3–4 min.
  - In **petit mal epilepsy**, spike and dome pattern is obtained of amplitude 50 mV. There will be blinking of eyes, twitching of facial muscles, etc. This can progress to grand mal type.
  - **Psychomotor seizure**—Low-amplitude abnormal wave pattern is obtained in EEG. It is very difficult to distinguish between these people and normal people without taking EEG.

Simple type of fits occurring while falling asleep is normal and is of the petit mal type.

SLEEP

Sleep is defined as a state of unresponsiveness or unconsciousness from which a person can be aroused by appropriate sensory stimulation or any other type of stimuli. *If the person cannot be aroused, the condition is known as coma*.

Sleep and wakefulness shows **circadian periodicity** of about 24 hours (an average of 8 hours sleep and 16 hours of wakefulness). It is controlled by **suprachiasmatic nucleus** of hypothalamus, which forms the **biological clock**. There

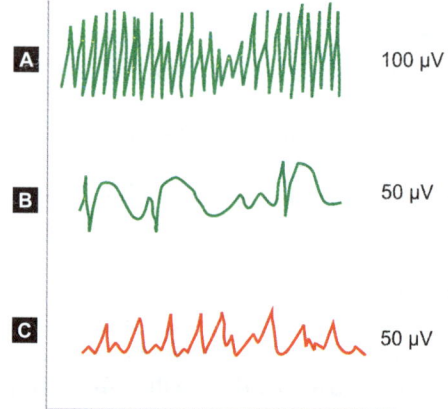

Figs. 95.4A to C: EEG pattern in different types of epilepsy: (A) Grand mal epilepsy (high frequency, high amplitude waves); (B) Petit mal epilepsy (spike and dome pattern); (C) Psychomotor epilepsy.

are two kinds of sleep; rapid eye movement (REM) sleep and non-REM sleep. Several episodes of REM sleep and NREM sleep are observed each night and dreams occur mostly during REM sleep.

Importance of Sleep

The purpose of sleep is unclear, but it is seen that lack of sleep can be debilitating. Sleep is a state of inactivity or period of rest for the nervous system where there is suppression of cortical neuronal activity. This period of rest is a must for a normal person, otherwise he becomes irritable. Chemicals that accumulate in the brain during wakefulness are metabolized during sleep.

Experimental animals completely deprived of sleep for long periods, lose weight despite increased caloric intake and eventually die. So, sleep has important homeostatic role. Secretion of growth hormone and gonadotropins is increased during sleep.

Sleep is also necessary for learning and memory consolidation. Performance following learning improves only if a period of slow wave and REM sleep has occurred without interruption.

Physiological Changes during Sleep

- During sleep, somatic nervous system is completely suppressed with little cortical neuronal activity. Muscle tone is decreased, reflexes are suppressed and receptor function is also suppressed. A nearly complete paralysis of skeletal muscle occurs during rapid eye movement (REM) sleep to prevent the person from physically acting out the dreams.
- The sympathetic system is suppressed and para-sympathetic activity predominates. Pupils will be constricted.
- A 30% reduction in general metabolism (BMR) is seen during sleep.
- There is a reduction in heart rate and blood pressure in NREM sleep.
- In the GIT, secretion and digestion continue and there is increase in gastrointestinal motility.
- Urine formation is less than that of waking hours. Urine is highly concentrated with more phosphate.
- In the respiratory system, there is a reduction in the rate and depth of respiration and slight hypoxemia is seen during sleep. There is a reduction in the sensitivity of respiratory centers to CO_2. In a very small percentage of people, periods of **sleep apnea** are seen due to suppression of respiratory center (*refer* 'sleep apnea in respiratory system' page 376).
- Towards the onset of sleep, thoughts become illogical and incoherent. The transition from wakefulness to sleep tends to produce a **retrograde amnesia**. For example, it is difficult to remember the time when we fell asleep. This is because sleep onset inactivates the consolidation of short-term memory into long-term memory.

Classification of Sleep Depending on EEG Pattern

Depending on EEG pattern, sleep is divided into two stages:
1. **Slow-wave sleep or spindle sleep or NREM sleep**
2. Fast-wave sleep or paradoxical sleep or REM sleep.

Distribution of Sleep Stages

In normal adults, sleep mostly begins with NREM sleep. (In infants, entry into sleep occurs through REM sleep.) Thereafter, NREM sleep and REM sleep alternate cyclically through the night. The average duration of a sleep cycle is 90 min. In a night's cycle, we get 75 min slow wave sleep then, 15 min REM sleep; then again 75 min of slow wave sleep. This cycle is repeated about 4–5 times throughout the night. Thus, 4–6 REM periods occur per night. Towards waking hours, REM sleep pattern is seen more. The proportion of NREM to REM sleep varies with age. Newborn children spend half of their sleep time in REM sleep, whereas elderly have little REM sleep. About 20–25% of sleep of young adults is REM sleep (**Table 95.2**). *REM sleep accounts for about 80% of total sleep duration in premature infants.*

The transition from wakefulness to sleep is always through stage 1 of NREM sleep. The transition from sleep to the awake state occurs either at the end of REM sleep or at the end of stage 2.

Changes in EEG Pattern during Different Stages of Sleep

NREM Sleep

According to EEG pattern, there are four stages of NREM sleep. Stages 1 and 2 are of short duration.
- **First stage**: This is the stage of drowsiness and falling asleep. EEG pattern obtained is β rhythm.
- **Second stage**: In this stage, β rhythm is interspersed with α rhythm. Appearance of α rhythm in between β rhythm is known as **sleep spindles**. Occasional high voltage biphasic waves called **K-complexes** are also seen in this stage.
- **Third stage**: Sleep deepens and the predominant rhythm is θ. In between, some α waves and β waves are also seen occasionally in this stage. *Sleep spindles are seen only up to third stage.*
- **Fourth stage**: It is the stage of deep sleep in which it is difficult to arouse the person. Here, we get δ rhythm with marked synchronization.

> Gamma and delta rhythms are normal during sleep but their appearance during wakefulness is a sign of brain dysfunction.

Slow-wave sleep or NREM sleep is not associated with dreams. During stage 2 of NREM sleep, **bruxism** or grinding of teeth is usually seen in children. There is some activity of skeletal muscles throughout NREM sleep, but no eye movements occur.

REM Sleep

The high amplitude slow waves (δ waves) seen in EEG during the fourth stage of NREM sleep are periodically replaced by rapid, low voltage EEG activity (β rhythm) which resembles that seen in the awake aroused state. This is **REM sleep or paradoxical sleep**. But sleep is not interrupted in this stage and the threshold for arousal is increased. Rapid roving movements of eyes occur during paradoxical sleep and hence called **rapid eye movement (REM) sleep**. The pattern changes to β rhythm from δ rhythm due to presence of dreams in REM sleep.

Features of REM Sleep (Table 95.2)
- EEG becomes desynchronized, i.e., low-voltage fast activity seen.
- Large spikes are seen in the EEG called ponto-geniculo-occipital (PGO) waves in between fast activity. **PGO spikes** are characteristic of REM sleep. They are large phasic potentials, in groups of 3–5 that originate in the cholinergic neurons in the pons and pass rapidly to the lateral geniculate body and from there to the occipital cortex.
- Autonomic changes such as loss of temperature regulation, penile erection, irregularities in heart rate and respiration, etc., are also seen depending on the type of dream.
- Muscle tone is lost, the tone of the skeletal muscles of the neck, tongue and pharynx is markedly reduced during REM sleep leading to falling back of tongue and snoring in some individuals. But phasic contractions occur in some muscles such as eye muscles. The rapid rolling movement seen in the eyes in this stage of sleep gave this phase the name rapid eye movement sleep (REM).
- Even though the EEG pattern in REM sleep resembles that seen in awake, aroused state, it is more difficult to arouse a person from REM sleep and hence the term **paradoxical sleep**.
- REM sleep and dreaming are closely associated. REM sleep is more towards morning and hence dreams are more frequent towards waking hours. Activity in the visual association areas is increased in REM sleep but there is decreased activity in the primary visual cortex.
- *REM sleep occurs only after a period of slow-wave sleep.*

Mechanism of Sleep

The mechanism of sleep is incompletely understood. Two theories have been put forward:
1. Passive mechanism
2. Active mechanism

Passive Mechanism

There is a circuitous connection between the cerebral cortex and intralaminar nuclei of thalamus. Wakefulness is due to reverberating circuits in the brain. If the reverberation is continuing for a long time, there will be fatigue of the synapses between cortex and intralaminar nuclei of thalamus and sleep sets in.

The ascending reticular activating system (ARAS) is stimulated by impulses reaching it through collaterals from specific sensory pathways. The RAS, in turn, sends a strong facilitatory drive to the cerebral cortex, increasing the excitability of cortical neurons. Thus, the RAS is responsible for the wakefulness, full consciousness and alertness of the individual. In the passive mechanism of sleep, minimum number of sensory stimuli passes through the ARAS leading to sleep.

Active Mechanism

According to active mechanism, there is a **sleep center** in the intralaminar nuclei of thalamus and anterior hypothalamus and a **waking center** in the reticular formation and posterior hypothalamus. It is seen that lesions of posterior hypothalamus result in coma. Activation of neurons which inhibit reticular activating system (RAS) will induce sleep. Certain neurons in the limbic system when stimulated induce sleep. Suprachiasmatic nucleus of hypothalamus is responsible for circadian control of sleep.

Repeated stimulation of afferents from mechano-receptors in the skin at rates of 10 Hz or less also induces sleep.

Hypnotoxin, a chemical substance when injected into the CSF of an animal will induce sleep. Hypnotoxin is produced in the nervous system of animals which are kept awake for a long time. At the onset of sleep there is a slight increase in growth hormone level.

Other substances that induce sleep are **acetylcholine, lactic acid, etc.**

Concentrations of **adenosine** in some sleep areas increase during sleep. So it is considered as a sleep producing factor. This is supported by the fact that caffeine which is an adenosine antagonist leads to alertness.

Mechanism of Slow-wave Sleep (NREM Sleep)

Stimulation of three subcortical regions produces slow-wave sleep. They are:

Table 95.2: Difference between NREM and REM sleep.

Slow wave sleep (NREM sleep)	Rapid eye movement sleep (REM)
Accounts for 75–80% of sleep time	20–25% of normal sleep time
Rapid roving movements of eye absent	Rapid roving movements of eye present hence called REM sleep
Muscle tone reduced	Muscle atonia
Associated with sleep spindles	Not associated with sleep spindles
Hypnic jerks occur	Hypnic jerks absent
People are disoriented and confused when awakened from NREM sleep	People are oriented when awakened from REM sleep
20% of dreams occur in this stage	80% of dreams occur in REM sleep
Dreams difficult to be recalled	Dreams easier to be recalled
10–30% decrease in BP, BMR, heart rate and respiratory rate seen	HR, RR and BP change intermittently
Apnea not observed in NREM sleep	Periods of apnea seen
Easy to arouse the person	Highest threshold for awakening by sensory stimuli
CNS activity is depressed	CNS activity is increased
Reflexes normal or diminished	Deep tendon reflexes absent
PGO spikes absent in EEG	PGO spikes present
Parasympathetic activity predominates	Sympathetic activity increases intermittently
Cerebral blood flow and cerebral metabolic rate decreased by 5–25% in NREM sleep	Cerebral blood flow and metabolic rate increase by 10–40% above waking levels
Thermoregulatory response depressed	Thermoregulation absent

- **Diencephalic sleep zone** in the posterior hypothalamus and nearby intralaminar and anterior thalamic nuclei. Only low-frequency stimulation of this area produces sleep.
- **Medullary synchronizing zone** in the reticular formation of medulla oblongata at the level of nucleus tractus solitarius. Only low-frequency stimulation produces sleep. If frequency is high, it produces arousal.
- **Basal forebrain sleep zone** which includes the **preoptic area and the diagonal band of Broca**. Whether the stimulating frequency is high or low, this area produces slow wave sleep. There is inhibition of ARAS inputs by the descending pathways arising from these areas.

Mechanism of REM Sleep

The mechanism that triggers REM sleep is located in the **pontine reticular formation**. Pontogeniculooccipital (PGO) spikes originate in the pons. The spikes are due to discharge of cholinergic neurons. **Cholinergic PGO spike** discharge initiates REM sleep. PGO spike is a characteristic feature of REM sleep. These spikes activate the reticular inhibiting area in the medulla oblongata producing the marked hypotonia seen in REM sleep. Firing of these cholinergic neurons is blocked by the noradrenergic neurons originating in locus coeruleus and serotonergic neurons of raphe nuclei.

Neurotransmitters Involved in Sleep-wake Cycles

- The posterior hypothalamic neurons involved in sleep-wake cycles release **histamine** as the neurotransmitter. These histaminergic neurons stimulate the ARAS and increase cortical neuronal activity. These neurons are inhibited by a group of GABAergic neurons in the anterior hypothalamus. *Thus, histamine released by posterior hypothalamic neurons induces wakeful state while GABA released by preoptic neurons in anterior hypothalamus induces NREM sleep.*
- The pontine reticular formation contains groups of neurons which release norepinephrine, serotonin and acetyl choline as neurotransmitters.
- Locus coeruleus contain **norepinephrine** containing neurons while, raphe nuclei contain **serotonin** secreting neurons. The pontine neurons responsible for the generation of PGO spikes in REM sleep release **acetyl choline** (ACh) as the neurotransmitter. *Cholinergic system is necessary for shifting NREM sleep to REM sleep.*
- When the activity of norepinephrine and serotonin containing neurons in reticular formation is dominant, there is inhibition of activity in ACh containing neurons in the pontine reticular formation. This leads to a wakeful state. In contrast, when there is decreased activity in the norepinephrine and serotonin containing neurons, there is increased activity of acetylcholine containing neurons which leads to REM sleep. When there is a balance in the activity of aminergic and cholinergic neurons, NREM sleep occurs.
- The preoptic area of the basal forebrain sleep zone release prostaglandin D_2 (**PGD_2**) which causes increase in NREM and REM sleep.

Theories of Sleep

Pavlov's Theory of Sleep

According to this theory, sleep occurs as a conditioned reflex. To prove this, Pavlov showed a circular object and an elliptical object to an animal. The animal was conditioned to salivate on seeing the circular object but not with the elliptical one. When the circular object was made more elliptical and elliptical object more circular, the animal became either neurotic or due to confusion it went to sleep. This is an example of **conditioned inhibition**.

Cerebral Anemia Theory

Cerebral anemia theory states that cerebral vasoconstriction occurs during sleep causing cerebral hypoxia and sleep.

Kleitman's Theory

Kleitman's theory states that decrease in the number of sensory stimuli reaching the sensorium induces sleep.

PHYSIOLOGY OF SLEEP-WAKE CYCLES

Role of Brainstem Reticular Formation and Hypothalamic Neurons

Nuclei in the brainstem and hypothalamus are responsible for the sleep-wake cycles which manifest a circadian rhythm. Brainstem reticular formation is composed of several groups of neurons that release norepinephrine, serotonin or acetylcholine as neurotransmitters. Norepinephrine is produced by **locus coeruleus**, serotonin by **raphe nuclei** and acetyl choline by **ponto-mesencephalo-tegmental complex** of brainstem reticular formation.

The hypothalamic neurons involved in the control of sleep-wake cycles are the **preoptic neurons** in the hypothalamus which release GABA and **posterior hypothalamic neurons** which release histamine.

Transitions from sleep to wakefulness may involve alternating reciprocal activity of different groups of reticular activating system neurons. Increased activity of norepinephrine and serotonin containing neurons in locus coeruleus and raphe nuclei leads to inhibition of acetyl choline containing neurons in the pontine reticular formation. This leads to the wakeful state. When norepinephrine and serotonergic neurons are inhibited there is increased secretion of acetyl choline from the pontine neurons which leads to REM sleep. *Cholinergic system is necessary for shifting NREM sleep to REM sleep. When there is a balance between the activity of aminergic and cholinergic neurons, NREM sleep occurs* (**Flowchart 95.1**).

Posterior hypothalamic neurons release histamine which activates the thalamus and cortex leading to wakeful state. Stimulation of preoptic neurons in hypothalamus leads to increased release of GABA which inhibits the secretion of histamine from posterior hypothalamus leading to NREM sleep. When there is decreased secretion of GABA from the preoptic neurons, there is increased secretion of histamine from posterior hypothalamus leading to increased activity in the thalamus and cortex producing wakeful state.

Flowchart 95.1: Sleep-wake cycle.

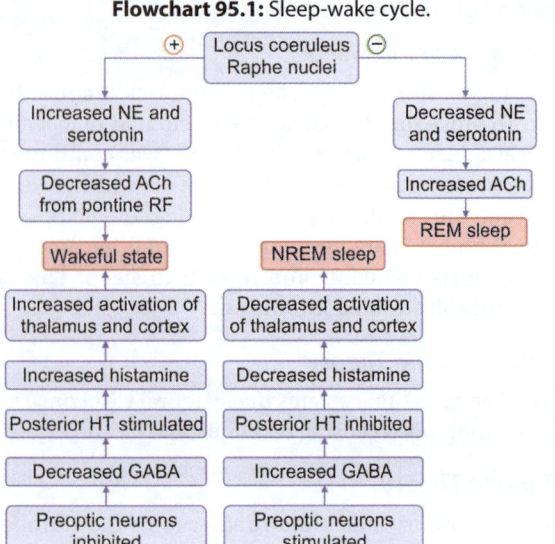

(HT: hypothalamus; NE: norepinephrine; RF: reticular formation; ACh: acetyl choline; '+' sign denotes stimulation and '–' sign denotes inhibition)

Role of Melatonin in Sleep-wake Cycle

Melatonin released from the pineal gland also plays a role in sleep-wake mechanism. Melatonin synthesis and secretion are increased during the dark period of the day and decreased during day time. The sympathetic nerves to the pineal gland are stimulated by light signals. The information reaches the suprachiasmatic nucleus of hypothalamus via the retinohypothalamic tract **(Flowchart 95.2)**.

From the hypothalamus, descending pathways converge onto preganglionic sympathetic neurons which reach the superior cervical ganglion. The postganglionic neurons which release norepinephrine innervate the pineal gland and stimulate melatonin synthesis and secretion. *The diurnal change in melatonin secretion may function as a timing signal to coordinate events with the light-dark cycle in the environment including the sleep-wake cycle.*

Sleep Abnormalities or Parasomnia

Parasomnia is disturbing sleep disorders essentially seen during the REM stage and sometimes during NREM stage of the sleep cycle. Sleep abnormalities include insomnia, bed-wetting, bruxism (tooth grinding), sleep walking, sleep apnea, snoring and narcolepsy.

Insomnia is lack of sufficient, restful sleep. It may be due to medical or psychiatric causes.

Bed wetting or nocturnal enuresis is involuntary voiding of urine during deep sleep. It occurs in some children during slow wave sleep. It is a normal phenomenon in infants.

Sleep bruxism is an involuntary, unconscious mandibular movement with tooth grinding during sleep. It occurs mainly during stages 1 and 2 of NREM sleep and also during REM sleep and to a lesser degree in stages 3 and 4 of NREM sleep.

Sleep walking or somnambulism is common in children than adults. These individuals walk during sleep with their eyes open and also avoid obstacles while walking. But when awakened, they cannot recall the episode.

Snoring occurs due to the hypotonia associated with sleep which results in the soft palate falling back to partially occlude the nasopharynx.

Narcolepsy is irresistible desire to sleep during day time. It is characterized by several brief bouts of REM-onset sleep in a day. It is due to the inability to inhibit REM sleep in the wakeful state. In normal individuals, REM sleep never occurs without previous NREM or slow-wave sleep. But in narcolepsy, there is sudden onset of REM sleep.

It is seen that people with this defect have very low levels of orexins in their CSF. **Orexins** are hormones synthesized in the lateral hypothalamus. Orexin receptors are present in hypothalamus. Orexin deficiency also leads to hyperphagia and obesity.

REM Behavior Disorder or Hypnic Myoclonia

Hypnic myoclonia is a generalized or localized muscle contraction often associated with vivid visual imagery. In REM sleep, there is a reduction in skeletal muscle tone due to impulses coming from **locus coeruleus**. When there is a lesion in locus coeruleus, hypotonia fails to occur during REM sleep. So in this condition REM sleep is associated with voluntary activity to dream events. It appears that they are acting out their dreams. This condition is known as REM behavior disorder or **hypnic myoclonia**.

YOGA AND MEDITATION

PY11.12: Discuss the physiological effects of meditation.

Physiology of Yoga

The term yoga is derived from the Sanskrit word **"yuj"** which means '**union**' or harness. Yoga is a profound physical, emotional and cognitive experience, each of which is capable of influencing the human body. Various techniques in yoga aim at attaining a conscious state in which mental activities such as perception, analysis and imagination are suspended and a *mindless state is reached*.

Flowchart 95.2: Role of suprachiasmatic nucleus of hypothalamus (HT) in sleep-wake cycle.

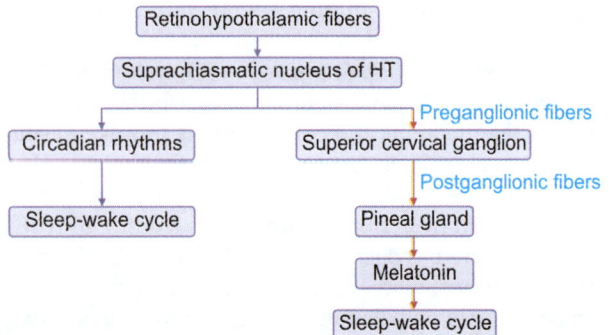

Yoga Techniques

Yoga is classified in terms of the means adopted to reach the final aim. Some of the experimentally investigated yogic techniques include:
a. Asana (postures)
b. Pranayama (breathing techniques)
c. Krias (cleansing techniques)
d. Mudras (attitudes)
e. Bandhas (neuromuscular influences).

Importance of Asana

The term **asana** means a steady, comfortable posture. Properly performed asanas are associated with relaxation of the related skeletal muscles as assessed from EMG recording. The activity in CNS is predominantly cerebellar, and postural equilibrium is achieved at a new resting muscle length.

With proper practice, proprioceptive and visceroceptive inputs become stronger and stronger in intensity so as to suppress the inputs coming from the sense organs. The end result is the development of a *pleasant type of internalized awareness free of disturbance, pain or tension*. In yoga, such a turning away of awareness from sense organ is called **'pratyahara.'**

The physiological basis of the above state is that there is a change in the nature of sensory inputs as well as the processing of the sensory information in the cerebral cortex. There is a shift in the processing of information to sub-cortical levels involving cerebellum, brainstem and limbic system. Long-term training in asanas leads to improvement in the fine coordination of movements, flexibility of joints and an overall improvement in physical and mental fitness.

Breathing and Relaxation Techniques

Breathing techniques include:
- **Abdominal breathing**, which is slow and deep with proper usage of the diaphragm.
- **Intercostal breathing** involves expansion of ribs and the chest wall with proper usage of intercostal muscles.
- **Clavicular breathing**—During inhalation, the shoulders and clavicle are raised as the abdomen is drawn in.

Pranayama involves more advanced breathing techniques such as alternate nostril breathing, alternate nostril breathing with retention, without retention, etc. If properly and regularly performed, breathing techniques lead to the following changes in the body:
- Increase in resting tidal volume
- Decrease in the resting respiratory rate
- Increase in vital capacity
- Increase in breath-holding time
- Increase in the tone of abdominal muscles
- In energy metabolism, there is a reduction in O_2 consumption and CO_2 production by about 30%.

Relaxation Techniques

Uncontrolled emotions such as anger, frustration, hostility, etc., use up as much energy as physical activity. The act of relaxation is very important in yoga. Asanas are used for physical relaxation and release of muscular tension. Sitting in a meditational posture for some time changes the tonic equilibrium between antagonistic muscles. Even simple relaxation techniques like sitting in a quiet environment with eyes closed, keeping on repeating a simple sound in order to block out word-related thoughts, etc, can decrease muscle tension, heart rate, blood pressure and respiratory rate. This type of *mental and physical relaxation is of great benefit in coping up with stress and stress related disorders.*

Effect of Yoga on Brain

There is a preponderance of alpha waves in EEG in yogis. It is also observed that sensory stimuli which normally block the alpha rhythm could not do so in yogis while on meditation. The explanation for this is **neuronal plasticity**. Plasticity includes formation of new synapses and circuits in the nervous system and also reorganizes and reinforces them in response to new stimuli and learning experiences. Plasticity also involves changes in neurotransmitter release and changes in the structure of their receptors. Neuronal plasticity is of three types:
1. Developmental plasticity
2. Experience-related plasticity
3. Regeneration-related plasticity.

The influence of yoga on brain is due to **experience-related plasticity**. Yoga can be considered as an experience and the changes seen in yoga have remarkable similarities to learning. It involves changes in synaptic function such as long-term potentiation, long-term depression, change in the number of synapses, change in neurotransmitter profile, etc. Thus *yogic practices bring about sustained changes in the structure and function of brain.*

Influence of Yoga on Cardiovascular System

Cardiovascular efficiency increases after regular yoga practice. Properly performed yoga techniques bring about changes in heart rate, blood pressure and regional blood flow. The resting heart rate as well as the increase in heart rate during exercise will decrease due to *increase in the vagal tone*. The blood pressure decreases. Well-trained yogis can control their heart voluntarily such as inducing tachycardia, bradycardia, or they can even reduce venous return to heart to such an extent that the pulse could not be felt.

Other Physiological Benefits of Yoga

- Sleep improves
- Immunity increases
- Pain decreases
- Mood improves and subjective well-being increases
- Social adjustments increase
- Anxiety and depression decrease
- Hostility decreases
- Psychomotor functions improve
- Depth perception improves
- Integrated functioning of body parts improves

- Cognitive function improves
- Attention and concentration improves
- Memory increases
- Learning efficiency improves.

Biochemical Effects

- Blood glucose, sodium, total cholesterol, triglycerides, LDL cholesterol and VLDL cholesterol decrease
- HDL cholesterol increases
- Catecholamine level decreases
- Thyroxine level increases and so is of benefit in hypothyroidism
- Oxytocin and prolactin level increases
- Oxygen level in the brain increases.

Hematological Changes

- Hematocrit value increases
- Hemoglobin level increases
- Lymphocyte count increases, but total white blood cell count decreases.

MULTIPLE CHOICE QUESTIONS

1. **Chemical transmitter in REM sleep is:**
   a. Dopamine   b. GABA
   c. Serotonin   d. Acetyl choline

2. **Night terror is called:**
   a. Somnambulism   b. Somniloquy
   c. Pavor nocturnus   d. Bruxism

3. **All the following are sleep disorders of REM sleep, *except*:**
   a. Night mares
   b. Narcolepsy
   c. Nocturnal penile tumescence
   d. Somnambulism

4. **What are the EEG waves recorded from parieto-occipital region with the subject awake and eyes closed?**
   a. Alpha waves   b. Beta waves
   c. Delta waves   d. Theta waves

5. **EEG rhythm having highest frequency is:**
   a. Alpha   b. Beta
   c. Theta   d. Delta

6. **Epileptic attacks beginning in the inferior parts of precentral gyrus is referred to as:**
   a. Petitmal epilepsy
   b. Grandmal epilepsy
   c. Jacksonian epilepsy
   d. Psychomotor epilepsy

7. **Muscle tone is markedly reduced in:**
   a. First stage of NREM sleep
   b. REM sleep
   c. Second stage of NREM sleep
   d. Third stage of NREM sleep

8. **All the following neurotransmitters maintain wakeful state, *except*:**
   a. Norepinephrine   b. Serotonin
   c. Histamine   d. Adenosine

9. **The pacemaker responsible for maintaining circadian sleep-wake cycles is:**
   a. Paraventricular nucleus
   b. Suprachiasmatic nucleus
   c. Supraoptic nucleus
   d. Median raphe nucleus

10. **Beta waves in EEG designate which of the following states of the subject?**
    a. Deep anesthesia
    b. Surgical anesthesia
    c. Eyes closed and relaxed
    d. Awake and alert

11. **Sleep spindles and K complex in EEG occur in which stage of sleep?**
    a. Stage I   b. Stage II
    c. Stage III   d. Stage IV

12. **The wave in EEG that reflects synchronized brain activity is:**
    a. Alpha wave   b. Beta wave
    c. Theta wave   d. Delta wave

13. **True statement regarding paradoxical sleep is:**
    a. Prominent beta waves
    b. Prominent alpha waves
    c. Also known as NREM sleep
    d. Low amplitude, mixed frequency waves

14. **Which one of the following phenomena is closely associated with slow wave sleep?**
    a. Dreaming   b. Atonia
    c. Sleep walking   d. Irregular heart rate

15. **Dreams registered in the memory occurs in:**
    a. REM sleep
    b. Stage I NREM sleep
    c. Stage II NREM sleep
    d. Stage III NREM sleep

16. **Sleep talking is called:**
    a. Somnambulism   b. Somniloquy
    c. Pavor nocturnes   d. Bruxism

17. **Normal adult human EEG:**
    a. Will show high frequency waves during stage III sleep
    b. Shows alpha rhythm when a person is awake but inattentive
    c. Has lower frequency waves during mental activity
    d. Is predominated by large amplitude waves during REM sleep

18. **Hypnic jerk is a very common sleep related movement during:**
    a. Dreaming   b. Transition to sleep
    c. REM sleep   d. Waking

19. All the following neurotransmitters maintain wakeful state, *except*:
    a. Norepinephrine
    b. Serotonin
    c. Histamine
    d. Adenosine
20. In deep sleep, EEG shows:
    a. Alpha waves
    b. Beta waves
    c. Theta waves
    d. Delta waves
21. The EEG curves are called:
    a. Delta waves
    b. Berger's rhythm
    c. Neurogenic rhythm
    d. REM rhythm
22. Berger waves (alpha waves) of EEG have the rhythm per second of:
    a. 0–4
    b. 4–7
    c. 8–13
    d. 13–30
23. EEG with spike and dome pattern is characteristic of which type of epilepsy?
    a. Jacksonian
    b. Grandmal
    c. Petitmal
    d. Temporal lobe
24. During light sleep, the sleep spindles that appear have the frequency of:
    a. 1–2/sec
    b. 6–12/sec
    c. 14–16/sec
    d. 21–26/sec
25. Delta waves in EEG are seen in:
    a. Deep sleep
    b. REM sleep
    c. Awake with eyes open
    d. Awake with eyes closed
26. The condition known as REM sleep is:
    a. That point at which the individual becomes aware and alert
    b. Referred to as paradoxical sleep
    c. Characterized by total lack of all muscular activity
    d. Characterized by appearance of sleep spindles
27. EEG rhythm recorded from the surface of the scalp during REM sleep is:
    a. Alpha
    b. Beta
    c. Delta
    d. Theta
28. Nightmares are seen in:
    a. REM sleep
    b. NREM stage II
    c. NREM stage III
    d. NREM stage IV
29. Arousal response is mediated by:
    a. Dorsal column
    b. Reticular activating system
    c. Spinothalamic tract
    d. Vestibulo-cerebellar tract
30. EEG rhythm having lowest frequency is:
    a. Alpha
    b. Beta
    c. Theta
    d. Delta
31. An EEG:
    a. Provides indication of intelligence
    b. Tends to show waves of smaller amplitude during sleep than of alert state
    c. Show waves with a lower frequency during intense thought than during sleep
    d. Is bilaterally symmetrical
32. The frequency of beta waves in EEG is:
    a. 0–4/sec
    b. 4–7/sec
    c. 7–13/sec
    d. 13–30/sec
33. All the following are seen in REM sleep, *except*:
    a. Bruxism
    b. Hypotonia
    c. Tachycardia
    d. Dreams
34. The usual voltage of alpha rhythm is:
    a. 50 mV
    b. 10 mV
    c. 5 mV
    d. 100 mV
35. Alpha waves in EEG is seen in:
    a. Sleep
    b. REM sleep
    c. Awake state
    d. Mental work
36. The EEG rhythm in a person who is awake, eyes closed, mind wandering is:
    a. Beta
    b. Theta
    c. Delta
    d. Alpha
37. In the hippocampus, EEG waves are:
    a. Alpha wave
    b. β wave
    c. Theta wave
    d. Delta wave

ANSWERS

1. d	2. c	3. d	4. a	5. b
6. c	7. b	8. d	9. b	10. d
11. b	12. a	13. d	14. c	15. a
16. b	17. b	18. b	19. d	20. d
21. b	22. c	23. c	24. c	25. a
26. b	27. b	28. a	29. b	30. d
31. d	32. d	33. a	34. a	35. c
36. a	37. c			

Higher Functions of Brain

CHAPTER 96

LEARNING OBJECTIVES

Must know
- Differentiate between unconditioned and conditioned reflexes
- Classify the different forms of memory and describe the theories of memory
- Explain the role of synaptic plasticity, long-term potentiation, long-term depression, habituation and sensitization in learning and memory
- Summarize the differences between categorical and representational hemisphere
- Classify aphasia and explain the pathophysiology of each type
- Explain intercortical transfer of learning

Desirable to know
- Explain the abnormalities of learning and memory
- Explain cortical plasticity

INTRODUCTION

PY10.9: Describe and discuss the physiological basis of memory, learning and speech.

Reflex is an involuntary response to an adequate stimulus. Study of conditioned reflex is one of the methods for the study of higher functions of brain. Reflexes can be broadly classified into two **(Table 96.1)**:
1. Conditioned reflex
2. Unconditioned reflex.

UNCONDITIONED REFLEX

These are inborn or inherent reflexes present **from birth** onwards. Examples are:
- When we touch a hot object, there is sudden withdrawal of the hand.
- When food is placed in the mouth, there will be salivation.
- When light is flashed into the eye, pupil constricts.

Table 96.1: Difference between unconditioned and conditioned reflexes.

Unconditioned reflexes	Conditioned reflexes
Inborn	Acquired
No training required, can be elicited in infants	Requires training, cannot be elicited in infants
Stable	Unstable
Limited in number	Unlimited
Lower centers like spinal cord or brainstem are sufficient	Higher center, i.e., cerebralcortex is essential
Special pathways present	No special pathway

CONDITIONED REFLEX

Conditioned reflex is not inborn, but is **acquired** by training. For example, smell, sight or even thought of delicious food will produce salivation in adults, but not in infants. This is a conditioned reflex. Conditioned reflexes are built upon the basis of unconditioned reflexes and require previous experience. They are reflexes conditioned by previous exposure to the same situation.

Definition

A **conditioned reflex** may be defined as a reflex response to a stimulus which previously elicited little or no response, acquired by repeatedly pairing the stimulus with another stimulus, which normally produces the response.

Types of Conditioned Reflexes

Ivan Petrovich Pavlov, a Russian neurophysiologist was the first person to describe conditioned reflex and he classified them into two:
1. Pavlovian type I (classical conditioning)
2. Pavlovian type II (instrumental conditioning or operant conditioning).

Another classification is:
- **Natural conditioned reflexes** which are established under normal circumstances of life.
- **Artificial conditioned reflexes** which are established experimentally or by special methods.

Classical Conditioning

Classical conditioning was studied by Pavlov on dogs. The salivary reflex is employed because, the response can be quantitatively expressed in terms of volume of saliva secreted.

A bell is rung and meat is placed in the dog's mouth. There will be salivation. After repeatedly pairing the two, ringing of bell alone without giving meat will produce salivation. Here, meat is the **unconditioned stimulus** and ringing of bell is the **conditioned stimulus**. The response obtained, i.e., salivation, is the **conditioned response**. Here, we can say that the conditioned reflex is established.

The bell is an indifferent or **neutral stimulus** and salivation is an **unconditioned response**. After training is over, the neutral stimulus acquires fresh properties because of its past association with food. Thus, it can elicit salivation by itself, i.e., without food.

Instead of a bell, a flash of light or some other stimulus can be used. Removal of a stimulus can also act as a conditioned stimulus. For example, a bell is first rung then stops ringing the bell and after that, give food. Thus, stoppage of ringing of bell can become a conditioned stimulus.

A number of somatic and visceral changes can be made to occur as conditioned reflex responses. Conditioning of visceral response is known as **biofeedback**. For example, trained persons can alter their blood pressure, heart rate, etc., as conditioned responses (*refer* yoga).

Criteria for Establishing a Conditioned Reflex

- Animal should be alert, healthy and free from all simultaneously acting nervous influences, i.e., there should be no distractions. Special sound-proof room is required and minimum training sessions required is around 30.
- A conditioned reflex can be built up only on the basis of unconditioned reflex. The conditioned stimulus should precede the unconditioned stimulus and both must overlap for some time. For example, first ring bell, then give food while continuing to ring bell.
- After establishing the conditioned response, the unconditioned stimulus must be provided occasionally for **reinforcement**. Otherwise, the conditioned response will gradually disappear. If the conditioned reflex is reinforced from time to time by pairing the conditioned stimulus and the unconditioned stimulus, the conditioned reflex persists indefinitely.
- Conditioned responses are easily formed if the unconditioned stimulus is associated with some pleasant or unpleasant effects.
- If the response is purely motor, the conditioned reflex is difficult to form since motor activities are mainly under voluntary control.

Special Features of Conditioned Reflex

- Summation
- Conditioned inhibition
- Discrimination.

Summation: If in the same animal, two different conditioned reflexes are built upon the basis of a single unconditioned reflex, and then if the two conditioned stimuli are applied simultaneously, the response will be greater. For example:
Light → Salivation
Bell → Salivation
Light + bell → Greater response, i.e., salivation is more.

Conditioned inhibition

- *External inhibition*: If the animal is distracted by some factor in the environment, there is inhibition of conditioned response. For example, along with ringing of bell, if there is the sound of a gramophone the conditioned reflex cannot be established.
- *Internal inhibition or extinction:* Periodic reinforcement is necessary for maintaining the conditioned reflex.

If the conditioned stimulus is repeatedly applied without unconditioned stimulus the response decreases which is called **decay** of conditioned reflex. Finally, the reflex disappears and is called **extinction**.

Discrimination: The animal can be taught to discriminate between closely related stimuli. For example, the animal is conditioned to respond to sound stimulus of tone A. Then if sound of tone B is applied and not followed by food, the animal will learn to discriminate between these two frequencies. So, there will be salivation for tone A and no salivation for tone B. For differential inhibition, there should be wide variation between tone A and tone B. But, when the difference becomes very close, it becomes a problem for the animal. A conflict between inhibition and excitation occurs and depending on which gains upperhand it either goes to sleep or becomes neurotic.

Operant or Instrumental Conditioning

Operant conditioning involves the use of some instruments. This can be studied under three systems:
1. Reward/approach system
2. Avoidance/punishment system
3. Maze learning.

The animal is taught to do some task in response to a stimulus. If it does the task correctly it is rewarded with food or it can avoid a punishment. Here, the unconditioned stimulus is the reward or punishment, and conditioned stimulus is the signal which alerts the animal to perform the task. Conditioned motor responses that permit an animal to avoid an unpleasant event is called **conditioned avoidance reflex**.

In maze learning, there is a complicated circuit, at the end of which food is kept. Learning is said to be complete when the animal reaches the food through the shortest path in the shortest time.

Physiological Basis of Conditioned Reflex

Conditioned reflex is established by the opening up of new functional neural connections between the cortical area receiving impulses from the conditioned stimulus and the neural center controlling the unconditioned response. For example, in the Pavlov's experiment, connections are made between auditory cortex and subcortical center for salivation. *Cerebral cortex is essential for establishing conditioned reflex.*

Importance of Conditioned Reflex

- **Learning** depends to a great extent on the process of conditioning.
- **Biofeedback** is a technique to control autonomic functions of the body by conditioning technique or in other words

conditioning of visceral responses is called biofeedback. Treatment of hypertension by yoga, meditation, etc. is an example.
- Operant conditioning is used to study effects of drugs like tranquilizers, antidepressants, etc.
- Pitch discrimination by conditioning has practical application in hearing mechanism for the appreciation of frequency.

Intercortical Transfer of Learning

If an animal is conditioned to respond to a visual stimulus with one eye covered and then tested with the blindfold transferred to the other eye, it performs the conditioned response. This occurs if the optic chiasma is cut so that visual input can go only to the ipsilateral cortex. If in addition to optic chiasma, the anterior and posterior commissures and corpus callosum are sectioned, no transfer of learning occurs. This animal is called **split-brain animal**. This proves that intercortical transfer of learning occurs through the commissures. Split brain animal can be trained to respond to different and conflicting stimuli, one with one eye and another with another eye. This is an example of *not letting the right side know what the left side is doing*. Similar results have been obtained in humans in whom corpus callosum is congenitally absent or in whom it has been sectioned surgically to control epileptic seizures.

LEARNING AND MEMORY

Learning

Learning is a neural mechanism by which the individual changes his behavior as the result of past experience. It is the process by which new experiences are acquired and integrated with previous experience. It is the acquisition of knowledge and skills. One important basis of learning is conditioned reflex. Learning is also impossible without memory. **Memory** is defined as the ability to recall past experience or the storage mechanism of what is learned through past experiences. So, memory is an integral part of learning. New neuronal circuits or neural connections between different parts of the brain, especially the various association areas are formed in the process of learning.

Learning is classified into two types:
1. Non-associative learning
2. Associative learning.

Non-associative Learning

In **non-associative learning**, the subject learns about the properties of a single stimulus. It results when a person is repeatedly exposed to a single type of stimulus. There are two types of non-associative learning:
1. Habituation
2. Sensitization.

In **habituation**, a repeated stimulus causes a response that gradually diminishes. This is because the individual learns that the stimulus is not important. For example, the sound of a new fan kept in the study room may be annoying at first, but after a few days it no longer bothers. Habituation is due to inactivation of Ca^{2+} channels in the presynaptic nerve endings which leads to a decrease in the neurotransmitter released at the synapse.

Sensitization is opposite to habituation. Here, a repeated stimulus which is strong, distinctly pleasant or unpleasant, results in greater response to later similar stimuli. When the stimulus is first given, the response may be minimal. With repetition of the stimulus the response increases. If the stimulus is unpleasant, the behavior of the individual is directed towards escape from the stimulus. This occurs in cases of threatening stimuli.

Associative Learning

Associative learning occurs when the learning process involves a consistent relationship in the timing between stimuli. Examples are classic conditioning, operant conditioning, etc. (*refer* 'conditioned reflex').

Mechanisms of Learning

- **Habituation and sensitization**: At cellular level, the presynaptic endings of the sensory neuron can change the amount of neurotransmitter released during learning. In **habituation**, the amount of transmitter released in successive responses gradually decreases. There will be a decrease in the number of Ca^{2+} channels in the presynaptic membrane. In long-term habituation, there will be reduction in the number of synaptic endings in the nerve terminal.
- **Sensitization** is opposite to habituation. It is due to increased release of neurotransmitter from axonal endings.
- **Long-term potentiation (LTP)**: It is seen in neocortex and some other parts of nervous system like hippocampus. The neurotransmitter involved in long-term potentiation includes excitatory amino acid that acts on **N-methyl-D-aspartate (NMDA) receptors**. The effects are due to:
  - Second messenger pathways and also due to increased influx of Ca^{2+} into postsynaptic neuron.
  - Increase in the release of neurotransmitter from presynaptic endings. This is mainly by a **retrograde messenger**, NO or CO, released from postsynaptic neurons to act on presynaptic ending so as to increase transmitter release.
  - Changes in gene expression are also involved.
  - The dendritic spines increase in number during development. The number of spines increases rapidly from birth to 8 months of age. They also appear, change and even disappear within a short time. A special type of cell adhesion membrane protein on the postsynaptic membrane called **neurolignin** controls synapse formation. Neurolignins act as ligands for neurexins which are cell adhesion proteins located presynaptically. The selective changes in the dendritic spines contribute to learning and long-term potentiation.
- **Long-term depression (LTD)**: Long-term depression is opposite to that of LTP. Here, stimulation of presynaptic neuron is associated with a smaller rise in intracellular

calcium. There is also decrease in the number of receptors synthesized by the endoplasmic reticular–Golgi apparatus system in the postsynaptic neuron. LTD is also involved in learning.

Memory

Memory is the ability to store information and to recall it at a later time. It is a function of synapses. Each time certain types of sensory signals pass through sequence of synapses, these synapses become more capable of transmitting the same type of signal the next time. This is due to the property of the synapse called **facilitation**. After a particular type of sensory signal has passed through the synapses a large number of times, the synapses become so facilitated that signals generated in the brain itself can also cause transmission of impulses through the same sequence of synapses, even when the sensory input is not excited. This gives the feeling of the original sensations although the perceptions are only memories of the sensation.

Once memories have been stored in the nervous system, they become part of the thinking process. This helps to compare new sensory experiences with stored memories so that the new sensory information can be channelled into appropriate memory storage areas for future use or into motor areas to cause immediate responses.

Classification of Memory

- Primary, secondary, tertiary and remote memory
- Reflexive and declarative memory
- Short-term memory and long-term memory.

Reflexive or habit memory or **implicit memory** is unconscious memory and includes associative and non-associative learning.

Declarative or recognition memory or explicit memory is conscious memory and involves evaluation and comparison established by a single experience. Explicit memory is initially required for learning skills such as driving and it will become implicit memory when thoroughly learned.

According to the duration of storage, memory is classified into long-term memory and short-term memory.

Short-term Memory

Short-term memory includes ability to recall names, numbers, few words, etc, immediately after exposure to such information. It lasts for a maximum of few hours. **Working memory** is a form of short-term memory which keeps information available for very short periods while the individual plans actions based on it. For example, looking at the telephone number and remembering it to dial the number immediately.

Mechanism of short-term memory

- **Reverberating circuit theory**: Information reaching cortical area will set up reverberating circuit in the cortex. As long as the reverberation is continuing the memory will be there. When there is fatigue in the circuit, the memory will be lost.
- **Post-tetanic potentiation**: Post-tetanic potentiation occurs after a brief tetanizing stimulation of presynaptic neurons. Repeated firing of impulses reaching a neuron increases the excitability of the neuron. It is due to accumulation of Ca^{2+} in the presynaptic neuron and the resulting increased neurotransmitter release. It lasts for about 4–60 sec.
- **Presynaptic facilitation**: Information reaching a neuron produces presynaptic facilitation and this forms the basis of short-term memory. **Serotonin** released at the axo-axonic ending increases the intra neuronal cAMP and the resulting phosphorylation of one group of K^+ channel closes these channels. This slows repolarization and prolongs action potential. Ca^{2+} channels will be open for a longer period in the presynaptic membrane. This increases the neurotransmitter release from the presynaptic ending.

Long-term Memory

Long-term memory is the ability to recall information after a long time, sometimes lifelong. Some physical or chemical change must occur in the neuron for long-term memory. Long-term memory involves structural changes in the nervous system because this memory remains intact even after events that disrupt short-term memory.

Mechanism of long-term memory

- **Long-term potentiation** has a very important role in establishing long-term memory. At the synaptic level the changes increase in the number of synaptic terminals or increase in the thickness of the postsynaptic membrane. The number of terminals in any neuron increases with age and experience. The more frequently a sensory process is repeated or recalled, the long-term memory of it can be established easily. **Repetition** is the most effective method by which long-term memory can be established. If a person is blind, the visual cortex becomes thinned up because no sensory inputs are reaching this area.
- Another view is that long-term memory is due to **biochemical change** in neuron. A stable alteration of RNA probably involving a protein synthesis is occurring in long-term memory.

Cortical Areas Involved in Learning and Memory

Experiments have shown that prefrontal areas, temporal lobe and hippocampus play an important role in memory.

Temporal lobes play an important role in memory. If temporal lobe is stimulated, it evokes memory of recent past, and this was studied by **Penfield**. Excessive stimulation of temporal lobe gives a strange feeling in familiar surrounding or a familiar feeling in strange surrounding. This is called **deja vu syndrome**. Temporal lobe acts like a key to unlock the memory stored elsewhere in the cortex.

The **hippocampal formation** is important for recent memory because bilateral removal of hippocampal formation disrupts recent memory. Here, short-term and long-term memories are unaffected, but new long-term memories can no longer be stored. Hippocampus is the primary structure involved in the conversion of short-term memory to long-term memory. Consolidation occurs mostly during REM sleep. *Hippocampus is the area in brain where neurons can divide and regenerate.*

Kluver-Bucy Animal

Kluver and Bucy did **bilateral temporal lobectomy** in monkeys and such an animal was called Kluver-Bucy animal. Parts of limbic system were also removed. Manifestations are hyperphagia, hypersexuality and signs of loss of memory. The animal puts anything into the mouth and if it is not edible, it will throw it away. Again it will take the same substance into the mouth due to loss of memory.

In **prefrontal lobectomy** also, loss of memory is a feature.

Drugs facilitating long-term memory increase the excitability of neurons and temporarily improve neuronal function. They include **caffeine, amphetamine, nicotine**, etc.

Pathological Conditions Affecting Memory

Loss of memory is called **amnesia**. It is of two types:
1. Retrograde amnesia
2. Anterograde amnesia.

Retrograde Amnesia

Retrograde amnesia is seen in complete loss of memory following brain concussion, shock therapy, etc. This may last for a period of few weeks, months or years.

Anterograde Amnesia

Inability to establish any new long-term memory due to lesion of hippocampus and associated areas is called **anterograde amnesia**. Here, short-term memory is intact.

Progressive Loss of Memory and Comprehensive Power

Comprehensive power refers to the ability to understand. **Dementia** means loss of general cognitive function with loss of short-term memories. If progressive loss of memory is seen in middle-aged people it is called **Alzheimer's disease**. If it occurs in older individuals it is called **senile dementia**. This may be due to decrease in cholinergic fibers in the hippocampal formation and other areas. Improvement may occur temporarily by anticholinesterase, physostigmine. **Nucleus basalis of Meynert** in basal forebrain sends cholinergic projection to neocortex, amygdala and hippocampus.

Confabulation

Confabulation or 'honest lying' is seen in patients with lesions of ventromedial portions of frontal lobes. They perform poorly in memory tests and spontaneously describe events that never occurred.

Deja vu Phenomenon

This is a condition where the patient shows inappropriate familiarity in new surroundings or with new events. Deja vu means already seen. This condition occurs as an aura in patients with temporal lobe epilepsy.

THOUGHT

Mechanism of thought is not known. It may be due to simultaneous signals arising from different parts of cortex, thalamus, limbic system areas, reticular formation, etc. This is called **holistic theory of thought**. Nature of thought depends on the area from where signals come.

NEUROPLASTICITY OR CORTICAL PLASTICITY

Neuroplasticity or cortical plasticity or cortical remapping refers to the brain's malleability and its ability to change and adapt as a result of experience. Experiences reorganize neural pathways in the brain. Long lasting functional changes occur in the brain when we learn new things or memorize new information. These changes in neural connections are referred to as neuroplasticity. Neurons, glial cells and vascular cells are involved in neuroplasticity.

Brain continues to create new neural pathways and alter existing ones in order to learn new information and create new memories. Recent research proves that the brain has the capacity to create new connections, reorganize pathways and even create new neurons. Plasticity occurs as a result of learning and memory formation or as a result of damage to the brain.

❖ Number of synapses per neuron in the cerebral cortex at birth is 2,500
❖ By 3 years of age it comes to about 15,000 synapses.

In adults, the number of synapses decrease to half because as we gain new experiences, some connections are strengthened and others get eliminated which is called **synaptic pruning.** Frequently used neurons develop stronger connections and those that are never used eventually die. By making new connections and pruning away weak ones, the brain is able to adapt to the changing environment. Use, disuse and lesions are the strong stimuli for plasticity and reorganization in the adult cortex (use it or lose it).

Types of Plasticity

Functional Plasticity

Brain has the ability to move functions from damaged area of brain to other undamaged areas. For example, if the cortical area representing a digit is removed, the somatosensory map of the digit moves to the surrounding cortex.

Structural Plasticity

Brain can change its physical structure as a result of learning (*refer* synaptic plasticity).

Neurogenesis

Neurogenesis is seen throughout life in the following areas:
❖ Hippocampus associated with learning, memory and emotions create new cells till old age
❖ Olfactory receptors (bipolar neurons)
❖ Cerebellum
❖ Prefrontal region which has a role in decision making

- Inferior temporal region concerned with visual recognition
- Posterior parietal region concerned with 3-D representation.

Due to neuronal plasticity, even after a stroke, the brain can often heal itself over time and form new connections and reroute functions through healthy brain areas. If the cortical map is deprived of its input, it will become activated at a later time in response to other inputs, usually adjacent inputs (**remapping of the somatosensory cortex**). That is, only those regions bordering a certain area will invade it to alter the cortical map. For example, in some individuals who had an arm amputated, stroking different parts of the face gives a feeling of being touched in the area of the missing limb.

Cortical reorganization plays an important role in the phantom limb phenomenon following amputation of hands, arm, legs etc. The cells that are close in the sensory periphery are also close in the cortical representation. Plasticity also occurs in the motor cortex.

Positive Plasticity and Negative Plasticity

- Neuroplasticity can be positive plasticity or negative plasticity. For example, if an individual recover after a stroke to normal levels of performance, that adaptiveness could be considered as an example of **positive plasticity**.
- But if the changes lead to excessive neuronal growth leading to spasticity or an excessive release of neurotransmitter which could kill nerve cells it is considered as negative plasticity. Drug addiction, obsessive-compulsive disorder etc. are examples of **negative plasticity.** Thus negative plasticity is due to maladaptive reorganization of the neuronal system.

Physiotherapy, pharmacotherapy and electrical stimulation therapy help to speed up the plastic changes in the brain in response to injury.

Neurotrophins like brain derived neurotrophic factor, neurotrophin-3, nerve growth factor, and insulin like growth factor (IGF-1) are found to be elevated in the area of representation of the area of lesion. The related neurotrophin receptors are also elevated. Enhanced synaptic plasticity is accompanied by changes in the intracellular Ca^{2+} concentration. There is increase in the resting Ca^{2+} concentration and stimulus evoked Ca^{2+} influx into neurons which are undergoing plastic changes.

It is seen that females in the reproductive age group recover from traumatic brain injury faster. This is because of the effect of progesterone. It reduces edema, inflammation and neuronal cell death after stroke. If a three day progesterone treatment is given to stroke patients immediately after the injury, recovery is found to be fast and mortality rate is also found to be reduced.

SPEECH AND LANGUAGE

The ability to communicate with each other is present in all living organisms. Language is an important aspect of human intelligence and a key part of human culture. The most sophisticated form of communication is present in humans in the form of speech. **Speech** is the ability to express one's ideas and thoughts symbolically in the form of language. Reading and writing are immediate relatives of speech and this ability is seen only in humans. The two aspects of speech are:
1. Sensory speech
2. Motor speech.

The ability to understand what is written and spoken is sensory aspect of speech. Motor aspect of speech is the ability to speak and write, where muscular activity is necessary.

Mechanism of Speech (Flowchart 96.1)

Two centers are present in the cortical area of brain concerned with speech.
1. Sensory speech center
2. Motor speech center.

Sensory Speech Center

Sensory speech center is located in the general interpretative area or **Wernicke's area or Brodmann's areas 22 and 39** in the posterior end of superior temporal gyrus and parietal lobe on either side of lateral sulcus. It is well developed only on the dominant side. This area is concerned with comprehension of auditory and visual information. The spoken speech stimulates the auditory receptors and through the auditory pathway the impulses reach the auditory cortex (**Flowchart 96.1**). From there the information reaches the Wernicke's area and is processed. The written speech which is read goes through the visual pathway to the visual cortex and the information is processed in the angular gyrus behind the Wernicke's area. The angular gyrus process information from words that are read in such a way, that they are converted into the auditory forms of the words in the Wernicke's area. Wernicke's area interprets the meaning of written and spoken words.

Motor Speech Center

Motor speech center is located in the **Broca's area or Brodmann's area 44** in the frontal lobe immediately in front of the inferior end of motor cortex close to lateral cerebral sulcus. This center processes the information received from the Wernicke's area through the arcuate fasciculus and controls the muscles of speech. Planning and programming of speech occurs in Broca's area and the processed information

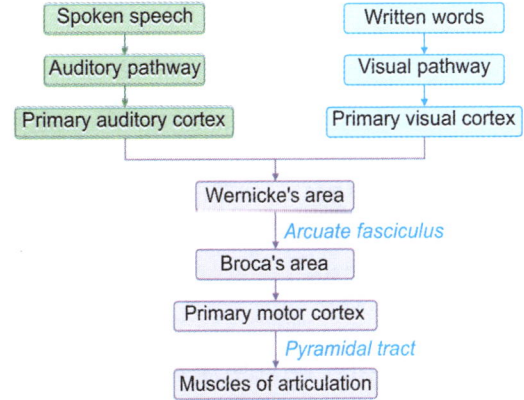

Flowchart 96.1: Mechanism of speech.

is fed to the primary motor area or area 4 that controls the muscles of larynx, pharynx, tongue and lips, and coordinated action of speech muscles occurs. Simultaneously, impulses propagate from the Broca's speech area to the primary motor area that controls the muscles of respiration to regulate the flow of air past the vocal cords. *In 97% of population, the language areas are localized in the left hemisphere.*

The faculty of speech develops during childhood. The child associates the sound of the word with the concerned object. If the child is deaf it cannot develop the faculty of speech. Association occurs in the Wernicke's area. During development, new pathways appear from Wernicke's area to Broca's area and the tract is known as **arcuate fasciculus (Fig. 96.1)**.

Speech is an act of **respiration**. Vocal cords play an important role in speech. Sound is produced by vibration of vocal cords as air is expelled out of the lungs. The extent of vibration depends on the tension in the vocal cord, which in turn is controlled by the degree of contraction of laryngeal muscles. Sound is modulated into words by the action of laryngeal, pharyngeal, lingual and labial muscles. Coordinated contraction of these muscles is necessary for normal speech mechanism. **Vision, hearing**, **motor pathways**, **cerebellar control, basal ganglia, reticular formation**, etc, should function normally for normal speech.

Speech Abnormalities

- Anarthria
- Dysarthria
- Aphasia.

Anarthria

Defective speech can occur due to damage of pyramidal tract, extrapyramidal tract, etc. Defective speech due to damage of motor tract is called anarthria.

Dysarthria

Defective speech due to motor defects in the muscles of articulation as seen in cerebellar lesion or basal ganglia lesion is dysarthria.

Aphasia

Aphasia or dysphasia is abnormality in language functions such as speech, writing or reading due to lesions in the speech centers of cerebral cortex. There is loss of production or comprehension of spoken and/or written language. *It is not due to defects of vision or hearing or due to motor paralysis.*

Classification of Aphasia

- **Sensory aphasia** or fluent aphasia—Wernicke's area or arcuate fasciculus affected.
- **Motor aphasia** or non-fluent aphasia—Broca's area affected.
- **Global aphasia**, where both motor and sensory speech centers are affected.
- **Anomic aphasia**—there is a lesion in the angular gyrus.

Sensory aphasia or fluent aphasia: *Sensory aphasia or receptive aphasia* can be due to a lesion in the Wernicke's area or auditory association area (area 22) or visual association area (area 18, 19) in the categorical (dominant) hemisphere. Here, the ability to understand what is heard or read is absent depending on the area involved. In sensory aphasia, the person is not able to communicate with others but he can say something without any meaning, i.e., the speech is fluent and the patient may speak a lot. So it is called fluent aphasia.

It is of two types—word deafness and word blindness. Inability to understand spoken speech is **word deafness**. Inability to understand written language is **word blindness or alexia**.

Auditory agnosia or word deafness: In this condition the hearing is perfect but the subject does not understand what is talked to him. If he is asked to show his teeth he will not do it because he does not understand the meaning of what is said. Such a state is produced when there is damage to the auditory center situated in the temporal lobe.

Visual agnosia or word blindness or alexia: In this condition the vision is perfect but written words mean nothing to him, as if he has not learned those words. Confirm the person is not blind and he has learnt to read and understand. Write down simple commands and observe his response. A person

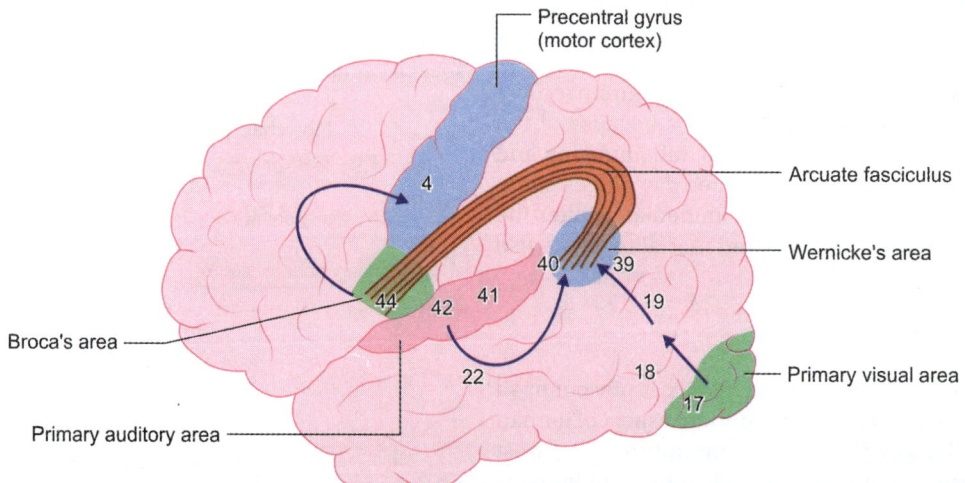

Fig. 96.1: Lateral view of left cerebral hemisphere showing the pathway for speaking a heard word and a written word. Numbers denote Brodmann's areas.

with visual agnosia will not be able to execute the task. Such a state is caused by damage to visual word center situated in front of the visual area in the angular gyrus.

Motor aphasia or non-fluent aphasia:
In **motor aphasia**, the person is not able to speak or write or both but there is fairly good comprehension of speech. Inability to write is **agraphia**. Damage to the Broca's speech area in the categorical hemisphere (dominant hemisphere) results in non-fluent aphasia or motor aphasia. The patient is not able to properly articulate and form words. Speech is limited and effortful. They know what they wish to say but cannot speak.

Global aphasia: Global aphasia combines the features of sensory and motor aphasias. Comprehension and speech are completely lost.

Anomic aphasia: When there is a lesion in the angular gyrus in the categorical hemisphere without affecting Wernicke's or Broca's areas, there is no difficulty in speech or the understanding of auditory information. But there is difficulty in understanding written language or pictures because visual information from the primary visual area is not processed in the angular gyrus. This condition is called anomic aphasia.

Head's Classification of Aphasia
- Verbal aphasia
- Nominal aphasia
- Semantic aphasia
- Syntactic aphasia.

Verbal aphasia: The person is not able to speak out an idea. He can say some words. He is able to understand what is heard and he can write. The lesion is in the Broca's area.

Nominal aphasia: The affected person is not able to say the name of objects, but he can describe the object. Lesion is in the angular gyrus in the categorical hemisphere.

Semantic aphasia: Person is able to say something but he cannot understand or say the general meaning of what is said or heard. The lesion is in the Wernicke's area. The meanings of the words and sentences are called semantics.

Syntactic aphasia: The person can say something without any grammar. Several words are strung together using certain rules (grammar) called the syntax. The syntax can change the semantics.

Cerebral Dominance and Language

In majority of individuals, **left hemisphere** is the dominant hemisphere with respect to language. Lesions of the left hemisphere produce defects in language function called aphasia. The right hemisphere is dominant for functions other than language. For example, left-handedness reflects dominance of right hemisphere. But in these individuals also left hemisphere is dominant when language is concerned. A part of brain called **planum temporale**, located in the floor of the lateral fissure, is mainly involved in language dominance. It is seen that left planum temporale is larger than that of the right.

Dyslexia is a developmental disorder where there is difficulty in learning to read. Dyslexic children do not have a well-developed **planum temporale** on the left hemisphere. This suggests that the basic defect in them may be absence of hemispheric specialization for language.

Several areas in the left hemisphere are involved in language. For example, Wernicke's area in the posterior part of superior temporal gyrus near auditory cortex, Broca's area in the posterior part of inferior temporal gyrus close to face area of motor cortex, etc, are very important in language development. Sensory or motor aphasia is not associated with alterations in sensation or motor functions and it is a deficit in the reception or planning of language expression. But if a large part of dominant hemisphere is affected as in hemiplegia, sensory and motor changes are present such as paralysis of muscles of speech.

INTERCORTICAL TRANSFER OF LEARNING

The two cerebral hemispheres can function independently if the corpus callosum and other association fibers are cut. Such an animal is called **split-brain animal**. For normal functioning of the body, information must be transferred between the hemispheres to coordinate activities on the two sides of the body.

Each hemisphere must know what the other is doing. Much of the intercortical transfer of information occurs through the corpus callosum although some are transmitted through other commissures like anterior commissure or hippocampal commissure. If both optic chiasma and corpus callosum are cut before training the animal, the information is not transferred intercortically and each hemisphere must learn the task independently.

Split-brain animal can be trained to respond to different stimuli, one with one eye and another with the other, i.e., not letting the right side know what the left side is doing.

Apraxia

Apraxia is inability to control voluntary movement and is seen in split-brain animal. There will be lack of coordination of movement. For example, while the person is dressing, one hand may button the shirt while the other hand tries to unbutton it. So, when corpus callosum is cut and there is no interconnection between the two hemispheres, each hemisphere can operate independently. But in this case only one hemisphere can express itself with language and the other hemisphere can communicate only nonverbally.

MULTIPLE CHOICE QUESTIONS

1. Salivation by dog seen when food is given along with ringing of bell is:
   a. Conditioned reflex
   b. Reinforcement
   c. Habituation
   d. Innate reflex

2. All the following are properties of spinal cord reflex, except:
   a. Memory
   b. Summation
   c. Delay
   d. Fatigue

3. Aluminium toxicity leads to:
   a. Parkinson's disease
   b. Alzheimer's disease
   c. Hemiplegia
   d. Sub-acute combined degeneration

4. The part of the brain involved in emotions is:
   a. Neocortex
   b. Thalamus
   c. Limbic system
   d. Basal ganglia

5. Motor aphasia refers to defect in:
   a. Peripheral speech apparatus
   b. Verbal expression
   c. Auditory comprehension
   d. Verbal comprehension

6. Efferent connections of the hippocampus travel through the:
   a. Stria terminalis
   b. Medial longitudinal stria
   c. Stria medullaris thalami
   d. Fornix

7. True regarding Broca's area is:
   a. Present bilaterally in the brain
   b. Supplied by middle cerebral artery
   c. Lesion causes laryngeal palsy
   d. Present in the temporal lobe

8. Memory is processed in:
   a. Sensory cortex
   b. Motor cortex
   c. Cerebellum
   d. Hippocampus

9. Storage of memory is the function of:
   a. Cerebellum
   b. Neocortex
   c. Hippocampus
   d. Limbic system

10. True about retrograde amnesia:
    a. Abolished by prefrontal lobotomy
    b. Commonly precipitated by a blow on the head
    c. Is increased by vasopressin administration
    d. Is due to damage to brain stem

11. Cognition is:
    a. Skill
    b. Practice
    c. Knowledge
    d. Feeling

12. Affect is the:
    a. Feeling
    b. Action
    c. Thought
    d. Knowledge

13. Human brain is more intelligent than monkey's brain due to:
    a. Larger brain
    b. Increased convolutions
    c. Increased brain area compared to surface area
    d. More blood supply

14. Broca's area (area 44) lies at:
    a. Superior border of frontal lobe
    b. Inferior border of frontal lobe
    c. Posterior border of temporal lobe
    d. Anterior border of occipital lobe

15. Wernicke's area is located at:
    a. Posterior end of superior temporal gyrus
    b. Anterior end of superior temporal gyrus
    c. Inferior end of motor cortex in frontal lobe
    d. Anterior border of occipital lobe

16. The area in the superior temporal gyrus that is involved in language-related auditory processing is called:
    a. Broca's area
    b. Planum temporale
    c. Arcuate fasciculus
    d. Wernicke's area

17. Lesions producing agnosia are generally in the:
    a. Frontal lobe
    b. Temporal lobe
    c. Parietal lobe
    d. Occipital lobe

18. Decreased blood flow in the angular gyrus in the categorical hemisphere usually leads to:
    a. Dyslexia
    b. Agnosia
    c. Astereognosis
    d. Aphasia

19. Lesion of the right inferior temporal lobe in right handed individuals leads to:
    a. Agnosia
    b. Dyslexia
    c. Prosopagnosia
    d. Aphasia

20. Inability to recognize faces is called:
    a. Agnosia
    b. Prosopagnosia
    c. Aphasia
    d. Amnesia

21. The percentage of left handers who have left hemisphere dominance is:
    a. 15%
    b. 50%
    c. 70%
    d. 85%

22. Broca's area is present in:
    a. Superior temporal gyrus
    b. Precentral gyrus
    c. Postcentral gyrus
    d. Inferior frontal gyrus

23. A stimulus event is called a reinforce only if it can be shown to:
    a. Produce reduction of a homeostatic need
    b. Lead to increased probability of response
    c. Serve as an unconditioned response for operant behavior
    d. Elicit the response that follows it

24. Consolidation of long term memory occurs in the:
    a. Hippocampus
    b. Amygdala
    c. Prefrontal cortex
    d. Hypothalamus

25. Motor speech area is in:
    a. Brodmann's area 22
    b. Brodmann's area 44
    c. Brodmann's area 4
    d. Brodmann's area 42

ANSWERS

1. d	2. a	3. b	4. c	5. b
6. d	7. b	8. d	9. b	10. b
11. c	12. a	13. a	14. b	15. a
16. b	17. c	18. a	19. c	20. b
21. c	22. d	23. b	24. a	25. b

Cerebrospinal Fluid

CHAPTER 97

LEARNING OBJECTIVES
- Describe the mechanism of formation of cerebrospinal fluid its circulation and drainage
- Discuss the role of CSF in protecting the brain
- Explain the structure and functions of blood-brain barrier
- Describe lumbar puncture and its uses

INTRODUCTION

The neuronal microenvironment of the brain includes the brain extracellular fluid (BECF), capillaries and the glial cells. The BECF composition should be kept constant for normal neuronal functioning. The neurons should maintain steep ion gradients on which neuronal excitability depends. The concentration of solutes in the BECF fluctuates with neuronal activity because of its high metabolic rate. But the brain effectively controls this composition within the normal range by three ways: (1) the blood brain barrier protects the BECF from fluctuations in blood composition (2) the cerebrospinal fluid strongly influences the composition of BECF (3) the glial cells surrounding the neurons also maintains the composition of BECF.

The brain has a very soft consistency and it is protected from mechanical injury by the skull bones and the cerebrospinal fluid (CSF) in which it floats. The cavity enclosing the brain and spinal cord has a volume of approximately 1650 mL and about 130–150 mL of this volume is occupied by CSF. This fluid is found in the **ventricles** of brain, in the **cisterns** around the brain, in the **subarachnoid space** around the brain and spinal cord, and in the **central canal** of spinal cord. All these chambers are interconnected. Of the 150 mL, about 30 mL is present in the ventricular system and rest in the subarachnoid space.

ANATOMY OF THE VENTRICLES OF BRAIN AND THEIR CONNECTIONS

Central nervous system develops as a hollow **neural tube** in the embryo and is surrounded by and filled with a fluid which later develops into CSF and ECF of brain and spinal cord.

Brain and spinal cord are covered by **dura mater, arachnoid and pia mater**. Arachnoid is thin and does not dip into the sulci of brain. Pia mater which is very thin dips into the sulci and covers the brain closely. The dura mater is thick and inelastic which has two layers that split to form the intracranial venous sinuses. Substances from the dural capillaries cannot diffuse into the CSF because of the existence of blood-CSF barrier created by the arachnoid.

In the vertebral column, dura mater and arachnoid mater comes to the level of second sacral vertebra. The spinal cord and pia mater end at the level of L_1 vertebra (*refer* **Chapter 78, Fig. 78.4**). CSF is present in the subarachnoid space. The subarachnoid space freely communicates with the ventricles of brain and with the central canal of spinal cord. Prolongations of the subarachnoid space extend along the sheaths of spinal and cranial nerve to the point where they leave the skull and then fuse with the perineurium of each nerve, especially optic nerve and olfactory nerve. The arachnoid and pia mater extend around the optic nerve to the back of the eyeball where they fuse with the sclera. Thus, the subarachnoid space extends around the optic nerve as far as the eyeball. *This is the reason why the fundus of the eye is examined when raised intracranial tension is suspected.*

Brain tissue is insensitive to pain. Headache is due to stimulation of pain receptors situated in the dura mater and blood vessels of brain. Sensory supply to the dura mater is through the trigeminal nerve and first three cervical nerves.

Ventricles of Brain

The ventricles of the brain are four small compartments located within the brain. The ventricles are connected together by channels or foramina, which allow CSF to move easily between them. There are **two lateral ventricles** one in each cerebral hemisphere. Each lateral ventricle is divided into anterior horn, posterior horn, inferior horn and a central body. The **third ventricle** is situated in the diencephalon between the thalami. Lateral ventricle communicates with the third ventricle through **interventricular foramen of Monro**, one on each side. The **fourth ventricle** is situated in the brainstem. It is bounded by the cerebellum superiorly and by the pons and medulla inferiorly. The third ventricle is connected to the fourth ventricle through the narrow

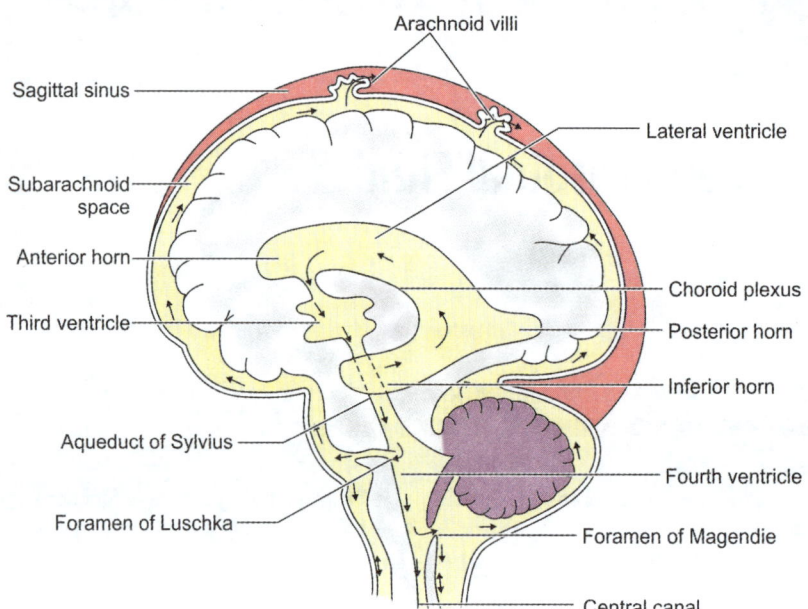

Fig. 97.1: Formation and circulation of CSF through the ventricular system and subarachnoid space.

aqueduct of Sylvius or cerebral aqueduct which is about 1.8 cm long. The fourth ventricle is continuous with the central canal of spinal cord. Through the three foramina in its roof the fourth ventricle is connected to the subarachnoid space. They are **foramen of Magendie** and two **foramina of Luschka (Fig. 97.1)**. The ventricles, the central canal of spinal cord and the subarachnoid space are filled with CSF. Thus, CSF surrounds the whole CNS being both inside and outside it. The ventricles and the central canal are lined with ependyma. The subarachnoid space also contains cerebral arteries, veins and cranial nerves.

The fourth ventricle communicates with the **cisterna magna or cerebellomedullary cistern** through foramen of Magendie. Cisterna magna is found in the area between medulla and undersurface of cerebellum. In some places, subarachnoid space is enlarged where the contour of brain is angular and there is more space between bone and brain substance. These expanded subarachnoid spaces are called cisterns. Other important cisterns are **pontine cistern and interpeduncular cisterns**. The two foramina of Luschka situated laterally in the roof of fourth ventricle open into the pontine cistern on the basal aspect of the brainstem.

CEREBROSPINAL FLUID

Cerebrospinal fluid (CSF) is a clear, colorless watery fluid with a pH of 7.35–7.4. It is similar to other body fluids, especially interstitial fluid. CSF forms part of the ECF compartment of the body. It fills the ventricles of the brain and also forms a thin layer around the brain and spinal cord in the subarachnoid space. The composition of CSF is highly regulated, and because it directly mixes with brain extracellular fluid (BECF), it helps to regulate the composition of BECF. The differences between CSF and plasma are shown in **Table 97.1**.

Table 97.1: Composition of CSF compared to that of plasma.

Substance	Composition in CSF	Composition in plasma
Protein	20–30 mg/dL	6000 mg/dL
Glucose	60 mg/dL	100 mg/dL
Uric acid	1.5 mg/dL	3 mg/dL
Urea	12 mg/dL	20 mg/dL
Creatinine	1.5 mg/dL	0.6–1.5 mg/dL
Na^+	145 mEq/L	145 mEq/L
Cl^-	113 mEq/L	100 mEq/L
HCO_3^-	25 mEq/L	24 mEq/L
K^+	3 mEq/L	4.5 mEq/L
Inorganic phosphate	3.4 mg/dL	4 mg/dL

The pressure of CSF is maintained at a constant level.
❖ Normal CSF pressure is 10 mm Hg or 60–150 mm of water.
❖ Osmolarity of CSF is 289 mOsm/L of water.
❖ Total volume of CSF is about 150 mL (30 mL in the ventricles and 120 mL in the subarachnoid space of brain and spinal cord.
❖ Rate of formation of CSF is 500–600 mL/day (0.5 mL/min) which means that it undergoes rapid turnover. Turn over time is 5 hours.

Formation of CSF

❖ More than 2/3rd of CSF is secreted by the choroid plexus
❖ Secreted from ependymal cells
❖ Diffuse from the capillaries with in the brain (30% of CSF).
CSF is formed at a rate of 500 mL/day. The 2/3rd of CSF is produced by the **choroid plexus** present in the ventricles especially by the large plexus present in the lateral ventricles **(Fig. 97.1)**. Choroid plexus is also present in the posterior part of third ventricle and roof of fourth ventricle.

Choroid plexus is a cauliflower-like growth seen in the walls of the ventricles. As blood vessels pass into the brain parenchyma, they take a sheath of pia mater along with them. When they reach the ventricles, they break up into capillaries and also get covered by ependymal cells. The tuft of blood vessels projecting into the ventricles and their lining epithelium constitute the choroid plexus.

The blood vessels of the choroid plexus of lateral ventricle and third ventricle are formed from the choroidal branches of the **internal carotid and basilar arteries**. Venous blood drains into the internal cerebral veins. The choroidal plexus of fourth ventricle is from the **posterior inferior cerebellar arteries**. The central canal of spinal cord contains no choroid plexus, but is filled with CSF.

CSF is also secreted by the **ependymal cells** lining the ventricles. Small amount of CSF is produced by the brain tissue itself and comes through the perivascular spaces which surround the blood vessels entering brain.

Previously, CSF was considered to be a protein-free filtrate of plasma. Now it is known that it is the **active secretion of choroid epithelium**. CSF has lower concentrations of K^+ and amino acids than plasma. The secretion of fluid by choroid plexus depends mainly on the active transport of Na^+ through the epithelial cells into the ventricles via the Na^+-K^+ activated ATPase system. To maintain electrical neutrality, Cl also accompanies Na^+ into the ventricle. This increases the number of osmotically active substances in the CSF. This leads to passage of water into the CSF by **osmosis**. Small amount of glucose also **diffuse** into the CSF, and K^+ and HCO_3^- move out from the CSF into the capillaries by active transport. Ca^{2+} is actively transported from CSF to plasma, whereas Mg^{2+} is actively transported into CSF.

Inhibitors like ouabain and dinitrophenol which block active Na^+ transport into the CSF, decrease CSF production.

Circulation of CSF

The CSF formed in the lateral ventricle passes through the foramen of Monro into the third ventricle. This mixes with the fluid in the third ventricle and goes to the fourth ventricle through aqueduct of Sylvius. Through the openings in the fourth ventricle, CSF circulates through the entire subarachnoid space and central canal of spinal cord **(Fig. 97.1)**.

CSF circulation is aided by the **arterial pulsations** of choroid plexus and by the **action of cilia** of the ependymal cells lining the ventricles.

Absorption of CSF

CSF is returned to circulation at a rate equal to its rate of production. CSF pressure is maintained constant by a balance between CSF formation and absorption. It is absorbed through **arachnoid villi** that project into the dural venous sinuses, especially superior sagittal sinus which lies between the two cerebral hemispheres. The arachnoid villi (microscopic) are grouped together to form elevations known as **arachnoid granulations** (0.5 to 1 cm in diameter) **or pacchionian bodies.** Meningiomas arise from the arachnoid villi found along the dural venous sinuses. The absorption of CSF into the venous sinuses occurs when the CSF pressure exceeds the venous pressure in the sinus. When the CSF pressure exceeds 70 mm H_2O, absorption commences and increases in a graded fashion with further increase in intracranial pressure. Absorption of CSF through the arachnoid villi controls CSF pressure **(Fig. 97.2)**. There are two reasons for the movement of fluid from subarachnoid space to the dural venous sinuses:

1. The hydrostatic pressure is high in the arachnoid granulations than in the dural sinuses. The osmotic pressure is higher in the dural sinuses than in the arachnoid granulations. So, according to Starling's forces, fluid moves from arachnoid villi to the dural sinuses.
2. The endothelial cells lining the arachnoid villi have large vesicular holes and these are large enough to allow free flow of CSF, protein molecules and particles as large as red blood cells into the venous blood by transcytosis. The endothelial cells of the villi act as **one-way valves**, allowing substances to move only from CSF to the venous side and not in the reverse direction. Thus, it prevents reflux of blood from the venous sinuses into the subarachnoid space.

Functions of CSF

- CSF acts as a cushion for the brain and protects the CNS from mechanical trauma.
- Provides mechanical buoyancy and support for the brain. The CSF that surrounds the brain reduces the effective weight of the brain from 1400 g to less than 50 g and the

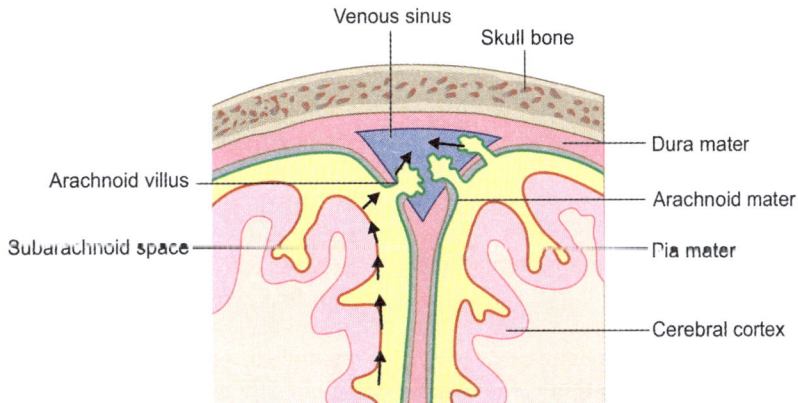

Fig. 97.2: Drainage of CSF through the arachnoid villi into the venous sinus.

brain floats in the CSF. This buoyancy (fluid suspension system) is due to the difference in the specific gravities of brain (1.040) and CSF (1.007). When an extremely severe blow is given to one side of head the brain moves to the opposite side. So no injury occurs in the side where blow is given but the opposite side may be damaged. This is called **contrecoup injury**.

- CSF acts as reservoir for regulating the contents of the cranial vault. If the brain volume is decreased or blood volume decreased, more of CSF is produced.
- It nourishes the brain.
- CSF helps to remove neuronal metabolites from CNS. Substances can be freely exchanged between the CSF and BECF. Products of metabolism and other substances released by neurons for signaling purposes can diffuse into the CSF and can be ultimately removed by bulk reabsorption into the venous sinuses or by active transport across the choroid plexus into the blood. For example, the choroid plexus actively absorbs the breakdown products of the neurotransmitters serotonin (5-hydroxyindoleacetic acid) and dopamine (homovanillic acid).
- It is the route through which pineal secretions reach the pituitary gland.
- There are no lymphatics in the CNS. So if proteins and large molecular weight substances escape from blood into the brain interstitial space, its return to blood is brought about by diffusion into CSF first and then via arachnoid villi into the dural venous sinuses.

Measurement of CSF Pressure: Lumbar Puncture

CSF pressure is measured by **lumbar puncture or spinal tap**. This is done by introducing the lumbar puncture needle below the level of L_1 vertebra. Usually, the third or fourth lumbar intervertebral space is selected for safety. The needle is connected to a special glass tube which is connected to a manometer. The CSF pressure is measured in mm of water. The patient is kept in the horizontal position so that the spinal fluid pressure is same as the pressure in the cranial vault.

CSF pressure can be indirectly assessed by ophthalmoscopy, where there will be **papilledema** in the optic disc. Papilledema is due to compression of the retinal vein as it crosses the extension of the subarachnoid space to enter the optic nerve.

Uses of Lumbar Puncture

- Diagnostic
- Therapeutic
- Spinal anesthesia.

Diagnostic Uses

- Take out a little fluid collected by lumbar puncture and examine it.
- Gross appearance:
  - Normally CSF is a clear and colorless fluid.
  - **Cloudy or turbid** appearance when there is increase in the number of neutrophils as in bacterial meningitis and encephalitis or it may be due to increase in the protein content of CSF as in tuberculous meningitis and poliomyelitis.
  - **Reddish** in color due to subarachnoid hemorrhage.
  - **Yellow** in xanthochromia.
- Microscopic examination
- Biochemical examination
- Culture to isolate organisms and sensitivity tests.
- LP is also used to measure CSF pressure when raised intracranial tension is suspected.

Therapeutic Uses of Lumbar Puncture (LP)

- Therapeutically cytotoxic drugs in case of leukemia, penicillin in pyogenic meningitis, streptomycin in tuberculous meningitis, etc., can be instilled into the subarachnoid space by LP. CSF in the ventricles and the subarachnoid space can exchange freely with the brain ECF across two borders, the pia mater and the ependymal cells. The pia mater has paracellular gaps through which substances can equilibrate between sub-arachnoid space and BECF.
- LP is also done to relieve raised intracranial pressure as in meningitis provided the foot end of the bed is kept raised for some time to prevent medullary coning and herniation of cerebellum.
- The side effects of morphine when given by systemic injection can be minimized by injecting morphine into the subarachnoid space. Long-term cancer pain can be treated by continuous infusion of morphine into the subarachnoid space.
- In infants, spinal cord reaches up to the level of third lumbar vertebra. This point should be considered while doing LP in infants, otherwise it may damage the spinal cord.

Use of LP in spinal or caudal anesthesia: In spinal anesthesia, drugs are introduced into the subarachnoid space especially in the first and second stages of labor to reduce pain. The advantage is that, the anesthetic drugs do not affect the baby.

Caudal anesthesia is also used in operations of sacral regions like hysterectomy, anorectal surgery, etc.

Abnormalities in CSF Pressure

- Large brain tumor, cerebral edema and cerebral abscess increase CSF pressure.
- Tumor of choroid plexus leads to excessive formation of CSF.
- Hemorrhage or infection in cranium increases CSF pressure.
- If CSF pressure is very high, lumbar puncture is contraindicated because a sudden fall in intracranial pressure when CSF is withdrawn leads to medullary coning into foramen magnum. This compresses the medulla oblongata and since all the vital centers are located in the medulla this condition becomes fatal.
- Fall in CSF pressure is seen in dehydration especially in children.

Blood-Brain Barrier (BBB)

The existence of this barrier was first demonstrated by **Paul Ehrlich** in 1885. Aniline dyes like trypan blue when injected intravenously stained most of the body tissues except brain tissue. This proves the presence of a barrier between blood and brain tissue called BBB. The blood-brain barrier prevents certain blood constituents from entering the brain extracellular space. For normal neuronal functioning, the BECF solute and ion concentration should be kept constant. The concentration of these substances in blood varies greatly depending on factors such as diet, metabolism, etc. For example, after a protein-rich meal, the concentration of many amino acids increases in blood. Some of these amino acids may act as neurotransmitters within the brain and may disturb normal neurotransmission. Severe exercise can increase plasma concentrations of K^+ and H^+ that could disrupt neural activity. Other substances like hormones, other ions, cytokines etc. present in blood can influence the behavior of neurons and glial cells. This shows the need for a blood brain barrier for the brain to function efficiently. A stable environment is provided for the CNS by isolating the brain tissue from blood due to the existence of BBB.

Substances from blood reach the brain tissue by two ways:
1. From blood to brain interstitial fluid
2. From blood to CSF, and from CSF, substances pass readily to the brain tissue. There is no physiological barrier between CSF and brain extracellular compartment.

Blood-brain barrier exists in all areas of brain except circumventricular organs which include hypothalamus.

Hypothalamus is very important in maintaining body homeostasis and it should respond to changes in the composition of body fluids for the feedback regulation of each of the factors. Hence, it is outside the BBB.

Blood-brain barrier is highly permeable to water due to the presence of aquaporin-4 in the astrocytic end feet, CO_2, O_2, lipid-soluble substances like alcohol, anesthetics, caffeine, nicotine, etc. It is impermeable to plasma proteins, protein-bound metabolites such as bilirubin, ions such as Mg^{2+}, K^+, etc. The barrier isolates the brain tissue from blood in the capillaries. Only lipid-soluble substances can cross the BBB. It is not well developed in newborn. In newborn babies with very high serum bilirubin level as in hemolytic disease of newborn, bilirubin crosses the BBB and gets deposited in basal ganglia. The condition is known as kernicterus and is associated with extrapyramidal symptoms.

Factors Contributing to BBB

The tight junction between the endothelial cells of the blood capillaries in the CNS is the main factor responsible for the formation of BBB. Other factors are:
❖ Presence of a continuous basement membrane outside the endothelial cells.
❖ The foot processes of the astrocytes that adhere to the outer surface of the capillary wall.
❖ Absence of vesicular transport across vascular endothelium of choroid plexus.

Parts of Brain Outside the Blood-brain Barrier (Circumventricular Organs)

The small brain areas that lack a BBB are called circumventricular organs because they surround the ventricular system.
❖ Posterior lobe of pituitary
❖ Median eminence of hypothalamus
❖ Tuber cinereum
❖ Subfornical organ and supraoptic crest (organum vasculosum laminae terminalis)—angiotensin II acts on these areas and increases water intake.
❖ Vascular area postrema, which is an area of medulla on the floor of fourth ventricle just rostral to the opening into the central canal. It initiates vomiting in response to chemical changes in plasma. Angiotensin II acts on area postrema to increase blood pressure.

Parts coming under 4 and 5 are also called **chemoreceptor zones**.

Pineal gland and anterior pituitary are outside the BBB, but both are endocrine glands and are not part of the brain.

Blood-CSF Barrier

Blood-CSF barrier is created by the arachnoid mater. The arachnoid is composed of layers of cells held together by tight junctions. The arachnoid isolates the CSF in the subarachnoid space from blood in the overlying vessels of the dura mater. The arachnoid and the pial layers are relatively avascular and they derive nutrition from the CSF that they enclose. The blood-CSF barrier also exists in the choroid plexus. The tight junction between the choroidal epithelial cells serves as the barrier.

Importance of BBB and Blood-CSF Barrier

❖ These barriers protect the brain and spinal cord from potentially harmful substances like norepinephrine, acetylcholine, dopamine, etc., which are powerful neurotransmitters, while permitting gases and nutrients to enter the nervous tissue.
❖ Provides a controlled environment for the brain tissue.
❖ Maintains a low potassium concentration so that the neurons generate very high electrical potentials.
❖ If we give a drug intravenously it does not cross the BBB. But if the drug is injected into the CSF it will have the desired effect on the brain. Substances from CSF can easily diffuse to the interstitial fluid of brain.
❖ BBB also prevents the escape of neurotransmitters from brain into the general circulation.

Cerebrospinal Fluid-Brain Interface

Substances in the CSF easily enter the brain interstitial fluid. There is no physiological barrier between CSF and brain extracellular compartment.

Applied Physiology

❖ **Raised intracranial tension and papilledema**: A rise in intracranial tension will compress the thin walls of the retinal vein as it crosses the extension of the subarachnoid space to enter the optic nerve. This results in congestion of retinal vein, bulging forward of optic disc and edema of the disc which is referred to as **papilledema**. Papilledema is bilaterally seen if it is due to raised intracranial tension. This can be visualized using an **ophthalmoscope**. If papilledema persists, it leads to blindness.

- **Hydrocephalus**: Hydrocephalus is an abnormal increase in the volume of CSF within the skull. Hydrocephalus means excess water in the cranial vault. When there is a block in the absorption of CSF, excess fluid collects in the ventricular system or in the subarachnoid space.

Types

- Communicating or external hydrocephalus
- Non-communicating or internal hydrocephalus.

Communicating Hydrocephalus

In this condition, fluid flows readily from the ventricular system into the subarachnoid space. Here, obstruction is at the level of arachnoid granulation. This may be due to blockage of arachnoid villi by large particulate matter or due to fibrosis. Fluid collects both inside the ventricles and in the subarachnoid space. In infants, the sutures of the skull have not fused and so, the head swells tremendously and the brain will be compressed due to pressure, leading to damage to the brain.

Non-communicating Hydrocephalus

In this type, the obstruction is in any of the foramina or in the aqueduct of Sylvius. So, fluid formed in the choroid plexus will accumulate in the ventricles and their volumes increase significantly. This compresses the brain so that brain tissue is reduced to a thin shell against the skull if the condition is not treated promptly. The obstruction may be due to brain tumor.

The site of obstruction can be determined by injecting **phenolsulfonphthalein (Psp test)** into the lateral ventricle. Normally, this dye appears in the fluid from spinal tap in 2–3 min and in the urine in 10–12 min. If it does not appear in the spinal fluid or appear after a long delay, the hydrocephalus is non-communicating. If the dye appears in the spinal fluid normally, but appears in the urine after an undue delay, the hydrocephalus is communicating type. The block may be in the arachnoid villi or in the dural venous sinuses (e.g., thrombosis of dural sinus).

Queckenstedt's sign: This test is done to find out whether there is a block in the flow of CSF. When pressure is applied on the internal jugular vein, while doing lumbar puncture, if there is no obstruction to the flow of CSF there will be increase in CSF pressure. If there is obstruction, there will be no rise in pressure.

Pneumoencephalography: CSF is removed from the ventricle and air is injected into the ventricle, and X-ray pictures are taken. This helps to diagnose **tumor of ventricle**. When CSF is removed, the brain hangs on blood vessels and nerves, and this stimulates the pain fibers leading to severe headache. Injecting isotonic saline into the ventricle can relieve this.

MULTIPLE CHOICE QUESTIONS

1. **Normal volume of CSF in an adult man is about:**
   a. 50 mL
   b. 100 mL
   c. 150 mL
   d. 250 mL

2. **Rate of CSF production per day is about:**
   a. 150 mL
   b. 250 mL
   c. 350 mL
   d. 550 mL

3. **CSF is absorbed through:**
   a. Arachnoid villi
   b. Choroid plexus
   c. Ependymal cells
   d. Lymphatics

4. **CSF is formed by:**
   a. Active transport
   b. Filtration and secretion
   c. Diffusion
   d. Passive transport

5. **Normal pH of CSF is:**
   a. 7.13
   b. 7.23
   c. 7.33
   d. 7.40

6. **Blood brain barrier is maximally permeable to:**
   a. Na^+
   b. K^+
   c. Cl^-
   d. CO_2

7. **Cerebral aqueduct connect:**
   a. Third and fourth ventricle
   b. Fourth ventricle and central canal of spinal cord
   c. Third and lateral ventricle
   d. The two lateral ventricles

8. **Normal adult CSF pressure is:**
   a. 1–2 mm Hg
   b. 6–12 mm Hg
   c. 15–30 mm Hg
   d. 730 mm Hg

9. **CSF/plasma glucose ratio is:**
   a. 0.2–0.4
   b. 0.6–0.8
   c. 1.2–1.6
   d. 1.6–2.2

10. **The large mass of egg shaped gray matter that lies on either side of third ventricle is:**
    a. Caudate nucleus
    b. Globus pallidus
    c. Lentiform nucleus
    d. Thalamus

11. **Normal CSF pressure in the supine position is:**
    a. 150 mm H_2O
    b. 18 mm H_2O
    c. 100 mm H_2O
    d. 30 mm H_2O

12. **The ion that is present in higher concentration in CSF than in blood is:**
    a. Na^+
    b. K^+
    c. Cl^-
    d. Ca^{2+}

13. **Length of cerebral aqueduct is:**
    a. 5.2 cm
    b. 1 cm
    c. 1.8 cm
    d. 8 cm

14. **Normal CSF pressure is:**
    a. 10 mm Hg
    b. 150 mm Hg
    c. 30 mm Hg
    d. 5 mm Hg

15. The following structures are outside the blood brain barrier, *except*:
    a. Hypothalamus   b. Area postrema
    c. Pineal gland   d. Anterior pituitary
16. Blood-brain-barrier is present in all of the following sites, *except*:
    a. Habenular nucleus b. Subfornical organ
    c. Cerebellum   d. Pontine nucleus
17. The cavity of the midbrain filled with CSF is called:
    a. Cerebral aqueduct b. Fourth ventricle
    c. Lateral ventricle d. Third ventricle
18. Normal cerebrospinal fluid pressure is:
    a. 30 cm of H_2O b. 6–15 cm of H_2O
    c. 30–40 mm of H_2O d. 18 mm H_2O
19. Compression of internal jugular vein in the neck raises the CSF pressure by:
    a. Inhibiting the absorption of CSF into the venous system
    b. Increasing the production of CSF
    c. Decreasing the flow of CSF through the subarachnoid space
    d. Increasing the intracranial arterial pressure
20. The cavity present in each cerebral hemisphere is called:
    a. Lateral ventricle b. Third ventricle
    c. Fourth ventricle   d. Cisterna magna
21. Blood brain barrier is maximally permeable to:
    a. Na^+ b. K^+
    c. Cl^- d. CO_2
22. Subarachnoid space ends at the level of which vertebra?
    a. S4   b. S2
    c. L2   d. L3

ANSWERS

1. c	2. d	3. a	4. b	5. c
6. d	7. a	8. b	9. b	10. d
11. a	12. c	13. c	14. a	15. d
16. b	17. a	18. b	19. a	20. a
21. d	22. b			

FILL IN THE BLANKS/NAME THE FOLLOWING/GIVE THE NORMAL VALUE (NERVOUS SYSTEM)

1. The structural and functional unit of nervous system is neuron.
2. Weight of human brain: **1400 g.**
3. The process of the neuron that carries information towards the cell body is **dendrite** and the process that carries information away from the cell body is **axon.**
4. Nissl granules are absent in the **axon hillock** of neuron.
5. **Astrocytes** are the neuroglial cells that help in the formation of blood brain barrier.
6. The collective term used to describe astrocyte and oligodendrocyte: **macroglia.**
7. Normally glucose is the exclusive brain fuel but in starvation brain can use **ketone bodies**.
8. Normal cerebral blood flow: **750 mL/min.**
9. Name the three major association areas of human brain—*frontal association area* in front of premotor area, *parietal-temporal-occipital association area* between somesthetic and visual cortex and *temporal association area* from lower portion of temporal lobe to limbic system.
10. The ascending tract that carries proprioceptive information that does not reach consciousness is **spinocerebellar** tract.
11. The ability to identify an object by touching it utilizing past experience: **stereognosis.**
12. Golgi type II neurons are often **inhibitory** in function.
13. The junction between two neurons: **synapse.**
14. The normal synaptic delay: **0.5 ms.**
15. **Gap** junctions are present in electrical synapse.
16. During IPSP, the excitability of the neuron to other stimuli is **decreased** and during EPSP, the excitability of the neuron to other stimuli is **increased**.
17. IPSP can be produced by increasing the influx of **chloride** ions through the plasma membrane.
18. When the frequency of stimuli is increased it leads to **temporal** summation.
19. When the strength of stimulus is increased more synaptic knobs are activated and it leads to **spatial** summation.
20. Low intensity benign stimuli given for a prolonged period result in **habituation.**
21. Cranial nerves which are purely sensory in function: **olfactory, optic and vestibulo-cochlear nerves.**
22. Cranial nerves which are purely motor in function: **oculomotor, trochlear, abducens, spinal accessory and hypoglossal nerves.**
23. The basic unit of integrated reflex activity: **reflex arc.**
24. The neurotransmitter in the central integrating station in stretch reflex: **glutamate.**
25. The receptor for stretch reflex: **muscle spindle.**
26. Examples of bisynaptic reflexes: **inverse stretch reflex and reciprocal innervation.**
27. Withdrawal reflex is an example of **polysynaptic** reflex.
28. Receptor for inverse stretch reflex is **Golgi tendon organ**.
29. The muscle spindles (intrafusal fibers) are positioned in **parallel** to extrafusal fibers (muscle fibers) whereas; Golgi tendon organs are arranged in **series** with the muscle fibers.
30. The reaction time for knee jerk (stretch reflex): **19–24 ms.**
31. **Neurotendinous spindle (Golgi tendon organ)** is activated by changes in muscle tension and inhibits muscle contraction.
32. The inhibitory interneuron involved in reciprocal innervation: **Golgi bottle neuron.**
33. The only receptor that has a motor supply of its own: **muscle spindle.**
34. **Gamma efferents** determine the sensitivity of muscle spindle to stretch.
35. Percentage of the fibers in the ventral root constituted by γ-motor neurons: **30%.**

36. **Muscle spindle** informs the CNS continuously about the length of the muscle and rate of change of its length.
37. Areas in the brain that give information to the gamma motor neurons in spinal cord include **reticular formation, basal ganglia** and **cerebellum**.
38. The acetyl choline receptors on the postsynaptic membrane of neuromuscular junction are of the **nicotinic** type.
39. Synaptic stripping is seen in **neuronal injury**.
40. Loss of memory is termed **amnesia** and disorder of speech is called **aphasia**.
41. The last sensations to return after neuronal regeneration are **light touch** and **tactile discrimination**.
42. The area of the skin supplied by a single spinal nerve i.e. a single segment of spinal cord is called a **dermatome**.
43. Non-repetitive, quick, jerky movements are called **choreiform** movements.
44. Alternating contraction of the agonists and antagonists of a joint: **tremor.**
45. Sudden, involuntary contraction of the muscles of the trunk and extremities on falling asleep: **myoclonic jerk.**
46. The main excitatory neurotransmitter in brain and spinal cord: **glutamate. It is responsible for 75% of excitatory transmission in brain.**
47. The major inhibitory transmitter in brain: **GABA.**
48. Pain receptors show little or no adaptation.
49. Fast pain is carried by **A**δ fibers and slow pain is carried by **C** fibers.
50. Central analgesic system act by inhibiting the release of **substance P** in the posterior gray column of spinal cord.
51. Central analgesia system inhibits pain sensation by the liberation of **enkephalin, endorphin** and **serotonin** in the posterior gray columns.
52. Name three pain producing substances which stimulate free nerve endings: **serotonin, bradykinin, histamine.**
53. The law that explains the intensity of sensation is determined by the amplitude of the stimulus applied to the receptor: **Weber-Fechner law.**
54. **Bell-Magendie** law states that, in the spinal cord, the dorsal root is sensory and ventral root is motor.
55. Pyramidal cells are located in the **fifth** layer of cerebral cortex.
56. Percentage of fibers in the pyramidal tract are unmyelinated: **50%.**
57. Paralysis of one half of the body: **hemiplegia.**
58. Paralysis of all the four limbs: **quadriplegia.**
59. paralysis of both lower limbs: **paraplegia.**
60. In decerebrate rigidity the lesion is made at **mid-collicular** level.
61. Name the important extrapyramidal tracts: **rubrospinal, tectospinal, reticulospinal, vestibulospinal tracts and medial longitudinal bundle.**
62. Tectospinal and tectobulbar tracts arise from **superior colliculus.**
63. Medial longitudinal fasciculus connect **oculomotor, trochlear** and **abducens nerve nuclei.**
64. The parasympathetic part of the oculomotor nucleus: **Edinger-Westphal nucleus.**
65. Each cerebellar hemisphere controls muscular movements on the **same** side of the body.
66. The main afferents to cerebellar cortex: **climbing fibers and mossy fibers.**
67. Climbing fibers come from **inferior olivary nuclei**.
68. The only output neurons from cerebellar cortex: **Purkinje cells.**
69. The output of Purkinje cell is inhibitory to **deep cerebellar nuclei**.
70. Output from the flocculonodular lobe is concerned with **maintenance of equilibrium**.
71. **Granule** cells of cerebellar cortex are excitatory.
72. Name the inhibitory interneurons of cerebellar cortex: **basket cells, stellate cells and Golgi cells.**
73. Muscle atrophy, sensory changes and paralysis are **absent** in cerebellar lesions.
74. The main pathway linking the cerebral cortex to the cerebellum: **cortico-ponto-cerebellar pathway.**
75. inability to perform rapid alternate successive movements: **dysdiadochokinesia.**
76. The part of the brain between the cerebral cortex and the hypothalamus forms the **limbic system**.
77. Largest commissure of the brain: **corpus callosum.**
78. The function of **sympathetic nervous system** is to prepare the body for an emergency.
79. Muscarine is a poison obtained from **toad stools**.
80. Most common cause of cerebral hemorrhage is rupture of the **lenticulostriate artery**, a branch of middle cerebral artery.
81. The main blood supply to the internal capsule is from the central branches of **middle cerebral artery.**
82. Longest cranial nerve: **10th cranial nerve or vagus.**
83. Papez circuit connects limbic system with **hypothalamus** and **thalamus**.
84. Name the parts of the limbic system: **cingulate gyrus, septal nuclei, hippocampus and amygdala.**
85. Primary somatosensory area (SSA-I) is Brodmann's area **1,2,3** in postcentral gyrus.
86. Name the suppressor strips in the cerebral cortex - Brodmann's areas 4s, 2s, 8s, 19s and 24s.
87. Stimulation of the suppressor strips in the cerebral cortex causes **inhibition** of stretch reflex.
88. Motor aphasia is due to lesion of **Broca's area**.
89. Sensory aphasia is due to lesion of **Wernicke's area**.
90. Name the parts of basal ganglia: **caudate nucleus, putamen, globus pallidus, subthalamic nucleus and substantia nigra.**
91. Corpus striatum is formed of **caudate nucleus** and **putamen**.
92. Lenticular nucleus is formed of **globus pallidus** and **putamen**.
93. The main output from basal ganglia goes to the **thalamus**.
94. Dopaminergic fibers pass from **pars compacta** of substantia nigra to the corpus striatum.
95. Degeneration of nigrostriatal dopaminergic system causes **Parkinson's disease**.
96. Neurotransmitter in striatonigral pathway: **GABA.**

97. The part of brain concerned with short term memory: **hippocampus**.
98. Parts of brain outside the blood brain barrier which have fenestrated capillaries: **circumventricular organs**.
99. Name the circumventricular organs: **median eminence of hypothalamus, subfornical organ, organum vasculosum of lamina terminalis (OVLT), area postrema and posterior pituitary**.
100. Mutation of one of the orexin receptor gene has been linked to **narcolepsy**.
101. Subdural space is filled with **tissue fluid**.
102. Total volume of CSF: **150 mL**.
103. Rate of CSF formation: **550 mL/day**.
104. CSF in the subarachnoid space is absorbed through the **arachnoid villi** into the cerebral venous sinuses.
105. Normal CSF pressure in the supine position: **10 mm Hg or 130 mm of water**.
106. The structure in the inner ear responsible for maintenance of equilibrium: **vestibular apparatus**.
107. Receptors in the semicircular canals detect **rotational** acceleration.
108. Receptors in the utricle and saccule detect **linear** acceleration.
109. The sense organ in the semicircular canal: **crista ampullaris**.
110. The sense organ in utricle and saccule: **macula**.
111. Receptors for hearing and equilibrium: **hair cells**.
112. Jerky movement of the eye ball is called **nystagmus**.

CLINICAL CASE SCENARIO

1. **A 60-year-old man complains of irregular swaying gait, tendency to drift to the right while walking and difficulty in keeping balance when standing still. On examination, the tone of the muscles of right upper and lower limbs was diminished when compared to the left side, inability to perform finger-nose test correctly with the right hand and there was also inability to pronate and supinate the right forearm quickly and had wide-based gait. CT scan revealed a tumor in the brain.**
   Answer the following questions.
   a. Which part of the brain is involved in the lesion?
   b. Indicate the side of lesion giving proper explanation of the pathway involved with the help of a diagram.
   c. Give the physiological basis of the given signs and symptoms.

   Ans:
   a. Cerebellum
   b. Right side of cerebellum is involved, because in cerebellar lesion, effects are seen on the same side of lesion due to double decussation (explain)

2. **A 50-year-old man undergoing treatment for hypertension was brought to the casualty with c/o inability to move the right upper and lower limbs and inability to speak. On examination, there was complete paralysis of the right side of the body. Only the right lower half of the face was affected. Babinski sign was positive, and other superficial reflexes were absent on the right side. He responded to painful stimuli and was conscious. Answer the following questions:**
   a. Where can be the side and the probable site of lesion?
   b. Explain with the help of a diagram the pathway involved from its origin to termination.
   c. What is the cause for positive Babinski sign?

   Ans:
   a. Left internal capsule

3. **A 15-year-old girl was clinically diagnosed as suffering from malignant tumor of the right cerebellar hemisphere. Answer the following questions:**
   a. What will be the important manifestations in this girl?
   b. Specify the side of the body affected giving proper explanation.
   c. Enumerate the functions of cerebellum and explain one function in detail.
   d. Mention two tests that can be performed in this girl to determine loss of cerebellar function.

4. **A man was brought to the casualty with history of fall from a height. On examination, there was paralysis of both lower limbs. X-ray spine revealed fracture and dislocation of vertebral column at T10 level.**
   b. Identify the probable condition.
   c. What will be the immediate clinical manifestations in this patient?
   d. Explain the progress of the condition.
   e. What is mass reflex?

   Ans:
   a. Paraplegia due to complete transection of spinal cord at T10 level.
   b. All manifestations of stage of spinal shock (explain).

SECTION 11 SPECIAL SENSES

Vision

CHAPTER 98

LEARNING OBJECTIVES

- Describe the functions of various parts of the eye
- Describe the formation, circulation, drainage and functions of aqueous humor
- Mechanism of image formation in the retina
- Define visual acuity and explain the process of accommodation
- Define the errors of refraction and their correction
- Explain the functional anatomy of retina
- Enumerate the events involved in photosensory transduction in eye
- Explain visual pathway with the help of a diagram
- List the visual field deficits that occur when there is a lesion in specific areas of the visual pathway
- List the eye movements and the role of extraocular muscles
- Explain the mechanisms involved in color perception
- Define color blindness and the tests to identify it

INTRODUCTION

PY10.17: Describe and discuss functional anatomy of eye, physiology of image formation, physiology of vision including color vision, refractive errors, color blindness, physiology of pupil and light reflex.

Light is a very useful source of information about the world. Eyes gather information from the environment to form images in the retina which is interpreted by the brain and converted to conscious visual images. Maximum information regarding the environment is brought to the central nervous system by the eyes and vision is very essential for the survival of most mammals.

Eye has two parts:
1. An **optical part** which gather and focus light and form an optical image on the retina.
2. A **neural part** called the retina, which converts the image into a sensation by sending impulses to the visual cortex. The visible spectrum is between **400 nm and 700 nm**.

Light from external objects passes through transparent media in the eye, and by the image-forming mechanism in the eye, images of external objects fall on the retina. In the retina, there are receptors called photoreceptors sensitive to light, and photochemical changes take place by absorbing photons. Through the visual pathway, nerve impulses reach the visual cortex and we can see the objects in the external environment.

The study of the structure, functions and diseases of the eye is called **ophthalmology**.

FUNCTIONAL ANATOMY OF EYEBALL

The eyeball is spherical in shape, about 2.5 cm in diameter and is well protected by the bony walls of the orbit. Structure of the eye is shown in **Figure 98.1**. Eye has two major components: an **optical part** to gather light and to focus it to form an image and a **neural part**, the retina which convert the image into a sensation. The eyeball consists of three layers:
1. Outermost layer is the transparent **cornea** in front and opaque **sclera** behind.
2. Middle layer is the **uvea** (iris and ciliary body in front and vascular choroid behind).

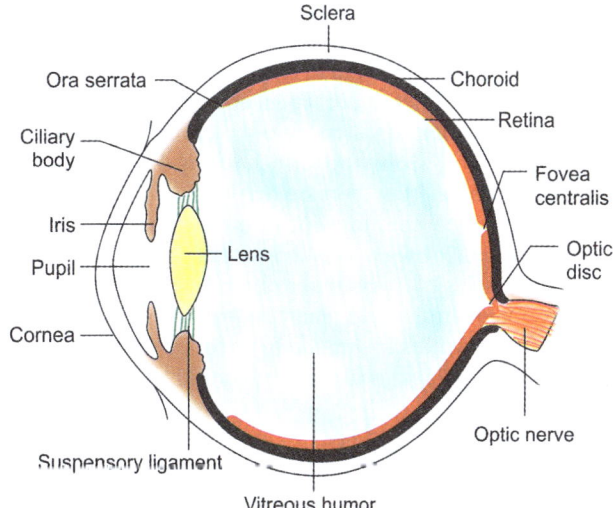

Fig. 98.1: Longitudinal section of eyeball.

3. Innermost layer is the **retina** which is the neural layer. It stops at ora serrata anteriorly and is continued as the epithelial lining of ciliary body and iris.

Contents of the eye are:
- Lens
- Aqueous humor
- Vitreous humor.

Layers of the Eyeball

Sclera

The outer protective layer of the eyeball is sclera. It contains white fibrous tissue, elastic fibers, fibroblasts, etc. The extraocular muscles are inserted in various parts of the sclera (*see* **Fig. 98.5**).

Sclera is modified anteriorly to form the transparent cornea. The junction of the cornea with the sclera is called the **limbus**.

Conjunctiva

Conjunctiva is a layer of thin stratified mucous membrane that covers the sclera on the exposed part of the eyeball. It is reflected onto the inner surface of the eyelids. It protects the sclera.

Cornea

Light rays enter the eye only through the transparent cornea.

Causes for Corneal Transparency

- Regular and parallel arrangement of stromal collagen fibrils in the cornea.
- Cornea is devoid of blood vessels and lymph vessels and water content of cornea is also less. Relative dehydration of cornea is maintained by active transport of Na^+ and fluid outward through the epithelium and corneal endothelium. An edematous cornea loses its transparency and hence should be kept dehydrated.
- Absence of pigments in cornea.
- Absence of myelin sheath in corneal nerve fibers.
- Uniform arrangement of corneal epithelial cells.

Cornea is richly supplied by unmyelinated, free nerve endings derived from the ophthalmic division of the **trigeminal nerve**. The fibers belong to C and Aδ type. The only sensory receptors present in the cornea are the **free nerve endings**. Cornea is sensitive to touch and temperature changes. It is highly sensitive to pain sensation. Its outer surface is kept moist and clear by tear secreted from the lacrimal gland, which is situated in the upper lateral portion of each orbit. Corneal avascularity minimizes corneal graft rejection.

Cornea consists of five layers:
1. Epithelium
2. Bowman's membrane
3. Substantia propria (stroma)
4. Descemet's membrane
5. Endothelium.

Epithelium is stratified and is the continuation of conjunctiva over the cornea.

Substantia propria (90% of total corneal thickness) or stroma is the forward continuation of sclera. It is composed of regularly arranged thin fibrils of collagen and the transparency of cornea is related to the regularity of the stromal components.

Descemet's membrane is a thin elastic membrane covered on its posterior surface by endothelium. Function of corneal endothelium is stromal dehydration. Endothelial cells become less in number with age.

Nutrition of cornea is from aqueous humor, which provides amino acid and glucose. 65% of corneal metabolism is by glycolysis and the rest is by Krebs cycle and hexose monophosphate (HMP) shunt. Products of metabolism like lactic acid diffuse into the aqueous humor. O_2 to cornea is obtained by diffusion from air and CO_2 diffuses to the atmospheric air.

The corneal epithelium undergoes complete turnover in a week and if the epithelium is damaged, since it is highly proliferative, it heals rapidly. But if the Bowman's membrane is damaged, the cornea develops scar that leads to corneal opacity.

Injury to cornea → Loss of corneal transparency → Loss of vision.

Transparency of cornea is also lost in severe vitamin A deficiency (*refer* xerophthalmia) and in metabolic diseases like uncontrolled diabetes mellitus.

Uveal Tract (Uvea)

Just inner to sclera is the highly vascular uvea concerned with the nutrition of the eye. The iris, ciliary body and the choroid are collectively called the uvea. The **choroid** and the **ciliary body** line the sclera, while the **iris** forms a free circular diaphragm in the anterior part. The central aperture in the diaphragm forms the pupil. The uvea is innervated by sensory fibers of trigeminal nerve as well as by vasomotor fibers.

Choroid and Ciliary Body

Just inside the sclera is the choroid. It is a highly vascular and pigmented layer present over the posterior 2/3rd of the eyeball, in contact with the sclera. The capillary plexus in the choroid nourishes the visual receptors. The pigment in the choroid absorbs light, prevents back scattering of light and prevents entry of light through areas other than cornea and lens (Reflection of light rays back through the retina would produce blurring of the visual images).

Ciliary Body

The thickened anterior part of the choroid forms the ciliary body.

Functions of the ciliary body
- Keeps the lens in position
- Secretes aqueous humor.

The ciliary body has an outer and an inner part. The outer part is composed of circular and longitudinal smooth muscle fibers. The longitudinal muscle fibers are attached near the corneoscleral junction. The lens is attached by **ciliary zonule or lens suspensory ligament** to the ciliary muscles. Thus this part keeps the lens in position. The inner part has tufts of blood capillaries. The anterior surface of the inner part of the ciliary body is thrown into folds called **ciliary processes**, which secrete aqueous humor **(Fig. 98.2)**.

Iris and Pupil

Iris is known as the diaphragm of eye and it is a pigmented disc visible through the cornea. It controls the diameter of the **pupil**, which is the central aperture in the iris. Both circular and radial muscle fibers are present in the iris, which are ectodermal in origin **(Fig. 98.3A to C)**.

Circular fibers (sphincter pupillae) are present at the inner most rim of iris running round the pupillary margin. It is supplied by postganglionic parasympathetic cholinergic nerve fibers from the ciliary ganglion, which on stimulation produce constriction of pupil or **miosis.** Radial fibers (dilator pupillae) are supplied by postganglionic sympathetic adrenergic fibers from the superior cervical ganglion, which on stimulation produce dilatation of pupil or **mydriasis.** The balance of tone between these two antagonistic autonomic innervations maintains the pupil at its normal size. The sphincter pupillae tone is more than that of radial muscles. The regulation of pupillary size by ambient light levels is called pupillary light reflex.

- ❖ **Miotics** are drugs that produce pupillary constriction, e.g., pilocarpine, physostigmine.
- ❖ **Mydriatics** are drugs producing pupillary dilatation, e.g., atropine.

Functions of the pupil

- ❖ Pupils regulate the amount of light that enters the eyes
- ❖ Diameter of the pupil affects the quality of the retinal image. A smaller pupil diameter gives a greater depth of focus.

Depending on the background illumination, pupillary size varies. Variations in the diameter of the pupil can produce up to 16-fold change in the amount of light reaching the retina. By decreasing the size of pupil, chromatic and spherical aberration is decreased and depth of focus is increased. But very small pupil leads to blurred vision and diffraction.

- ❖ Normal size of pupil is 2–3 mm.
- ❖ In near vision, pupil constricts.
- ❖ The pupils are of equal size on the two sides normally. The condition in which unequal pupils are seen is called **anisocoria**. Anisocoria can be due to unilateral pontine tumor, excess intraocular pressure in one eye, aneurysm in brain, inflammation of the iris, direct trauma to the eye, unilateral application of medications like pilocarpine and neurological disorders like Horner's syndrome.

Retina

Retina is, histologically and embryologically, a part of the central nervous system. It is the neural layer lining the posterior two thirds of the choroid and is ~200 μm thick in humans. It contains the light sensitive cells, the **photoreceptors, rods and cones**. Photoreceptors capture photons and the light energy is used to generate action potentials in the optic nerve. Rods are responsible for dim light vision and black and white vision while cones are responsible for bright light vision and color vision. Number of cones is more toward the center and rods are more at the periphery of the retina.

The photoreceptors are present on the outer surface of retina, that is, the side facing away from the vitreous humor and incoming light. The receptor layer rests on the pigment epithelium next to the choroid. So the light rays must pass through the ganglion cell and bipolar cell layers of the retina to reach the rods and cones. This path does not affect the image quality because of the thinness and transparency of the neural layers. Rods and cones undergo a continuous process of renewal (sloughing off membrane from their outer segments and rebuilding them). Since the photoreceptors are close to the pigment epithelium, the renewal process occurs easily.

In addition to rods and cones, nerve cells like bipolar cells, ganglion cells, horizontal cells, amacrine cells, etc., are present in the retina. Rods and cones synapse with bipolar cells and bipolar cells synapse with ganglion cells. The axons of the ganglion cells leave the eye as the optic nerve at the **optic disc** of eye.

Optic disc is about 3 mm medial to and slightly above the posterior pole of the eyeball. All the layers of retina except the layer of optic nerve fibers are absent in this region. There are no photoreceptors at the optic disc and consequently this spot is blind, as image falling here cannot be detected. Hence, it is referred to as **blind spot** since it is totally insensitive to light.

Retinal blood vessels enter the eye through the optic disc. The central retinal artery supplies bipolar cells and ganglion cells, i.e., the inner layers of the retina. *But the receptor cells are nourished by the capillary plexus of choroid since the outermost layer of retina is adherent to the choroid. This is*

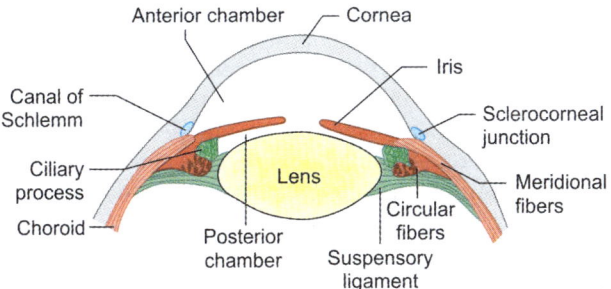

Fig. 98.2: Anterior parts of eyeball.

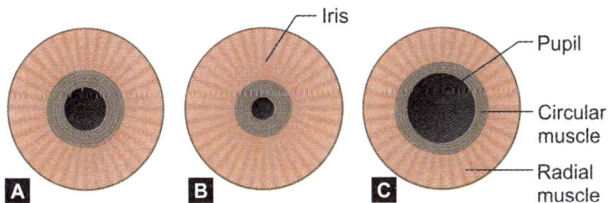

Figs. 98.3A to C: Structure of iris: (A) Normal pupil; (B) Constriction of pupil (miosis); (C) Dilatation of pupil (mydriasis).

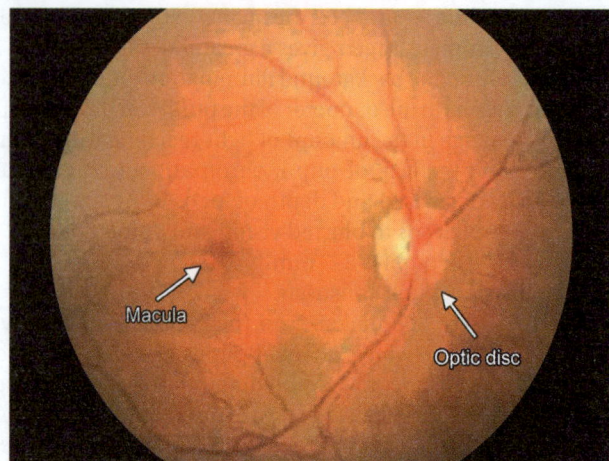

Fig. 98.4: Appearance of normal fundus of eye.

the reason for the destruction of photoreceptors in retinal detachment and the resulting blindness. The retina sometimes gets detached from the pigment epithelium when there is injury to the eyeball.

Fovea Centralis and Macula Lutea (Fig. 98.4)

At the posterior pole of the eye, 3 mm to the temporal side of the optic disc is a pit or depression where the inner retinal layers are thinned out exposing the cones better to light. This is the **fovea centralis**, which is the most sensitive part of retina. It is about 300–700 µm in diameter. Here the neurons in the inner layer of retina are displaced laterally to the side of fovea to minimize light scattering on the way to the photoreceptors. There are no blood vessels at the very center of fovea. *Fovea centralis contains only cones.* If image falls here, maximum acuity of vision is obtained.

A yellowish-pigmented spot, the **macula lutea or the yellow spot** surrounds it. Yellow color is due to the presence of the pigment xanthophyll. Macula lutea is about 1 mm² in diameter.

> Since the receptor layer of retina rests on the pigment epithelium next to the choroid, light rays entering the eye must pass through the ganglion cell and bipolar cell layers to reach the rods and cones except for fovea centralis, where the light reaches the cones directly.

OPHTHALMOSCOPY

The arteries, arterioles and veins in the superficial layers of retina near its vitreous surface can be seen clearly using an instrument called **ophthalmoscope** invented by Helmholtz in 1851. **Fundus** of the eye is the interior surface of the eye opposite to the lens. It includes the retina, optic disc, macula and fovea. Retina is the only place in the body where arterioles are readily visible. The optic disc can also be seen clearly by ophthalmoscopy. The ophthalmoscopic observations in a normal eye are as follows:

* Optic disc is creamy pink and the center of the disc is pale and hollowed out.
* Retina is pinkish red.
* Blood vessels consist of four main arteries and their accompanying veins.
* Macula appears slightly darker than the surrounding retina.

Cupping of the optic disc is seen in ocular hypertension and optic disc is bulged in raised intracranial tension. Ophthalmoscopic examination helps not only in the diagnosis of eye diseases like retinitis pigmentosa, papilledema, etc. but also in detecting systemic disorders which affect the blood vessels of the eye leading to retinopathy. Thus, diseases affecting blood vessels like diabetes mellitus, hypertension, etc., can be evaluated by ophthalmoscopic examination. Twisting and kinking of tiny retinal blood vessels is a finding in hypertension.

CONTENTS OF THE EYEBALL

Aqueous Humor

Aqueous humor is a thin, clear, colorless, protein-free, transparent fluid with a pH of 7.1-7.3 present in the anterior and the posterior chambers of the eye. It is secreted from the ciliary processes in the ciliary body by ultrafiltration and active secretion and is formed at an average rate of 2-3 µL/min. This fluid exerts a pressure known as **intraocular pressure (IOP)**.

Composition

Electrolytes—Na^+, K^+, HCO_3^-, Cl^-
* Glucose, urea, uric acid
* Ascorbic acid, lactic acid and hyaluronic acid
* Dissolved oxygen.

Active transport of Na^+, Cl^-, HCO_3^- and other ions occurs into the space enclosed by the ciliary processes, followed by oozing out of H_2O. The solution thus formed is aqueous humor, which enters the posterior chamber first. Glucose, amino acids, ascorbic acid, etc., are transported actively or by facilitatory diffusion into the aqueous humor.

Aqueous humor flows from the posterior chamber (part between iris and lens) into the anterior chamber through the pupil. Anterior chamber is bounded in front by cornea and behind by the iris and it is 2.5 mm deep in the center. Its peripheral recess is called angle of the anterior chamber, which contains a circular venous sinus called **canal of Schlemm**. Aqueous humor escapes through the canal of Schlemm and from there, into the episcleral veins **(Fig. 98.2)**. It is a continuous process. The canal of Schlemm is a thin walled highly porous vein that extends circumferentially all the way around the eye. The endothelium of the canal of Schlemm is so porous that even large protein molecules, as well as particulate matter up to the size of red blood cells, can enter the canal of Schlemm. So much aqueous humor normally flows into it that it is filled with aqueous humor rather than with blood.

Normal intraocular pressure is 10-20 mm Hg and the pressure in the canal of Schlemm and episcleral veins is only 10-15 mm Hg. This difference helps in continuous drainage of aqueous humor into the venous plexus.

Functions of Aqueous Humor

- It maintains normal intraocular pressure (IOP).
- It contributes to maintaining the spherical shape of the eyeball and its transparency.
- It forms one of the refracting media of the eye, which has a refractive index of 1.34.
- It supplies nutrition to lens and cornea and drains metabolites like lactic acid from the surrounding structures.
- IOP helps in appropriate spacing and alignment of the optical contents, which is very essential for normal vision.

INTRAOCULAR PRESSURE

The pressure exerted by the aqueous humor in the anterior chamber of the eye is called intraocular pressure (IOP). Normal intraocular pressure is 10–20 mm Hg (15 mm average). Intraocular pressure is important in spacing of the refractive media in the eyeball, which is essential for normal vision. IOP increases with age, especially after 40 years. Myopes (those having shortsightedness) and those taking glucocorticoids tend to have a higher IOP. IOP is decreased in severe dehydration, uveitis and in retinal detachment.

Measurement of IOP—Tonometry

Intraocular pressure is measured using **tonometer**. Local anesthesia is used to anesthetize the cornea. Place the footplate of tonometer onto the center of cornea. By the central plunger, a depression is made in the central part of cornea and the deflection produced is measured in terms of millimeters of Hg. This gives the IOP. Regular measurement of IOP is very important as age advances especially after the age of 40.

Ocular Hypertension

Increase in IOP is called **ocular hypertension**. It is mainly due to accumulation of aqueous humor inside the anterior chamber of eye. The lens will be pushed backward into the vitreous body, and the vitreous body in turn compresses the blood vessels and the neurons of retina. Eyeball feels abnormally hard in this condition. The retinal artery, which enters the eyeball at the optic disc, is compressed causing retinal degeneration leading to glaucoma. In this condition, ophthalmoscopic examination shows cupping of the optic disc. *A chronic elevation of IOP will lead to characteristic degenerative changes in the optic disc.* If the IOP is greater than 30 mm Hg, and if it is maintained for a long time (chronic glaucoma), there will be destruction of neurons in the retina and degeneration of optic disc leading to blindness. The optic nerve fibers have no neurilemma and hence cannot regenerate. Glaucoma is one of the most common causes of blindness. Usually, it is seen as age advances.

Causes for Increased IOP

- Increased production of aqueous humor
- Improper drainage of aqueous humor due to blockage of canal of Schlemm.
- Drugs like glucocorticoids increase IOP.
- Increase in venous pressure outside the eye, e.g., obstruction to superior vena cava causes ocular hypertension secondary to increased venous pressure.

GLAUCOMA

Glaucoma is a degenerative disease in which there is loss of ganglion cells of the retina. It is the second most common cause of blindness next to cataract. Raised intraocular pressure is only one of the risk factors for developing glaucoma. But ocular hypertension may worsen glaucoma. If left untreated may lead to blindness. So, intraocular pressure should be reduced to prevent complications associated with glaucoma.

Types of Glaucoma

- Open-angle glaucoma
- Angle-closure glaucoma.

In **open-angle glaucoma**, the increased IOP is due to the increased resistance of the trabeculae of canal of Schlemm to aqueous outflow. It is due to deposition of pigments and mucopolysaccharides from the iris and lens capsule in the trabecular meshwork. In inflammatory diseases of the eye, white blood cells and tissue debris can block the trabecular spaces and cause increase in the intraocular pressure. In some cases, this type of glaucoma occurs due to a genetic defect. When drainage is decreased, there will be accumulation of aqueous humor in the anterior chamber leading to increased IOP. Surgical treatment of open angle glaucoma involves trabeculectomy, i.e., the creation of a fistula between the anterior chamber and the sub-conjunctival space.

In **angle-closure glaucoma**, the sclera-corneal angle (angle of anterior chamber) is narrow and therefore easily occluded by the peripheral part of the iris. Here there is forward movement of iris, which obliterates the angle between the iris and the cornea (anterior chamber angle). This leads to block in the opening of the trabecular meshwork at the angle and pooling of aqueous humor and a rise in the IOP.

Treatment

Glaucoma is treated with drugs that decrease the secretion of aqueous humor or that which increase the outflow of aqueous humor. Beta adrenergic blockers like timolol and carbonic anhydrase inhibitors like acetazolamide decrease the production of aqueous humor and thus reduce IOP. Parasympathomimetic drugs (miotics) like pilocarpine and some prostaglandins are also helpful to increase the outflow of aqueous humor by causing ciliary muscle contraction. Usually a combination of beta blocker and prostaglandin is used to treat increased intraocular pressure. The drugs are given in the form of eye drop solution. If the block to the drainage of aqueous humor persists, it is removed by surgery.

LENS

Lens is situated behind the iris and in front of the vitreous humor. It is a transparent, biconvex, avascular structure consisting of collagen fibers enclosed within a thin, tough, transparent capsule made of epithelial cells. Lens is circular, about 11 mm in diameter. The lens fibers are arranged in a regular and orderly pattern. There is continuous growth of lens fibers throughout life, like an onion. Older fibers seen toward the center is called nucleus of lens and this is thick and dense. The periphery is called cortex, which is soft and consists of the youngest cells or fibers. The cells of the lens have a high concentration of proteins called α-**crystallins**, which help increase the density of the lens and enhance its focusing power.

The lens is held in place by a circular **lens suspensory ligament or ciliary zonule** composed of connective tissue fibers. Medially, it is attached to the periphery of the lens capsule and laterally it is attached to the inner surface of the ciliary body. The anterior curvature of lens is flattened in the relaxed eye and this is due to the tension in the suspensory ligament by which it is attached to the ciliary body.

Movements of the ciliary body can alter the tension in the suspensory ligament. When the ciliary muscles contract, the suspensory ligament becomes lax and the lens bulges and increases its curvature especially on the anterior surface.

For near vision, the anterior curvature of the lens is increased, thereby increasing the refractive power of the lens. Capacity to change the refractory power of the lens decreases with age. The elasticity of lens also decreases with age and the lens becomes opaque. The condition is called **cataract**. These changes occur at an early age in uncontrolled diabetes mellitus and also in injury to lens and exposure of eye to ionizing radiation. Removal of the lens and substituting it by a biconvex lens outside the eye or by an implantable intraocular lens is the treatment for cataract. An eye without a lens is called **aphakic eye**.

VITREOUS BODY

Vitreous body or vitreous humor is a transparent gel-like substance containing thin fiber like strands made up of a hygroscopic protein called **vitrein**. It is present behind the lens and forms ¾ of the volume of the eyeball. Vitreous forms a semisolid support to the retina and prevents detachment of retina. Small collagen fibrils produced by fibrocytes in the vitreous can be seen and forms one of the refractive media in the eye. Sometimes, the fine collagenous fibrils in the vitreous humor undergo contracture, pulling parts of retina toward the interior of the globe. This leads to retinal detachment, which is a medical emergency since it leads to degeneration of retina and blindness.

Lens absorbs all the ultraviolet rays entering the eye. Most of the large waves are absorbed by aqueous and vitreous humor.

EXTRAOCULAR MUSCLES

The skeletal muscles attached to the eyeball externally are called extraocular muscles (the intraocular muscles or the intrinsic muscles of the eye, i.e., the muscles of ciliary body and iris are smooth muscles). The extraocular muscles originate from the bone of the orbit and are inserted on the sclera. The eyeball can be moved in all directions by six extraocular muscles that are inserted in various parts of the sclera. These muscles are supplied by 3rd, 4th and 6th cranial nerves. The muscles are **medial and lateral recti, superior and inferior recti, and superior and inferior oblique (Fig. 98.5).** Superior oblique is supplied by 4th cranial nerve; lateral rectus by 6th cranial nerve and the rest of the extraocular muscles are supplied by the 3rd cranial nerve.

Functions of the Extraocular Muscles

- Extraocular muscles control eye movements
- They control direction of gaze
- They help in the coordination of the two eyes to keep their retinal images on corresponding retinal points when the eye, head and visual world move about.
- When there is weakness or paralysis of any of these muscles, it leads to a condition called **squint or strabismus.** This causes double vision.

Eye Movements

The movements of eyeball are adduction (medial rotation), abduction (lateral rotation), elevation, depression, intortion (inward rotation), extortion (outward rotation), convergence, saccades, smooth pursuit movements and vestibular movements. The muscles and their actions are:

- Medial rectus: Adduction or medial rotation
- Lateral rectus: Abduction or lateral rotation
- Superior rectus: Elevation when the eyeball is abducted
- Inferior rectus : Depression when the eyeball is abducted

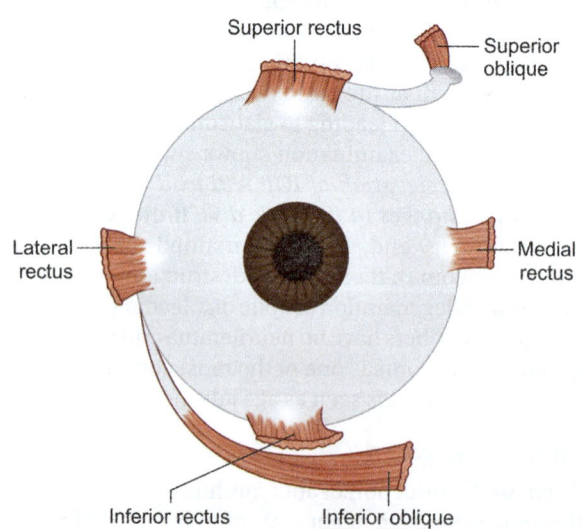

Fig. 98.5: Extraocular muscles of eye seen attached to sclera.

- Superior oblique: Depresses the eyeball when the eye is adducted
- Inferior oblique: Elevates the eyeball when the eye is adducted.

Intortion is due to contraction of superior oblique and superior rectus muscles. Extortion is due to combined action of inferior oblique and inferior rectus muscles.

Convergence movements of the eyeball bring the visual axes toward each other when the person focuses his attention on a nearby object. Saccades are sudden jerky movements that occur as the gaze shifts from one object to another. They bring new objects of interest onto the fovea. Smooth pursuit movements are tracking movements of the eyes as they follow moving objects.

Vestibular movements occur due to stimulation of semicircular canals and it helps to maintain visual fixation as the head moves.

There is close coordination between the muscles of the two eyes. This is necessary for the images to fall on corresponding points of the two retinas. The eye muscles show reciprocal innervation and inhibition so that coordination of eye movements is achieved. The opposite muscle, i.e., the muscle that opposes the movement relaxes while the muscle that is stimulated contracts. Otherwise, diplopia will result.

Movements of the eyeball can be brought about voluntarily by impulses arising from the motor areas of the cerebral cortex. Frontal eye fields are involved in voluntary eye movements. The fibers descend in the pyramidal tract to end in the nuclei of III, IV and VI cranial nerves, which supply the extraocular muscles. In involuntary eye movements, the impulses arise from the retina and reach the occipital cortex. From there, via the superior colliculus, impulses reach the III, IV and VI cranial nerve nuclei (*refer* 'visual body reflexes' page 932 of this chapter).

Effects of Unilateral Lesion of Oculomotor Nerve

- Eye cannot be moved upward, downward and inward.
- At rest, the eye looks laterally due to the activity of lateral rectus and downward due to the activity of superior oblique.
- Diplopia occurs, i.e., the patient sees double.
- Drooping of upper eyelid (ptosis) due to paralysis of levator palpebrae superioris.
- Pupil is widely dilated and non-reactive to light due to paralysis of sphincter pupillae and unopposed action of dilator pupillae.
- Accommodation reflex will be absent.

Lesion of the Trochlear and Abducens Nerve

- The **trochlear nerve** supplies the superior oblique muscle of eye whose action is depression and intortion of the eye. Lesion leads to diplopia (double vision) and the affected eye drifts upwards due to the unopposed action of the other extraocular muscles. There will be inability to move the adducted eye downwards
- The **abducens nerve** supplies the lateral rectus whose function is abduction of the eyeball. Lesion produces double vision and the affected eye will be medially rotated due to the unopposed action of medial rectus. Convergent squint is also a feature.

LACRIMAL APPARATUS

The cornea and conjunctiva are kept moist by tears produced by the **lacrimal gland** which is drained by the **lacrimal ducts** into the nose. Together, they form the lacrimal apparatus. Tear is an ultrafiltrate of plasma and it lines the cornea in a layer that is <10 μm thick. Tear is composed of 98% water and 1.5% NaCl. It contains antibacterial agents like lysozyme and lactoferrin. Tear also contains mucus secreted by conjunctival goblet cells. Vitamin A deficiency leads to malfunctioning of the goblet cells leading to dryness of cornea and the condition is called **xerophthalmia.** It leads to corneal damage and repeated infections. The **meibomian glands** in the eyelids secrete the outermost lipid layer of the tear. Tear secretion is increased by parasympathetic stimulation and decreased by sympathetic nerve stimulation.

Functions of Tears

- Cornea is avascular and it gets O_2 from atmospheric air. O_2 dissolves in the tear and is made available to the cornea.
- Tear keeps the cornea and conjunctiva moist. Blinking helps in keeping the cornea moist. Dryness of cornea leads to ulcer formation and impaired vision.
- In times of irritation of eye due to foreign substances, there is increased secretion of tear, which washes away the irritants from the eye.
- Tear contains mucus secreted by conjunctival goblet cells that lubricates the eye for the smooth movement of eyelids.
- Antibacterial agents like lysozyme, lactoferrin, antibodies etc., present in the tear prevent eye infections to a certain extent.
- The outermost lipid layer of the tear film is secreted by the meibomian glands in the eyelids. It slows evaporation of tears and keeps the eye always moist.

PHYSICAL OPTICS

Visible spectrum is the part of the electromagnetic spectrum to which the photoreceptors in the retina are sensitive. Wavelength range of visible spectrum is 400–700 nm and the color ranges from violet to red.

- Rays with wavelength less than violet are ultraviolet rays (UV).
- Rays with wavelength greater than red are infrared rays (causes heating of tissues).

Both UV and infrared rays are injurious to the tissues.

Eye acts as a camera with optical lens system for image formation. Pupil acts as the aperture and retina as the film. Light passes through various refractive media before it reaches the retina. The path of light before it reaches the visual receptors is shown in **Flowchart 98.1**.

Flowchart 98.1: Path of light rays through the eye.

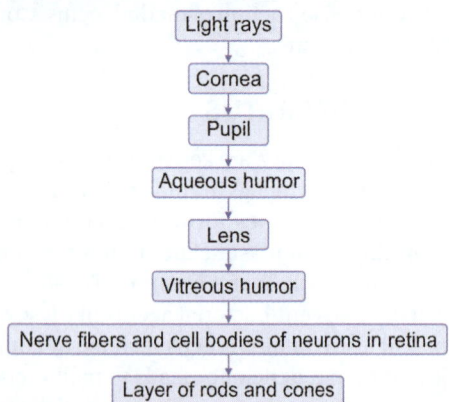

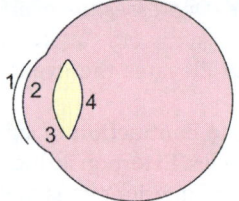

Fig. 98.6: Sites of refraction of light rays in the eye.

- Difference in refractive index is maximum here, i.e.,1 and 1.38
- Curvature of cornea is greater.

REFRACTIVE INDEX

Light rays bend as they pass obliquely from air into a denser medium or from one medium into another medium of different density. This bending of light rays is known as **refraction** and the extent to which it bends while passing in and out of the medium is expressed as the **refractive index** of the medium. The extent to which a light ray is refracted depends on two factors:
a. The difference in the refractive indices of the two media
b. The angle between the incident light and the interface between the two media. No refraction occurs when the light rays strike perpendicular to the interface.

$$\text{Refractive index of the medium} = \frac{\text{Velocity of light in air}}{\text{Velocity of light in the medium}}$$

Refractive index for a substance is essentially a measure of the speed of light within it. It is relative to the speed of light rays in air. Speed of light in air is approximately 300,000 km/s. Refractive index is calculated by dividing the speed of light in air by the speed of light in the medium. If light travels through a medium at a speed of 150,000 km/s, then it has a refractive index of, 2, i.e., 300,000/150,000.

Refractive indices for air and the different refractive media of the eye are:
- Air—1
- Cornea—1.38
- Aqueous humor—1.33
- Lens—1.4
- Vitreous body—1.34.

Interphases for Refraction of Light in the Eye (Fig. 98.6)

1. Between air and tear covered anterior surface of cornea
2. Posterior surface of cornea and aqueous humor
3. Aqueous humor and anterior surface of lens
4. Posterior surface of lens and vitreous body.

Thus in the eye, light is refracted at the anterior surface of the cornea, at the anterior surface and posterior surface of the lens. But maximum refraction occurs at the first interphase, i.e., between air and anterior surface of cornea because of the following reasons:

REFRACTIVE POWER

The refractive power of a lens is expressed in diopters (D), the number of diopters being the reciprocal of the principal focal length in meters (1/f). For example, a lens with principal focal length of 25 cm (0.25 m) has a refractive power of 1/0.25 or 4 diopters. The greater the curvature of lens, the greater will be its refractive power. The refractive power of a biconvex lens is expressed in positive values and power of biconcave lens is expressed in negative values (minus diopters). The intraocular lens is biconvex. When two co-axial lenses are placed together, their dioptric powers get added algebraically. This forms the basis of correction of refractory errors by using external lenses.

The refractive power of the anterior surface of cornea: +48 D Posterior surface of cornea: -4 D

Biconvex lens: +15 D

> About 2/3rd of the 59 D of refractive power of the relaxed eye is provided by the anterior surface of the cornea and not by the lens. Refractive index of lens in air is six times more than that in fluid. Even though lens has a greater refractive power than cornea, within the eye, lens is surrounded by fluid. Because of the small difference in the refractive index between the lens and the aqueous and vitreous humors surrounding it, the effective refractive power of the lens is much lower than that of cornea i.e., +15D.

Reduced Eye of Listing

For convenience, combined refractory power of cornea, aqueous humor, lens and vitreous humor is taken. If the refractive powers of all the refractive surfaces of the eye are algebraically added together and then considered to be one single lens, the optics of the normal eye can be simplified and represented schematically as a reduced eye. Algebraic sum of the various refractive powers is taken and is given by [(+48) + (-4) + (+15)], i.e., +59 diopters. Thus, eye is represented as a single lens with a total refractive power of +59 D when the eye is fully relaxed. This concept of **reduced eye of Listing** helps to simplify the complex refractive processes occurring in the different refractive layers of the eye. Or in other words, in the Listing's reduced eye, the nodal point is 17 mm anterior to the retina (focal length of the optical system). Hence the power of the single lens of Listings eye is 1/0.017 = 59 D.

Optical System of Eye

The anterior surface of cornea is almost spherical with radius of curvature 8 mm. The centers of curvature of the cornea and the two surfaces of the lens are on the same straight line, which is called **optic axis**. From optical point of view, the entire system can be regarded as one lens with one optical center called the **nodal point** (concept of reduced eye of Listing). In other words, central point of single lens surface is the nodal point at which light rays pass without refraction. It is about 17 mm in front of the retina or 7.2 mm behind the anterior surface of cornea in the reduced eye. It is situated a little behind the center of lens in the eye **(Fig. 98.7)**.

Principal axis is the line joining the centers of curvatures of the lens.

Principal focus: Parallel rays striking a biconvex lens are refracted to a point on the principal axis behind the lens, called principal focus or focal point.

REFRACTION IN THE EYE

Objects at Infinity

Objects at infinity produce a parallel beam of light, which after refraction, is brought to a focus on the retina in a fully relaxed eye with a power of +59 D. Fully relaxed eye is called an **unaccommodated eye**. The center of the retina is ~24 mm behind the center of cornea.

Object at infinity is greater than 6 m (20 ft) distant from the eye. Inverted images are formed in the retina, as the lens is convex **(Fig. 98.8)**. Re-inversion of images is a function of cerebral cortex. So, objects are seen erect.

Near Object

As the objects come less than 6 meters from the eye, a divergent beam of light passes through the eye from the object. If the eye is fully relaxed with +59 D, the image will be formed behind the retina. But this will not happen because the optical system increases the refractive power of the lens and the divergent beam of light is brought into focus clearly

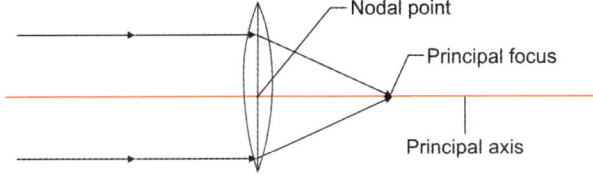

Fig. 98.7: Principal axis and principal focus in a convex lens.

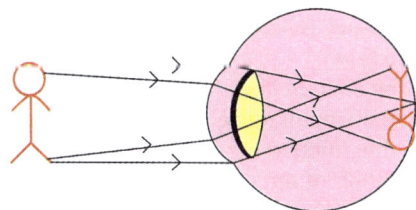

Fig. 98.8: Image formation on the retina on viewing a distant object.

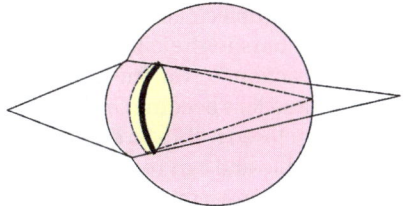

Fig. 98.9: Accommodation on viewing a near object. Note the change in the curvature of lens.

on the retina by the mechanism of **accommodation** and the image will be formed on the retina **(Fig. 98.9)**.

Near Point

Nearest point to the eye at which an object can be brought to a focus clearly on the retina with maximum accommodation is called near point of vision. In other words, it is the minimum distance at which the eye can see objects clearly. The near point recedes slowly as age advances. It is 9 cm at the age of 10 and 83 cm at the age of 60. This is due to hardening of lens substance and loss of elasticity of lens. In young adults, the power of accommodation of lens is 15D, but around age 45, it decreases to about 2 diopters. This makes reading and close work difficult in the middle age. Distant vision, which requires very little accommodation, remains unaffected. The condition is called **presbyopia**.

Far Point

Far point is the farthest point from the eye where an object can be placed and its image can be focused clearly in the retina. It is at infinity. **Range of accommodation** is the difference between far point and near point.

ACCOMMODATION

Accommodation is defined as the process by which the curvature of the lens is increased to bring into focus a near object clearly on the retina. The refractive power of the lens of eye is about 20 D. In children the refractive power can be increased from 20 D to about 34 diopters during near vision which gives an accommodation of 14 D. To achieve this accommodation, the lens becomes more convex. The power of accommodation decreases with age from about 14 D in a child to less than 2 D in a person about 50 years of age.

It is the anterior curvature of lens that increases significantly during accommodation (*see* **Fig. 98.9**). Changes in the anterior curvature occur by the contraction and relaxation of the circular and meridional fibers of the ciliary body.

Circular Fibers

Circular fibers of the ciliary body form a ring around the inner part of the ciliary body and are attached to the lens by the **suspensory ligament or ciliary zonule**. When the eye is relaxed, the lens capsule is stretched and relatively flattened due to the tension in the lens ligament. The zonal fibers or the suspensory ligament pull the edges of the lens toward the periphery because the circular fibers of ciliary body are relaxed.

On looking at a near object, i.e. during accommodation, the circular muscle fibers in the ciliary body contract and exert a sphincter-like action. So, the tension in the suspensory ligament is reduced and lens becomes more spherical. This is because the lens is enclosed within an elastic capsule and the lens fibers are malleable and can remold themselves. When the lens becomes more convex the refractive power increases and shifts the focal point closer to the eye. But there is a limit to accommodation which is age dependent as stated above.

Increase in curvature occurs exclusively at the central part of the anterior surface of the lens. *The anterior surface becomes more convex than the posterior part of the lens because the lens capsule is thinnest at the center of the anterior curvature of lens.*

Meridional Fibers

Meridional fibers or radial fibers of the ciliary body are attached to the corneoscleral junction. When they contract, they pull the ciliary body forward and downward. This movement also helps in relaxing the tension in the ciliary zonule. Thus, contraction of both circular and meridional fibers of the ciliary body relaxes the suspensory ligament and helps in increasing the anterior curvature of lens.

Stimulation of parasympathetic fibers coming through the third cranial nerve contracts both sets of ciliary smooth muscle fibers. This relaxes the lens ligaments and the lens becomes more spherical increasing its refractive power.

Experiment to Prove that Anterior Curvature of Lens is Increased During Accommodation

An experiment was done by **Helmholtz** using an instrument called **phakoscope**. It is a hexagonal box having six sides and a set of prisms. There are three apertures in the box— one for the subject's eye, another for the examiner's eye and a third aperture for the object. The apertures are arranged in such a way that the examiner can see the eye of the subject. The experiment is carried out in a fully darkened room.

Experiment

Ask the subject to look through the hole. Keep lighted candle in front of the prism. Ask the subject to look at a distant object through the third hole. Look at the subject's eye through the examiner's aperture. Three reflected images are seen in subject's eye. The images are:
1. Bright erect image reflected from anterior surface of cornea.
2. Erect but dim image reflected from anterior surface of lens.
3. Bright inverted image reflected from posterior surface of lens.

These images are known as **Purkinje-Sanson images** (**Figs. 98.10A and B**). Next ask the subject to look at a near object. A small object, usually a needle, is used.

The examiner can see that the second image becomes smaller and moves toward the first image, while there is only negligible change in the other two images.

It means that the anterior curvature of the lens changes during accommodation and that it becomes more convex during accommodation.

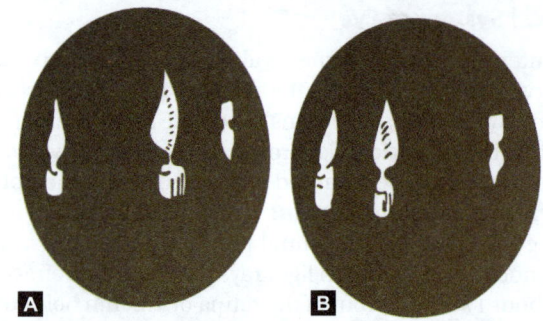

Figs. 98.10A and B: Purkinje-Sanson images: (A) During distant vision; (B) During accommodation for near vision (Note that the second image has come closer to the first one during accommodation).

NEAR RESPONSE OR NEAR REFLEX

The three-part response occurring in the eye when an individual looks at a near object is called near response or near reflex or accommodation-convergence reaction. It is a reflex action.

When a person changes his gaze from a distant object to a near object three adjustments occur in the eyeball. They are:
1. **Constriction** of pupil
2. **Convergence** of eyeball
3. **Curvature** of the anterior surface of lens increases (accommodation).

Pathway for Accommodation Reflex (Flowchart 98.2 and Fig. 98.11) or Near Response

Afferent Pathway

Receptors are rods and cones. Up to visual cortex, pathway is same as that of visual pathway (*see* visual pathway, **Fig. 98.36**). From the primary visual area (area 17), visual information concerned with accommodation is relayed to the frontal eye field (area 8) in the frontal lobe through the long association fibers.

Efferent Pathway

From area 8 of frontal cortex, some of the corticobulbar fibers pass through the anterior limb of the internal capsule to the Edinger-Westphal nucleus of the third cranial nerve of both sides. From here, the preganglionic fibers pass through the third cranial nerve to the ciliary ganglion. The post ganglionic parasympathetic fibers from the ciliary ganglion pass via short ciliary nerves and supply the ciliary muscle and sphincter pupillae. This causes constriction of pupil and relaxation of suspensory ligament leading to increase in the anterior curvature of lens. (The oculomotor nerve has two motor nuclei in the midbrain, the **main motor nucleus and the accessory parasympathetic nucleus or Edinger-Westphal nucleus).**

Some of the efferent fibers from the frontal eye field go to the somatic main motor nucleus of the third nerve. The motor fibers from this nucleus supply the medial rectus of both sides. Stimulation of the main motor nuclei stimulates the medial recti. Contraction of medial recti causes convergence of eyeball. *The effect in near response is bilateral increase*

Flowchart 98.2: Pathway for accommodation reflex (the main changes that occur in the eye while viewing a near object is shown in bold letters).

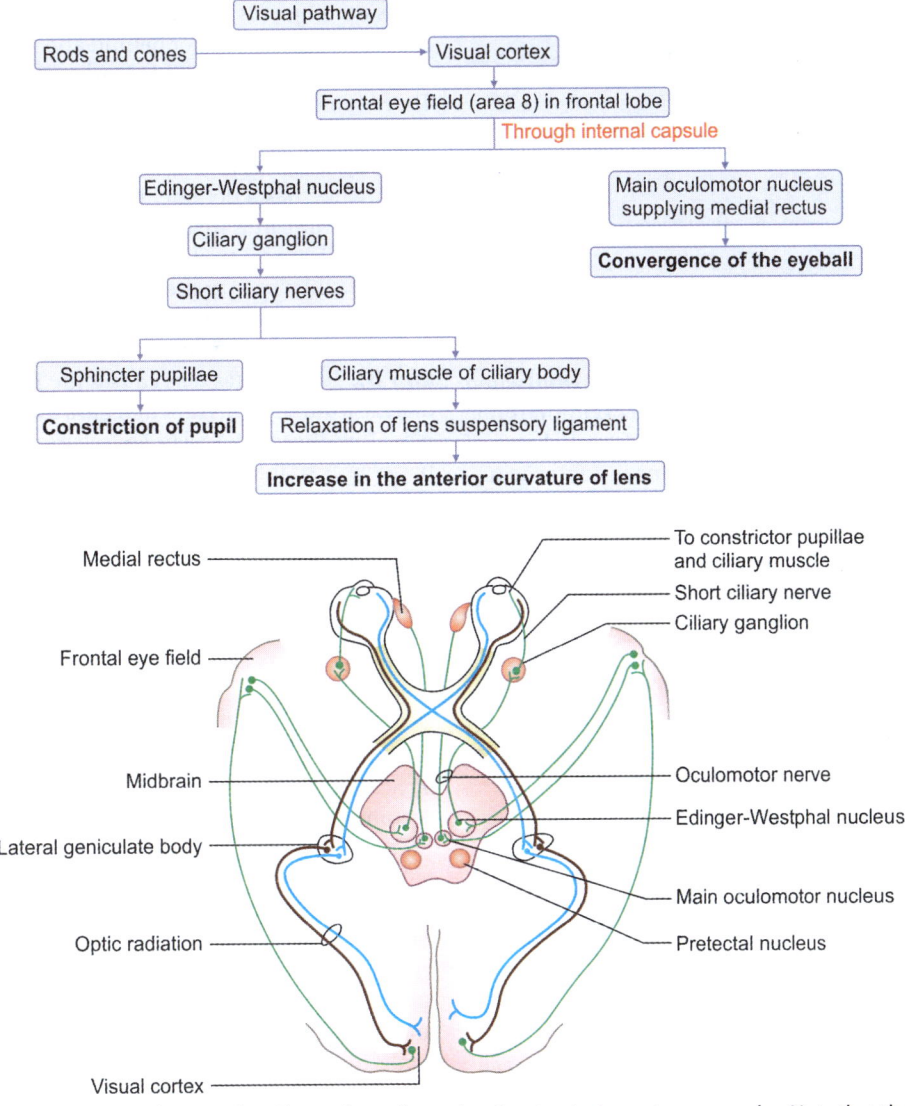

Fig. 98.11: Pathway for accommodation reflex. The pathway from visual cortex is shown in green color. Note that the accommodation pathway also includes the visual pathway up to the visual cortex since it starts from the visual receptors.

in the anterior curvature of lens, pupillary constriction and convergence of eyeball.

Amplitude of Accommodation

Amplitude of accommodation is the difference in refractive power of the eye between far point and near point of the eye, i.e., the difference between the dioptric powers of the eye when the eye is completely relaxed and when the eye is fully accommodated for near vision. For example, if the refractive power of the eye is 69 D to view clearly an object at a distance of 15 cm, then the amplitude of accommodation is 10 D (69 D minus 59 D). The refractive power of the completely relaxed eye is 59 D.

The amplitude of accommodation decreases as age advances from 11 diopters at the age of 10 to 1 D at 70 years **(Table 98.1)**. The lens capsule becomes less elastic leading

Table 98.1: Comparison of age and amplitude of accommodation.		
Age (year)	Amplitude of accommodation	Near point of vision (cm)
10	11 Diopters	9
30	7.5 D	12
50	2 D	50
70	1 D	100

to a decrease in the ability to change the curvature of lens so that near vision becomes difficult at old age. There is also slow denaturation of lens proteins. For comfortable reading, the distance is 25 cm from the eye, where an accommodation of 4 D is needed. If it becomes less than 4 D, then near vision becomes difficult. The condition is called **presbyopia or receding of near point**. This can be corrected using a convex lens. If distant vision is also affected, then a bifocal lens should be used. The upper part of glass (spectacle) is for distant vision and lower part for near vision.

OPTICAL DEFECTS IN THE EYE

Errors of Refraction

- Ametropia
  - Myopia
  - Hypermetropia
  - Anisometropia
  - Astigmatism
- Presbyopia.

Ametropia

Normal eye is called **emmetropic eye (Fig. 98.12)** and when the refractive state of the eye differs from that of emmetropia, it is known as **ametropia**. In other words, if parallel rays of light are not brought to a focus on the retina in a relaxed unaccommodated eye, the condition is known as ametropia. If the image falls in front of the retina, it is called myopia and if the image falls behind the retina, it is called hypermetropia. Astigmatism is a type of ametropia in which refractive error changes with meridian.

Myopia or Short-sightedness or Near-sightedness

In myopia, parallel rays from a distant object are brought to a focus in front of the retina. So the image will be blurred. It may be due to:

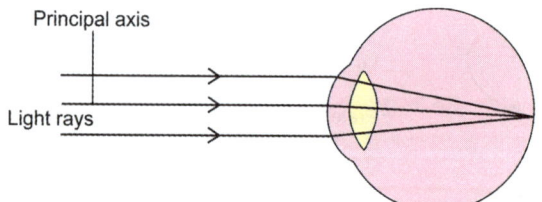

Fig. 98.12: Normal eye (emmetropic eye) parallel rays of light are brought to a focus on the retina in normal eye.

- Abnormally long eyeball
- Very strong lens.

As the object is brought closer to the eye, the image will move further and further behind and at a particular distance from the eye, image will be focused clearly on the retina. There is no mechanism in the eye by which the lens can decrease its strength. So the object should be brought nearer to the eye to focus it.

A myope has a definite limiting far point and near point. The far point in a myope is not at infinity, but there is a limiting distance. In the case of near point, if the object is brought still closer to the eye, image falls behind the retina but by accommodation, image can be brought to the retina. It is corrected using a spectacle with concave lens **(Figs. 98.13A and B)**. The *concave lens causes the peripheral light rays to diverge* from the light rays that pass through the center of the lens. Thus the image will be shifted from the front of the retina backwards so that it will fall on the retina.

Hypermetropia or Hyperopia or Long-sightedness or Far-sightedness

In hypermetropia, parallel rays from a distant object are brought to a point behind the retina in a relaxed, unaccommodated eye. Causes may be:

- Short eyeball
- Weak lens.

Initially, image can be brought to a focus on the retina by accommodation. As the person becomes older, power of accommodation decreases and image cannot be brought to a focus on the retina. These people do not have a definite far point. The condition is corrected using a convex lens **(Figs. 98.14A and B)**. Parallel light rays passing through the convex lens get refracted except those passing through the center of the lens. The peripheral rays converge that is they bend more and more towards the center. By converging the light rays, the image will be shifted from behind the retina forwards so that it falls on the retina. Contact lens can also be used to correct myopia and hypermetropia.

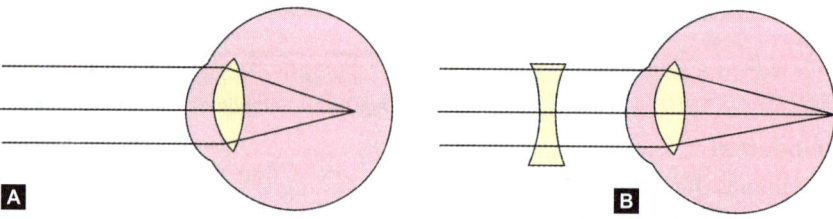

Figs. 98.13A and B: (A) Myopia; (B) Myopia corrected using biconcave lens.

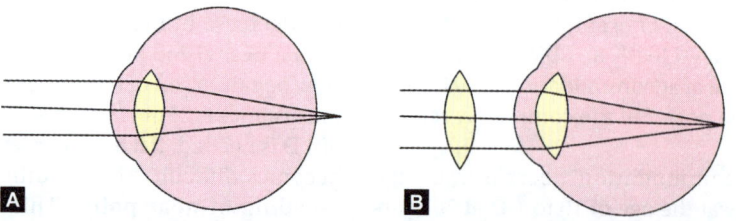

Figs. 98.14A and B: (A) Hypermetropia; (B) Hypermetropia corrected using biconvex lens.

Anisometropia

When the refractions of the two eyes are different, the condition is called anisometropia.

Astigmatism

In astigmatism, the light rays are not brought to a point focus on the retina and the focus for rays in the horizontal plane differs from that for rays in the vertical plane. This is because the cornea or the lens has different curvatures in the different planes at right angles to each other. For example, it resembles the surface of spoon, egg, etc. So, different degrees of refraction occur in different planes since refractive index of astigmatic cornea is different in different meridians. Parallel light rays passing through the meridian of greater curvature will reach a focus before those passing through the meridian of lesser curvature.

So, a point image is not obtained for a point object. For every point, a line image is obtained so that image becomes blurred **(Fig. 98.15)** due to diffuse focusing. In the case of a line object, a distorted image is obtained for a straight object **(Fig. 98.16)**.

Astigmatism is corrected using cylindrical lens, which has two different focal lengths in the two different planes (transverse and vertical planes). An astigmatic surface can be compared to two cylindrical surfaces having different curvatures placed at right angles to each other. If astigmatism has to be corrected in one plane, the cylindrical lens has to be placed with its axis at right angles to the plane, which is to be corrected. This arrangement causes convergence of the light rays from an object, passing through the two perpendicular planes of varying curvatures, into a single image.

Presbyopia

Receding of near point due to decrease in the power of accommodation with advancing age is called **presbyopia** (or loss of accommodation with age). There is loss of elasticity of the lens due to denaturation of lens proteins as age advances. As a result, the lens becomes hard and the near point of vision increases and the power of accommodation decreases.

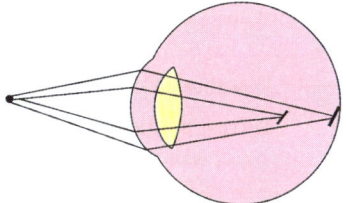

Fig. 98.15: Astigmatism in the case of a point object.

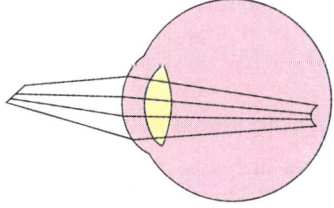

Fig. 98.16: Astigmatism in the case of a line object.

During accommodation, though the ciliary muscles are contracting, curvature of the lens does not change and the person cannot see near objects when held at normal distance. It is a progressive condition. At the age of 20, near point of vision is 10 cm whereas at the age of 40, it becomes 18 cm. In presbyopia, loss of accommodation is sufficient to make reading and close work difficult. The effect is similar to that occurring in hypermetropia. Presbyopia is also corrected by wearing spectacles with convex lens for near vision.

Keratoconus

There are conditions in which cornea shows different shapes or abnormal curvatures. For example, in keratoconus the curvature of cornea is different in different planes. This condition cannot be corrected using glasses. It is better to use a contact lens in this case. A thin film of tear will be present between the contact lens and cornea. Refraction takes place between contact lens and air and the irregularities of cornea are not considered.

OPTICAL ABERRATIONS

❖ Spherical aberration
❖ Chromatic aberration.

Spherical Aberration

The refractive power of the intraocular lens at the periphery and the central part is not the same. Normally, refractive power at the periphery of the lens is less than that at the center of the lens and therefore light rays are more divergent at the periphery. In spherical aberration, the peripheral rays of light are affected. Normally, this is eliminated by the iris that acts as a diaphragm cutting off the peripheral rays falling on the cornea. If pupillary constriction is not proper, rays farther away from the principal axis are refracted too much causing a blurring of the edges of the image **(Fig. 98.17)**. This is spherical aberration. The iris reduces this effect to a minimum. *The smaller the pupil, the less is the spherical aberration and sharper the image.*

Chromatic Aberration

Chromatic aberration is due to imperfect refraction of the different colors comprising white light at spherical surfaces. White light is made up of all the colors of the spectrum. The component rays are refracted differently depending on their

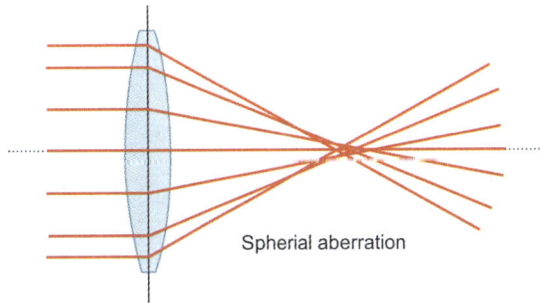

Fig. 98.17: Spherical aberration.

wavelength and hence there is a tendency for the white light to be split up into its components especially at the periphery of the lens. This causes the image to have a colored edge **(Fig. 98.18)**. This is chromatic aberration. Normally, this effect in the eye is small. It occurs in dilated eyes when exposed to bright light.

CATARACT

In old age, lens becomes opaque and degeneration of lens fibers occurs. Thus, the transparency of lens is lost. Calcium deposition also occurs in the lens so that it becomes opaque and obstructs the entry of light **(Fig. 98.19B)**. Cataract occurs at an earlier age in diabetics. Removing the lens and replacing it using an intraocular lens or extraocular lens treat it. An eye without lens is referred to as **aphakic eye**.

> The source of energy for the lens is glucose, which is metabolized normally through glycolysis. In hyperglycemia as in uncontrolled diabetes mellitus, the sorbitol pathway metabolizes large amounts of glucose. The sorbitol produced gets trapped inside the lens because the lens capsule is impermeable to sorbitol. The sorbitol absorbs water osmotically causing swelling of the lens which results in cataract formation.

VISUAL ACUITY (RESOLVING POWER OF EYE)

Visual acuity is the ability of the eye for spatial resolution, i.e., the ability to perceive detailed forms and contours of an object. It is defined in terms of the shortest distance which two lines can be separated and still be perceived as two lines. It is a function of cones and of bright light. Visual acuity is maximal in the fovea where cones are tightly packed and minimum in the peripheral part of retina where the number of cones is very few.

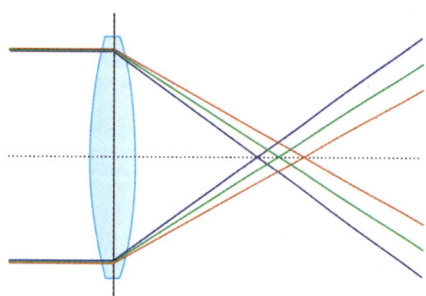

Fig. 98.18: Chromatic aberration.

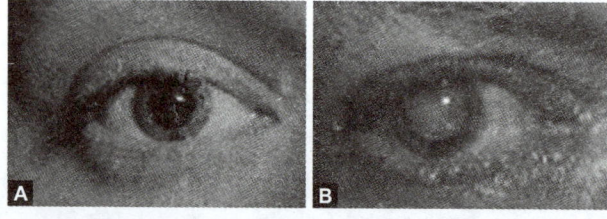

Figs. 98.19A and B: Appearance of pupil: (A) Normal pupil; (B) Cataract (the opaque lens is clearly visible).

For every point object, image will not be a sharp focus. There will be a halo around each point. The resolving power of eye is limited by imperfections in lens and diffraction defects. Normal eye sees two points as separate points when visual angle is 1 minute, i.e., 60 seconds and the distance between the two points should be 1 mm. When the two points are placed 10 m from the eye, the retinal images will be separated by 2 to 4 micrometer. As the visual angle increases, the visual acuity diminishes. When the visual angle is 1, the visual acuity is 1. If the visual angle is increased to 1.36 minutes, the visual acuity is reduced to 0.67.

Visual acuity can be denoted in two ways:
1. By expressing the minimum distance between two points seen separately as **minimum separable distance.**
2. By expressing as **reciprocal of visual angle**. Visual angle is the angle subtended by an object at the nodal point of the eye.

Test for Near Vision

Near vision is tested using **Jaeger's chart** which contains sentences of letters of different sizes. The subject is asked to read it from normal reading distance.

Test for Distant Vision

Visual acuity is tested using **Snellen's chart**. The subject is seated 6 meters away from the chart. This is because light rays incident on the eye from a distance of 6 m or more can be considered parallel. The chart consists of block letters printed in black on a white board. There are about 7 rows of letters. Their size decreases from above downward. A normal subject should be able to read every letter from the topmost line to the last line at a distance of 6 m. If the subject can read all the 7 rows from 6 m, his vision is 6/6. Normal vision is 6/6. Numerator is the distance at which subject reads the chart (usually he is seated at a distance of 6 meters from the chart). Denominator is the greatest distance in meters from the chart at which a healthy individual can read the line. If he can read only up to the 6th row, his vision is 6/9. If he can read only the first line, then his vision is 6/60 **(Fig. 98.20)**. This means that a normal person can read the first row at a distance of 60 m.

$$\text{Visual acuity} = \frac{\text{Distance of the subject from the chart}}{\text{Maximum distance at which the letter can be read by the normal eye}}$$

Width of the letter in the first row of the Snellen's chart subtends an angle of 1 minute at the nodal point if it is placed 60 m from the eye. While the letters from second to the eighth row subtends an angle of 1 minute at the nodal point of the eye at 36, 24, 18, 12, 9, 6 and 5 meters respectively **(Table 98.2)**.

Factors Influencing Visual Acuity

- **Optical factors** like the image-forming mechanism of the eye which include curvature of cornea and the lens, integrity of ciliary muscle and suspensory ligament, etc.

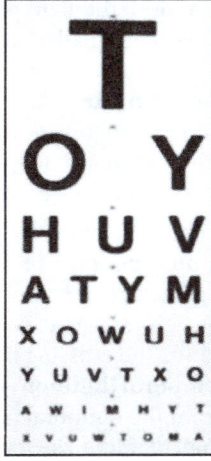

Fig. 98.20: Snellen's chart for testing distant vision.

Table 98.2: Rows in the Snellen's chart (left) and the distance at which a person with normal visual acuity can read the line (e.g., first row can be read at a distance of 60 meters by a normal person).

Row	Distance at which a normal person can read (meters)
1	60
2	36
3	24
4	18
5	12
6	9
7	6
8	5

- **Retinal factors** like the functioning of the photoreceptors and density of cones (visual acuity is highest at the fovea).
- **Stimulus factors** like illumination, size and color of the object, brightness of the stimulus, contrast between the stimuli and the background and length of application of stimulus.

Modifications in the Fovea for Maximum Acuity of Vision

- In the fovea, light falls directly on the layer of rods and cones. Other layers are displaced at the fovea. In the center of fovea, only cones are present.
- Fovea contains the smallest cones packed at the highest density. So, visual acuity is maximal if the image falls on the center of the fovea. Rods are more numerous in the periphery and cones are more numerous in the center of the retina. So visual acuity decreases as the image moves towards the periphery of the retina.
- Most of the foveal photoreceptors synapse on only one bipolar cell, which synapses on only one ganglion cell **(Fig. 98.21)**. Thus the ratio of receptor to optic nerve fiber is 1:1 at the fovea.
- The receptive field of a foveal ganglion cell is very small and this increases visual acuity. At the periphery of the retina,

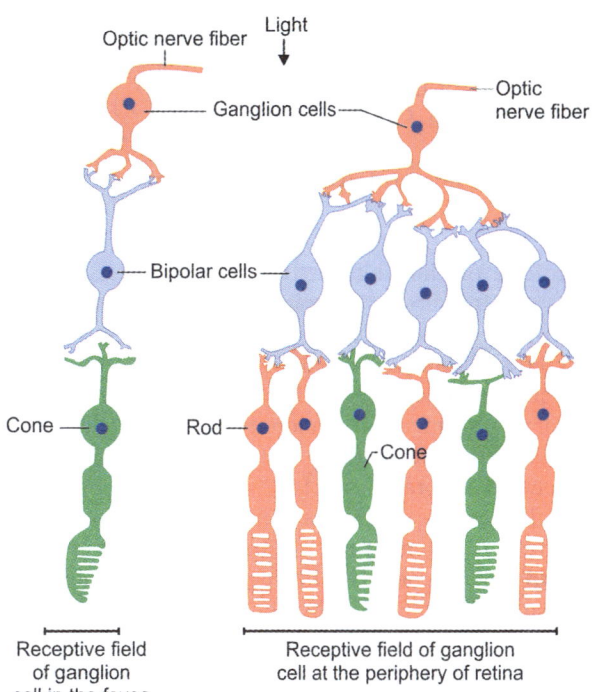

Fig. 98.21: Receptive fields in the fovea and the periphery of retina. In the first figure, one photoreceptor is connected to a single ganglion cell (1:1 ratio) whereas in the second figure, there is considerable convergence from several photoreceptors to a single ganglion cell.

the ratio of receptors to ganglion cells is high and thus each ganglion cell has a large receptive field **(Fig. 98.21)**. The large receptive field reduces the spatial resolution of the peripheral portion of retina.

FIELD OF VISION OR VISUAL FIELD

Field of vision or visual field of eye is defined as the entire extent of the external world, which can be seen by the eye in all directions at any given moment without moving the eye, with the gaze fixed at a point. The part of the external world seen by one eye with the other eye closed without moving the eye, with the gaze fixed in one direction is called the field of vision of that eye. The eye can see clearly only an extremely small area at a time when the eye is focused at a point. This point-sized area is called **fixation point**.

The visual field is divided into the nasal and temporal halves by a vertical line passing through the fixation point in the **visual field**. The area seen to the nasal side is called the nasal field of vision and the area seen to the lateral side is called **temporal field** of vision. The images of objects in the temporal half of the visual field are formed in the nasal half of retina, while those in the nasal field fall on the temporal half of retina. Similarly, objects in the upper half of the visual field form images in the lower part of retina and vice versa. This is because the image of the field of vision is inverted on the retina by the optical system of the eye.

If the eyeballs were protruding out, field of vision would be a complete circle. In human beings, eye is kept in a socket and

so the field of vision is not circular **(Fig. 98.22)**. Boundaries of the eyeball which limits the visual field are:
- Above: Eyelid and roof of orbit
- Below: Maxilla
- Medially: Nose
- There is no obstruction on the lateral side

Perimetry

Technique of charting out the field of vision is called perimetry. Instrument is **perimeter**. There is a test object, which can be moved from periphery to the center of the perimeter. A point is marked on the chart paper when the subject sees the object at different positions. The normal field of vision with a white colored object 5 mm in diameter is 50° superiorly, 60° medially (nasally), 70° inferiorly and 90° laterally or temporally **(Figs. 98.23A and B)**.

As the test object moves from periphery to center, it disappears and then appears again. The disappearance is due to **blind spot**. It is obtained 15° lateral to the central point on the chart. This is because the photoreceptors are absent at the region of optic disc. Occasionally, blind spots are found in portions of the field of vision other than the optic disc area. Such blind spots are called **scotomas** or **scotomata**. It may be due to allergic reactions in retina, lead poisoning, excessive use of tobacco, etc. It can also be due to damage of optic nerve fibers as a result of glaucoma.

In tubular field of vision, the field of vision is narrowed to a tubular shape. It is seen in advanced glaucoma and in retinitis pigmentosa. In retinitis pigmentosa, a degenerative condition of retina, melanin is deposited in the degenerated areas of retina. It produces progressive decrease in the visual field. Loss of vision first occurs in the peripheral portion of retina leading to tubular vision and gradually it spreads to the center leading to complete loss of vision.

Effect of lesions in the optic pathway in the field of vision
- Optic nerve lesion produces ipsilateral blindness or **anopia.**
- Central part of optic chiasma gets compressed by tumors of the pituitary gland. The crossing fibers will be affected and it leads to **bitemporal (heteronymous) hemianopia**. Since the image from the temporal half of the visual field falls on the nasal half of retina, the temporal field of vision of both eyes are blinded. This is because the image of the field of vision is inverted on the retina.
- Optic tract lesion of one side produces **contralateral homonymous hemianopia**
- Lesion in the optic radiation and visual cortex produces **contralateral homonymous hemianopia with macular sparing.**

Binocular Vision and Depth Perception

If the field of vision of both eyes is charted in the same sheet, there will be overlap of visual fields. This is called binocular vision **(Fig. 98.24)**.

If the object is in binocular field of vision, two images are formed which send impulses to the cortex. At the cortex, the images fuse to give a single impression. For fusion to take place, certain conditions should be satisfied:
- Images should fall on corresponding points in the retina.
- Images should be almost identical.

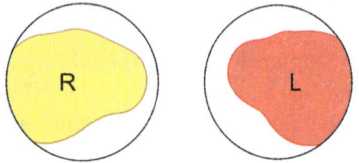

Fig. 98.22: Extent of visual field in right (R) and left (L) eyes.

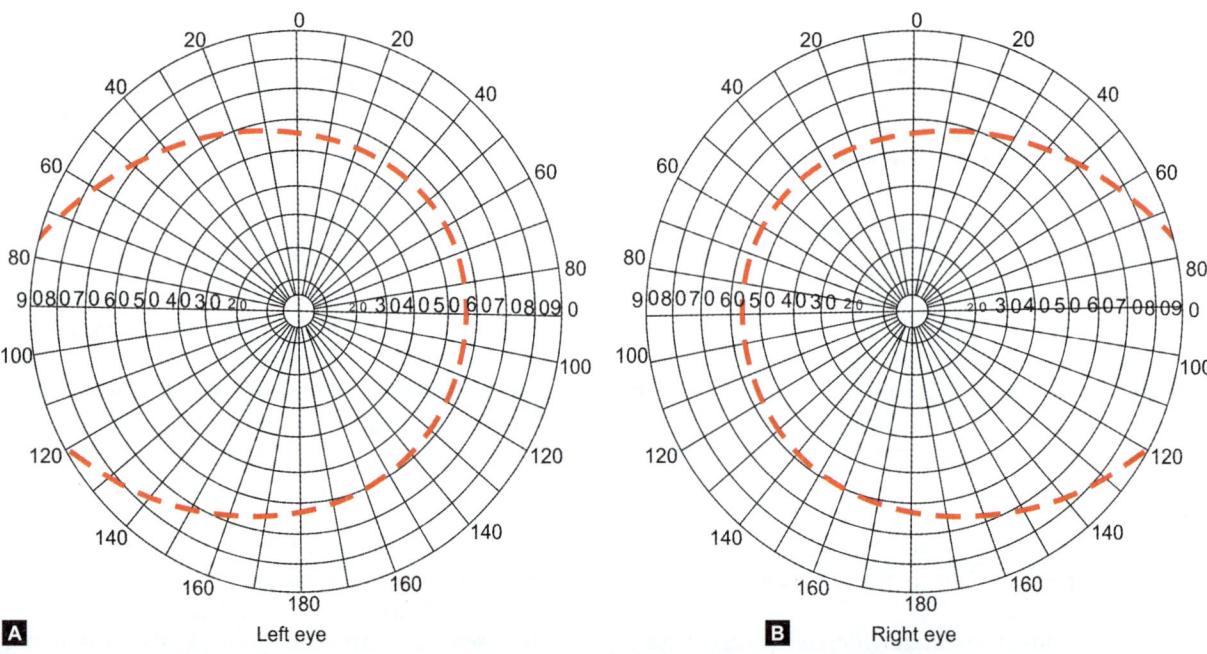

Figs. 98.23A and B: Normal field of vision of left eye and right eye charted in a perimeter.

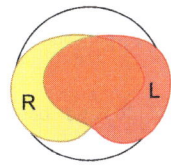

Fig. 98.24: Binocular vision (charted from both eyes in the same chart). Note the overlap of fields of vision of both eyes.

Corresponding Retinal Points

There is a set of points on the retina called corresponding retinal points. They are:
- The two fovea
- Upper halves of two retinas
- Lower halves of retina
- Right halves of retina
- Left halves of retina

These retinal areas are coordinated visually in the occipital cortex so that, such an object is seen with both eyes as a single object. Therefore, they are called **corresponding points**. For example, if the image falls on the fovea of one retina, it should fall on the fovea of the other retina also at the same time. If this does not occur, diplopia or double vision results.

In **strabismus or squint** (crossed eyes), there is defective action of extraocular muscles and the visual images do not fall on corresponding retinal points. Diplopia is the result. If we press the eyeball, two images of objects can be seen. This is because the images do not fall on the corresponding points on retina. Diplopia can be corrected by treating the cause like eye muscle training exercises, use of glasses with prisms, surgical shortening of extra-ocular muscles, etc.

If diplopia is long standing, especially in children below 6 years, one of the images is suppressed and the child sees only one image at the expense of the other. This condition is called **suppression scotoma**. It is a cortical phenomenon and is not seen in adults.

Advantages of Binocular Vision

- Field of vision of the two eyes together is larger than that of a single eye.
- Optical defects in one eye will be made less obvious.
- Defects in visual field of one eye can be compensated by the other eye.
- Stereoscopic vision is possible, i.e., depth perception is possible. For example, appreciation of the solidity of objects, appreciation of distance, etc., depends on good vision with both eyes simultaneously. This type of assessment is called **stereopsis**.

Depth Perception

The ability to determine the distance of an object from the eye is called depth perception. Depth perception is possible due to three causes:
1. Stereopsis or binocular vision
2. By moving parallax
3. From the sizes of retinal images of known objects.

Stereopsis

Stereopsis is defined as binocular depth perception, i.e., judgment of solidity and recognition of depth and distance. It is a function of cerebral cortex and it depends on the inputs from both eyes. It is caused by slight differences in the retinal images formed in the two eyes. Such disparities give different perspectives that lead to visual signals about depth. Thus a person with functioning two eyes has a greater ability to judge relative distances of nearby objects than by a person having only one eye. However, stereopsis alone is not useful to judge distances beyond 100 ft. The large ganglion cells (M cells) of the retina are concerned with stereopsis.

Moving Parallax

Another method of depth perception is that of **moving parallax**. When a person moves his head sideways, the images of close-by objects move rapidly across the retinas, while the images of distant objects remain stationary or the movement cannot be perceived. By this mechanism of moving parallax, the relative distances of different objects can be assessed even with one eye.

Retinal Images of Known Objects

Distance can be assessed from experience. If the size of the object's image on the retina is known already, the brain has learned to automatically calculate the distance of the object from the eye. The person already knows the dimensions of the object. Thus people with only one eye can also judge the dimensions, and distance of an object from the eye.

■ RETINA

The retina lies in the inner surface of the choroid. It contains six types of cells, which are the photoreceptor cells, bipolar cells, ganglion cells, horizontal cells, amacrine cells and Muller cells. These cells are organized into 10 layers.

Layers of Retina

The retina contains 10 layers except at the optic disc and fovea centralis. The layer of rods and cones are seen outward towards the choroid layer. The layers of retina from outside to inside are **(Fig. 98.25)**:
- Pigment epithelium
- Layer of rods and cones
- Outer limiting membrane
- Outer nuclear layer
- Outer plexiform layer
- Inner nuclear layer
- Inner plexiform layer
- Ganglion cell layer
- Layer of optic nerve fibers
- Inner limiting membrane

Pigment Epithelium

The pigment epithelium, which is the outermost layer in the retina, is a sheet of heavily pigmented epithelial cells. It

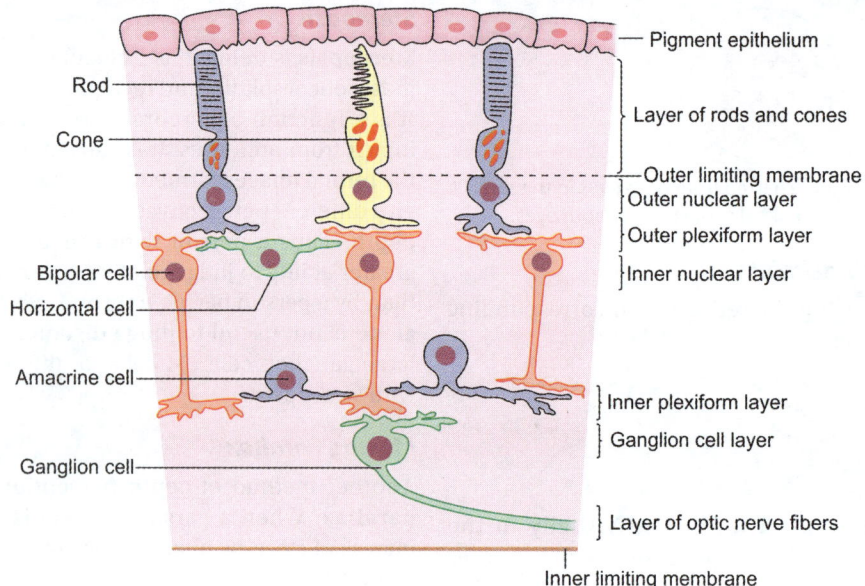

Fig. 98.25: Layers of retina.

contains melanin pigment and is in close contact with the receptor layer of retina. Light rays must pass through the ganglion cells and bipolar cells to reach the rods and cones. The pigment epithelium along with the choroid layer absorbs light rays, thereby preventing back reflection of light rays. Otherwise, the image will be blurred. By preventing scattering of light, visual acuity is increased. Visual acuity is decreased in albinos due to the absence of melanin.

Functions

- Pigment epithelium contains the pigment melanin which absorbs light and prevents its reflection back through the retina.
- Pigment epithelial cells store vitamin A in the membranes of smooth endoplasmic reticulum which is necessary for the synthesis of retinene in the visual pigments.
- Tight junctions between the pigment epithelial cells protect retina from toxic metabolites present in the choroid capillaries.
- The pigment epithelium also has phagocytic function. During renewal of rods, the cells of the pigment epithelium remove the old discs from the outer segment by phagocytosis. This phagocytic function is defective in a disease called **retinitis pigmentosa**. Blindness in this condition is due to accumulation of debris in between the receptor layer and the pigment epithelium.

Layer of Rods and Cones

The two main types of photoreceptors, **rods and cones,** are named for their characteristic shapes. The distribution of photoreceptors in the retina is non-uniform, having greatest concentration of cones in the fovea and parafoveal regions. Foveal photoreceptors consist of only the smallest cones packed at the highest density. The concentration of rods increases from the area outside the fovea and maximum is seen at a distance of 20° from the foveal center. Ratio of rods and cones in retina is 20:1. Optic disc is devoid of photoreceptors.

Rod is long and slender, whereas cone is short and stout in general. But the morphology of cones varies from place to place in the retina. For example, cones are thin and elongated at the fovea. Diameter of cones in the fovea is only 1.5 µm whereas the cones in the peripheral portion of the retina are 5-8 µm in diameter. Rods have thin, rod-like outer segment, and cones have thick inner segment and conical outer segment, and hence the names. But the cones in the fovea have long slender outer segments with thousands of photoreceptive discs. Difference between rods and cones is given in **Table 98.3**.

Rods and cones have two parts **(Fig. 98.26)**:
1. Outer segment
2. Inner segment that includes a nuclear region and a synaptic terminal zone.

Outer Segment

Outer segment consists of folds of cell membrane (discs) arranged in a pile. There are as many as 1000 discs in each rod or cone. The outer segments are highly modified cilia. The photosensitive pigment that reacts to light is present in the outer segment.

Pigment of rod is called rhodopsin.

Pigment of cones is called iodopsin (three types of color pigments).

These pigments are present in the discs in the outer segment of the photoreceptors. Actually the pigments are conjugated proteins incorporated into the disc membrane as transmembrane proteins. In the outer segment of cones, the discs are formed by infoldings of the cell membrane itself. The outer segment of the rod has tightly packed stacks of disc membranes which are flattened, membrane-bound

Table 98.3: Differences between rods and cones.	
Rods	**Cones**
• 120 million rods in each eye	• Only 6 million cones in each eye
• Thin with rod like outer segment	• Thick with conical outer segment
• The discs in the outer segment are separated from the cell membrane	• Discs are formed by infoldings of cell membrane
• Predominate in the peripheral portion of retina	• Concentrated in the fovea centralis
• There is good deal of convergence on bipolar cell	• Convergence to a lesser extent
• Visual receptors for dim light vision (scotopic vision)	• Visual receptors for bright light vision (photopic vision) and color vision
• Respond to low levels of illumination	• Respond to high levels of illumination
• Has lower threshold and lesser acuity	• Has higher threshold and greater acuity
• Contains only one pigment which is rhodopsin or visual purple	• Pigments are erythrolabe, chlorolabe and cyanolabe (iodopsins or color pigments)
• Gene for rhodopsin is located on chromosome 3	• Genes for color pigments are located in X chromosome (for red & green) and chromosome 7 (for blue-sensitive pigment)
• Protein is scotopsin	• Protein is photopsin
• Cannot detect color	• Can detect as many as 160 different colors
• Loss of function leads to night blindness	• Loss of function leads to loss of vision
• Respond maximally to light of wavelength 505 nm	• The blue, green and red cones respond maximally to light at wavelengths of 445, 535 and 570 nm respectively
• Rod receptor potential rise and decay slowly	• Cone receptor potentials rise and decay more rapidly than rod receptor potentials
• Rods detect absolute illumination	• Do not represent absolute illumination. Cones generate good responses to changes in light intensity above background illumination
• Rods are highly sensitive to light	• Cones are about 30-300 times less sensitive to light than the rods

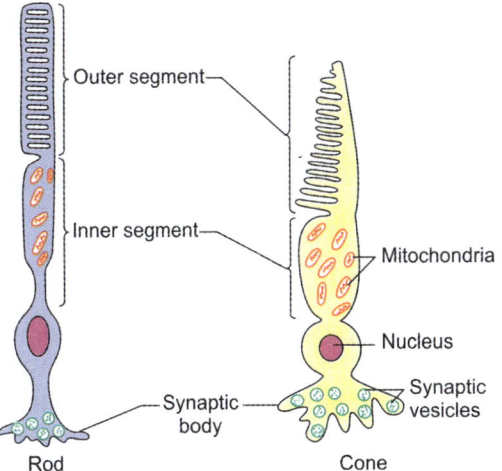

Fig. 98.26: Structure of rod and cone.

intracellular organelles that have pinched off from the outer cell membrane. They are free floating discs in rods.

The discs of membranes are constantly being renewed. Cells in the pigment epithelium will phagocytose older discs from the tip of rod and new discs will be formed at the inner edge of the segment. Cone renewal is a more diffuse process and occurs at multiple sites in the outer segment.

Inner Segment

Inner segment includes the nuclear region containing cytoplasm with organelles. The nuclear region of rods and cones forms outer nuclear layer of retina. A thin ciliary stalk connects the inner segment to the outer segment.

Large number of mitochondria in the inner segment provides energy for the function of the photoreceptors. Photosensitive pigments are synthesized in the inner segment. The photo pigments move from the inner segment through the stalk into the outer segment and get incorporated in the disc membranes.

Inner segment also includes the synaptic body. The synaptic body contains synaptic vesicles that store the neurotransmitter **glutamate**. The synaptic terminal synapses with the bipolar cells and horizontal cells.

Other Layers of Retina

Functionally, there are four types of neurons in the retina:
1. Bipolar cells
2. Ganglion cells
3. Horizontal cells
4. Amacrine cells.

Horizontal cells are present in the outer plexiform layer and connect receptor cells to other receptor cells. Inner nuclear layer contains bipolar cells and amacrine cells. The synapse between the axon of bipolar cells with the dendrites of ganglion cell is seen in the inner plexiform layer. Amacrine cells connect ganglion cells to one another in the inner plexiform layer. They are also connected with the terminals of bipolar cells. It is the site of major processing of visual image. Amacrine cells and horizontal cells are interneurons. Thus the circuitry of the retina is very complex. The four types of neurons are in turn divided into at least 10 to 20 distinct subtypes, each with different physiological and morphological features.

Ganglion cell layer contains a single layer of ganglion cells. There are different types of ganglion cells and they are the only output neurons of the retina. Axons of the ganglion cells form the layer of optic nerve fibers.

In addition to neurons, retina also contains glial cells or supporting cells called **Muller cells**. These glial cells bind the neural elements of the retina together and give physical support to the retina. Processes of these cells are responsible for the formation of inner limiting membrane and outer limiting membrane of retina. Inner limiting membrane is a thin basement membrane that separates the retina from the vitreous humor.

> All the layers of retina except the layer of optic nerve fibers are absent in the region of optic disc. It is totally insensitive to light and is called blind spot. The optic nerve fibers have no neurilemma and hence cannot regenerate.

Potentials Developed in the Neurons of Retina

One unique feature in the retina is that the electrical responses in all the neurons in the retina are graded potentials except in the ganglion cells. Ganglion cells alone can generate action potentials. The responses in the rods, cones and horizontal cells are hyperpolarizing. The response in the bipolar cells may be hyperpolarizing or depolarizing depending on the type stimulated. Amacrine cells produce depolarizing potentials that can generate action potentials in the ganglion cells.

Convergence and Divergence in the Visual Pathway

There are 120 million rods and 6 million cones in each human eye (ratio of rods and cones is 20:1). Number of optic nerve fibers is only 1.2 million in each optic nerve.

So, there is convergence from receptor through bipolar cells to ganglion cells in the ratio 105:1 (105 receptors per ganglion cell).

But there is divergence from ganglion cell onward. There are twice as many fibers in the geniculocalcarine tract as in the optic nerves, and in the visual cortex, the number of neurons concerned with vision is 1000 times the number of fibers in the optic nerves.

> At the region of fovea, a single cone is connected to a single bipolar cell that is connected to one ganglion cell and the ratio is 1:1:1. That is, each foveal cone is connected to a single fiber in the optic nerve. Thus the receptive field of a foveal ganglion cell is small. This is one reason for maximum acuity of vision at the fovea. At the periphery, the ratio of receptors to ganglion cell is high and so each ganglion cell has a large receptive field (**Fig. 9.23**). The large receptive field reduces the spatial resolution of the peripheral portion of the retina but increases its sensitivity because more photoreceptors collect light for a ganglion cell.

Reasons for Maximum Acuity at the Fovea

- Light falls directly on the cones at the fovea because the inside layers of the retina are displaced to one side rather than resting directly on the top of the cones.
- Cones are densely aggregated in the center of fovea (there are no rods in the fovea).
- The fovea contains only fine arteries, capillaries and veins. Blood vessels are absent at the very center of fovea.
- Receptor and optic nerve fiber ratio is 1:1, i.e., there is no convergence of the nerve fibers of the foveal cones.
- There is a disproportionately large area of representation for the fovea in the visual cortex.

Duplicity Theory of Vision

- *Rods aid in dim light (twilight) vision or night vision, i.e., scotopic vision.*
- *Cones aid in bright light vision and color vision, i.e., photopic vision.*

Functions of Rods

Rods are involved in dim light vision or night vision (scotopic vision). They are extremely sensitive to light and they detect absolute illumination. They cannot function at high levels of illumination. In dim light, objects appear in shades of gray. Shades of color are not appreciated in dim light.

Functions of Cones

- Bright light vision and to some extent dim light vision
- Acuity of vision
- Color vision.

Cones have a much higher threshold to light than rods but have a much greater acuity. They generate good responses to changes in light intensity above background illumination but do not represent absolute illumination. Their responses are proportional to stimulus intensity at high levels of illumination.

This division of labor by the two visual receptors is called **duplicity of vision**. Each type of receptor works at a particular light intensity. The existence of two kinds of inputs, each working maximally under different conditions of illumination is called the duplicity theory.

■ VISUAL RECEPTOR MECHANISM

It is divided into two:
1. Photochemistry of vision
2. Electrophysiological aspects.

Photochemistry of Vision

Visual Pigments

Rods—**Rhodopsin** or visual purple is the pigment in rods Cones—There are three types of pigments in cones: cyanolabe (blue-sensitive pigment), chlorolabe (green-sensitive pigment) and erythrolabe (red-sensitive pigment). They are collectively called **iodopsin.**

Rhodopsin-Retinene Visual Cycle or Visual Phototransduction (Fig. 98.27)

When light is absorbed by the photosensitive pigments in the rods and cones, their structure changes and leads to a sequence of events that initiates neural activity in the visual pathway. Phototransduction involves a cascade of chemical and electrical events in response to light. The process by which light is converted into electrical signals in rods and cones and ganglion cells of retina is called **Wald's visual cycle.** George Wald was awarded Nobel Prize in 1967 for this discovery. The receptor potential of photoreceptors is a hyperpolarizing potential. Rods have been studied to a greater extent and so the changes occurring in rods are described below.

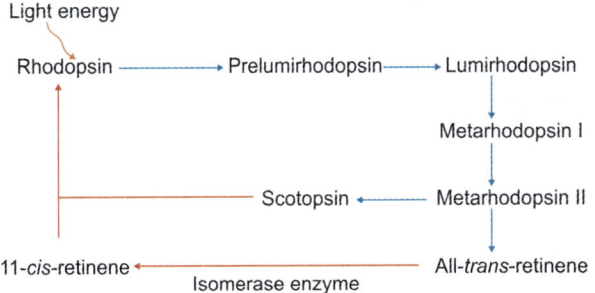

Fig. 98.27: Rhodopsin-retinene visual cycle in the rod showing decomposition of rhodopsin on exposure to light and resynthesis of rhodopsin.

Rhodopsin is one of the most tightly packed proteins in the body, with a density of about 30,000 molecules per square micrometer in the disc membrane. One rod contains ~10^9 rhodopsin molecules. Rhodopsin consists of a protein part called **scotopsin** and **retinene or retinal**, the aldehyde of vitamin A (retinol refers to vitamin A which is an alcohol). The protein part of photosensitive pigments of rods and cones are called **opsins** in general. Opsin is part of the large family of G-protein-coupled receptors (GPCR). Opsin is a single polypeptide which passes 7 times around the disc membrane from inside to outside. Retinene is attached to 3 of the loops of the protein and is seen parallel to the membrane surface. Retinene is found in the 11-cis configuration in the dark. Only the 11- cis retinene (or 11-cis retinal) can bind with scotopsin to form rhodopsin. Because of its instability, the cis form of retinene can exist only in the dark.

When light falls on rhodopsin, photons are absorbed by **11-cis retinene** and the rhodopsin begins to decompose within a very small fraction of a second. Photoactivation of electrons in the retinene portion of rhodopsin leads to instantaneous change of 11-cis-retinene (11-cis retinal) to its isomer **all-trans-retinene** within 1 picosecond, which is more stable. Chemical structure of cis form and all-trans form is the same but physical structure is different. 11-cis-retinene is a curved molecule, whereas all-trans-retinene is a straight one. The reactive sites on all-trans-retinene do not fit in on the reactive sites on the protein (opsin). So, all-trans retinene tries to pull away from scotopsin. The intermediate product formed is called **bathorhodopsin**, which is a partially split combination of all-trans retinene and scotopsin. Bathorhodopsin is extremely unstable and decays in nanoseconds to form **lumirhodopsin**. This product decomposes in microseconds to form **metarhodopsin I**. The configuration of the opsin changes when it gets separated from retinene and triggers a series of conformational changes in the opsin that lead to the formation of **metarhodopsin II** in about a millisecond. Then slowly i.e., within seconds, metarhodopsin II completely splits to the products **scotopsin and all-trans retinene**. The process of complete separation of all- trans retinene and opsin from metarhodopsin II is called **bleaching (Fig. 98.27)**. This separation causes the color of rhodopsin to change from a rosy red color of rhodopsin to the pale yellow color of opsin. *11-cis retinene is responsible for rhodopsin's rosy red color.*

It is the metarhodopsin II which is also called **activated rhodopsin** that excites electrical changes in the rods which in turn transmit the visual image in the form of action potential in the optic nerve to the central nervous system (**Flowchart 98.3**).

Metarhodopsin II activates its associated heterotrimeric G-protein, **transducin or Gt$_1$**. This causes a decline in the cytoplasmic cGMP concentration by activation of **phosphodiesterase** enzyme by transducin. Phosphodiesterase increases hydrolysis of cGMP to form 5´-guanylate monophosphate. cGMP normally acts directly on Na$^+$ channels on the outer segment of photoreceptors to maintain them in the open state. So, decrease in cytoplasmic cGMP concentration causes cGMP gated Na$^+$ channels to close. The decreased Na$^+$ influx produces the hyperpolarizing potential in the receptor and a reduction in the neurotransmitter (glutamate) output from the synaptic zone of the receptor (**Flowchart 98.3**).

Absorption of 1 photon activates 1 metarhodopsin II molecule, which can activate approximately 700 transducin molecules within 100ms. cGMP is synthesized in the photoreceptor by guanylyl cyclase and broken down by phosphodiesterase.

Resynthesis of Rhodopsin

Resynthesis of rhodopsin can occur in the dark as well as in the presence of light (11-cis-retinene to all-trans- retinene occurs only in the presence of light). Resynthesis of rhodopsin is a prolonged process. It takes more time because all-trans-retinene cannot combine with scotopsin to form rhodopsin.

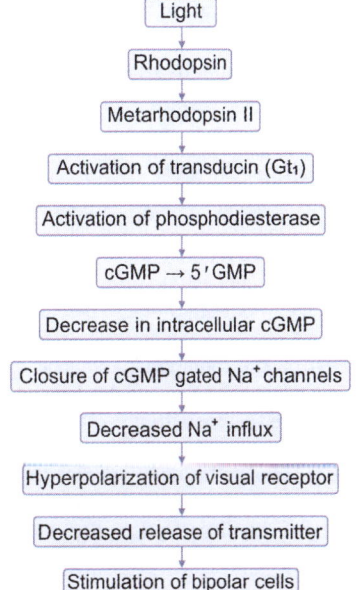

Flowchart 98.3: Events involved in phototransduction in rods (electrophysiological changes in the photoreceptors).

Flowchart 98.4: Alternate route of formation of retinene.

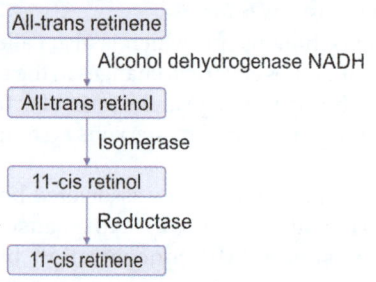

It has to be first converted to 11-cis- retinene by **retinal isomerase** enzyme and the process requires energy. Once the 11-cis-retinene is formed, it automatically recombines with scotopsin to form rhodopsin directly. This cycle of rhodopsin regeneration takes a few minutes.

There is an alternate route by which all-trans-retinene can be converted to 11-cis-retinene. This is by conversion of all-trans-retinene to **all-trans-retinol**, which is one form of vitamin A by the enzyme **alcohol dehydrogenase or retinal reductase** in the presence of NADH. Under the influence of **isomerase** enzyme, all-trans-retinol is converted to 11-cis-retinol or 11-cis-vitamin A. Finally, 11-cis-retinol is converted to 11-cis-retinene by the enzyme **reductase** (**Flowchart 98.4**). 11-cis-retinene combines with scotopsin to form rhodopsin.

Role of Vitamin A in the Formation of Rhodopsin

Vitamin A stored in the pigment epithelium is also used in restoring the level of rhodopsin but it is a slow process while the synthesis of rhodopsin from retinene is a fast process. Vitamin A is also present in the cytoplasm of rods. Thus vitamin A is always available to form new retinene when needed. When there is excess retinene in the retina, it is converted back into vitamin A and stored in the pigment epithelial cells. This helps to reduce the amount of light- sensitive pigment in the retina. The interconversion of retinene and vitamin A is very important for the retina to adapt to different light intensities. In bright sunlight, rods become ineffective because most of their rhodopsin remains inactivated or bleached.

Vitamin A Deficiency
Vitamin A, which is very essential for the synthesis of retinene, is present in the cytoplasm of the photoreceptors and in the pigment layer of the retina. In vitamin A deficiency, night vision or dim light vision is impaired because there will be degeneration of rods. Vitamin A deficiency is due to inadequate intake of vitamin A rich foods like meat, liver, whole egg, etc. It can also be due to inadequate intake of beta carotene (a precursor of vitamin A) rich foods like green leafy vegetables, yellow or orange fruits and vegetables like carrot. The condition is known as night blindness or nyctalopia. Giving large doses of vitamin A before the receptors are destroyed can cure this condition.

Prolonged deficiency of vitamin A can cause degeneration of rods as well as cones followed by degeneration of the neural layers of retina. Once this occurs, retinal function cannot be restored. Vitamin A deficiency can also lead to dryness of cornea and ulceration, a condition called xerophthalmia. This can also lead to blindness.

ELECTROPHYSIOLOGICAL CHANGES IN RETINAL RECEPTORS

Receptor Potential

The responses of rods and cones to light are local hyperpolarizing potentials. Light causes a decrease in amount of transmitter released at the synaptic terminals.

Rod Receptor Potential

In the Dark

The K^+ channels in the inner segment of the photoreceptor, which are not regulated by light, are leak channels and K^+ moves to the outside from the inner segment. Na^+-K^+ pump is located in the inner segment of the photoreceptor. Na^+ is actively pumped out from the inner segment of the receptor cell by Na^+-K^+ ATPase in exchange for K^+.

But the outer segment of the receptor cell contains cGMP-gated Na^+ channels which are leaky to Na^+ in the dark. These channels are kept open by cyclic GMP in the dark. (In the dark, the active **guanylyl cyclase** synthesizes cGMP from GTP and keeps cGMP levels high within the photoreceptor) Thus, the Na^+ pumped out from the inner segment by the Na^+-K^+ pump returns into the rods continuously through the outer segment. Thus in the dark, each photoreceptor produces an ionic current that flows steadily into the outer segment and out of the inner segment. This is called the **dark current**. The electrical circuit for this dark current is completed by K^+ leaving the inner segment. The dark current decreases interior negativity and depolarizes the photoreceptor leading to constant neurotransmitter (glutamate) release at the synaptic ending in the dark (**Fig. 98.28A**).

The potential of the rod in the dark is –40 mV, i.e., the resting potential is a depolarizing potential. In the visual receptors, the synaptic endings release the neurotransmitter **glutamate** that inhibits the bipolar cells indirectly in the dark (**Flowchart 98.5**). Glutamate stimulates the horizontal cells, which are inhibitory interneurons, which in turn inhibit the bipolar cells. This inhibition is removed when light falls on the photoreceptors.

Flowchart 98.5: Changes occurring in the outer segment of rods in the dark.

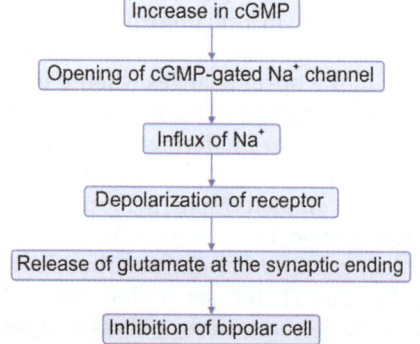

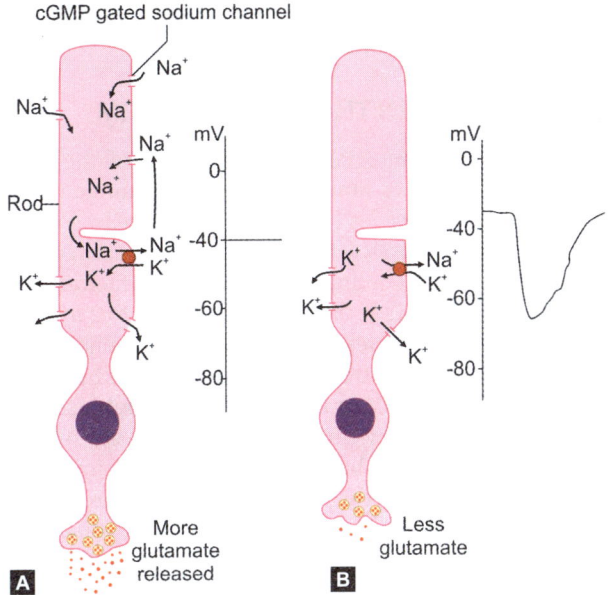

Figs. 98.28A and B: Potential changes in a photoreceptor: (A) In dark; (B) When light falls on retina. Note the resting membrane potential of -40 mV in dark and photoreceptor potential (hyperpolarizing) -70 mV in light.

Photochemical Changes When Light Falls on the Receptor

When light falls on the receptor, rhodopsin is converted to metarhodopsin II (activated rhodopsin) which splits to form all-trans retinene and scotopsin **(Fig. 98.28B)**. Meta-rhodopsin II causes closure of cGMP-gated sodium channels of the outer segment by the following mechanism. Metarhodopsin II activates a G-protein, **transducin (Gt_1)**, which in turn reduces cyclic GMP level. Transducin activates **cGMP phosphodiesterase** enzyme, which catalyzes the hydrolysis of cGMP to 5′ guanylate monophosphate (5′ GMP). One photon leads to the hydrolysis of ~1400 cGMP molecules. When cGMP level decreases, Na^+ channels in the outer segment close since these are kept open by cGMP. The total conductance of the outer segment decreases. The number of cation channels that close depends on the number of photons that are absorbed. Studies have shown that absorption of one photon suppresses the entry of more than 10^6 Na^+ ions into the outer segment.

Recent view is that change in the configuration of opsin when it gets separated from retinene is responsible for the activation of transducin. *Inner segment is continuously active both in light and darkness. But, the outer segment is leaky to Na^+ only in the darkness.*

Because the K^+ channels of the inner segment are not regulated by light, they remain open, and K^+ continues to flow out. This outward current causes the cell to hyperpolarize. Moreover, by the activity of Na^+-K^+ ATPase, more Na^+ moves out from the inner segment. When 3 Na^+ move out, only two K^+ enter the cell and so the interior negativity again increases. The potential goes to a level of –70 to –80 mV, i.e., it is a hyperpolarization potential. Thus, *the receptor potential in rod is hyperpolarization.* Electrotonic conduction of the hyperpolarizing potential through the rod occurs and it reaches the synaptic border. This causes decrease in the synaptic transmitter released at the synapse **(Figs. 98.28A and B)**. Synaptic transmitter is glutamate released in large quantities in the dark. In light, the bipolar cells that were inhibited by glutamate become excited when the glutamate output from the photoreceptor decreases.

> The retinene portion of all the visual pigments is exactly the same in rods as well as in the cones. The only difference between the pigments in rods and cones is that of the protein portion or opsins, photopsin in cones and scotopsin in rods. The color sensitive pigments of cones are combinations of retinene and photopsins. The details of the responses of cones to light are almost similar to those in rods. The cones are about 30–300 times less sensitive to light than the rods. The G protein that is activated in cones by light is Gt_2 which is different from rod transducin, Gt_1.

EXPERIMENTAL EVIDENCE TO SHOW THAT RODS ARE RESPONSIBLE FOR DIM LIGHT VISION

Scotopic Visibility Curve

- Subjects were kept in dim light and sensitivity of retinal surface to low levels of illumination was tested for various wavelengths of light. A graph was plotted with wavelength on X-axis and sensitivity on Y-axis. The curve is called scotopic visibility curve. A correction factor was applied to eliminate the effect of optical surfaces. Maximum sensitivity was obtained at a wavelength of 505 nm **(Fig. 98.29)**.
- The above experiment was done in an aphakic eye (eye without lens) in dim light. A similar graph was plotted and a similar graph was obtained.
- In vitro experiment—retina was taken out in an experimental animal, macerated and rhodopsin from outer segment of rods was isolated by differential centrifugation. Thus, rhodopsin solution is obtained in vitro. The absorption characteristics of this pigment at various wavelengths of light were studied. This study also showed maximal absorption occurred at a wavelength of 505 nm.

These three experiments proved that 505 nm corresponds to dim light vision and rods are responsible for dim light vision.

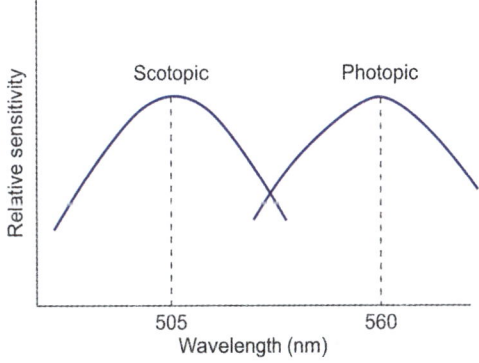

Fig. 98.29: Spectral sensitivity curves.

Photopic Visibility Curve

Under photopic conditions, the above experiments were done. Subject was exposed to various wavelengths of bright light, and sensitivity of his retinal surface was studied. Shift in the visibility curve when illumination changed from scotopic field to photopic field is **Purkinje shift or Purkinje phenomenon (Fig. 98.29)**.

Same experiments can be performed in cones also. Retina is macerated and cones are isolated, and the pigment is studied for their absorption characteristics. Three types of curves are obtained with their peaks at 445, 535 and 570 nm **(Fig. 98.30)**.

This shows that there are three different types of cones with three different pigments, and they are concerned with color vision. Curve at 560 nm **(Fig. 98.29)** is a composite curve obtained from the three different types of cones in the retina.

Melanopsin

A group of ganglion cells in the retina contain a photo pigment called **melanopsin**. It is different from rhodopsin and iodopsin. These photosensitive retinal ganglion cells function independent of rods and cones. They depolarize in response to light even in subjects who lack functional rods and cones. The axons of these melatonin-containing photosensitive retinal ganglion cells project via two pathways.

- Information from these receptors projects to the suprachiasmatic nucleus of hypothalamus, which controls all the circadian photoentrainment responses to light–dark changes.
- Some of the axons can travel via the optic nerve, optic chiasma and optic tract (bypassing the lateral geniculate nucleus) to terminate in the pretectal nucleus. From here neurons synapse on the parasympathetic preganglionic neurons in the Edinger-Westphal nucleus to mediate the pupillary light reflex. When the gene for melanopsin is knocked out, circadian photoentrainment is abolished and the pupillary light reflex is reduced.

ADAPTATION IN THE VISUAL SYSTEM

One of the most important characteristics of the visual system is its ability to function over a wide range of light intensity. When one goes from darkness to bright sunlight, light intensity increases very much. The fluctuation in light intensity reaching the retina is reduced by two factors: (i) by reducing the diameter of the pupil from 8 mm to 2 mm, and (ii) presence of two types of receptors whose sensitivity to light varies. Rods are extremely sensitive to light because of low threshold and function maximally in dim light (scotopic vision). Cones have a much higher threshold and are responsible for vision in bright light (photopic vision).

Adaptation means the change in retinal threshold to different levels of illumination. It requires time for adaptation before the eye can respond optimally. There are two types of adaptation:
1. Dark adaptation
2. Light adaptation.

Dark Adaptation

When a person goes from bright light to a dark room, initially he cannot see anything clearly. But gradually, retinal threshold decreases and vision becomes clearer and this decline in visual threshold is called dark adaptation. The retina slowly becomes more sensitive to light as the individual becomes accustomed to the dark. Time taken for full dark adaptation is about 20 minutes.

In bright light, rhodopsin as well as the cone pigments are broken down to retinene and opsins and it takes time for resynthesis of the visual pigments. So the sensitivity of retina to light is reduced very much and we cannot see initially in the dim light. Actual mechanism for dark adaptation is not fully understood.

Studies have been carried out by plotting time taken for dark adaptation on X-axis and log of the intensity of minimal effective stimulus on the Y-axis. The graph obtained is called **dark adaptation curve**.

The dark adaptation response has two components. First part of the dark adaptation curve **(Fig. 98.31)** is due to the adaptation by cones. This is because resynthesis of visual pigments occurs about four times rapidly in cones than in rods but ceases adapting after a few minutes. The second prolonged part of the curve is due to adaptation by rods which continue to adapt for many minutes and even hours. This can be proved by the following experiment. When the foveal part alone of retinal surface is illuminated, only the first part of the graph is obtained. This proves that the initial drop in visual threshold is due to dark adaptation of the cones (fovea contains only cones). But when the peripheral part of retinal surface is illuminated, the second part of graph is obtained which proves that it is due to adaptation of the rods. Rods are mainly responsible for dim light vision and cones play only a minor role in dim light.

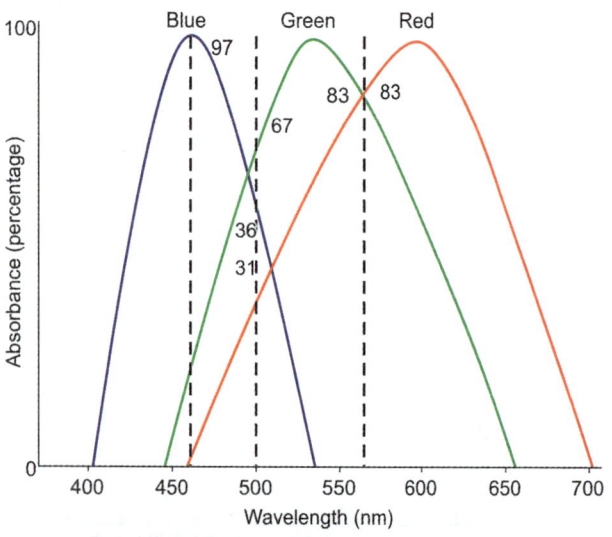

Fig. 98.30: Absorbance spectra of cones.

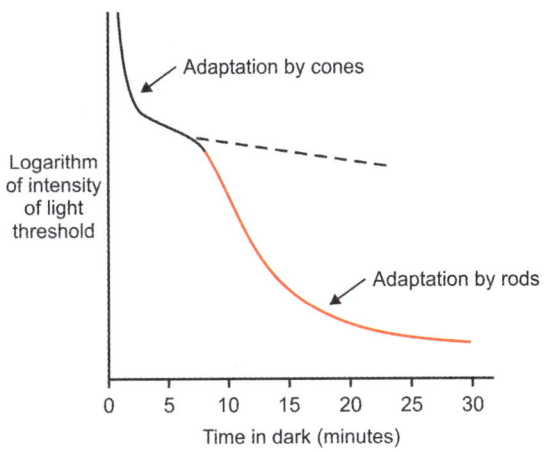

Fig. 98.31: Effects of dark adaptation on the visual threshold.

Another mechanism of dark adaptation is that the pupils dilate in darkness so that more light enters the eyes.

Changes in Dark Adaptation
- Pupil dilates to a diameter of 8 mm in full dark adaptation.
- Increased sensitivity of retina
- Regeneration of visual pigments in the photoreceptors, first in the foveal cones and then in the rods
- Purkinje shift toward blue end of the spectrum

> Red light wavelength (650 nm) does not produce change in rhodopsin than does white light. However, red light stimulates cones reasonably well and can see in bright light. This is the principle behind aircraft pilots and radiologists wearing red goggles while on duty in bright light. These people need maximum visual sensitivity in dim light. Normally, it takes 20 minutes for full dark adaptation. If they wear red goggles in bright light, they need not wait for long time in the dark to become dark-adapted.
> Red light stimulates the rods to only a slight degree while permitting the cones to function reasonably well. So, minimum bleaching of rods occurs in bright light with red goggles, i.e., the amount of rhodopsin broken down is less and that necessary for optimal rod function in dim light will be remaining. So, dark adaptation occurs without delay.

Light Adaptation

Light adaptation is the ability of visual threshold to increase at higher levels of illumination after it is adapted to lower illumination. The light appears too bright when stepped out from a dark room since the threshold is high.

In darkness, rhodopsin is synthesized and stored and retina is very sensitive. When light falls on retina, rhodopsin is broken down and this contributes to rise in visual threshold.

Actually, light adaptation is merely the disappearance of dark adaptation and it occurs over a period of about 5 minutes.

Along with light adaptation, there is pupillary change. The pupil constricts in light adaptation so that less light enters the eye. Regulation of the size of the pupil by iris can change light sensitivity by approximately 16 fold.

Changes in Light Adaptation
- Pupillary constriction
- Decreased sensitivity of retina
- Bleaching of rhodopsin
- Purkinje shift toward red end of the spectrum.

Night Blindness or Nyctalopia

Night blindness or nyctalopia is a condition in which dim light vision is lost. Main cause of night blindness is deficiency of fat-soluble vitamin A in the diet or due to defective absorption of vitamin A as a result of liver diseases like cirrhosis. Night blindness is due to interference with the function of rods in the retina due to deficiency of the pigment visual purple or rhodopsin. Impairment of cone function occurs later. Vitamin A is necessary for the synthesis of retinene. Prolonged deficiency of vitamin A is associated with damage to both rods and cones followed by degeneration of the neural layers of retina.

Vitamin A deficiency also contributes to blindness by causing thickening of the corneal epithelium and malfunctioning of the goblet cells of the conjunctiva leading to decreased mucus in the tears. As a result, the cornea becomes dry and its epithelium becomes keratinized (xerophthalmia) leading to corneal damage and repeated infections. In cases of malnutrition, cod liver oil is indicated and the condition improves rapidly. Treatment with vitamin A restores retinal function only if administered before the receptors are destroyed.

Critical Fusion Frequency

At very low frequencies if intermittent flashes of light are presented to the eye, separate flashes of light are seen. When the frequency of the intermittent flashes is increased, at a particular frequency, fusion of the images occurs to produce a continuous sensation and the flicker disappears. Critical fusion frequency (CFF) is the rate at which stimuli can be presented to the eye and still be perceived as separate stimuli. In other words, the rate of stimuli above which it is perceived as continuous stimuli is the critical fusion frequency. Stimuli presented at a rate higher than the CFF are perceived as continuous stimuli. This is the principle behind motion pictures where the picture frames are projected at a frequency greater than CFF, which is about 16–24 frames/sec. When the projector slows down, movies begin to flicker because the rate becomes less than CFF.

Visual Processing and Image Formation in the Retina

Three types of visual processing occur in the retina. This involves the formation of three images in the retina:
1. The first image is formed by the action of light on photoreceptors.
2. Signal is modified by horizontal cells and a second type of image is formed in the bipolar cells.
3. Third type of image is formed in the ganglion cell after the signal is modified by amacrine cells. The impulse pattern

passing from the ganglion cell is not much changed in the lateral geniculate bodies. So, the third image reaches the occipital cortex without further modification.

Receptive Field of Neurons in the Visual Pathway

Except in the fovea, there is a great degree of convergence from receptors to bipolar cell and bipolar cells to ganglion cell. This is because bipolar cells and ganglion cells are much fewer than receptor cells. Each bipolar cell and ganglion cell shows change in its activity in response to visual stimulation of a fairly wide area of the retina. The part of the retina in which a stimulus alters the activity of a bipolar cell or ganglion cell is called its receptive field, respectively. This is true for neurons in the lateral geniculate body and the neurons in the striate cortex.

The receptive field or receptor field for any neuron in the visual pathway is defined as that area of the retina or that corresponding part of the visual field from which the discharge of that neuron is most effectively influenced. The area of the receptor field depends on the degree of convergence in the visual pathway. The receptive field near the central retina is smaller than those of the periphery. At the fovea, the area of receptor field of a ganglion cell is very small since receptor: ganglion cell ratio is 1:1. At the periphery of the retina, many receptor cells converge on a single bipolar cell and several bipolar cells converge on a single ganglion cell. So the receptive field of this ganglion cell is very large (*refer* **Fig. 98.21**). Similarly, the receptive fields of neurons in the lateral geniculate body and striate cortex also vary in size.

Types of Bipolar and Ganglion Cells

On-center and Off-center Bipolar Cells

The receptor fields of the bipolar cells are organized into central and peripheral portions that generate opposite reactions, i.e., on-center and off-center responses. There are two types of bipolar cells, viz, hyperpolarizing and depolarizing bipolar cells. Hyperpolarizing bipolar cells are inhibited by light and depolarizing cells are stimulated by light. In some cells, hyperpolarizing potentials are produced by a spot of light, whereas depolarization is produced by an annulus of light around the center. Cells with opposite patterns are also observed.

On-center bipolar cells: If central spot is excitatory and surrounding bipolar cells are inhibitory, it is an on-center bipolar cell. An on-center cell is stimulated when light falls on the center of its receptor field and inhibited when light falls on the periphery of the field. The central bipolar cell is depolarizing bipolar cell and the surrounding cells are hyperpolarizing cells.

Off-center bipolar cells: If central spot is inhibitory and surrounding cells are excitatory, it is off-center bipolar cell. An off-center cell is stimulated when light falls on the periphery of the field and inhibited by light on its center.

On-center and Off-center Ganglion Cells

At the level of ganglion cells also, there are "on center" and "off center" cells and also small and large ganglion cells. An on-center cell is stimulated when light falls on the center of its receptor field and inhibited when light falls on the periphery of the field. Conversely, an off-center cell is stimulated when light falls on the periphery of the field and inhibited by light falling on its center.

The receptive field of the ganglion cell has two parts:
1. The center of the receptive field where one ganglion cell is connected to several receptor cells via bipolar cells.
2. The surround of the receptive field where ganglion cell is connected to receptor cells via horizontal cells.

When light strikes the receptive field of this ganglion cell, two types of responses may occur.
1. When light strikes the center of the receptor field, excitation (depolarization) of the ganglion cells occur while light striking the surround of the center causes inhibition (hyperpolarization) of the ganglion cells of the surround. This is called on-center off-surround pattern.
2. If light inhibits the center and excites the surround, it is called off-center on-surround pattern.

These patterns (on-off patterns) are present not only in the ganglion cells and bipolar cells, but also in the cells of the lateral geniculate body and fourth layer of the visual cortex. This is a form of lateral inhibition, which facilitates sensory perception and spatial discrimination.

Large Ganglion Cells, Small Ganglion Cells and Amacrine Cells

Large ganglion cells, Y-cells or M-cells add up the responses obtained from different cones. This type of ganglion cell is concerned with appreciation of movement and stereoscopic vision.

Small ganglion cells, X-cells or P cells subtract the signal from one cone and signal from another cone. They are concerned with color texture and shape of visual images.

Action potential is generated at the level of ganglion cells which is transmitted along their axons to the lateral geniculate body. In the resting stage or in darkness, the ganglion cells fire at a low rate called **resting discharge**.

Amacrine cells are of different types, 30 types have been identified. Some amacrine cells respond to change in the level of illumination, i.e., they respond when a light is turned on or off. Another type responds strongly at the onset of a continuing visual signal, but the response dies rapidly. Other amacrine cells respond strongly at the offset of visual signals, but the response fades quickly. In general, the amacrine cells help to analyze visual signals before they leave the retina.

LATERAL INHIBITION IN THE VISUAL PATHWAY

Lateral inhibition or afferent inhibition is that form of inhibition in which activation of a particular neural unit is associated with inhibition of the activity of nearby units **(Figs. 98.32 and 98.33)**. The center of the receptive field of neurons in the visual pathway can be excitatory or inhibitory depending on the type of neurons.

The bipolar cells, ganglion cells, lateral geniculate cells and cells of layer 4 of visual cortex respond best to a small circular

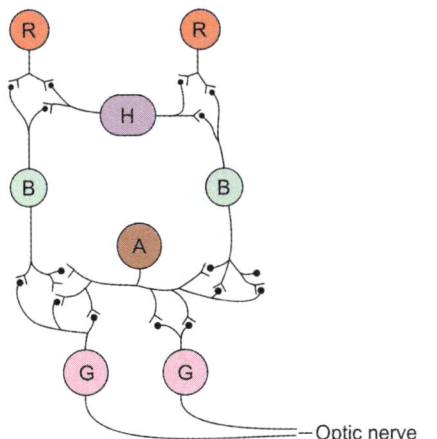

Fig. 98.32: Schematic representation of the connections of different cells of retina.
(A: amacrine cell; B: bipolar cell; G: ganglion cell; H: horizontal cell; R: rod cell)

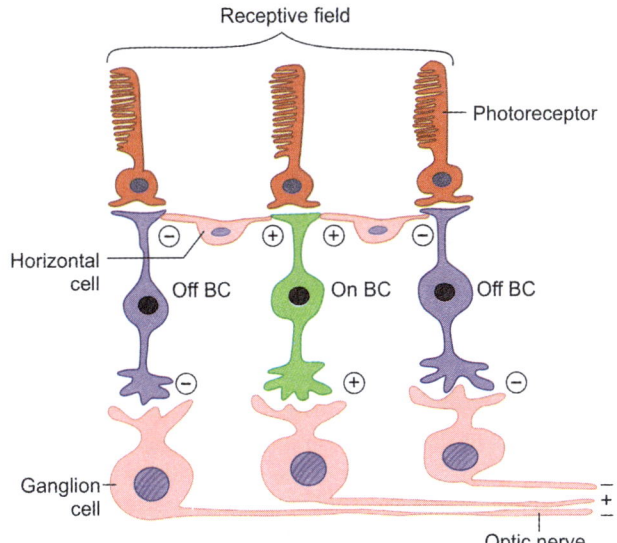

Fig. 98.33: Lateral inhibition in retina. When light falls on the photoreceptors in the receptive field the on centre bipolar cell as well as the inhibitory horizontal cells supplying the surrounding bipolar cells are stimulated. Thus the on center bipolar cell is stimulated while the surrounding BC in the receptive field is inhibited.
(BC: bipolar cell. Minus sign (−) denotes inhibition and plus sign (+) denotes stimulation).

stimulus of light within their receptive field. The surround illumination, i.e., an annulus of light around the central spot inhibits the response to the central spot.

The center can be excitatory with an inhibitory surround where the concerned neuron is an on-center cell or the center can be inhibitory with an excitatory surround where it is an off-center cell. The inhibition of the center response by the surround is probably due to inhibitory feedback from one photoreceptor to another mediated by horizontal cell. Thus, activation of nearby photoreceptors around the center of the receptor field stimulates horizontal cells, which in turn inhibit the response of the centrally activated photoreceptors. The inhibition of the response to central illumination by an increase in the surrounding illumination is an example of lateral inhibition. This phenomenon helps to sharpen the edges of a stimulus and improve spatial discrimination.

The horizontal cells connect laterally between the synaptic bodies of the rods and cones, as well as with the dendrites of bipolar cell in the outer plexiform layer. The output of the horizontal cell is always inhibitory. In the plexiform layer, because of the spreading dendritic and axonal trees, there is a tendency for the excitatory signal to spread widely in the retina. Transmission through the horizontal cells puts a stop to this by providing lateral inhibition in the surrounding areas.

■ VISUAL PATHWAY

The area of the field of vision seen to the nasal side of the eye is called the nasal field of vision and the area seen to the lateral side is called temporal field of vision. Nasal field objects will form images in the temporal half of retina and objects in temporal field of vision will form images in the nasal half of retina **(Table 98.4)**. This is because the image of the field of vision is inverted on the retina by the optical system of the eye. The rods and cones in the retina convert energy in the visible spectrum into action potentials in the optic nerve which are conducted to the cerebral cortex where they produce the sensation of vision **(Fig. 98.34)**.

Stimulus: Light rays
Receptors: Rods and cones

First order neuron: Bipolar cells of retina. One of its processes synapses with synaptic body of photoreceptor and the other process synapses with the cell body of ganglion cells.

Second order neuron: Ganglion cells of retina. Axons of ganglion cells form the optic nerve. From the retina, fibers have a topographical arrangement in the optic nerve. The fibers from the upper half of retina will lie above; fibers from lower half of retina will lie below, medial fibers on medial side and lateral fibers laterally in the optic nerve. The optic nerve fibers are myelinated and the myelin sheath is formed from **oligodendrocytes** rather than Schwann cells.

Optic nerve leaves the orbital cavity through the optic canal and unites with the optic nerve of the opposite side to form the optic chiasma. In the region of optic chiasma, the fibers from the nasal half of retina cross to the opposite side and the temporal half fibers go uncrossed, thus forming the optic tract of that side. Thus, each optic tract contains both crossed and uncrossed fibers. For example, the left optic tract contains fibers from the nasal half of retina of opposite side (right side) and from the temporal half of retina of the same side (left side) or from the left halves of both retinas. Since each half of retina receives light rays from opposite half of the

Table 98.4: Image formation in the retina.

Position of object	Position of image
• Upper half of visual field	• Lower half of retina
• Lower half of visual field	• Upper half of retina
• Nasal half of visual field	• Temporal half of retina
• Temporal half of visual field	• Nasal half of retina

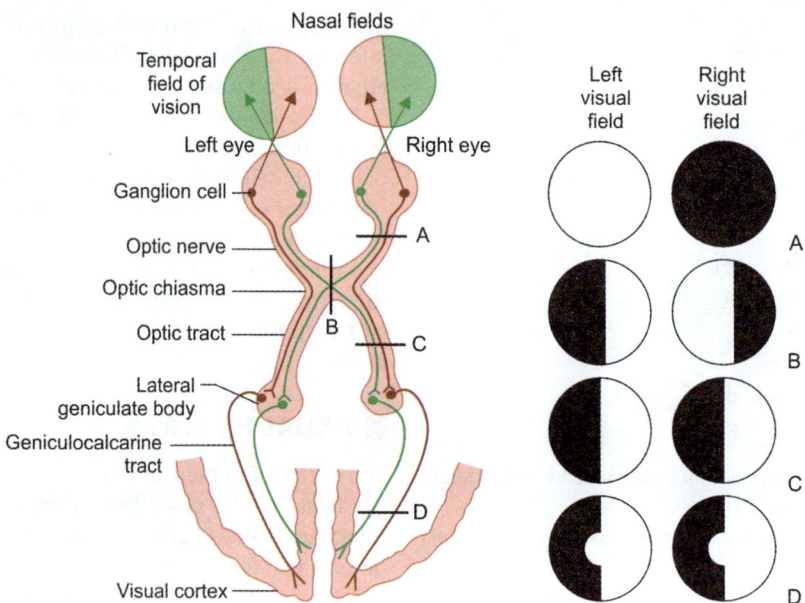

Fig. 98.34: Visual pathway and effects of lession at various levels of visual pathway: A. Lesion of right optic nerve causes blindness of right eye, B. Lesion of optic chiasma (central part, mainly by pituitary tumor) destroy fibers from both nasal hemiretinas and produce bitemporal hemianopia or heteronemous hemianopia, C. Lesion of right optic tract causes left homonymous hemianopia (same side of both visual fields affected), D. Lesion of right occipital cortex may spare the fibers from macula and produce left homonymous hemianopia with macular sparing.

field of vision, the left optic tract represents the right halves of the visual fields.

In the optic tract, fibers from upper half of retina are seen medially and end in medial part of lateral geniculate body. Fibers from lower half of retina are seen laterally and end in the lateral part of lateral geniculate body.

Third order neurons are present in the lateral geniculate body of thalamus (**Fig. 98.34**). In each geniculate body, the fibers from the temporal half of one retina and the nasal half of the other retina synapse on the lateral geniculate body cells.

From lateral geniculate body, the axons of the third order neurons go as optic radiation or geniculocalcarine fibers to the occipital cortex (visual cortex or calcarine cortex) close to the calcarine fissure. The geniculocalcarine fibers from the medial half of the lateral geniculate body terminate on the superior lip of the calcarine fissure, and those from lateral half terminate on the inferior lip. The fibers that are responsible for macular vision separate from the other fibers and terminate more posteriorly on the lips of the calcarine fissure.

1. Primary visual area—Brodmann's area 17
2. Visual association area—area 18, 19 (responsible for recognition of objects and perception of color)

The primary visual area receives the visual information, but it is analyzed and interpreted in the visual association areas. Area 19 (occipital eye field) projects to the frontal eye field (area 8) concerned with eye movements. In the occipital cortex, fourth layer is called koniocortex, which receives specific thalamocortical fibers.

The visual cortex is divided into eight visual projection areas, which are designated as V_1 to V_8. V_1 is the primary visual cortex, which receives input from the lateral geniculate body and it processes information in terms of orientation, edges, etc. The primary visual cortex (area V_1) projects to areas V_2 to V_8. Color information is projected mainly to area V_8 of visual cortex (**Fig. 98.35**).

Fate of the Medial and Lateral Fibers in the Optic Tract

Lateral fibers in the optic tract end in the lateral geniculate body of thalamus. Majority of the medial fibers in the optic tract ends in the superior colliculus and pretectal nucleus. These fibers mediate visual reflexes like visual righting reflex, light reflex, etc. Rest of the medial fibers goes to the suprachiasmatic nucleus of hypothalamus.

❖ The pretectal nuclei in the midbrain control pupillary light reflexes.
❖ The superior colliculus, controls rapid directional movements of the two eyes (*refer* visual body reflexes).

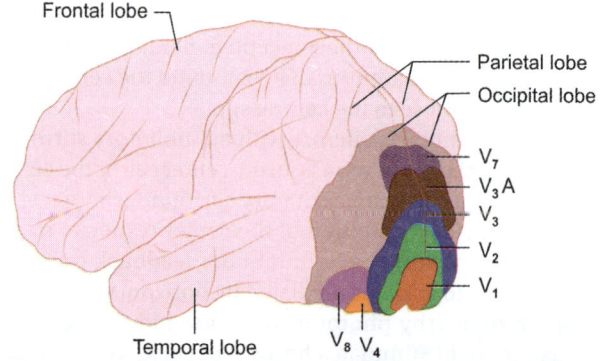

Fig. 98.35: Posterolateral view of brain showing the visual areas in the occipital cortex.

- The suprachiasmatic nucleus of hypothalamus (retinohypothalamic pathway) is concerned with control of circadian rhythms.

Lateral Geniculate Body (LGB)

Lateral geniculate body has six layers **(Table 98.5)**. Layers 2, 3 and 5 receive the temporal fibers from same eye and layers 1, 4 and 6 receive crossed fibers (nasal fibers from opposite side).

LGB receives the fibers which bring impulses from the corresponding retinal points of two eyes. These fibers reach the adjacent layers of lateral geniculate body. They act as pairs, which can process information from corresponding retinal points in the eye. Fusion of images is necessary for stereoscopic vision of the eye.

Layers 3-6 of LGB have small cells and are called **parvocellular** layers, whereas layers 1 and 2 have large cells and are called **magnocellular** layers. Large (M) cells have large dendritic field and thick axon while the small (P) cells have small dendritic field and thin axon. M cells have higher sensitivity to light contrast while P cells have higher sensitivity to color contrast.

LGB also receives inputs from layer 6 of the primary visual cortex and other brain areas. The feedback pathway from the visual cortex is involved in visual processing related to the perception of orientation and motion.

The M ganglion cells (large ganglion cells) of the retina project to the magnocellular portion of the LGB, whereas the P ganglion cells (small ganglion cells) project to the parvocellular portion. From the LGB, a magnocellular pathway (from layer 1 and 2) and a parvocellular pathway (from layers 3-6) project to the visual cortex. The **magnocellular pathway** is concerned with detection of movement, depth and flicker. The **parvocellular pathway** is concerned with color vision, texture, shape and fine details. Cells in the interlaminar region of the LGB also receive input from P ganglion cells. The interlaminar cells project via a separate component of parvocellular pathway to the blobs in the visual cortex concerned with color vision.

Macular Sparing

Macular sparing is loss of peripheral vision with intact macular vision, since the macular representation is separate from that of peripheral fields and the area of representation is very large.

- In the occipital cortex, the central portion of retina (macular region) is represented in a larger area at the posterior pole of the primary visual cortex (area 17). The macular area occupies nearly one-third of area 17.
- In addition, the macular area of visual cortex is supplied by the posterior and middle cerebral arteries, both of which are seldom blocked at the same time. Hence, only extensive lesions of occipital cortex will damage the macular vision (central vision).
- Macular fibers are also widespread in their course in the optic radiations and so, small lesions in the optic radiation also spare macular vision.

Retinohypothalamic Pathway

Few retinal fibers in the optic tract project bilaterally to the suprachiasmatic nucleus (SN) of hypothalamus above the optic chiasma. This forms the retinohypothalamic pathway. This pathway provides information about light-dark cycles to the suprachiasmatic nucleus. Supra-chiasmatic nucleus is concerned with control of circadian rhythms like one day long cyclic rhythms in sleep and wakefulness, food intake, melatonin secretion by the pineal gland and adrenal cortisol secretion. Bilateral ablation of SN eliminates circadian controls and interferes with reproductive behavior.

Visual Areas in the Occipital Cortex

The visual areas in the occipital cortex are divided into eight functional areas viz visual area 1 (V_1) to visual area 8 (V_8) as shown in **Figure 98.35.**

1. V_1 is the primary visual cortex (Brodmann area 17) concerned with perception of orientation, edges, etc.
2. V_2 occupies much of area 18 concerned with processing in terms of depth perception, visual orientation, edges, etc. of larger visual fields.
3. V_3 is a narrow strip adjoining the anterior margin of V2 within area 18 concerned with perception of motion.
4. V_4 lies within area 19 and may include parts of area 20 (function unknown). It is called occipital eye field and may be responsible for conjugate movement of eye to the opposite side.
5. V_5 corresponds to the junction of the parietal, temporal and occipital cortices lying in area 19 concerned with perception of motion.
6. V_6 is seen anterior to V_5 and is concerned with recognition of large objects.
7. V_7 is located superior to V_3 and its function is unknown.
8. V_8 is seen inferiorly anterior to V_4 and is concerned with color vision **(Fig. 98.35)**.

Primary Visual Cortex (V_1)

The primary visual cortex or striate cortex (area 17) is located largely in the medial surface of the occipital lobe. It is made up of 6 layers of cells numbered 1 to 6. Layer 4 is further subdivided into four sub layers: 4A, 4B, 4Cα and 4Cβ. Afferents from the lateral geniculate body enter layer 4 (koniocortex). The magnocellular afferents enter layer 4Cα. The parvocellular afferents enter layer 4Cβ from where they project to the blobs concerned with color vision. Axons from

Table 98.5: Layers of LGB.

Layer	Type of fibers
1	Nasal fibers
2	Temporal
3	Temporal
4	Nasal
5	Temporal
6	Nasal

the interlaminar region of lateral geniculate body end in layers 2 and 3. Layers 1, 2, 3, 4A and 4B of V_1 project to V_2, V_4 and V_5 and through the corpus callosum to the contralateral visual areas. Layer 5 projects to superior colliculus and layer 6 project back to the LGB. The feedback pathway from the visual cortex to LGB is involved in visual processing related to the perception of orientation and motion.

LESIONS OF VISUAL PATHWAY

> **PY10.18:** Describe and discuss the physiological basis of lesion in visual pathway.

Lesions of the visual pathway occur due to expanding tumors of the brain and neighboring structures such as the pituitary gland and the meninges; and cerebrovascular accident is another common cause (*see* **Fig. 98.34**).

- Lesion of one optic nerve leads to loss of vision (anopia) of that eye.
- Lesion at the level of optic chiasma can be of two types:
  1. Lesion of central part of optic chiasma as in the case of a pituitary tumor pressing on the central part of optic chiasma, causes damage of the nasal fibers from both eyes, i.e., temporal field of vision of both eyes is affected (heteronymous). This is known as **bitemporal hemianopia** or heteronymous hemianopia.
  2. Nasal hemianopia occurs in partial lesion of optic chiasma on its lateral side. It may be due to aneurysm of carotid artery of one side. In damage to the lateral parts of optic chiasma on both sides, the temporal fibers from both eyes are damaged or the nasal field of vision is lost on both eyes. This is known as **binasal hemianopia** (heteronymous hemianopia). This occurs rarely and may be due to aneurysm of carotid artery of both sides or due to dilated third ventricle.
- Lesion of the optic tract leads to contralateral homonymous hemianopia. The nasal field of vision of same side and temporal field of vision of opposite eye is lost. If right optic tract is affected, nasal field of right side and temporal field of left side are lost, i.e., a left temporal hemianopia and right nasal hemianopia will occur. This is called left homonymous hemianopia, i.e., left halves of field of vision is affected in both eyes **(Table 98.6)**. Similarly, if left optic tract is affected, it leads to right homonymous hemianopia. Direct pupillary light reflex may be affected.
- Lesions of the LGB and geniculocalcarine tract or optic radiation also produce homonymous hemianopia as above. Pupillary reflexes will be intact. If the lesion is small, homonymous quadrant anopia may also occur. Here, corresponding quadrants of each field will be lost. For example, the upper or lower half of one temporal and the upper or lower half of the other nasal field will be lost. This is also caused by cortical partial lesions of one occipital lobe.
- Partial lesion of the occipital cortex produces homonymous hemianopia or homonymous quadrantanopia with macular sparing. But, if the cortical lesion is very extensive involving the posterior lip of calcarine fissure, then macular sparing will be absent.

> Blindness is referred to the visual field and not to the retina. Complete blindness of one eye is called anopia (both the nasal field and temporal field of vision of that eye are affected). Blindness of one-half of the visual field is called hemianopia. If opposite sides of the visual field are affected, i.e., nasal field of one eye and temporal field of the opposite eye, it is called homonymous hemianopia (right homonymous hemianopia means temporal field of right eye and nasal field of left eye are affected). If the same halves of the field of vision of both eyes are affected, it is called heteronymous hemianopia (bitemporal or binasal hemianopia).

Cortical Blindness

Cortical blindness or visual agnosia is seen in lesions of visual association areas (areas 18 and 19).

The affected patients can see an object but may not identify it. If they can identify the object, they may not know its usage.

PUPILLARY REFLEXES

The size of the pupil can be varied by stimulation of the sympathetic or parasympathetic nerve fibers to the eye.

Stimulation of parasympathetic fibers causes pupillary constriction (miosis) and sympathetic stimulation produces pupillary dilatation (mydriasis). Pupillary reflexes are:
- Pupillary constrictor reflex
- Pupillary dilator reflex or psycho-sensory reflex.

Pupillary Constrictor Reflex

- Direct light reflex
- Indirect light reflex or consensual light reflex
- Accommodation reflex or near reflex.

Direct Light Reflex

When light is thrown into one eye, pupil of that eye constricts. This response is direct light reflex.

Indirect Light Reflex

When light is thrown into one eye, pupil of the other eye also constricts. This is indirect light reflex or consensual light reflex. Direct and indirect light reflexes together constitute pupillary light reflex.

Pathway for Pupillary Light Reflex (Flowchart 98.6 and Fig. 98.36)

Stimulus—Light Receptors—Rods and cones

Pathway is same as visual pathway up to LGB. At the LGB, without relaying in the LGB, the pupillary fibers separate and go to the pretectal nucleus. This region is close to aqueduct and third ventricle. So, any rise in intracranial pressure will damage this region and affect the pupillary response. This is an important test to test pupil and to some extent intracranial pressure.

Fresh fibers arise from pretectal nucleus and go to Edinger-Westphal nucleus (EWN) of same side and opposite side. EWN is a part of third cranial nerve nucleus. From EWN,

Table 98.6: Effect of lesions in the visual pathway.

Site of lesion	Visual field defect	Accommodation reflex	Pupillary light reflex of same side
Optic nerve of one side	Anopia of same side	Absent	Direct lost, indirect present
Central part of optic chiasma being pressed by pituitary tumor	Bitemporal hemianopia	Present	May or may not be present
Temporal part of optic chiasma (both sides)	Binasal hemianopia	Present	Wernicke's pupillary reaction
Optic tract (one side)	Contralateral homonymous hemianopia	Absent	Wernicke's pupillary reaction
Pretectal nucleus both sides	No defect	Present	Both direct and indirect lost (ARP)
Optic radiation (one side)	Contralateral homonymous hemianopia	Absent	Present
Occipital cortex (small lesion on one side)	Contralateral homonymous hemianopia with macular sparing	Depends on the extent of lesion	Present
Occipital cortex (extensive lesion on one side)	Contralateral homonymous hemianopia without macular sparing	Absent	Present

(ARP: Argyll Robertson pupil)

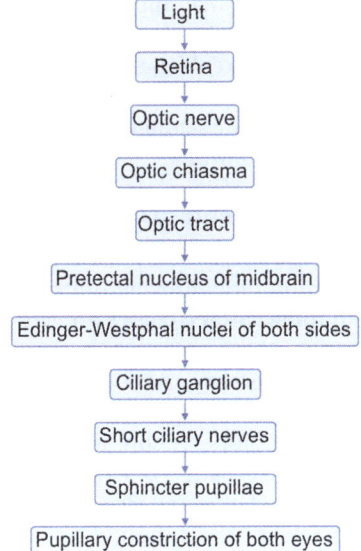

Flowchart 98.6: Pathway for pupillary light reflex.

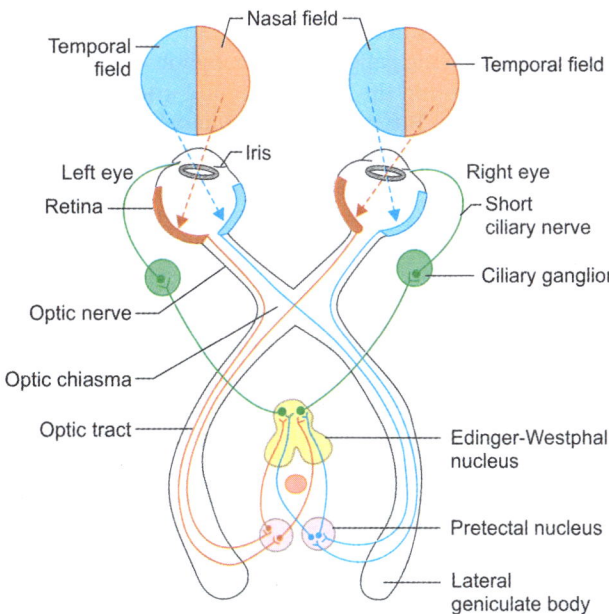

Fig. 98.36: Pathway for direct and indirect pupillary light reflex.

fibers go through oculomotor nerve to ciliary ganglion in the orbit. From there, short ciliary nerves pass to the eyeballs and supply the sphincter pupillae of iris and causes pupillary constriction.

Consensual light reflex occurs due to the following reasons:
❖ Because of the partial decussation of the fibers from the pretectal nuclei in the midbrain going to the Edinger-Westphal nuclei, if light is thrown into one eye, the pupil of that eye as well as the pupil of the opposite eye constricts (consensual light reflex).
❖ The optic fibers from each eye reach the pretectal nuclei of both sides due to incomplete decussation of fibers at the optic chiasma.

Function of pupillary light reflex is to help the eye to adapt to rapidly changing conditions of light. When exposed to bright light, the pupillary diameter may decrease to a minimum of 1.5 mm and in the darkness, the pupillary diameter may increase to a maximum of 8 mm.

Drugs causing pupillary constriction are called miotics, e.g., acetylcholine, pilocarpine, etc.

Lesions of Pupillary Light Reflex Pathway

❖ *Lesion of optic nerve of one side:* Direct light reflex lost and indirect light reflex in the same eye present since the opposite optic nerve is intact.
❖ *Lesion of optic chiasma and optic tract:* When light falls on the sound half of retina; both direct and indirect light reflexes are present. If light falls on the blind half of retina, both direct and indirect light reflexes will be absent. This is known as **Wernicke's hemianopic pupillary reaction**.
❖ *Lesion of pretectal nuclei:* Both direct and indirect pupillary light reflexes will be absent. Accommodation reflex will be present since the visual pathway to the visual cortex is unaffected. This condition is called **Argyll Robertson pupil**

(ARP), seen in tabes dorsalis or neurosyphilis (tertiary syphilis).

Pupillary Dilator Reflex

Pupillary dilatation is seen in the following conditions:
- Withdrawal of light.
- Cervical sympathetic stimulation by pinching the skin of neck region (ciliospinal reflex or pupillodilator reflex).
- Emotional disturbances like anger, fear, anxiety, etc.
- Drugs that cause pupillary dilatation are called mydriatics, e.g., epinephrine, cocaine, etc.

Pathway for Pupillodilator Reflex or Ciliospinal Reflex

When the skin of neck region is pinched, afferent sensory fibers make connection with the preganglionic sympathetic neurons in the lateral gray column of the first and second thoracic segments of spinal cord. The preganglionic fibers pass to the sympathetic trunk and end in the superior cervical sympathetic ganglion. Postganglionic fibers travel in the plexus around the internal carotid artery and enter the cranial cavity. Through the long ciliary nerves that are branches of the ophthalmic division of trigeminal nerve, the fibers reach the dilator pupillae muscle of iris leading to pupillary dilatation. Lesion of the cervical sympathetic fibers causes **Horner's syndrome**.

Visual Body Reflexes

The fibers of the optic tract reaching the superior colliculi after relaying there pass to the tectospinal and tectobulbar tracts. These tracts synapse with the neurons in the anterior gray matter of spinal cord and cranial motor nuclei (III, IV and VI). This pathway is responsible for the reflex actions like simultaneous movement of eyes and head while reading; the automatic movement of eyes, head and neck toward the source of the visual stimulus and the protective closing of the eyes.

Horner's Syndrome

Horner's syndrome occurs due to damage to the cervical sympathetic fibers. The sympathetic innervation of the eye originates in the intermediolateral horn cells of the first and second thoracic spinal cord segments. The efferent preganglionic fibers enter the sympathetic chain and synapse with the postganglionic neurons in the superior cervical ganglion. Postganglionic sympathetic fibers travel in the plexus around the internal carotid artery and enter the cranial cavity and reach the eye. They supply the radial fibers of iris (dilator pupillae) via the long ciliary nerves. Cervical sympathetic fibers also supply the levator palpebrae superioris (Muller muscle), the smooth muscle of the upper eyelid. In Horner's syndrome, the effects on the affected side are:
- Pupillary constriction **(miosis)** because of interruption of sympathetic fibers supplying the dilator pupillae.
- Drooping of upper eyelid **(ptosis)**. This is due to paralysis of the smooth muscle embedded in the upper eyelid innervated by the cervical sympathetic which maintain the upper eyelid in an open position.
- Absence of sweating on the ipsilateral side of face and head **(anhydrosis)**.
- The blood vessels on the affected side of face and head become persistently dilated.
- **Enophthalmos** (recession of the eyeball) due to reduced intraocular pressure.

COLOR VISION

Characteristics of Color

Colors have three attributes or qualities: hue, intensity (brightness) and saturation.
- **Hue** depends entirely on the wavelength. Depending on the wavelength hue will be any of the colors, i.e., blue, green, yellow, etc.
- **Brightness** depends on the intensity of the light rays. Same wavelength color may appear brighter or less bright depending on the intensity of the rays.
- **Saturation** or purity of a color is the degree of freedom from dilution with white, i.e., it varies with the amount of white mixed with it. Red is more saturated than pink because pink has more white mixed with it.

Primary and Complementary Colors

Red, green and blue are called **primary colors** because they give a sensation of white when mixed in the proper proportion. **Complementary colors** are two colors which when mixed in a particular proportion give the sensation of white. A complementary color exists for every color. For example, yellow and blue, red and greenish blue, etc., are complementary colors. Yellow when properly mixed with blue produces a sensation of white, thus yellow is the complementary color of blue and vice versa.

Contrast Phenomena in Color Vision

Sense of contrast is the ability of the eye to perceive slight changes in the luminance between regions which are not separated by definite borders. When a colored object is viewed, the background color or the color of other objects in the visual field or the color of illumination used influences the color of the object. For example, if a red colored object is viewed in red illumination, the object is seen as pink or white. But if the red colored object is viewed in green or blue light it will be seen as red. This is known as contrast effect. The types of contrast effects are:
- Simultaneous contrast
- Successive contrast.

Simultaneous Contrast

For the eyes to perceive a particular color, the color of the object and the color of illumination used in the field of vision are important factors. When a black object is placed against white background, black appears blacker and white appears pure white. If black object is placed against any other color, this much of contrast is not seen. If a red colored object is viewed in green or blue light, it will be seen as red. But if red light is used to illuminate the field of vision, the red object will appear as pink or white. This is simultaneous color contrast. Other colors exhibiting simultaneous contrast are yellow and blue.

If a lemon is held in bright light, a hue of blue color is seen at the periphery of the lemon which is due to simultaneous contrast. This is because when one part of the retina is stimulated, the part surrounding it tends to discourage a similar stimulus but favors a complementary color. This is an extension of the after-image phenomenon to the region of retina outside the area of original stimulus. Simultaneous contrast is important in color vision because it is related to the color of the object seen.

Successive Contrast

If we look at bright light for some time and then if we look at a white wall, then a dark image appears on the wall against the white background.

Instead of white light, if we look at a colored light for some time and then look at the white background, an image of the complementary color is formed on the white wall. If the colored object is small, then a small image is formed on the white wall. This is successive contrast. This is because, on stimulation of the retina, another stimulus of a similar nature is inhibited, while a complementary color is favored and is due to negative after-image. Successive contrast is not so important in color vision.

After-images

After-images are images that persist after a stimulus ceases to act, and disappear gradually. It may be negative after image or positive after image.

Negative After-image

If after looking at an object, the eyes are fixed on a white or bright surface, the after-image appears dark and is of a complementary color. This is called negative after-image.

Positive After-image

If we look at bright object for some time and then turn to a dark background, the image of the object appears on the dark background and then fades away. This is positive after-image. Positive after-images are the cause for visual persistence. If a series of flashes of light are presented to the eye, when the rate of flickering is increased beyond a critical frequency, then the light appears continuous. This is because the positive afterimages fuse together and is known as **flicker fusion frequency** or critical fusion frequency. This is the basis of cinema where we see continuous pictures.

■ MECHANISM OF COLOR VISION

Retinal Mechanism

Color vision is a function of cones and is better appreciated in photopic vision. In scotopic or dim light vision, all colors are seen as gray. There are three different types of cones in the retina containing three different pigments located in the outer segment as evidenced by absorption spectrum. Photopigment in each cone is highly sensitive to one of the three primary colors. Each pigment is a combination of retinene and photopsin. Photopsin is different in the different cone pigments, but retinene is the same (**Table 98.7**). The three types of cones operate in different wavelengths of the spectrum. Peak light sensitivity of blue cone (S-cone) is to 445 nm wavelength, green cone (M-cone) is 535 nm and red cone (L-cone) is 570 nm, respectively.

■ THEORIES OF COLOR VISION

❖ Trichromatic theory or pigment theory
❖ Opponent color theory.

Young-Helmholtz Trichromatic Theory

Thomas Young put forward the theory of color vision and **Von Helmholtz** later modified it. According to this theory, referred to as **Young-Helmholtz theory**, color vision is trichromatic at the level of photoreceptors. There are three types of cones namely, the L cone for red (650 nm wavelength) color, M cone for green (530 nm) and S cone for blue (440 nm) color. They have different absorbance spectrum. The letters L, M and S denote long, middle and short wavelength of light absorbed by these cones. Erythrolabe is the long wavelength sensitive (**LWS**) cone pigment, chlorolabe is the medium wavelength sensitive (**MWS**) pigment and cyanolabe is the short wavelength sensitive (**SWS**) cone pigment. The genes for green sensitive and red sensitive pigments are located in the short arm of X chromosome. Gene for blue sensitive pigment is present on chromosome 7 (the gene for rhodopsin is located in the chromosome 3).

The different shades of color that we perceive are due to differential stimulation of three types of cones sensitive to the three primary colors. Light of a single wavelength stimulates each of the three cones to different degrees, and light of any other wavelength stimulates these cones with a distinctly different pattern. White sensation is due to the stimulation of the three cones equally The sensation of any given color depends on the relative frequency of impulses being sent from each of the cone systems. The nervous system can compare the relative stimulation of the 3 cone types to decode the wavelength. At least two types of cones are required for color vision.

An orange monochromatic light, having a wavelength 580 nm stimulates red cone 99%, green cone 42% and does not stimulate the blue cone. The nervous system interprets this set of ratios as the sensation of orange.

Therefore, for orange sensation, the ratio of Red: Green: Blue = 99: 42:0.

Table 98.7: Pigments in cones.	
Red-sensitive pigment (L pigment)	Erythrolabe
Green-sensitive pigment (M pigment)	Chlorolabe
Blue-sensitive pigment (S pigment)	Cyanolabe

- Yellow monochromatic light of wavelength 550 nm stimulates as 83:83:0.
- Green monochromatic light of wavelength 490 nm stimulates as 31:67:36.
- Blue monochromatic light of wavelength 450 nm stimulates as 0:0:97 (Fig. 98.30).

Opponent Color Theory or Hering's Theory of Opposite Color Pairs

Color vision is trichromatic at the level of photoreceptors. Some colors appear to be mutually exclusive and this phenomenon cannot be explained by trichromatic theory. Hering's theory explains color discrimination from ganglion cell onward. He observed that there is no greenish-red or bluish-yellow color.

According to this theory, there are two types of color opponent ganglion cells. Some of the ganglion cells are stimulated by only one color type of cone but inhibited by a second type. This type of reciprocal effect occurs between red and green cones; between blue cones on the one hand and a combination of red and green cones (yellow signal) on the other hand. In the first case, red light cause excitation and green cause inhibition or vice versa i.e. red and green colors oppose each other. Both cannot excite the same ganglion cell. The red-green opponent color ganglion cells use signals from red and green cones. In the second case, there exists a reciprocal excitation-inhibition relation between blue and yellow colors. Yellow signal occurs from the summed output of red and green cones. So blue-yellow opponent color cells obtain a yellow signal from the summed output of red and green cones, which is contrasted with the output from blue cones within the receptive field. Neurons excited by blue may be inhibited by yellow.

Such color opponent neurons are found both in the retina and at other areas in the visual pathway like lateral geniculate body and visual cortex. Electrical responses at the level of LGB show that in some units, turning off a red stimulus is similar to turning on a green stimulus. LGB contains color opponent cells that respond with red-on, green-off; green-on, red-off; yellow-on, blue-off or blue-on, yellow-off. This mechanism serves to increase the ability of the eye to see the contrast between opposing colors. For example, greenish red or bluish yellow color does not exist. Opposing colors are green and red, black and white, yellow and blue.

Thus, each color-contrast type of ganglion cell is excited by one color but inhibited by the opponent color, i.e., red-green opponent color cells and blue-yellow color opponent ganglion cells. This is opponent color theory.

The mechanism of this opposing effect of colors is that, one color type of cone excites the ganglion cell by the direct excitatory route through depolarization of bipolar cells. The other color type inhibits the same ganglion cell by the indirect inhibitory route through hyperpolarization of bipolar cells through horizontal cell (Flowchart 98.7).

Neural Mechanism of Color Vision

Color processing starts in the retina. Mechanism of color processing is not fully understood. Ganglion cells that subtract or add input from one type of cone to input from another type mediate color sensation. For example, in the red-green opponent mechanism, there is subtraction of signals of the L (red) and M (green) cones, i.e., L − M. Large ganglion cells or M (magno) cells add responses from different kinds of cones while small ganglion cells or P (parvo) cells function to subtract information from one type of cone and input from another cone. On-center cells and off-center cells are present in the ganglion layer.

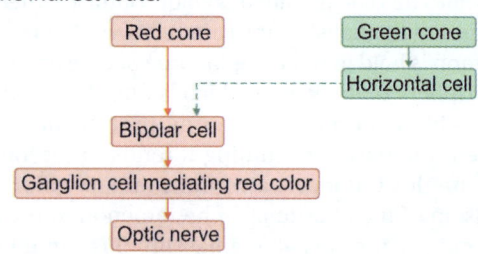

Flowchart 98.7: Opponent color theory (dashed lines indicate inhibition) Note that the red cone stimulates the bipolar cell by the direct excitatory route while the green cone inhibits the same bipolar cell by the indirect route.

The M ganglion cells project to the magnocellular portion of the lateral geniculate body (layers 1 and 2). The P ganglion cells project to the parvocellular portion (layers 3, 4, 5 and 6) of the LGB. In the LGB, color vision is by layers 3, 4, 5 and 6 and also by the interlaminar area cells. The axons from the interlaminar region of the LGB end in layers 2 and 3 of visual cortex (color blobs). The parvocellular pathway carries information for color vision which reaches layer 4 of the primary visual cortex, goes to the complex layers 1 and 2 and to visual association areas where processing of visual information takes place. The parvocellular pathway also carries color opponent data to the deep part of layer 4. The final area of color vision is the anterior edge of visual cortex.

Layers 2 and 3 of the primary visual cortex (V_1) contain clusters of cells about 0.2 mm in diameter called **blobs**. Unlike neighboring cells, these cells contain a high concentration of the mitochondrial enzyme, cytochrome oxidase. The blobs are arranged in a mosaic in the visual cortex and are concerned with color vision. The interlaminar area of the LGB contains interlaminar cells which project via a separate component of the parvocellular pathway to the blobs in the visual cortex (Flowchart 98.8).

Color opponent cells are also present in the lateral geniculate nucleus. Electrical responses at the level of LGB show that in some units turning off a red stimulus is similar to turning on a green stimulus. LGB contains color-opponent cells that respond with red-on, green off; green-on, red-off; yellow-on, blue-off or blue-on, yellow off.

Processing in the ganglion cells and LGB produces impulses that pass along three types of neural pathways that project to the primary visual cortex. This is color opponent theory.

- A red-green pathway that signals differences between L and M-cone responses.
- A blue-yellow pathway that signals differences between S-cone and the sum of L and M-cone responses.

Flowchart 98.8: Neural mechanism of color vision

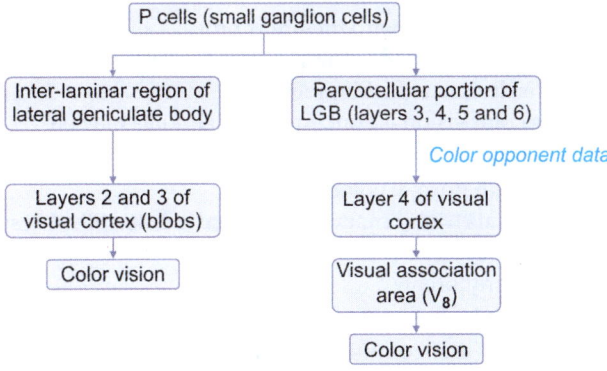

- A luminance pathway that signals the sum of L and M-cone responses.

These pathways project to the blobs and the deep portion of layer 4 of primary visual cortex or V_1. From the blobs and layer 4, color information is projected to V_8 of visual cortex. V_8 converts color input into the sensation of color. Lesion of V_8 area (projection area for color vision) affect color vision and the defect is called **achromatopsia.**

TESTS FOR COLOR VISION

- Ishihara charts
- Colored wool tests
- Edridge green lantern test

Ishihara charts are printed with numbers or designs in colored circles on a background of similarly shaped color circles. The figures are intentionally made of colors that are likely to look the same as the background to an individual who is color blind **(Fig. 98.37)**. A color blind person reads them differently. It is the most commonly used test for color blindness.

In **Holmgren's colored wool test**, the subject is asked to identify the wool of various colors. He is given one type of wool and is asked to pick out from a large number of colored wool pieces of different shades, those that match the given color.

Edridge color lantern is used to test would-be engine drivers for evidence of color blindness. The subject is asked to identify the color of a small illuminated area, the size of which can be varied. A lantern is shown through colored glass pieces fixed on a rotation disc and the subject should name the color **(Fig. 98.38)**.

Test for color blindness is a must for people engaged in driving, traffic services, and professionals working in railways, armed forces, pilots and doctors.

COLOR BLINDNESS

Color blindness is the failure to appreciate one or more of the three primary colors. In this condition, people may be unable to distinguish certain colors or have weakness to distinguish colors. Color blindness is 20 times more common in males than in females. Individuals with normal color vision have three types of cones and are called **trichromats**. In **anomalous trichromats**, there is no complete blindness for any color but one of the cones will be weak and the

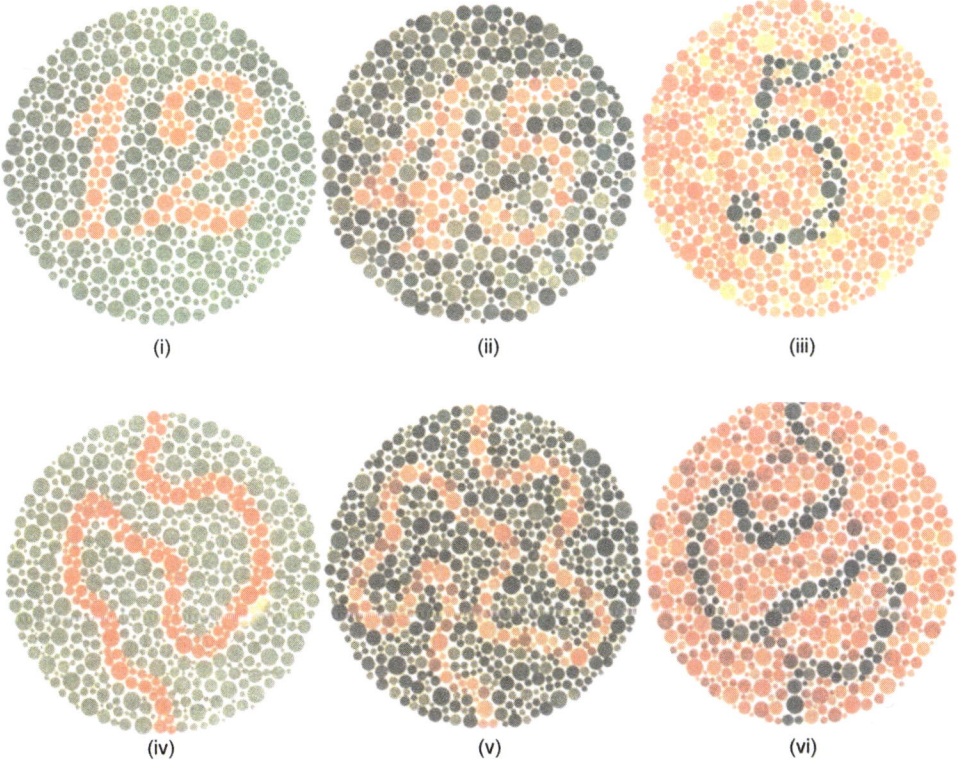

Fig. 98.37: Ishihara's chart to test color vision.

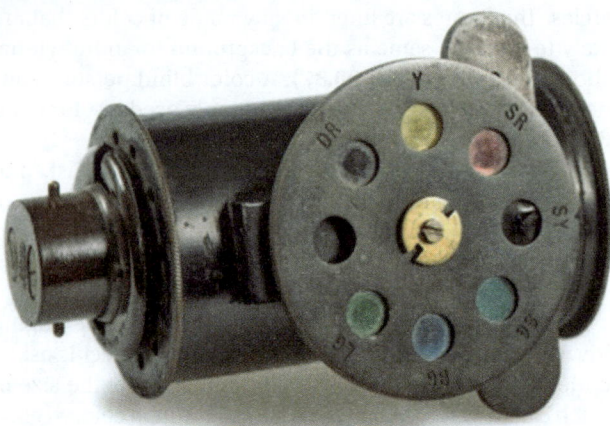

Fig. 98.38: Edridge color lantern.

appreciation of that color will be less. Persons with only two types of cones are called **dichromats** and those with only one type of cone are called **monochromats**.

Some colorblind individuals are unable to distinguish certain colors (anopia) and the condition is called dichromatic or monochromatic color blindness, whereas others have only a color weakness (anomaly) and is referred to as trichromatic color blindness.

Color blindness may be congenital or acquired. Acquired color blindness may be due to damage to the macula or optic nerve. It can also occur in lesions of area V_8 of the visual cortex since this area is concerned with color vision in humans. This type of defect is called **achromatopsia**. Individuals taking the drug viagra for the treatment of erectile dysfunction can also show transient blue-green defect since the drug interacts with retinal phosphodiesterase enzyme.

Inheritance

Inheritance of red and green color blindness is similar to that of hemophilia, and is inherited through X-linked recessive gene (X-linked recessive trait). 80% of color blind is men and females are usually carriers. Males suffer from color blindness if the X chromosome has the abnormal gene. Females will suffer from color blindness only when both X-chromosomes carry the defective gene. However, all the daughters of a man with X-linked color blindness are carriers of color blindness and pass the defect to half of their sons. Thus, X-linked color blindness skips generations and appears in males of every second generation as in the case of hemophilia.

Blue color blindness affects both males and females equally because the gene responsible is located on chromosome 7. Presence of color blind individuals is a proof of trichromatic theory of color vision.

> Gene for red and green are carried in the X-chromosome. The gene for blue is in chromosome 7 and that for rhodopsin is in chromosome 3.

- If **anomaly** is suffixed, it means weakness
- If **anopia** is suffixed, it means blindness
- Red is designated with the prefix prot
- Green is designated with the prefix deuter
- Blue is designated with prefix trit

As far as color vision is concerned, individuals may be:

Trichromats
- Those with normal color vision
- Anomalous trichromacy (**trichromatic color blindness**)
  - Protanomaly
  - Deuteranomaly
  - Tritanomaly

Dichromats (dichromatic color blindness)
- Protanopes (red-blind)
- Deuteranopes (green-blind)
- Tritanopes (blue-blind)

Monochromats (monochromatic color blindness)

Trichromats

Normal individuals with all the three cones functioning normally are referred to as trichromats. Anomalous trichromatic vision (**anomalous trichromacy or trichromatic color blindness**) is one form of partial color blindness. There is no complete blindness for any color but appreciation of one color is less.

Anomalous trichromats can see all the three colors, but there is weakness for one color. More of stimulation of that cone is necessary for the synthesis of white sensation. It may be due to abnormal pigments.
- If the red cone is weak, the condition is called protanomaly
- If green cone is weak it is called deuteranomaly
- If blue cone is weak the condition is tritanomaly

Dichromats

In these individuals, any one of the cones is absent and the color blindness is called dichromatic color blindness. About 2% of affected males are dichromats.
- Red cone absent—Protanopia (red-blind)
- Green cone absent—Deuteranopia (green-blind)
- Blue cone absent—Tritanopia (blue-blind, rare)

Monochromats

- Those affected have only one type of cone and they cannot appreciate any color. Minimum of two cone systems are required to appreciate a color.
- By changing the intensity of stimulation of a particular cone, they may identify colors by experience.
- They have only black and white vision. Sometimes, they can recognize shades of gray.

Deuteranomaly accounts for 50% of the total cases of color blindness. It is seen in approximately 5% of male population. The decreasing order of occurrence is deuteranopia, protanopia and least is protanomaly. Tritanomaly and tritanopia are extremely rare.

Transient blue-green color weakness occurs as a side effect in individuals taking viagra for the treatment of erectile dysfunction. cGMP which is produced by nitric oxide (NO) is a potent vasodilator leading to penile erection. Viagra (sildenafil) inhibits the breakdown of cGMP by inhibiting phosphodiesterases. The action of phosphodiesterase is to convert cGMP to non-signaling form, 5'-GMP. Since the phosphodiesterases of retina are also inhibited by viagra, this drug produces transient blue-green color blindness.

ELECTRORETINOGRAM

Electroretinogram (ERG) records the electrical activity from eye, and is not of much diagnostic value. It is of some help in diagnosing diseases in which visualization of retina is difficult. It is done by stimulating the retina with a flash of light and recording the electrical activities.

Procedure

The pupil is dilated fully and after the application of local anesthetic, a recording electrode is placed on the cornea. Keep the reference electrode on the skin of scalp behind retina or on the forehead. In the resting state, potential difference of 6 mV is obtained between the front and back of eye. Apply a light stimulus and switch it off.

The electrode records a series of changes and the record obtained is called electroretinogram **(Fig. 98.39)**.

- First wave is **"a" wave**. It is a negative wave which is due to the activity in the photoreceptors (rods and cones).
- First negative wave is followed by **"b" wave** which is a positive wave. It is due to activity in the inner nuclear layer.
- **"c" wave** is also a positive wave and is due to activity in the pigment epithelium of retina. It is a prolonged slow wave.
- When light is switched off, a small downward deflection occurs before the "c" wave.

Types of ERG

- **Extinguished**—the response is extinguished, resulting in the complete failure of functioning of rods and cones like pigmentary retinal dystrophy, complete occlusion of retinal artery, retinal detachment, vitamin A deficiency etc.
- **Subnormal**—where a large area of retina does not function.
- **Negative**—in gross disturbance of retinal circulation.

VISUAL EVOKED POTENTIAL

Visual evoked potentials (VEP) are electrical responses recorded from the scalp in response to visual stimuli. The responses are generated in the visual pathway from the retina to the visual cortex in response to alternating checkerboard pattern stimulation of the eye. Different wave forms are recorded at various latencies on a computer screen. This test is very useful for detecting optic nerve problems. It is also useful to check vision in children and in inarticulate adults. Abnormality in the latency and amplitude of the waves helps in the diagnosis of diseases like optic neuritis, optic atrophy, multiple sclerosis, refractive errors etc. The test also helps to confirm that the visual pathway is intact. VEP measures the time taken by the visual stimulus to travel from the eye to the occipital cortex. For example, in multiple sclerosis since there is destruction of myelin sheath in the nerve fibers, it takes a longer time for the impulses to be conducted from the eye to the occipital cortex.

Procedure

Electrodes are placed on the scalp over the occipital cortex. Visual stimuli are presented to the subject. The stimulation of the visual pathway generates electrical responses in the visual cortex. The responses which originate from the occipital cortex are amplified and are displayed as a reading on an electroencephalogram. Each eye is tested separately.

The typical VEP wave form contains an initial negative peak (N1 or N75), followed by a positive peak (P1 or P100), which is followed by a second negative peak (N2 or N135) and a second positive peak (P2). 75, 100 and 135 denotes the time in milliseconds when the peak is reached. The latency of onset of a peak after the light stimulus and the amplitude of the peak are the features analyzed (**Fig. 98.40**). Demyelination of the optic nerve results in increased latency of the P100 waveform, without significant effect on amplitude. Compression of the optic nerve by tumors reduces the amplitude primarily, with less effect on latency.

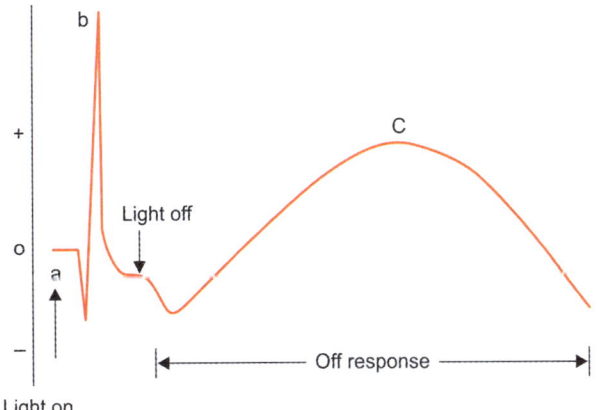

Fig. 98.39: Electroretinogram.

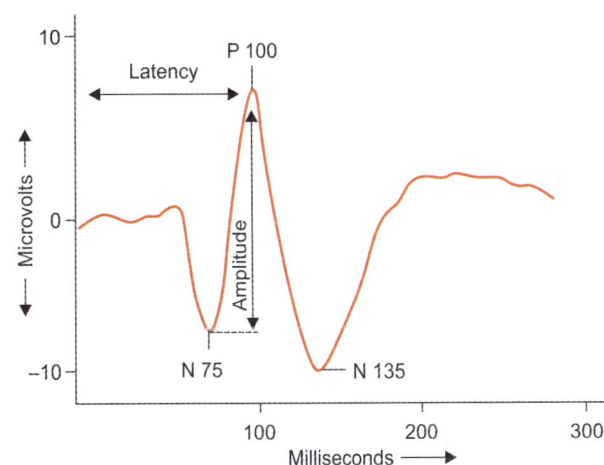

Fig. 98.40: Normal pattern of visual evoked potential.

MULTIPLE CHOICE QUESTIONS

1. Visible range of electromagnetic spectrum of human eye is:
   a. 370-740 nm
   b. 740-1140 nm
   c. 200-340 nm
   d. 200-370 nm

2. Which part of the eye has the greatest concentration of rods?
   a. Iris
   b. Optic disc
   c. Fovea centralis
   d. Parafoveal region

3. Intraocular pressure normally is:
   a. 10-20 mm H_2O
   b. 40-50 mm H_2O
   c. 40-50 mm Hg
   d. 10-20 mm Hg

4. All are actions of superior oblique, *except*:
   a. Extorsion
   b. Intorsion
   c. Lateral rotation
   d. Downward movement

5. In a tumor which compresses the optic chiasma the color affected first is:
   a. White
   b. Red
   c. Blue
   d. Green

6. Maximum refraction of light occurs in the:
   a. Air-corneal interphase
   b. Anterior surface of lens
   c. Posterior surface of lens
   d. Vitreous humor

7. Accommodation is brought about by:
   a. Dilation of iris
   b. Dilation of pupil
   c. Ciliary body contraction
   d. Suspensory ligament made tense

8. Binasal hemianopia occur due to lesion in:
   a. Central portion of optic chiasma
   b. Outer margins of optic chiasma
   c. Optic tract
   d. Optic radiation

9. True stereopsis is perceived due to the following:
   a. Overlay of contours
   b. Motion parallax
   c. Binasal disparity
   d. Linear perspective

10. The fibers from the contralateral hemi retina project to the following layers of the lateral geniculate body:
    a. Layers 2,3 and 5
    b. Layers 1,2 and 6
    c. Layers 1,4 and 6
    d. Layers 4,5 and 6

11. Most afferent fibers from the lateral geniculate nucleus terminating in the primary visual cortex is from:
    a. Layer 1
    b. Layers 2 and 3
    c. Layer 4
    d. Layers 5 and 6

12. The blobs of the visual cortex are associated with:
    a. Ocular dominance
    b. Color processing
    c. Orientation
    d. Saccadic eye movements

13. The parvocellular pathway from the lateral geniculate nucleus to the visual cortex carries signals for the detection of:
    a. Movement, depth and flicker
    b. Color vision, shape and fine details
    c. Temporal frequency
    d. Luminance contrast

14. The parvocellular pathway from lateral geniculate nucleus to the visual cortex is most sensitive for the stimulus of:
    a. Color contrast
    b. Luminance contrast
    c. Temporal frequency
    d. Saccadic eye movements

15. The following extraocular muscle is not supplied by III cranial nerve:
    a. Medial rectus
    b. Superior rectus
    c. Superior oblique
    d. Inferior oblique

16. Visual acuity of 6/24 using Snellen's chart indicates:
    a. Normal subject can read the first line at 6 meter and the subject can read it at 24 meter
    b. Normal person can read the last line at 6 meter whereas the subject can read it at 24 meter
    c. Normal person can read the third line at 24 meter and subject reads it at 6 meter only
    d. Normal person can read the third line at 6 meter but the subject can read it at 24 meter

17. The B wave in electroretinogram is due to activity in:
    a. Bipolar cells
    b. Rods
    c. Cones
    d. Pigment epithelium

18. Vitamin-A is associated with all the following, *except*:
    a. Rhodopsin synthesis
    b. Scotopic vision
    c. Prevention of nyctalopia
    d. Accommodation reflex

19. A patient presented with normal eye sight and absence of direct and consensual light reflexes. Which of the following cranial nerves is suspected to be affected?
    a. Optic
    b. Oculomotor
    c. Trochlear
    d. Abducens

20. Relative color and luminosity of photoreceptive input under changing light conditions are regulated and maintained by:
    a. Muller cells
    b. Amacrine cells
    c. Ganglion cells
    d. Retinal astrocytes

21. During the dark phase of visual cycle, which form of vitamin A combines with opsin to make rhodopsin?
    a. All trans-retinaldehyde
    b. All trans-retinol
    c. 11 cis-retinaldehyde
    d. 11 cis-retinol
22. Right optic tract lesion leads to:
    a. Bitemporal hemianopia
    b. Binasal hemianopia
    c. Right homonymous hemianopia
    d. Left homonymous hemianopia
23. Lesion of right optic nerve produces:
    a. Right anopia
    b. Left anopia
    c. Right homonymous hemianopia
    d. Left homonymous hemianopia
24. A lesion at the left optic tract level leads to:
    a. Complete blindness in the right eye
    b. Complete blindness in the left eye
    c. Blindness in the right temporal and left nasal fields
    d. Blindness in the left temporal and right nasal fields
25. The defect in the refracting mechanisms in the case of myopia is:
    a. Failure of accommodation to near response
    b. Increased antero-posterior diameter of eyeball
    c. Uneven curvature of cornea
    d. Thickening of lens capsule fibers
26. Major part of refractive power of eye is provided by:
    a. Crystalline lens   b. Cornea
    c. Aqueous humor   d. Vitreous humor
27. Bifocal lens can be used for the correction of:
    a. Myopia   b. Hypermetropia
    c. Cataract   d. Presbyopia
28. Lens of eye develop from:
    a. Mesoderm
    b. Ectoderm
    c. Endoderm
    d. Ectoderm and endoderm
29. The term anisometropia indicates:
    a. Refractive error   b. Long sight
    c. Short sight   d. Aging process
30. The part of the eye that has the maximum refractive power is:
    a. Anterior surface of lens
    b. Posterior surface of lens
    c. Anterior surface of cornea
    d. Posterior surface of cornea
31. Snellen's chart is used to test:
    a. Vision   b. Refraction
    c. Color blindness   d. Presbyopia
32. Color vision is the function of:
    a. Rods   b. Cones
    c. Bipolar cells   d. Occipital cortex
33. The layer of retina that is affected by laser therapy is:
    a. Layer of rods and cones
    b. Pigment layer
    c. Inner plexiform layer
    d. Nerve fiber layer
34. Greatest concentration of rods is found in:
    a. Optic disc   b. Iris
    c. Fovea   d. Parafoveal region
35. Near point of a five-year-old child is:
    a. 5 cm   b. 10 cm
    c. 15 cm   d. 25 cm
36. Which part of the eye continues to grow in the life time?
    a. Cornea   b. Lens
    c. Retina   d. Ciliary body
37. Frontal eye field is Brodmann's area:
    a. Area 8   b. Area 18
    c. Area 19   d. Area 4
38. All the following are true regarding accommodation reflex, *except*:
    a. Accommodation reflex is bilateral
    b. Anterior curvature of lens increases by relaxation of ciliary muscle
    c. Spherical and chromatic aberrations are decreased by constriction of pupil
    d. Convergence of visual axes is due to contraction of medial rectus muscles
39. The correct statement regarding Argyll-Robertson pupil is:
    a. Accommodation reflex is present
    b. Accommodation reflex is absent
    c. Pupillary reflex is present
    d. It is due to lesion in the occipital cortex
40. The condition in which there is receding of near point of vision with age is called:
    a. Myopia   b. Astigmatism
    c. Hypermetropia   d. Presbyopia
41. The light that is least refracted in the eye is:
    a. Blue light   b. Green light
    c. Red light   d. yellow light
42. Parallel rays of light from distant object are focused in front of the retina in:
    a. Emmetropia   b. Myopia
    c. Hypermetropia   d. Presbyopia
43. The neurotransmitter released by horizontal cells in the retina is:
    a. GABA   b. Glycine
    c. Glutamic acid   d. Acetylcholine

44. Weakness to recognize red color is called:
    a. Protanopia   b. Protanomaly
    c. Deuteranomaly   d. Trianomaly
45. The most common defect of color blindness is:
    a. Protanopia   b. Protanomaly
    c. Deuteranomaly   d. Tritanomaly
46. Fovea of the eye:
    a. Has the lowest light threshold
    b. Is the region of highest visual acuity
    c. Contains only red and green cones
    d. Contains only rods
47. Myopia can be corrected by:
    a. Biconcave lens b. Biconvex lens
    c. Bifocal lens   d. Cylindrical lens
48. Color blindness is more common in men than women because it is caused by an abnormal:
    a. Dominant gene on Y chromosome
    b. Recessive gene on Y chromosome
    c. Recessive gene on the X chromosome
    d. Dominant gene on X chromosome
49. Trichromats are individuals with:
    a. Normal color vision
    b. Weakness to two colors
    c. Two cone system
    d. One cone system
50. Achromatopsia is due to lesion of :
    a. Area V_8 of visual cortex
    b. Frontal eye field
    c. Lateral geniculate body
    d. Edinger-Westphal nucleus
51. In lesion of trochlear nerve:
    a. Patient cannot move his eye downwards and outwards
    b. There will be no diplopia
    c. There is lateral deviation of the eye
    d. Patient cannot move his eye upwards
52. Lateral deviation of the eye is seen when there is paralysis of:
    a. Superior oblique muscle
    b. Inferior oblique
    c. Lateral rectus
    d. Medial rectus
53. Ishihara charts are used to test:
    a. Acuity of vision   b. Color vision
    c. Field of vision   d. Accommodation
54. After removal of the lens, the dioptric power of the eye is reduced by:
    a. 4 diopters   b. 8 diopters
    c. 16 diopters   d. 32 diopters
55. All the following structures of eye are transparent, *except*:
    a. Cornea   b. Sclera
    c. Aqueous humor   d. Vitreous humor
56. Fovea centralis is a part of retina having:
    a. Maximum number of rods
    b. No rods or cones
    c. Equal number of rods and cones
    d. Only cones
57. In Argyll-Robertson pupil:
    a. Pupillary light reflex is lost
    b. Accommodation reflex is lost
    c. Both accommodation and light reflexes are lost
    d. Both accommodation and light reflex normal
58. Accommodation in the eye involves the following:
    a. Decrease in the curvature of lens
    b. Relaxation of constrictor pupillae
    c. Increased intraocular pressure
    d. Contraction of the ciliary muscle
59. Hypermetropia is corrected using:
    a. Biconcave lens b. Biconvex lens
    c. Bifocal lens   d. Cylindrical lens
60. Vitamin A is necessary for the synthesis of:
    a. Choroid pigment b. Scotopsin
    c. Aqueous humor   d. Retinene$_1$
61. The percentage of change in light intensity for visual discrimination is:
    a. 1%   b. 30%
    c. 5%   d. 3%
62. Most of the refraction that occurs in the eye occurs at the:
    a. Anterior surface of cornea
    b. Posterior surface of cornea
    c. Anterior surface of lens
    d. Posterior surface of lens
63. Which one of the following is most likely to decrease intraocular pressure of glaucoma patient?
    a. High dose of vitamin C
    b. Decreased pressure in jugular vein
    c. Dark environment
    d. Carbonic anhydrase inhibitor
64. Red color blindness is called:
    a. Deuteranopia   b. Protanopia
    c. Protanomaly   d. Deuteranomaly
65. If the red cones and green cones are stimulated approximately equally, what color will the person see?
    a. Red   b. Yellow
    c. Purple   d. Green
66. The receptors in retina for those of blue, green and red wave lengths are called:
    a. Modulators   b. Trichromators
    c. Dominators   d. None of the above
67. Under resting conditions, the ganglion cells of the retina discharge at approximately what rate?
    a. 5/sec   b. 25/sec
    c. 125/sec   d. 1250/sec

68. The medium with highest refractive index in the eye is:
    a. Cornea
    b. Nucleus of the lens
    c. Cortex of the lens
    d. Aqueous humor
69. Rhodopsin is most sensitive to:
    a. Green light
    b. Red light
    c. Blue light
    d. Violet light
70. Rhodopsin is least sensitive to:
    a. Green light
    b. Red light
    c. Blue light
    d. Violet light

ANSWERS

1. a	2. d	3. d	4. a	5. b
6. a	7. c	8. b	9. c	10. c
11. c	12. b	13. b	14. c	15. c
16. c	17. a	18. d	19. b	20. b
21. c	22. d	23. a	24. c	25. b
26. a	27. d	28. b	29. a	30. c
31. a	32. b	33. b	34. d	35. a
36. b	37. a	38. b	39. d	40. d
41. c	42. b	43. a	44. b	45. c
46. b	47. a	48. c	49. a	50. a
51. a	52. d	53. b	54. c	55. b
56. d	57. a	58. d	59. b	60. d
61. a	62. a	63. d	64. b	65. b
66. b	67. b	68. b	69. a	70. b

■ FILL IN THE BLANKS/GIVE THE NORMAL VALUE/NAME THE FOLLOWING

1. Receptors for vision in the retina: **rods and cones present**.
2. Name the photosensitive pigment contained in rods: **rhodopsin or visual purple**.
3. Name the components of rhodopsin: **opsin called scotopsin combined with retinene, which is the aldehyde of vitamin A (11 cis- retinaldehyde)**.
4. The photosensitive pigment of cones: **iodopsin**.
5. Name the components of iodopsin: **opsin called photopsin and retinene**.
6. Iodopsin is maximally sensitive to greenish: **yellow light of wave length 560 nm**.
7. Name the four types of neurons present in retina: **bipolar cells, ganglion cells, horizontal cells and amacrine cells**.
8. Name the neurotransmitter released by cones: **glutamic acid**.
9. Name the neurotransmitter released by horizontal cells: **GABA**.
10. Name the neurotransmitter released by amacrine cells: **acetylcholine**.
11. The axons of the ganglion cells form the optic nerve and optic tract that end in the **lateral geniculate body** in the thalamus.
12. The overall convergence of receptors through bipolar cells on ganglion cells: **105:1**.
13. Name the subcortical structures stimulated by visual stimuli: **lateral geniculate body, superior colliculus, pulvinar, caudate nucleus, putamen and claustrum**.
14. Name the vascular layer of the eye: **choroid**.
15. The area where the optic nerve leaves the eye is called **blind spot or optic disk**.
16. The area in the retina where there are only cones and no rods and blood vessels: **fovea centralis**.
17. Maximum visual acuity is obtained if the image falls on **fovea centralis**.
18. Constrictor pupillae of iris is supplied by **parasympathetic** fibers while dilator pupillae is supplied by **sympathetic** fibers.
19. Sympathetic stimulation produces **mydriasis** and parasympathetic stimulation produces **miosis** in the pupil.
20. Name the extraocular muscle supplied by fourth cranial nerve: **superior oblique**.
21. Name the extraocular muscle supplied by fourth cranial nerve: **lateral rectus**.
22. Name the cranial nerves that innervate the extraocular muscles: **3rd, 4th and 6th cranial nerves**.
23. Aqueous humor is produced by ciliary body by **diffusion** and **active transport from plasma**.
24. Aqueous humor is drained through **canal of Schlemm**.
25. The lens is held in place in the eye by the **lens suspensory ligament (zonule)**.
26. The centre point of the lens is known as its **nodal point or optical center**.
27. The **focal length** of a lens is the distance between nodal point and principal focus.
28. Normal intraocular pressure: **10–20 mm Hg**.
29. Name a degenerative condition where there is loss of retinal ganglion cells and intraocular pressure is found to be increased: **glaucoma**.
30. The condition where the lens becomes opaque: **cataract**.
31. In myopia the image is formed **in front of** the retina and is corrected by concave lens.
32. In hypermetropia, the image is formed **behind** the retina and can be corrected by **accommodation or by using convex lens**.
33. Name the condition where the accommodation of lens is reduced for near vision due to increasing hardness of lens with advancing age: **presbyopia**.
34. The changes during near response: **constriction of pupil, convergence of eyeball and change in the anterior curvature of lens (accommodation)**.
35. The process by which the curvature of lens is increased in the eye: **accommodation**.
36. Name the refractive error of eye due to altered curvature of cornea: **astigmatism**.
37. Astigmatism is corrected by **cylindrical** lens.
38. Near point of a 5 year old child: **5 cm**.
39. Deficiency of vitamin A produces **nyctalopia or night blindness** and **xerophthalmia**.

40. Receptor for dim light vision: **rod**.
41. The receptor for bright light vision and color vision: **cone**.
42. Normal refractive power of relaxed eye: **+60 D**
43. Distant vision and visual acuity is tested using **Snellen's chart**.
44. Normal visual acuity in an adult: **6/6**.
45. Ishihara's chart is used to test **color vision**.
46. Binocular vision has most important role in **depth perception**.
47. Parvocellular pathway which arise from layer 3, 4, 5 and 6 of LGB carries signals for **color vision, texture, shape and fine details**.
48. Both magnocellular and parvocellular pathways end in **layer 4** of visual cortex.
49. Clusters of cells that contain high concentration of mitochondrial cytochrome oxidase present in layer 2 and 3 of visual cortex: **blobs**.
50. Blobs are concerned with **color vision**.
51. Primary visual cortex corresponds to Brodmann's area **17**
52. Visual association area corresponds to Brodmann's area **18 and 19**
53. Amacrine cells of retina increases visual acuity by **lateral inhibition**
54. Visible range of electromagnetic spectrum: **397 nm to 723 nm**.
55. Dim light vision is referred to as **scotopic** vision and bright light vision is called **photopic vision**.
56. When light strikes the outer segment of rods and cones sodium channels close and the cells are **hyperpolarized**.
57. The decline in visual threshold in a dimly lit room is called **dark adaptation**.
58. Primary colors of vision: **red, blue and green**.
59. The **Young-Helmholtz** theory of color vision postulates the existence of three kinds of cones, each containing a different photopigment that are maximally sensitive to one of the three primary colors.
60. Area **V8** of the visual cortex appears to be uniquely concerned with color vision.
61. Color blindness caused due to lesion of area V_8 is called **achromatopsia**.
62. Blindness for red color is called **protanopia**, for green color is **deuteranopia** and for blue color is **tritanopia**.
63. Weakness for red, green and blue is referred to as **protanomaly, deuteranomaly and tritanomaly** respectively.
64. The most common form of color blindness: **deuteranomaly**.
65. Name the condition where accommodation reflex is present and pupillary reflex absent: **argyll Robertson pupil**.
66. Name one disease that produces Argyll Robertson pupil: **neurosyphilis due to lesion in the pretectal area.**
67. The technique done to map the visual fields: **perimetry**.
68. **Anopia** means complete blindness of an eye.
69. **Hemianopia** means blindness of half of the visual field.
70. Lesion of one optic nerve causes **anopia** of that eye.
71. The fibers from each nasal hemi retina decussate in the **optic chiasma**.
72. Lesion of optic tract and optic radiation of right side produces **left homonymous hemianopia**.
73. In pituitary tumors that cause destruction of the fibers from the nasal half of retina of both eyes in the region of optic chiasma produce **heteronymous hemianopia or bitemporal hemianopia**.
74. Lesion of outer margins of the optic chiasma damages fibers from the temporal half of both retina causes **binasal hemianopia**.
75. Loss of peripheral vision with intact macular vision—**macular sparing**.
76. Pupillary light reflex will be preserved if the lesion to the visual pathway is beyond the **optic tract**.
77. Lesion of visual association areas, area 18 or 19 leads to **visual agnosia**.
78. Name the four types of eye movements—**saccades, smooth pursuit movements, vestibular movements and convergence movements.**

Audition

CHAPTER 99

LEARNING OBJECTIVES
- Describe the functions of the different parts of the ear
- Mention the properties of sound waves
- Explain the mechanism of transmission of sound waves in the ear
- Explain the theories of hearing
- Mechanism of stimulation of auditory hair cells
- Explain cochlear microphonics
- Explain physiology of tympanic reflex
- Describe the auditory pathway
- Explain the types and causes of deafness and the tests used to distinguish between them
- Describe and discuss auditory evoked potential
- Mention the mechanism of hearing aids
- Draw the diagram of organ of Corti

■ INTRODUCTION

Ear has two functions, one to detect sound and the second to help us maintain balance. To accomplish this, receptors for two sensory modalities are present in the ear, **hearing and equilibrium**. The external ear, the middle ear and the cochlea of inner ear are concerned with hearing. The semicircular canals, utricle and saccule of the inner ear are concerned with equilibrium. The receptors for both hearing and equilibrium are called **hair cells**. There are six groups of hair cells in the inner ear: (1) one group in each of the semicircular canals, (2) one in the utricle, (3) one in the saccule and (4) one in the cochlea.

Hearing is a mechanoreceptor sense. Learning and past experience are necessary for normal hearing and hence it is called a **subjective sensation**. Hearing is more important than vision with respect to language development. Deafness imposes severe social and communicative disability.

■ FUNCTIONAL ANATOMY OF THE EAR

PY10.15: Describe and discuss functional anatomy of ear and auditory pathways and physiology of hearing.

Ear has three parts: (1) external ear, (2) middle ear, and (3) internal ear **(Fig. 99.1)**. The external ear collects sound waves, middle ear conveys sound vibrations to the oval window and inner ear contains the receptors for hearing and equilibrium. The ear converts sound waves in the external environment into action potentials in the auditory nerves.

External Ear
External ear consists of three parts:
1. Pinna or auricle
2. External auditory meatus
3. Tympanic membrane or ear drum

Pinna
Pinna is a flap of elastic cartilage covered with skin.

Functions of Pinna
- Direct sound waves towards the auditory canal
- Helps in localization of sound
- Amplification of sound to a small extent

External Auditory Canal
It is a curved tube which lies in the temporal bone. It channels sound waves to the tympanic membrane. It also protects the tympanic membrane from external injury. It is about 2.5 cm long, directed medially and anteriorly and ends in the tympanic membrane. It is lined by skin containing sebaceous glands and special type of glands called **ceruminous glands**. Hairs are present near the outer part of external auditory canal. *Ear wax or cerumen* is a product of secretions of ceruminous glands as well as sebaceous glands. Hair and cerumen prevent dust and insects from entering the ear. Excessive accumulation of ear wax can lead to conduction deafness.

Tympanic Membrane
The tympanic membrane (ear drum) marks the beginning of the middle ear. It is a thin, whitish glistening membrane which separates external ear from middle ear. It is 9–10 mm in diameter and 0.1 mm thick. Its outer side is lined by skin and the middle ear side by mucous membrane. Handle of malleus is attached to the inner aspect of tympanic membrane and hence it appears cone shaped. The outer surface is concave and the inner surface convex. The tympanic membrane can be visualized by an **auroscope**. A red or bulging tympanic membrane indicates middle ear disease. Perforation of the

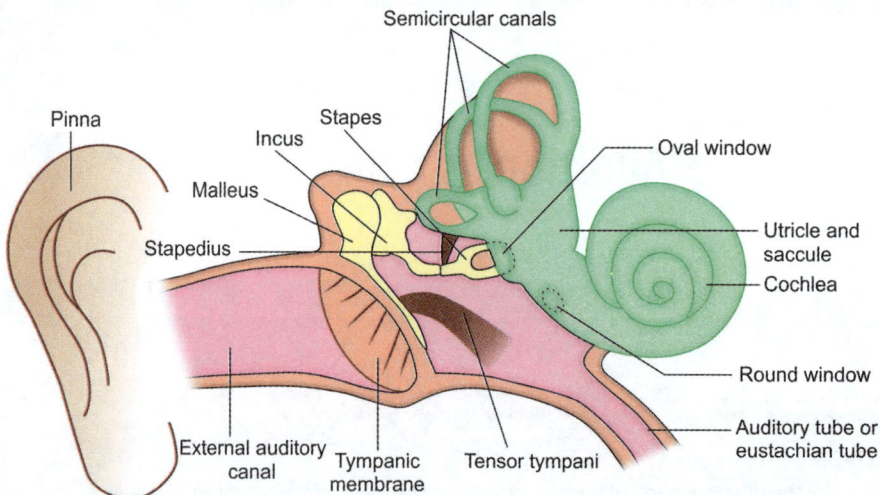

Fig. 99.1: Structures of the external, middle and inner ear.

tympanic membrane due to infection of middle ear or injury leads to hearing loss of about 5–50 dB.

Surface area of tympanic membrane is 60–70 mm², but only 3/4 of this area function physiologically, i.e., 55 mm².

When the sound wave strikes the tympanic membrane, it vibrates thus functioning as a **resonator** that reproduces the vibrations of the sound source. This vibration is transmitted through the middle ear ossicles which function as a lever system that converts the resonant vibrations of the tympanic membrane into movements of the foot plate of the stapes. The foot plate of stapes transmits the vibrations through the oval window to the fluid filled scala vestibuli in the inner ear. When the sound reaches the oval window, the sound pressure is amplified 22 times (refer 'functions of middle ear'). The vibration of the ear drum stops almost immediately when the sound wave stops.

Functions of Tympanic Membrane
* Separates middle ear from external ear
* Functions as a resonator

Middle Ear
Middle ear is the small air-filled cavity in the temporal bone. It is separated from the external ear by the ear drum and from the internal ear by a thin bony partition that contains two small membrane covered openings, the oval window and the round window. Middle ear cavity is connected to pharyngeal cavity through the **eustachian tube or auditory tube**.

Contents of the Middle Ear
* *Middle ear ossicles*: Malleus (hammer), incus (anvil) and stapes (stirrup).
* *Middle ear muscles*: Tensor tympani and stapedius.

Middle Ear Ossicles
The auditory ossicles, which are the three *smallest bones in the body* extend across the middle ear and is attached to it by ligaments. The bony attachment in the middle ear is such that it exerts a lever mechanism by which it can amplify sound waves. The **handle of malleus** (manubrium) is attached to the back of the tympanic membrane and the head of malleus is attached by ligaments to the wall of the middle ear and its short process is attached to the **incus**. The incus in turn articulates with the head of the **stapes (Fig. 99.1)**. The base or foot plate of the stapes is attached by annular ligament to the walls of the oval window of cochlea. Oval window marks the beginning of the inner ear.

When sound waves strike the tympanic membrane, it moves in and out to function as a resonator that reproduces the vibrations of the sound. The tympanic membrane movements are imparted to the manubrium of the malleus, which moves and through the short process of malleus it transmits the vibrations of manubrium to the incus. Incus in turn moves and the vibrations are transmitted to the head of stapes. This movement makes the foot plate of stapes to swing to and fro on the oval window. Thus the auditory ossicles function as a lever system that converts vibrations of the tympanic membrane into movements of the stapes against the perilymph in the scala vestibuli of cochlea. In some diseases, such as **otosclerosis**, sclerosis of the bony ossicles of middle ear occurs and the lever mechanism does not function properly leading to partial deafness.

Functions of middle ear ossicles
* Conduction of sound from external ear to internal ear
* Amplification of sound

Middle Ear Muscles
The middle ear muscles are the two small skeletal muscles, **tensor tympani** and **stapedius** attached to the malleus and stapes respectively **(Fig. 99.1)**. Tensor tympani is innervated by mandibular branch of the trigeminal nerve (V cranial nerve) and stapedius by facial nerve (VII cranial nerve). *Stapedius is the smallest of all skeletal muscles*. Loud sounds initiate reflex contraction of these muscles, dampening the movements of the ossicular chain. Contraction of tensor tympani pulls the manubrium of malleus medially and decreases the vibrations of the tympanic membrane. Contraction of stapedius muscle

pulls the foot plate of stapes out of the oval window. The reflex is called the tympanic or acoustic reflex.

Tympanic reflex or acoustic reflex: The **tensor tympani** is inserted into the handle of the malleus **(Fig. 99.1)**. When it contracts, it can tense the tympanic membrane by pulling the handle of malleus inwards and thus can reduce the amplitude of vibration of the ear drum. Thus, the ear drum is protected from injury when the pressure of sound wave is too high. It also prevents damage to the inner ear from loud noises. Stapedius is inserted into the stapes. Contraction of **stapedius** pulls the foot plate of the stapes out of the oval window towards the middle ear so that sound waves are not conducted to the internal ear. This reduces the impact on the organ of Corti in the internal ear by very loud sounds.

Contraction of both the middle ear muscles presses the ossicles against one another, thereby increasing the rigidity of the ossicular lever system. As a result, very loud sound waves are not conducted to the internal ear. When the amplitude of sound is very high, these two muscles contract reflexly and prevent entry of very loud sound into the internal ear. Thus, these muscles protect the internal ear as well as the tympanic membrane from damage due to very loud sounds of low frequency **(Flowchart 99.1)**. This reflex contraction of the middle ear muscles when the person hears a loud sound is called **tympanic reflex**. The reaction time for this reflex is 40–80 millisec and so very loud sounds very close to the ear fail to protect the inner ear. The duration from the time of application of stimulus to the time when response is obtained is called reaction time. *Sound reaching one ear elicits contralateral as well as ipsilateral reflex contraction of the middle ear muscles.*

Contraction of stapes is of much functional importance in humans since acoustic reflex is absent in paralysis of stapedius but not when diseases affect the tensor tympani. Tympanic reflex involves four neurons – *cochlear afferent neuron in the spiral ganglion, ventral cochlear nuclei, medial superior olive and the motor nuclei of V and VII cranial nerves.*

Functions of middle ear muscles

* Attenuation (attenuate means to make weaker) of loud sound through tympanic reflex in order to protect the cochlea from damaging vibrations caused by excessively loud sound.
* Middle ear muscles especially stapedius contract prior to and during vocalization, thus attenuating acoustic responses to one's own voice before as well as during vocalization. Thus, it decreases the hearing sensitivity of a person for his own speech and protects him from the disturbing effect of his own voice. This effect is activated by collateral nerve signals transmitted to these muscles at the same time when the brain activates the voice mechanism. Paralysis of the stapedius muscle is associated with **hyperacusis,** i.e., abnormally sensitive hearing.
* Middle ear muscles can also mask low-frequency sounds in a loud environment. This removes a major share of the background noise and allows a person to concentrate on sounds above 1,000 cycles/sec. Normal voice communication occur at about this frequency.
* The tensor tympani muscle keeps the tympanic membrane tense which allows sound vibrations on any portion of the tympanic membrane to be transmitted to the ear ossicles. This would not have been possible if the membrane was lax.

Eustachian Tube or Auditory Tube

The **eustachian tube** or pharyngotympanic tube or the auditory tube, which consists of both bone and hyaline cartilage, connects the middle ear cavity to the nasopharynx **(Fig. 99.1)**. It is about 4 cm long and its diameter is more (3 times) at its middle ear opening than at its nasopharyngeal opening.

Functions of Auditory Tube

* Auditory tube is responsible for equalization of pressure between the middle ear cavity and the atmosphere especially when the atmospheric pressure decreases (at high altitude) or increases (in deep sea diving). It usually remains collapsed at its pharyngeal end so that debris and infectious agents cannot pass from the oral cavity to the middle ear. The auditory tube opens during yawning, chewing, swallowing, etc., allowing air to enter or leave the middle ear until the pressure in the middle ear equals the atmospheric pressure. This is very essential for normal hearing.
* Auditory tube prevents fluid from collecting in the middle ear. It drains the fluid into the nasopharynx.

In conditions, such as common cold, infections of nasopharynx, etc., there will be obliteration of the nasopharyngeal opening of eustachian tube due to inflammation and swelling of mucosal cells. Thus, the tube fails to open even during swallowing. O_2 in the air trapped in the middle ear cavity will be absorbed by the mucosa and the middle ear pressure falls. This leads to unequal pressures on the two sides of the tympanic membrane. This causes retraction of tympanic membrane into the middle ear cavity resulting in pain in the ear and partial deafness. Infections in the nasopharynx can reach the middle ear through the eustachian tube and cause **otitis media.** At high altitudes, the air in the middle ear cavity expands if there is a block in the auditory tube, leading to discomfort in the ear.

Functions of Middle Ear

* Transmission of sound waves to the inner ear through the tympanic membrane and the ossicular chain

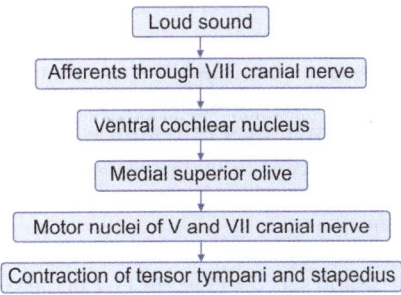

Flowchart 99.1: Mechanism of attenuation of loud sound (tympanic reflex).

- Amplification of sound and acoustic transformer function
- Impedance matching between air and fluid
- Attenuation of loud sound
- Equalization of pressure

Amplification of Sound and Acoustic Transformer Function

- In the middle ear, the force of sound waves is amplified **22 times** which is equivalent to an increase of 27 dB. This is achieved by two mechanisms.
- The surface area of oval window is only 1/17th that of the tympanic membrane. Area of tympanic membrane is 55 mm^2 and that of oval window is only 3.2 mm^2. Thus, the force of sound wave falling on tympanic membrane is amplified 17 times.
- Since the malleus is longer than the incus, the incus is displaced less than the malleus but with a greater force. Ear ossicles thus perform a lever mechanism by which sound is amplified 1.3 times (mechanical advantage of the ossicular chain is 1.3).

So, the total amplification is 17 × 1.3 = 22 times. This much amplification of sound energy is necessary for proper impedance matching. The force exerted on the fluid in the cochlea by the foot plate of stapes is about 22 times the force exerted by the sound waves against the tympanic membrane.

Fluid in the inner ear is perilymph. When sound reaches this fluid from air, there will be loss of sound energy. The sound waves tend to be reflected from the air-liquid interface due to mismatch of the mechanical properties of the two media and is called mismatching of impedance. To compensate for this loss, sound is amplified in the middle ear.

Since force = Pressure × Area, when a sound falling on the tympanic membrane with a given force is transmitted to the stapes, its pressure is much higher at the stapes. Movement of fluid in the cochlea depends on the pressure rather than force. Since the major mechanism for impedance matching is change of pressure level of sound energy, which is analogous to change in voltage of an electrical signal, the middle ear is said to function as a **transformer**.

Impedance Matching Between Air and Fluid

When sound wave is transmitted from one medium to another, which differs in their acoustic impedance (which is comparable to resistance), most of the sound energy is lost due to mismatch between the acoustic impedance of the two media. In the ear, since fluid in the cochlea has far greater inertia than air does, increased amount of force is necessary to cause vibration of the fluid. If the sound waves strike the oval window directly without passing through the ossicular chain, only 0.5% of the sound energy would have reached the fluid in the inner ear. Amplification of sound in the middle ear helps to compensate for the loss.

Because of amplification of sound in the middle ear, there is impedance matching to about 75% in the range of frequency between 300 and 3,000 Hz. Some sound energy is lost as a result of resistance and this is the reason why only 75% of sound energy incident on the tympanic membrane is transmitted to the fluid in the cochlea. Because of amplification of sound energy in the middle ear, the inner ear can be stimulated sufficiently in spite of its higher impedance. This is the reason why middle ear is said to match the impedance of the external ear to that of the inner ear.

> In **otosclerosis**, abnormal growth of middle ear bone anchors the foot plate of stapes so that it cannot move the oval window. The ossicular system becomes more rigid. Here, the bony ossicles do not vibrate and the receptors for hearing have to depend solely on the vibrations transmitted to the temporal bone through air in the middle ear. Hearing loss is severe in this case because there is very poor impedance matching between air and bone. Modern hearing aids can restore considerable hearing since they apply electromagnetically driven vibrations by placing the aid directly over a bone (usually over the mastoid process).

Attenuation of Loud Sound

This is achieved by the **tympanic reflex or acoustic reflex**. When ear is exposed to a loud sound, there is reflex contraction of tensor tympani and stapedius. Sound waves having frequency >1,000 Hz can damage the auditory receptors. So, these sounds are attenuated and thus the cochlea is protected. By tympanic reflex, the hearing sensitivity can be decreased by 30–50 dB. Since there is a latent period of about 10–15 milliseconds for reflex contraction of middle ear muscles, they cannot protect the inner ear from abrupt, unexpected sounds such as pistol shot, bomb blast, etc., which are very near to the ear.

Middle ear muscles can also mask low-frequency sounds in a loud environment. It also decreases the hearing sensitivity of a person for his own speech (*refer* 'functions of middle ear muscles').

Equalization of Pressure

Equalization of pressure is achieved by the eustachian tube which connects middle ear to nasopharynx so that the pressure on both sides of the tympanic membrane will be the same. This is very important for normal hearing. For example, if there is a block to the eustachian tube, the air in the middle ear cavity gets absorbed and the pressure falls, leading to retraction of tympanic membrane into the middle ear and discomfort.

Inner Ear or Labyrinth

Structurally inner ear has two parts:
1. Outer bony labyrinth
2. Inner membranous labyrinth

Bony labyrinth is a series of channels in the petrous part of temporal bone. It is lined by periosteum. **Membranous labyrinth** is enclosed within the bony labyrinth. It consists of a series of sacs and tubes lined by epithelium.

Endolymph which is a K$^+$ rich fluid is present inside the membranous labyrinth. **Perilymph** which is chemically similar to cerebrospinal fluid or plasma is present between membranous and bony labyrinth. Perilymph has a low concentration of K$^+$.

Labyrinthine apparatus includes cochlea, semicircular canals, utricle and saccule (**Fig. 99.1**). Cochlea is concerned

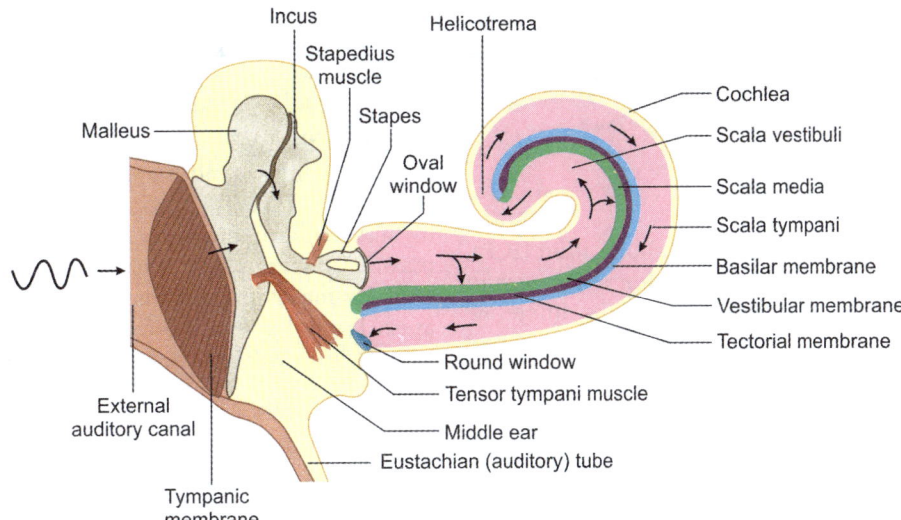

Fig. 99.2: Structure of middle ear and uncoiled cochlea. Note the transmission of sound waves through the ear denoted by arrows.

with hearing and the other three structures, collectively called the vestibular apparatus are concerned with maintenance of equilibrium.

Cochlea

Cochlea has the shape of a snail and hence the name. It is a coiled tube wound round a central bony structure called **modiolus**. It takes 2 and 3/4 turns from base to apex. If the tube is elongated, it has a length of 35 mm and diameter 3 mm. The coiled structure has three compartments or scalae separated by two membranes which stretch from the upper surface of spiral lamina (a bony edge projecting from the modiolus) to the bony wall. The two membranes fuse towards the apex of the cochlea **(Fig. 99.2)**. The membranes are:

1. **Vestibular membrane or Reissner's membrane** which separates scala vestibuli from scala media.
2. **Basilar membrane** (BM) forms the partition between scala media and scala tympani.

The three compartments are:
1. Scala vestibuli
2. Scala media or cochlear duct
3. Scala tympani

The functional interphase between middle ear and inner ear is provided by two small openings in the temporal bone, the **oval window and the round window**. The foot plate of stapes fits into the oval window. The scala tympani end at the **round window** which is closed by the flexible **secondary tympanic membrane** at the base of the cochlea. Wedged between these two spiraling canals, i.e., scala vestibuli and scala tympani is the scala media or **cochlear duct**. At the base of the cochlea the scala media is connected to the saccule through the ductus reuniens. The BM constitutes the partition between scala media and scala tympani. The **vestibular membrane or Reissner's membrane** separates scala vestibuli from scala media and it is a very thin membrane. The only function of vestibular membrane is to separate the perilymph in the scala vestibuli from endolymph in scala media.

Displacement of oval window against fluid in scala vestibuli is compensated by the reciprocal displacement of the secondary tympanic membrane of the round window into the middle ear cavity **(Fig. 99.3)**. Thus, the secondary tympanic membrane plays an important role in the proper vibration of the BM.

The scala vestibuli and scala tympani connect freely with one another via a wide opening at the apex of the cochlear spiral, the **helicotrema (Fig. 99.3)**. These two chambers contain perilymph, which resembles cerebrospinal fluid or extracellular fluid (ECF) in composition (high Na^+ and low K^+). The scala media does not communicate with the other two chambers of the cochlea. It ends blindly at the apex of the cochlea and contains endolymph which bathes the acoustic neuroepithelium. Endolymph has a distinctive

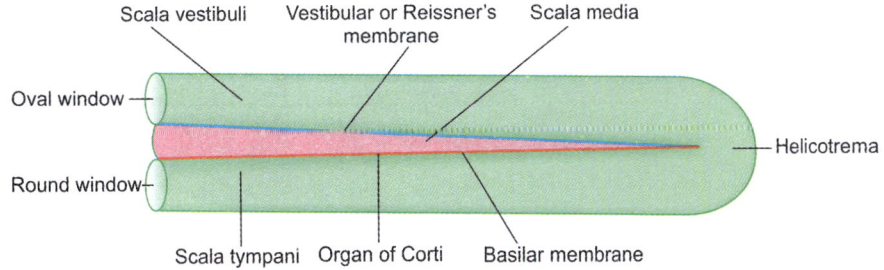

Fig. 99.3: Compartments of cochlea; scala vestibuli, scala media and scala tympani.

Table 99.1: Composition of ions in mEq/L in the different compartments of cochlea.			
Ion	Scala tympani	Scala media	Scala vestibuli
Na⁺	150	1	150
K⁺	5	150	3
Cl⁻	125	130	125

chemical composition similar to intracellular fluid (ICF), being relatively higher in K⁺ concentration and lower in Na⁺, Cl⁻ and protein content **(Table 99.1)**. This difference in electrolyte and protein composition is established and maintained by the vascular structure called **stria vascularis** which lies along the outer wall of the scala media. The scala media communicates with the saccule (which also contains endolymph) through a minute canal called **Hensen's duct** or canalis reunions.

The difference in chemical composition between endolymph and perilymph creates a steady potential across the BM, approximately double that across ordinary cell membranes. The cochlea including the stria vascularis receives autonomic innervation. Autonomic sympathetic fibers release norepinephrine to control the vascular supply.

Basilar Membrane

The BM constitutes the partition between scala media and scala tympani. It becomes broader towards the apex of the cochlea and it becomes progressively less stiff towards the apex. It is 32 mm long and 40–80 μm wide at the base and 500 μm wide at the apex of the cochlea.

The BM is a sheet of radially oriented collagen fibers of varying lengths stretched between bony partitions that extends partway across the cochlea from its origin in the bony modiolus, to the outer wall of cochlea. *The differences between the two ends of the BM is that it is narrow, thick and stiff at the base and wide, thin and relatively flaccid at the apex.* The elastic fibers of BM are thick and short at the base of the cochlea (portion closer to the oval window), whereas at the apex they are long and slender.

Almost all the sound energy transmitted to the cochlea is absorbed by the BM near its stiff basal region, i.e., the base of cochlea responds to all frequencies of sound stimuli while the apex responds only to low frequencies of sound. Each segment of the BM is tuned for a particular frequency (pitch). High-frequency sound is appreciated at the base and low-frequency sound is appreciated at the apex of the BM. The highest audible frequency of 20,000 Hz makes the BM vibrate maximally near its base while the lowest audible frequency of 20 Hz makes the membrane vibrate maximally near its apex. The BM does not oscillate in response to waves with frequencies lower than 20 Hz.

Organ of Corti

Basilar membrane contains the sense organ for hearing called the **organ of Corti (Fig. 99.4)**. The organ of Corti also takes a spiral turn and hence called spiral organ of Corti and it extends from the apex to the base of the cochlea. It bears the **acoustic neuroepithelium**, which has special receptors for hearing (auditory receptors) called **hair cells** surrounded by supporting cells (phalangeal cells). Hair cells are modified cuboidal epithelial cells. The tip of each hair cell consists of 30–100 stereocilia that extend into the endolymph in the scala media. **Stereocilia** are long hair like microvilli arranged in several rows of graded height. They have cores composed of parallel filaments of actin.

The components of the organ of Corti include hair cells, afferent and efferent nerve terminals, supporting cells, rods of Corti, BM, tectorial membrane and reticular lamina **(Fig. 99.4)**.

There are two types of auditory receptors:
1. Outer hair cells
2. Inner hair cells

Outer hair cells are 20,000 in number, arranged in 3 rows and each hair cell has about 100 **stereocilia**. Inner hair cells are 3,500 in number arranged in a single row and have only 50 stereocilia or hairs per receptor. (Differences between inner hair cells and outer hair cells are given in **Table 99.2**).

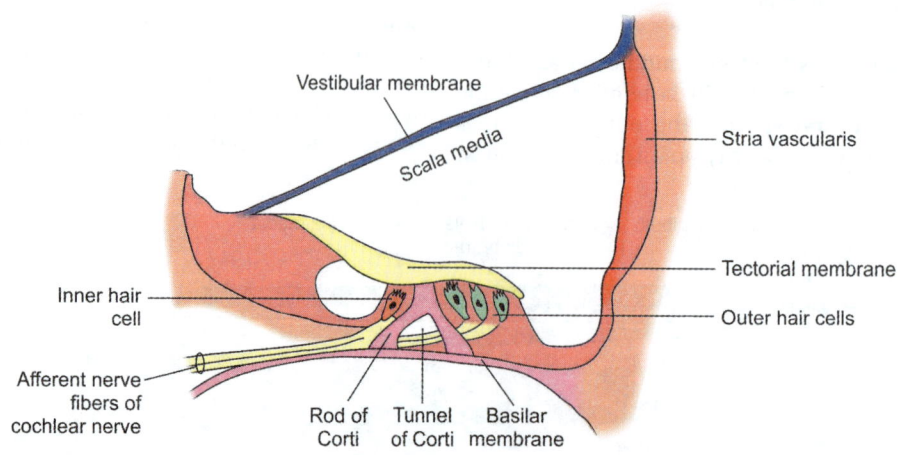

Fig. 99.4: Organ of Corti.

Table 99.2: Differences between inner hair cells and outer hair cells in the organ of Corti.

Outer hair cells	Inner hair cells
Arranged lateral to the tunnel of Corti and each cell is tube shaped	Arranged medial to tunnel of Corti and are flask shaped
About 20,000 in number arranged in 3 to 4 rows	About 3,500 in number arranged in a single row
About 100 stereocilia per hair cell	About 50 stereocilia per hair cell
Embedded in the thin, viscous, elastic tectorial membrane	Not embedded in the tectorial membrane
Only 5% of sensory nerves innervate outer hair cells	Receives 90–95% of sensory innervation
One sensory nerve fiber (afferent fibers) innervates several outer hair cells	One sensory nerve fiber innervates single inner hair cell
90% of efferent nerve fibers supply outer hair cell	Receives only 10% of efferent nerve supply
Function is to control the sensitivity of inner hair cell	Function is auditory perception and discrimination
Outer hair cells when depolarized do not generate action potentials in the afferent fiber, instead they shorten and amplify sound vibrations reaching inner ear	Inner hair cell when depolarized generates action potentials in the afferent nerve

In each hair cell the stereocilia increases progressively in height. Very fine processes called **tiplinks** connect the tip of each stereocilium to the side of its higher neighbor where there are mechanically sensitive cation channels in the taller process. When the shorter stereocilia move towards the taller ones, the channels open. K⁺ and Ca²⁺ in the endolymph enter via the channel into the hair cell and induce depolarization (*refer* **Fig. 89.4**). A myosin based molecular motor in the taller stereocilia moves the channels towards the base, releasing tension in the tiplink. This causes the channel to close and restores the resting state.

The K⁺ that enters the hair cells via the cation channel is recycled. It enters the supporting cells and eventually reaches the stria vascularis and is secreted back into the endolymph. K⁺ is the most abundant cation in the endolymph.

On the BM, the hair cells are arranged in such a way that outer hair cells are arranged lateral to a structure called **tunnel of Corti**. The inner hair cells are arranged medial to the tunnel of Corti **(Fig. 99.4)**. Tunnel of Corti is a triangular space formed by two **rods of Corti or pillar cells**. They are pillar-like structures found in the BM which supports a tough membrane called **reticular lamina**. The processes of the hair cells pierce the reticular lamina. (According to some authors, reticular lamina is the surface formed by the tight junctions, which connect the hair cells and the supporting cells to one another at their apices. The hairs of the hair cells seem to project out of the reticular lamina.) The hairs at the tip of outer hair cells are embedded in the thin, viscous but elastic **tectorial membrane** while, the hairs of the inner hair cells remain free **(Fig. 99.4)**.

*The entire assembly of the BM, the tectorial membrane, the tunnel of Corti, supporting cells and the hair cells with their sensory afferents is called the **spiral organ of Corti**.*

Tight junctions between the hair cells and the adjacent supporting cells prevent endolymph from reaching the bases of the hair cells. But the BM is permeable to perilymph in the scala tympani and so, the tunnel of Corti and the bases of the hair cells below the tight junctions are bathed in perilymph. Hence, there is a very high potential difference between the upper and lower surfaces of the hair cells.

Innervation of the Hair Cells

Maximum sensory innervation is to the inner hair cells, i.e., about 90–95% of sensory neurons (**afferent fibers** in the auditory nerve) innervate the inner hair cells. Each inner hair cell receives one sensory nerve fiber, whereas one sensory nerve fiber innervates many outer hair cells. The inner hair cells when depolarized release glutamate which in turn generates action potentials in the afferent nerve fiber. On the other hand, the outer hair cells when depolarized do not generate action potentials in the afferent fiber. Instead a membrane motor protein called **prestin** present in it makes them shorten. Hyperpolarization makes them lengthen and this action increases the amplitude and clarity of sounds. Thus the outer hair cells amplify sound vibrations entering the inner ear from the middle ear. The axons of the afferent neurons that innervate the hair cells form the auditory (cochlear) division of the eighth cranial nerve.

The hair cells also receive **efferent fibers** through the cochlear division of the VIII cranial nerve. 90% *of the efferent fibers in the auditory nerve synapse on the outer hair cells rather than the inner hair cells.* The **olivocochlear bundle** forms the efferent fibers which arise from the superior olivary complex in the brain stem. They end around the bases of the outer hair cells. Acetyl choline is the neurotransmitter released and the activity of the efferent fibers modulates the sensitivity of the hair cells. The effect is inhibition and the function is to block background noise so that the other sounds can be heard clearly.

The inner hair cells are mainly involved in auditory perception and discrimination. The outer hair cells are believed to control the sensitivity of inner hair cells to sound. Both inner hair cell and outer hair cell contribute to integrated responses in auditory afferents.

PHYSIOLOGY OF HEARING OR AUDITION

Sound

Sound is the sensation produced when longitudinal alternate condensation and rarefaction of the molecules of the external environment strike the tympanic membrane. Sound waves originate from a vibrating object. Sound never travels through vacuum. The medium can be air, liquid or solid.

Velocity of sound in air is 344 m/sec at 20°C at sea level. Velocity increases when density of medium increases. The speed of sound increases with temperature and altitude.

Properties of Sound

- ❖ Frequency (determines the pitch of sound)
- ❖ Amplitude or intensity (determines the loudness of sound).

Frequency of Sound

Frequency of sound is the number of waves per unit time or it is the number of waves produced in 1 sec. Unit of frequency is **cycles/sec or Hertz (Hz) (Fig. 99.5A)**. **Pitch** or tone of the sound is the psychophysiological appreciation of frequency and it is directly related to its frequency. *The greater the frequency, higher will be the pitch. The greater the amplitude louder will be the sound.* Although the pitch of a sound depends primarily on the frequency of the sound wave, loudness also plays a part. Duration also affects pitch to a small extent. The pitch of a tone cannot be perceived unless it lasts for more than 0.01 second and the pitch rises as the duration increases to 0.1 second.

Sound waves contain a mixture of different frequencies. If there is only one frequency, it is called **pure tone**. If it is a mixture of different frequencies, then it is called a **complex tone (Fig. 99.5B)**. Complex waves form the basis of quality or **timbre** of sound waves. Repetition of complex tone at periodic intervals is **music (Fig. 99.5C)**. If complex tone occurs at irregular intervals, it is **noise (Fig. 99.5D)**.

In musical sound, the wave with the minimum frequency is called the **fundamental frequency**. The high frequency waves are called **harmonics or overtones** which are multiples of fundamental frequency. Fundamental frequency determines the pitch of the sound and overtones determines the quality or timbre of sound. Variations in timbre allow us to distinguish the sounds of different musical instruments even though they are playing notes of the same pitch. A person can differentiate approximately 2,000 pitches this is more in musicians.

Audible frequency for human ear is 20-20,000 cycles/ sec. During normal aging, sensitivity to higher frequencies is gradually lost and by middle age hearing is limited to less than 5,000 Hz.

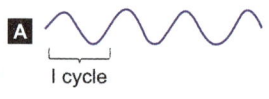

Figs. 99.5A to D: Characteristics of sound wave: (A) Pure tone; (B) Complex tone; (C) Music; (D) Noise.

Pitch discrimination is maximal between the frequency ranges 1,000–3,000 cycles/sec and is poor at high and low frequencies. This is because maximum amplification of sound occurs in the middle ear at this frequency range.

During normal conversation, the frequency range is between 200 and 4,500 Hz. The pitch of average male voice in conversation is about 120 Hz and that of average female voice is about 250 Hz. An average man can distinguish about 2,000 pitches and it is still higher for musicians.

*Frequency greater than 20,000 Hz is called **ultrasonic sound** and sounds having frequencies less than 20 Hz are called **infrasonic sounds**.*

Amplitude or Intensity of Sound

Intensity or amplitude of sound determines the loudness of sound. When the sound waves reach the tympanic membrane, they exert some amount of pressure on the tympanic membrane. The tympanic membrane can respond to very low sound energy as well as to massive sound pressure without any damage to the ear.

Unit of measurement of intensity of sound is **Bel** after **Alexander Graham Bel**, the inventor of telephone. The intensity of sound in Bel is the logarithm of the ratio of the intensity of that sound and a standard sound. 1/10 of a Bel is **decibel (dB)** and it is taken as the unit of intensity in hearing. The minimum pressure for hearing is 0.0002 dyne/cm² at 20°C which corresponds to 0 dB as adopted by the **Acoustical Society of America**. A value of 0 dB does not mean the absence of sound but it denotes a sound level of intensity equal to that of the standard. Each 10 dB represents a 10-fold increase in sound intensity.

$$1 \text{ Bel} = \log \frac{\text{Intensity of a given sound}}{\text{Intensity of the standard sound}}$$

Hearing Threshold

Lowest intensity that will give just the sound sensation is known as **threshold intensity** which varies with the frequency (pitch) of sound. The greatest sensitivity is in the 1,000–3,000 Hz range. Hearing threshold is the point at which an average young adult can just distinguish sound from silence. It is 0 dB at a frequency of 1,000 Hz.

From **Table 99.3**, it is clear that 120 dB is the limit of tolerance of the human ear. Continued exposure to high intensity sounds is one cause of deafness. The louder the

Table 99.3: Intensity of different types of sounds.	
Type of sound	Intensity (dB)
Just audible sound	0
Whispering sound	30
Normal conversation	60
Heavy traffic	90
Sound producing slight pain in the ear	120
Sound which is extremely painful to the ear	>140
Sound that damages the tympanic membrane	200–300

sound, the more rapid is the hearing loss. Animals, such as dogs, bats, etc., can appreciate ultrasonic sound.

MECHANISM OF HEARING

Ear acts as a **transducer**. It converts mechanical energy (sound) to electrical impulses in the auditory nerve which reaches the auditory cortex, where sound is appreciated.

* When sound waves strike the eardrum, it vibrates. This vibration is transmitted through the ear ossicles to the oval window.
* The oval window vibrates 22 times more vigorously than the ear drum due to amplification of sound energy in the middle ear.
* As the oval window bulges inwards, it pushes on the perilymph in the scala vestibuli.
* This pressure wave pushes the vestibular membrane back and forth creating pressure waves in the endolymph in the scala media.
* This cause the BM to vibrate, which moves the hair cells of the organ of Corti against the tectorial membrane by creating a shearing force between BM and tectorial membrane.
* This produces receptor potentials in the hair cells that ultimately lead to the generation of nerve impulses in the auditory nerve.
* The impulses reach the auditory cortex and we appreciate the sound.

Effects of Displacement of Basilar Membrane

The upper part of hair cells in the organ of Corti is held rigid by the **reticular lamina** which is a tough membrane into which the processes of the hair cells pierce. The hairs (stereocilia) of the outer hair cells are embedded in the **tectorial membrane** which is a thin, viscous, elastic membrane which has a free border. On the BM, rods of Corti and reticular lamina function as a single unit. Depending on the intensity of displacement of BM, the reticular lamina is displaced. When the stapes moves inwards, the pressure in the perilymph of scala vestibuli increases and this depresses the Reissner's membrane which in turn depresses the BM **(Fig. 99.6)**. When the stapes move outwards the BM moves upward. The up and down movements of the BM produce movements of the hair cells of the organ of Corti in different directions.

When the stapes moves, both tectorial membrane and reticular membrane move in the same direction. But they are hinged on different axes, so there is a **shearing motion** that bends the stereocilia leading to stimulation of the hair cells. The hairs of the inner hair cells are probably not attached to the tectorial membrane, but they are apparently bent by the movement of fluid between the tectorial membrane and the underlying hair cells.

When the BM is displaced downwards, reticular lamina is also displaced downwards and outwards, whereas when BM is displaced upwards, the reticular lamina moves upwards and inwards.

The outward and inward movement of reticular lamina produces a shearing force on the hair cells where they are embedded in the tectorial membrane. Because of the high potential difference between the endolymph and the interior of the hair cell, changes in membrane conductance induced by shearing force is accompanied by rapid flux of ions. This generates a receptor potential that initiates release of neurotransmitter at the synaptic junctions between hair cells and the afferent nerve terminals. This initiates action potential in the cochlear nerve which is propagated **(Flowchart 99.2)**.

Displacements of fluid in the scala tympani due to depression of BM into the fluid will be dissipated into the air at the round window.

Endocochlear Potential

The hair cells are already sensitized because the tips of the hairs are dipping into endolymph. Stria vascularis secretes K^+ continuously into scala media. One of the K^+ channel proteins in the stria vascularis called **KVLQT1** is essential for maintaining the high K^+ concentration in the endolymph. The potential difference existing between perilymph in the scala vestibuli and scala tympani and endolymph in scala media is +80 mV. The scala media is electrically positive by 80 mV relative to scala vestibuli and scala tympani. This potential difference is called **endolymphatic potential** or **endocochlear potential**. Endocochlear potential is

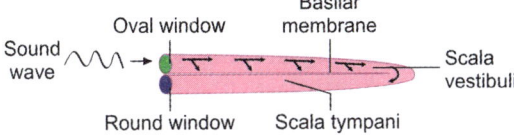

Fig. 99.6: Displacement of basilar membrane by sound energy.

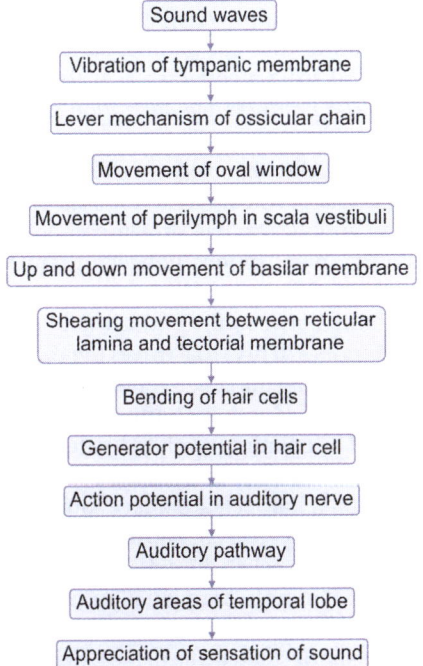

Flowchart 99.2: Physiology of hearing.

generated by continual secretion of K⁺ into the scala media by stria vascularis.

The endocochlear potential is given a positive sign showing that the endolymph is positive with respect to perilymph. The endocochlear potential is abolished by anoxia, blocking of circulation to stria vascularis or when cyanide is injected into the endolymph.

The potential difference between the ICF of hair cell and perilymph is –70 mV. Inside of the cell is more negative than outside. The interior of the hair cell is strongly negative with respect to the endolymph. The potential difference between interior of the hair cell and tip of hair cell which is bathed in endolymph is –150 mV. Hence, the opening of ion channels results in an influx of K^+ from the endolymph into the cells, for which there is a marked electrical gradient even though there is no significant concentration gradient.

The base of the hair cell is bathed in perilymph. The hair cells have a negative intracellular potential of –70 mV with respect to perilymph, but –150 mV with respect to the endolymph at their upper surfaces where the hairs are dipped in endolymph. The high potential difference at the tip of the hair cell (where the stereocilia are located) and the base of the hair cell makes the cell very sensitive. This increases the ability of the hair cell to respond to the slightest sound.

Receptor Potential and Genesis of Action Potentials in Afferent Nerve Fibers

Maximum sensory innervation is to the inner hair cells. Innervation is diffuse for the outer hair cells. Discrimination of sound is mainly by inner hair cell. The hair cells are already sensitized. The potential difference existing between the interior of hair cell and tip of hair is –150 mV. Minimal bending at the tip can stimulate the hair cells and action potentials are transmitted through the cochlear division of VIII cranial nerve.

When pressure is applied against the oval window by inward motion of the foot plate of stapes, fluid in the scala vestibuli and scala media displaces the BM. *Upward displacement of BM produces depolarization and downward displacement produces hyperpolarization of hair cells.*

Bending of hair cells when BM is moved upwards causes some change in the permeability of the cell. Since the ICF of hair cell and endolymph has similar composition, there is no diffusion gradient of ions between them. When the transduction channels open, it is the large potential difference of 150 mV existing between the endolymph (+80 mV) and the hair cell interior (–70 mV) that drives the cations into the stereocilia, depolarizing the cell. K^+ enters the interior of the hair cell through **transduction channels** in the stereocilia, which is followed by opening of voltage-gated Ca^{2+} channels and Ca^{2+} enters the cell.

Rows of cilia on a hair cell are linked laterally. Very fine processes called **tiplinks** (Ch 89, **Fig. 89.4**) tie the tip of each stereocilium of the hair cell to the side of its higher neighbor. There are cation channels (transduction channels) in the higher stereocilium at the junction that are **mechanically gated**. When the shorter stereocilia of the hair cell are pushed towards the longer ones, the membrane potential is decreased to –50 mV from –70 mV and the cell gets depolarized. This generates a receptor potential that initiates release of neurotransmitter, glutamate at the synaptic junction between hair cell and the afferent nerve terminal. This initiates action potential in the cochlear afferents. *The inner hair cells are the primary sensory cells that generate action potential in the auditory nerve.*

The K^+ that enters the hair cell is recycled. It enters the sustentacular cells and through gap junctions in the sustentacular cells eventually reaches the stria vascularis and is secreted back into the endolymph, completing the cycle. The efflux of K^+ restores the hair cell to its resting potential. The Ca^{2+} that enters the cell during depolarization is pumped out to the exterior by a Ca^{2+} pump.

Whereas when the hairs are pushed in the opposite direction (shorter one away from the longer one), the cell is hyperpolarized. That is, when BM moves downwards, resting permeability of K^+ is decreased and causes hyperpolarization.

> The conduction of sound waves to the inner ear via the tympanic membrane and ear ossicles is called **air conduction or ossicular conduction**. Transmission of vibrations of the bones of the skull to the fluid of the inner ear is called **bone conduction**. Extremely loud sounds and vibrations as that of tuning fork applied directly to the skull occur by bone conduction.

MECHANISM OF APPRECIATION OF FREQUENCY, INTENSITY AND LOCALIZATION OF SOUND

Mechanism of Appreciation of Frequency of Sound Waves

Vibrations delivered to the oval window through the stapes directly impact fluid in the scala vestibuli. To reach the round window, the kinetic energy must pass along two membranes, vestibular membrane and BM.

Theories of Hearing and Pitch Discrimination

Each auditory nerve fiber gets maximally stimulated at a particular frequency and the pathways from the various parts of the cochlea to the brain are separate. Frequency of the sound waves determines the pitch.

Many theories have been postulated to explain the mechanism of hearing and pitch discrimination. The important are:
❖ Traveling wave theory
❖ Telephone theory of Rutherford
❖ Resonance theory of Helmholtz
❖ Volley theory

Of the various theories put forward, *traveling wave theory is the most accepted one.*

Traveling Wave Theory or Place Theory

Traveling wave theory was put forward by **George Von Bekesy** in 1960 and he got Nobel Prize for physiology or medicine for his study. When sound waves reach the oval window, they are

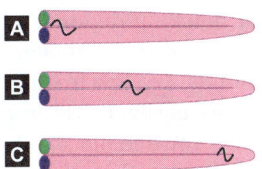

Figs. 99.7A to C: Sites of maximum displacement of basilar membrane: (A) By high frequency sound waves; (B) Medium frequency; (C) Low frequency sound waves.

transmitted to scala vestibuli. The movement of stapes is so fast that the vibrations are imparted on the BM and causes displacement of BM (**Figs. 99.7A to C**). The initial part of BM is the first part that is displaced. This produces elastic tension on the base of BM which in turn produces a wave in the BM. The pattern of vibration of the BM shows a traveling wave of transverse displacement similar to the movement seen on shaking a piece of ribbon from one end. *The transverse wave that travels along the BM in response to the pressure wave in the scala vestibuli is called the traveling wave.*

The traveling wave set up by a particular tone produces peak depression of the BM at that point which is tuned to that particular frequency and consequently maximal receptor stimulation occurs at this point of cochlea. The distance from the stapes to this point of maximum height varies with the frequency of the vibrations initiating the wave. High-pitched sounds generate waves that reach maximum height near the base of the cochlea. Low-pitched (low frequency) sounds generate waves that peak near the apex of cochlea (**Figs. 99.7 and 99.8**). The pathways from the various parts of cochlea to the brain are distinct. There are different areas in the auditory cortex that can respond to different frequencies of sound.

If the hair cells at the base of the cochlea are destroyed, appreciation of high frequency sound is completely lost which proves that the base of the cochlea responds to high frequency sounds.

> According to **place theory**, the entire cochlea is a tuned structure, with different parts of the BM responding to different frequencies. The basal part of the BM is the narrowest part which has the greatest stiffness and responds best to high frequencies. The apical part near the helicotrema is the widest part and is less stiff and responds best to low frequency. According to this theory, discrimination of pitch is a function of cochlea.

Telephone Theory

Telephone or frequency theory was put forward by Rutherford in 1886. According to this theory, the BM vibrates as a whole at the same frequency as the sound wave and sets up action potentials of the same frequency. Since this is similar to the diaphragm of a telephone, it is called telephone theory. This theory was not accepted because nerve fibers cannot transmit impulses faster than 1,000/sec due to refractory period.

Resonance Theory

According to the **resonance theory**, there are a series of resonators in the cochlea each responding to a different frequency. The shorter fibers at the base of the BM respond to higher frequencies and the longer fibers at the apex respond to lower frequencies.

Volley Principle

From the place theory it is difficult to explain the mechanism of appreciation of very low frequency sound waves, i.e., less than 2,000 cycles/sec. These low frequencies have been postulated to be discriminated by volley or frequency principle. Since the auditory nerve has a very large number of fibers, impulses are discharged over separate fibers as a scattered volley, so that a group of fibers may discharge at a particular frequency.

When the frequency is low, the nerve fibers begin to respond with one impulse to each cycle of a sound wave. Low frequency sounds from 20 to 2,000 cycles/sec can cause volleys of nerve impulses at the same frequencies in the cochlear nerve which is transmitted into the cochlear nuclei of the brain. Cochlear nuclei can distinguish the different frequencies of the volleys. This is called **volley principle of frequency discrimination**.

*Thus, traveling wave theory is responsible for the discrimination of sound frequencies from 2,000 to 20,000 Hz and volley principle accounts for the discrimination of sound frequencies from 20 to 2,000 Hz. Together it is called **duplex theory of pitch discrimination**.*

Mechanisms of Appreciation of Intensity (Loudness) of Sound

- By increasing or decreasing the number of nerve fibers stimulated.
- Different intensities produce different frequencies of sounds. There are different areas in the auditory cortex that can respond to different frequencies of sound.

The frequency of firing in an auditory nerve fiber increases as the intensity of the sound wave increases. As the sound becomes louder, the amplitude of vibration of the BM increases and a large portion of the BM is vibrated. It causes stimulation of more and more hair cells so that more auditory nerve fibers are stimulated. This causes spatial summation of impulses, i.e., transmission through many nerve fibers rather than through only a few. Normally, the outer hair cells are not stimulated but when the intensity of vibration of BM becomes very high, the outer hair cells become stimulated. Stimulation of the outer hair cells informs the nervous system that the sound is loud.

Thus sound intensity is discriminated by the frequency of impulses in the afferent nerve fiber and also by the number of afferent nerve fibers in the auditory nerve that are stimulated.

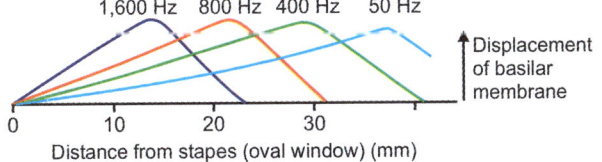

Fig. 99.8: Mechanism of appreciation of frequency of sound waves: Traveling wave theory.

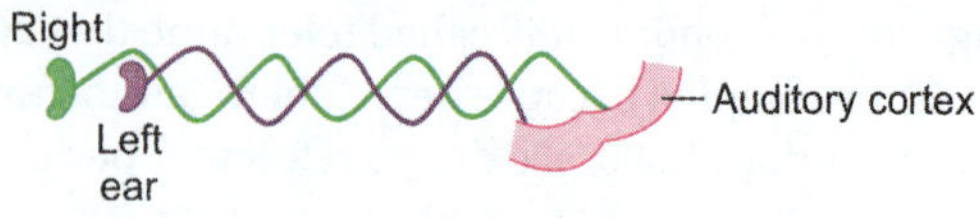

Fig. 99.9: Time lag mechanism of localization of sound.

Localization of Sound

A person is able to locate the source of sound by three mechanisms:

1. *Time lag mechanism*: The direction, from which a sound comes in the horizontal plane, depends on the difference in the time between the arrivals of the sound stimulus in the two ears. For example, when the source of sound is from the right, the hair cells in the organ of Corti on the right side are stimulated earlier than that of the left. Eventually, the action potentials from right cochlear nerve reach brain earlier. This helps to locate the direction from which the sound comes **(Fig. 99.9)**. Slight differences in the timing of impulses coming from the two ears to the olivary nuclei allow us to locate the source of the sound. The detectable time difference is said to be the most important factor at frequencies below 3,000 Hz.

2. Difference in the **intensity** of sound: The sound is louder on the side closest to the source. Intensity or loudness of sound reaching the right ear in the above example is more than that in the left ear. Loudness difference plays an important role at frequencies above 3,000 Hz.

3. Sounds coming from front of the individual differ in quality from those coming from behind. If sound is reaching exactly at an area in between the two ears, its direction cannot be localized without moving the head. Normally, a person rotates his head reflexly to locate the sound. Pinna also plays an important role in locating the sound in the vertical plane. Reflections of the sound waves from the pinnal surface change as sounds move up or down.

Masking

Masking is a phenomenon by which presence of one sound decreases an individual's ability to hear other sounds. Weaker sounds are completely inaudible in the presence of loud sounds. This is due to refractoriness of previously stimulated auditory receptors and nerve fibers to other stimuli. The degree of masking depends on the pitch of sounds. Low frequency sounds have greater masking effect than high frequency sounds, i.e., low frequency tones mask high frequency tones more easily. For example, we have to raise our voice in a noisy, crowded place to become audible to another person. Masking tends to be greater for tones of approximately similar frequency than for tones widely different in frequency. The Weber and Schwabach's tests demonstrate the important masking effect of environmental noise on the auditory threshold.

■ AUDITORY PATHWAY

Receptors are the hair cells in the organ of Corti.

First order neurons in the spiral ganglion in the modiolus are bipolar cells. Each has a short dendrite ending on hair cells and a long central process which goes as the cochlear division of VIII cranial nerve **(Fig. 99. 10)**.

Second order neurons are in the cochlear nuclei.

Further order neurons are in the trapezoid body, superior olivary nuclei, nucleus of lateral lemniscus, inferior colliculi and medial geniculate body of thalamus.

From medial geniculate body, the final order neurons arise and terminate in the area 41 of temporal lobe which is called **primary auditory cortex**. Each auditory cortex receives extensive connections from both the ears.

Axons of the afferent neurons (first order neurons) in the spiral ganglion go in a group, forming auditory nerve or **cochlear nerve** which passes through the axis of the modiolus. The fibers enter medulla and end in the second order neurons of the **dorsal and ventral cochlear nuclei** in the upper part of medulla on the same side **(Fig. 99.11)**. Majority of fibers arising from here, cross to the opposite side and reach the **trapezoid body**. The trapezoid body is formed by decussating auditory fibers in the medulla. From the trapezoid body, fibers project to the **superior olivary nucleus** in pons. Most of the fibers relay here. Slight differences in the timing of impulses coming from the two ears to the olivary nuclei allow us to locate the source of the sound. Fibers that have not crossed to the opposite side go to the ipsilateral olivary nucleus and relay there. Thus, the superior olivary nuclei receive inputs from both ears.

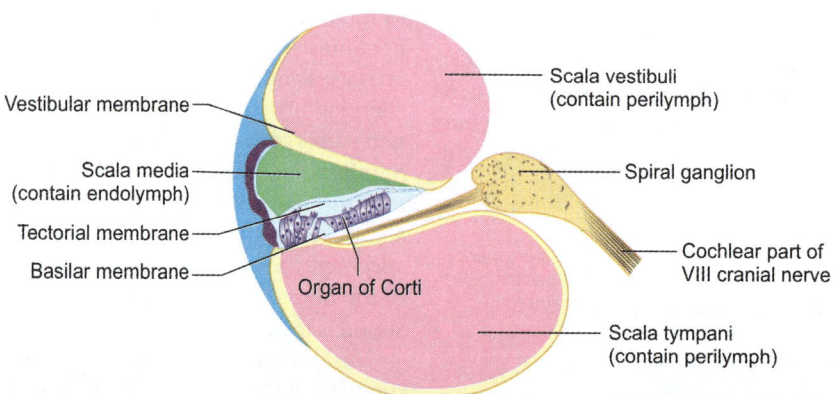

Fig. 99.10: Section through cochlea.

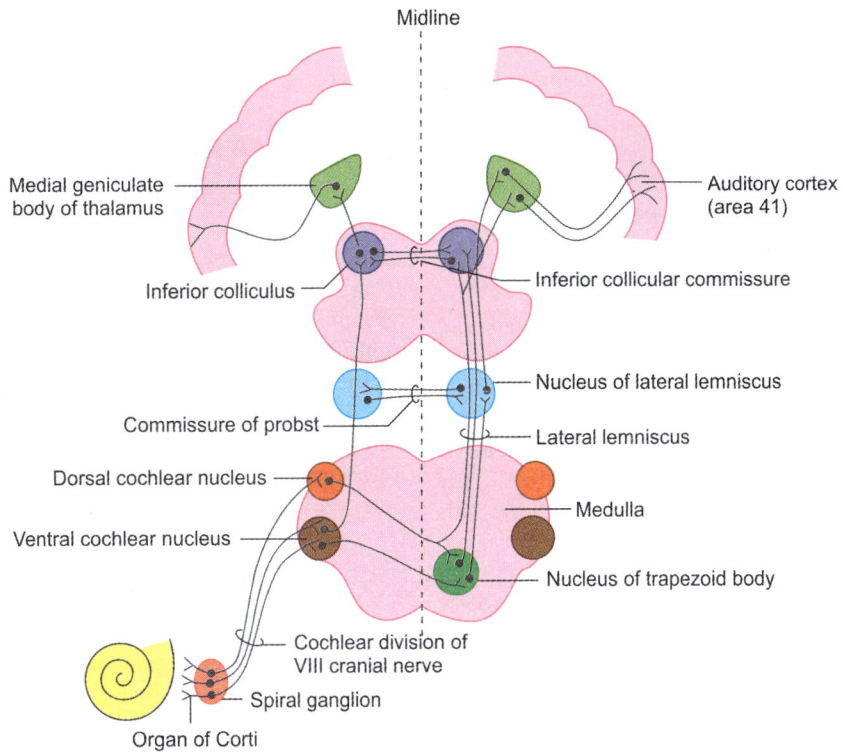

Fig. 99.11: Auditory pathway.

The ascending auditory projections pass through pons and midbrain as a major dense bundle called **lateral lemniscus**. A number of nuclei are scattered along the path of lateral lemniscus just below the level of inferior colliculus. Some ascending fibers relay in the **nucleus of lateral lemniscus** and the rest reach the **inferior colliculus** (center for auditory reflexes) and synapse there. Some cells in the lateral lemniscal nuclei cross the midline to ascend to the inferior colliculus on the opposite side. They also send collaterals to contralateral lateral lemniscal nuclei. These crossing fibers constitute the **commissure of Probst**. *The inferior colliculus has the highest metabolic rate per unit weight of any region in the nervous system.*

Many contralateral fibers in the auditory pathway pass directly into the reticular activating system of brain stem.

From the inferior colliculus, fibers reach the **medial geniculate body** of the thalamus. All the auditory fibers relay in the medial geniculate body. From here, fibers project to the primary **auditory cortex** in the **superior temporal gyrus** (Brodmann's area 41) of the cerebral cortex. Both ears have representation on both sides of auditory cortex. In the primary auditory cortex, the anterior part receives impulses arising from the apex of the cochlea (low frequency sounds) and the posterior part of the gyrus receives impulses arising from the base of the cochlea (high frequencies).

The primary auditory cortex projects to the **auditory association area** or area 42 (**Flowchart 99.3**) in the temporal lobe. With the help of the auditory association area, sounds are interpreted and given proper meaning and recognition. Fibers also reach the Wernicke's area (area 22) located behind areas 41 and 42 in the superior temporal gyrus in

Flowchart 99.3: Summary of auditory pathway.

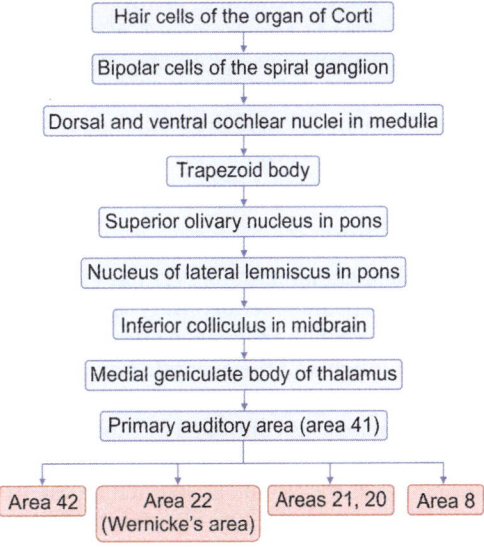

the categorical hemisphere, i.e., the dominant hemisphere. This area process the auditory signal related to speech and is concerned with the interpretation of sounds and comprehension of spoken language. Areas 21 and 20 located in the middle and inferior temporal gyrus are concerned with interpretation and integration of auditory impulses. Lesion of this area impairs auditory short term memory. The temporal lobe also projects to the frontal lobe (frontal eye field or area 8). This is involved in turning the gaze towards the origin of sound.

Since many of the auditory axons cross over in the medulla while others remain on the same side, the right and the left primary auditory areas receive nerve impulses from both ears.

> Many collateral fibers from the auditory tract pass directly into the reticular activating system of brainstem. Because of this connection with the ascending reticular activating system (ARAS), the entire nervous system is activated in response to loud sounds.

Hemispheric Specialization of Auditory Areas

The auditory areas show marked hemispheric specialization. For example, area 22 is much more active on the left side than on the right side during language processing. Area 22 on the right side is concerned with melody, pitch and sound intensity. A portion of the posterior superior temporal gyrus known as **planum temporale** is larger in the left than in the right cerebral hemisphere in right handed individuals. This area is involved in language-related auditory processing. Dyslexic children do not have a well-developed planum temporale on the left hemisphere. This suggests that the basic defect in them may be absence of hemispheric specialization for language.

Descending Auditory Pathways

Parallel to the ascending auditory pathway is a descending auditory projection system from auditory cortex to the cochlear outer hair cells. 95% of the neurons in the cochlear nerve are afferents originating in the inner hair cells. The remaining 5% of the neurons are efferent fibers that innervate several outer hair cells. Auditory cortex sends three descending tracts:
1. Directly to thalamus, i.e., to the medial geniculate body
2. To inferior colliculus of midbrain
3. To the olivary nucleus in pons

Olivocochlear Bundle

The olivocochlear cholinergic fibers in the VIII cranial nerve arise bilaterally from the superior olivary complex in pons and this bundle of efferent fibers is called **olivocochlear bundle**. The efferents branch and the synaptic terminals innervate all the 20,000 outer hair cells. The sensitivity of the cochlea to specific frequencies is controlled by olivocochlear fibers. The olivocochlear efferent fibers which innervate principally the outer hair cells play a role in sharpening the frequency response of the BM. Activity of efferent fibers causes inhibition of the afferent fibers by liberating a hyperpolarizing mediator which is probably acetylcholine. Stimulation of these efferent fibers attenuates outer hair cell responses to improve the sharpness of impulses of each auditory afferent. These efferent influences represent *presynaptic inhibition*.

The efferent fibers do not synapse directly with the inner hair cells as it does with the outer hair cells. They synapse with afferent neurons close to their synaptic junctions. At these junctions, efferent signals attenuate or block afferent nerve impulse generation. This represents *postsynaptic inhibition*.

By means of the olivocochlear bundle, the central nervous system can exert control over peripheral acoustic receptors. This system allows the nervous system both to be more selective about what it hears and to hear better what it wants to hear.

COCHLEAR MICROPHONICS

Cochlea can function as a microphone. Besides its role in detecting sounds, the cochlea has the ability to produce sounds. The study was conducted by *Wever and Bray in 1930*. An active needle electrode is introduced through the tympanic membrane and placed near the cochlea and an indifferent electrode is placed on some other part of the ear. Connect these electrodes to an audio amplifier. When the amplifier is connected to a loud speaker, click stimuli put into the ear or music played could be heard with the same frequency and amplitude of the input sound waves. This proves that the wave form of cochlear microphonic potential is an exact replica of the sound wave that produces it. This is called *Wever-Bray phenomenon*. The same effect is obtained when an electrode is placed in the scala media and another in the scala tympani and the output signal connected to the amplifier. Since the original sound is accurately reproduced, the electrical activity generated in the cochlea in response to the click stimulus is called **cochlear microphonics**.

These potentials are not nerve action potentials and cannot be obtained from the auditory nerve or auditory pathway. The source of the cochlear microphonic potentials is the summed activity of many outer hair cells at the level of reticular lamina. The outer hair cells vibrate in response to sound waves and to signals from efferent neurons. As the outer hair cells depolarize and repolarize, they rapidly shorten and lengthen. This vibratory behavior changes the stiffness of the tectorial membrane and is thought to enhance the movement of the BM. The antibiotic kanamycin, which destroys outer hair cells selectively, reduces the cochlear microphonic response markedly. This proves that the cochlear microphonics arise mainly in the outer hair cells.

Cochlear microphonics develops in the hair cells of the cochlea before the development of action potentials in the auditory nerve fibers. They are due to electrical changes that occur in the hair cells due to distortion, similar to Piezo-electric potentials developed in the crystal of a microphone, i.e., the hair cells can generate electricity when subjected to mechanical stresses. Since they originate in the cochlea, which appears to behave like a microphone, they are called **cochlear microphonics**. If the acoustic stimulus polarity is reversed from condensation-rarefaction to rarefaction-condensation, the cochlear microphonics reverse polarity as does a microphone but action potentials do not. This proves that cochlear microphonics is analogous to functions of microphone.

The cochlear microphonic potentials are not of biological origin and they do not have a significant role in the hearing mechanism. They are preliminary to nerve action potentials and probably boost receptor excitation. Clinically, cochlear microphonics is used for testing the integrity of cochlea since they disappear when the hair cells are damaged. If local degeneration of the organ of Corti occurs by prolonged exposure to a loud sound, the cochlear microphonic potential produced by this particular band of frequency is abolished. In deaf babies, these potentials are not produced or are greatly reduced in size.

Features of Cochlear Microphonics

- Cochlear microphonic potentials can be recorded from any part of the inner ear, whereas action potentials can be recorded only from the auditory nerve.
- Unlike action potential, cochlear potential do not exhibit all or none phenomenon but shows gradation.
- Their latent period is only 1/8th of action potentials.
- They do not have a refractory period.
- They do not undergo fatigue.
- They are resistant to ischemia, hypoxia and anesthesia.
- Their frequency can be unusually high, i.e., they follow stimulus rates in excess of those that can be followed by the auditory neurons.
- They persist several hours after death.

APPLIED ASPECTS

Effect of Constant Exposure of the Ear to a Particular Frequency of Sound

If the ear is exposed to a particular frequency constantly, the auditory nerve cells become refractory for some time to that frequency. The second stimulus cannot stimulate the nerve endings. People working in certain factories will be exposed to a particular frequency and the hair cells which are responding to that particular frequency get damaged. If the duration of exposure is more, the damage will also be more. An example of acoustic trauma is **boiler maker's disease**. If the hair cells responding to 4,000 Hz are damaged, he may not be able to appreciate that frequency. Regeneration is not possible once the hair cells are damaged. The cochlear microphonic potentials generated by this particular band of frequency are found to be abolished.

Tinnitus, Hyperacusis and Auditory Hallucinations

Tinnitus is a sensation of sound in the absence of auditory stimulus. The sound may be ringing, buzzing or humming in character. It is usually associated with conductive deafness. Tinnitus can also occur due to hypersensitivity of the hair cells. Injury to the inner hair cell can produce random electrical impulses that are relayed to the auditory cortex producing intermittent or steady high pitched ringing in the ear known as tinnitus.

In **hyperacusis**, the intensity of even slight sounds is greatly increased and may even be painful. It may occur when there is paralysis of stapedius muscle due to facial nerve lesion or in nerve deafness due to lesions in the cochlea.

Auditory hallucinations or delusions are hearing of voices when it is not there and may occur in psychological disorders. In temporal lobe epilepsy, auditory halluci- nations may occur as an aura.

Types of Hearing Impairment

Hearing loss is the most common sensory defect in humans. The causes of deafness can be considered in five groups:
1. If the hearing defect is due to interference to the conduction of sound to the cochlea it is called conduction deafness.
2. If the hearing defect is associated with damage to cochlea or to the auditory nerve, it is called nerve deafness or sensorineural deafness.
3. Central deafness if the defect is in the auditory cortex.
4. **Diplacusis**, a false sense of pitch.
5. Gradual hearing loss associated with aging is called *presbycusis*. It affects those over 75 years of age and is probably due to gradual loss of hair cells and neurons.

Deafness

> **PY10.16:** Describe and discuss pathophysiology of deafness. Describe hearing tests.

Conduction Deafness

Conduction deafness may be caused by anything that interferes with the sound waves reaching the acoustic neuroepithelium.

Causes:
- Water or wax or foreign bodies in the external auditory canal
- Otitis media and perforation of tympanic membrane
- Loss of mobility (otosclerosis) or destruction of the ossicular chain can cause deafness. In otosclerosis, bone is resorbed and replaced with sclerotic bone that overgrows and prevents movement of stapes against the oval window.

Characteristic feature of conductive deafness are:
- Hearing impairment
- Rinne test negative
- In Weber's test, patient hears better by the diseased ear
- In Schwabach's test bone conduction is better than normal

Nerve Deafness or Sensorineural Deafness

Nerve deafness occur either due to defects in the internal ear or due to lesions of auditory pathways.

Causes:
- Presbycusis due to gradual loss of hair cells and cortical neurons at old age
- Hereditary
- Injury to VIII cranial nerve
- Tumors of VIII cranial nerve (acoustic neuroma)
- *Drug induced*: Drugs, such as streptomycin, gentamicin, quinine, etc., affect the mechanosensitive channels in the stereocilia of hair cells and leads to degeneration of hair cells
- Infections, such as measles and meningitis may lead to degeneration of VIII cranial nerve
- *Industrial hazards*: Prolonged exposure to loud sound damages hair cells
- Autoimmune disorders and destruction of hair cells

Features of Sensorineural Deafness

- In unilateral nerve deafness, air conduction is longer than bone conduction.
- In Weber's test, the patient hears better by the normal ear.
- In Schwabach's test, bone conduction is worse than normal.
- The patient talks loudly in nerve deafness.

Central Deafness

Central deafness is due to lesions in the auditory cortex. Unilateral damage to the auditory cortex does not result in deafness because the auditory pathways are extensively crossed at all levels above cochlear nuclei. Thus, the ear is bilaterally represented in the auditory pathway. The affected person may have difficulty in localizing sounds. Extensive damage to the auditory cortex of the dominant hemisphere leads to difficulties in speech recognition.

Tests to Distinguish Between Nerve Deafness and Conduction Deafness (Table 99.4)

Tuning Fork Tests

- Rinne's test
- Weber's test
- Schwabach's test

In tuning fork tests, a tuning fork of frequency 512 Hz is used. Tuning fork tests help to distinguish between conductive deafness and sensorineural deafness. Both air conduction and bone conduction are tested. To test air conduction, the prongs of the vibrating tuning fork are held in front of the ear to be tested so that the sound passes through the air to the tympanic membrane and across the middle ear to reach the cochlea. To test bone conduction, the base of the vibrating tuning fork is placed firmly against the skull so that the sound is transmitted through the bones of the skull to the cochlea bypassing the middle ear.

Rinne's Test

The base of the vibrating tuning fork is placed on the mastoid process until the subject no longer hears the sound, then it is held in front of the ear on the same side. A normal subject hears the vibration in air after bone conduction is over, i.e., normally *air conduction is better than bone conduction*. Then *Rinne's test is said to be positive*. In conduction deafness, air vibration is not heard after bone conduction is over, i.e., bone conduction is better than air conduction and *Rinne's test is said to be negative*. In sensorineural deafness, even though both air conduction and bone conduction are affected, air conduction remains better than bone conduction and therefore Rinne's test remains positive in partial nerve deafness. In complete nerve deafness, both air conduction and bone conduction are absent.

Weber's Test

The base of vibrating tuning fork is placed on the center of the forehead or on the vertex of the skull so that the sound is conducted through bone to both ears. A normal subject hears equally on both sides, i.e., there is no lateralization to one side. In unilateral conduction deafness, sound appears louder in the affected ear because the masking effect of environmental noise is absent on the affected side. This is called *lateralization of sound to the affected side*. The sound is less clearly heard in the normal ear due to the masking effect of background noise. In unilateral nerve deafness, the sound appears louder in the normal ear, i.e., 'lateralized' to the healthy ear.

Schwabach's Test

Bone conduction of patient is compared with that of normal subject or with that of the examiner assuming that the examiner has normal hearing. The base of the vibrating tuning fork is placed first on the mastoid process of the patient till he stops hearing the sound. The examiner then places the base of the tuning fork on his mastoid. If he still hears the sound, it indicates that the patient's bone conduction is impaired which may be due to sensorineural deafness. In conduction deafness, bone conduction of the subject is better than that of the examiner. In nerve deafness, bone conduction of the subject is worse than the examiner's.

HEARING AIDS

Since the cochlea is embedded in the bony cage of temporal bone, vibration of the skull can cause vibration of fluid in the cochlea. So if a special electromechanical sound transmitting device is applied directly to the mastoid process of a person suffering from conduction deafness he can hear the sound. But this is of limited use in a person suffering from

Table 99.4: Tuning fork tests to distinguish between conduction deafness and nerve deafness.

Test	Normal	Conduction deafness (unilateral)	Nerve deafness (unilateral)
Rinne's test: Base of vibrating tuning fork placed on mastoid process, until subject no longer hear it, then held in front of ear	Air conduction is better than bone conduction (Rinne positive)	Bone conduction is better than air conduction (Rinne negative)	• In partial nerve deafness Rinne test is positive on the affected side • In complete nerve deafness, both air and bone conduction are absent on affected side
Weber's test: Base of vibrating tuning fork placed on the vertex of the head	Sound heard equally on both sides (no lateralization)	Sound lateralized to effected side	Lateralized to the healthy ear
Shwabach's test: Bone conduction of patient is compared with that of a healthy subject	Both examiner and subject hear the sound equally well	Subject's bone conduction is better than the examiner's	Subject's bone conduction is worse than the examiner's

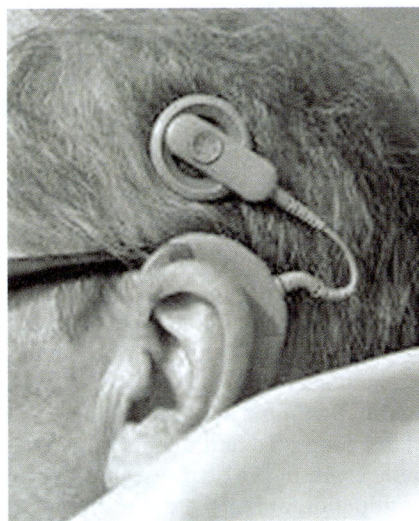

Fig. 99.12: Hearing aid.

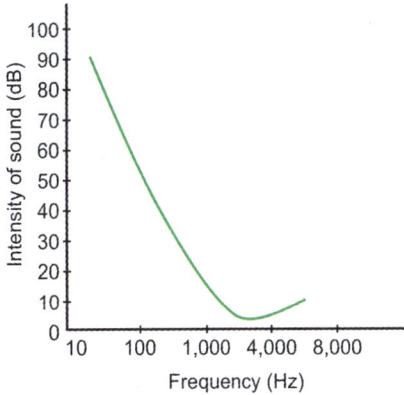

Fig. 99.13: Audibility curve.

sensorineural deafness. In such cases if the deafness is due to destruction of hair cells then cochlear implants are of benefit provided the auditory pathway is intact.

A **hearing aid** is an electroacoustic device which fits in or behind the ear and is designed to amplify and modulate sound **(Fig. 99.12)**. The basic components of hearing aid include a microphone, an amplifier, a receiver and a power supply. The microphone picks up the sound signals from the environment and converts them into electrical signals. Amplifier is a transformer that increases the amplitude of the electrical signal that is sent to the receiver. The receiver or the loud speaker changes the modified electrical signal back into sound energy that is directed into the ear. Battery serves as the power source for the hearing aid.

> **Cochlear implant** is a device that translates sounds into electrical signals that can be interpreted by the brain. This device is advised to patients having severe sensorineural deafness in both ears that is caused by damage to hair cells in the cochlea. The auditory nerves should be functional. Parts of the cochlear implant are a microphone, a sound processor, a transmitter, an internal receiver and electrodes. The electrodesare implanted in the cochlea which triggers nerve impulses in the sensory neurons of the cochlear division of the VIII cranial nerve. The artificially induced nerve impulses pass through thenormal auditory pathway and reach the auditory areas of the cerebral cortex and thus the sound is perceived.

AUDIOMETRY

Auditory acuity, i.e., sharpness of hearing is measured using an instrument called **audiometer** and the record obtained is called **audiogram**. The test should be performed in a soundproof room. While one ear is being tested, the opposite ear must be masked to exclude it from the test. There are different types of audiometric tests like pure tone audiometry and speech audiometry.

In **pure tone audiometry**, there are two controls in the instrument by which both the frequency and intensity of sound can be varied. The electronic oscillator can generate pure tones of varying frequencies. The intensity dial helps to adjust the threshold intensity of hearing for each frequency. The subject wears a headphone.

The audiometer presents the subject with pure tones of different frequencies between 10 to 8,000 Hz and of different intensities between 0 to 100 dB through the ear phone. The intensity is initially kept low at 0 dB. If the sound is inaudible to the subject, the intensity is gradually increased until the subject can hear the sound. At each frequency, the audible intensity is determined and plotted on a graph as percentage of normal hearing showing intensity against frequency. The curve obtained is called **audibility curve (Fig. 99.13)**. The threshold for hearing sound at different frequencies is obtained and it is seen that for lower frequencies to be heard, the intensity of sound should be high. From the graph, it is seen that maximum hearing is recorded at frequencies between 1,000 and 3,000 Hz because the threshold intensity is minimum between these frequencies. Amplification of sound energy in the ear is greatest between frequencies of 1,000–3,000 Hz.

Audiometric Tests to Distinguish Between Conduction Deafness and Nerve Deafness

Audiometry can be made use of *to distinguish between conduction deafness and nerve deafness (sensorineural deafness)*. Here, graphs for air conduction and bone conduction are plotted separately. The audiometer, in addition to being equipped with an ear phone for testing air conduction by the ear, is equipped with a mechanical vibrator for testing bone conduction from the mastoid process of the skull into the cochlea.

Usually, air conduction thresholds are measured for tones of frequencies 125, 250, 500, 1,000, 2,000 and 4,000 Hz and bone conduction thresholds for 250, 500, 1,000, 2,000 and 4,000 Hz. For each frequency, a series of tone pips (short high pitched sounds) are delivered at increasing intensities (beginning from sub-threshold) and the subject is instructed to signal every time he hears a sound. Each frequency is tested in the intensity range of 0–100 dB. Graphs can be plotted with frequency of sound in Hertz on the *x*-axis and hearing loss in decibels on the *y*-axis for air conduction and bone conduction separately. The results are charted and the record obtained is called **audiogram** and it helps to distinguish between nerve deafness and conduction deafness.

The instrument is calibrated in such a way that zero intensity-level sound at each frequency is the loudness that can barely be heard by the normal ear. Thus, 0 dB means the person can just hear the sound at all the frequencies tested. If the loudness (intensity) must be increased to 30 dB above normal before it can be heard, the person is said to have a hearing loss of 30 dB at that frequency.

In normal audiogram, the threshold for hearing through air conduction is 0 dB and the threshold for bone conduction is slightly higher may be about 5 dB which means that air conduction is slightly better than bone conduction **(Fig. 99.14)**. The threshold of bone conduction is a measure of cochlear function.

In sensorineural deafness, both air conduction and bone conduction are impaired with equal severity. The threshold for bone conduction remains slightly higher than air conduction **(Fig. 99.15A)** and the air bone gap is normal. Thus, audiogram provides an objective measurement of the degree of deafness. The tonal range most affected can also be found out.

In conduction deafness, air conduction is impaired but bone conduction is normal **(Fig. 99.15B)**. The threshold for air conduction is higher than bone conduction here and there is a wide air-bone gap. Difference in the thresholds of air and bone conduction (air-bone gap) is a measure of the degree of conduction deafness.

In **conduction deafness**, bone conduction is normal and air conduction is impaired and the hearing loss is more for lower frequencies. In **nerve deafness**, both air conduction and bone conduction are affected and the hearing loss is more for higher frequencies.

Brain Stem Auditory Evoked Responses

> **PY10.19:** Describe and discuss auditory and visual evoked potentials.

Brain stem auditory evoked response (BAER) records potentials from the auditory pathway in response to a brief auditory stimulation, using clicking sounds.

Uses:
- It helps to assess the integrity of the auditory pathway up to the midbrain.
- It helps in diagnosing and localizing early lesions of the auditory system. Auditory evoked responses help to distinguish and localize peripheral and brainstem interferences along the auditory pathway.
- It helps in the interpretation of various types of coma, trauma, neurological diseases and effects of drugs.

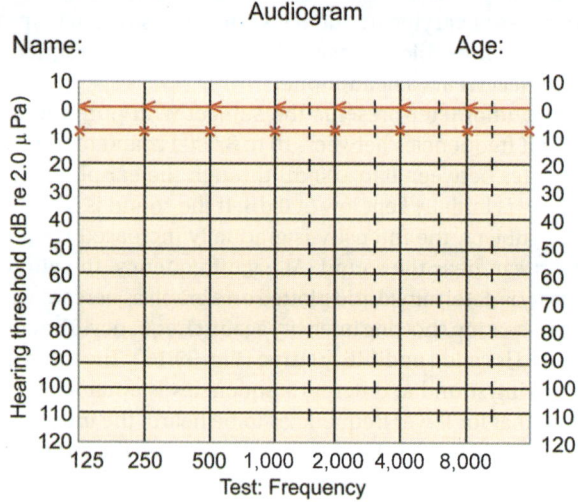

Fig. 99.14: Normal audiogram recorded from the left ear: (<) denotes air conduction; (x) denotes bone conduction.

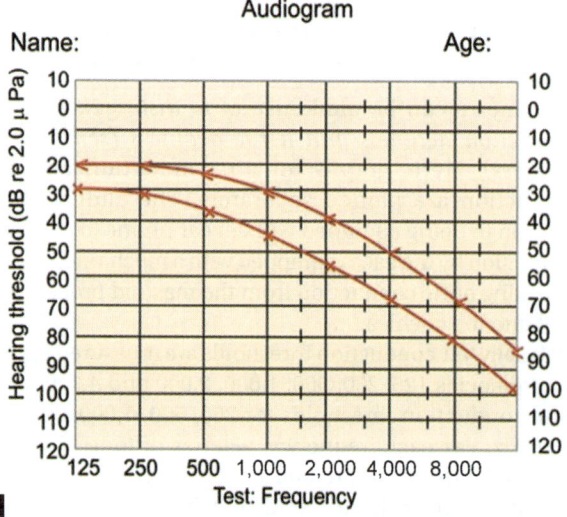

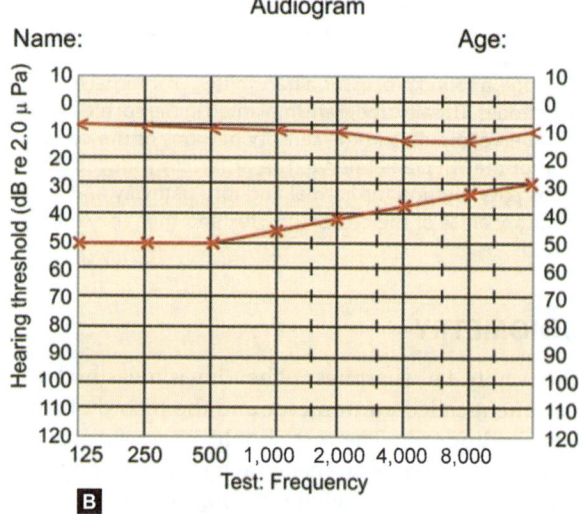

Figs. 99.15A and B: Audiogram showing: (A) Sensorineural deafness; (B) Conductive deafness recorded from the left ear. Note that in sensorineural deafness, both air and bone conduction are equally affected and hearing loss is more for higher frequencies. In conductive deafness, bone conduction is normal and the hearing loss for air conduction is about 50 dB at frequency 500 Hz; whereas at higher frequencies, the hearing loss is less. Symbol '<' denotes bone conduction and symbol 'x' denotes air conduction.

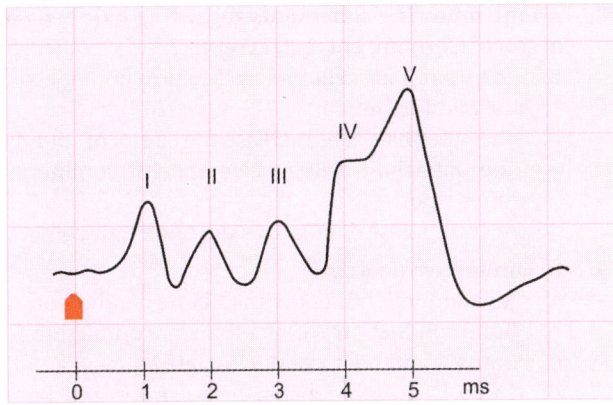

Fig. 99.16: Brainstem auditory evoked response curves.
(1) Wave I is produced by action potential generated in the peripheral portion of the eighth cranial nerve; (2) Wave II arises from cochlear nuclei; (3) Wave III is generated by action potential in superior olivary nucleus; (4) Wave IV arises from lateral lemniscus; (5) Wave V originates from inferior colliculi.

* BAER test can help to diagnose hearing loss and nervous system disorders, especially in premature infants, newborns, young children, and others who may not be able to participate in a standard hearing test.
* It also helps to diagnose acoustic neuroma, multiple sclerosis, Meniere's disease, stroke, etc.

Procedure

Electroencephalography (EEG) electrodes are placed on the scalp. A clicking sound is introduced into the ear using a set of ear phones and the responses referred to as auditory evoked potentials are recorded with EEG electrodes. A print out of the result is obtained. If it shows spikes in the brain activity each time the clicking sound is heard it is normal. If the results show flat lines when the clicking sound was made, it may indicate hearing loss. Then further tests should be performed to determine the cause. Five wave forms are obtained in BAER **(Fig. 99.16)**.

Absence or reduced amplitude of the wave form indicates lesion in that specific region.

■ MULTIPLE CHOICE QUESTIONS

1. **All the following are contents of middle ear, *except*:**
   a. Ear ossicles   b. Tensor tympani
   c. Stapedius   d. Hair cells
2. **The ear ossicles that is attached to back of tympanic membrane is:**
   a. Stapes   b. Handle of malleus
   c. Head of malleus   d. Incus
3. **Stapes rest in:**
   a. Round window
   b. Oval window
   c. Tympanic membrane
   d. Basilar membrane
4. **Attenuation reflex is due to:**
   a. Contraction of tensor tympani
   b. Contraction of stapedius
   c. Contraction of both tensor tympani and stapedius
   d. Inward movement of oval window
5. **The ion that is present in higher concentration in the endolymph:**
   a. K^+ b. Na^+
   c. Ca^{2+} d. Cl^-
6. **The length of the cochlear portion of labyrinth in humans:**
   a. 23 mm   b. 40 mm
   c. 35 mm   d. 15 mm
7. **Perilymph is present in:**
   a. Scala vestibuli and scala tympani
   b. Scala media
   c. Scala media and scala tympani
   d. Scala media and scala vestibuli
8. **Scala tympani end in:**
   a. Helicotrema   b. Round window
   c. Oval window   d. Organ of Corti
9. **Raised ECF K^+ levels is seen in:**
   a. Endolymph   b. Ectolymph
   c. Aqueous humor   d. Vitreous humor
10. **Secondary tympanic membrane covers:**
    a. Eustachian tube
    b. Round window
    c. Oval window
    d. The junction of middle ear and external ear
11. **Organ of Corti is located on the:**
    a. Basilar membrane
    b. Reissner's membrane
    c. Tectorial membrane
    d. Reticular lamina
12. **The part of the organ of Corti which is pierced by the processes of the hair cells:**
    a. Tectorial membrane
    b. Reticular lamina
    c. Rods of Corti
    d. Stria vascularis
13. **All the following statements regarding the hair cells of organ of Corti are correct, *except*:**
    a. The processes of the hair cells are bathed in endolymph, whereas the bases are bathed in perilymph
    b. There are 20,000 outer hair cells and 3,500 inner hair cells in each cochlea
    c. 90% of sensory neurons innervate the outer hair cells
    d. The tips of the outer hair cells and not the inner hair cells are embedded in the tectorial membrane
14. **The cell bodies of the sensory neurons of the hair cells in organ of Corti are located in the:**
    a. Spiral ganglion
    b. Inferior colliculus
    c. Dorsal cochlear nucleus
    d. Ventral cochlear nucleus

15. All the following statements are correct, *except*:
    a. Perilymph is formed from plasma
    b. Endolymph is formed by the stria vascularis
    c. Endolymph has a high concentration of K⁺ and low concentration of Na⁺
    d. Scala media is electrically negative by 85 mV relative to scala vestibuli and scala tympani

16. Impedance matching is the function of:
    a. External ear
    b. Middle ear
    c. Inner ear
    d. Utricle and saccule

17. In humans, primary auditory cortex is located in the:
    a. Precentral gyrus
    b. Post central gyrus
    c. Superior part of temporal lobe
    d. Posterior part of occipital lobe

18. Organ of Corti is found in:
    a. Macula
    b. Cochlea
    c. Niddle ear
    d. Semicircular canal

19. The speed of sound waves in air at 20°C at sea level is:
    a. 344 m/s
    b. 770 m/s
    c. 1,450 m/s
    d. 1,000 m/s

20. Audible frequency range in humans is:
    a. 120–160 Hz
    b. 20–20,000 Hz
    c. 1,000–3,000 Hz
    d. 120–250 Hz

21. Tympanic membrane develops from:
    a. Ectoderm
    b. Endoderm
    c. Mesoderm
    d. All of the above

22. Conduction deafness results if there is damage to:
    a. Pinna
    b. Basilar membrane
    c. Incus
    d. Auditory nerve

23. Human ear is most sensitive to:
    a. 0–200 Hz
    b. 200–600 Hz
    c. 1,000–4,000 Hz
    d. 6,000–10,000 Hz

24. Pitch discrimination is best in the frequency range of:
    a. 0–200 Hz
    b. 200–600 Hz
    c. 1,000–4,000 Hz
    d. 1,000–3,000 Hz

25. The lever mechanism of the ear ossicles amplifies the sound waves:
    a. 1.3 times
    b. 21 times
    c. 10 times
    d. 19 times

26. The reaction time for tympanic reflex is:
    a. 40–50 ms
    b. 40–160 ms
    c. 200 ms
    d. 10–20 ms

27. Motor protein of the outer hair cells in the organ of Corti is:
    a. Prestin
    b. Kinesin
    c. Dynein
    d. Myosin

28. All the following statements regarding hair cells of organ of Corti are correct, *except*:
    a. The inner hair cells generate action potentials in the auditory nerve
    b. The outer hair cells increase the clarity of sounds
    c. The outer hair cells receive efferent cholinergic innervation
    d. Acetyl choline depolarizes the outer hair cells

29. In conductive deafness:
    a. Air conduction is better than bone conduction
    b. Bone conduction is better than air conduction
    c. Both air and bone conduction are equal
    d. There is no relationship between air and bone conduction

30. Center for auditory reflexes is:
    a. Inferior colliculi
    b. Medial geniculate body
    c. Spiral ganglion
    d. Auditory cortex

31. The primary auditory cortex is Brodmann's area:
    a. 42
    b. 41
    c. 22
    d. 39

32. The efferent fibers in the auditory nerve supplying the outer hair cells of the organ of Corti arises from:
    a. Primary motor area
    b. Auditory cortex
    c. Superior olivary complex
    d. Auditory association area

33. The second order neurons in the auditory pathway are located in the:
    a. Cochlear nuclei
    b. Spiral ganglion
    c. Medial geniculate body
    d. Inferior colliculi

34. In certain diseases damaging the hair cells of organ of Corti, if the damage to the outer hair cell is greater than the damage to inner hair cell:
    a. Clarity of sound decreases
    b. There is severe hearing loss
    c. Leads to conduction deafness
    d. Leads to both sensorial and conduction deafness

35. Language related auditory processing occurs in the:
    a. Primary auditory cortex
    b. Auditory association area
    c. Planum temporale
    d. Brodmann's area 22

36. Gradual hearing loss associated with aging is called:
    a. Presbyopia
    b. Presbycusis
    c. Conductive deafness
    d. Sensorineural deafness

37. The test of hearing that demonstrates the masking effect of environmental noise on auditory threshold is:
    a. Rinne's test
    b. Watch test
    c. Weber and Schwabach's tests
    d. Audiometry
38. Sound intensity is measured in:
    a. Diopters
    b. Decibels
    c. Daltons
    d. Hertz
39. Medial geniculate body is concerned with:
    a. Hearing
    b. Vision
    c. Smell
    d. Taste
40. Organ of Corti is situated in:
    a. Scala media
    b. Scala tympani
    c. Scala vestibuli
    d. Saccule
41. Endolymph is present in:
    a. Scala vestibuli
    b. Scala media
    c. Scala tympani
    d. Helicotrema
42. In humans the primary auditory cortex is located in:
    a. Post central gyrus
    b. Precentral gyrus
    c. Inferior part of frontal lobe
    d. Superior part of temporal lobe
43. Impedance matching is a function of:
    a. External ear
    b. Middle ear
    c. Internal ear
    d. Hair cells
44. Sense organ of hearing is:
    a. Organ of Corti
    b. Crista ampullaris
    c. Ear
    d. Hair cells
45. The receptor for hearing is:
    a. Organ of Corti
    b. Crista ampullaris
    c. Otoconia
    d. Hair cells
46. For diagnosing middle ear deafness the following test is done:
    a. Testing Babinski reflex
    b. Eliciting Bhvosted's reflex
    c. Finger-nose test
    d. Weber's test

ANSWERS

1. d	2. b	3. b	4. c	5. a
6. c	7. a	8. b	9. a	10. b
11. a	12. b	13. c	14. a	15. d
16. b	17. c	18. b	19. a	20. b
21. d	22. c	23. c	24. d	25. a
26. b	27. a	28. d	29. b	30. a
31. b	32. c	33. a	34. a	35. c
36. b	37. c	38. b	39. a	40. a
41. b	42. d	43. b	44. a	45. d
46. d				

NAME THE FOLLOWING/FILL IN THE BLANKS/GIVE THE NORMAL VALUE

1. Name the two sensory modalities whose receptors are housed in the ear: **Hearing and equilibrium.**
2. Cochlea of the inner ear is concerned with **hearing**.
3. The receptors for hearing and equilibrium: **Hair cells**
4. The middle ear opens into the nasopharynx via the **auditory (eustachian) tube**.
5. Name the three auditory ossicles located in the middle ear: **Malleus, incus and stapes.**
6. Foot plate of stapes is attached to the **oval window**.
7. Magnification of sound intensity by the lever mechanism of ear ossicles is **1.2–1.3** times.
8. The effective surface area of the tympanic membrane: 50 mm^2.
9. Sound is amplified **17** times when it reaches the oval window from tympanic membrane.
10. The impedance matching in the middle ear: **22 times amplification of sound.**
11. The reflex that protects the auditory receptors from excessive stimulation by loud sounds: **Tympanic reflex.**
12. Reaction time of tympanic reflex: **40–160 msec.**
13. Duplex theory of pitch discrimination: **Volley principle and place theory together.**
14. Perilymph is present between the **bony labyrinth** and **membranous labyrinth**.
15. Length of cochlea: **35 mm**.
16. Scala vestibuli and scala media are separated by **Reissner's** membrane.
17. Scala tympani and scala media are separated by **basilar** membrane.
18. The fluid contained in scala tympani and scala vestibuli: **Perilymph**.
19. Scala media contain **endolymph** secreted by stria vascularis.
20. The fluid in the inner ear that has a high concentration of K$^+$ and a low concentration of Na$^+$: **Endolymph**.
21. Scala media is electrically positive by **85** mV relative to the scala vestibuli and scala tympani.
22. Sense organ for hearing: **Organ of Corti.**
23. There are **20,000** outer hair cells and **3,500** inner hair cells in each cochlea.
24. The percentage of the sensory neurons which innervate the inner hair cells: **90–95%.**
25. The processes of the hair cells in the organ of Corti are bathed in **endolymph**, whereas their bases are bathed in **perilymph.**
26. The potential difference between endolymph and perilymph is called **endolymphatic potential**.
27. The longest hair like process of the hair cells in the inner ear is called **kinocilium**.
28. Bending of hair cells toward kinocilium produce **depolarization** of hair cells.

29. Bending of hair cells away from kinocilium results in **hyperpolarization of hair cells**.
30. Sound waves travel through air at a speed of **344 m/sec** at 20°C at sea level.
31. The quality or timbre of a sound is determined by its .
32. Sound becomes painful to the ear above **140 dB**.
33. Audible frequency in humans range from about **20** to a maximum of **20,000** cycles per second.
34. Greatest sensitivity of the ear to sound: **Between 1,000–4,000 Hz range**.
35. The primary sensory cells that generate action potentials in the auditory nerve: **The inner hair cells**.
36. The nucleus of thalamus that is concerned with hearing: **Medial geniculate body**.
37. The primary auditory cortex: **Brodmann's area 41**.
38. In lesion of auditory association areas, the person can perceive sound information but fails to understand the **meaning** of the sound.
39. Centre for auditory reflex: **Inferior colliculi**.
40. Auditory acuity (sharpness of hearing) is commonly measured with **audiometer**.
41. In a normal person **air** conduction is better than **bone** conduction.
42. Sound of minimal intensity that the human ear can perceive: **0 dB**.
43. Types of deafness: **Conductive and sensorineural hearing loss**.
44. Gradual hearing loss associated with aging is called **presbycusis**.

Gustation or Taste Sensation

CHAPTER 100

LEARNING OBJECTIVES
- With the help of a diagram describe taste bud
- Discuss the primary taste sensations
- Explain the mechanism of taste perception
- Describe the taste pathway
- Discuss the pathophysiology of altered taste sensation

INTRODUCTION

PY10.13: Describe and discuss perception of smell and taste sensation.

Flavors of various foods are a combination of taste and smell with contributions from temperature, pain and touch sensations. Most of the spicy foods, which give a hot or pungent taste, do so by stimulating the receptors of general sensation of the tongue.

Texture of food also contributes to taste. Physiologically, taste and smell are interrelated but anatomically, they are different. For example, when there is a nasal block, food does not taste good. Onion may taste as apple when there is a complete nasal block. These sensory inputs combine to create a sense of pleasure as well as give information regarding the consistency and chemical composition of food. Usually, bitter substances are avoided because most of them are highly toxic as in the case of alkaloids.

Gustation and olfaction are considered as **visceral senses** because of their close relation to gastric function. Both are **chemical senses**. These sensations also affect secretion of digestive juices and gastrointestinal motility. Flavor also leads to associative learning or conditioned learning leading to preference for certain foods and aversion to certain others. Differences between taste and smell are shown in **Table 100.1**.

TASTE BUDS

Taste is mainly a function of taste buds in the mouth which form the **sense organ of taste**. The gustatory receptors are located in these oval structures. There are about 10,000 taste buds in man. Most of them are distributed over the tongue, but a few are seen in the mucous membrane covering the soft palate, epiglottis, larynx and pharynx.

Taste buds are ovoid structures measuring about 50–70 µm. In the tongue, the taste buds are located in the walls of **fungiform, foliate** and **circumvallate papillae**. The fungiform papillae are rounded structures, present mainly near the tip and the margins of the anterior 2/3rd of tongue and contain about 5 taste buds per papilla. They are innervated by **chorda tympani** nerve, branch of VII cranial nerve. The circumvallate papillae are arranged in the form of alphabet "V" on the back of the tongue. It contains about 100 taste buds per papilla. Foliate papillae are located in the posterior 1/3rd of tongue and are innervated by the **glossopharyngeal nerve** (IX cranial nerve). Pharyngeal and laryngeal taste buds are innervated by **vagus** (X cranial nerve). Palatal taste buds are innervated by greater petrosal branch of **facial nerve**.

Structure of Taste Bud

Each taste bud is made up of four types of cells. They are **basal cells**, two types of **sustentacular cells** and **gustatory receptor cells**. There are about 40 cells altogether in each taste bud. The taste bud opens into the oral cavity by a **taste pore or gustatory pore**. The receptor cell has microvilli that projects into the taste pore (**Fig. 100.1**). The tips of the

Table 100.1: Differences between taste and smell.	
Smell	Taste
Receptor is a telereceptor as well as chemoreceptor	Chemoreceptor; taste can be appreciated only if the substance is in contact with taste buds
No direct relay in the thalamus	Has direct relay in the thalamus
Substance can be in any form to appreciate smell but should be volatile	Substance should be in liquid form or should get dissolved in saliva to appreciate taste

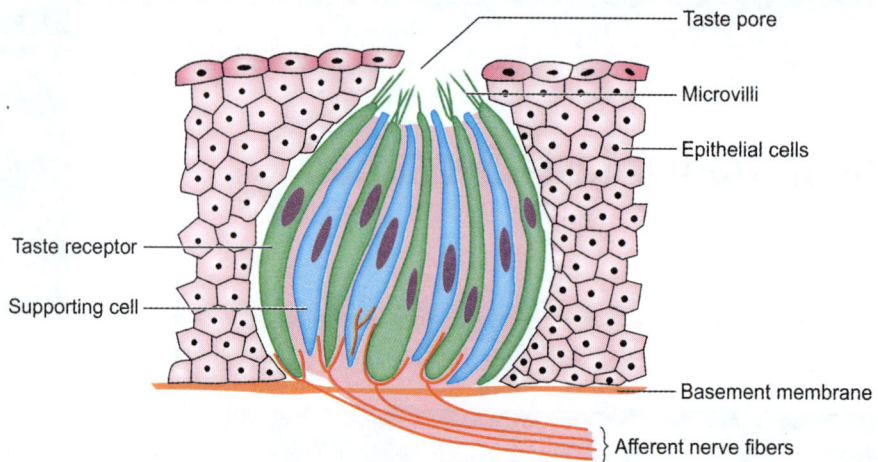

Fig. 100.1: Structure of a taste bud.

gustatory cells and the sustentacular cells are connected to each other and to the surrounding epithelial cells by tight junctions. The only part of the receptor cell exposed to oral fluid is the microvillus.

Innervation of Taste Buds

The receptor cell makes synaptic contact with afferent nerve terminals at various points. Each taste bud is innervated by about 50 nerve fibers, and each nerve fiber receives input from about 5 taste buds. New receptor cells are formed by differentiation from the basal cells. Half-life of receptor cell is 10 days. If the sensory nerve supplying a taste bud is cut, the taste bud degenerates. If the nerve regenerates, new taste bud will be formed from the neighboring cells.

■ TASTE PATHWAY

The sensory nerve fibers from the taste buds of anterior two-thirds of tongue pass through the chorda tympani branch of **facial nerve** and reach the brainstem. The sensory taste fibers from the posterior 1/3rd of tongue pass through the **glossopharyngeal nerve,** and sensory fibers from areas other than tongue pass through the **vagus** nerve to reach the brainstem. The cell bodies of the first order neurons of taste pathway are located in the ganglia of 7th (geniculate ganglion), 9th (petrosal ganglion) and 10th (nodose ganglion) cranial nerves. The taste fibers from these three nerves reach the gustatory portion of the **nucleus of tractus solitarius** in the medulla oblongata and synapse with the second order neurons. From there, axons of second order neurons ascend in the *ipsilateral medial lemniscus* and reach the **ventral posteromedial nucleus** of **thalamus**. From the thalamus, axons of third order neurons pass through the thalamic radiation and the posterior limb of internal capsule to reach the face area of somatosensory cortex in the **ipsilateral postcentral gyrus (gustatory cortex) (Fig. 100.2).** The gustatory cortex is in the anterior insula and the frontal operculum (inferior part of postcentral gyrus).

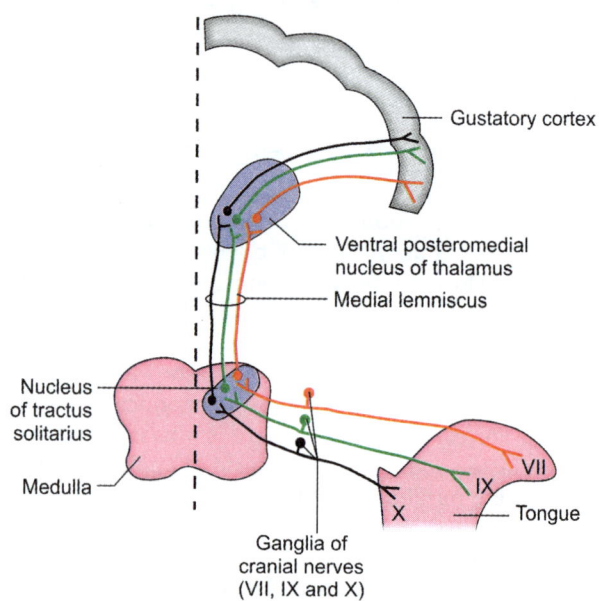

Fig. 100.2: Taste pathway from one half of tongue.

The sensations of touch, hot, cold, pain, etc., from the tongue are carried by the lingual branch of 5th cranial nerve. It has a similar course and end in the inferior part of postcentral gyrus. These sensations contribute to the flavor of food. The burning sensation experienced when food containing capsaicin is taken is due to the stimulation of these sensory fibers in the trigeminal nerve.

Mechanism of Taste Perception

The chemoreceptor respond to substances dissolved in the oral fluids. This stimulus evokes a generator potential in the taste receptor cell. Receptors for taste are present in the microvilli of the gustatory cell. The substance producing taste sensation forms a weak bond to the receptor protein. Taste is abolished by washing the tongue with water.

The membrane of taste cell, such as any other sensory receptor is negatively charged on the inside with respect to

Table 100.2: Different taste modalities and their receptors.		
Taste modality	Substances producing the taste	Receptor
Sour	Organic and inorganic acids, such as HCl, citric acid, etc.	ENaCs, HCN
Salt	NaCl, dipeptides, such as lysyl taurine, ornithotaurine, etc.	ENaC
Sweet	Glucose, sucrose, fructose, saccharin, alcohol, glycerol, aldehyde, esters, etc.	G-protein linked receptor
Bitter	Alkaloids, such as strychnine, quinine, morphine, nicotine, caffeine, etc. inorganic salts of Mg, NH_4, Ca^{2+}, etc.	G-protein linked gustducin
Umami	Monosodium glutamate	Glutamate receptor, mGluR4

(ENaC: epithelial sodium channel; HCN: hyperpolarization-activated cyclic nucleotide-gated cation channel or receptor)

outside. Application of a taste producing substance to the microvillus produces partial loss of this negative potential. The microvillus becomes more permeable to Na^+ and Na^+ enters the cell and causes depolarization. This change in potential is proportional to the logarithm of concentration of the stimulating substance. This change in potential in the gustatory receptor is the receptor potential for taste. The mechanism of production of generator potential in different taste receptor varies **(Table 100.2)**. The receptor potential generates action potential in the sensory fiber innervating the gustatory cell.

> At any H^+ concentration, organic acids, such as acetic acid taste sourer than inorganic acids, such as HCl. This is due to the greater ability of organic acids to penetrate the cell.

■ BASIC TASTE MODALITIES OR PRIMARY TASTE SENSATIONS

There are five primary taste sensations. They are **sour, salt, sweet, bitter and umami**. There are no special areas on the surface of the tongue for each of these sensations. They are sensed from all parts of the tongue. The afferent nerves to nucleus tractus solitarius contain fibers from all types of taste buds, without any localization. About 100 different tastes can be sensed by the tongue, which are combinations of these primary taste sensations and other sensations, such as pain and temperature.

For example, peculiar taste of ginger is due to the taste, burning sensation and smell.

Certain substances in the blood will cause peculiar taste in the tongue. For example, intravenous injection of histamine produces a metallic taste in the tongue, and in patients with jaundice a bitter taste is felt on the tongue due to bilirubin.

Bitter taste has a protective function. **Deadly toxins** found in poisonous plants are alkaloids and they have an intensely bitter taste. Bitter taste serves as a warning and so these plants are usually avoided by animals.

Two proteins isolated from African berries, **thaumatin I** and **monellin**, etc., are identified to be extremely sweet. They are 200–300 times as sweet as sucrose.

Saccharin, dulcin, cyclamate, etc., are synthetic sweeteners and are used in diabetic and obese patients. **Saccharin** is 600 times as sweet as sucrose. There is a substance called **P-4000** which has a sweet index 5000 times as great as that of sucrose. But it is very toxic.

Miraculin is a taste-modifying protein obtained from the miracle fruit seen in Africa. After eating this fruit, sour substances (acids) taste sweet. For example, after placing this substance over the tongue, lemon tastes like orange.

Taste Threshold and Intensity Discrimination

Taste threshold is the minimum concentration of the substance necessary to arouse a primary taste sensation. Taste threshold varies for different substances. Taste receptor cells are most sensitive to bitter. Bitter substances have the lowest threshold. The bitter taste at very low concentration helps to prevent accidental ingestion of these toxic substances. Sweet substances have a very high threshold. For example, the threshold concentration for glucose is 80,000 µmol/L whereas, for strychnine hydrochloride (bitter) it is only 1.6 µmol/L. **Intensity** discrimination for a particular taste is relatively crude. A 30% change in the concentration of the substance being tasted is necessary before an intensity difference can be detected.

Factors Influencing Taste Sensation

- **Area** of stimulation—threshold for taste decreases as the area of application of stimulus increases.
- **Duration**—the more the duration of stimulation, less is the reaction time or the response is quick.
- **Temperature** of the substance—maximum sensitivity to taste is obtained at 30–40°C.
- **Olfaction**—flavors of various foods are a combination of taste and smell.
- **Individual variations**—there is a general reduction in taste sensitivity in older people. This is due to atrophy of taste buds.
- **Sex**—women are more sensitive to sweet and salt and less sensitive to sour than men.
- **Affective nature** of taste—pleasantness and unpleasantness are called the affective attributes of a sensation. These make an individual select or reject food. For example, sweet taste is unpleasant at very low concentration, but very pleasant at high concentration. Sour and bitter are pleasant at low concentration, but very unpleasant at high concentration.
- **Taste preference** and control of diet—taste preference means that an animal will choose certain types of food in preference to others. It depends on the needs of the body. For example, in adrenalectomized animals, salt and water content is lost. So, they prefer salt water to pure water.
- **Adaptation**—taste buds quickly adapt to a particular taste. If we continuously apply a substance on the tongue, the intensity of taste decreases and threshold increases.
- **Interaction** between taste-producing substances affects taste sensation. For example, if lemon juice which is very sour is mixed with sugar it tastes good.

ABNORMALITIES OF TASTE SENSATION

PY10.14: Describe and discuss pathophysiology of altered smell and taste sensation.

❖ **Ageusia** is absence of sense of taste. It can be due to lesions of facial nerve, glossopharyngeal nerve, etc., or it may be congenital. Ageusia can also be an adverse side effect of drugs like captopril. Vitamin B_3 or zinc deficiency also causes ageusia.

❖ **Hypogeusia** is diminished taste sensitivity due to certain diseases.

❖ **Dysgeusia** is altered taste sensation. It is usually associated with temporal lobe lesion.

❖ **Parageusia** is unpleasant perception of taste (foul or rancid taste).

There are two clinical conditions in which there are clearly identifiable taste defects:
1. Familial dysautonomia
2. Selective taste blindness

Familial dysautonomia is a rare condition. Here, very high concentration of sugar fails to produce sweet sensation. It may be associated with other sensory defects.

Selective taste blindness is inherited as a Mendelian recessive trait. There is a very high increase in the threshold to bitter taste of phenylthiourea. They are called **non-tasters**. All other taste sensations are normal to them.

MULTIPLE CHOICE QUESTIONS

1. **Taste sensation from the anterior part of tongue is mediated by:**
   a. 10th cranial nerve   b. 7th
   c. 12th   d. 5th cranial nerve

2. **General sensation from the anterior 2/3 of tongue is carried by:**
   a. 10th cranial nerve   b. 7th
   c. 12th   d. 5th cranial nerve

3. **Tip of tongue is highly sensitive to:**
   a. Bitter taste   b. Sour taste
   c. Sweet taste   d. Salt taste

4. **Bitter taste is mediated by action of:**
   a. Guanylyl cyclase
   b. G-protein
   c. Tyrosine kinase
   d. Epithelial Na^+ channel

5. **The basal cells in the taste bud arise from:**
   a. Epithelial cells   b. Receptor cells
   c. Sensory neurons   d. Supporting cells

6. **Sense organ for taste is:**
   a. Taste bud   b. Circumvallate papilla
   c. Hair cell   d. Tongue

7. **Dysgeusia is:**
   a. Disturbed sense of taste
   b. Absent taste sensation
   c. Diminished taste sensation
   d. Increased taste sensation

8. **Salt sensation is perceived maximum at the:**
   a. Tip of tongue
   b. Sides of tongue
   c. Posterior part (base) of tongue
   d. Centre of tongue

9. **Bitter substance is tasted normally at the:**
   a. Tip of tongue
   b. Sides of tongue
   c. Posterior part (base) of tongue
   d. Centre of tongue

10. **Dryness of mouth is called:**
    a. Xerostomia   b. Xerophthalmia
    c. Sialorrhea   d. Anhydrosis

ANSWERS

| 1. b | 2. d | 3. c | 4. b | 5. a |
| 6. a | 7. a | 8. b | 9. c | 10. a |

Olfaction

CHAPTER 101

LEARNING OBJECTIVES
- Describe the features of olfactory epithelium
- Explain the mechanism of perception of smell
- Trace the olfactory pathway
- Mention the factors affecting olfaction
- Discuss the pathophysiology of altered smell

■ INTRODUCTION

PY10.13: Describe and discuss perception of smell and taste sensation.

Sense of smell or olfaction is the most primitive of all our senses. Sense of smell is a **chemical sense** like taste.

Physiologically, taste and smell are related to each other. Flavors of different foods are a combination of gustation and olfaction. These two are also known as **visceral senses** because of their close association to gastrointestinal system. For appreciation of taste, the substance must be in the liquid form. For smell it must be in the gaseous form. Volatile substances generally have strong odors. After reaching the nose, the vapors get dissolved in mucus secreted by olfactory epithelium. The olfactory receptors are stimulated by the molecules in solution.

The importance of smell
- Nutritive function—olfaction helps in the search for food, and it also help in enjoying the taste of food.
- Increases gastrointestinal secretion and motility.
- Protective function—sense of smell makes the animal aware of environmental hazards, like the smell of smoke.
- Helps in reproduction. Olfaction has an important role in the reactions of sex. Male gypsy moth can be attracted by the female at a distance of three miles!
- Pleasurable olfactory memories are very resistant to decay and are retained lifelong. For example, the emotional tie between the mother and the baby is retained lifelong.
- Certain odors can awaken long time old memories associated with it

Olfaction is unique among other sensations because of the following reasons:
- Olfactory receptor cell (bipolar neuron) is the only nerve cell that is exposed to the external environment.
- Olfactory cells are not only receptors but also neurons. Bipolar olfactory sensory neuron function both as receptor and ganglion cell (first order neuron).
- Olfactory receptor cells (sensory neurons) undergo rapid turnover by proliferation and differentiation of the basal cells of olfactory mucosa (exception to the statement that neurons cannot regenerate).
- Olfaction has no direct relay in the thalamus. The fibers from the primary olfactory cortex (piriform cortex, entorhinal cortex, amygdala etc.) pass through the dorsomedial nucleus of thalamus to reach the neocortex which is concerned with discrimination of odors.
- Olfaction has *no direct* neocortical projection. The olfactory sensation reaches the orbitofrontal and frontal cortex only after projecting to the primary olfactory cortex.
- In contrast to all other sensory pathways, the olfactory afferent pathway has only two neurons.

■ THE OLFACTORY APPARATUS

The Olfactory Epithelium/Olfactory Mucosa

Olfactory epithelium is the only place where the nervous system is very close to the external environment. The olfactory mucosa is a yellowish pigmented epithelium which covers an area of 9 cm^2 in the roof of the nasal cavity. It lines the superior turbinate and upper 1/3rd of the nasal septum **(Fig. 101.1)**.

Structure

Olfactory epithelium is composed of three types of cells:
1. Olfactory receptor cells (olfactory sensory neurons)
2. Supporting cells or sustentacular cells
3. Basal stem cells.

Olfactory Receptor Cell

Olfactory receptor is a **bipolar sensory neuron,** which lies between the supporting cells. There are about 10–20 million olfactory sensory receptor cells in man. The olfactory receptor cell has a cell body, an axon and a dendrite. The dendrite, which is short and thick, extends to the free surface of the

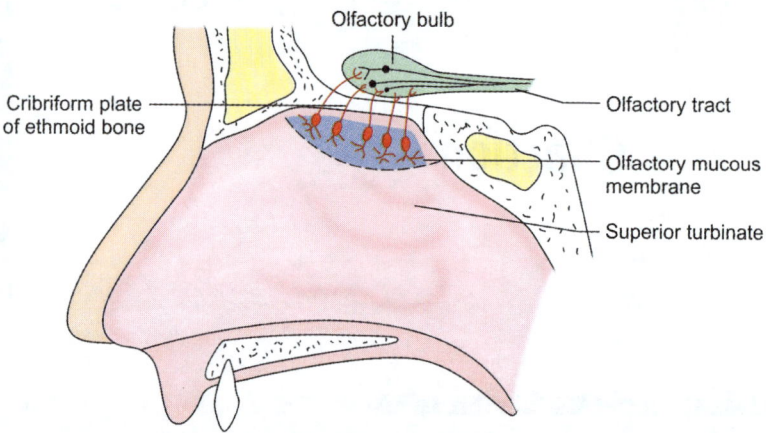

Fig. 101.1: Location of olfactory mucosa.

olfactory epithelium where it expands to form the olfactory rod or knob, which bears **olfactory cilia**. There are about 6–12 cilia for each rod which projects into the mucus secreted by the supporting cells overlying the epithelium. The cilia are unmyelinated, 2 micrometer long and 0.1–0.3 micrometer in diameter. Cilia contain odorant receptor proteins which are GPCRs. There are more than 1000 different types of odorant receptor proteins. The odorant receptors bind to odor-producing molecules (odorants) dissolved in the mucus. Odorant binding proteins are present in the mucus which facilitates the diffusion of odorants to the odorant receptors.

The olfactory sensory neurons survive for about 1-2 months. Then they are replaced by new olfactory sensory neurons generated from the basal stem cells by mitosis. *A peculiar feature of olfactory neuron is that it is one of the neurons in the adult nervous system that can be regenerated. Neurons of hippocampus can also regenerate.*

The axon of the olfactory receptor cell (bipolar neuron) is unmyelinated and it forms the olfactory nerve which passes through the cribriform plate of the ethmoid bone and enters the olfactory bulbs on the inferior surface of the frontal lobe. Here, the **first order neuron** ends. Actually there is no olfactory nerve as such. The axons of many receptors run in small bundles or fascicles not as a discrete nerve, and they pierce the basal lamina, where each bundle becomes ensheathed by Schwann cells.

Supporting Cell or Sustentacular Cell

Supporting cells are large, irregular, columnar cells that separate the bipolar neurons. The free surface bears numerous microvilli, which secrete **mucus,** which cover the olfactory epithelium.

Basal Cells

Basal cells are irregular polygonal stem cells confined to the basal lamina. New receptor cells are formed from the basal cells.

Olfactory Gland or Bowman's Gland

Olfactory glands are branched, tubular structures beneath the olfactory epithelium. It secretes a serous fluid containing both water and oil, which lines the olfactory epithelium. Odoriferous substances that are soluble in water and oil produce strong odors. These glands also secrete the yellow pigment.

Olfactory Bulb

Olfactory bulb is a flattened ovoid strip of gray matter seen on the cribriform plate of ethmoid bone. The different types of cells in the olfactory bulb are:
1. Mitral cells
2. Tufted cells
3. Interneurons
❖ Granule cells
❖ Periglomerular short axon cells.

Mitral Cells

The axons of bipolar cells synapse with dendrites of mitral cells to form complex glomerular synapse called **olfactory glomerulus (Fig. 101.2)**. About 1000 olfactory neurons synapse on the dendrites of a single mitral cell.

Tufted Cells

Tufted cells are small triangular cells whose dendrites form olfactory glomeruli. Mitral cells and tufted cells form **second order** neurons of olfactory pathway. Their axons constitute the olfactory tract.

Granule Cells

Granule cells are inhibitory interneurons that have no axons (anaxonic neuron).

They synapse with dendrites of mitral cells and tufted cells. The synapses are **dendro-dendritic reciprocal synapses**. Mitral cells stimulate granule cells while granule cells inhibit mitral cells. In reciprocal synapse, the presynaptic and the postsynaptic membranes contain receptors for the neurotransmitter and vesicles that release neurotransmitters. So this synapse does not obey the property of one-way conduction of impulses. Gamma-amino butyric acid (GABA) is the neurotransmitter in the granule cell.

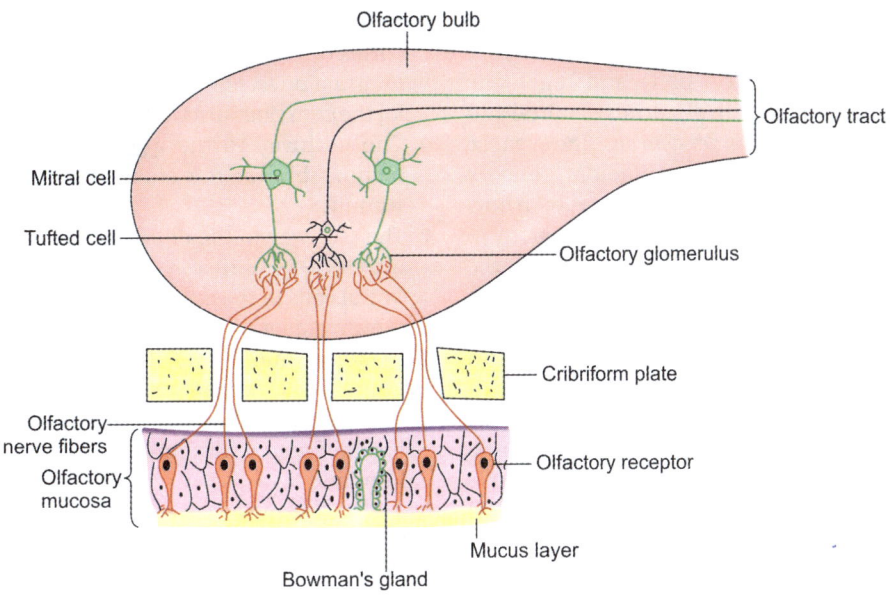

Fig. 101.2: Details of olfactory mucosa and olfactory bulb.

Periglomerular Short Axon Cells

Periglomerular short axon cells connect glomeruli and inhibit mitral cells. The olfactory glomeruli demonstrate lateral inhibition mediated by periglomerular cells and granule cells. This sharpens and focuses olfactory signals.

It shows a regional projection from olfactory epithelium; upper part neurons are projected to upper part of olfactory bulb and lower part neurons are projected to lower part of olfactory bulb.

Mechanism of Stimulation of Olfactory Receptors (Fig. 101.3)

- An odorant molecule binds to the specific olfactory receptor protein in the cilium of the olfactory receptor cell.
- The olfactory receptors are G-protein coupled receptors (GPCRs) which has 3 subunits α, β and γ. When the odorant binds to the receptor, the receptor gets activated and stimulates the heterotrimeric G protein attached to it and the subunits (*refer* **Fig. 61.1**).
- The α-subunit of G-protein in turn activates adenylyl cyclase present in the cell membrane and increases the production of cAMP from ATP.
- The cAMP acts as a second messenger and binds to cAMP gated cation channels on the cell membrane.
- Cation channels open and Na⁺ and Ca²⁺ diffuse into the cilium
- The increased positivity inside produces membrane depolarization and graded potential in the receptor.
- The increased Ca²⁺ opens Ca²⁺ activated Cl⁻ channels. Cl⁻ moves out of the receptor cell which further depolarizes the cell **(Fig. 101.3)**.
- When the receptor potential exceeds its threshold it triggers action potential in the olfactory neuron that travel along the axon of the sensory neuron to the olfactory bulb (receptor itself is modified olfactory neuron).

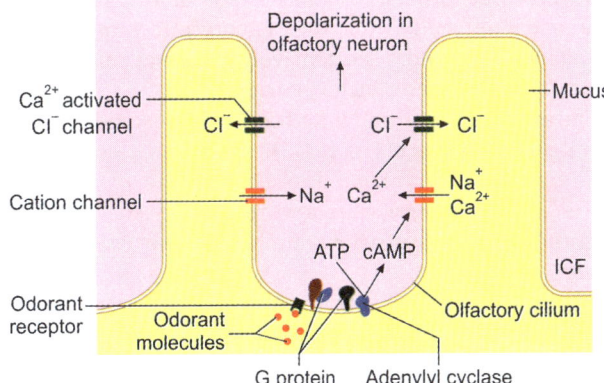

Fig. 101.3: Signal transduction in an odorant receptor.

Innervation of Olfactory Mucosa

Olfactory nerve (I cranial nerve) carries the sense of smell from the olfactory mucosa. General sensations from the mucosa are carried by trigeminal nerve (V cranial nerve). If irritant substances like ammonia are used to test the sense of smell, it stimulates both the cranial nerves. So such substances should not be used to test the sense of smell.

OLFACTORY PATHWAY

Olfactory receptors are **chemoreceptors** as well as **telereceptors**. The olfactory receptor proteins are located in the cilia of the bipolar cells. The odorant molecule which reaches the olfactory epithelium from inspired air should be *volatile and water or lipid soluble*. It dissolves in the mucous layer covering the olfactory mucosa. The interaction of the odorant molecule with its receptor induces conformational change in the receptor protein. The receptor potential generates an action potential in the olfactory sensory neuron which is transmitted to the olfactory bulb.

Bipolar olfactory sensory neuron is the *first order neuron*. Axons of bipolar cells (unmyelinated) form the olfactory nerve which pierce the cribriform plate and reach the olfactory bulb. Here, it synapses with dendrites of mitral and tufted cells which form the *second order neurons*. The synapse forms the **olfactory glomeruli**. Each olfactory sensory neuron with one type of odorant receptor synapses with only one or two glomeruli so that the pathway becomes unique to the odorant. Thus the central olfactory system can decode the identity of the odorant precisely.

Olfactory bulb also contains periglomerular cells and granule cells which are inhibitory neurons that release GABA as the transmitter. The periglomerular cells connect one glomerulus to another. The granule cells are anaxonic cells which make reciprocal synapses with the dendrites of mitral and tufted cells. The mitral and tufted cells excite the granule cell by releasing glutamate and the granule cells in turn inhibit the mitral and tufted cells by releasing GABA. This is an example of **lateral inhibition** mediated by periglomerular cells and granule cells and this helps to sharpen the olfactory signals. There are also multiple inputs from olfactory areas of the cerebral cortex as well as from basal forebrain to the olfactory glomeruli. Thus, the sensory information from the olfactory receptors is extensively processed and refined before it is sent to the olfactory cortex.

The axons of mitral and tufted cells pass posteriorly as the lateral **olfactory tract (Fig. 101.2)**.

Some of the axons of tufted cells cross to the opposite side in the anterior commissure and reach opposite olfactory bulb and make synapse with granule cells. The rest reach the olfactory tubercle.

Axons of the mitral cells terminate on the dendrites of pyramidal cells in five areas of the olfactory cortex:
1. Anterior olfactory nucleus
2. Piriform cortex
3. Olfactory tubercle
4. Amygdala
5. Entorhinal cortex.

- From these regions information reaches the frontal cortex or via the thalamus to the orbitofrontal cortex. The information reaching the orbitofrontal cortex is responsible for the conscious discrimination of odor (**Flowchart 101.1**).
- The pathway to the amygdala and hypothalamus is responsible for the emotional responses to olfactory stimuli.
- The pathway to the entorhinal cortex is concerned with olfactory memories.
- Mitral cells in the accessory olfactory bulb project only to the amygdala.
- In some mammals, the sensory neurons from the Vomeronasal organ project to the accessory olfactory bulb and from there to amygdala and hypothalamus. It is concerned with reproduction. It is usually absent in humans.

> From the olfactory cortex, information is relayed to the frontal cortex directly and to the orbitofrontal cortex via the thalamus. Olfactory pathway is the only sensory pathway that does not have an obligatory synaptic relay in the thalamus. All other sensations are first processed in the thalamus before projecting to the cerebral cortex.

Processing of Olfactory Information

It is in the prepiriform cortex that the more complex aspects of olfaction are integrated. Entorhinal cortex is concerned with **olfactory memories**. From the entorhinal cortex, fibers are projected to hippocampus, insula and orbitofrontal cortex which are the areas of **olfactory discrimination**. The orbitofrontal cortex, part of neocortex is concerned with conscious discrimination of odors. In lesion of the orbitofrontal cortex, the capacity to discriminate odors is lost. Amygdala and hypothalamus are concerned with emotional and behavioral responses to olfactory stimuli.

If the anterior commissure is cut, olfaction of both sides is impaired. If olfactory tract is cut, olfaction of opposite side is lost.

Flowchart 101.1: Schematic representation of olfactory pathway.

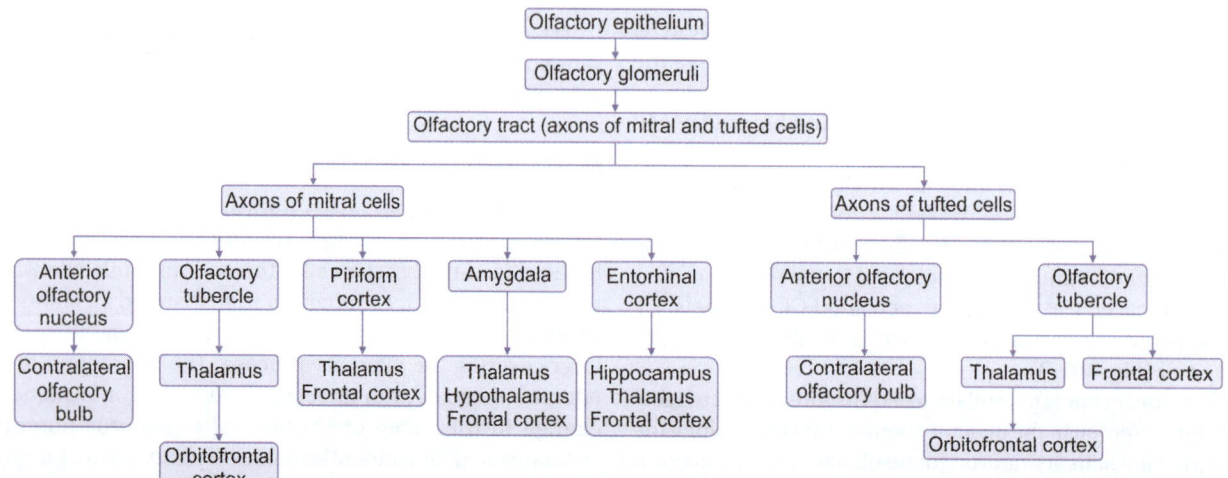

Another phylogenetically more recent olfactory pathway passes through the dorsomedial nucleus of thalamus and terminates in the posterolateral quadrant of the orbitofrontal cortex. This pathway is involved in the conscious perception of odor.

Inhibitory Pathways

Large number of *corticofugal inhibitory fibers* passes from the olfactory regions of brain backward along the olfactory tract and terminate on special inhibitory cells, the granule cells in the olfactory bulb. The granule cells in turn inhibit the mitral and tufted cells.

This contributes to the lateral inhibition occurring in the olfactory glomeruli.

Factors Influencing Olfactory Function

1. Threshold of olfactory receptors
2. Concentration of the odorant substance
3. Solubility of the odorant—substances having high water and lipid solubility have strong odors
4. Olfactory adaptation.

Olfactory Threshold

High lipid and water-soluble substances have strong odors. Substances with same number of carbon atoms but different structures have different odors. Humans can distinguish about 10,000 different odors. Common odors are aromatic, fragrant, garlic, burning, nauseating odor, etc.

Olfactory threshold for various substances are different. **Odor detection threshold** is the lowest concentration of a chemical that can be detected. Substances that can be detected at very low concentration include hydrogen sulfide, acetic acid, kerosene etc. Olfactory threshold can be measured by an **olfactometer** called **Zwaardimaker's olfactometer**. According to Zwaardimaker, odors are classified into alliaceous, e.g., H_2S; ambrosial (amber, musk); aromatic (camphor, clove); caprillic (cheese); empyreumatic (coffee); ethereal (fruit, ether); fragrant (flower, vanilla); nauseating (feces); and repulsive (bed bug).

Olfactory threshold of *methyl mercaptan* present in garlic is 1/million of a mg/L of air and for chloroform it is 3.3 mg/L of air. *Methyl mercaptan is usually mixed with natural gas to detect leak from the pipeline.*

It is seen from the study of the structure of odorous substances that each smell is evoked by characteristic structure of the molecule which has a particular shape. According to Amoore, smells are a mixture of 7 primary smells—camphorous, musky, floral, peppermint, ethereal, pungent and putrid. Recent studies indicate that there are as many as 50 or more primary sensations of smell in contrast to 3 primary colors detected by the eye and 5 primary taste sensations.

Olfactory Adaptation

Olfactory pathway shows adaptation. For example, when a person is continuously exposed to a particular smell, the perception of odor decreases and finally it ceases. This is due to the fairly rapid adaptation or desensitization occurring in the olfactory pathways. Adaptation is specific for that particular odor and the threshold for other odors remains unchanged. This is due to a central phenomenon and also due to changes occurring at the level of receptors. 50% of olfactory adaptation is due to changes occurring in the receptors. Rest occurs in the CNS. Central phenomenon is due to the strong inhibitory feedback to the olfactory bulb from the olfactory cortex. Large number of nerve fibers passes from the olfactory areas of brain backwards along the olfactory tract and terminate on special inhibitory cells in the olfactory bulb called granule cells.

The **olfactory coefficient or minimum identifiable odor (MIO)** of a substance can be determined using olfactometer. The degree of adaptation for a particular odor can be measured by the rise in the threshold concentration required to excite the sense of smell.

Masking of Odors

An offensive odor can be masked by a pleasant odor. This principle is made use of in perfume industry. Deodorants do not remove the offensive odor; they only mask it with the pleasant odor. Weaker odors are masked by the stronger ones.

VOMERONASAL ORGAN

1. **Vomeronasal organ or Jacobson's organ** is a patch of olfactory epithelium located along the anterior third of the nasal septum. It is well developed in rodents and other mammals. This structure is concerned with the perception of odors related to pheromones. Vomeronasal sensory neurons project to the accessory olfactory bulb and from there to areas in the amygdala and hypothalamus that are concerned with reproduction and feeding behavior.
2. **Pheromones** are hormone-like substances produced by animals during the mating season which emit specific odor that can attract another animal of the same species even from a distance. Pheromones can produce hormonal and behavioral changes in another animal of the same species. There is evidence for the existence of pheromones in humans, and there is close relationship between smell and sexual function.

VARIATIONS IN THE SENSE OF SMELL

> **PY10.14:** Describe and discuss pathophysiology of altered smell and taste sensation.

1. Sex—females are more sensitive to smell especially at the time of ovulation and pregnancy.
2. Age—olfactory sensitivity decreases with advancing age.
3. **Hyperosmia** is increased sensitivity to sense of smell. For example, in hysteria, raised intracranial pressure, adrenal insufficiency, menopause, neurasthenia, etc., sensitivity to smell and taste is increased.
4. **Hyposmia** is decreased sensitivity to smell, may be due to constant exposure to that particular smell (adaptation)

or it may be pathological as in hypogonadism, vitamin A deficiency, etc.
5. **Anosmia** is absence of sense of smell. Bilateral anosmia is seen in common cold, fracture of cribriform plate, prolonged use of snuff, bilateral mechanical obstruction in the nasal cavity, etc. Unilateral anosmia may be due to diseases affecting olfactory nerve, olfactory bulb or tract of one side. Lesion of the olfactory cortex of one side does not produce anosmia of that side because fibers from each olfactory tract travel to both cerebral hemispheres.
6. **Parosmia** is altered sense of smell. It occurs in sinusitis.
7. **Olfactory hallucinations,** i.e., perception of non-existing odors occur as an aura of temporal lobe epilepsy, secondary to temporal lobe lesion, psychiatric disorders, etc. Amygdaloid complex is situated in the temporal lobe and the olfactory aura which precedes an epileptic attack is due to involvement of the temporal lobe of cerebral cortex. **Aura** is a movement, a sensation or a mental disturbance which precedes an epileptic convulsion.

MULTIPLE CHOICE QUESTIONS

1. The place in the body where a neuron is closest to external environment:
    a. Taste bud
    b. Skin
    c. Cornea
    d. Olfactory mucous membrane
2. The type of neuron in the olfactory bulb which connects one glomerulus to another and serves as an inhibitory interneuron:
    a. Mitral cell
    b. Periglomerular cell
    c. Tufted cell
    d. Granule cell
3. The first order neurons in the olfactory pathway are:
    a. Receptor cells
    b. Mitral cells
    c. Granule cells
    d. Tufted cells
4. Olfactory bulb contains all the following cells, *except:*
    a. Mitral cells
    b. Tufted cells
    c. Granule cells
    d. Golgi cells
5. Odorant receptors are located in the:
    a. Olfactory bulb
    b. Sustentacular cells of olfactory epithelium
    c. Cilia of the olfactory sensory neuron
    d. Olfactory mucus lining the olfactory epithelium
6. All the following statements are true regarding olfactory transmission, *except:*
    a. An olfactory sensory neuron expresses a wide range of odorant receptors
    b. Lateral inhibition within the olfactory glomeruli helps in olfactory discrimination
    c. Conscious discrimination of odor is dependent on the pathway to orbitofrontal cortex
    d. Olfactory adaptation is due to stimulation of descending fibers from olfactory cortex ending in granule cells
7. Which of the following sensory deficits is likely to be experienced if there is damage to the brain including periamygdaloid, piriform and entorhinal cortices?
    a. Hyperosmia
    b. Taste and odor abnormalities
    c. Visual disturbance
    d. Hearing defect
8. All the following statements regarding olfaction are true, *except:*
    a. It has no relay in the thalamus
    b. Its receptors are in direct contact with the external environment
    c. Olfactory sense is poorly developed in man
    d. Olfactory receptors are telereceptors as well as chemoreceptors.
9. Olfactory stimuli are relayed to all the following regions of brain, *except:*
    a. Anterior olfactory nucleus
    b. Pyriform cortex
    c. Medial geniculate body
    d. Amygdala
10. All the following statements related to olfactory pathway are true, *except:*
    a. Medial olfactory stria contains axons of tufted cells
    b. Mitral cells stimulate granule cells while granule cells inhibit mitral cells
    c. Lateral inhibition occurs in the olfactory bulb
    d. Orbitofrontal cortex is concerned with the emotional responses to olfactory stimuli
11. The true statement regarding olfactory adaptation is:
    a. Adaptation develops within seconds or minutes
    b. Olfactory receptors are tonic receptors
    c. Adaptation does not occur to irritant chemical sense
    d. Degree of adaptation cannot be measured
12. Difference in the intensity of a given odor can be detected by changing the concentration of the odor producing substance by:
    a. 1%
    b. 30%
    c. 5%
    d. 3%
13. All the following statements regarding olfaction are true, *except:*
    a. It has neocortical projection
    b. The ability to identify smells decreases as age advances
    c. Lateral inhibition in olfactory glomeruli is mediated by periglomerular cells and granule cells
    d. Alzheimer disease does not affect the olfactory nerves
14. The substance that is mixed with natural gas to detect leak from the pipe line is:
    a. Methyl mercaptan
    b. Methanol
    c. Chloroform
    d. Camphor

15. The substance with the least olfactory threshold is:
    a. Artificial musk
    b. Methyl mercaptan
    c. Propyl mercaptan
    d. Chloroform
16. All the following directly relay in the sensory cortex, except:
    a. Pain
    b. Touch
    c. Temperature
    d. Olfaction
17. Smell receptors are seen in:
    a. Lower 1/3 of nasal mucosa
    b. Upper 1/3 of nasal mucosa
    c. Amygdaloid body
    d. Cribriform plate
18. Receptor which itself is the dendrite of a nerve:
    a. Olfactory
    b. Gustatory
    c. Visual
    d. Auditory

ANSWERS

1. d	2. b	3. a	4. d	5. c
6. a	7. b	8. a	9. c	10. d
11. a	12. b	13. d	14. a	15. b
16. d	17. b	18. a		

FILL IN THE BLANKS/NAME THE FOLLOWING/ GIVE THE NORMAL VALUE

1. Smell and taste are classified as **visceral** senses.
2. Smell and taste receptors are **chemoreceptors**.
3. Name the only place in the body where the nervous system is closest to the external worldL: **olfactory epithelium**.
4. Olfactory bipolar sensory neurons have the ability to regenerate by differentiation from basal cells.
5. Life span of olfactory receptor cells: **60 days**.
6. Axons of the olfactory sensory neurons form the **first cranial nerve or olfactory nerve**.
7. The cells contained in the olfactory bulb: **mitral and tufted cells, periglomerular cells and granule cells**.
8. Orbitofrontal cortex is concerned with **conscious discrimination** of odors.
9. Humans can recognize more than **10,000** different odors.
10. The concentration of the odor producing substance must be changed by about **30%** before a difference in intensity can be detected.
11. All the odorant receptors are coupled to **heterotrimeric G proteins**.
12. Vomeronasal organ is concerned with the perception of odors that act as **pheromones**.
13. The sense of smell is most acute at the time of **ovulation** in females.
14. Inability to smell: **anosmia**.
15. Alteration in the character of smell: **parosmia**.
16. Primary taste sensations: **sweet, salty, sour, bitter and umami**.
17. Taste sensation from the anterior 2/3rd of tongue is carried by **facial** nerve.
18. Taste sensation from posterior 1/3rd of tongue is carried by **glossopharyngeal** nerve.
19. The sense organ of taste: **taste bud**.
20. Name the papilla that does not contain taste buds: **filiform papilla**.
21. The standard reference substance for sweetness: **sucrose**.
22. Second order neurons of taste pathway is located in the **nucleus of tractus solitarius** in the medulla.
23. Absence of sense of taste: **ageusia**.
24. Disturbed sense of taste: **dysgeusia**.
25. Name the taste modifier protein extracted from miracle fruit when applied to the tongue makes acids taste sweet: **miraculin**.

CLINICAL CASE SCENARIO

1. A 10-year old boy had difficulty in interpreting graphs in the class room. He was advised to consult an ophthalmologist. On examination his visual acuity was found to be normal. But he could not identify numbers correctly in the ishihara chart. Answer the following:
    a. Identify the defect.
    b. State the mode of inheritance of the condition.
    c. Describe the tests done to come to a diagnosis.
    d. Explain the pathway for accommodation.

SECTION 12 INTEGRATED PHYSIOLOGY

CHAPTER 102: Integrated Physiology

LEARNING OBJECTIVES

Desirable to know
- Describe the physiology of infancy
- Discuss the physiology of aging

Must Know
- Describe the concept and criteria for brain death
- Describe the cardiorespiratory and metabolic adjustments during exercise and the effects of physical training
- Compare the cardiorespiratory changes in isotonic and isometric exercise
- Explain the effects of free radicals and antioxidants in the body
- Explain the effects of exercise under different environmental conditions like heat and cold
- Explain the consequences of sedentary lifestyle

PHYSIOLOGY OF INFANCY

PY11.6: Describe physiology of infancy.

For the first year after birth, a baby is called an **infant.** The term **baby** can be used to refer to any child from birth to the age of 4 years. Early childhood begins at age two, when a child may be referred to as a toddler. Childhood continues until adolescence, which is the period of transition into adulthood. For the first month after birth, an infant is called a **newborn**. A newborn has a distinctive appearance.

Features of a Newborn

- During labor and birth, the infant's skull changes shape to fit through the birth canal, sometimes causing the child to be born with a deformed or elongated head. It will usually return to normal on its own within a few days or weeks.
- A newborn's head is very large in proportion to the body.
- Normal head circumference for a full-term infant is 33–36 cm at birth. At birth, many regions of the newborn's skull have not yet been converted to bone, leaving soft areas known as fontanels. Later in the child's life, these bones will fuse together in a natural process. A protein called noggin is responsible for the delay in an infant's skull fusion.
- A newborn's shoulders and hip are wide, the abdomen protrudes slightly, and the arms and legs are relatively long with respect to the rest of their body.
- The average birth weight of a full-term newborn is in the range of 2.7–4.2 kg. Over the first 5–7 days following birth, the body weight of a term neonate decreases by 3–7%. It is as a result of the resorption and urination of the fluid that initially fills the lungs. After the first week, healthy term neonates should gain 10–20 grams/day.
- Immediately after birth, a newborn's skin is often greyish to dusky blue in color. As soon as the newborn begins to breathe, usually within a minute or two, the skin's color reaches its normal color.
- A newborn's genitalia are enlarged and reddened, with male infants having an unusually large scrotum. The breasts may also be enlarged, even in male infants. This is caused by naturally occurring maternal hormones. Vaginal discharge or bleeding may occur in female babies and is a temporary condition.
- After birth, the umbilical cord is normally cut, leaving a 1–2 inch stump. The umbilical stump will dry out, shrivel, darken, and spontaneously fall off within about 3 weeks. This will later become umbilicus after it heals.
- The infant lacks in the newborn period vitamin K putting it at the risk for hemorrhagic disease. To prevent this, all infants born should be given vitamin K prophylaxis.

Changes in the Cardiovascular System

Refer fetal circulation (Chapter 32).

Respiratory System

- During intrauterine life, the fetal lungs are filled with amniotic fluid. After birth the lung requires the clearance of the lung amniotic fluid with sufficient surfactant secretion. Infants that are born via vaginal deliveries are squeezed as they pass through the vaginal canal which allows removal of much of the fluid from the lungs by compressing it.

- Regular and automatic breathing should start.
- Once the baby is out of the uterus, several external environmental factors, such as light, change in temperature, and noise, activate the nervous system and prompt the infant to take the first breath. Internal factors, such as stimulation of central chemoreceptors, also play a role in stimulating respiration due to hypoxia.
- In the newborn, the work of breathing is high and breathing is usually labored using accessory muscles to overcome the high surface tension. As the fluid leaves the alveoli in the lungs, the effort of breathing is reduced. This is also one of the reasons why newborns have an increased respiratory rate of 30 to 60 breaths per minute. Other reasons include high metabolic rate and perfusion-ventilation differences.
- Due to immature central drive responses, newborns may have periods of apnea lasting less than 5 seconds. While this is considered abnormal in adults, it is normal for newborns to have apneic episodes.

Hematological System

- Adult hemoglobin is hemoglobin A. **Hb F** is the primary hemoglobin produced by the fetus. Its role is to transport oxygen adequately at low oxygen tension. It has a high affinity for oxygen, making it suitable for oxygen extraction from maternal blood across the placenta. HbF is important in the newborn period due to impairment of oxygen delivery to the tissues.
- Around six months of age, Hb F is replaced with Hb A, also known as adult hemoglobin.
- Infants lack vitamin K due to immature hepatocyte function and lack of enteric bacteria that produce vitamin K. Vitamin K is used in the synthesis of clotting factors II, VII, IX, X and proteins C and S. Therefore, those who lack vitamin K have an increased risk of hemorrhage. So a prophylactic injection of vitamin K is given to every newborn to protect against hemorrhagic disease.

Metabolism and Thermoregulation

- Intrauterine temperature is that of the normal maternal temperature. Fetal body temperature is 0.5°C above the maternal temperature.
- At birth, the newborn loses its heat due to the dramatic drop in environmental temperature. The newborn's heat is mostly lost via radiation.
- For the newborn to be able to thermo-regulate, the newborn's sympathetic system should be activated in response to the cold stimulus. The main mediators to cope up with the new environment are cortisol and catecholamine.
- The sympathetic stimulation activates thermogenesis via brown adipose tissue. Brown adipose tissue is present around the kidneys and muscles of the back. Brown adipose tissue generates heat by uncoupling oxidative phosphorylation in the mitochondria. The newborn also can produce heat by shivering.
- The high heart rate (120 to 160 beats per minute) seen in newborn infants can be attributed to the high rate of metabolic activity mainly due to labored breathing, feeding, and thermogenesis.

Infancy

Infancy is defined as the first year of life after birth. Infants are born with certain abilities already developed. For example, they have a well-developed sense of smell. They can also communicate their needs by crying when they are hungry, uncomfortable, etc. During their first year, they develop many other abilities:

- By 6 weeks after birth, babies start smiling and make sounds.
- By 6 months, they spend a lot of time babbling. They have also learned to sit and are start to crawl.
- By 12 months, they will say their first words. They can stand with support and can walk with help.
- Infancy is the period of most rapid growth after birth. Growth during infancy is even faster than growth during puberty. By the end of the first year, the average baby is twice the length it was at birth and three times its birth weight. Infancy is also the period when most of the deciduous teeth erupt. The front teeth erupt first, usually starting around six months after birth. There are 20 deciduous teeth altogether, and they continue to erupt until about three years of age.
- Newborns need about 18 hours of sleep each day. They usually sleep in long naps throughout the day and night. As infants get older they need less sleep. They also start to sleep through the night and just take short naps during the day.

APPLIED PHYSIOLOGY

Cardiovascular System

The cardiovascular shunts present in the fetus in the intrauterine life take time to close. If they fail to close, they can cause complications for the infant. There are two different types of shunts: left-to-right and right-to-left.

Left-to-right Shunts

These are usually benign and symptoms present later in the child's life. They are:
- Atrial septal defect
- Ventricular septal defect
- Patent ductus arteriosus

Right-to-left Shunts

These are usually present earlier in infancy and can be associated with other cardiac abnormalities such as:
- Persistent truncus arteriosus
- Transposition of the great vessels
- Tricuspid atresia
- Tetralogy of Fallot

Hematological System

Around six months of age, Hb F of the fetus is replaced with Hb A. However, Hb F disappears much quicker than HbA is produced. This leads to a physiological anemia of infancy at 7 to 11 weeks of life.

Infants lack vitamin K due to immature hepatocyte function and lack of enteric bacteria that produce vitamin K. Infants that do not receive the vitamin K supplementation at the time of birth are at increased risk of bleeding disorder known as vitamin K deficiency bleeding.

Metabolism and Thermoregulation

Preterm infants are at a particular disadvantage when it comes to thermoregulation because the brown adipose tissue has not fully developed and does not provide adequate heat response.

PHYSIOLOGY OF AGING

PY11.7: Describe and discuss physiology of aging; free radicals and antioxidants.

Aging (senescence) is a natural process that begins at conception and continues for as long as we live. Physiological changes occur with aging in all organ systems with progressive degeneration of organ systems and tissues. With advancing age, all of the body systems show reduced efficiency. The basic mechanism of aging is the long-term imbalance between tissue damage and repair. During development, there is a brief adult period when damage and repair are in balance, and then begins long-term imbalance in favor of damage. Current concept of old age is the **young-old** as being around 65–74 years of age, the **middle-old** 75–84 and the **old-old** more than 85 years.

Changes in the Different Systems during Aging

Nervous System

Aging is associated with many neurological disorders as the capacity of the nervous system to transmit signals decreases. There is loss of neurons in both the brain and spinal cord. There is loss of neuronal dendrites which reduces the amount of synaptic transmission. Depression can be the result of impaired synaptic activity.

Alzheimer's and Parkinson's diseases are the progressive neurodegenerative diseases associated with aging. Alzheimer's is characterized by progressive cognitive deterioration along with a change in behavior and a decline in the activities of daily life. It causes nerve cell death and tissue loss throughout the brain, affecting all its functions. The cortex atrophies and this damages the areas involved in thinking, planning and remembering. The shrinkage of nerve cells is especially severe in the hippocampus which plays an important role in the formation of new memories. The disease leads to memory loss, changes in personality, depression, apathy, social withdrawal, mood swings, and distrust in others, irritability and aggressiveness.

Skin and Temperature Regulation

The primary function of the skin is to protect the organism from the environment. As we age, the dermis decreases in thickness by about 20%. The epidermis of the skin atrophies with age and due to changes in collagen and elastin, the skin loses its tone and elasticity. As it thins it loses vascularity, cellularity and sensitivity. The skin's ability to dissipate or retain internal heat is diminished. The skin becomes thin, fragile and slow to heal. Subcutaneous fat deposition is altered in the elderly. Muscle, blood vessels and bone become more visible beneath the skin due to thinning of subcutaneous fat on the extremities. Fat deposition occurs mainly on the abdomen and thighs.

Sweat glands undergo atrophy and temperature regulation by heat loss by evaporation of sweat becomes less efficient. Cutaneous circulation is also diminished. Decreased temperature sensitivity can increase the risk of injury from hyperthermia and hypothermia.

Musculoskeletal System

Normal aging is characterized by a decrease in bone and muscle mass and an increase in adiposity. As early as the third decade of life there is a general reduction in the size, elasticity and strength of all muscle tissue. The loss of muscle mass continues throughout life. Muscle fibers continue to become smaller in diameter due to a decrease in reserves of ATP, glycogen, myoglobin and the number of myofibrils. As a result, as the body ages, muscular activity becomes less efficient and requires more effort to accomplish a given task. Heat production by muscular contraction decreases. A decline in muscle mass and a reduction in muscle strength lead to risk of fractures, weakness, reduction in the quality of life and loss of independence. Osteoporosis is frequently seen due to a linear decline in bone mass after the fourth decade. Lean body mass declines with age and this is primarily due to loss and atrophy of muscle cells. Degenerative changes occur in many joints and this, combined with the loss of muscle mass, affects elderly patients' locomotion.

Respiratory System

Lung function diminishes with age. The lungs show impaired gas exchange, a decrease in vital capacity and slower expiratory flow rates. The major contributing factors are the progressive loss of elastic recoil within lung tissue, the chest wall becomes stiff, and there is a decrease in alveolar surface area. These changes diminish the efficiency of gas exchange and make it more difficult to exercise.

Gastrointestinal System

Functional changes, largely related to altered motility patterns, occur in the gastrointestinal system with senescence, and atrophic gastritis and altered hepatic drug metabolism are common in the elderly. There is a reduction in the secretion of digestive enzymes which leads to a decline in the capacity to digest and absorb nutrients.

Cardiovascular System

The heart becomes stiffer and so its efficiency as a pump decreases. The arteries lose their elasticity and offer greater resistance to blood flow. The cardiac output decreases, blood pressure increases and arteriosclerosis develops. Cardiac output of healthy exercising elders can usually be maintained, allowing moderate continued physical activity throughout their lives. The major disadvantage of the elderly seems to lie in their relatively reduced blood flow to the periphery, demonstrated by their slow increase in skin temperature, and reduced efficiency of evaporation of sweat during exercise.

Renal System

The number of nephrons decreases as age advances. Blood flow to the kidneys is also decreased and the efficiency of the kidney to remove waste products decreases. The creatinine clearance decreases with age although the serum creatinine level remains relatively constant due to a proportionate age-related decrease in creatinine production.

Endocrine System and Metabolism

Old age is accompanied by a generalized reduction in hormone production and activity. This reduction affects most metabolic functions of the body. Water, mineral, electrolyte, carbohydrate, protein, lipid and vitamin related disorders are more common in the elderly. Nutrition and the ability to use food for energy are seriously affected in the elderly. Diabetes is common in the elderly. Over time, skeletal muscle becomes less responsive to insulin. Recent research indicates that the elderly are at risk for nutritional deficiencies due to anorexia which may be due to decreased taste sensation. Progressive elevation of blood glucose occurs with age on a multifactorial basis. Decline in the levels of growth hormone and sex hormones like estrogen, progesterone and dehydroepiandrosterone as age advances also contribute to aging process.

Special Senses

The sense of smell, taste, sight, touch and hearing are all diminished over time.

- **Hearing loss**, particularly of high-frequency sound, is seen as age advances. This impairment is usually caused by loss of hair cells of the organ of Corti, but it can also result from loss of nerve cells of the auditory nerve or from reduced blood supply to the cochlea.
- **Vision** also deteriorates with increasing age. A progressive loss in the power of accommodation (**presbyopia**) occurs during adult life. Almost all elderly persons have a reduced number of retinal cones, decreased ability for accommodation and decreased ability of retinal rods to adapt to low-intensity light. In addition, age-associated diseases like cataract, glaucoma, and macular degeneration can markedly decrease vision in many elderly persons.
- The ability to detect and discriminate among sweet, sour, salty, and bitter **taste** qualities deteriorates somewhat at advanced ages, along with a marked reduction in **olfaction**. Because taste involves both gustation and olfaction, many elderly persons have anorexia which leads to weight loss.

Changes at the Cellular Level

- Random mutations occurring in the DNA of somatic cells, with consequent introduction of cumulative DNA abnormalities.
- Non-enzymatic combination of glucose with the amino groups of collagen and other proteins produce increased cross linkage between these molecules. This also leads to cumulative abnormalities.
- Free radicals formed in the tissues during metabolism damage them. It is seen that species with longer life spans produce more superoxide dismutase, an enzyme that inactivates oxygen-free radicals.
- DNA helicase is an enzyme that helps to split the DNA strand before replication. Mutation of a gene coding for this enzyme is seen in **Werner's syndrome** which is characterized by aging at a markedly accelerated rate.
- Increased caloric intake also leads to accelerated aging.
- Caloric restriction leads to decreased metabolism and decreased formation of protein cross links.

FREE RADICALS AND ANTIOXIDANTS

> **PY11.7:** Describe and discuss physiology of aging; free radicals and antioxidants.

A **free radical** is an electrically charged atom or group of atoms with an unpaired electron in its outermost shell. A free radical is highly unstable and is not normally present in the body e.g., superoxide (O_2^-). Substances that generate free radicals can be found in the food we eat, the medicines we take, the air we breathe and the water we drink. These substances include fried foods, alcohol, tobacco smoke, pesticides and air pollutants. Free radicals are the natural by-products of chemical processes, such as metabolism. Free radicals can be either harmful or helpful to the body. Free radicals include hydroxyl radical ($OH^\bullet$), superoxide (O_2^-), nitric oxide (NO), nitrogen dioxide ($NO_2^\bullet$), peroxyl (ROO^-) and lipid peroxyl (LOO^-). Also, hydrogen peroxide (H_2O_2), ozone (O_3), singlet oxygen ($^1O_2$), hypochlorous acid (HOCl), nitrous acid (HNO_2), peroxynitrite ($ONOO^-$), dinitrogen trioxide (N_2O_3), lipid peroxide (LOOH), are not free radicals and are generally called **oxidants**, but can easily lead to free radical reactions in living organisms.

There are mechanisms operating in the body called antioxidant defense mechanism to remove these free radicals as soon as they are formed. **Free radical scavengers** include vitamin E (α-tocopherol), urate, ascorbate, glutathione, β-carotene, flavonoids, etc.

Formation of Free Radicals

When cells use oxygen to generate energy, free radicals are created as a consequence of ATP (adenosine triphosphate) production by the mitochondria. These by-products are generally **reactive oxygen species (ROS)** as well as **reactive nitrogen species (RNS)** that result from the cellular redox process. These substances have both toxic and beneficial effects. The delicate balance between their two antagonistic effects is very essential for homeostasis. At low or moderate levels, ROS and RNS exert beneficial effects on cellular responses and immune function. At high concentrations, they generate oxidative stress, a deleterious process that can damage all cell structures.

Formation of ROS and RNS can occur in the cells by two ways: enzymatic and non-enzymatic reactions. **Enzymatic reactions** generating free radicals include those involved in the respiratory chain, phagocytosis, prostaglandin synthesis and the cytochrome P450 system. For example, the superoxide anion radical (O_2^-) is generated via several cellular oxidase systems such as NADPH oxidase, xanthine oxidase, peroxidases. Once formed, it participates in several reactions yielding various ROS and RNS such as hydrogen peroxide, hydroxyl radical (OH^-), peroxynitrite ($ONOO^-$), hypochlorous acid (HOCl), etc. H_2O_2 (a non-radical) is produced by the action of several oxidase enzymes, including amino acid oxidase and xanthine oxidase. Xanthine oxidase catalyses the oxidation of hypoxanthine to xanthine and xanthine to uric acid. Hydroxyl radical (OH^-), the most reactive free radical in vivo, is formed by the reaction of O_2^- with H_2O_2 in the presence of Fe^{2+} or Cu^+ (catalyst). Hypochlorous acid (HOCl) is produced by the neutrophil-derived enzyme, myeloperoxidase, which oxidizes chloride ions in the presence of H_2O_2. Nitric oxide radical (NO^-) is formed in biological tissues from the oxidation of L-arginine to citrulline by nitric oxide synthase.

Free radicals can be produced from **non-enzymatic reactions** of oxygen with organic compounds as well as those initiated by ionizing radiations. The non-enzymatic process can also occur during oxidative phosphorylation (i.e., aerobic respiration) in the mitochondria.

Beneficial Effects of Free Radicals

- At low or moderate concentrations, ROS and RNS are necessary for the maturation process of cellular structures and can act as weapons for the host defense system.
- Phagocytes (neutrophils, macrophages, monocytes) release free radicals to destroy invading pathogenic microbes as part of the body's defense mechanism against disease.
- ROS and RNS have physiological roles in the function of a number of cellular signalling systems. Their production by non-phagocytic NADPH oxidase isoforms plays a key role in the regulation of intracellular signalling cascades in various types of non-phagocytic cells including fibroblasts, endothelial cells, vascular smooth muscle cells, cardiac myocytes, and thyroid tissue. For example, the highly reactive signalling molecule nitric oxide (NO) which is a free radical is an intercellular messenger for modulating blood flow and neural activity. NO is also important for nonspecific host defense, and for killing intracellular pathogens and tumors. ROS also play important physiological roles in the oxidation of iodide anions by thyroid peroxidase in the formation of thyroid hormone as well as in the destruction of certain bacteria by NADPH oxidase and myeloperoxidase in phagocytic cells. Thus ROS/RNS at low or moderate levels are vital to human health.

Deleterious Effects of Free Radicals

Free radical in excess can be injurious to the body tissues and is responsible for producing gene mutations. Since all other molecules have electron pairs in their outer shell, when a free radical reacts with such a molecule, it forms another free radical. The first free radical pulls an electron from a molecule, which destabilizes the molecule and turns it into a free radical. That molecule then takes an electron from another molecule, destabilizing it and turning it into another free radical. This cascade effect can eventually disrupt and damage the whole cell.

Oxidative stress occurs when there are too many free radicals and too much cellular damage. Thus a chain reaction is initiated resulting in formation of numerous free radicals. The free radical chain reaction may change the structure of a lipid, making it more likely to become trapped in an artery. The damaged molecules may mutate and lead to formation of tumors or can damage the DNA or change the DNA code.

- Free radicals can lead on to cancer development, atherosclerosis and other chronic conditions.
- Produce oxidative stress. Symptoms of oxidative stress include fatigue, headache, memory loss, muscle and joint pain, wrinkles and gray hair, and decreased immunity.
- Oxidative stress is associated with damage of proteins, lipids and nucleic acids. Oxidative stress plays a role in the development of many conditions, including macular degeneration, cardiovascular disease, certain cancers, emphysema, Alzheimer's disease, Parkinson's disease, ulcers and all inflammatory diseases, such as arthritis and lupus.
- Free radicals are also associated with aging. Free radicals can damage DNA's instructional code, causing our new cells to grow incorrectly, leading to aging.

Antioxidants

Antioxidants are compounds that can deactivate free radicals and also can prevent free radicals from taking electrons and causing damage. Antioxidants keep free radicals in check. Antioxidants are able to give an electron to a free radical without becoming destabilized themselves, thus stopping the free radical chain reaction. Many of the antioxidants are natural substances whose job is to clean up free radicals. The important antioxidants include *beta-carotene and other carotenoids, lutein, resveratrol, vitamin C, vitamin E, lycopene and other phytonutrients. Antioxidant enzymes in the body include glutathione peroxidase which requires selenium for its formation, superoxide dismutase (manganese, zinc and copper) and catalase (iron).*

Our body produces some antioxidants on its own, but it is insufficient to neutralize the free radicals formed in the body. **Oxidative stress** occurs when there is an imbalance of free radicals and antioxidants (too many free radicals and too few antioxidants). Antioxidants can be acquired through diet.

Antioxidants are plentiful in fruits and vegetables, especially colorful fruits and vegetables like berries, tomatoes, broccoli, spinach, nuts and green tea. Studies showed that a combination of vitamin C, vitamin E, beta-carotene and zinc offered some protection against the development of advanced age-related macular degeneration.

BRAIN DEATH

PY11.11: Discuss the concept and criteria for diagnosis of brain death and its implications.

Brain death is the complete stoppage of brain function which cannot be reversed and so brain death is death. All neurological functions including autonomic functions will be absent. All vital centers are located in the brain stem. In brain death there is death of cerebrum and the brain stem. If cerebrum alone is dead, there will be spontaneous breathing. Once the diagnosis of brain death is confirmed, the individual is declared legally dead. This is the time that should appear in the death certificate. Brain death is the principal prerequisite for the donation of organs for transplantation.

Causes

- Serious trauma or massive irreversible injury to the brain of identifiable cause.
- Blood supply to the brain gets blocked and brain cannot survive in anoxia and the brain tissue dies.

Criteria for the Diagnosis of Brain Death

- Diagnosis of brain death is based on legally accepted medical guidelines.
- The three essential findings in brain death are **coma, absence of brain stem reflexes and apnea**.
- Clinical examination should show that the individual has no brain reflexes and cannot breathe on his own.
- Spinal reflexes may be present even though the brain is dead. A complete neurological examination should be performed.
- The patient whose brain is dead will be on ventilator support since he cannot breathe and medications will be provided to maintain blood pressure. These supports should be maintained while testing for brain death.
- The blood level of sedatives and muscle relaxants should be checked and it may be necessary to wait till their level comes down
- Since the ventilator provides enough oxygen to the heart, the heart continues to beat for several hours. The heart will stop beating if the ventilator is removed
- Look for pupillary reaction to light and corneal reflex.
- Both will be absent. Cough and gag reflexes will also be absent.
- **Electroencephalogram (EEG)** should be recorded using 16-channel EEG instrument for at least 30 minutes. In brain death, an isoelectric EEG, i.e., absence of any electrical activity in the EEG is obtained **(Fig. 102.1)**. An isoelectric EEG alone should not be taken as a criterion for diagnosing brain death. It is also present in hypnotic overdose, severe hypothermia, hepatic coma, cerebral lesions, etc.

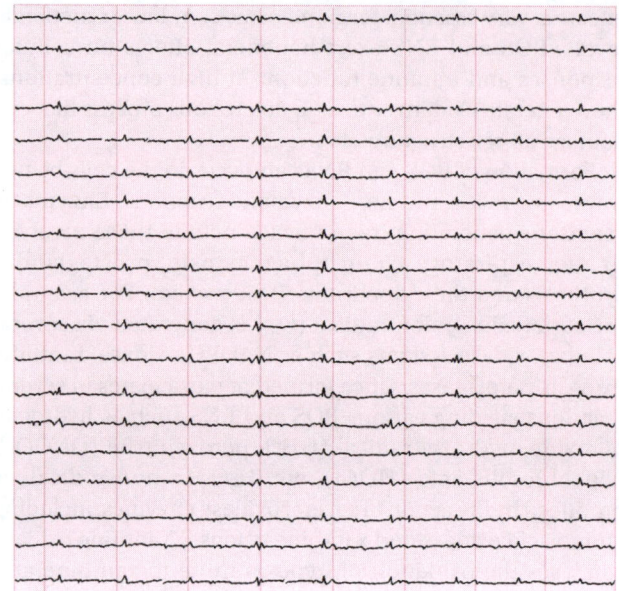

Fig. 102.1: Flat EEG indicating brain death.

- Standard **apnea test** and a 10 minute apnea test should be performed. Connect a pulse oximeter and disconnect the ventilator. Deliver 100% oxygen into the trachea. Look closely for any respiratory movements. Measure arterial PO_2, PCO_2 and pH after 8 minutes and reconnect the ventilator. If respiratory movements are absent and arterial PCO_2 is more than 60 mm Hg, the apnea test result is positive. If respiratory movements are observed, the apnea test result is negative.
- Failure of heart rate to increase by more than 5 beats per minute after giving 1–2 mg of atropine intravenously is an indication for brain death.
- Brain death is different from coma state. A patient in coma continues to have brain activity.

After confirming brain death the relatives can be informed that the patient is legally dead and if the ventilator is removed, the patient will stop breathing and the heart will stop. If the relatives are willing for organ donation brain death should be diagnosed with utmost accuracy and urgency. If the relatives give consent for organ donation, it can be informed to the authorities. If organ transplant is to be done, the ventilatory support is withdrawn in the operating room.

CARDIORESPIRATORY AND METABOLIC ADJUSTMENTS DURING EXERCISE

PY11.4: Describe and discuss cardiorespiratory and metabolic adjustments during exercise; physical training effects.

Many factors affect the physiology of the human body. Exercise is one of the most important of these factors. During exercise, all the systems of the body play a role. Skeletal muscle contraction is the primary physiological event. All the other systems of the body play supportive roles. The initiation, coordination and maintenance of movement depend upon nervous system, cardiovascular system and respiratory system. These adjustments are initiated by chemical, mechanical and thermal stimuli associated with the neuromuscular activity. They are carried out through the nervous and endocrine systems. The skin blood supply is increased in order to dissipate the extra heat generated during exercise. Thus all the systems of the body work together in a coordinated manner to meet the increased demand of tissues during exercise. The adaptation of exercise depends on the type and severity of exercise that is performed and the state of training of the individual.

Respiratory and metabolic adjustments in exercise is dealt with in detail in Chapter 41.

Cardiovascular Adjustments in Exercise

Regular physical activity is beneficial for cardiovascular health. Frequent exercise is associated with a decrease in cardiovascular mortality as well as the risk of developing cardiovascular disease. Physically active individuals have lower blood pressure, higher insulin sensitivity, and a more favorable plasma lipoprotein profile. Regular physical activity is shown to suppress atherosclerosis and increases the availability of vasodilator mediators such as nitric oxide. Aerobic exercises like brisk walking, running, swimming, etc. are effective for improving cardiovascular health than anaerobic exercises.

Effect of Exercise on Heart Rate

There is a linear **increase in heart rate** with the physical effort in exercise. Maximum heart rate that can be achieved during exercise is 220 beats/minute. This is due to AV nodal delay. Increase in heart rate is due to:

- Psychic stimuli arising from the limbic system which act on the cardiac centers in the medulla.
- Impulses coming from proprioceptors in the muscle and joints.
- Increased release of hormones like catecholamines and thyroxine.
- Increase in body temperature (for every 1°F increase in body temperature, there is an increase of 10 beats/minute).
- Stimulation of chemoreceptors due to decrease in pH and PO_2 and increase in PCO_2.

Effect on Stroke Volume

There is **increase in stroke volume** twice the normal value during exercise. This increase is due to:

- Increase in venous return due to the skeletal muscle pump, venous pump and negative intrathoracic pressure.
- Increase in myocardial contractility due to sympathetic stimulation and release of catecholamines from the adrenal medulla.

Effect on Cardiac Output and Blood Pressure

- During exercise, increases in stroke volume and heart rate lead to four-fold to five-fold **increase in cardiac output**. The increase in stroke volume is partly due to an increase in end-diastolic cardiac size (Frank-Starling mechanism) and secondarily due to increased contractility of the myocardium, mediated by beta-adrenergic stimulation.
- The increased cardiac output is distributed preferentially to the exercising muscles including the heart. Blood flow to the heart increases fourfold to five-fold due to increased metabolic requirements of the myocardium as a result of increase in heart rate and contractility. The heart has to do more work.
- The systolic blood pressure increases linearly with the severity of the exercise. There is not much change in the diastolic blood pressure in mild and moderate exercise due to vasodilatation in the working muscles. Increase in cardiac output with a transient increase in systemic vascular resistance elevates the mean arterial blood pressure. However, long-term exercise can promote a net reduction in blood pressure at rest and a lower resting heart rate.

Effect of Exercise on Blood Flow

- Resting **muscle blood flow** is 3–4 mL/100 g/minute. During heavy exercise it increases by 25–30 times. This increase is due to recruitment of closed capillaries and vasodilation. There is also stimulation of the sympathetic vasodilator system to the skeletal muscles during exercise. In isometric contraction of muscles, when the muscle develops 70% of its maximum tension, blood flow is completely stopped due to compression of blood vessels. This leads to accumulation of metabolites.
- **Coronary blood flow** increases in exercise. This is due to coronary vasodilation caused by metabolites like lactic acid, K^+, ATP and ADP; hypoxia, fall in pH and release of catecholamines.
- There is a linear increase in **pulmonary blood flow** with increase in cardiac output. In mild to moderate exercise there is no increase in pulmonary arterial pressure because pulmonary circulation is a low pressure, low resistance high capacitance system. But in heavy exercise, the pulmonary arterial pressure increases markedly.
- **Cutaneous blood flow** increases up to 7 times due to cutaneous vasodilation produced by increase in body temperature. In severe exercise there is cutaneous vasoconstriction inorder to divert blood to the exercising muscles.
- Due to autoregulation, there is no change in **brain blood flow** during exercise.
- **Blood flow to viscera** like kidney and gastrointestinal tract is maintained during severe exercise due to local autoregulatory mechanisms operating in these organs. However, if the oxygen-carrying capacity of the blood is decreased as in anemia, visceral blood flow is reduced drastically and blood is diverted to the exercising musculature.

Effect of Exercise on Blood Volume

In exercise, blood volume decreases by 15% leading to hemoconcentration. Reduction in blood volume is due to:

- Accumulation of fluid in the tissue spaces due to increase in the hydrostatic pressure of capillaries.

- Increase in the hydrostatic pressure of interstitial fluid due to accumulation of metabolites.
- Increased sweating during exercise leads to loss of body water.

Cardiorespiratory Endurance

For increasing cardiorespiratory endurance regular physical activity is required. Aerobic exercises that cause increase in heart rate is better than isometric exercise. **Cardiorespiratory endurance** is the level at which the heart, lungs, and muscles work together while exercising for an extended period of time. It is an indicator of how physically fit and healthy a person is. Increasing cardiorespiratory endurance has a positive effect on the overall health. The lungs and heart will be able to use oxygen in a better way. Exercise can be performed for longer periods without getting tired. Most people can increase their cardiorespiratory endurance by doing regular exercise. Cardiorespiratory endurance is measured by maximum oxygen uptake (VO_2 max) and how it is used during intense exercise. Higher amounts of oxygen uptake show that more oxygen is being used and that cardiorespiratory system is functioning efficiently. Submaximal exercise tests are used to measure cardiorespiratory endurance. The tests can help provide information about how well the heart and lungs are working to provide oxygen to the muscles during exercise. It includes:

- Treadmill test
- 2.4 km run test
- Multistage bleep test

Changes in Trained Athletes

- Cardiorespiratory responses reach a steady state early in trained athletes.
- O_2 debt falls.
- VO_2 max increases to 70–80 mL/kg/min from 45 mL/kg/min
- When lactate level is 70 mg/100 mL of blood, the person stops exercise normally. This is the **breaking point in exercise**. Breaking point can be increased to 110 mg/100 mL of blood by training. Normal blood lactate level is 20 mg/100 mL of blood at rest.
- Blood flow distribution will be optimal. Capillary density in the muscles increases and there will be recruitment of closed capillaries.
- Hypertrophy of the left ventricle and skeletal muscles occurs after training. The enlargement of muscles is due to increased synthesis of protein filaments like actin and myosin.
- The ligaments and tendons also increase in strength to support the muscles.
- Bradycardia is seen due to increased vagal tone.

CARDIORESPIRATORY CHANGES IN ISOTONIC AND ISOMETRIC EXERCISES

Isotonic and Isometric Exercise

There are two types of exercise:
- Isotonic or dynamic exercise
- Isometric or static exercise

Most forms of exercise contain both types of contractions, although some are mostly isotonic (jogging, cross-country skiing, and swimming) and others isometric (weightlifting).

Cardiovascular Changes in Isotonic Exercise

- In isotonic exercise, rhythmic muscular contractions with changes in muscle length, using a relatively small force occurs.
- Isotonic exercise causes a volume overload of the heart and an increase in oxygen consumption, heart rate, stroke volume, cardiac output, and systolic blood pressure.
    - Increase in heart rate and stroke volume produces a four-fold to six-fold increase in cardiac output in healthy individuals. The increase in heart rate is due to decrease in vagal tone and an increase in sympathetic tone. Heart rate gradually rises during exercise to a maximal level that can be predicted by the following formula:

        Maximum predicted heart rate = 220 − Age in years
    - Stroke volume increases by 20 to 50% as a result of both increased venous return from exercising muscles and increased left ventricular emptying due to enhanced myocardial contractility and to decreased peripheral vascular resistance due to vasodilation in exercising muscle.
    - Vascular beds other than in the heart, brain, and exercising muscle constrict during exercise. This vasoconstriction along with the increase in cardiac output, results in a rise in systolic blood pressure.
- Owing to the decrease in peripheral resistance, the diastolic blood pressure may fall or remains unchanged during isotonic exercise.

Benefits of Isotonic Exercise

- Isotonic exercise helps to strengthen the cardiovascular system, as it results in increased oxygen consumption, heart rate, stroke volume, cardiac output, and muscular endurance while reducing the risk of heart disease.
- Isotonic exercise also improves bone density and causes
- new bone formation reducing the risk of fracture.
- Isotonic exercise also burns calories and decreases cholesterol and blood sugar levels.
- It also helps to build bigger, stronger muscles, which help to resist injury from strains, sprains, fractures, and falls.

Cardiovascular Changes in Isometric Exercise

- Isometric exercise needs a relatively large force with little or no change in muscle length.
- Isometric exercise, which causes mainly pressure overload, induces a sudden increase of blood pressure
- The increase in oxygen consumption and cardiac output is limited.
- The volume load on the heart in isometric exercise may be difficult to control.
- Isometric exercise results in a moderate increase in cardiac output, predominantly as a result of an increase in heart rate.

- Contracting muscle produces a rise in peripheral vascular resistance and may result in an increase in both systolic and diastolic blood pressure.

Benefits of Isometric Exercise

- Isometric exercises build muscle, strength, and bone density while improving cholesterol levels and digestive function.
- Isometric exercise helps to lower blood pressure.
- However, if the blood pressure is high, the person should exercise at a lower level of intensity. Exercising at a higher level of intensity can cause a dramatic increase in blood pressure during the activity.
- Isometric exercise involves remaining in a static position while engaging the muscles. The joint doesn't move, but it can help to stabilize injured or weak joints. It is good for people suffering from arthritis.
- Avoid holding the breath and straining during any weight training exercise, as this may cause a dangerous rise in blood pressure.

Respiratory Changes in Isotonic and Isometric Exercise

- There is increase in the rate and depth of breathing in both isotonic and isometric exercise. At a given level of pulmonary gas exchange, ventilation is appreciably higher during isometric exercise than during isotonic exercise.
- The isotonic exercise produces metabolic (lactic) acidosis with partial respiratory compensation. In contrast, isometric exercise consistently resulted in a respiratory alkalosis, with little or no increase of blood lactate concentration.
- At the end of the isometric exercise, ventilation falls abruptly and then rise again after a short interval (20 seconds). This secondary stimulation is as a result of the increased blood lactate concentration (3–5 mmol) which occurs in the recovery phase.
- Respiratory alkalosis occurs during isometric exercise.
- This is due to ventilatory stimulation by the metabolites released during isometric contraction which are trapped within the contracting muscles as a result of impeded blood flow. The initial rapid reduction of ventilation which occurred at the cessation of the isometric exercise is consistent with a washing-out of metabolites that stimulate the chemoreceptors.

EFFECT OF EXERCISE UNDER DIFFERENT ENVIRONMENTAL CONDITIONS (HEAT AND COLD)

Effect of Exercise when Exposed to Heat

- Increased sweating due to stimulation of hypothalamus by a rise in body temperature.
- Increased production of aldosterone and antidiuretic hormone lead to increase in blood volume and increased absorption of sodium chloride by the sweat ducts and renal tubules.
- Core temperature is reduced by cutaneous vasodilation and thermal sweating.
- As the core temperature decreases, the heart rate also falls.
- Onset of fatigue is delayed as muscle glycogen is spared. Free fatty acids are mobilized rapidly and are used for energy.

Effect of Exercise when Exposed to Cold

- The utilization of glycogen by the muscles is more in lower temperature.
- Muscle contraction is adversely affected by cold. The velocity and strength of muscle shortening is decreased in cold. Muscle functions best at a temperature of 40°C.
- Hormonal changes like increased secretion of catecholamines occur in the cold.
- There is very little rise in the plasma free fatty acid level as the subcutaneous blood flow is less in cold.

CONSEQUENCES OF SEDENTARY LIFE STYLE

PY11.5: Describe and discuss physiological consequences of sedentary life style.

A **sedentary lifestyle** is a type of lifestyle involving **little or no physical activity**. A person living a sedentary lifestyle is often sitting or lying down while engaged in activities like reading, watching television, playing video games, or using a computer for much of the day. Sedentary lifestyle is one of the biggest threats to our health. It can contribute to ill health and many preventable causes of death. Physical activity and regular exercise are essential for optimum health. But many fail to add enough exercise to their daily schedule.

Effects of a Sedentary Lifestyle

- One of the most prominent effects of a sedentary lifestyle is an increased body mass index (**BMI**) leading to **obesity**. Fewer calories are burnt out and this leads to weight gain. The risk is higher among those who sit still for more than 5 hours per day. Being obese has its own side effects. Obesity is linked with many serious diseases and health conditions such as sleep apnea, joint pain, risk of stroke, heart disease, hypertension, etc.
- There will be loss of muscle strength and endurance, because muscles are not used much.
- Bones may get weaker and lose some mineral content.
- Metabolism of carbohydrates and fats may be affected
- leading to hyperglycemia and dyslipidemia.
- Immunity may get affected and the body becomes more prone for inflammation.
- Many with sedentary lifestyle develop hormonal imbalance like metabolic syndrome and type 2 diabetes mellitus.

Diseases that can be caused by Sedentary Lifestyle and Lack of Physical Activity

- Anxiety, dementia and depression.
- Cardiovascular disease like coronary artery disease and heart attack.

- Migraine
- Being physically inactive and long hours of sitting can increase the risk of certain cancers including colon, breast and lung cancer.
- Diabetes mellitus
- Gout
- Hypertension
- Dyslipidemia (there will be increase in LDL cholesterol and triglyceride level and decrease in HDL cholesterol).
- Sedentary life can make the bones weaker which is associated with a higher risk of osteoporosis.
- There can also be pressure on the vertebral disks in the lower back which is a common reason for spinal disc herniation producing low back pain.
- Premature death.

Prevention of the Health Effects of Sedentary Lifestyle

- If a person has been inactive for long, exercise should be started slowly by adding more exercise gradually till the recommended amount of exercise for the age and health is attained. Exercise daily for at least 30 minutes a day.
- Do more physical activity- go for brisk walking, running, cycling or play an outdoor sport.
- Housework, gardening, etc. are all physical work.
- Get some exercise equipment at home. Treadmills can be used if affordable.
- Those who are working on the computer should get up from the chair and move around at least once an hour.
- Take the stairs instead of the elevator.

Important Questions

SECTION 1: GENERAL PHYSIOLOGY

■ REVIEW QUESTIONS

1. What are the differences between mitosis and meiosis?
2. What is cell cycle? How is it regulated?
3. What is apoptosis?
4. What are cell adhesion molecules?
5. What are the types of intercellular connections?
6. State the law of laplace. What are its clinical applications?
7. What is Gibbs-Donnan equilibrium? Give the importance of Donnan effect in the body.
8. What is the reason for swelling of cells after death?
9. What is the difference between osmotic pressure and oncotic pressure?
10. What are the main causes of aging?
11. What are molecular motors? Give examples.
12. How is total body water measured? Give its normal value.
13. Name the trans-cellular fluids in the body. Why are they called so?
14. Define pH of a solution.
15. What is meant by neutral pH? What is the normal pH of blood?
16. What is a buffer? What are the important buffer systems in the body?
17. What are the compensatory responses of the body in acid-base disturbances?
18. Define homeostasis.
19. What is a negative feedback system?
20. What is positive feedback system? Give examples.
21. What are the functions of cell membrane proteins?
22. What is the difference between semipermeable and selectively permeable membrane? Give example.
23. Define osmosis.
24. What is diffusion?
25. Explain facilitated diffusion.
26. What is nonionic diffusion?
27. What is active transport?
28. What is the importance of active transport in the body? Give the significance of Na^+-K^+ pump.
29. Describe secondary active transport.
30. What is the difference between primary active transport and secondary active transport?
31. What is meant by receptor-mediated pinocytosis (endocytosis)? What is its significance?
32. Name the excitable cells in the body.
33. Write briefly on sodium-potassium pump. Why is it called electrogenic pump?
34. What is the difference between monophasic and biphasic recording of membrane potentials?
35. Define resting membrane potential (RMP). What is its ionic basis?
36. Define action potential. Explain its ionic basis in nerve fiber.
37. What are the salient features of action potential?
38. What is threshold strength of stimulus?
39. Define refractory period?
40. What is all-or-none phenomenon regarding membrane potentials?
41. What are the sites of impulse production in motor and sensory neurons?
42. What is meant by saltatory conduction of action potential? Give its significance.
43. What is maximal stimulus?
44. Explain compound action potential?
45. What is voltage inactivation of Na^+ channel?
46. What are the main differences between action potential and graded potential or local response?
47. Enumerate the properties of nerve fibers.
48. What are the factors that influence the velocity of conduction in a nerve fiber?
49. What is the difference between EPSP and IPSP?
50. Name the cells that are responsible for myelination in the peripheral nervous system and central nervous system.
51. What are the functions of myelin?
52. Which type of nerve fibers is found maximally in the peripheral nerves?
53. What is the difference between Golgi type I and Golgi type II neurons?
54. What is the difference between orthodromic conduction and antidromic conduction of impulse?
55. Describe Wallerian degeneration or orthograde degeneration? Why does it occur?
56. What is chromatolysis?
57. What are the conditions for regeneration in an injured nerve?
58. Explain nerve regeneration after nerve section.
59. What is a neuroma?
60. What are the properties of skeletal muscle tissue?

61. What is a motor unit?
62. What is meant by size principle?
63. What is a sarcomere?
64. Describe excitation-contraction coupling in skeletal muscle?
65. Enumerate the sequence of events occurring in skeletal muscle contraction.
66. What is the mechanism of skeletal muscle relaxation?
67. Name the calcium-binding proteins in the body.
68. What is meant by resting heat, initial heat and recovery heat in skeletal muscle?
69. What are the causes of muscle fatigue?
70. Define Starling's law?
71. What is Frank-Starling's law?
72. Name the regulatory or relaxing proteins of skeletal muscle?
73. What is the difference between isotonic and isometric contraction?
74. Mention the differences between fast muscle and slow muscle?
75. What is rigor mortis?
76. What is meant by reaction of degeneration?
77. Explain fibrillation and fasciculation in skeletal muscle.
78. Explain the ionic basis of ventricular muscle action potential.
79. What are the causes of pacemaker potential or pre-potential?
80. What is functional refractory period in cardiac muscle?
81. What are the main differences between visceral smooth muscle and multiunit smooth muscle?
82. What is tonus or tone in smooth muscle?
83. Explain the mechanism of contraction and relaxation in smooth muscle.
84. What is the role of calmodulin in smooth muscle contraction?
85. Describe the property of plasticity in smooth muscle?
86. Explain muscle hypertrophy?
87. Describe the events occurring at the neuromuscular junction (NMJ)?
88. What is miniature end plate potential (MEPP)?
89. What are the main differences between endplate potential and action potential?
90. What is meant by safety factor for neuromuscular transmission?
91. Classify the drugs acting on the neuromuscular junction and briefly mention their mechanism of action.
92. Describe the mechanism of action of curare at the NMJ? How is it treated?
93. What is the mechanism of action of botulinum toxin? Mention its clinical significance.
94. What is the role of succinylcholine in anesthesia?
95. Discuss the difference between myasthenia gravis and Lambert-Eaton myasthenic syndrome?
96. What is synapse en passant?
97. Explain denervation hypersensitivity or denervation supersensitivity of muscle?

GIVE THE PHYSIOLOGICAL BASIS

1. When K^+ concentration is decreased in ECF, there is a decrease in excitability.
2. p53 is called guardian angel of the genome.
3. The role of sodium pump is very significant in excitable tissues.
4. $Na^+ K^+$ pump is called an electrogenic pump.
5. Hypertonic solution like mannitol is given intravenously in cerebral edema.
6. Hypotonic solution can be used to treat patients with dehydration.
7. Salted rice water (kanji water) is given in times of dehydration or diarrhea.
8. Paralysis is sometimes experienced after eating shellfish.
9. Oral rehydration solution (ORS) is given in times of dehydration.
10. Solutes such as urea do not affect osmotic pressure.

IMPORTANT DIAGRAMS

1. Intercellular connections or cell junctions
2. Events occurring in endocytosis and exocytosis
3. Na^+-K^+ pump
4. Structure of a typical neuron
5. Nerve action potential (monophasic) and its ionic basis
6. Absolute and relative refractory period in nerve action potential
7. Saltatory conduction in axon
8. Compound action potential
9. Electron microscopic structure of sarcomere
10. Neuromuscular junction in skeletal muscle
11. Ventricular muscle action potential and its ionic basis
12. Correlate mechanical and electrical events in ventricular muscle fiber
13. Length-tension relationship in skeletal muscle and cardiac muscle
14. Pacemaker potential
15. Types of membrane potentials in smooth muscles
16. Cystometrogram or plasticity in smooth muscle

SECTION 2: HEMATOLOGY

REVIEW QUESTIONS

1. Enumerate the functions of blood.
2. Name the plasma proteins giving the normal value.
3. What are the functions of plasma proteins?
4. Give examples of conditions producing hyperproteinemia.
5. What is the significance of albumin-globulin ratio?
6. What is the normal morphology of RBC?
7. How is the biconcave shape of RBC maintained?

8. What are the advantages of biconcave shape of RBC?
9. What is anisocytosis and poikilocytosis?
10. What is meant by MCV, MCH and MCHC? Give their normal values and variations.
11. What is meant by rouleaux formation of RBCs? Why it does not occur in the body under normal conditions? Give one condition where it occurs in the body during life.
12. What are hematinic principles? Give examples.
13. What are the functions of RBC?
14. Define ESR giving the normal value.
15. What are the factors affecting ESR?
16. Enumerate the sites of RBC production in the intrauterine life and after birth.
17. What is the life span of RBC? How is it determined? Give examples where the life-span of RBC is decreased.
18. Name the main protein of RBC. Give its normal value in blood.
19. Enumerate the functions of hemoglobin.
20. What is the normal hemoglobin content of blood in newborn, adult male and female?
21. What happens if hemoglobin is present freely in the plasma?
22. Name the plasma proteins that combine with hemoglobin in circulation. What is its significance?
23. What is the normal structure of adult hemoglobin? What is meant by hemoglobinopathy?
24. Name the maturation factors in erythropoiesis. What are their functions?
25. Describe the stages of erythropoiesis in bone marrow.
26. Give the duration of various phases in erythropoiesis.
27. What are the factors affecting erythropoiesis?
28. Name the sites of production of erythropoietin. Mention its functions.
29. Write a note on reticulocyte.
30. What is polycythemia? Mention the types of polycythemia.
31. What is the difference between primary polycythemia and secondary polycythemia?
32. Define anemia. How is anemia graded?
33. What are the causes of iron deficiency anemia?
34. What are the features of iron deficiency anemia?
35. What are the causes of megaloblastic anemia? Mention its features.
36. Write a note on pernicious anemia?
37. Enumerate the causes of vitamin B_{12} deficiency.
38. What is the role of intrinsic factor in vitamin B_{12} absorption?
39. Define anemia. How will you investigate a case of anemia?
40. What is the fate of hemoglobin after destruction of RBC?
41. What is physiological jaundice? How is it treated?
42. What is cyanosis? Mention the types.
43. Mention the properties of leukocytes.
44. What is meant by margination of neutrophils?
45. What are the functions of neutrophils and monocytes?
46. What is agranulocytosis or granulocytopenia?
47. What is the difference between leukocytosis and leukemia?
48. What are the functions of eosinophils?
49. What is eosinophilia? Give examples of conditions where eosinophilia is seen.
50. Name the sites of lymphocyte production after birth.
51. What are the types of T lymphocytes? Give their functions.
52. Define immunity. What is the role of lymphocytes in immunity?
53. Explain innate immunity.
54. What is acquired immunity or adaptive immunity or specific immunity?
55. What are the differences between cellular and humoral immunity?
56. What functions do B, T and natural killer cells perform?
57. What are immunoglobulins? Mention the types and their functions.
58. What are the functions of platelets?
59. Explain the properties of platelets.
60. What is thrombocytosis and thrombocytopenia? Give examples.
61. Enumerate the consequences of low platelet count.
62. What is the difference between hemostasis and homeostasis?
63. What are the main processes that prevent bleeding after damage to a blood vessel?
64. What are the mechanisms involved in producing vascular spasm at the site of injury?
65. What are the mechanisms by which platelet plug or temporary hemostatic plug is formed after injury to a blood vessel? Or write a note on temporary hemostasis or primary hemostasis.
66. Enumerate the clotting factors.
67. What are the three main stages of coagulation (secondary or permanent hemostasis)?
68. Explain the intrinsic and extrinsic mechanisms of coagulation.
69. What are the main differences between intrinsic and extrinsic pathways of coagulation?
70. Which are the steps in coagulation that do not require calcium ions? Or what is the role of Ca^{2+} in coagulation?
71. What are the differences between plasma and serum?
72. What are the differences between plasma and serum?
73. What is the mechanism of clot retraction? Give the normal bleeding time, clotting time and clot retraction time.
74. What are the factors favoring and retarding coagulation of blood in the body?
75. Which are the clotting factors and components of the fibrinolytic system that require vitamin K for their synthesis in the liver?
76. What is protein C and protein S?
77. What is the reason for uncontrolled bleeding in obstructive jaundice?

Important Questions

78. What do you mean by fibrinolytic system?
79. What are the factors that prevent intravascular coagulation?
80. What is the mechanism of action of intravascular anticoagulants?
81. Name the activators of plasminogen to plasmin.
81a. Ans. Thrombin, XIIa and tissue plasminogen activator (t-PA)
82. Explain fibrinolytic system.
83. What is fibrinolysis? How does plasmin produce fibrinolysis?
84. What is the difference between thrombus and embolus?
85. What are anticoagulants? What is the mechanism of action?
86. What is the mechanism of action of warfarin and phenindion as anticoagulants?
87. Name the anticoagulants present in blood in vivo. Mention their mechanism of action.
88. Give the differences between hemophilia and purpura.
89. Enumerate the tests of coagulation giving the normal values.
90. Write a note on hemophilia. Name the blood tests to confirm hemophilia.
91. State Landsteiner's laws.
92. What is cross matching? What is dangerous "O" group?
93. How is ABO blood group system inherited? What is Bombay group?
94. Why Rh system is called so? How is Rh system inherited?
95. What are the main differences between ABO system and Rh blood group system?
96. What are the indications for blood transfusion?
97. What are the precautions to be taken before blood transfusion?
98. What is autologous transfusion?
99. What are the possible complications of blood transfusion?
100. Name some diseases transmitted through blood transfusion.
101. What are the causes of renal shut-down in incompatible blood transfusion? How can it be treated?
102. What is preservation injury?
103. What is kernicterus?
104. Explain erythroblastosis fetalis?
105. What are the functions of lymphatic system?
106. What are the factors affecting lymph formation and lymph flow?
107. Name the areas in the body where lymphatic vessels are absent.
108. Write a note on Starling's forces.
109. State Starling's law.
110. What is edema? What are the types of edema?
111. Name the important hormones that maintain osmotic pressure and blood volume relatively constant.
112. What is the normal blood volume? How is it regulated?
113. What is meant by reticuloendothelial system or tissue macrophage system of the body?
114. What are the functions of reticuloendothelial system?

GIVE THE PHYSIOLOGICAL BASIS

1. Edema occurs in hypoproteinemia.
2. ESR is decreased in spherocytic anemia.
3. Rouleaux formation does not occur in the body during life under normal conditions.
4. Hematocrit value is higher in males when compared to females of the same age.
5. MCHC is normal in megaloblastic anemia.
6. Anemia can never be hyperchromic
7. MCHC remains relatively constant even though the erythrocyte size varies greatly.
8. Increased size of RBCs is seen in macrocytic anemia (B_{12} or folic acid deficiency).
9. Anemia occurs in premature newborns.
10. Edema occurs in nephrotic syndrome.
11. Physiological jaundice in newborn is treated by phototherapy with white light.
12. Anti-D injection should be given to an Rh-negative woman who has given birth to an Rh-positive baby.
13. ABO incompatibility between mother and her fetus rarely causes problems.
14. ABO incompatibility can to some extent prevent Rh incompatibility.
15. Hydrops fetalis is a feature of hemolytic disease of newborn.
16. Removal of Ca^{2+} from blood prevents coagulation.
17. Blood does not clot in vivo normally.
18. In thrombocytopenia, the clot formed is soft and friable.
19. Anticoagulants like sodium citrate are added to blood (in vitro) to maintain the fluidity of blood.
20. Warfarin is prescribed to prevent intravascular coagulation in conditions like atrial fibrillation.
21. Streptokinase is used in the treatment of myocardial infarction.
22. In purpura bleeding time is prolonged but clotting time is normal.
23. Cross matching should be done before blood transfusion even if the blood groups are same.
24. Clotting time is prolonged in liver diseases.
25. Transfusion of blood stored in the blood bank at 4°C leads to hyperkalemia.
26. Anemia occurs after gastrectomy.
27. Generalized edema occurs in hypoproteinemia.
28. Edema usually develops in the dependent parts of the body.
29. Absence of cyanosis in anemia
30. Aspirin is given to prevent thromboembolism and to treat myocardial infarction.
31. Serum does not clot.
32. Leukocytosis occurs after splenectomy.
33. Polycythemia may occur in renal artery stenosis.

34. Opsonization aids phagocytosis.
35. Hemolytic anemia is referred to as acholuric jaundice.
36. Reticulocyte count increases after vitamin B_{12} therapy in pernicious anemia.
37. Anemia occurs after gastrectomy.
38. After splenectomy there will be an increase in reticulocyte count.
39. Anemia occurs in hereditary spherocytosis.

IMPORTANT DIAGRAMS

1. Structure of hemoglobin
2. Degradation of hemoglobin
3. Stages of erythropoiesis
4. Morphology of leukocytes
5. Structure of platelet
6. Inheritance of hemophilia

SECTION 3: CARDIOVASCULAR SYSTEM

REVIEW QUESTIONS

1. What is the difference between lesser circulation and greater circulation?
2. What are the functions of pericardium?
3. What is the importance of intercalated disc in cardiac muscle?
4. Define apex beat.
5. What is the difference between stenosis and insufficiency of heart valves? Give examples.
6. Mention the parts of conducting system of heart and their rate of impulse production.
7. What are the peculiarities of the conduction system of heart?
8. Give the location and innervation of SA node and AV node.
9. Which part of the heart has the maximum speed of conduction of impulse and minimum speed?
10. What is the importance of Purkinje fibers in the conducting system of heart?
11. Give the causes of pacemaker potential or prepotential.
12. Name the pacemaker of heart. Why is it called pacemaker?
13. What is sinus rhythm, nodal rhythm and idioventricular rhythm?
14. Enumerate the factors that affect the rate of firing from the SA node.
15. What is the role of vagus in controlling heart rate?
16. What is extrasystole?
17. What is meant by postextrasystolic potentiation?
18. What is bundle of Kent? Mention its significance.
19. What is AV nodal delay? What is its importance?
20. What are the causes of AV nodal delay? Give its normal value.
21. Explain the origin and spread of cardiac impulse. Or, explain the spread of cardiac impulse from SA node to the ventricular muscle.
22. Give the speed of conduction of impulse in different parts of the heart.
23. Name the last parts of the heart to be depolarized during spread of cardiac impulse.
24. What is the normal duration of cardiac action potential?
25. What are the differences between absolute refractory period (ARP) and relative refractory period (RRP) in cardiac muscle?
26. What is the importance of long refractory period in AV node?
27. Enumerate the properties of cardiac muscle.
28. Who is the father of modern ECG?
29. Which are the clinically used leads in ECG?
30. Explain the different waves, their causes, duration and amplitude in ECG lead II.
31. What is R-R interval? What is its significance?
32. What is PR interval? Give its significance.
33. What is Wolff-Parkinson-White (WPW) syndrome?
34. What is the clinical significance of ST segment?
35. What does an abnormal T-wave indicate?
36. What is mean electrical axis?
37. What is meant by axis deviation in ECG? Give examples.
38. What is sinus arrhythmia? Give its cause.
39. What is sick sinus syndrome?
40. What is first degree heart block?
41. What is Wenckebach's phenomenon?
42. Explain Stokes-Adams syndrome?
43. What is meant by re-entry phenomenon or circus movement?
44. What is meant by arrhythmias? What are the different types of arrhythmias?
45. What is the reason for AV block in atrial flutter?
46. What is the indication for cardiopulmonary resuscitation? How is it performed?
47. Name two ions that depress myocardium.
48. Define cardiac cycle and give its normal duration.
49. Name the different phases of cardiac cycle according to Wigger's classification and give their normal duration.
50. Enumerate the events occurring in the aorta during cardiac cycle. Or explain the aortic pressure curve during cardiac cycle.
51. What is the reason for the incisura in aortic pressure curve?
52. What is end-diastolic volume and end-systolic volume? Give the normal values at rest.
53. What is ejection fraction? How is it measured? Give its significance.
54. What is the significance of atrial systole?
55. How many heart sounds can be recorded by phonocardiography and by auscultation?
56. Explain the causes of heart sounds.

57. Which are the areas of auscultation of heart sounds?
58. What is the difference between murmur and bruit?
59. What is the difference between stenosis and incompetence of heart valves?
60. Classify murmur. Mention few causes of cardiac murmur?
61. What is the difference between resistance vessels and capacitance vessels?
62. What is shear rate and shear stress?
63. What are Newtonian and non-Newtonian fluids?
64. State Poiseuille-Hagen formula. What is its clinical application?
65. Give the differences between laminar flow and turbulent flow.
66. What is the relationship between flow, pressure and resistance in the vascular system?
67. State Bernoulli's principle. What is its significance in cardiovascular physiology?
68. What is Reynolds number?
69. What is the cause for turbulence when velocity of flow is increased?
70. What is circulation time?
71. What is Poiseuille's law?
72. What are the main factors that convert pulsatile flow in large arteries to continuous flow in capillaries?
73. Enumerate the factors affecting viscosity of blood in circulation.
74. What is Fahraeus-Lindqvist effect?
75. Explain law of Laplace and its application in the body?
76. What is critical closing pressure in blood vessels?
77. Define total peripheral resistance. What are the factors affecting TPR directly?
78. What is Windkessel effect?
79. Define stroke volume and cardiac output giving normal values.
80. What is cardiac index? Give its normal value.
81. State Fick's principle. What is its application in CVS?
82. How is cardiac output measured?
83. What is the mechanism of regulation of cardiac output?
84. How is stroke volume regulated?
85. Explain heterometric regulation of stroke volume.
86. Explain homometric regulation of stroke volume.
87. What is meant by preload and afterload on the heart? Give conditions where these are increased.
88. State Frank-Starling's law.
89. Give an account of the innervation of heart.
90. Explain the location, structure and innervation of baroreceptors.
91. Explain the regulation of heart rate.
92. What is the effect of chemoreceptor stimulation on heart rate? Or write a note on chemoreceptor reflex.
93. What are the causes for variation in heart rate during inspiration and expiration?
94. What is CNS ischemic response?
95. State Marey's law?
96. Write a note on Cushing reflex or Cushing reaction.
97. What is sino-aortic reflex? Or Explain baroreceptor mechanisms for regulation of blood pressure.
98. What are the causes of increased heart rate in exercise?
99. Define arterial pulse.
100. Mention few abnormalities of arterial pulse.
101. What are the main differences between venous and arterial pulse?
102. What is jugular venous pulse? Which vein is observed? Give reason.
103. What are the causes of different waves of JVP? What are the alterations in JVP?
104. Give the clinical importance of JVP.
105. Define blood pressure. What is its normal value?
106. What is pulse pressure?
107. What is mean arterial pressure? Give its significance.
108. What are the factors that maintain normal arterial blood pressure? Or what are the determinants of arterial blood pressure?
109. What is the effect of posture and gravity on blood pressure?
110. What is the effect of stimulation of pain fibers on blood pressure?
111. What is the mechanism of action of baroreceptors when there is increase in blood pressure?
112. Explain the regulation of peripheral resistance.
113. How is blood pressure regulated?
114. Describe the short-term regulation of blood pressure.
115. Explain the long-term regulation of blood pressure.
116. What is critical closing pressure?
117. What is postural hypotension or orthostatic hypotension?
118. What are the compensatory mechanisms that operate in the body when there is a fall in the mean arterial pressure?
119. What are the direct effects of hypercapnia and hypoxia on the vasomotor areas in the medulla oblongata?
120. What are the actions of nitric oxide (NO) in the body?
121. Define circulatory shock.
122. What are the clinical features of circulatory shock?
123. What is rapid thready pulse?
124. What are the causes of circulatory shock? Classify shock.
125. Explain the stages of circulatory shock?
126. What are the immediate and delayed compensatory mechanisms in circulatory shock?
127. Explain the pathophysiology of progressive stage of circulatory shock.
128. Write a note on sympathetic vasodilator fibers.
129. Classify the capillaries in the body.
130. Explain autoregulation of blood flow.
131. What is meant by sympathetic tone of blood vessels?
132. What is triple response?
133. Explain the phasic variation in coronary blood flow with the help of a diagram (Variation of coronary blood flow in different phases of cardiac cycle).

134. Describe the special features of coronary circulation.
135. Explain the chemical and neural factors regulating coronary blood flow?
136. Explain the factors affecting cerebral blood flow (regulation of cerebral blood flow)
137. What is Cushing reflex?
138. Name the important blood reservoirs in the body.
139. What are the factors that contribute to the distensibility and reservoir function of veins?
140. How does placenta act as the fetal lung?
141. What are the changes that occur in the fetal circulation after birth?
142. What is the normal resting blood flow to skeletal muscles?
143. What are the mechanisms of increase in skeletal muscle blood flow during exercise?
144. What is vasovagal syncope?
145. Explain the effects of positive "g" on circulatory system.

GIVE THE PHYSIOLOGICAL BASIS

1. Normally the left ventricular wall is thicker than the right ventricular wall.
2. Extrasystole is followed by a compensatory pause.
3. Sub-endocardial region of left ventricle is more prone for myocardial infarction.
4. Cardiac muscle cannot be tetanized.
5. Severe tachycardia diminishes left ventricular blood supply.
6. Bradycardia and elevation of blood pressure occur in raised intracranial tension.
7. Steady blood flow occurs in certain organs despite changes in systemic blood pressure.
8. Pulsatile flow in arteries is converted to continuous flow in capillaries.
9. Norepinephrine produces reflex bradycardia or Decrease in cardiac output occur following norepinephrine administration.
10. Fall in blood pressure and fainting occurs during intense emotional states like fear.
11. Oxygen consumption by the heart can be increased only by increasing coronary blood flow.
12. Angina pectoris occurs in coronary insufficiency.
13. A patient in heart failure is often treated with digitalis and a diuretic.
14. A patient in shock should not be warmed or covered with a blanket.
15. Dopamine is usually used to treat circulatory shock.
16. Palpatory method is done before auscultatory method while recording blood pressure.
17. In standing posture, systolic blood pressure decreases and diastolic blood pressure increases.
18. Cerebral vessels do not rupture when exposed to negative 'g'.
19. Gray out is sometimes experienced by pilots during looping or when exposed to + 'g'.
20. There is increase in pulse pressure during severe isotonic exercise.
21. Heart rate increases during exercise.
22. There is increase in the heart rate and BP in times of hypoxia.
23. There is a fall in the diastolic pressure in severe exercise.
24. In some individuals, sudden standing from lying down position causes a fall in blood pressure, dizziness, dimness of vision and even fainting.
25. During diastole blood pressure in the arteries does not fall to zero level.
26. Depolarization and repolarization waves are in the same direction in ECG.
27. There is increased affinity of fetal hemoglobin for O_2.
28. The foramen ovale closes to form fossa ovalis after birth.
29. Ductus arteriosus of fetus closes after birth.
30. Cardiac murmur occurs in anemia.
31. Brief period of apnea is seen following adrenaline injection.
32. In the capillaries, hematocrit value is less than that of total blood hematocrit value.
33. Reddening and warming are seen along the line of stroke in triple response.
34. When a hard stroke is made on the skin with a pointed object, there is swelling or edema along the line of stroke.
35. Coronary blood flow is decreased during systole.
36. Cardiac output is regulated in transplanted heart during exercise.
37. Stroke volume is increased during exercise.
38. Stroke volume is more in athletes at rest.
39. Normally ventricular systole starts after the completion of atrial systole.
40. Following sympathectomy, there is a reduction in the heart rate.
41. Heart rate is increased in deep inspiration.

IMPORTANT DIAGRAMS

1. Conducting system of heart
2. Origin and spread of cardiac impulse
3. Normal ECG pattern obtained in lead II giving normal values of different waves, segments and intervals
4. Ventricular extrasystole
5. Phases of cardiac cycle
6. Left ventricular pressure change in Wigger's diagram
7. Aortic pressure changes during different phases of cardiac cycle
8. Left ventricular volume changes
9. Recording of jugular venous pulse
10. Phasic variation in coronary blood flow

SECTION 4: RESPIRATORY SYSTEM

REVIEW QUESTIONS

1. Define respiration.
2. What are the functions of the nasal cavity?
3. What are the non-respiratory functions of the lung?
4. Describe the conducting zone and respiratory zone (physiological unit) of lung?
5. Explain the importance of bronchial smooth muscle
6. Explain the innervation of lung.
7. What are the functions of pleural fluid? What is pleural effusion?
8. What is pneumothorax? What are the causes and types of pneumothorax?
9. Explain the terms eupnea, tachypnea, apnea, dyspnea and orthopnea.
10. Name the muscles of respiration.
11. Give an example where quiet expiration becomes an active process.
    Ans. In emphysema, expiration becomes an active process due to loss of elasticity of lung.
12. Briefly explain the mechanism of ventilation of lungs.
13. Explain the mechanism of increase in vertical dimension of the thoracic cage during inspiration.
14. Explain the mechanism of increase in antero-posterior and transverse diameter of the thoracic cage.
15. What is the cause of breath sounds? Mention the types of breath sounds.
16. How will you distinguish between bronchial and vesicular breath sounds?
17. What are the adventitious sounds in lungs?
18. What is the normal intrapleural pressure? What are the causes of negative intrapleural pressure?
19. What is the importance of negative intrapleural pressure?
20. Explain the variations in intrapleural pressure during phases of respiration.
21. Discuss the Regional variation in intrapleural pressure in the erect posture.
22. What are the reasons for recoil of lung?
23. What is surfactant? Give its composition.
24. What are the functions of surfactant?
25. What are the factors affecting surfactant production?
26. What is hyaline membrane seen in the lungs in infant respiratory distress syndrome?
27. State the application of law of Laplace in lung.
28. Which are the different lung volumes and capacities?
29. Define residual volume? What is its significance?
30. What is minimal volume?
31. Define functional residual capacity? What is its importance?
32. Name the lung volumes and capacities that cannot be measured using a spirometer.
33. Define vital capacity? What are the factors affecting vital capacity?
34. Define vital index?
35. What is the importance of vital capacity?
36. What is forced expiratory volume (FEV) or timed vital capacity (TVC)?
37. State the importance of timed vital capacity (TVC).
38. What is pulmonary ventilation or respiratory minute volume (RMV) or minute ventilation?
39. Define breathing reserve and dyspneic index? Give the normal values.
40. Define respiratory dead space? What are the types? Give its significance.
41. What is alveolar ventilation?
42. What is the effect of respiratory rate in alveolar ventilation?
43. What is closing capacity and closing volume? Give the normal value.
44. What is transmural or transpulmonary pressure? What is its significance?
45. Explain Bohr's equation?
46. What is compliance in respiratory system?
47. What are the factors affecting compliance? Give its variations.
48. What is specific compliance?
49. What is work of breathing?
50. What is the work done during breathing?
51. What is the normal airway resistance? Give an example where it is increased.
52. Define dyspnea.
53. What are the special features of pulmonary circulation?
54. What is meant by shunt in lungs? What is the difference between physiologic shunt and pathologic shunt?
55. Explain the factors that keep the alveoli dry?
56. What is pulmonary edema and pulmonary hypertension?
57. What is ventilation-perfusion ratio? What is its importance? State the regional variation in V/P ratio.
58. What is meant by partial pressure of a gas? What is the importance of partial pressure in gas exchange?
59. What are the reasons for the difference in the composition of atmospheric air and alveolar air?
60. What are the mechanisms by which composition of alveolar air is kept constant?
61. Explain the factors affecting diffusion across the respiratory membrane.
62. Explain the diffusing capacity of lungs?
63. What is the normal oxygen consumption and carbon dioxide output by the body at rest?
64. What is respiratory quotient (RQ) or respiratory exchange ratio?

65. Give example of the organ where RQ is negative. Give reason.
66. What are the factors that determine the amount of O_2 in the blood?
67. How is O_2 transported in blood?
68. What are the advantages of oxygenation of hemoglobin?
69. What is heme-heme interaction?
70. What is oxygen-carrying capacity of hemoglobin?
71. What is oxygen content of blood?
72. What is the normal O_2 consumption at rest?
73. What is meant by percentage saturation of hemoglobin?
74. Explain oxygen-dissociation curve with the help of a diagram.
75. What is P_{50}?
76. What are the factors affecting ODC?
77. What is the normal 2,3-BPG level (2,3-DPG)? Give few conditions where 2,3-BPG level is increased.
78. Give examples where 2,3-DPG is decreased.
79. Ans. Fetal blood and stored blood
80. What is Bohr effect?
81. What is the role of 2,3-DPG in oxygen transport?
82. Explain the significance of fetal hemoglobin?
83. What is meant by coefficient of utilization?
84. Write briefly on myoglobin
85. State the main differences between hemoglobin and myoglobin.
86. Explain the mechanism of CO_2 transport in blood?
87. What is meant by Hamberger phenomenon and water shift in RBC?
88. What is the mechanism by which CO_2 is eliminated at the lung level?
89. What is Haldane effect (CDH effect) or what is the role of O_2-Hb reaction in CO_2 transport?
90. What is the importance of CDH effect or Haldane effect?
91. Explain the neural control of respiration.
92. Explain pulmonary chemoreflex or J-reflex.
93. What is meant by breaking point in respiration?
94. How expiration is made smooth and not spasmodic?
95. What is inspiratory ramp signal (IRS)?
96. Explain Hering-Breuer inflation reflex.
97. Explain Hering-Breuer deflation reflex.
98. State the importance of Hering-Breuer inflation reflex.
99. What is meant by chemical control of respiration?
100. Explain the mechanism of action of central chemoreceptors?
101. Describe the location, structure and innervation of peripheral chemoreceptors (PCR).
102. Explain the mechanism of action of peripheral chemoreceptor (PCR).
103. What is the effect of increased PCO_2 in ventilation? What is CO_2 narcosis?
104. What are the ventilatory responses to decreased PCO_2?
105. What is the effect of hypoxia on respiration?
106. What is the effect of increased H^+ concentration (acidosis) on respiration?
107. Describe respiratory acidosis?
108. What is alkalosis? What are the respiratory adjustments in alkalosis?
109. What is the relation between hypercapnia, acidosis and hypoxia on ventilation?
110. Enumerate the abnormalities in regulation of respiration.
111. Explain Cheyne-Stokes respiration?
112. Explain Biot's breathing?
113. What is sleep apnea and sleep apnea syndrome? What are the theories put forward to explain sleep apnea?
114. What is the explanation for the periodicity in voluntary hyperventilation?
115. What is hypercapnia? Mention its causes.
116. Define asphyxia. What are the causes of asphyxia?
117. Describe the stages of asphyxia?
118. Define hypoxia. What are the types of hypoxia?
119. Explain hypoxic hypoxia.
120. What is anemic hypoxia? Explain carbon monoxide poisoning.
121. What is stagnant hypoxia?
122. What is histotoxic hypoxia?
123. What is the cause for hypoxia in cyanide poisoning? How will you treat the condition?
124. What is O_2 toxicity?
125. Write briefly on hyperbaric O_2 therapy?
126. Define cyanosis. How is it classified?
127. What is the differential diagnosis for cyanosis?
128. Describe acute mountain sickness and its management
129. Explain chronic mountain sickness
130. Explain acclimatization at high altitude.
131. What is natural acclimatization of inhabitants at high altitude (18,000 ft)?
132. What is meant by hyperbarism?
133. What is nitrogen narcosis or raptures of the depth?
134. What are the advantages of using Helium over N_2 in the inhaled air at depths?
135. What is high pressure nervous syndrome?
136. Explain decompression sickness or dysbarism or diver's paralysis or bends or caisson disease.
137. What is the treatment of decompression sickness? How can it be prevented?
138. How can you prevent O_2 toxicity at high barometric pressure?
139. Explain the respiratory adjustments in exercise.
140. What is oxygen debt?
141. What are the changes that occur in trained athletes?

142. What is VO$_2$ max (maximal O$_2$ consumption)?
143. Define fatigue. What are the causes of fatigue in exercise?
144. What are the indications for artificial respiration?
145. What is the importance of immediate respiratory resuscitation when there is arrest of respiration?
146. Explain the most effective method of manual artificial respiration.
147. Explain the different pulmonary function tests (PFT.)

GIVE THE PHYSIOLOGICAL BASIS

1. Before reaching the alveoli inhaled air is warmed and humidified.
2. Left ventricular output is about 1–2% greater than the right ventricular output.
3. Transection of the spinal cord above the third cervical segment is fatal but transection below the 5th cervical segment maintains life.
4. Syncopial attacks follow continuous severe bouts of cough.
5. Respiratory distress syndrome occurs in premature infants.
6. Apnea occurs following voluntary hyperventilation.
7. Right ventricular output is a little less than that of left ventricular output.
8. The blood in the systemic arteries has a PO$_2$ about 2 mm Hg less than that of blood that has equilibrated with alveolar air and the saturation of hemoglobin is 0.5% less.
9. Pulmonary tuberculosis affects apex of the lung first or apex of lung is more prone for pulmonary tuberculosis.
10. Patient with non-functioning lung on one side is advised to lie on the side in which the lung is functioning.
11. Tobacco smokers often cough.
12. Even though the pressure gradient for CO$_2$ across the respiratory membrane is only 6 mm Hg, it is adequate for CO$_2$ transfer. Or diffusion defects causes hypoxemia but not CO$_2$ retention.
13. The volume of dissolved O$_2$, although very less is of great functional importance.
14. Respiratory quotient (RQ) for fat is less than that of carbohydrate.
15. The combination of O$_2$ with hemoglobin is called oxygenation and not oxidation.
16. The oxygen-dissociation curve (ODC) of hemoglobin is sigmoid shaped or S-shaped.
17. Stored blood is not safe to be transfused to a hypoxic patient.
18. The size of RBCs is larger in venous blood than in arterial blood and there is increased fragility of red blood cells in venous blood.
19. pH of venous blood is lower than that of arterial blood.
20. There is 3% increase in the hematocrit value in venous blood.
21. In anemic hypoxia as in anemia, carbon monoxide poisoning, etc., there is no stimulation of respiration through peripheral chemoreceptors (PCR).
22. Asthma attacks are more severe in early morning and exercise triggers asthmatic attacks.
23. O$_2$ administration should be done with caution in patients with acute respiratory failure.
24. Hypercapnia is rarely a problem in pulmonary fibrosis.
25. Tetany occurs in hyperventilation.
26. An anemic person with 50% of normal amount of HbO$_2$ can do moderate work but an individual whose HbO$_2$ is reduced to 50% due to formation of carboxy-hemoglobin cannot.
27. Cyanosis is not seen in anemic hypoxia.
28. The problem of N$_2$ narcosis can be avoided by breathing O$_2$-He mixture.
29. There is an abrupt increase in ventilation at the start of exercise.
30. Oxygen-dissociation curve is shifted to the left in newborn.
31. RBC count is high in fetus.
32. Alveoli are always kept dry.
33. In left ventricular failure or in mitral stenosis there is collection of fluid in the alveoli.
34. Orthopnea occurs in cardiac failure.
35. Normal intrapleural pressure is negative
36. He-O$_2$ mixture is used in SCUBA.
37. Tetany can occur in hyperventilation.
38. Heart rate is increased in deep inspiration.
39. Atelectasis or collapse of lung occurs in respiratory distress syndrome.
40. RQ of carbohydrate is 1 and that of fat is 0.7.
41. Fetal blood and stored blood has high affinity for O$_2$.

IMPORTANT DIAGRAMS

1. Tracheobronchial tree
2. Intrapleural pressure changes in inspiration and expiration
3. Intrapulmonary pressure changes during respiration
4. Normal spirogram giving the normal values
5. Structure of respiratory membrane
6. Oxygen-hemoglobin dissociation curve
7. CO$_2$ dissociation curve
8. Medullary and pontine respiratory centers
9. Structure of carotid body
10. Pattern of respiration in voluntary hyperventilation
11. Changes in ventilation in exercise

SECTION 5: GASTROINTESTINAL SYSTEM

■ REVIEW QUESTIONS

1. Define digestion.
2. What are the layers of gastrointestinal tract.
3. Mention the merits and drawbacks of the mucosal layer lining the gut wall.
4. Mention the innervation of gut.
5. Describe enteric nervous system (ENS).
6. Name the excitatory and inhibitory transmitters released by the ENS.
7. Explain the extrinsic innervation of gut.
8. What is the mechanism of action of catecholamines and acetylcholine in intestinal smooth muscle?
9. What is the significance of NO and VIP secreted by neurons in ENS?
10. What is vago-vagal reflex?
11. What is meant by basic electrical rhythm? Or, explain the electrical responses of smooth muscles.
12. Write a note on migrating motor complex (MMC).
13. What is the function of migrating motor complexes?
14. Mention the different types of gastrointestinal glands or give the structural classification of gastrointestinal glands.
15. What is the functional classification of exocrine glands?
16. Explain the basic mechanism of secretion from the gastrointestinal glands.
17. What are the sources of saliva? Name the ducts that drain the major salivary glands.
18. What is meant by sialography?
19. Explain the parasympathetic innervation of the salivary glands.
20. Write a note on the sympathetic supply to the salivary glands.
21. What are the effects of stimulating the nerves supplying the salivary glands?
22. Mention the rate of secretion, pH, specific gravity and viscosity of saliva?
23. What is the composition of saliva? Give the functions of the organic constituents.
24. What is the importance of HCO_3^- and H_2CO_3 ratio in saliva?
25. What are the functions of saliva?
26. Explain the regulation of salivary secretion.
27. Explain the salivary reflexes.
28. What are the disturbances of salivary secretion?
29. What is chorda-tympani syndrome?
30. What is paralytic salivary secretion?
31. Write a note on lower esophageal sphincter (LES).
32. Enumerate the factors that prevent regurgitation of gastric contents into esophagus.
33. Lower esophageal sphincter which is tonically contracted
34. Angulation of esophagus as it passes through the diaphragm
35. A rosette-like formation of loose gastric mucosa at the cardia
36. Diaphragmatic crura which surround the lower esophageal sphincter.
37. What are the functions of esophagus?
38. Enumerate the functions of stomach.
39. Name the different parts of the stomach.
40. Name the gastric glands. Add a note on their structure and functions.
41. Explain the structure and functions of oxyntic gland.
42. What are mucins? What is their function?
43. Explain the factors that contribute to the mucosal barrier of stomach. Or, what are the factors that prevent autodigestion of gastric mucosa?
44. What is the pH, rate of secretion and composition of gastric juice? State the functions of each component.
45. Explain the mechanism of secretion of HCl by the parietal cells of stomach with the help of a diagram.
46. Write briefly on postprandial alkaline tide
47. What are the factors affecting HCl secretion in the stomach?
48. What is the mechanism of release of gastrin from G-cells of pylorus?
49. What is the mechanism of action of acetylcholine in increasing gastric secretion?
50. Explain the phases of gastric juice secretion.
51. What is enterogastric reflex?
52. Name the sources of gastrin.
53. Discuss the synthesis, chemistry and inactivation of gastrin.
54. Enumerate the actions of gastrin.
55. What are the factors that affect gastrin secretion?
56. What are gastrinomas?
57. What is the pathophysiology of achalasia cardia?
58. What is meant by sham feeding? What is its importance?
59. Give examples of hyposecretion of gastric juice or hypochlorhydria.
60. Give examples of hypersecretion of gastric acid.
61. What is peptic ulcer or acid-peptic disease (APD)? Enumerate the causes of peptic ulcer.
62. What are the complications of peptic ulcer?
63. How will you investigate and diagnose a case of peptic ulcer?
64. Explain the management of peptic ulcer.
65. What is dumping syndrome?
66. What is Zollinger-Ellison syndrome?

67. What are the differences between duodenal ulcer and gastric ulcer?
68. Describe the physical properties, composition and functions of pancreatic juice.
69. What is the difference between endopeptidases and exopeptidases?
70. Write a note on trypsin inhibitor.
71. What is the importance of phospholipase A_2 and pancreatic amylase in pancreatitis?
72. Explain the regulation of secretion of pancreatic juice.
73. Explain the phases of pancreatic juice secretion.
74. Name the conditions that lead to pancreatic insufficiency. What is steatorrhea?
75. Write a note on pancreatitis.
76. Enumerate the pancreatic function tests.
77. Enumerate the functions of liver.
78. Name the plasma proteins synthesized in the liver.
79. Trace the biliary system.
80. What is the composition of hepatic bile?
81. Name the bile acids and bile salts. What is the mechanism of formation of bile salts?
82. What is enterohepatic circulation of bile salts?
83. Name the substances that undergo enterohepatic circulation in the body.
84. What are the properties and functions of bile salts?
85. Mention the importance of bile salts in the intestine.
86. Name the bile pigments. What is their significance?
87. Explain the mechanism of formation of bile pigment.
88. Define jaundice or icterus. What is the differential diagnosis of jaundice?
89. Describe the different types of jaundice
90. What are the complications of biliary tract obstruction?
91. What are cholagogues and choleretics? Or what is the mechanism of regulation of biliary secretion?
92. What are the functions of gallbladder?
93. Mention the difference between hepatic bile and gallbladder bile
94. What is the mechanism of contraction of gallbladder? How is it controlled?
95. Enumerate the investigations of gallbladder and liver.
96. What is cholelithiasis? Mention the causes.
97. What is cholecystectomy? What are the indications?
98. Mention are the parts of small intestine?
99. Name the small intestinal glands.
100. What is the structure and function of Brunner's gland?
101. Give the composition and functions of small intestinal juice or succus entericus.
102. Enumerate the functions of small intestine.
103. What is the importance of ileocecal valve? What is gastroileal reflex?
104. Explain the functions of large intestine.
105. Mention the composition of feces?
106. Write a note on intestinal bacteria. What are the advantages and disadvantages of them?
107. What is dietary fiber? What is its importance in daily life?
108. Define mastication. Explain the mechanism of mastication.
109. What are the functions of mastication?
110. Define deglutition or swallowing. Describe the stages of deglutition.
111. What is dysphagia and odynophagia? Give examples of conditions producing dysphagia in different stages of deglutition.
112. What is the difference between achalasia cardia and chalasia?
113. What is aerophagia?
114. Write a note on the control of deglutition.
115. What are the types of gastric movements?
116. Briefly describe the movements of empty stomach.
117. What is meant by receptive relaxation of stomach?
118. Explain gastric mixing and emptying movements.
119. Explain the factors affecting gastric emptying.
120. What is meant by gastroparesis?
121. What is vomiting?
122. What is central vomiting?
123. What are the complications of gastrectomy?
124. What are the movements exhibited by the small intestine?
125. Write a short note on peristalsis.
126. What is gastroenteric or gastroileal reflex?
127. What are the movements of intestinal villi? State their functions.
128. What is adynamic ileus or paralytic ileus?
129. What are peristaltic rushes?
130. What is malabsorption syndrome?
131. Which are the movements exhibited by the large intestine?
132. Write a note on mass action contraction or mass peristalsis? Where is it seen?
133. Mention the transit time in the gastrointestinal tract.
134. What is defecation? Describe the mechanism of defecation.
135. Define constipation and diarrhea.
136. Explain the pathophysiology of Hirschsprung's disease or adynamic colon
137. Explain the digestion and absorption of carbohydrates. Write a note on its abnormality.
138. Explain defective carbohydrate digestion and absorption
139. Explain protein digestion and absorption. Write a note on its disturbance.
140. Explain the digestion and absorption of fat.
141. What is steatorrhea? Mention its causes.
142. Name the essential fatty acids.
143. What is the mechanism of absorption of iron in the gastrointestinal tract?
144. Mention the distribution of iron in the body.
145. Which are the factors that regulate iron absorption?
146. What are the effects of iron deficiency and iron overload?
147. Name a condition where anti-peristalsis is seen.
148. Write a note on incretins.
149. Which is the 'gut factor' for insulin secretion?

GIVE THE PHYSIOLOGICAL BASIS

1. After a meal, the blood flow to the gut increases as much as 8-fold during the next one hour.
2. People with dry mouth have a tendency to develop infections of the oral cavity.
3. Mouth becomes dry during fear and stress.
4. Salivary digestion is completed in the stomach.
5. Continuous secretion of saliva occurs in the absence of any stimulus.
6. In the early phase of vomiting there is increased salivation and a catch in the respiration.
7. Oral administration of vitamin B_{12} is ineffective in pernicious anemia (due to absence of intrinsic factor).
8. Iron deficiency anemia is a frequent complication of partial gastrectomy.
9. Pernicious anemia occurs after gastrectomy.
10. The respiratory quotient of stomach is negative.
11. After a heavy meal urine becomes alkaline.
12. Stress is often associated with peptic ulcer.
13. Gastric acid secretion is increased after the removal of large parts of the small intestine.
14. Ranitidine and omeprazole are given in gastritis and peptic ulcer.
15. Following meals, dizziness and sweating occur after partial or total gastrectomy.
16. Steatorrhea is seen in diseases of terminal ileum or after resection of terminal ileum.
17. Hemolytic jaundice is also called acholuric jaundice.
18. Urine is deep yellow and stool is clay colored (pale) in obstructive jaundice.
19. Length of small intestine is 300 cm during life and 700 cm after death.
20. Absorptive capacity of large intestine is considerably less when compared to that of the small intestine.
21. Normally, duodenal contents do not regurgitate into the stomach.
22. Travelling in a ship usually produces vomiting or vomiting occurs in motion sickness.
23. Defecation is a rule in infants after meals.
24. Urobilinogen is normally present in urine.
25. Gallbladder bile is different from hepatic bile.
26. Dumping syndrome is seen after gastrectomy.
27. Food is prevented from entering the respiratory passage during deglutition.
28. Vitamin B_{12} is administered parenterally in pernicious anemia.
29. Vagotomy is indicated in severe cases of peptic ulcer:
30. Autodigestion of gastric mucosa does not occur normally.
31. Histamine is a necessary cofactor for significant acid secretion in the stomach.
32. Peptic ulcer is frequently seen in people with strong emotional stimuli like business executives.
33. Destruction of pancreatic tissue in pancreatitis
34. High cholesterol-lecithin ratio leads to formation of gall stones.
35. Plasma has a milky appearance after a heavy fatty meal.

IMPORTANT DIAGRAMS

1. Structural organization of the gastrointestinal tract or cross section of intestine
2. Microscopic structure of seromucinous acinus
3. Parasympathetic innervation of salivary glands
4. Structure of oxyntic or fundic gland of stomach
5. Structure of small intestinal villus
6. Segmentation contraction and peristalsis in small intestine
7. Steps of fat absorption in intestine

SECTION 6: RENAL PHYSIOLOGY

REVIEW QUESTIONS

1. How does kidney contribute to homeostasis?
2. What are the functions of kidney?
3. Name the constituents of blood that are not present in the glomerular filtrate.
4. Give the differences between cortical and juxtamedullary nephron
5. Mention the type of epithelium lining the different segments of the nephron.
6. Describe the structure of the filtration membrane of kidney
7. Mention the location of juxtaglomerular apparatus? Give its structure.
8. Enumerate the functions of juxtaglomerular apparatus.
9. What are the functions of mesangial cells? What is its clinical importance?
10. What is tubuloglomerular feedback mechanism?
11. What is glomerulotubular balance? What is its significance?
12. Explain the mechanism of glomerulotubular balance.
13. Briefly outline the blood supply of kidney
14. How is renal blood flow measured?
15. What are the criteria for the substance to be used to measure renal plasma flow?
16. What are the special features of renal circulation?
17. What is renorenal reflex?
18. What is effective filtration pressure or net filtration pressure in the kidney?
19. What is glomerular filtration and glomerular filtration rate?

20. Explain the factors that affect GFR
21. What is the mechanism of action of ANP in increasing GFR?
22. What is the mechanism of action of angiotensin II in decreasing GFR?
23. Which branch of ANS innervates renal blood vessels? What is the effect of sympathetic stimulation on GFR?
24. What is meant by clearance of a substance?
25. What is the difference between maximal urea clearance and standard urea clearance?
26. How is GFR measured?
27. What are the criteria of the substance used for the measurement of GFR?
28. What is filtration fraction?
29. Which are the main mechanisms by which GFR is regulated?
30. Explain renin-angiotensin system in regulation of GFR.
31. What is ANP? Mention its clinical significance.
32. What is meant by transport maximum of a substance?
33. What is meant by renal threshold of a substance?
34. What are the different mechanisms by which Na^+ is reabsorbed in the different segments of the nephron? What is the importance of sodium reabsorption?
35. What is the fate of Na^+ inside the tubular cell?
36. Explain the factors affecting sodium reabsorption in the renal tubules?
37. What is the mechanism of action of angiotensin converting enzyme (ACE) inhibitors in decreasing blood pressure?
38. How is filtered glucose reabsorbed in the renal tubules?
39. What is splay phenomenon in glucose reabsorption?
40. How is water reabsorbed by the renal tubules?
41. What is the difference between obligatory water reabsorption and facultative water reabsorption in renal tubules?
42. What are aquaporins?
43. Name the hormones that regulate renal tubular reabsorption.
44. What is meant by tubular secretion? Give examples of substances secreted by renal tubules.
45. What is the normal K^+ excretion? How is K^+ secretion regulated?
46. What are the mechanisms by which H^+ is secreted by renal tubules?
47. What is a countercurrent system? What is its role in maintaining medullary osmotic gradient?
48. Which are the factors that are responsible for the production and maintenance of medullary osmotic gradient?
49. What is the role of urea in maintaining the medullary interstitial gradient?
50. What is the mechanism of action of ADH in the collecting duct of nephron?
51. What is urea recycling? Mention its importance.
52. Explain the mechanism of excretion of dilute and concentrated urine.
53. Describe the renal mechanisms of maintenance of normal specific gravity of urine.
54. How is ADH secretion regulated?
55. Discuss the abnormalities of ADH secretion.
56. What are vasa recta? Mention their importance?
57. What is the mechanism of acidification of urine? Or summarize the renal regulation of pH. Or what are the renal buffer systems?
58. How does renal tubule secrete ammonia? What is its role in acidification of urine?
59. What is titrabtale acidity?
60. What are the factors that affect H^+ secretion in the renal tubules?
61. What is anion gap?
62. Discuss few abnormalities of renal function.
63. What are the indications for dialysis?
64. Describe the types of dialysis. What are the complications of dialysis?
65. What is meant by diuresis and what are diuretics?
66. What is the difference between water diuresis and osmotic diuresis?
67. What is the role of kidney in the long-term regulation of blood pressure?
68. Explain the innervation of the urinary bladder with the help of a diagram.
69. What is meant by micturition? Describe micturition reflex.
70. Discuss the control of micturition by higher centers.
71. What is the difference between continence and incontinence of urine?
72. What are the abnormalities of bladder function?
73. Explain how micturition is affected in spinal shock.
74. What is residual urine?
75. Mention the significance of plasticity in urinary bladder. Or explain how the structure of urinary bladder is suited to its function.
76. What is cystometrogram? What is the application of law of Laplace in urinary bladder?
77. Explain the important renal function tests.

GIVE THE PHYSIOLOGICAL BASIS

1. Urinary bladder can store considerable amount of urine without much discomfort.
2. Chronic renal diseases result in anemia
3. Albuminuria and edema occur in nephrotic syndrome. Or Edema is seen in proteinuria.
4. Osteomalacia or abnormal bone formation occurs in chronic renal failure.
5. Splay in glucose titration curve.
6. Hyperosmolarity of medullary interstitium.
7. Plateau phase is seen in cystometrogram. Or in cystometrogram, the second component of the graph is a long nearly flat segment.

8. Renal medulla is vulnerable to hypoxic damage than the cortex.
9. Micturition can be stopped once it has been initiated or micturition can be initiated even if there is no desire to void urine.
10. Polyuria and polydipsia occurs in pituitary diabetes insipidus.
11. Hypokalemia is seen following administration of loop diuretics.
12. Vasa recta are referred to as countercurrent exchangers. Or, vasa recta preserves medullary osmotic gradient.
13. Dopamine infusion is advised for the treatment of severe hypotension (shock).
14. Glomerular capillary pressure is very high when compared to other capillaries OR renal blood pressure is comparatively high.
15. Tubular fluid entering the distal tubule of juxtamedullary nephron is always hypotonic.
16. Renal blood flow does not change within a systolic pressure range of 90 to 220 mm Hg.
17. PAH is used to measure renal plasma flow.
18. Reflux of semen into the urinary bladder does not occur during ejaculation.
19. Blood flow to the renal medulla is less than that of cortex.
20. Na^+ excretion cannot be regulated by changes in GFR alone.
21. The volume of fluid filtered by the renal glomerulus is much larger than in other capillaries of the body.
22. Parathyroid hypertrophy is seen in chronic renal disease.
23. In water diuresis, the maximal urine flow possible is about 16 mL/min, whereas osmotic diuresis can produce much larger urine flow rate.
24. Even though hyperglycemia in uncontrolled diabetes mellitus increases ADH secretion, there will be polyuria in DM.
25. A high-protein diet increases the ability of kidneys to concentrate the urine.

IMPORTANT DIAGRAMS

1. Structure of a juxtamedullary nephron.
2. Microscopic structure of different segments of nephron.
3. Longitudinal section of kidney showing the arterial blood supply.
4. Structure of renal filtration membrane.
5. Juxtaglomerular apparatus.
6. Draw a labelled diagram to demonstrate the phenomenon of splay in glucose reabsorption.
7. Diagrammatically represent countercurrent system in kidney.
8. Innervation of urinary bladder.
9. Spinal reflex arc for micturition.
10. Cystometrogram or pressure-volume curve of urinary bladder.

SECTION 7: SKIN AND TEMPERATURE REGULATION

REVIEW QUESTIONS

1. What are the important functions of skin?
2. What is meant by constitutional hyperthermia?
3. What is the difference between albinism and vitiligo?
4. Name two important hormones that increase heat production in the body.
5. What are the types by which water is evaporated from the body?
6. Name the sweat glands of the body. What is thermal sweating and non-thermal sweating?
7. Name the areas in the skin where sweat glands are absent.
8. Which is the most effective means of heat loss during exercise?
9. Name the centers concerned with temperature regulation.
10. What will happen if anterior hypothalamus is destroyed locally?
11. What are the responses of the body when exposed to hot climate?
12. Discuss the adjustments that occur in the body when exposed to cold
13. What is the cause of death in acute heat stress or heat exhaustion?
14. What is meant by acclimatization of sweating mechanism?
15. What is the role of brown fat in thermogenesis?
16. What is hyperthermia and hypothermia? Mention the common causes.
17. What is malignant hyperthermia?
18. What is the mechanism of production of fever?
19. Explain the pathogenesis of fever
20. What are the advantages of fever?

GIVE THE PHYSIOLOGICAL BASIS

1. Regulation of body temperature is very essential for life
2. One feels hotter on a humid day.
3. Shivering in a cold environment.
4. Shivering occurs in fever.
5. Aspirin is given to decrease fever.
6. Induced hypothermia is made use of in cardiac and brain surgeries.
7. Body temperature is subnormal in old age.
8. Hypothyroid patients prefer hot environment and cannot tolerate cold.

SECTION 8: ENDOCRINE SYSTEM

REVIEW QUESTIONS

1. Define hormone.
2. What are the differences between endocrine, paracrine and autocrine secretions?
3. Enumerate the endocrine glands.
4. What is the chemical nature of hormones?
5. What are hormone receptors?
6. What are the types of intercellular communications?
7. Write a note on the regulation of hormone receptors. Or what is meant by up-regulation and down-regulation of receptors?
8. What is meant by internalization and desensitization of receptors?
9. What is receptor specificity and crossing over of hormones?
10. What are the mechanisms by which combination of hormone with receptor trigger cellular function?
11. Explain the action of hormones through second messengers. Or write short note on second messengers.
12. Explain adenylyl cyclase-cAMP system.
13. What are G proteins? How are they classified?
14. Enumerate the ligands that exert their effects through heterotrimeric G proteins.
15. Give examples of G protein diseases.
16. Explain calcium-calmodulin second messenger system.
17. Explain the action of phosphatidylinositol derivatives as second messengers.
18. Name the water-soluble hormones that do not act through adenylate cyclase.
19. What are the causes for the specificity of hormonal action?
20. Explain hormonal action by activation of genetic mechanism.
21. What is meant by non-genomic actions of steroid hormones?
22. Explain the regulation of hormone secretion.
23. What is meant by negative feedback regulation?
24. What is meant by positive feedback mechanism?
25. Give examples of positive feedback mechanisms occurring in the body.
26. What is meant by permissive action of hormones?
27. What is circadian rhythm? Give examples.
28. Write briefly on growth factors.
29. Mention the relation of pituitary gland to hypothalamus.
30. What are the parts of pituitary gland?
31. Name the hormones secreted by the pituitary gland.
32. Explain the action of growth hormone on somatic growth.
33. Explain the mechanism of growth-promoting action of growth hormone. Or write a note on somatomedins.
34. Explain the actions of growth hormone on metabolism.
35. How is growth hormone secretion regulated?
36. Enumerate the factors causing hypersecretion of growth hormone.
37. What is the effect of hypersecretion of growth hormone before puberty?
38. What is the effect of hypersecretion of growth hormone after puberty?
39. What is the effect of hyposecretion of growth hormone before puberty?
40. What are the causes of dwarfism?
41. What is the effect of growth hormone deficiency in adults?
42. Define growth.
43. What are the factors that influence growth?
44. What is pituitary insufficiency or panhypopituitarism or Simmond's disease?
45. What is Sheehan's syndrome?
46. Explain hypothalamic control of the anterior pituitary Or hypothalamo-hypophysial axis.
47. Name the hormones released from posterior pituitary.
48. What are the actions of vasopressin or ADH?
49. Explain the regulation of ADH secretion.
50. What are the abnormalities in ADH secretion?
51. What are the actions of oxytocin? Which are the factors that increase oxytocin secretion?
52. What is neuroendocrine reflex?
53. What are the functions of melatonin?
54. What are the unique features of thyroid gland?
55. Name the hormones produced by the thyroid gland.
56. Explain the steps in the biosynthesis of thyroid hormones. Mention the action of antithyroid drugs in the different stages of synthesis.
57. Name the iodotyrosines and the iodothyronines.
58. Name the areas other than thyroid gland where iodide trapping is seen.
59. Write a note on thyroglobulin.
60. What is the mechanism of secretion of thyroid hormones?
61. Give the normal plasma levels of thyroid hormones. How are they transported in blood?
62. Why T_3 is more active physiologically than T_4?
63. Compare and contrast T_3 and T_4.
64. Explain the actions of thyroid hormones.
65. How is thyroid function assessed?
66. What is metathyroid diabetes?
67. Explain the regulation of secretion of thyroid hormones.

68. Describe Wolff-Chaikoff effect
69. What are the effects of TSH on thyroid gland?
70. Explain the cause of enlargement of thyroid gland in simple goitre.
71. What is the effect of deficiency of thyroid hormones in childhood?
72. Enumerate the causes of dwarfism.
73. Distinguish between pituitary dwarf and cretin.
74. What is the effect of thyroid deficiency in adults?
75. Describe Graves disease or exophthalmic goitre
76. Explain the management for hyperthyroidism
77. What are goitrogens?
78. Enumerate the functions of ionic calcium in the body.
79. Give the value of total body phosphorus and its plasma concentration. What are the functions of phosphorus in the body?
80. What is meant by solubility product?
81. What is the normal plasma calcium level? Name the three hormones that affect calcium and phosphorus metabolism.
82. Which are the other hormones regulating calcium metabolism?
83. What is the mechanism of calcium homeostasis by parathormone (PTH)?
84. Explain the actions of parathormone.
85. What are the features of hypoparathyroidism?
86. What is accoucheur's hand and laryngeal stridor?
87. What is latent tetany? How can you diagnose the condition?
88. What is tetany? Name some conditions where tetany is seen.
89. What are the features of hyperparathyroidism? How can the condition be diagnosed?
90. Explain the actions of calcitonin
91. Name the sites of production of calcitriol.
92. Discuss the steps in the synthesis of calcitriol. Give its normal plasma value.
93. Enumerate the actions of calcitriol or 1,25-dihydroxy-cholecalciferol. Add a note on its deficiency.
94. Explain the regulation of secretion of calcitriol.
95. Name the layers of adrenal cortex and mention the hormones secreted by each layer.
96. Name the most potent glucocorticoid.
97. Explain the physiological actions of cortisol or glucocorticoids.
98. What is meant by permissive action of glucocorticoids? Give examples.
99. What is the role of glucocorticoids in reactions to stress situation?
100. Discuss the anti-inflammatory action of glucocorticoids.
101. What is the anti-allergic action of glucocorticoids?
102. What is the anti-immunity effect of glucocorticoids?
103. What are the pharmacological actions of glucocorticoids?
104. What is gluconeogenesis?
105. Explain the regulation of secretion of glucocorticoids.
106. Describe the effect of hypersecretion of glucocorticoids
107. How is Cushing's syndrome diagnosed?
108. Name the most potent mineralocorticoid.
109. Explain the actions of aldosterone.
110. Explain aldosterone escape
111. How is secretion of aldosterone regulated?
112. Describe the abnormalities in aldosterone secretion
113. What are the features of primary adrenal insufficiency or Addison's disease?
114. What is meant by sympatho-medullary system?
115. Name the hormones of adrenal medulla.
116. What are the steps in the biosynthesis of catecholamines?
117. Discuss the metabolism of catecholamines.
118. Explain the mechanism of action of catecholamines.
119. Discuss the effects of stimulation of different adrenergic receptors.
120. What is the importance of a_2 adrenergic receptors?
121. Compare the effects of α-adrenergic receptor and β-adrenergic receptor stimulation?
122. Explain the actions of catecholamines.
123. What is biphasic action of adrenaline?
124. What is meant by adrenaline apnea?
125. What is the importance of adrenal medulla in the body?
126. What is Dale's vasomotor reversal?
127. What is pheochromocytoma?
128. Mention the cell types in the islets of Langerhans and the hormones produced by each.
129. Name the most important hypoglycemic hormone in the body. Mention its target organs.
130. Name the important hyperglycemic hormones in the body.
131. Mention the insulin-like substances in the body.
132. Name the areas in the body that do not require insulin for the transport of glucose into the cell.
133. Explain the actions of insulin.
134. Explain the action of insulin on carbohydrate metabolism
135. What is the mechanism of action of insulin?
136. Explain the regulation of insulin secretion.
137. What is the difference between diabetes mellitus and diabetes insipidus?
138. What are the types of diabetes mellitus?
139. List the causes of diabetes mellitus.
140. What are the effects of lack of insulin in diabetics?
141. Name the ketone bodies that are formed in the body.
142. What is ketoacidosis? Name the conditions that lead to ketoacidosis.

143. How is diabetes mellitus diagnosed?
144. Mention the treatment of diabetes mellitus.
145. What is metabolic syndrome or syndrome-X? What is the importance of leptin in obesity?
146. Explain the actions of glucagon
147. What are the actions of somatostatin?
148. Explain the paracrine function of the hormones of the islets of Langerhans.
149. Enumerate the actions of angiotensin-II.
150. What are the actions of atrial natriuretic peptide (ANP)?
151. Enumerate the actions of histamine.
152. Enumerate the actions of serotonin.
153. Enumerate the functions of prostaglandins
154. Name the prostaglandin inhibitors.
155. What are the actions of bradykinin?
156. Name the sites where acetylcholine is found in the body.
157. Mention the types of cholinergic receptors. State their location.
158. Name the hormones that promote uptake of K^+ into the cells when there is a rise in plasma K^+ level.

GIVE THE PHYSIOLOGICAL BASIS

1. In adrenal insufficiency and in Cushing's syndrome there will be hyperpigmentation.
2. Puberty is delayed in blind girls. Or precocious puberty occurs in deficiency of melatonin in girls.
3. Lugol's iodine is administered before thyroidectomy in hyperthyroidism.
4. Transport of iodide into the thyroid cell is called iodide trapping.
5. T_3 is physiologically more active than T_4.
6. Even though physiologically less active, T_4 is produced in larger amounts than T_3 by the thyroid gland.
7. Exophthalmos is a feature of Graves disease.
8. Exophthalmos is not relieved by thyroidectomy.
9. There is increase in pulse pressure in hyperthyroidism.
10. Vitamin deficiency is seen in hyperthyroidism.
11. Cretins have short stature and mental defect.
12. Edema and carotenemia is seen in hypothyroidism.
13. Puffiness, slowing of tendon reflexes and intolerance to cold are seen in myxedema.
14. People who consume lot of cabbage and cauliflower are prone to develop goitre.
15. Lack of iodine in the diet leads to goitre.
16. Measurement of plasma TSH levels is one of the best tests for assessing thyroid functions.
17. There is increased risk of osteoporosis and fracture after menopause.
18. In hyperparathyroidism, Ca^{2+} excretion is increased.
19. Blood calcium level increases after administration of parathyroid extract.
20. Tetany occurs in hyperventilation.
21. Carpopedal spasm occurs in tetany.
22. Plasma calcium level is low in chronic renal disease.
23. Secondary hyperparathyroidism is seen in chronic renal disease and rickets.
24. Parathyroid hypertrophy is seen in chronic renal disease.
25. Patients with alkalosis are more susceptible to hypocalcemic tetany.
26. Cortisol increases blood glucose.
27. Cortisol is contraindicated in diabetes mellitus.
28. Moon face and buffalo hump are features of glucocorticoid excess.
29. Hyperglycemia occurs in Cushing syndrome.
30. About 85% of patients with Cushing syndrome are hypertensive.
31. Purplish striae are seen in the trunk in Cushing's syndrome.
32. Tomato cheeks (red cheeks) are a feature of Cushing syndrome.
33. Adrenocortical insufficiency is characterized by hypotension.
34. Hyperglycemia occurs in glucocorticoid excess.
35. Eosinopenia is seen in glucocorticoid excess.
36. Glucocorticoids are prescribed in hypersensitivity reactions.
37. Long-term therapy with glucocorticoids should not be stopped suddenly.
38. The actions of glucocorticoids in patients with bacterial infections are dramatic but dangerous.
39. Absence of edema in primary hyperaldosteronism or Conn's syndrome
40. Diarrhea and dehydration occur in aldosterone deficiency.
41. Hyperpigmentation of skin and mucosa occurs in primary adrenal insufficiency.
42. There is hyperpigmentation in primary adrenal insufficiency (Addison disease) as well as in Cushing syndrome due to ACTH-secreting tumors.
43. Bilateral adrenalectomy results in death.
44. Epinephrine is not produced in postganglionic sympathetic nerve endings.
45. Epinephrine does not produce reflex bradycardia whereas norepinephrine does.
46. Exaggerated manifestations of cardiovascular symptoms are seen in pheochromocytoma.
47. Pancreas is referred to as a dual gland.
48. Diabetic patients are advised to do exercise regularly to lower blood sugar level even though there is deficiency of insulin.
49. Cortisol is contraindicated in diabetes mellitus.
50. Muscle glycogen cannot be converted to glucose in between meals.
51. Failure to grow is a symptom of diabetes mellitus in children.
52. In diabetes mellitus, there will be muscle wasting and weight loss even if there is increased food intake.
53. Insulin is called "the hormone of abundance."
54. Orally administered glucose exerts a greater insulin-stimulating effect than intravenously administered glucose.

55. Polyuria, polydipsia and polyphagia occur in diabetes mellitus.
56. Diabetes is called a condition of starvation in the midst of plenty.
57. Diabetic patients are more prone for infections.
58. Ketoacidosis and Kussmaul breathing are features of severe diabetes mellitus.
59. Food intake increases in untreated diabetes mellitus.
60. Hyperprolactinemia leads to sterility in males.

SECTION 9: REPRODUCTIVE SYSTEM

REVIEW QUESTIONS

1. Define reproduction.
2. What are the major factors that differentiate adult male and female?
3. What are the functions of sex chromosomes?
4. What is meant by Barr body? What is its significance?
5. What are the criteria for the development of a normal ovary?
6. Which is the main factor responsible for sex differentiation?
7. What is testis-determining factor?
8. What are the different stages of sex differentiation?
9. What is the structure of the primitive gonad?
10. What is the importance of hormones in sex differentiation?
11. Write a note on Turner's syndrome.
12. Does hormonal treatment to the mother affect gonadal differentiation in fetus? Support your answer.
13. What are the functions of mullerian inhibiting substance or mullerian regression factor?
14. What is the role of dihydrotestosterone in the development of external genitalia?
15. What is psychological sex?
16. What is the difference between true hermaphroditism and pseudo-hermaphroditism?
17. What is meant by genetic screening?
18. What is amniocentesis?
19. What is the role of testosterone in fetal life?
20. Enumerate the factors causing male pseudo-hermaphroditism.
21. What is cryptorchidism?
22. Define puberty. What is precocious puberty?
23. Enumerate the pubertal changes in males.
24. Enumerate the pubertal changes in females.
25. What is the role of leptin in puberty?
26. What is spermatogenesis?
27. What is the importance of the arrangement of testicular vessels in spermatogenesis?
28. Explain the stages of spermatogenesis?
29. What is spermiogenesis?
30. What is spermiation?
31. What are the main functions of sertoli cells?
32. What is blood-testis barrier (BTB)?
33. Enumerate the functions of blood-testis-barrier (BTB).
34. What is the role of sertoli cells in spermatogenesis?
35. Name the substances produced by Sertoli cells and their functions.
36. Name the transport proteins secreted by Sertoli cells.
37. Enumerate the hormones stimulating and inhibiting spermatogenesis.
38. What is the effect of the temperature of scrotum in spermatogenesis? How is it maintained?
39. What is the complication of undescended testes?
40. What are the functions of androgen binding protein (ABP) in testis? What is the stimulus for its production?
41. What is the composition of seminal fluid (secretion of seminal vesicle)?
42. What is the composition of prostatic secretion?
43. What do you mean by erection of penis? What is the mechanism?
44. Name the neurotransmitters responsible for penile erection.
45. What is the mechanism of action of Viagra? What is the cause for the transient color blindness observed following Viagra administration?
46. What is the difference between emission and ejaculation?
47. What is semen?
48. What is the function of acrosome?
49. What is capacitation? What are the changes that occur in the sperm during capacitation?
50. What are the factors that stimulate capacitation in the male genital tract?
51. How is polyspermy prevented?
52. Name the hormones secreted by testis.
53. Briefly mention the actions of testosterone.
54. What are the secondary sexual characters in male?
55. What is penis-at-12 syndrome?
56. What is testicular feminizing syndrome?
57. What are the effects on subsequent sexual development when normal testes fail to develop in a human, genetically male fetus?
58. Name the hormones secreted by Sertoli cells, Leydig cell, Graafian follicle and corpus luteum.
59. What are the main causes of infertility in males?
60. What is eunuchoidism?
61. List four important functions of testosterone.
62. What is the significance of episodic bursts of GnRH secretion in female?
63. Give the composition of liquor folliculi.

Important Questions

64. What is the difference between luteinization and luteolysis? Or how is corpus luteum and corpus albicans formed?
65. Enumerate the tests of ovulation.
66. What is meant by ferning of cervical mucus?
67. Name the progestogens.
68. Name the sources of progesterone
69. What are the forms of naturally occurring estrogens?
70. What is mid-cycle LH surge?
71. Summarize hormonal control of ovarian function.
72. Give the composition of normal menstrual blood.
73. What are the differences between the actions of estrogen and progesterone in female?
74. What is menopause? What is its mechanism?
75. What are the physiological effects of menopause?
76. Explain the mechanism of fertilization of ovum.
77. What is meant by implantation of blastocyst? What are the events occurring during implantation?
78. Which is the source of progesterone in the initial weeks of gestation?
79. What are the functions of placenta?
80. Briefly describe the functions of the hormones produced by the placenta
81. What is the role of hCG as a tumor marker?
82. What is fetoplacental unit?
83. What is the double Bohr effect occurring in the placenta?
84. How is immunological test for pregnancy or Gravindex test done?
85. What is hCG? What are its functions?
86. Which are the hormones which cause increased uterine contractility during parturition?
87. What is the role of cortisol on fetus towards term?
88. What is the role of oxytocin in parturition?
89. Which is the hormone that has both growth hormone and prolactin secretion capabilities?
90. What are the changes that occur in the breasts during menstrual cycle?
91. Mention the hormones acting on mammary gland.
92. How is lactation initiated and maintained?
93. What is the cause for lactation amenorrhea?
94. What are the principal stimuli and drugs that affect prolactin secretion?
95. What are the effects of breastfeeding on mother and baby?
96. Which are the hormones responsible for galactogenesis?
97. What is galactorrhea?
98. What is meant by contraception? What are the different contraceptive methods?
99. What is safe period?
100. What is the mechanism of action of oral contraceptive pill? What are its side effects and contraindications?
101. Which are the methods of contraception in women?
102. What are IUCDs? What is its mechanism of action?
103. What are the causes of sterility or infertility?
104. What is impotence?
105. What are the fertility tests in male?

GIVE THE PHYSIOLOGICAL BASIS

1. 5α-reductase deficiency during intrauterine life leads to pseudohermaphroditism.
2. Administration of androgens to the mother during the first trimester of pregnancy leads to female pseudohermaphroditism.
3. Only one Graafian follicle is formed in one menstrual cycle normally.
4. Menstrual blood does not clot normally.
5. HCS is referred to as human placental lactogen and the maternal growth hormone of pregnancy.
6. hCG is not absolutely specific for pregnancy.
7. Fetal adrenal cortex is very large.
8. ESR is increased in pregnancy.
9. There is no milk secretion during pregnancy even though the prolactin level is high.
10. Rejection reaction produced when other foreign tissues are transplanted fail to occur in the case of fetal graft in the mother.
11. There is increased extraction of O_2 from the maternal blood to the fetal circulation.
12. Onset of labor can be delayed by administration of drugs like aspirin.
13. Gynecomastia occurs in liver diseases and following digitalis therapy.
14. There is slight male preponderance in the population.
15. It is seen that well nourished girls attain puberty at an earlier age.
16. Oral contraceptives prevent pregnancy.
17. Implantation of copper-T prevents pregnancy.
18. A low temperature is maintained in the testis and sterility is seen in cryptorchidism.
19. Sterility is seen in males who suffer from mumps in adult life.
20. Removal of ovary is not advisable in the first trimester of pregnancy. Or, removal of corpus luteum before the 7th week of pregnancy results in spontaneous abortion.
21. Double Bohr effect is seen in the placenta.
22. Polyspermy is prevented during fertilization of ovum.
23. Hot flushes occur in women at the time of menopause.
24. The drug Viagra produces transient color blindness.
25. Vasectomy is done in males for sterilization and not orchidectomy.
26. Systemic administration of testosterone is used for male contraception.

IMPORTANT DIAGRAMS

1. Structure of testis.
2. Structure of a sperm.
3. Structure of ovary.

4. Graafian follicle.
5. Uterine changes during a menstrual cycle.
6. Hormonal changes in menstrual cycle.
7. Milk ejection reflex.

SECTION 10: NERVOUS SYSTEM

REVIEW QUESTIONS

Sensory System

1. Define nervous system.
2. Name the neuroglial cells of CNS.
3. Name the neuroglial cells of peripheral nervous system.
4. What are the functions of astrocytes?
5. What are satellite cells in nervous system?
6. Which are the unmyelinated fibers in the nervous system?
7. Name the important neural centers in the medulla oblongata.
8. Name the areas where new neurons are formed throughout life.
9. Define synapse
10. What is the morphological classification of synapse?
11. Name the most common type of transmission at the synapses?
12. Define neurotransmitters. Give examples.
13. Mention the names of some excitatory and inhibitory transmitters.
14. Explain the mechanism of transmission of impulse in an excitatory chemical synapse.
15. Give the differences between chemical and electrical synapse.
16. Write briefly on electrical synapse. Name the sites where electrical synapses are present in the nervous system.
17. Mention five properties of synaptic transmitters.
18. What are neurohormones?
19. Enumerate the properties of synapses.
20. Explain any three properties of synapses.
21. What is synaptic inhibition? What is its ionic basis? What are the types of synaptic inhibition?
22. Explain postsynaptic inhibition.
23. What is presynaptic inhibition? Explain the mechanism involved.
24. Explain the terms summation, occlusion and subliminal fringe effect in terms of synaptic transmission.
25. What is the mechanism and significance of after-discharge?
26. Write a note on post-tetanic potentiation.
27. Write a note on synaptic plasticity. What is its significance?
28. What are the causes for synaptic fatigue? Mention its clinical significance.
29. Compare neuronal synapse with myoneuronal junction (neuromuscular junction)
30. Name the different types of inhibition in the CNS.
31. Compare and contrast pre-synaptic and postsynaptic inhibition.
32. What is Renshaw cell inhibition or feedback inhibition?
33. State an example of lateral inhibition occurring in the spinal cord?
34. Enumerate the functions of synapse.
35. What is a reciprocal synapse?
36. Write a brief note on postsynaptic potential.
37. Define reflex activity. Give examples.
38. What is a reflex arc? What are its components?
39. Classify reflexes
40. What are muscle spindles and Golgi tendon organs?
41. Describe stretch reflex or myotatic reflex. Mention its pathway.
42. Describe withdrawal reflex or flexor reflex and mention its functional significance?
43. What is crossed extensor reflex?
44. Trace the pathway for knee jerk.
45. What is the physiological basis of exaggerated knee jerk and absent knee jerk?
46. Describe reciprocal innervation? Give its functional importance.
47. What is the difference between agonist and antagonist muscles?
48. What are the flexor and extensor responses of plantar reflex?
49. What is the difference between stretch reflex and inverse stretch reflex?
50. What are the mechanisms by which muscle spindle is stimulated?
51. What is the role of muscle spindle in the regulation of muscle length?
52. What is the physiological basis of Jendrassik's maneuver?
53. Mention three differences between monosynaptic and polysynaptic reflexes.
54. How reflexes are useful in clinical examination?
55. Explain the function of gamma motor neuron
56. What is meant by α-γ linkage?
57. Why α-motor neurons are called so?
58. Mention the inputs to α-motor neurons
59. Define muscle tone. Describe the physiological basis and regulation of muscle tone.
60. What is clonus seen in hypertonia?
61. Explain the physiological basis of clonus?
62. What is clasp knife effect or lengthening reaction?
63. What is crossed extensor response? What is its functional importance?

Important Questions

64. What is a sensory receptor?
65. Classify sensory receptors. Give examples of each.
66. Describe five properties of sensory receptors.
67. What is the difference between tonic and phasic receptors?
68. Write a note on generator potential or receptor potential.
69. Differentiate between receptor potential and action potential.
70. What is Bell-Magendie law?
71. All sensory nerve fibers transmit only action potentials. Then what is the mechanism by which different nerve fibers transmit different modalities of sensation?
72. Give the explanation for phantom limb phenomenon?
73. What is Muller's doctrine of specific nerve energies?
74. Write a note on sensory unit and receptive field.
75. Explain the mechanism of appreciation of intensity of a sensation.
76. What is Weber-Fechner law?
77. What are the differences between epicritic and protopathic sensations?
78. Write a note on synthetic senses or cortical sensations.
79. Explain stereognosis.
80. What is a dermatome?
81. Name the important ascending and descending tracts of spinal cord.
82. Give the main differences between dorsal column and spinothalamic tracts.
83. What do you mean by perception?
84. Name the sensations carried by dorsal column pathway.
85. Name the sensations carried by spinothalamic pathway.
86. Write a note on somatic sensory area I (SSA I).
87. Write a note on sensory homunculus.
88. Write briefly on sensory association area.
89. What is amorphosynthesis?
90. What are the differences between touch, pressure and vibration sense?
91. Explain touch pathway.
92. What are the mechanisms of two point discrimination and tactile localization?
93. What is graphesthesia?
94. What are the effects of damage to the dorsal column?
95. Explain the pathway for proprioception.
96. What are the functions of spinocerebellar pathway?
97. Explain the pathway for superficial pain sensation.
98. What are the differences between fast pain and slow pain?
99. What are the differences between referred pain and radiating pain?
100. Describe endogenous pain inhibiting mechanism Or Explain endogenous analgesia system.
101. What is meant by visceral pain? Briefly outline the pathway for visceral pain.
102. What are the characteristic features of deep pain or visceral pain?
103. Explain referred pain giving examples.
104. What is gate control theory of pain perception?
105. How is pricking pain and burning pain produced?
106. Mention ways by which pain sensation can be blocked.
107. Differentiate between substance P and Lewis P-factor.
108. What is the physiological basis of relief of itching sensation by scratching?
109. What is meant by muscle guarding?
110. What is the mechanism by which morphine produces analgesia?
111. What is stress analgesia?
112. What is allodynia?
113. What is the mechanism by which acupuncture relieves pain?
114. Give the functional classification of thalamic nuclei.
115. Enumerate the functions of thalamus.
116. Write a note on thalamic syndrome.
117. What is meant by thalamocortical system?

Motor System

1. What is the difference between lower motor neuron and upper motor neuron?
2. Differentiate between UMN and LMN lesion.
3. Mention the origin of pyramidal tract.
4. Describe the origin, course and termination of corticospinal tract.
5. Enumerate the functions of pyramidal tract.
6. What is the effect of lesion in the left internal capsule?
7. What are the effects of lesion of the pyramidal tract in the right internal capsule?
8. What is the role of corticospinal pathway in the control of posture and movement?
9. Write briefly on hemiplegia. What are the signs of upper motor neuron lesion?
10. What happens when there is damage to the lower motor neuron (LMN)?
11. What is the difference between contralateral hemiplegia and crossed hemiplegia?
12. Name the cranial nerves that do not originate from the brainstem.
13. Comment on facial palsy.
14. Differentiate between pyramidal tract and extra-pyramidal tract.
15. How can you produce a pure pyramidal tract lesion?
16. Name the conditions where hypertonia is present.
17. What is the difference between spasticity and rigidity?
18. What is the difference between lead pipe and cogwheel rigidity?
19. Give a few conditions which produce hypotonia.
20. What is the effect of complete transection of spinal cord at the mid-thoracic level?
21. What are the features of spinal shock?

22. What are the causes of spinal shock? What are the precautions to be taken during this stage?
23. Describe the neurological changes that are seen four weeks after complete transection of spinal cord at L1 level.
24. What is mass reflex?
25. What happens in stage of degeneration in spinal cord lesion?
26. What are the causes of bed sores in complete section of spinal cord?
27. What is the difference between hemiplegia, paraplegia and quadriplegia?
28. Write a note on Brown-Sequard syndrome?
29. Enumerate the complications of spinal cord transection.
30. Enumerate the effects below the level of lesion in Brown-Sequard syndrome. What are the causes of Brown-Sequard syndrome?
31. What is the effect of cutting posterior nerve root of spinal cord or what are the features of tabes dorsalis?
32. What is Argyll Robertson pupil?
33. Give the anatomical divisions of cerebellum.
34. What are the different parts of cerebellum based on its connections or what are the functional divisions of cerebellum?
35. Mention the phylogenetic divisions of cerebellum.
36. What are the parts of neocerebellum?
37. Write a note on deep cerebellar nuclei.
38. What are the afferent and efferent connections of cerebellum?
39. Name the fibers going through the different peduncles of cerebellum.
40. Explain the functions of cerebellum.
41. What is meant by damping action of cerebellum?
42. Describe the signs of cerebellar disease
43. Write a note on decomposition of movement.
44. Explain four tests to identify cerebellar lesion.
45. Name the parts of basal ganglia.
46. Explain the connections of basal ganglia.
47. Explain the effect of substantia nigra on corpus striatum.
48. Describe the functions of basal ganglia
49. What is Parkinson's disease? Mention the features of this disease giving the physiological basis.
50. What is the treatment for Parkinson's disease?
51. Mention four abnormal gaits, stating the diseases associated with them.
52. Name the diseases affecting basal ganglia and mention the cause of each.
53. What is the difference between chorea and athetosis?
54. What is Sydenham's chorea?
55. What is hemiballism?
56. Enumerate the sequence of events occurring in voluntary motor activity.
57. Write briefly on reticular formation.
58. What is ascending reticular activating system (ARAS)? Give its functions and clinical significance.
59. Name the neurotransmitters of reticular formation.
60. Write a note on reticulospinal tracts stating its functions.
61. Enumerate the functions of reticular formation in general.
62. What are the components of vestibular apparatus?
63. Which are the synergistic pairs of semicircular canals?
64. Write a note on crista ampullaris. Explain the mechanism of stimulation of vestibular afferent fibers.
65. What is the mechanism of stimulation of macula?
66. What is the mechanism of detection of linear and rotational acceleration?
67. Name the vestibular reflexes.
68. Describe the vestibular pathway.
69. Explain vestibulo-ocular reflex (VOR)
70. Write a short note on nystagmus.
71. Write briefly on motion sickness.
72. Define vertigo.
73. Enumerate the functions of vestibular apparatus.
74. Define posture.
75. What is the effect of section of midbrain at the mid-collicular level?
76. What is decerebrate rigidity? What is the cause of rigidity?
77. Explain the reflexes present in a decerebrate cat?
78. Name the postural reflexes.
79. Name the reflexes integrated at the level of spinal cord, medulla, midbrain and cerebral cortex.
80. Write a note on righting reflexes?
81. What is the difference between positive and negative supporting reaction?
82. What is cerebral dominance?
83. What are the functional asymmetries in the structurally symmetrical cerebral hemispheres? What is its significance?
84. Name the different layers in the cerebral cortex.
85. Mention the important functional areas in the frontal lobe giving their significance.
86. What is the importance of cortical Brodmann's area 3, 1 and 2?
87. What are the functions of prefrontal areas of brain? What are the effects of lesion to this area?
88. What are the effects of lesion of postcentral gyrus?
89. Enumerate the importance of temporal lobe.
90. Write a note on parietal cortex.
91. Describe cortical plasticity
92. What are the differences between decerebrate and decorticate preparations?
93. Explain the functions of hypothalamus.
94. What is the importance of satiety and feeding center?
95. What is the role of hypothalamus in water intake?
96. Name the areas of hypothalamus which control body temperature.

97. Write a note on circadian rhythm
98. What is sham rage?
99. Name the components of limbic system.
100. Describe the functions of limbic system
101. Explain Papez circuit and its importance
102. State the differences between muscarinic and nicotinic actions of acetylcholine.
103. Name the drugs that block acetylcholine receptors.
104. What are the functions of autonomic nervous system?
105. Mention the effects of parasympathetic stimulation.
106. Enumerate the effects of sympathetic stimulation.
107. What are the differences between sympathetic and parasympathetic divisions of ANS?
108. Name the adrenergic and cholinergic neurons of ANS.
109. Give examples of autonomic reflexes.
110. What is EEG? Mention the different waves in EEG and their causes.
111. What are the clinical uses of EEG?
112. What are the changes in EEG during different stages of sleep?
113. What is alpha block?
114. Compare NREM and REM sleep.
115. What is the cause for atonia in REM sleep?
116. What is the role of thalamus in producing EEG rhythm?
117. Name the neurotransmitters that induce wakeful state.
118. Give examples of sleep-inducing substances or somnogens.
119. What is sleep cycle?
120. Explain paradoxical sleep
121. What is meant by cataplexy?
122. What is hypnoeic myoclonia?
123. What is hypnoeic jerk?
124. What is the difference between coma and sleep?
125. What is the difference between persistent vegetative state and coma?
126. What is the physiological basis of epilepsy?
127. Name the type of epilepsy where non-convulsive attacks are seen.

Higher Functions of Brain

1. Which are the parts of cerebral cortex related to speech?
2. What are the connections and functions of Broca's area?
3. Explain the importance of Broca's area?
4. What is the importance of Wernicke's area?
5. Define and classify aphasias.
6. Explain Head's classification of aphasia
7. What is dysarthria?
8. What is anomia?
9. What is agnosia and prosopagnosia?
10. Write briefly on dyslexia
11. Define learning.
12. Define conditioned reflex. Give its important features.
13. What is the physiological basis of conditioned reflex?
14. What are the differences between unconditioned and conditioned reflexes?
15. Enumerate the importance of conditioned reflex.
16. Mention the conditions essential for the development of conditioned reflexes.
17. What is operant or instrumental conditioning?
18. What is conditioned avoidance reflex? What is its clinical significance?
19. What is meant by biofeedback?
20. What is discriminate conditioning?
21. Write a note on inter-cortical transfer of learning. What is split brain animal?
22. Define memory. What are the types of memory?
23. What are the mechanisms of short-term memory?
24. Explain the mechanisms of long-term memory
25. What is the difference between retrograde amnesia and anterograde amnesia?
26. What is déjà vu phenomenon?
27. What is meant by dementia?
28. Write a note on Alzheimer's disease.
29. What is the physiological basis of depression and mania?
30. Mention the beneficial effects of meditation in the body.
31. What is the normal CSF pressure? Give the normal composition of CSF.
32. Explain the mechanism of formation, circulation and drainage of CSF.
33. What are the functions of CSF?
34. Describe Monro-Kellie doctrine and its significance
35. What is contre-coup injury?
36. Write short note on choroid plexus.
37. Write a note on hydrocephalus
38. Describe lumbar puncture or spinal tap. Mention its uses.
39. What is blood-brain barrier? What is its significance?
40. Explain circumventricular organs?

GIVE THE PHYSIOLOGICAL BASIS

1. Sensory receptors are referred to as biological transducers.
2. Strychnine poisoning produces spasm of skeletal muscles or convulsions.
3. Phenomenon of phantom limb in amputated individuals.
4. Tactile localization and discrimination are precise in the lips and fingertips.
5. Precise localization is possible for fine touch sensation but not for crude touch.
6. Lumbar and sacral spinal nerves have long roots.
7. Lumbar puncture is done below the level of L1 vertebra.
8. Wounded soldiers in the battlefield and accident victims often feel no pain at the time of accident.

9. Rubbing an injured area reduces pain. Or acupuncture reduces pain.
10. Pain perception is possible even if cortex is removed.
11. Prefrontal lobotomy or leucotomy is done in untreatable cases of pain.
12. In myocardial infarction pain is felt along the medial aspect of left arm.
13. Pain in angina pectoris.
14. Visceral pain is poorly localized.
15. Antidromic impulses transmitted through the axon stops in the soma of most of the neurons.
16. Cessation of fits during an epileptic attack without treatment.
17. Positive Babinski sign occurs in pyramidal tract lesion.
18. Babinski sign is positive in infants.
19. When a muscle is overstretched, it relaxes.
20. Clasp knife phenomenon occurs in pyramidal tract lesion.
21. Cerebellar lesion produces motor effects on the same (ipsilateral) side of the body.
22. Tremor occurs in cerebellar disease OR Nystagmus is seen in cerebellar disease.
23. Pendular knee jerk is seen in cerebellar lesion.
24. Execution of speech is lost in lesion of frontal lobe in the dominant (categorical) hemisphere.
25. L-dopa is given instead of dopamine to treat Parkinson's disease.
26. Along with L-dopa, carbidopa is used to treat Parkinson's disease.
27. Rigidity occurs in basal ganglia lesion.
28. Stimulation of gamma efferent system causes reflex contraction of muscle.
29. Atonia is associated with REM sleep.
30. REM sleep is called paradoxical sleep.
31. Lesion of the ventromedial nucleus of hypothalamus causes hyperphagia.
32. Unilateral supranuclear lesions of V, VIII, X and XII cranial nerves do not produce much impairment of functions.
33. Supranuclear lesion of VII cranial nerve nucleus causes paralysis of only the lower part of the face.

IMPORTANT DIAGRAMS

1. Pain pathway from the right upper limb
2. Structure of a chemical synapse
3. Reflex arc
4. Muscle spindle
5. Pathway for stretch reflex
6. Inverse stretch reflex
7. Diagrammatically represent a bi-synaptic reflex to show reciprocal innervation
8. Section of spinal cord at the thoracic level showing different nuclei in grey matter
9. Draw a section of spinal cord showing the descending tracts
10. Ascending tracts in spinal cord
11. Pyramidal pathway
12. Thalamic nuclei
13. Fine touch pathway
14. Crude touch pathway
15. Pathway for touch and pain sensation from face
16. Connections of basal ganglia
17. Motor and sensory homunculus
18. Structure of cerebellar cortex
19. Double crossing in cerebellar connection
20. Crista ampullaris
21. Important functional areas in cerebral cortex

SECTION 11: SPECIAL SENSES—VISION

REVIEW QUESTIONS

1. Mention the various parts of the eyeball and list the functions of each.
2. Tabulate the extraocular muscles, their actions and innervation.
3. Distinguish between rods and cones.
4. What is the importance of coordination of eye movements? How is it achieved?
5. What are the effects of section of III cranial nerve?
6. What is meant by blind spot and fovea centralis? Give their significance.
7. Describe the formation, circulation, drainage and functions of aqueous humor.
8. Enumerate the functions of tears.
9. What are the causes of corneal transparency?
10. What is meant by miosis, mydriasis and anisocoria?
11. What are scotomas?
12. What is the importance of ophthalmoscopic examination?
13. What is the normal intraocular pressure? How is it measured? What is its significance?
14. What is glaucoma?
15. Name the extraocular muscles and mention their innervation.
16. Name the interphases for refraction of light in the eye.
17. What is meant by refractive index of a medium?
18. Mention the range of visible spectrum
19. What is meant by power of a lens?
20. What is a diopter?
21. What is the normal refractive power of the eye? What is the concept of reduced eye of Listing?
22. How can you compare the eye to a camera?

Important Questions

23. Explain the process by which light rays are brought to a focus on the retina.
24. What is accommodation in the eye? What is the mechanism of accommodation?
25. What is near response? Trace the pathway for near response.
26. Mention the mechanisms by which anterior curvature of lens is increased in accommodation.
27. What are the errors of refraction? How can it be corrected?
28. What is meant by near point and far point?
29. What is meant by amplitude of accommodation?
30. What is presbyopia? How can it be corrected?
31. What are the optical aberrations?
32. What are Purkinje-Sanson images? What do they demonstrate?
33. Write a note on cataract
34. Describe visual acuity
35. Name the factors that affect visual acuity
36. What is meant by field of vision? Why is it not circular? What are the limits of field of vision in different meridians?
37. What is perimetry? What is the significance of blind spot?
38. What is binocular vision?
39. What are the advantages of binocular vision?
40. What is meant by corresponding retinal points?
41. What is strabismus?
42. What is duplicity theory of vision?
43. Draw the flow chart showing rhodopsin-retinene cycle.
44. Describe the photochemistry of vision.
45. Discuss the visual processing and image formation in the retina.
46. What is Purkinje shift or Purkinje phenomenon?
47. What is the effect of vitamin-A deficiency in the eye?
48. Define and explain dark adaptation.
49. Explain the mechanism of light adaptation
50. Name the layers of retina
51. What are the functions of bipolar, horizontal, amacrine and ganglion cells in retina?
52. Explain lateral inhibition in the eye.
53. Describe the visual pathway from rods and cones to the visual cortex. Write a note on the lesions of the pathway.
54. What is the difference between homonymous and heteronymous hemianopia?
55. Trace the pathway for pupillary light reflex. Write a note on the lesions of the pupillary reflex pathway.
56. Explain the effect of lesions in the visual pathway at various levels, in a tabular column.
57. What is Argyll-Robertson pupil? Name the site of lesion producing it.
58. Which are the cortical areas concerned with vision?
59. What is meant by macular sparing?
60. What is the role of superior colliculi in vision?
61. What is meant by stereopsis?
62. Explain the function of melanopsin
63. Name the primary colors. What is meant by complementary color?
64. What are the theories of color vision? Explain briefly trichromatic theory of color vision. Describe the neural mechanism of color vision.
65. What are blobs in the visual cortex?
66. Write a note on color blindness. Mention the most common type.
67. What is the peculiarity of inheritance of color blindness?
68. What are the tests for detecting color blindness?
69. What is critical fusion frequency in vision?
70. What are the four types of eye movements? Mention their functions.

GIVE THE PHYSIOLOGICAL BASIS

1. Cones are not activated in dim light
2. Rods of retina are very effective in dim light.
3. Aircraft pilots wear red goggles in bright light.
4. A person entering a dark room from a bright area, experiences difficulty in seeing objects immediately but can see clearly after some time.
5. For sharp image, decreased size of pupil is necessary.
6. Blindness occurs in long standing raised intraocular pressure.
7. Retinal detachment leads to blindness.
8. Change in curvature of the lens occurs during near response.
9. Macular sparing is seen in lesions of occipital cortex.
10. Ophthalmoscopic examination is useful in detecting vascular complications associated with diabetes mellitus, hypertension etc.
11. Bitemporal hemianopia occurs in pituitary tumors.
12. When light is thrown into one eye, the pupil of the opposite eye constricts.
13. Three primary colors are responsible for the perception of a variety of colors.
14. Presbyopia occurs in normal individuals as age advances, usually after the age of 40 years.
15. Field of vision is not circular in humans.
16. Examination of visual field is important in pituitary tumors.

IMPORTANT DIAGRAMS

1. Longitudinal section of eyeball
2. Draw diagram to show image formation in hypermetropia, myopia and astigmatism. Show their corrections also.
3. Structure of rods and cones
4. Dark adaptation curve
5. Visual pathway
6. Pupillary light reflex pathway

SECTION 11: SPECIAL SENSES—AUDITION

REVIEW QUESTIONS

1. Define sound. What is the velocity of sound in air?
2. What are the properties of sound?
3. What does 0 decibel mean?
4. Define pitch of sound. What is meant by ultrasonic and infrasonic sound?
5. What is the difference between pure tone, complex tone, music and noise?
6. What is meant by quality or timbre of a sound?
7. What are the contents of middle ear?
8. Enumerate the functions of tympanic membrane
9. What is the lever mechanism operating in the ear? Give its significance. Or, describe the functions of middle ear ossicles.
10. What are the functions of middle ear muscles? Or What is tympanic reflex
11. What is the function of eustachian tube? Mention its clinical importance.
12. Describe the functions of middle ear
13. Write briefly on tympanic reflex or attenuation reflex.
14. Write a note on basilar membrane and organ of Corti.
15. Explain traveling wave theory.
16. What are the effects of displacement of basilar membrane? Or how is action potential generated in the auditory nerve?
17. Write briefly on endolymphatic or endocochlear potential
18. What is the significance of the resting potential of the hair cells of the organ of Corti?
19. Explain the auditory pathway.
20. Name the descending auditory pathways or the efferent fibers in the auditory nerve. Mention its importance.
21. Mention the special features of auditory pathway.
22. Name the center for auditory reflexes.
23. Explain the physiology of hearing.
24. Mention the uses of auditory evoked responses.
25. Write a note on cochlear microphonics.
26. What is the effect of constant exposure of the ear to a particular frequency of sound?
27. Write a note on masking related to hearing.
28. What are the types of hearing impairment?
29. What are the causes of conduction deafness? Give its features.
30. Give the causes of nerve deafness. What are its features?
31. Describe the tests to distinguish between nerve deafness and conduction deafness?
32. Write a note on audiometry.
33. What are the advantages of audiometry?

GIVE THE PHYSIOLOGICAL BASIS

1. Loud sounds do not normally damage the ear drum.
2. A bomb explosion in the vicinity can lead to deafness.
3. Obstruction to the auditory tube produces pain in the ear.
4. A person is able to locate the source of sound.
5. Appreciation of intensity of sound is possible.
6. Sound is amplified in the middle ear.
7. Deafness is not caused by unilateral auditory cortex lesions.
8. Sound appears louder in diseased ear when Weber's test is performed in conduction deafness.

IMPORTANT DIAGRAMS

1. Parts of middle ear.
2. Structure of organ of Corti.
3. Auditory pathway.
4. Audiogram showing conduction deafness and nerve deafness.

SECTION 11: SPECIAL SENSES—OLFACTION AND TASTE

REVIEW QUESTIONS

1. What are the similarities between sense of smell and taste?
2. What is the importance of chemical senses in humans?
3. Describe olfactory epithelium.
4. What are the unique features of olfaction?
5. Describe the olfactory pathway.
6. What is the mechanism of olfactory discrimination?
7. Comment on the processing of olfactory information in the brain.
8. How can olfactory pathways be inhibited?
9. What is the role of pain fibers in the olfactory epithelium?
10. Write a note on vomeronasal organ. What are pheromones?
11. Describe olfactory adaptation?
12. What is the importance of sniffing?
13. Write a note on the abnormalities of odor detection.
14. What is meant by flavor of a substance?
15. Describe the structure and innervation of taste bud.
16. Mention the nerve supply of tongue which carries the general sensations and taste sensations from the tongue.
17. Explain the taste pathway with the help of a diagram. Or how is taste information conveyed from the tongue to the brain?

18. What are the basic taste modalities or primary taste sensations?
19. What is the relation between chemical nature of a substance and the basic taste sensations? Name the receptors involved.
20. What is the importance of bitter taste?
21. Which is the standard reference substance for sweetness?
22. Name a taste-modifying protein. Why is it called so?
23. Enumerate the factors influencing taste sensation.
24. What are the abnormalities of taste sensation?

IMPORTANT DIAGRAMS

1. Structure of taste bud
2. Taste pathway
3. Olfactory pathway

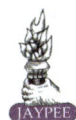

TOP DOC BANE WOHI JISKA GUIDE HO SAHI | **diginerve** — A Jaypee Initiative

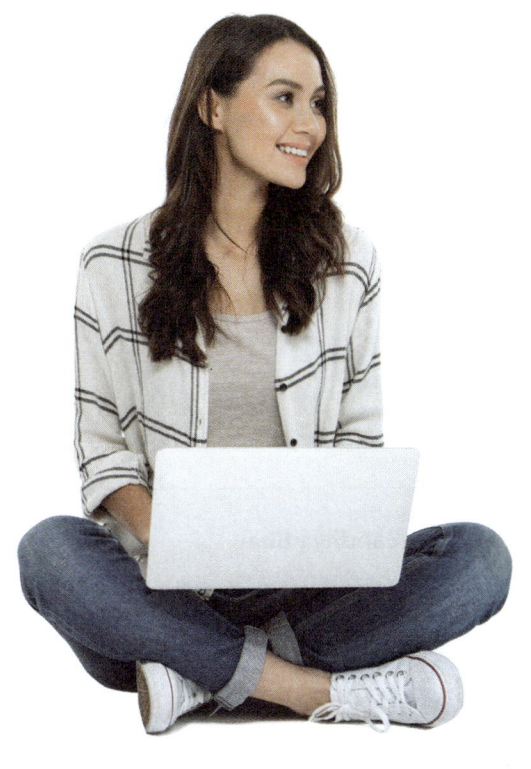

YOUR GUIDE AT EVERY STEP

Expert Knowledge Anytime, Anywhere

SCAN QR CODE FOR MORE DETAILS

WHY CHOOSE US

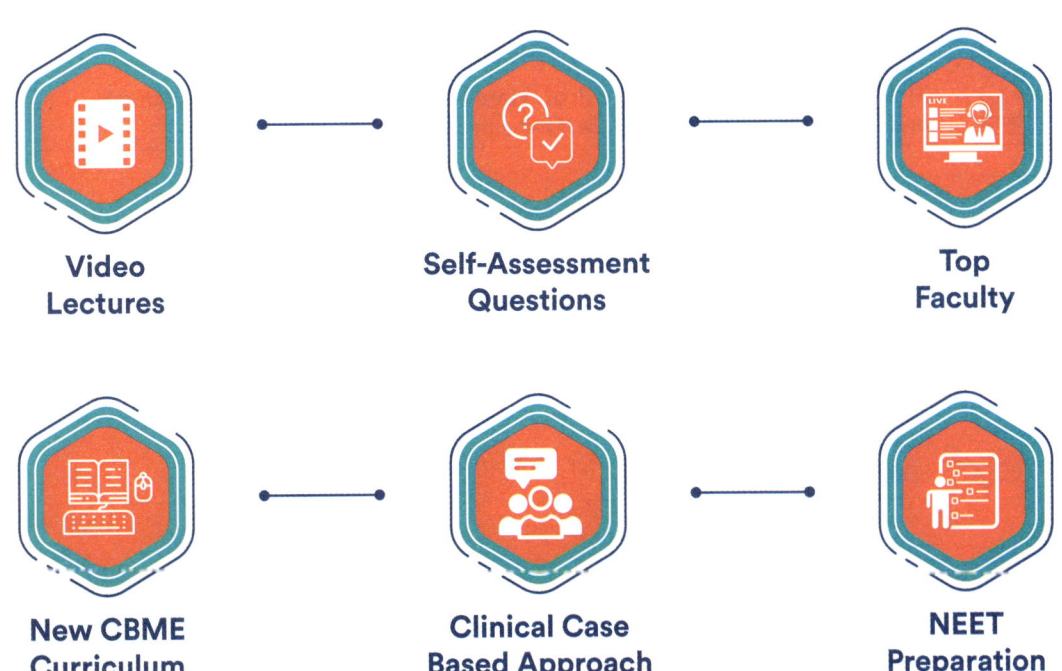

- Video Lectures
- Self-Assessment Questions
- Top Faculty
- New CBME Curriculum
- Clinical Case Based Approach
- NEET Preparation

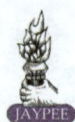
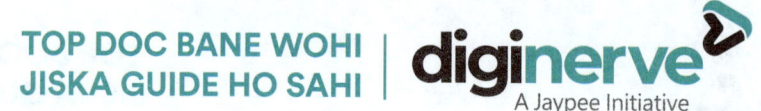

TOP DOC BANE WOHI | JISKA GUIDE HO SAHI

Video Lectures | Notes | Self-Assessment
UnderGrad Courses Available

Community Medicine for UnderGrads — by Dr. Bratati Banerjee

Forensic Medicine & Toxicology for UnderGrads — by Dr. Gautam Biswas

Medicine for UnderGrads — by Dr. Archith Boloor

Microbiology for UnderGrads — by Dr. Apurba S Sastry, Dr. Sandhya Bhat & Dr. Deepashree R

OBGYN for UnderGrads — by Dr. K. Srinivas

Ophthalmology for UnderGrads — by Dr. Parul Ichhpujani & Dr. Talvir Sidhu

Orthopaedics for UnderGrads — by Dr. Vivek Pandey

Pathology for UnderGrads — by Prof. Harsh Mohan, Prof. Ramadas Nayak & Dr. Debasis Gochhait

Pediatrics for UnderGrads — by Dr. Santosh Soans & Dr. Soundarya M

Pharmacology for UnderGrads — by Dr. Sandeep Kaushal & Dr. Nirmal George

Surgery for UnderGrads — by Dr. Sriram Bhat M (SRB)

Download the App.

*T&C Apply

Contact:
+91 8800 418 418
marketing@diginerve.com

Index

Page numbers followed by *f* refer to figure, *fc* refer to flowchart, and *t* refer to table.

A

A wave, causes of 283
Abdomen 865
  hypophysis of 451
Abducens nerve 907
  lesion of 907
ABO
  blood group system 186, 187*f*, 188*t*, 190, 191, 191*t*
  incompatibility 196
  system, inheritance of 186
Abortion 718
Absorption, disturbances of 471
Accommodation reflex 911*f*
  pathway for 910, 911*fc*
Accoucher's hand 613, 613*f*
Acetic acid 411
Acetone-free methyl alcohol 131
Acetylcholine 17, 79, 82, 245, 250, 268, 296, 318, 408, 411, 420, 427, 428, 428*f*, 447, 465, 556, 656, 658, 743, 784, 817-819, 855, 866, 867, 876-878
  degradation of 658
  esterase 80
  receptors 80
  release of 867
  synthesis of 658
Achalasia cardia 431, 431*f*, 461, 461*f*
Achilles reflex time 599
Aching pain 781, 784
Achlorhydria 426
Acholic stools 456
Achondroplasia 574
Achromatopsia 935, 936
Acid 1
  citrate dextrose 194, 360
  peptic disease, surgical management of 434
  phosphatase 19, 132, 609
  secretion 427, 428
    inhibition of 434
  sources of 510
Acid-base
  balance 99, 103, 314, 483
  disorders 2
  disturbances 3, 512
Acid-citrate dextrose 172
Acidic gastric 433*f*
Acidic substances 418
Acidophils 567
Acidosis 2*t*, 248, 257, 373, 510, 513, 742
  causes of 373*t*, 510*t*, 513
Acid-pepsin mixture 432
Acid-resistant trefoil peptides 425
Acid-sensing ion channel 781
Acini 413, 591
  microscopic structure of 414*f*
Acoustic neuroepithelium 948

Acoustic neuroma 726
Acoustic reflex 945, 946
Acquired immune system, development of 148*f*
Acquired immunity 150
  characteristics of 150
  types of 150
Acquired immunodeficiency syndrome 40, 137, 157
Acromegalic facies 571
Acromegaly 572*f*
Acromicria 573
Acrosin 697, 701
Acrosomal cap 675
Acrosomal reaction 701
Acrosome 675
Actin-based molecular motors 18
Activated partial thromboplastin time 171, 173
Actomyosin 160
Adaptation 764
  mechanism of 764
  stage of 871
Addison's disease 627, 631, 632
Addisonian crisis 274, 632
Addisonian pernicious anemia 124
Adenocorticotrophic hormone 556
Adenomatous goiter, simple 600
Adenosine 296, 297
  concentrations of 876
  diphosphate 74, 557
  monophosphate 74
  triphosphate 73, 194, 313, 555, 557, 626, 781, 980
Adenylyl cyclase 428, 507, 555, 612, 626
Adenylyl cyclase-cAMP system 557
Adequate adrenocorticotropic hormone 621
Adequate stimulus 762
Adiadochokinesis 832
Adiponectin 648, 858
Adipose tissue 549
  brown 535, 978
Adiposogenital syndrome 680
Adrenal androgens 631
  actions of 631
  secretion of 631
Adrenal cortex 621, 621*t*, 628*fc*
  enlargement of 871
  hormone of 621
  hypofunctioning of 631
Adrenal cortical hormones, synthesis of 621, 622*fc*
Adrenal crisis 632
Adrenal gland 620, 620*f*
  functional anatomy of 620
  innervation of 621
Adrenal insufficiency 631, 632
Adrenal medulla 621, 621*t*, 632, 636, 867

chromaffin cell of 633*f*
  hormone of 632
  innervation of 621*f*
  regulation of secretion of 636
Adrenaline 448, 621*f*, 635*t*
  apnea 370
Adrenarche 631, 670
Adrenergic agonists 634
  uses of 634
Adrenergic receptors 634*t*, 868
Adrenergic transmission 867
Adrenocortical steroids 121
Adrenocorticotropic hormone 121, 410, 531, 557, 562, 566, 567, 578, 588, 626, 628, 648
Adrenogenital syndrome 631
Adrenoleukodystrophy, neonatal 20
Adult respiratory distress syndrome 274, 326
Adventitia 407
Aerobic glycolysis 74, 396
Aerobic system 74
Aerophagia 462
Aerosols 314
Afibrinogenemia 173
Agammaglobulinemia 104
Aganglionic megacolon 466, 467
A-gene 187
Ageusia 968
Agglutination 146, 189, 196
Agglutinins 188
Agglutinogens 186
Agranular chromophobes 567
Agranulocytes 131, 133
Agranulocytosis 138
Agraphesthesia 778
Agraphia 889
Air
  conditioning function 313
  conduction 952
Airway
  cartilage-free 316
  divisions of 316*f*
  resistance 334
  respiratory function of 314
  temperature, lowers 317
Akinesia 820
Alarm reaction 871
Albinism 531, 578
Albumin 102, 622, 679
Albumin-globulin ratio 104
Albuminuria 495, 513
Alcohol dehydrogenase 922
Alcoholism 441
Aldosterone 184, 456, 473, 501, 506, 516, 621, 628
  deficiency of 631
  escape 628
  mechanism of action of 629
  regulation of secretion of 629, 629*fc*

  secretion 630
  sensitive sodium transporters 473
  synthase 622, 628
  synthesis of 628*fc*
Alexia 888
Algal polysaccharides 456
Alimentary canal, functional anatomy of 406
Alimentary system 597
Alkaline
  fluid 677
  medium 678
  mucus 452
  phosphatase 132, 439, 608
Alkalosis 2*t*, 374, 613, 742
  causes of 373*t*
Allergen 157
Allergy 157
Allocortex 849, 850, 860
Allodynia 790
Allopurinol 503
All-*trans*-retinol 922
Alpha-agglutinin 188
Alpha-block 874*f*
Alpha-cells 477
Alpha-motor neuron 753*t*
Alpha-receptor blockers, uses of 634
Alpha-waves 873*f*
Alveolar air 344, 351, 351*f*, 352
Alveolar capillary
  diffusion block 378
  membrane 353
Alveolar dead space 336, 349
Alveolar epithelial cells 325
Alveolar epithelium 317
Alveolar sacs 316
Alveolar stability 326, 327
Alveolar ventilation 335, 336
Alveolar vessels 347
Alveoli 316, 317
  dry 326, 327, 344
Alzheimer's disease 20, 22, 419, 886, 979, 981
Amelognosia 797
Amenorrhea 694, 695
  galactorrhea syndrome 578
  primary 668, 671, 695
  secondary 695
Ametropia 912
Amine precursor uptake and decarboxylation cell 318, 423, 424, 477
Amino acid 430, 469, 644, 650, 677
  absorption of 471
  decarboxylase 477
  essential 469
  reabsorption of 503
  transmitters 743
Amino peptidases, actions of 471
Amnesia 886
  retrograde 875, 886

Amniocentesis 669, 706
    advantages of 706
Amoeboid movement 134
Amorphosynthesis 775
A-motor neurons 748
Amphetamine 857, 886
Ampulla 673, 838
Amygdala 429, 972
    bilateral lesion of 862
Amygdaloid nucleus 860
    stimulation of 862
Amylase 414, 416
Amylopectin 469
Amylose 469
Amyotrophic lateral sclerosis 135, 805
Anabolic functions 20
Anabolic hormone 569, 595
Anabolic nervous system 869
Anacrotic limb 281
Anaerobic glycolysis 74, 272, 396
Anaerobic metabolism 74
Anal canal 304, 455
Anal sphincter
    external 466
    internal 466
Analgesia 790
    stress-induced 788
    system, activation of 789
Analgesics 790
Anaphylaxis 137
    eosinophil chemotactic factor of 132
Anarthria 888
Anasarca 181
Anatomical dead space 316, 336, 337f
Anaxonic neuron 45
Androgen 121, 574, 676, 686
    binding protein 676
    resistance 670, 713
    secrete small amounts of 685
    source of 678
    synthesis of 679fc
Andropause 696
Androstenedione 678
Androsterone 679
Anemia 111, 122, 122f, 123, 193, 474
    destructive 125
    etiological classification of 122, 123fc
    mild 122
    moderate 122
    severe 122, 122f
    signs of 122
    symptoms of 122
Anemic hypoxia 372, 378, 381
Anesthesia 777
    dissociated 778, 812
    general 401
Anesthetic accidents 398
Aneurysmal murmur 232
Angina pectoris 297
Angioblasts 261
Angiogenesis 261, 576
Angiogram 298f
Angiography 852
Angioneurotic edema 181
Angiotensin 296
    converting enzyme 299, 314, 344, 497, 498, 501, 630, 655
    receptor 277
    sources of 515
Angiotensinase 655
Angiotensinogen 515
Anhydrosis 932

Anion gap 513
    concept of 513f
Anisocoria 903
Anisocytosis 106
Anisometropia 913
Anisopoikilocytosis 106f
Ankle
    clonus 755
    jerk 752
Ankyrin 107
Annexins 171
Annuli fibrosi 203
Annulospiral nerve endings 749
Anomalous trichromats 935
Anomic aphasia 888, 889
Anopia 916, 936
Anosmia 974
Anovulatory cycle 694
Ansa lenticularis 816
Anterograde amnesia 886
Anterolateral system 771
Antiallergic action 625
Anti-androgens 695
Antibody 153, 188, 550, 602, 907
    classes of 154
    complete 192
    functions of 155
    incomplete 192
    mechanism of action of 155
    titer 155
    warm 155
Anticholine esterases 81
Anticholinergic agents 434
Anticoagulant
    natural 172
    protein C 162
Anti-D serum 192
Antidepressants 884
Antidiuresis 506
Antidiuretic action 583
Antidiuretic hormone 184, 497, 498, 556, 562, 567, 582, 583, 857
    secretion 508t
    regulation of 583
Antidromic conduction 56
Antiemetic drugs 844
Anti-estrogenic action 692
Antigen 147
    antibody complex 146, 153
    hidden 157
    recognition 150
Antiglobulin test 192
Antigravity muscle 752, 836
    tone 845
Anti-H antibodies 188
Anti-H serum 188
Antihuman globulin reagent 192
Antihypertensive drug 379
Anti-inflammatory
    action 625
    drugs 429
Anti-insulin 623
    hormone 649
Antimullerian hormone 666, 667, 676, 677fc
Antioxidant 299, 589, 981
Antipernicious factor 121
Antiplasmin 162
Antiport 40, 427, 499
Anti-Rh gamma globulin 192
Antiseptic action 446
Antithrombin 170, 172
Antithyroid
    drugs 606
    peroxidase 599

Antitrypsin 328
Antitumor 589
Antral follicle 687
Antral systole 463
Antrum 687
Anuria 272, 513
Anus 455
Aorta 262
    abdominal 865
    maximum pressures in 229t
Aortic arch baroreceptors 246
Aortic area 231
Aortic body 371, 371f, 372t
Aortic component 231
Aortic impedance 255, 256
Aortic pressure changes 229
Aortic stenosis 295
Aphakic eye 906, 914
Aphasia 888
    classification of 888
    non-fluent 888, 889
Apnea 321, 373, 375, 982
    deglutition 370, 461
    irregular periods of 376
    test 982
Apneusis 321, 367
Apneustic center 367
Apocrine gland 411, 530, 530t
Apoferritin 116
Apoptosis 29, 156
    antigen 157
    mechanism of 29
    significance of 29
Apoptotic bodies 29
Appearance time 254
Appetite juice 429
Apraxia 889
Aptyalism, permanent cessation of 419
Aquaporins 34, 505, 507, 583
Aqueous humor 904
    functions of 905
Arachidonic acid 558, 657
Arachnoid 891
    granulations 893
    villi 893
Archicerebellum 826
Arcuate arteries 488
Arcuate fasciculus 888
Arcuate fibers, internal 771, 773
Areflexia 810
Arginine 644, 650, 744
    vasopressin 184, 509, 582
Argyll Robertson pupil 813, 931
Arm lift-back pressure method 399
Aromatherapy 871
Aromatic L-amino acid decarboxylase 633
Arrector pili 529
Arrhenoblastoma 678
Arrhythmia 217
    ventricular 218
Arsenic 473
Arterial blood 351f, 361
    pressure 261, 263, 271, 864
        determinants of 266
        measurement of 264
Arterial pressure 285, 301, 491
Arterial pulse 281, 283t
    abnormalities of 282, 282f
    recording of 281
    tracing 282f
Arteriole
    afferent 485, 489
    efferent 485, 489

Arterioles 262, 290
Arterioluminal vessels 294
Arteriosinusoidal vessels 294
Arteriovenous anastomotic channels 263
Arteriovenous fistula 514
Artery
    basilar 299, 689
    brachial 264
    celiac 303
    facial 415
    functions of 261
    interlobar 488
    posterior descending 294
    pulmonary 345t
    segmental 488
    spiral 689
    straight 689
    subclavian 281
    sublingual 415
    umbilical 305
Artificial respiration 398
    method of 398
    principles of 380
    prolonged application of 398
Aryl sulfatase 132
Arylalkylamine-N-acetyltransferase 588
Asana 879
Ascending reticular activating system 740, 773, 783, 784, 796, 835, 836, 836f, 851, 852, 869, 876
    functions of 836
Ascorbic acid 677, 904
Asexual reproduction 663
Asparagine 24
Aspartate aminotransferase 448
Asphyxia 377
    stages of 377
Aspirin 424, 429, 657, 790
Assisted reproductive technology, type of 717
Astereognosis 768, 778, 796
Asthenia 831
Astigmatism 913, 913f
Astrocytes 725
    functions of 725
Astrocytoma 726
Asynchronous muscle contraction 75
Ataxia 831, 870
Atelectasis 338
Atherosclerosis 327, 647
Athetosis 820
Atmospheric air 352
Atonic bladder 521
Atrial arrhythmia 217
    consequences of 218
Atrial baroreceptors 248
Atrial branch 294
Atrial contraction 231, 256
Atrial depolarization 213
Atrial diastole 224, 226
Atrial extrasystole 218
Atrial fibrillation 218, 218f
Atrial flutter 218, 218f
Atrial gallop 231
Atrial natriuretic peptide 184, 185, 497, 502, 516, 549, 554, 558, 628, 656
Atrial pressure changes 227
Atrial repolarization 214
Atrial septal defect 232, 255, 978
Atrial syncytium 205
Atrial systole 224, 225, 228, 229, 295

Index

Atrial tachycardia 217, 218
Atrial volume changes 229
Atrioventricular bundle 205
Atrioventricular node 205
Atrioventricular valve 204, 204f, 225, 230
Atrophy 758
Atropine 448, 658, 867
Audibility curve 959, 959f
Audiogram 959, 960, 960f
Audiometric tests 959
Audiometry 959
Audition, physiology of 949
Auditory agnosia 888
Auditory canal, external 531, 943
Auditory cortex 951, 955
   primary 954
Auditory hallucinations 957
Auditory meatus, external 943
Auditory pathway 954, 955f, 955fc
   descending 956
Auditory tube 944, 945
   functions of 945
Auerbach's plexus 407, 408, 430
Augmented unipolar limb leads 211
Aura 974
Auricular artery, posterior 415
Auriculotemporal branch 415
Auroscope 943
Auscultatory gap 264
Auscultatory method 264
Autocrine secretion 547, 547f
Auto-digestion 441
Autoimmune 604
   disease 82, 151, 157
   disorder 104, 957
   hemolytic anemia 157
Autoimmunization, prevention of 155
Autologous transfusion 195
Autolysis 19
Automatic bladder 521
Automatic pharyngeal muscle 460
Automatic spinal reflex 520
Autonomic activities, regulation of 856
Autonomic disturbances 858
Autonomic effector organs 864
Autonomic efferent 864
   pathways 722t
Autonomic function 853
   control of 861
Autonomic nervous system 245, 318, 407, 409, 548, 722, 748, 786, 798, 835, 856, 863, 866, 869
   disorders of 870
   divisions of 722fc
   functions of 869
   parasympathetic divisions of 866f
   sympathetic division of 865f, 866f
Autonomous bladder 521
Autophagosomes 119
Autophagy 19
Autosomal inheritance 22
Autosomes 665
   nonisjunction of 669
Avian influenza 145
Axial velocity 235
Axo-axonal synapse 738
Axon 46
   hillock 46
   reflex 268, 293, 748, 748f
Axonotmesis 58
Azotemia 504, 513

Azur granules 133
Azurophilic granule 132

B

Bachmann's bundle 206
Bacteria, overgrowth of 456
Bacteruria 514
Bainbridge reflex 249, 249fc
Ballism 820
Barany chair 843f
Barany test 843
Barometric pressure 386, 388, 390
   effects of 386
Baroreceptor 246, 369, 370, 509
   afferents 268
   location of 246
   mechanism of action of 247
   reflex 246f, 247, 269, 271, 274, 289
      mechanism 247fc
   stimulation inhibits 372
   structure and innervation of 246
   ventricular 248
Barotrauma 390
Barr body 132, 666, 666f
Barrel shaped chest 388
Bartholin ducts 413
Bartter's syndrome 37
Basal forebrain sleep zone 877
Basal ganglia 815, 816f, 818fc, 888
   connections of 816, 819, 819fc
   functions of 820
   lesion of 820
   parts of 818
   role of 820
Basal lamina 46, 47
Basal metabolic rate 396, 534, 595, 635
Basal metabolism 595
Basal nuclei 815
Basal secretion 418
Basement membrane 486
Basic electrical rhythm 411, 411f, 462, 464
Basilar membrane 947, 948, 953f
   displacement of 951, 951f
Basopenia 137
Basophilia 137
Basophilic normoblast 118
Basophils 132, 133f, 135, 137, 146, 567
   functions of 135
Bathmotropic effect, positive 244
Bathorhodopsin 921
B-dystroglycan 66
Beatty's protein 107
Becker muscular dystrophy 76
Bed sores 811
Bed wetting 878
Behavior, motivation of 862
Behavioral thermoregulation 537
Belching 462
Bell's palsy 419, 807
Bell-Magendie law 268, 727
Bence-Jones proteins 104
Beri-beri 778
Bernoulli's principle 235
Bertin column 484
Beta-blockers, uses of 634
Beta-chains, synthesis of 112
Beta-glucuronidase 132
Betamethasone 632
Beta-waves 873
Bezold-Jarisch reflex 249, 269, 273
Bicuspid valve 204
Big-big gastrin 430

Biguanides 647
Bile 444
   acidification of 448
   canaliculi 443f
   concentrations of 447
   pigment 446
   secretion of 469
   storage of 447
Bile acids
   primary 445
   secondary 445
Bile duct 444f, 786
   common 444
Bile salt 439, 445, 446
   act 446
   activated lipase 472
   enterohepatic circulation of 445
   formation of 445fc
   functions of 445
   secondary 445
Biliary canaliculi 444
Biliary secretion, regulation of 447
Biliary system 443, 444, 448
Bilirubin 114f, 446
   conjugated 114, 446
   diglucuronide 114, 446
   fate of 115f
Biliverdin 446
Binasal hemianopia 930
Binocular vision 916, 917f
   advantages of 917
Bioassay 549
Biochemical liver function tests 448
Biochemical methods 548
Bioelectrical potentials 48
Biogenic amine transmitters 743
Biological anticoagulants 172
Biological clock 858, 874
Biological hemolysins 110
Biological tests 705
Biopsy 434
Biosynthesis 633, 692
Biot's breathing 375, 376
Biot's respiration 376f
Bipolar cell 926, 927
   center 927f
   types of 926
Bipolar leads 210, 211
Bipolar neuron 45, 969, 970
Bird beak appearance 431f, 461f
Bisferiens pulse 283
Bisphosphoglycerate 359
Bisphosphonates 616
Bisynaptic reflex 753, 754f
Bitemporal hemianopia 570, 916, 930
Bladder
   function, abnormalities of 521
   innervation of 519, 520f
   neck 519
   sensations 773
   trigone 519
Blastocyst 702
   implantation of 702f
Bleaching 921
Bleeding disorders 172
Bleeding time 171
Blind spot 903, 916
Blindness 380
Blood 99, 201, 625
   anticoagulant function of 314
   banks 194
   brain barrier 191, 540, 587, 676, 857, 895

cell
   agglutination of 189f
   growth factors 577
cholesterol, reduction in 596
clotting 165
coagulation 13, 103, 162, 165, 168f, 562
collection of 193
colloidal osmotic pressure 495
composition of 100, 100fc
examination 123, 525
filtration of 314
functions of 99
indices 113
islands 261
lactate, normal 397
normal viscosity of 103
occurs, pulsatile flow of 347
oxygen tension 399
physical properties of 100
picture 122, 124
prevent coagulation of 169t
reservoir 531
storage of 193, 360
stream enters cells 396
substitutes 195
testis barrier 157, 676
tests 173
type B 186
viscosity of 109, 238, 266
Blood flow 295f, 301, 346f, 409, 433, 983
   counter current 303
   direction of 202f
   distribution of 349
   measuring 235
   turbulence of 236
   velocity of 234t, 236f, 238
Blood glucose 623fc, 650, 874
   control of 650
   level 644, 650t
Blood group 186, 189
   antigens 186
      structure of 188f
   parents 190, 190t
   proper 193
   substances 426
Blood loss 195
   prevention of 99
Blood pressure 99, 234, 236, 247fc, 271, 271fc, 483, 658, 861, 879, 980, 983
   classification of 265t
   diastolic 263, 983, 984
   high 265
   normal range of 263
   regulation of 270, 270fc, 314
   systolic 263, 984
   variations in 264
Blood transfusion 186, 193
   complications of 195
   exchange 191
   incompatible 189f
   indications of 193
Blood vessel 201, 603
   classification of 262
   constriction of 236f
   cross-section of 235f
   development of 261
   endothelial lining of 161f
   great 248
   structure of 262
   vasoconstrictors of 270t
   vasodilators of 270t

Index

Blood volume 183, 256, 266, 390, 483, 983
    measurement of 183
    regulation of 184, 314
    variations in 183
Blood-gas barrier, structure of 352
Blood-testis barrier, functions of 676
Blue green color blindness 678
B-lymphocytes 133, 148t
Body
    calcium 609
    control systems of 11
    disequilibrium of 832
    electrolytes 8
    immune response 157
    inverted representation of 774
    mass index 985
    on-body righting reflex 847
    on-head righting reflex 847
    parts of 240
    surface area 255, 334
    systems 534t
    water, total 7
    weight 336
Body fluid
    compartments 7
    distribution of 7, 8fc
    volumes, measurement of 8
Body temperature 109, 238, 539fc
    chemical regulation of 534
    maintenance of 534
    measurement of 533
    physical regulation of 535
    regulation of 100
    variations in 540
Bohr's effect 360, 362
Bohr's equation principle 337
Boiler maker's disease 957
Bombay group 188
Bombay phenotype 187, 188
Bone
    conduction 952, 960f
    cysts 613
    deformity 616f
    deposition of 608
    physiology of 608
    resorption 608, 609, 611
    smallest 944
    structure of 609f
Bone marrow 117, 119, 393
    hyperplasia of 124
    littoral cells of 142
    osteoclasts of 142
    stem cells 117
Bony labyrinth 946
Bony walls 901
Borborygmi sounds 462
Borelli's experiment 237, 238f
Botulinum toxin 82
Botzinger complex 367
Bound ribosomes 19
Bowel sounds 465
Bowman's capsule 485, 486, 494
Bowman's gland 970
Bowman's membrane 902
Boyle's law 389
Brachium conjunctivum 825
Bradycardia 217, 243, 248, 397, 984
Bradykinesia 820, 821, 870
Bradykinin 268, 296, 412, 492, 656, 658, 784
Brain 301, 667, 879
    anatomy of ventricles of 891
    arterial supply of 300f
    blood flow 983

death 874, 982, 982f
    diagnosis of 982
    development 596
    extracellular fluid 891, 892
    functional anatomy of 724
    higher functions of 882
    microglia in 142
    natriuretic peptide 656
    nuclei of 45
    parts of 724f, 895
    posterolateral view of 928f
    sagittal section of 587f, 836f, 856f, 860f
    sand 587
    stem reflexes, absence of 982
    surgery 543
    thalamus in 794f
    tumors 874
    ventricles of 724, 891
Brainstem 864
    auditory evoked response curves 960, 961f
    regulate muscle tone 800
    reticular formation, role of 877
Braxton-Hicks contractions 706
Breast 690, 691
    carcinoma of 716
    suckling of 584
Breath method, single 336
Breath sounds 322
    causes of 322
Breathing
    abdominal 322, 879
    capacity, maximum 335, 336
    clavicular 879
    normal 375
    patterns of 321
    reserve 336
    stage of exaggerated 378
    technique 879
    types of 322
Broca's area 852, 887
Brodmann's area 801, 850, 850f, 887, 888f, 929
Brodmann's classification 774
Bronchi 315
    primary 316
Bronchial arteries 343
Bronchial asthma 321, 335
Bronchial blood flow 344
Bronchial breath sound 323, 323f
Bronchial obstruction 349
Bronchial smooth muscle 317
Bronchial tone 317
Bronchial vessels 319
Bronchiectasis 314
Bronchioles 316
Bronchodilation 318
Bronchogram 318, 318f
Bronchopulmonary dysplasia 380
Bronchoscopy 318
Brown-Sequard syndrome 811, 812f
Bruit 232
Brunner's glands 452
Brush border hydrolases 451, 452
Bruxism 875
Buccal glands 413
Bucket handle movement 322, 323f
Buffy coat layer 108
Bulbar poliomyelitis 461
Bulboreticular facilitatory area 804, 836
    fibers, larger 836
Bulbourethral gland 677
Burning pain 781, 784

Burst forming units 116
Burst promoting activity 118, 120
Butyryl trihexyl citrate 193
Bypass surgery 299

C

C cells 477
C wave, causes of 283
Cadherins 30, 31
Caffeine 886
Caisson disease 388, 389
Calbindin 615
Calcarine sulcus 849
Calcitonin 503, 515, 516, 574, 592, 614
    actions of 614
    gene-related peptide 296, 744, 782
Calcitriol 473, 503, 515, 516, 615
    actions of 615
    deficiency of 616
    regulation of secretion of 616
    synthesis of 612, 615fc
Calcitropic hormones 516
Calcium 41, 473
    bilirubinate stones 448
    calmodulin system 557
    channel 36, 36f
    homeostasis 377
        mechanism of 611fc
    sensing receptors 611
Calmodulin 92
Caloric test 843
Calorigenic action 595, 635
Calorigenic hormones 535, 539
Calpain 685, 688
Calsequestrin 67, 70
Camphor 781
Cancers 981
Capacitance vessels 234, 262, 263
Capillary basket 343
Capillary circulation 290, 291f
    regulation of 292, 292t
Capillary endothelium 486
Capillary fluid shift mechanism 270
Capillary hydrostatic pressure 178, 180
Capillary pressure 291
Capillary surface area 180
Capsaicin 781
    receptors 781
Capsular hydrostatic pressure 495
Captopril 516
Carbamino compounds 361
Carbaminohemoglobin 112, 361
Carbaminoprotein 361
Carbidopa 821
Carbohydrate
    absorption of 469
    digestion of 469, 470
    metabolism 396, 569, 595, 623, 635, 643, 858
    splitting enzyme 439, 452
Carbon dioxide 17, 34, 314
    dissociation curve 361, 362f
    response curve 375f
    transport 361
Carbon monoxide 659, 678
    poisoning 372, 398
Carbonic acid bicarbonate 2
Carbonic anhydrase 361, 426, 427, 503, 511
    inhibitors 502
Carbonmonoxyhemoglobin 112, 379
Carboxyhemoglobin 112, 379

Carboxypeptidase 439, 471
Carcinoid syndrome 477
Carcinoid tumors 477
Cardiac arrest 506
Cardiac catheterization 227
Cardiac centers 246, 248
Cardiac conducting system 205
    components of 205
Cardiac cycle 224, 227, 229
    duration of 226
    phases of 224, 224f, 225t, 228f, 295
Cardiac depression 275
Cardiac edema 181
Cardiac excitation, ectopic foci of 207
Cardiac failure 275
    acute 276
    causes of 276
    severe 277
Cardiac function 242
    tests to assess 240
Cardiac glands 420, 423
Cardiac impulse
    causes of 220
    spread of 207, 207f
Cardiac index 255
Cardiac murmurs 236
Cardiac muscle 39f, 85-88, 88f, 88t, 93, 94, 94t
    action potential 86f
    different values for 85
    electrical activity of 85
    fiber 85f
    hypertrophy 83
    properties of 88, 208
    relaxation of 87
    structure of 85, 85f, 205f
Cardiac output 253, 255, 266, 269, 271, 286, 288, 345, 596, 980, 983, 984
    decreases, maximum 391
    determinants of 254f
    distribution of 253, 253t
    homometric regulation of 257t
    measurement of 253
    pathological variation of 255
    regulation of 255, 257
    variations in 255
Cardiac plexus, superficial 243
Cardiac reserve 255
Cardiac sphincter 423
Cardiac tamponade 203
Cardiac veins, anterior 294
Cardio-acceleratory center 244
Cardioinhibitory center 217, 244, 245, 250, 807, 835
Cardiolipin 21
Cardiology 201
Cardiometer 229
Cardiopulmonary resuscitation 398, 399
Cardiospasm 461
    causes of 461
Cardiovascular adjustments 285, 710, 983
Cardiovascular disease 981, 983, 985
Cardiovascular system 201, 357, 390, 596, 624, 879, 977-979
Carotid angiogram 300, 300f
Carotid artery, internal 299
Carotid body 371, 372t
    microscopic structure of 371f
    structure of 371
Carotid pulse 399
Carotid sinus nerve 246

Carotinemia 446
Carpopedal spasm 377, 613
Carrier protein 17, 38
Caspases 29
Castle intrinsic factor 121, 124, 426
Catabolic nervous system 869
Catabolism 595
Catacrotic limb 281
Catalase 115, 135, 299
Catalytic cyclase 556
Catalytic receptors 554
Catalytic unit 555
Cataract 646, 906, 914
Catecholamine 249, 257, 296, 557, 632, 633, 707, 743
   mechanism of action of 634
   metabolism of 633fc
   O-methyltransferase 633, 867
   release of 274
   secretion 637
   synthesis of 633f
Cathepsin 132
Cathode ray oscilloscope 48, 50, 50f, 212, 873
Catsper 676
Cauda equina 727
Caudal anesthesia 894
Caudal inhibitory
   area 804, 836
   fibers, smaller 836
Caudal ventrolateral medulla 247, 267
Caudate circuit 819
Causalgia 790
Caveolin 41
Celiac ganglion 641
Celiac plexus 425, 865
Cell 54, 567t
   acinar 440
   adhesion molecules 17, 30, 134
   adrenal cortical 626
   amacrine 925-927
   aneuploid 668
   antigen presenting 150-152
   argentaffin 424, 452
   attached patch clamp 35
   basal 965, 970
   basket 737, 826-828
   Betz 801, 850, 852
   biology 15, 45
   body 59, 60
   cajal 411, 850
   chief 423
   chromaffin 621, 632, 633f, 867
   clara 315
   columnar epithelial 405
   cycle 26, 27f
   dark 674
   decarboxylation 314, 317, 406, 408, 424, 430, 477
   decidual 703
   dendritic 152
   desquamated mucosal 456
   division 26
   duct 440
   dust 142, 317
   electron microscopic structure of 16f
   endocrine 423, 478
   endothelial 495
   enterochromaffin 424, 428, 452
   enteroendocrine 424
   ependymal 726, 893
   epithelial 425, 525f
   excitable 54

   fusiform 850
   glial 44, 373, 726
   glomus 371
   goblet 314, 315, 411, 452
   granular 488
   granulosa 686
   groups 728
   growth, control of 29
   gustatory receptor 965
   histamine containing 406
   identity markers 17
   inhibitory 768
   intercalated 487
   intestinal epithelial 40f
   junctions 30
   juxtaglomerular 488
   lacis 485, 488
   leydig 667, 673, 678
   lines stimulated 118
   martinotti 850
   membrane 49t, 159, 642
      functions of 16
      proteins, functions of 17
      structure of 15, 16f
   mesangial 485, 496
   microfold 452
   mitral 733, 970
   monosomic 668
   myoepithelial 414
   neighboring 966
   neuroglial 725f
   nucleated 603
   null 133
   older 138
   olfactory 969
   organelles 17, 19
   osteogenic 608
   outside 5
   oxyphil 610
   pale 674
   paneth 452
   parafollicular 592
   parts of 15
   peptic 420, 423, 432
   periglomerular 971
   physiology 15
   pillar 949
   plasma 153
   postsynaptic target 867
   principal 487, 505, 507
   produce pepsinogen 423
   progenitor 117
   protein free 104
   pus 135
   renal tubular 40f
   rod 927
   satellite 65, 724
   scavenger 726
   secretory 41f, 411f, 488
   specialized 762
   sperm 675
   stellate 826-828, 850
   supporting 372, 970
   sustentacular 372, 965, 970
   target 547, 679
   theory 15
   trisomic 668
   trophoblast 702
   tufted 970
   types of 641t, 850
   virus-infected 147
   worn out 19
   younger 138
Cellular metabolism 596, 870
Cellulose 456

Central analgesia system 789, 789f
Central excitatory state 739, 758
Central inhibitory state 739, 758
Central nervous system 44, 46, 179, 248, 269, 373, 393, 407-409, 537, 567, 597, 625, 722, 726, 731, 748, 770, 789, 800, 829, 841, 866, 891, 903
   structure of 724
Central sulcus 849
Central thermoreceptors 537
Central venous pressure 283
Centrifugal acceleration 288
Centrioles 19
Centromere 27
Centrosome 19
Cephalic phase 429, 441
Cerebellar arteries, posterior inferior 893
Cerebellar ataxia 831
Cerebellar control 888
Cerebellar cortex 826-828
   histology of 827f
Cerebellar disease 831, 832
Cerebellar dysarthria 832
Cerebellar functions 830f
Cerebellar gait 870
Cerebellar hemispheres 825
Cerebellar nystagmus 832
Cerebellar peduncle
   inferior 773, 780, 825, 829, 829t
   middle 825, 829
   superior 774, 780, 825, 829, 829t
Cerebellohypothalamic
   circuits 831
   pathway 829
   projections 831
Cerebellomedullary cistern 892
Cerebellum 825, 828, 828f
   connections of 828
   flocculonodular lobe of 841, 843
   functional divisions of 826f
   functions of 830
   in muscle tone, role of 830
   lesion of 831
   non-somatic functions of 831
   parts of 825, 825f, 826f
   peduncles of 829
   predictive functions of 830
   role of 831
Cerebral anemia theory 877
Cerebral aqueduct 724, 892
Cerebral arterioles, state of 301
Cerebral artery, posterior 796
Cerebral autoregulation, myogenic hypothesis of 302
Cerebral blood flow 289, 301
   measurement of 300
   regulation of 302
Cerebral circulation 299, 302
Cerebral cortex 245, 247, 459, 765, 766, 800, 801, 830, 849, 850, 852, 860, 864
   afferent connections of 851
   connections of 851
   efferent connections of 851
   functional anatomy of 849
   histology of 850
Cerebral dominance 849, 889
Cerebral edema 288, 387
   acute 387
   high altitude 387
   resolution of 388
Cerebral gas embolism 380

Cerebral gray matter 849
Cerebral hemispheres 974
Cerebral lesions 982
Cerebral palsy 419
Cerebral vascular resistance 301
Cerebral vessels, innervation of 300
Cerebrocerebellum 826
Cerebrocortical function 851
Cerebrohepatorenal syndrome 20
Cerebro-olivocerebellar pathway 828
Cerebro-reticulocerebellar pathway 828
Cerebrospinal fluid 2, 7, 288, 370, 387, 724, 726, 891, 892, 895
   absorption of 893
   circulation of 893
   formation of 892
   functions of 893
   osmolarity of 892
   pressure, measurement of 894
Ceruloplasmin 823
Cerumen 943
Ceruminous glands 531, 943
Cervical
   cap 714
   enlargement 727
   esophagus 420
   ganglion 415, 864, 865
   mucus 696
   secretion 689
   vertebra 420
Cervix 684, 691
Chalasia 461
Chalone 429
Channelopathy 37
Charcot joints 813
Charcot-Leyden crystals 132
Charcot-Marie-Tooth disease 31, 47
Chemical digestion 406
Chemical irritation 412
Chemical regulation 430
Chemical sense 965, 969
Chemical synapse 732, 733t
   functional anatomy of 733
   structure of 733f
Chemical thermogenesis 539
Chemically sensitive nociceptors 781
Chemokines 134, 144
Chemoreceptor 369, 370, 762, 863, 971
   central 370, 371f
   mechanism 269
   reflex 271
   stimulation 274, 369
   trigger zone 464
   zones 895
Chemotactic cytokines 149
Chemotaxis 134, 144, 146, 701
   defective 136
Chenodeoxycholic acid 445
Chest
   fluoroscopy 331
   leads 215
   wall, compliance of 338
Cheyne-Stokes breathing 321, 376, 376f
   causes of 376
Cheyne-Stokes respiration 375
Chiari-Frommel syndrome 713
Chief sensory nucleus 728, 772-774, 777, 780
Childbirth 562
Chloride
   channels 37, 426
   shift 361

Chloromycetin 137
Cholecalciferol 612
Cholecystectomy 448
Cholecystokinin 304, 406, 410, 426, 440, 556
  actions of 440t
Cholelithiasis 448
Cholera 467
  toxin 557
Cholesterol 16
  alpha-monooxygenase 602
  desmolase 622
  esterase 472
  lecithin ratio 448
  metabolism 596
  stones 448
Cholesterol-lecithin ratio, high 448
Cholesteryl ester hydrolase 626
Cholic acid 445
Cholinergic neurons 857, 877
Cholinergic receptors 658
Cholinergic system 877
Cholinergic transmission 867
Chondrogenesis 568
Chondroitin sulfate 608
  proteoglycan 486
Chorda tympani
  nerve 419, 965
  syndrome 419, 420
Chordae tendineae 204, 204f
Chorea 820
Choreoathetosis 797, 820
Choriocarcinoma 604
Chorionic growth hormone prolactin 705
Chorionic villus sampling 669
Choroid 902
  capillary plexus of 903
  epithelium, active secretion of 893
  plexus 892, 893
Christmas disease 173
Chromaffin granules 633
Chromatic aberration 913, 914f
Chromatids 27
Chromatin 22
Chromatolysis 46
Chromium 473
Chromogranin A 633
Chromosomal abnormalities 577
  detection of 669
Chromosomal disorders 668, 669
Chromosomal mosaicism 669
Chromosomal pattern 668
Chromosomal sex 664
Chromosome 822, 936
  number of 668
  parts of 668, 669
  single 663
Chronaxie 55
Chronaxie, values of 55
Chronotropic effect, positive 244
Chvostek's sign 377, 613
Chylomicrons 472
Chyme 422
Chymosin 425
Chymotrypsin 471
Chymotrypsinogen 439
Cilia 18
  actions of 893
Ciliary body 902
  functions of 902
Ciliary ganglion 865
Ciliary processes 903
Ciliary zonule 903, 906, 909

Ciliated secretory epithelium 685
Ciliospinal reflex 932
Ciliotoxins 328
Cingulate gyrus 782, 861
Circadian pacemaker 589
Circadian rhythm 429, 588, 589, 858
Circulatory shock 272, 562
  causes of 272
  end stages of 272
Circulatory system 288, 629
  functions of 201
Circumventricular organs 587
Cisterna magna 892
Citrate phosphate dextrose 172, 194, 360
Citric acid cycle 396
Clarke's column 728, 773, 780
Clasp knife effect 755
Clathrin 41
  coated pits 40
  coated vesicle 40
Claudins 30
Clonal anergy 156
Clonal deletion 155, 156
Clonal selection 150
Clonus 755
Clostridium botulinum 82
Clot retraction 162, 167, 171
Clotting, stages of 165
Coagulation, tests of 171
Cobalt 473
Cocaine 430
Cochlea 838, 947
  compartments of 947f, 948t
Cochlear duct 947
Cochlear implant 959
Cochlear microphonics 956, 957
Codon, deletion of 24
Cofactor protein S 172
Cogwheel rigidity 821
Coiled glands 423
Coitus 696
  interruptus 714
Colchicine 503, 665
Cold
  antibody 155
  saline 254
  sweat 537
Colicky pain 781
Colipase 439, 472
Collagenase 423
Collateral vessels 294
Collecting system 261
Colliculus
  inferior 301, 955
  superior 774, 805, 846, 853
Colloid 195, 591
  bismuth compounds 434
  goiter 600
  osmotic pressure 103, 177
Colon 455f
  ascending 455
  descending 455, 866
  storage 456
Colonic bacteria 456
Colony forming unit 116, 138, 162
Colony stimulating factors 116, 118, 138, 162, 576
Color blindness 666, 935
  dichromatic 936
  monochromatic 936
  trichromatic 936
Color Doppler 240
Color flow Doppler 241
Color vision 932

neural mechanism of 933, 934, 935*fc*
  tests for 935
  theories of 933
Colostrum 711
Columnar epithelium 487
Coma 646, 874, 982
  stage of 378
Combined pill 715
  mechanism of action of 716
  side effects of 716
Committed hematopoietic stem cell 118
Compensatory cardiovascular adjustments 289
Complement system 147
  functions of 146
Complete androgen resistance syndrome 670
Complex tone 950
Computed axial tomography 441, 852
Concentration dilution tests 525
Condom 714
Conduction deafness 957-960, 960f
Cones
  absorbance spectra of 924f
  functions of 920
  pigments in 933t
Congenital central hypoventilation syndrome 870
Congenital disease 314
Congestive cardiac failure 180, 182f, 273, 276, 317, 334, 339, 376, 379, 387, 630
Conjoint synapse 733
Conjunctiva 902
Conn syndrome 630
Connective tissue 142
Conscious proprioception 779
Conscious senses 761
Consciousness 861
Consensual light reflex 931
Constipation 466
  symptoms of 467
Constrictors renal vessels 491t
Continuous sampling technique 352
Continuous wave Doppler 240, 241
Contraception 714
  female 717
  male 717
Contractile proteins 66
Contracting muscle 985
Contralateral hemiplegia 806, 807
Contralateral homonymous hemianopia 916
Conus medullaris 727
Convergence projection theory 788
Convex lens 909f, 913
Coombs' reagent 192
Coombs' test 192
  direct 192, 192f
  indirect 192, 193f
  types of 192
  uses of 192
Copper 473
  deficiency 113
  metabolism 823
  T 715f
Cornea 901, 902
Corona radiata 771, 802
Coronary angiography 298
Coronary artery 202, 293
  bypass grafting 299
  disease 241, 297, 647, 985

  diagnosis of 298
  risk factors for 298
  left 293t, 294
  right 293t, 294
Coronary blood flow 294-296, 983
  measurement of 294
  regulation of 296
  variation of 295
Coronary chemoreflex 249
Coronary circulation 293, 296
  defects of 297
Coronary perfusion 399
Coronary sinus 202, 294
Coronary vascular disease 328
Coronary vessels, functional anatomy off 293
Corpora cavernosa 677
Corpus
  albicans 688
  callosum 849, 851
  hemorrhagicum 688
  luteum 688, 692
  spongiosum 677
  striatum 818
Cortex 429
Cortical blindness 930
Cortical hormones, biosynthesis of 621
Cortical nephron 487, 487f
Cortical neuronal excitability 836
Cortical plasticity 766, 886
Cortical sensations 767
Corticobulbar tract 800, 802, 803f
Corticonuclear tract 802, 803f
Cortico-pontocerebellar
  pathway 828
  tract 829
Corticospinal disorders 870
Corticospinal tract 802, 803f
  anterior 800, 802
  direct 802
  functions of 803
  lateral 800, 802
Corticosterone 622
Corticostriatal system 816
Cortico-striato-pallido-thalamo-cortical pathway 817
Corticotropin-releasing hormone 410, 556, 580, 626, 632, 648, 706
Cortisol 82, 621, 622, 650
  antigrowth effects of 626
  binding globulin 622, 629
  metabolic effects of 623
  role of 707
Cortisone 622, 623, 711
Cosmic radiation 392
Costal breathing 322
Cough reflex 369
Counter current multiplier system 507, 507f, 508
COVID-19 145
Cowper's gland 678
Cranial nerve 724, 725t, 961f
  ganglia 723
  neuritis 461
Craniosacral outflow 409, 863
C-reactive protein 104, 147, 298
Creatine
  kinase 605
  phosphate 74
  phosphokinase 298
Cresyl violet 666
Cretinism 601f
  causes of 601

Crigler-Najjar syndrome 115
Crista ampullaris 839
    structure of 839f
Critical air temperature 540
Critical closing pressure 239, 291
Critical fusion frequency 75, 925
Critical micellar concentration 446, 472
Crude sensations 774
Crude touch 773
    pathway for 777
Crush syndrome 273
Cryptorchidism 673, 680
Crystalline zinc insulin 647
Crystalloids 195
C-type natriuretic peptide 656
Cuboidal cells, waldeyer formed of 684
Cuboidal epithelium 487
Cumulus oophorus 687
Cuneocerebellar tract 828, 829
Cupula 839
Curare poisoning, treatment for 81
Cushing's disease 137, 627
Cushing's reaction 248
Cushing's reflex 248, 249fc, 269, 301
Cushing's syndrome 137, 266, 374, 624, 627, 627f
Cutaneous blood flow 983
    measurement of 292
    regulation of 292
Cutaneous thermoreceptors 537
Cutaneous vascular responses 292
Cyanide
    absorption of 379
    metabolism of 379
    poisoning 370, 379
    sources of 379
Cyanocobalamin 121
Cyanosis 112, 381, 531
    central 381, 381f
    peripheral 381, 381f
Cyanotic heart disease, congenital 381
Cyclic adenosine monophosphate 505, 555, 556, 588, 626
    role of 557fc
Cyclopentanoperhydrophenanthrene ring 621
Cystic duct 444
Cystic fibrosis 24, 37, 332, 441
Cystinuria 471
Cystometrogram 93, 93f, 521, 521f
Cystoscopy 525
Cytochrome
    C 29, 112
    oxidase 115, 379, 934
Cytokeratin 17
Cytokines 118, 118t, 138, 144, 145, 145t, 540, 576
    functions of 144
    receptors 781
    storm 145
Cytokinesis 27, 29
Cytopempsis 41
Cytoplasm 15, 17, 132, 160
Cytoplasmic division 27
Cytoskeleton 17
    proteins 19
Cytosol 15, 17
Cytotoxic
    drugs 137
    T cells 149, 150t, 157
Cytotrophoblast 702

D

D-agglutinogen 190
Dale's phenomenon 734
Dalton's law 351
Damping effect 830
Dark adaptation 925
Daughter chromosomes 27
Daytime sleepiness 376
Dead space 336
    physiological 336, 337
Deafness, central 958
Decompression sickness 389, 390
    prevention of 390
    treatment of 390
Decubitus ulcers 813
Deep brain stimulation 822
Deep cerebellar nuclei 826f, 827, 828
Deep pain 782, 782t, 785, 787
Deep pressure 773
Deep somatic pain 785
Deep tendon reflexes 752
Deep tubular glands 411
Defecation 466
    reflex 466, 467f
Defensins 132, 134
Deglutition
    center 807, 835
    control of 462
    esophageal stage of 461
    oral stage of 460f
    pharyngeal stage of 460f
Dehydration exhaustion 542
Dehydroepiandrosterone 631, 678, 695
    sulfate 695, 704
Deiodinase 595
Deiters' nucleus 841
Deja vu syndrome 885
Delta waves 873f
Dementia 886
Dendrites 45, 46, 48, 827
Dendritic spines 48
Dendrodendritic reciprocal synapses 970
Dendrodendritic synapse 733
Denervation hypersensitivity 82, 420
Dense bodies 90
Dense granules 160, 371
Dentato-rubro-thalamo-cortical fibers 829
Dentatothalamic pathway 828
Deoxycholic acid 445
Deoxygenated blood passes 710
Deoxyhemoglobin 362
Deoxyribonuclease 439
Deoxyribonucleic acid 160, 557
    technology, recombinant 25
Dephosphorylation 92
Depolarization 50, 52, 207
Depolarizing neuromuscular blocker 81
Depo-provera 716
Depression, long-term 741, 884
Dermatomal rule 787
Dermatome 727, 770
Dermis 529
Dermographism 293, 293f
Descemet's membrane 902
Desmin 66
Desmosomes 31
Desynchronization 874
Detrusor muscle 519, 521
Deuterium oxide 8
Dexamethasone 632

Dextrose-normal saline 9
Diabetes insipidus 583
    central 509
    nephrogenic 505, 509, 584
Diabetes mellitus 298, 374, 441, 570, 645, 646fc, 986
    adrenal 623, 627
    bronze 116, 474
    diagnosis of 647
    non-insulin dependent 645
    signs of 645
    symptoms of 645
    treatment of 647
    type 1 645t
    type 2 457, 645t, 985
Diabetic ketoacidosis 646
Diacylglycerol 558, 867
Dialysate 514t
Dialysis 514
    types of 514
Diameter 132, 133
Diapedesis 134
Diaphragm 322
    activity of 322
    contraction of 323f
Diarrhea 466, 467
Diastasis 226
Diastolic pressure 227, 265
Dichromats 936
Dicoumarol 172
Dicrotic notch 281
Diencephalon 724
Diet, control of 967
Dietary fiber 456
    advantages of 457
    amount of 457
Diffusion 4, 34, 178, 291, 472
DiGeorge syndrome 612
Digestion 459
Digestive apparatus 19
Digestive enzymes, activation of 13
Digestive function 417, 422, 452
Digestive system 405
Digitalis 87, 257
    therapy 713
Dihydrocortisol 623
Dihydropyridine
    channels 87
    receptor 69, 70
Dihydrotestosterone 667, 679
Diiodothyronine 592
Diiodotyrosine 593
Di-isopropyl fluorophosphate 81
Dilute urine, excretion of 508
Dilution syndrome 584
Dinitrogen trioxide 980
Dipalmitoyl lecithin 325
Dipalmitoylphosphatidyl-choline 325
Dipeptidases 471
Dipeptidyl peptidase-4 inhibitors 478
Diphosphoglycerate 111, 359
Diphtheria 461
Diplacusis 957
Disaccharidase deficiency 470
Disaccharide maltose 417
Disequilibrium 831
Disseminated intravascular coagulation 175, 274, 562
Distal convoluted tubule 184, 499, 504
Distant vision 910f
    test for 914
Distension, prevents undue 203

Disuse osteoporosis 617
Diuresis 185, 506, 522, 629, 656
Diuretics 522
Diurnal variation 265, 540, 588
Divalent metal transporter-1 474
Diver's paralysis 389
Dominant hemisphere 849, 852
Donnan membrane equilibrium 4, 4f
Donor's plasma 189t
Dopa decarboxylase 633
Dopamine 408, 484, 492, 515, 516, 636, 743, 818
    B-hydroxylase 633
    receptors 372, 818, 819
Doppler echo 241
Doppler study 240
Dorsal column pathway 770, 771, 771f, 773, 775
Double Bohr effect 703
Down's syndrome 669, 704
Drinker's method 399
Drinker's respirator 399
Drugs, detoxification of 444
Drunken gait 832
Dry spoon-shaped nails 123
D-tubocurarine 80, 81, 867
Dual gland 640
Duchenne's muscular dystrophy 24, 75
Duct, collecting 504, 511
Ductless glands 547
Ductus
    arteriosus 305, 306
    venosus 305
Dull aching pain 783
Dumping syndrome 435, 464
Duodenal bulb 451
Duodenal cap 451
Duodenal factors 463
Duodenal hormones 429
Duodenal mucosa, I cells of 440
Duodenal papilla 444
Duodenal ulcers 433, 433t
Duodenocolic reflexes 466
Duodenum 451, 474
Dura mater 891
Dwarfism 572, 572f, 668
Dye dilution method 183, 254f
Dynamic lung volumes 332, 334
Dynein 18, 46
Dysarthria 393, 888
Dysdiadochokinesis 832
Dysgeusia 968
Dyskinesia 820
Dyslexia 889
Dyslipidemia 986
Dysmenorrhea 694, 695
Dysmetria 831
Dyspnea 321
Dyspneic index 336
Dystonia 820
Dystrophia adiposogenitalis 858
Dystrophin 22, 66, 75, 87

E

Ear
    drum 943
    dust 840
    external 943
    functional anatomy of 943
    wax 943
Early dumping syndrome 435
Ebner's glands 416, 471
Ecchymosis 288

Index

Eccrine 530t
   gland 530
Echocardiography 241, 254, 255
Echoencephalography 852
Ectopic beat, ventricular 219, 219f
Eddy currents 236
Edema 181
   generalized 181
   localized 181
   non-pitting 181
   types of 181
Edinger-Westphal nucleus 864, 865, 910, 924, 930
Edridge color lantern 936f
Enckebach phenomenon 219f
Eestergren's stand 109f
Effector organ 748, 749
Egg retrieval 717
Einthoven's law 211
Einthoven's triangle 210f, 211, 216f
Ejaculation 677, 678
Ejaculatory duct 673
Elastases 471
Elastic lamina, internal 262
Elasticity 69
Elastin 262
Electric pain 781, 784
Electrical stimulus, characteristics of 54
Electrical synapse 732, 733t
Electrocardiogram 210, 212, 210
Electrodes 49, 73, 210
Electrodiagnostic test 61
Electroencephalogram 873, 873f, 982
Electrogenic pump 39
   role of 49
Electrolyte 469
   absorption of 473
   balance 484
   functions of 8
   loss 273
   mechanism of secretion of 440
   metabolism 569, 596, 692
Electromagnetic flow meter 235, 253, 300
Electromagnetic receptors 762
Electromyogram 73
Electromyography 73
Electroneuronography 368
Electrophoresis 103
Electrophysiological methods 851
Electroretinogram 937, 937f
Electrotonic conduction 56
Electrotonic potentials 56
Elephantiasis 182f
Embden-Meyerhof pathway 110, 360
Embolus 174
Embryo 665
   transfer 717
Emeiocytosis 41f, 80, 412, 440
Emission 678, 697
Emotion 796
   expression of 861
   genesis of 861
   role in 861
Emotional behavior, role in 858
Emotional brain 861
Emotional disturbances 575
Emotional excitement 255
Emotional expression, manifestations of 862
Emotional state 265, 429
Emotional stimuli 370
Emphysema 328, 374
Empty stomach, movement of 462

Enalapril 516
Encapsulated receptors 763
Encephalitis lethargica 837
End-diastolic volume 227, 230, 253, 255, 256
Endemic colloid goiter 600, 602
Endocardium 203, 204, 207
Endocochlear potential 951
Endocrine 547, 577
   control 406
   disorders 266, 433
   function 314, 405, 452, 483, 550, 671, 673, 676, 703, 855, 858,
   orchestra, master of 579
   organs 626
   pancreas 640, 641t
   secretion 547, 547f
   secretory organ 438
Endocrine gland 548, 549t, 636, 691, 692
   function, assessment of 549
   location of major 549f
Endocrine system 547, 548, 721t, 980
   peripheral 855
Endocytosis 40, 498, 594
   receptor-mediated 40, 41f
Endogenous
   analgesia system 789
   antigen 151
   pain inhibition, pathway for 790fc
   pyrogens 540
   toxins 540
Endolymph 946
Endolymphatic potential 951
Endometrial biopsy 696
Endometrial cycle 688
Endometrium 44, 46, 685, 689, 691, 692, 702f
Endonucleases 439
Endopeptidases 439
Endoplasmic reticulum 19, 65, 67, 70, 87
Endoscopic retrograde cholangiopancreatography 441, 442f, 449
Endoscopy 305f, 434
Endosteal niche 116
Endothelial capsular membrane 486f
Endothelial surface factors 169
Endothelin 492, 516, 659, 659t
Endothelium 204, 658, 902
   derived relaxing factor 268, 270, 296, 658
   types of 262
Endotoxins 275
Endotracheal tube 398
End-plate potential 70, 80
End-systolic volume 227, 253
Energy 41
   expenditure 38
   stored 69
Enkephalin 632, 633
Enophthalmos 932
Enteric nervous system 406, 407, 408f, 409, 420, 428, 430, 461, 465, 863
Enterobacter aerogenes 456
Enterocytes 451
Enterogastric reflex 429, 463
Enterogastrones 432, 452
Enterohepatic circulation 114, 115, 445, 446
Enterokinase 439, 452, 453, 471

Enteropancreatic reflex 441
Enteropeptidase 439, 452
Enterotoxins 452
Entorhinal cortex 972
Environmental temperature 255, 535
Enzymatic reactions 981
Enzyme 17, 452
   cascade hypothesis 165
   fat-splitting 439
   methyl transferase 867
   rhodanase 379
   types of 675
Enzyme-linked immunosorbent assay 550
Eosinopenia 137
Eosinophil 132, 132f, 137, 147
   cationic protein 132
   functions of 135
   secrete lysophospholipase 132
Eosinophilia 137
Ependymoma 726
Epicardium 203, 207
Epicritic sensation 766
Epidermal growth factor 576
Epidermis 529
Epididymis 673
Epiglottis, horizontal deflection of 461
Epilepsy 874
   types of 874f
Epinephrine 269, 411, 430, 535, 650, 743, 789, 835
   intravenous infusion of 636f
Epineurium 44
Episodic
   ataxia 37
   bursts 693
Epithalamus 794
Epithelial podocytes 495
Epithelial sodium channel 37, 266, 499, 501, 967
Epithelioid 488
Epithelium 407, 519, 902
   derived relaxing factors 317
Epitopes 150
Equilibrium 943
   control of 831
Erb's sign 613
Erectile dysfunction 697
Erection 677
Erythema 392
Erythroblastosis fetalis 191
Erythrocyte 106
   mature 119
   sedimentation rate 108, 109
   special properties of 108
Erythroid
   cells die 120
   series 117
Erythron 117
Erythropoiesis 116, 117, 119, 120, 120t, 121
   sites of 117
   stages of 117, 118f, 120fc
Erythropoietin 116, 119, 121, 483, 576, 577, 656
   actions of 120
Esophageal adenocarcinoma 434
Esophageal lead 212
Esophageal reflux 420
Esophageal sphincter, inferior 420
Esophageal stage 460, 461
Esophageal varices 304, 305f
Esophagitis 433f
Esophago-salivary reflex 419

Esophagus 413, 420, 433f
   abdominal 420
   carcinoma of 462
   conducts food 405
   diffuse spasm of 461
   functions of 420
   innervation of 420
   lower end of 432
Esrite method 109
Esterase 132
Estrogen 121, 574, 617, 631, 688-690, 706
   actions of 691, 711
   forms of 690
   functions of 704
   level 696
   receptor-alpha 691
   receptor-beta 691
   secreting tumors 713
   sources of 690
   synthesis of 690, 690fc, 704
   therapy 713
   transport of 691
Etanercept 145
Ethinyl estradiol 691, 715
Ethylene diamine tetra acetic acid 172
Etiocholanolone 679, 692
Eunuchoidism 671, 713, 680
Eupnea 321
Eupneic breathing 321
Eustachian tube 944, 945
Euthyroid 600
Evans blue 183, 254
Eve's rocking method 398
Exchange vessels 262, 290
Excitability 48, 54, 68, 208
Excitation 51
Excitation-contraction coupling 69, 87
Excitatory postsynaptic potential 48, 735, 742, 748, 763
   production of 736f
Excretory function 99, 417, 456, 483, 703
Excretory organ 531
Exenatide 478
Exercise 575
   effects of 983, 985
   mild 395
   moderate 395
   recovery phase of 396
   severe 395
   stoppage of 396
   sweating in 537
Exocrine
   glands, functional classification of 411
   pancreas 438
   pancreatic acini 641f
Exocytosis 41, 80, 472, 734f
Exogenous antigens 151
Exons 22
Exopeptidase 439
Exophthalmic goiter 604
Exophthalmos 605, 605f
Expiration, accessory muscles of 322
Expiratory reserve volume 332, 333
External genitalia 667, 667f
Exteroceptive information 770
Exteroceptors 763
Extra-alveolar
   blood vessels 347
   capillaries feed 346
Extracardiac anastomosis 294

Index

Extracellular buffering 3, 512
Extracellular edema 181
Extracellular fluid 3, 7, 8, 11, 13, 54, 69, 151, 183, 484, 499, 501, 514t, 547, 555, 583, 608, 624, 626, 630, 734, 857, 947
Extracellular ligands 35
Extracorpuscular defects 122
Extraglomerular mesangial cells 485, 488
Extramedullary hematopoiesis 117
Extraocular muscles 906, 906f
   functions of 906
Extrapyramidal neurons 798, 800
Extrapyramidal pathways 800
Extrapyramidal tracts 804, 830
Extrasystole 208, 219
Eye
   crossed 917
   emmetropic 912, 912f
   extraocular muscles of 906f
   movements 906
   normal 912f
      fundus of 904f
   optical
      defects in 912
      system of 909
   reduced 908
   refraction of 909
   resolving power of 914
   third 587
Eyeball
   anterior parts of 903f
   contents of 904
   convergence of 910
   functional anatomy of 901
   layer of 902
   longitudinal section of 901f

F

Fabricius, bursa of 138
Fabry disease 20
Facial muscles 861
Facial nerve 409, 415, 865, 966
   nucleus, part of 800
   greater petrosal branch of 965
Facial puffiness 602f
Facilitation theory 788
Facilitatory drugs 80, 81
F-actin 75
Facultative water reabsorption 504, 505
Fahraeus-Lindqvist effect 238
Fainting 266, 268, 289
Fallopian tube 684, 685, 691, 692, 701
   ampulla of 702
Fallot's tetralogy 232
Familial dysautonomia 968
Far point 909
Far sightedness 912
Fas gene 157
Fas ligand 702
Fascia, superficial 529
Fascicle, posterior 207
Fasciculations 83
Fasciculus gracilis 520, 771
Fast axonal transport system 46
Fast muscle 72, 72t
Fast pain 783t
   pathway for 784
Fast-wave sleep 875
Fat
   absorption of 471, 472f
   brown 535
   digesting enzymes 406
   digestion of 471
   emulsification of 445
   metabolism 569, 596, 624, 643
   redistribution of 624
   regulation of 858
Fatigue 397
   causes of 397
Fatty acid 34, 472, 644
   free 472
   short-chain 472
Fecal fat estimation 441, 448
Fecal stercobilinogen estimation 448
Feedback system 12
Feed-forward inhibition 827
Feeding center 856
Feminizing hormone 691
Fern pattern 689
Ferritin 115, 474
Ferroportin 474
Ferrous sulfate 124
Fertilin 701
Fertilization 665f, 685, 701, 702
Fetal capillaries, endothelium of 702
Fetal circulation 305, 306fc
Fetal hemoglobin 360
Fetal lung, maturation of 624
Fetal membrane 702, 702f
Fetal ovary 667
Fetoplacental unit 704, 704fc
Fetus, role of 706
Fever 540
   advantages of 541
   characteristics of 541, 541f
   production of 540, 541fc
Fiberoptic bronchoscopy 401
Fiberoptic catheter 438
Fibers 829, 851
   adrenergic 267
   afferent 46, 485, 779, 780, 949
   autonomic 531
   band 59
   cerebellar
      afferent 828
      efferent 828
   cervical 771f
   cholinergic 536
   circular 909
   climbing 827, 828
   commissural 829, 851
   corticobulbar 800, 803
   corticofugal 789, 973
   corticonuclear 803
   corticopontine 851
   cortico-pontocerebellar 829
   corticospinal 803
   descending reticular system of 835
   diameter 57
   dynamic nuclear bag 749
   efferent 46, 829, 949
   extrafusal 749
   extrapyramidal 804, 851
   facilitatory 804
   hypothalamo-cerebellar 828
   inhibitory 804
   intrafusal 749, 750f
   meridional 910
   mossy 827, 828
   motor 66
   myelinated 46
   nuclear
      bag 749
      chain 749
   olivocerebellar 803
   parasympathetic
      afferent 415
      preganglionic 866
   peripheral nerve 47f
   pontocerebellar 803
   postganglionic
      sympathetic 409
   preganglionic parasympathetic 728
   projection 851
   pyramidal 851
   serotonergic 836
   soluble 457
   sympathetic 267, 268, 318, 865, 866
   thalamic projection 851
   type B 864
   type C 837
   uncrossed 774
   unmyelinated 46
   vasoconstrictor 267
   vestibulocerebellar 828
   vestibulo-reticular 841
Fibrillation 82
Fibrin
   degradation product 170, 175
   monomer 167
   threads 170
Fibrinogen 102-104, 327
   soluble 167f
Fibrinolysin 170
Fibrinolysis 170
   coagulation of 103
   extrinsic mechanism of 170fc
   inhibitors 171
   intrinsic mechanism of 170f
Fibrinolytic system 170, 171, 175
Fibroblast 603
   growth factor 576
Fibrous
   astrocyte 725
   pericardium 203
Fick's law 4, 34
Fick's method 253
Fick's principle 253, 345, 489
   modified 294
Filaments, intermediate 17
Filtering membrane
   structure of 486, 486f
   surface area of 496
Filtration 177, 291
   fraction 496
Filum terminale 727
Fine granules 132
Fine needle aspiration cytology 526
First order neuron 727, 770, 771, 775, 777, 927, 954, 970
First polar body 685
Fissure 849
   primary 825
Fistulous murmur 232
Fixation point 915
Fixed macrophages 142
Flaccid paralysis 82, 805, 811
Flagella 18
Flare 268, 292
Flatus 462
Flavin pigments 677
Flexible gel 424
Flexor group 805
Flexor reflex 756
Flicker fusion frequency 933
Flocculonodular lobe 825, 841, 843
Fluent aphasia 888

Fluid
   connective tissue 99
   dynamics 234
   loss, substitutes for 195
   metabolism 596
   mosaic model 16
   overload 9
   suspension system 894
   therapy, precautions in 9
Fluorescein 237
Fluorine 473
Fluoroscopy 331
Folic acid 121, 121f, 122, 456
   actions of 121
   deficiency 121, 125
Folium 825
Follicle, primary 686
Follicle-stimulating hormone 549, 556, 557, 562, 567, 578, 589, 624, 686
Follicular cells 591
   functions of 592
Follicular phase 686, 693
Food
   absorption of 469
   allergy, incidence of 471
   chemical composition of 463
   digestion of 469
   intake
      glucostatic hypothesis of 857
      regulation of 856
      role in 861
   specific dynamic action of 534
   texture of 965
Foramen magnum 724, 726
Foramen ovale 305
Forced expiratory
   flow rate 335
   volume 332, 335
Forced vital capacity 332, 335
Forebrain 724
Fornix 861
Forrel's decussation 805
Fossa ovalis 305, 710
Foul smelling stools 446
Fovea
   centralis 904
   modifications in 915
Fowler's method 336
Fragility 110
Frame shift mutation 25
Frank-Starling
   law 88, 256
   mechanism 257, 286, 983
Free bilirubin 446
Free radical
   beneficial effects of 981
   formation of 980
   scavengers 980
Fresh frozen plasma 194
Frog's sartorius muscle 48
Frohlich's syndrome 680
Frontal lobe 849, 852
   syndrome 853
Frost bite 542
Fulcrum 203
Functional plasticity 766, 886
Functional refractory period 86
Functional residual capacity 332, 333, 346
Functional syncytium 85, 90, 205
Fundic gland 423
Fundoplication 462
Fundus 422, 904
Fungiform 965

G

G actins 67
G cell 424
  morphology of 430
G protein
  coupled receptor 612
  small 554, 560
  stimulating 555
Gait 832
Galactopoietic hormone 577
Galactosyltransferase 187
Galanin 410, 641
Gallbladder 447
  bile 444, 444t
  capacity of 447
  contraction of 447, 448
  functions of 447
  investigations of 448
  normal appearance of 449f
Gallop rhythm 231
Gallstones
  formation of 448
  treatment of 448
Gamete
  intrafallopian transfer 717
  production of 685
Gametogenesis 671
Gametogenic function 671
Gamma scintillation camera 295
Gamma-amino butyric acid 35, 247, 410, 554, 733, 743, 817, 818, 828, 970
Gamma-motor neurons 748, 753t, 798
  activity, modulation of 804f
Ganglia 724
Ganglion cell 926, 927, 969
  large 926, 929
  small 926, 929
  types of 926
Ganglioside 20
Gap junctions 31, 85, 90, 205
Gas
  chromatography 352
  diffusion coefficient of 353
  exchange of 313f
  partial pressure of 351, 351f
  solubility of 353
  transport of 313, 357, 357f
Gastrectomy 116
  complications of 464
  partial 434
Gastric acid 461
  hypersecretion of 432
  neutralization of 434
  secretion 428f
    regulation of 427, 428f
Gastric amylase 426
Gastric content
  consistency of 463
  osmolality of 463
  pH of 463
  prevent regurgitation of 420
  volume of 463
Gastric emptying movement 462
Gastric epithelium 423
Gastric factors 463
Gastric filling movement 462
Gastric foveolae 423
Gastric gland
  feedback inhibition of 429
  structure of 423f
Gastric inhibitory
  peptide 478
  polypeptide 650
Gastric irritation 424
Gastric juice 425
  composition of 425t
  secretion 429, 432
Gastric lipase 426, 472
Gastric lumen stimulate 430
Gastric mixing movement 462
Gastric movements 459, 462
  types of 462
Gastric mucosa 406, 432, 432t
  atrophy of 124
  barrier 424
  normal 432f
Gastric mucus 433
Gastric phase 429, 430, 441
Gastric pits 423
Gastric secretion 431
Gastric secretory function, abnormalities of 432
Gastric ulcer 432f, 433t
Gastrin 428-430
  chemistry of 430
  functions of 430
  induced juice 430
  receptors 428
  releasing peptide 408, 427, 431
  secretion 430, 431, 431t
  stimulate acid 428f
Gastrinomas 431, 435
Gastritis 433
Gastrocolic reflex 466
Gastroenteric reflex 465
Gastroesophageal reflux disease 434, 457, 461, 466
Gastroesophageal sphincter 420
Gastroileal reflex 455, 465
Gastrointestinal blood flow 412
Gastrointestinal function 405
  control of 406
  regulation of 407
Gastrointestinal glands 411
Gastrointestinal hormones 477, 478, 479t, 656, 857
Gastrointestinal secretions 7
Gastrointestinal system 405, 625, 979
  functions of 405
  parts of 405f
Gastrointestinal tract 132, 133, 149, 405, 459, 466, 477, 617
  movements of 459
  structure of 407f
Gastropancreatic reflex 440, 441
Gastroparesis 463
  diabeticorum 463
Gastro-salivary reflex 419
Gaucher's disease 20
Gelatinase 423, 426, 471
  granules 132
Gender sex 664
Genes 22
  deletion, large 24
  histocompatibility 151
  single 669
  therapy 25
  X determining 666
General adaptation syndrome 870, 871
Genetic 22
  defects 696
  disorders, carriers of 717
  engineering 25
  factors 574
  mechanism, activation of 559
  mutation 24
  phenomenon 665
  predisposition 298, 433
  sex 664, 668
Geniculate body
  lateral 795, 796, 929
  medial 795, 796, 955
Geniculate cells, lateral 926
Genital ducts, formation of 667
Genital ridge 666
Genital sex 664
Genitalia 668
  development of 667
  internal 667f
Genome 22
Genomic action 598
Genotype 22, 187, 667
Germinal angiotensin converting enzyme 675, 677
Germinal epithelium 673, 684
Gestagens 692
Ghrelin 410, 424, 569, 580, 857
  stimulates 857
Giant edema 181
Giant pyramidal cells 852
Gibbs-Donnan equation 4
Gigantism 568, 570, 571f
Gilbert's syndrome 115
Gland
  complex 411
  hormones of 622fc
  innervation of 587
Glandular secretions 477
Glaucoma 905
  angle-closure 905
  chronic 905
  open-angle 905
  types of 905
Glicentin 453
Glioma 726
Gliptins 478
Global aphasia 888, 889
Globulin 102, 104, 439
Globus pallidus 815-817
Glomerular blood hydrostatic pressure 495
Glomerular filtration rate 485, 494, 495, 498, 626, 656
Glomerular membrane 486, 494
Glomeruli 828
Glomerulonephritis 495, 514, 519
Glomerulotubular balance 499-501
Glomerulus 485, 489
Glossitis 122f
Glucagon 257, 424, 557, 649, 649t, 650
  actions of 649
  peptide 478
  polypeptide 644
  regulation of secretion of 649
  secretion 649t
Glucocorticoid 444, 492, 574, 617, 621, 622, 711, 712
  excess, consequences of 624t
  mechanism of action of 623
  permissive action of 625
  physiological actions of 623
  production of 626f
  regulation of secretion of 626, 626fc
  role of 625
  secretion 627
  sites of actions of 624t
  symptoms of 623
  synthesis of 622fc
  therapeutic uses of 628
  transport of 622
Gluconeogenesis 444, 596, 623, 624
Glucoreceptors 646
Glucose
  6-phosphate dehydrogenase deficiency 110, 114, 135
  absorption across intestinal epithelial cell, mechanism of 470f
  dependent insulinotropic polypeptide 478
  facilitated diffusion of 38f
  intolerance 630
  reabsorption 502
  sodium symport 40f
  transport maximum for 503
  transporter 17, 40, 470, 642, 644
  tubular maximum for 502
Glucostats 857
Glucosuria 502
Glucuronic acid 623
Glucuronidase 132
Glucuronides 595, 691
Glucuronosyl transferase 114
Glucuronyl transferase 446
Glutamate 245, 247, 744, 749, 783, 784, 819, 922
Glutamine 744
Glycentin-related polypeptide 649
Glycine 737, 743
Glycocalyx 486
Glycocholic acid 445
Glycogen 17
  granules 160
  lactic acid system 74
  synthesis 444, 623
Glycogenolysis 444, 596
Glycolysis 110, 596
Glycoprotein 16, 159, 161
  rapidly migrating 426
Glycosaminoglycans 596, 603
Glycosuria 502, 645, 646
Glycosyl phosphatidylinositol 16
Goiter 600, 603, 606
  simple 600, 600f
Goitrogens 606
Goldblatt hypertension 509
Goldman-Hodgkin-Katz equation 5
Golgi apparatus system 19, 885
Golgi bottle neuron 737, 754
Golgi cells 826-828
Golgi tendon organ 754, 755f, 755t
Golgi vesicles 19
Gonadal dysgenesis 668, 671
Gonadal growth curve 576
Gonadal sex 664, 668
Gonadal steroid binding globulin 679, 691
Gonadogenesis 666
Gonadotropin-independent precocity 671
Gonadotropin-releasing hormone 556, 579, 580, 589, 670, 680, 693, 716
Gonads 663, 668
Gorilla facies 571
Gossypol 716
G-protein
  coupled receptors 554, 556, 584, 745, 971
  types of 554
Graafian follicle 687
  structure of 687f
Gram-negative bacteria 433
Grand mal epilepsy 874, 874f
Granular cast 525f

Index

Granular chromophils 567
Granular layer 827
Granule cell 733, 826-828, 850, 970, 971, 973
   axons of 851
   layer 826, 850
Granule, secondary 132
Granulocyte 116, 118, 131, 132, 577
   colony stimulating factor 116, 139
   formation of 138
   macrophage colony stimulating factor 116
   monocyte 138
      colony stimulating factor 139
Granulocytopenia 138
Granulomatous
   disease, chronic 135
   thyroiditis, sub-acute 602
Graves' disease 604, 605
Gravindex test 705
Gravity 324
   effects of 178, 288, 345, 346
   force of 288
Growth and development
   physiology of 573
   stages in 573
Growth curves 575, 575f
Growth factor 549, 576, 887
Growth hormone 121, 444, 567, 568, 573, 617, 650, 677, 711, 712
   binding protein 568, 572
   deficiency 573
   hypersecretion of 570
   hyposecretion of 572
   inhibiting hormone 569, 570, 580
   insensitivity 572
   physiological actions of 568
   receptor 568
   releasing hormone 556, 557, 569, 570, 572, 580
   secretion 570
      regulation of 569, 570f
   stimulates secretion of 580
Growth-promoting action,
      mechanism of 568
Guanosine
   diphosphate 554, 555, 560
   triphosphate 554, 555, 558
Guanylin 452
Guanylyl cyclase 744, 922
Guillain-Barre syndrome 47, 104
Gums 456
Gunshot injuries 810
Gustatory cortex 966
Gustatory pore 965
Gustatory salivary reflex 419
Gustatory sweating 537
Gut
   extrinsic innervation of 409
   innervation of 407, 408f
   wall, distension of 412
Gut-brain-immune system
      interactions, dysfunctional 410
Gynecomastia 605, 713
Gyrus 849

H

H antigen 188
H band 66
Haddad syndrome 870
Hair 529
   bulb 529
Hair cell 840, 943, 948
   depolarization of 841f
   inner 949t
   innervation of 949
   outer 949t
   structure of 839f
Hair distribution 679
   abnormal 669
Hair follicle 529
   receptors 775
Haldane's effect 362, 362f
   causes of 362
Haldane's gas analyzer 352
Haldane-Priestly method 351
Hamberger phenomenon 110, 361
Hamilton's method 254
Haploid number 674
Hapten 147
Haptocorrin 426
Haptoglobin 104, 196
Harmful substances, fat-soluble 444
Hartnup disease 471
Hashimoto's thyroiditis 601, 604
Headache 570
Health effects, prevention of 986
Hearing 943
   aid 958, 959, 959f
   impairment, types of 957
   loss 960f, 980
   mechanism of 951
   physiology of 949, 951fc
   theories of 952
Heart 201, 202, 298, 603, 656
   anastomosis of 294
   attack 985
   burns 420
   conducting system of 205, 206f
   contraction of 208
   coverings of 203
   different chambers of 227t
   electrical activity of 210
   fibrous skeleton of 203, 203f
   functional anatomy of 201, 202
   innervation of 243, 244f, 246f
   musculature of 203
   papillary muscles of 204
   parasympathetic innervation of 244, 425
   parts of 207t
   valves 204
   venous drainage of 294
   volume changes in 229t
Heart block
   complete 219
   first-degree 219
   third-degree 219
Heart disease
   chronic 108
   ischemic 297, 716
   prevents 457
Heart failure 179, 275, 277, 277fc, 376, 381
   cells 142, 317
   compensated 276
   decompensated 277
   left 179, 276
   pathophysiology of 276
   right 276
   treatment of 277
Heart rate 208, 217, 217f, 243, 245, 269, 596, 983
   central influences on 245, 257
   effects of 295
   regulation of 250, 257
   variations in 243, 243t
Heart sound 225f, 230, 230t
   abnormalities of 231
   auscultation of 231
   first 230
   fourth 231
   intensity of 232t
   second 231
   third 231
Heat balance 534
Heat cramps 542
Heat edema 181
Heat exhaustion 542
Heat gain 534, 538
   mechanism of 534f
Heat loss 534, 535, 538, 539
Heat production 74, 534, 538
Heat shock protein 692
Heat stroke 542
Heavy fatty meal 472
Helicobacter pylori 433, 434
Helicotrema 947
Helper T cell 149, 150t
   stimulation of 151
Hematocrit 107, 238
   significance of 108
   value 100, 880
Hematological system 978
Hematology 99
Hematopoiesis 116, 116f, 117, 118t
Hematopoietic stem cell 116
Hematuria 514
Heme oxygenase 114
Heme-heme interaction 358
Hemianesthesia 778, 796
Hemiballism 820, 823
Hemic murmur 232
Hemicelluloses 456
Hemidesmosomes 30, 31
Hemiplegia 807, 810
   stages of 807
Hemochromatosis 116, 195, 474
Hemocytometer 111
Hemodialysis 514
Hemoglobin 2, 106, 111, 114f, 305, 357, 360t, 531
   based products 195
   concentration 358
   content, normal 111
   derivatives of 112
   falls 122
   functions of 112
   glycated 112
   oxygen dissociation curves for 360f
   oxygenation of 358
   percentage saturation of 358
   production, abnormalities of 113
   reaction of 112, 358
   reduced 112, 358, 361
   structure of 112
   synthesis of 113
Hemoglobinopathy 113
Hemolysins 110
Hemolysis 196
Hemolytic anemia 122, 125
Hemolytic disease 191
   of newborn, treatment of 191
Hemolytic reactions 195, 196
Hemophilia 24, 172, 173, 193, 666
   inheritance of 173, 173f
Hemopoiesis 117f
Hemopoietic function 422, 453
Hemorrhage, postpartum 193
Hemosiderin 116, 474
Hemosiderosis 474
Hemostasis 160, 164
   permanent 165
   primary 162, 164, 164fc
   secondary 165
   temporary 164
Henle loop 500, 500f, 504, 507f
Hensen's duct 948
Heparin 135, 170, 172, 314
   sulfate proteoglycans 486
Heparinase 172
Hepatic artery 304
   branches 444f
Hepatic bile 444, 444t
   composition of 445
Hepatic coma 982
Hepatic ducts 444
Hepatic portal circulation 304, 304fc
Hepatitis 193
Hepatocytes 443
Hepatopancreatic duct system 438f
Hephaestin 474
Hereditary methemoglobinemia 112
Hering's nerve 246, 371
Hering's theory 934
Hering-Breuer reflexes 368, 369
Hermaphroditism 669
Herpes zoster 790
Herring bodies 582
Hesche's gyrus 853
Heterocrine gland 640
Heterometric regulation 255
Heteronemous hemianopia 928f
Heterotrimeric G-protein 555, 555f
Heterozygous disorders 125
Hexamethonium 430, 867
Hexose monophosphate 111, 902
High pressure
   nervous syndrome 389
   neurological syndrome 389
   receptors 509
Hilus 484
Hindbrain 724
Hippocampal formation 885
Hirschsprung's disease 408, 466, 467, 659, 870
His-bundle 203, 205, 207
   electrogram 217, 217f
Histamine 132, 135, 296, 424, 428, 448, 656, 743, 877
   actions of 656
   fate of 656
Histidine 469
   decarboxylase 656
Histones 22
Histotoxic hypoxia 379, 380
Hodgkin's cycle 13
Hodgkin's disease 136, 138
Holger-Nielsen method 398, 399
Holmgren's colored wool test 935
Holocrine
   glands 411
   secretion 452
Holter technique 213
Homeostasis 11, 201, 483, 722
Homogenous semi-fluid mass 422
Homologous chromosomes 26, 668
Homovanillic acid 894
Homozygous disorder 125
Hormonal abnormalities 669
Hormonal control 292, 668
Hormonal disorders 668
Hormonal factors 292, 304, 326, 345, 428, 463, 501, 573, 676, 706
Hormonal feedback 463
Hormonal mechanism 491

Hormonal regulation 296, 430, 447, 453, 497, 644
Hormone 429, 547, 548, 549t, 556t
  actions of 650t
  assay of 549
  characteristics of 548
  deficiency 550
  degradation of 554
  effects of 375
  estimation of 599
  excess 551
  functions of 548
  genomic effects of 561
  mechanism of
    action of 556fc
    secretion of 582
  nongenomic effects of 561
  paracrine function of 650
  radioimmunoassay of 550f
  reserve, dynamic test of 550
  resistance 551
  secretion 12fc, 594
    regulation of 561, 562f
  sensitive receptor 555, 556
  sources of 678
  storage of 633
Horn
  anterior 727
  cells 243, 246, 728
  gating, dorsal 788
  posterior 772
Horner's syndrome 870, 903, 932
Hot flashes 696
Hot spots 295
Human chorionic
  gonadotropin 556, 557, 666, 680, 688, 702-704, 717
  somatomammotropin 577, 703, 705
  thyrotropin 703, 705
Human genome
  mapping of 23
  project 23, 24
Human growth hormone 572
Human heart 244
Human immunodeficiency virus 40, 149, 157, 807
Human leukocyte
  antigens 515
  associated antigen 151
Human milk, composition of 712t
Human physiology 1
Human placental lactogen 705
Human sexual responses, physiology of 696
Human tissue type plasminogen activator 171
Humidity, effects of 388
Humoral immunity 150, 153, 155t, 462
  mechanism of 154f
Hunger contractions, functions of 462
Huntington's disease 822
Hutchinson devised spirometer 331
Hyaline cast 525f
Hyaline membrane disease 326
Hyaluronic acid 608, 904
Hyaluronidase 675
Hydrocephalus, communicating 896
Hydrocholeretics 447
Hydrogen ions 371f
  buffering of 112
Hydrogen peroxide 980
Hydrops fetalis 191
Hydrostatic pressure 177, 498, 983

Hydrotropic effect 445
Hydroxy dehydroepiandrosterone sulfate 704
Hydroxyapatite crystals 608
Hydroxyindoleacetic acid 894
Hydroxyl radical 980, 981
Hydroxyl-indole-o-methyltransferase 743
Hymen 685
Hyoglossus muscle, strong contraction of 460
Hyperacusis 945, 957
Hyperaldosteronism
  primary 266, 374, 630
  secondary 630
Hyperalgesia 782, 790
  primary 790
  secondary 790
Hyperbaric chamber 390
Hyperbaric O_2 therapy 380, 390
  complications of 380
Hyperbarism 389
Hyperbola, rectangular 360, 360f
Hypercalcemia 613, 614
Hypercalciuria 613
Hypercapnia 248, 250, 257, 377, 710
  causes of 377
Hyperemia 288
  reactive 293, 297
Hypereosinophilia 137
Hyperesthesia 778, 812
Hyperfibrinogenemia 104
Hypergammaglobulinemia 104
Hyperglycemia 645, 646, 648, 650
  causes of 646fc
  temporary 464
Hyperhidrosis 537
Hyperimmune reaction 157
Hyperinsulinemia 647, 648
Hyperkalemia 506
Hyperkalemic periodic paralysis 37
Hyperkinetic movements, abnormal 820
Hyperlipidemia 298, 647, 912f
Hypermetropia 912
Hypernatremia 630
Hyperopia 912
Hyperosmia 973
Hyperosmolar medullary interstitium 507
Hyperparathyroidism 612, 613
  primary 613
  secondary 613
Hyperpigmentation 578
Hyperplasia 83
Hyperpolarization 50, 86
Hyperproteinemia 104
Hypersalivation 419
Hypersensitivity 137, 157
  causes of 82
  reaction 9, 135
Hypersexuality 862
Hypertension 265, 298, 716, 986
  essential 265
  malignant 265
  primary 265
  secondary 265
  types of 265
Hyperthermia
  constitutional 540
  malignant 76, 542
Hyperthyroidism 604, 713
  diagnosis of 606
  treatment of 606

Hypertonia 755, 799, 804, 810
Hypertonic solution 4
Hyperventilation 369, 377
Hypervitaminosis
  A 473
  D 473
  K 473
Hypervolemia 184
Hypesthesia 778
Hypnic myoclonia 878
Hypnotoxin 876
Hypoadrenalism 631
Hypoalbuminemia 104
Hypocapnia 377
  effects of 377
Hypochlorhydria 432
Hypochlorous acid 980, 981
Hypoesthesia 778
Hypogastric plexus 865
Hypogeusia 968
Hypoglycemia 428, 647, 648
  reactive 435, 464
Hypogonadism 680
  male 680
  primary 680
  secondary 680
Hypohidrosis 870
Hypokalemia 374, 464, 506, 630
  causes of 506
Hypokalemic nephropathy 630
Hypomenorrhea 695
Hyponatremia 9
Hypo-osmolarity 508
Hypoparathyroidism 612, 613
Hypophosphatemia 613
Hypophyseal arteries, inferior 566
Hypophyseal pouch 565
Hypophyseal stalk 565
Hypophysiotropic hormones 579
Hypoproteinemia 104, 496
Hypoprothrombinemia 173
Hyporeninemic hypoaldosteronism 631
Hyposecretion 432
Hyposmia 973
Hypotension 247, 266, 269
Hypothalamic disorders, features of 858
Hypothalamic eunuchism 680
Hypothalamic hypophyseal-thyroid axis 598
Hypothalamic neurons 877
Hypothalamic nucleus 855, 856f
Hypothalamic obesity 856
Hypothalamic pituitary-gonadal axis 670
Hypothalamic regions 856
Hypothalamic thermostat 540, 541
Hypothalamo-cerebellar circuits act 831
Hypothalamo-hypophyseal
  axis 580
  portal system 304, 565, 566, 566f
  tract 565, 566f, 582, 582f, 858
Hypothalamus 245, 247, 429, 538, 541, 548, 562, 565, 570, 579, 712, 794, 828, 853, 855, 864, 878
  anterior 268, 292
  connections of 855
  functions of 856
  paraventricular nuclei of 858
  release of 862
  role of 598, 693, 858
  ventromedial nuclei of 862

Hypothalamus-pituitary-adrenal axis 626
  central branch of 410
Hypothermia 388, 542
  advantages of 543
  severe 388
Hypothyroid iodide goiter 599
Hypothyroidism 600, 601
  central 600, 602, 604
  congenital 601
  pathophysiology of 603
  primary 600, 603
  secondary 600
  severe 602
  tertiary 600
  treatment of 604
Hypotonia 799, 807, 810, 813, 831
Hypotonic solution 4
Hypovolemia 183, 271fc
Hypoxia 58, 250, 257, 296, 378, 380, 710
  acute 377
  clinical features of 380
  direct effects of 248
  effects of 58, 373, 386, 742
  ischemic 379
  physiological adjustments to 387
  produces vasodilation 345
  severe 380
  types of 378
Hypoxic hypoxia 378, 386
Hypoxic pulmonary vasoconstriction 346
Hysteresis loop 338, 338f

I

I band 66
Ibuprofen 790
Ice water test 843
Icterus 446
Idiopathic non-toxic colloid goiter 600
Idiopathic thrombocytopenic purpura 174
Idioventricular rhythm 245
Ileocecal
  sphincter 455
  valve 451, 455
Ileum 451
Iliac artery, internal 865
Imminent rupture, point of 256
Immune
  function 103, 181
  modulation, transfusion-related 193
  response 146
  system 11, 144, 410, 625
    development of 148
  tolerance 149
Immunity 146
  acquired 150
  active 148
  adaptive 150
  cell mediated 150, 154f, 155t
  cellular 150, 152f
  innate 147
  natural 147
  passive 148
  specific 150
Immunization, passive 192
Immunoglobulin 147, 148, 153, 439
  A 325
  classes of 154
  molecule, structure of 154f
Immunological disorders 157

Index

Immunological function 703
Immunological memory 155, 156f
Immunological synapse 152, 153, 153f
Immunological tests 402, 705
Immunological tolerance 151, 156
Impulse
    production, ectopic foci of 219
    velocity of conduction of 207t
In vitro fertilization 16, 717
    therapy, complications of 9
Incretins 477, 650
Indomethacin 657
Inedible dry powder 418
Infancy, physiology of 977
Infantile Refsum disease 20
Infarction 174
Infectious mononucleosis 136, 137
Infertility 714, 717
Inflamed pleural surfaces 324
Inflammatory edema 181
Information
    storage of 721
    transmission of 761
Infundibulum 565, 855
Inhibition theory 822
Inhibitory enkephalinergic interneurons 788
Inhibitory interneurons 827
Inhibitory neurotransmitters 742
Injury
    effects of 758
    severe 58
Inorganic constituents 416, 438, 452
Inorganic phosphate 69
Inositol 1,4,5-triphosphate 867
Inositol triphosphate 556, 558
Insoluble fibrin 167, 167f
Insomnia 878
Inspiration, muscles of 321
Inspiratory capacity 332, 333
Inspiratory ramp signal 367, 367f, 368, 369
Inspiratory reserve volume 332, 333
Inspired air 351f
Insular gyrus 782
Insulin 440, 574, 617, 641, 649t, 650, 711, 858
    actions of 642, 643
    dependent diabetes mellitus 645
    effects of 642t
    like growth factor 549, 556, 568, 571, 575, 576, 608, 642, 644
    mechanism of action of 644
    metabolism 642
    receptor 643
        substrate 644, 645
        structure of 644f
    resistance 648
    secretion 642, 644t
        abnormalities of 645
        regulation of 644
    sensitivity, higher 983
    structure of 641f
Integral proteins 16, 17
Integrins 30, 31, 549
    deficiency of 135
Integumentary system 11
Intensity 765
    discrimination 53, 765, 967
Intention tremor 797, 831
Intercalated disc 85, 205
Intercellular communication 554
Intercellular connections 30, 31f
Intercostal muscles, external 322

Interferon-gamma 605
Interleukin 116, 118, 120, 138, 150, 163, 502, 540, 617
Interlobular ducts 414
Intermittent claudication 781
Internal capsule, posterior limb of 802
International sensitivity index 171
Interneurons 45, 729, 970
Internodal atrial pathways 206
Internodal pathways 206
Interoceptors 763
Interpeduncular cisterns 892
Intersegmental tract 805
Interstitial cell 685
    stimulating hormone 566, 676, 578
Interstitial edema 496
Interstitial fluid 201
    buffer system 2
    colloid osmotic pressure 180
    volume, measurement of 8
Interventricular septum, activation of 207f
Intestinal bacteria 456
    advantages of 456
Intestinal blood flow 303
Intestinal factors 429
Intestinal flora, harmful effects of 456
Intestinal functions, peripheral 409
Intestinal gastrin 431
Intestinal glands, small 452
Intestinal lipase 446
Intestinal lumen 470
Intestinal microcirculation 303
Intestinal mucosa 446
Intestinal obstruction 465
Intestinal phase 429, 431, 441
Intestinal smooth muscle cells 409
Intestinal villus 303
    movements of 465
Intestine 612, 615, 629
    law of 465
Intra-abdominal pressure, positive 256
Intra-alveolar pressure 324
Intracardiac lead 212
Intracellular buffering 3, 512
Intracellular canaliculi 426
Intracellular component 733
Intracellular edema 181
Intracellular fluid 5, 7, 69, 555, 624, 626, 838, 948
    buffer systems 2
Intracellular ligands 35
Intracorpuscular defects 122
Intracranial pressure 301
Intracranial tension 248, 895
Intracytoplasmic sperm injection 717
Intra-cytoplasmic tyrosine kinases 559
Intraesophageal pressure 324
Intralaminar nuclei 815
Intralobular duct 414
Intraocular fluid 7
Intraocular muscles 906
Intraocular pressure 904, 905
Intrapericardial pressure 256
Intrapleural pressure 324, 325, 327, 338f, 347
    measurement of 324
Intrapulmonary pressure 324, 325, 338f
Intrastriatal cholinergic system 822

Intrauterine contraceptive devices 714, 715f
Intrauterine devices 714
Intrauterine insemination 717
Intrauterine life 117, 568, 667, 669, 673, 685, 710
Intravascular anticoagulants 169
Intravascular clot 165
Intravascular coagulation 169
Intravenous cholangiography 449
Intravenous fluid 8
    therapy 8
Intravenous pyelography 525, 525f
Introns 22
Inulin 496
    clearance 496
Inverse stretch reflex 753, 754, 754f
Involuntary motor activity, role in 830
Involuntary muscles 90
Iodide
    administration of 419
    pump 593
    role of 599
    trapping 593
Iodine 473, 606
Iodopsin 920
Iodotyrosine
    coupling of 593
    deiodinase 594
Ion 473
    channels 35
    types of 36
Ionic calcium, functions of 610
Ionized calcium 377
Ionizing radiation 388, 392
Ionotropic receptor 554, 733, 735
Ipsilateral blindness 916
Ipsilateral ophthalmoplegia 807
Ipsilateral postcentral gyrus 966
Iris 903
    forms 902
    structure of 903f
Iron 473, 474
    absorption, regulation of 474
    deficiency 122
        anemia 111, 113, 116, 122, 123, 124f, 422, 464
    dextran complex 124
    distribution of 115t
    transport protein transferrin 115
Irradiation 677, 757
    clinical manifestation of 392
Irritable bowel syndrome 410, 466
Ischemic pain 781
Ischemic tissues 275
Ishihara's chart 935, 935f
Islet hormones, concentrations of 440
Isoantigens 186
Isoleucine 469
Isomerase enzyme 922
Isometric contraction 71, 225, 228, 229, 230
Isometric exercise 984, 985
    benefits of 985
Isometric muscle contraction 71t
Isometric relaxation phase 226, 228, 230
Isotonic contraction 71
Isotonic exercise 984, 985
    benefits of 984
Isotonic muscle contraction 71t
Isovolumetric contraction phase 226, 230

Isovolumetric relaxation phase 226
Isthmus 591, 794
Itching 769, 773, 780

J

Jacobson's organ 973
Jaeger's chart 914
Janus tyrosine kinases 559, 560, 569
Jaundice 114, 125, 446, 446f, 531
    acholuric 111, 115, 447
    cholestatic 447
    hemolytic 446
    hepatic 446, 447
    hepatocellular 446
    obstructive 446
    physiological 111, 115
    posthepatic 446, 447
    prehepatic 446
    prolonged neonatal 601
    types of 446, 447t
Jaw bone, lower 571
Jejunum 451, 470
Jendrassik's maneuver 750, 799
Jod-Basedow effect 599
J-receptors 368
J-reflex 369
Jugular pulse tracing 283
Jugular vein, internal 283, 300
Jugular venous pulse 283, 283f
Juxtaglomerular apparatus 487, 488, 488f, 501
    functions of 488
Juxtaglomerular hypothesis 491
Juxtamedullary nephron 487, 487f
    structure of 485f
Juxtapulmonary capillary receptors 369

K

K cells 478
Kallidin 412
Kallmann's syndrome 696
Kaposi's sarcoma 157
Kartagener's syndrome 314
Karyokinesis 27
Kaspar Hauser syndrome 577
K-complexes 875
Kent bundle 221
Keratin 31
Keratoconus 913
Keratopathy 605
Kernicterus 191, 823
Ketoacidosis 646
    production of 646fc
Ketogenic hormone 569
Ketone bodies 646
Ketosteroids 679
Kety's method 294, 300
Kidney 483, 488, 611, 616, 628, 655
    artificial 514, 514f
    blood supply of 488, 489fc
    functional anatomy of 483, 484
    goldblatt hypertension 509
    nerve supply of 484
    regional blood flow to 490
    role of 185
Kinesin 18, 46
Kinesthesia 779
Kinesthetic sensation 779
Kinetic energy 240
Kinins 484
Kinocilium 839
Kisspeptin 687
Kleitman's theory 877
Klinefelter's syndrome 668, 669

Kluver-Bucy syndrome 862
Knee jerk 752, 831
    absence of 752
    pendular 832
Kolliker-Fuse nucleus 367
Korotkoff's sounds 236, 264
Krause's end bulb 778
Krenein 547
Kupffer cells 134, 142, 152, 304, 443, 444
Kussmaul breathing 3, 321, 512, 646
Kyphoscoliosis 333

L

Labor contractions 706
Labyrinthectomy, bilateral 844
Labyrinthine
    apparatus 946
    righting reflex 842, 847
Lacrimal apparatus 907
Lacrimal ducts 907
Lacrimal gland 907
Lactase 470
    deficiency 470
Lactate dehydrogenase 298
Lactation 711, 712
    amenorrhea 577, 713, 714
    initiation of 712
    maintenance of 712
Lactic acid 296, 396, 876, 904
Lactic acidosis 250, 272, 397
Lactobacilli 456
Lactoferrin 139, 416, 907
Lactose intolerance 470
Lactotrophs, tumor of 578
Lactrodectus mactans 82
Lambert-Eaton
    myasthenic syndrome 82
    syndrome 37
Lamina 235
    fenestra 486
    propria 407, 685
    terminalis, organum vasculosum of 541, 857
Laminins 30, 31, 60
Landsteiner's laws 188
Langerhans dendritic cells 152
Langerhans islets 438, 640, 641f, 650
Laparoscopy 716
Laplace law 239, 240, 327, 522
Large artery, dilatation of 658
Large intestine 455
    functions of 455
    movements of 459, 466
    parts of 455f
L-arginine 484
    oxidation of 981
Laron dwarfism 572
Laryngeal stridor 613
Larynx 314, 315
Late dumping syndrome 435, 464
Lateralis dorsalis 795
Laurence-Beidel-Moon syndrome 858
Learning 741, 884
    intercortical transfer of 884, 889
    mechanisms of 884
Lee-Jones test 380
Left bundle branch 207
Left ventricular
    contraction 256
    pressure changes 228
    wall 204
Leishman's stain 118, 131, 132
Lemniscal system, medial 771

Lens 906
    biconcave 912f
    biconvex 912f
    suspensory ligament 903, 906
Leptin 648, 670, 857, 858
    receptors 535
Lesions, storage 194
Lethal temperature 540
Leucine 469, 650
Leucotomy, prefrontal 853
Leuenkephalin 408, 789
Leukemia 136
Leukemoid reaction 136
Leukocytes 131, 131f, 136t
    functions of 134
    properties of 134
Leukocytosis 136
Leukopenia 136
Leukopoiesis 116, 138
    control of 138
    stages of 138fc
Leukotrienes 516
Liddle's syndrome 37, 266
Lieberkuhn crypts 411, 452
Ligament, suspensory 909
Ligamentum
    arteriosum 306, 710
    teres 305, 710
    venosum 305, 710
Light adaptation 925
Light reflex 930
Lignin 456
Lignocaine 791
Limb
    ascending 486, 487
    descending 486, 487
    efferent 748, 752
    leads 210, 211
    thick ascending 487
Limb-girdle muscular dystrophies 76
Limbic cortex 247, 267, 849
Limbic lobe 849, 860
Limbic system 429, 860, 861, 864
    components of 860f
    connections of 861
    functions of 861
    parts of 860
    role of 861
Linear acceleration 288, 838
Lingual lipase 416, 471
Lingula 825
Lipase 132, 452
Lipid 121
    complex mixture of 325
    matrix 34
    metabolism 635
    peroxide 980
    peroxyl 980
    profile estimation 599
    soluble 971
Lipofuscin 46
    granules 19
Lipogenesis 624
Lipolysis 596
Lipolytic hormones 635
Lipoprotein 16, 159
Lipostatic hypothesis 857
Lippes loop 714, 715f
Lips, bluish discoloration of 381f
Liquor folliculi 687
Lissauer's tract 772, 773
Lithium carmine 142
Litocholic acid 445
Little brain 408

Liver
    biopsy 449
    cells 549, 642
    cirrhosis of 304, 447, 713
    diseases, chronic 104
    function tests 448
    functions of 443
    investigations of 448
    lobule, histology of 443f
    role of 170
    structural organization of 444f
    system 443
Lobe
    anterior 825
    posterior 825
Lobectomy, prefrontal 853, 886
Lobules, number of 443
Lobulus centralis 825
Lobulus simplex 825
Local enteric reflex 408f, 430
Local hormones, synthesis of 656t
Local reflex 268, 408, 453
Local skin temperature reflexes 539
Lochia 707
Locus coeruleus 816, 877, 878
Loop diuretics 502
Loud sound, attenuation of 945fc, 946
Low body temperature 874
Low glucocorticoid level 874
Low-density lipoprotein 40, 457, 621, 688
Lower esophageal
    incompetence 461
    sphincter 420, 431, 461
    functions of 420
Lower motor neuron 798, 799, 801, 805, 806t, 812
Lower urinary tract 519
Low-ionic-strength saline 192
Low-pitched rustling sound 323
Low-pressure receptors 509
Lumbar puncture 727, 894
    therapeutic uses of 894
    uses of 894
Lumbar vertebra 727
Lumirhodopsin 921
Lumirubin, water-soluble 115
Lung 327
    amniotic fluid 977
    blood supply of 319
    cancer 328, 986
    capacity 332, 333
    collapse of 338
    compliance of 326, 334, 338
    constitute ventilation 321
    diffusing capacity of 322, 354
    diseases 108, 381
    elastic
        behavior of 325
        recoil 366
    elasticity of 334
    fibrosis of 328, 374
    hyperinflation of 327
    innervation of 318
    level 361
    lobectomy of 338
    mechanism of ventilation of 322
    parts of 348
    physiological unit of 317
    primary lobule of 317
    respiratory unit of 317
    rupture of 319
    synthesize surfactant 314

    tumors 333
    volume 332, 338, 347, 401
Luschka foramen 892
Luteinizing hormone 549, 556, 557, 562, 566, 567, 578, 589, 624, 688
    releasing hormone 693
    role of 688
Luteolysis 688
Lymph 99, 179, 179t
    capillary, structure of 179f
    flow 180
    formation 180
    functions of 180
    movement of 180
    rate of flow of 180
    valve 179
Lymph node 142, 595
    number of 179
Lymphadenopathy 181
Lymphatic pump 180
Lymphatic system 179, 180
Lymphedema 181
Lymphocyte 133, 133f, 137
    clone of 149
    count 880
    formation of 138
    functions of 135
    large 133
    majority of 133
    small 133
    stem cells 138
Lymphocytosis 137
Lymphoid growth curve 576
Lymphoid leukemia, chronic 136f
Lymphoid organs 141
Lymphoid progenitor cell, common 118
Lymphopenia 137
Lymphotoxin 153
Lysine 469, 644
Lysophospholipid 558
Lysosomal enzyme 439
Lysosomal storage disorders 20
Lysosome 19, 20t, 132, 147, 416, 907
    functions of 19

M

Macrocytes 106
Macrocytic anemia 124f, 124f
Macrocytic normochromic anemia 124
Macroglobulin 170
Macula densa cells 488, 497
Macula lutea 904
Macular sparing 916, 929
Magendie foramen 892
Magnet reaction 846
Magnocellular pathway 929
Malabsorption syndrome 466
Malleus, handle of 944
Malnutrition 181
Malpighian corpuscle 485
Maltase 470
Mammary gland 531
    development of 711f
    pair of 684
Mammillary body 856f
Mammillothalamic tract 861
Mammotropin 567
Mandibular prognathism 571
Manganese 473
Mannose-binding lectin pathway 146
Manteaux test 402
Marble bone disease 617

Index

Marey's law 247
Masklike facies 821
Mass
    peristalsis 466
    reflex 811
    spectrometer 352
    sympathetic discharge 869
Mast cell 133, 318
    activation of 146
    degranulation 146
Master gene 870
Masticatory salivary reflex 419
Maternal behavior 861
Maternal blood across 978
Maternal origin, active X
        chromosome of 666
Mcardle syndrome 76
Mean aortic pressure, effects of 295
Mean blood pressure 263f
Mean corpuscular hemoglobin 113
Mechanical fragility 110
Mechanical stimuli 292
Mechanoreceptors 419
Medulla 459, 802, 807, 835
    hypothalamus 245
    inner 620, 654, 666, 684
    oblongata 245, 370f
    reticular formation of 245
Medullary lamina 794
Medullary lesions 376
Megakaryoblast 162
Megakaryocyte 162
    erythroid progenitor 116
Megaloblastic anemia 121, 122
Megaloblasts 124, 426
Meibomian glands 907
Meiosis 27, 28f, 674
    significance of 29
Meissner's corpuscle 762, 763, 764, 768
Meissner's plexus 407-409, 430
Melanin 17, 529, 815
Melanocyte 529, 531
    stimulating hormone 531, 556
Melanopsin 587, 924
Melanotropins 578
Melatonin 587, 878
    functions of 588
    role of 878
    secretion 588fc
        regulation of 588, 588fc
    synthesis of 588, 588fc
    uses of 588
Membrane permeability 556
Membrane phospholipase-
        phospholipid system 558
Membrane stabilizer 54
Membranous labyrinth 946
Memory 724, 741, 796, 884, 885
    B cells 149, 153
    cells 153f
    classification of 885
    immunologic 150
    implicit 885
    long-term 885
    loss of 862
    pleasurable olfactory 969
    progressive loss of 886
    recognition 885
    response 146
    short-term 741, 885
    T cells 149
    working 885
Meniere's disease 844
Meninges 727f

Meningioma 726
Meningitis 376
Menopause 617, 690, 696
Menorrhagia 695
Menstrual cycle 686, 689f, 693f, 694f
Menstrual induction 718
Menstrual regulation 717
Menstruation 712
    abnormalities of 694
Mental confusion 288
Mental sweating 537
Menthol 781
Mercury salts 419
Merkel's disc 762, 764
    found 775
Merocrine glands 411
Mesenteric artery, superior 303
Mesenteric ganglia 409, 865
Mesocortex 849
Mesoderm 702
Messenger ribonucleic acid 22, 557
Metabolic acidosis 2, 373, 374, 511
    causes of 374
Metabolic adjustments 983
Metabolic alkalosis 2, 374, 464, 630
Metabolic function 483
Metabolic myopathies 76
Metabolic syndrome 266, 648, 695
Metabolic theory 270
Metabolism 568, 623, 633, 649, 978, 979
Metamorphosis 596
Metaphase, stage of 685
Metathyroid diabetes 595
Metencephalin 408, 789
Methemoglobin 112, 378
Methemoglobinemia 381
Methionine 469
Methyl mercaptan 973
Methyl tetrahydrofolate 125
Methylene blue 131, 132
Metrorrhagia 695
Metyrapone test 550
Micelle 446, 472
    formation 446
Microbial metabolites, role of 410
Microbiota-gut-brain axis 410
Microcytes 106
Microcytic hypochromic anemia 122
Microglia 726
Micro-hematocrit tube 107
Microneurography 763
Micropill 716
Micropipettes 498
Micropuncture technique 498
Microvascular bed 290
Micturition 520
Midbrain 724, 802, 807, 835
    animal 847
Mid-collicular section 846
Middle ear 944
    contents of 944
    disease 943
    functions of 944, 945
    muscles 944
        functions of 945, 946
    ossicles 944
        functions of 944
Mifepristone 692, 718
Migrating motor complex 462, 464
Migrating myoelectrical complex 462
Miliaria 542, 543f
Milk
    producing effect 711
    secretion 711, 712, 712f

Milk ejection 711, 712, 712f
    reflex 584, 585, 585fc
Miller-Abbot's tube 452
Mineral 473
    absorption of 473
    metabolism 635, 643
Mineralocorticoids 621, 628
Minilaparotomy 716
Minimal air volume 333
Minipill 716
Minisatellites 26
Minus sign 48, 927
Minute ventilation 335
Minute volume 253
Miosis 903, 903f
Mirror neurons 801
Misoprostol 718
Missense mutation 24
Mitochondria 21, 46
    functions of 21
Mitochondrial enzyme 934
Mitochondrial membrane 535
Mitochondrial metabolic myopathy 76
Mitogen 576
    activated protein kinase 560
Mitral area 230, 231
Mitral valve 204
Mixed acini 413, 414
Modiolus 947
Molecular layer, external 826
Molecular motors 18, 46
Molecular motors, functions of 18
Molecule transmitter, large 742, 744
Molybdenum 473
Monge's disease 387
Monoamine oxidase 633, 822, 867
Monocyte 133, 134f, 137, 147
    colony stimulating factor 139
    formation of 138
    functions of 135
Monocytopenia 137
Monoglyceride 472
Monoiodothyronine 592
Monoiodotyrosine 593
Monophasic recording 48, 51
Monoplegia 806
Monosaccharides 469
Monosynaptic reflex 748, 749, 749f
Monosynaptic stretch reflex 749
Monro foramen 891
Monro-Kellie doctrine 301
Morning headache 376
Morula 702
Motility 406
Motion sickness 844
Motor activity, segmental loss of 813
Motor aphasia 888, 889
Motor area, secondary 802
Motor cortex 267, 366, 801, 826
Motor function 44, 721, 796
Motor neuron 758, 864
    disease 419
    pool 748
    structure of 45f
Motor nucleus, dorsal 250
Motor pathway 800
Motor speech 887
Motor unit recruitment 75
Mountain sickness
    acute 386
    chronic 387
Mouth-to-mouth method 398
Movement
    decomposition of 832

sense, rate of 779
    types of 459
Mucin 416, 424
Mucociliary transport 314
Mucopolysaccharide metabolism 596
Mucosa 406
Mucous acini 413, 414
Mucous cells 423, 424, 470
Mucous glands 411, 413, 420
Mucous neck cells 424
Muller's cells 919
Muller's doctrine 766
Muller's maneuver 324, 325
Muller's muscle 932
Mullerian duct 667
    regression factor 666
Mullerian inhibiting substance 666, 667
Mullerian regression factor 667, 676
Multinodular goiter 600
Multiple myeloma 104
Multiple sclerosis 20, 47
Multiplication-stimulating activity 577
Multipolar neurons 45, 45f
Multistage bleep test 984
Multiunit smooth muscle 90, 90f, 91f, 91t
Mumps 419
Murmur 232
    causes of 232t
    classification of 232t
    continuous 232
    diastolic 232
    types of 232
Muscarinic receptors, sites of 867
Muscle
    abdominal 322
    accessory 321
    atrophy 83, 831
    blood flow 395, 983
    cells, atrophy of 979
    denervation of 82
    extensor group of 846
    fatigue 75
    flexor group of 845
    functions best 985
    growth 679
    heaviness of 397
    hypertrophy 83
    metabolism 73
    proteins 66
    relaxation, mechanism of 70
    secondary 321
    twitch, simple 68, 68f
    wasting 83, 646
    weakness 630
Muscle contraction
    mechanism of 70f
    types of 71
Muscle fiber 72, 72f, 755f
    groups of 83
    ventricular 86f, 89f
Muscle spindle 749, 750, 751f, 755f, 755t, 799
    functions of 751
    innervation of 749, 750f
    role of 799f
    structure of 750f
Muscle tone 68, 798, 804, 846
    control of 836
    higher control of 804f
    loss of 813
    maintenance of 820

Muscular activity 534
  gradation of 75
Muscular component 230, 462
Muscular dystrophy 75
Muscular exercise 250, 265
Muscular pain, ischemic 786
Muscular system 391, 597
Muscularis
  externa 406
  mucosa 407
Musculoskeletal system 624, 979
Mushroom poison 867
Mutant genes 669
Mutation
  effects of 24
  types of 24
Myasthenia gravis 82, 104, 419, 461
Mycobacterium leprae 135
Mydriasis 903, 903f
Myelin
  functions of 47
  protein zero 47
  sheath 46, 47
Myelinated axon 57f
Myelination 57, 597, 726
Myelinogenesis 46
Myelitis, transverse 393, 810
Myeloid
  leukemia, chronic 137
    phase 117
  progenitor cell, common 118
  series 117
Myeloperoxidase 132, 135
  deficiency, congenital 136
Myeloproliferative disorders 137
Myenteric plexus 407, 408
  neurons of 409
  neurotransmitters of 408t
  stimulation, effects of 408
Myenteric reflex 465
Myobril, structure thick filament
    of 67f
Myocardial cell, working 85
Myocardial compliance 256
Myocardial infarction 171, 221, 276,
    297, 298f, 376, 399
  acute 222f, 277f
  causes of 297
  treatment of 299
Myocardial ischemia 295
Myocardial necrosis 542
Myocardial oxygen demand 294
Myocardium 203
Myofibril 65f
  electron microscopic structure
    of 66, 66f
  thin filament of 68f
Myogenic contraction 165
Myogenic hypothesis 497
Myogenic theory 270, 491
Myogenic tone, intrinsic 421
Myoglobin 112, 115, 360, 360f, 360t
Myomesin 66
Myometrium 685, 691
Myoneural junction 79
Myopathy 75
Myopia 18, 66, 90, 912, 912f
Myosin
  head, re-cocking of 69
  light chain
    kinase 92
    phosphatase 92
  regulatory chain of 92
  structure of 67, 67f
Myotatic reflex 749

Myotome 727
Myxedema 596, 602, 602f
  coma 603
  madness 602

N

N-acetyl galactosaminyltransferase
    187
Narcolepsy 858, 878
Nasal bones 571
Nasal cavity 313, 314
Natriuresis 185, 656
Natriuretic peptide, B-type 656
Natural killer 148
  cell 133, 145, 147, 148, 157
  T cells 148
Nausea, sensations of 429
Nauseating pain 781, 784
Near point 909
  receding of 911
Near reflex 910
Near vision 910f
  test for 914
Near-sightedness 912
Neck righting reflex 847
Neck, position of 336
Necrosis appear, areas of 690
Neocerebellum 826
Neocortex 849, 850
Neospino-thalamic pathway 784
Neostigmine 82
Nephrin 486
Nephron 485
  different segments of 487f, 499t
  functions of 485
  parts of 485
  proximal tubule of 500f
  segments of 504
  types of 487
Nephrotic syndrome 495, 513
Nerve 46
  action potential latent period 52f
  aortic 371
  auditory 957
  buffer 246
  cardiac 243
  cell body 45, 58
  cochlear 954
  deafness 957-959, 960
  gas 81
  glossopharyngeal 965, 966
  growth factor 61, 416, 576, 781
  hypogastric 519
  impulse, conduction of 56, 56f, 57f
  pelvic 304, 409, 520
    splanchnic 866
  peripheral 44, 58
  physiology 44
  pudendal 466
  root 813
  sinoaortic 247, 371
  sinus 371
  somatic 407
  splanchnic 409, 438, 621
  trigeminal 779
  tympanic 415
  vagus 304, 409, 410, 966
  vasomotor 484
  X cranial 965
Nerve fiber 89f
  afferent 952
  classification of 57, 57t
  myelinated 56
  properties of 48
  single 54

Nerve injury
  classification of 58
  types of 58
Nervous system 243, 548, 603, 721,
    721t, 722, 875, 979
  centers of 723
  functions of 721
  integrative function of 723
  intrinsic 407
  motor part of 723
  organization of 722fc
  peripheral 46, 59f, 722
  physiology of 731
  sensory
    division of 761
    portion of 723
Neural activity, basis of 722
Neural crest 654
Neural factors 243, 257, 267, 292,
    491, 501
Neural growth curve 575
Neural hormones 582
Neural mechanism 430
Neural regulation 250, 296, 304, 440,
    447, 453, 497, 645
Neural tube 891
Neurexins 734
Neurilemma 46
Neuroeffector junction 91
Neuroendocrine
  reflex 578, 584, 585, 588, 712
  tumor 477
Neurofibrils 46
Neurogenesis 886
Neurogenic diabetes insipidus 509,
    583
Neurogenic edema 782
Neurogenic hypertension 265
Neuroglia 724
Neuroglobin 112
Neurohormones 744
Neurohypophyseal bud 565
Neurohypophysis 855
Neuro-immuno-endocrine
    mediators 410
Neuroligin 884
Neurological disorders 903
Neuroma 61
Neuromodulators 742
Neuromuscular blocking drugs 81
Neuromuscular junction 75, 79, 79f,
    91, 867
Neurons 45, 724
  afferent 747, 749
  classification of 44
  dorsal respiratory group of 366
  efferent 45
  lack centrosome 19
  length of 45
  myelination of 46
  postganglionic 867
  postsynaptic 731, 735, 866
  preganglionic parasympathetic
    865
  processes of 46
  types of 45f
  unipolar 44
Neuronal plasticity 879
Neuropathic pain 790
Neuropathy, peripheral 47
Neuropeptide 742, 744, 744t
  Y 302, 410, 580, 744
Neurophysin 582
Neuroplasticity 742, 886
Neuropraxia 58

Neurosyphilis 813
Neurotendinous spindle 754
Neurotensin 304, 408
Neurotmesis 58
Neurotransmitter 36, 80, 548, 656,
    742
  actions of 735
  classification of 742
  gaba 850
  glutamate 919
Neurotrophic factor 887
Neurotrophin 60, 887
Neurovascular hilus 72
Neutral stimulus 883
Neutropenia 136
Neutrophil 132, 132f, 136, 147, 666f
  diapedesis of 134f
  functions of 134
  hypomotility syndrome 135
  phagocytose bacteria 317
Neutrophilia 136
Newborn's skull 977
Newborn's sympathetic system 978
Newtonian fluids 238
Nicotine 867, 886
Nicotinic acetylcholine receptors
    80, 82
Nicotinic receptors 80, 658, 867
Niemann-Pick disease 20
Nifedipine 36, 387
Night blindness 925
Nigrostriatal dopaminergic system
    822
Nissl bodies 46
Nissl granules 46
Nitrates 296
Nitric oxide 112, 161, 169, 268, 273,
    492, 516, 658, 697, 744,
    867, 980, 981
  actions of 658
  radical 981
  reaction with 113
  synthase 658
Nitrogen
  balance 624, 679, 812
  dioxide 980
  meter 336
  narcosis 389
  species, reactive 980
Nitroglycerine 296
Nitrous acid 980
N-methyl-d-aspartate receptors 884
Nociceptive afferents 485
Nociceptors 369, 762, 863
Nocturia 513
Nocturnal enuresis 521, 878
Nodes of Ranvier 46
Nodulus 825
Noise 950
Nominal aphasia 889
Non-depolarizing neuromuscular
    blocker 81
Non-dominant hemisphere 849
Non-genomic action 598
Non-hemolytic reactions 195, 196
Non-hormonal
  disorders 660, 670
  factors 270
Nonionic diffusion 4, 506, 512
Non-newtonian fluid 234, 235
Non-rapid eye movement 570, 876t
Nonsense mutation 25
Nonsensory tracts 772, 773
Non-shivering thermogenesis 535,
    539

Index

Non-ST elevation myocardial infarction 298, 298f
Non-steroidal anti-inflammatory drugs 424, 433
Non-viral vectors 26
Non-volatile acids 510
Noradrenaline 635t, 656, 697, 867
Norepinephrine 121, 262, 269, 318, 408, 409, 484, 492, 535, 538, 650, 743, 789, 819, 835, 855, 867, 877
    combination of 869
    intravenous infusion of 636f
Nose, mucous membrane of 315
Nuchal translucency 669
Nuclear
    cholescintigraphy 449
    division 27
    envelope 22
    pores 22
    receptors 554
    sex 664
Nucleic acid 471
    absorption of 471
    digestion of 471
    metabolism 643
    splitting enzymes 439
Nucleosidase 132, 471
Nucleosome 22
Nucleotidase 471
Nucleus 15, 22, 46, 132, 795
    ambiguus 245, 367, 462
    anterior 795
    arcuate 856f
    basalis 886
    caudate 803, 815
    cochlear 961f
    cranial nerve 803f, 930
    cuneatus 771, 773, 775, 779
    dentate 825
    dorsalis 728
    dorsolateral 795, 796
    dorsomedial 795, 856f
    emboliformis 825
    fastigial 825
    globosus 825
    gracilis 771, 773, 775, 779
    hypoglossal 800
    lateroventral 795, 796
    lenticular 815
    lentiform 815
    magnus 835
    parabrachialis medialis 367
    paraventricular 505, 563, 582, 585, 856f
    posterolateral 795, 796
    posteroventral 781, 795
    proprius 728
    raphe 789, 816, 877
    red 803, 835, 846
    retroambigualis 367
    sensory 780
    subthalamic 815, 816
    suprachiasmatic 587, 589, 856f, 929
    supraoptic 563, 856f
    tractus solitarius 245, 247, 248, 265, 400, 462, 864
    ventral posterior 771
    ventral posterolateral 771, 773, 775, 777-779, 784
    ventromedial 856f
    visceral afferent 728
Nutritional deficiency disorder 123
Nutritive function 99, 180, 405, 969

Nyctalopia 925
Nystagmus 832, 842, 843

O

O gene 187
Obesity 648
Obstructive lung disease 335f
Obstructive pulmonary disease, chronic 336, 345, 349, 401
Occipital cortex 929
Occipital lobe 849, 853, 885
Ocular hypertension 905
Oculocardiac reflex 249
Oculomotor nerve, unilateral lesion of 907
Odor 524
    detection threshold 973
    masking of 973
Odynophagia 460
Ohm's law 235, 304
Olfaction 967, 969, 980
Olfactometer 973
Olfactory adaptation 973
Olfactory apparatus 969
Olfactory bulb 970, 971f
Olfactory cilia 970
Olfactory discrimination, areas of 972
Olfactory epithelium 969
Olfactory function 314, 973
Olfactory gland 970
Olfactory glomerulus 970, 972
Olfactory hallucinations 974
Olfactory information, processing of 972
Olfactory memories 972
Olfactory mucosa 969, 971f
    innervation of 971
    location of 970f
Olfactory neuron, peculiar feature of 970
Olfactory nucleus, anterior 972
Olfactory pathway 971, 972fc
Olfactory receptor cell 764, 969
Olfactory sensory neuron 971
Olfactory threshold 973
Olfactory tract 972
Olfactory tubercle 972
Oligodendrocytes 46, 47, 726, 927
Oligodendroglioma 726
Oligomenorrhea 695
Oligosaccharides 456
Oliguria 513
Olivary nucleus
    inferior 803, 805, 828
    superior 954, 961f
Olivocochlear bundle 949, 956
Olivospinal tract 805
Omeprazole 434
Oncotic pressure 103
Ondine's curse 366
One-way valves 893
Oocyte
    maturation inhibitor 685
    primary 685
    secondary 685
Oogenesis 668f, 685, 686fc
Oogonia 685
Ophthalmology 901
Ophthalmoscope 896, 904
Opioid peptides 744
Opponent color theory 934fc
Opposite color pairs 934
Opsins 921
Opsonins 134

Opsonization 134, 146
Optic axis 909
Optic chiasma, lesion of 928f, 931
Optic disc 903, 904
Optic nerve, lesion of 931
Optic tract 928, 931
Optical aberrations 913
Oral cholecystography 449, 449f
Oral contraceptive pills 715, 715f
Oral glucose tolerance test 647
Oral rehydration solution 473
Orbitofrontal cortex 853, 972
Orchitis 157, 419, 677, 878
Orcin stain 666
Organ and tissues 654t
Organ of corti 948, 948f, 949t
Organelles 15
Organic acids 456
Organic constituents 416, 438, 445, 452
Orgasm, time of 697
Oropharyngeal airway 398
Oropharynx, normal anatomy of 460f
Orthodromic conduction 56
Orthopnea 321
Orthostatic albuminuria 513
Orthostatic hypotension 266
Osmolality 3
Osmolarity 3
Osmoreceptors 408, 508, 857, 863
Osmosis 3, 34, 498, 504, 893
    law of 473
Osmotic diuresis 522, 646
Osmotic fragility 110
Osmotic pressure 3, 34, 99
Ossicular conduction 952
Osteitis fibrosa 613
Osteoblasts 608
Osteocalcin 608
Osteoclastic activity 611
Osteocytes 609
Osteocytic osteolysis 609, 611
Osteomalacia 616
Osteonectin 608
Osteopetrosis 605, 616, 617, 627
Osteoprotegerin, stimulation of 691
Ota ring 714
Otic ganglion 866
Otitis media 945
Otoconia 840
Otolith organ 840
Otosclerosis 944, 946
Ovarian agenesis 668
Ovarian cycle 686
Ovarian follicle and testes 692
Ovarian function, control of 693
Ovarian hormones 690t
Ovarian tumors 696
Ovariectomy 617
Ovary
    endocrine function of 690
    functions of 685
    structure of 685f
Overcome elastic resistance 339
Ovulation 687
    induction 717
    mechanism of 687
    tests of 696
Oxidants 135, 980
Oxidase 135
Oxidative phosphorylation 21, 74, 313
Oxidative stress 981
Oxygen 314
    carrying capacity of hemoglobin 358

    dissociation curve 388
    hemoglobin dissociation curve 358, 359f, 513
    species, reactive 980
    therapy 380
    toxicity 389
        symptoms of 380, 390
    transport of 357
Oxygenation, advantages of 358
Oxygen-hemoglobin dissociation curve, shift of 359f
Oxyhemoglobin 112, 358, 361
Oxyntic gland 423, 423t
Oxytocin 584, 706
    actions of 584
    release of 697
    secretion 584
    uses of 585
Ozone 980

P

P cells 205
P wave 213
    abnormalities 218
Pacchionian bodies 893
Pacemaker 205, 218
    abnormal 207
    cells 85, 411
    ectopic 207
    tissue 86
    waves 411
Pacinian corpuscle 762-764
Packed cell volume 107, 107f
Packed red cell 193
    volume 107, 108
Pain
    acute 125, 784
    affective nature of 796
    causes of 781
    chronic 784
    control 789
    pathway 782
    perception
        gate control theory of 788, 788f, 789
        theory of 788
    radiating 787
    reaction to 785
    receptors 762, 781
    reference 787, 788f
    referred 787
    sensation 781, 790
        components of 782
        control of 788
        pathway for superficial 783
        types of superficial 783
    sharp pricking 783
    superficial 782, 782t
    types of 782
Paleocerebellum 826
Paleospinothalamic pathway 784
Pallidotomy 822
Palpatory method 264
Palpebral conjunctiva, appearance of 122f
Palpitation 870
Pancreas
    cystic fibrosis of 441
    histological structure of 641f
Pancreatic amylase 439
    acts 470
Pancreatic carcinoma 441
Pancreatic duct cells 440f
Pancreatic function tests 441
Pancreatic insufficiency 470

Pancreatic islet hormones 651t
Pancreatic juice 438, 469
　　cephalic phase of 440
　　composition of 438
　　mechanism of secretion of 440
　　nucleases of 471
　　regulation of secretion of 440
　　secretion 441
Pancreatic lipase 439, 472
Pancreatic polypeptide 441, 650
　　regulation of secretion of 650
Pancreatitis 441
　　acute 439, 441
　　chronic 441
Pancreozymin 426, 440
Pancytopenia 137
Panhypopituitarism 570, 579
Pap stain 666
Paper recording 212
Papez circuit 853, 860, 861, 861fc
Papilla 529
Papillary duct 487
Papillary muscles 204
Papilledema 894-896
Paraaminohippuric acid 490
Paracrine
　　control 406
　　secretion 547, 547f
Paradoxical sleep 875, 876
Parageusia 968
Parahippocampal gyrus 860
Paralysis 758, 805
　　agitans 820
Paralytic ileus 465
Paralytic salivary secretion 420
Paralytic secretion 420, 453
Paraplegia 806, 810
Parasomnia 878
Parasympathetic defecation reflex 466
Parasympathetic fibers 438, 677
　　mechanism of action of 245
Parasympathetic nervous system 418fc, 863, 869
　　functional anatomy of 865
Parasympathetic nucleus, accessory 910
Parasympathetic reflex 678
Parasympathetic stimulation 257, 296, 418, 425
　　effects of 409
Parasympathetic supply 300, 409, 415, 420
Parasympathetic system, functions of 409
Parasympathetic tone 244, 866
Parasympathetic vasodilator fibers 268
Parathormone 503, 516, 574, 610, 712
Parathyroid
　　glands 610
　　hormone 515, 556, 557, 610
　　　　regulation of secretion of 612
Paravertebral ganglia 865
Parenchymatous goiter 600
Paresis 758
Paresthesia 778, 814
Parietal cells 406, 423, 426
　　autoimmune destruction of 124
Parietal gland 423
Parietal layer 203, 486
Parietal lobe 849, 853
Parietal pain 788
Parietal pleura 318, 786
Parieto-occipital sulcus 849

Parkinson's disease 20, 22, 419, 743, 820-822, 979, 981
　　treatment of 821
Parkinsonism 870
Parosmia 974
Parotid gland 413, 415
　　sialogram of 415f
Parotin 416
Paroxysmal atrial tachycardia 220
Paroxysmal hypertension 637
Paroxysmal tachycardia 208, 220
Paroxysmal ventricular tachycardia 218
Pars compacta 815
Pars distalis 565f
Pars intermedia 565, 565f, 566, 567
Pars reticularis 815, 817
Pars reticulata 815
Pars tuberalis 565f
Parturition 585, 706
　　reflex 13
Parvocellular pathway 929
Patch clamp 35f
　　technique 35
　　types of 35
Patellar clonus 755
Patent ductus arteriosus 255, 657, 710, 978
Pavlov's theory of sleep 877
Peak expiratory flow rate 332, 335, 401
Pectins 456
Pedicels 486
Pelvis 865
Pendrin 593
Penicillamine 823
Penicillin 137
Penile erection 658
Penis-at-12 syndrome 679
Pentagastrin 430
Pentose phosphate pathway 111
Pepsin
　　actions of 425
　　hydrolyses 471
Peptic disease 432
Peptic ulcer
　　causes of 433
　　complications of 434
　　management of 434
　　signs of 434
　　symptoms of 434
Peptide hormone 441, 587
　　mechanism of action of 557f
Perchlorate 606
Percutaneous transluminal coronary angioplasty 299
Perforins 146, 153, 346
　　pressure, effective 235, 301
Periaqueductal gray 791
　　matter 789, 837
　　region 784
Pericardial cavity 203
Pericardial effusion 203
Pericardial fluid 203
Pericardial rub 203
Pericarditis 203
Pericardium 203
Pericytes 90
Periglomerular short axon cells 970, 971
Perilymph 946
Perimenopause 696
Perimetrium 44, 685
Periodic abstinence 714
Periodic breathing 375

Peripheral chemoreceptor 370-372, 396
　　innervation of 371
　　location of 371f
　　mechanism of action of 372
　　stimulation of 372fc
Peripheral pulse 282
　　examination of 282
　　tracing 281
Peripheral resistance 271, 272
　　hormonal regulation of 269
Peristalsis 465f, 466
　　mechanism of 465
　　primary 461
　　reverse 464
　　secondary 461
Peristaltic activity 408
Peristaltic constrictor rings 463
Peristaltic reflex 465
Peristaltic rushes occur 465
Peristaltic wave 461
　　second degree 461
Peritoneal dialysis 514
　　advantages of 515
Peritubular capillaries 489
Peritubular venules 489
Perivascular niche 116
Pernicious anemia 111, 121, 124, 157, 422, 426, 464, 814
　　causes of 124
　　treatment of 125
Peroxidase 115, 132, 135, 981
Peroxins 20
Peroxisome 20, 20t
　　biogenesis disorders 20
　　functions of 20
Peroxynitrite 980, 981
Persistent truncus arteriosus 978
Pertussis toxin 557
Pest control 379
Pesynaptic inhibition, mechanism of 738
Petit mal epilepsy 874, 874f
Petrosal nerve
　　greater superficial 300
　　lesser superficial 415
Peyer's patches 452
Phagocytes 40
Phagocytic barrier 147
Phagocytic function, disorders of 135
Phagocytic vacuoles 134
Phagocytosis 40, 134, 146, 162, 726
Phagolysosome 594
Phagosome 41, 134
Phakoscope 910
Phantom
　　eye syndrome 766
　　limb 766, 790
　　tooth pain 766
Pharyngeal muscles relax 376
Pharyngitis 461
Pharynx 314, 315
　　carcinoma of 461
　　inferior constrictor of 421
Phasic coronary blood flow 297
Phasic postural reflexes 845, 846
Phasic reflexes 846
Phasic smooth muscles 92
Phenacetin 381
Phenobarbitone 192
Phenolsulfonphthalein 896
Phenotype 22, 668
Phenybutazone 657
Phenylalanine 469, 633
　　hydroxylase 633

Phenylbutazone 503
Phenylethanolamine n-methyltransferase 624, 633
Pheochromocytes 632
Pheochromocytoma 266, 637
Pheromones 530, 973
Phlorizin 470, 502
Phonocardiograph 230
Phosphate
　　buffer system 511
　　reabsorption 504
Phosphatidyl inositol diphosphate 558
Phosphatidylcholine 16
Phosphatidylethanolamine 16
Phosphatidylserine 16
Phosphocreatine 74
Phosphodiesterase 557, 678
　　enzyme 921
Phospholamban 87
Phospholipid 16, 168, 472
　　phospholipase system, mechanism of action of 558fc
Phosphoprotein phosphatase 557
Phosphorus metabolism 610
Phosphoryl choline 677
Phosphorylase kinase 558
Photophthalmia 388
Photopic visibility curve 924
Phototherapy 115, 192
PHOX2B gene 870
Phylogenetic classification 826
Physiologic prolactin releasing hormone 580
Pia mater 891
Pigment epithelium 917
Pill
　　hypertension 266
　　male 716
　　morning-after 716
　　post-coital 716
Pillrolling tremor 821
Pilocarpine 903
Piloerection 529
Piloerector muscle 529
Pineal gland 587, 588f, 589
　　location of 587f
　　secretion of 587
Pinealocytes 587
Pinna 943
　　functions of 943
Pinocytic channel 291
Pinocytosis 41, 412, 471
Piriform cortex 969, 972
Pitch discrimination 952
　　duplex theory of 953
Pitting edema 181
Pituicytes 566
Pituitary diabetes
　　insipidus 509
　　mellitus 570
Pituitary dwarf 601t
Pituitary gland 565, 566f, 567fc
　　anterior 565
　　development of 565, 566f
　　disorders of 579fc
　　hormone of 566
　　hypothalamic control of 579
　　parts of 565, 565f
　　types of anterior 567t
Pituitary hormones, anterior 567
Pituitary hyperglycemia 569
Pituitary insufficiency 579

Pituitary ischemia 579
Pituitary stalk 565
Pituitary tumor 604
Place theory 952, 953
Placenta
    functions of 703
    structure of 703f
Placental barrier 702
Placental growth hormone 705, 712
Plain muscles 90
Planum temporale 889, 956
Plasma 102, 179t
    colloid osmotic pressure 180
    expanders 195
    glucose level 503f
    glycated hemoglobin 647
    layer 108
    lipids 109
    membrane 15, 16
    osmolality 184
    parathormone 613
    pH 609
    platelet-rich 194
    skimming 239f
    testosterone level, total 679
    thromboplastin antecedent 165
    values, normal 102
Plasma protein 2, 102, 103, 103f, 104, 109, 180, 238, 513f
    estimation 449
    functions of 103
    level 104
    separation of 103
    solution 193
Plasma renin
    activity 655
    concentration 655
Plasma volume 100
    determination of 183
    measurement of 8
Plasmapheresis 103
Plasmin 170
Plasminogen 132, 170
    activator inhibitor 171
Plastic rigidity 821
Plasticity 93, 521
    negative 887
    positive 887
    property of 462
    types of 886
Platelet 159
    activating factor 161, 159
    aggregation 161, 161t
    concentrate 194
    count 160, 171
    defects 174
    derived growth factor 160, 162, 576
    factor 159, 160
    formation of 163fc
    function 162, 163
    phospholipid 165
    plug formation 165
    properties of 160, 165
    structure of 159, 159f
Platelet-to-platelet adhesion 161
Plethysmography 229, 235
Pleura 318
Pleural anatomy 318f
Pleural cavity 318, 324f
Pleural effusion 318, 338
    causes of 318
Pleural fluid, functions of 318
Pleural rub 324
Pleural space rises 319

Plexus 566
Pneumoencephalography 852, 896
Pneumography 331
Pneumonia 401
Pneumotaxic center 367
Pneumothorax 319, 319f, 333, 338, 401
    causes of 319
    closed 319
    open 319
    types of 319
Podocin 486
Podocytes 486
Poikilocytosis 106
Poiseuille's law 237
Poiseuille-Hagen formula 237
Poliomyelitis 814
Polychromatophilic normoblast 118
Polycystic ovary syndrome 695
Polycythemia 108f, 111, 379, 387
    relative 111
    secondary 111
    severe 266
    vera 111
Polydipsia 584, 645, 646
Polymenorrhea 694
Polymerase chain reaction 23
Polymodal nociceptors 781
Polymorphs 132
Polypeptide 25, 430
    chains 125
Polyphagia 645, 646
Polysaccharides 469
Polyspermy 701, 702
    prevention of 702
Polysynaptic reflex 748, 756, 756f
Polyuria 513, 584, 630, 645, 646
Pompe disease 76
Pons 802, 807
    and medulla 366, 460
Pontine
    centers 367, 892
    reticular formation 877
    reticular nuclei 835
Ponto-mesencephalo-tegmental complex 877
Poor brain development 601
Porphyrin 112
    derivative 112
Portal hypertension 304
    complications of 304
Portal venous blood 412
Postcentral gyrus 782
    inferior part of 966
Post-conceptional fertility control 717
Post-hemorrhagic anemia 123
Postmenopausal hormone replacement therapy 691
Postpartum thyroiditis 602
Postprandial alkaline tide 427
Post-rotatory nystagmus test 843
Postsynaptic inhibition 737, 956
    types of 737
Postsynaptic membrane 867
Post-tetanic facilitation 741
Post-tetanic potentiation 741, 885
    causes of 741
Postural reflexes 845, 846t
Posture 821, 845
    and equilibrium 845
    and gravity 256, 265
    maintenance of 845
Pot belly 601

Potassium
    channel 36, 36t
    glycocholate 445
    ions 784
    leak channel 36f
    taurocholate 445
Potential energy 240
Power stroke 69
Pranayama 879
Pratyahara 879
Pre-botzinger complex 366
Pre-capillary sphincter 262, 290
Precocious pseudopuberty 671
Precocious puberty 631, 670, 671f, 681f, 696
Prednisolone 632
Prefrontal lobe 864
Prefrontal syndrome 853
Preganglionic sympathetic
    efferent fibers 728
    fibers synapse 621f
Pregnancy 701
    immunological test of 705
    maternal growth hormone of 705
    medical termination of 718
    tests 705
Pregnanediol 692
Prekallikrein 165
Premature beat 219
Premature death 986
Premenstrual syndrome 691, 695
Premenstrual tension 691
Premotor cortex 801, 802
Preoptic neurons 877
Preoptic nucleus, medial 856f
Preprogastrin 430
Preproglucagon 649
    structure of 649fc
Preproinsulin 641
Preproparathormone 611
Presbycusis 957
Presbyopia 909, 911, 913, 980
Preservation injury 194, 360
Pressure
    curve, relaxation 337
    equalization of 448, 946
    gradient 180, 235, 256
    natriuresis 629
    wave 953
Prestin 949
Presynaptic facilitation 738, 741, 885
Presynaptic inhibition 738, 956
Presynaptic membrane 79
Presynaptic neuron 731, 738f
Presynaptic nicotinic cholinergic receptors 658
Pretibial edema 605
Pricking pain 781, 784
Primordial follicle 685, 686
Prison population 669
Probenecid 503
Probiotics 456
Procarboxypeptidase 438, 439
Procoagulants 171
Proelastase 439
Proenkephalin 789
Proerythroblast 118
Progesterone 688, 689, 692, 706
    actions of 692, 711
    synthesis of 704
Progestin 692
Programmed cell death 29
Proinsulin 641
    structure of 641f

Prolactin 567, 577, 617, 711
    actions of 577, 712
    hypersecretion of 578
    inhibiting hormone 578, 580, 712, 743
    lactogenic effect of 711
    release of 712
    factor 580
    hormone 580
    secretion 578
    stimulating 580
Proline-rich protein 416
Pro-megakaryocyte 162
Promptness 398
Pronormoblast 118
Proopiomelanocortin 565, 567, 578, 632, 789
Proparathormone 611
Properdin 146
Propionic acid 411
Proprioception 779
Proprioceptive sense 779
Propriofascicular tract 774
Proptosis 605
Prosopagnosia 854
Prostacyclin 170, 484, 658
Prostaglandins 139, 408, 424, 432, 433, 484, 492, 515, 541, 617, 656, 690, 697, 706, 784, 877
    functions of 657
    inhibitor 657
    synthesis of 657fc
Prostanoid receptors 781
Prostate 678
    secretion of 677
    specific antigen 677
Prostatic hypertrophy, benign 634
Protamine 514
    sulphate 172
Proteasomes 21, 152
Proteins 107, 121, 614
    absorption of 471
    act 17
    acute phase 104, 110
    basic 132, 135
    bound iodine 595, 599
    C 168, 172
        deficiency 174
    complex 103, 325
    digestion 471
    histocompatibility complex 17, 151
    kinase 556, 559, 626
    metabolism 569, 623, 643, 691
    peripheral 16
    reserve 103
    S 168
    splitting enzymes 439, 452
    structural 17, 66
    synthesis 623, 679
    uncoupling 535
Protein-rich meal 895
Proteinuria 495, 513
Proteoglycans 608
Proteolytic enzyme 167, 685, 784
Prothrombin activator 167
Prothrombinase 167
    formation of 165
Protodiastole 226, 228
Proton pump 427
Protopathic sensations 766
Protoplasmic astrocytes 725
Protruded umbilicus 601
Proximal convoluted tubule 487, 499, 506f

Pruritus 769
Pseudo-hemophilia 174
Pseudohermaphrodite 669
Pseudohermaphroditism 631
Pseudohypertrophic muscular dystrophy 76
Pseudohypoaldosteronism 631
Pseudohypoparathyroidism 613
Pseudopodia 486
Pseudoreflex 268, 748, 748f
Psychic blindness 862
Psychic phase 429
Psychic reaction 785
Psychological sex 664, 668
Psychomotor
   epilepsy 874f
   seizure 874
Psychosocial dwarfism 575, 577
Pterygoid venous plexuses 300
Pterygopalatine ganglion 866
Ptosis 870, 932
Ptyalin, actions of 469
Pubarche 670
Puberty 570, 572
Puerperium 707
Puffy face 601
Pulmonary alveolar macrophages 142, 317
Pulmonary arteriolar vasoconstrictors 345
Pulmonary artery 229, 229t, 343
   pressure 347
      changes in 229
Pulmonary blood flow 345, 346, 396, 401, 983
   measurement of 345
   regulating 345t
   regulation of 345
Pulmonary blood pressure 344
Pulmonary capillary 352
   blood flow 347
   hydrostatic pressure 327
Pulmonary chemoreflex 249, 369
Pulmonary circulation 201, 202, 202f, 319, 343, 343fc, 344f, 346
   system 324
Pulmonary congestion 333
Pulmonary conus 207
Pulmonary edema 323, 326, 333, 338, 344, 345, 349, 353
   acute 387
   development of 326
   high altitude 387
Pulmonary function tests 401
Pulmonary gas exchange 351
Pulmonary hypertension 265, 345, 376, 380
Pulmonary irritant receptors 368, 369
Pulmonary pressure 401
Pulmonary systolic pressure 346
Pulmonary tuberculosis 348
Pulmonary vascular resistance 345
Pulmonary venous pressure 347
Pulmonary ventilation 313, 335, 336, 387
Pulmonary venules, constriction of 345
Pulmonary vessels 319
Pulmonary wedge pressure 227
Pulse 568
   damping of 281
   pressure 263
   rate 282
   rhythm of 282
   tracing, central 281
   wave 281
      Doppler 240, 241
      velocity of 281
Pulsus alternans 282
Pulsus bigeminus 283
Pulsus paradoxus 283
Pump-handle movement 323f
Pumping blood 283
Pumps, accessory 202
Pupil 903
   appearance of 914f
   constriction of 903f, 910
   dilatation of 903f
   functions of 903
Pupillary constriction 870, 932
Pupillary constrictor reflex 930
Pupillary dilator reflex 932
Pupillary light reflex 931fc
   pathway for 930, 931
Pupillary reflexes 930
Pupillodilator reflex, pathway for 932
Pure tone audiometry 959
Purinergic receptors 781
Purkinje cell 737, 826-828
   dendrites of 827
   layer 827
Purkinje fibers 207
Purkinje phenomenon 924
Purkinje-Sanson images 910f
Purpura 174, 174f
   hemorrhagica 163
Putamen circuit 819
Pyelography, retrograde 525
Pyloric antrum 423
   G cells of 406
Pyloric area 422, 423
Pyloric canal 423
Pyloric glands 423, 424
Pyloric pump 463
Pyloric sphincter 423
   tone of 463
Pyramidal cell 850, 851
Pyramidal lobe 591
Pyramidal pathways 803f
Pyramidal tract 520, 801
   course of 802
   divisions of 802fc
   lesion 806
   origin of 802
   termination of 802
Pyrexia 540
Pyridinolines 611
Pyrogens 540
   mechanism of action of 540
Pyruvate kinase deficiency 114
Pyuria 514

Q

QT syndrome, long 37, 219
Quadriplegia 806, 810
Qualitative defect 163, 174
Quantitative defect 163, 174
Queckenstedt's sign 896

R

Rab family 554
Rab protein 734
Radiation 535, 536
   biologic effects of 392
   cancer 393
   dermatitis
      acute 392, 392f
      chronic 392, 393
   poisoning 456
   sources of 392
   therapy 460
Radioactive xenon gas, breath of 348
Radio-femoral delay 282
Radioimmunoassay 550, 595
Radioisotope method 114
Radionuclide technique 295
Radio-receptor assay 550
Raloxifene 692
Rapid eye movement 376, 391, 570, 875
   behavior disorder 878
   sleep 875, 876, 876t
Rare skin manifestation 393
Ratchet mechanism 69
Rathke's pouch 565, 566
Raynaud's disease 870
Raynaud's phenomenon 379
Reabsorption lacunae 592, 594
Reaction
   positive supporting 845, 846
   time 749, 757
   white 292
Rebound phenomenon 832, 832
Receptive relaxation, property of 422
Receptor proteins 733
Recipient's serum 189t
Reciprocal inhibition 754
   circuit 739
Reciprocal synapse 733
Recompression chamber 390
Recording
   device 50
   electrode 49
Rectum 304, 455
Recurrent collateral inhibition 737
Red blood cell 100, 110fc, 124f, 141, 189f, 353, 525f, 642
   combines 361
   count 109, 111
   fragility of 110
   shape of 109, 238
   size of 109
Red blood corpuscle 106
   morphology of 106f
Red blood substitutes 195
Red bone marrow 111
Red cell
   central pallor of 124f
   fragility 110
   mass decreases 391
   mature 119
   membrane 107
   produce 117
   volume 108
Red marrow 117
Red muscle 845
Red pulp 141
Referred pain, mechanism of 787
Reflex
   acquired 418
   action 747
   activity, stage of 810, 811, 846
   arc 722, 723f, 747, 747f, 845
   attitudinal 845, 847
   bradycardia 269
   classification of 748
   conditioned 418, 429, 882, 882f, 883
   control 296
   dynamic 846
   grading of 757
   hypertension 248
   increase 269
   loss of 813
   modification of 758
   motor reaction 785
   natural conditioned 882
   nervous 165
   ovulation 696
   pathological 753
   responses, sensitization of 758
   righting 846, 847
   segmental loss of 813
   sympathetic dystrophy 790
   tachycardia 269
   thermoregulation 537
   types of conditioned 882
   vestibular 842
   withdrawal 756
Reflux 417, 519
Refraction 908
   errors of 912
Refractive index 908
Refractive power 908
Refractory period 48, 55, 55f, 68
Regeneration
   signs of 60
   tube 60
Regional blood flow, measurement of 301
Regulate blood volume 184
Regurgitation 204
Reissner's membrane 947, 951
Relaxation
   point of 68
   technique 879
   volume 338
Relaxin 692, 703, 705
Relaxing proteins 66
Renal angiography 526
Renal arteries 488
Renal biopsy 526
Renal blood flow
   measurement of 489
   regulation of 490
Renal calculi 613
Renal catheterization 525
Renal circulation 490
Renal column 484
Renal compensation 277
Renal corpuscle 485
   structure of 488f
Renal cortex 484
Renal diseases 104, 181
Renal failure 374
   acute 514
   chronic 514
Renal function
   abnormalities of 513
   tests 524
Renal hypertension 266, 509
Renal mechanism 3, 512
Renal medulla 484, 507
Renal nerves, functions of 485
Renal papilla 484
Renal pelvis 484
Renal plasma flow 490
Renal plexus 484
Renal shutdown, causes of 196
Renal system 980
Renal threshold 499
Renal tomography 526
Renal transplantation 514, 515
Renal tubular functions 498
Renal tubule 486, 503t, 985
   histology of 487
Renal vessels, dilatation of 491t
Renin 484, 488, 491, 515, 610, 655
   actions of 655

Index

Renin-angiotensin
  mechanism 271
  system 497
Renin-angiotensin-aldosterone
  mechanism 269, 491, 498fc, 501, 501fc, 629
  system 630fc
Rennin 423, 425
  acts 471
Renorenal reflex 485
Renshaw cell 737, 768
  inhibition 737
Reperfusion damage 299
Replacement therapy 193
Representational hemisphere 850
Reproductive cell division 27, 28f
Reproductive cloning 25, 26
Reproductive cycle, female 686
Reproductive organs, female 684f
Reproductive system 597, 603, 663
  female 684
  male 673, 674f
Resonance theory 953
Respiration 313, 367
  chemical regulation of 370
  external 313
  internal 313, 354
  muscles of 321
  neural control of 366
  phases of 265, 336, 338, 345
  reflex control of 368
  regulation of 366, 375
  rhythm of 367
Respiratory acidosis 2, 373, 374, 511
Respiratory alkalosis 2, 374, 387, 985
Respiratory center 368, 369, 372, 807, 835
  depression 374, 375
Respiratory compensation 374
Respiratory control mechanism 376
Respiratory cycle 324
Respiratory dead space 336
Respiratory disease 401
Respiratory distress syndrome 326, 706
Respiratory failure 389
Respiratory function 703
Respiratory gases, transport of 99
Respiratory infections 323
Respiratory membrane 352, 353
Respiratory movements 331
Respiratory muscles, paralysis of 377
Respiratory pump 256, 258
Respiratory rate 336, 879
Respiratory system 313, 315, 386, 391, 624, 692, 875, 977, 979
  functional anatomy of 315
  receptors 368, 369
  structure and functions of 313
  structure of 315f
Respiratory tract 313
  functions of 313
  lining epithelium of 315
Respiratory zone 316
Restiform body 825
Resting discharge 926
Resting membrane potential, recording of 48
Rete testis 673
Reticular activating system 876
  functions of 835
Reticular formation 801, 803, 835, 851, 878, 888
  connections of 835
  functions of 836

Reticular lamina 949, 951
Reticular nuclei 835
Reticulocyte 119, 119f
  count 119
  crisis 119, 125
  response 119, 125
Reticulocytopenia 119
Reticulocytosis 119
Reticuloendothelial cells 141, 114f, 142, 180
Reticuloendothelial system 114, 141, 142
Reticulospinal tract 799, 800, 804, 835, 836
  anterior 804
  functions of 836
  part of 864
Retina 902, 903, 917
  formation in 925, 927t
  layers of 917, 918f, 919
  neurons of 920
  periphery of 915f
Retinal factors 915
Retinal images 917
Retinal isomerase enzyme 922
Retinal mechanism 933
Retinal receptors 922
Retinal reductase 922
Retinitis pigmentosa 918
Retinoblastoma 726
Retinohypothalamic pathway 929
Retinohypothalamic tract 587
Retrolental fibroplasia 380
Retroperitoneal organ 438
Reverberating circuit theory 885
Rexed's laminae 729
Reynolds number 236
Rh
  blood group systems 190, 191t
  factor 190
  incompatibility 191, 196
  null 191
  system 186, 190, 191
RHD gene 190
Rheobase strength 55
Rhesus monkey 190
Rheumatic fever 157, 205
Rhodopsin
  formation of 922
  resynthesis of 921, 921f
  retinene visual cycle 920, 921f
  rosy red color 921
Rh-positive blood transfusion 191
Rhythmic muscular contractions 984
Rhythmicity 208
Ribonuclease 439
Ribonucleic acid 160
Ribosomal RNA 19
Ribosome 19, 46
Rickets 616, 616f
Ridges 30
Riedel's thyroiditis 602
Right bundle branch 207
Right vagus 205, 641
Rigor mortis 71
Ringer lactate 9
Ringer-locke fluid 104
Rinne's test 958
Riva-Rocci cuff 264
Rivinus ducts 413
Road accidents 810
Rod and cone 918, 919t
  layer of 918
  structure of 919f
Rods of corti 949

Romanowsky stains 132
Romberg's sign 780
Romberg's test 780, 813
Root ganglion, dorsal 723, 74, 749, 754, 756f, 771, 775, 778, 781, 784
Rough endoplasmic reticulum 19, 22
Rouleaux 109
  formation 108, 108f, 109, 132f
  prevention of 103
Round ligament 305
R-protein 426
Rubrospinal tract 800, 803, 805
Ruffini endings 762
Ruffini's end organ 778
Ryanodine receptor 37, 69, 70

S

SA node 205
Saccule 838, 840
Saline 9
  antibody 192
Saliva
  acts 417
  composition of 416
  functions of 416
  mechanism of secretion of 417
  nature of 418
  pH of 416
  secreted, volume of 882
Salivary amylase 417fc
Salivary digestion 417
Salivary ducts 418
Salivary gland 413, 414t, 415, 416f, 629
  duct system of 414f
  histology of 413
  innervation of 415
  location of 413f
Salivary reflexes 418
Salivary secretion
  disturbances of 419
  hormonal regulation of 418
  modification of 417f
  regulation of 418, 418fc
  stages of 417f
Salivation
  permanent cessation of 419
  temporary cessation of 419
Salivatory nucleus 415
Salmonella bacteria 456
Saltatory conduction 57f
Santorini duct 438
Sarcoglycan 66, 75
Sarcoidosis 401
Sarcolemma 66
Sarcomere 66
  structure of 67f
Sarcoplasm 65
Sarcoplasmic reticulum 70, 85f
Sarcotubular system 67, 67f, 87, 91
Satiety center 856
Saxagliptin 478
Saxitoxin 36
Scala media 947f
Scala tympani 947f
Scala vestibule 947f
Scammon's growth curves 575
Scanning speech 832
Scarpa's ganglion 841
Scattered endocrine cells 423
Schafer's method 398, 399
Schilling index 138
Schlemm canal 904
Schwabach's test 958

Schwann cells 46, 724, 927, 970
Sclera 901, 902, 916
  yellowish discoloration of 446f
Scotomata 916
Scotopic visibility curve 923
Scotopsin 921
Scratch reflex 769, 781
Sea sickness 844
Sebaceous glands 529
Sebum 529
Second order neuron 770-772, 777, 927, 954, 972
Secrete acid 430
Secrete mucus 970
Secretin 429, 440, 547
  actions of 440t
Secretin-pancreozymin test 441
Secretion, rate of 416, 691
Secretory activity 19
Sedentary lifestyle 985
  consequences of 985
  effects of 985
Selectins 30, 134
Selective estrogen receptor
  modulators 692
Selegiline 822
Selenium 473
Semantic aphasia 889
Semen 678
  analysis 678
Semenogelin 677
Semicircular canal 831, 838, 843
  external 838
  tests for 843
Semilunar valve 204, 226, 230, 231
Seminal vesicle 673
  secretion of 677, 678
Seminiferous tubule 673
  cross-section of 675f
  dysgenesis 669
Senile dementia 886
Sensation 761
  appreciation of 837
  double 783
  subcortical perception of 795
  subjective 943
Sense
  organ 531, 762
  static position 779
  superficial 766
Sensitization 741, 758, 884
Sensorimotor cortex 852
Sensorineural deafness 957, 958, 960f
Sensory
  aphasia 854, 888
  association area 768, 775, 853
  ataxia 780, 796, 813, 831
  coding 765
  cortex 774, 826
  cortical area 774
  decussation 773
  discriminative component 782
  fibers 66, 409, 485
    lamination of 771f
  function 44, 721
  homunculus 774, 774f
  information
    coding of 765
    processing of 723
  loss 812, 813
    dissociated 812, 813
  modality 761, 767t
  nerve fibers, classification of 57
  neurons 765f, 969
  pathways 766

receptors 723, 762
    classification of 762
    functions of 762
speech 887
    area 853
    center 887
supply 749
system 53
tracts 728, 772, 773
unit 764
    recruitment of 765
Sensory-motor
    area 801
    coordination 729, 796
Septal defect, ventricular 255, 978
Septicemia 456
Seromucinous acini 414
Serosa 407, 685
Serotonin 121, 408, 424, 430, 452, 538, 656, 738, 743, 784, 819, 855, 877, 885
    actions of 657
    reuptake inhibitor 743
Serotonin-N-acetyltransferase 588
Serous
    acini 413, 414
    demilunes 414
    glands 413
    pericardium 203
Sertoli cells 667, 673, 675, 676
    endocrine function of 676
    functions of 676, 677
    role of 676, 677
    secrete estrogen 678
Serum 167, 448
    albumin, radioiodinated 183
    alkaline phosphatase, estimation of 448
    amylase 441
    creatinine 514
    glutamate-O-methyl transferase 298
    glutamic
        oxaloacetic transaminase 448
        pyruvic transaminase 448
    lipase level 441
Sese genes 186
Sex characters, secondary 663, 663t, 664
Sex chromatin 132, 666
    test 668
Sex chromosomes 665, 668
    functions of 665
    nondisjunction of 668, 668f, 669
Sex determining region 666
Sex differentiation 666
Sex organs
    accessory 663, 663t
    primary 663, 663t
    secondary 663
Sex phenotype 664
Sex steroids 609, 621
Sex-linked
    inheritance 23
    inherited disease 172
    recessive disorders 173
Sexual behavior 858, 861
    role in 861
Sexual characteristics, secondary 668
Sexual characters, secondary 691
Sexual development 665
Sexual function, disorders of 858
Sexual identity 668
Sexual organs, secondary 685
Sexual reproduction 663

Shallow breaths 375
Shearing motion 951
Sheehan's syndrome 579, 602
Sheep's red blood cell 705
Sherrington's classification 763
Shivering 538
Shock
    anaphylactic 274
    burn 273
    cardiogenic 273
    classification of 273
    cold 273
    electric 398
    hemorrhagic 273
    hypovolemic 273
    lung syndrome 195, 274, 275, 379
    neurogenic 273
    obstructive 274
    pathophysiology of 273
    septic 273
    stages of 274
    surgical 273
    traumatic 273
    treatment of 275
    types of 272t
    vasogenic 273
    wound 273
Short loop reflexes 408
Short reflex 408
Short stature, causes of 577
Short-sightedness 912
Shuffling gait 821
Shunt 263
    pathological 344
    physiological 344, 358
    right-to-left 978
    vessels 262, 263
Shy-Drager syndrome 870
Sialic acid, presence of 108
Sialography 414
Sialolithiasis 419
Sialorrhea 419
Sick sinus syndrome 205, 218
Sickle cell
    anemia 113, 125, 125f
    disease 717
    trait 125
Silent mutation 24
Silvester method 398
Simian sarcoma 576
Simmonds disease 579
Simple goiter, development of 600fc
Single smooth muscle cell, structure of 90f
Singlet oxygen 980
Sinoaortic reflex 246f, 247, 247fc, 269
Sinoatrial node 205
    pacemaker potential of 86
Sinus
    arrhythmia 217, 248
    bradycardia 217, 217f
    dural 300
    of Valsalva 230
    rhythm 217
    tachycardia 217, 217f
Sinusoids 291, 443
Sitagliptin 478
Sjogren's syndrome 419, 645
Skeletal disorders 333
Skeletal growth 568
Skeletal maturation 596
Skeletal muscle 61, 65, 65f, 66, 67f, 68, 68f-70f, 71, 72f, 88, 88t, 94, 94t, 267, 391, 650

contraction 70fc
    mechanism of 69
fiber 65f, 89f, 749
    structure of 65f
innervation of 65
properties of 68
pump 256, 258
relaxation, mechanism of 71fc
tone 269
types of 72
Skeletal system 391, 597
Skin 529, 543f, 597
    and temperature regulation 979
    appendages of 529
    blood supply of 531
    cherry-red discoloration of 379f
    color 531
    functions of 531
    pigmentation 578
    prick test 402
    purplish striae in 624
    structure of 529, 530f
    types of vessels in 292
Skull, plain X-ray of 852
Sleep 589, 874, 875
    abnormalities 878
    bruxism 878
    center 876
    depending, classification of 875
    mechanism of 876
    spindles 875
    theories of 877
    walking 878
Sleep apnea 375, 376
    causes of 376
    complications of 376
    obstructive 376
    periods of 875
    prolonged 377
    symptoms of 376
    syndrome 376
Sleep-wake cycle 877, 878, 878fc
    physiology of 877
Sleep-wakefulness cycle 858
Slit membrane 486
Slow muscle 72, 72t
Slow pain 783t
    pathway 784, 785
Slow postsynaptic potentials 736
Slow reacting substance 657
Slow-wave sleep 875
    mechanism of 876
Sludged blood 275
Slurring 832
Small arteries 262
Small intestine 451, 452, 565f
    diseases of 465
    functions of 452
    juice 452
    lumen 456
    movements of 459, 464
    mucosa 451
    parts of 451
    secretion, regulation of 453
Small molecule
    neurotransmitters 743, 744t
    transmitters 742, 743
Smell 965t
    sense of 969, 973
Smoke destroys lung tissue 328
Smoker's lungs 317
Smokers often cough 328
Smooth endoplasmic reticulum 19
Smooth muscle 90, 91, 315, 345t, 411
    activity of 830

contraction 92
innervation of 91f
nerve supply of 91
relaxation of 92, 93fc
single-unit 90
structure of 91f
types of 90
Snake venom 172
Snare proteins 734
Sneezing reflex 314, 369
Snellen's chart 914, 915f, 915t
Snoring 878
Sodium 473
    channel 36, 36f
        activation 52
    chloride 985
        solution 110
    dependent glucose transporter 40, 470
    fluoride 172
    glycocholate 445
    nitroprusside 379
    potassium
        adenosine triphosphatase 38
        pump 39f
    reabsorption 499, 500, 500f, 504f
        regulation of 501fc
    taurocholate 445
    tetraiodo-phenolphthalein 449
Soft tissues 568
Sole plate 79
Soluble mucus 424
Solvent drag 469
Somatic cell division 26, 28f
Somatic chromosomes 665
Somatic efferent pathways 722t
Somatic growth 568
Somatic motor pathways, classification of 800
Somatic nervous system 722, 798, 863, 867, 875
Somatic responses 861
Somatic sensations 795
Somatic sensory area 768, 771, 774, 777-779, 853
Somatomedin 568, 570, 577
    impaired hepatic synthesis of 572
Somatosensory
    cortex 887
    map 770
Somatostatin 408, 424, 447, 453, 569, 649
    actions of 649
    secretion 650
Somatostatin-containing cells 424
Somatotropin 568
    release inhibiting factor 569
Somesthetic cortex 774
Somnambulism 878
Sound 236
    abnormal 231
    amplification of 946
    energy 951f
    frequency of 950
    infrasonic 950
    intensity of 231, 950, 954
    localization of 954
    properties of 950
    splitting of 231
    types of 950t
    wave
        characteristics of 950f
        high frequency 953f
        low frequency 953f
        timbre of 950

Index

Spastic hemiplegic gait 808
Spastic neurogenic bladder 521
Spastic paralysis 805
Spasticity 799, 810
Special sensations 761, 795
Special senses 901, 980
Spectral sensitivity curves 923f
Spectrin 107
Spectrophotometry 379
Speech 416, 796, 887
    abnormalities 888
    and language 887
    disturbances of 832
    mechanism of 887, 887fc
Sperm 675f
    before fertilization 701
    development of 675f
Spermatic veins, pampiniform plexus of 673
Spermatids 674
Spermatocytes 674
    primary 674
    secondary 674
Spermatocytogenesis 674
Spermatogenesis 673, 674, 675fc, 676, 676t
    normal duration of 675
    stages of 674
Spermatogonia 674, 675f
Spermatozoa, maturation of 676
Spermatozoon, structure of 675f
Spermicides 714
Spermine 677
Spermiogenesis 674-676
Spherical aberration 913f
Sphincter
    contraction of 409
    vessels 262
Sphingomyelin 16
Sphygmograph 231
Sphygmomanometer 264
Spinal anesthesia 894
Spinal animal 757, 846
Spinal cardioacceleratory center 245
Spinal cat 757
Spinal cord 245, 268f, 771f, 802, 813, 814, 864, 748
    ascending tracts of 772
    central canal of 891
    complete section of 810
    cross-section of 727, 728f, 772f
    descending tracts of 800f
    gray matter of 728, 728f, 729f
    hemisection of 811, 812f
    incomplete section of 811
    lesion of 810
    level 245, 723
    lower extent of 727f
    posterior horn of 773
    structure of 726
    transection, complications of 812
    types of lesions of 810
Spinal fillet 773
Spinal lemniscus 772, 773, 781
Spinal motor neurons 5t
Spinal nerve, mixed 727
Spinal shock 810, 812, 846
    causes of 811
    stage of 810, 811
Spinal tap 894
Spindle sleep 875
Spinocerebellar pathway, functions of 780
Spinocerebellar tract 773, 780, 828, 829
Spinocerebellum 826
Spino-olivary
    pathway 829
    tract 774
Spinoreticular pathway 782, 784, 829, 835
Spinoreticular tract 773
Spinotectal tract 774, 829
Spinothalamic pathway 770, 771, 772t
Spinothalamic tract
    anterior 772, 773, 777
    lateral 769, 772, 773, 781, 784
Spino-visual reflex, pathway for 805fc
Spirogram 332f
Spirometer 331, 332f
Splanchnic blood flow 412
Splanchnic circulation 303, 412
Spleen 141, 142
    functions of 141
    surgical removal of 141
Splenectomy, effects of 141
Splenic cords 141
Splenic pulp 141
Splenic sinuses 141
Split-brain animal 884, 889
Sports injuries 810
Squamous epithelium 315, 487
Square wave pulse 54
Squeeze 390
Squint 906, 917
SRY gene 665, 666
SRY protein 665, 666
Staggering gait 832
Stagnant hypoxia 372, 379
    causes of 379
Stamping gait 813
Stannous pyrophosphate 295
Stapedius muscle, contraction of 944
Stapedius pulls, contraction of 945
Staphylococcus aureus 514
Starch
    cooked 416, 439
    uncooked 439, 470
Starling's forces 177, 178f, 270, 291, 495, 502
    balance of 178
Starling's law 72
Static
    compliance 337
    contraction 751
    equilibrium 842
    lung volumes 332
    nuclear bag fibers 749
    postural reflexes 845
    reflexes 845
    tremor 821
Steatorrhea 441, 446, 472
Stein-Leventhal syndrome 695
ST-elevation myocardial infarction 298
Stellate ganglion 865
Stenosis 231
Stensen's duct 413
Stercobilinogen 115
Stereocilia 839, 948
Stereognosis 767, 768
Stereopsis 917
Sterility 419, 678, 680
Sterilization 716
Steroid hormone 17, 34, 559
    actions of 559fc
    mechanism of action of 559f
    non-genomic actions of 561
Steroidogenesis 704
    two-cell theory of 687
Stethogram 331
Stethography 331
Stilbestrol 691
Stimulate gastric juice secretion 431
Stimulate granule cells 970
Stimulate respiration 369
Stimulate sensory receptors 762
Stimulates erythropoiesis 597
Stimulatory G protein 428, 626
Stimulus 50, 464, 749, 775, 846
    artifact 51
    duration of 55
    supra-maximal 55
    types of 762
    unconditioned 883
Stokes-Adams syndrome 219
Stomach 422
    abnormal movements of 463
    carcinoma of 124
    functions of 422
    fundus of 423f
    innervation of 425
    lesser curvature of 432
    mucosal barrier of 424f
    oxyntic cells of 857
    parts of 422f
    respiratory quotient of 427
Stone
    bone 617
    presence of 448
Stop flow technique 498
Strabismus 906, 917
Stratified squamous epithelium 420, 529
Stratum basale 529, 689
Stratum corneum 529
Streamline flow 235
Streptococcus
    bacteria 171
    pneumoniae 141
Streptokinase 171, 299
Streptomycin therapy, long-term 844
Stress 625, 870
    analgesia 791
    electrocardiogram 217
    relaxation 93
        mechanism 270
        reverse 93
    response 869
    symptoms of 870
    test 217
    ulcers 625
    volume 261
Stressors 625, 870
Stretch receptors 368, 464, 583
Stretch reflex 749, 749f, 750f, 753, 799
    clinical importance of 753
    higher control of 753
Stretch sensitive sodium channels 763
Stria terminalis 861
Stria vascularis 948
Striatum 815
Stroke 303
    output 253
Stroke volume 227, 253, 983
    heterometric regulation of 256
    hometric regulation of 257
    regulation of 255
Strychnine poisoning 737
Strychnos nux-vomica 737
ST-segment elevation myocardial infarction 298f
Stupor 389
Subarachnoid space 891
Subcortical white matter 849
Subcutaneous venous plexus 292
Subdural hematoma 874
Subfornical organ 857, 895
Subliminal fringe 741, 788
    summation of 757, 757f, 758
Sublingual gland 413, 415
    salivary 415f
Submandibular ganglion 415, 866
Submandibular gland 413
    salivary 415f
Submaxillary gland 415
Submucosa 406
    plexus 407
Subneuronal clefts 79
Substance
    P 465, 656, 782-784
    temperature of 967
Substantia gelatinosa 788
    of Rolando 728, 772, 773, 781, 784, 788, 789, 837
Substantia nigra 815, 817
    effects of 818
    pars compacta 818, 819
    pars reticulata 818, 819, 823
Substantia propria 902
Sub-threshold stimulus 54
Sucralfate 434
Sucrase 470
Sudden infant death syndrome 328, 377
Sulcus 849
Sulfate 595, 623
Sulfhemoglobin 112
Sulfonylurea 647
Superficial senses, Head's classification of 766
Superoxide 980
    anion 380
    dismutase 299, 981
Supraoptic crest 895
Supra-threshold stimulus 54
Suprathyroid mechanism 598
Surfactant deficiency 338
Sweat gland 530, 629
    innervation of 536
Sweat pore 530
Sweating, types of 537
Swimming 984
Sydenham's chorea 820
Sylvius aqueduct 724, 892
Sympathetic activity 537
Sympathetic discharge 535
Sympathetic effects 870t
Sympathetic ganglion 246
Sympathetic innervation 243, 425, 519
Sympathetic nervous system 536, 863, 864, 867, 869
Sympathetic reflex 678
Sympathetic stimulation 208, 257, 415, 418, 429
Sympathetic stress response 870
Sympathetic tone 244, 267, 866
Sympathetic vasoconstrictor tone 246
Sympathetic vasodilator system 268fc
    pathway of 268f
Sympathoadrenal system 636
Sympathomedullary system 632
Synapse 721, 731
    en passant 91
    functional classification of 732
    properties of 736, 757

Index

structural classification of 731, 732f
  types of 731, 732f
Synapsins 734
Synaptic after-discharge 739
Synaptic cleft 79, 733, 869
Synaptic delay 736
Synaptic fatigue 741
Synaptic inhibition 736
Synaptic knobs 46
Synaptic modulation 734
Synaptic plasticity 741, 886
Synaptic pruning 886
Synaptic specificity 734
Synaptic transmitters 46, 408
Synaptic web 733
Synaptobrevin 734
Syncope 266, 268, 273
Syncytiotrophoblast 702
Syndrome X 648, 695, 648
Syngamy 702
Synovial fluid 8
Syntactic aphasia 889
Syntaxin 734
Synthetic anticoagulants 169
Synthetic cutaneous senses 768
Synthetic estrogens 691
Synthetic progesterone 692
Syntrophins 66
Syringomyelia 813
Systemic actions 635
Systemic circulation 201, 202, 203f
Systemic hypertension 265, 380
Systemic lupus erythematosus 104, 109, 136, 137, 157, 345, 628, 645
Systolic discharge 253
Systolic failure 276
Systolic murmur 232
Systolic pressure 227, 265

T

T cell 149, 205
  receptor 152
  regulatory 156
  suppressor 149
T lymphocyte 148
  activation of 152
T wave 213, 220
  inversion 220f
  tall 221
Tabes dorsalis 813
Tabetic bladder 521
Tachycardia 217, 243, 380
Tachypnea 321
Tactile 419
  acuity 767
  agnosia 768
  discrimination 773
  localization 767, 773
  stimuli 412
Tamoxifen 692
Tank respirator 399, 399f
Tape recorder recording 213
Taste 965t
  affective nature of 967
  appreciation of 459
  blindness, selective 968
  modalities 967t
  pathway 966, 966f
  perception, mechanism of 966
  pore 965
  preference 967
  sense organ of 965
  threshold 967

Taste bud 965
  innervation of 966
  structure of 965, 966f
Taste sensation 965, 967
  abnormalities of 968
  primary 967
Taurocholic acid 445
Tay-Sachs disease 20
T-cell
  activation 153f
  receptors 151
Tears, functions of 907
Technetium-99 295, 401
Tectocerebellar tract 829
Tectorial membrane 949, 951
Tectospinal tract 800, 805, 805fc
Telencephalon 724
Telephone theory 953
Telophase 27, 28
Temperature regulation 533
  mechanisms 539t
Temperature sensation, pathway for 778
Temporal gyrus, inferior 854
Temporal lobe 849
Temporal lobectomy, bilateral 886
Temporal summation 735, 740
Teniae coli 455
Tension
  pneumothorax 319
  total 71
Tensor tympani 944, 945
Teratogen 670
Terminal bronchiole 316
Terminal cisterns 67
Terminal lymphatics 179
Terminator codon mutation 25
Tertiary granules 132
Testes determining factor 666, 667
Testicular feminizing syndrome 670
Testicular hormones 678t
Testicular vessels 673
Testis 673
  endocrine function of 678
  histology of 674f
  structure of 673
  undescended 680
Testosterone 666, 667, 673, 676, 678, 716
  actions of 679
  acts 667
  administration of 716
  chemistry of 678
  mechanism of action of 679
  metabolism of 679
  receptor complex 679
  regulation of secretion of 680, 680fc
  stimulates erythropoiesis 679
  transport of 679
Tetanus 75
Tetraethyl ammonium 36
Tetrahydrobiopterin 633
Tetrahydrocortisol 623
Tetrahydrofolate 125
Tetraiodothyroacetic acid 595
Tetralogy of Fallot 978
Tg cell 430
Th17 cells 149
Thalamic hand 797
Thalamic nucleus 795f
  anatomical classification of 794
  functional classification of 795
Thalamic overreaction 796
Thalamic pain 796

Thalamic phantom limb 797
Thalamic preparation 847
Thalamic syndrome 790, 796
Thalamocortical system 794
Thalamo-geniculate branch 796
Thalamostriatal system 816
Thalamus 779, 794, 835, 851
  connections of 795
  functional anatomy of 794
  functions of 795
  lesion of 796
Thalassemia 113, 125, 717
Thallium-201 295
Theca externa 686
Theca interna 686
Thelarche 670
T-helper cells, functions of 149
Theodor Schwann 15
Therapeutic cloning 25, 26
Thermal nociceptors 781
Thermal sweating 537
Thermistor 254
Thermosensitive 212
Thermodilution method 254
Thermogenesis 534
Thermogenic action 692
Thermogenin 21, 535
Thermoreceptors 369, 408, 762, 863
Thermoregulation 537
Thermoregulatory centers 538
Thermoregulatory responses 538
Thermostat 538
Theta waves 873, 874
Thiazides 502
Thiocarbamides 606
Thiocyanate 593, 606
Thionamides 606
Thiouracil 606
Thoracic breathing 322
Thoracic cage
  boundaries of 321
  movements of 322, 323f
Thoracic esophagus 420
Thoracolumbar outflow 863
Thorax 865
Thoroughfare
  channels 290
  vessels 263
Thought 886
Threonine 469
Threshold core temperatures 538
Threshold intensity 55, 950
Threshold stimulus 54
Throbbing headache 288
Throbbing pain 781, 784
Thrombasthenia 163
Thrombasthenic purpura 163, 174
Thrombin 167
  functions of 167
  positive feedback of 167
Thrombocytopenia 160, 163, 174, 193
Thrombocytopenic purpura 174
Thrombocytosis 160, 163
Thromboembolic conditions 174
Thrombomodulin 169
Thrombomodulin-thrombin complex 169, 170
Thrombopoiesis 116, 162
Thrombopoietin 116, 163
Thrombosis 174
  causes of 174
Thrombospondin 160 161
Thrombosthenin 160, 162, 167
Thromboxane 161, 170, 299, 496, 658
Thrombus 165, 174

Thymopoietin 654
Thymosin 148, 654
Thymus 654
  atrophy of 871
Thyrocalcitonin 614
Thyrocytes 591
  functions of 594
Thyroglobulin 591, 594
  antibodies 602
  synthesis of 592
Thyroid
  artery 592
  dwarf 601t
  function tests 599
  peroxidase 593, 602
  stimulation test 599
  storm 605
  suppression test 599
Thyroid gland 477, 591, 591f
  diseases of 600
  functional anatomy of 591
  histology of 592f
  hormone of 592
  non-malignant enlargement of 600fc
  peculiarities of 591
Thyroid hormone 250, 574, 598, 617
  actions of 595
  biosynthesis of 592
  effects of 597t
  metabolism of 595
  regulation of secretion of 598
  release of 593f
  secretion, regulation of 598f
  structure of 593f
  synthesis of 592
Thyroid stimulating
  hormone 556, 557, 562, 566, 578, 580, 594, 598, 624, 626
  immunoglobulin 604, 606
Thyrotoxic crisis 605
Thyrotoxic myopathy 597, 605
Thyrotoxicosis 266, 604, 605f
Thyrotropin-releasing hormone 556, 569, 579, 580, 598
Thyroxine 121, 535, 650, 711
  mechanism of action of 598
Thyroxine-binding
  albumin 594
  globulin 594, 605
  pre-albumin 594
Tidal volume 332, 333
Timed vital capacity 332, 335, 401
Tinel's sign 60
Tinnitus 957
Tissue 1
  cells, formation of 142
  conductance 536, 539
  culture 25, 26
  Doppler 241
  elasticity 325
  factor pathway 165, 169
  fluid 177, 178f
  ischemia 125
  lymph 177
  macrophage 134, 142, 147
  perfusion theory 270
  phase 359
  plasminogen activator 170
  resistance work 339
  thromboplastin 166, 175
Titrable acid 511
Titrable acidity 511
T-lymphocytes 133, 148t

Index

Tobacco amblyopia 328
Tomato cheeks 627
Tongue
    atrophy of papillae of 122
    bluish discoloration of 381f
    inflammation of 122f
    protruded 601
Tonic contraction 285, 464
Tonic labyrinthine 846
    reflexes 842, 843, 846
Tonic muscle contraction 411
Tonic neck reflexes 846, 847
Tonic postural reflexes 845
Tonic receptors 763
Tonic reflexes 845
Tonic smooth muscles 92
Tonic vagal 429
Tonic vestibular reflexes 846
Tonicity 3
Tonometer 358, 905
Tonsillitis 461
Tonus 92
Tortuous glands 424
Total blood
    volume, determination of 183
    water, measurement of 8
Total pancreatectomy, effects of 441
Touch sensation
    abnormalities of 777
    from face 776
Touch, sense of 775
Toxemia 266
Toxic adenoma 604, 605
Toxic multinodular goiter 604, 604f
Toxins 444
    release of 275
TPlasma 892t
Trachea 315
Tracheobronchial tree 315, 316f
Tract 46
    of Goll 771
    of Lissauer 778
Tractus cuneatus 773
Tractus dorsolateralis 773
Tractus gracilis 771, 773
Tractus solitaries, nucleus of 244, 366, 966
Tranquilizers 853, 884
Transcellular fluid 7
Transcobalamin 121, 426
Transcutaneous electrical nerve stimulation 789
Transcytosis 41, 290, 471
Transducin 923
Transduction channels 952
Trans-esophageal echo 241
Transferrin 474
Transfusion
    medicine, centers of 194
    reactions 196t
Transgenderism 668
Transmembrane protein channel 16, 35, 36f
Transmit diseases 666
Transmural pressure 239, 324, 325
Transneuronal degeneration 61
Transplantation 822
    tolerance 157
Transplanted heart 257
    regulation of 250
Transpulmonary pressure 324, 325
Transverse tubules 66
Trapezoid body 954
Tread mill test 217, 240, 984

Trefoil peptides 433
Trehalase 452, 470
Treitz ligament 451
Tremor, physiological 751
Triaxial reference system 216, 216f
Tributerase 426
Trichromats 935, 936
Trigeminal ganglia 300, 776
Trigeminal lemniscus 777
Trigeminal nerve 415, 902
    mesencephalic nucleus of 780f
    sensory nucleus of 776
Trigeminal neuralgia 790
Trigeminothalamic tract 777, 779
Trigger zone 46
Triggers asthmatic attacks 317
Triglycerides 17, 472
Triiodothyroacetic acid 595
Triiodothyronine 598
Trinucleotide expansion 24
Trisodium citrate 172
Trochlear nerve 907
    lesion of 907
Tropomyosin 66, 68, 90
Troponin 66, 68, 298
    C 68
    T 221, 298
Troublesome psychological disorders 853
Trousseau's sign 613
Truncal adiposity 627
Trypan blue 142
Trypsin 471
    inhibitor 439
Trypsinogen 439
Tryptophan 469, 657
    metabolism, role in 410
T-snare protein 734
Tube
    geometry of 239
    method 706
Tubectomy 716
Tubercle bacilli 348
Tubular colloid osmotic pressure 495
Tubular secretion 498, 505
Tubular structures beneath 970
Tubules 511
Tubulin 18, 19
Tubulovesicular structures 427
Tumor
    malignant 680
    marker 594
    necrosis factor 29, 133, 138, 139, 145
    suppressor genes 29, 30
Tunica
    adventitia 262
    albuginea 684
    intima 262
    media 262
Tuning fork tests 958, 958t
Turbulence, causes of 236
Turbulent flow 236
Turner's syndrome 577, 668, 669, 671
Two-bag technique 352
Tympanic membrane 943, 949
    functions of 944
    rupture of 380
    secondary 947
Tympanic plexus 415
Tympanic reflex 945, 945fc
Typhoid 444
Tyrosine 531, 633
    hydroxylase 633

U

U wave 214
Ubiquitin 22
Ubiquitination 22
Ultra-microelectrode 49
Ultrasonic sound 950
Ultrasonography 441, 449
Ultraviolet
    radiation 386
    rays 907
Umbilical cord 703f
Umbilical ligament, medial 305, 710
Unconscious proprioception 779, 780
Unconscious senses 761
Unilateral labyrinthectomy, effects of 844
Uniport 40
Upper esophageal sphincter 420, 461
Upper eyelid, drooping of 932
Upper motor neuron 798-800, 805, 812
    lesion 806t
    pathways 799
Urate oxidase 20
Urea
    clearance, maximum 504
    reabsorption 504
    recycling 508
Uremia 504, 513
Ureter 484, 519
Urethra 519, 673
Urethral glands 678
Urethral sphincter 519, 520
Urethrography 526
Urethroscopy 526
Uric acid 503
Uridine diphosphoglucuronic acid 114
Urinary acid excretion 512
Urinary amylase, estimation of 439
Urinary bilirubin estimation 448
Urinary bladder 93f, 484, 519, 866
Urinary buffers 511
Urinary retention 521
Urinary tract 484
Urine 2, 524
    abnormal constituents of 524
    analysis 524
    concentrations of 498, 507f
    dilatation of 506
    limiting pH of 511
    mechanism of formation of 494
    microscopic examination of 524, 525f
    normal osmolality of 505
    tasteless 583
    volume, renal regulation of 506
Urobilinogen 114
Urokinase 170, 171
Urology 483
Uropepsinogen 425
Ursodeoxycholic acid 445
Uterine bleeding, dysfunctional 691
Uterine cycle 688
    phases of 689
Uterus 684, 685, 691
    lower portions of 866
Utricle 838, 840
    and saccule, test for 843
Uvea 901, 902

Uveal tract 902
Uvula 825

V

Vagal escape 245
Vagal influences 367
Vagal tone 244, 245, 879
Vagina 684, 691
Vaginal epithelial cells, cornification of 690
Vaginal ring 716
Vaginal smear 696
Vagotomy 434
    effects of 431
Vagovagal reflex 409, 462
    long 428, 430, 461
Vagus 87, 409, 420, 965
    dorsal motor nucleus 244, 245, 430
    stimulation of 440
Valine 469
Valsalva's maneuver 324, 325
Valves, movements of 230
Valvulae conniventes 451
Valvular component 230
Valvular murmur 232
Van Allen's hematocrit tube 107
Van den Bergh test 114
Vanilloid receptors 762
Vanillylmandelic acid 549, 633, 634, 637
Vapor pressure 352
Vas deferens 673
Vasa recta 485f, 507f
Vasa vasorum 262
Vascular smooth muscle 262
    relaxation of 658
Vascular spasm 164, 379
    parts of 234, 263f
Vasectomy 677, 716
Vasoactive intestinal polypeptide 317, 318, 408, 415, 580
Vas-occlusive plugs 716
Vasoconstrictor 270, 303
Vasodilators 270, 303, 345
Vasomotor center 245, 267, 269, 807
    failure of 275
    higher control of 267
Vasomotor tone 262
Vasopressin 121, 269, 505, 582
    actions of 582
    escape 584
Vasovagal syncope 268
Vater ampulla 438
Vector cardiogram 217
Vegetative nervous system 863
Veins 263
    arcuate 489
    deep 300
    functions of 261
    hepatic 443
        portal 303, 304
    interlobular 489
    portal 304, 412, 444f
    pulmonary 345t
    renal 489
    Thebesian 294, 344
    umbilical 305
Vena cava
    inferior 202, 203, 305
    superior 202, 203
Venous blood 351f, 361
Venous drainage 489, 566
Venous plexus 531, 904
Venous pressure 301

Venous pulse 281, 283t
Venous tone 256, 269
Venous valves, mechanism of action of 263f
Ventilation 3, 395, 512
    measurement of 348
    mechanics of 321
    tests to assess 401
    wasted 337
Ventilation-perfusion
    imbalance 378
    inequality 377
    mismatch 378
    ratio 348, 401
Ventilators 399
Ventilatory volume, maximum 335
Ventral cochlear nuclei 954
Ventral median fissure 727
Ventral respiratory group 366
Ventral spinocerebellar tracts 829
Ventricular gallop 231
Ventricular muscle 86
Ventricular syncytium 205
Ventricular systole 224, 226, 295
Ventrolateral sulcus 727
Venules 290
Verapamil 36
Veratridine 249
Verbal aphasia 889
Vermis, lobules of 825f
Vertebrae, portions of 571
Vertebral arteries 299
Vertigo 831, 832, 844
Vesicles 733
Vesicular breath sound 323, 323f
Vesicular follicle 687
Vesicular transport 41, 291
Vessel wall
    condition of 282
    elasticity of 266
Vestibular apparatus 838, 947
    connections of 841f
    functional anatomy of 838
    functions of 842
    removal of 844
Vestibular dysfunction 844
Vestibular function tests 843
Vestibular ganglion 841
Vestibular membrane 947
Vestibular nuclear complex 841
Vestibular nucleus 803, 826, 835
Vestibular nystagmus 842, 843
Vestibular pathway 841
Vestibular system 391
Vestibulocerebellar tract 803, 829
Vestibulocerebellum 826
Vestibulo-fastigial tract 841
Vestibulo-ocular reflex 842
Vestibulospinal tract 800, 803, 804, 841
Vestibulo-thalamo-cortical fibers 841
Viagra 677
Vibration sense 768
Vildagliptin 478
Villus
    epithelial cells 451
    lashing movement of 465f
    of small intestine, structure of 451f

Vimentin 17
Vincristine 18
Violent respiratory efforts 710
Virilizing congenital adrenal hyperplasia 631
Viruses, neutralization of 146
Viscera 983
    reflex control of 787
Visceral blood flow 983
Visceral brain 861
Visceral control system 870
Visceral disease 788
Visceral epithelium 486
Visceral functions 863
Visceral nervous system 863
Visceral pain 786, 787, 787f
    causes of 786
    pathway for 786
Visceral peritoneum 407
Visceral pleura 318
Visceral sensations 781
Visceral senses 965, 969
Visceral smooth muscle 90, 90f, 91f, 91t, 93, 94, 94t
Visceroceptors 369, 370, 863
Viscosity 100, 101, 238, 301, 416
Vision 391, 901
    duplicity theory of 920
    field of 915
    maximum acuity of 915
    normal field of 916f
    photochemistry of 920
Visual acuity 914
Visual agnosia 862, 888
Visual angle, reciprocal of 914
Visual area 929
    primary 853, 928
Visual association area 853, 928
Visual body reflexes 907, 928, 932
Visual cortex 911f
    primary 876, 929
Visual defects 380
Visual evoked potential 937, 937f
Visual field 915
    extent of 916f
Visual pathway 920, 926, 927, 928f, 931t
    lesion of 930
Visual phototransduction 920
Visual pigments 920
Visual processing 925
Visual reflex 842
Visual righting reflex 847
Visual system 924
Vital index 334
Vital staining 142
Vitamin 473, 474, 474t
    A 473
        deficiency 922
        role of 922
        absorption of 473
    B 121
        complex 456
    B12 121, 121f, 122, 426, 496
        absorption of 121
        actions of 121
        deficiency 426
    B6 473
    C 121, 981

    D 121, 473, 531, 574, 615
        deficiency 613
    E 121, 473, 981
    K 456, 473
        antagonists 172
        deficiency 168, 173
        dependent 168
        epoxide 168
        hydroquinone 168
        prophylaxis 977
        role of 168, 168f
        metabolism 596
        synthesis of 456
        water-soluble 473
Vitiligo 531, 531f, 578
Vitreous
    body 906
    humor 906
Vocal cords, approximation of 460f
Volatile acid 509, 510
Voltage clamp technique 51
Voluntary hyperventilation 375, 375f
Voluntary motor activity 800, 802
    control of 830
Voluntary ventilation, maximum 332, 335, 401
Vomeronasal organ 973
Vomiting
    central 464
    mechanism of 464
von Willebrand disease 162, 174
von Willebrand factor 159-162, 164
V-snare protein 734

W

Wakefulness, state of 837
Wald's visual cycle 920
Wallerian degeneration 59
Wandering macrophages 142
Warfarin sodium 172
Water
    balance 99, 417, 453, 484, 857
    diffusion of 531
    diuresis 522
    excretion, controlling rate of 184
    hammer pulse 282
    intake, regulation of 857
    intoxication 505
    loss 536
    pump-handle effect 322
    reabsorption 473, 504
Water-soluble substances 973
Watery saliva, secretion of 418
Watery stools 466
Wave theory, traveling 952
Weber and Schwabach's tests 954
Weber's test 958
Weber-Fechner law 765
Weibel's model 316
Weight loss 391, 645, 646
Weightlessness, physiological effects of 390
Wenckebach's phenomenon 219
Werner's syndrome 980
Wernicke's area 854, 887
Wernicke's hemianopic pupillary reaction 931

Westergren's method 109
Westergren's pipettes 109f
Wever-Bray phenomenon 956
Wharton's duct 413
White blood cell 142
    count 136
    types of 131f
White commissure
    anterior 728
    posterior 728
White pulp 141
Whole-cell patch 35
Wigger's diagram 224, 225f
Willis circle 299, 300f
Wilson disease 473, 823
Windkessel effect 262
Windkessel vessels 262
Wintrobe's hematocrit tube 107, 107f
Wintrobe's method 109
Wintrobe's mixture 172
Wirsung duct 438
Wolff-Chaikoff effect 599, 606
Wolffian duct 667
Wolff-Parkinson-White syndrome 221, 221f
Woltman's sign 603
Word
    blindness 888
    deafness 888
Wright's peak expiratory flow meter 335

X

X chromosome 172, 665, 666, 936
Xanthine 257, 502
    oxidase 981
Xerophthalmia 902, 907, 925
Xerostomia 416, 419

Y

Y chromosome 663, 665, 666
    absence of 666
Yellow fever 444
Yoga
    and meditation 878
    effects of 879
    influence of 879
    physiology of 878, 879
    techniques 879
Young-Helmholtz theory 933

Z

Zellweger spectrum disorders 20
Zellweger syndrome 20
Zero gravity 390
Zinc 439, 473
Zollinger-Ellison syndrome 432, 435
Zona
    fasciculata 621
    glomerulosa 621, 628fc
    pellucida 686, 701
    reticularis 621
Zonula adherens 30
Zonula occludens 30
Zwaardimaker's olfactometer 973
Zygote 702
    genotypes 665f
Zymogen granules 412, 414